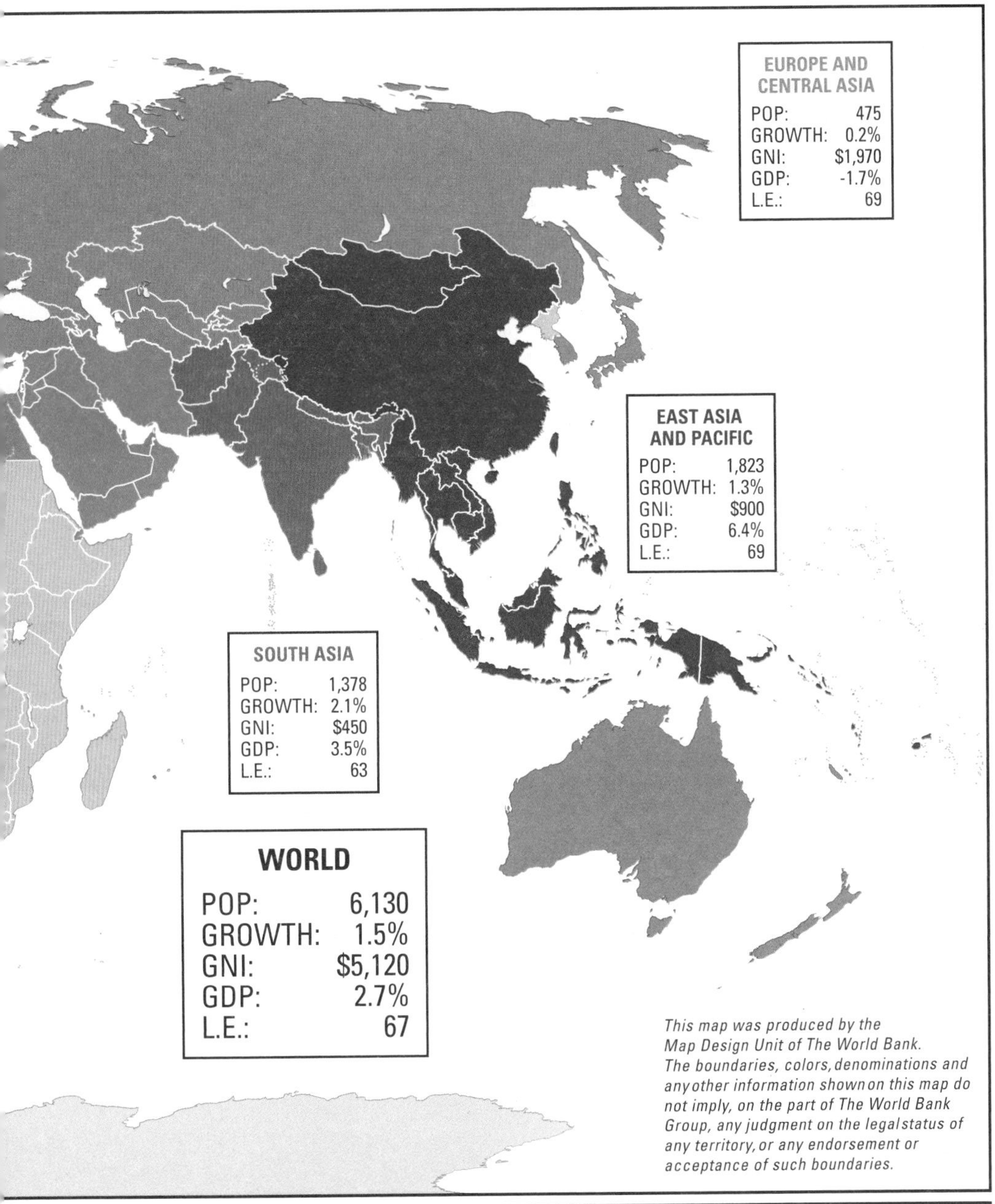
EUROPE AND CENTRAL ASIA
POP: 475
GROWTH: 0.2%
GNI: $1,970
GDP: -1.7%
L.E.: 69
EAST ASIA AND PACIFIC
POP: 1,823
GROWTH: 1.3%
GNI: $900
GDP: 6.4%
L.E.: 69
SOUTH ASIA
POP: 1,378
GROWTH: 2.1%
GNI: $450
GDP: 3.5%
L.E.: 63
WORLD
POP: 6,130
GROWTH: 1.5%
GNI: $5,120
GDP: 2.7%
L.E.: 67

This map was produced by the Map Design Unit of The World Bank. The boundaries, colors, denominations and any other information shown on this map do not imply, on the part of The World Bank Group, any judgment on the legal status of any territory, or any endorsement or acceptance of such boundaries.

omies

LATIN AMERICA AND THE CARIBBEAN — **REGION**

POP:	524	POP:	Population in millions
GROWTH:	1.8%	GROWTH:	Population Growth Rate (1991-2001) in percent
GNI:	$3,580	GNI:	GNI per Capita (US$)
GDP:	1.2%	GDP:	GDP Growth Rate (1990-2001) in percent per year
L.E.:	71	L.E.:	Life Expectancy at Birth (Average male and female)

SOURCE: World Development Indicators, 2003.

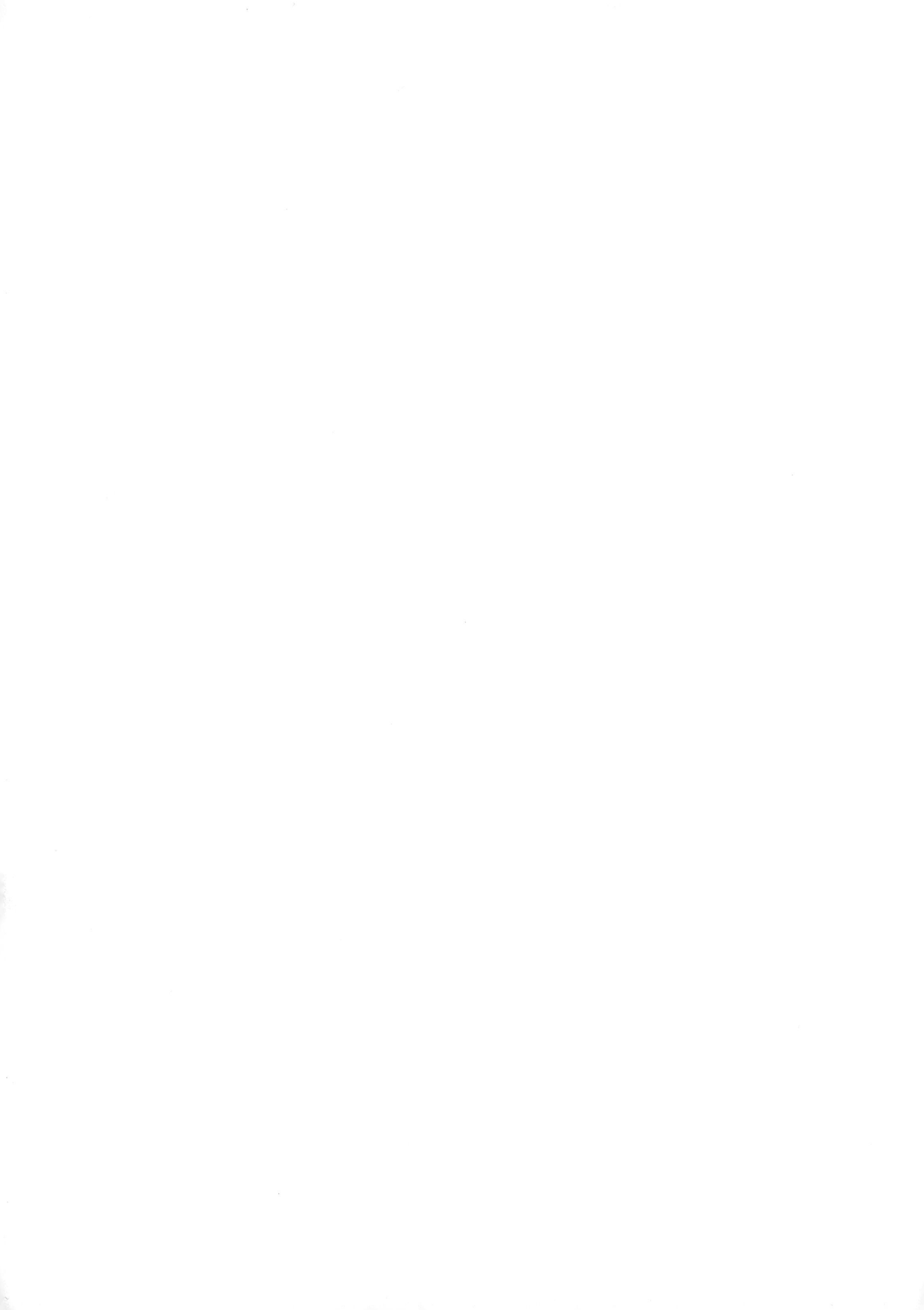

Disease Control Priorities in Developing Countries

SECOND EDITION

Disease Control Priorities in Developing Countries

SECOND EDITION

Editors

Dean T. Jamison

Joel G. Breman

Anthony R. Measham

George Alleyne

Mariam Claeson

David B. Evans

Prabhat Jha

Anne Mills

Philip Musgrove

A copublication of Oxford University Press and The World Bank

Dedication

This book is dedicated to Bill and Melinda Gates, whose vision, leadership, and financing over the past decade have catalyzed global support for transforming the lives of the world's poor through inexpensive but powerful health interventions.

Contents

Foreword

The 1993 publication of the now classic book, *Disease Control Priorities in Developing Countries,* by Oxford University Press and of its companion document, the *World Development Report 1993: Investing in Health,* published by the World Bank that same year, constitute a landmark in the public health literature. For the first time, decision makers and public health practitioners had a comprehensive review of the cost-effectiveness of available interventions to address the most common health problems in the developing world. They were also provided with the useful metric known as disability-adjusted life years to calculate the burden of disease and the cost-effectiveness of interventions more accurately than in the past.

As was the case with the first edition, this second edition of *Disease Control Priorities in Developing Countries* will serve an array of audiences. One primary audience consists of people working in the health sector, ranging from those who are responsible for making evidence-based decisions to those who practice medicine and public health under often suboptimal field conditions. A second audience consists of people working in finance and planning ministries, who will benefit from the solid recommendations for improving the health of populations through sound resource reallocation and cost-effective practices.

PURPOSE

The purpose of this book is to provide information about what works—specifically, the cost-effectiveness of health interventions in a variety of settings. Such information should influence the redesign of programs and the reallocation of resources, thereby helping to achieve the ultimate goal of reducing morbidity and mortality.

FUNDAMENTAL POLICY CONSIDERATIONS

Although economic and budgetary constraints are clearly important considerations, money is not the only limitation. Additional factors fundamental to improving outcomes are the particular circumstances in each country, as well as the individual institutional capacities to deliver goods and services and to implement policies and processes.

Context-specific strategies and responses are essential, because application of the Disease Control Priorities Project's findings will vary according to each country's circumstances: one size does not fit all. Understanding that most health interventions require a minimum level of institutional capacity to deliver goods and services is equally important, and such capacity may have to be built up before money or physical inputs can yield any benefits. Accordingly, goals and priorities should be established and tailored to each country's context.

TRANSITION IN HEALTH

Every developing region is facing a transition in its epidemiological profile from an environment with high fertility rates and high mortality from preventable causes to one in which a combination of lower fertility rates and changing lifestyles has led to aging populations and epidemics of tobacco addiction, obesity, cardiovascular disease, cancers, diabetes, and other chronic ailments. The 20th century will be remembered for, among other things, witnessing the largest universal increase in life expectancy in history. While life expectancy is highest in the richest countries, the upward trend is apparent in almost every society. Moreover, in the past 50 years, variations in this health indicator across and within countries have decreased. This convergence of improved life expectancy and reduced variations, which has occurred even in the presence of widening income gaps in many regions, can be explained solely by the impact of knowledge expansion and direct public health interventions.

The increase in life expectancy worldwide will, however, soon reach a plateau, and a retraction has occurred in many countries. HIV/AIDS and civil unrest in Africa, vaccine-preventable diseases and alcoholism in Eastern Europe, and obesity in the United States have reduced—or will soon do so—the years of life their populations can expect.

SCALING UP EFFECTIVE INTERVENTIONS

The late Jim Grant, former executive director of the United Nations Children's Fund, was one of the first leaders with a vision for setting specific health goals and priorities within a time frame and on a global scale. He recognized the need to raise awareness of the dramatic disparities in children's health and to mobilize political will accordingly. His missionary zeal for universal child immunization and for organizing the first summit of world leaders for children's health and rights in 1990 permitted the scaling up of interventions of proven efficacy. The Millennium Development Goals are a natural consequence of that vision and an extremely useful instrument for maintaining both focus and social pressure. Achieving these ambitious goals will require not only the universal implementation of effective interventions that are currently available, but also the development of new interventions.

NEED FOR ONGOING RESEARCH

Today, most vaccines, medical devices, diagnostic tools, and drugs have been subjected to careful investigation in the laboratory, at the bedside, and in the field. However, not enough investment has gone into research to increase well-being and development globally. We need more epidemiological and health systems research to improve the efficiency of available interventions, technological research to reduce their costs, and biomedical research to develop new tools for dealing with as yet unsolved and emerging health problems.

OPPORTUNITIES AND CHALLENGES OF GLOBALIZATION

One of the greatest opportunities and challenges for international public health is globalization. We live in an era when the explosion of trade, travel, and communications is spreading new cultural influences and lifestyles faster than ever before, and the division between domestic and international health problems is becoming increasingly obsolete. At the same time, globalization also permits the spread of risks, pathogens, and other threats. The ever-increasing movement of people everywhere increases the potential for epidemics. Travelers, refugees, and displaced people are more vulnerable to infectious diseases, and their movement contributes to spreading pathogens into new areas. Overall, however, the positive consequences outweigh the negative ones, and cautious optimism about this irreversible trend is justified. Certainly, one of the most valuable contributions of globalization is the rapid accrual and spread of knowledge about useful tools for controlling disease and ways to implement those tools on a large scale.

In recent years, the huge advances in information technology have greatly boosted the globalization of knowledge.

Ideally, this should become a tide that lifts all boats to yield global benefits. The challenge is to harness the information technology revolution to foster the growth of economies. One step in the right direction is the open access movement, which promotes and permits free and immediate access to research results and other components of knowledge transfer.

SPENDING MORE AND SPENDING BETTER

It is indeed a paradox to observe that even though the money spent on health worldwide has reached 10 percent of overall global income, that amount is both insufficient and poorly allocated. The World Health Organization's Commission on Macroeconomics and Health and several other global initiatives make a persuasive plea for a larger investment in health. At the same time, this book is dedicated to making the case for better spending—that is, deriving more health benefits from every dollar spent. The aim should be to reduce inequalities in health investment between and within countries: a 100-fold difference between the rich and the poor in money spent on health services still persists in many places. Despite a lack of clarity about what constitutes the optimum balance of health spending, a larger share should go to prevention. This book looks at several prevention options and clinical interventions that are not being fully implemented.

SELECTING INTERVENTIONS

This book persuasively makes the case that both clinical and public health interventions depend on the capacity of a given country's health system to deliver, noting that some interventions are more demanding than others in terms of infrastructure and human resources. Therefore, both the costs and the likelihood of success of the more complex interventions are a function of the health capacity in place. In addition, decisions about which interventions should be given priority will depend on assessments of the local burden of disease, local health infrastructure, and other social factors as well as on cost-effectiveness analyses. The following chapters identify the health system capacity needed for scaling up a given intervention. Even middle-income countries with relatively better health infrastructure often pursue sophisticated approaches to medical care that result in fewer health gains per amount of money invested. Every country, regardless of level of development, could benefit from the recommendations presented here.

DIAGONAL APPROACH

The medical literature has long debated which approach to delivering health interventions is more effective: vertical programs or horizontal programs. *Vertical programs* refer to focused, proactive, disease-specific interventions on a massive scale, whereas *horizontal programs* refer to more integrated, demand-driven, resource-sharing health services. This is a false dilemma, because both need to coexist in what could be called a *diagonal approach*—that is, the proactive, supply-driven provision of a set of highly cost-effective interventions on a large scale that bridges health clinics and homes. This approach often starts vertically (polio vaccination, for instance) but moves toward an increasing number of interventions (for example, oral rehydration, other vaccines, residual spraying and bednets for malaria control, micronutrient supplementation, and supervised tuberculosis treatment), making full use of field health workers and existing infrastructure. This could well be the equivalent of a public health polypill.

MULTIDISCIPLINARY ORIENTATION

What makes this book unique, in addition to its comprehensive scope, is its truly multidisciplinary approach to disease control, which merges the best of the medical and economic sciences. Every recommendation has been carefully researched and documented. Evidence-based approaches must be the foundation for allocating scarce resources. The poor cannot afford anything but the most efficient methods for organizing and implementing health care. This book is a fundamental component for fostering equitable outcomes in health and development. It will inspire all those who seek the highly complex but attainable goal of universal good health for all members of the global community.

FACILITATING PROGRESS

We all share global responsibility: governments and international agencies, public and private sectors, and society and individuals all have specific tasks. We must all strive toward more equitable distribution of the benefits of new knowledge to reduce health and development gaps between rich and poor, between countries, and within countries. The second edition of *Disease Control Priorities in Developing Countries* is a new step in precisely the right direction. If we succeed in conveying the main lessons and messages of this book, public health in developing countries will progress farther and faster.

Jaime Sepúlveda, *Director, National Institutes of Health of Mexico, Mexico City, Mexico*
Chair, Advisory Committee to the Editors

Preface

In the late 1980s, the World Bank initiated a review of priorities for the control of specific diseases and used this information as input for comparative cost-effectiveness estimates of interventions addressing most conditions important in developing countries. The purpose of the comparative cost-effectiveness work was to inform decision making within the health sectors of highly resource-constrained low- and middle-income countries. This process resulted in the 1993 publication of the first edition of *Disease Control Priorities in Developing Countries* (*DCP1*) (Jamison and others 1993). That volume's preface stated its purpose as follows:

> Between 1950 and 1990, life expectancy in developing countries increased from forty to sixty-three years with a concomitant rise in the incidence of the noncommunicable diseases of adults and the elderly. Yet there remains a huge unfinished agenda for dealing with undernutrition and the communicable childhood diseases. These trends lead to increasingly diverse and complicated epidemiological profiles in developing countries. At the same time, new epidemic diseases like AIDS are emerging; and the health of the poor during economic crisis is a source of growing concern. These developments have intensified the need for better information on the effectiveness and cost of health interventions. To assist countries to define essential health service packages, this book provides information on disease control interventions for the commonest diseases and injuries in developing countries.

To this end, *DCP1* aimed to provide systematic guidance on the selection of interventions to achieve rapid health improvements in an environment of highly constrained public sector budgets through the use of cost-effectiveness analysis.

DCP1 provided limited discussion of investments in health system development. Other major efforts undertaken at the World Bank at about the same time, including the *World Development Report 1993: Investing in Health,* used the findings of *DCP1* and dealt more explicitly with the financial and health systems aspects of implementation (Feachem and others 1992;

World Bank 1993). Closely related efforts in collaboration with the World Health Organization led to the first global and regional estimates of numbers of deaths by age, sex, and cause and of the burden (including the disability burden) from more than 100 specific diseases and conditions (Murray, Lopez, and Jamison 1994; World Bank 1993).

This second edition of *Disease Control Priorities in Developing Countries* (*DCP2*) seeks to update and improve guidance on the "what to do" questions in *DCP1* and to address the institutional, organizational, financial, and research capacities essential for health systems to deliver the right interventions. *DCP2* is the principal product of the Disease Control Priorities Project, an alliance of organizations designed to review, generate, and disseminate information on how to improve population health in developing countries. In addition to *DCP2*, the project produced numerous background papers, an extensive range of interactive consultations held around the world, and several additional major publications. The other major publications are as follows:

- *Global Burden of Disease and Risk Factors* (Lopez and others 2006), undertaken in collaboration with the World Health Organization
- *Millions Saved: Proven Successes in Global Health* (Levine and the What Works Working Group 2004), undertaken in collaboration with the Center for Global Development
- "The Intolerable Burden of Malaria: II. What's New, What's Needed" (Breman, Alilio, and Mills 2004), undertaken in collaboration with the Multilateral Initiative on Malaria
- *Priorities in Health* (Jamison and others 2006), a brief and nontechnical companion to this volume.

Each product of the Disease Control Priorities Project marries economic approaches with those of epidemiology, public health, and clinical medicine.

While general lessons emerge from the Disease Control Priorities Project, they result from careful consideration of individual cases. The diversity of health conditions necessitates specificity of analysis. Arrow clearly stated the need for technical analyses to underpin health economics: "Another lesson of medical economics is the importance of recognizing the specific character of the disease under consideration. The policy challenges that arise in treating malaria are simply very different from those attached to other major infectious scourges (Arrow, Panosian, and Gelband 2004, xi–xii)." Chapters in this volume address this need for specificity, yet use cost-effectiveness analysis in a way that makes findings on the relative attractiveness of interventions comparable.

DCP2 goes beyond *DCP1* in a number of important ways as follows:

- While virtually all chapters of *DCP1* were structured around clusters of conditions, *DCP2* provides integrative chapters—for example, on school health systems, surgery, and integrated management of childhood illness—that draw together the implementation-related responses to a number of conditions. These and other chapters reflect *DCP2*'s inclusion of implementation and system issues.
- *DCP2* includes explicit discussions of research and product development opportunities.
- Although *DCP1* dealt with policy mechanisms to change behavior (or the environment), *DCP2* attempts to do so in a more systematic way. In particular, a number of chapters assess in depth the public sector instruments for influencing behavior change that were described briefly in *DCP1*: information, education, and communication; laws and regulations; taxes and subsidies; engineering design, such as speed bumps; and facility location and characteristics.
- Different interventions place different levels of demand on a country's health system capacity. *DCP2* builds on earlier work (Gericke and others 2005) in attempting, in some chapters, to identify which interventions require relatively less system capacity for scaling up and which require more.
- Although *DCP1* briefly discussed the nonhealth outcomes of interventions, *DCP2* does so in a more systematic way, including looking at the consequences of interventions (and intervention financing) for reducing financial risks at the household level. Other important nonhealth outcomes include, for example, the time-saving value of having piped water close to the home, the increased labor productivity of healthy workers, and the amenity value of clean air.
- An important element of *DCP1* was its assumption that to inform broad policy, major changes from the status quo need to be considered, not just marginal ones. For cost-effectiveness analysis, any major change needs to be informed by burden of disease assessments in a way not required for judging the attractiveness of marginal change, because the size of the burden affects total costs and the feasibility of extending the intervention to all who would benefit. This is particularly true when considering research and

development priorities, but also applies to control priorities. In this regard, *DCP2* continues in the spirit of *DCP1* in assessing cost-effectiveness analyses of major changes, but it does so more systematically for each of the six regional groupings of low- and middle-income countries used throughout this volume (see map 1, inside the front cover).

What was becoming clear in 1990 is clearer today: focusing health system attention on delivering efficacious and often relatively inexpensive health interventions can lead to dramatic reductions in mortality and disability at modest cost. A valuable dimension of globalization has been the diffusion of knowledge about what these interventions are and how to deliver them. The pace of this diffusion into a country determines the pace of health improvement in that country much more than its level of income. Our purpose is to help speed this diffusion of life-saving knowledge.

The Editors

REFERENCES

Arrow, K. J., C. Panosian, and H. Gelband, eds. 2004. *Saving Lives, Buying Time: Economics of Malaria Drugs in an Age of Resistance.* Washington, DC: National Academies Press.

Breman, J. G., M. S. Alilio, and A. Mills, eds. 2004. "The Intolerable Burden of Malaria: II. What's New, What's Needed." *American Journal of Hygiene and Tropical Medicine* 71 (2 Suppl): 1–282.

Feachem, R. G. A., T. Kjellstrom, C. J. L. Murray, M. Over, and M. Phillips, eds. 1992. *Health of Adults in the Developing World.* New York: Oxford University Press.

Gericke, C. A., C. Kurowski, M. K. Ranson, and A. Mills. 2005. "Intervention Complexity: A Conceptual Framework to Inform Priority-Setting in Health." *Bulletin of the World Health Organization* 83 (4): 285–93.

Jamison, D. T., J. G. Breman, A. R. Measham, G. Alleyne, M. Claeson, D. B. Evans, P. Jha, A. Mills and P. Musgrove, eds. 2006. *Priorities in Health.* Washington, DC: World Bank.

Jamison, D. T., W. H. Mosley, A. R. Measham, and J. L. Bobadilla, eds. 1993. *Disease Control Priorities in Developing Countries.* New York: Oxford University Press.

Levine, R., and the What Works Working Group. 2004. *Millions Saved: Proven Successes in Global Health.* Washington, DC: Center for Global Development.

Lopez A. D., C. D. Mathers, M. Ezzati, D. T. Jamison, and C. J. L. Murray, eds. 2006. *Global Burden of Disease and Risk Factors.* New York: Oxford University Press.

Murray, C. J. L., A. D. Lopez, and D. T. Jamison. 1994. "The Global Burden of Disease in 1990: Summary Results, Sensitivity Analysis, and Future Directions." In *Global Comparative Assessments in the Health Sector: Disease Burden, Expenditures, and Intervention Packages*, ed. C. J. L. Murray, and A. D. Lopez, 97–138. Geneva: World Health Organization.

World Bank. 1993. *World Development Report 1993: Investing in Health.* New York: Oxford University Press.

Editors

Dean T. Jamison is a professor of health economics in the School of Medicine at the University of California, San Francisco (UCSF), and an affiliate of UCSF Global Health Sciences. Dr. Jamison concurrently serves as an adjunct professor in both the Peking University Guanghua School of Management and in the University of Queensland School of Population Health.

Before joining UCSF, Dr. Jamison was on the faculty of the University of California, Los Angeles, and also spent many years at the World Bank, where he was a senior economist in the research department; division chief for education policy; and division chief for population, health, and nutrition. In 1992–93, he temporarily rejoined the World Bank to serve as director of the World Development Report Office and as lead author for the Bank's *World Development Report 1993: Investing in Health.*

His publications are in the areas of economic theory, public health, and education. Dr. Jamison studied at Stanford (B.A., philosophy; M.S., engineering sciences) and at Harvard (Ph.D., economics, under K. J. Arrow). In 1994, he was elected to membership in the Institute of Medicine of the U.S. National Academy of Sciences.

Joel G. Breman, M.D., D.T.P.H., is senior scientific adviser, Fogarty International Center of the National Institutes of Health, and comanaging editor of the Disease Control Priorities Project. He was educated at the University of California, Los Angeles; the Keck School of Medicine, the University of Southern California; and the London School of Hygiene and Tropical Medicine. Dr. Breman trained in medicine at the University of Southern California–Los Angeles County Medical Center; in infectious diseases at the Boston City Hospital, Harvard Medical School; and in epidemiology at the U.S. Centers for Disease Control and Prevention.

Dr. Breman worked in Guinea on smallpox eradication (1967–69); in Burkina Faso at the Organization for Coordination and Cooperation in the Control of the Major Endemic Diseases (1972–76); and at the World Health Organization, Geneva (1977–80), where he was responsible for orthopoxvirus research and the certification of smallpox eradication. In 1976, in the Democratic Republic of Congo (formerly Zaire), Dr. Breman investigated the first outbreak of Ebola hemorrhagic fever.

Following the confirmation of smallpox eradication in 1980, Dr. Breman returned to the U.S. Centers for Disease Control, where he began work on the epidemiology and control of malaria. Dr. Breman joined the Fogarty International Center in 1995 and has been director of the International Training and Research Program in Emerging Infectious Diseases and senior scientific adviser. He has been a member of many advisory groups, including serving as chair of the World Health Organization's Technical Advisory Group on Human Monkeypox and as a member of the World Health Organization's International Commission for the Certification of *Dracunculiasis* (guinea worm) Eradication. Dr. Breman has written more than 100 publications on infectious diseases and research capacity strengthening in developing countries. He was guest editor of two supplements to the *American Journal of Tropical Medicine and Hygiene*: "The Intolerable Burden of Malaria: A New Look at the Numbers" (2001) and "The Intolerable Burden of Malaria: What's New, What's Needed" (2004).

Anthony R. Measham is co-managing editor of the Disease Control Priorities Project at the Fogarty International Center of the National Institutes of Health; deputy director of the Communicating Health Priorities Project at the Population Reference Bureau, Washington, DC; and a member of the Working Group of the Global Alliance for Vaccines and Immunization on behalf of the World Bank.

Born in the United Kingdom, Dr. Measham practiced family medicine in Dartmouth, Nova Scotia, before devoting the remainder of his career to date to international health. He spent 15 years living in developing countries on behalf of the Population Council (Colombia), the Ford Foundation (Bangladesh), and the World Bank (India). Early in his international health career (1975–77), he was deputy director of the Center for Population and Family Health at Columbia University, New York. He then served for 17 years on the staff of the World Bank, as health adviser from 1984 until 1988 and as chief for policy and research of the Health, Nutrition, and Population Division from 1988 until 1993.

Dr. Measham has spent most of his career providing technical assistance, carrying out research and analysis, and helping to develop projects in more than 20 developing countries, primarily in the areas of maternal and child health, family planning, and nutrition. He was an editor of the first edition of *Disease Control Priorities in Developing Countries* and has authored approximately 60 monographs, book chapters, and journal articles.

Dr. Measham graduated in medicine from Dalhousie University, Halifax, Nova Scotia. He received a master of science and a doctorate in public health from the University of North Carolina in Chapel Hill and is a diplomat of the American Board of Preventive Medicine and Public Health. His honors include being elected to the Alpha Omega Alpha Honor Medical Society; being appointed as special professor of International Health, University of Nottingham Medical School, Nottingham, United Kingdom; and being named Dalhousie University Medical Alumnus of the Year in 2000–1.

George Alleyne, M.D., F.R.C.P., F.A.C.P. (Hon.), D.Sc. (Hon.), is director emeritus of the Pan American Health Organization, where he served as director from 1995 to 2003. Dr. Alleyne is a native of Barbados and graduated from the University of the West Indies in medicine in 1957. He completed his postgraduate training in internal medicine in the United Kingdom and did further postgraduate work in that country and in the United States. He entered academic medicine at the University of the West Indies in 1962, and his career included research in the Tropical Metabolism Research Unit for his doctorate in medicine. He was appointed professor of medicine at the University of the West Indies in 1972, and four years later he became chair of the Department of Medicine. He is an emeritus professor of the University of the West Indies. Dr. Alleyne joined the Pan American Health Organization in 1981, in 1983 he was appointed director of the Area of Health Programs, and in 1990 he was appointed assistant director.

Dr. Alleyne's scientific publications have dealt with his research in renal physiology and biochemistry and various aspects of clinical medicine. During his term as director of the Pan American Health Organization, he dealt with and published on issues such as equity in health, health and development, and international cooperation in health. He has also addressed several aspects of health in the Caribbean and the problems the area faces. He is a member of the Institute of Medicine and chancellor of the University of the West Indies.

Dr. Alleyne has received numerous awards in recognition of his work, including prestigious decorations and national honors from many countries of the Americas. In 1990, he was made Knight Bachelor by Her Majesty Queen Elizabeth II for his services to medicine. In 2001, he was awarded the Order of the Caribbean Community, the highest honor that can be conferred on a Caribbean national.

Mariam Claeson, M.D., M.P.H., is the program coordinator for AIDS in the South Asia Region of the World Bank since January 2005. She was the lead public health specialist in the Health, Nutrition, and Population, Human Development Network, of the World Bank (1998–2004), managing the Health, Nutrition, and Population Millennium Development Goals work program to support accelerated progress in countries.

Dr. Claeson coauthored the call for action by the Bellagio study group on child survival in 2003, *Knowledge into Action for Child Survival,* and the World Bank's 2005 report on *The Millennium Development Goals for Health: Rising to the Challenges.* She was a member of the What Works Working group hosted by the Center for Global Development that resulted in the report *Millions Saved: Proven Successes in Global Health* (2005). Dr. Claeson coauthored the health chapter of the *Poverty Reduction Strategy* source book, promoting a life-cycle approach to maternal and child health and nutrition. As a coordinator of the public health thematic group (1998–2002), she led the development of the strategy note *Public Health and World Bank Operations* and promoted multisectoral approaches to child health within the World Bank and in Bank-supported country operations, analytical work, and lending.

Prior to joining the World Bank, Dr. Claeson worked with the World Health Organization from 1987 until 1995, in later years as program manager for the Global Program for the Control of Diarrheal Diseases. She has several years of field experience working in developing countries; in clinical practice at the rural district level in Bangladesh, Bhutan, and Tanzania; in national program management of immunization and diarrheal disease control programs in Ethiopia; and in health sector development projects in middle- and low-income countries.

David B. Evans, Ph.D., is an economist by training. Between 1980 and 1990, he was an academic, first in economics departments and then in a medical school, during which time he undertook consultancies for the World Bank, the World Health Organization, and governments. From 1990 until 1998, he sponsored and conducted research into social and economic aspects of tropical diseases and their control in the United Nations Children's Fund, United Nations Development Programme, World Bank, and World Health Organization Special Programme on Research and Training in Tropical Diseases. He subsequently became director of the Global Programme on Evidence for Health Policy and then the Department of Health Systems Financing of the World Health Organization, where he is now responsible for a range of activities relating to the development of appropriate health financing strategies and policies. These activities include the World Health Organization's CHOICE project, which has assessed and reported the costs and effectiveness of more than 700 health interventions, the costs of scaling up interventions, the levels of health expenditures and accounts, and the extent of financial catastrophe and impoverishment caused by out-of-pocket payments for health and which has assessed the impact of different ways to raise funds for health, pool them, and use them to provide or purchase services and interventions. He has published widely in these areas.

Prabhat Jha is Canada research chair of health and development at the University of Toronto. He is also the founding director of the Centre for Global Health Research, St. Michael's Hospital; associate professor in the Department of Public Health Sciences, University of Toronto; research scholar at the McLaughlin Centre for Molecular Medicine; and professeur extraordinaire at the Université de Lausanne, Switzerland.

Dr. Jha is lead author of *Curbing the Epidemic: Governments and the Economics of Tobacco Control* and coeditor of *Tobacco Control in Developing Countries*. Both are among the most influential books on tobacco control. He is the principal investigator of a prospective study of 1 million deaths in India, researching mortality from smoking, alcohol use, fertility patterns, indoor air pollution, and other risk factors among 2.3 million homes and 15 million people. This work is currently the world's largest prospective study of health. He also conducts studies of HIV transmission in various countries, focusing on documenting the risk factors for the spread of HIV and interventions to prevent the spread of the HIV/AIDS epidemic. His studies have received more than $5 million in peer-reviewed grants.

Dr. Jha has published widely on tobacco, HIV/AIDS, and health of the global poor. His awards include a Gold medal from the Poland Health Promotion Foundation (2000), the Top 40 Canadians under Age 40 Award (2004), and the Ontario Premier's Research Excellence Award (2004). Dr. Jha was a research scholar at the University of Toronto and McMaster University in Canada. He holds an M.D. from the University of Manitoba and a D. Phil. in epidemiology and public health from Oxford University, where he studied as a Rhodes Scholar at Magdalen College.

Anne Mills, Ph.D., is professor of health economics and policy at the London School of Hygiene and Tropical Medicine. She has more than 20 years of experience in research pertaining to health economics in developing countries and has published widely in the fields of health economics and health planning, including books on the role of government in health in developing countries, health planning in the United Kingdom, decentralization, health economics research in developing countries, and the public-private mix. Her most recent research interests have been in the organization and financing of health systems, including the evaluation of contractual relationships between the public and private sectors and the application of economic evaluation techniques to improve the efficiency of disease control programs.

Dr. Mills has had extensive involvement in supporting the health economics research activities of the World Health Organization's Tropical Disease Research Programme. She founded, and is head of, the Health Economics and Financing Programme, which has become one of the world's leading groups in developing and applying theories and techniques of health economics to increase knowledge on how best to improve the equity and efficiency of developing countries' health systems. She has acted as adviser to a number of multilateral and bilateral agencies—notably, the United Kingdom Department for International Development and the World Health Organization. She guided the creation of the Alliance for Health Policy and Systems Research and chairs its board. Most recently, she has been a member of the Commission for Macroeconomics and Health and cochair of its working group on improving the health outcomes of the poor.

Philip Musgrove is deputy editor—global health for *Health Affairs,* which is published by Project HOPE in Bethesda, Maryland. He worked for the World Bank (1990–2002), including two years on secondment to the World Health Organization (1999–2001), retiring as a principal economist. He was previously an adviser in health economics at the Pan American Health Organization (1982–90) and a research associate at the Brookings Institution and at Resources for the Future (1964–81).

Dr. Musgrove is an adjunct professor at the School of Advanced International Studies, Johns Hopkins University, and has taught at George Washington University, American University, and the University of Florida. He holds degrees from Haverford College (B.A., 1962, summa cum laude); Princeton University (M.P.A., 1964); and Massachusetts Institute of Technology (Ph.D., 1974).

Dr. Musgrove has worked on health reform projects in Argentina, Brazil, Chile, and Colombia and has dealt with a variety of issues in health economics, financing, equity, and nutrition. His publications include more than 50 articles in economics and health journals and chapters in 20 books.

Advisory Committee to the Editors

J. R. Aluoch
Professor, Nairobi Women's Hospital, Nairobi, Kenya

Jacques Baudouy
Director, Health, Nutrition, and Population, World Bank, Washington, DC, United States

Fred Binka
Executive Director, INDEPTH Network, Accra, Ghana

Mayra Buvinić
Director, Gender and Development, World Bank, Washington, DC, United States

David Challoner, Co-Chair
Foreign Secretary, Institute of Medicine, U.S. National Academies, Gainesville, Florida, United States

Guy de Thé, Co-Chair
Research Director and Professor Emeritus, Institut Pasteur, Paris, France

Timothy Evans
Assistant Director General, Evidence and Information for Policy, World Health Organization, Geneva, Switzerland

Richard Horton
Editor, *The Lancet*, London, United Kingdom

Sharon Hrynkow
Acting Director, Fogarty International Center, National Institutes of Health, Bethesda, Maryland, United States

Gerald Keusch
Provost and Dean for Global Health, Boston University School of Public Health, Boston, Massachusetts, United States

Kiyoshi Kurokawa
President, Science Council of Japan, Kanawaga, Japan

Peter Lachmann
Past President, U.K. Academy of Medical Sciences, Cambridge, United Kingdom

Mary Ann Lansang
Executive Director, INCLEN Trust International Inc., Manila, Philippines

Christopher Lovelace
Director, Kyrgyz Republic Country Office and Central Asia Human Development, World Bank, Bishkek, Kyrgyz Republic

Anthony Mbewu
Executive Director, Medical Research Council of South Africa, Tygerberg, South Africa

Rajiv Misra
Former Secretary of Health, Government of India, Haryana, India

Perla Santos Ocampo
President, National Academy of Science and Technology, San Juan, Philippines

G. B. A. Okelo
Secretary General and Executive Director, African Academy of Sciences, Nairobi, Kenya

Sevket Ruacan
General Director, MESA Hospital Ankara, Turkey

Pramilla Senanayake
Chairman, Foundation Council of the Global Forum for Health Research, Colombo, Sri Lanka

Jaime Sepúlveda, Chair
Director, National Institutes of Health of Mexico, Mexico City, Mexico

Chitr Sitthi-amorn
Director, Institute of Health Research, and Dean, Chulalongkorn University, College of Public Health, Bangkok, Thailand

Contributors

Taghreed Adam
World Health Organization

Sarah Adomakoh
Chronic Disease Research Centre, University of the West
    Indies Associates for International Development

Olu Akinyanju
Sickle Cell Foundation, Nigeria
University Teaching Hospital, Nigeria

Mark A. Anderson
U.S. Centers for Disease Control and Prevention

Sevgi O. Aral
U.S. Centers for Disease Control and Prevention

Samira Asma
U.S. Centers for Disease Control and Prevention

Cristian Baeza
World Bank

Rob Baltussen
Erasmus MC

Delia Barcelona
United Nations Population Fund

Scott Barrett
Johns Hopkins University

John H. Barton
Stanford University

Jane Batt
University of Toronto
St. Michaels Hospital

Angela Bayer
Johns Hopkins University Bloomberg School of Public Health

Kathleen Beegle
World Bank

Geneviève Begkoyian
United Nations Children's Fund

Jere R. Behrman
University of Pennsylvania

Nicole Bellows
University of California, Berkeley

Sandra E. Bendeck
University of Texas at Southwestern

Stefano Bertozzi
Instituto Nacional de Salud Pública

Jeff Bethony
George Washington University

Alok Bhargava
University of Houston

Sohinee Bhattacharya
University of Aberdeen

Zulfiqar A. Bhutta
Aga Khan University

Nancy Birdsall
Center for Global Development

David Bishai
Johns Hopkins University

Robert E. Black
Johns Hopkins Bloomberg School
    of Public Health

Barry R. Bloom
Harvard School of Public Health

Stephen B. Blount
U.S. Centers for Disease Control and Prevention

Cynthia Boschi-Pinto
World Health Organization

Douglas Bratthall
World Health Organization Collaborating Centre
Centre for Oral Health Sciences, Malmo University

Carol Brayne
University of Cambridge

Joel G. Breman
Fogarty International Center, National Institutes of Health
Disease Control Priorities Project

Logan Brenzel
World Bank

Dan W. Brock
Harvard Medical School

Simon Brooker
London School of Hygiene and Tropical Medicine

Peter Brooks
University of Queensland

Claire V. Broome
U.S. Centers for Disease Control and Prevention

L. Jackson Brown
American Dental Association

Martin L. Brown
National Cancer Institute, National Institutes of Health

Nigel Bruce
University of Liverpool

Jennifer Bryce
Independent consultant

Colin H. W. Bullough
University of Aberdeen

Donald A. P. Bundy
World Bank

Alexander Butchart
World Health Organization

Mayra Buvinić
World Bank

Sandy Cairncross
London School of Hygiene and Tropical Medicine

John Cairns
London School of Hygiene and Tropical Medicine

Balla Camara
Ministry of Public Health, Guinea
Ministry of Education, Guinea

Pierre Cattand
Association against Trypanosomiasis

Laura E. Caulfield
Johns Hopkins University Bloomberg School of Public Health

Frank J. Chaloupka
University of Illinois at Chicago

Vijay Chandra
World Health Organization, Regional Office for
  South-East Asia

Heng Leng Chee
National University of Singapore

Suephy Chen
Emory University
Atlanta Veterans Administration Medical Center

Thomas Cherian
World Health Organization

Tom M. Chiller
U.S. Centers for Disease Control and Prevention

Dan Chisholm
World Health Organization

Lester Chitsulo
World Health Organization

Jeffrey Chow
Resources for the Future

Mushtaque Chowdhury
Bangladesh Rural Advancement Committee
Columbia University

Mariam Claeson
World Bank

Luke B. Connelly
University of Queensland

Joseph Cook
International Trachoma Initiative

Rodrigo Correa-Oliveira
Centro de Pesquisas Rene Rachou—FIOCRUZ

Mark Cullen
Yale University

Patricia M. Danzon
Wharton School, University of Pennsylvania

Haile T. Debas
University of California, San Francisco

Louisa Degenhardt
University of New South Wales

Lisa M. DeMaria
Instituto Nacional de Salud Pública

Nilanthi de Silva
University of Kelaniya, Sri Lanka

Phillippe Desjeux
Institute for OneWorld Health

Claude de Ville de Goyet
Independent consultant

John Dirks
International Society of Nephrology
University of Toronto

Jane Doherty
University of the Witwatersrand, South Africa

Chris Doran
University of Queensland

Ogobara K. Doumbo
University of Bamako, Mali

Gerrit Draisma
Erasmus MC

Lesley Drake
St. Mary's Medical School

Maureen S. Durkin
University of Wisconsin Medical School
University of Wisconsin-Madison

Adriano Duse
University of the Witwatersrand, South Africa
National Health Laboratory Service

Courtenay Dusenbury
Emory University

Christopher Dye
World Health Organization

Michael M. Engelgau
U.S. Centers for Disease Control and Prevention

Dirk Engels
World Health Organization

Mike English
Kenya Medical Research Institute
University of Oxford

Victoria Espitia-Hardeman
U.S. Centers for Disease Control and Prevention

Roberto Estrada
Universidad Autónoma de Guerrero, Mexico

David B. Evans
World Health Organization

Timothy Evans
World Health Organization

Qiu Fang
World Bank

Piet Feenstra
Royal Tropical Institute, Netherlands

Becca Feldman
Harvard School of Public Health
Instituto Nacional de Salud Pública

Alan Fenwick
Imperial College

Elisa Fernández
Inter-American Development Bank

Marilyn Fingerhut
National Institute for Occupational Safety
    and Health, United States

Katherine Floyd
World Health Organization

Kathleen M. Foley
Memorial Sloan-Kettering Cancer Center
Weill Medical College of Cornell University

Olivier Fontaine
World Health Organization

Susan Foster
Boston University School of Public Health

Julia Fox-Rushby
Brunel University, United Kingdom

Julio Frenk
Secretaria de Salud de Mexico

Kevin D. Frick
Johns Hopkins Bloomberg School of Public Health

Suthat Fucharoen
Mahidol University, Thailand

Vendhan Gajalakshmi
Epidemiological Research Center, India

Rae Galloway
World Bank

Helene Gayle
Bill & Melinda Gates Foundation

Thomas A. Gaziano
Brigham and Women's Hospital
Harvard Medical School

Hellen Gelband
Institute of Medicine, National Academies

Amaya Gillespie
United Nations Study on Violence against Children

Julian Gold
Prince of Wales Hospital, Australia

Sue J. Goldie
Harvard School of Public Health

Chuck Golmar
World Health Organization

Richard Gosselin
University of California, Berkeley

Pablo Gottret
World Bank

Eduardo Gotuzzo
Universidad Peruana Cayetano Heredia
Hospital Nacional Cayetano Heredia, Peru

Wendy J. Graham
University of Aberdeen
London School of Hygiene and Tropical Medicine

Robert Grant
J. David Gladstone Institutes, United States

Brian Greenwood
London School of Hygiene and Tropical Medicine

Prakash C. Gupta
Healis-Sekhsaria Institute of Public Health, India
Arnold School of Public Health, United States

M.G. Guzmán
Pedro Kouri Tropical Medicine Institute, Cuba

Anne Haddix
Rollins School of Public Health, Emory University

Wayne Hall
University of Queensland

Neal A. Halsey
Johns Hopkins University Bloomberg School of Public Health

Joe Harford
National Cancer Institute, National Institutes of Health

Roderick Hay
Queen's University Belfast

Robert M. Hecht
International AIDS Vaccine Initiative

D. A. Henderson
University of Pittsburgh Medical Center

Martin Hensher
Department of Health, United Kingdom

Susan Herman
University of Pennsylvania

Eduardo Romero Hicks
Secretaria de Salud Guanajuato, Mexico
University of Guanajuato, Mexico

Anna-Maria Hoffman
United Nations Educational Scientific, and Cultural
    Organization

Karen J. Hofman
Fogarty International Center, National Institutes of Health

King K. Holmes
University of Washington
Harborview Medical Center

Charles Hongoro
London School of Hygiene and Tropical Medicine
Aurum Health Research Institute

Susan Horton
Wilfrid Laurier University, Canada

Peter J. Hotez
George Washington University

Fleur Hourihan
University of Newcastle, Australia

Guy Hutton
Swiss Tropical Institute

Adnan A. Hyder
Johns Hopkins Bloomberg School of Public Health

Steven Hyman
Harvard University
Harvard Medical School

Giuseppina Imperatore
U.S. Centers for Disease Control and Prevention

Rubina Imtiaz
U.S. Centers for Disease Control and Prevention

Michael T. Isbell
Independent consultant

Dean T. Jamison
University of California, San Francisco
Disease Control Priorities Project

Jean Jannin
World Health Organization

Philip Jenkins
World Health Organization

Prabhat Jha
University of Toronto
Centre for Global Health Research

T. Jacob John
Christian Medical College (retired)
National HIV/AIDS Reference Center, India (retired)

Jack Jones
World Health Organization

David E. Joranson
University of Wisconsin Comprehensive Cancer Center
World Health Organization

Manjul Joshipura
Academy of Traumatology, India
Apollo Hospitals, India

Matthew Jukes
Imperial College London

Alka M. Kanaya
University of California, San Francisco

Scott Kasner
University of Pennsylvania

Ronald Kessler
Harvard Medical School

Gerald T. Keusch
Boston University Medical Campus
Boston University School of Public Health

Peter Kilima
International Trachoma Initiative

Sally Kingsland
National Centre for Epidemiology and Population Health,
Australian National University

Tord Kjellström
Australian National University
National Institute of Public Health, Sweden

Keith P. Klugman
Rollins School of Public Health, Emory University

Felicia Knaul
Fundación Mexicana para la Salud
Secretaria de Educación Pública de Mexico

Rudolf Knippenberg
United Nations Children's Fund

James C. Knowles
Independent consultant

Olive C. Kobusingye
World Health Organization Regional Office for Africa

Jeffrey P. Koplan
Emory University

Daniel Kress
Bill & Melinda Gates Foundation

A. Kroeger
World Health Organization

Richard Laing
Boston University School of Public Health, now World Health
    Organization

John R. La Montagne (Deceased)
National Institute of Allergy and Infectious Diseases,
    National Institutes of Health

Claudio F. Lanata
Instituto de Investigación Nutricional, Peru

Ana Langer
EngenderHealth

Carlene M. M. Lawes
University of Auckland

Joy E. Lawn
Save the Children–USA
Institute of Child Health

Ramanan Laxminarayan
Resources for the Future

Seung-Hee Frances Lee
Save the Children–USA

Christian Lengeler
Swiss Tropical Institute

P. R. Lever
Royal Tropical Institute, Netherlands

Ruth Levine
Center for Global Development

Joseph Lipscomb
Rollins School of Public Health, Emory University

Madhumita Lodh
Commonwealth Department of Transport and Regional
    Services, Australia

Alan Lopez
University of Queensland
Harvard School of Public Health

Elizabeth Lule
World Bank

Antoine Mahé
Programme National de Lutte Contre le SIDA

Adel Mahmoud
Merck & Company Inc.
Case Western Reserve University

Margaret Maier
RAND Corporation

Lisa Manhart
University of Washington

Bala Manyam
Texas A&M University HSC School of Medicine

Paola Marchesini
World Health Organization

Maureen S. Marshall
Task Force for Child Survival and Development

John B. Mason
Tulane University School of Public Health
    and Tropical Medicine

Gaverick Matheny
University of Maryland

Colin McCord
Columbia University

Martin McKee
London School of Hygiene and Tropical Medicine

Tonya McLeod
Emory University

Tony McMichael
Australian National University

Anthony R. Measham
World Bank (retired)
Disease Control Priorities Project

Jeffrey Mecaskey
Axios International

André Médici
Inter-American Development Bank

Carol Ann Medlin
University of California, San Francisco

Sumi Mehta
World Health Organization
Health Effects Institute

Bjørn Melgaard
World Health Organization

David Meltzer
University of Chicago

Kamini Mendis
World Health Organization

James Mercy
U.S. Centers for Disease Control and Prevention

Catherine Michaud
Harvard School of Public Health

Mark Miller
Fogarty International Center, National Institutes
    of Health

Anne Mills
London School of Hygiene and Tropical Medicine

Andrew Mitchell
Harvard School of Public Health

Arlene Mitchell
World Food Programme

Charles Mock
University of Washington
Harborview Medical Center

Antonio Montresor
World Health Organization

James Moore
U.S. Centers for Disease Control and Prevention

Chantal Morel
London School of Hygiene and Tropical Medicine
Oxford Outcomes

Luis Morillo
Javeriana University

Roy D. Mugerwa
Makerere University, Uganda
Case Western Reserve University

Jo-Ann Mulligan
London School of Hygiene and Tropical Medicine

Philip Musgrove
Health Affairs
Disease Control Priorities Project

Vasant Narasimhan
Novartis Pharma AG, Switzerland

K. M. Venkat Narayan
Centers for Disease Control and Prevention
Rollins School of Public Health at Emory
    University

Mike B. Nathan
World Health Organization

Karin B. Nelson
National Institute for Neurological Disorders and Stroke,
   National Institutes of Health

Isaac Ngugi
KEMRI/Wellcome Trust Programme, Kenya

Mounkaila Noma
African Programme for Onchocerciasis Control

Charles Normand
University of Dublin, Trinity College
London School of Hygiene and Tropical Medicine

Robyn Norton
George Institute for International Health
University of Sydney

Peter Nsubuga
U.S. Centers for Disease Control and Prevention

Rachel Nugent
Population Reference Bureau
Fogarty International Center, National Institutes
   of Health

Thomas O'Brien
Brigham and Women's Hospital

Adesola Ogunniyi
University of Ibadan
University College Hospital, Nigeria

Iruka N. Okeke
Haverford College
Eidgenossische Technische Hochschule, Switzerland

Nancy Olivieri
Hemoglobinopathy Research Program, University Health
   Network, Canada

Claudio Osorio
Pan American Health Organization

Mead Over
World Bank

Ariel Pablos-Mendez
World Health Organization
Columbia University

Fred Paccaud
University of Lausanne
University of Montreal

Nancy S. Padian
University of California, San Francisco

Rajesh Pandav
World Health Organization, Regional Office for
   South-East Asia

Vikram Patel
London School of Hygiene and Tropical Medicine

Vikram S. Pathania
University of California, Berkeley

John W. Peabody
University of California, San Francisco
University of California, Los Angeles

Richard Peck
University of Illinois at Chicago

Margie Peden
World Health Organization

Poul Erik Petersen
World Health Organization

Ndola Prata
University of California, Berkeley

Alexander S. Preker
World Bank

Max Price
University of the Witwatersrand, South Africa

Pekka Puska
National Public Health Institute, Finland

Zahidul Quayyum
University of Aberdeen

Sadanand Rajkumar
University of Newcastle
Bloomfield Hospital

Ambady Ramachandran
M.V. Hospital for Diabetes, India
Diabetes Research Centre, India

K. D. Ramaiah
Vector Control Research Centre, India

Geetha Ranmuthugala
Australian National University

Fawzia Rasheed
Independent consultant

K. Srinath Reddy
All India Institute of Medical Sciences
Initiative for Cardiovascular Health in the
   Developing Countries

Eva Rehfuess
World Health Organization

Jürgen Rehm
Centre for Addiction and Mental Health, Canada
ISGF/ARI, Switzerland

Jan H. F. Remme
World Health Organization

Giuseppe Remuzzi
Mario Negri Institute for Pharmacological Research, Italy
Azienda Ospedaliera Ospedali Riuniti di Bergamo, Italy

Serge Resnikoff
World Health Organization

Stephanie A. Richard
Johns Hopkins University Bloomberg School of
    Public Health

Frank Richards
U.S. Centers for Disease Control and Prevention
The Carter Center of Emory University

Juan A. Rivera
Instituto Nacional de Salud Pública, Mexico

S. Adibul Hasan Rizvi
Sindh Institute of Urology and Transplantation

David A. Robalino
World Bank

Anthony Rodgers
University of Auckland

Khama Rogo
World Bank

Robin Room
Stockholm University

James E. Rosen
World Bank

Mark L. Rosenberg
Task Force for Child Survival and
Development

Linda Rosenstock
University of California, Los Angeles

David Sanders
University of the Western Cape

Lorenzo Savioli
World Health Organization

Richard M. Scheffler
University of California, Berkeley

George Schieber
World Bank

Arrigo Schieppati
Mario Negri Institute for Pharmacological
    Research, Italy
Azienda Ospedaliera Ospedali Riuniti di Bergamo, Italy

Gabriel Schmunis
Pan American Health Organization

Helen Schneider
University of the Witwatersrand, South Africa

C. J. Schofield
London School of Hygiene and Tropical Medicine

A. Seketeli
African Programme for Onchocerciasis Control

Malick Sembene
Ministry of National Education, Senegal

Sheldon Shaeffer
United Nations Educational, Scientific, and
    Cultural Organization

Raj J. Shah
Bill & Melinda Gates Foundation

Sonbol A. Shahid-Salles
Disease Control Priorities Project
Population Reference Bureau

Brian Sharp
Medical Research Council

Alexandra Shaw
AP Consultants

Donald Shepard
Schneider Institute for Health Policy, Heller School,
    Brandeis University

Rupendra Shrestha
Australian National University

Xiao Shu-Hua
National Institute of Parasitic Diseases, China

Donald Silberberg
University of Pennsylvania

Eric A. F. Simoes
University of Colorado Health Sciences Center
Children's Hospital

Lone Simonsen
National Institute of Allergy and Infectious Diseases,
    National Institutes of Health

Susheela Singh
Alan Guttmacher Institute, United States

Arthur S. Slutsky
St. Michael's Hospital
University of Toronto

Andrew Smith
World Health Organization

Kirk Smith
School of Public Health, University of California, Berkeley

Peter C. Smith
Centre for Health Economics, University of York

Robert W. Snow
Centre for Tropical Medicine, University of Oxford
Kenya Medical Research Institute

Soekirman
Institut Pertanian Bogor, Indonesia

Geoffrey C. Solarsh
Monash University, Australia

Dan Sosin
U.S. Centers for Disease Control and Prevention

Frank E. Speizer
Harvard Medical School
Harvard School of Public Health

Sally K. Stansfield
Bill & Melinda Gates Foundation
University of Washington

Richard W. Steketee
PATH

Jayanthi Ramanathan Stjernswärd
Malmø University

Stephen E. Straus
National Center for Complementary and Alternative
    Medicine, National Institutes of Health

Donna F. Stroup
U.S. Centers for Disease Control and Prevention

Mario M. Taguiwalo
Department of Health, Republic of the
    Philippines

Tsutomu Takeuchi
School of Medicine, Keio University, Japan

Caroline Tanner
Parkinson's Institute

Robert V. Tauxe
U.S. Centers for Disease Control and
    Prevention

Stephen B. Thacker
U.S. Centers for Disease Control and Prevention

William Theodore
National Institute for Neurological Disorders and Stroke,
    National Institutes of Health

Amardeep Thind
University of Western Ontario
University of California, Los Angeles

Stephen Tollman
Medical Research Council
University of the Witwatersrand, South Africa

Ana Cristina Torres
World Bank

Murray Trostle
U.S. Agency for International Development

Vivian Valdmanis
University of the Sciences in Philadelphia

W. H. van Brakel
Royal Tropical Institute, Netherlands

Anna Vassall
Royal Tropical Institute, Netherlands

Cesar G. Victora
Universidade Federal de Pelotas, Brazil

Maya Vijayaraghavan
U.S. Centers for Disease Control and Prevention

Theo Vos
University of Queensland

Judith L. Wagner
Institute of Medicine, United States

Adam Wagstaff
World Bank

Julia Walsh
University of California, Berkeley

Prawese Wasi
Siriraj Hospital
Mahidol University

Hugh Waters
Johns Hopkins University Bloomberg
    School of Public Health

David Weatherall
University of Oxford

Jeny Wegbreit
University of California, San Francisco

Mark E. White
U.S. Centers for Disease Control and Prevention

Nicholas J. White
Mahidol University, Thailand
University of Oxford

Harvey Whiteford
University of Queensland

Daniel Wikler
Harvard School of Public Health

Suwit Wilbulpolprasert
Ministry of Public Health, Thailand

Walter C. Willett
Harvard School of Public Health
Harvard Medical School

Desmond E. Williams
U.S. Centers for Disease Control and Prevention

Lara J. Wolfson
World Health Organization

Anthony Woolf
Peninsula Medical School, United Kingdom
Royal Cornwall Hospital, United Kingdom

Cream Wright
United Nations Children's Fund

Merrick Wright
Independent consultant

Michel Zaffran
World Health Organization

Ricardo Zapata Marti
United Nations Economic Commission for Latin America
    and Caribbean

Witold Zatonski
Cancer Center and Institute of Oncology, Poland
Health Promotion Foundation

Ping Zhang
U.S. Centers for Disease Control and Prevention

Zhen-Xin Zhang
Peking Union Medical College Hospital
Chinese Academy of Medical Science

Jelka Zupan
World Health Organization

Disease Control Priorities Project Partners

The Disease Control Priorities Project is a joint enterprise of the Fogarty International Center of the National Institutes of Health, the World Health Organization, the World Bank, and the Population Reference Bureau.

The Fogarty International Center is the international component of the U.S. National Institutes of Health. It addresses global health challenges through innovative and collaborative research and training programs and supports and advances the mission of the U.S. National Institutes of Health through international partnerships.

The World Health Organization is the specialized agency for health of the United Nations. Its objective, as set out in its constitution, is the attainment by all peoples of the highest possible level of health, with *health* defined as a state of complete physical, mental, and social well-being and not merely the absence of disease or infirmity.

The World Bank Group is one of the world's largest sources of development assistance. The Bank, which provides US$18 billion to US$22 billion each year in loans to its client countries, provided US$1.27 billion for health, nutrition, and population in 2004. The World Bank is working in more than 100 developing economies, bringing a mix of analytical work, policy dialogue, and lending to improve living standards—including health and education—and reduce poverty.

The Population Reference Bureau informs people around the world about health, population, and the environment and empowers them to use that information to advance the well-being of current and future generations. For 75 years, the bureau has analyzed complex data and research results to provide objective and timely information in a format easily understood by advocates, journalists, and decision makers; has conducted workshops around the world to give key audiences the tools they need to understand and communicate effectively about relevant issues; and has worked to ensure that policy makers in developing countries base policy decisions on sound evidence.

Acknowledgments

Preparation of this volume required efforts over four years by many institutions and almost 1,000 individuals: chapter coauthors, advisory committee members, peer reviewers, copy editors, and research and staff assistants. We have many contributions to acknowledge. We particularly thank our chapter authors, who worked extremely hard through a long and exacting process of writing, review, and revision. We also owe much gratitude to the institutional sponsors of this effort:

- *The Fogarty International Center (FIC) of the U.S. National Institutes of Health.* The FIC supported both the senior editor and one of the co-managing editors of this project, as well as support staff. Gerald Keusch, former director of the FIC, initiated and facilitated this effort, and FIC's acting director, Sharon Hrynkow, continued to provide support and counsel.
- *The World Bank.* Successive directors of the World Bank's Health, Nutrition, and Population Department, Christopher Lovelace and Jacques Baudouy, provided support, guidance, and critical reactions and facilitated the involvement of Bank staff as coauthors and reviewers.
- *The World Health Organization.* Successive leaders of the World Health Organization's Evidence and Information for Policy Cluster, Christopher Murray and Timothy Evans, coordinated the involvement of the World Health Organization, which had been agreed by Gro Harlem Brundtland, then the director-general.
- *The Bill & Melinda Gates Foundation.* Richard Klausner, Sally Stansfield, and Beth Peterman arranged for the foundation to provide major financial support and interacted closely with us throughout the past four years. Initial conversations with and encouragement from William Gates Senior are gratefully acknowledged.

In undertaking the work leading to this volume, we benefited from the close engagement of three institutions that helped organize and host consultations and arranged for background analyses to be undertaken. These institutions were the London School of Hygiene and Tropical Medicine (Anne Mills), the University of Toronto's Center for Global Health (Prabhat Jha), and Resources for the Future (Ramanan Laxminarayan). The Center for Global Development (Ruth Levine) collaborated with the chapter authors in an effort to identify proven successes in global health, the results of which were used both in this book and in a separate publication. We are grateful to each of these institutions and individuals.

We were particularly fortunate to have the strong collaboration of the Inter-Academies Medical Panel (IAMP), an association of the medical academies or medical divisions of the scientific academies of 44 countries. David Challoner and Guy de Thé cochaired the Steering Committee of the IAMP and invested much time and effort into facilitating the collaboration. In particular, the IAMP helped establish the productive Advisory Committee to the Editors, chaired by Jaime Sepúlveda, on which many members of the IAMP Steering Committee served. The IAMP's second global meeting hosted the launch of this volume in Beijing in April 2006, and the IAMP also sponsored the peer review process for all the chapters. We are most grateful to David Challoner and Guy de Thé, as well as to Jaime Sepúlveda and other members of the Advisory Committee to the Editors. The U.S. member of the IAMP, the Institute of Medicine of the National Academy of Sciences, played a critical role in facilitating all aspects of the IAMP's collaboration. Patrick Kelley, Patricia Cuff, Dianne Stare, Stacey Knobler, and Leslie Baer at the Institute of Medicine and Mohamed Hassan and Muthoni Fanin at the IAMP managed this effort and provided critical, substantive inputs.

The Office of the Publisher at the World Bank provided outstanding assistance, enthusiastic advice, and support during every phase of production of this volume and helped coordinate publicity and initial distribution. We particularly wish to thank Dirk H. Koehler, the publisher; Carlos Rossel; Mary Fisk; Santiago Pombo-Bejarano; Nancy Lammers; Randi Park; Valentina Kalk; Alice Faintich; Joanne Ainsworth; Enid Zafran; Deepa Menon; and Janice Tuten for their timely, high-quality professionalism.

Donald Lindberg, director of the National Library of Medicine (NLM) of the U.S. National Institutes of Health, and Julia Royall, chief, International Programs, NLM, graciously offered the competent services of the NLM's Information Engineering Branch of the National Center for Biotechnology Information to convert the text into an electronic product available to all visitors to the National Library of Medicine's PubMed Web site. We would like to extend our gratitude to the National Center for Biotechnology Information team members—David Lipman, Jo McEntyre, and Mohammad Al-Ubaydli, and Belinda Beck—for their technical expertise and commitment.

With this volume now in the dissemination phase, the Population Reference Bureau is charged to communicate its findings in formats likely to be of use to a range of audiences. We greatly value the work of the bureau's William P. Butz, president, and Nancy Yinger, director of international programs, in rapidly initiating this effort.

Multiple institutions from around the world contributed to organizing and hosting meetings that facilitated the preparation of this book and providing background for such meetings. We greatly appreciate the contributions and hospitality of these institutions, including the following:

- Chinese Academy of Engineering and Chinese Academy of Sciences, Disease Control Priorities Project Launch and Inter-Academies Medical Panel Global Meeting, Beijing, China (April 2006)
- Italian Ministry of Health, Veneto Region, consultation on child health and nutrition, Venice, Italy (January 2004)
- Instituto Nacional de Salud Pública, Advisory Committee to the Editors meeting, Cuernavaca, Mexico (June 2002)
- Institut Pasteur, Advisory Committee to the Editors meeting, Paris, France (March and December 2004)
- Johns Hopkins Bloomberg School of Public Health, consultation on maternal and child health, Annapolis, Maryland (May 2002)
- Johns Hopkins Paul H. Nitze School of Advanced International Studies, consultation on elimination and eradication of disease, and vaccinations, Washington, DC (October 2004)
- Merck & Company Inc., consultation on research and product development priorities, Whitehouse Station, New Jersey (September 2004)
- Multilateral Initiative on Malaria, consultations on the burden of malaria:
  - National Institute of Medical Research, Arusha, Tanzania (November 2002)
  - University of Yaoundé, Cameroon (November 2005)

- National Cancer Institute, National Institutes of Health, consultation on cancer prevention, treatment, and pain control, Bethesda, Maryland (June 2003)
- Oswaldo Cruz Foundation, World Health Organization, and Pan-American Health Organization, consultation on tropical infectious diseases, Rio de Janeiro, Brazil (April–May 2003)
- Université de Lausanne, consultation on cardiovascular disease, Lausanne, Switzerland (March 2002)
- University of California, Berkeley, consultation on learning and developmental disorders, Berkeley, California (August 2003)
- University of California, San Francisco, consultation on surgery, San Francisco, California (July 2003)
- University of Queensland, School of Population Health, authors' meeting on psychiatric disorders, neurology, and alcohol and other substance abuse, Brisbane, Australia (August 2003)
- University of Washington, consultation on sexually transmitted infections, Seattle, Washington (July 2003)
- University of the Witwatersrand, consultations on health systems and on capacity strengthening and management reform, Johannesburg, South Africa (July 2004)
- World Health Organization, Division of Mental Health, and National Institutes of Health, National Institute of Mental Health, consultation on mental health economics, Geneva, Switzerland (March 2004).

Coordination of the work leading to this publication and background research were undertaken by a small secretariat. Nancy Hancock, Pamela Maslen, and Sonbol A. Shahid-Salles provided outstanding research assistance; Andrew Marshall ably managed the budget and process; Candice Byrne provided key communications guidance, staff and editorial assistance; and Mantra Singh and Cherice Holloway provided staff assistance. Richard Miller, Lauren Sikes and Tommy Freeman of the FIC provided excellent administrative support to the Disease Control Priorities Project. Their work was absolutely essential in producing this book, and we are deeply grateful for their commitment and productivity. With so many authors and institutions involved, we are aware that many more people gave countless hours to this endeavor. We thank them also for their dedication.

The Editors

Abbreviations and Acronyms

ACE	angiotensin-converting enzyme
ACER	average cost-effectiveness ratio
ACT	artemisinin combination therapy
AD	Alzheimer's disease
ADB	Asian Development Bank
ADHD	attention deficit and hyperactivity disorder
AED	antiepileptic drug
AHEAD	applied health education and development
AIDS	acquired immunodeficiency syndrome
AIN-C	atención integral a la niñez comunitaria
ALRI	acute lower respiratory infection
AMI	acute myocardial infarction
ANW	*anganwadi* worker
aP	acellular pertussis vaccine
APOC	African Programme for Onchocerciasis Control
ARF	acute rheumatic fever
ARI	acute respiratory infection
ART	atraumatic restorative treatment
ASD	autism spectrum disorder
ATLS	advanced trauma life support
AUD	alcohol-use disorder
AZT	Zidovudine
BCC	behavior-change communication
BCG	Bacillus Calmette-Guérin
BEmOC	basic emergency obstetric care
BINP	Bangladesh Integrated Nutrition Program
BMI	body mass index
BMT	buprenorphine maintenance treatment
BOD	burden of disease
BRAC	Bangladesh Rural Advancement Committee
BRFSS	behavioral risk factor surveillance system
BZA	benzimidazole anthelmintic
CABG	coronary artery bypass graft
CAD	coronary artery disease
CAM	complementary and alternative medicine
CAPP	Country/Area Profile Programme
CBA	cost-benefit analysis
CBE	clinical breast examination
CBHI	community-based health insurance

CBR	cost-benefit ratio
CDC	U.S. Centers for Disease Control and Prevention
CDD	control of diarrheal diseases
CEA	cost-effectiveness analysis
CEmOC	comprehensive emergency obstetric care
CER	cost-effectiveness ratio
CFR	case-fatality rate
CHA	community health aide
CHD	coronary heart disease
CHF	congestive heart failure
CHNP	community-based health and nutrition program
CHNW	community health and nutrition worker
CHOICE	choosing interventions that are cost-effective
CI	confidence interval
CKD	chronic kidney disease
CL	cutaneous leishmaniasis
CL/P	cleft lip and palate
CM	cerebral malaria
CMH	Commission on Macroeconomics and Health
CML	chronic myeloid leukemia
CO	carbon monoxide
COBRA	combination therapy for rheumatoid arthritis
COHRED	Council on Health Research for Development
COM	chronic otitis media
COPCORD	Community-Oriented Program for Control of Rheumatic Disease
COPD	chronic obstructive pulmonary disease
CoV	coronavirus
COX	cyclo-oxygenase
CRA	comparative risk analysis
CT	computed tomography
CVD	cardiovascular disease
CVS	chorionic villus sampling
CYP	couple-year of protection
DAH	development assistance for health
DALY	disability-adjusted life year
dBHL	decibel hearing level
DCP1	*Disease Control Priorities in Developing Countries*, first edition

DCP2	*Disease Control Priorities in Developing Countries*, second edition
DCPP	Disease Control Priorities Project
DDT	dichlorodiphenyltrichloroethane
DEET	N,N-diethyl-meta-toluamide
DF	dengue fever
DHF	dengue hemorrhagic fever
DHS	demographic and health survey
DMARD	disease-modifying antirheumatic drug
DMFT	decayed, missing, and filled teeth
DNA	deoxyribose nucleic acid
DOT	directly observed therapy
DOTS	directly observed therapy short course
DRC	Democratic Republic of Congo
DSM-IVTR	*Diagnostic and Statistical Manual of Mental Disorders*
DSS	dengue shock syndrome
DTP	diphtheria-tetanus-pertussis
EAP	economically active population
EBM	evidence-based medicine
ED	emergency department
EFA	education for all
EFM	electronic fetal monitoring
EHCAP	Effective Health Care Alliance Programme
EIR	entomological inoculation rate
ELISA	enzyme-linked immunosorbent assay
EMR	electronic medical record
EMS	emergency medical services
EPI	Expanded Program on Immunization
ESRD	end-stage renal disease
EUROSTAT	European Statistical Office
FA	folic acid
FBD	food-borne disease
FCTC	Framework Convention on Tobacco Control
FDA	U.S. Food and Drug Administration
FDC	fixed-dose combinations
FEFO	first expiry, first out
FETP	Field Epidemiology Training Program
FEV1	forced expiratory volume in one second
FGM	female genital mutilation
FHP	family health program
FIC	fully immunized child
FRESH	focusing resources on effective school health
FTE	full-time equivalent
G6PD	glucose-6-phosphate dehydrogenase
G-7	Group of Seven
GATB	Global Alliance for TB Drug Development
GAVI	Global Alliance for Vaccines and Immunization
GDP	gross domestic product
GET 2020	World Health Organization Alliance for the Global Elimination of Trachoma
GFHR	Global Forum on Health Research
GIS	geographic information system
GM	genetic modification
GMP	good manufacturing practice
GNI	gross national income
GNP	gross national product
GSE	glutathione S-transferase
GUSTO	global use of strategies to open occluded coronary arteries
HAART	highly active antiretroviral therapy for the treatment of HIV/AIDS
Hb	hemoglobin
HBV	hepatitis B virus
HDL	high-density lipoprotein
HepB	hepatitis B
HHV	human herpes virus
Hib	*Haemophilus influenzae* type B
HIC	high-income country
HIS	health information system
HIV	human immunodeficiency virus
HMN	Health Metrics Network
HPLC	high-performance liquid chromatography
HPS	health promoting school
HPV	human papillomavirus
HR	human resource
HRT	hormone replacement therapy
HSV-1	herpes simplex virus type 1
HSV-2	herpes simplex virus type 2
IAEA	International Atomic Energy Agency
IAP	indoor air pollution
IAVI	International AIDS Vaccine Initiative
ICD-10	*International Statistical Classification of Diseases and Related Health Problems*, 10th revision
ICDS	integrated child development services
ICER	incremental cost-effectiveness ratio
ICPD	international conference on population and development
ICT	information and communication technologies
IDA	International Development Association
IDD	iodine deficiency disorders
IDSR	integrated disease surveillance and response
IEC	information, education, and communication
IFF	International Finance Facility
IHD	ischemic heart disease
ILO	International Labour Organisation
IMCI	integrated management of infant and childhood illness
IMF	International Monetary Fund
IMR	infant mortality rate
INCB	International Narcotics Control Board

INDEPTH	International Network of Field Sites with Continuous Demographic Evaluation of Populations and Their Health in Developing Countries	MR	mental retardation
		MRI	magnetic resonance imaging
		MSF	Médecins Sans Frontières (Doctors Without Borders)
INFECTOM	information, feedback, contracting with providers to adhere to practice guidelines, and ongoing monitoring	MTCT	mother-to-child transmission
		MVA	modified vaccinia virus Ankara
		NAFTA	North American Free Trade Agreement
IPT	intermittent preventive treatment	NAP	nonaffective psychosis
IPTi	intermittent preventive treatment in infancy	NCCAM	National Center for Complementary and Alternative Medicine
IPV	inactivated polio vaccine	NCE	new chemical entity
IRB	institutional review board	NDP	national drug policy
IRR	internal rate of return	NGO	nongovernmental organization
IRS	indoor residual spraying	NHA	national health account
ISDR	international strategy for disaster reduction	NHS	national health service
ISIC	international standard industrial classification of all economic activities	NIH	National Institutes of Health
		NIOSH	National Institute for Occupational Safety and Health
ITN	insecticide-treated net	NIPA	national income and product accounts
IUATLD	International Union against Tuberculosis and Lung Disease	NMR	neonatal mortality rate
		NO_2	nitrogen dioxide
IUD	intrauterine device	NORA	national occupational research agenda
IUGR	intrauterine growth retardation	NOx	nitrogen oxide and nitrogen dioxide
JE	Japanese encephalitis	NRA	national regulatory authority
LAAM	levo-alpha-acetyl-methadol	NRT	nicotine replacement therapies
LBW	low birthweight	NSAID	nonsteroidal anti-inflammatory drug
LDD	learning and developmental disability	NSO	national statistics office
LDL	low-density lipoprotein	NTD	neural tube defect
LE 20	life expectancy at age 20	OA	osteoarthritis
LF	lymphatic filariasis	OCP	Onchocerciasis Control Program
LIC	low-income country	ODA	official development assistance
LMICs	low- and middle-income countries	OECD	Organisation for Economic Co-operation and Development
LPG	liquid petroleum gas		
LRI	lower respiratory tract infection	OEPA	Onchocerciasis Elimination Program for the Americas
LSD	lysergic acid diethylamide		
MBB	marginal budgeting for bottlenecks	OP	osteoporosis
MCE	multi-country evaluation of IMCI effectiveness, cost, and impact	OPV	oral polio vaccine
		ORS	oral rehydration solution
MCH	maternal child and health	ORT	oral rehydration therapy
MDA	mass drug administration	PAHO	Pan American Health Organization
MDG	Millennium Development Goal	PAL	practical approach to lung health
MDMA	methylenedioxymethamphetamine	PARIS21	Partnership in Statistics for Development in the 21st Century
MDR-TB	multidrug-resistant tuberculosis		
MDT	multidrug therapy	PCBs	polychlorinated biphenyls
MEASURE	monitoring and evaluation to assess and use results	PCD	Partnership for Child Development
		PCP	*Pneumocystis carinii* pneumonia
MIC	middle-income country	PCR	polymerase chain reaction
MMR	measles-mumps-rubella	PCV	protein-conjugated polysaccharide vaccine
MMT	methadone maintenance treatment	PD	Parkinson's disease
MMV	Medicines for Malaria Venture	PDOH	Philippine Department of Health
MNCH	maternal, neonatal, and child health	PDSA	plan-do-study-act
MOH	ministry of health		

PFGE	pulsed-field-gel-electrophoresis		TB	tuberculosis
PHC	primary health care		TCA	tricyclic antidepressant
PHSWOW	public health school without walls		TDR	Special Programme for Research and Training in Tropical Diseases
PLACE	Priorities for Local AIDS Control Effort			
PM	particulate matter		TEHIP	Tanzania Essential Health Interventions Program
PMTCT	prevention of mother-to-child transmission			
PopEd	population and family life education		THC	tetrahydrocannabinol
ppm	parts per million		TINP	Tamil Nadu Integrated Nutrition Program
PPPs	public-private partnerships		TLTI	treatment for latent tuberculosis infection
PRSC	poverty reduction support credit		TLV	threshold limit value
PRSP	Poverty Reduction Strategy Paper		TM	traditional medicine
PSV	polysaccharide vaccine		TRIPS	Agreement on Trade-Related Aspects of Intellectual Property Rights
PTA	parent-teacher association			
PTCA	percutaneous transluminal coronary angioplasty		UN	United Nations
PTSD	posttraumatic stress disorder		UNAIDS	Joint United Nations Programme on HIV/AIDS
PZQ	Praziquantel		UNEP	United Nations Environment Programme
QALY	quality-adjusted life year		UNESCO	United Nations Education, Scientific, and Cultural Organization
RA	rheumatoid arthritis			
R&D	research and development		UNFPA	United Nations Population Fund
RCT	randomized clinical trial		UNICEF	United Nations Children's Fund
RDI	recommended dietary intake		UNIDO	United Nations Industrial Development Organization
RESU	regional epidemiology and surveillance unit			
RHD	rheumatic heart disease		URI	upper respiratory tract infection
RNA	ribonucleic acid		USAID	U.S. Agency for International Development
ROP	retinopathy of prematurity		VAD	vitamin A deficiency
RRT	renal replacement therapy		VC	vital capacity
RSV	respiratory syncytial virus		VCT	voluntary counseling and testing
RTI	road traffic injury		VERC	village education resource center
rt-PA	recombinant tissue plasminogen activator		VF	ventilation factor
SAFE	surgery, antibiotics to control the infection, facial cleanliness, and environmental improvements		VIA	visual inspection after application of an acetic acid solution
			VL	visceral leishmaniasis
SAR	search and rescue		VOI	value-of-information (techniques)
SARS	severe acute respiratory syndrome		VSL	value of a statistical life
SBP	systolic blood pressure		WFP	World Food Programme
SCC	short-course chemotherapy		WHA	World Health Assembly
SD	standard deviation		WHO	World Health Organization
SiC	significant caries (index)		WHO/TDR	WHO Special Programme for Research and Training in Tropical Diseases
SMA	severe malarial anemia			
SO_2	sulfur dioxide		WHOCC	WHO Collaborating Center
SP	sulfadoxine-pyrimethamine		WISE	work improvement in small enterprises
SSO	social security organization		WTO	World Trade Organization
SSRI	selective serotonin reuptake inhibitor		YF	yellow fever
STATCAP	statistical capacity building		YLD	year of life lived with disability
STH	soil-transmitted helminth		YLL	year of life lost
STI	sexually transmitted infection		YLS	year of life saved
SWAp	sectorwide approach			

All dollar amounts are U.S. dollars unless otherwise indicated.

Part **One**

Summary and Cross-Cutting Themes

- Summary
- Cross-Cutting Themes

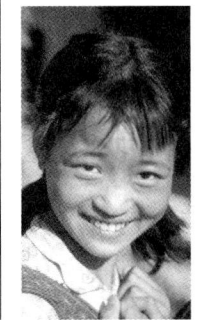

Chapter **1**

Investing in Health

Dean T. Jamison

A girl born in Chile in 1910 could expect to live only to age 33. Since then, her life expectancy has more than doubled to its current level of 78 years. What has this increase meant for her? The probability that she will die before her fifth birthday has declined from 36 percent to less than 2 percent. Throughout middle age the likelihood that she will die is also far lower: death in childbearing or from tuberculosis (TB) as a young adult are no longer threats, and she is less likely to die in middle age from cancer. Mirroring this mortality reduction—but less easily quantified—are marked improvements in health-related quality of life. She will be able to choose to have fewer children and thus spend less time in pregnancy and child rearing. From an average of about 5.3 children at midcentury, Chilean women's fertility rate has dropped to its current level of 2.3. She will have fewer infections, less anemia, greater strength and stature, and a quicker mind. Her life is not only much longer; it is much healthier as well.

Chile's history of health improvements is unusually well documented but typifies changes that have occurred in much of the world. These dramatic improvements in health have, moreover, been possible without major increases in income. In the early 1900s, income levels in the United States were roughly the same as they are in Chile today, yet U.S. life expectancy then was 25 years shorter. New knowledge, new vaccines, and new drugs have inexpensively enabled major gains in health that were not possible before, even for those whose incomes were high. Although those gains are now *possible*, they do not occur unless health systems and policies effectively realize the available potential.

Although the magnitude of possible gains in health was clear by the early 1990s, it is even clearer today: focused attention by health systems on delivering powerful but often inexpensive interventions can lead to dramatic improvements in health at modest cost. Globalization has helped diffuse knowledge about what those interventions are and how health systems can deliver them. The pace of diffusion of such knowledge into a country—much more than its level of income—determines the pace of health improvement in that country. Our purpose in *Disease Control Priorities in Developing Countries*, 2nd edition (*DCP2*), is to help speed the diffusion of policy-relevant knowledge.

This introductory chapter to *DCP2* serves two purposes:

- First, it provides the context for the rest of the book by discussing broad trends in health conditions, by summarizing health conditions of the world at the dawn of the 21st century, and by pointing to recent research suggesting that the economic benefits from successful investments in health are likely to be exceptionally high.
- Second, it highlights some of the main messages for policy that emerge from the 37 chapters that deal with conditions and risk factors and the 21 chapters that deal with strengthening health systems. These highlights are deliberately brief because chapters 2 and 3 summarize the remainder of the book: chapter 2 summarizes findings about intervention cost-effectiveness from across the book, and chapter 3 synthesizes findings on strengthening health systems.

Box 1.1 summarizes the main messages of this chapter.

3

Box 1.1

Disease Control Priorities

Chapters in this volume convey compact distillations of current knowledge concerning interventions to improve health and the related delivery systems. Chapter 2 summarizes main messages of the chapters dealing with interventions, and chapter 3 summarizes the main messages concerning health systems. Chapter 1 provides context and conveys examples of the range of findings from across the volume. Here, in brief, are the main messages of chapter 1:

1. *Average life expectancy in low- and middle-income countries increased dramatically in the past half-century, while cross-country health inequalities decreased.* In the countries with the best health indicators, life expectancy increased a substantial two and one-half years per decade since 1960; low- and middle-income countries on average, with life expectancy gains of about five years per decade, have been converging toward the countries with the longest life expectancy. Improvement in average income and education levels contributed to these worldwide gains in health. Of much greater quantitative significance, however, have been the generation and diffusion of new knowledge and of low-cost, appropriate technologies. Increased access to knowledge and technology has accounted for perhaps as much as two-thirds of the impressive 2 percent per year rate of decline in under-five mortality rates.

2. *Improved health has contributed significantly to economic welfare.* Per capita GNP rose rapidly in developing countries in the decades following 1960, and economic research suggests that health improvements led to perhaps 10 percent to 15 percent of that GNP growth. Although GNP includes the costs of providing medical care and reflects changes in health-related consumption, such as the quantity and quality of food, it omits altogether the value that mortality reduction represents for countries. Recent economic research has extended measurement to a broader indicator, known as *full income,* that reflects reasonable valuation of changes in mortality. For many countries, recent mortality changes exceed in value the growth of GNP. More widespread use of full-income measures to calculate the rate of return to investments in health—and health research—will almost certainly conclude that, today, most countries substantially undervalue those investments.

3. *Although health improvements constituted an enormous success for human welfare in the 20th century, four critical challenges face developing countries (and the world) at the beginning of the 21st century:*
   - high levels and rapid growth (for mostly demographic reasons) of noncommunicable conditions in the disease profiles of developing countries
   - the still unchecked HIV/AIDS pandemic
   - the possibility of a successor to the influenza pandemic of 1918
   - the persistence in many countries and many population subgroups of high but preventable levels of mortality and disability from diseases such as malaria, TB, diarrhea, and pneumonia; from micronutrient malnutrition; and, for both mothers and infants, from childbirth.

The main purpose of this volume is to facilitate diffusion of appropriate approaches for addressing those problems.

4. *The volume's conclusions concerning interventions include the following:*
   - Although 50 percent of deaths (including stillbirths) of children under age five occur at ages younger than 28 days, relatively little attention has been paid to this age group. Cost-effective interventions exist.
   - Treatment of HIV-positive mothers, treatment of sexually transmitted infections, free distribution of condoms, and other interventions can cost-effectively interrupt HIV transmission. These preventive interventions continue to receive inadequate attention from health systems and workers.
   - Controlling tobacco use, particularly through taxation, is feasible in developing countries and is the single most important intervention for reducing noncommunicable disease.
   - Lifelong medical management of risk factors in individuals at high risk for heart attacks or strokes, using aspirin and other drugs, is cost-effective and would benefit tens of millions of individuals.

5. *This volume's findings concerning health services and systems include the following:*
   - Provider incentives matter. Financial or other recognition for timely, responsive service increases the likelihood of such services. Conversely, financial incentives for excessive or inappropriate use of

drugs or diagnostic tests is an all-too-common cause of high costs and poor health outcomes.

- Provider experience matters. Having providers do a few things frequently, rather than attempting to provide diverse services, facilitates quality improvement with potentially major improvements in health outcomes.
- Strengthening surgical capacity at district hospitals is likely to be cost-effective and would address broad needs.
- In low-income countries, targeting the very limited public sector resources for health to control of diseases—such as TB—that particularly affect the poor would be efficient.
- In middle-income countries, public finance—or publicly mandated finance—of a substantial package of clinical care for all would be not only equitable but also efficient in terms of meeting health needs, controlling costs, and providing financial protection to populations.

6. *The generation and diffusion of new knowledge and products underpinned the enormous improvements in*

Source: Author.

health in the 20th century. Every reason exists to believe that continued progress—meeting the challenges of noncommunicable disease, HIV/AIDS, potential pandemics, and neglected populations—will also rely heavily on new knowledge. The rapidly growing commitment of high-income countries to providing development assistance for health would be more effectively used if a larger share were devoted to research and development. Public-private partnerships provide a promising institutional mechanism for new product development. A particularly important—and much neglected—type of knowledge results from tight evaluations of interventions and systems.

This volume represents an attempt to learn systematically from the enormous successes of the past half-century in improving human health. Knowledge that has been gained—and that this volume pulls together—creates a platform for addressing the problems that remain.

THE 20TH CENTURY TAKEOFF IN HUMAN HEALTH

The 20th century differed markedly from previous history in two critical domains:

- First, the rapid economic growth that had begun in the 19th century in countries of the North Atlantic diffused widely around the globe while continuing in the countries where it originated (DeLong 2000; Maddison 1999).
- Second, human mortality rates plummeted, and other dimensions of health improved dramatically. These changes also began in the North Atlantic countries in the 19th century but remained modest until the 20th century, during which the rate of improvement increased and spread to most of the rest of the world (Easterlin 1996, 1999; Oeppen and Vaupel 2002).

Improvements in Health

This section briefly documents the magnitude of health improvements and then points to the challenges that remain. For the past 160 years, life expectancy in the healthiest countries has increased steadily. At the same time, differences in life expectancy between those countries and much of the rest of the world have narrowed. Figure 1.1 depicts trends in female life expectancy in the country with the *highest* estimated level of

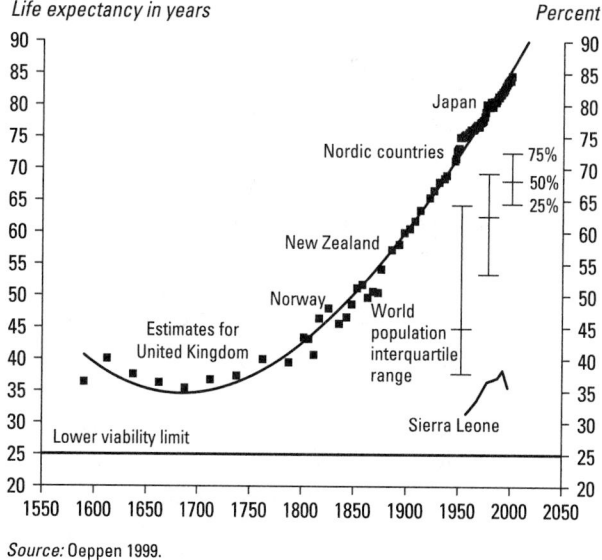

Source: Oeppen 1999.

Figure 1.1 Trends in Maximum Female Life Expectancy, 1600–2000

life expectancy. From about 1600 to about 1840, there is fluctuation but no clear trend; after 1840, the graph turns upward at a surprisingly uniform rate of improvement: maximum life expectancy increased by about two and one-half years per decade for 160 years.

Table 1.1 Levels and Changes in Life Expectancy, 1960–2002, by World Bank Region

Region	Life expectancy (years)			Rate of change (years per decade)	
	1960	1990	2002	1960–90	1990–2002
Low- and middle-income countries	44	63	65	6.3	1.7
East Asia and the Pacific	39	67	70	9.3	2.5
(China)	(36)	(69)	(71)	(11)	(1.7)
Europe and Central Asia	—	69	69	—	0.0
Latin America and the Caribbean	56	68	71	4.0	2.5
Middle East and North Africa	47	64	69	5.7	4.2
South Asia	44	58	63	4.7	4.2
(India)	(44)	(59)	(64)	(5)	(4.6)
Sub-Saharan Africa	40	50	46	3.3	−3.3
High-income countries	69	76	78	2.3	1.7
World	50	65	67	5.0	1.7

Source: World Bank 2004 (CD-ROM version).
— = not available.
Note: Entries are the average of male and female life expectancies.

Table 1.1 shows progress in life expectancy by World Bank region between 1960 and 2002. (Map 1 on the inside front cover depicts the World Bank regions.) For the first three decades of this period, progress was remarkably fast—a gain of 6.3 years in life expectancy per decade on average, albeit with substantial regional variation. Progress continued between 1990 and 2002 in the low- and middle-income countries but at a much slower pace. This slower pace is due, in great part, to mortality increases from HIV/AIDS. Sub-Saharan Africa actually lost more than four years of life expectancy.

Since 1950, life expectancy in the median country has steadily converged toward the maximum and cross-country differences have decreased markedly. This reduction in inequality in health contrasts with long-term *increases* in income inequality between and within countries. Despite the magnitude of global improvements, many countries and populations have failed to share in the overall gains or have even fallen behind. Some countries—for example, Sierra Leone—remain far behind (figure 1.1). China's interior provinces lag behind the more advantaged coastal regions. Indigenous people everywhere probably lead far less healthy lives than do others in their respective countries, although confirmatory data are scant.

Reasons for remaining health inequalities lie only partially in income inequality: the experiences of China, Costa Rica, Cuba, Sri Lanka, and Kerala state in India, among many others, conclusively show that dramatic improvements in health can occur without high or rapidly growing incomes. The experiences of countries in Europe in the late 19th and early 20th centuries similarly show that health conditions can improve without prior or concomitant increases in income (Easterlin 1996). A recent review, undertaken in part as background for this volume,

identified many specific examples of low-cost interventions leading to large and carefully documented health improvements (Levine and others 2004). The public sector initiated and financed virtually all of these interventions. The goal of this book is to assist decision makers—particularly those in the public sector—to realize the potential for low-cost intervention to rapidly improve the health and welfare of their populations.

Remaining Challenges

Four central challenges for health policy ensue from the pace and unevenness of the progress just documented and from the evolving nature of microbial threats to human health.

Epidemiological Transition. First, the next two decades will see continuation of trends resulting from the dramatic mortality declines of recent decades. The key phenomenon is that the major noncommunicable diseases—circulatory system diseases, cancers, and major psychiatric disorders—are fast replacing (or adding to) the traditional scourges—particularly infectious diseases and undernutrition in children. This phenomenon results in substantial part from rapid relative population growth at the older ages, when noncommunicable diseases become manifest. Additionally, injuries resulting from road traffic are replacing more traditional forms of injury. Using data from Chile, figure 1.2 illustrates the huge increase in the relative importance of injuries, cancers, and cardiovascular disease between 1909 and 1999. Responding to this epidemiological transition with sharply constrained resources is a key challenge. Tables 1.A1 and 1.A2 (see annex 1.A) provide cause-specific summaries of death and disease burden, measured in DALYs, in 2001 for the world as a whole and for low- and

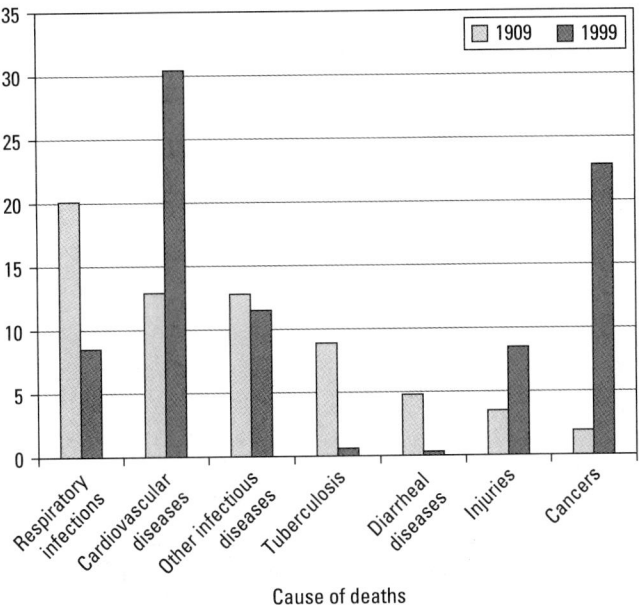

Percentage distribution

Source: WHO 1999, 13.

Note: For 1909, 35.1 percent of deaths were categorized as "other," and for 1999, the corresponding percentage was 17.5. The cause-specific percentages shown in the figure are the number from the indicated cause as a percentage of the total number classified into a specific cause for that year.

Figure 1.2 Distribution of Deaths by Cause in Chile, 1909 and 1999

middle-income countries as a group as well as for high-income countries. Those summaries indicate that noncommunicable disease already accounts for over half of all deaths in the low- and middle-income countries, although nearly 40 percent of deaths continue to be from infection, undernutrition, and maternal conditions, creating a "dual burden" that Julio Frenk and colleagues have pointed to (Bobadilla and others 1993).

HIV/AIDS Epidemic. A second key challenge is the HIV/AIDS epidemic. Control efforts and successes have been very real but, with only a few exceptions, limited to upper-middle-income and high-income countries. Poorer countries remain in the epidemic's deadly path.

New Pandemics. The global influenza pandemic of 1918 resulted in more than 40 million human deaths, exceeding the 20th-century toll of HIV/AIDS or of World Wars I and II. Continued evolution of the influenza virus leaves the world at risk of another such pandemic—as has been much discussed in the press as this book goes to print. If the H5N1 strain of avian influenza, for example, evolved so that (like the human flu) it could be efficiently transmitted from human to human, a major pandemic would be likely. Preparing for such an eventuality is the third great challenge to global health.

Unequal Progress. A fourth key challenge results from continued high levels of inequality in health conditions across

and within countries. Bourguignon and Morrisson (2002) have stressed that global inequalities are declining if one properly accounts for convergence across countries in health conditions, which more than compensates for income divergence. However, in far too many countries health conditions remain unacceptably—and unnecessarily—poor. This factor is a source of grief and misery, and it is a sharp brake on economic growth and poverty reduction. From 1990 to 2001, for example, the under-five mortality rate remained stagnant or increased in 23 countries. In another 53 countries (including China), the rate of decline in under-five mortality in this period was less than half of the 4.3 percent per year required to reach the fourth Millennium Development Goal (MDG-4) (see map 2 on the inside back cover of this book). Meeting the MDG for under-five mortality reduction by 2015 is not remotely possible for these countries. Yet the examples of many other countries, often quite poor, show that with the right policies dramatic reductions in mortality are possible. A major goal of this volume is to identify strategies for implementing interventions that are known to be highly cost-effective for dealing with the health problems of countries remaining behind—for example, treatment for diarrhea, pneumonia, TB, and malaria; immunization; and other preventive measures against a large proportion of those diseases.

THE ECONOMIC BENEFITS OF BETTER HEALTH

The dramatic health improvements globally during the 20th century arguably contributed as much or more to improvements in overall well-being as did the equally dramatic innovation in and expansion of the availability of material goods and services. To the substantial extent that appropriate investments in health can contribute to continued reductions in morbidity and mortality, the economic welfare returns to health investments are likely to be exceptional and positive—with previously unrecognized implications for public sector resource allocation. These returns go far beyond the contribution better health makes to per capita income, which itself appears substantial (see Bloom, Canning, and Jamison 2004; Lopez-Casasnovas, Rivera, and Currais 2005). This section first summarizes the evidence concerning health's effect on per capita income and then turns to more recent literature concerning the effect of health changes on a broader measure of economic well-being than per capita gross domestic product (GDP).

Health and Income

How does health influence GDP per person? Healthy workers are more productive than workers who are similar but not healthy. Supporting evidence for this plausible observation comes from studies that link investments in health and nutrition of the young to adult wages (Strauss and Thomas 1998). Better health also raises per capita income through a number of other channels. One involves altering decisions about expenditures and savings over the life cycle. The idea of planning for retirement occurs only when mortality rates become low enough for retirement to be a realistic prospect. Rising longevity in developing countries has opened a new incentive for the current generation to save—an incentive that can dramatically affect national saving rates. Although this saving boom lasts for only one generation and is offset by the needs of the elderly after population aging occurs, it can substantially boost investment and economic growth rates while it lasts.

Encouraging foreign direct investment is another channel: investors shun environments in which the labor force suffers a heavy disease burden. Endemic diseases can also deny humans access to land or other natural resources, as occurred in much of West Africa before the successful control of river blindness.

Boosting education is yet another channel. Healthier children attend school and learn more while they are there. A longer life span increases the returns on investment in education.

Demographic channels also play an important role. Lower infant mortality initially creates a "baby-boom" cohort and leads to a subsequent reduction in the birth rates as families choose to have fewer children in the new low-mortality regime. A baby-boom cohort thereby affects the economy profoundly as its members enter the educational system, find employment, save for retirement, and finally leave the labor market. The cohorts before and after a baby boom are much smaller; hence, for a substantial transition period, this cohort creates a large labor force relative to overall population size and the potential for accelerated economic growth (Bloom, Canning, and Malaney 2000).

If better health improves the productive potential of individuals, good health should accompany higher levels of national income in the long run. Countries that have high levels of health but low levels of income tend to experience relatively faster economic growth as their income adjusts. How big an overall contribution does better health make to economic growth? Evidence from cross-country growth regressions suggests the contribution is consistently substantial. Indeed, the initial health of a population has been identified as one of the most robust and potent drivers of economic growth—among such well-established influences as the initial level of income per capita, geographic location, institutional environment, economic policy, initial level of education, and investments in education. Bloom, Canning, and Sevilla (2004) found that one extra year of life expectancy raises GDP per person by about 4 percent in the long run. Jamison, Lau, and Wang (2005) estimated that reductions in adult mortality explain 10 to 15 percent of the economic growth that occurred from 1960 to 1990. Not all countries benefit equally from this link. Bhargava and others (2001) found that better health matters more for income growth in low-income countries than in high-income ones. Although attribution of causality is never unequivocal in analyses like these, different types of evidence point consistently to a likely causal effect of health on growth.

Health declines can precipitate downward spirals, setting off impoverishment and further ill health. For example, the effect of HIV/AIDS on per capita GDP could prove devastating in the long run. An enormous waste of human capital occurs as prime-age workers die. A high-mortality environment deters the next generation from investing in education and creating human capital. The creation of a generation of orphans means that children may be forced to work to survive and may not get the education they need. High rates of mortality may reduce investment. Saving rates are likely to fall, and retirement becomes less likely. A foreign company is less likely to invest in a country with a high HIV prevalence rate because of the threat to the firm's own workers, the prospect of high labor turnover, and the loss of workers who have gained specific skills by working for the firm. The International Monetary Fund recently published a collection of important studies of the multiple mechanisms through which a major AIDS epidemic can be expected to affect national economies (Haacker 2004).

Health and Economic Welfare

Judging countries' economic performance by GDP per person fails to differentiate between situations in which health conditions differ: a country whose citizens enjoy long and healthy lives clearly outperforms another with the same GDP per person but whose citizens suffer much illness and die sooner. Individual willingness to forgo income to work in safer environments and social willingness to pay for health-enhancing safety and environmental regulations provide measures, albeit approximate, of the value of differences in mortality rates. Many such willingness-to-pay studies have been undertaken in recent decades, and their results are typically summarized as the *value of a statistical life* (VSL). Chapter 7 discusses these issues in the context of assessing the economic returns to investments in health research and development.

Although the national income and product accounts include the value of inputs into health care (such as drugs and physician time), standard procedures do not incorporate information on the value of changes in longevity. In a seminal paper, Usher (1973) first brought the value of mortality reduction into national income accounting. He did this by generating estimates of the growth in what Becker, Philipson, and Soares (2003) have called *full income*—a concept that captures the value of changes in life expectancy by including them in an assessment of economic welfare. Estimates of changes in full income are typically generated by adding the value of changes in annual mortality rates (calculated using VSL figures) to changes in annual GDP per person. These estimates of change in full income are conservative in that they incorporate only the value of mortality changes and do not account for the total value of changes in health status. Valuation of changes in mortality, it should be noted, is only one element—albeit a quantitatively important one—of potentially feasible additions to national account to deal with nonmarket outcomes. The U.S. National Academy of Sciences has recently proposed broad changes for the United States that would include but go beyond valuation of mortality change (Abraham and Mackie 2005).

For many years, little further work was done on the effects of mortality change on full income although, as Viscusi and Aldy (2003) document, the number of carefully constructed estimates of VSLs increased enormously. Bourguignon and Morrisson (2002) address the long-term evolution of inequality among world citizens, starting from the premise that a "comprehensive definition of economic well-being would consider individuals over their lifetime." Their conclusion is that rapid increases in life expectancy in poorer countries had resulted in declines in inequality (broadly defined) beginning sometime after 1950, even though income inequality had continued to rise. In another important paper, Nordhaus (2003) assessed the growth of full income per capita in the United States in the 20th century. He concludes that more than half of the growth in full income in the first half of the century—and less than half in the second half of the century—had resulted from mortality decline. In this period, real income in the United States increased sixfold and life expectancy increased by more than 25 years.

Three lines of more recent work extend those methods to the interpretation of the economic performance of developing countries. All reach conclusions that differ substantially from analyses based on GDP alone. Two of those studies—one undertaken for the Commission on Macroeconomics and Health (CMH) of the World Health Organization (WHO) (Jamison, Sachs, and Wang 2001) and the other at the International Monetary Fund (Crafts and Haacker 2004)—assessed the impact of the AIDS epidemic on full income. Both studies conclude that the AIDS epidemic in the 1990s had far more adverse economic consequences than previous estimates of effects on per person GDP growth would suggest. Accounting for mortality decline in Africa before the 1990s, on the other hand leads to estimates of much more favorable overall economic performance than does the trend in GDP per person. Figure 1.3 shows that in Kenya, for example, full income grew more rapidly in GDP per person before 1990 (and far more rapidly in the 1960s). After 1990 the mounting death toll from AIDS appears to have only a modest effect on GDP per person but a dramatically adverse impact on changes in full income. Becker, Philipson, and Soares (2003) extended the earlier work of Bourguignon and Morrisson (2002) in finding strong absolute convergence in full income across countries over time, in contrast to the standard finding of continued divergence (increased inequality) of GDP per person. Finally,

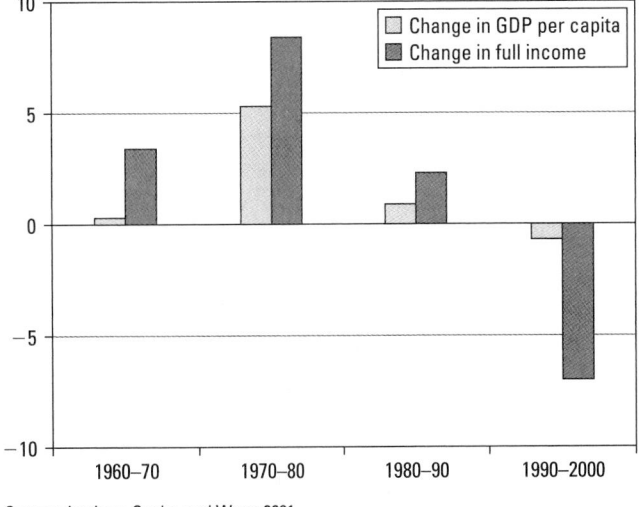

Annual change as percentage of initial year GDP per capita

Source: Jamison, Sachs, and Wang 2001.

Figure 1.3 Changes in GDP and Full Income in Kenya, 1960–2000

Jamison, Jamison, and Sachs (2003) have adapted standard cross-country growth regressions to model determinants of full income (rather than GDP per person). Like Becker, Philipson, and Soares (2003), they conclude that inequalities have been decreasing.

The dramatic mortality declines of the past 150 years—and their reversal in Africa by AIDS subsequent to 1990—have had major economic consequences. The effect of health on GDP is substantial. The intrinsic value of mortality changes—measured in terms of VSL—is even more substantial. What are the implications of these findings for development strategy and for benefit-cost analyses of public sector investment options? Using full income in benefit-cost analyses of investments in health (and in health-related sectors such as education, water supply and sanitation, and targeted food transfers) would markedly increase estimates of net benefits or rates of return. A careful, quantitative reassessment of competing policies for improving a country's living standards would probably conclude that development assistance and budgetary allocations to health deserve greater relative priority.

WHY HAS MORTALITY DECLINED AT SUCH DIFFERENT RATES IN DIFFERENT COUNTRIES?

This section explores some of the reasons mortality has declined so rapidly and at such different rates in different countries. It considers the question of whether income levels or growth rates play an important role in achieving better health or whether good policies can potentially lead to good health for low-income populations. The section concludes with a snapshot of health conditions in the world at the dawn of the 21st century.

The 20th century witnessed huge and unprecedented declines in mortality rates at all ages and in most parts of the world. Easterlin (1996) and Crafts (2000) place an emphasis on mortality transformation that is comparable to their emphasis on economic growth in their retrospectives on the unprecedented changes in the human condition during the 20th century. Understanding the sources of mortality changes is important for understanding one of the defining events of world history and also for devising policies to address the needs of the perhaps 25 percent of the world's population whose mortality rates remain far higher than those of the rest of humanity.

Several approaches shed light on the sources of mortality decline. Epidemiologists and demographers have carefully tracked specific communities for many years to assess levels of mortality and causes of death. In rural Senegal, rapid mortality decline followed introduction of interventions addressing specific conditions (Pison and others 1993).

Another approach is historical. Easterlin (1996, 1999) examined the interplay of economic growth, urbanization, and mortality in 19th- and 20th-century Europe. He concluded that although income growth in the 19th century probably did play a role in reducing mortality (through its influence on food availability and environmental conditions), the magnitude of the effect was small. Fogel (1997) stressed the importance of increases in food availability during this period. Positive effects of income growth were partially offset by increased infectious disease transmission resulting from urbanization. Easterlin (1999) concludes that 20th-century mortality decline, which was much more rapid than that of the 19th century, had its origin in technical progress, and Powles (2001) has pointed to the importance and nature of the institutional changes required to translate technical change and economic improvements into mortality reduction. Mosk and Johansson's (1986) assessment of the interplay between income and mortality in Japan illustrates the role that adoption of public health knowledge and institutional development played in mortality decline in the country that now has the world's lowest mortality rates.

Most analysts agree that advances in science and technology have underpinned the 20th-century transformations both of income and of mortality levels. Models of economic growth rely heavily on technological progress to account for economic change (Boskin and Lau 2000; Easterly and Levine 1997; Solow 1957). Preston (1975, 1980) and Fuchs (1974) provided early quantitative assessments of the central importance of technical progress in accounting for 20th-century increases in life expectancy. [Economists use the term *technical progress* to denote advances in knowledge that lead to new products, like vaccines, or that can inform behavior change, like knowledge of the germ theory of disease (Preston and Haines 1998).] Davis (1956) had already concluded that the unprecedented reduction in mortality in underdeveloped areas since 1940 is the result primarily of the discovery and dissemination of new methods of disease treatment that can be applied at reasonable cost. The reduction was rapid because it did not depend on general economic development or social modernization (Davis 1956, 306–7, 314). Some strands of the literature, however, attribute the high correlation of income and life expectancy at any given time to a significant causal effect of income on health (see, for example, Pritchett and Summers 1996).

Background work for this volume (Jamison, Sandbu, and Wang 2004) attempted to provide a better sense of the importance of income as a determinant of mortality by exploring the relationships among income, technical progress (or diffusion), and mortality decline. Previous econometric research either has given little emphasis to technical progress—in part simply because much of the research is cross-sectional and therefore fails to address developments over time—or has assumed the rate of technical progress or technology adoption to be constant across countries. The background work for this volume relaxed the assumption that the rate of technology adoption is constant across countries. Allowing for cross-country variation in the rate of adapting new methods resulted in weaker estimated effects of income on infant mortality rates than previously found, although education's estimated effect was robust with respect to this change.

Much of the variation in country outcomes results from the very substantial cross-country variation in the rate of technical progress—from essentially no decline in infant mortality rate caused by technical progress to reductions of up to 5 percent per year from that source. Deaton (2004) provides a complementary and extended discussion of the importance of technological diffusion for improvements in health. Many factors from outside the health sector also affect the pace of health improvement; the education levels of populations are most important. Box 1.2 briefly discusses the multisectoral nature of health's determinants. The importance of technical progress and diffusion should be viewed in this larger context.

However technical progress or diffusion may be manifested, the large differences in its magnitude across countries suggest important effects of a country's health-related policies (Fuchs 1980; Oeppen 1999). This point bears reiterating in a slightly different way: income growth is neither necessary nor sufficient for sustained improvements in health. Today's tools for improving health are so powerful and inexpensive that health conditions can be reasonably good even in countries with low incomes.

CHILD HEALTH

A small number of conditions accounts for most of the (large) differences in health between the poor and the not so poor. Less than 1 percent of all deaths from AIDS, TB, and malaria, for example, occur in the high-income countries. Available technical options—exemplified by but going well beyond immunization—can address most of the conditions that affect

Box 1.2

The Multisectoral Determinants of Health

Malnourished children easily acquire diseases, and they easily die from the diseases that they acquire. Dwellings and neighborhoods without sanitation provide fertile environments for transmission of intestinal infections. Cooking with wood and coal results in air dense with particulates and gases, which destroy lungs and lives. Hopeless life circumstances thrust young girls (and boys) into commercial sex work with its attendant risks of violence and sexually transmitted infections, including HIV/AIDS. Manufacturers of tobacco and alcohol profit enormously from advertising and promotion that spread addiction. Rapid growth in vehicular traffic—often with untrained drivers on unsafe roads—generates a rising toll of injury. Poorly designed irrigation creates breeding grounds for vectors of disease. The point is clear: determinants of health are truly multisectoral.

WHO coordinated a group of more than 100 individuals to generate estimates of the percentage of deaths, by region and globally, associated with a range of 26 risk factors (Ezzati and others 2004). Those estimates were revised and updated for the Disease Control Priorities Project. The results give a sense of the extent to which multisectoral factors contributed to mortality and disease burden in low- and middle-income countries in 2001. The following, for example, are estimates of the percentage of disease burden (and, in parentheses, of deaths) in those countries attributable to the indicated risk factors:

- tobacco smoking—4.7 percent (8.5 percent)
- indoor air pollution—2.7 percent (3.2 percent)
- inadequate water and sanitation—3.4 percent (2.8 percent)

- risky sexual activity—5.3 percent (5.1 percent)
- alcohol use—3.6 percent (3.4 percent).

Underlying most proximal risks are more general determinants of health, such as education and, to a lesser extent, income. The effects of income and education operate for the most part through influencing risk (and permitting effective use of health services). If an important fraction of ill health results from poverty and low educational levels—or from their consequences in inadequate food or sanitation or other specific risks—then ought the task of the health professional lie principally in addressing these underlying problems? In one sense, the answer is surely yes: the health community should measure the effects on health of actions outside the health sector. It should ensure that these findings are communicated and are considered by those making policy choices. The magnitude of the demonstrated effect of girls' education on health and fertility outcomes, for example, provides one powerful argument for investing in expansion of educational access to girls. Millions of premature deaths, to take another example, could be averted in Africa alone in the next quarter century with appropriate policies toward supply of energy for household use (Bailis, Ezzati, and Kammen 2005). It is essential that the health sector document and advocate opportunities such as these.

The health community has limited capacity for direct action outside the health sector, however. It will make more of a difference if it focuses its energy, expertise, and resources on ensuring that health systems efficiently deliver the powerful interventions provided by modern science.

Source: Author.

Note: The estimates reported here of DALYs and deaths that are attributable to various risk factors come from Ezzati and others (2006).

---

children, and can do so with great efficacy and at modest cost. That short list of conditions, including undernutrition, relates directly to achieving the MDGs for health. Public expenditures to address those conditions have, in the past, benefited the relatively well off, albeit within poor countries (although global inequities have decreased because many poor countries have made much progress).

Under-Five Health Problems and Intervention Priorities

MDG-4 for under-five mortality (reducing its level in 2015 by two-thirds relative to what it was in 1990) is highly ambitious. Yet its implication of an average 4.3 percent per year decline is well within recent experience. In the first half of the MDG period (1990–2002), 46 countries achieved rates of decline in under-five mortality greater than 4.3 percent per year. Figure 1.4 displays trends in the rate of decline in under-five mortality relative to the requisite 4.3 percent per year for China, India, Latin America and the Caribbean, and Sub-Saharan Africa. Africa's slowed progress probably stems mostly from HIV/AIDS and the spread of resistance to previously effective and widely used antimalarial drugs. Map 2 (on the inside back cover of this

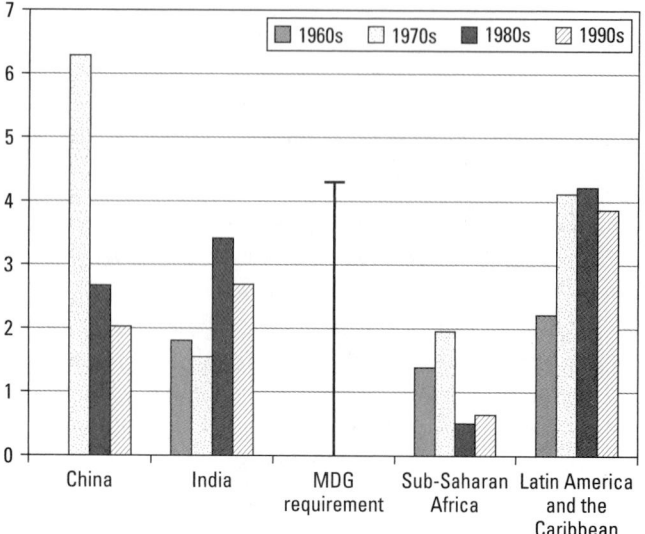

Rate of decline of under-five mortality rates (percent)

Legend: ☐ 1960s ☐ 1970s ☐ 1980s ☐ 1990s

China, India, MDG requirement, Sub-Saharan Africa, Latin America and the Caribbean

Source: Calculations based on data in World Bank 2004 (CD-ROM version).

Note: The black bar in the center shows the 4.3 percent per year rate of decline required for the period 1990–2015 to meet MDG-4 of reducing under-five mortality by two-thirds.

Figure 1.4 Rate of Progress in Reducing Under-Five Mortality, 1960–2000: China, India, Latin America and the Caribbean, and Sub-Saharan Africa

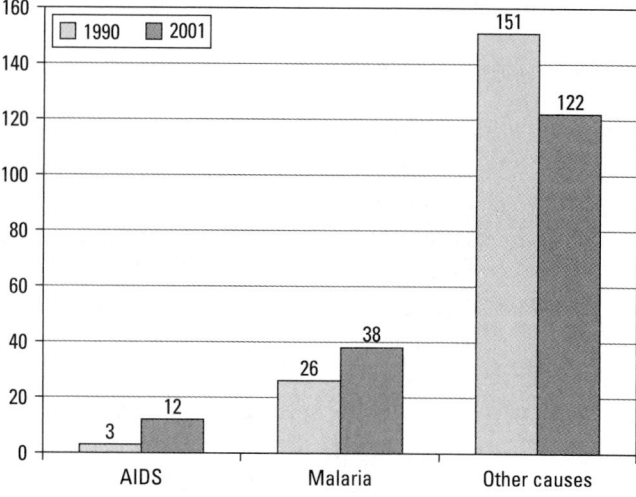

Under-five deaths per 1,000 births

Legend: ☐ 1990 ■ 2001

AIDS (3, 12), Malaria (26, 38), Other causes (151, 122)

Source: Lopez, Begg, and Bos 2006, table 2.4.

Figure 1.5 Under-Five Deaths from AIDS, Malaria, and Other Causes, per Thousand Births, 1990 and 2001, Sub-Saharan Africa

book) shows country-specific progress in reducing under-five mortality:

- Countries colored in green experienced annual rates of decline greater than 4.3 percent in the first half of the MDG period (1990–2002).
- Countries colored in red saw no decrease (or an increase) in their under-five mortality.
- Countries colored in yellow and orange depict countries in between—with yellow indicating performance in the top half of the range between 0 and 4.3 percent, and orange indicating poorer performance in the bottom half of the range.

Basic knowledge about the cost-effectiveness of interventions to address maternal and child health has been available from the 1980s. *DCP2*'s work provides a reassessment with few surprises but some additions. It makes two important relatively new points. The first results from noting that half of under-five deaths occur at ages less than 28 days, when the substantial but usually neglected problem of stillbirth is considered. *DCP2* identifies some highly cost-effective approaches to intervention against stillbirth and neonatal death (chapter 27). The second new point results from the rapid spread of resistance of the malaria parasite to chloroquine and sulfadoxine-pyrimethamine (SP). These inexpensive, highly effective, widely available drugs provided an important partial check on the high levels of malaria mortality in Africa. Their loss is

leading to an even greater rise in malaria mortality and morbidity that could be substantial. Figure 1.5 illustrates increases in malaria death rates in under-five children in Sub-Saharan Africa in the period from 1990 to 2001. The design of instruments for financing a rapid transition to effective new treatments—artemisinin combination therapies (ACTs)—is a high priority (chapter 21; Arrow, Gelband, and Jamison 2005).

The other intervention priorities for addressing under-five mortality are for the most part familiar:

- Expand immunization coverage.
- Expand the use of the simple and low cost but highly effective treatments for diarrhea and child pneumonia through integrated management of childhood illness or other mechanisms.
- Prevent transmission of and mortality from malaria by expanding coverage of insecticide-treated bednets, by expanding use of intermittent preventive treatment for pregnant women, and, particularly, by financing the adoption of ACTs to replace the now widely ineffective drugs chloroquine and SP.
- Ensure widespread distribution of key micronutrients.
- Expand the use of a package of measures to prevent mother-to-child transmission of HIV (further discussed in the next section on HIV/AIDS).

In addition to interventions to reduce under-five mortality, one other priority is clear. The world's most prevalent infections are intestinal helminth (worm) infections, and children of all ages are among the most heavily affected. Chapter 24 discusses these infections, which a low-cost drug (albendazole), taken every six months to a year, can control effectively. Chapter 58 on school health services points to both the importance to children's school progress of taking albendazole where needed and the potential efficacy of school health programs as a vehicle for delivery. In the long run, improved sanitation and water supplies will prevent transmission. Use of albendazole is only an interim solution, but it is one that may be required for decades if the experience of the currently high-income countries is relevant.

Delivering Child Health Interventions

The list of potential interventions is far from exhaustive, and different regions, countries, and communities will face different mixes of the problems these interventions address. However, there can be little dispute that any short list of intervention priorities for under-five mortality in low- and middle-income countries would include many on the list in the preceding section. Why not, then, simply put money into scaling up these known interventions to a satisfactory level?

To greatly oversimplify—and these issues are discussed more substantially in chapter 3—two schools of thought exist. One line of thinking—often ascribed to macroeconomist Jeffrey Sachs and his work as chair of the WHO CMH— concludes that more money and focused effort *are* the solutions. Although acknowledging dual constraints—of money and of health system capacity—Sachs and his colleagues (WHO CMH 2001; Sachs 2005) contend that money can buy (or develop, or both) relevant system capacity even over a period as short as five years. Major gains are affordable and health system capacity constraints can be overcome. Immunization provides an example of where, even in the short term, money can substitute for system capacity. Adding antigens for *Haemophilus influenzae* type B (Hib) and hepatitis B (HepB) to the immunization schedule is costly (although still cost-effective). In some environments, however, it proves less demanding of system capacity than expanding coverage does. Money can be effectively spent by adding antigens at the same time as investing in the capacity to extend coverage.

A second school of thought acknowledges the need for more money but asserts that health system capacity is often a binding short- to medium-term constraint on substantial scaling up of interventions. Critical priorities are, therefore, system reform and strengthening while ensuring that such reforms focus clearly on achieving improved health outcomes and financial protection.

Chapter 3, as indicated, discusses these issues further in the context of all the problems facing a health system, and chapter 9 provides a thoughtful assessment of how to overcome the constraints facing achievement of the MDGs for health. From an individual country's perspective, however, if financial resources are available, the question is very much an empirical one: to what extent can those resources be effectively deployed in buying interventions, in buying out of prevailing system constraints, and in investing in relevant system capacity for the future? What needs to be constantly borne in mind throughout this continued controversy is that *something* works: under-five mortality rates have plunged by more than half since 1960 in the low- and middle-income countries.

HIV/AIDS

For dozens of countries around the world—including several of the most populous—the AIDS epidemic threatens every aspect of development. No other threat comes close, with the possible exceptions of use of nuclear weapons in densely populated areas or a devastating global pandemic similar to the 1917–18 influenza episode. Most governments of affected low- and middle-income countries and most providers of development assistance have only recently begun to respond more than minimally. Creation of the Global Fund to Fight AIDS, Tuberculosis, and Malaria can be viewed as an attempt of the world's top political leaders to improve on the records of existing institutions. The Global Fund's initial years have seen substantial success, but that success is potentially undermined by sharp constraints on resource availability (Bezanson 2005).

Tools to Control the Epidemic

In contrast to the initially slow programmatic movement of most national leaders and international institutions, the research and development community—public and private— has made rapid progress in developing tools to control the HIV/AIDS epidemic, although both a vaccine and a curative drug remain distant objectives. Sensitive, specific, and inexpensive diagnostics are available; means of prevention have been developed and tested; modes of transmission are well understood; and increasingly powerful drugs for controlling viral load allow radical slowing of disease progression. Tools for dealing with HIV/AIDS are thus available: As emphasized in chapter 18, a number of countries show by example that those tools can be put to effective use. Most of the high-income countries have done so, and Brazil and Mexico provide examples of upper-middle-income countries that have forestalled potentially serious epidemics. Mexico succeeded, for example, with a policy of responding both early and forcefully to the epidemic (del Rio and Sepúlveda 2002). The major successes of Thailand and Uganda demonstrate that countries with fewer financial resources can also succeed—and succeed against more established epidemics that had already penetrated deeply into their populations.

Prevention and Management

Prevention underpins success. At the time the World Bank's *World Development Report: Investing in Health* (World Bank

1993) was being written in 1992 and 1993, the only tool for dealing with the epidemic was prevention. In collaboration with the then–Global Programme against AIDS at WHO, the *World Development Report* commissioned very approximate estimates of the consequence for the new infection rate of fully implementing available preventive measures (its optimistic case scenario) or of doing very little (worst case). Actual incidence numbers for 2000, unfortunately, fall very close to the worst-case projection, and chapter 18 points out that even by 2003 fewer than one in five people at high risk of infection had access to the most basic preventive services. In much of the world, little has been spent on prevention, and little has been achieved. In addition, the current U.S. administration may be partially responsible for discouraging condom use in some countries and in stigmatizing and alienating commercial sex workers who are particular priorities for prevention programs. Despite those problems, the potential for prevention is very real, and a number of successful countries have shown the possibility of using that potential well. Chapter 17 on sexually transmitted infections (STIs) and chapter 18 on AIDS discuss a broad menu of preventive measures and experiences with their implementation. Among them, treatment of STIs may be of particular salience both because the diseases are well worth treating in their own right and because the absence of STIs greatly reduces transmission of HIV.

In addition to prevention, better management of patients with AIDS could avert much misery, both by treating opportunistic infections and by ameliorating the often excruciating pain associated with many AIDS deaths. Medically inappropriate restrictions on the use of inexpensive but powerful opiates for pain control continue to deny dignity and comfort to millions of patients with AIDS and cancer in their final days (chapter 52).

Antiretroviral Treatment

Intensive research and development efforts have led in the past decade to the availability of well over a dozen antiretroviral drugs that can greatly reduce the quantity of HIV in an infected person. This reduction in viral load slows or halts progression of AIDS and can return individuals from serious illness to reasonable health. Available drugs leave a residual population of HIV in the body, however, and this population grows if the drugs are stopped. At present the drugs must be taken for life. Widespread use of these drugs in high-income (and some middle-income) countries has transformed the life prospects of HIV-infected individuals.

Early generation antiretroviral drugs suffered notable shortcomings: they were enormously costly; regimens for their use were complicated, making adherence difficult; their use generated unpleasant side effects; and rapid evolution of HIV led to

resistant mutants that undermined the efficacy of therapy. In a remarkably short time, scientific advances have substantially attenuated those problems, making feasible, at least in principle, antiretroviral therapy in low-income settings. WHO's "3 by 5" program had as its objective, for example, to reach 3 million people in low- and middle-income countries with antiretroviral therapy by 2005. Although that goal was far from being met, the global effort to make treatment widely available is well under way.

Despite the indicated progress against the problems with antiretroviral drugs, challenges to their effective use in low-income environments remain formidable. The complexity of patient management is very real. Management requires high levels of human resources and other capacities in many of the countries where those capacities need to be most carefully rationed. Perhaps in consequence, achieving effective implementation has been difficult on even a limited scale. Chapter 18 reviews those problems and how they might be addressed.

Three points concerning widespread antiretroviral drug use are particularly noteworthy:

- Poor implementation (low adherence, development of resistance, interruptions in drug supplies) is likely to lead to very limited health gains, even for individuals on therapy. (This outcome is unlike that of a weak immunization program in which health gains still exist in the fraction of the population that is immunized.) Poorly implemented antiretroviral drug delivery programs could divert substantial resources from prevention or from other high-payoff activities in the health sector. Even worse, they could lead to a false sense of complacency in affected populations: evidence from some countries suggests that treatment availability has led to riskier sexual behavior and increased HIV transmission. The injunction to "do no harm" holds particular salience.

- Unless systematic efforts are made to acquire hard knowledge about which approaches work and which do not, the likelihood exists that unsuccessful implementation efforts will be continued without the appropriate reallocation of resources to successful approaches. Learning what works will require major variations in approach and careful evaluation of effects. Failing to learn will lead to large numbers of needless deaths. Most efforts to scale up antiretroviral therapy unconscionably fail to commit the substantial resources required for evaluation of effects. Such evaluations are essential if ineffective programs are to be halted or effective ones are to receive more resources.

- Many programs rely exclusively on the cheapest possible drugs, thereby risking problems with toxicity, adherence, and drug resistance. From the outset a broader range of drug regimens needs to be tested.

NONCOMMUNICABLE DISEASE AND INJURY

At the same time that most low- and middle-income countries need to address health problems that are now effectively controlled in high-income countries, they are increasingly sharing the high-income countries' heavy burdens of cardiovascular system disease (chapters 33, 44, and 45); cancers (chapter 29); psychiatric disorders (chapter 31); and automobile-related injuries (chapter 39). The public health research and policy community has been surprisingly silent about these epidemics even though, for example, cardiovascular disease (CVD) in low- and middle-income countries killed over twice as many people in 2001 as did AIDS, malaria, and TB combined (table 1.A1). An important early exception is Feachem and others (1992), who indicated approaches to treatment and prevention of these conditions that can be adapted to the tighter budget constraints of developing countries. The World Health Organization provides a valuable and more up-to-date discussion that emphasizes prevention (WHO 2005). In addition, low-cost but effective approaches to long-term management of chronic conditions need to be developed and implemented.

The remainder of this section briefly discusses, as examples, the prevention and management of cardiovascular diseases, psychiatric disorders, and injuries.

Cardiovascular Disease

Cardiovascular diseases in low- and middle-income countries result in about 13 million deaths each year, over a quarter of all deaths in those countries. Most cardiovascular deaths result from ischemic heart disease (5.7 million) or cerebrovascular disease (4.6 million). Because such deaths occur at older ages, they account for a substantially smaller fraction of total disease burden in disability-adjusted life years (DALYs)—12.9 percent—than they do of deaths (table 1.A2).

Growing tobacco use accounts for a substantial and avoidable fraction of CVD and of cancers. Reasonable projections show the number of tobacco-related deaths to be not only large but also growing, particularly in developing countries. In 2000, the number of tobacco-related deaths in developing countries about equaled the number in high-income countries; projections suggest that by 2030 developing countries will have more than twice as many. For those reasons, controlling smoking is a key element of any national strategy for preventing CVD or for promoting health more generally. Preventing the initiation of smoking is important because addiction to tobacco makes smoking cessation very difficult, even for the numerous individuals who would like to do so. However, helping people quit smoking is at least as important as preventing initiation. Figure 1.6 portrays estimates showing that far more lives could be saved between now and 2050 with successful efforts to help people stop smoking than with efforts to keep them from

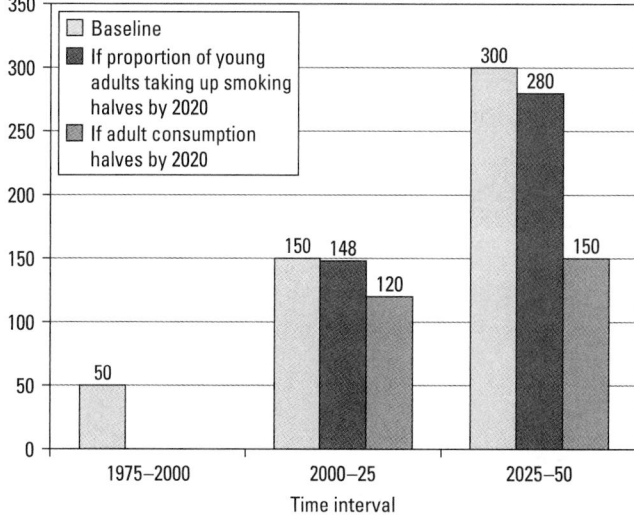

Tobacco deaths worldwide in the indicated quarter century (millions)

Source: Chapter 46, figure 46.2. Adapted from Jha and Chaloupka 2000; Peto and Lopez 2001.

Figure 1.6 Increase in Tobacco-Related Deaths as Populations Age

starting. Reducing smoking levels is well demonstrated to be within the control of public policy. The principal instrument is through taxation: Complementary measures discussed in chapter 46 are important as well.

The main risk factors for CVD account for very large fractions of the deaths (and even more of the burden) from those diseases. For ischemic heart disease, they collectively account for 78 percent of deaths in low- and middle-income countries; for stroke, they account for 61 percent (Ezzati and others 2006). Measures to reduce the levels of those risk factors—high blood pressure, high cholesterol, smoking, obesity, excessive alcohol use, physical inactivity, and low fruit and vegetable consumption—are the goals for prevention. Unlike the favorable experience with controlling tobacco use, attempts to change the behaviors leading to obesity, hypertension, high cholesterol, or physical activity appear to have had little success at a population level. However, as chapter 44 documents, many promising approaches remain to be tried. Common sense suggests that they should be initiated even while more systematic efforts to develop and evaluate behavior-change packages are ramped up.

Pharmaceutical interventions to manage two major components of cardiovascular risk—hypertension and high cholesterol levels—are well established and are highly cost-effective for individuals at high risk of a stroke or heart attack. From at least the time of publication of *Disease Control Priorities in Developing Countries*, 1st edition (*DCP1*), researchers have recognized that the low cost and high effectiveness of drugs to prevent the reoccurrence of a cardiovascular event made their long-term use potentially cost-effective in low-income environments (Pearson, Jamison, and Trejo-Gutierrez 1993). Even if sustained behavior change proves difficult to achieve, medications have the potential to reduce CVD risks by 50 percent or more. Chapters 33 and 45 develop the current evidence on that point. A key problem, however, concerns the health care personnel and systems requirements associated with the need for lifelong medication use, a problem also faced with antiretroviral therapy for AIDS and the use of medications to target several major psychiatric disorders. How to achieve effective long-term management of lifesaving drugs is a key delivery and research challenge for health system reformers.

In contrast to the lifelong requirement for drug use associated with CVD risk reduction in high-risk individuals, treatment of acute heart attacks with inexpensive drugs is both less demanding of system resources and highly cost-effective (chapter 45). Given the high incidence of these problems, systemwide efforts to achieve high rates of appropriate drug use in response to acute heart disease are a high priority.

Psychiatric Disorders

Although neurological and psychiatric disorders lead to only about 1.4 percent of deaths in low- and middle-income countries (1.8 percent in high-income countries), they cause suffering and disability far beyond what the mortality numbers suggest. About 10 percent of disease burden in DALYs in low- and middle-income countries results from these conditions; three major psychiatric diseases—unipolar major depression (3.1 percent of DALYs), bipolar disorder (0.6 percent), and schizophrenia (0.8 percent)—account for much of it (table 1.A2).

Chapter 31 provides a concise overview of advances made in recent years in treating these conditions (as well as panic disorder), summarizes information on their burden, and develops estimates of the cost-effectiveness of drug-based and cognitive behavioral therapies in different settings (hospital based and community based). Although the cost-effectiveness estimates reported in chapter 31 suggest interventions are only moderately cost-effective, the authors suggest that a fuller analysis of benefits than is captured by a health metric such as the DALY would justify substantial investments. They analyze a basic package of mental health services that could provide a practical vehicle for providing these interventions in environments with tightly constrained financial and implementation resources. A continuing theme in this volume—and one of particular relevance here—is that without careful evaluations of the effects of alternative approaches to large-scale intervention against psychiatric disorders, the world will fail to develop hard knowledge of what does—and does not—work. Without that knowledge, far less health and financial security will be gained than is potentially possible from the inevitably limited resources available.

Injuries

Injuries constitute an additional major and neglected component of disease burden in developing countries. This volume's chapters on injury (chapters 39 and 40) emphasize prevention. Timely treatment is also important, and chapters 67 (on surgery) and 68 (on emergency medical services) point to the potential, at low cost, for much better treatment of injury victims than is typical today.

The great diversity of both causes and consequences of injury precludes an attempt in this chapter to do more than highlight their importance. Chapter 2 and the injury-related chapters just mentioned provide a rich menu of practical options. It is worth pointing out here the central importance of two specific categories of injury—road-traffic injuries (1.07 million deaths in 2001 in low- and middle-income countries) and suicides (0.75 million deaths). Safer roads, safer driving, safer vehicles, and better emergency care have sharply reduced the toll from road-traffic injuries in high-income countries, but unless dramatic action is taken in developing countries, the toll will surely rise. Although there has been less success in reducing suicide rates, the improved treatments now available for psychiatric disorders are proving to be one important approach in suicide prevention.

This discussion of noncommunicable diseases and injury highlights the huge and growing burden from those conditions and conveys a consistent message that constructive action is feasible at relatively modest cost. No attempt has been made to be comprehensive (chapters 29 through 38 all deal with non-communicable diseases); rather the discussion points to the need for health systems to systematically incorporate effective responses to noncommunicable diseases and injuries as their capacities grow.

HEALTH SYSTEM DEVELOPMENT AND FINANCE

DCP1 focused principally on intervention priority. What mix of public health and clinical interventions would best respond to important disease conditions in highly resource constrained environments? Given the results of those assessments, where were the most important overall best buys? Where were resource commitments likely to be of low value? *DCP2* returns to those questions but goes beyond them in assessing the steps required for strengthening of health services and systems in ways that will allow the appropriate mix of interventions to be delivered equitably and well. De Savigny and others (2004) describe a specific example from Tanzania that links system reform to intervention selection.

Part 3 of the volume addresses strengthening of health systems. For valuable discussions of the goals of health systems, see WHO's *World Health Reports* for 1999 and 2000 (WHO 1999, 32–33; 2000, 23–25) and Roberts and others (2003).

Part 3 first reviews options for public health services with chapters on surveillance and information (chapters 53 and 54), drug resistance (chapter 55), community health and nutrition programs (chapter 56), contraception (chapter 57), school-based health (chapter 58), adolescent health (chapter 59), occupational health (chapter 60), natural disaster relief (chapter 61), and disease elimination and eradication (chapter 62). A major point implied by the simple number of chapters devoted to public health is that health system strengthening and reform efforts need to commit substantial financial resources and political and managerial attention to public health.

A second cluster of chapters in part 3 deals with strengthening personal health services. The first of those chapters deals with an important facet of community-level health services, the integrated management of the sick child (chapter 63). Chapters 64 to 66 deal with levels of care: general primary care, the district hospital, and the referral hospital, respectively. Three chapters address services offered at multiple levels of the system: surgery (chapter 67), emergency medical services (chapter 68), and complementary and alternative medicine (chapter 69). The final cluster of four chapters addresses capacity strengthening and management reform: quality of care (chapter 70), the health workforce (chapter 71), supplies of drugs and vaccines (chapter 72), and management of clinical services (chapter 73).

This overview of the topics on health systems provides a sense of the breadth of the issues considered. Chapter 3 provides a concise and integrated statement of the main findings. The remainder of this section deals briefly with assessing the performance of health systems and with the key issue of finance. Before we turn to those topics, however, it is worth highlighting several particular points.

First, in low-income countries, limited health system capacity has sometimes led governments (and development assistance agencies) to focus their capacity on a few high-priority items—such as immunization or control of HIV/AIDS. The objective may be a reasonable one: a greater reduction in disease burden in the population and more financial protection for it are likely to be achieved by doing a few important things well than by doing many things poorly. Yet if this focused effort is undertaken by establishing vertical structures outside the health system, then important opportunities for increasing capacity may be missed. Chapter 3 stresses a critical point: a focused program should be designed so that it contributes to, rather than detracts from, long-term system strengthening. Second, quality of care is important; it can be measured, and it can be improved (box 1.3). Third, providing basic surgical services, particularly at the district hospital level appears to offer major but neglected opportunities for addressing

---

Box 1.3

Tangible Approaches to Improving Quality of Care

A 2001 report from the Institute of Medicine of the U.S. National Academy of Sciences (Institute of Medicine 2001b) highlights great variation in the quality of clinical care in the United States. Its publication catalyzed reform efforts. In a recent evaluation, Leape and Berwick (2005) found that those reform efforts had a major effect on professional attitudes and organizational culture, although less effect, so far, on mortality. Chapter 70 on quality of care documents the similarly large variation in quality in low- and middle-income countries and the associated cost in lives and money. Improving quality of care amplifies the effect of investments in health. Promising approaches in improving the quality of care include the following:

- Invest in measuring quality and feeding that information back into the system. This approach has been shown to be possible (for example, clinical vignettes) and effective.

- Use evidence-based criteria to link quality of care to outcomes. This approach can be implemented by training and creating incentives for adapting clinical guidelines or by using the collaborative improvement model.

- Improve system-level and provider incentives. Minimally, do no harm with the structure of financial incentives facing providers, for example, by establishing a legal and ethical environment where care providers do not profit personally from sale of drugs, diagnostic procedures, or referrals to expensive specialized care.

- Emphasize high-volume care for selected surgical procedures and prevalent medical conditions. Such an approach can lead to higher quality and lower cost even while, in some cases (for example, cataract removal), allowing lower-level workers to substitute for more expensive and scarcer physicians.

Source: This box was prepared with input from John Peabody.

significant sources of disease burden. An important substantive component of health sector reforms should often involve strengthening surgical capacity.

Health System Performance

Since about 1940, the publication of economic performance indicators in national income and product accounts has made it possible to hold political leaders accountable for economic management. Additionally, measures of economic performance—such as GDP growth rates and unemployment rates—have allowed economists to move toward evidence-based assessments of which policies facilitate good economic performance and which do not.

In many ways, unfortunately, the assessment of health system performance remains where economic performance measures were before the development of national income and product accounts in the United Kingdom in the late 1930s. Chapter 3 observes, for example, that "The body of knowledge [on health systems] represents a largely ad hoc and disjointed collection of facts, figures, and points of view. Making confident recommendations relevant to strengthening health system capacity is thus difficult." In its 2000 *World Health Report*, WHO made an ambitious effort to provide the performance measures for health systems that would enable progress toward more systematic knowledge of the policies to improve health systems (WHO 2000). Such knowledge could replace what is now frequently simply ideology and opinion. The 2000 *World Health Report* proved to be highly controversial, and its ranking of health system performance may in the end be judged as more of a first attempt than an initial approximation (Jamison and Sandbu 2001). WHO set an agenda that will certainly continue to be advanced.

Despite current inability to judge health system performance and the consequently ad hoc character of knowledge, much is in fact known that bears on health policy. Chapters 2 and 3 of this volume summarize very specific knowledge about intervention characteristics and system design that can inform policy. Although broad prescriptions may still elude us, particular knowledge is still important. Additionally, the perform-ance of countries is better understood even though relating country performance to performance of its health systems may remain only judgmental for the moment. For example, Brazil and China had under-five mortality rates that were quite close in 2002: 37 per 1,000 for Brazil and 38 per 1,000 for China. In 1990, however, Brazil's rate was 60 per 1,000 and China's was 49 per 1,000: the rate of improvement in Brazil was far more rapid than in China. This measure is only one dimension of outcome, and many explanations are possible. Yet hard numbers on country perform do exist to initiate discussions of policy.

Financing Health Services

Chapters 12 and 13 in this volume discuss domestic and external financing of health systems. Different issues arise in low-income countries than in middle-income ones, and the discussion that follows is so divided. Table 1.2 provides context by conveying the level of health expenditures in 2001 in different income groupings of countries, the fraction of GDP spent on health, and the extent to which those expenditures are publicly financed. Almost 10 percent of the total product of the world pays for health services. In the low-income countries, about three-quarters of expenditures are from private, out-of-pocket payment. In the high-income European countries, only about one-quarter of expenditures is private. Middle-income countries spend about 5 times as much per capita on health services as do low-income ones and over 10 times as much through the public sector. Although available data sets (for example, from the World Bank or WHO) provide no direct evidence on trends over time in health expenditures (for more than very short periods), current levels of expenditure are likely to substantially exceed those of several decades ago, even as a percentage of growing incomes. The availability of physicians provides one indicator: in a large sample of countries the number of physicians per 100,000 population increased from 54 in the mid 1960s to 116 in the early 1990s, an annual rate of increase of 2.8 percent.

Before we turn to questions of financing health services (or insurance), briefly discussing related issues concerning the public sector's financial role is worthwhile. Those issues address

Table 1.2 Health Expenditures by Country Income Level, Public and Total, 2001

Country group	Health expenditure per capita (2001 US$)	Health expenditure (percentage of GDP)	Public sector expenditures (percentage of total health expenditures)
Low income	23	4.4	26.3
Middle income	118	6.0	51.1
High income	2,841	10.8	62.1
(Countries in the European Monetary Union)	(1,856)	(9.3)	(73.5)
World	500	9.8	59.2

Source: World Bank 2004, table 2.14.

what chapter 11 calls "healthy fiscal policy and fiscal policy for health." An example of unhealthy fiscal policy was the Polish government's subsidy of fatty animal products. Elimination of that subsidy was a gain for the treasury and resulted in improved diets and health. Minimally, a healthy fiscal policy identifies and corrects such inappropriate subsidies. Fiscal policy for health is exemplified by tobacco taxation, which chapter 46 deals with at length and chapter 11 deals with more briefly. Fiscal policy for health involves taxes whose principal purposes lie more in changing health-related behaviors than in generating revenue (although the latter can be important as well).

Financing Health in Middle-Income Countries. A major cause of poverty (and economic insecurity more generally) results from highly uneven and unpredictable needs to finance health expenditures. In consequence, most societies have moved toward prepaid care as income rises. The current high-income countries, with only two exceptions, have decided in favor of universal public financing (rather than private voluntary insurance) as the principal means of meeting the demand for prepaid care. Taiwan (China) and the Republic of Korea, several years ago, and Mexico and Thailand more recently, have also taken the path toward universal public, financing. The health sector is exceptional: no one in the mature capitalist democracies would contemplate substantial public financing for food or housing, and public subsidies and protection for agriculture result from unusually powerful interest groups.

Public financing for health, including for clinical services for well-off individuals, has been the result of the democratic process in all the major capitalist countries except Switzerland and the United States. (Public financing is, of course, consistent with private provision of services, and the countries of the Organisation for Economic Co-operation and Development (OECD) display substantial diversity in this regard.) Efficiency as well as equity concerns underlie this pattern. Barr (2001) examines in detail the efficiency rationales that have underpinned major public sector financial involvement in health, education, and social protection in the high-income countries.

Why do market economies choose public sector financing (either public spending or publicly mandated social insurance) for many of their personal clinical services? The case for publicly financing interventions that are shared by all (for example, antitobacco advertising or water fluoridation) or where significant externalities exist (such as interruption of transmission of TB by treatment of infections) is widely accepted. Providing personal clinical services, like hernia repair, has none of those attributes. Nonetheless, as Arrow (1963) articulated in a now-classic article, the pervasiveness of incomplete information for decision makers (patients, providers, insurers) dominates private health insurance and delivery of clinical services. These personal clinical services account for the bulk of health expenditure. The evidence is increasingly clear that a strong government presence in finance is the least bad way of dealing with these problems. Such a presence is necessary to achieve universal access to health care and makes it easier to impose the hard budget constraints that impose discipline in resource allocation. Additional evidence indicates that introducing universal mandatory health coverage favorably affects both wages and employment levels. Gruber and Hanratty (1995) provide thorough documentation of these effects in Canada. Some combination of these factors likely underpins the choices of the high-income democracies to fund a large fraction of private clinical services with public resources.

Public financing of services for all does not imply that all services can be provided. Indeed, given their resource constraints, countries face hard choices about what to include (and exclude) in the universal benefits package—choices that this volume seeks to inform.

Middle-income countries vary substantially in the extent to which health care providers are financed on a fee-for-service basis—that is, by direct payment for specific services. Although that is traditionally the chief way to pay for *private* care, it is worth clarifying that *government* providers can also be financed (legally or illegally) on a fee-for-service basis—as is increasingly the case in China, for example. Similarly, providers are sometimes compensated through other means, such as capitation, and individual physicians in the private sector are sometimes on salary or a combination of salary plus capitation. Out-of-pocket payments to a public sector provider are usually called *user fees,* but they differ little from fee-for-service compensation of private providers.

What is the OECD experience with user fees? Basically, it is that both providers and patients respond strongly to the incentive environment. Indeed, a problem exists of providers being too responsive: much low-value or useless surgery, diagnosis, and drug use is, in some systems, highly profitable to the provider, and often the provider must, as agent for the patient, decide what to do. This conflict of interest has led to cost escalation and to inappropriate care. A case may be made for divorcing provider compensation from the delivery of individual services, drugs, or diagnostic tests unless a need exists to accelerate coverage of critical services by giving bonuses to providers for providing them, as the United Kingdom's National Health Service has done with immunization.

If fee-for-service financing can generate a perverse incentive environment, does that imply that a system must forgo charging beneficiaries for services they receive? Not at all: other ways exist to ensure that funds are adequate for costs—ways that may be more effective. Earmarking payroll taxes to finance health care for workers and their dependents (usually called *social insurance*) is one approach for recovering costs that is consistent with provider compensation mechanisms relying principally on salaries or capitation rather than fee-for-service. It has been argued that cost recovery through payroll taxes will generate more economic distortions than do income, consumption, or sin taxes—although recent evidence suggests that may not be true (Blanchard and Katz 1997). Nonetheless, when general revenue mechanisms are incapable of financing the nationally defined basic package of services for all, the option of cost recovery through payroll taxes for the privileged workers in the formal sector is clearly desirable on equity grounds. This form of taxation also links contributions to a specific service, which increases its acceptability.

Financing Health in Low-Income Countries. Approximately 2.5 billion people live in countries the World Bank classifies as low-income—that is, with a per capita gross national income in 2002 of less than US$735 per year. These countries include India but not China. Table 1.2 reflects that the estimated average per capita health expenditure for these 2.5 billion people is about US$23 per year, of which US$5 or US$6 comes from public sources. Chapter 12, on financing health systems, points to the severe challenges in setting priorities that these resource limitations imply. Not only are expenditure levels currently very low, but also the fiscal space needed to increase them is, in most low-income countries, sharply constrained. Fiscal space results from an excess of potential government revenues, including reasonable projections of official development assistance (ODA), over public expenditures. The concept of fiscal space combines both short-term fiscal balance and long-term debt sustainability. Grant ODA can help with short-term balance, and soft loans (such as International Development Association credits from the World Bank) can reduce the repayment burden from a given level of incurred debt. Health financing policy for low-income countries must focus heavily on mobilizing public sector resources and concentrating resources on true priorities (although the broader range of issues just discussed that middle-income countries must address is relevant to low-income countries with large formal sectors).

The chapters in this volume make clear that incremental resources for health, well spent, could have an enormous effect: resource mobilization is important. Increasing public sector expenditures in health by 0.5 percent or more of GDP will be possible in some countries, but not in all, and even where it is possible other investment priorities will also be pressing. However, increases of as much as 1 percent of GDP may possible where the political will exists, as is now being attempted in India. Cost estimates for meeting just the health-related MDGs, as reported in chapter 9, can exceed that amount, and other estimates have run higher. Development assistance for health, discussed in chapter 13 and here, can expand the available resource envelope, but even multiples of current levels of development assistance would likely prove insufficient to finance attainment of the MDGs in some countries.

Achieving gains for health (and frequently concomitant gains in financial protection) requires that critical decisions be made on how to allocate highly limited public sector resources. Much of this volume deals with resource allocation across interventions. Public finance must address an additional set of decisions. Do interventions with substantial positive externalities have a particular claim on public resources—beyond the amount of health and financial protection they buy per million dollars spent? Should public resources be spent only on individuals with low income? Or should health systems provide universal public finance for the very limited range of interventions that can be afforded? Should public finance emphasize providing interventions that maximize financial protection or improvements in health? What patterns of public sector resource allocation are likely to prove politically sustainable? Fewer tradeoffs may exist among these criteria than at first seems to be the case.

A starting point for thinking about these criteria is the availability of an increasing number of good benefit incidence studies—that is, studies of how the benefits of a public intervention distribute across income (or asset) quintiles of the population. Those studies find that in a great majority of countries wealthier people are more likely to benefit from public programs than are the poor, at least where benefits are measured in expenditures. The World Bank's 1993 *World Development Report* pointed to that pattern some time ago (although noting a number of important exceptions), and more recent studies add support to that conclusion. The caveat "measured in expenditures" is important and insufficiently noted. The value or welfare benefit to the poor of a given level of transfer may well exceed the value received by the well off from the same level of transfer. A landmark benefit incidence study of the U.S. Medicare program, a mandatory health insurance for the elderly, found it to be regressive in dollar terms but pro-poor in welfare outcomes (McClellan and Skinner 1997).

Public programs that are not universal appear to systematically benefit the better off, and that pattern is understandable from a political perspective. It follows that if an immunization program, for example, is differentially benefiting the well off, then making immunization universal would be pro-poor in terms of incremental public expenditures. Figure 1.7 uses data from a careful benefit incidence assessment in the Philippines (Gwatkin and others 2000) to illustrate this point for immunization and for attended deliveries.

Making coverage universal for cost-effective interventions *for conditions important to the poor* is thus likely to prove to be an efficient way of both improving health outcomes and enhancing equity. Many of these interventions address infectious disease where control has significant externalities, and implementing universal coverage is likely to prove more politically sustainable than targeting population subgroups. Lindert (2004) extensively discusses the experience in high-income countries with universalization of public financing of education, health, and old-age pensions and concludes not only that

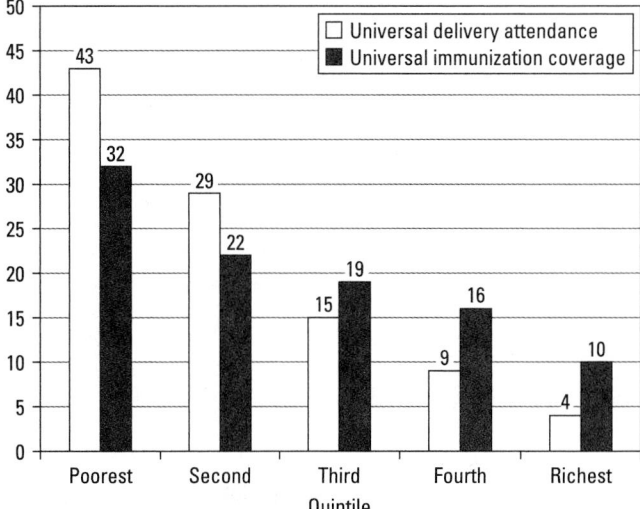

Percentage of incremental benefit received by each quintile

Legend: □ Universal delivery attendance ■ Universal immunization coverage

Poorest: 43 / 32
Second: 29 / 22
Third: 15 / 19
Fourth: 9 / 16
Richest: 4 / 10

Quintile

Source: Calculations based on data reprinted in Gwatkin and others (2000).

Notes: Universal immunization coverage means complete coverage with the standard immunization schedule. The Philippines achieved 75 percent coverage overall in 1998, and Gwatkin and others (2000) show the coverage level by quintile. The black bar shows what the percentage distribution of benefits by population quintile would be of moving from the 1998 status quo to universal coverage. *Universal delivery attendance* means that all births would be attended by a doctor, nurse, or nurse-midwife. The Philippines achieved 63 percent coverage overall, and the white bar shows what the percentage distribution of benefits by population quintile would be of moving from the current pattern of coverage to universal coverage.

Figure 1.7 Equity Implications of Providing Universal Coverage for Immunization and Attended Delivery in the Philippines, 1998

it is politically sustainable but also that no evidence indicates that the resulting higher taxes have harmed economic growth.

Two final points are worth stating about making coverage universal:

• First, early adoption of universalization of coverage for publicly financed interventions—even if only a few can be financed—sets the stage for expansion, in a middle-income environment, to universal public financing of health care, the overwhelming choice of the democratic process in high-income countries.

• Second, the implementation capacity of health systems in low-income countries will often be highly constrained. Capacity is likely to grow most rapidly by building on a base of doing a few things well rather than many things poorly. Universal coverage implies tight focus in highly resource-constrained environments.

RESEARCH AND DEVELOPMENT

Why has health improved so dramatically after controlling for income and, hence, the availability of commodities that, like food, are essential for health? Although no unambiguous

answer to this question exists, an important factor has been advance in scientific knowledge and its application both in creating powerful interventions and in guiding behavior. Acquisition and use of health research and development or its products becomes, then, an essential function of a country's health system. Moreover, it is important that research extend beyond development of new products to encompass knowledge generation on health system financing and performance.

Much knowledge is embodied in global public goods: once a vaccine against hepatits B has been developed anywhere, it becomes, in some sense, available everywhere. Although monopoly pricing made possible by patents may slow the diffusion of some innovations, the temporary nature of patent-induced monopoly pricing limits that effect. However, an innovation's being cheap, powerful, and globally available in no way assures its global use. The implication is clear: globally available knowledge and products offer enormous opportunities to countries, but national policies and national health systems determine whether that knowledge is put to local use. Additionally, although some information for improving outcomes is principally local and must be locally produced, making the results available contributes to a growing evidence base. Chapter 4 on health research stresses the value of contributing to a global evidence base and summarizes with the observation that "all health care is national" and "all health research is global."

What are the implications for policy? One is that if knowledge gains prove even partially as important for future health improvements as they have in the past century—and chapters in this volume point to a number of reasons for expecting this to be so—then investments in health research and development will continue to have high payoffs in health status and economic productivity. Chapter 7 points to the potential for enormous economic returns. Ensuring an adequate level of research and development investment, therefore, holds strong claim on health budgets—a claim for more than the approximately 3 percent now committed. Equally important—or more important—is that the investments be efficient in generating useful new knowledge and products. Fauci (2005) discusses the need for greater efficiency in conducting research and development in an environment of tightening budgets in U.S. agencies, and he points to a number of specific directions for doing so.

In some cases, additional resources (probably from growth within national health budgets or health aid budgets) will be required to meet these research and development needs adequately. In many cases, institutional change will be necessary to create the information and incentives required for efficient resource allocation. At the international level, resource allocation has often lacked focus, failing to bring results to the point of application, and has neglected important conditions and issues while providing, often generously, for less important ones. Reform is needed. Successful models of competitively driven international funding and experience-sharing networks should be applied to currently neglected clusters of conditions.

Just as the quality and productivity of research efforts vary dramatically from one institution to another within the high-income countries, they vary in the low- and middle-income countries. Exemplary work is done in a number of institutions and countries; but in general, the obstacles to high quality are greater when countries' incomes are lower. Inadequate training, insufficient staff motivation, and lack of competition prevent many institutions from attaining their potential. The instability of short-term funding, isolation from peers, and poor access to the research literature all compound the problem and prevent researchers from responding rapidly to ever-changing demands. Given the shortage of good researchers, an argument exists for the talent to move to countries (including low- and middle-income countries) whose policies are likely to facilitate productive research (WHO 1996). Donor funding should reflect this possibility.

Institutions are more likely to succeed not only if they receive stable core funding but also if a proportion of their work is funded competitively. Some institutions, such as the Oswaldo Cruz Foundation in Brazil, have already moved in these directions with great success—for example, by freeing up intramural resources for competitive allocation between groups and within the institution, with assessments being made by an external review group. Notable successes have occurred in assisting with capacity strengthening, such as the Special Programme for Research and Training in Tropical Diseases collaboratively supported by WHO, the World Bank, and the United Nations Development Programme.

The failure of current incentive structures, essentially the patent system, to produce health products for the lowest income groups demands remedial action (chapter 5). In essence, either the public sector must harness the skills, energy, and capacity of the private sector to develop and bring promptly to market products for the lowest income groups, or it must take responsibility for doing so itself. In reality, a combination of the two is likely, as is exemplified in successful public-private partnerships such as the Medicines for Malaria Venture or the International AIDS Vaccine Initiative. Recently proposed precommitments by the public sector to purchase specific new products are an additional potential instrument to generate incentives for private sector investment (Kremer and Glennerster 2004). Developing countries that participate in private sector innovation will be positioned to more quickly learn of and have access to the technical progress that is critical in driving health improvements.

Global challenges demand, in some sense, a global response. All nations share the fruits of research and development. Even though each country may invest a relatively modest sum toward collective goals, the aggregate effort potentially benefits all substantially. Collective action is the economically rational approach to public goods such as research and development; here, responsibility for catalyzing collective action lies principally in the hands of the global community. Far from overshadowing action at the national level, global efforts help both to make national research and development efforts more productive and to lead to a global result that exceeds the sum of national ones. Thus, among the many competing demands on the funds allocated to international assistance for health, those contributing to generation of new knowledge, products, and interventions that can be shared by all have special merit.

DEVELOPMENT ASSISTANCE FOR HEALTH

Development assistance, wisely focused, has the potential for unusual effect. First, because health gains for the poor can be relatively inexpensive (compared to the cost of achieving significant effect in other sectors), development assistance itself can achieve much, particularly if it serves as a channel for diffusion of new technologies and best practices. Second, evidence suggests that development assistance in health can be more effective than other development assistance in poor policy and weak institutional environments. Third, the economic benefits of investing in health can be exceptionally high. Finally, because research and development have had high impact (chapter 7) and are an international public good, development assistance has a particular comparative advantage in ensuring their finance.

Those conclusions point to a proactive strategy within development assistance agencies and governments for achieving major shifts in staffing and budgetary allocations toward specific high-payoff investments in health. They also point to the need, in order to achieve the potential benefits, for a focused concentration of health system development on a limited set of priority health goals—for example, controlling AIDS, controlling smoking, meeting the health-related MDGs, and—for middle-income countries—implementing finance reforms that lead toward universal public financing. The section argues that although financial fungibility—the capacity to redirect government resources away from areas supported by external financing—can dilute the effect of development assistance in health, as in other sectors, designing development assistance for health that minimizes the fungibility problem is possible. Performance-based budget support will be one instrument.

In 2003, the world committed to ODA of almost US$100 billion, and news reports in May 2005 suggested the possibility of substantial increases by European donors. Approximately 10 percent of ODA is spent for health, a percentage that has grown rapidly. Table 13.1 in chapter 13 shows recent trends in external financing for health, of which ODA (that is, grant or highly concessional loans) is only a part: these numbers are for commitments, not actual disbursements, which are smaller and lag behind commitments. (The Global Fund to Fight AIDS, Tuberculosis, and Malaria is one of the few providers of developmental finance that reports disbursements as well as commitments.) External financing for health has grown from about US$6.7 billion in 1998 to US$9.3 billion in 2002 (Michaud 2003). For some countries, development assistance constitutes a significant and growing fraction of health expenditures. Economists have recently returned to the question of the returns to expenditures on development assistance, and several recent trends have important potential implications for health.

Aid Effectiveness

Recent work has been reassessing aid effectiveness and has focused on the following questions: Is there any evidence that infusions of development assistance have affected economic growth rates? Is there any evidence that infusions of economic assistance have affected mortality rates or levels of poverty? These questions are clearly not easy to answer. Nonetheless, some data provide insights. Burnside and Dollar (2000) conclude, for example, that development assistance does seem to work in countries where a good policy environment and a good institutional environment exist, but not in countries lacking those elements. Recent work focuses on aid directed to economic development and greatly strengthens the inclusiveness of the conclusion that aid boosts growth (Clemens, Radelet, and Bhavnani 2004). The effect of development assistance on growth is quantitatively important even in countries with poor policies and institutions, although the effect is stronger in countries with better policies. Interestingly, aid's effect appears larger in countries with higher life expectancy. That development assistance contributes broadly to growth does not, of course, imply that development assistance for health will accelerate health improvements. However, it is certainly suggestive of the potential in health to know that development assistance works for growth.

Even if development assistance is viewed as working better in strong institutional and policy environments, a dilemma exists in that the countries that most need aid are often ones that have weak policies and weak institutions (Radelet 2003, 194). Experiences with ODA in health complement the recent research on aid for growth in suggesting that ODA can pay off despite limited institutional or absorptive capacity. Polio has certainly been eliminated in countries with good health systems, but it has also been eliminated from most countries with weak ones. No smallpox exists today in countries with bad policies and bad institutions. A number of those countries have immunization rates of 60 or 70 percent, or as high as in the United States. An important question concerns the extent to which other development assistance for health, particularly

highly targeted development assistance, can be as successfully implemented as immunization programs where health systems are weak.

Project Support versus Budget Support

Development assistance is tending to move away from project support—for example, of an immunization program, an AIDS control program, or an extension of a road network—and toward general budgetary support, often to be provided through pooling of donor assistance. There are many reasons for this tendency, some of which are good (Kanbur and Sandler 1999, 106). The usefulness (and even propriety) of budget support is contingent, however, on adequacy of the policy and institutional environments. Chapter 3 points to arguments that as health systems evolve, development assistance should move from project assistance toward program assistance. The Global Alliance for Vaccines and Immunization (GAVI) is pointing to ways that support for immunization programs can be advanced within the context of this tendency to move toward general budget support. GAVI's innovation is to support immunization programs based on performance—US$20 for a fully immunized child. The country gets the US$20 for immunizing the child in whatever way it decides; thus, GAVI provides general budget support that is conditioned on performance. GAVI's concern has been with transitional financing (rather than with sustained assistance), but its approach points the way for designing long-term budget support conditioned on measurable performance with respect to specific health goals. Jamison (2004) outlined design of long-term development assistance for health that could meet this objective, maintaining incentives for countries to increase coverage (or performance) while scaling back the volume of aid as a country's income increased. Adequate measurement underpins assessment of performance and can be difficult even for immunization coverage. Measurement requires resources that must be planned for and budgeted.

Macroeconomic Consequences of Aid

Another concern in the aid community—particularly in the International Monetary Fund—is that development assistance could have adverse domestic macroeconomic consequences—essentially inflationary consequences (see WHO 2002, chapter 8). This argument needs to be taken seriously. It is in essence an argument about the generation of domestic inflationary pressures—of projects chasing after those few good engineers or doctors with an increasing amount of foreign money and creating an inflationary spiral in that way. However, if the principal proposed use for the money is for drugs or vaccines—for example, the US$10 increment for adding Hib and HepB vaccines to the Expanded Program on Immunization schedule—that money is almost all foreign exchange, and the macroeconomic arguments about inflationary consequences simply would not apply. Careful project design can respond to what on the whole are serious concerns from the macroeconomic part of the development assistance community. Economic analysis can provide information—such as this volume attempts to provide—on getting the maximum health and financial protection outcomes from the development assistance available and for designing interventions (tradable and commodity intensive) that will minimize potentially adverse macroeconomic consequences.

The Millennium Development Goals

An additional and significant direction in thinking about ODA concerns achievement of the MDGs (chapter 9). The MDGs are very specific targets for improvement in education, health, and income-related poverty. Interestingly, focusing development assistance on achieving the MDGs stands in at least partial opposition to the move toward budget support.

These considerations point to several directions for the design of development assistance for health. Radelet (2003, 194) provides detailed quantitative examples to show that, even under very favorable circumstances, in a lower-middle-income country development assistance is likely to be needed for decades. Some conclusions follow that are drawn from the preceding discussion and from the need for predictability and long time horizons in donor behavior. ODA should move toward the following:

- providing aid over long-term perspectives (10 or more years)
- ensuring predictability in assistance commitments
- emphasizing demand-side support (with concomitant country control of resources)
- providing incentives for countries to maintain high coverage for cost-effective programs
- avoiding perverse incentives
- including a transparent exit strategy (for example, reduced grant support with per capita GDP growth).

There is a strong analogy to within-country programs like Mexico's Progresa, which provides cash transfers to poor households contingent on getting children immunized or into school. Gertler (2004) has reported evaluation results indicating a high degree of effectiveness. The effectiveness of coverage incentives is well exemplified by the Bill & Melinda Gates Foundation in its work on polio with both GAVI and the World Bank in providing a financial incentive for enhanced coverage (chapter 13). Although donors increasingly state a commitment to providing aid predictably and over long periods, the reality for many countries is that aid flows will be volatile and

of uncertain duration. Jamison and Radelet (2005) point to ways of using such aid that can be minimally disruptive.

CONCLUSIONS

A volume as large as this one can provide only a sampling of opportunities and potential pitfalls for investments in health. Indeed, the *International Statistical Classification of Diseases* (WHO 2003a) takes more than 1,500 pages simply to list the conditions that a health system must address. Yet the diseases accounting for most of the burden can be listed in perhaps half a dozen pages, and the diseases that account for most of the differences in outcome between high- and low-mortality countries can be listed on a page. Chapters in this volume assess 115 population interventions and 204 personal interventions that address most conditions of importance. The conclusions listed in this final section of the chapter simply highlight important conclusions for policy without attempting to summarize the volume as a whole. Chapters 2 and 3 complement this one with a fuller summary.

Table 1.3 provides a sense of the nature of the findings in much of the book, and box 1.4 provides a brief description of the methods. The table shows the number of DALYs that we estimate could be averted (or years of healthy life that could be bought) by spending a million dollars on a few of the interventions addressing major sources of disease burden. If we think of these numbers as the prices for buying health by different means, the price variation is enormous, ranging from one or two DALYs per million dollars up to well over 100,000. All the standard caveats more than apply to these numbers. Nonetheless, they do convey information relevant for policy. Expanding coverage of the currently used mix of vaccines, for example, appears more attractive than does adding new vaccines (except when the lower demands on system capacity of adding new vaccines are considered). Bypass surgery used even in the most appropriate circumstances is an expensive way to buy a year of healthy life, but for many common indications it is inordinately expensive. Findings from table 1.3 exemplify findings of the cost-effectiveness analyses from throughout the book that are summarized in chapter 2.

A general conclusion follows from the preceding discussion. There are many inexpensive ways to reduce mortality rates and improve health. A country that focuses on those interventions can expect to achieve major improvements—even with very limited resources. There are also ways to spend money on health that can dissipate even a substantial budget with almost no return—either for better health or for the financial protection of populations. Intervention selection matters. Many of the good and bad buys are now well known. Some are not, and our main purpose in this volume has been to assemble the evidence based on what is known.

We now turn to more specific conclusions. Different items on the list are relevant in different countries. (Chapter 2

Table 1.3 How Much Health Will a Million Dollars Buy?

Service or intervention	Cost per DALY (US$)	Estimated DALYs averted per million US$ spent
Reducing under-five mortality		
Improving care of children under 28 days old (including resuscitation of newborns)	10–400	2,500–100,000
Expanding immunization coverage with standard child vaccines	2–20	50,000–500,000
Adding vaccines against additional diseases to the standard child immunization program (particularly Hib and HepB)	40–250	4,000–24,000
Switching to the use of combination drugs (ACTs) against malaria where resistance exists to current inexpensive and previously highly effective drugs (Sub-Saharan Africa)	8–20	50,000–125,000
Preventing and treating HIV/AIDS		
Preventing mother-to-child transmission (antiretroviral-nevirapine prophylaxis of the mother; breastfeeding substitutes)	50–200	5,000–20,000
Treating STIs to interrupt HIV transmission	10–100	10,000–100,000
Using antiretroviral therapy that achieves high adherence for a large percentage of patients	350–500	2,000–3,000
Using antiretroviral therapy that achieves high adherence for only a small percentage of patients		Because of very limited gains by individual patients and the potential for adverse changes in population behavior, it is possible that more life years would be lost than saved.
Preventing and treating noncommunicable disease		
Taxing tobacco products	3–50	24,000–330,000
Treating AMI (heart attacks) with an inexpensive set of drugs	10–25	40,000–100,000
Treating AMI with inexpensive drugs plus streptokinase (costs and DALYs for this intervention are in addition to what would have occurred with inexpensive drugs only)	600–750	1,300–1,600
Treating heart attack and stroke survivors for life with a daily polypill combining four or five off-patent preventive medications	700–1,000	1,000–1,400
Performing coronary artery bypass grafting (bypass surgery) in specific identifiable high-risk cases—for example, disease of the left main coronary artery (incremental to treatment with polypill)	>25,000	<40
Using bypass surgery for less severe coronary artery disease (incremental to treatment with polypill)	Very high	Very small
Other		
Detecting and treating cervical cancer	15–50	20,000–60,000
Operating a basic surgical ward at the district hospital level that focuses on trauma, high-risk pregnancy, and other common surgically treatable conditions	70–250	4,000–15,000

Source: Authors.
AMI = acute myocardial infarction.

suggests, for example, major differences between the priorities for South Asia and those for Sub-Saharan Africa.) Many interventions or policy changes that are important are not on this list, but they are included in the more extensive discussions in chapters 2 and 3, which synthesize messages from the rest of the book on setting intervention priorities and strengthening health system capacity. Given often quite limited availability of money or political leadership or health system capacity, it will often be necessary to focus the available resources on a few key priorities. Chapter 12 makes it disappointingly clear that, for the low-income countries, not only are financial resources sharply limited now, but prospects for more than modest increases seem unlikely for many years. (Financial constraints in the middle-income countries, although real, are less

Cost-Effectiveness Analysis in This Volume

A starting point for cost-effectiveness analysis is to observe that health systems have two objectives: (a) to improve the level and distribution of health outcomes in the population and (b) to protect individuals from financial risks that are often very substantial and that are frequent causes of poverty. Financial risk results from illness-related loss of income as well as expenditures on care; the loss can be ameliorated by preventing illness or its progression and by using appropriate financial architecture for the system.

For the purposes of this book, we consider two classes of resources to be available: financial resources and health system capacity. To implement an intervention in a population, the system uses some of each resource. Just as some interventions have higher dollar costs than others, some interventions are more demanding of system capacity than others. In countries with limited health system capacity, it is clearly important to select interventions that require relatively little of such capacity. Human resource capacity constitutes a particularly important aspect of system capacity, discussed in chapter 71 and in a recent report of the Joint Learning Initiative (2004).

Although in the very short run little tradeoff may exist between dollars and human resources or system capacity more generally, investing in the development of such capacity can help make more of that resource available in the future. Chapter 3 discusses different types of health system capacity and intervention complexity, and it points to the importance of and potential for responding to low capacity by selecting interventions that are less demanding of capacity and by simplifying interventions. Chapter 3 also explores the extent to which financial resources can

substitute for different aspects of system capacity (see also Gericke and others 2003). An important mechanism for strengthening capacity, inherent in highly outcome-oriented programs, may simply be to use it successfully—learning by doing. Several chapters discuss capacity strengthening at different levels of the clinical system, in public health, and in health research and development.

The literature on economic evaluation of health projects typically reports the cost per unit of achieving some measure of health outcome—quality-adjusted life years (QALYs) or DALYs or deaths averted—and at times addresses how that cost varies with the level of intervention and other factors. Pritchard (2004) provides a valuable introduction to this literature. *DCP1* reported such cost-effectiveness findings for a broad range of interventions; *DCP2* does so as well. *DCP2* authors were asked to use methods described in Jamison (2003); chapter 15 discusses actual implementation. Cost-effectiveness calculations provide important insights into the economic attractiveness of an intervention, but other considerations—such as consequences for financial protection and demands on health system capacity—are also relevant.

DCP2 also makes a preliminary attempt to accumulate information about the extent to which interventions place demands on health system capacity; this information is qualitative. *DCP2* provides only an initial effort, but qualitative information does provide helpful input to policy. Kim (2005) develops a more quantitative approach in an analysis dealing with cervical cancer. Much less has been done on the extent to which specific interventions provide financial protection for patients and their families.

Source: Author.

---

binding.) Selecting priorities will be hard. This section provides a starting point for discussing which activities should be high priorities. The conclusions are grouped under four headings: interventions; health services, systems, and financing; research and development; and development assistance.

Interventions

1. Standard interventions for reducing under-five mortality have long been known to be highly cost-effective. The challenge is to scale up while conserving and strengthening scarce health system capacity. These interventions include immunization; micronutrient supplement delivery;

treatment for diarrhea, malaria, and acute respiratory infections; and improved prenatal and delivery care. In cases of sharply limited resources—financial or health system capacity—often the single highest priority will be expansion of immunization coverage with the basic antigens: poliomyelitis, measles, diphtheria, tetanus, pertussis, and perhaps BCG.

2. Cost-effective interventions exist to address the 50 percent of under-five deaths that occur under 28 days of age, including stillbirths. These are underused relative to interventions for older children, and correcting this neglect is a priority.

3. Standard interventions to treat TB are also known to be highly cost-effective, although probably more demanding of health system capacity than are some of the child health interventions. Scaling up by using already developed models for strengthening relevant health system capacity is a priority.

4. Many well-tested preventive interventions for AIDS are effective and cost-effective. Such interventions include treating STIs, promoting condom use, providing voluntary counseling and testing, promoting peer intervention, using antiretroviral therapies to prevent mother-to-child transmission, ensuring safe blood supplies, and encouraging the use of breast milk alternatives by HIV-positive mothers. Scaling up treatment for STIs may prove particularly important. Much more rapid implementation of these interventions is of highest priority and needs to be accompanied by effective mechanisms of surveillance and evaluation. The appropriate mix and distribution of interventions depends on the stage of the epidemic. In particular, limited financial and institutional resources imply focusing effort on populations at high risk early in an epidemic.

5. Antiretroviral drugs have been successful on a wide scale in high-income countries (and in some upper-middle-income countries—notably Brazil and Mexico) in sharply reducing viral load and extending the life expectancy of patients who are HIV positive. Health system capacity for achieving durable benefits from antiretroviral drug use at scale in resource-constrained environments, however, remains to be demonstrated. Failure to achieve good adherence in such an environment would provide minimal benefits to the patient, increase risks of drug resistance, and incur substantial costs: the financial and human losses could be enormous. Multiple approaches to successful maintenance on antiretroviral drugs should be tried and evaluated in large-scale pilots or as part of implementation scale-up. Given the magnitude of the AIDS problem, undertaking and evaluating variations in implementation (including possible variation in the choice of first-line drugs) in parallel rather than serially is important. This approach is not now being used. Similarly important is being rigorous in dropping unsuccessful implementation models before they consume substantial resources that could otherwise have greatly affected AIDS prevention or other priorities in the health sector.

6. Control of tobacco use is the cornerstone of proven approaches to primary prevention of heart disease, stroke, chronic pulmonary disease, and many types of cancer. Instruments for control of tobacco use centering on taxation and improved public information are well established.

7. A range of potential approaches to changing dietary and exercise patterns of populations would, if successful, reduce problems of obesity, hypertension, and dyslipidemia and their consequences for vascular disease. Successes are rare but suggestive that large-scale efforts could be worthwhile. Careful impact evaluation will be essential to ascertain whether these investments deliver value for money.

8. Lifetime medical management—eventually using variants of the polypill—of individuals at high risk for stroke or ischemic heart disease is cost-effective and important for tens of millions of individuals. The clearest indications of high risk are a previous vascular event or diabetes.

Health Services, Systems, and Financing

9. Focused funding for particular diseases or programs—for example, TB or immunization—is a fact of life in many low-income countries. Using such funding to build health system capacity is feasible as well as desirable, but it is far from automatic. As capacity grows, the potential advantages of categorical programs are likely to fade while a more integrated (but still outcome-oriented) health system assumes responsibility for dealing with the relevant conditions.

10. Quality of clinical care makes an enormous difference, both to the cost of care and to health outcomes. Tangible actions can be taken to improve quality: important among them is having each provider do a few things well rather than many things poorly.

11. Strengthening capacity for surgery at the district hospital level is a frequently neglected priority. Major important uses of this capacity will be to deal with injuries and obstetrical emergencies.

12. In low-income countries public funding for health will remain highly constrained as a percentage of GDP for the foreseeable future. Targeting these funds to provide universal access to a limited number of interventions that are high priority for poor people is both efficient and equity enhancing, but it will require clear setting of priorities, particularly for incremental resources as they become available.

13. Middle-income countries can learn from the OECD experience that universal public financing of a substantial package of clinical care is both efficient and equity enhancing.

Research and Development

14. Impact evaluation of interventions in many domains is an essential priority and should be done around planned variations in implementation. One specific area of importance is evaluation of effective ways to manage lifelong drug use—for example, for AIDS, secondary prevention of vascular disease, diabetes, and major psychiatric disorders.

15. Public-private partnerships such as the Medicines for Malaria Venture and the International AIDS Vaccine

Initiative provide promising models for developing important new drugs, vaccines, and diagnostic products to deal with the major diseases of poverty as well as the problem of drug resistance and microbial evolution more generally.

Development Assistance

16. Development assistance for health has begun to become performance based, and this trend should accelerate, along with making development assistance more stable and long term (contingent on performance). This change may involve at least a partial shift away from the sectorwide approaches to development assistance that recent evidence suggests may lead to neglect of focus on outcomes. It will require renewed attention to outcome measurement.

17. Resistance of the malaria parasite that is responsible for most deaths to chloroquine and SP is now widespread and rapidly increasing. A particular challenge is overcoming financial and institutional barriers to virtually complete replacement of those drugs with ACTs, which minimize resistance and can decrease transmission. Absent such an effort, malaria mortality is likely to continue rising. A centralized procurement mechanism receiving subsidies from development assistance agencies and making low-cost ACTs available to public and private supply chains globally would address this problem.

18. Investing in global capacity to respond effectively to a new influenza pandemic, particularly within the resource constraints of low-income countries, is a priority for the international system. Such capacity would include effective surveillance, surge manufacturing capacity for drugs and vaccines, stockpiles of drugs that could be used to attempt to contain epidemics, and mass media messages and public policies prepared in advance to be deployed if needed.

19. Because research and development is so important for health and because it is a classic international public good, a substantial fraction of incremental development assistance for health should go to research and development.

The content of these specific recommendations, and of recommendations throughout this volume, point to the enormous potential we now have to reduce further the human and financial burden of ill health. Scientific advance created this potential. Its more widespread realization requires the focused attention of health systems to finance and deliver priority interventions.

ANNEX 1.A: THE BURDEN OF DISEASE IN 2001

This annex provides estimates of the burden of different diseases and injuries in 2001. Alan Lopez, Colin Mathers, Christopher Murray, and their colleagues at WHO generated the estimates, aggregated them by World Bank regions, and provided final updates. A companion volume (Lopez and others 2006) will provide more comprehensive tables of results for a much finer disaggregation of conditions, a full exposition of methods and data sources, and sensitivity analyses (including assessments of the sensitivity of results to including stillbirth). All numbers in this annex are consistent with those in the companion volume.

This annex first provides a brief background on assessments of deaths by cause and disease burden and then an overview of the uses of such measures for health policy. It concludes with aggregated tables on deaths and on disability-adjusted life years (DALYs) by selected causes or groups of causes. The tables present estimates both with and without stillbirths, which constituted approximately 5.5 percent of deaths globally in 2001. Estimates are provided separately for high-income countries and for the low- and middle-income countries as a group.

Background

Many countries, including all high-income ones, maintain vital registration systems that provide data (usually annual) on the number of deaths by cause, age, sex, and sometimes race. Some countries additionally compute years of life lost (or YLL) by cause, which assigns a number of years of life lost attributable to each cause that depends on the age of death and some relevant measure of life expectancy. As of the early 1990s, no similar estimates existed for many developing countries or for regional groupings of them. Experts on individual conditions or the relevant disease program at WHO generated estimates for the diseases of interest to them. When added up across diseases, however, such estimates exceeded, often by a factor of 2 or more, any plausible estimate of the total number of deaths occurring in each age group. *DCP1* and the *World Development Report 1993* (Lopez 1993 and World Bank 1993) generated estimates of the number of deaths by cause that were consistent with demographically determined death totals for eight regional groupings of countries. WHO collaborated closely on this work. The number of deaths from a disease is one measure of the magnitude of its burden, and YLL constitutes for many purposes a better measure. Neither takes account of the disability or suffering associated with a nonfatal disease.

The 1993 *World Development Report* also developed a variant of the quality-adjusted life year (QALY) from the health economics literature to add a disability dimension to YLLs in order to generate a more comprehensive measure of burden. The result, called a *disability-adjusted life year*, measures burden from a specific cause as the sum of years of life lost from that cause and the equivalent years of life lost (in a sense that is made quite specific) from the disability caused by the condition. Original publications on disease burden included estimates that discounted future events at 0 percent or at 3 percent per year. They also included estimates that weighted the value of a year of life uniformly across all age groups and estimates that placed greater value on middle-aged groups. These are labeled DALYs (r,k) with the first number indicating the discount rate in percent per year and the second indicating whether uniform or nonuniform age weights were used. The most widely reported variant on the DALY is the DALY (3,1)— that is, one that uses a 3 percent discount rate and nonuniform age weighting. This chapter and the companion volume report DALYs (3,0)—that is, with discounting but uniform age weighting.

Estimates of DALYs by cause for 1990 first appeared as appendix B of the 1993 *World Development Report* and, in expanded form, in Murray, Lopez, and Jamison (1994). Christopher Murray, Alan Lopez, and colleagues later produced updated estimates for 1990 and a fuller account of the methods used (Murray and Lopez 1996a, 1996b). The relative burden of different conditions as measured by numbers of deaths correlates highly with DALYs, but important exceptions exist. The massive burden of major psychiatric conditions, for example, is captured by DALYs but missed in estimates of deaths by cause or YLLs. Table 1.A1 summarizes the current estimates of deaths by cause in 2001 from Mathers, Murray, and Lopez (2006). Table 1.A2 shows disease burden in DALYs. Additional columns in these tables show the effect of including stillbirths on the percentage distribution of burden across conditions while leaving unchanged the other numbers (see Jamison and others 2006).

Disease burden can be assessed by risk factor as well as by disease or condition. An initial assessment of risk factor burden appeared in the 1993 *World Development Report* and later in Murray and Lopez (1997) and WHO (1996). WHO published a much fuller set of estimates in its 2003 *World Health Report* (WHO 2003b). Ezzati and others (2006) provided a substantial update adjusted to the same methodological assumptions as for deaths and DALYs, including use of DALYs (3,0).

Uses of Disease Burden Measures

DALYs are useful for informing health policy in at least six ways. Estimates of deaths by cause or YLL serve these same purposes, but for some uses less well.

1. *Assessing performance.* A country-specific (or regional) assessment of the burden of disease provides an outcome indicator that can be used over time to judge progress or across countries or regions to judge relative performance. The most natural comparison is to the development of national income and product accounts (NIPAs) by Simon Kuznets and others in the 1930s, which culminated in 1939 with a complete NIPA for the United Kingdom prepared by James Meade and Richard Stone at the request of the U.K. Treasury. NIPAs have, in the subsequent decades, transformed the empirical underpinnings of economic policy analysis. One leading scholar has put it this way:

The national income and product accounts for the United States (NIPAs), and kindred accounts in other nations, have been among the major contributions to economic knowledge over the past half century. . . . Several generations of economists and practitioners have now been able to tie theoretical constructs of income, output, investment, consumption, and savings to the actual numbers of these remarkable accounts with all their fine detail and soundly meshed interrelations. (Eisner 1989, 1)

Disease burden measures have the potential of serving a similar purpose for health policy.

2. *Generating a forum for informed debate of values and priorities.* The assessment of disease burden in a country in practice involves participation of a broad range of national disease specialists, epidemiologists, and, often, policy makers. Debating the appropriate values, say, for disability weights or for years of life lost at different ages helps clarify values and objectives for national health policy. Discussing the interrelations among diseases and their risk factors in the light of local conditions sharpens consideration of priorities.

3. *Identifying national control priorities.* Many countries now identify a relatively short list of interventions, the full implementation of which becomes an explicit priority for national political and administrative attention. Examples include interventions to control TB, poliomyelitis, HIV infection, smoking, and specific micronutrient deficiencies. Because political attention and high-level administrative capacity are in relatively fixed and short supply, the benefits from using those resources will be maximized if they are directed to interventions that are both cost-effective and aimed at problems associated with a high burden. Thus, national assessments of disease burden are one input in establishing a potential short list of control priorities. In the summary of the cost-effectiveness analyses reported in this volume, chapter 2 pays particular attention to identifying cost-effective interventions capable of averting a large disease burden.

4. *Allocating training time for clinical and public health practitioners.* Medical schools offer a fixed number of instructional hours; training programs for other levels and types of practitioners are likewise limited. A major instrument for implementing policy priorities is allocating this fixed-time resource well. Again that means allocation of time to training in cost-effective interventions in which disease burden is high.

5. *Allocating research and development resources.* Whenever a fixed effort will have a benefit proportional not only to the size of the effort but also to the size of the problem being addressed, estimates of disease burden become essential for formulating policy. Developing a vaccine for a broad range

Table 1.A1 Causes of Deaths in Low- and Middle-Income and High-Income Countries and the World, 2001
(percent)

	Low- and Middle-Income		High-Income		World	
	Stillbirths excluded	Stillbirths included	Stillbirths excluded	Stillbirths included	Stillbirths excluded	Stillbirths included
Population (thousands)	5,221,572		928,660		6,150,233	
Births (thousands)	118,505	121,733	11,371	11,416	129,878	133,150
Total deaths (thousands)	48,377	51,605	7,936	7,981	56,268	59,542
Causes of death (percent)						
I. COMMUNICABLE DISEASES, PREGNANCY OUTCOMES, AND NUTRITIONAL DEFICIENCIES	**36.4**	**34.1**	**7.0**	**6.9**	**32.3**	**30.5**
A Infectious and parasitic diseases	22.1	20.7	1.9	1.9	19.3	18.2
1 Tuberculosis	3.3	3.1	0.2	0.2	2.9	2.7
2 STIs excluding HIV	0.4	0.3	0.0	0.0	0.3	0.3
3 HIV/AIDS	5.3	4.9	0.3	0.3	4.6	4.3
4 Diarrheal diseases	3.7	3.4	0.1	0.1	3.2	3.0
5 Childhood diseases	2.8	2.6	0.0	0.0	2.4	2.3
a Pertussis	0.6	0.6	0.0	0.0	0.5	0.5
b Poliomyelitis	0.0	0.0	0.0	0.0	0.0	0.0
c Diphtheria	0.0	0.0	0.0	0.0	0.0	0.0
d Measles	1.6	1.5	0.0	0.0	1.4	1.3
e Tetanus	0.6	0.6	0.0	0.0	0.5	0.5
6 Meningitis	0.3	0.3	0.1	0.1	0.3	0.3
8 Malaria	2.5	2.3	0.0	0.0	2.1	2.0
Other I.A. (7, 9–15)	3.8	3.6	1.3	1.3	3.5	3.3
B Respiratory infections	7.2	6.7	4.4	4.4	6.8	6.4
C Maternal conditions	1.0	1.0	0.0	0.0	0.9	0.9
D Perinatal conditions	5.1	4.8	0.4	0.4	4.5	4.2
1 Low birth weight	2.7	2.5	0.1	0.1	2.3	2.2
2 Birth asphyxia and birth trauma	1.5	1.4	0.1	0.1	1.3	1.2
3 Other perinatal conditions	1.0	0.9	0.1	0.1	0.9	0.8
E Nutritional deficiencies	0.9	0.9	0.2	0.2	0.8	0.8
II. NONCOMMUNICABLE CONDITIONS	**53.8**	**50.5**	**86.5**	**86.0**	**58.5**	**55.3**
A Malignant neoplasms	10.2	9.6	26.0	25.9	12.5	11.8
C Diabetes mellitus	1.6	1.5	2.6	2.5	1.7	1.6
E Neuropsychiatric disorders	1.4	1.4	4.8	4.7	1.9	1.8
1 Unipolar major depression	0.0	0.0	0.0	0.0	0.0	0.0
2 Bipolar disorder	0.0	0.0	0.0	0.0	0.0	0.0
3 Schizophrenia	0.0	0.0	0.0	0.0	0.0	0.0
Other II.E. (4–16)	1.4	1.3	4.7	4.7	1.9	1.8
G Cardiovascular disease	27.6	25.9	38.3	38.1	29.1	27.5
3 Ischaemic heart disease	11.8	11.0	17.2	17.1	12.6	11.9
4 Cerebrovascular disease	9.5	8.9	9.8	9.8	9.6	9.1
Other II.G. (1, 2, 5, 6)	6.3	5.9	11.3	11.2	7.0	6.6
H Respiratory diseases	6.5	6.1	6.0	6.0	6.4	6.1
I Digestive diseases	3.3	3.1	4.2	4.2	3.4	3.3
M Congenital anomalies	1.0	0.9	0.4	0.4	0.9	0.9
Other II. (B, D, F, J–L, N)	2.2	2.0	4.3	4.3	2.5	2.3
III. INJURIES	**9.8**	**9.1**	**5.9**	**5.9**	**9.2**	**8.7**
A Unintentional	6.6	6.2	4.0	4.0	6.3	5.9
1 Road traffic accidents	2.2	2.1	1.5	1.5	2.1	2.0
Other III. A. (2–6)	4.4	4.2	2.5	2.5	4.2	3.9
B Intentional	3.1	2.9	1.9	1.9	2.9	2.8
1 Self-inflicted	1.5	1.5	1.6	1.6	1.6	1.5
Other III.B. (2–4)	1.6	1.5	0.3	0.3	1.4	1.3

Sources: Estimates in the columns excluding stillbirths come from Mathers, Lopez, and Murray (2006). Estimates in the columns including stillbirths come from Jamison and others (2006), which uses the estimates from Mathers, Lopez, and Murray (2006) while adding in stillbirths.

Table 1.A2 The Burden of Disease in Low- and Middle-Income and High-Income Countries and the World, 2001 *(percent)*

	Low- and Middle-Income		High-Income		World	
	DALYs[a]	DALYs$_{SB}$[b]	DALYs[a]	DALYs$_{SB}$[b]	DALYs[a]	DALYs$_{SB}$[b]
Total DALYs (thousands)	**1,387,426**	**1,260,643**	**149,161**	**148,316**	**1,536,587**	**1,412,600**
Causes of death (percent)						
I. COMMUNICABLE DISEASES, PREGNANCY OUTCOMES, AND NUTRITIONAL DEFICIENCIES	**39.8**	**33.6**	**5.7**	**5.4**	**36.5**	**30.5**
A Infectious and parasitic diseases	23.1	21.0	2.3	2.2	21.1	18.9
1 Tuberculosis	2.6	2.8	0.1	0.1	2.3	2.5
2 STIs excluding HIV	0.7	0.7	0.1	0.1	0.6	0.6
3 HIV/AIDS	5.1	5.3	0.4	0.4	4.7	4.8
4 Diarrheal diseases	4.2	2.6	0.3	0.3	3.9	2.6
5 Childhood diseases	3.1	2.4	0.1	0.1	2.8	2.4
a Pertussis	0.8	0.7	0.1	0.1	0.8	0.6
b Poliomyelitis	0.0	0.0	0.0	0.0	0.0	0.0
c Diphtheria	0.0	0.0	0.0	0.0	0.0	0.0
d Measles	1.7	1.5	0.0	0.0	1.5	1.4
e Tetanus	0.6	0.5	0.0	0.0	0.5	0.4
6 Meningitis	0.4	0.4	0.1	0.1	0.4	0.3
8 Malaria	2.9	2.1	0.0	0.0	2.6	1.8
Other I.A. (7, 9–15)	4.1	4.2	1.1	1.1	3.8	4.2
B Respiratory infections	6.3	4.6	1.7	1.7	5.8	4.3
C Maternal conditions	1.9	2.1	0.3	0.3	1.7	1.9
D Perinatal conditions	6.4	3.7	0.9	0.6	5.9	3.4
1 Low birth weight	3.1	1.4	0.3	0.2	2.8	1.5
2 Birth asphyxia and birth trauma	2.3	1.5	0.4	0.4	2.1	1.4
3 Other perinatal conditions	1.1	0.6	0.3	0.3	1.0	0.5
E Nutritional deficiencies	2.1	2.2	0.6	0.6	2.0	2.0
II. NONCOMMUNICABLE CONDITIONS	**48.9**	**52.4**	**86.7**	**87.2**	**52.6**	**56.4**
A Malignant neoplasms	5.4	5.9	17.4	17.4	6.6	7.1
C Diabetes mellitus	1.1	1.3	2.8	2.8	1.3	1.4
E Neuropsychiatric disorders	9.9	10.8	20.9	21.0	11.0	11.9
1 Unipolar major depression	3.1	3.4	5.6	5.7	3.4	3.7
2 Bipolar disorder	0.6	0.7	0.7	0.7	0.6	0.7
3 Schizophrenia	0.8	0.8	0.7	0.8	0.8	0.8
Other II.E. (4–16)	5.4	5.9	13.8	13.9	6.2	6.7
G Cardiovascular disease	12.9	14.2	20.0	20.1	13.6	14.7
3 Ischaemic heart disease	5.2	5.7	8.3	8.4	5.5	6.0
4 Cerebrovascular disease	4.5	5.0	6.3	6.3	4.7	5.1
Other II.G. (1, 2, 5, 6)	3.2	3.5	5.4	5.5	3.4	3.7
H Respiratory diseases	4.2	4.5	6.6	6.6	4.4	4.7
I Digestive diseases	3.8	4.0	4.4	4.4	3.8	4.1
M Congenital anomalies	1.7	1.3	1.0	0.8	1.6	1.3
Other II. (B, D, F, J–L, N)	9.9	10.9	13.7	13.8	10.3	11.2
III. INJURIES	**11.2**	**12.1**	**7.5**	**7.5**	**10.9**	**11.6**
A Unintentional	8.2	8.8	5.3	5.3	7.9	8.4
1 Road traffic accidents	2.3	2.5	2.0	2.0	2.3	2.5
Other III. A. (2–6)	5.9	6.3	3.2	3.3	5.6	6.1
B Intentional	3.1	3.4	2.3	2.3	3.0	3.2
1 Self-inflicted	1.3	1.4	1.7	1.7	1.3	1.4
Other III.B. (2–4)	1.8	2.0	0.5	0.5	1.7	1.8

Sources: Mathers, Lopez, and Murray (2006) provide the reported estimates of DALYs. Jamison and others (2006) provide the estimates for DALYs$_{SB}$.

a. The burden of disease is measured in DALYs. DALYs form a class of measures that aggregate years of life lost from premature mortality with years of life lost due to disability. The DALYs reported here are calculated at a 3 percent per year discount rate with no age-weights, i.e. a year of life at any age is valued the same. These are referred to as DALYs (3,0) in the accompanying volume on burden of disease and risk factors (Lopez and others, 2006).

b. The DALYs$_{SB}$ is analagous to the DALY except that it includes stillbirths in the estimates of burden and assumes a gradual "acquisition of life potential" that allows the burden associated with a death near the time of birth to grow gradually with age rather than instantaneously increasing from 0 to a high value at birth or some earlier time. Jamison and others (2006) provide the estimates used here, which they label DALYs$_{SB}$ (3,0,0.54).

of viral pneumonias, for example, would have perhaps hundreds of times the effect of a vaccine against Hanta virus infection. Thus, information on disease or risk factor burden is one vital input (of several) to inform research and development resource allocation, as discussed in chapters 4 and 5.

6. *Allocating resources across health interventions.* Here disease burden assessment often plays a minor role; the task is to shift resources to interventions, which, at the margin, will generate the greatest reduction in DALY loss. When there are major fixed costs in mounting an intervention, as is the case with political and managerial attention for national control priorities, burden estimates are required to improve resource allocation. Likewise, major fixed costs may be associated with making the use of an intervention universal (or expanding it to cover a major percentage of the population), and if so, the cost-effectiveness of the expansion will depend in part on the size of the burden.

Results

Tables 1.A1 and 1.A2 convey summaries of deaths by cause and burden of disease in 2001, respectively.

ACKNOWLEDGMENTS

Sonbol Shahid-Salles provided invaluable research support and critical advice during preparation of this chapter. Mantra Singh expertly provided word-processing support. Candice Byrne provided valuable comments. The other editors of *Disease Control Priorities in Developing Countries*, 2nd edition, provided extensive critical reactions to the messages and text, and the chapter is consequently very different than it would have been. The Advisory Committee to the editors of this volume, chaired by Jaime Sepúlveda, provided invaluable comments and reaction during a meeting at the Institut Pasteur, Paris, in December 2004.

In the early 1990s, the World Bank initiated efforts to understand and disseminate policies to address the remaining large burden of disease affecting the world's poor. The World Bank's (1993) *World Development Report: Investing in Health* reported the results of that assessment, which drew on a second publication, *Disease Control Priorities in Developing Countries,* 1st edition (*DCP1*) (Jamison and others 1993). Enormous changes both in the world and in our knowledge base occurred during the subsequent decade, leading to the conclusion that a major revision, update, and expansion of *DCP1* would be of value. In a collaborative undertaking, the World Bank, the World Health Organization, and the Fogarty International Center of the U.S. National Institutes of Health sponsored this new effort (*DCP2*) with substantial financial support from the Bill & Melinda Gates Foundation. This book results from that collaboration.

REFERENCES

Abraham, K. G., and C. Mackie, eds. 2005. *Beyond the Market: Designing Nonmarket Accounts for the United States.* Washington, DC: The National Academies Press.

Arrow, K. J. 1963. "Uncertainty and the Welfare Economics of Medical Care." *American Economic Review* 53 (5): 851–83.

Arrow, K. J., H. Gelband, and D. T. Jamison. 2005. "Making Antimalarial Agents Available in Africa." *New England Journal of Medicine* 353: 333–35.

Bailis, R., M. Ezzati, and D. M Kammen. 2005. "Mortality and Greenhouse Gas Impacts of Biomass and Petroleum Energy Futures in Africa." *Science* 308: 98–103.

Barr, N. 2001. *The Welfare State as Piggy Bank: Information, Risk, Uncertainty, and the Role of the State.* Oxford: Oxford University Press.

Becker, G. S., T. J. Philipson, and R. R. Soares. 2003. "The Quantity and Quality of Life and the Evolution of World Inequality." NBER Working Paper 9765, National Bureau of Economic Research, Cambridge, MA.

Bezanson, K. 2005. "Replenishing the Global Fund: An Independent Assessment." http://www.theglobalfund.org/en/files/about/replenishment/assessment_report_en.pdf.

Bhargava, A., D. T. Jamison, L. J. Lau, and C. J. L. Murray. 2001. "Modeling the Effects of Health on Economic Growth." *Journal of Health Economics* 20 (May): 423–40.

Blanchard, O., and L. F. Katz. 1997. "What We Know and Do Not Know about the Natural Rate of Unemployment." *Journal of Economic Perspectives* 11 (1): 51–72.

Bloom, D. E., D. Canning, and D. T. Jamison. 2004. "Health, Wealth and Welfare." *Finance and Development* 41 (1): 10–15.

Bloom, D. E., D. Canning, and P. Malaney. 2000. "Demographic Change and Economic Growth in Asia." *Supplement to Population and Development Review* 26: 257–90.

Bloom, D. E., D. Canning, and J. Sevilla. 2004. "The Effect of Health on Economic Growth: A Production Function Approach." *World Development* 32: 1–13.

Bobadilla, J. L., J. Frenk, R. Lozano, T. Frejka, and C. Stern. 1993. "The Epidemiologic Transition and Health Priorities." In *Disease Control Priorities in Developing Countries,* ed. D. T. Jamison, W. H. Mosley, A. R. Measham, and J. L. Bobadilla, 746. New York: Oxford University Press.

Boskin, M. J., and L. J. Lau. 2000. "Generalized Solow-Neutral Technical Progress and Postwar Economic Growth." NBER Working Paper 8023, National Bureau of Economic Research, Cambridge, MA.

Bourguignon, F., and C. Morrisson. 2002. "Inequality among World Citizens: 1820–1992." *American Economic Review* 92: 727–44.

Burnside, C., and D. Dollar. 2000. "Aid, Policies and Growth." *American Economic Review* 90: 847–68.

Clemens, M., S. Radelet, and R. Bhavnani. 2004. "Counting Chickens When They Hatch: The Short-Term Effect of Aid on Growth." Working Paper 44, Center for Global Development, Washington, DC.

Crafts, N. 2000. "Globalization and Growth in the Twentieth Century." IMF Working Paper WP/00/44, International Monetary Fund, Washington, DC.

Crafts, N., and M. Haacker. 2004. "Welfare Implications of HIV/AIDS." In *The Macroeconomics of HIV/AIDS,* ed. M. Haacker, 182–97. Washington, DC: International Monetary Fund.

Davis, K. 1956. "The Amazing Decline of Mortality in Underdeveloped Areas." *American Economic Review* (Papers and Proceedings) 46 (2): 305–18.

Deaton, A. 2004. "Health in an Age of Globalization." NBER Working Paper 10669, National Bureau of Economic Research, Cambridge, MA.

DeLong, J. B. 2000. "Cornucopia: The Pace of Economic Growth in the Twentieth Century." Working Paper 7602. Cambridge, MA: National Bureau of Economic Research.

del Rio, C., and J. Sepúlveda. 2002. "AIDS in Mexico: Lessons Learned and Implications for Developing Countries." *AIDS* 16: 1445–57.

de Savigny, D., H. Kasale, C. Mbuya, and G. Reid. 2004. *Fixing Health Systems.* Ottawa: International Development Research Centre.

Easterlin, R. A. 1996. *Growth Triumphant: The Twenty-First Century in Historical Perspective.* Ann Arbor: University of Michigan Press.

———. 1999. "How Beneficent Is the Market? A Look at the Modern History of Mortality." *European Review of Economic History* 3: 257–94.

Easterly, W., and R. Levine. 1997. "Africa's Growth Tragedy: Policies and Ethnic Divisions." *Quarterly Journal of Economics* 112: 1203–50.

Eisner, R. 1989. *The Total Incomes System of Accounts.* Chicago: University of Chicago Press.

Ezzati, M., A. D. Lopez, A. Rodgers, and C. J. L. Murray, eds. 2004. *Comparative Quantification of Health Risks: Global and Regional Burden of Disease Attributable to Selected Major Risk Factors.* Vols. 1–2. Geneva: World Health Organization.

Ezzati, M., S. vander Hoorn, A. D. Lopez, G. Danaei, A. Rodgers, C. D. Mathers, and C. J. L. Murray. 2006. "Comparative Quantification of Mortality and Burden of Disease Attributable to Selected Major Risk Factors." In *Global Burden of Disease and Risk Factors,* ed. A. D. Lopez, C. Mathers, M. Ezzati, D. T. Jamison, and C. J. L. Murray. New York: Oxford University Press.

Fauci, A. S. 2005. "The Global Challenge of Infectious Diseases: The Evolving Role of the National Institutes of Health in Basic and Clinical Research." *Nature Immunology* 6 (8): 743–47.

Feachem, R. G. A., T. Kjellstrom, C. J. L. Murray, M. Over, and M. Phillips (Eds.). 1992. *Health of Adults in the Developing World.* New York: Oxford University Press.

Fogel, R. W. 1997. "New Findings on Secular Trends in Nutrition and Mortality: Some Implications for Population Theory." In *Handbook of Population and Family Economics*, Vol. 1A, ed. M. Rosenzweig and O. Stark, 433–81. Amsterdam: Elsevier Science.

Fuchs, V. 1974. "Some Economic Aspects of Mortality in Developed Countries." In *The Economics of Health and Medical Care*, ed. M. Perlman, 174–93. London: Macmillan.

———. 1980. "Comment." In *Population and Economic Change in Developing Countries*, ed R. Easterlin, 348–51. Chicago: University of Chicago Press.

Gericke, C. A., C. Kurowski, M. K. Ranson, and A. Mills. 2003. "Feasibility of Scaling-up Interventions: The Role of Intervention Design." Working Paper 13, Disease Control Priorities Project, Bethesda, MD.

Gertler, P. 2004. "Do Conditional Cash Transfers Improve Child Health? Evidence from PROGRESA's Control Randomized Experiment." *Health, Health Care, and Economic Development* 94 (2): 336–41.

Gruber, J., and M. Hanratty. 1995. "The Labor-Market Effects of Introducing National Health Insurance: Evidence from Canada." *Journal of Business and Economic Statistics* 13 (2): 163–73.

Gwatkin, D. R., S. Rustein, K. Johnson, R. P. Pande, and A. Wagstaff. 2000. "Socio-Economic Differences in Health, Nutrition, and Population in the Philippines." Washington, DC: World Bank.

Haacker, M., ed. 2004. *The Macroeconomics of HIV/AIDS.* Washington, DC: International Monetary Fund.

Institute of Medicine. 2001. *Crossing the Quality Chasm.* Washington, DC: National Academies Press.

Jamison, D. T. 1993. "Investing in Health." *Finance and Development* 30 (2): 2–5.

———. 2003. "Cost-Effectiveness Analysis: Concepts and Applications." In *The Oxford Textbook of Public Health*, ed. R. Detels, J. McEwen, R. Beaglehole, and H. Tamaka, 2: 903–19.

———. 2004. "External Finance of Immunization Programs: Time for a Change in Paradigm?" In *Vaccines: Preventing Disease and Protecting Health*, ed. C. de Quadros, 325–32. Scientific and Technical Publication 596. Washington, DC: Pan American Health Organization.

Jamison, D. T., E. A. Jamison, and J. D. Sachs. 2003. "Assessing the Determinants of Growth When Health Is Explicitly Included in the Measure of Economic Welfare." Paper presented at the 4th World Congress of the International Health Economics Association, San Francisco, June.

Jamison, D. T., L. J. Lau, and J. Wang. 2005. "Health's Contribution to Economic Growth in an Environment of Partially Endogenous Technical Progress." In *Health and Economic Growth: Findings and Policy Implications,* ed. G. Lopez-Casasnovas, B. Rivera, and L. Currais, 67–91. Cambridge, MA: MIT Press.

Jamison, D. T., W. H. Mosley, A. R. Measham, and J. L. Bobadilla, eds. 1993. *Disease Control Priorities in Developing Countries.* New York: Oxford University Press.

Jamison, D. T., and S. Radelet. 2005. "Making Aid Smarter." *Finance and Development* 42 (2): 42–46.

Jamison, D.T., J. Sachs, and J. Wang. 2001. "The Effect of the AIDS Epidemic on Economic Welfare in Sub-Saharan Africa." CMH Working Paper WG1:13, Commission on Macroeconomics and Health, World Health Organization, Geneva.

Jamison, D. T., and M. E. Sandbu. 2001. "The WHO Ranking of Health Systems." *Science* 293: 1595–96.

Jamison, D. T., M. Sandbu, and J. Wang. 2004. "Why Has Infant Mortality Decreased at Such Different Rates in Different Countries?" Working Paper 21, Disease Control Priorities Project, Bethesda, MD.

Jamison, D. T., S. Shahid-Salles, J. S. Jamison, J. Lawn, and J. Zupan. 2006. "Incorporating Deaths Near the Time of Birth into Estimates of the Global Burden of Disease." In *Global Burden of Disease and Risk Factors*, ed. A. D. Lopez, C. D. Mathers, M. Ezzati, D. T. Jamison, and C. J. L. Murray. New York: Oxford University Press.

Jha, P., and F. J. Chaloupka, eds. 2000. *Tobacco Control in Developing Countries.* Oxford, U.K.: Oxford University Press.

Joint Learning Initiative. 2004. *Human Resources for Health: Overcoming the Crisis.* Washington, DC: Communications Development.

Kanbur, R., and T. Sandler. 1999. *The Future of Development Assistance: Common Pools and International Public Goods.* Washington, DC: Overseas Development Council.

Kim, J. J. 2005. "Using Mathematical Modeling to Evaluate the Public Health Impact and Cost-Effectiveness of Cervical Cancer Screening Strategies in Different World Regions." Ph.D. dissertation, Program in Health Policy, Harvard University, Cambridge, MA.

Kremer, M., and R. Glennerster. 2004. *Strong Medicine: Creating Incentives for Pharmaceutical Research on Neglected Diseases.* Princeton, NJ: Princeton University Press.

Leape, L. L., and D. M. Berwick. 2005. "Five Years after to Err Is Human: What Have We Learned?" *Journal of American Medical Association* 293 (19): 2384–90.

Levine, R. and the What Works Working Group. 2004. *Millions Saved: Proven Successes in Global Health.* Washington, DC: Center for Global Development.

Lindert, P. H. 2004. *Growing Public: Social Spending and Economic Growth since the Eighteenth Century.* Vol. 1. Cambridge, U.K.: Cambridge University Press.

Lopez, A. D. 1993. "Causes of Death in Industrial and Developing Countries: Estimates for 1985–90." In *Disease Control Priorities in Developing Countries,* eds. D. T. Jamison, W. H. Mosley, A. R. Measham, and J. L. Bobadilla, 35–50. New York: Oxford University Press.

Lopez, A. D., S. Begg, and E. Bos. 2006. "Demographic and Epidemiological Characteristics of Major Regions of the World, 1990 and 2001." In *Global Burden of Disease and Risk Factors*, ed. A. D. Lopez,

C. D. Mathers, M. Ezzati, D. T. Jamison, and C. J. L. Murray. New York: Oxford University Press.

Lopez, A. D., C. D. Mathers, M. Ezzati, D. T. Jamison, and C. J. L. Murray, eds. 2006. "Measuring the Global Burden of Disease and Risk Factors." In *Global Burden of Disease and Risk Factors,* ed. A. D. Lopez, C. D. Mathers, M. Ezzati, D. T. Jamison, and C. J. L. Murray. New York: Oxford University Press.

Lopez-Casasnovas, G., B. Rivera, and L. Currais, eds. 2005. *Health and Economic Growth: Findings and Policy Implications.* Cambridge, MA: MIT Press.

Maddison, A. 1999. "Poor until 1820." *Wall Street Journal Europe,* July 11.

Mathers, C. D., C. J. L. Murray, and A. D. Lopez. 2006. "The Burden of Disease and Mortality by Condition: Data, Methods and Results for the Year 2001." In *Global Burden of Disease and Risk Factors,* ed. A. D. Lopez, C. D. Mathers, M. Ezzati, D. T. Jamison, and C. J. L. Murray. New York: Oxford University Press.

McClellan, M., and J. Skinner. 1997. "The Incidence of Medicare." NBER Working Paper 6013, National Bureau of Economic Research, Cambridge, MA.

Michaud, C. 2003. "Development Assistance for Health: Recent Trends and Resource Allocation." Paper prepared for the Second Consultation Commission on Macroeconomics and Health, World Health Organization, Geneva.

Mosk, C., and S. R. Johannson. 1986. "Income and Mortality: Evidence from Modern Japan." *Population and Development Review* 12: 415–40.

Murray, C. J. L., and A. D. Lopez. 1996a. *Global Health Statistics: A Compendium of Incidence, Prevalence and Mortality Estimates for Over 200 Conditions.* Cambridge, MA: Harvard University Press.

———. 1996b. *The Global Burden of Disease,* Volume 1. Cambridge, MA: Harvard University Press.

———. 1997. "Global Mortality, Disability and the Contribution of Risk Factors: Global Burden of Disease Study." *Lancet* 349 (9063): 1436–42.

Murray, C. J. L., A. D. Lopez, and D. T. Jamison. 1994. "The Global Burden of Disease in 1990: Summary Results, Sensitivity Analysis and Future Directions." In *Global Comparative Assessments in the Health Sector: Disease Burden, Expenditures and Intervention Packages,* ed. C. J. L. Murray and A. D. Lopez, 97–138. Geneva: World Health Organization. (A shorter version of this paper appeared in *Bulletin of the World Health Organization* 72: 495–509.)

Nordhaus, W. 2003. "The Health of Nations: The Contributions of Improved Health to Living Standards." In *Measuring the Gains from Health Research: An Economic Approach,* ed. K. M. Murphy and R. H. Topel, 9–40. Chicago: University of Chicago Press.

Oeppen, J. 1999. "The Health and Wealth of Nations since 1820." Paper presented at the Social Science History Conference, Fort Worth, TX, November.

Oeppen, J., and J. W. Vaupel. 2002. "Demography. Broken Limits to Life Expectancy." *Science* 296 (5570): 1029–31.

Pearson, T. A., D. T. Jamison, and J. Trejo-Gutierrez. 1993. "Cardiovascular Disease." In *Disease Control Priorities in Developing Countries,* ed. D. T. Jamison, W. H. Mosley, A. R. Measham, and J. L. Bobadilla, 746. New York: Oxford University Press.

Peto, R. S., and A. D. Lopez. 2001. "The Future Worldwide Health Effects of Current Smoking Patterns." In *Critical Issues in Global Health,* ed. C. E. Koop, C. E. Pearson, and M. R. Schwarz. New York: Jossey-Bass.

Pison, G., J. F. Trape, M. Lefebvre, and C. Enel. 1993. "Rapid Decline in Child Mortality in a Rural Area of Senegal." *International Journal of Epidemiology* 22(1): 72–80.

Powles, John. 2001. "Healthier Progress: Historical Perspectives on the Social and Economic Determinants of Health." In *The Social Origins of Health and Well-Being,* ed. R. Eckersly, J. Dixon, and B. Douglas, 3–24. Cambridge, U.K.: Cambridge University Press.

Preston, S. H. 1975. "The Changing Relation between Mortality and Level of Economic Development." *Population Studies* 29 (2): 231–48.

———. 1980. "Causes and Consequences of Mortality Declines in Less Developed Countries during the Twentieth Century." In *Population and Economic Change in Developing Countries,* ed. R. Easterlin, 289–360. Chicago: University of Chicago Press.

Preston, S. H., and M. Haines. 1991. *Fatal Years: Child Mortality in Late 19th Century America.* Princeton, NJ: Princeton University Press.

Pritchard, C. 2004. "Developments in Economic Evaluation in Health Care: A Review of HEED." OHE Briefing 40, Office of Health Economics, London, March 2004.

Pritchett, L., and L. H. Summers. 1996. "Wealthier Is Healthier." *Journal of Human Resources* 31(4): 841–68.

Radelet, S. 2003. *Challenging Foreign Aid.* Washington, DC: Center for Global Development.

Roberts, M., W. Hsiao, P. Berman, and M. Reich. 2003. *Getting Health Reform Right: A Guide to Improving Performance and Equity.* New York: Oxford University Press.

Sachs, J. D. 2005. *The End of Poverty: Economic Possibilities for Our Time.* New York: The Penguin Press.

Solow, R. 1957. "Technical Change and the Aggregate Production Function." *Review of Economics and Statistics* 39: 312–20.

Strauss, J., and D. Thomas. 1998. "Health, Nutrition, and Economic Development." *Journal of Economic Literature* 36: 766–817.

Usher, D. 1973. "An Imputation to the Measure of Economic Growth for Changes in Life Expectancy." In *The Measurement of Economic and Social Performance,* ed. M. Moss, 193–226. Chicago: Columbia University Press for the National Bureau of Economic Research.

Viscusi, W. K., and J. E. Aldy. 2003. "The Value of a Statistical Life: A Critical Review of Market Estimates from Around the World." *Journal of Risk and Uncertainty* 27: 5–76.

World Bank. 1993. *World Development Report: Investing in Health.* New York: Oxford University Press.

———. 2004. *World Development Indicators.* New York: Oxford University Press. Available annually.

World Health Organization. 1996. "Investing in Health Research and Development." Report of the Ad Hoc Committee on Health Research Relating to Future Intervention Options (Document TDR/GEN/96.1). Geneva: WHO.

———. 1999. *The World Health Report: Making a Difference.* Geneva: WHO.

———. 2000. *The World Health Report: Health Systems.* Geneva: WHO.

———. 2002. *The World Health Report: Reducing Risks, Promoting Healthy Life.* Geneva: WHO.

———. 2003a. *International Statistical Classification of Diseases and Related Health Problems, 10th revision.* Geneva: WHO.

———. 2003b. *The World Health Report 2003: Shaping the Future.* Geneva: WHO.

———. 2005. *Preventing Chronic Diseases: A Vital Investment.* Geneva: WHO.

WHO CMH (World Health Organization Commission on Macroeconomics and Health). 2001. *Macroeconomics and Health: Investing in Health for Economic Development.* Geneva: WHO.

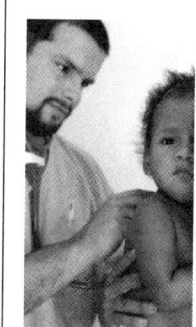

Chapter **2**

Intervention Cost-Effectiveness: Overview of Main Messages

Ramanan Laxminarayan, Jeffrey Chow, and Sonbol A. Shahid-Salles

Deeper understanding of the role of human health as a critical component of economic development has stimulated interest in improving the efficiency with which the modest health resources available in low- and middle-income countries (LMICs) are spent. In recent years, exponential growth in the number of economic evaluations of health interventions, spurred in part by the first edition of this volume (Jamison and others 1993), has created a wider knowledge base for evaluating the costs and benefits of interventions to enable better targeting of financial resources in the health sector (box 2.1). Although efficient spending on health has always been a desirable goal, it is particularly critical in the face of recent threats, such as HIV/AIDS and drug-resistant bacteria, as well as the problems presented by increasing prevalence of chronic diseases, such as diabetes and cardiovascular disease (CVD), that threaten to roll back the significant health gains achieved in the past two decades. This book is an opportunity to assess anew the costs associated with and the health gains attainable from specific interventions and thereby better inform the allocation of new health funding.

Drawing from the collective knowledge and analytical work of the many experts who have contributed to this volume, this chapter provides a broader perspective on the relative efficiency and effect on health of a number of interventions than is possible in a single, condition-specific chapter.[1] The objective is to provide information on the cost-effectiveness estimates for 319 interventions covering nearly every disease condition considered in the volume, and the resulting avertable burden

of disease.[2] This chapter provides broad conclusions on the economic efficiency of using these interventions to improve health.

PRIORITY SETTING

Information on the costs of purchasing health in conjunction with regional or national realities regarding disease priorities, private willingness to pay for health, and public budget constraints can be used to identify widely prevalent investments that are not cost-effective (shaded in figure 2.1) and highly cost-effective opportunities to improve health that policy makers are currently neglecting. Throughout the chapter, "not cost-effective" describes an intervention that has a relatively high ratio of costs to effectiveness. The information provided also may be helpful in identifying interventions that are not cost-effective and are rarely used and cost-effective interventions that are justifiably widely used (unshaded in figure 2.1). The broad objective of this exercise is to help improve global population health by improving understanding of the implications of investing in different interventions. Some of the interventions considered are widely prevalent, whereas others are less well known. Although some interventions are personal, others are population-based (see annex 2.A for definitions). They encompass the spectrum of disease conditions covered in this book but are by no means exhaustive of the universe of possible interventions.

Box 2.1

Use of Cost-Effectiveness to Set Policy: The Directly Observed Treatment Strategy

Nearly 2 million people die from tuberculosis (TB) each year, 98 percent of whom live in developing countries and most of whom are 15 to 49 years old. Meanwhile, anti-TB medicines are 95 percent effective in curing TB, even in low-income countries, and cost as little as US$10 for a six-month course of treatment or directly observed therapy short course (DOTS). The TB chapter of the first edition of this book (Murray, Styblo, and Rouillon 1993) and studies by Joesoef, Remington, and Jiptoherijanto (1989) and Kamolratanakul and others (1993) describe treatment of smear-positive TB with short-course chemotherapy as an extremely cost-effective intervention for TB.

Since 1980, the World Health Organization (WHO) has collaborated closely with many countries in East Asia and the Pacific to introduce short-course chemotherapy and then the DOTS strategy to achieve global targets, with a cure rate of 85 percent and a case-detection rate of 70 percent. In 1990, 10 countries were using short-course chemotherapy. In 1993, as a result of growing TB prevalence rates, WHO's declaration of a global emergency,

and studies showing DOTS' cost-effectiveness, the DOTS strategy was established worldwide as the most effective response to TB. By 1995, DOTS had expanded to 73 countries, and by 2003, it had reached more than 180 countries worldwide (WHO 2004).

As of 1999, DOTS has been implemented with the collaboration of WHO in 13 provinces of China and has achieved a cure rate of 90 percent. The population in East Asia and the Pacific with access to DOTS increased from 44 percent in 1995 to 57 percent in 1997, with the proportion of registered TB patients who are enrolled in a DOTS program also increasing, from 30 percent in 1995 to 46 percent in 1997 (WHO 1999). The progress is mainly attributable to high-prevalence countries in the region, which include Cambodia, China, and the Philippines.

By 2002, national TB programs reported that 69 percent of the world's population lived in countries or parts of countries with DOTS coverage. DOTS programs treated a total of 13.3 million TB patients and 6.8 million smear-positive patients between 1995 and 2002.

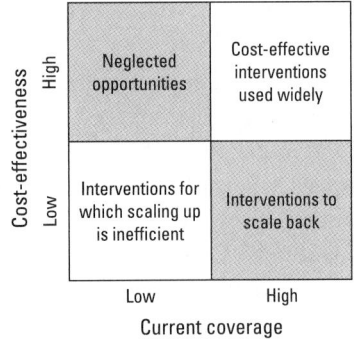

Source: Authors.

Figure 2.1 Efficiency of Interventions

Cost-Effectiveness

The specific measure of cost-benefit analysis adopted in this volume is cost-effectiveness. Effectiveness is measured in natural units (deaths averted and years of life saved) and in disability-adjusted life years (DALYs), a composite measure that combines years lived with disability and years lost to premature death in a single metric (see chapter 15 for an explanation of how DALYs are calculated). Nevertheless, dollars per DALY averted can at best be only one consideration in the allocation of resources to different diseases and interventions. This

chapter also focuses on the total burden of disease avertable by expanding population coverage of an intervention. The delivery of many interventions, including those that are relatively cost-effective, may require a certain degree of institutional and organizational capacity on the part of a health system, and countries will have to pay attention to this important consideration.[3] These factors, in combination with other considerations such as equity, social justice, medical suitability, and epidemiological appropriateness, should guide where money may be spent most effectively (Cookson and Dolan 1999, 2000).

Cost-effectiveness ratios can be used to set health priorities in two ways. One approach is to use a cutoff level of cost-effectiveness beyond which interventions are no longer used. This cutoff can vary from place to place depending on the availability of health resources, the disease burden, and the local preferences for health spending. The World Bank has described health interventions that cost less than US$100 per year of life saved as highly cost-effective for poor countries, but this benchmark is arbitrary, as chapter 15 makes clear by noting the interaction with income, budget levels, and the disease burden (Jamison and others 1993).

An alternative approach to using cost-effectiveness data to set intervention priorities is to interpret the cost-effectiveness ratio as the "price" of equivalent units of health using different interventions (box 2.2 explains this approach). Reinterpreted

Box 2.2

A Framework for Using Cost-Effectiveness Information to Set Health Priorities

A frequent, often justified, criticism of cost-effectiveness analyses is that they address only one of many criteria that could be used to evaluate health interventions. Epidemiological, medical, political, ethical, and cultural factors often also play important roles in the decision to allocate resources to a specific health condition or intervention; however, determining how one might weigh cost-effectiveness ratios alongside these other considerations when setting priorities for spending is difficult. Musgrove (1999) shows how to take some of these connections into account, including circumstances in which cost-effectiveness is an adequate criterion by itself. One approach is for the policy maker to think of cost-effectiveness ratios as the relative "price" of purchasing a unit of health (a DALY, for instance) using different interventions. These costs, along with the budget constraint, can help determine the optimal allocation of resources among a given set of interventions.

Consider, for instance, a policy maker in a country in Sub-Saharan Africa facing the choice between treating Parkinson's disease and expanding malaria treatment programs while constrained by a fixed budget allocated by the ministry of finance. The cost per DALY averted of treating Parkinson's disease using carbidopa is vastly greater than that for the malaria control program. A simplistic interpretation of the cost-effectiveness information would be to expand the malaria treatment program to the maximum extent possible before turning to the treatment of Parkinson's disease. This solution could be desirable in some situations, particularly if the budget is large enough to deal fully with the malaria problem and still allow for some treatment of Parkinson's. Emphasizing as complete coverage as possible of a particular problem may be especially appropriate in an epidemic situation, in which turning to another disease first can mean the epidemic will be worse in the future. Devoting some resources to each problem instead of concentrating on either may be more sensible when neither presents the threat of a growing epidemic.

Asking policy makers to make a binary choice between two sets of interventions on the basis of cost-effectiveness ratios alone may be unrealistic and misleading. Rather, policy makers should first determine their willingness to trade off health improvements in children (malaria) versus the elderly (Parkinson's). Policy makers may want to avert at least some burden from Parkinson's even if these cases are relatively expensive to treat for each unit of health gained because of such considerations as the target age group, the

socioeconomic status of target populations (including the extent to which they can obtain treatment from their own resources), and the ministry of health's ability to deliver the program effectively. After the tradeoffs have been made and can be represented by an indifference curve (see the figure and explanation), the cost-effectiveness information is useful in determining how much of the policy makers' fixed budget should be allocated to each intervention— that is, at what coverage of one problem should they start devoting resources to the other? The indifference curve represents health planners' willingness to trade off between investment in antimalarial drugs and treatment for Parkinson's based on all the relevant factors and independent of the budget constraint.

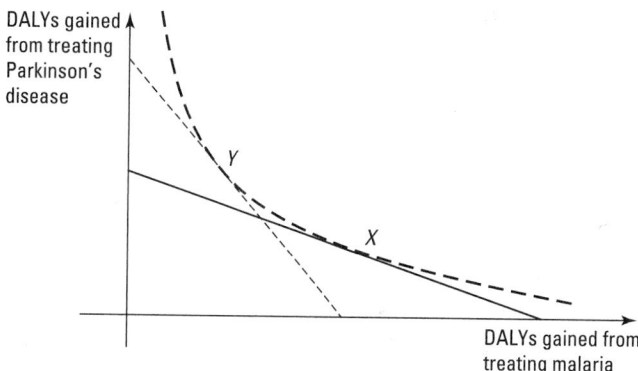

The solid line represents the budget, and its slope is the ratio of the cost-effectiveness ratios of the two interventions. The dashed line represents an alternative scenario in which the cost-effectiveness of treating Parkinson's is better (more DALYs can be gained) than the ratio represented by the solid line. The axes show how many DALYs can be gained from each treatment, so a large number of DALYs corresponds to a low "price" of health or cost per DALY. The figure shows the simple case, in which these prices are constant for either budget line—that is, expanding either program does not raise the unit cost—although this case is unlikely when part of the population is difficult to reach, is harder to treat, or has more severe disease, in which case the rise in unit cost means that an intervention becomes relatively less cost-effective, giving a further reason to start devoting resources to an alternative intervention.

When the price of buying a unit of health to treat Parkinson's is relatively high in terms of cost per DALY averted, the relatively flat (solid) budget line applies, and the optimal balance of investment in the two interventions is at

Box 2.2

Continued

point *X*. If the cost of buying a unit of health to treat Parkinson's is relatively low, then the steeper (dashed) budget line applies and the relative allocation of resources is represented by point *Y*. Therefore, policy makers would allocate relatively more resources to treating Parkinson's when the price of buying a unit of health through this intervention is relatively low, and they would allocate fewer resources when the price of health obtained through this intervention is relatively high. The figure shows the general likely shape of an indifference curve, but one possibility is

that policy makers' willingness to trade off between buying health from the two approaches is just a straight line, in which case they would want to invest the maximum amount possible in the lower-cost intervention (malaria) before turning to the higher-cost intervention (Parkinson's). The role of the cost-effectiveness information is to make policy makers aware of differences in the price of improving health using different interventions. Interventions with a high price should, all else being equal, be used less, whereas those with a low price should be used to a greater extent.

this way, there is no one-dimensional economic criterion that interventions must attain to be declared economically fit, and cost-effectiveness plays the more useful function of informing tradeoffs that policy makers are forced to make when investing in a portfolio of health interventions.

Target Audiences

The general notion of efficiency in how resources, both public and private, are spent on improving health is of interest not only to severely resource-constrained countries that each year spend only a few public dollars on health for each individual, but also to relatively wealthier nations with many competing priorities for public and private resources. The primary audiences for cost-effectiveness information are ministries of health and finance and policy makers in other branches of government in LMICs, both to help reallocate existing outlays in the health sector and to allocate new monies efficiently. Other audiences include aid agencies, international development lending institutions, nongovernmental organizations, and private health care providers.

Priority Setting in the Private Sector

The use of the efficiency criterion in priority setting should not be limited to public resources. A large proportion of health care in developing countries is paid for out of pocket, and greater clarity on interventions that are efficient from an economic perspective is no less urgent when the payer is private: inefficient private spending on health care in developing countries is wasteful as well. Much of this inefficiency may be attributed to significant differences in knowledge—termed *information*

asymmetries—between profit-making providers and patients. Private providers may encourage unnecessary procedures and excessively invasive procedures that, in some instances, can be more dangerous than no treatment at all. Governments have a role to play in lowering these information asymmetries, partly by providing information to populations, for instance, on the importance of childhood vaccinations. Moreover, even if government expenditures are not directly influenced by the lack of efficiency in privately delivered health care, they are affected by the inefficiency of private health systems if private patients seek public emergency care or require other state assistance. In their role as large purchasers of health care, governments—even in largely privately financed health care systems, such as in the United States—exercise enormous influence over the choices of drugs used and interventions provided and can play an important role in promoting policies to facilitate greater efficiency in health care systems.

The costs and efficacy of interventions may vary greatly, even within a single geographical region, depending on local health system capacity, cultural context, disease epidemiology, and a host of other factors. Greater efficiency in how countries spend their health care resources can have a tremendous effect on the health of their populations. Box 2.3 discusses gains from improved priority setting found in the lifesaving study by Harvard University (Tengs 1997; Tengs and others 1995).

METHODOLOGY

This chapter compares the cost-effectiveness of interventions that cover a broad spectrum of health conditions prevalent in developing countries. All results are presented in U.S. dollars discounted to the year 2001 using a 3 percent annual discount

The Harvard Lifesaving Study

A study by Harvard University in the United States showed potential gains of life years saved by choosing interventions on the basis of their cost-effectiveness. The study's authors assessed more than 500 types of lifesaving interventions, defined as any behavioral or technological strategy that reduces the probability of premature death among a specified target population. The study focused on 185 interventions and the extent to which each intervention was currently being implemented, without taking its cost-effectiveness into account.

The authors estimated that the selected 185 interventions would cost US$21.4 billion per year and would save 592,000 life years. The same amount of money could have saved another 636,000 life years had funds been redirected from less to more cost-effective interventions. Following an assessment of varying factors regarding interventions—those that affect the most people and are the most effective, least cost, and most cost-effective—the study reports that if the goal is to save the most life years, cost-effectiveness is a useful approach that will result in the most efficient allocation of resources. The study indicates that choosing the most cost-effective interventions could double the life years saved.

Sources: Tengs 1997; Tengs and others 1995.

rate. Chapter 15 summarizes the general guidelines governing the analysis leading to the results reported for all LMICs.

Regional Variations

Where possible and appropriate, intervention cost-effectiveness ratios and other information have been disaggregated by World Bank region. In discussing the estimates, this chapter focuses on differences in the costs of interventions rather than on differences in their effectiveness in specific regional settings, although both contribute to differences in cost-effectiveness estimates across regions. Cost-effectiveness estimates also differ among regions because of variations in underlying mortality, age structure, disease prevalence, and efficiency with which interventions are implemented. The analyses take all but the last of these considerations into account.

Interregional cost differences are attributable to differences in the local costs of goods and services that are not easily tradable. For components that are tradable, such as patented drugs and specialized medical equipment typically imported from industrial nations, the analyses assume uniform international costs for all LMICs, usually adjusted for local transportation and distribution costs. By using a single composite set of resource costs for each region, the analyses mask intraregional differences in the costs of nontradable goods, such as physician time or hospitals, but this methodology is appropriate because results are presented only at the level of the region.[4] Interventions may differ in cost-effectiveness because they are targeted more appropriately to some age groups rather than others, and important gender differences may also exist in cost-

effectiveness for some conditions, but data to estimate such differences are lacking.

Caveats

The findings in this chapter are subject to a number of caveats. First, despite efforts to ensure the consistency of cost-effectiveness numbers across chapters, the approaches taken in arriving at these numbers vary significantly. Although some chapters rely on cost-effectiveness numbers drawn from the literature, other chapters have analyzed these numbers afresh using the standardized resource costs described elsewhere. Table 2.1 contains definitions of indicators used to assess the

Table 2.1 Quality of Cost-Effectiveness Evidence for Interventions

Level	Source of cost-effectiveness evidence
1	Literature review of one cost-effectiveness study in one country
2	Literature review of several cost-effectiveness studies for multiple countries
3	Literature review of several cost-effectiveness studies for a single intervention in a single region
4	Original economic analysis by authors following the volume editors' guidelines in one country
5	Original economic analysis by authors following the volume editors' guidelines in one region

Source: Authors.

Note: Standard region-specific age structures and underlying mortality rates were used to calculate DALYs. Nontradable inputs were converted into U.S. dollars at the market exchange rate. The costs of tradable inputs were assumed to be internationally consistent, as were the costs associated with surgical treatments.

quality of evidence on which the cost-effectiveness estimates are based. The tables in annex 2.B and annex 2.C indicate the quality of evidence associated with each intervention.

Second, almost without exception, the cost-effectiveness numbers do not vary with the scale at which the intervention is undertaken, and this is probably not the case in reality (Birch and Donaldson 1987; Johns and Torres 2005). Some interventions, such as vaccination programs, have large setup costs but marginal costs of extending coverage that decline at least initially. Other interventions, such as educational campaigns for condom use, may be easy to target to urban populations, but the marginal costs of expanding such interventions to relatively inaccessible populations increase with coverage. Therefore, many of the cost-effectiveness ratios presented here are useful only for modest increments in coverage, and separate analyses may have to be conducted to determine their applicability to program start-ups and larger-scale intervention changes.

Third, the cost-effectiveness numbers presented apply to countries whose institutional and technical capacity in relation to health is close to the average for the region. This evaluation is restricted to what countries could do more (or less) of, and clearly a more ambitious analysis would also cover what countries could do better. This issue is discussed in detail in chapters 3 and 70.

Finally, the estimates are based on the best available data, which in many cases are somewhat weak. Statistically derived confidence bounds for the cost-effectiveness estimates are not provided, and in most cases, uncertainty analysis has not been carried out. Readers are encouraged to pay attention to the order of magnitude of each estimate rather than to the specific number presented.

ASSESSING THE EVIDENCE ON THE COST-EFFECTIVENESS OF INTERVENTIONS

Figures 2.2 and 2.3 display results gathered from other chapters on cost-effectiveness ratios. In some cases, interventions are grouped on the basis of their similarity and whether they were personal interventions or population-based interventions. For instance, all population-based programs to prevent HIV transmission via contaminated blood and needles were grouped as a single intervention. Note that the cost-effectiveness ranges should not be interpreted as statistical confidence intervals but rather as a range of "best estimates" of cost-effectiveness incorporating variation across interventions included in the cluster. Ranges for the cost-effectiveness ratios are also attributable to variations in the epidemiological settings in which these interventions were evaluated. For example, a population-based primary intervention in an area of low prevalence is likely to be less cost-effective than the same intervention in a region of

high prevalence. Figure 2.2 reflects sets of interventions dealing with high-burden diseases, and figure 2.3 deals with relatively low-burden diseases.

Within each figure, intervention clusters are displayed in the order of increasing cost-effectiveness. Additional information on the setting, objective, and target population of each intervention cluster for which cost-effectiveness has been calculated is provided in annex 2.B. The tables in annex 2.B also provide information on the quality of the evidence on which the data presented are based. Furthermore, the annex tables present information on potentially avertable deaths and DALYs if the coverage of these interventions were expanded by a further 20 percentage points of the relevant population (scaling up from 62 percent means reaching 82 percent, not 74 percent, of the pertinent population). Care should be taken not to confuse this information with the current burden of the underlying disease, on which basis interventions were divided into high-burden and low-burden diseases (figures 2.2 and 2.3, respectively).[5] For example, a cost-effective treatment for CVD has only limited scope for increased scale of intervention in countries with a low burden of this disease. At the same time, in many parts of Asia and Sub-Saharan Africa, even though HIV treatment is not a highly cost-effective intervention, it deserves attention because of its sizable potential for lowering the disease burden.

The tables in annex 2.C summarize information on intervention clusters for which cost-effectiveness was evaluated with a metric other than DALYs. For these interventions too, details of setting, objective, target population, and quality of the evidence have been provided. Given the difficulty in comparing these intervention clusters with those evaluated using DALYs, they are excluded from figures 2.2–2.5.

Observations about specific interventions follow. Ranges of cost-effectiveness estimates shown reflect geographical variations across regions.

Prevention and Control of Tuberculosis

The treatment of all forms of active tuberculosis (TB) using the directly observed treatment strategy based on short-course chemotherapy is among the most cost-effective of all interventions available to improve health in LMICs (US$5 to US$35 per DALY averted except in Europe and Central Asia) (box 2.1). The bacillus Calmette-Guérin (BCG) vaccination for children is also cost-effective (US$40 to US$170 per DALY averted), but its main effect is to reduce the burden of severe TB in children (TB meningitis and miliary TB). Because BCG has relatively little effect on the huge burden of pulmonary TB in adults—which constitutes the major cause of ill health resulting from *Mycobacterium tuberculosis*—development of a new vaccine that targets adults is highly desirable. The treatment of latent TB in patients uninfected with HIV is relatively cost-ineffective (US$4,000 to US$25,000 per DALY averted), but it is more cost-effective for groups of patients who are coinfected with TB

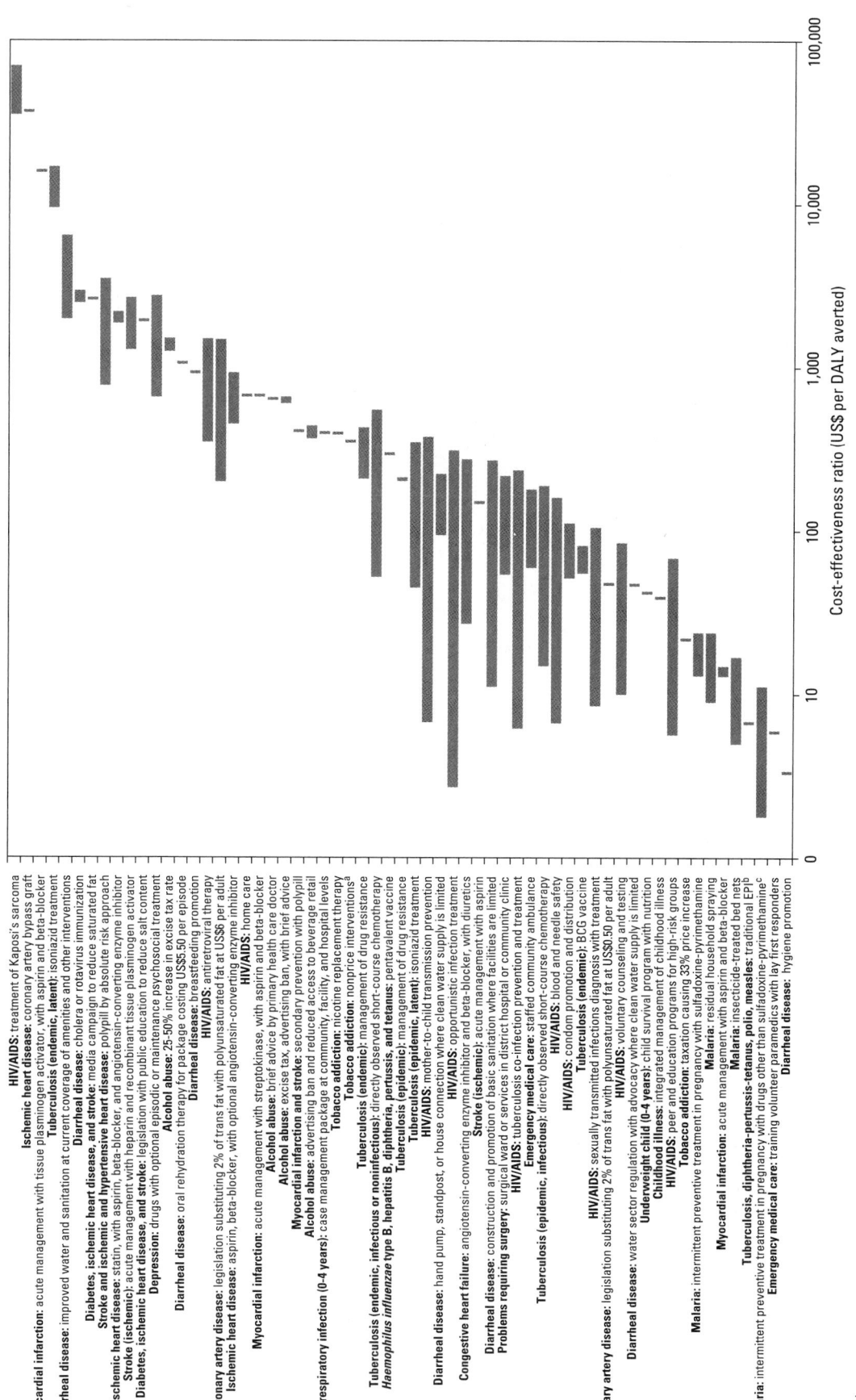

Source: Authors.

Note: Diseases were considered high burden for LMICs if their total avertable burden was greater than 35 million DALYs. Bars represent the range in point estimates of cost-effectiveness ratios for specific interventions included in each intervention cluster and do not represent variation across regions or statistical confidence intervals. Point estimates for LMICs were obtained directly from the relevant chapters, calculated as the midpoint of range estimates reported in the chapters, or calculated from a population-weighted average of the region-specific estimates reported in the chapters. For details of these intervention clusters, including the specific interventions covered in each, see annex tables 2.B.1 and 2.B.2. Only interventions with cost-effectiveness reported in terms of DALYs are included in this figure. For interventions with cost-effectiveness reported in other units, see annex tables 2.C.1 and 2.C.2.

a. Nonprice interventions for tobacco addiction include advertising bans, smoking restrictions, supply reduction, and information dissemination.

b. EPI = Expanded Program on Immunization.

c. Chloroquine as first-line drug, artemisinin combination therapy as second-line drug and sulfadoxine-pyrimethamine as first- or second-line drug.

Figure 2.2 Cost-Effectiveness of Interventions Related to High-Burden Diseases in LMICs

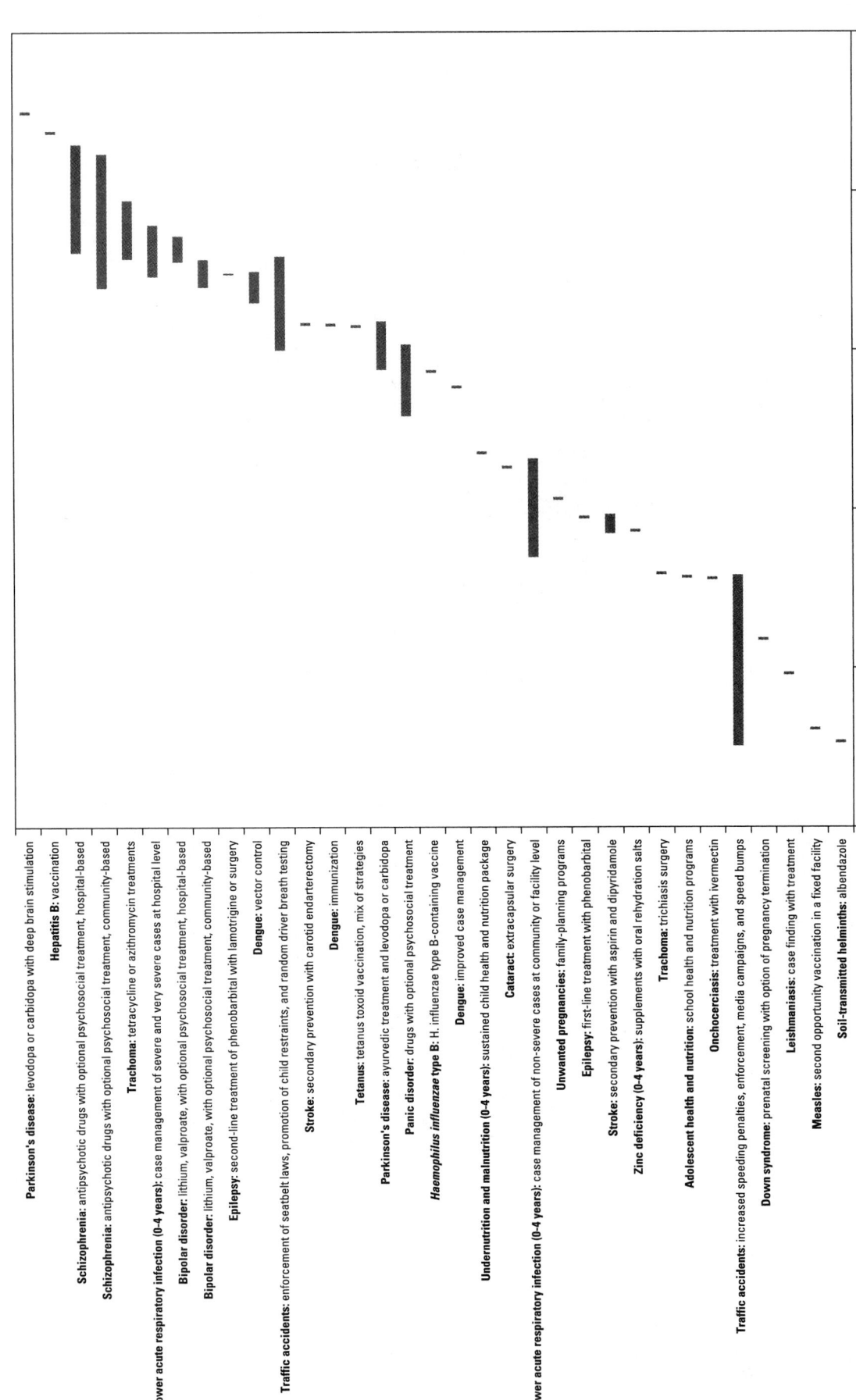

Figure 2.3 Cost-Effectiveness of Interventions Related to Low-Burden Diseases in LMICs

Source: Authors.

Note: Diseases were considered low burden for LMICs if their total avertable burden was less than 35 million DALYs. Bars represent the range in point estimates of cost-effectiveness ratios for specific interventions included in each intervention cluster and do not represent variation across regions or statistical confidence intervals. Point estimates for LMICs were obtained directly from the relevant chapters, calculated as the midpoint of range estimates reported in the chapters, or calculated from a population-weighted average of the region-specific estimates reported in the chapters. For details of these intervention clusters, including the specific interventions covered in each, see annex tables 2.C.1 and 2.C.2. Only interventions with cost-effectiveness reported in terms of DALYs are included in this figure. For interventions with cost-effectiveness reported in other units, see annex tables 2.B.1 and 2.B.2.

and HIV. In the context of TB control, antiretroviral therapy for HIV/AIDS is likely to be useful in extending the lives of patients successfully treated for TB.

Multidrug-resistant TB is much more expensive to treat than drug-susceptible TB—2 to 10 times the cost of standard first-line regimens for drug-susceptible TB—and this is one reason why priority should be given to preventing its emergence and spread. The management of drug resistance through the use of a standardized regimen that includes second-line drugs costs roughly US$70 to US$450 per DALY averted. Individualized treatment regimens for multidrug-resistant TB—that is, with drug combinations adjusted to the resistance pattern of each patient—are more costly but usually yield higher cure rates. Individualized treatment is harder to implement on a large scale but may not be less cost-effective than standardized treatment with regimens that include second-line drugs. The set of interventions needed to manage drug-resistant TB and TB associated with HIV requires higher levels of investment than the basic directly observed treatment strategy, but its cost is still typically less than US$1 for each day of healthy life gained. Thus, a strong economic argument exists for integrating such interventions into an enhanced strategy for TB control.

Prevention and Treatment of HIV/AIDS

Despite the scale and relentless progression of the HIV/AIDS epidemic, important strides have been made in developing cost-effective interventions for both prevention and treatment.

Prevention. Although remarkably little rigorous evaluation has been conducted, population-based programs to prevent HIV/AIDS appear to be highly cost-effective approaches in countries with high HIV/AIDS prevalence where the epidemic is generalized. These programs include voluntary testing and counseling (US$14 to US$261 per DALY averted); peer-based programs to educate high-risk groups, including sex workers and injecting drug users (US$1 to US$74 per DALY averted); and social marketing, promotion, and distribution of condoms (US$19 to US$205 per DALY averted). Programs to improve blood and needle safety, while highly cost-effective (US$4 to US$51 per DALY averted), are limited in terms of the burden of disease they can avert.

Prevention of mother-to-child transmission using a single dose of nevirapine in generalized epidemic settings (US$6 to US$12 per DALY averted) stands out for its combination of well-documented high cost-effectiveness and significant avertable infections and deaths. Treatment of sexually transmitted infections to lower the risk of HIV transmission, although less well proven, also appears to be highly cost-effective (US$16 to US$105 per DALY averted).

Treatment. For care of people living with HIV/AIDS, treatment of most infectious opportunistic infections is cost-effective (US$10 to US$500 per DALY averted), with treatment becoming significantly more cost-effective for patients who also have access to antiretroviral treatment. Few studies evaluate the cost-effectiveness of providing antiretroviral treatment, and even these are limited to clinical trial settings and are not directly applicable to the resource-poor settings in which antiretroviral treatment is being expanded. Economic evaluation of the cost-effectiveness of antiretroviral treatments based only on health outcomes for the treated patient is incomplete because of the large nonhealth impacts of HIV/AIDS and the effect of treatment on prevention of HIV transmission.

The cost-effectiveness of antiretroviral treatments is highly variable across settings as a function of drug prices and adherence rates. In low-cost settings with high adherence rates, antiretroviral treatment is moderately cost-effective (US$350 to US$500 per DALY averted); however, it can be a significantly poor value for resources spent in low-adherence settings if drug resistance is allowed to emerge and proliferate. Little is known about how to achieve necessary adherence levels (80 to 90 percent) at large scale at an affordable cost in low-income settings. To this end, research on effective, low-cost interventions to achieve long-term adherence to antiretroviral treatments (using support groups and other complementary interventions) in resource-poor settings is an urgent priority.

Childhood Illnesses and Mortality among Children under Five

Neonatal mortality rates and mortality rates for children under five can be reduced by large margins, at an affordable cost, by using interventions proven effective in low-income settings. Improvements are likely to come from increasing the coverage of preventive measures, such as breastfeeding, and from expanding the scope of existing childhood vaccines beyond the traditional six antigens in areas where existing coverage is relatively high and where new antigens address diseases of significant burden, particularly pneumococcal vaccines. Curative interventions—including case management of acute respiratory infections, malaria, and diarrhea—hold promise for lowering the 6 million preventable deaths each year in this age group.

Neonatal Mortality. An estimated 4 million deaths occur during the first 28 days of life, accounting for 38 percent of all deaths of children under five. Causes include infections (36 percent, including neonatal sepsis, pneumonia, diarrhea, and tetanus), preterm birth (27 percent), and asphyxia (23 percent). Intensive care is not required to save most of these babies. Developed countries and some low-income countries—for instance, Sri Lanka—have achieved neonatal mortality rates of 15 per 1,000 without intensive care, which is less than a third of current neonatal mortality rates in Sub-Saharan Africa.

Adding a set of community-based interventions—including promoting healthy behaviors, such as breastfeeding, and providing extra care of moderately small babies at home through cleanliness, warmth, and exclusive breastfeeding, plus community-based management of acute respiratory infections—to the standard maternal and child health package is likely to be highly effective. The cost of a year of life saved using this approach could be as low as US$100 to US$257 in India (US$221 to US$568 per DALY averted) and US$100 to US$270 in Sub-Saharan Africa (US$183 to US$493 per DALY averted). Use of these approaches is feasible now in most countries. Adding a clinical package that includes essential newborn care (warmth, cleanliness, and immediate breastfeeding); neonatal resuscitation; facility-based care of small newborns; and emergency care of ill newborns to the maternal and child health package has been shown to be highly cost-effective in India (US$11 to US$265 per year of life saved, or US$24 to US$585 per DALY averted) and Sub-Saharan Africa (US$25 to US$360 per year of life saved, or US$46 to US$657 per DALY averted); however, clinical care will require significant initial investment to raise coverage.

Basic resuscitation of newborns using a self-inflating bag that is available for as little as US$5 in LMICs can save lives at low cost in areas where a midwife is available. Providing two tetanus toxoid immunizations costing less than US$0.20 each to all pregnant women would avert more than 250,000 deaths at low cost and is eminently achievable. Improving maternal and child health services delivered through a combination of family- and community-level care, outreach, and clinical care will improve the survival of newborns and children and reduce stillbirths and maternal deaths.

Vaccinations. Childhood vaccinations, long recognized as among the most cost-effective uses of limited health resources in low-income countries, prevented more than 3 million deaths in 2001. National immunization programs traditionally have included vaccines against TB, diphtheria, tetanus, pertussis, poliomyelitis, and measles at a cost per fully immunized child of US$13 to US$24, depending on coverage levels and type of delivery strategy. The total cost in developing countries for national programs in 2001 ranged from US$717 million to US$1.4 billion, with an estimated cost per death averted ranging by region from under US$275 (under US$10 per DALY averted) in Sub-Saharan Africa and South Asia to US$1,754 (US$20 per DALY averted) in Europe and Central Asia.

The cost-effectiveness of scaling up immunization coverage with the traditional Expanded Program on Immunization (EPI) vaccines is highly dependent on the underlying prevalence of illness, starting coverage levels and trajectories, and mix of delivery strategies (whether facility-based strategies, campaigns, or mobile and outreach modalities). The cost per death averted varies by region, from US$162 in Africa to more than US$1,600 in Eastern Europe. Cost-effectiveness ratios are less than US$20 per DALY averted in all regions other than Europe and Central Asia. The cost-effectiveness of the tetanus toxoid vaccine also varies widely by region from under US$400 per death averted and under US$14 per DALY averted in Sub-Saharan Africa and South Asia to more than US$190,000 per death averted and more than US$15,000 per DALY averted in Europe and Central Asia.

Adding additional antigens to national programs has been successfully accomplished in many countries. Expanding the vaccination schedule to include a second opportunity for measles through either routine or campaign-based approaches costs between US$23 and US$228 per death averted and under US$4 per DALY averted in regions other than Europe and Central Asia. Other new vaccines are less cost-effective because of their high unit costs per dose, but they may be worthwhile, especially in regions of high disease prevalence. For instance, the pentavalent vaccine (diphtheria, pertussis, tetanus, hepatitis B, and *Haemophilus influenzae* type B) was estimated to have a cost per death averted ranging from US$1,433 to greater than US$40,000 and cost-effectiveness of US$42 per DALY averted in Sub-Saharan Africa and greater than US$245 per DALY averted in other regions. The cost of adding a yellow fever vaccine ranges from US$834 per death averted and US$26 per DALY averted in Sub-Saharan Africa to US$2,810 per death averted and US$39 per DALY averted in Latin America and the Caribbean.

Because certain regions and countries contain the largest burden of disease, such as measles in India and Nigeria, targeting scarce public health resources to those geographic areas could potentially yield high returns to investment. Although immunization may have relatively low incremental cost-effective ratios, the total budget requirements for maintaining or increasing coverage rates, as well as for introducing new vaccines, can account for a large share of government health budgets.

The cost-effectiveness ratios of vaccination interventions presented here are based on estimates of their current costs and effectiveness; but they could change substantially with changing costs and the development of new interventions. For instance, multivalent pneumococcal conjugate vaccines have shown the potential to reduce the incidence of invasive pneumococcal disease while lowering the need for antibiotic use and the likelihood of drug resistance. The current price of these vaccines makes them expensive to most people in the developing world. However, with future price decreases, these vaccines could be adopted widely and could markedly lower the impact of the most common causes of morbidity and mortality in children under five (excluding the neonatal period). Moreover, new vaccines being developed could be included in the EPI schedule, including vaccines that protect against rotavirus, malaria, human papilloma virus associated with cervical cancer, HIV/AIDS, and dengue. With future demonstrations of reasonable cost-effectiveness, these vaccines could become a component of the set of attractive interventions.

Acute Respiratory Infections. Even though vaccination strategies can be cost-effective in lowering the disease burden related to acute respiratory infections, case management may also be an efficient use of financial resources, although more demanding of health system capacity. Moreover, community case management and case management at a health care facility may be of comparable cost-effectiveness. In fact, treating nonsevere pneumonia at health care facilities using a combination of oral antimicrobials and acetaminophen (US$24 to US$424 per DALY averted) is more cost-effective than a similar treatment administered at home by a health care worker (US$139 to US$733 per DALY averted). Treating severe pneumonia in a hospital facility is more expensive (US$1,486 to US$14,719 per DALY averted).

Diarrheal Disease. Among interventions against diarrheal disease during the first year of life, breastfeeding promotion programs (US$527 to US$2,001 per DALY averted), measles immunization (US$257 to US$4,565 per DALY averted), and oral rehydration therapy (US$132 to US$2,570 per DALY averted) are relatively cost-effective compared with rotavirus immunizations (US$1,402 to US$8,357 per DALY averted) and cholera immunizations (US$1,658 to US$8,274 per DALY averted). The cost-effectiveness of oral rehydration therapy is extremely sensitive to the cost of the package. The cost-effectiveness of this intervention can be as low as US$132 per DALY averted for an assumed cost per child of US$0.70. An important reason for the relatively unfavorable cost-effectiveness ratios for diarrheal disease is that significant reductions in mortality from this condition have already been achieved and further gains are likely to be more expensive.

Further improvements in water and sanitation (US$1,118 to US$14,901 per DALY averted from diarrheal disease) are generally less cost-effective in regions where access to these amenities is adequate and other interventions against diarrheal disease exist. However, in areas with little access to water and sanitation facilities, improving access can be highly cost-effective (US$94 per DALY averted for installation of hand pumps and US$270 per DALY averted for provision and promotion of basic sanitation facilities).

Inherited Disorders of Hemoglobin. Inherited hemoglobin disorders, including sickle cell anemia and the thalassemias, affect roughly 500,000 babies born each year and cause early death for many of them. Prenatal screening for sickle cell disease, which is expensive, can be replaced by much cheaper newborn screening. Antibiotic prophylaxis is moderately cost-effective at preventing death in the first few years (US$8,000 to US$12,000 per death averted, or US$300 to US$400 per DALY averted). Expensive interventions, such as bone marrow transplantation or repeated transfusions, are seldom needed. At US$10,000 or more per DALY averted, treatment for transfusion-dependent thalassemias is expensive and probably unaffordable to all but the rich in LMICs. A feasible strategy to deal with the thalassemias is to screen couples to determine their risk of having an affected child, followed by prenatal testing—a relatively expensive proposition—of couples at high risk. Information is then available to parents to help them determine whether to terminate the pregnancy. Such strategies appear to have worked in Cyprus, Greece, and Italy, all countries that formerly had a high incidence of thalassemias.

Ongoing Challenges: Malaria and Other Tropical Diseases

Despite health researchers' relative neglect of diseases predominantly found in the tropics, interventions to control—and in some cases even eliminate—these diseases rank among the most cost-effective of all available options.

Malaria. In countries where malaria is prevalent, both prevention and effective treatment of this disease are highly cost-effective and can result in large health gains. Prevention tools include insecticide-treated bednets (US$5 to US$17 per DALY averted) and indoor residual spraying where DDT, malathion, deltamethrin, or lambda-cyhalothrin is applied to surfaces inside homes as a spray or deposit for prolonged action (US$9 to US$24 per DALY averted for Sub-Saharan Africa).

Intermittent preventive treatment of malaria during pregnancy using sulfadoxine-pyrimethamine is a highly cost-effective intervention (US$13 to US$24 per DALY averted) to decrease neonatal mortality and reduce severe maternal anemia. Changing first-line treatment for malaria from chloroquine, a drug that is ineffective in many parts of the world, to artemisinin-based combinations offers the advantage of faster cures and potential reductions in transmission, with cost-effectiveness ratios of less than US$150 per DALY averted. Changing to sulfadoxine-pyrimethamine may be slightly more cost-effective initially because of the lower cost of this drug relative to artemisinin-based combinations; however, this advantage is likely to be eroded quickly because of the rapid expected growth of parasite resistance.

Lymphatic Filariasis, Onchocerciasis, and Chagas Disease. Annual mass drug administration to treat the entire population at risk for a period long enough to interrupt transmission is a cost-effective approach for eliminating lymphatic filariasis in areas of high prevalence (US$4 to US$8 per DALY averted). An alternative approach is to fortify salt with diethylcarbamazine (US$1 to US$3 per DALY averted) and to use ivermectin in countries where onchocerciasis is coendemic. Onchocerciasis control programs have been highly successful in West Africa: investigators have estimated the cost-effectiveness of community-directed ivermectin treatment programs at roughly US$6 per DALY averted when the drug has been provided free of charge. The cost of vector control to prevent—and perhaps eliminate—Chagas disease has been estimated at US$260 per DALY averted.

Leishmaniasis and African Trypanosomiasis. Feasible intervention opportunities exist even for tropical diseases for which control measures are relatively less effective. Improved case management and immunization (currently undergoing clinical trials) for dengue (US$587 to US$1,440 per DALY averted) are relatively cost-effective compared with environmental vector control (more than US$2,000 per DALY averted). Leishmaniasis treatment is also extremely cost-effective (US$315 per death averted and US$9 per DALY averted), as is treating African trypanosomiasis patients in the second stage of the disease using melarsoprol or eflornithine (US$10 to US$20 per DALY averted).

Helminthic Infections. Helminthic infections, although not a major contributor to deaths in tropical regions, have a significant effect on health, growth and physical fitness, school attendance, worker productivity, and earning potential. Mass school-based treatment of soil-transmitted helminths (*Ascaris, Trichuris,* and hookworm) using albendazole costs US$2 to US$9 per DALY averted. Although the cost of treating schistosomiasis with praziquantel is significantly greater (US$336 to US$692 per DALY averted), a combination of albendazole and praziquantel is extremely cost-effective (US$8 to US$19 per DALY averted).

Maternal and Neonatal Health

Given the hugely disproportionate burden of maternal and neonatal deaths in LMICs, identifying affordable, easy-to-implement interventions to prevent these deaths is a priority. Evidence from South Asia and Sub-Saharan Africa suggests that improved primary-level coverage with a package of interventions is extremely cost-effective (US$3,337 to US$6,129 per death averted and US$92 to US$148 per DALY averted). Improvements in the quality of prenatal and delivery care are of similar cost-effectiveness (US$2,729 to US$5,107 per death averted and US$82 to US$142 per DALY averted). An important finding is that improving the quality of care and expanding coverage are of comparable cost-effectiveness.

Improving Nutrition

The direct and indirect effects of undernutrition and micronutrient deficiencies account for a significant propor-tion of the overall burden of disease in LMICs. For the most part, interventions to provide micronutrient supplementation can prevent malnutrition in children at a fairly low cost. They include breastfeeding support programs (US$3 to US$11 per DALY averted and US$100 to US$300 per death averted) and growth monitoring and counseling (US$8 to US$11 per DALY averted). Specific micronutrient supplementation programs can be implemented either by distributing capsules or by fortifying sugar, salt, water, or other essentials. In addressing vitamin A deficiencies, capsule distribution (US$6 to US$12 per DALY averted) is more cost-effective than sugar fortification (US$33 to US$35 per DALY averted), especially in countries where the prevalence of vitamin A deficiency is low. However, fortification of salt, sugar, and cereal in the case of iron deficiency and fortification of water and salt in the case of iodine deficiency is less expensive than distributing supplements for mild deficiency, though pregnant women and severely anemic or iodine-deficient people may still require supplementation. Overall cost-effectiveness is US$66 to US$70 per DALY averted for iron fortification programs and US$34 to US$36 per DALY averted for iodine fortification programs.

Cancer Prevention and Treatment

Screening for breast cancer using clinical breast examination (CBE) is estimated to be cost-effective at US$552 per life year saved for biennial screening of women from age 40 to 60. This efficacy of CBE is related to the large percentage of tumors with a poor prognosis observed in developing countries. In this setting, CBE is estimated to be more cost-effective than mammography: mammograms every two years result in 10 percent more life years saved than annual CBE, but the cost is more than 100 percent greater. As with any screening program, cost-effectiveness is greater with higher underlying prevalence of disease.

In general, cancer prevention, when feasible, is far more cost-effective than treatment. The cost-effectiveness of initial treatment is between US$1,300 and US$6,200 per year of life saved for the more treatable cancers of the cervix, breast, oral cavity, colon, and rectum and between US$53,000 and US$163,000 per year of life saved for the less treatable cancers of the liver, lung, stomach, and esophagus. Postmastectomy radiation might be more cost-effective in developing countries, where the cost of radiation treatment can be relatively low compared to developed countries. Palliative care for terminally ill cancer patients can be a challenge in resource-constrained settings, where opioid drugs, a cost-effective option, may be in short supply. Studies from developed countries indicate that more advanced treatments to relieve pain and side effects of chemotherapy may be cost-effective under certain conditions.

Mental and Neurological Disorders

Mental disorders are a heterogeneous group of conditions with considerable variation in both the cost of the interventions and the burden reduction associated with such interventions. Interventions to treat depression, bipolar disorder, and schizophrenia rank among the least cost-effective of interventions considered in this volume. However, the potentially significant benefits to family members and to society as a whole are not captured by the DALY methodology and should be balanced against the relatively high cost of improving health of people with these disorders. For many disorders, drug treatment has been shown to be effective, especially when combined with psychosocial treatment that includes cognitive-behavioral approaches to managing symptoms and improving adherence to medications, group therapy, and family interventions.

Schizophrenia and Bipolar Disorder. Drug treatment accompanied by psychosocial treatment delivered through a community-based service was found to be the most cost-effective approach for severe mental disorders such as schizophrenia and bipolar disorder. Newer antipsychotic and mood-stabilizing drugs have recently become less expensive; even so, they are less cost-effective than drugs that have been available for many years. For example, family psychoeducation was much more cost-effective with haloperidol (US$1,743 to US$4,847 per DALY averted) compared with a newer antipsychotic drug (risperidone) in treating schizophrenia (US$10,232 to US$14,481 per DALY averted). For bipolar affective disorder, the combination of family psychoeducation with the older medication lithium (US$1,587 to US$4,928 per DALY averted) is more cost-effective than the combination of family psychoeducation with the newer sodium valproate (US$2,765 to US$5,908 per DALY averted).

Depression and Panic Disorder. Treating the more common depressive and anxiety disorders was more cost-effective than treating the more severe disorders; the interventions were less expensive, and the reduction in disability was greater. For depression, drug therapy with tricyclic antidepressants (imipramine or amitriptyline) costs US$478 to US$1,288 per DALY averted. Managing depression as a chronic illness with case management to reduce relapses did not greatly decrease the cost-effectiveness (US$749 to US$1,760 per DALY averted). Using newer medications with fewer side effects and potentially greater compliance (an advantage if medications need to be taken long term)—for example, a generic selective serotonin reuptake inhibitor (SSRI) such as fluoxetine—increased the cost somewhat (US$1,229 to US$2,459 per DALY averted). Finally, the treatment of panic disorder using tricyclic antidepressants (US$305 to US$619 per DALY averted) and SSRIs (US$567 to US$865 per DALY averted) was

more cost-effective than when combined with psychosocial treatment. Psychosocial treatment without drug treatment was of comparable cost-effectiveness (US$338 to US$927 per DALY averted).

The use of tricyclic antidepressants was more cost-effective than benzodiazepines, which are still commonly prescribed for anxiety disorders and produce dependence in many patients. Overall, the cost-effectiveness of a package of mental health interventions that addressed all four sets of disorders is between US$1,429 and US$2,902 per DALY averted, depending on the region.

Parkinson's Disease and Epilepsy. Ayurvedic treatment, a form of traditional medicine used in India, is relatively cost-effective in treating Parkinson's disease (US$750 per DALY averted). Less cost-effective interventions include a combination of levodopa and carbidopa (US$1,500 per DALY averted), which are used to treat the debilitating symptoms and delay the progress of the disease, and deep-brain stimulation (US$31,000 per DALY averted).

Cost-effective options for treating epilepsy are available, especially the use of phenobarbital to help control seizures (US$89 per DALY averted), but few eligible patients receive treatment. More expensive options, such as lamotrigine or surgery, are significantly less cost-effective than phenobarbital for first-line treatment; however, they are cost-effective for the small proportion of epilepsy patients who do not respond to phenobarbital.

Multipronged Strategy to Prevent and Treat CVD

CVD, including ischemic heart disease, congestive heart failure, and stroke, is the single most important cause of death worldwide; interventions to treat CVD are likely to account for increasingly greater proportions of health care expenditures in developing countries.

Population-Based Primary Prevention. Interventions to modify lifestyles can effectively lower the risk of coronary artery disease and stroke without expensive health infrastructure. They include lowering the fat composition of the diet, limiting sodium intake, avoiding tobacco use, and engaging in regular physical activity. The costs and the effectiveness of these approaches vary widely with the socioeconomic and cultural context in which they are contemplated.

Replacing dietary trans fat from partial hydrogenation with polyunsaturated fat is likely to be extremely effective in populations in South Asia, where the intake of trans fat is high. If such replacement is done during manufacture at a relatively low cost rather than through changes in individual behavior, a cost-effectiveness ratio of US$25 to US$73 per DALY averted can be attained. Replacing saturated fat with monounsaturated fat in manufactured foods accompanied by a public education campaign is relatively expensive in the base case (US$1,865 to US$4,012 per DALY averted), although the cost per DALY averted is highly sensitive to both the relative risk reduction in CVD events as well as the cost per individual. Reducing salt in manufactured foods through a combination of legislation and education campaigns is also relatively expensive in the base case (US$1,325 to US$3,056 per DALY averted), but could be much more cost-effective in high-density populations with a high salt intake. Little evidence is available on the cost-effectiveness of programs to encourage exercise and other behavior changes by individuals.

Personal Interventions. Prevention strategies targeted at individuals at high risk for CVD—measured as a combination of nonoptimal blood pressure and cholesterol, lifestyle, and genetic risk factors—can be effective, especially when implemented in tandem with population-based measures. A previous cardiovascular event is a reliable predictor of a second event. The cost-effectiveness of primary prevention of CVD may vary greatly depending on the underlying risk factors, the age of the patient, and the cost of medications.

Single-pill combinations of blood pressure–lowering medications, statins, and aspirin offer the potential dual benefit of being highly effective at lowering the risk of CVD and facilitating patient compliance with the ongoing drug regimen. A hypothetical multidrug regimen that includes generic aspirin, a beta-blocker, a thiazide diuretic, an angiotensin-converting enzyme (ACE) inhibitor, and a statin may be implemented at a cost-effectiveness ratio of US$721 to US$1,065 per DALY averted compared with a baseline of no treatment in a population with an underlying 10-year CVD risk of 35 percent. The use of the multidrug regimen for prevention in patients with a lower underlying CVD risk improves health benefits, but costs increase more than proportionately.

Acute Management of CVD. The cost of treating acute myocardial infarction using aspirin and beta-blockers is less than US$25 per DALY averted in all regions. Relatively more expensive interventions that offer marginally greater effectiveness include the use of thrombolytics such as streptokinase (US$630 to US$730 per DALY averted) and tissue plasminogen activator (US$16,000 per DALY averted).

The combination of aspirin and the beta-blocker atenolol has been shown to be highly cost-effective in preventing the recurrence of a vascular event. The incremental cost-effectiveness ratio of sequentially adding an ACE inhibitor such as enalapril (US$660 to US$866 per DALY averted), a statin such as lovastatin (US$1,700 to US$2,000 per DALY averted), and coronary artery bypass graft (more than US$24,000 per DALY averted) to the baseline therapy is greater when hospital facilities are available. In regions with poor access to hospitals,

the combination of aspirin and a beta-blocker is highly cost-effective (US$386 to US$545 per DALY averted). In all regions, treating congestive heart failure using enalapril and the beta-blocker metoprolol is also highly cost-effective (approximately US$200 per DALY averted).

Acute Management and Secondary Prevention of Stroke. The cost of treating acute ischemic stroke using aspirin is US$150 per DALY averted. Relatively cost-ineffective interventions involve the use of a tissue plasminogen activator (US$1,300 per DALY averted) and anticoagulants such as heparin or warfarin (US$2,700 per DALY averted). Aspirin is the lowest-cost option for secondary prevention of stroke (US$3.80 per single percentage point decrease in the risk of a second stroke within two years or US$70 per DALY averted). The combination of the antiplatelet medication dipyridamole and aspirin is equally cost-effective (US$93 per DALY averted). In contrast, carotid endarterectomy is expensive for secondary prevention (US$1,500 per DALY averted).

Strategies for Injury Prevention

Increasing economic development and use of motor vehicles has resulted in increases in traffic-related deaths and injuries; these events account for roughly a third of the burden from all unintentional injuries in LMICs.

Speed bumps appear to be the most cost-effective and cost less than US$5 per DALY averted in all regions if installed at the most dangerous junctions that account for 10 percent of junction deaths. Increased speeding penalties, media coverage, and enforcement of traffic laws are only slightly less cost-effective. Motorcycle helmet legislation (US$467 per DALY averted in Thailand), bicycle helmet legislation (US$107 per DALY averted in China), and improved enforcement of traffic codes through a combination of enforcement and information campaigns (US$5 to US$169 per DALY averted) are relatively more expensive but deserve greater attention, given the growing health burden associated with rising levels of vehicle ownership. Research has demonstrated that seat belts and child restraints are effective in the developed world, and lowering their costs and encouraging their routine use may improve their cost-effectiveness in LMICs.

Key interventions to reduce intentional violence, both self-inflicted (suicides) and interpersonal (homicides and war-related deaths), include changing cultural norms, reducing access to guns, and improving criminal justice and social welfare systems, but these interventions are difficult to evaluate using a cost-effectiveness framework, and a cost-benefit analysis is more appropriate. Studies of interventions targeting interpersonal violence in developed countries show that behavioral, legal, and regulatory interventions cost less than the money they save, in some cases by an order of magnitude. Providing shelters for victims of domestic violence in the United States has a benefit-cost ratio of 6.8 to 18.4. Implementing a gun registration law in Canada involved a one-time cost of US$70 million, compared with annual health-related costs of US$50 million for firearm-related injuries in that country. Interventions for troubled youths to reduce criminal activity include mentoring (with net benefits ranging from US$231 to US$4,651 per participant), family therapy (US$14,545 to US$60,721), and aggression replacement therapy (US$8,519 to US$34,071).

Policy Interventions to Lower Alcohol and Tobacco Use

The growing prevalence of smoking, especially among women in LMICs, is a serious threat to health. Interventions to reduce tobacco use are noteworthy not just because they are highly cost-effective but also because the burden of deaths and disability that they can avert is large. Tobacco control through tax increases often has dual benefits of increasing tax revenues as well as discouraging smoking initiation and encouraging smokers to quit. The cost-effectiveness of a policy to increase cigarette prices by 33 percent ranges from US$13 to US$195 per DALY averted globally, with a better cost-effectiveness ratio (US$3 to US$42 per DALY averted) in low-income countries. In comparison, nicotine replacement therapy (US$55 to US$751 per DALY averted) and nonprice interventions, including banning advertising, providing health education information, and forbidding smoking in public places, are relatively less cost-effective (US$54 to US$674 per DALY averted) in low-income countries but are still important components of any tobacco control program.

In regions with a relatively high prevalence of high-risk alcohol use—that is, Europe and Central Asia, Latin America and the Caribbean, and Sub-Saharan Africa—tax increases to lower alcohol use are extremely cost-effective (US$105 to US$225 per DALY averted). However, in regions with a lower prevalence of high-risk use—namely, East Asia and the Pacific and South Asia—tax-based policies can be among the least cost-effective interventions (more than US$2,500 per DALY averted). Advertising bans are among the most cost-effective (but least studied) of all interventions to reduce high-risk drinking in all regions (US$134 to US$280 per DALY averted). In East Asia and the Pacific, a comprehensive ban on advertising and reduced access to retail outlets are highly cost-effective interventions (US$123 to US$146 per DALY averted). Random breath testing is one of the least cost-effective interventions to reduce the alcohol-related disease burden (US$973 to US$1,856 per DALY averted). In Sub-Saharan Africa, however, averting the burden of disease associated with drunk driving is an important priority and is addressed effectively through such policies as random breath testing and stricter enforcement of drunk-driving laws (US$531 per DALY averted). Providing high-risk drinkers with brief advice from a physician in primary care settings is of intermediate cost-effectiveness

(US$480 to US$819 per DALY averted) in all regions, but combining this intervention with a tax on alcohol increases cost-effectiveness (US$260 to US$533 per DALY averted) in all regions except Sub-Saharan Africa.

Packaging of Interventions and Services

This section examines the overall cost-effectiveness of a service level, including all conditions addressed as part of a package of services, rather than evaluating individual interventions separately.

Emergency and Hospital Care. The cost per death averted of training lay first responders and volunteer paramedics is between US$130 and US$283 (or US$5 to US$11 per DALY averted) depending on the region. Ambulances outfitted with trained paramedics can avert deaths at a cost of US$1,148 to US$3,479 (US$46 to US$137 per DALY averted) in urban settings and US$3,457 to US$10,449 (US$140 to US$410 per DALY averted) in rural settings. Although the evidence for the cost-effectiveness of district and referral hospitals is very limited, it does indicate that basic hospital care at the district level could be highly cost-effective (US$13 to US$104 per DALY averted).

Surgery. Some types of surgery are highly cost-effective as part of a country's health strategy. These include providing surgical care to injury victims, including those suffering from head trauma and burns; handling obstetric complications, such as obstructed labor or hemorrhage; and undertaking elective surgery to address conditions such as cataracts and otitis media that have a significant impact on the quality of life. In areas of high prevalence, cataract surgery can be extremely cost-effective at roughly US$100 per DALY averted.

Many of these surgical interventions—including improved resuscitation and airway management using relatively simple procedures such as chest tubes and tracheostomy, improved fracture management, and improved management of burns covering less than 30 percent of the body—require only the basic facilities offered by district hospitals. The quality of surgery and the risk of complications vary widely, and adequate health system capacity is an important consideration. For the typical surgical facility located in a district hospital in an LMIC, the average cost per DALY averted for a representative set of surgical procedures is between US$70 and US$230. General surgery at the district hospital is cost-effective relative to other interventions in South Asia and Sub-Saharan Africa because of the relatively low input costs related to infrastructure and the high level of the avertable disease burden. Examples of surgical interventions with poor cost-effectiveness include first-line treatment of epilepsy with surgery, which is useful only to patients who do not respond to drug treatment, and percutaneous transluminal coronary angioplasty for cardiovascular events.

Integrated Management of Childhood Illnesses. An intervention package consisting of exclusive breast feeding; vitamin A and zinc supplementation; screening for immunization; and case management of pneumonia, malaria, and diarrhea, including oral rehydration therapy, costs approximately US$4.10 per child in Sub-Saharan Africa and is a cost-effective approach (US$38 per DALY averted) to improving the health of children under five when program coverage is 50 percent.

Value of Doing Things Better

Intervention quality is an important determinant of cost-effectiveness, and improving quality can be an efficient way to use resources. Community health status tends to be correlated with the quality of health service facilities, which can be enhanced even in resource-constrained settings. Indeed, resource-poor settings have the greatest potential for improving quality at low cost. In the case of acute respiratory infections, for example, the cost-effectiveness of improving the quality of care by implementing an educational activity for providers ranges from US$132 to US$800 per life saved (US$4 to US$28 per DALY averted) when initial intervention quality is poor and infections are widespread. Quality improvements can cost between US$2,000 and US$5,000 per life saved (US$70 to US$176 per DALY averted) with improved baseline quality, low disease prevalence, or both. Educational interventions to improve the quality of diarrhea treatment can be extremely cost-effective (less than US$18 per DALY averted) depending on these two factors.

Regional Analyses for South Asia and Sub-Saharan Africa

Given the significant health burden borne by countries in South Asia and Sub-Saharan Africa, cost-effectiveness information for interventions related to high-burden health conditions is presented for these two regions. In South Asia (figure 2.4), CVD-related interventions, including tobacco taxes, treatment of acute myocardial infarction with aspirin and beta-blockers, and increasing coverage of the EPI program, rank among the most cost-effective interventions. Treatment of latent TB, coronary artery bypass graft for ischemic heart disease, treatment of depression, and cholera immunization to prevent diarrheal disease rank among the least cost-effective. Vitamin A deficiency, leprosy, and epilepsy are important conditions that impose a relatively lower burden of DALYs on this region, but a number of highly cost-effective interventions to deal with each of these conditions could be scaled up.

In Sub-Saharan Africa (figure 2.5), HIV/AIDS and malaria rank among the highest-burden conditions. Of the 16 most cost-effective interventions addressing high-burden diseases, 8 are associated with these two sources of ill health alone. Other interventions that are both cost-effective and address high-burden diseases include nutritional support (including breast-feeding advice for mothers) for children under the age of four, and increasing coverage of the EPI. Oral rehydration therapy for diarrheal disease can be cost-effective if the cost of the package is relatively low (that is, less than US$1 per child per treatment).

Table 2.2 identifies interventions relevant to South Asia and Sub-Saharan Africa that have been evaluated in this volume and have the greatest potential to reduce the burden of disease in those regions at an affordable price.[6] The table also highlights interventions that address conditions that account for a moderate to high burden of disease but at a relatively high cost.

Personal versus Population-based Interventions

Figure 2.6 displays a histogram of intervention clusters categorized as either population based or personal (see annex 2.A for definitions). A greater number of personal intervention clusters than population-based intervention clusters are categorized as being highly cost-effective. Although this result may be partly an artifact of the way in which we have grouped interventions into clusters, it lends some support to the observation first made in the first edition of *Disease Control Priorities in Developing Countries* (Jamison and others 1993) that personal interventions are not necessarily less cost-effective than population-based interventions. Population-based interventions are cost-effective when effectively targeted to populations in which disease prevalence (or the potential prevalence and subsequent mortality if the interventions are not implemented) is high. For example, primary prevention of acute myocardial infarction using aspirin is not nearly as cost-effective as secondary prevention in patients who have already suffered a stroke or myocardial infarction, because this latter category has, by virtue of the first event, identified itself as being at higher risk than the general population. Similarly, malaria prevention programs will be highly cost-effective in areas where malaria is a serious problem but less so in countries where the burden of this disease is less and people are better served by treatment with an effective antimalarial.

DISCUSSION

Since the publication of the previous edition of this book, the epidemiological and demographic profiles of many LMICs and the range of available health interventions have changed significantly. This edition has the benefit of hindsight in looking back at the variety and affordability of interventions that were evaluated in the previous edition, both to see how the optimal mix of strategies may have changed in the intervening period and to ascertain trends.

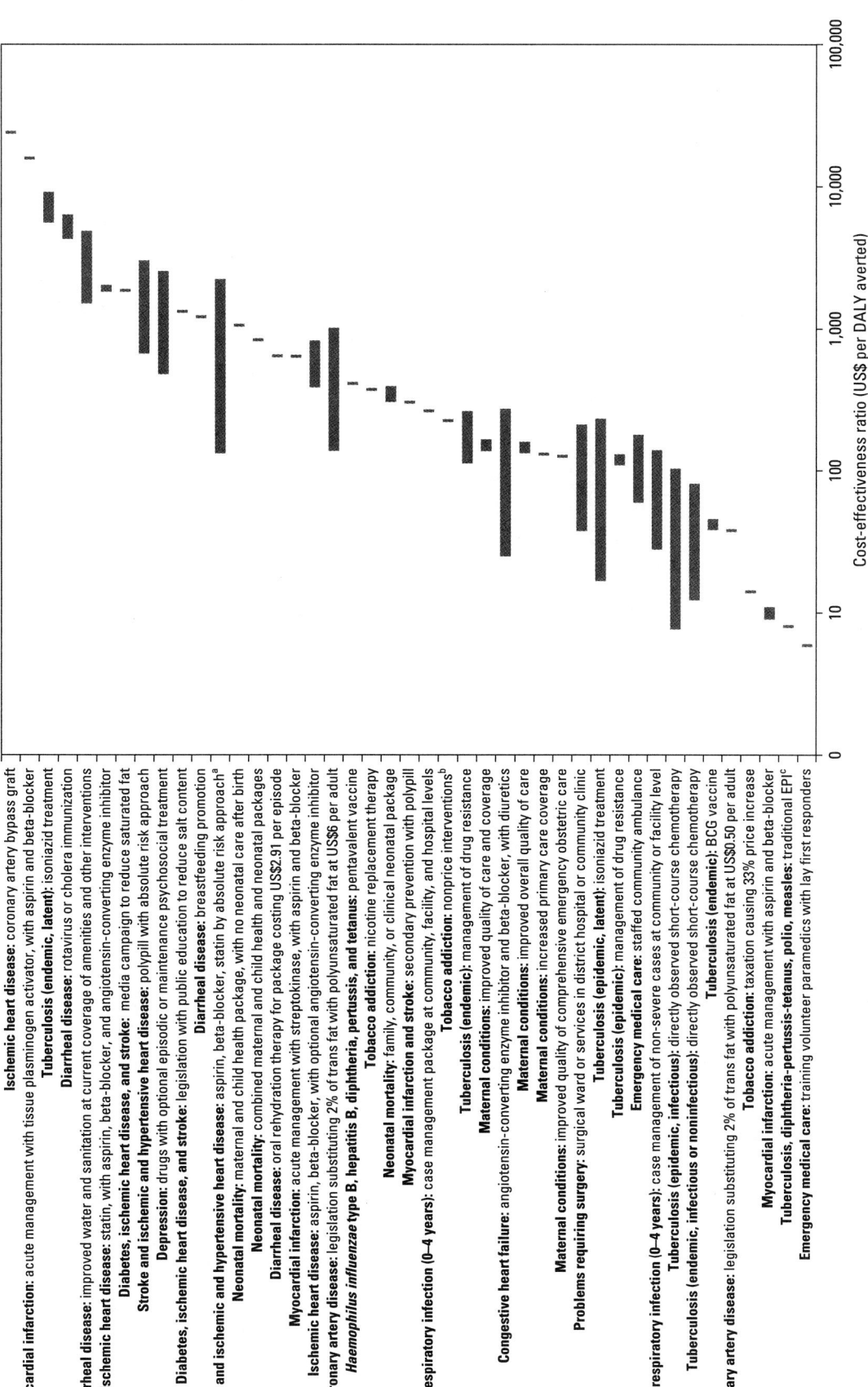

Source: Authors.

Note: Diseases were considered high burden for South Asia if their total avertable burden was greater than 10 million DALYs. Bars represent the range in point estimates of cost-effectiveness ratios for specific interventions included in each intervention cluster and do not represent variation across regions or statistical confidence intervals. Point estimates for LMICs were obtained directly from the relevant chapters, calculated as the midpoint of range estimates reported in the chapters, or calculated from a population-weighted average of the region-specific estimates reported in the chapters. For details of these intervention clusters, including the specific interventions covered in each, see annex tables 2.B.1 and 2.B.2. Only interventions with cost-effectiveness reported in other units, see annex tables 2.C.1 and 2.C.2.

a. Cost-effectiveness range of aspirin, beta-blockers, and statin to prevent stroke and ischemic and hypertensive heart disease is incremental to salt reduction legislation and health education.

b. Nonprice interventions for tobacco addiction include advertising bans, smoking restrictions, supply reduction, and information dissemination.

c. EPI = Expanded Program on Immunization.

Figure 2.4 Cost-Effectiveness of Interventions Related to High-Burden Diseases in South Asia

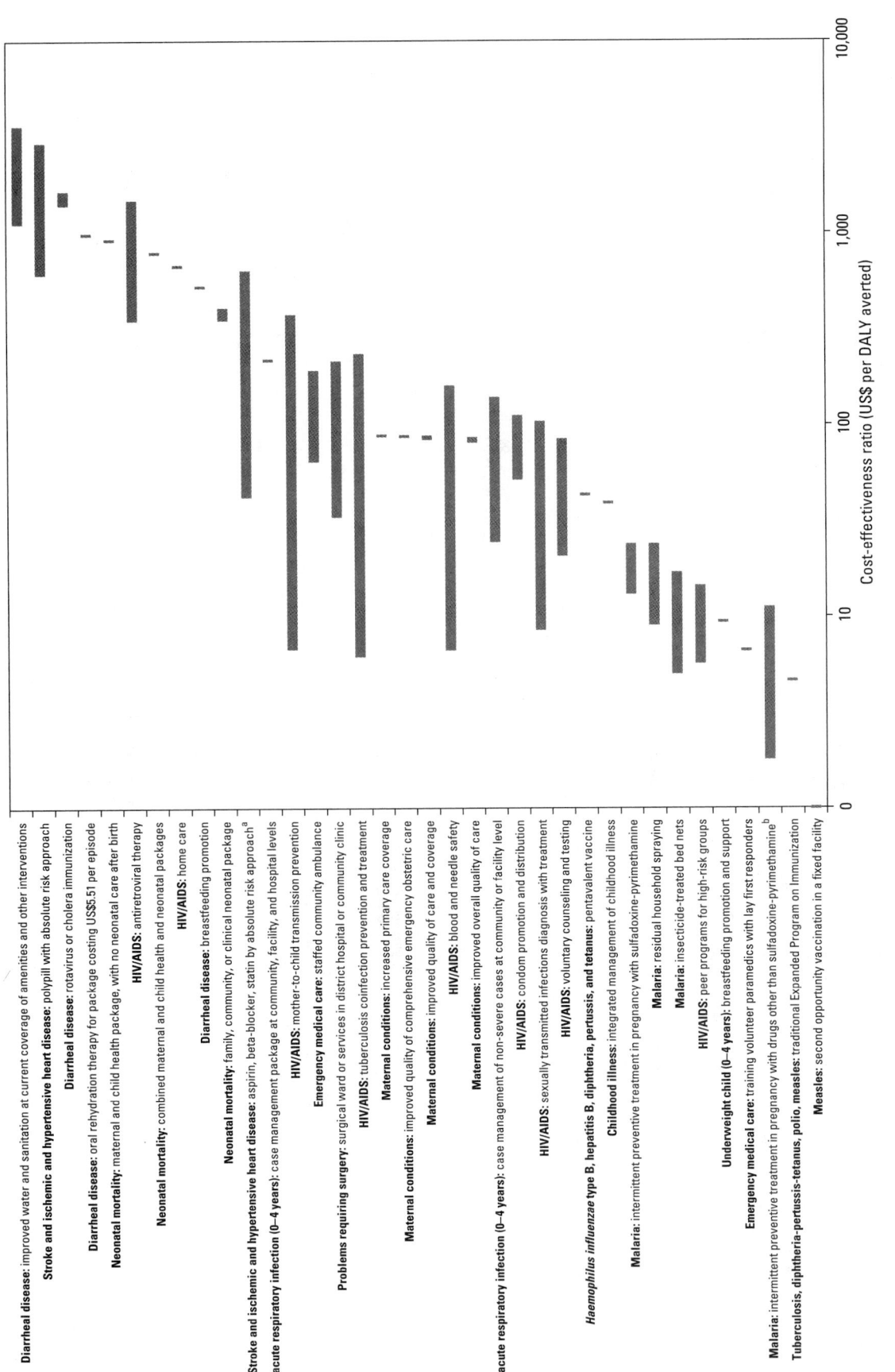

Cost-effectiveness ratio (US$ per DALY averted)

Diarrheal disease: improved water and sanitation at current coverage of amenities and other interventions

Stroke and ischemic and hypertensive heart disease: polypill with absolute risk approach

Diarrheal disease: rotavirus or cholera immunization

Diarrheal disease: oral rehydration therapy for package costing US$5.51 per episode

Neonatal mortality: maternal and child health package, with no neonatal care after birth

HIV/AIDS: antiretroviral therapy

Neonatal mortality: combined maternal and child health and neonatal packages

HIV/AIDS: home care

Diarrheal disease: breastfeeding promotion

Neonatal mortality: family, community, or clinical neonatal package

Stroke and ischemic and hypertensive heart disease: aspirin, beta-blocker, statin by absolute risk approach[a]

Lower acute respiratory infection (0–4 years): case management package at community, facility, and hospital levels

HIV/AIDS: mother-to-child transmission prevention

Emergency medical care: staffed community ambulance

Problems requiring surgery: surgical ward or services in district hospital or community clinic

HIV/AIDS: tuberculosis coinfection prevention and treatment

Maternal conditions: increased primary care coverage

Maternal conditions: improved quality of comprehensive emergency obstetric care

Maternal conditions: improved quality of care and coverage

HIV/AIDS: blood and needle safety

Maternal conditions: improved overall quality of care

Lower acute respiratory infection (0–4 years): case management of non-severe cases at community or facility level

HIV/AIDS: condom promotion and distribution

HIV/AIDS: sexually transmitted infections diagnosis with treatment

HIV/AIDS: voluntary counseling and testing

Haemophilus influenzae type B, hepatitis B, diphtheria, pertussis, and tetanus: pentavalent vaccine

Childhood illness: integrated management of childhood illness

Malaria: intermittent preventive treatment in pregnancy with sulfadoxine-pyrimethamine

Malaria: residual household spraying

Malaria: insecticide-treated bed nets

HIV/AIDS: peer programs for high-risk groups

Underweight child (0–4 years): breastfeeding promotion and support

Emergency medical care: training volunteer paramedics with lay first responders

Malaria: intermittent preventive treatment in pregnancy with drugs other than sulfadoxine-pyrimethamine[b]

Tuberculosis, diphtheria-pertussis-tetanus, polio, measles: traditional Expanded Program on Immunization

Measles: second opportunity vaccination in a fixed facility

Source: Authors.

Note: Diseases were considered high burden for Sub-Saharan Africa if their total avertable burden was greater than 10 million DALYs. Bars represent the range in point estimates of cost-effectiveness ratios for specific interventions included in each intervention cluster and do not represent variation across regions or statistical confidence intervals. Point estimates for LMICs were obtained directly from the relevant chapters, calculated as the midpoint of range estimates reported in the chapters, or calculated from a population-weighted average of the region-specific estimates reported in the chapters. For details of these intervention clusters, including the specific interventions covered in each, see annex tables 2.B.1 and 2.B.2. Only interventions with cost-effectiveness reported in other units, see annex tables 2.C.1 and 2.C.2.

a. Cost-effectiveness range of aspirin, beta-blockers, and statin to prevent stroke and ischemic and hypertensive heart disease is incremental to salt reduction legislation and health education.

b. Chloroquine as first-line drug, artemisinin combination therapy as second-line drug and sulfadoxine-pyrimethamine as first- or second-line drug.

Figure 2.5 Cost-Effectiveness of Interventions Related to High-Burden Diseases in Sub-Saharan Africa

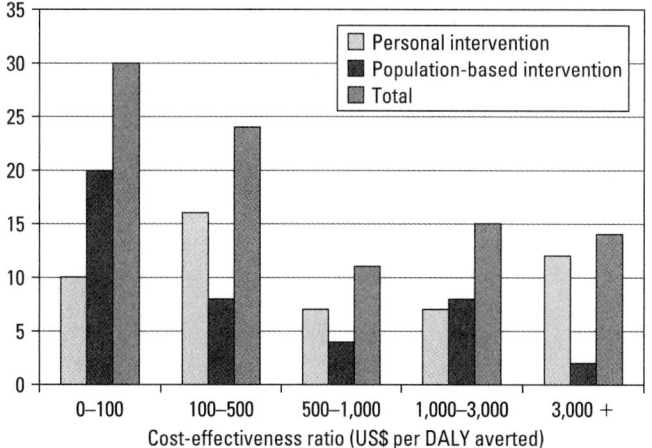

Number of intervention clusters

Legend:
- Personal intervention
- Population-based intervention
- Total

Cost-effectiveness ratio (US$ per DALY averted)

Source: Authors.

Note: Point estimates for the LMICs were obtained directly from the relevant chapters, calculated as the midpoint of range estimates reported in the chapters, or calculated from a population-weighted average of the region-specific estimates reported in the chapters.

Figure 2.6 Distribution of Interventions in LMICs by Cost-Effectiveness Ratio

Lessons

Three lessons are broadly applicable. They relate to communicable diseases, noncommunicable diseases, and technological progress.

Communicable Diseases. Interventions to treat communicable diseases have been highly cost-effective in the past and remain so despite new challenges, such as drug-resistant pathogens and vectors. Although much progress has been made in lowering the burden of disease associated with vaccine-preventable illnesses, diarrhea, and to a lesser extent with acute respiratory infections, progress made on other diseases, such as malaria and TB, has been rolled back by such challenges as parasite resistance in the case of malaria and the HIV epidemic in the case of TB. An important exception may be diseases for which vaccines have been available, where significant gains in health have been achieved. In general, discerning a link between the availability of effective, affordable interventions in 1993 and a significant effect on the disease burden since that time is difficult because of the problem in defining the appropriate counterfactual of what would have happened in the absence of interventions that were implemented.

Noncommunicable Diseases. Compared with 13 years ago, many more cost-effective interventions have been evaluated and are being used for noncommunicable diseases, which continue to grow in importance as populations undergo the epidemiological transition. Many of these interventions have been available for more than a decade; however, their costs have

dropped as key drugs have gone off patent. Acute management of stroke and myocardial infarction using aspirin, beta-blockers, and nitroglycerin costs as little as US$15 to US$30 per DALY averted and ranks among the most cost-effective interventions available in LMICs. Even though many of the interventions were first developed in the industrial world, their benefits are now largely available in the developing world. Thus, the challenge lies in the ability of health care systems in LMICs to adopt these interventions on a large scale.

Technological Progress. Much progress has been made in scientific understanding and in the availability of affordable, population-based and personal interventions for preventing and treating HIV/AIDS; however, adequate scaling up of these interventions remains a challenge, with a few notable exceptions. The international health system has shown remarkable technological agility in responding to this epidemic, demonstrating that the world's scientific-industrial machinery is capable of rising to the challenge of emerging diseases when there is sufficient economic motivation for doing so. For instance, combination antiretroviral treatments are currently available for as little as US$150 for a year's supply in some countries. In contrast, monotherapy with zidovudine, or AZT, which was the standard of care 10 years ago, was less effective, more expensive, and much more prone to drug resistance. As before, the challenge does not appear to be in the availability of interventions either to prevent infection in adults or to effectively ensure against transmission from infected mothers to newborns. Rather, the challenge lies in the willingness and ability to fund and deploy the interventions effectively. Clearly, much more remains to be done to develop affordable treatments. However, without a vaccine, the only feasible solution appears to be to aggressively prevent further transmission while treating patients under well-implemented programs that can achieve the high rates of treatment adherence required to maintain the continued effectiveness of drug therapy.[7] More generally, the challenge of motivating technological advances for diseases that do not threaten the developed world remains to be addressed.

Importance of Health Systems

In describing efficient means of producing health, this chapter has said little about how such efficiency may be translated into practice. The overall cost-effectiveness of a service level or package of interventions, rather than the cost-effectiveness of individual interventions, is the appropriate indicator to determine which interventions should be used. From a planning point of view, taking the infrastructure as fixed, at least in the immediate future, and then asking how it can best be used to deliver the most cost-effective interventions might be sensible. Where infrastructure is limited, expanding access will have to take priority. Other factors related to health system

Table 2.2 Neglected Low-Cost Opportunities and High-Cost Interventions in South Asia and Sub-Saharan Africa

Neglected low-cost opportunities in South Asia	Cost per DALY averted[a] (US$)	Thousands of DALYs averted[a,b] per 20% increase in coverage	Burden of target diseases[a] (millions of DALYs)
CHILDHOOD IMMUNIZATION			
Additional coverage of traditional Expanded Program on Immunization (tuberculosis, diphtheria-pertussis-tetanus, polio, measles)	8	n.e.	28.4
HIV AND AIDS			
Voluntary counseling and testing			
Peer-based programs targeting at-risk groups (e.g., commercial sex workers) to disseminate information and teach specific skills	9–126	n.e.	7.4
School-based interventions that disseminate information to students			
Prevention of mother-to-child-transmission with antiretroviral therapy			
SURGICAL SERVICES AND EMERGENCY CARE			
Surgical ward in a district hospital, primarily for obstetrics, trauma and injury	6–212	at least 1.8	48.0–146.3
Staffed community ambulance			
Training of lay first responders and volunteer paramedics			
TUBERCULOSIS			
Childhood vaccination against endemic TB			
Directly observed short-course chemotherapy	8–263	n.e.	13.9
Isoniazid treatment of epidemic TB			
Management of drug resistance			
LOWER ACUTE RESPIRATORY ILLNESSES OF CHILDREN UNDER FIVE			
Community- or facility-based case management of non-severe cases			
Case management package including community- and facility-based care for non-severe cases and hospital-based care for severe cases	28–264	0.7–1.8	9.7–26.4
CARDIOVASCULAR DISEASE			
Management of acute myocardial infarction with aspirin and beta-blocker			
Primary prevention of coronary artery disease with legislation substituting 2% of trans fat with polyunsaturated fat, at $0.50 per adult			
Secondary prevention of congestive heart failure with angiotensin-converting enzyme inhibitors and beta-blockers incremental to diuretics	9–304	at least 0.1	25.9–39.1
Secondary prevention of myocardial infarction and stroke with polypill containing aspirin, beta-blocker, thiazide diuretic, angiotensin-converting enzyme inhibitor, and statin			
TOBACCO USE AND ADDICTION			
Tax policy to increase price of cigarettes by 33 percent			
Non-price interventions such as advertising bans, health information dissemination, tobacco supply reductions, and smoking restrictions	14–374	at least 2.5	15.7
Nicotine replacement therapy			
MATERNAL AND NEONATAL CARE			
Increased primary care coverage			
Improved quality of comprehensive emergency obstetric care	127–394	at least 1.3	37.7–47.8
Improved overall quality and coverage of care			
Neonatal packages targeted to families, communities, and clinics			

Table 2.2 *(Continued)*

Neglected low-cost opportunities in Sub-Saharan Africa	Cost per DALY averted[a] (US$)	Thousands of DALYs averted[a,b] per 20% increase in coverage	Burden of target diseases[a] (millions of DALYs)
CHILDHOOD IMMUNIZATION			
Second opportunity measles vaccination[c]			
Additional coverage of traditional Expanded Program on Immunization (tuberculosis, diphtheria-pertussis-tetanus, polio, measles)	1–5	n.e.	13.5–31.3
TRAFFIC ACCIDENTS			
Increased speeding penalties, media, and law enforcement	2–12	n.e.	6.4
Speed bumps at the most dangerous traffic intersections			
MALARIA			
Insecticide-treated bed nets[c]			
Residual household spraying[c]	2–24	20.8–37.6	35.4
Intermittent preventive treatment during pregnancy[c]			
SURGICAL SERVICES AND EMERGENCY CARE			
Surgical ward in a district hospital, primarily for obstetrics, trauma and injury	7–215	1.6–21.2	25–134.2
Staffed community ambulance			
Training of lay first responders and volunteer paramedics			
CHILDHOOD ILLNESSES			
Integrated management of childhood illnesses[c]			
Case management of non-severe lower acute respiratory illnesses at the community or facility level			
Case management package including community- or facility-based care for non-severe cases and hospital-based care for severe lower acute respiratory illnesses	9–218	at least 1.2	9.6–45.1
Breastfeeding support to prevent underweight children[c]			
CARDIOVASCULAR DISEASE			
Management of acute myocardial infarction with aspirin and beta-blocker			
Primary prevention of coronary artery disease with legislation substituting 2% of trans fat with polyunsaturated fat, at $0.50 per adult			
Secondary prevention of congestive heart failure with angiotensin-converting enzyme inhibitors and beta-blockers incremental to diuretics	9–273	at least 0.04	4.6
Secondary prevention of myocardial infarction and stroke with polypill containing aspirin, beta-blocker, thiazide diuretic, angiotensin-converting enzyme inhibitor, and statin			
HIV AND AIDS			
Peer-based programs targeting at-risk groups (e.g., commercial sex workers) to disseminate information and teach specific skills			
Voluntary counseling and testing			
Diagnosis and treatment of sexually-transmitted diseases[c]	6–377	n.e.	56.8
Condom promotion and distribution[c]			
Prevention and treatment of tuberculosis co-infection[c]			
Blood and needle safety programs[c]			
Prevention of mother-to-child transmission with antiretroviral therapy			
MATERNAL AND NEONATAL CARE			
Increased primary care coverage			
Improved quality of comprehensive emergency obstetric care	82–409	at least 2.8	29.8–37.7
Improved overall quality and coverage of care			
Neonatal packages targeted to families, communities, and clinics			

(Continues on the following page.)

Table 2.2 *(Continued)*

High-cost interventions in South Asia	Cost per DALY averted[a] (US$)	Thousands of DALYs averted[a,b] per 20% increase in coverage	Burden of target diseases[a] (millions of DALYs)
DEPRESSION			
Episodic treatment with newer antidepressant drug (selective serotonin reuptake inhibitors)	1,003–1,449	0.4–0.8	14.6
Episodic or maintenance psychosocial treatment plus treatment with newer antidepressant drug (selective serotonin reuptake inhibitors)			
HIGH BLOOD PRESSURE AND CHOLESTEROL			
Primary prevention of stroke and ischemic and hypertensive heart disease with aspirin, beta-blocker, and statin, incremental to policy-induced behavior change, at 15 percent risk of CVD event over 10 years	1,120–1,932	at least 6.7	48.6
Primary prevention of stroke and ischemic and hypertensive heart disease with a polypill, containing aspirin, beta-blocker, thiazide diuretic, angiotensin-converting enzyme inhibitor, and statin, at 15 percent risk of CVD event over 10 years			
LIFESTYLE DISEASES			
Primary prevention of diabetes, ischemic heart disease, and stroke through policy that replaces saturated fat with monounsaturated fat in manufactured foods, accompanied by a public education campaign	1,325–1,865	1.3–1.8	39.5
Primary prevention of diabetes, ischemic heart disease, and stroke through legislation that reduces salt content plus public education			
STROKE (ISCHEMIC)			
Acute management with recombinant tissue plasminogen activator with 48 hours of onset			
Acute management with heparin within 48 hours of onset	1,630–2,967	0.03–0.4	2.2–9.2
Secondary prevention with carotid endarterectomy			
DIARRHEAL DISEASES			
Oral rehydration therapy if the package cost is greater than US$2.30 per child per episode	500–6,390	0.02–2.5	22.3
Rotavirus or cholera immunization			
TUBERCULOSIS			
Isoniazid treatment for latent endemic TB in patients uninfected with HIV	5,588–9,189	n.e.	13.9
SCHIZOPHRENIA AND BIOPOLAR DISORDER			
Antipsychotic medication and psychosocial treatment for schizophrenia	1,743–17,702	0.02–0.12	2.2–2.9
Valproate and psychosocial treatment for bipolar disorder			
CARDIOVASCULAR DISEASE			
Management of acute myocardial infarction with streptokinase or tissue plasminogen activator, incremental to aspirin and beta-blocker			
Secondary prevention of ischemic heart disease with statin, incremental to aspirin, beta-blocker, and angiotensin-converting enzyme inhibitor	638–24,040	0.04–0.3	25.9
Secondary prevention of ischemic heart disease with coronary artery bypass graft			

Table 2.2 *(Continued)*

High-cost interventions in Sub-Saharan Africa	Cost per DALY averted[a] (US$)	Thousands of DALYs averted[a,b] per 20% increase in coverage	Burden of target diseases[a] (millions of DALYs)
DIARRHEAL DISEASES			
Oral rehydration therapy if the cost per episode is greater than US$2.80 per child	500–1,658	0.1–4.6	22
Rotavirus or cholera immunization			
HIV AND AIDS			
Home care treatment[c]	673–1,494	n.e.	56.8
Antiretroviral therapy in populations with low adherence[c]			
TRAFFIC ACCIDENTS			
Random driver breath tests			
Enforcement of seatbelt laws	973–2,146	at least 0.05	6.2–6.4
Child restraint promotion			
HIGH BLOOD PRESSURE AND CHOLESTEROL			
Primary prevention of stroke and ischemic and hypertensive heart disease with aspirin, beta-blocker, and statin, incremental to policy-induced behavior change, at 15 percent risk of CVD event over 10 years	1,920	n.e.	10.6
LIFESTYLE DISEASES			
Primary prevention of diabetes, ischemic heart disease, and stroke through policy that replaces saturated fat with monounsaturated fat in manufactured foods, accompanied by a public education campaign	1,766–2,356	1.4–1.8	9.6
Primary prevention of diabetes, ischemic heart disease, and stroke through legislation that reduces salt content plus public education			
STROKE (ISCHEMIC)			
Acute management with recombinant tissue plasminogen activator within 48 hours of onset	1,284–2,940	0.02–0.3	0.9–3.6
Acute management with heparin within 48 hours of onset			
Secondary prevention with carotid endarterectomy			
TUBERCULOSIS			
Isoniazid treatment for latent endemic TB in patients uninfected with HIV	4,129–5,506	n.e.	8.1
CARDIOVASCULAR DISEASE			
Management of acute myocardial infarction with streptokinase or tissue plasminogen activator, incremental to aspirin and beta-blocker			
Secondary prevention of ischemic heart disease with statin, incremental to aspirin, beta-blocker, and angiotensin-converting enzyme inhibitor	634–26,813	0.03–0.2	4.6
Secondary prevention of ischemic heart disease with coronary artery bypass graft			

Source: Authors.

n.e. = not evaluated.

a. Ranges represent variation in point estimates of cost-effectiveness, DALYs averted, or burden of disease among the different interventions listed in each group. Point estimates of cost-effectiveness and DALYs averted were obtained directly from the relevant chapters or calculated as the midpoint of range estimates reported in the chapters. Burden of disease were obtained from the relevant chapters and from Mathers and others 2006.

b. Avertable DALYs per 20% increase in treatment coverage in a hypothetical sample population of one million people.

c. Only evaluated for Sub-Saharan Africa.

capacity and infrastructure may play a key role in determining the adoption of interventions. The current evidence on the cost-effectiveness of service levels such as district or referral hospitals is weak. Even though part of the problem lies with the difficulty of valuing the health benefits these facilities produce, more could be done. Chapter 3 presents a more detailed discussion of issues pertaining to health systems, but the broader questions of why some cost-effective interventions are used while others are not is a subject for future inquiry.

Even though much of the technology to significantly reduce the burden of disease already exists, few cost-effective interventions are available for some diseases. Shaping research priorities in a manner that is responsive to the treatment needs of the millions of HIV/AIDS patients and of people suffering from mental disorders across the range of LMICs is a challenge.

Setting intervention priorities efficiently can make a dollar go farther in improving health and can substantively increase available resources. Moreover, without demonstrably improved efficiency in health spending, aid agencies and development partners are unlikely to be persuaded to dig deeper into their pockets to pay for further expansions of health programs. Improving efficiency should not, however, detract from the importance of increasing resources that are available for implementing these interventions and of meeting broader internationally agreed-upon development goals such as the Millennium Development Goals. These objectives are complementary.

The lack of reliable data on costs and effectiveness is an important obstacle to efficient priority setting. Despite the relatively good data on the efficacy of interventions in clinical trial settings, reliable effectiveness data are generally lacking. Furthermore, not enough is known about the costs, extent of coverage, and institutional capacity requirements of interventions in developing countries. The messages presented in this chapter represent the best available information about the relative costs of purchasing health through a wide range of interventions. The challenge that lies ahead is for these messages to move beyond the academic realm: ultimately, it is the extent to which policy makers make the commitment to act on them that will save lives.

ACKNOWLEDGMENTS

We are grateful to the many authors and the nine editors of this volume, whose work, guidance, and feedback were essential inputs to this chapter. Pamela Maslen provided valuable assistance in compiling annex tables. Any remaining errors are ours alone.

ANNEX 2.A: INTERVENTION CATEGORIES AND PERTINENT POLICY INSTRUMENTS

The term *intervention* is used to denote actions taken by or for individuals to reduce the risk, duration, or severity of an adverse health condition. Policy instruments encourage, discourage, or undertake interventions. Stopping smoking, for example, is an intervention that an individual can take to reduce his or her risk of a range of diseases, and taxing tobacco products is a potential instrument of government policy to encourage this intervention. Interventions are divided into those that are *population based* and those that are *personal* as follows:

- Population-based primary prevention is directed toward entire populations or population subgroups. These interventions fall into three broad categories: personal behavior change, control of environmental hazards, and population-oriented medical interventions (for example, immunization, mass chemoprophylaxis, and screening and referral).
- Personal interventions are directed toward individuals and can be provided at home; at clinics (community, private, work-based, or school-based); at district hospitals; or at referral hospitals.

Primary prevention aims at reducing the level of one or more identified risk factors to reduce the probability of the initial occurrence of a disease (for instance, providing medication for established hypertension to prevent stroke or myocardial infarction).

Cure of a condition aims at removing the cause and restoring function to what it was before.

Acute management consists of time-limited interventions that decrease the severity of acute events or the level of established risk factors to minimize their long-term effect (for instance, providing thrombolytics for acute myocardial infarction or angioplasty to reduce stenosis in coronary arteries).

Secondary prevention (or *chronic care*) consists of ongoing interventions aimed at decreasing the severity and frequency of recurrent events of chronic or episodic diseases (for instance, providing selective serotonin reuptake inhibitors for severe unipolar depression).

Rehabilitation aims at restoring or partially restoring physical, psychological, or social function resulting from a previous condition.

Palliation aims at reducing pain and suffering from a condition for which no cure or means of rehabilitation is currently available. It may range from the use of aspirin for headaches to the use of opiates to control terminal cancer pain.

Policy instruments are activities that governments or other entities that wish to encourage or discourage interventions or to expand the potential interventions could undertake. The following are five major instruments of policy:

- Information, education, and communication seek to improve the knowledge of individuals and service providers about the consequences of their choices.
- Taxes and subsidies on commodities, services, and pollutants seek to effect appropriate behavioral responses.
- Regulation and legislation seek to limit the availability of certain commodities, to curtail certain practices, and to define the rules governing the financing and provision of health services.
- Direct expenditures seek to provide or to finance the provision of selected interventions (such as immunizations); to provide infrastructure (for instance, medical schools) that facilitates the provision of a range of interventions; or to alter infrastructure so as to influence behavior (for example, by installing speed bumps).
- Research and development, either undertaken directly or encouraged through subsidies, are central to the goal of expanding the range of interventions available and reducing their costs.

Source: This annex was prepared by Thomas Gaziano, Dean Jamison, and Sonbol Shahid-Salles.

ANNEX 2.B: SUMMARY OF INTERVENTIONS

Table 2.B.1 summarizes personal interventions. A summary of population-based interventions is shown in table 2.B.2.

ANNEX 2.C: SUMMARY OF OTHER INTERVENTIONS

Table 2.C.1 summarizes personal interventions for which cost-effectiveness is evaluated using a measure other than US$/DALY averted. A summary of population-based interventions evaluated using measures other than DALYs is shown in table 2.C.2.

Table 2.B.1 Summary of Personal Interventions

Condition	Intervention	Intervention description	Intervention setting	Objective	Target population[a]	Cost-effectiveness[b] (US$/DALY)	Cost-effectiveness range[b] (US$/DALY)	Number of DALYs averted[b] (hundreds)	Number of deaths averted[b]	Quality of cost-effectiveness analysis evidence[c]
African trypanosomiasis	Case finding and treatment	Identification and treatment of *Trypanosoma brucei gambiense* using the card agglutination trypanosomiasis test with parasitological confirmation, allowing for rapid diagnosis and treatment	Clinic	Primary prevention, cure	All ages	15 (Sub-Saharan Africa)	—	—	—	2 (Sub-Saharan Africa)
African trypanosomiasis	Melarsoprol	Used in the second stage of the disease	Clinic	Secondary prevention	All ages	10 (Sub-Saharan Africa)	—	—	—	2 (Sub-Saharan Africa)
African trypanosomiasis	Eflornithine	Used in the second stage of the disease	Clinic	Secondary prevention	All ages	20 (Sub-Saharan Africa)	—	—	—	2 (Sub-Saharan Africa)
Alcohol abuse	Brief advice to heavy drinkers by primary health care providers	During primary health care visits, provision of advice by physicians through education sessions and psychosocial counseling	Clinic	Primary prevention	Adolescents and adults	642	—	1.75	—	5
Bipolar disorder	Lithium, valproate, with optional psychosocial treatment, hospital-based	Episodic treatment in a hospital setting with lithium or valproate with or without maintenance or episodic psychosocial treatment	District or referral hospital	Secondary prevention	Adults over 15	4,417	3,590–5,244	1.00	—	5
Bipolar disorder	Lithium, valproate, with optional psychosocial treatment, community-based	Episodic treatment of bipolar disorder in a community setting using lithium or valproate with or without maintenance or episodic psychosocial treatment	District or referral hospital	Secondary prevention	Adults over 15	3,113	2,498–3,728	1.35	—	5
Cataract	Extracapsular surgery	Extracapsular cataract extraction with implantation of a posterior chamber intraocular lens; removal of the lens and the front portion of the capsule, which are then replaced with an artificial lens	District or referral hospital	Cure	Adults over 40	183	—	—	—	3
Congestive heart failure	ACE inhibitor and beta-blocker, with diuretics	Use of ACE inhibitor and an optional beta-blocker (metoprolol), incremental to diuretics	District hospital	Secondary prevention	Adults	150	27–274	11.59	—	5

Disease	Intervention	Description	Setting	Type	Target group				
Dengue	Improved case management	No specific treatment: early recognition of symptoms such as intense continuous abdominal pain, persistent vomiting, restlessness or lethargy; supportive treatment includes fluid replacement and electrolytic therapy	Clinic or district hospital	Acute management	All ages	587	—	—	2
Depression	Drugs with optional episodic or maintenance psychosocial treatment	Antidepressant drugs (tricyclic antidepressant or selective serotonin reuptake inhibitor) used alone or in combination with psychosocial treatment for episodic depression or maintenance treatment	District or referral hospital	Secondary prevention	Adults over 15	1,699	657–2,741	3.96	5
Diarrheal disease	Oral rehydration therapy for package costing US$5.50 per episode	Case management of acute diarrheal infection with oral rehydration salt solutions, for package costing US$5.50 per child per episode	Clinic	Acute management	Children	1,062	—	16.57	5
Epilepsy	First-line treatment with phenobarbital	First line treatment with phenobarbital to treat epilepsy patients	District hospital	Secondary prevention	All ages	89	—	2.99	5
Epilepsy (refractory)	Second-line treatment with phenobarbital and lamotrigine or surgery	Antiepileptic drugs, phenobarbital and lamotrigine, or a combination of phenobarbital and surgery to treat epilepsy patients unresponsive to phenobarbital	Referral hospital	Secondary prevention	All ages	3,027	2,994–3,060	0.29	5
HIV/AIDS	Mother-to-child transmission prevention	All pregnant women offered screening to prevent mother-to-child transmission; administration of a short-course of AZT, lamivudine, or nevirapine to mothers prepartum and intrapartum and to newborns postpartum and to reduce the risk of mother-to-child transmission; also includes breastfeeding advice	Clinic	Primary prevention	Mothers and infants	192	7–377	—	2
HIV/AIDS	Sexually transmitted infection diagnosis and treatment	Sexually transmitted infection screening and treatment promotion to prevent future infection and to identify and treat high-risk populations	Clinic	Primary prevention, cure	Adolescents and adults	57 (Sub-Saharan Africa)	9–105 (Sub-Saharan Africa)	—	2 (Sub-Saharan Africa)

(Continues on the following page.)

Table 2.B.1 *(Continued)*

Condition	Intervention	Intervention description	Intervention setting	Objective	Target population[a]	Cost-effectiveness (US$/DALY)	Cost-effectiveness range[b] (US$/DALY)	Number of DALYs averted[b] (hundreds)	Number of deaths averted[b]	Quality of cost-effectiveness analysis evidence[c]
HIV/AIDS	Treatment of Kaposi's sarcoma	Treatment before or after antiretroviral treatment, including failed antiretroviral treatment; local or systemic treatment of lesions to provide largely cosmetic benefit	Clinic or district hospital	Primary prevention, palliation	All ages	52,449	34,968–69,930	—	—	3
HIV/AIDS	Treatment of opportunistic infections	Opportunistic infection prophylaxis; necessary for patients without access to antiretroviral treatment, for immunosuppressed patients waiting for antiretroviral treatment to take effect, for patients who refuse or cannot take antiretroviral treatment, for patients for whom antiretroviral treatment fails, and for groups of patients who are unable to recover sufficient CD4 cells despite good inhibition of viral replication	Clinic or district hospital	Primary prevention, cure	All ages	156	3–310	—	—	3
HIV/AIDS	Tuberculosis coinfection prevention and treatment	Preventive therapy, short-course chemotherapy, or co-trimoxazole prophylaxis	Clinic	Primary prevention, cure	All ages	121 (Sub-Saharan Africa)	6–235 (Sub-Saharan Africa)	—	—	2 (Sub-Saharan Africa)
HIV/AIDS	Home care	Home visits providing basic care to sick AIDS patients or comprehensive schemes that provide palliative care, nutrition, psychosocial support and counseling, and links to primary and secondary health care	Household	Secondary prevention, palliation	All ages	673 (Sub-Saharan Africa)	—	—	—	2 (Sub-Saharan Africa)
HIV/AIDS	Antiretroviral therapy	Combination therapy with multiple antiretroviral drugs associated with prolonged survival in treated patients	Clinic	Primary prevention	All ages	922 (Sub-Saharan Africa)	350–1,494 (Sub-Saharan Africa)	—	—	3 (Sub-Saharan Africa)

Integrated management of childhood illness	Integrated management of childhood illness	Integration of effective interventions to improve child health and nutrition into a coordinated strategy by improving health worker performance, child health service delivery, and family and community practices	Clinic	Primary prevention, secondary prevention, cure	Children	39 (Sub-Saharan Africa)	—	—	—	3 (Sub-Saharan Africa)
Ischemic heart disease	Aspirin, beta-blocker, and optional ACE inhibitor	Aspirin plus beta-blocker (atenolol) with optional ACE inhibitor (enalapril), with or without hospital availability	District or referral hospital	Secondary prevention	Adults	688	451–926	8.40	—	5
Ischemic heart disease	Statin, with aspirin, beta-blocker and ACE inhibitor	Statin (lovastatin), incremental to aspirin, beta-blocker (atenolol), and ACE inhibitor (enalapril), with or without hospital availability	District or referral hospital	Secondary prevention	Adults	2,028	1,864–2,193	3.54	—	5
Ischemic heart disease	Coronary artery bypass graft	Placement of grafts (usually saphenous vein or internal mammary artery) to bypass stenosed coronary arteries, while maintaining cerebral and peripheral circulation by cardiopulmonary bypass	Referral hospital	Secondary prevention	Adults	36,793	—	0.76	—	5
Leishmaniasis	Case finding and treatment	Combination of identification and treatment, vector control where feasible, and (in zoonotic foci) control of animal reservoirs	Clinic or district hospital	Primary prevention	All ages	9	—	—	—	2
Lower acute respiratory infections (nonsevere)	Case management at community or facility level	Nonsevere infection diagnosed by breath rate and treated by a community health worker or at a health facility, with amoxicillin, acetaminophen, and possibly salbutamol	Clinic, community	Cure	Children under 5	129	50–208	5.15	17.36	5
Lower acute respiratory infections (severe and very severe)	Case management at hospital level	Severe or very severe infection diagnosed by breath rate and with x-ray tests and treated at a hospital with antibiotics and possibly salbutamol, oxygen, and prednisolone	District hospital	Cure	Children under 5	4,530	2,916–6,144	0.48	1.57	5

(Continues on the following page.)

Table 2.B.1 *(Continued)*

Condition	Intervention	Intervention description	Intervention setting	Objective	Target population[a]	Cost-effectiveness[b] (US$/DALY)	Cost-effectiveness range[b] (US$/DALY)	Number of DALYs averted[b] (hundreds)	Number of deaths averted[b]	Quality of cost-effectiveness analysis evidence[c]
Lower acute respiratory infections	Case-management package at community, facility, and hospital levels	Comprehensive case-management strategy covering nonsevere infection being treated by a community health worker or at a health facility, severe infection treated at a hospital, and very severe infection treated at a hospital	Clinic or district hospital	Cure	Children under 5	398	—	11.26	37.86	5
Malaria	Intermittent preventive treatment in pregnancy with sulfadoxine-pyrimethamine	Intermittent preventive treatment in areas with high and stable transmission of *Plasmodium falciparum* malaria; two curative doses of sulfadoxine-pyrimethamine given during the second and third trimesters of pregnancy during prenatal care visits	Clinic	Primary prevention	Pregnant women	19 (Sub-Saharan Africa)	13–24 (Sub-Saharan Africa)	208.00 (Sub-Saharan Africa)	827.80 (Sub-Saharan Africa)	5 (Sub-Saharan Africa)
Malaria	Intermittent preventive treatment in pregnancy with drug other than sulfadoxine-pyrimethamine	Intermittent preventive treatment in areas with high and stable transmission of *Plasmodium falciparum* malaria; two curative doses of antimalarial treatment given with a possible change in first-line therapies from chloroquine to sulfadoxine-pyrimethamine, chloroquine to artemisinin combination therapy, or sulfadoxine-pyrimethamine to artemisinin combination therapy	Clinic	Primary prevention	Pregnant women	7 (Sub-Saharan Africa)	2–11 (Sub-Saharan Africa)	—	77,500.00 (Sub-Saharan Africa)	5 (Sub-Saharan Africa)
Maternal mortality	Increased primary care coverage	Increased percentage of women accessing routine prenatal, intranatal, and postnatal care	Clinic or district hospital	Primary prevention	Pregnant women	132 (South Asia), 88 (Sub-Saharan Africa)	—	13.09 (South Asia), 27.88 (Sub-Saharan Africa)	32.00 (South Asia), 77.00 (Sub-Saharan Africa)	5 (South Asia), 5 (Sub-Saharan Africa)
Maternal mortality	Improved quality of comprehensive emergency obstetric care	Increased percentage of women with severe complications receiving comprehensive emergency obstetric care	Clinic or district hospital	Acute management	Pregnant women	127 (South Asia), 87 (Sub-Saharan Africa)	—	13.28 (South Asia), 28.28 (Sub-Saharan Africa)	32.00 (South Asia), 78.00 (Sub-Saharan Africa)	5 (South Asia), 5 (Sub-Saharan Africa)

Maternal mortality	Improved overall quality of care	Improvements to quality of prenatal and delivery care; enhanced package including availability of doctor and full range of basic and comprehensive emergency obstetric care (all six essential obstetric functions: administering antibiotics intravenously or intramuscularly, administering oxytocics intravenously or intramuscularly, administering anticonvulsants intravenously or intramuscularly, manually removing the placenta, carrying out instrumental delivery, and removing retained products of conception; optional nutritional supplementation	Clinic	Primary prevention, acute management	Pregnant women	147 (South Asia), 83 (Sub-Saharan Africa)	133–160 (South Asia), 82–85 (Sub-Saharan Africa)	21.90 (South Asia), 53.05 (Sub-Saharan Africa)	56.20 (South Asia), 153.20 (Sub-Saharan Africa)	5 (South Asia), 5 (Sub-Saharan Africa)
Maternal mortality	Improved quality of care and coverage	Improvements to quality of prenatal and delivery care and increase in the proportion of women receiving needed care; enhanced package including availability of doctor and full range of basic and comprehensive emergency obstetric care (all six essential obstetric functions noted above); optional nutritional supplementation	Clinic	Primary prevention, acute management	Pregnant women	152 (South Asia), 86 (Sub-Saharan Africa)	138–167 (South Asia), 85–86 (Sub-Saharan Africa)	23.51 (South Asia), 56.93 (Sub-Saharan Africa)	60.29 (South Asia), 164.14 (Sub-Saharan Africa)	5 (South Asia), 5 (Sub-Saharan Africa)
Myocardial infarction	Aspirin and beta-blocker	Aspirin with or without beta-blocker (atenolol)	District or referral hospital	Acute management	Adults	14	13–15	1.04	—	5
Myocardial infarction	Streptokinase, with aspirin and beta-blocker	Incremental use of streptokinase, in addition to aspirin and beta-blocker (atenolol)	District or referral hospital	Acute management	Adults	671	—	1.04	—	5
Myocardial infarction	Tissue plasminogen activator, with aspirin and beta-blocker	Incremental use of tissue plasminogen activator in addition to aspirin and beta-blocker (atenolol)	District hospital	Acute management	Adults	15,869	—	0.42	—	5
Myocardial infarction and stroke	Polypill	Combination treatment with aspirin, beta-blocker, thiazide diuretic, ACE inhibitor and statin, based on 10-year risk of cardiovascular disease	District hospital	Secondary prevention	Adults	409	—	—	—	5

(Continues on the following page.)

Table 2.B.1 *(Continued)*

Condition	Intervention	Intervention description	Intervention setting	Objective	Target population[a]	Cost-effectiveness[b] (US$/DALY)	Cost-effectiveness range[b] (US$/DALY)	Number of DALYs averted[b] (hundreds)	Number of deaths averted[b]	Quality of cost-effectiveness analysis evidence[c]
Neonatal mortality	Maternal and child health package with no neonatal care after birth	Mother and child health package that includes family planning, prenatal care, and comprehensive obstetric care	Clinic or district hospital	Primary prevention	Mothers and infants	1,060 (South Asia), 924 (Sub-Saharan Africa)	—	—	—	4 (South Asia), 5 (Sub-Saharan Africa)
Neonatal mortality	Family, community, or clinical neonatal package	Healthy home care practices, including exclusive breastfeeding, warmth protection, clean cord care, care seeking for emergencies; if birth outside a facility, then clean delivery kit	Clinic, community or household	Primary prevention	Mothers and infants	349 (South Asia), 345 (Sub-Saharan Africa)	305–394 (South Asia), 338–351 (Sub-Saharan Africa)	—	—	4 (South Asia), 5 (Sub-Saharan Africa)
Neonatal mortality	Combined maternal and child health with neonatal packages	Family planning, prenatal care, and comprehensive obstetric care packages, as well as healthy home care practices, including exclusive breastfeeding, warmth protection, clean cord care, care seeking for emergencies; if birth outside a facility, then clean delivery kit	Clinic, community or household	Primary prevention	Mothers and infants	839 (South Asia), 789 (Sub-Saharan Africa)	—	—	—	4 (South Asia), 5 (Sub-Saharan Africa)
Panic disorder	Drugs with optional psychosocial treatment	Anxiolytic drugs (benzodiazepine), tricyclic antidepressants or selective serotonin reuptake inhibitor used with or without psychosocial treatment	District or referral hospital	Secondary prevention	Adults over 15	734	384–1,084	0.83	—	5
Parkinson's disease	Ayurvedic treatment and levodopa or carbidopa	Levodopa (l-dopa), carbidopa, or ayurvedic therapy for partial relief of symptoms	District hospital or referral hospital	Secondary prevention	Adults over 45	1,132	752–1,512	0.13	—	5
Parkinson's disease	Levodopa or carbidopa and deep brain stimulation	Levodopa or carbidopa and deep brain stimulation	District hospital or referral hospital	Secondary prevention	Adults over 45	31,114	—	0.15	—	5

Schizophrenia	Antipsychotic drugs with optional psychosocial treatment, hospital-based	Maintenance treatment in a hospital setting with antipsychotic drugs, neuroleptic antipsychotic drug, or an atypical antipsychotic drug, with or without psychosocial treatment	District hospital or referral hospital	Secondary prevention	Adults over 15	11,920	4,105–19,736	0.60	—	5
Schizophrenia	Antipsychotic drugs with optional psychosocial treatment, community-based	Maintenance treatment in a community-based setting with antipsychotic drugs, neuroleptic antipsychotic drug, or an atypical antipsychotic drug, with or without psychosocial treatment	Community	Secondary prevention	Adults over 15	9,834	2,472–17,197	0.70	—	5
Stroke (ischemic)	Aspirin	Aspirin dose within 48 hours of onset of acute stroke	Clinic or district hospital	Acute management	Adults over 15	149	—	1.62	0.12	5
Stroke (ischemic)	Heparin and recombinant tissue plasminogen activator	Heparin within 48 hours of onset of stroke or thrombolytic therapy using recombinant tissue plasminogen activator within 3 hours of onset	District hospital	Acute management	Adults over 15	1,977	1,278–2,675	1.22	1.70	5
Stroke (recurrent)	Aspirin and dipyridamole	Daily aspirin dose or combination of aspirin and extended release dipyridamole	Clinic or district hospital	Secondary prevention	Adults over 15	81	70–93	1.77	14.29	5
Stroke (recurrent)	Carotid endarterectomy	Carotid endarterectomy surgery to remove harmful plaque from the carotid arteries	Referral hospital	Secondary prevention	Adults over 15	1,458	—	4.93	39.82	5
Stroke and ischemic and hypertensive heart disease	Polypill by absolute risk approach	Combination treatment with aspirin, beta-blocker, thiazide diuretic, ACE inhibitor, and statin based on 10-year risk of cardiovascular disease	District or referral hospital	Primary prevention	Adults	2,128	773–3,483	61.65	—	5
Tobacco addiction	Nicotine replacement therapy	Smoking cessation treatments in the form of nicotine replacement therapy	Clinic	Primary prevention	Adults	396	—	37.14	452.05	5
Trachoma	Trichiasis surgery	Trichiasis surgery (eyelid correction) to prevent blindness and reduce likelihood of other conditions	District hospital or referral hospital	Secondary prevention	Adults over 40	39	—	—	—	3

(Continues on the following page.)

Table 2.B.1 *(Continued)*

Condition	Intervention	Intervention description	Intervention setting	Objective	Target population[a]	Cost-effectiveness[b] (US$/DALY)	Cost-effectiveness range[b] (US$/DALY)	Number of DALYs averted[b] (hundreds)	Number of deaths averted[b]	Quality of cost-effectiveness analysis evidence[c]
Trachoma	Tetracycline or azithromycin	Tetracycline or azithromycin to treat the initial trachoma infection through either mass treatment of all children younger than 10 or through targeted treatment of infected children and household members	Clinic	Primary prevention	Children and adults	6,269	3,752–8,785	—	—	3
Tuberculosis (endemic)	Management of drug resistance	Introduction of resistance testing, second-line drugs, longer treatment regimen (12–18 months), and rigorous bacteriological and clinical monitoring; standardized or individualized regimen	District hospital	Secondary prevention, cure	Adults over 15	318	208–429	—	—	5
Tuberculosis (endemic, infectious or noninfectious)	Directly observed short-course chemotherapy	Short-course chemotherapy of infectious or noninfectious tuberculosis (with or without transmission, non-HIV-positive), diagnosed via directly observed treatment strategy	Clinic	Primary prevention, cure	Adults over 15	301	84–551	—	—	5
Tuberculosis (endemic, latent)	Isoniazid treatment	Isoniazid treatment of latent infection (with or without x-ray exclusion of active cases; non-HIV-infected population)	District hospital	Secondary prevention	Adults over 15	13,158	9,450–16,867	—	—	5
Tuberculosis (epidemic)	Management of drug resistance	Management of drug resistance (standard regimen) for epidemic TB conducted via introduction of resistance testing, second-line drugs, longer treatment regimen (12–18 months), and rigorous bacteriological and clinical monitoring	District hospital	Secondary prevention, cure	Adults over 15	207	201–212	—	—	5
Tuberculosis (epidemic, infectious)	Directly observed short-course chemotherapy	Short-course chemotherapy of infectious TB (allowing for transmission, non-HIV positive) carried out for epidemic TB	Clinic	Primary prevention, cure	Adults over 15	102	15–189	—	—	5

Tuberculosis (epidemic, latent)	Isoniazid treatment	Isoniazid treatment of latent infection (x-ray exclusion of active cases; non-HIV-positive population) is conducted for epidemic tuberculosis	District hospital	Secondary prevention	Adults over 15	197	45–348	—	5
Unwanted pregnancy	Family-planning programs	Intrauterine devices, voluntary sterilization, condoms and other barrier methods, implants, and oral contraceptives	Clinic	Primary prevention	Women of childbearing age	117	—	—	3
Zinc deficiency	Supplements with oral rehydration salts	Provision of zinc as an adjunct to oral rehydration salts in treating diarrhea in young children	Clinic or district hospital	Primary prevention	Children under 5	73	—	—	3

Source: Authors.

ACE = angiotensin — converting enzyme

Note: — = not available.

a. Refers to the age group to whom the intervention is targeted and not necessarily the one that is benefiting.

b. Ranges in cost-effectiveness reflect the variation in point estimates for specific interventions included in each intervention cluster and do not represent either variation across regions or statistical confidence intervals. Point estimates were obtained directly from the relevant chapters, calculated as the midpoint of range estimates reported in the chapters, or calculated from a population-weighted average of the region-specific estimates reported in the chapters. DALYs and deaths potentially avertable are for a 20 percentage point increase in intervention coverage in a hypothetical sample population of 1 million.

c. See table 2.1.

Table 2.B.2 Summary of Population-Based Interventions

Condition	Intervention	Intervention description	Intervention setting	Objective	Target population[a]	Cost-effectiveness (US$/DALY)	Cost-effectiveness range[b] (US$/DALY)	Number of DALYs averted[b] (hundreds)	Number of deaths averted[b]	Quality of cost-effectiveness analysis evidence[c]
Adolescent health and nutrition	School health and nutrition programs	Inclusion of deworming of intestinal worms and schistosomiasis; prompt recognition and treatment of malaria; insecticide-treated bednets; micronutrient supplements; breakfast, snacks, other meals; first-aid kits; referral to youth-friendly clinics; and counseling and psychosocial support	Community, school	Population-oriented medical intervention	School-age children	37	—	—	—	3
Alcohol abuse	Excise tax	25 to 50 percent increase in the current excise tax rate on alcoholic beverages	Policy level	Instrument of policy	Adolescents and adults	1,377	1,249–1,504	0.62	—	5
Alcohol abuse	Advertising ban and reduced access to beverage retail	Reduced access to alcoholic beverage retail outlets by reducing the hours of sale or advertising bans on television, radio, and billboards	Policy level	Instrument of policy	Adolescents and adults	404	367–441	0.44	—	5
Alcohol abuse	Excise tax, advertising ban, with brief advice	50 percent increase in the current excise tax rate on alcoholic beverages, combined with advice, education sessions, and psychosocial counseling; possible inclusion of random driver breath testing and advertising bans	Policy level	Instrument of policy	Adolescents and adults	631	601–661	2.85	—	5
Chagas disease	Vector control	Vector control activities including spraying combined with housing improvement, community involvement in surveillance, and strong programs of health education	Community	Control of environmental hazard	All ages	284 (Latin America and the Caribbean)	—	—	—	1 (Latin America and the Caribbean)

(Continues on the following page.)

Coronary artery disease	Legislation substituting 2% of trans fat with polyunsaturated fat at US$0.50 per adult	Legislation replacing 2% of dietary trans fat from partial hydrogenation in manufactured foods with polyunsaturated fat, at a cost of US$0.50 per adult, and assuming a 7% reduction in coronary artery disease	Policy level	Instrument of policy	Adults	48	—	—	—	5
Coronary artery disease	Legislation substituting 2% of trans fat with polyunsaturated fat at US$6 per adult	Legislation replacing 2% of dietary trans fat from partial hydrogenation in manufactured foods with polyunsaturated fat, at a cost of US$6 per adult, and assuming a 7–40% reduction in coronary artery disease	Policy level	Instrument of policy	Adults	838	199–1,478	—	—	5
Dengue	Vector control	Chemical vector control using larvicides and insecticide space sprays (including emephos, permethrin, methoprene, pyriproxyfen, and *Bacillus thuringiensis israelensis*) to protect drinking water, or environmental vector control, such as removal of standing water	Community or district hospital	Control of environmental hazard	All ages	2,566	1,992–3,139	—	—	2
Dengue	Immunization	Dengue immunization (a vaccine is currently undergoing clinical trials in Southeast Asia)	Community clinic or district hospital	Population-oriented medical intervention	Children	1,440	—	—	—	2
Diabetes, ischemic heart disease, and stroke	Legislation with public education to reduce salt content	Legislated reduction in salt content of manufactured foods and an accompanying public education campaign	Policy level	Instrument of policy	All ages	1,937	—	18.73	—	5
Diabetes, ischemic heart disease, and stroke	Media campaign to reduce saturated fat	Media campaign to reduce saturated fat content in manufactured foods and replace part of the saturated fat with polyunsaturated fat	2,617	Instrument of policy	All ages	2,617	—	13.86	—	5
Diarrheal disease	Breastfeeding promotion	Promotion of exclusive breastfeeding (recommended for six months) to new mothers, in which no other food or drink, including water, is permitted, except for supplements of vitamins and minerals and necessary medicines	Community, clinic, or district hospital	Personal behavior change	Adult women	930	—	0.43	1.33	5

Table 2.B.2 *(Continued)*

Condition	Intervention	Intervention description	Intervention setting	Objective	Target population[a]	Cost-effectiveness (US$/DALY)	Cost-effectiveness range[b] (US$/DALY)	Number of DALYs averted[b] (hundreds)	Number of deaths averted[b]	Quality of cost-effectiveness analysis evidence[c]
Diarrheal disease	Cholera or rotavirus immunization	Immunization for endemic cholera with live oral vaccine or rotavirus immunization with rhesus-human rotavirus reassortant-tetravalent vaccine (currently under development) in populations at risk of an outbreak	Clinic	Population-oriented medical intervention	Children	2,712	2,478–2,945	0.62	1.98	5
Diarrheal disease	Improved water and sanitation at current coverage of amenities and other interventions	Improved water supply and excreta disposal where established infrastructure currently exists, in urban or rural settings for at least five years	Community	Control of environmental hazards	All ages	4,185	1,974–6,396	3.52	315.30	5
Diarrheal disease	Hand pump, standpost, or house connection where clean water supply is limited	Installation of hand water pump, standpost, or house connection where clean water supply is limited and associated infrastructure currently do not exist	Community	Control of environmental hazards	All ages	159	—	—	—	1
Diarrheal disease	Water sector regulation with advocacy where clean water supply is limited	Surveillance of drinking water quality and quality of service by the water supply utility in terms of coverage, quantity, continuity, control of sanitary hazards, and cost, as well as advocacy of lower connection charges	Policy level, community	Instrument of policy, control of environmental hazards	All ages	47	—	—	—	1
Diarrheal disease	Construction and promotion of basic sanitation where facilities are limited	Construction of low-cost excreta disposal facilities such as household pit latrines, ventilation-improved latrines, or pour-flush toilets, combined with public promotion of sanitation and hygiene	Policy level, community	Instrument of policy, control of environmental hazards	All ages	141	11–270	—	—	1

Down syndrome	Prenatal screening with option of pregnancy termination	Prenatal genetic screening program, incorporating maternal serum triple screening of all pregnant women, for trisomy of chromosome 21, to allow parents to determine whether to continue with an affected pregnancy	Clinic, district hospital	Population-oriented medical intervention	Pregnant women	15	—	—	—	5
Emergency medical care	Training volunteer paramedics with lay first responders	Identification and training of community member first responders and paramedics to act in health emergencies, recognize life- or limb-threatening situations, transport patients, and provide basic first aid	Policy level	Instrument of policy	All ages	6	—	18.42	74.00	5
Emergency medical care	Staffed community ambulance	Introduction or promotion of training programs for emergency responders and ambulance drivers in urban or rural settings for countries that lack ambulances and training programs	Policy level	Instrument of policy	All ages	120	60–179	34.84	140.00	5
Haemophilus influenzae type B (Hib)	Vaccine containing Hib	Hib vaccination (three or four doses), given concurrently with diphtheria-pertussis-tetanus	Clinic	Population-oriented medical intervention	Infants and children	733[d]	—	29.25	113.83	5
Hib, and hepatitis B, diphtheria, pertussis, and tetanus	Pentavalent vaccine	Hib vaccination (three or four doses) and hepatitis B (three or four doses) given concurrently with diphtheria-pertussis-tetanus vaccine	Clinic	Population-oriented medical intervention	Infants and children	296[d]	—	—	—	5
Hepatitis B	Hepatitis B vaccination	Hepatitis B (three or four doses) given through intramuscular injection	Clinic	Population-oriented medical intervention	Infants and children	23,520[d]	—	—	—	5

(Continues on the following page.)

Table 2.B.2 *(Continued)*

Condition	Intervention	Intervention description	Intervention setting	Objective	Target population[a]	Cost-effectiveness (US$/DALY)	Cost-effectiveness range[b] (US$/DALY)	Number of DALYs averted[b] (hundreds)	Number of deaths averted[b]	Quality of cost-effectiveness analysis evidence[c]
HIV/AIDS	Condom promotion and distribution	Targeted distribution and placement of condoms in locations such as bars or brothels; distribution linked to voluntary counseling and testing and sexually transmitted infection care to ensure universal access; information, education, and communication, including education through literature, classroom, and clinical settings and radio, newspapers, and television	Community or Community, clinic	Personal behavior change	Adolescents and adults	82 (Sub-Saharan Africa)	52–112 (Sub-Saharan Africa)	—	—	1 (Sub-Saharan Africa)
HIV/AIDS	Blood and needle safety	Screening of all blood for transfusions; sterilization for all injections; harm reduction for injecting drug users, including needle exchange and drug substitution programs	All levels, including community clinics to referral hospitals	Population-oriented medical intervention	All ages	84 (Sub-Saharan Africa)	7–161 (Sub-Saharan Africa)	—	—	2 (Sub-Saharan Africa)
HIV/AIDS	Voluntary counseling and testing	Routine and voluntary confidential HIV counseling and testing	Clinic	Population-oriented medical intervention	Adults	47	10–85	—	—	2
HIV/AIDS	Peer and education programs for high-risk groups	Targeting community members (for example, students or commercial sex workers) to disseminate information and teach specific skills	Community	Personal behavior change	Adolescents and adults	37	6–68	—	—	2
Lymphatic filariasis	Annual mass drug administration	Two annual, single-dose, two-drug regimens are recommended: ivermectin plus albendazole in African countries that are coendemic for onchocerciasis, and diethylcarbamazine plus albendazole for all other endemic countries	Clinic, community	Population-oriented medical intervention	All ages	15 (South Asia)	4–27 (South Asia)	—	—	4 (South Asia)

Disease	Intervention	Description	Policy level	Type	Age group					
Lymphatic filariasis	Diethyl carbamazine salt	Fortification of salt with diethyl carbamazine	Policy level	Instrument of policy	All ages	22 (South Asia)	1–43 (South Asia)	—	—	4 (South Asia)
Lymphatic filariasis	Vector control	Integrated vector control to reduce overall prevalence of microfilaria parasites, such as polystyrene beads in vector (mosquito) breeding habitats	Policy level	Instrument of policy	All ages	160 (South Asia)	43–277 (South Asia)	—	—	4 (South Asia)
Malaria	Insecticide-treated bednets	Impregnation of bednets with deltamethrin, one treatment of permethrin, or two treatments of permethrin, with the bednets either purchased or subsidized	Household	Control of environmental hazards	All ages	11 (Sub-Saharan Africa)	5–17 (Sub-Saharan Africa)	376.00 (Sub-Saharan Africa)	1,429.60 (Sub-Saharan Africa)	5 (Sub-Saharan Africa)
Malaria	Residual household spraying	One or two doses of malathion, DDT, deltamethrin, or lambda-cyhalothrin applied to household surfaces	Household	Control of environmental hazards	All ages	17 (Sub-Saharan Africa)	9–24 (Sub-Saharan Africa)	376.00 (Sub-Saharan Africa)	1,429.60 (Sub-Saharan Africa)	5 (Sub-Saharan Africa)
Measles	Second opportunity vaccination in a fixed facility	Second opportunity to receive a dose of measles vaccine (either through routine or supplemental immunization activities) at a fixed facility	Clinic	Population-oriented medical intervention	Infants and children	4	—	—	—	5
Meningitis	Neisseria meningitidis vaccine	Neisseria meningitidis vaccine for serogroups A, C, Y, W135 only; unconjugated polysaccharides given subcutaneously; one dose with repeat three to five years later for those at high risk	Clinic	Population-oriented medical intervention	Children	12,632 (Sub-Saharan Africa)	—	—	—	5 (Sub-Saharan Africa)
Problems requiring surgery	Surgical ward or services in district hospital or community clinic	Surgical ward in a district hospital or community clinic to provide care for a wide range of conditions, such as trauma, childbirth, and abdominal conditions	District hospital, clinic	Instrument of policy	All ages	136	54–217	—	—	5
Onchocerciasis	Ivermectin	Annual dose of ivermectin	Clinic, community	Population-oriented medical intervention	Adults over 40	37	—	—	—	3
Soil-transmitted helminthic infections	Albendazole	Annual albendazole anti-helminthic drug treatment to reduce morbidity through the deworming of *Ascaris, Trichuris,* and hookworm in school-age children	Community, school	Population-oriented medical intervention	School-age children	3	—	—	127.76	1.98	5

(Continues on the following page.)

Table 2.B.2 *(Continued)*

Condition	Intervention	Intervention description	Intervention setting	Objective	Target population[a]	Cost-effectiveness (US$/DALY)	Cost-effectiveness range[b] (US$/DALY)	Number of DALYs averted[b] (hundreds)	Number of deaths averted[b]	Quality of cost-effectiveness analysis evidence[c]
Tetanus	Tetanus toxoid vaccination, mix of strategies	Tetanus toxoid vaccination via a mix of strategies depending on local needs, including fixed facilities, immunization campaigns, mobile delivery, and community outreach	Clinic, community	Population-oriented medical intervention	Infants and children	1,411	—	—	—	5
Tobacco addiction	Taxation causing 33% price increase	A 33 percent price increase due to tobacco taxes to discourage tobacco use, prevent initiation (and subsequent addiction) among youths, increase the likelihood of cessation among current users, reduce relapse among former users, and reduce consumption among continuing users	Policy level	Instrument of policy	Adolescents and adults	22	—	37.27	1,905.99	5
Tobacco addiction	Nonprice interventions	Advertising bans on television, radio, and billboards; health information and advertising in the form of health warning labels on tobacco products; interventions to reduce tobacco supply, such as smuggling control; restrictions on smoking	Policy level	Instrument of policy	Adolescents and adults	353	—	—	—	5
Traffic accidents	Increased speeding penalties, enforcement, media campaigns, and speed bumps	Minimizing exposure to high-risk scenarios by installation of speed bumps at hazardous junctions, increased penalties for speeding, and other effective road-safety regulations combined with media coverage and better enforcement of legislation	Policy level	Instrument of policy	Adults	21	3–38	0.67	197.16	5
Traffic accidents	Enforcement of seatbelt laws, promotion of child restraints and random driver breath testing	Mandatory seat belt and child-restraint laws, enforcement of drunk-driving laws, and random breath testing of drivers	Policy level	Instrument of policy	Adults	2,449	999–3,899	0.32	93.87	5

Condition	Intervention	Description	Setting	Type	Target population					
Tuberculosis (endemic)	BCG vaccine	Live attenuated vaccine, BCG; recommended at birth or at first contact with health services in areas of high incidence	Clinic or district hospital	Primary prevention Population-oriented medical intervention	Children	68	55–82	—	—	5
Tuberculosis, diphtheria, pertussis, tetanus, polio, measles	Traditional Expanded Program on Immunization (EPI)	Scaling up of EPI; a fixed increment of coverage added for each year 2002–11 to reach 90 percent; coverage increases assumed to result from switching to more effective and intensive implementation strategies rather than additional infrastructure investments	Community	Population-oriented medical intervention	Infants and children	7	—	—	—	5
Undernutrition and malnutrition	Sustained child health and nutrition program	Possible inclusion of prenatal care, women's health and nutrition, breastfeeding promotion and counseling, complementary feeding, growth monitoring and promotion, micronutrient supplementation, micronutrient fortification, supplementary feeding using local supplies, oral rehydration, and immunization and deworming; actual mix depends on local capabilities and conditions	Community, clinic	Population-oriented medical intervention	Children under five	225	—	—	—	3
Underweight children	Child survival program with nutrition component	Community-based nutrition programs to prevent growth faltering, control morbidity, and improve survival by promoting breastfeeding, providing education and counseling on optimal child feeding, preventing diarrheal disease, and monitoring growth	Community	Population-oriented medical intervention	Children under five	42	—	—	—	2

Source: Authors.

BCG = bacillus Calmette – Guérin; DDT = dichlorodiphenyl trichloroethane; EPI = Expanded Program on Immunizations

Note: — = not available.

a. Refers to the age group to whom the intervention is targeted and not necessarily the one that is benefiting.

b. Ranges in cost-effectiveness reflect the variation in point estimates for specific interventions included in each intervention cluster and do not represent either variation across regions or statistical confidence intervals. Point estimates were obtained directly from the relevant chapters, calculated as the midpoint of range estimates reported in the chapters, or calculated from a population-weighted average of the region-specific estimates reported in the chapters. DALYs and deaths potentially avertable are for a 20 percentage point increase in intervention coverage in a hypothetical sample population of 1 million.

c. See table 2.1.

d. Cost-effectiveness ratio calculated from deaths averted only.

Table 2.C.1 Cost Effectiveness of Other Personal Interventions

Condition	Intervention	Intervention description	Intervention setting	Objective	Target population	Cost-effectiveness estimate (US$)[a]	Quality of CEA evidence[b]
Breast cancer	Clinical breast exam	Examination of the breast performed by doctors or other trained health care professionals; annually, biennially, or every five years; for women ages 40–60	Clinic	Secondary prevention	Women ages 40–60	7,125–9,907 per death prevented (India); 522–722 per LYS (India)	4
Breast cancer	Screening mammography	Examination of the breasts performed by compressing the breast firmly between a plastic plate and an X-ray cassette that contains special X-ray film; one lifetime or biennially	Clinic	Secondary prevention	Women ages 40–70	12,262–24,493 per death prevented (India); 902–1846 per LYS (India); 2,450–14,790a per YLS (Europe); 28,600–47,900 (USA)	2 (USA, Europe); 4 (India)
Breast cancer	Chemotherapy and/or tamoxifen	Tamoxifen and/or chemotherapy for 45-year-old premenopausal women with early-stage breast cancer; for node-positive, node-negative, estrogen-receptor-positive, and estrogen-receptor-negative patients	District hospital	Secondary prevention	Women age 45	12,820–171,700 (USA)	3
Breast cancer	Radiation therapy	Radiation therapy following mastectomy and chemotherapy for node-positive breast cancer in premenopausal women	District hospital	Secondary prevention	Premenopausal women	23,300–44,000 per QALY (USA)	2
Cervical cancer	Nationwide Pap screening program based on five-year intervals	Nationwide Pap screening program based on five-year intervals	District hospital	Secondary prevention	Adult women	769 per YLS (Vietnam)	2
Cervical cancer	Conventional or liquid-based cytology testing	Conventional cytology using the Papanicolaou (Pap) smear and HPV testing every 1 to 10 years; or Liquid-based cytology using the Papanicolaou (Pap) smear and HPV testing every 1 to 5 years	District hospital	Secondary prevention	Adult women	126,500 (USA); 162,400 (Thailand)	2
Cervical cancer	Two-visit HPV testing	HPV DNA testing during the first visit followed by treatment of screen-positive women during the second visit	District hospital	Secondary prevention	Adult women	122 per YLS (Brazil); 167 per YLS (Madagascar); 41 per YLS (South Africa); 117 per YLS (Zimbabwe)	1
Cervical cancer	One-visit VIA	Cervix is viewed after the application of an acetic acid solution; screening and treatment conducted during the same visit	District hospital	Secondary prevention	Women age 35–42	56 per YLS (Brazil); 54 per YLS (Madagascar); 43 per YLS (Zimbabwe)	1
Cervical cancer	Three-visit cytology	Cytology sample obtained during the first visit, colposcopy for screen-positive women conducted during the second visit, and treatment provided during the third visit	District hospital	Secondary prevention	Women age 35–48	589 per YLS (Brazil); 379 per YLS (Madagascar); 331 per YLS (Zimbabwe)	1

Disease	Intervention	Description	Facility level	Category	Population	Cost-effectiveness	Priority
Cervical cancer	Chemoradiation therapy	Cisplatin-based chemoradiation regimens on the basis of published and estimated survival	District hospital	Secondary prevention	Adult women	337–31,400 per LYS (USA)	1
Chronic obstructive pulmonary disease	Inhaled medication	Inhaled ipratropium bromide or corticosteroid such as fluticasone propionate	Clinic/district hospital	Palliation	Adults	7,800–13,400 per QALY (High-income countries)	1
Chronic obstructive pulmonary disease	A-1 antitrypsin augmentation therapy	Intravenous treatment of chronic obstructive pulmonary disease related to severe deficiency; ranges with age and efficacy	Clinic/district hospital	Palliation	Adults	14,400–215,000 per QALY (High-income countries)	1
Chronic obstructive pulmonary disease, asthma, and cardiovascular disease	Mechanical ventilation or oxygen therapy	Mechanical ventilation with inspiratory support, invasive respiration in intensive care unit, or long-term home oxygen therapy	Clinic/district hospital	Palliation	Adults	15,000–19,000 per YLS (High-income countries); 32,350–47,850 per QALY (High-income countries)	1
Colorectal cancer	Flexible sigmoidoscopy every 5 years with or without fecal occult blood test	Flexible sigmoidoscopy enables the physician to look at the inside of the large intestine from the rectum through the last part of the colon, called the sigmoid or descending colon; fecal occult blood test checks stool samples for traces of blood.	District hospital	Secondary prevention	Adults	18,700–25,954 (USA)	2
Colorectal cancer	Double-contrast barium enema every 5 years	A series of x-rays of the colon and rectum taken after the patient is given an enema, followed by an injection of air. The barium outlines the intestines on the x-rays, allowing many abnormal growths to be visible. This is conducted every 5 years.	District hospital	Secondary prevention	Adults	11,503–26,393 per YLS (USA)	2
Colorectal cancer	Colonoscopy every 10 years	Colonoscopy allows the physician to look inside the entire large intestine, from the lowest part, the rectum, all the way up through the colon to the lower end of the small intestine. The procedure is used to look for early signs of cancer in the colon and rectum.	District hospital	Secondary prevention	Adults	9,309–22,672 per YLS (USA)	2
Colorectal cancer	Chemotherapy	Adjuvant chemotherapy for stage three colon cancer	District hospital	Secondary prevention	Adults	3,000–7,000 per YLS (High-income countries)	1
Colorectal cancer	Radiation therapy	Preoperative radiation therapy for rectal cancer patients; with varying rates of recurrence and survival advantage with and without radiation treatment	District hospital	Secondary prevention	Adults	908–15,228 per YLS (Sweden)	1

(Continues on the following page.)

Table 2.C.1 (*Continued*)

Condition	Intervention	Intervention description	Intervention setting	Objective	Target population	Cost-effectiveness estimate (US$)	Quality of CEA evidence
Diabetes	Smoking cessation	Counseling and medication such as the nicotine patch	Clinic	Primary prevention	Adolescents and adults	870 per QALY (EAP); 1,170 per QALY (ECA); 1,450 per QALY (LAC); 1,230 per QALY (MNA); 730 per QALY (SAR); 660 per QALY (SSA)	5
Diabetes	Annual eye examination	Dilated eye examination to detect proliferative diabetic retinopathy and macular edema followed by appropriate photocoagulation therapy to prevent blindness	Clinic	Secondary prevention	Adults	420 per QALY (EAP); 560 per QALY (ECA); 700 per QALY (LAC); 590 per QALY (MNA); 350 per QALY (SAR); 320 per QALY (SSA)	5
Diabetes	ACE inhibitor	ACE inhibitors for blood pressure control	Clinic	Secondary prevention	Adults	620 per QALY (EAP); 830 per QALY (ECA); 1,020 per QALY (LAC); 870 per QALY (MNA); 510 per QALY (SAR); 460 per QALY (SSA)	5
Diabetes	Metformin intervention for preventing type 2 diabetes	Metformin therapy for preventing type 2 diabetes among people at high risk, such as those with prediabetes	Clinic	Primary prevention	Adults	2,180 per QALY (EAP); 2,930 per QALY (ECA); 3,630 per QALY (LAC); 3,080 per QALY (MNA); 1,820 per QALY (SAR); 1,640 per QALY (SSA)	5
Diabetes	Cholesterol control	Cholesterol control for people with total cholesterol higher than 200 milligrams/deciliter	Clinic	Secondary prevention	Adults	4,420 per QALY (EAP); 5,940 per QALY (ECA); 7,350 per QALY (LAC); 6,240 per QALY (MNA); 3,680 per QALY (SAR); 3,330 per QALY (SSA)	5
Diabetes	Intensive glycemic control	Intensive glucose control to lower the level of glucose in the person with diabetes to a level close to that of a person without diabetes, for people with HbA1c higher than 8 percent, in order to prevent or delay long-term diabetes complications	Clinic	Secondary prevention	Adults	2,410 per QALY (EAP); 3,230 per QALY (ECA); 4,000 per QALY (LAC); 3,400 per QALY (MNA); 2,000 per QALY (SAR); 1,810 per QALY (SSA)	5
Kidney disease	Hemodialysis	Most common method used to treat advanced and permanent kidney failure; conducted in a treatment center or home.	Clinic, home	Secondary prevention	Adults	42,700–70,000 per YLS (USA); 61,000–99,400 per QALY (USA)	1

Kidney disease	Kidney transplant	Kidney transplant surgery	District or referral hospital	Cure	Adults	10,000 per LYS (USA); 11,000 per QALY (USA)	2
Kidney disease	ACE inhibitors	ACE inhibitors for all type-1 diabetics with macroproteinuria and all type-2 diabetics	Clinic	Secondary prevention	Adults	1,100–7,700 per QALY (USA)	4
Mild to moderate asthma	Quick-relievers in addition to inhaled corticosteriods	Rapid-acting bronchodilators that act to relieve bronchoconstriction and accompanying acute symptoms of wheeze, chest tightness, and cough, e.g., salbutamol; incremental to inhaled corticosteroid treatment	Clinic or district hospital	Palliation	Adults	10,600-13,900 per QALY (High-income countries)	1
Opioid abuse	Naltrexone induced rapid opioid detoxification under sedation (RODS)	Patient is given naltrexone under general anesthetic.	District hospital	Rehabilitation	Adults	2,498 per week of abstinence (Australia)	1
Opioid abuse	Conventional outpatient detoxification	Conventional outpatient detoxification is supervised withdrawal from a drug of dependence that attempts to minimize withdrawal symptoms.	Clinic	Rehabilitation	Adults	12,764 per abstinent patient (Australia)	1
Opioid abuse	Drug-free treatments	Residential or outpatient drug-free treatments as well as self-help group attendance	Clinic	Rehabilitation	Adults	7,000–13,000^a (USA)	1
Opioid abuse	Methadone maintenance substitution	Substitution of short-acting heroin with long-acting orally administered opioid Methadone; includes heroin users living in communities with high HIV prevalence	Clinic	Rehabilitation	Adults	6,800 per LYS (High-income countries); 9,000 per QALY (High-income countries, high-HIV prevalence)	1
Opioid abuse	Buprenorphine maintenance substitution	Buprenorphine substitution maintenance treatment for non-methadone patients.	Clinic	Rehabilitation	Adults	49,000 per QALY (High-income countries)	1
Osteoarthritis	Lifestyle change	Exercise (aquatic) and calcium supplements	Clinic	Primary/secondary prevention	Adults age 55–75; post-menopausal women	96,119–498,700 per QALY (High-income countries)	1
Osteoarthritis	Replacement surgery	Synovial fluid replacement (hylan G-F 20) for patients with osteoarthritis of the knee; or complete hip joint or knee replacement with implant	Clinic, district hospital	Secondary prevention; tertiary intervention	Elderly men and women	5,233–6893 per QALY (High income countries)	1
Osteoporosis	Hormone replacement therapy	Estrogen replacement from age 50, 60, or menopause for healthy women; 5-year to lifetime treatment	Clinic	Primary/secondary prevention	Postmenopausal women and women age 50 and up	5,088–23,734 per QALY	1

(Continues on the following page.)

Table 2.C.1 *(Continued)*

Condition	Intervention	Intervention description	Intervention setting	Objective	Target population	Cost-effectiveness estimate (US$)[a]	Quality of CEA evidence[b]
Osteoporosis	Calcium supplements with or without vitamin D	Calcium with or withouth vitamin D supplements, based on evidence that it reduces appendicular fractures; assumes a compliance rate of 70%	Clinic	Primary prevention	Women age 50 to 80	37,633–149,705 per QALY	1
Osteoporosis	Nonestrogen drug treatments	Raloxifene or calcitonin to reduce bone fractures; with or without 5 years of therapy	Clinic	Secondary prevention	Postmenopausal women age 50 to 80	34,166–835,622 per QALY (High income Countries)	1
Osteoporosis	Fluoride	Fluoride appears to decrease the risk of vertebral fracture for women with established osteoporosis; assumes neutral effect on hip fractures	Clinic	Secondary prevention	Postmenopausal women	46,684 per QALY (UK)	1
Pain	Morphine	Providing oral morphine and necessary associated drugs	Clinic	Palliation	All ages	210–408 per year of pain free life added (Chile, Romania, Uganda)	4
Primary care ailments	Limited care	Includes treatment of infection and minor trauma; for more complicated condition, includes diagnosis, advice and pain relief, and treatment as resources permit	Clinic	Cure	All ages	253–380 per DALY (Low income countries); 507–760 per DALY (Middle income countries)	1
Respiratory disease (end stage)	Lung transplant	Surgical replacement with donor lung	District hospital	Cure	Adults	238,200–464,000 per QALY (High-income countries)	1

Source: Authors.

a. Currency units in US$, but not necessarily 2001.

b. See table 2.1.

Table 2.C.2 Cost-Effectiveness of Other Population-Based Interventions

Condition	Intervention	Intervention description	Intervention setting	Objective	Target population	Cost-effectiveness estimate (US$)[a]	Quality of CEA evidence[b]
Asthma	Education	Education in addition to exercise program	Clinic	Personal behavior change	Adults	71,500/QALY (High-income countries)	1
Colorectal cancer	Fecal occult blood test	Fecal occult blood test to check stool samples for traces of blood; conducted annually or biennially	District hospital	Secondary prevention	Adults	3,200–12,100 per YLS (High-income countries)	2
Diarrhea	Improved quality of care	Educational interventions to improve quality of care and encourage oral rehydration therapy in hospitals; varies with marginal improvement; low to average prevalence	Clinic/district hospital	Instrument of policy	All ages	14–6000[a] per death averted	4
Diabetes	Lifestyle intervention (type 2 prevention)	Behavioral change for weight reduction by means of a combination of a low-calorie diet and moderate physical activity	Clinic	Personal behavior change	Adults	80 per QALY (EAP); 100 per QALY (ECA); 130 per QALY (LAC); 110 per QALY (MNA); 60 per QALY (SAR); 60 per QALY (SSA)	5
Diabetes	Influenza and pneumococcal vaccinations	Influenza and pneumococcal vaccinations for elderly individuals with type 2 diabetes	Clinic	Population-oriented medical intervention	Elderly	220 per QALY (EAP); 290 per QALY (ECA); 360 per QALY (LAC); 310 per QALY (MNA); 180 per QALY (SAR); 160 per QALY (SSA)	5
Diabetes	Screening	Screening of individuals at increased risk for undiagnosed diabetes	Clinic, district hospital	Population-oriented medical intervention	Adults over 25	5,140 per QALY (EAP); 6,910 per QALY (ECA); 8,550 per QALY (LAC); 7,260 per QALY (MNA); 4,280 per QALY (SAR); 3,870 per QALY (SSA)	5
Diabetes	Annual screening for microalbuminuria	Screening for microalbuminuria and treating those who test positive	Clinic, district hospital	Population-oriented medical intervention	Adults	3,310 per QALY (EAP); 4,450 per QALY (ECA); 5,510 per QALY (LAC); 4,680 per QALY (MNA); 2,760 per QALY (SAR); 2,500 per QALY (SSA)	5
Indoor air pollution-related illness	Liquefied petroleum gas	Substitution of wood, dung, and crop residues with liquefied petroleum gas for cooking and heating	Policy level	Instrument of policy	All ages	103–1,746 per healthy year (EAP); 1,258–1,361 per healthy year (ECA); 806–1,447 per healthy year (LAC); 779–785 per healthy year (MNA); 321–558 per healthy year (SA); 534–736 per healthy year (SSA)	5

(Continues on the following page.)

Table 2.C.2 *(Continued)*

Condition	Intervention	Intervention description	Intervention setting	Objective	Target population	Cost-effectiveness estimate (US$)[a]	Quality of CEA evidence[b]
Indoor air pollution-related illness	Kerosene	Substitution of wood, dung, and crop residues with kerosene for cooking and heating	Policy level	Instrument of policy	All ages	12–232 per healthy year (EAP); 172–188 per healthy year (ECA); 109–650 per healthy year (LAC); 98 per healthy year (MNA): 37–65 per healthy year (SAR); 62–87 per healthy year (SSA)	5
Indoor air pollution-related illness	Improved stove	Replacement of traditional open stoves with enclosed stoves that are more efficient and/or have flues for ventilation	Policy level	Instrument of policy	All ages	306–605 per healthy year (EAP); 975–1,134 per healthy year (LAC); 379–471 per healthy year (MNA): 13–15 per healthy year (SAR); 21–26 per healthy year (SSA)	5
Indoor air pollution-related illness	Improved stove with kerosene or LPG	Replacement of traditional open stoves with enclosed stoves that use kerosene or liquified petroleum gas (LPG)	Policy level	Instrument of policy	All ages	26–85 per healthy year (EAP); 522–1,416 per healthy year (ECA); 305–784 per healthy year (LAC); 227–624 per healthy year (MNA): 27–182 per healthy year (SAR); 46–304 per healthy year (SSA)	5
Lung cancer	Early detection screening	Screening of high-risk individuals, such as current and former smokers, for lung cancer using helical computed tomography	District hospital	Population-oriented medical intervention	Adults	20,000–100,000 per YLS (USA)	3
Pneumonia	Improved quality of care	Improved quality of care, including education for health providers and treatment of non-severe and severe pneumonia; varies with marginal improvement; low to average prevalence	Clinic/district hospital	Instrument of policy	Children	132–5,000[a] per death averted	4
Pollution-related illness	Control of toxins related to energy industry	Interventions include coal-fired power plant emissions controls, gasoline lead reduction, and desulphuring of residual fuel oil	Policy level	Instrument of policy	All ages	less than 0 per LYS (USA)	1
Pollution-related illness	Control of toxins related to agriculture and forestry	Interventions include targeted pesticide bans and emissions standards at processing facilities	Policy level	Instrument of policy	All ages	less than 0 per LYS (USA)	1
Pollution-related illness	Control of toxins related to residential sector	Interventions include radon remediation and sedimentation, filtration, and chlorination of drinking water	Policy level	Instrument of policy	All ages	5320–7730 per LYS (USA)	1

Pollution-related illness	Control of toxins related to industrial sector	Interventions include arsenic emissions standards at copper smelters and asbestos ban for brake linings	Policy level	Instrument of policy	All ages	less than 45,600 per LYS (USA)	
Silicosis	Engineering control	Wet method e.g. spraying a surface or wetting a blade to reduce dust; local exhaust ventilation; total plant ventilation	Policy level	Control of environ-mental hazards	Working adults	105[a] per DALY (USA and Canada); 109[a] per DALY (Western Pacific)	3
Silicosis	Comfort or dust mask	Comfort or dust mask with associated training	Policy level	Instrument of policy	Working adults	111–191[a] per DALY (USA and Canada); 117–174[a] (Western Pacific)	3
Silicosis	Respirator	Half-face or full-face respirator and asso-ciated training	Policy level	Instrument of policy	Working adults	300–305[a] per DALY (USA and Canada); 266–274[a] per DALY (Western Pacific)	3

Source: Authors.
a. Currency units in US$, but not necessarily 2001.
b. See table 2.1.

NOTES

1. Few other cost-effectiveness studies have covered a similarly extensive set of health interventions (Dixon and Welch 1991; Jamison and others 1993; Tengs and others 1995), and only one of those studies makes these comparisons on a global scale (Jamison and others 1993). The current World Health Organization project CHOICE (Choosing Interventions That Are Cost-Effective) is a parallel effort to make such global comparisons (Murray and others 2000; http://www.who.int/evidence/cea).

2. Of these 319 cost-effectiveness estimates, 257 were in terms of U.S. dollars per DALY and therefore comparable. Interventions with cost-effectiveness in terms of dollars per DALY were grouped into 121 intervention clusters to facilitate analyses and presentation.

3. *Health system capacity* is often used to describe both the level of care (primary, secondary, and tertiary) and the institutional and organizational capacities. We use the term to refer to the latter.

4. Chapter 15 presents a fuller discussion of these methods. Note that not all chapters have used these standardized costs. Furthermore, the analyses have used U.S. dollars rather than purchasing-power parity dollars (which provide a better measure of input resource intensity and are less susceptible to exchange rate fluctuations) in order to provide a monetary estimate that may be more useful to policy makers and donors.

5. Noneconomic reasons for maintaining certain interventions can include retaining key technical skills that may be required in the future and may lead to the development of new methods that may be more cost-effective (see chapter 66 on referral hospitals for a more in-depth discussion).

6. Some interventions with high potential to reduce the burden of disease may have been excluded due to the way their cost-effectiveness ratios were calculated. For example, nutrition-related interventions are excluded from the table because those evaluated in the volume address either vitamin A deficiency or iodine deficiency both of which are associated with low avertable burden. Also, only the burden of children age 0 to 4 was considered, further lowering the avertable burden. Another example is of the integrated management of infant and childhood illness, which is evaluated for Sub-Saharan Africa but not for the South Asia Region.

7. The second and third observations speak more generally to the global public goods nature of health research (see chapter 4 for an in-depth discussion). In relation to both HIV/AIDS and noncommunicable diseases, the responsiveness of the medical research system to threats to populations in developed countries has the potential to bring great benefits to people living in LMICs.

REFERENCES

Birch, S., and C. Donaldson. 1987. "Cost-Benefit Analysis: Dealing with the Problems of Indivisible Projects and Fixed Budgets." *Health Policy* 7 (1): 61–72.

Cookson, R., and P. Dolan. 1999. "Public Views on Health Care Rationing: A Group Discussion Study." *Health Policy* 49 (1–2): 63–74.

———. 2000. "Principles of Justice in Health Care Rationing." *Journal of Medical Ethics* 26 (5): 323–29.

Dixon, J., and H. G. Welch. 1991. "Priority Setting: Lessons from Oregon." *Lancet* 337 (8746): 891–94.

Jamison, D. T., W. H. Mosley, A. R. Measham, and J. L. Bobadilla. 1993. *Disease Control Priorities in Developing Countries.* New York: Oxford University Press.

Joesoef, M. R., P. L. Remington, and P. T. Jiptoherijanto. 1989. "Epidemiological Model and Cost-Effectiveness Analysis of Tuberculosis Treatment Programs in Indonesia." *International Journal of Epidemiology* 18 (1): 174–79.

Johns, B., and T. T. Torres. 2005. "Costs of Scaling up Health Interventions: A Systematic Review." *Health Policy and Planning* 20 (1): 1–13.

Kamolratanakul, P., B. Chunhaswasdikul, A. Jittinandana, V. Tangcharoensathien, N. Udomrati, and S. Akksilp. 1993. "Cost-Effectiveness Analysis of Three Short-Course Anti-tuberculosis Programs Compared with a Standard Regimen in Thailand." *Journal of Clinical Epidemiology* 46 (7): 631–36.

Mathers, C. D., C. J. L. Murray, and A. D. Lopez. 2006. "The Burden of Disease and Mortality by Condition: Data, Methods and Results for the Year 2001." In *Global Burden of Disease and Risk Factors,* ed. A. D. Lopez, C. D. Mathers, M. Ezzati, D. T. Jamison, and C. J. L. Murray. New York: Oxford University Press.

Murray, C. J. L., D. B. Evans, A. Acharya, and R. M. P. M. Baltussen. 2000. "Development of WHO Guidelines on Generalized Cost-Effectiveness Analysis." *Health Economics* 9: 235–51.

Murray, C. J. L., K. Styblo, and A. Rouillon. 1993. "Tuberculosis." In *Disease Control Priorities in Developing Countries,* ed. D. T. Jamison, W. H. Mosley, A. R. Measham, and J. L. Bobadilla, 233–59. New York: Oxford University Press.

Musgrove, P. 1999. "Public Spending on Health Care: How Are Different Criteria Related?" *Health Policy* 47 (3): 207–23.

Tengs, T. O. 1997. "Dying Too Soon: How Cost-Effectiveness Can Save Lives." NCPA Policy Report 204, National Center for Policy Analysis, Dallas, TX.

Tengs, T. O., M. E. Adams, J. S. Pliskin, D. G. Safran, J. E. Siegel, M. C. Weinstein, and J. G. Graham. 1995. "Five Hundred Life Saving Interventions and Their Cost-Effectiveness." *Risk Analysis* 15 (3): 369–90.

WHO (World Health Organization). 1999. *TB Advocacy: A Practical Guide 1999.* Geneva: WHO Global Tuberculosis Program.

———. 2004. *Global Tuberculosis Control: Surveillance, Planning, Financing.* Geneva: WHO.

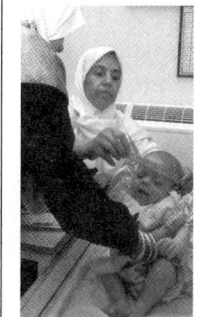

Chapter **3**

Strengthening Health Systems

Anne Mills, Fawzia Rasheed, and Stephen Tollman

Interventions are not generally provided as freestanding activities but are delivered in a variety of packages and through different levels of a health system.[1] For this reason, this book—in addition to including the disease- and program-specific chapters—addresses not only the cost-effectiveness of levels of care, packages of care, and services but also the strengthening of the management of health systems as a whole.

Cost-effectiveness data reflect largely what can be achieved in a reasonably well-functioning health system. In that sense, they can be considered to represent potential cost-effectiveness and need to be supplemented with evidence and guidance on how health systems can be strengthened to provide interventions effectively, efficiently, and equitably. This argument is given added weight by evidence on inadequacies in the performance of health institutions in countries at all levels of development (Hensher 2001; Preker and Harding 2003). Hensher (2001) documents the extensive inefficiencies in low- and middle-income countries, including the following:

- failure to minimize the physical inputs used—for example, prescribing excessive quantities of drugs
- failure to use the mix of inputs that costs the least—for instance, allocating a high proportion of expenditure to staff salaries and only a small share to operating costs and maintenance
- failure to operate at the appropriate scale—for example, running extremely large hospitals that suffer from scale inefficiencies
- failure to pay staff enough to encourage good performance.

Hensher estimates that hospital inefficiencies could easily account for up to 10 percent of total health spending.

Such inefficiencies have two main causes. First, they may occur because decision makers lack incentives to behave efficiently; for example, their promotion chances may not depend on how well they perform in managing a hospital. Second, decision makers may be constrained in their ability to make efficient choices; for instance, they may lack knowledge or experience of what to do or political factors may affect whether they can dismiss underperforming staff members or determine which company they must buy drugs from. Evidence on the quality of care (chapter 70) demonstrates that health systems may not merely be inefficient in failing to minimize costs but may also fail to deliver effective care.

The extent of inequities is also a major concern. Recent analyses show that even when interventions are provided, the poorest members of society usually have the least access to them (Gwatkin and others 2000). In many countries, gaps in child mortality between the poor and the better off widened during the 1990s (World Bank 2004). Thus, health systems need to have the capacity not only to deliver interventions efficiently but also to sustain high levels of coverage, especially of the poorest and most vulnerable.

Awareness has grown that international targets, such as the Millennium Development Goals (MDGs) and the provision of antiretroviral treatment for HIV/AIDS patients cannot be achieved without the key elements of a functioning health system. The example of the reduction of maternal mortality in Sri Lanka (chapter 8) demonstrates the improvements in health outcomes that are possible once a basic platform of functioning health services is available on which targeted initiatives can build (Levine 2004).

Thus, the aim of this chapter is to review how health systems can be strengthened in differing country contexts to deliver interventions effectively, efficiently, and equitably. The chapter is mainly concerned with strengthening health services: issues in managing core public health functions are reviewed elsewhere (Khaleghian and Das Gupta 2004). Although the chapter seeks to draw valuable lessons from all parts of the world, it focuses on countries with the least capacity, especially the poorer countries in Sub-Saharan Africa and Asia.

HISTORY AND CURRENT THEMES

Efforts to improve health in low- and middle-income countries over the past 50 years can be divided into a number of periods, with pendulum swings between focused, disease-specific support and broader health service or health system support. The 1950s, 1960s, and 1970s witnessed a number of successful disease control efforts, often termed *mass campaigns*—notably smallpox eradication, but also, for example, malaria and yaws control (Walt 2001). These mass campaigns built on earlier efforts, including those of the Rockefeller Foundation from the 1920s in controlling hookworm, yellow fever, and malaria. Despite regional differences in the degree of progress—for example, malaria control was not attempted in most of Sub-Saharan Africa—successes in regional and global control of diseases such as Chagas disease and measles in Latin America and the Caribbean and, more recently, polio worldwide have continued since the 1960s.

From early in the history of mass campaigns, the terminology used was of *vertical* and *horizontal* approaches (Gonzalez 1965), referring essentially to two key dimensions in program organization (Mills 2005): the extent to which program management was integrated into general health systems management, especially at lower management levels, as opposed to kept strictly separate, and the extent to which health workers had one function as opposed to many functions. Vertical programs (also known as *categorical programs*) had their own financing, management structures, and staff, even down to the service delivery level, instead of relying on existing systems. In contrast, horizontal programs delivered a number of services through the general health service structure.

In malaria control, for example, the World Health Organization defined a process whereby an initial vertical approach would evolve into a horizontal approach as the incidence of malaria fell. Initially, the effort required to detect and treat cases demanded dedicated and mobile workers. As transmission was reduced, these workers would detect fewer and fewer cases, so on efficiency grounds, detection and treatment activities needed to be handed over to the general health service infrastructure. However, this approach faced the dilemma that such services were often not strong enough to carry the control efforts forward.

The Alma Ata Declaration of 1978 was a turning point. The increasing emphasis on building networks of peripheral health services in a number of postindependence Sub-Saharan African countries and the health successes of countries such as China and Cuba influenced a new international emphasis on a broadly based definition of primary health care. Quickly, however, the advocates of more focused disease-specific efforts responded with the notion of selective primary health care (Walsh and Warren 1980), focused on a limited number of presumed cost-effective interventions.

Since 1980, this tension in international health policy has persisted, with four main strands, namely:

1. The health care reform movement of the 1990s, which has continued into the new millennium in a somewhat attenuated form, has focused almost exclusively on financing and organizational changes, largely neglecting the question of whether improved health outcomes have been achieved.
2. The definition and development of cost-effective packages of care has progressed, as reviewed in chapter 64, with some attention given to their implications for services and systems.
3. The emphasis on specific disease-focused international programs, as reflected in the Global Fund for AIDS, Tuberculosis, and Malaria, has been increasing, and resources for such programs have been expanding.
4. The effort to encourage investment in integrated health services has continued.

Recent events indicate that these tensions remain unresolved. For example, Molyneux and Nantulya (2004) call for combining community-driven, global health initiatives (including drug distribution for schistosomiasis, filariasis, and onchocerciasis; trachoma control; bednet distribution for malaria control; and immunization), with little mention of how community-based efforts might link with the general health infrastructure. In contrast, Unger, de Paepe, and Green (2003) examine how best to implement disease control programs so as to strengthen existing health systems and propose a code of best practice for such programs.

This debate is being given a new urgency by the introduction of treatment for HIV/AIDS. Immunization can be delivered using either a vertical or a horizontal approach. HIV/AIDS treatment, which requires continuing care, calls for strong health service backup. Nonetheless, such treatment services could be organized so that they isolate themselves from the broader health system—say, through separate clinics with their own workers and separate laboratories—or they could contribute to a greater degree of integration by sharing resources.

The implications of these different approaches for health system change are not purely academic. Table 3.1 compares the responses to health system constraints that derive from a

Table 3.1 Typical Health System Constraints and Possible Disease-Specific and Health System Responses

Constraint	Disease-specific response	Health system response
Financial inaccessibility: inability to pay, informal fees	Allowing exemptions or reducing prices for focal diseases	Developing risk-pooling strategies
Physical inaccessibility: distance to facility	Providing outreach for focal diseases	Reconsidering long-term plans for capital investment and siting of facilities
Inappropriately skilled staff	Organizing in-service training workshops to develop skills in focal diseases	Reviewing basic medical and nursing curricula to ensure that basic training includes appropriate skills
Poorly motivated staff	Offering financial incentives for the delivery of particular priority services	Instituting performance review systems, creating greater clarity about roles and expectations, reviewing salary structures and promotion procedures
Weak planning and management	Providing ongoing education and training workshops to develop planning and management skills	Restructuring ministries of health, recruiting developing a cadre of dedicated managers
Lack of intersectoral action and partnership	Creating disease-focused, cross-sectoral committees and task forces at the national level	Building systems of local government that incorporate representatives from health, education, and agriculture, promoting the accountability of local governance structures to the people
Poor-quality care among private sector providers	Offering training for private sector providers	Developing accreditation and regulation systems

Source: Travis and others 2004.

disease-specific focus as opposed to a health systems focus. A disease-specific focus leads to solutions for the specific program, whereas a health systems focus identifies a somewhat different set of reform priorities that relate to system-level changes and affect disease management across multiple diseases and conditions. The disease-focused responses can generally be implemented relatively quickly, whereas the systems-focused actions take longer. However, numerous, separate disease-specific responses can rapidly overwhelm frontline workers and managers.

HEALTH SYSTEM CONSTRAINTS ON THE DELIVERY OF PUBLIC AND PERSONAL HEALTH SERVICES

The challenge of scaling up services to meet the health-related MDGs and concerns that the multiple international efforts may overwhelm countries' fragile infrastructures have encouraged efforts to think systematically about health system constraints on achieving the MDGs, and the extent to which additional funding can readily and quickly improve services (Ranson, Hanson, and Mills 2003; Travis and others 2004). Weaknesses in service delivery—for example, at the health center level—may stem from problems at that level, such as staff shortages, or may be affected by factors higher up the system, such as a poor drug distribution system. Ranson and others (2003) therefore analyze constraints by five different levels: community and household, health services delivery, health sector policy and strategic management, public policies cutting across sectors, and environmental and contextual characteristics (see table 3.2).

At the community and household level, lack of demand can limit coverage. This lack may stem from cultural factors, such as low acceptability of immunization or prenatal care, but it may also result from financial and physical barriers to access. For example, estimates indicate that, in Niger, children under five average only 0.5 visits to a health provider per year, and in Bangladesh, only 8 percent of ill children were taken to a qualified provider (see chapter 63). Many barriers can be reduced by increasing accessibility, for example, by expanding the service infrastructure closer to communities. In Cameroon, Litvack and Bodart's (1993) study finds that a combination of user fees and improved quality, including a better drug supply and improved geographic access, led to increased use despite the user fees.

Low use may stem less from inaccessibility than from low quality at the level of health care delivery. Low quality can result from human resource shortages, limited incentives for the staff to provide good quality care, training inappropriate to local needs, poor drug supply systems, and lack of simple equipment such as that needed to measure blood pressure (Southern Africa Stroke Prevention Initiative Project Team 2004). In Tanzania, an analysis of the treatment-seeking decisions of those who later died from malaria showed that the great majority had preferred modern medicine, even for cerebral malaria, which according to a substantial body of evidence mothers view as a condition best treated by traditional healers (de Savigny and others 2004). Yet despite high rates of seeking modern medicine, malaria mortality remained high, whether because of delay in seeking treatment, poor quality care, or poor patient adherence. Treatment quality can be improved by increasing resources, although it may also demand change

Table 3.2 Constraints on Improving Access to Essential Health Interventions, by Level

Level of constraint	Types of constraints
Community and household	Lack of demand for effective interventions
	Barriers to the use of effective interventions (physical, financial, social)
Health services delivery	Shortages and inadequate distribution of appropriately qualified staff
	Weak technical guidance, program management, and supervision
	Inadequate drugs and medical supplies
	Lack of equipment and infrastructure, including poor accessibility of health services
Health sector policy and strategic management	Weak and overly centralized planning and management systems
	Weak drug policies and drug supply system
	Inadequate regulation of pharmaceutical and private sectors and improper industry practices
	Lack of intersectoral action and partnership for health between government and civil society
	Weak incentives to use inputs efficiently and to respond to users' needs and preferences
	Reliance on aid agency funding, which reduces flexibility and ownership
	Aid agency practices that overload country management capacity
Public policies cutting across sectors	Government bureaucracy (civil service rules and remuneration, centralized management system)
	Poor availability of communications and transportation infrastructure
Environmental and contextual characteristics	Governance and overall policy framework:
	• Corruption, weak government, weak rule of law, weak enforceability of contracts
	• Political instability and insecurity
	• Low priority attached to social sectors
	• Weak structures for public accountability
	• Lack of a free press
	Physical environment:
	• Climatic and geographic predisposition to disease
	• Physical environment unfavorable to service delivery

Source: Hanson and others 2003.

higher up the system; for example, better health worker performance may not be possible without reforming human resource management systems.

Performance at the third level, health sector policy and strategic management, can have a pervasive influence on performance at lower levels and is less easy to address through additional funding alone. Some improvements, such as orienting management more toward good performance and reduced corruption, may require a change in organizational culture or a change in structures—for instance, decentralizing authority or creating autonomous agencies. Such changes can be difficult and may take time to implement (Preker and Harding 2003). Other improvements require action outside the country—for example, a change in aid agency practices so that weak country management structures are not overloaded by multiple demands and reporting structures.

Finally, at the highest levels, broad multisectoral public policies and environmental and contextual characteristics set limits on what the health sector can change without help. For exam-

ple, wage policies for the public sector health staff are usually set centrally and linked to overall levels of pay for the public sector. Even if funds are available, increasing the wages of only health staff members may not be possible.

At this highest level, constraints also reflect much broader institutional influences, as was demonstrated by recent analyses of the results of efforts to build state capacity in Africa. Levy's (2004) review points out that the results are mixed at best. For example, of all World Bank civil service reform projects completed by 1997, only 29 percent were rated as satisfactory by the operations evaluation department. Levy argues that a key reason for the limited success was an implicit presumption that the weakness of public administration was managerial and could be remedied through organizational change and financial support for technical advice, hardware, and training. However, public administrations are part of political institutions and of social, economic, and political interests more broadly, and they do not change readily or quickly. Nevertheless, windows of opportunity may open that drastically affect the chances of change within a few years. Consider the cases of Mozambique, Rwanda, and Uganda, all countries that experienced many years of conflict and economic collapse but that have since made significant progress in reforming government institutions and performance. Apart from those exceptional cases, Levy argues that the way forward for administrative reform is likely to be an incremental one.

In general, straightforward shortages of buildings, equipment, and drugs and a lack of specific skills on the part of health workers and managers can be addressed fairly rapidly with additional funding. Remedying staff shortages takes somewhat longer, especially if the education system is producing insufficient numbers of people with the qualifications needed to enter health training programs. The constraints most impervious to additional funding are likely to relate to broader systems and institutional deficiencies, such as a bureaucratic culture that does not reward good performance and political systems that ignore the voices of the poor. Long-term and carefully phased capacity building in the broadest sense, including political development and strengthened governance structures, is likely to be required to relax these constraints (Mills and others 2001).

ASSESSMENT OF APPROACHES TO STRENGTHEN HEALTH SYSTEM CAPACITY

Strengthening health system capacity to improve performance is a wide-ranging subject, likely to require action—often simultaneously or appropriately sequenced—on many fronts. In particular, it requires attention to the various functions of the health system, especially to the various dimensions of management, as well as to the relationships between the health system, its patients (clients), and their communities. Evidence on which approaches work best is limited. The coverage of this section is therefore selective, drawing on chapters in part III and focusing on stewardship and regulation, organizational structures and their financing, and general management functions—namely, human resources and quality assurance.

When possible, we identify general lessons and note instances of relevant country experiences. In interpreting them, readers will need to keep in mind the strengths and weaknesses of their own country's health system. For example, in South Africa, where basic hospital supplies are good, improved training of health staff members reduced case-fatality rates for severe malnutrition, whereas in settings that experience shortages of antibiotics, potassium, and milk powder and that lack a doctor, training alone is highly unlikely to reduce high case-fatality rates (Ashworth and others 2004).

Stewardship and Regulation

Saltman and Ferroussier-Davis (2000, 735) explain stewardship as a "function of governments responsible for the welfare of populations and concerned about the trust and legitimacy with which its activities are viewed by the general public." The importance of the stewardship role is indicated by analyses that suggest that, in countries with good governance, a relationship is apparent between increased health spending and reduced child mortality (chapter 9), but that such a relationship is not apparent in countries that scored less well on indicators of good governance.

Strengthening structures of accountability to communities and introducing mechanisms to ensure that users have a voice in the local health system and can influence priorities are likely to be important in encouraging good performance. Methods to increase the transparency of resource allocation to peripheral services are also needed. In Burkina Faso, participation by community representatives in public primary health care clinics has increased the coverage of immunization, the availability of essential drugs, and the percentage of women who get two or more prenatal visits. In Ceara, Brazil, strengthened community accountability mechanisms helped improve service delivery (chapter 9). Factors identified as important to the success of community-based health and nutrition programs in chapter 56 include the existence of an effective, respected, and socially inclusive organization at the community level that builds on established community procedures.

Because of the substantial role that private sources of care play in almost all low- and middle-income countries, regulating and developing creative ways to work with the private sector are important. This effort needs to be seen as part of the stewardship role. Even though most countries have a network of regulations controlling private providers and products such as drugs, the regulations are often outdated and poorly enforced and can even be counterproductive (box 3.1).

Evidence is growing that using a mix of measures to influence both consumers and providers can improve the quality of care obtained through private providers. Chapter 70 provides several examples, including introducing total quality management practices and training with peer review feedback. Providers in the informal sector are some of the hardest to reach because of their wide distribution, small scale, and minimal education; however, some evidence indicates that their dispensing practices can be improved (box 3.2).

Regulation can be used as an intervention in its own right, as well as a way to improve health service delivery. The list of interventions identified as success stories (chapter 8) includes these in which a change in regulation was at the root of success:

- regulations requiring all sex workers in brothels to use condoms in Thailand
- tobacco control legislation in Poland and South Africa
- provision of a legal and regulatory framework for adding fluoride to salt in Jamaica
- legislation banning the sale of noniodized salt in China.

Bringing de Jure and de Facto Regulations in Line

In Tanzania, local drug shops are important sources of drugs. They are required to obtain a permit each year and to meet certain conditions related to premises, qualifications of the seller, and products (nonprescription medicines only). A study in three districts found that, despite regular inspections of drug shops, infringement of the regulations was widespread—including the sale of prohibited or inappropriately packaged drugs, which inspectors must have known about. Illegal drug sales may have contributed to poor-quality treatment and encouraged the development of drug resistance, but they had important benefits in terms of accessibility, because drug supplies in drug shops were more reliable than those in government facilities. Revising the regulations to permit drug shops to stock a small set of oral antibiotics, for example, would allow more constructive engagement between sales staff members and regulators, including the provision of information on essential drugs, registered brands, appropriate dosing, and consumer advice. The Strategies for Enhancing Access to Medicines Project is experimenting with allowing a wider range of drugs to be provided in one region using accredited outlets for dispensing drugs (drug shops that meet specified quality criteria and whose staff members have been trained by the project).

Source: Goodman 2004.

Improving the Quality of Drug Dispensing by Private Sector Shops

In Kilifi district, Kenya, an education program piloted by the Kenya Medical Research Institute–Wellcome Trust Collaborative Research Programme worked with district health managers to train and inform rural drug retailers and communities. Its effect was evaluated by means of annual household surveys of drug use and shop surveys in an early and a late implementation area. The program showed major improvements in drug-selling practices. Between 1998 and 1999, the proportion of antimalarial drug users obtaining an adequate dose rose from 8 to 33 percent, and by 2001, with a national change to sulfadoxine pyrimethamine, to 64 percent. The proportion of those with malarial fevers who received an adequate dose of a recommended antimalarial drug within 24 hours rose from 1 to 28 percent by 2001.

Source: Marsh and others 2004.

Given that enforcement is the Achilles heel of regulation, a noteworthy point is that these countries are all middle-income countries with a reasonable level of enforcement capacity. In other countries, approaches such as that outlined in box 3.2, where the authorities work with the private sector rather than seeking to control it, may have a better chance of succeeding.

Organizational Structures and Financing

The appropriate configuration of health system structures can ensure a clear delineation of responsibilities and accountabilities inside organizations, linking performance with rewards. Governance and organizational structures can also help ensure organizations' accountability to the public.

In recent years, the approach known as *new public management,* explained further in chapter 73, has encouraged a rejection of traditional, hierarchical forms of public sector management, whereby a single organization both finances and provides health services. For example, the U.K. health service has introduced a clear separation between the entities purchasing services (deciding what services are required for a given population and allocating funds for them) and those providing services. One aim of such arrangements is to ensure that providers' interests—as opposed to users' interests—do not dominate decisions on what services are funded. In addition, separating purchasers and providers allows competition to be introduced in service provision. Although introducing competition is widely considered desirable to encourage efficiency, debate continues on the magnitude of potential adverse effects.

Examples of new organizational structures include removing national health services from civil service control, introducing executive agencies to manage health services, and using contracts to govern relationships, both within the public sector (between public purchasers and public providers) and between the public and private sectors (Preker and Harding 2003). Colombian reforms introducing competition in both insurance and provider markets are among the most comprehensive. Another reform example is Ghana's creation of the Ghana Health Service, which is separate from the Ministry of Health.

The high transaction costs involved in creating and managing these types of arrangements and the lack of evidence that competition improves the quality of care have moderated initial enthusiasm for new forms of public management. In addition, critics argue that such arrangements are more demanding on management capacity than is direct service provision (Mills and others 2001). Moreover, implementation has proved challenging. For example, in Trinidad and Tobago and in Zambia, reforms to create new health service agencies have run into major opposition from public sector workers, who oppose changes in their terms and conditions of service.

Some of the more successful elements of new public management reforms are those that involve contracting out services, especially to nongovernmental organizations (NGOs). Early evaluation of contracting experiences indicated that, even though contracting had been perceived as a way to avoid the inefficiencies inherent in public sector provision, it nonetheless required public sector capacity to manage the contracting process (Mills 1998). This situation was particularly a problem if the contractor was a commercial firm or individual provider with incentives to maximize profits (box 3.3). Contracting with individuals and firms that are strongly influenced by a profit motive requires a certain level of state capacity to ensure that the arrangements work in the interests of the state and the general public. In some countries, therefore, NGOs may be more appropriate service providers (Palmer and Mills 2003). A number of quite positive results from contracting with NGOs are now available (World Bank

---

Box 3.3

The Importance of Government Capacity: Contracting Out Health Services in South Africa

Successive studies have evaluated experiences in contracting out hospital care and primary care services in South Africa. The hospital study compared three district hospitals whose management had been contracted out to the same private company with three nearby, comparable, publicly managed district hospitals. Overall, the contractor hospitals were able to provide care of more or less equivalent quality at significantly lower cost to themselves—in major part because their productivity was more than double that of the public hospitals as a result of their effective human resource policies. However, the contractor captured all the efficiency gains as profit, leading to a situation where contracting out was actually more costly for the government than direct provision. The contractor's capacity to profit from the arrangement was due mainly to its ability to secure highly favorable contract terms and prices and to ensure a high total number of days of care. Interview data confirmed a substantial imbalance between the government and the contractor in relation to the skills, capacities, and information required to negotiate contracts. In addition, government officials underestimated the extent of potential competition for contracts and therefore overestimated their dependence on the one contractor.

A similar study evaluated the performance of contracts with general practitioners for primary care in two provinces and compared their performance with that of public clinics. General practitioners' costs were similar to those of small public clinics, but the service was generally of poorer quality. Exploration of the relationship between purchasers and providers found that the contract was incomplete and open to interpretation and that monitoring was constrained both by a lack of capacity and resources and by the difficulty of monitoring a complex service delivered in remote locations. Sanctions were vaguely specified and rarely used because of a sense of mutual dependence between parties to the contract that lessened their willingness to enter into disputes. In addition, the two provinces varied in terms of their capacity to monitor performance. The province with lesser capacity had little information about general practitioners' performance and little contact with them, which seemed to increase suspicions of what general practitioners were doing. In contrast, the province with greater capacity had a better information system and a decentralized management system that led to greater contacts between managers and general practitioners and an apparently greater degree of understanding between the parties.

Sources: Broomberg, Masobe, and Mills 1997; Mills and others 2004; Palmer and Mills 2003.

2004), and the example of Cambodia is one of the most frequently quoted (chapter 13). Nevertheless, most evidence comes from programs with substantial external financial and technical resources, and long-term experience of sustainability is lacking.

Management decentralization has been another continuing theme in recent years. One variant is its application to hospital management, which involves giving hospitals autonomous or corporate status along with much greater responsibilities for raising income and managing their own affairs. A second variant is the creation of autonomous government agencies, and a third is decentralization to general management structures at lower levels, such as a health authority or local government.

Some pushing down of the locus of control over decision making is a prerequisite for effective management at the local and facility levels. However, without the necessary resources and management expertise at these levels and the right incentives, adverse consequences may arise for both efficiency and equity. For example, experience with hospital autonomy in low-capacity settings suggests that making the hospital partially dependent on fees for its income will restrict access by the poor to the hospital and also worsen the care they receive when admitted (Castaño, Bitrán, and Giedion 2004). However, for nonpatient care services, whose functions are easier to specify and monitor, autonomous agencies may have some advantages. For example, the Tamil Nadu Medical Supply Corporation has greatly improved the efficiency and effectiveness of drug purchasing and distribution (Mills and others 2001).

For decentralization of general health service management to succeed, attention must be paid to the entire management system, including management skills, information, analytical tools, and accountability mechanisms both to the community and to higher levels of management. Because decentralization is a complex process, takes a variety of forms, and is affected by the local context, research on its merits and demerits has been inconclusive (Alliance for Health Policy and Systems Research 2004). Some evidence indicates that decentralization to local governments can lead to neglect of broader public health functions and disease control, because these types of care are less visible to the public than curative care, as Khaleghian and Das Gupta (2004) indicate occurred in the Philippines.

Reviews of the merits of integrating services and of the effect of vertical programs on health systems have also been inconclusive. Some positive examples are available, such as the strengthening of health infrastructure and surveillance systems by the polio elimination campaign in Latin America and the Caribbean (Levine 2004). Nonetheless Briggs, Capdegelle, and Garner's (2001) review of the effects of strategies for integrating primary health care services on performance, costs, and patient outcomes finds too few studies of good enough quality to draw firm conclusions.

Human Resources

Achieving health policy goals depends on being able to train, recruit, and retain a staff with the necessary bundles of skills. In planning for human resource needs, countries must relate the numbers and levels of each category of staff members to health policy goals and the priorities that are set, given the overall availability of resources and local labor market constraints.

In recent years, concerns about the international brain drain have increased greatly, with evidence indicating that migration by doctors and nurses is severely affecting health services in some Sub-Saharan African countries (Physicians for Human Rights 2004). Actions by developing countries to improve recruitment and retention should either raise the rewards, both financial and nonfinancial, of local employment or reduce the attractiveness of alternative employment—for example, by making qualifications less portable across countries (chapter 71). Raising the remuneration of health workers may be difficult because it is likely to lead to demands for increased pay from other public sector employees. There is a long history of making use of local cadres, which can also allow training that is more specific to the needs of the local health system and its priorities.

Examples include nurses with extended training and roles and people working at subnurse levels with training of a few weeks to three years. For example, Bangladesh employs family welfare visitors, health assistants, and medical assistants; Uganda provides three years of training to clinical officers, who function as subdoctors, and three months of training to nursing aides; and Malawi trains clinical officers, who carry out surgical procedures and administer anesthetics in addition to providing medical care. Despite widespread use of such workers, evidence on how they perform relative to more qualified staff members is limited, though a study of clinical officers in Malawi suggests that well-trained clinical officers can safely substitute for doctors in performing cesarean deliveries (Fenton, Whitty, and Reynolds 2003).

The salaries necessary to recruit and retain staff members will depend on the opportunities they have for other employment both within the country and in other countries. Salary levels will also depend on health workers' preferences between financial and nonfinancial incentives. Evidence suggests that influences on motivation, though reflecting universal principles, will vary considerably from place to place (Brown 2002). Therefore, compensation and incentive structures need to be adapted to countries' circumstances; however, evidence is scanty on how countries have attempted to adapt such structures and whether they have been successful in improving recruitment and retention.

One approach to improving health workers' performance is to link performance and remuneration. The Chinese national tuberculosis (TB) program, identified as a success story (chapter 8), provided village doctors with incentives to treat TB patients. However, performance-related pay requires a good regulatory framework, skilled managerial resources, and careful monitoring to counter adverse effects—all features that are unlikely to be available in countries with limited capacity. Even in China, other experiences are much less positive because managers were not required to take likely adverse health consequences into account (box 3.4). Similar comments apply to the widespread practice of allowing doctors to work in both the public and the private sectors to increase their incomes. Doctors may exploit their private practice rights by encouraging patients to attend privately if they want better quality care—or even by diverting government resources, such as drugs, to private patients. Thus, the effects of private practice on incentives in public practice tend to be negative unless carefully monitored and controlled.

Nonmonetary rewards to encourage staff retention can be useful in such settings, as well as easier to manage. They include the availability of facilities and materials; of opportunities for learning and career progression; of subsidized housing and education for dependents; and of a culture that values the contribution of health workers to the achievement of organizational and system goals. In addition, the methods and levels of funding, the extent of organizational autonomy, the nature of support and supervisory systems, the role of the organization and of providers in the health system, and the regulation and accountability structures all influence how organizations and individuals function. Thailand provides an example in which the provision of both monetary and nonmonetary rewards has improved the recruitment, retention, and status of rural doctors (box 3.5).

The introduction of well-funded disease control programs runs the risk of attracting the most able staff members away from other positions. Past programs have successfully used combinations of financial and other incentives to encourage

---

Box 3.4

Incentive Payments in China

China has made wide use of incentive payments in hospitals—and even in public health programs. Research suggests that such payments have deleterious effects when their ability to skew behavior is not controlled. In Shandong province, studies found that a change in the bonus system for hospital doctors from one that was tied to the quantity of services provided to one that was tied to revenue generated was associated with a significant increase in hospital revenue. About 20 percent of hospital revenue was generated by the provision of unnecessary care. Although data did not permit linking bonus type to quality of care, the bonus system was clearly designed to achieve financial goals rather than quality goals. Furthermore, during the 1980s and 1990s, the government provided a decreasing share of the income of public health institutions, and the share of service charges greatly increased. As a result, public health institutions became heavily dependent on generating their own income. Negative effects included duplicate inspections of factory premises by different public health units, excessively frequent inspections, and neglect of less profitable factories that were less able to pay inspection charges.

Source: Liu and Mills 2002, 2003.

Box 3.5

The Role of Financial and Nonfinancial Incentives in Thailand

Thailand has experienced periods of severe medical brain drain from the public to the private sector and has had great difficulties in staffing hospitals in rural areas. Since the late 1970s, policies have been directed at making service in rural areas more attractive. Measures include substantial salary increases, good working conditions in district hospitals, and provision of housing. Professional self-esteem has been increased by providing career opportunities up to the post of deputy director general, an annual award for rural doctors, and membership in the rural doctor society. Substantial experience as a rural doctor is explicitly valued by leading public health specialists, who themselves have spent substantial periods working as rural doctors.

Source: Wibulpolprasert and Pengpaiboon 2003.

Improving Staff Performance in Cambodia

An NGO contracted to manage a district in Cambodia introduced contracts between the NGO's managers and facility staff members involving a monthly incentive payment, a punctuality incentive, and a performance bonus. The contracts were initially introduced in three facilities, which subsequently experienced significantly higher use levels than those that did not have the incentive payments. Because individual contracts were too demanding to manage and excluded health center and hospital directors from staff management, the system was changed to one of subcontracting with facility managers. Output improved even more. Subcontracts were made competitive: if a health center's management or output was poor, other health workers or managers were asked to apply to take over the contract. During 2001, four contracts were replaced. Monitoring activities, especially spot checks at the household level to verify that recorded visits had taken place, were considered vital to ensuring quality and transparency. Soeters and Griffiths (2003) argue that outsiders—in this case the NGO—are better able to introduce new management procedures than a ministry of health, which tends to be risk averse.

Source: Soeters and Griffiths 2003.

good worker productivity and program performance (chapter 71). Incentives have included better salaries; field and transportation allowances; and nonfinancial incentives such as streamlined management, specialized training, availability of facilities and material resources, and results-oriented management that provides effective administrative and technical support. Governments need to find ways of benefiting and learning from these experiences. For example, governments might allow periods of secondment to externally funded programs, after which staff members return to the government with enhanced skills. The success of such an approach will depend on remuneration not differing too greatly and on government bureaucracies providing the scope for staff members to use their new skills.

However, the history of civil service reform is not encouraging (Nunberg 1999). Reforms have sought to reduce the size of the civil service and to improve productivity using incentive schemes such as performance-based pay and promotion structures. Such reforms have been largely unsuccessful because of the political difficulties of reducing the size of the civil service. Structural and organizational changes are typically unpopular with labor unions, especially if they perceive such changes as threatening workers' well-being. Experience demonstrates the difficulties of aligning system and organizational objectives with individual workers' objectives (Martineau and Buchan 2000) and suggests that solutions need to be sought that do not involve radical reform of employment patterns unless the country setting is particularly propitious.

Where contracting with NGOs or other private providers is an option, doing so may permit changed employment patterns and improved performance without the widespread disruption that can result from attempting to change government workers' terms and conditions of service. In Cambodia, a project contracted to an NGO (HealthNet) obtained some improvements in staff performance by establishing clear agreements with staff members concerning issues such as the working hours that would be expected and the informal charges that staff members were not to demand from patients. In return, staff members received substantial incentive payments (box 3.6).

Quality Assessment and Assurance

The quality of health services has a number of important implications. It affects the outcomes that a health system can achieve—both directly, through patient treatment, and indirectly, by encouraging or discouraging use of the services. It also affects staff morale, because working in an environment where employees know the treatment quality is poor is not motivating.

Substantial evidence, reviewed in chapter 70, indicates that the quality of care is often suboptimal and varies widely within countries. In part this suboptimal quality is attributable to resource constraints, but providing good-quality care is possible even in resource-poor settings.

Evidence on how providers' practices can be improved can be grouped into two categories: policies that indirectly affect providers' practices by changing structural conditions, including the practice environment, and policies that directly affect individual and group practices.

In the first category, legal mandates and administrative regulations can be used to bar unqualified workers from practicing; professional oversight and clinical guidelines can encourage good practices; contracts can specify and monitor quality standards, such as immunization coverage targets; and accreditation can stimulate quality improvements. Among policies that directly affect providers' behavior, training with peer review feedback has been shown to improve quality, as have total quality management approaches; remuneration can be made dependent on performance subject to the caveats raised earlier. Measures that improve quality can increase use, strengthen the public sector's capabilities, and be highly cost-effective—even cost saving.

TARGETING RESOURCES

An important dimension of health system capacity that has not been considered explicitly so far, is the ability to ensure that resources are used in ways that meet health system objectives. As noted earlier, many health systems fail to perform as well as they might on effectiveness, efficiency, and equity criteria. This section addresses what policy instruments might be available to ensure that additional resources are used to the greatest effect, first at the systems level and then at the level of service delivery.

Systems-Level Mechanisms

At the systems level, tools available to decision makers include regulation and legislation, resource allocation formulas, and financial incentives.

Decision makers can use regulation and legislation to set minimum standards of care that insurance packages must cover, for instance. They can influence the availability of drugs by, for example, liberalizing prescribing and introducing accompanying measures to educate providers and users so as to increase the use of certain drugs that are safe to distribute on a large scale. One approach that has worked in Uganda is a social-marketing program making subsidized and clearly packaged drugs for sexually transmitted diseases available through the retail sector (Mills and others 2002).

In some settings, explicit rationing of the provision of care in the public and private sectors can be used to prioritize the most cost-effective interventions and limit the provision of less cost-effective ones. However, regulatory controls are unlikely to be effective in low-capacity settings and will simply encourage illicit activities. Moreover, explicit rationing requires a high degree of public acceptance and public involvement in the pri-oritization process. A more acceptable strategy in most settings is to constrain the overall public sector resource envelope in terms of staff, buildings, equipment, and drugs and to leave rationing decisions within the envelope to clinical discretion (Segall 2003). However, clinicians may implicitly ration services in inequitable ways—for example, on the basis of age or social status—and supplementary measures are likely to be needed to ensure that health workers do not discriminate against poorer and marginalized members of society.

Resource allocation formulas have an important role to play in the public sector in directing resources to underserved geographic areas and population groups and to underfunded programs (Musgrove 2004). Given the typical shortages of health workers in more remote areas, such formulas should include remote area allowances or allow for the higher costs of delivering services in such areas. A formula in Zambia, for example, used distance from the railway line as a proxy for remoteness.

A similar approach to ensuring that resources go where they are most needed is the "marginal budgeting for bottlenecks" approach of the World Bank (see chapter 9). This country-based planning and budgeting approach assesses health sector impediments to faster progress toward the MDGs, identifies ways to remove them, and estimates both the costs and the likely effects of their removal on MDG outcomes.

In targeting resources to specific programs, expansion of one area of health provision should not occur at the expense of another priority area. For example, where staff capacity and facilities are limited, targeting additional funding to TB case detection and treatment may simply take staff time away from child health. This problem of the systemwide effects of disease-specific programs was discussed earlier. Addressing this problem requires empowering a central body, such as a ministry of health or a regional or district health authority, to take an overall view of priorities so that resource conflicts can be resolved.

Even though financial incentives need to be used cautiously, they can be powerful tools for influencing providers' behavior, as indicated earlier. They can also be an important influence on users' behavior. Experience in South Africa and Uganda (box 3.7)

Box 3.7

Removal of Fees at the Primary Care Level in Uganda

In February 2001, the government of Uganda abolished cost sharing in public facilities at the community level. This move was followed by a marked increase in the use of health services by all population groups. For villages near public health centers, the increase was greatest among the poorest groups. The frequency with which centers ran out of drugs worsened during the first year of implementation but gradually improved during the second year. A study concluded that before the policy change user fees were probably a major deterrent to the use of public health services and that their removal was especially beneficial to the poor.

Source: Nabyonga and others 2005.

suggests that, in some settings, removing or reducing user fees at the primary care level may be an important element in encouraging greater take-up of primary care. Further studies of the effects of fee removal are needed.

Service-Level Mechanisms

At the service level, evidence suggests the value of providing a framework of resources and guidance within which managers and health workers can prioritize their efforts. The experience of the Tanzania Essential Health Interventions Program (chapter 54) highlights the health gains that a decentralized management structure can achieve when district managers are provided with the information, tools, and training to enable them to match services and additional resources with the local burden of disease. Berwick (2004) draws similar lessons from the experience of several highly successful projects in resource-poor settings: set clear aims and targets, use a team approach, build an infrastructure of human resources and data systems, engage with the policy environment, and develop simple approaches to rapid scaling up.

Patient education on major causes of ill health is also important to ensure that people know when to seek care (for example, in the case of childhood illness); understand their rights to various services and the official level of charges; and can make appropriate decisions about drug purchases. Patient charters may play a role in making explicit what patients have the right to expect from their health services and what level of service providers should achieve. Local policies on service provision need to relate to community preferences: if they do not, clients' confidence in the public health system will be undermined. One simple example is the pervasive view in some South African communities that public clinics water down medicines, thereby rendering them ineffective (Schneider and Palmer 2002). Indeed, generic medicines used by the public sector are often perceived as less effective than name brand drugs. Accurate public information is needed to counter that perception.

SOLUTIONS IN LOW-CAPACITY ENVIRONMENTS

Developing countries possess a range of capacities to improve the functioning of their health systems, but one group of countries faces the greatest constraints to doing so. Analyses undertaken for the Commission on Macroeconomics and Health used the framework presented in table 3.2 to understand the dimensions of the constraints problem in 79 low-income countries. Using proxies for the various types and levels of constraints—gross domestic product per capita, female literacy rate, number of nurses per population ratio, diphtheria-pertussis-tetanus immunization coverage, access to health services, control of corruption, and government effectiveness—countries can be classified as more or less constrained. Table 3.3

shows key indicators for the most constrained and other countries.

The most constrained group has significantly worse health indicators and much worse access to health resources. For example, countries in this group have almost twice the infant mortality rate and more than twice the maternal mortality rate of other countries but only one-sixth as many nurses. In absolute terms, the most constrained group represents a relatively small share of the total population of countries analyzed and consists, for the most part, of small countries (more than half have populations of less than 10 million) in Sub-Saharan Africa.

The key question in relation to improving health outcomes is what financing and delivery strategy might work best in these settings. Should it take the form of a limited number of programs, each addressing one or a few diseases? Or should efforts be devoted to building up the basic health service infrastructure on which targeted efforts to address specific health problems can then be built? Given the lack of evidence, providing guidance is difficult, and the chapters in this book present different views. Chapter 63 firmly dismisses the option of bypassing organized health services altogether in the poorest countries and promoting the delivery of child health interventions directly to households through, for example, community-based projects dispensing antimalarials or antibiotics. It argues that, though this approach may be a short-term solution, successes using it largely occur in small-scale pilots with strong managerial backup. Chapter 56 suggests that in the poorest societies basic preventive services should be introduced first—especially immunization, access to basic drugs, and management of the most severe threats to health such as emergency care for traffic injuries. At slightly higher levels of development, the introduction of community-based activities may be cost-effective if coverage by the formal health service is poor. Both chapters imply that the issue is not which approach to use but how to phase approaches and use a mix that depends on the intervention and the local context. Accomplishing this requires not only service delivery capacity but also management capacity to plan and evaluate the mix of approaches and make adjustments over time.

Molyneux (2004) suggests that disease control programs can be used to build capacity for the long term and that, with time, such programs can become more advisory and less managerial. For example, in Pakistan, primary health care was built on the experience of TB and leprosy clinics. In China, the vertical programs for disease control purchased time from health service operational staff members, thereby ensuring that funds flowed into the health service infrastructure (Dean Jamison, personal communication, 2004). In seven countries in southern Africa, a successful combined strategy for measles immunization started with a single, nationwide catch-up campaign in which mobile teams vaccinated all children in a particular age group (Levine 2004), an action that can sharply

Table 3.3 Health Indicators by Country Level of Constraint

Indicator	Unit	Most constrained countries[a]	Other countries
Total population (in 2000)	Millions	401	3,525
Population living on less than US$1/day	Millions	123 (9 countries)	886 (29 countries)
Population living on less than US$1/day	Percent[b]	30	25
Population living on less than US$2/day	Millions	192 (9 countries)	2,128 (30 countries)
Population living on less than US$2/day	Percent[b]	48	60
Physicians	Per 100,000 population	8.9	101.7
Nurses	Per 100,000 population	39.6	208.7
Hospital beds	Per 1,000 population	0.78	3.00
Maternal mortality	Per 100,000 births	1,134	565
Births with skilled attendant	Percent	30.6	59.8
Low birthweight infants	Percent	16.4	13.9
Infant mortality (in 1998)	Per 1,000 live births	105.3	61.2
Mortality among children under five	Per 1,000 live births	171.2	91.9
Measles immunization coverage	Percent	48.4	75.3
Diphtheria-pertussis-tetanus immunization coverage	Percent	40.3	76.3
TB Directly observed therapy short course (DOTS) detection	Percent	31.15	42.10
TB DOTS treatment success	Percent	68.4	77.1
Number of countries included	n.a.	20	59

Source: Ranson, Hanson, and Mills 2003.

n.a. = not applicable.

Note: Calculations were performed for a constraints index with up to three missing variables. Values for missing variables were imputed using a method described in the source.

a. These are the bottom quartile of countries, according to the constraints indicators, compiled into an index. The constraints index was calculated by normalizing each of the variables (subtracting the mean and dividing by the standard deviation) and then summing the normalized values. This calculation gives each variable equal weight in the index.

b. These averages are population weighted, whereas all other means in the table are unweighted.

reduce the spread of the virus. Routine services were used to continue measles immunization but with a follow-up campaign three to four years later to prevent the number of susceptible cases from rising to the level required for transmission. Over five years, measles virtually disappeared from southern Africa. However, maintaining this achievement requires that routine services be able to reach more than 80 percent coverage, a level many countries find hard to sustain. Moreover, in low-capacity environments, campaigns can divert attention and resources from routine primary health care services. Schreuder and Kostermans (2001) indicate that this problem occurred in southern Africa, particularly with respect to diverting scarce management capacity, implying that reducing deaths from one cause may risk worsening services for other diseases and conditions.

Victora and others (2004) suggest that the most appropriate mix of vertical and horizontal approaches depends on the human and financial resources available, the urgency with which results need to be achieved, the existing organization of health services, and the natural development of programs over time. Within a horizontal approach, the weaker the health system setting is, the more important the provision of good technical and management backup will be to service delivery. The authors ascribe some of the difficulties that integrated management of infant and childhood illness (IMCI) faced in several countries to the absence of full-time IMCI coordinators, operational plans, and specific budget lines. They suggest that, when health systems are extremely weak, vertical programs may be required; however, as health systems strengthen, financing and delivery strategies can become less vertical and more horizontal and less selective and more integrated.

RESEARCH PRIORITIES

A notable paucity of evidence is apparent in relation to most key areas discussed in this chapter. This lack of evidence is illustrated by a recent review of the evidence on the equity of utilization and financing strategies (box 3.8). This and other reviews of the available evidence have led the *Lancet* to call for a new health systems research specialty ("Mexico 2004: Global Health Needs a New Research Agenda" 2004).

Gaps in the Evidence on Equity of Health Financing and Utilization in Low-Income Settings

A recent review evaluated evidence on the effect of various financing strategies on use of health care. It found that most research was small scale and had findings of limited applicability. Well-designed, large-scale evaluations of the effect of alternative financing interventions were lacking, and a multitude of case studies described specific experiences but with little methodological rigor. The review recommended larger-scale, more systematic studies in a range of settings, including nonrandomized designs when randomization is impossible or inappropriate and multicenter case studies that examine why arrangements do or do not work in different settings. The study proposed developing and applying quality criteria for quantitative and case study research along the lines of guidelines recently developed for randomized group trials.

Source: Palmer and others 2004.

Areas where evidence is especially limited that are identified in this chapter—where research is a high priority—include the following:

- Evidence on most health system reforms—for example, hospital autonomy reforms and decentralization—is inadequate to draw conclusions about the circumstances under which reforms are likely to improve the efficiency and equity of service delivery.
- Few studies relate a reform to health outcomes, and even evidence on intermediate outcome measures, such as costs and quality of service provision, is often lacking.
- Virtually no information is available about the costs of strengthening capacity or the effectiveness of different approaches to capacity strengthening, even though the lack of system capacity is widely noted.
- Evidence is largely lacking on the characteristics of delivery strategies capable of achieving and maintaining high coverage for specific interventions in various epidemiological, health system, and cultural contexts.
- Evidence is lacking on what types of governance and institutional arrangements will support the achievement of widespread health improvements, especially for the poorest members of society.

Addressing the deficiencies in the evidence base requires developing better study designs and analytical methods and building expertise in and understanding of health systems research. Capacity for research and analysis in health policy and health systems is currently limited. A recent survey (Alliance for Health Policy and Systems Research 2004) estimated that project funding for health systems research accounted for less than 0.02 percent of the total annual health expenditure of developing countries. More than half of research projects had budgets of less than US$25,000. Of institutions identified as engaged in health systems research, a third had no staff qualified at the doctoral level, and researchers with doctoral degrees made up only a quarter of the research workforce. An analysis of studies cited in Medline showed that only 5 percent of the health systems research literature concerned developing countries.

Given the importance of influencing policy and practice, the approach to research needs to encompass solving operational problems in real-life settings. Ethical issues arise in using limited supplies of talent to study problems unrelated to the local context when the human resources and systems required to improve operational programs are lacking. Moreover, the quality and effect of investigations are much improved when they are based on dialogue with the primary users and set in real-life contexts. The concept of the cycle from research to policy and practice needs to be emphasized more strongly. It encompasses not only generating knowledge but also managing the research agenda, including setting priorities, and promoting the use of evidence through means such as advocacy channels and specific mechanisms designed to link producers and users of research (Alliance for Health Policy and Systems Research 2004). Given the importance of context in translating research evidence into service and system practice, operational research and program evaluation capacity must be built among country-based scientists and practitioners.

CONCLUSIONS

This chapter has sought to address the question of how health systems can be strengthened to deliver cost-effective and equitable interventions and services. Recent cross-country analysis on the association between health expenditure by government and health outcomes has suggested that the effectiveness of increased health expenditure depends heavily on governments adopting the right policies (World Bank 2004). What are the right policies, and what are effective implementation processes? The review in this chapter suggests that in many areas not enough is known to recommend particular approaches and also that recommendations need to be adapted to local contexts. Nonetheless, six key points can be identified in relation to improving health systems:

- Health systems face numerous constraints in low-income countries, but they are the basis for the long-term future of sustained health improvements. The health of the system must, therefore, be carefully considered whenever major new programs are put in place.
- If capacity constraints are such that a focused disease- or program-specific effort is desirable to address an urgent problem, the effort should be designed to contribute to the long-term system strengthening, rather than detracting from it. Countries must avoid having multiple vertical programs competing for limited human resources and managerial capacity. Over time, as horizontally organized services strengthen, the need for more vertical financing and delivery strategies will lessen.
- Reforms affecting organizational structures and human resource management are likely to play an important role in improved performance. However, emerging evidence suggests in most settings that changes are most likely to be successfully implemented if they are incremental and gradual rather than "big bang" reforms. Stability of policies and consistent implementation are also required.
- Linking financial incentives to performance, whether through contracts with health care providers or through performance-related pay, may bring rewards if careful monitoring is possible; however, evidence on the sustainability of such arrangements is lacking, and effective monitoring may require long-term external involvement. Evidence is needed on alternative approaches to improving performance.
- Organizational reforms must keep the goal of improved health outcomes, equity, and responsiveness in sight. Doing so requires paying special attention to users' demands, to primary care and first-level hospitals, to quality of care, and to technical backup for disease control programs.
- Capacity-strengthening efforts in most settings must encompass action at all levels, from increasing leadership of the ministry of health at the national level through strengthening support for peripheral levels.

The current body of knowledge represents a largely ad hoc and disjointed collection of facts, figures, and points of view. Making confident recommendations relevant to strengthening health system capacity is thus difficult. Although international financing is vital, countries need flexibility to develop solutions based on local assessments and experience and to progress at a pace commensurate with their situations. Sustained investment in analytical and operational research capacity is needed as part of program and systems support, to serve national priority setting and policy formulation.

ACKNOWLEDGMENTS

Discussions at a workshop sponsored by the Disease Control Priorities Project in South Africa during June 30–July 3, 2004, contributed considerably to the development of ideas for this chapter.

NOTE

1. The health system is understood to encompass all activities whose prime intent is to improve health.

REFERENCES

Alliance for Health Policy and Systems Research. 2004. *Strengthening Health Systems: The Role and Potential of Policy and Systems Research.* Geneva: Alliance for Health Policy and Systems Research.

Ashworth, A., M. Chopra, D. McCoy, D. Sanders, D. Jackson, N. Karaolis, and others. 2004. "WHO Guidelines for Management of Severe Malnutrition in Rural South African Hospitals: Effect on Case Facility and the Influence of Operational Factors." *Lancet* 363: 1110–15.

Berwick, D. M. 2004. "Lessons from Developing Nations on Improving Health Care." *British Medical Journal* 328: 1124–29.

Briggs, C. J., P. Capdegelle, and P. Garner. 2001. "Strategies for Integrating Primary Health Services in Middle- and Low-Income Countries: Effects on Performance, Costs, and Patient Outcomes. *Cochrane Database of Systematic Reviews* (4) CD003318.

Broomberg, J., P. Masobe, and A. Mills. 1997. "To Purchase or to Provide? The Relative Efficiency of Contracting Out versus Direct Public Provision of Hospital Services in South Africa." In *Private Health Providers in Developing Countries: Serving the Public Interest?*, ed. S. Bennett, B. McPake, and A. Mills, 214–36. London: Zed Press.

Brown, K. 2002. "Improving Organisational and Individual Performance for Service Delivery: How Can Officials Become More Responsive to the Needs of the Poor?" Paper presented at the Department for International Development workshop on Improving Service Delivery in Developing Countries, Eynsham Hall, Oxfordshire, U.K., November 24–30.

Castaño, R., R. Bitrán, and U. Giedion. 2004. *Monitoring and Evaluating Hospital Autonomization and Its Effects on Priority Services.* Bethesda, MD: Partners for Health Reform Plus Project, Abt Associates.

de Savigny, D., E. Mwageni, C. Mayombana, H. Masanja, A. Minhaj, D. Momburi, and others. 2004. "Care-Seeking Patterns in Fatal Malaria." Background paper prepared for the Institute of Medicine study on the Economics of Antimalarial Drugs, Washington, DC.

Fenton, P. M., C. J. Whitty, and F. Reynolds. 2003. "Caesarean Section in Malawi: Prospective Study of Early Maternal and Perinatal Mortality." *British Medical Journal* 327 (7415): 587–91.

Goodman, C. 2004. "An Economic Analysis of the Retail Market for Fever and Malaria Treatment in Rural Tanzania." Ph.D. thesis, University of London.

Gonzalez, C. L. 1965. "Mass Campaigns and General Health Services." Public Health Paper 29. Geneva: World Health Organization.

Gwatkin, D., S. Rutstein, K. Johnson, R. Pande, and A. Wagstaff. 2000. *Socioeconomic Differences in Health, Nutrition, and Population: 45 Countries.* Washington, DC: World Bank.

Hanson, K., K. Ranson, V. Oliveira-Cruz, and A. Mills. 2003. "Expanding Access to Health Interventions: A Framework for Understanding the Constraints to Scaling Up." *Journal of International Development* 15 (1): 1–14.

Hensher, M. 2001. "Financing the Health System through Efficiency Gains." Background paper prepared for Working Group 2 of the Commission on Macroeconomics and Health, World Health Organization, Geneva. http://www.cmhealth. org/docs/wg3_paper2.pdf.

Khaleghian, P., and M. Das Gupta. 2004. "Public Management and the Essential Public Health Functions." Working Paper 25, Disease Control Priorities Project, Bethesda, MD.

Levine, R. 2004. *What's Worked? Accounting for Success in Global Health.* Washington, DC: Center for Global Development.

Levy, B. 2004. "Governance and Economic Development in Africa: Meeting the Challenge of Capacity Building." In *Building State Capacity in Africa: New Approaches, Emerging Lessons,* ed. B. Levy and S. Kpundeh, 1–42. Washington, DC: World Bank Institute.

Litvack, J., and C. Bodart. 1993. "User Fees plus Quality Equals Improved Access to Health Care: Results of a Field Experiment in Cameroon." *Social Science and Medicine* 37 (3): 369–83.

Liu, X., and A. Mills. 2002. "Financing Reforms of Public Health Services in China: Lessons for Other Nations." *Social Science and Medicine* 54 (11): 1691–98.

———. 2003. "The Influence of Bonus Payments to Doctors on Hospital Revenue: Results of a Quasi-Experimental Study." *Applied Health Economics and Health Policy* 2 (2): 91–98.

Marsh, V. M., W. M. Mutemi, A. Willetts, K. Bayah, S. Were, A. Ross, and K. Marsh. 2004. "Improving Malaria Home Treatment by Training Drug Retailers in Rural Kenya." *Tropical Medicine and International Health* 9 (4): 451–60.

Martineau, T., and J. Buchan. 2000. "Human Resources and the Success of Health Sector Reform." *Human Resources Development Journal* 4 (3): 174–83.

"Mexico 2004: Global Health Needs a New Research Agenda." 2004. *Lancet* 364: 1555–56.

Mills, A. 1998. "To Contract or Not to Contract? Issues for Low- and Middle-Income Countries." *Health Policy and Planning* 13 (1): 32–40.

———. 2005. "Mass Campaigns versus General Health Services: What Have We Learnt in 40 Years about Vertical versus Horizontal Approaches." *Bulletin of the World Health Organization* 83 (4): 315–16.

Mills, A., S. Bennett, S. Russell, with N. Attanayake, C. Hongoro, V. E. Muraleedharan, and P. Smithson. 2001. *The Challenge of Health Sector Reform: What Must Governments Do?* Oxford, U.K.: Macmillan Press.

Mills, A., R. Brugha, K. Hanson, and B. McPake. 2002. "What Can Be Done about the Private Health Sector in Low-Income Countries?" *Bulletin of the World Health Organization* 80 (4): 325–30.

Mills, A., N. Palmer, L. Gilson, D. McIntyre, H. Schneider, E. Sinanovic, and H. Wadee. 2004. "The Performance of Different Models of Primary Care Provision in Southern Africa." *Social Science and Medicine* 59 (5): 931–43.

Molyneux, D. 2004. "'Neglected' Disease but Unrecognised Successes: Challenges and Opportunities for Infectious Disease Control." *Lancet* 364: 380–83.

Molyneux, D., and V. Nantulya. 2004. "Linking Disease Control Programmes in Rural Africa: A Pro-Poor Strategy to Reach Abuja Targets and Millennium Development Goals." *British Medical Journal* 328 (7448): 1129–32.

Musgrove, P. 2004. "Compensatory Finance in Health: Geographic Equity in a Federal System." In *Health Economics in Development,* ed. P. Musgrove, 133–42. Health, Nutrition, and Population Series. Washington, DC: World Bank.

Nabyonga, J., M. Desmet, H. Karamagi, P. Y. Kadama, F. G. Omaswa, and O. Walker. 2005. "Abolition of Cost-Sharing Is Pro-Poor: Evidence from Uganda." *Health Policy and Planning* 20 (2): 100–8.

Nunberg, B. 1999. "Rethinking Civil Service Reform." Poverty Reduction and Economic Management Notes 31, World Bank, Washington, DC. http://www1.worldbank.org/ prem/PREMNotes/premnote31.pdf.

Palmer, N., and A. Mills. 2003. "Classical versus Relational Approaches to Understanding Controls on a Contract with GPs in South Africa." *Health Economics* 12: 1005–20.

Palmer, N., D. Mueller, L. Gilson, A. Mills, and A. Haines. 2004. "Health Financing and Equity of Utilisation in Low-Income Settings: Is There an Evidence Base?" *Lancet* 364 (9442): 1365–70.

Physicians for Human Rights. 2004. *An Action to Prevent Brain Drain: Building Equitable Health Systems in Africa.* Boston: Physicians for Human Rights.

Preker, A. S., and A. Harding. 2003. *Innovations in Health Service Delivery.* Washington, DC: World Bank.

Ranson, K., K. Hanson, and A. Mills. 2003. "Constraints to Expanding Access to Health Interventions: An Empirical Analysis and Country Typology." *Journal of International Development* 15 (1): 15–40.

Saltman, R. B., and O. Ferroussier-Davis. 2000. "On the Concept of Stewardship in Health Policy." *Bulletin of the World Health Organization* 78 (6): 732–39.

Schneider, H., and N. Palmer. 2002. "Getting to the Truth? Researching User Views of Primary Health Care." *Health Policy and Planning* 17: 32–41.

Schreuder, B., and C. Kostermans. 2001. "Global Health Strategies versus Local Primary Health Care Priorities: A Case Study of National Immunization Days in Southern Africa." *South African Medical Journal* 91 (3): 249–54.

Segall, M. 2003. "District Health Systems in a Neoliberal World: A Review of Five Key Policy Areas." *International Journal of Health Planning and Management* 18 (S1): S5–26.

Soeters, R., and F. Griffiths. 2003. "Improving Government Health Services through Contract Management: A Case from Cambodia." *Health Policy and Planning* 18 (1): 74–83.

Southern Africa Stroke Prevention Initiative Project Team. 2004. "Secondary Prevention of Stroke: Results from the Southern Africa Stroke Prevention Initiative (SASPI) Study." *Bulletin of the World Health Organization* 82 (7): 503–8.

Travis, P., S. Bennett, A. Haines, T. Pang, Z. Bhutta, A. Hyder, and others. 2004. "Overcoming Health Systems Constraints to Achieve the Millennium Development Goals." *Lancet* 364: 900–6.

Unger, J.-P., P. de Paepe, and A. Green. 2003. "A Code of Best Practice to Avoid Damaging Health Care Services in Developing Countries." *International Journal of Health Planning and Management* 18 (S1): S27–40.

Victora, C., K. Hanson, J. Bryce, and J. P. Vaughan. 2004. "Achieving Universal Coverage with Health Interventions." *Lancet* 364: 1541–48.

Walsh, J., and K. Warren. 1980. "Selective Primary Health Care: An Interim Strategy for Disease Control in Developing Countries." *New England Journal of Medicine* 301: 967–74.

Walt, G. 2001. "Global Cooperation in Global Public Health." In *International Public Health,* ed. M. Merson, R. Black, and A. Mills, 667–99. Gaithersburg, MD: Aspen Publishers.

Wibulpolprasert, S., and P. Pengpaiboon. 2003. "Integrated Strategies to Tackle the Inequitable Distribution of Doctors in Thailand: Four Decades of Experience." *Human Resources for Health* 1: 12.

World Bank. 2004. *The Millennium Development Goals for Health: Rising to the Challenges.* Washington, DC: World Bank.

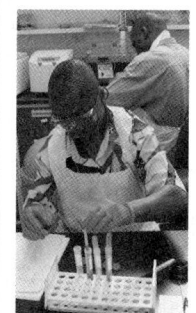

Chapter **4**

Priorities for Global Research and Development of Interventions

Barry R. Bloom, Catherine M. Michaud, John R. La Montagne,
and Lone Simonsen

It is a profound and necessary truth that the deep things in science are not found because they are useful;
they are found because it was possible to find them.
—J. Robert Oppenheimer
In R. Rhodes, *The Making of the Atomic Bomb*

NEEDS, CONTEXT, OPPORTUNITIES, AND MAJOR CHALLENGES

Half of the entire increase in human life expectancy—a crude but easily defined measure of the health of populations—realized over recorded history occurred in the 20th century. From 1900 to 2000, life expectancy at birth increased from 48.0 to 77.1 years in the United States and from 48.0 to 77.7 years in the United Kingdom, gains of almost 30 years. However, improvements in life expectancy were not limited to the industrial nations. For example, between 1900 and 1990, life expectancy in India increased from 27 to 59 years, a gain of 32 years (Fogel 2004). These increases are largely attributable to a better understanding of biology, medicine, and public health—that is, to the benefits of research.

Research is traditionally defined as the generation of new knowledge and the development of new and enabling technologies to identify or respond to major gaps in current knowledge. Research includes the development of new tools, methodologies, and strategies. The World Health Organization (WHO) and its Advisory Committee on Health Research have suggested two other defining aspects of health research—namely, the verification of knowledge in different contexts and the creation and dissemination of products of knowledge. The Institute of Medicine (1997, page 1) in

the United States has defined the realm of global health research as "problems, issues, and concerns that transcend national boundaries and may best be addressed by sharing knowledge and cooperative action."

An important corollary of this definition is that global health research is derived from individuals and institutions rather than from nation states. Thus, global health knowledge should be available to everyone, not just to the country in which it is done or that sponsored it. As a result, knowledge derived from health research is a true public good, which by definition possesses the following two special properties (Commission on Macroeconomics and Health 2001):

- *Nonexclusivity.* Thus, when supplied it does not require payment to benefit individuals or groups (for example, the benefit to the world community of eliminating smallpox).
- *Nonrivalry.* Hence, the use of the benefits by an individual, group, or country will not diminish others' ability to benefit from the same good or service.[1]

Investments in research have produced remarkable improvements in global health, especially over the past 20 years. Immunization programs have led to unprecedented progress in the fight against common childhood diseases (such as measles, pertussis, poliomyelitis, and tetanus) and in the eradication of smallpox. At the same time, vaccination programs have catalyzed the construction of a global infrastructure for epidemiological monitoring and research, especially in the Americas and in Asia. Moreover, researchers are rapidly developing many preventive, diagnostic, and therapeutic tools, and the growing power of genomics and proteomics will accelerate the pace.

The 21st century will see a continuation of the inexorable trend toward the globalization of travel, trade, and communications. At one level, economic globalization has increased disparities between countries in terms of gross domestic product per capita. On a population basis, however, economic gains by China, India, and other developing countries have made vast numbers of people substantially wealthier than ever before (Fischer 2003). Cell phones and radios are ubiquitous, even in the most remote parts of Africa and Asia, and the Internet has permitted the transmission of data across long distances rapidly, accurately, reliably, and cheaply. With these technologies, global research relationships that once would have been impossible are now commonplace. For example, in a matter of weeks, researchers in China could sequence the gene for the surface protein of the coronavirus associated with severe acute respiratory syndrome (SARS) and then produce the surface protein as diagnostic antigen. Such speedy reaction would have been inconceivable just a decade ago.

Daunting challenges remain, however, that health research alone is unlikely to solve. The context for health is very complex and varies in different countries of the world (box 4.1). The predictable outcome of current trends is an increase in the health and technology gaps between the rich and poor countries. Tip O'Neill, the colorful speaker of the U.S. House of Representatives for 10 years, often said that "all politics is local." A provocative thesis we present here is that (a) all health care is national, and (b) all health research is global.

Box 4.1

Context of Global Health

Advances include the following:

- the globalization of knowledge and the increased mobility of the world's population
- the expansion of knowledge about disease problems in most of the developing world
- the remarkable progress achieved in the control of infectious diseases in most parts of the world
- the worldwide penetration of new forms of communication
- the promise of new technologies in biomedical research (for example, in the fields of genomics, transgenic organisms, informatics, robotics, and nanotechnology)
- the increasing flow of private resources devoted to understanding health problems related to development.

The following concerns are pertinent:

- The world's population continues to grow, numbering 6.3 billion people in 2004, with 200,000 added each day. In at least 68 countries, more than 40 percent of the population is younger than 15, whereas in wealthy countries, the proportion of elderly people in the population is expanding quickly.
- Despite falling global poverty rates, progress is uneven: 1.2 billion people still live on less than US$1 a day, and 2.8 billion live on less than US$2 a day. One in six children is chronically hungry.

- Disparities have increased. The richest 20 percent of the world's population now accounts for 150 times the income of the poorest 20 percent. The ratio of the income of the top 20 percent to that of the poorest 20 percent rose from 30 to 1 in 1960 to 61 to 1 in 1991 and to 78 to 1 in 1994. Evidence of global environmental degradation is apparent, especially in the developing world. For example, 45 percent of tropical rain forest has already been lost, at least 20 percent of current species will be extinct by 2030 and 50 percent by the end of the century, and half of China's and many other countries' cities already face water shortages.
- With global warming, temperatures will likely rise 1.0°C to 4.5°C this century, threatening coastal areas and changing patterns of vectorborne and epidemic disease.
- The pace of migration from rural to urban environments is speeding up, giving rise to more megacities.
- The period 1955–98 witnessed 31 civil and foreign wars, 35 million displaced people and refugees, and 127 instances of state failures—ethnic wars, revolutionary wars, and disruptive regime changes—in 96 states.
- Terrorism has become a global threat.
- Gender discrimination persists.

Sources: King and Zeng 2001, 2002; Wilson 2003; World Bank 2004; World Revolution (http://www.worldrevolution.org).

Global Burden of Disease

Tables 4.1 and 4.2 summarize some of the key findings that are most relevant to a discussion of global health research priorities. The magnitude and distribution of the burden of disease across different regions in 2001 reveals a great deal about unmet research needs (Mathers and others 2003), in particular:

- Communicable diseases and maternal, perinatal, and nutritional conditions remain the major contributors to the burden of disease in Sub-Saharan Africa and in parts of East Asia and the Pacific. These regions differ significantly from all the other low- and middle-income regions and call for a unique set of priorities in relation to global health research.
- Noncommunicable diseases are already the leading contributors to the disease burden in all other low- and middle-income regions, which are undergoing rapid demographic, economic, and epidemiological transitions. Not only does the world face an epidemic of cardiovascular

disease and major unipolar depressive disorders, for example, but also these two chronic conditions already account for an increasing burden of disease and death in developing countries. Demographic changes in many low- and middle-income countries are driving the observed transition toward patterns of disease previously seen only in the industrial countries. The incidence of both ischemic heart disease and cerebrovascular disease increases rapidly with age; thus, countries in which the proportion of elderly people in the population increases will also experience increases in the relative importance of noncommunicable illness. Unlike communicable illnesses among younger people, chronic illness associated with aging cannot be entirely prevented, only delayed. These factors must be considered when setting priorities for global health research.

Children under five still account for an unnecessarily large share of the disease burden in many low- and middle-income

Table 4.1 Broad Patterns of the Disease Burden, by World Bank Region, 2001

Category	East Asia and the Pacific	Europe and Central Asia	Latin America and the Caribbean	Middle East and North Africa	South Asia	Sub-Saharan Africa	High-income countries	World
Population (*millions*)	1,851	477	526	310	1,388	668	929	6,150
Communicable, maternal, perinatal, and nutritional conditions (*prevalence, percent*)	22.2	9.4	21.8	27.1	44.3	70.4	5.7	36.7
Noncommunicable diseases (*prevalence, percent*)	65.8	76.4	65.0	59.3	44.4	21.2	86.7	52.6
Injuries (*prevalence, percent*)	12.0	14.3	13.2	13.7	11.4	8.4	7.5	10.7

Source: Mathers and others 2003.

Table 4.2 Leading Causes of the Disease Burden, by World Bank Region, 2001

Rank	East Asia and the Pacific	Europe and Central Asia	Latin America and the Caribbean	Middle East and North Africa	South Asia	Sub-Saharan Africa	High-income countries
1	Cerebrovascular diseases	Ischemic heart disease	Perinatal conditions[a]	Ischemic heart disease	Perinatal conditions[a]	HIV/AIDS	Ischemic heart disease
2	Perinatal conditions[a]	Cerebrovascular diseases	Unipolar depressive disorders	Perinatal conditions[a]	Lower respiratory infections	Malaria	Cerebrovascular diseases
3	Chronic obstructive pulmonary disease	Unipolar depressive disorders	Homicide and violence	Traffic accidents	Ischemic heart disease	Lower respiratory infections	Unipolar depressive disorders
4	Ischemic heart disease	Self-inflicted injuries	Ischemic heart disease	Lower respiratory infections	Diarrheal diseases	Diarrheal diseases	Alzheimer's disease and other dementias
5	Unipolar depressive disorders	Chronic obstructive pulmonary disease	Cerebrovascular diseases	Diarrheal diseases	Unipolar depressive disorders	Perinatal conditions[a]	Tracheal and lung cancer

Source: Mathers and others 2003.
a. Perinatal conditions include low birthweight, birth asphyxia, and birth trauma.

regions where lower respiratory infections, diarrheal diseases, and perinatal conditions persist. Because these diseases can largely be prevented through relatively low-cost interventions, research into how best to implement these interventions and reduce the infectious disease burden in lower-income countries remains a priority.

The 10:90 Issue

Efforts over the past two decades by the Commission on Health Research in Development, the WHO human reproduction and tropical disease research programs, the WHO Ad Hoc Committee on Research Relating to Future Intervention Options, and—more recently—the Global Forum for Health Research have been largely responsible for the increasing focus on the role of health research in economic and social development. At a time when few health research resources were being devoted to the specific health problems of developing countries, these entities played a critical role in making the case that more should be done. The Global Forum for Health Research took the most effective advocacy position, arguing that 90 percent of the US$70 billion per year devoted to health research and development (R&D) was spent on diseases of the rich countries and only 10 percent was spent on the diseases uniquely afflicting poor countries. This advocacy has been effective and has galvanized global recognition that more research funding should be devoted to improving the health of the 85 percent of the world's population who live in developing or transition countries.

An absolute divergence in gross domestic product persists between industrial and developing countries and, thus, what they can reasonably devote to research. Infectious diseases continue to exact their highest tolls in the poorest countries, and new tools to prevent and treat HIV/AIDS, tuberculosis (TB), malaria, respiratory and diarrheal disease, SARS, influenza, and more exotic infections such as Ebola are urgently needed.

A longer-term view of global health problems recognizes the increasing convergence of health problems, particularly chronic diseases and injuries. It is no longer true that research on cardiovascular disease, diabetes, or depression, for example, is not relevant to developing countries. Vast knowledge is available on how to prevent a major portion of heart disease, lung cancer, type 2 diabetes, sexually transmitted infections, and injuries in the elderly, yet most countries do not implement that knowledge effectively. Thus, more research is needed to successfully transfer that knowledge from industrial to developing countries. For example, if monitored carefully, cost-effective, community-based antihypertensive, antiretroviral, and antidepressive treatments could have an enormous effect in most developing countries.

Increased surveillance and diagnostic capacity for emerging infectious diseases in developing countries will prevent enormous new disease burdens in those countries, while at the same time providing early warning to industrial countries to stimulate new research on vaccines and drugs. Even though industry in developing countries may currently be devoting more effort to creating look-alike drugs, which are unlikely to add a great deal to the duration or quality of life, than to creating drugs for major global killers, and even though market incentives for interventions in resource-poor countries are lacking for most diseases, the solution is not to balkanize research and science, but to stimulate scientific capacity in all countries. Local researchers and industries in developing countries might be able to create interventions that can find a niche in markets in developing countries or that public sector or public-private partnerships are prepared to support.

Global Health Agendas

Some major global health problems cannot be addressed with the available knowledge and existing tools. Major challenges for R&D remain to reduce the unfinished burden of infectious diseases; address the rapidly increasing burden of chronic diseases in aging populations; and reduce the unnecessary burden caused by injuries, casualties of war, and humanitarian emergencies.

The Unfinished Agenda of Infectious Diseases. In 1969, the U.S. surgeon general issued a now famous, if less than prescient, pronouncement: "The time has come to close the book on infectious diseases" (WHO 2000). In 2001, infectious diseases still accounted for 32 percent of the global burden of mortality and 37 percent of the global burden of disease. In Sub-Saharan Africa, they are responsible for 68 percent of deaths. The HIV/AIDS epidemic continues to spread, affecting large proportions of populations in Sub-Saharan Africa, but it is at only an early stage in Asia, when effective prevention efforts could make a difference, as they did in Thailand. AIDS is responsible for the decline in life expectancy to less than 40 years of age in five Sub-Saharan African countries. Yet recent promising results of public health efforts in Brazil, Senegal, Thailand, and Uganda demonstrate that HIV/AIDS can be prevented and controlled on a nationwide scale.

Even though the public in industrial countries often seems surprised by each new outbreak of infectious disease, the pattern of emerging infectious diseases worldwide is continuing and, at the same time, is constantly changing. Since 1970, people have been afflicted by 32 new diseases that had never previously been reported in humans, such as hepatitis C, Legionnaire's disease, Ebola, *Vibrio cholerae* 0139 epidemic, Nipah virus encephalitis, SARS, and the highly pathogenic avian influenza. The 1918 influenza epidemic killed 20 million to 40 million people worldwide. Precisely when human-to-human transmission of the avian influenza viruses will occur is impossible to predict, but it is likely to happen eventually. This eventuality underscores the importance of encouraging systematic collaboration on emerging and reemerging infections and strengthening global surveillance and laboratory capability. A syndromic approach to diagnosis and surveillance, as for the identification of flaccid paralysis, which accelerated the elimination of poliomyelitis in the Western hemisphere, may be crucial when laboratory diagnosis is not readily available.

Finally, the deliberate dissemination of anthrax spores in September and October 2001 in the United States has raised the specter of biological terrorism, either with pathogens natural to the environment that took years to eradicate, like smallpox, or genetically engineered pathogens of unknown capability.

Thus, the global infectious disease agenda remains unfinished. Given the continuing emergence of new infectious diseases and the increasing resistance of microbial pathogens to existing drugs and of insect vectors to pesticides, as well as low compliance with treatments, it is likely to remain so.

The Coming Epidemic: Chronic Diseases and Aging Populations. In 1998, for the first time, chronic diseases contributed more to the global burden of disease than infectious diseases, indicating the emergence of a convergence between the principal diseases of the developing countries and the industrial countries. Worldwide, cardiovascular disease is the major cause of mortality and morbidity (13.6 percent of total disability-adjusted life years) followed by cancer (6.6 percent of total disability-adjusted life years). Diabetes type 2 is increasing in most countries of the world at an alarming rate. An unanticipated finding from the global burden of disease analysis was that psychiatric illness, particularly depression, is a major cause of disability everywhere (Murray and Lopez 1996a, 1996b). Depression is now the most important disability among women in the United States, and globally it is projected to be the second largest contributor to the burden of disease by 2020.

The success of public health and childhood immunization in reducing the number of childhood deaths from infectious disease is partially responsible for the increasing burden of chronic diseases. However, part of the increase is caused by poor eating habits, lack of exercise, smoking, and other unhealthy lifestyle choices that tend to increase with a nation's income. Even though noncommunicable diseases associated with aging are increasingly contributing to the global burden of disease, the emergence of a highly virulent infectious disease pandemic could allow communicable illnesses to reassert their primacy.

The Unnecessary Epidemic: Injuries, Casualties of War, and Humanitarian Emergencies. Before the analysis of the global burden of disease, the contribution of injuries to the burden of disease and disability was unclear. The most rapidly rising category of injuries is that resulting from motor vehicle crashes. If present trends continue, by 2020 motor vehicle crashes will be the third largest contributor to the global burden of disease. Clearly public health sectors have a great deal to contribute in terms of reducing injuries from motor vehicle crashes, falls, and workplace injuries. Less amenable to intervention by public health systems will be wars and humanitarian emergencies. Obtaining accurate figures is difficult, but as Murray and others (2002) note, available statistics have greatly underestimated the burden of war and civil strife on health systems.

The Crisis in Health Systems

Unprecedented advances in the development of health care technologies, drugs, vaccines, and new diagnostics, which hold the promise of healthier and longer lives for many, have profound influences on health systems worldwide; in rich and poor countries alike, they raise expectations and demand for health services along with difficult issues relating to access to information, costs, quality of care, equity, organization, and accountability. All systems are challenged by the need for quality improvement and self-learning.

The overall cost of health care has increased so much that fewer individuals can afford to pay for the best available care; thus, the financing of health systems has become central to national policy debates worldwide. Access and equity considerations pose particularly daunting challenges in poor countries, where access to treatment may be a matter of life and death for entire populations. This situation now prevails in the Sub-Saharan African countries, where the continuing spread of the HIV/AIDS epidemic has resulted in a sharp drop in life expectancy.

Comparative analysis of health systems worldwide seeks to understand the determinants of their performance—for instance, financing, human resources, health information, and quality of care—and to find ways to correct failures. Strengthening such research is one obvious way to tackle the current crisis in health systems. Another less obvious but important implication of the current situation is the need to pursue the best possible science to develop new and better tools and the concomitant need to ensure the availability and affordability of drugs and technologies where they are needed to address major health problems.

New Frontiers for R&D

The extraordinary advances in science provide unprecedented opportunities for both industrial and developing regions. The following sections highlight promises as well as potential pitfalls of frontier research.

Genomics, Molecular Epidemiology, and Preventive Medicine. Probably the most exciting area of biomedical research for at least the next decade derives from the Human

Genome Project and other efforts to sequence entire genomes of mammals, birds, insects, and microbial pathogens. Examination of these genome sequences will allow investigators to define and understand intrinsic risks for disease as well as interactions between genes and environmental threats. The sequencing of the major microbial pathogens has given rise to molecular targets for new drugs against specific pathogens that are distinct from their host counterparts and unique antigenic fragments that may become effective components of new vaccines. Researchers have sequenced the genomes of virtually all major viral, bacterial, and parasitic infectious disease agents and placed the results in databases available to everyone, a true public good (see The Institute of Genomic Research at http://www.tigr.org).

The availability of these genome sequences has catalyzed ambitious research efforts. For example, a project is under way to genetically engineer the *Anopheles* mosquito to render it unable to transmit malaria. Even if this effort fails, knowledge of the mosquito's genome has given new life to medical entomology and will likely help reduce vectorborne diseases in other ways. In a second example, the growing number of available influenza virus sequences will greatly aid understanding of the epidemiology and evolution of pandemic and interpandemic influenza viruses and will be a powerful tool for guiding vaccine strain selection.

The genome project has already changed the understanding of health and disease (box 4.2). Until now, epidemiology has dealt largely with external and environmental risks for disease. What the Human Genome Project offers is knowledge of the other side of the health equation—that is, the intrinsic risks for disease. Previously undreamed of molecular and cellular tools to explore gene expression and function are becoming available to provide such knowledge on a scale that was inconceivable even five years ago.

The hope is that genomics and related biomedical research on stem cells will give rise to new therapies for repairing and remodeling tissue damaged by chronic disease, from heart disease to diabetes and chronic neurological diseases. The possibility of preventive treatment has now also arisen—that is, the identification of risks for chronic disease early in life and the implementation of preventive strategies—behavioral, nutritional, or medical—to avert or overcome intrinsic risks and thereby prevent disease.

Despite the optimism and enthusiasm, a darker side of the Human Genome Project is emerging. Because individuals face different risks, the focus on "boutique medicine" will increase—that is, the focus on risks for individuals and the development of niche interventions targeting those risks, rather than the focus on populations. Identification of those intrinsic risks at birth, for example, will for some time be a luxury available to better-off children in rich countries but not to babies in poor countries or to poor populations of rich countries. Ultimately the Human Genome Project and the rapid advances in biomedical research in the industrial world have the unintended potential to increase the gap between rich and poor. If, however, most complex diseases have multigenic susceptibilities, the magic bullet approach of boutique medicine may not fulfill current expectations of rich or poor countries.

New therapies, whether they arise from genomics or from more traditional pharmacology, must be tested carefully to ensure that people in developing countries are not unfairly treated in clinical trials. Contract research organizations now carry out 60 percent of clinical trials. Many of these organizations already test products in developing countries that will

---

Box 4.2

Uncovering Individual Risks for Specific Diseases

Genomic information makes possible predicting individual risks for certain diseases and to certain components of the environment. One level relates to polymorphisms in individual genes that represent intrinsic risks for certain conditions (for example, breast cancer). A second level relates to differences in the expression patterns of multiple genes on DNA chips that make it possible, for example, to distinguish melanomas from lymphomas from colon cancers or stages within these cancers that no pathologist could duplicate for accuracy. Within patterns for breast cancer or certain types of leukemia, experts can now distinguish those likely to survive five years from those with

a poor prognosis and are creating the first generation of drugs effective against mutated genes causing specific cancers.

The promise of the genome is first and foremost a greater knowledge about disease, risks for disease, and mechanisms of pathogenesis. The exploitation of knowledge from the genome is just beginning, and practical ramifications and many effective products have yet to be realized. Despite the hyperbole about its promise, the genome does represent a new frontier, beyond random testing of compounds, for rational and evidence-based design of effective interventions.

Source: Authors.

have anticipated markets in rich countries but are unlikely, should they be licensed, to be available or affordable to populations in developing countries. This practice is both an ethical and a practical health problem.

Finally, in countries where testing for genetic risks becomes available, the likelihood of risk adjustment—that is, the exclusion of people with some risks from insurance and discrimination in relation to jobs, marriage, and housing—can be anticipated. In this information age, personal genetic information will certainly present an unprecedented challenge to privacy and confidentiality.

A Faint Hope: Population-Based Research. The focus of future research in the rich countries will likely be on individual risks and on interventions tailored to those risks. Yet from the point of view of the world as a whole, the most effective interventions are population-based interventions, such as vaccines, insecticide-impregnated bednets, environmental modifications, antismoking campaigns, clean water, and safe sex. With knowledge derived from biomedical science and the Human Genome Project, it is hoped that some interventions will emerge that do not require knowing any individuals' intrinsic genetic risks and that may apply to entire populations at risk. The hope is that they could be comparable to existing population-based interventions—for example, vaccines recommended for all children to prevent major infectious diseases, treatment of schoolchildren once a year with ivermectin to prevent onchocerciasis, and antismoking campaigns.

In the rich countries, research has shown that aspirin and a combination of inexpensive antihypertensive drugs reduce deaths from heart attacks by 30 percent and from strokes by 50 percent. Even though they are off patent, these interventions are currently not widely used in developing countries. These findings are the products of basic research, but their effective use will depend on operational research.

The Next Frontier: Human Behavior and Social Determinants of Disease. Another revolution in research is emerging: understanding the functioning of the human brain and, ultimately, human behavior. Biomarkers for neuropsychiatric disease and environmental stresses are being sought, and with MRI and positron emission tomography technology, researchers can see areas of the brain that are thinking, remembering, or enjoying music. Within the next 50 years, science will have the technical ability to begin to untangle the processes of thinking in molecular terms, with exciting or frightening possibilities to alter or affect them. Anticipating quantifiable biomarkers for stresses and psychopathology as well as objective tools for measuring the effectiveness of new psychotropic interventions in changing behavior is not unreasonable.

The factors that lead people to engage in unhealthy or destructive behaviors are more complex than simple individual choices.

Many of the lessons of social epidemiology—and the flourishing world of advertising—indicate that most behaviors, including risky or unhealthy behaviors, are socially patterned. Science has unfortunately not done a good job of learning how to change social patterns. For example, merely targeting individuals at high risk for HIV/AIDS without changing the social context that might reinforce stigmatization is not the best way to prevent disease. Indeed, in many developing countries that now provide free counseling, testing, and antiretroviral drugs for people with HIV/AIDS, the biggest barrier remains the social stigma of being HIV positive. Health systems must widen their view beyond individual patients to target entire communities and the media to change unhealthy socially patterned behavior. In the United States, epidemiological estimates indicate that 50 percent of the 2.3 million annual deaths are preventable or postponable. McGinnis and Foege (2004) find that in 2000, 19 percent of deaths were caused by tobacco, about 14 percent were attributable to poor diet and lack of exercise, and about 12 percent to injuries. One of the great challenges is to learn how to communicate what is known about the prevention of such conditions as heart disease, obesity, and diabetes more effectively.

Reliable and comparative analysis of health risks is key for preventing disease and injury. A recently published study (Ezzati and others 2003) reports estimates of the disease burden caused by the joint effect of 20 selected leading risk factors in 14 subepidemiological regions of the world. In regions where high mortality persists, four risk factors—underweight in childhood, micronutrient deficiency, indoor smoke from solid fuels, and tobacco—caused 35 to 42 percent of lower respiratory infections in 2000. In the same regions, the combined risks of high blood pressure, high cholesterol, high body mass index, low fruit and vegetable intake, and physical inactivity caused 82 to 89 percent of the burden of ischemic heart disease. Important gaps in scientific evidence about the effects of multiple risk factors and risk factor interactions persist and require further exploration (Ezzati and others 2003). In this context, investigators should not underestimate social and behavioral determinants of disease, including poverty, environment, culture, and so on.

"Appropriate Science" for the Developing World

Although much discussion about "appropriate technology" for developing countries has taken place in recent decades, curiously little discussion has occurred about appropriate science. Much of the past debate assessed the imbalance of research relevant to developing countries' health problems largely as a function of the projected affordability of the products of the research—drugs, diagnostics, and new technologies developed in the industrial countries—rather than considering the potential contributions that scientists from developing countries could make both to advancing science and to addressing their countries' health problems. Although some technologies are more or less appropriate to contexts in developing countries for reasons of cost, maintenance, or skill requirements, no limitation exists on what science or knowledge is appropriate in developing countries.

Some might argue that people in developing countries should restrict their research focus to diseases that principally affect their countries. If that were generalized to all countries, rich countries would not carry out research on tropical diseases, and the developing countries would do little research on chronic diseases. This strategy would violate two fundamental principles of science. First, connectivity in science is unpredictable: research on one disease or problem often brings conceptual or technological advances that are vital to progress in others; therefore, to the extent possible, every country should support a relatively broad spectrum of research. Second, creative science requires the freedom to pursue ideas. Progress in science is not fostered by restricting freedom of inquiry. There is every reason to believe that scientists in developing countries will create knowledge of value to diseases that primarily afflict people in industrial countries, both because of the convergence of health problems and because scientific knowledge is a public good.

Epistemology is the formal study of knowledge, and theories of how knowledge is generated abound. One such theory particularly relevant in the context of health research holds that three basic kinds of knowledge exist:[2]

- *Public knowledge.* This knowledge is generally published in the scientific literature, available in principle to all (with the glaring exception of those who cannot afford the major scientific journals). Because this knowledge is available to the entire global scientific community, it is a true public good. Indeed, publication in such journals is the basis for most judgments of academic and scientific achievement and is a precondition for scientific support and advancement.
- *Contextual knowledge.* This kind of knowledge is absolutely essential to bringing the fruits of public knowledge to a particular country or people. It requires learning and experience and involves cultural, social, and economic knowledge of a place, without which effectively implementing public knowledge or scientific discoveries in that context or evaluating the success of programs within national contexts is often impossible. In this case, research may have to be carried out in relation to how to implement interventions, as WHO's Special Programme for Research and Training in Tropical Diseases programs in leprosy and malaria have done in the absence of full scientific evidence. As essential as it may be, the global scientific and academic communities do not widely recognize or value contextual knowledge.
- *Tacit knowledge.* In contrast to public knowledge and contextual knowledge, tacit or intrinsic knowledge is impossible to write down or teach because it depends on a special kind of communication between individuals that makes transmission of knowledge possible. One thinks of a few great clinical teachers who simply "know" the diagnosis without laboratory tests, or health care professionals who can put their colleagues in developing countries at ease and bring out the best in everyone being taught rather than being condescending or patronizing. Tacit knowledge is intuitive, breaks down barriers of culture or training, is highly motivating, and is often transformational in people's lives.

A few examples illustrate the importance of contextual knowledge. Many ideas and interventions are available, but knowledge on their effectiveness in different populations and on how to increase their usefulness is limited. The need to define best practices in different circumstances is urgent in relation to health. For example, data from the industrial countries indicate that providing a three-drug package containing aspirin to people with hypertension as preventive treatment might be possible on a population-based model as well as by individual physicians or medical personnel. However, Asians are more predisposed to hemorrhagic strokes than Europeans; therefore, treatment with such a regimen in Asia might have a significantly increased risk of adverse effects.

In another example, antiretroviral drugs are responsible for the 50 percent decline in mortality from HIV/AIDS in the United States, and the Global Fund to Fight AIDS, Tuberculosis, and Malaria; bilateral agencies; and the pharmaceutical industry are engaging in major efforts to make them available to resource-poor endemic countries. Despite encouraging examples in Brazil and Haiti, it is unclear whether—as in DOTS (directly observed treatment short course), a supervised method of administering drugs used for treating TB in resource-poor countries—these drugs can be given safely and effectively by community-based treatment programs, be appropriately monitored, and prevent the emergence of drug resistance or toxicity and thus provide cures for a high percentage of the patients in poor countries. However, if this method can be used, it will strengthen the fight against HIV/AIDS.

Research on community-based programs for treating children with epilepsy or adults with depression provides another example. The provision of ivermectin (Mectizan) to prevent and treat onchocerciasis revealed that even making a drug to be taken only once a year available and providing it free of charge had an almost negligible effect initially, because in some areas of Sub-Saharan Africa an effective health delivery system was simply not available. It is to Merck's credit that the Mectizan program invested considerable resources to create a delivery and monitoring system that has moved onchocerciasis to the category of diseases targeted for elimination as public health problems by WHO.

The flow of knowledge is not unidirectional. Reciprocity between research in different fields and different countries is vital for the expansion of knowledge, and the unique contributions of developing countries to global health research are often overlooked and not always appreciated. For example, DOTS was initially developed in Tanzania, where researchers found that the best drug combination given with supervision, even though more costly, was both more effective in preventing relapse and emerging drug resistance and more cost-effective than the cheapest combinations. Similarly, artemisinin, the most rapidly acting drug for treating cerebral malaria, derives from an ancient Chinese medicine, qinghaosu, and is now a major tool in the armamentarium of malaria treatments. Research on isolated populations in developing countries can further the understanding of some of the genetic determinants of a variety of diseases, and transnational research on almost any disease has the potential to provide important insights into differences in risk factors in different contexts.

Such reciprocity depends critically on the development of scientific capacity. In terms of resource allocation, research funders often appear to have overlooked the necessary connection between research and training the next generations of researchers. Scientific and health capacity building and training are inseparable from research, yet funders seldom recognize the training aspect, and it is difficult to ensure that funding for training will be recognized as integral to research.

"Appropriate Technology" for the Developing World

The development community has long debated the nature of appropriate technology for resource-poor countries. Innumerable instances exist of high-tech biomedical equipment standing unused in laboratories and hospitals throughout the developing world, serving as status symbols but not as tools to further knowledge or alleviate illness. However, the best tools appropriate for learning from the research should be made available when the primary purpose of research is to acquire knowledge, particularly if human subjects are engaged as volunteers in clinical studies to help develop that new knowledge. For example, researchers studying the effectiveness of antiretroviral drugs in resource-poor countries should have access to technology that can measure CD4 cells, viral loads, and antiviral drug resistance, which are critical for analyzing the drugs' effectiveness. Sophisticated technology may be vital to establish the scientific principle of effectiveness, thereby enabling implementation of the most cost-effective treatment program in settings where the high-tech methodology may no longer be necessary on a large scale but may remain useful for validating the effectiveness of lower-tech surrogate markers.

Strengthening Capacity and Institutions

A 1996 WHO report (Ad Hoc Committee on Health Research Relating to Future Intervention Options 1996) emphasizes three research needs that had not previously been articulated as essential to development.

- The first is a need for new knowledge through research to develop new tools for addressing continually emerging global health problems. Some of this knowledge will be generalizable, but much will be context specific and perhaps country specific.
- The second is the recognition that in many developing countries research capacity—that is, people with the training to carry out surveillance and laboratory and operational research—is limited, indicating an enormous need for training. Career structures and incentives to retain trained professionals in public health, medical sciences, and health systems in developing countries are also needed. An enormous brain drain is under way for nursing and other health professionals. The inducements to leave developing countries for higher salaries and better working conditions in the industrial world are compelling, even though many in the health field would prefer to help alleviate their own countries' health problems if it were feasible for them to do so.
- The third is that all the key priorities depend on the strengthening of institutions: universities, schools of public health and medicine, centers for disease control, and research institutions for health policy and economics. As the report indicates, remarkably few high-level institutions for research and training in public health have been created in developing countries during the past 25 years. Little progress has been made since the mid 1990s. Thus, their large needs for human capacity as well as laboratory and research infrastructure for public health are not surprising. For this situation to improve in a timely way, a new basis for cooperation in support of people and institutions must be forged between the developing and industrial countries.

Clearly governments should make greater commitments to health training and institutions. Whereas the international community has focused primarily on access to drugs in resource-poor countries, new partnerships in research are clearly needed. It is gratifying that programs that encourage and support cross-national, North-South, and South-South scientific collaborations and institutional links have been increasing, and the tremendous effect of the Bill & Melinda Gates Foundation in supporting research has emphasized the value of public and private commitments and partnerships in research. Regrettably, concomitant commitment has been lacking on the part of governments and many foundations to support training in research; career path opportunities; and institutions such as university science departments, medical schools, and schools of public health, all of which are critical for reducing the research and capacity gap between rich and poor countries.

No simple answer is available regarding the best ways to ensure effective collaboration in relation to global heath. Global

SARS and Influenza: A Paradigm Shift for Global Research Collaboration

Outbreaks of emerging infectious diseases are by their nature unpredictable. They can be contained when they are detected early and the number of cases is small. When they are not contained, they can have enormous human and economic consequences. Economic losses attributed to SARS, which infected 8,000 people and killed 774, have been estimated at US$30 million per day in Canada and a total of US$16 billion to US$30 billion in Asia.

The global response to the SARS epidemic demonstrated the power of international collaboration under leadership of WHO among public health professionals, researchers, and institutions in several countries to halt the progression of a new disease (La Montagne and others 2004). Another example is influenza: an existing international network of influenza research sites, which is critical for defining the strains to be used each year for immunization, was instrumental in developing an unprecedented rapid response to the potentially devastating bird H5N1 influenza A.

These examples represent an important paradigm shift in global research collaboration in that they required national surveillance at the epidemiological and laboratory levels; unprecedented sharing of information at all levels of the health system; and close cooperation among clinicians, epidemiologists, and bench scientists, as well as those involved in veterinary surveillance, for the rapid development of effective intervention strategies. Integrated global responses raise difficult issues pertaining to information sharing and ownership of specimens and reagents, which have profound implications for future global health R&D. They also underscore that, despite the political temptations of denial and the economic threats of epidemic disease, honest and accurate information is essential for early warning and for making effective health policy.

Source: Authors.

collaborations can be difficult, they are not inexpensive, and their successes are limited in number, but they can potentially have a major effect (box 4.3). Questions arise about how to develop economies of scale in R&D and institutional capabilities; how many research centers are optimal in a developing country; how much should be done by country partners and how much in the developing countries; and what the roles of basic scientific versus epidemiological, clinical, and operational research should be. The experience of working together in true partnerships appears to be generally rewarding for scientists in both industrial and developing countries and seems to be an effective way of increasing research capacity. One set of lessons still to be learned is what the best forms of collaboration are: individual scientist, institutional, transnational, or multinational.

PRIORITY SETTING

Setting priorities for R&D of interventions is both complex and critical in the context of severely constrained resources. A systematic approach that takes into account the disease burden as well as scientific opportunities has been proposed to guide decisions.

Approaches

The challenge is to ensure that available resources are targeted at major health problems.

Inherent Difficulties in Setting Priorities. The first part of this chapter underscored the immense scope of health problems and the potential of global health research to make a difference. Given the complexity of the task and the multiple participants involved in the process, defining priorities for the global health research agenda is daunting.

Scientists tend to argue that more research is urgently needed on the diseases they are studying. Their research may certainly include worthwhile issues, but they may not be priorities in the wider context of global health R&D.

Some hold the view that the choice of priorities should begin with a statement defining topics that should not be priorities—for example, the development of vaccines (such as a leprosy or hookworm vaccine) when cost-effective treatments are available. Others strongly disagree, given the interconnectedness and unpredictability of science.

The failure of the U.S. "war on cancer" offers a useful caution on the limitations of rational planning of science. In the 1960s, a group of distinguished scientists developed a set of future research priorities for the National Cancer Program. Despite the importance of the problem, the requisite scientific knowledge was not then available to develop the modern tools that have recently been successful in treating and preventing cancer. Planning for where the new innovations and discoveries will come from is hard, and planners have to be open to changing their priorities and incorporating new approaches.

A key challenge is the problematic nature of anticipating scientific connections in advance. For example, the sequencing of a mouse leukemia virus genome as part of the National Cancer Program is what enabled scientists years later to classify HIV as a related member of the retrovirus family. Indeed, who would have predicted that research on the once arcane coronavirus would become essential to control the spread of SARS? Or that the esoteric question of whether tumor cells extinguished differentiated functions of normal body cells would lead to the discovery of monoclonal antibodies? Or that the study of sex in bacteria would give rise to the entire genetic revolution of the past half century? The need to recognize the unpredictability of science and the limitations of scientists at any time is best illustrated by Oppenheimer's statement at the beginning of this chapter.

Systematic and Evidence-Based Approach to Priority Setting. The process of setting priorities for the global health research agenda is complex and includes accurate or perceived assessments of the burden of disease; developed countries' threat assessments, for example, in relation to bioterrorism and epidemic potential; scientific or technical opportunities; advocacy; political commitment; ethical considerations; and funding availability.

Using a systematic and evidence-based approach to priority setting, the WHO Ad Hoc Committee for Health Research Relating to Future Intervention Options (1996) undertook the first broadly based, systematic effort to formulate "best buys" for health R&D (table 4.3). The steps included assessments of the following:

- size of the disease burden
- reasons the disease burden persisted
- adequacy of the current scientific knowledge base
- cost-effectiveness of potential interventions and the probability of successful development of new tools
- adequacy of the current level of ongoing research and funding.

Table 4.3 R&D Best Buys

Category	Key R&D investments
Maternal and child health	
Strategic research	Understand the relative importance, in different environments, of increased nutrient intake and of control of infectious disease as a way to reduce malnutrition
Package development and evaluation	Evaluate and refine the package for the integrated management of the sick child
	Develop, evaluate, and refine the mother-baby package for pregnancy, delivery, and neonatal care
	Evaluate the implementation of a range of family planning packages offering a wide choice of methods
New tools to improve package content	Evaluate the efficacy and optimal dosage of candidate rotavirus vaccines in low-income countries
	Evaluate the efficacy of optimal dosage of candidate conjugate pneumococcal vaccines and the effectiveness of existing vaccine against influenza B in low-income countries
	Develop and evaluate ways to increase efficiency in the Expanded Program on Immunizations by simplifying delivery and maximizing use of opportunities for immunization
	Evaluate the promotion of insecticide-impregnated bednets for inclusion in a future healthy household package
	Develop new contraceptive methods, particularly to widen the choice of long-term but reversible methods, postcoital methods for regular and emergency use, and methods for men
Microbial threats	
Strategic research	Screen drugs on molecular targets predicted by the genome sequence of major pathogens
	Investigate influences on the spread of antimicrobial resistance and approaches to monitoring resistant strains with the aim of identifying ways of slowing their emergence
Intervention development	Develop an effective prophylaxis for TB—for example, depot (or long-acting), or a vaccine chemoprophylaxis
	Develop a malaria vaccine
	Develop an HIV vaccine
	Develop improved methods for the diagnosis, prevention, and treatment of sexually transmitted diseases, including vaginal microbicides
Noncommunicable diseases and injuries	Establish a special program for research and training on noncommunicable diseases and healthy aging
	Establish a special program or initiative for research, training, and capacity building on injuries
Health policy	Establish a special program for research and training on health systems and policy

Source: Ad Hoc Committee on Health Research Relating to Future Intervention Options 1996.

This five-step approach has been influential. The Global Forum for Health Research and the Special Programme for Research and Training in Tropical Diseases have endorsed it and further developed it. The Global Forum's combined approach matrix links the five steps with four actors or factors determining the health status (Global Forum for Health Research 2002):

- individual, family, and community
- health ministry, health research institutions, and health systems and services
- sectors other than health
- central government macroeconomic policies.

The five steps also provide the basis for the strategic emphases matrix for tropical diseases research (Remme and others 2002).

The individual disease chapters in this volume used a slightly modified version of the framework developed by the WHO Ad Hoc Committee to identify gaps and guide the formulation of research priorities on the basis of the following premise: even though the current mix of available cost-effective interventions averts a proportion of the burden of any particular disease and the remaining burden could be further reduced with improved application of existing technologies to affected populations, a fraction of disease remains that cannot be averted. Two reasons account for this fact. First, the cost for extending the existing technology to the remainder of the population would be prohibitive. Second, the existing interventions may simply not be sufficiently effective. These two categories define the magnitude of the need for new or better tools and, in essence, serve as a rationale and indicate priorities for research.

A clear example is the case of HIV/AIDS. Neither behavioral interventions, such as exhortations for abstinence and fidelity and the provision of condoms, nor antiretroviral therapy has stopped the global spread of HIV, which challenges the scientific community to undertake more research on preventive vaccines. The availability of highly active antiretroviral therapy challenges the research community to find ways of providing effective and life-saving treatment for HIV/AIDS patients in a manner that ensures proper use and compliance, averts the development of drug resistance, and thereby becomes a financially sustainable policy.

Participants and Decision Makers. Two main concerns lie at the core of most discussions of the priority-setting processes: the predominance of the industrial countries and the predominance of the scientific community in formulating research agendas. Two-thirds of respondents in a survey of researchers that was funded by the National Institute of Allergy and Infectious Diseases of the U.S. National Institutes of Health and was conducted in May 2004 were leading scientists from low- and middle-income developing countries and worked in the same region in which they held their citizenship. The survey highlighted their views about key factors influencing research priority setting as well as major barriers that hampered stronger participation by scientists from developing countries in global health research. According to the survey, the most important factors determining research priorities were the magnitude of disease burdens and the needs of the industrial countries. Major barriers to the success of research collaboration in global health were the lack of sustained funding; the difficulty of linking research, programs, and policy; the weak research leadership; and the absence of a science culture (Harley, Simonsen, and Breman 2004).

A more balanced participation of scientists from industrial and developing countries, a better gender mix, and the inclusion of major stakeholders are essential to the successful development of a truly global health research agenda. The challenge is to develop creative mechanisms for addressing current shortcomings.

The process for selecting the best research projects and programs within each priority area is well established and is grounded in scientific merit, based primarily on trust in peer review and expert judgment. Keeping this process independent from political pressures is extremely important. However, the peer review process has limitations, including a natural conservatism and risk aversion by scientists, given the responsibility for the allocation of public funding, their often narrow base of expertise in one discipline, and their specific cultural perspective. Alternative models of project selection from industry and other scientific, mission-oriented entities might offer interesting alternatives—for example, managerial systems or strategic planning processes, particularly for translating knowledge into successful interventions, an area that research is currently emphasizing.

Ethical considerations and pressures exerted by advocacy groups—such as public-private partnerships for targeted drug or vaccine development, fresh looks at "orphan drug" legislation, patent rules ensuring financial returns to industry as well as the affordability of new products in developing countries, and commitment before their development by the public and private sectors to subsidize their development or ensure markets for the products—are likely to counterbalance to some extent the lack of incentives for the pharmaceutical industry to develop drugs, diagnostics, and vaccines for which markets do not exist or are not profitable. In addition, one might hope that the growing pharmaceutical and vaccine industry in developing countries might place a higher priority on addressing nationally and regionally important health problems than do multinational companies.

The share of total R&D funds allocated to major causes of the disease burden in developing countries remains insufficient. As a result, the availability of funding to support global health R&D is ultimately the defining factor regarding the implementation of selected R&D priorities. Thus, the Bill & Melinda Gates Foundation has become a major driving force in defining priorities for global health R&D through its support of promising public-private partnerships. The new US$200 million it provided to finance the Grand Challenges in Global Health represents the newest large influx of funds in support of global health research (see Foundation of National Institutes of Health at http://www.grandchallengesgh.org).

Findings

Research agendas proposed in the various chapters fall into three broad categories:

- priorities that are already on the global health agenda
- important topics that are not yet on the global agenda, but should be pursued
- promising research topics that are not yet priorities, but should be pursued.

Michaud and others (2005) provide a more exhaustive account of the research priorities summarized here and recommended in the volume.

Priorities Already Part of the Global Health Agenda. Priorities that are already the most prominent part of the global health agenda relate almost exclusively to the unfinished agenda of infectious diseases and to the continuous threats of emerging infectious diseases, including bioterrorism. The largest investments pertain to the development of new drugs and vaccines that are needed to reduce the burden of HIV/AIDS, malaria, and TB; to the early detection and control of new highly pathogenic viral agents (for example, SARS); and to the prevention and treatment of infectious diseases resulting from microbial terrorism (for instance, anthrax and smallpox).

In 2001, the National Institute of Allergy and Infectious Diseases developed a global research plan for HIV/AIDS, malaria, and TB. The plan outlines a comprehensive approach for fighting infectious diseases that involves building a sustainable research capability domestically and internationally and enhancing global partnerships. It comprises short-, medium-, and long-term goals for research that "will lead to prevention and treatment strategies that are effective, feasible, and realistic for individual countries struggling with the burden of numerous infectious diseases" (National Institute of Allergy and Infectious Diseases 2001).

Since the mid 1970s, the WHO Special Programme for Research and Training in Tropical Diseases and a few other institutions have been key players in strengthening research and research capacity for tropical diseases that are endemic in specific developing regions—African trypanosomiasis, Chagas disease, dengue, leishmaniasis, leprosy, lymphatic filariasis, malaria, onchocerciasis, and schistosomiasis. As a result, effective control measures are now available for Chagas disease, leprosy, lymphatic filariasis, and onchocerciasis—but questions remain regarding effective implementation strategies. The other diseases still lack effective control measures and, thus, require further research to develop better tools and effective control strategies (http://www.who.int/tdr/grants/strategic-emphases/default.htm).

The process that led to the formulation of the Grand Challenges in Global Health represents two important departures from earlier approaches to priority setting. First, the announcement of the call for ideas in May 2003 had an unprecedented dissemination worldwide and resulted in over 1,000 submissions from scientists and institutions in 75 countries. Second, the formulation of a grand challenge, described as "a call for specific scientific or technological innovation that would remove a critical barrier to solving an important health problem in the developing world with a high likelihood of global impact and feasibility" (Varmus and others 2003) was broad and had a clear goal.

The research agendas proposed in chapters 16, 18, and 21 are extensive and encompass research on basic epidemiology and risk factors and the development of new or better drugs, vaccines, diagnostics, and intervention methods. The fact that these priorities do not represent a marked departure from previous research priorities for these conditions attests to the complexity of these diseases and their importance in the poorest countries. They will require a broadly based and sustained global research effort to overcome the rapid spread of antibiotic and insecticide resistance, limited human resources, and poorly developed health systems that severely constrain the health community's ability to reduce the burden of disease.

Important Topics That Are Not Yet on the Global Research Agenda but Should Be Pursued. Cardiovascular diseases, neuropsychiatric disorders, obesity, diabetes, and cancers are causing a rapidly increasing share of the disease burden in all developing regions, with the exception of Sub-Saharan Africa; however, they do not yet figure prominently on the global health research agenda. The research priorities recommended independently by the authors of various chapters pertaining to major causes of noncommunicable diseases converge. Indeed, diet, lifestyle, obesity, tobacco, and alcohol are common risk factors for cardiovascular diseases, certain cancers, and diabetes. These diseases and risk factors represent a cluster of conditions that pose similar research challenges.

The first important cross-cutting theme emerging from this cluster of chapters is the issue of portability, or how to bring knowledge and programs from one location and define how they can become best practices elsewhere. Cost-effective preventive strategies and therapeutic approaches to reduce the burden of cardiovascular diseases, cancer, diabetes, and mental disorders have been developed and tested in industrial countries. Much of the extensive knowledge base accumulated in industrial countries to prevent the development of cardiovascular diseases, diabetes, and cancers is likely to be relevant to developing countries, yet few epidemiological studies have quantified the impact of major risk factors for chronic diseases in developing regions, and few trials have been conducted to assess the effectiveness of different intervention strategies. Research to explore the transferability of cost-effective interventions from industrial to developing countries therefore figures prominently in several chapters.

The primary prevention for noncommunicable diseases in industrial countries rests on the reduction of major risk factors—namely, diet, lifestyles, and tobacco and alcohol consumption. Research priorities include the development of epidemiological databases and of intervention studies to identify cost-effective strategies to reduce the prevalence of major risk factors in different contexts in developing countries. The transfer of personal and population-based interventions to reduce the risk of cardiovascular disease, which are based on decades of research in the industrial countries, is particularly promising. Research priorities include evaluating a range of intervention strategies, from simple dietary interventions to reduce the risk of cardiovascular disease (for example, food supplementation with folic acid and linoleic acid and reduction in the salt, saturated fat, and trans fat content of processed foods), to the hypothetical "polypill," which would combine drugs to lower cholesterol, clotting, and blood pressure. Reducing the risk of cardiovascular disease is particularly important for diabetes, which is itself an important risk factor for cardiovascular disease.

The second theme pertains to lifelong medical management of chronic conditions that cannot be cured but could be improved through the development and testing of public health prevention and treatment algorithms. This issue has been little considered in past discussions of priorities for global health research but now appears to be reasonably cost-effective. Examples include unipolar depression, bipolar disorders, schizophrenia, epilepsy, diabetes, and secondary prevention of ischemic heart disease and stroke.

The third theme pertains to crucial implementation research that combines operations research and health services and systems research. Such research is becoming central to ensuring the success of the rapid scaling-up of cost-effective interventions that is required to meet the health targets of the Millennium Development Goals, particularly in resource-poor countries with weak health systems. In this context, further research is critical to elucidate neglected areas of health system reforms, including the following (Mills 2004):

- improving public service provision
- enhancing human resources
- ensuring accountability for health outcomes, funds, and medicines
- ensuring a functioning central government
- providing evidence for policy.

Promising Research Topics Not Yet Global Priorities. Other important research topics emerge from the various chapters that are not yet global priorities but that are nevertheless worthwhile pursuing. Major themes pertain to the following:

- epidemiology of injuries and cost-effective interventions to reduce the burden resulting from both intentional and unintentional injuries, particularly motor vehicle crashes and road and vehicle safety
- major risk factors for disease in different contexts (for example, tobacco, obesity, physical activity)
- medical and surgical errors
- occupational and environmental health
- risk analysis and risk communication
- delivery of care at different levels of the health system
- performance of health systems
- management of health research
- reproductive and sexual health
- health effects of global warming.

The importance of strengthening the research agenda in those and other areas and the resultant opportunities to make a real difference have not been sufficiently recognized in the past.

KEY RECOMMENDATIONS

The priority-setting process should focus initially on defining a small number of key priorities that have a reasonable chance of succeeding and yielding cost-effective outcomes in resource-constrained environments and that are, thus, least likely to divert limited resources from being more effectively directed elsewhere. Five broad recommendations emerge from this chapter.

Invest More Wisely in Health R&D

The focus should be on how best to invest limited resources for health R&D. This approach raises hard questions about selecting priorities and the extent to which the burden of disease and scientific opportunity to play a role. A telling example of the dilemma may be a vaccine against bird flu. Because bird flu, A (H5N1) or other strains, is not yet a major human disease, the setting of priorities by the disease burden criterion would not accord a bird flu vaccine high priority. But knowing that between 20 to 40 million people died in the 1918 influenza epidemic, and that with a transmission time of 1.5 days, there would be few public health measures other than a vaccine that would make a difference in preventing a pandemic, developing and testing multiple candidate vaccines should be an urgent research priority.

Despite the paucity of past analysis of the relationship between the cost of research in an area and its success in improving the level of health, the amount invested is unlikely to have been the most important determinant of success. The What Works Working Group has developed 17 case studies of success stories, all of which were supported by public finance mostly in resource-constrained settings (Levine and What Works Working Group 2004). A review of lessons learned from the 20 biggest research successes in improving health in low- and middle-income countries would be a worthwhile undertaking.

Shift the Paradigm for Priority Setting

The paradigm shift from dividing the world's health problems into those of the industrial countries and those of the developing countries toward creating a better understanding of the commonality of health problems between the industrial and most developing countries lies at the core of priority setting for global health research. Implicit in this shift is the recognition that the health problems of Sub-Saharan Africa are urgent and require special emphasis on the devastating burden of infectious diseases, particularly HIV/AIDS, and on the need to develop effective infrastructure for health. In time, the expectation is that the health needs of most Sub-Saharan African countries will similarly converge with those of other regions of the world and that knowledge developed in these regions will be transferable and helpful to accelerating development there.

As sociologists have long recognized, scientific and medical technology diffuses from the industrial to the developing countries, and it will, in the short term at least, increase the disparities between rich and poor countries—and perhaps to a comparable extent between the rich and the poor within countries—because more affluent and better-educated populations tend to have greater access to new technologies. However, even though disparities in health between affluent urban dwellers and poor rural populations in China and India have increased over the past decade, the overall quality of health of the entire population has increased during the same period. The hope is that information derived from research will be a great leveler over time and will contribute to reducing global inequities.

The shift in thinking in relation to the convergence of health burdens and research opportunities in both industrial and developing countries has far-reaching implications for the formulation of research priorities. In addition to emphasizing the commonality of health problems, it also emphasizes the importance of stronger global research collaboration in tackling major health problems and underscores the need for much stronger public-private partnerships to ensure that affordable drugs and vaccines will be developed and made available in resource-constrained environments.

Maximize the Potential of Information Technology

No advances in science have more potential for improving health globally than the information and communication sciences. At the scientific level, the ability to handle increasingly massive amounts of data, whether from genetics, epidemiology, or clinical trials, offers the opportunity to mine the world of knowledge in ways that could not be contemplated a decade ago. Knowledge can be transferred instantaneously through the Internet; through access to open databases; and through the new public libraries of science and medicine, such as the U.S. National Library of Medicine PubMed Central. With information technology, procedures can be put in place to minimize medical and pharmaceutical errors and to provide greater accounting for medical costs and outcomes. Finally, research with partners in many parts of the world can now be carried out in real or in lag time, as in the case of clinical research on malaria (Royall and others 2004). The tools, hardware, and software for this informatics revolution must be made available as widely as possible to universities and health systems in developing countries.

Increase Global Research Capacity

Research capacity continues to limit the successful implementation of those interventions most needed to improve health in resource-constrained environments. The number of people trained to carry out the surveillance and the laboratory and operational research that are so essential to the successful implementation of cost-effective interventions remains woefully inadequate. Redressing this limitation is a daunting task that will require substantial financial investment and creative approaches to create conditions that will reverse the brain drain and strengthen academic and research institutions in developing countries.

Create a Global Health Architecture

Health is not the sole provenance of the health sector, and yet there is no forum or architecture for coordinating the increasingly important multisectoral interactions to improve health.

Cardiovascular and pulmonary disease in Europe and the United States are increasingly determined by China's energy sector, and global warming is impacted by the policy of the U.S. President. Health is critically affected by education, energy, transport, finance, trade, immigration, communication, and the environment. Major health problems will be most successfully addressed if partnerships can be developed between sectors, governments, NGOs, business and industry, and academe.

Support Freedom of Scientific Inquiry

No country has a monopoly on ideas, and every country has something important to contribute to knowledge about health. The universality of science requires that scientists everywhere strive for the highest level of rigor and quality and that every country have some sustainable level of scientific research and problem-solving capacity. Encouraging and supporting scientists with the ability and passion to contribute to knowledge about health, globally or locally, must become one of the key aims of the global health and development agendas.

ACKNOWLEDGMENT

This chapter is dedicated to the memory of John La Montagne, who was a tireless supporter of health research into problems of developing countries, a good friend, and an inspiration to us all.

NOTES

1. Obviously, nonrivalry does not pertain to knowledge that is proprietary, as in the pharmaceutical industry, although the system of patents was created to make such enabling knowledge available to all by providing a limited monopoly for its exploitation by discoverers or inventors.

2. For this formulation, we are indebted to Suwit Wibulpolprasert, deputy permanent secretary of the Ministry of Health, Thailand.

REFERENCES

Ad Hoc Committee on Health Research Relating to Future Intervention Options. 1996. *Investing in Health Research and Development.* Geneva: World Health Organization.

Commission on Macroeconomics and Health. 2001. *Macroeconomics and Health.* Geneva: World Health Organization.

Ezzati, M., S. V. Hoorn, A. Rodgers, A. D. Lopez, C. D. Mathers, and C. J. Murray. 2003. "Estimates of Global and Regional Potential Health Gains from Reducing Multiple Major Risk Factors." *Lancet* 362 (9380): 271–80.

Fischer, S. 2003. "Socialist Economy Reform: Lessons of the First Three Years." *American Economic Review* 93 (May): 390–95.

Fogel, R. W. 2004. *The Escape from Hunger and Premature Death, 1700–2100.* Cambridge, U.K.: Cambridge University Press.

Global Forum for Health Research. 2002. *The 10/90 Report on Health Research 2001–2002.* Geneva: Global Forum for Health Research.

Harley, L., L. Simonsen, and J. Breman. 2004. "Perceptions of Health Research Priority Setting and Barriers: A Survey of International Health Researchers." Unpublished paper, National Institute of Allergy

and Infectious Diseases, U.S. National Institutes of Health, U.S. Department of Health and Human Services, Bethesda, MD.

Institute of Medicine. 1997. *America's Vital Interest in Global Health: Protecting Our People, Enhancing Our Economy, and Advancing Our International Interests.* Washington DC: National Academy Press.

King, G., and L. Zeng. 2001. "Improving Forecasts of State Failure." *World Politics* 53 (July): 623–58.

———. 2002. *Consolidated State Failure Events, 1955–2001.* College Park, MD: University of Maryland.

La Montagne, J. R., L. Simonsen, R. J. Taylor, and J. Turnbull. 2004. "SARS Research Working Group Co-Chairs—Severe Acute Respiratory Syndrome: Developing a Research Response." *Journal of Infectious Diseases* 189 (4): 634–41.

Levine, R., and What Works Working Group with Molly Kinder. 2004. *Millions Saved: Proven Successes in Global Health.* Washington, DC: Center for Global Development.

Mathers, C., A. Lopez, C. Stein, D. Ma Fat, R. Chalapati, M. Inoue, and others. 2005. "Death and Disease Burden by Cause: Global Burden of Disease Estimates for 2001 by World Bank Country Groups." Disease Control Priorities Project Working Paper No. 18. Fogarty International Center and National Institutes of Health, Washington, DC.

McGinnis, J. M., and W. H. Foege. 2004. "The Immediate versus the Important." *Journal of the American Medical Association* 291 (10): 1263–64.

Michaud, C. M., P. Maslen, S. Sahid-Salles, and J. Breman. 2005. "Synthesis of Priorities for Global Research and Development." Disease Control Priorities Project Working Paper, Fogarty International Center and National Institutes of Health, Washington, DC.

Mills, A. 2004. "Missing Areas in Health Sector Reform." Unpublished paper, London School of Hygiene and Tropical Medicine.

Murray, C. J., G. King, A. D. Lopez, N. Tomijima, and E. G. Krug. 2002. "Armed Conflict as a Public Health Problem." *British Medical Journal* 324 (7333): 346–49.

Murray, C. J., and A. D. Lopez, eds. 1996a. *The Global Burden of Disease: A Comprehensive Assessment of Mortality and Disability from Diseases, Injuries, and Risk Factors in 1990 and Projected to 2020.* Vol. 1 of *Global Burden of Disease and Injury.* Cambridge, MA: Harvard School of Public Health for the World Health Organization and the World Bank.

———. 1996b. *Global Health Statistics: A Compendium of Incidence, Prevalence, and Mortality for over 200 Conditions.* Vol. 2 of *Global Burden of Disease and Injury.* Cambridge, MA: Harvard School of Public Health for the World Health Organization and the World Bank.

National Institute of Allergy and Infectious Diseases. 2001. "NIAID Global Health Research Plan for HIV/AIDS, Malaria, and Tuberculosis." National Institute of Allergy and Infectious Diseases, National Institutes of Health, U.S. Department of Health and Human Services, Bethesda, MD.

Remme, J. H., E. Blas, L. Chitsulo, P. M. Desjeux, H. D. Engers, T. P. Kanyok, and others. 2002. "Strategic Emphases for Tropical Diseases Research: A TDR Perspective." *Trends in Parasitology* 18 (10): 421–26.

Royall, J., M. Bennett, I. van Schayk, and M. Alilio. 2004. "Tying up Lions: Multilateral Initiative on Malaria Communications: The First Chapter of a Malaria Research Network in Africa." *American Journal of Tropical Medicine and Hygiene* 71 (2 Suppl.): 259–67.

Varmus, H., R. Klausner, E. Zerhouni, T. Acharya, A. S. Daar, and P. A. Singer. 2003. "Grand Challenges in Global Health." *Science* 302 (5644): 398–99.

Wilson, E. O. 2003. *The Future of Life.* New York: Vintage Books.

WHO (World Health Organization). 2000. *Report on Global Surveillance of Epidemic-Prone Infectious Diseases.* WHO/CDS/CSR/ISR/2000.1. Geneva: WHO.

World Bank. 2004. *World Development Indicators.* Washington, DC: World Bank.

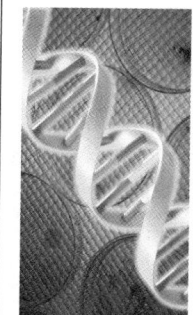

Chapter **5**

Science and Technology for Disease Control: Past, Present, and Future

David Weatherall, Brian Greenwood, Heng Leng Chee, and Prawase Wasi

As we move into the new millennium it is becoming increasingly clear that the biomedical sciences are entering the most exciting phase of their development. Paradoxically, medical practice is also passing through a phase of increasing uncertainty, in both industrial and developing countries. Industrial countries have not been able to solve the problem of the spiraling costs of health care resulting from technological development, public expectations, and—in particular—the rapidly increasing size of their elderly populations. The people of many developing countries are still living in dire poverty with dysfunctional health care systems and extremely limited access to basic medical care.

Against this complex background, this chapter examines the role of science and technology for disease control in the past and present and assesses the potential of the remarkable developments in the basic biomedical sciences for global health care.

MEDICINE BEFORE THE 20TH CENTURY

From the earliest documentary evidence surviving from the ancient civilizations of Babylonia, China, Egypt, and India, it is clear that longevity, disease, and death are among humanity's oldest preoccupations. From ancient times to the Renaissance, knowledge of the living world changed little, the distinction between animate and inanimate objects was blurred, and speculations about living things were based on prevailing ideas about the nature of matter.

Advances in science and philosophy throughout the 16th and 17th centuries led to equally momentous changes in medical sciences. The elegant anatomical dissections of Andreas Vesalius swept away centuries of misconceptions about the relationship between structure and function of the human body; the work of Isaac Newton, Robert Boyle, and Robert Hooke disposed of the basic Aristotelian elements of earth, air, fire, and water; and Hooke, through his development of the microscope, showed a hitherto invisible world to explore. In 1628, William Harvey described the circulation of the blood, a discovery that, because it was based on careful experiments and measurement, signaled the beginnings of modern scientific medicine.

After steady progress during the 18th century, the biological and medical sciences began to advance at a remarkable rate during the 19th century, which saw the genuine beginnings of modern scientific medicine. Charles Darwin changed the whole course of biological thinking, and Gregor Mendel laid the ground for the new science of genetics, which was used later to describe how Darwinian evolution came about. Louis Pasteur and Robert Koch founded modern microbiology, and Claude Bernard and his followers enunciated the seminal principle of the constancy of the internal environment of the body, a notion that profoundly influenced the development of physiology and biochemistry. With the birth of cell theory, modern pathology was established. These advances in the biological sciences were accompanied by practical developments at the bedside, including the invention of the stethoscope and an instrument for measuring blood pressure, the first use of x-rays, the development of anesthesia, and early attempts at the classification of psychiatric disease as well as a more humane approach to its management. The early development of the use of statistics for analyzing data obtained in medical practice also occurred in the 19th century, and the slow evolution of public health and preventive medicine began.

Significant advances in public health occurred on both sides of the Atlantic. After the cholera epidemics of the mid 19th century, public health boards were established in many European and American cities. The Public Health Act, passed in the United Kingdom in 1848, provided for the improvement of streets, construction of drains and sewers, collection of refuse, and procurement of clean domestic water supplies. Equally important, the first attempts were made to record basic health statistics. For example, the first recorded figures for the United States showed that life expectancy at birth for those who lived in Massachusetts in 1870 was 43 years; the number of deaths per 1,000 live births in the same population was 188. At the same time, because it was becoming increasingly clear that communicable diseases were greatly depleting the workforce required to generate the potential rewards of colonization, considerable efforts were channeled into controlling infectious diseases, particularly hookworm and malaria, in many countries under colonial domination.

However, until the 19th century, curative medical technology had little effect on the health of society, and many of the improvements over the centuries resulted from higher standards of living, improved nutrition, better hygiene, and other environmental modifications. The groundwork was laid for a dramatic change during the second half of the 20th century, although considerable controversy remains over how much we owe to the effect of scientific medicine and how much to continued improvements in our environment (Porter 1997).

This balance between the potential of the basic biological sciences and simpler public health measures for affecting the health of our societies in both industrial and developing countries remains controversial and is one of the major issues to be faced by those who plan the development of health care services for the future.

SCIENCE, TECHNOLOGY, AND MEDICINE IN THE 20TH CENTURY

Although rapid gains in life expectancy followed social change and public health measures, progress in the other medical sciences was slow during the first half of the 20th century, possibly because of the debilitating effect of two major world wars. The position changed dramatically after World War II, a time that many still believe was the period of major achievement in the biomedical sciences for improving the health of society. This section outlines some of these developments and the effect they have had on medical practice in both industrial and developing countries. More extensive treatments of this topic are available in several monographs (Cooter and Pickstone 2000; Porter 1997; Weatherall 1995).

Epidemiology and Public Health

Modern epidemiology came into its own after World War II, when increasingly sophisticated statistical methods were first applied to the study of noninfectious disease to analyze the patterns and associations of diseases in large populations. The emergence of clinical epidemiology marked one of the most important successes of the medical sciences in the 20th century.

Up to the 1950s, conditions such as heart attacks, stroke, cancer, and diabetes were bundled together as degenerative disorders, implying that they might be the natural result of wear and tear and the inevitable consequence of aging. However, information about their frequency and distribution, plus, in particular, the speed with which their frequency increased in association with environmental change, provided excellent evidence that many of them have a major environmental component. For example, death certificate rates for cancers of the stomach and lung rose so sharply between 1950 and 1973 that major environmental factors must have been at work generating these diseases in different populations.

The first major success of clinical epidemiology was the demonstration of the relationship between cigarette smoking and lung cancer by Austin Bradford Hill and Richard Doll in the United Kingdom. This work was later replicated in many studies; currently, tobacco is estimated to cause about 8.8 percent of deaths (4.9 million) and 4.1 percent of disability-adjusted life years (59.1 million) (WHO 2002c). Despite this information, the tobacco epidemic continues, with at least 1 million more deaths attributable to tobacco in 2000 than in 1990, mainly in developing countries.

The application of epidemiological approaches to the study of large populations over a long period has provided further invaluable information about environmental factors and disease. One of the most thorough—involving the follow-up of more than 50,000 males in Framingham, Massachusetts—showed unequivocally that a number of factors seem to be linked with the likelihood of developing heart disease (Castelli and Anderson 1986). Such work led to the concept of *risk factors*, among them smoking, diet (especially the intake of animal fats), blood cholesterol levels, obesity, lack of exercise, and elevated blood pressure. The appreciation by epidemiologists that focusing attention on interventions against low risk factors that involve large numbers of people, as opposed to focusing on the small number of people at high risk, was an important advance. Later, it led to the definition of how important environmental agents may interact with one another—the increased risk of death from tuberculosis in smokers in India, for example.

A substantial amount of work has gone into identifying risk factors for other diseases, such as hypertension, obesity and its accompaniments, and other forms of cancer. Risk factors defined in this way, and from similar analyses of the pathological role of environmental agents such as unsafe water, poor sanitation and hygiene, pollution, and others, form the basis of *The World Health Report 2002* (WHO 2002c), which sets out a program for controlling disease globally by reducing 10 conditions: underweight status; unsafe sex; high blood pressure; tobacco consumption; alcohol consumption; unsafe water, sanitation, and hygiene; iron deficiency; indoor smoke from solid fuels; high cholesterol; and obesity. These conditions are calculated to account for more than one-third of all deaths worldwide.

The epidemiological approach has its limitations, however. Where risk factors seem likely to be heterogeneous or of only limited importance, even studies involving large populations continue to give equivocal or contradictory results. Furthermore, a major lack of understanding, on the part not just of the general public but also of those who administer health services, still exists about the precise meaning and interpretation of *risk*. The confusing messages have led to a certain amount of public cynicism about risk factors, thus diminishing the effect of information about those risk factors that have been established on a solid basis. Why so many people in both industrial and developing countries ignore risk factors that are based on solid data is still not clear; much remains to be learned about social, cultural, psychological, and ethnic differences with respect to education about important risk factors for disease. Finally, little work has been done regarding the perception of risk factors in the developing countries (WHO 2002c).

A more recent development in the field of clinical epidemiology—one that may have major implications for developing countries—stems from the work of Barker (2001) and his colleagues, who obtained evidence suggesting that death rates from cardiovascular disease fell progressively with increasing birthweight, head circumference, and other measures of increased development at birth. Further work has suggested that the development of obesity and type 2 diabetes, which constitute part of the metabolic syndrome, is also associated with low birthweight. The notion that early fetal development may have important consequences for disease in later life is still under evaluation, but its implications, particularly for developing countries, may be far reaching.

The other major development that arose from the application of statistics to medical research was the development of the randomized controlled trial. The principles of numerically based experimental design were set out in the 1920s by the geneticist Ronald Fisher and applied with increasing success after World War II, starting with the work of Hill, Doll, and Cochrane (see Chalmers 1993; Doll 1985). Variations on this theme have become central to every aspect of clinical research involving the assessment of different forms of treatment. More recently, this approach has been extended to provide broad-scale research syntheses to help inform health care and research. Increasing the numbers of patients involved in trials and applying meta-analysis and electronic technology for updating results have made it possible to provide broad-scale analyses combining the results of many different trials. Although meta-analysis has its problems—notably the lack of publication of negative trial data—and although many potential sources of bias exist in the reporting of clinical trials, these difficulties are gradually being addressed (Egger, Davey-Smith, and Altman 2001).

More recent developments in this field come under the general heading of evidence-based medicine (EBM) (Sackett and others 1996). Although it is self-evident that the medical profession should base its work on the best available evidence, the rise of EBM as a way of thinking has been a valuable addition to the development of good clinical practice over the years. It covers certain skills that are not always self-evident, including finding and appraising evidence and, particularly, implementation—that is, actually getting research into practice. Its principles are equally germane to industrial and developing countries, and the skills required, particularly numerical, will have to become part of the education of physicians of the future. To this end, the EBM Toolbox was established (Web site: http://www.ish.ox.ac.uk/ebh.html). However, evidence for best practice obtained from large clinical trials may not always apply to particular patients; obtaining a balance between better EBM and the kind of individualized patient care that forms the basis for good clinical practice will be a major challenge for medical education.

Partial Control of Infectious Disease. The control of communicable disease has been the major advance of the 20th century in scientific medicine. It reflects the combination of improved environmental conditions and public health together with the development of immunization, antimicrobial chemotherapy, and the increasing ability to identify new pathogenic organisms. Currently, live or killed viral or bacterial vaccines—or those based on bacterial polysaccharides or bacterial toxoids—are licensed for the control of 29 common communicable diseases worldwide. The highlight of the field was the eradication of smallpox by 1977. The next target of the World Health Organization (WHO) is the global eradication of poliomyelitis. In 1998, the disease was endemic in more than 125 countries. After a resurgence in 2002, when the number of cases rose to 1,918, the numbers dropped again in 2003 to 748; by March 2004, only 32 cases had been confirmed (Roberts 2004).

The Expanded Program on Immunization (EPI), launched in 1974, which has been taken up by many countries with slight modification, includes Bacillus Calmette-Guérin (BCG) and oral polio vaccine at birth; diphtheria, tetanus, and pertussis at 6, 10, and 14 weeks; measles; and, where relevant, yellow fever at 9 months. Hepatitis B is added at different times in different communities. By 1998, hepatitis B vaccine had been incorporated into the national programs of 90 countries, but an estimated 70 percent of the world's hepatitis B carriers still live in countries without programs (Nossal 1999). Indeed, among 12 million childhood deaths analyzed in 1998, almost 4 million were the result of diseases for which adequate vaccines are available (WHO 2002a).

The development of sulfonamides and penicillin in the period preceding World War II was followed by a remarkable period of progress in the discovery of antimicrobial agents effective against bacteria, fungi, viruses, protozoa, and helminths. Overall, knowledge of the pharmacological mode of action of these agents is best established for antibacterial and antiviral drugs. Antibacterial agents may affect cell wall or protein synthesis, nucleic acid formation, or critical metabolic pathways. Because viruses live and replicate in host cells, antiviral chemotherapy has presented a much greater challenge. However, particularly with the challenge posed by HIV/AIDS, a wide range of antiviral agents has been developed, most of which are nucleoside analogues, nucleoside or nonnucleoside reverse-transcriptase inhibitors, or protease inhibitors. Essentially, those agents interfere with critical self-copying or assembly functions of viruses or retroviruses. Knowledge of the modes of action of antifungal and antiparasitic agents is increasing as well.

Resistance to antimicrobial agents has been recognized since the introduction of effective antibiotics; within a few years, penicillin-resistant strains of *Staphylococcus aureus* became widespread and penicillin-susceptible strains are now very uncommon (Finch and Williams 1999). At least in part caused by the indiscriminate use of antibiotics in medical practice, animal husbandry, and agriculture, multiple-antibiotic-resistant bacteria are now widespread. Resistance to antiviral agents is also occurring with increasing frequency (Perrin and Telenti 1998), and drug resistance to malaria has gradually increased in frequency and distribution across continents (Noedl, Wongsrichanalai, and Wernsdorfer 2003). The critical issue of drug resistance to infectious agents is covered in detail in chapter 55.

In summary, although the 20th century witnessed remarkable advances in the control of communicable disease, the current position is uncertain. The emergence of new infectious agents, as evidenced by the severe acute respiratory syndrome (SARS) epidemic in 2002, is a reminder of the constant danger posed by the appearance of novel organisms; more than 30 new infective agents have been identified since 1970. Effective vaccines have not yet been developed for some of the most common infections—notably tuberculosis, malaria, and HIV—and rapidly increasing populations of organisms are resistant to antibacterial and antiviral agents. Furthermore, development of new antibiotics and effective antiviral agents with which to control such agents has declined. The indiscriminate use of antibiotics, both in the community and in the hospital populations of the industrial countries, has encouraged the emergence of resistance, a phenomenon exacerbated in some of the

developing countries by the use of single antimicrobial agents when combinations would have been less likely to produce resistant strains. Finally, public health measures have been hampered by the rapid movement of populations and by war, famine, and similar social disruptions in developing countries. In short, the war against communicable disease is far from over.

Pathogenesis, Control, and Management of Noncommunicable Disease. The second half of the 20th century also yielded major advances in understanding pathophysiology and in managing many common noncommunicable diseases. This phase of development of the medical sciences has been characterized by a remarkable increase in the acquisition of knowledge about the biochemical and physiological basis of disease, information that, combined with some remarkable developments in the pharmaceutical industry, has led to a situation in which few noncommunicable diseases exist for which there is no treatment and many, although not curable, can be controlled over long periods of time.

Many of these advances have stemmed from medical research rather than improved environmental conditions. In 1980, Beeson published an analysis of the changes that occurred in the management of important diseases between the years 1927 and 1975, based on a comparison of methods for treating these conditions in the 1st and 14th editions of a leading American medical textbook. He found that of 181 conditions for which little effective prevention or treatment had existed in 1927, at least 50 had been managed satisfactorily by 1975. Furthermore, most of these advances seem to have stemmed from the fruits of basic and clinical research directed at the understanding of disease mechanisms (Beeson 1980; Comroe and Dripps 1976).

Modern cardiology is a good example of the evolution of scientific medicine. The major technical advances leading to a better appreciation of the physiology and pathology of the heart and circulation included studies of its electrical activity by electrocardiography; the ability to catheterize both sides of the heart; the development of echocardiography; and, more recently, the development of sophisticated ways of visualizing the heart by computerized axial tomography, nuclear magnetic resonance, and isotope scanning. These valuable tools and the development of specialized units to use them have led to a much better understanding of the physiology of the failing heart and of the effects of coronary artery disease and have revolutionized the management of congenital heart disease. Those advances have been backed by the development of effective drugs for the management of heart disease, including diuretics, beta-blockers, a wide variety of antihypertensive agents, calcium-channel blockers, and anticoagulants.

By the late 1960s, surgical techniques were developed to relieve obstruction of the coronary arteries. Coronary bypass surgery and, later, balloon angioplasty became major tools. Progress also occurred in treatment of abnormalities of cardiac rhythm, both pharmacologically and by the implantation of artificial pacemakers. More recently, the development of microelectronic circuits has made it possible to construct implantable pacemakers. Following the success of renal transplantation, cardiac transplantation and, later, heart and lung transplantation also became feasible.

Much of this work has been backed up by large-scale controlled clinical trials. These studies, for example, showed that the early use of clot-dissolving drugs together with aspirin had a major effect on reducing the likelihood of recurrences after an episode of myocardial infarction (figure 5.1). The large number of trials and observational studies of the effects of coronary bypass surgery and dilatation of the coronary arteries with balloons have given somewhat mixed results, although overall little doubt exists that, at least in some forms of coronary artery disease, surgery is able to reduce pain from angina and probably prolong life. Similar positive results have been obtained in trials that set out to evaluate the effect of the control of hypertension (Warrell and others 2003).

The management of other chronic diseases, notably those of the gastrointestinal tract, lung, and blood has followed along similar lines. Advances in the understanding of their pathophysiology, combined with advances in analysis at the structural and biochemical levels, have enabled many of these diseases to be managed much more effectively. The pharmaceutical industry has helped enormously by developing agents

such as the H2-receptor antagonists and a wide range of drugs directed at bronchospasm. There have been some surprises—the discovery that peptic ulceration is almost certainly caused by a bacterial agent has transformed the management of this disease, dramatically reducing the frequency of surgical intervention. Neurology has benefited greatly from modern diagnostic tools, while psychiatry, though little has been learned about the cause of the major psychoses, has also benefited enormously from the development of drugs for the control of both schizophrenia and the depressive disorders and from the emergence of cognitive-behavior therapy and dynamic psychotherapy.

The second half of the 20th century has witnessed major progress in the diagnosis and management of cancer (reviewed by Souhami and others 2001). Again, this progress has followed from more sophisticated diagnostic technology combined with improvements in radiotherapy and the development of powerful anticancer drugs. This approach has led to remarkable improvements in the outlook for particular cancers, including childhood leukemia, some forms of lymphoma, testicular tumors, and—more recently—tumors of the breast. Progress in managing other cancers has been slower and reflects the results of more accurate staging and assessment of the extent and spread of the tumor; the management of many common cancers still remains unsatisfactory, however. Similarly, although much progress has been made toward the prevention of common cancers—cervix and breast, for example—by population screening programs, the cost-effectiveness of screening for other common cancers—prostate, for example—remains controversial.

Many aspects of maternal and child health have improved significantly. A better understanding of the physiology and disorders of pregnancy together with improved prenatal care and obstetric skills has led to a steady reduction in maternal mortality. In an industrial country, few children now die of childhood infection; the major pediatric problems are genetic and congenital disorders, which account for about 40 percent of admissions in pediatric wards, and behavioral problems (Scriver and others 1973). Until the advent of the molecular era, little progress was made toward an understanding of the cause of these conditions. It is now known that a considerable proportion of cases of mental retardation result from definable chromosomal abnormalities or monogenic diseases, although at least 30 percent of cases remain unexplained. Major improvements have occurred in the surgical management of congenital malformation, but only limited progress has been made toward the treatment of genetic disease. Although a few factors, such as parental age and folate deficiency, have been incriminated, little is known about the reasons for the occurrence of congenital abnormalities.

In summary, the development of scientific medical practice in the 20th century led to a much greater understanding

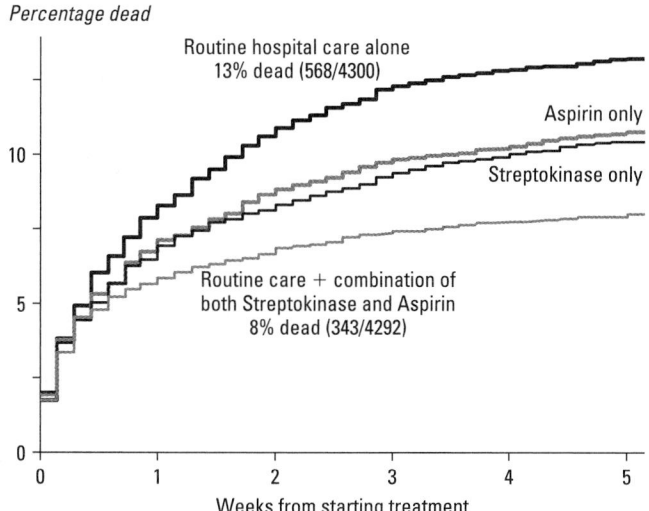

Percentage dead

Source: ISIS-2 Collaborative Group 1988 (with permission).

Figure 5.1 Effects of a One-hour Streptokinase Infusion Together with Aspirin for One Month on the 35-Day Mortality in the Second International Study of Infarct Survival Trial among 17,187 Patients with Acute Myocardial Infarction Who Would Not Normally Have Received Streptokinase or Aspirin, Divided at Random into Four Groups to Receive Aspirin Only, Streptokinase Only, Both, or Neither

of deranged physiology and has enabled many of the common killers in Western society to be controlled, though few to be cured. However, although epidemiological studies of these conditions have defined a number of risk factors and although a great deal is understood about the pathophysiology of established disease, a major gap remains in our knowledge about how environmental factors actually cause these diseases at the cellular and molecular levels (Weatherall 1995).

Consequences of the Demographic and Epidemiological Transitions of the 20th Century. The period of development of modern scientific medicine has been accompanied by major demographic change (Chen 1996; Feachem and others 1992). The results of increasing urbanization, war and political unrest, famine, massive population movements, and similar issues must have had a major effect on the health of communities during the 20th century, but there has been a steady fall in childhood mortality throughout the New World, Europe, the Middle East, the Indian subcontinent, and many parts of Asia during this period, although unfortunately there has been much less progress in many parts of Sub-Saharan Africa. Although much of the improvement can be ascribed to improving public health and social conditions, the advent of scientific medicine—particularly the control of many infectious diseases of childhood—seems likely to be playing an increasingly important part in this epidemiological transition. Although surveys of the health of adults in the developing world carried out in the 1980s suggested that many people between the ages of 20 and 50 were still suffering mainly from diseases of poverty, many countries have now gone through an epidemiological transition such that the global pattern of disease will change dramatically by 2020, with cardiorespiratory disease, depression, and the results of accidents replacing communicable disease as their major health problems.

Countries undergoing the epidemiological transition are increasingly caught between the two worlds of malnutrition and infectious disease on the one hand and the diseases of industrial countries, particularly cardiac disease, obesity, and diabetes, on the other. The increasing epidemic of tobacco-related diseases in developing countries exacerbates this problem. The global epidemic of obesity and type 2 diabetes is a prime example of this problem (Alberti 2001). An estimated 150 million people are affected with diabetes worldwide, and that number is expected to double by 2025. Furthermore, diabetes is associated with greatly increased risk of cardiovascular disease and hypertension; in some developing countries the rate of stroke is already four to five times that in industrial countries. These frightening figures raise the questions whether, when developing countries have gone through the epidemiological transition, they may face the same pattern of diseases that are affecting industrial countries and whether

such diseases may occur much more frequently and be more difficult to control.

Partly because of advances in scientific medicine, industrial countries have to face another large drain on health resources in the new millennium (Olshansky, Carnes, and Cassel 1990). In the United Kingdom, for example, between 1981 and 1989, the number of people ages 75 to 84 rose by 16 percent, and that of people age 85 and over by 39 percent; the current population of males age 85 or over is expected to reach nearly 0.5 million by 2026, at which time close to 1 million females will be in this age group. Those figures reflect the situation for many industrial countries, and a similar trend will occur in every country that passes through the epidemiological transition. Although data about the quality of life of the aged are limited, studies such as the 1986 General Household Survey in the United States indicate that restricted activity per year among people over the age of 65 was 43 days in men and 53 days in women; those data say little about the loneliness and isolation of old age. It is estimated that 20 percent of all people over age 80 will suffer from some degree of dementia, a loss of intellectual function sufficient to render it impossible for them to care for themselves. Scientific medicine in the 20th century has provided highly effective technology for partially correcting the diseases of aging while, at the same time, making little progress toward understanding the biological basis of the aging process. Furthermore, the problems of aging and its effect on health care have received little attention from the international public health community; these problems are not restricted to industrial countries but are becoming increasingly important in middle-income and, to a lesser extent, some low-income countries.

Although dire poverty is self-evident as one of the major causes of ill health in developing countries, this phenomenon is emphatically not confined to those populations. For example, in the United Kingdom, where health care is available to all through a government health service, a major discrepancy in morbidity and mortality exists between different social classes (Black 1980). Clearly this phenomenon is not related to the accessibility of care, and more detailed analyses indicate that it cannot be ascribed wholly to different exposure to risk factors. Undoubtedly social strain, isolation, mild depression, and lack of social support play a role. However, the reasons for these important discrepancies, which occur in every industrial country, remain unclear.

Economic Consequences of High-Technology Medicine

The current high-technology medical practice based on modern scientific medicine must steadily increase health expenditures. Regardless of the mechanisms for the provision of health care, its spiraling costs caused by ever more sophisticated technology and the ability to control most chronic illnesses, combined with greater public awareness and demand for medical care, are resulting in a situation in which most industrial countries are finding it impossible to control the costs of providing health care services.

The U.K. National Health Service (NHS) offers an interesting example of the steady switch to high-technology hospital practice since its inception 50 years ago (Webster 1998). Over that period, the NHS's overall expenditure on health has increased fivefold, even though health expenditure in the United Kingdom absorbs a smaller proportion of gross domestic product than in many neighboring European countries. At the start of the NHS, 48,000 doctors were practicing in the United Kingdom; by 1995 there were 106,845, of whom 61,050 were in hospital practice and 34,594 in general (primary care) practice. Although the number of hospital beds halved over the first 50 years of the NHS, the throughput of the hospital service increased from 3 million to 10 million inpatients per year, over a time when the general population growth was only 19 percent. Similarly, outpatient activity doubled, and total outpatient visits grew from 26 million to 40 million. Because many industrial countries do not have the kind of primary care referral program that is traditional in the United Kingdom, this large skew toward hospital medicine seems likely to be even greater.

The same trends are clearly shown in countries such as Malaysia, which have been rapidly passing through the epidemiological transition and in which health care is provided on a mixed public-private basis. In Malaysia, hospitalization rates have steadily increased since the 1970s, reflecting that use is slowly outstripping population growth. The number of private hospitals and institutions rose phenomenally—more than 300 percent—in the same period. In 1996, the second National Health and Morbidity Survey in Malaysia showed that the median charge per day in private hospitals was 100 times higher than that in Ministry of Health hospitals. Those figures reflect, at least in part, the acquisition of expensive medical technology that in some cases has led to inefficient use of societal resources. As in many countries, the Malaysian government has now established a Health Technology Assessment Unit to provide a mechanism for evaluating the cost-effectiveness of new technology.

Those brief examples of the effect of high-technology practice against completely different backgrounds of the provision of health care reflect the emerging pattern of medical practice in the 20th century. In particular, they emphasize how the rapid developments in high-technology medical practice and the huge costs that have accrued may have dwarfed expenditure on preventive medicine, certainly in some industrial countries and others that have gone through the epidemiological transition.

A central question for medical research and health care planning is whether the reduction in exposure to risk factors that is the current top priority for the control of common diseases in both industrial and developing countries will have a major effect on this continuing rise of high-technology hospi-

tal medical practice. The potential of this approach has been discussed in detail recently (WHO 2002c). Although the claims for the benefits of reducing either single or multiple risk factors are impressive, no way exists of knowing to what extent they are attainable. Furthermore, if, as seems likely, they will reduce morbidity and mortality in middle life, what of later? The WHO report admits that it has ignored the problem of competing risks—that is, somebody saved from a stroke in 2001 is then "available" to die from other diseases in ensuing years. Solid information about the role of risk factors exists only for a limited number of noncommunicable diseases; little is known about musculoskeletal disease, the major psychoses, dementia, and many other major causes of morbidity and mortality.

The problems of health care systems and improving performance in health care delivery have been reviewed in *World Health Report 2000—Health Systems: Improving Performance* (WHO 2000). Relating different systems of health care to outcomes is extremely complex, but this report emphasizes the critical nature of research directed at health care delivery. As a response to the spiraling costs of health care, many governments are introducing repeated reforms of their health care programs without pilot studies or any other scientific indication for their likely success. This vital area of medical research has tended to be neglected in many countries over the later years of the 20th century.

Summary of Scientific Medicine in the 20th Century

The two major achievements of scientific medicine in the 20th century—the development of clinical epidemiology and the partial control of infectious disease—have made only a limited contribution to the health of developing countries. Although in part this limited effect is simply a reflection of poverty and dysfunctional health care systems, it is not the whole story. As exemplified by the fact that of 1,233 new drugs that were marketed between 1975 and 1999, only 13 were approved specifically for tropical diseases, the problem goes much deeper, reflecting neglect by industrial countries of the specific medical problems of developing countries.

For those countries that have gone through the epidemiological transition and for industrial countries, the central problem is quite different. Although the application of public health measures for the control of risk factors appears to have made a major effect on the frequency of some major killers, those gains have been balanced by an increase in the frequency of other common chronic diseases and the problems of an increasingly elderly population. At the same time, remarkable developments in scientific medicine have allowed industrial countries to develop an increasingly effective high-technology, patch-up form of medical practice. None of these countries has worked out a way to control the spiraling costs of health care, and because of their increasing aged populations, little sign exists that things will improve. Although some of the diseases that produce this enormous burden may be at least partially preventable by the more effective control of risk factors, to what extent such control will be achievable is unclear, and for many diseases these factors have not been identified. In short, scientific medicine in the 20th century, for all its successes, has left a major gap in the understanding of the pathogenesis of disease between the action of environmental risk factors and the basic disease processes that follow from exposure to them and that produce the now well-defined deranged physiology that characterizes them.

These problems are reflected, at least in some countries, by increasing public disillusion with conventional medical practice that is rooted in the belief that if modern medicine could control infectious diseases, then it would be equally effective in managing the more chronic diseases that took their place. When this improvement did not happen—and when a mood of increasing frustration about what medicine could achieve had developed—a natural move occurred toward trying to find an alternative answer to these problems. Hence, many countries have seen a major migration toward complementary medicine.

It is against this rather uncertain background that the role of science and technology for medical care in the future has to be examined.

SCIENCE, TECHNOLOGY, AND MEDICINE IN THE FUTURE

Before considering the remarkable potential of recent developments in basic biological research for improvements in health care, we must define priorities for their application.

Priorities for Biomedical Research in the Future

In the setting of priorities for biomedical research in the future, the central objective is to restore the balance of research between industrial and developing countries so that a far greater proportion is directed at the needs of the latter. In the 1990s, it was estimated that even though 85 percent of the global burden of disability and premature mortality occurs in the developing world, less than 4 percent of global research funding was devoted to communicable, maternal, perinatal, and nutritional disorders that constitute the major burden of disease in developing countries (WHO 2002b).

The second priority is to analyze in much more detail methods of delivery of those aspects of health care that have already been shown to be both clinically effective and cost-effective. It is vital that the delivery of health care be based on well-designed, evidence-based pilot studies rather than on current fashion or political guesswork. It is essential to understand why there are such wide discrepancies in morbidity and mortality between different socioeconomic groups in many industrial countries and to define the most effective approaches to educating the public about the whole concept of risk and what is meant by risk factors. In addition, a great deal more work is required on mechanisms for assessing overall performance of health care systems.

The third priority must be to focus research on the important diseases that the biomedical sciences have yet to control, including common communicable diseases such as malaria, AIDS, and tuberculosis; cardiovascular disease; many forms of cancer; all varieties of diabetes; musculoskeletal disease; the major psychoses; and the dementias. Of equal importance is gaining a better understanding of both the biology and pathophysiology of aging, together with trying to define its social and cultural aspects.

In the fields of child and maternal health, the requirements for research differ widely in industrial and developing countries. Industrial countries need more research into the mechanisms of congenital malformation and the better control and treatment of monogenic disease and behavioral disorders of childhood. In developing countries, both child and maternal health pose different problems, mainly relating to health education and the control of communicable disease and nutrition. In many developing countries, some of the common monogenic diseases, notably the hemoglobin disorders, also require urgent attention.

In short, our priorities for health care research come under two main heads: first, apply knowledge that we already have more effectively; second, apply a multidisciplinary attack on diseases about which we have little or no understanding. These issues are developed further in chapter 4.

New Technologies

The sections that follow briefly outline some examples of the new technologies that should help achieve these aims.

Genomics, Proteomics, and Cell Biology. Without question the fields of molecular and cell biology were the major developments in the biological sciences in the second half of the 20th century. The announcement of the partial completion of the human genome project in 2001 was accompanied by claims that knowledge gained from this field would revolutionize medical practice over the next 20 years. After further reflection, some doubts have been raised about this claim, not in the least the time involved; nevertheless, considerable reason for optimism still exists. Although the majority of common diseases clearly do not result from the dysfunction of a single gene, most diseases can ultimately be defined at the biochemical level; because genes regulate an organism's biochemical pathways, their study must ultimately tell us a great deal about pathological mechanisms.

The genome project is not restricted to the human genome but encompasses many infectious agents, animals that are extremely valuable models of human disease, disease vectors, and a wide variety of plants. However, obtaining a complete nucleotide sequence is one thing; working out the regulation and function of all the genes that it contains and how they interact with each other at the level of cells and complete organisms presents a much greater challenge. The human genome, for example, will require the identification and determination of the function of the protein products of 25,000 genes (*proteomics*) and the mechanisms whereby genes are maintained in active or inactive states during development (*methylomics*). It will also involve the exploration of the roles of the family of regulatory ribonucleic acid (RNA) molecules that have been discovered recently (Mattick 2003). All this information will have to be integrated by developments in information technology and systems biology. These tasks may take the rest of this century to carry out. In the process, however, valuable fallout from this field is likely to occur for a wide variety of medical applications. Many of these are outlined in a recent WHO report, *Genomics and World Health 2002* (WHO 2002a).

The first applications of DNA technology in clinical practice were for isolating the genes for monogenic diseases. Either by using the candidate gene approach or by using DNA markers for linkage studies, researchers have defined the genes for many monogenic diseases. This information is being used in clinical practice for carrier detection, for prenatal diagnosis, and for defining of the mechanisms of phenotypic variability. It has been particularly successful in the case of the commonest monogenic diseases, the inherited disorders of hemoglobin, which affect hundreds of thousands of children in developing countries (Weatherall and Clegg 2001a, 2001b). Through North-South collaborations, it has been possible to set up screening and prenatal diagnosis programs for these conditions in many countries, resulting in a marked decline in their frequency, particularly in Mediterranean populations (figure 5.2). Gene therapy, that is, the specific correction of monogenic diseases, has been fraught with difficulties, but these are slowly being overcome and this approach seems likely to be successful for at least some genetic diseases in the future.

From the global perspective, one of the most exciting prospects for the medical applications of DNA technology is in the field of communicable disease. Remarkable progress has been made in sequencing the genomes of bacteria, viruses, and other infective agents, and it will not be long before the genome sequence of most of the major infectious agents is available. Information obtained in this way should provide opportunities for the development of new forms of chemotherapy (Joët and others 2003) and will be a major aid to vaccine development (Letvin, Bloom, and Hoffman 2001). In the latter case, DNA technology will be combined with studies of the basic immune mechanisms involved in individual infections in an attempt to

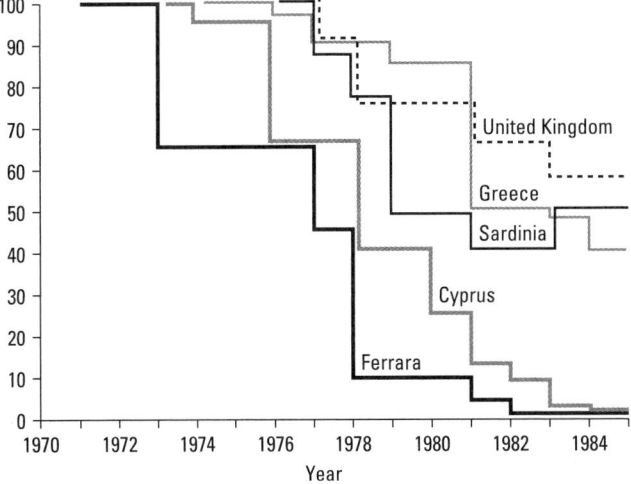

Expected % of births with thalassemia major

Source: Modified from Modell and Bulyzhenkov (1998, 244).

Figure 5.2 Decline in Serious Forms of Thalassemia in Different Populations after the Initiation of Prenatal Diagnosis in 1972 Following the Development of North-South Partnerships.

find the most effective and economic approach. Recombinant DNA technology was used years ago to produce pure antigens of hepatitis B in other organisms for the development of safe vaccines. More recently, and with knowledge obtained from the various genome projects, interest has centered on the utility of DNA itself as a vaccine antigen. This interest is based on the chance observation that the direct injection of DNA into mammalian cells could induce them to manufacture—that is, to express—the protein encoded by a particular gene that had been injected. Early experiences have been disappointing, but a variety of techniques are being developed to improve the antigens of potential DNA-based vaccines.

The clinical applications of genomics for the control of communicable disease are not restricted to infective agents. Recently, the mosquito genome was sequenced, leading to the notion that it may be possible to genetically engineer disease vectors to make them unable to transmit particular organisms (Land 2003). A great deal is also being learned about genetic resistance to particular infections in human beings (Weatherall and Clegg 2002), information that will become increasingly important when potential vaccines go to trial in populations with a high frequency of genetically resistant individuals.

The other extremely important application of DNA technology for the control of communicable disease—one of particular importance to developing countries—is its increasing place in diagnostics. Rapid diagnostic methods are being developed that are based on the polymerase chain reaction (PCR) technique to identify pathogen sequences in blood or tissues. These approaches are being further refined for identifying

Box 5.1

Chronic Myeloid Leukemia: The Path from Basic Science to the Clinic

1960 An abnormal chromosome, named the *Philadelphia chromosome,* was found in the white cells of most patients with chronic myeloid leukemia (CML).

1973 By the use of specific dyes to label chromosomes, notably quinacrine fluorescence and Giemsa staining, the Philadelphia chromosome was found to be the result of a translocation between chromosomes 9 and 22: t(9:22)(q34:q11).

1983 It was found that the translocation that causes the Philadelphia chromosome juxtaposes the c-abl oncogene from chromosome 9 with a breakpoint cluster (*bcr*) region on chromosome 22, resulting in an abnormal *bcr/abl* gene. The product of this gene, an abnormal tyrosine kinase, has increased tyrosine kinase activity compared with the product of the normal c-*abl* gene, a major fact in causing the uncontrolled white cell proliferation characteristic of CML.

1996 A selective inhibitor of the abnormal tyrosine kinase produced by the *bcr/abl* gene product was developed that results in a high remission rate in patients with CML and other tumors.

A major advance in the understanding of the mechanisms of malignant transformation followed the discovery that many forms of cancer result from the acquisition of mutations in cellular oncogenes—that is, normal housekeeping genes of cells that are involved in a variety of regulatory functions. In some cases, we may be born with a mutation of this kind, but the vast majority of cancers seem to be attributable to acquired mutations involving one or more oncogenes. The discovery of a drug that was able to interfere specifically with the activity of the product of an abnormal oncogene was a major advance in oncology, offering the hope that future research will make it possible to tailor-make agents directed at abnormal oncogene activity for the treatment of cancer.

Source: Bartram and others 1983; Druker and others 1996; Klein and others 1982; Nowell and Hungerford 1960; Rowley 1973.

---

organisms that exhibit drug resistance and also for subtyping many classes of bacteria and viruses. Although much remains to be learned about the cost-effectiveness of these approaches compared with more conventional diagnostic procedures, some promising results have already been obtained, particularly for identification of organisms that are difficult to grow or in cases that require a very early diagnosis (Harris and Tanner 2000). This type of technology is being widely applied for the identification of new organisms and is gaining a place in monitoring vaccine trials (Felger and others 2003). The remarkable speed with which a new corona virus and its different subtypes were identified as the causative agent of SARS and the way this information could be applied to tracing the putative origins of the infection are an example of the power of this technology (Ruan and others 2003).

Genomics is likely to play an increasingly important role in the control and management of cancer (Livingston and Shivdasani 2001). It is now well established that malignant transformation of cell populations usually results from acquired mutations in two main classes of genes:

- First are *oncogenes*—genes that are involved in the major regulatory processes whereby cells interact with one another, respond to environmental signals, regulate how and when they will divide, and control the other intricate processes of cell biology (box 5.1).
- Second are *tumor suppressor genes;* loss of function by mutation may lead to a neoplastic phenotype.

In the rare familial cancers, individuals are born with one defective gene of this type, but in the vast majority of cases, cancer seems to result from the acquisition during a person's lifetime of one or more mutations of oncogenes. For example, in the case of the common colon cancers, perhaps up to six different mutations are required to produce a metastasizing tumor. The likelihood of the occurrence of these mutations is increased by the action of environmental or endogenous carcinogens.

Array technology, which examines the pattern of expression of many different genes at the same time, is already providing valuable prognostic data for cancers of the breast, blood, and lymphatic system. This technology will become an integral part of diagnostic pathology in the future, and genomic approaches to the early diagnosis of cancer and to the identification of high-risk individuals will become part of clinical practice. It is also becoming possible to interfere with the function or products of oncogenes as a more direct approach to the treatment of cancer (box 5.1), although early experience indicates that drug resistance may be caused by mutation, as it is in more conventional forms of cancer therapy.

The genomic approach to the study of common diseases of middle life—coronary artery disease, hypertension, diabetes, and the major psychoses, for example—has been widely publicized (Collins and McKusick 2001). Except in rare cases, none of them is caused by a defective single gene; rather, they appear to be the result of multiple environmental factors combined with variation in individual susceptibility attributable to the action of several different genes. The hope is that if these susceptibility genes can be identified, an analysis of their products will lead to a better understanding of the pathology of these diseases and will offer the possibility of producing more definitive therapeutic agents. Better still, this research could provide the opportunity to focus public health measures for prevention on genetically defined subsets of populations.

Pharmacogenomics is another potential development from the genomics revolution (Bumol and Watanabe 2001) (table 5.1). Considerable individual variability exists in the metabolism of drugs; hence, clinical medicine could reach a stage at which every person's genetic profile for the metabolism of common drugs will be worked out and become part of their physicians' toolkit. This information will also be of considerable value to the pharmaceutical industry for designing more effective and safer therapeutic agents.

A word of caution is necessary: Although well-defined genetic variation is responsible for unwanted side effects of drugs, this information is still rarely used in clinical practice; a possible exception is screening for glucose-6-phosphate dehydrogenase (G6PD) deficiency for primaquine sensitivity, though the costs preclude its application in many developing countries. Furthermore, plasma levels after the administration of most common drugs follow a normal distribution, indicating that if genetic variation exists, a number of different genes must be involved. Hence, although the idea of all people having their genetic profile for handling drugs as part of their standard medical care will take a long time to achieve, if it ever happens, no doubt exists that this field will gradually impinge on medical research and clinical practice.

Many other potential applications of genomic research for medical practice wait to be developed. The role of DNA array technology for the analysis of gene expression in tumors has already been mentioned. Advances in bioengineering, with the development of biomicroelectromechanical systems, micro-level pumping, and reaction circuit systems, will revolutionize chip technology and enable routine analysis of thousands of molecules simultaneously from a single sample (Griffith and Grodzinsky 2001), with application in many other fields of research. Although somatic cell gene therapy—that is, the correction of genetic diseases by direct attack on the defective

Table 5.1 Pharmacogenomics

Gene	Drug	Clinical consequence
Drug metabolism		
NAT-2	Isoniazid, hydralazine, procainamide, sulfonamides	Neuropathy, lupus erythematosus
CYP2D6	Beta-blockers, antidepressants, codeine, debrisoquine, antipsychotics, many others	Arrhythmias, dyskinesia with antipsychotics, narcotic effects, changes in efficacy, many others
CYP2C9	Tolbutamide, phenytoin, nonsteroidal anti-inflammatories	Anticoagulant effects of warfarin modified
RYR-1	Halothane and other anesthetics	Malignant hyperthermia
Protection against oxidants		
G6PD	Primaquine, sulfonamides, acetanilide, others	Hemolytic anemia
Drug targets		
ACE	Captopril, enalapril	Modified response to treatment of cardiac failure, hypertension, renal disease
HERG	Quinidine	Cardiac arrhythmia (long Q–T syndrome)
HKCNE2	Clarithromycin	Drug-induced arrhythmia

Source: Modified from Evans and Relling (*Science* 286: 487 [2001], as quoted in WHO 2002a).
Note: Table shows examples of genetic polymorphisms that cause unwanted effects of drugs or modification of response. Currently, arrays are being developed for the rapid identification of families of polymorphisms related to infection-defense genotypes, drug-metabolism genotypes, and many others. Although many polymorphisms associated with variations to drug response or toxicity have been defined, the bulk of variation of response to drugs follows a multifactorial pattern of inheritance.
The examples shown are as follows: NAT-2 = N-acetyltransferase; CYP = cytochrome P450; RYR-1 = ryanidine receptor; G6PD = Glucose-6-phosphate dehydrogenase; and ACE = angiotensin-converting enzyme. HERG and HKCNE2 are potassium channels.

gene—has gone through long periods of slow progress and many setbacks, the signs are that it will be successful for at least a limited number of monogenic diseases in the long term (Kaji and Leiden 2001). It is also likely to play a role for shorter-term objectives—in the management of coronary artery disease and some forms of cancer, for example. DNA technology has already revolutionized forensic medicine and will play an increasingly important role in this field. Although it is too early to assess to what extent the application of DNA technology to the studies of the biology of aging will produce information of clinical value, considering the massive problem of our aging populations and the contribution of the aging process to their illnesses, expanding work in this field is vital. Current work in the field of evolution using DNA technology seems a long way from clinical practice; however, it has considerable possibilities for helping us understand the lack of adaptation of present day communities to the new environments that they have created.

Stem Cell and Organ Therapy. Stem cell therapy, or, to use its more popular if entirely inappropriate title, therapeutic cloning, is an area of research in cellular biology that is raising great expectations and bitter controversies. Transplant surgery has its limitations, and the possibility of a ready supply of cells to replace diseased tissues, even parts of the brain, is particularly exciting. Stem cells can be obtained from early embryos, from some adult and fetal tissues, and (at least theoretically) from other adult cells.

Embryonic stem cells, which retain the greatest plasticity, are present at an early stage of the developing embryo, from about the fourth to seventh day after fertilization. Although some progress has been made in persuading them to produce specific cell types, much of the potential for this field so far has come from similar studies of mouse embryonic stem cells. For example, mouse stem cells have been transplanted into mice with a similar condition to human Parkinson's disease with some therapeutic success, and they have also been used to try to restore neural function after spinal cord injuries.

Many adult tissues retain stem cell populations. Bone marrow transplantation has been applied to the treatment of a wide range of blood diseases, and human marrow clearly contains stem cells capable of differentiating into the full complement of cell types found in the blood. Preliminary evidence indicates that they can also differentiate into other cell types if given the appropriate environment; they may, for example, be a source of heart muscle or blood vessel cell populations. Although stem cells have also been found in brain, muscle, skin, and other organs in the mouse, research into characterizing similar cell populations from humans is still at a very early stage.

One of the major obstacles to stem cell therapy with cells derived from embryos or adult sources is that, unless they come from a compatible donor, they may be treated as "foreign" and rejected by a patient's immune system. Thus, much research is directed at trying to transfer cell nuclei from adult sources into an egg from which the nucleus has been removed, after which the newly created "embryo" would be used as a source of embryonic stem cells for regenerative therapy for the particular donor of the adult cells. Because this technique, called *somatic cell nuclear transfer,* follows similar lines to those that would be required for human reproductive cloning, this field has raised a number of controversies. Major ethical issues have also been raised because, to learn more about the regulation of differentiation of cells of this type, a great deal of work needs to be carried out on human embryonic stem cells.

If some of the formidable technical problems of this field can be overcome and, even more important, if society is able to come to terms with the ethical issues involved, this field holds considerable promise for correction of a number of different intractable human diseases, particularly those involving the nervous system (Institute of Medicine 2002).

Information Technology. The explosion in information technology has important implications for all forms of biomedical research, clinical practice, and teaching. The admirable desire on the part of publicly funded groups in the genomics field to make their data available to the scientific community at large is of enormous value for the medical application of genomic research. This goal has been achieved by the trio of public databases established in Europe, the United States, and Japan (European Bioinformatics Institute, GenBank, and DNA Data Bank of Japan, respectively). The entire data set is securely held in triplicate on three continents. The continued development and expansion of accessible databases will be of inestimable value to scientists, in both industrial and developing countries.

Electronic publishing of high-quality journals and related projects and the further development of telepathology will help link scientists in industrial and developing countries. The increasing availability of telemedicine education packages will help disseminate good practices. Realizing even these few examples of the huge potential of this field will require a major drive to train and recruit young information technology scientists, particularly in developing countries, and the financial support to obtain the basic equipment required.

Minimally Invasive Diagnostics and Surgery: Changes in Hospital Practice. Given the spiraling costs of hospital care in industrial countries and the likelihood of similar problems for developing countries in the future, reviewing aspects of diagnostics and treatment that may help reduce these costs in the future is important. Changes in clinical practice in the latter half of the 20th century have already made some headway on this problem. In the U.K. NHS, the number of hospital beds occupied daily halved between 1950 and 1990 even though the throughput of the service, after allowance for change of definition, increased from 3 million to 10 million inpatients per year. Remarkably, by 1996, of 11.3 million finished consultant episodes, 22 percent were single-day cases. How can this efficient trend be continued? A major development with this potential is the application of minimally invasive and robotic surgery (Mack 2001). Advances in imaging, endoscopic technology, and instrumentation have made it possible to convert many surgical procedures from an open to an endoscopic route. These procedures are now used routinely for gall bladder surgery, treatment of adhesions, removal of fibroids, nephrectomy, and many minor pediatric urological procedures. The recent announcement of successful hip replacement surgery using an endoscopic approach offers an outstanding example of its future potential. Although progress has been slower, a number of promising approaches exist for the use of these techniques in cardiac surgery and for their augmentation by the introduction of robotics into surgical practice. Transplant surgery will also become more efficient by advances in the development of selective immune tolerance (Niklason and Langer 2001).

These trends, and those in many other branches of medicine, will be greatly augmented by advances in biomedical imaging (Tempany and McNeil 2001). Major progress has already been made in the development of noninvasive diagnostic methods by the use of MRI, computer tomography, positron imaging tomography, and improved ultrasonography. Image-guided therapy and related noninvasive treatment methods are also showing considerable promise.

Human Development and Child and Maternal Health. Among the future developments in molecular and cell biology, a better understanding of the mechanisms of human development and the evolution of functions of the nervous system offer some of the most exciting, if distant, prospects (Goldenberg and Jobe 2001). In the long term, this field may well have important implications for reproductive health and birth outcomes. The role of a better understanding of the monogenic causes of congenital malformation and mental retardation was mentioned earlier in this chapter. Already thoughts are turning to the possibility of the isolation and clinical use of factors that promote plasticity of brain development, and specific modulators of lung and gut development are predicted to start to play an increasing role in obstetric practice. A better understanding of the mechanisms leading to vasoconstriction and vascular damage as a cause of preeclampsia has the potential for reducing its frequency and thus for allowing better management of this common condition. Similarly, an increasing appreciation of the different genetic and metabolic pathways that are involved in spontaneous preterm births should lead to effective prevention and treatment, targeting specific components of these pathways and leading to reduction in the frequency of premature births. An increasing knowledge of the mode of action of different growth factors and promoters of gut function will enhance growth and development of preterm infants.

Neuropsychiatry. Particularly because depression and related psychiatric conditions are predicted to be a major cause of ill health by 2020 and because of the increasing problem of dementia in the elderly, neuropsychiatry will be of increasing importance in the future (Cowan and Kandel 2001). Developments in the basic biomedical sciences will play a major role in the better diagnosis and management of these disorders. Furthermore, the application of new technologies promises to lead to increasing cooperation between neurology and psychiatry, especially for the treatment of illnesses such as mental retardation and cognitive disorders associated with Alzheimer's and Parkinson's diseases that overlap the two disciplines.

The increasing application of functional imaging, together with a better understanding of biochemical function in the brain, is likely to lead to major advances in our understanding of many neuropsychiatric disorders and, hence, provide opportunities for their better management. Early experience with fetally derived dopaminergic neurons to treat parkinsonism has already proved to be successful in some patients and has raised the possibility that genetically manipulated stem cell treatment for this and other chronic neurological disorders may become a reality. Promising methods are being developed for limiting brain damage after stroke, and there is increasing optimism in the field of neuronal repair based on the identification of brain-derived neuronotrophic growth factors. Similarly, a combination of molecular genetic and immunological approaches is aiding progress toward an understanding of common demyelinating diseases—notably multiple sclerosis.

Strong evidence exists for a major genetic component to the common psychotic illnesses—notably bipolar depression and schizophrenia. Total genome searches should identify some of the genes involved. Although progress has been slow, there are reasonable expectations for success. If some of these genes can be identified, they should provide targets for completely new approaches to the management of these diseases by the pharmaceutical industry. Recent successes in discovering the genes involved in such critical functions as speech indicate the extraordinary potential of this field. Similarly, lessons learned from the identification of the several genes involved in familial forms of early-onset Alzheimer's disease have provided invaluable information about some of the pathophysiological mechanisms involved, work that is having a major effect on studies directed at the pathophysiology and management of the much commoner forms of the disease that occur with increasing frequency in aged populations.

Nutrition and Genetically Modified Crops. By 2030, the world's population is likely to increase by approximately 2.5 billion people, with much of this projected growth occurring in developing countries. As a consequence, food requirements are expected to double by 2025. However, the annual rate of increase in cereal production has declined; the present yield is well below the rate of population increase. About 40 percent of potential productivity in parts of Africa and Asia and about 20 percent in the industrial world are estimated to be lost to pathogens.

Given these considerations, the genetic modification (GM) of plants has considerable potential for improving the world's food supplies and, hence, the health of its communities. The main aims of GM plant technologies are to enhance the nutritional value of crop species and to confer resistance to pathogens. GM technology has already recorded several successes in both these objectives.

Controversy surrounds the relative effectiveness of GM crops as compared with those produced by conventional means, particularly with respect to economic issues of farming in the developing world. Concerns are also expressed about the safety of GM crops, and a great deal more research is required in this field. The results of biosafety trials in Europe raise some issues about the effects of GM on biodiversity (Giles 2003).

Plant genetics also has more direct potential for the control of disease in humans. By genetically modifying plants, researchers hope it will be possible to produce molecules toxic to disease-carrying insects and to produce edible vaccines that are cheaper than conventional vaccines and that can be grown or freeze dried and shipped anywhere in the world. A promising example is the production of hepatitis B surface antigen in transgenic plants for oral immunization. Work is also well advanced for the production of other vaccines by this approach (WHO 2002a).

Social and Behavioral Sciences, Health Systems, and Health Economics. As well as the mainstream biomedical sciences, research into providing health care for the future will require a major input from the social and behavioral sciences and health economics. These issues are discussed in more detail in chapter 4.

The *World Health Report 2002* (WHO 2002c) emphasizes the major gaps in public perception of what is meant by health and, in particular, risk factors, in both industrial and developing countries. Epidemiological studies have indicated that morbidity and mortality may be delayed among populations that are socially integrated. Increasing evidence of this kind underlines the importance of psychosocial factors in the development of a more positive approach to human health, clearly a valuable new direction for research on the part of the social sciences.

Neither developing nor industrial countries have come to grips with the problems of the organization and delivery of health care. Learning more about how to build effective health delivery strategies for developing countries is vital. Similarly, the continuous reorganization of the U.K. NHS, based on short-term political motivation and rarely on carefully designed pilot studies, is a good example of the requirement for research into the optimal approaches to the provision of health care in industrial countries. Indeed, across the entire field of health provision and the education of health care professionals, an urgent requirement exists for research into both methodology and, in particular, development of more robust endpoints for its assessment.

Similar problems exist with respect to research in health economics. Many of the parameters for assessing the burden of disease and the cost-effectiveness of different parameters for the provision of health care are still extremely crude and controversial, and they require a great deal more research and development. These problems are particularly relevant to the health problems of the developing countries.

One of the main barriers to progress in these fields is the relative isolation of the social sciences and health care economics from the mainstreams of medical research and practice. Better integration of these fields will be a major challenge for universities and national and international health care agencies.

Integration of the Medical Sciences: Organizational Priorities for the Future

From these brief examples of the likely direction of biomedical research in the future, some tentative conclusions can be drawn about its effects on the pattern of global health care.

The control of communicable disease will remain the top priority. Although this goal can be achieved in part by improving nutrition and sanitation and applying related public health measures in developing countries, the search for vaccines or better chemotherapeutic agents must also remain a high priority. However, although optimism that new vaccines will become available is well founded, many uncertainties still exist, particularly in the case of biologically complex diseases like malaria. It is vital that a balance be struck between the basic biomedical science approach and the continued application of methods to control these diseases by more conventional and well-tried methods.

For the bulk of common noncommunicable diseases, the situation is even less clear. Although much more humane, cost-effective, and clinically effective approaches to their management seem certain to be developed, mainly by high-technology and expensive procedures, the position regarding prevention and a definitive cure is much less certain. Hence, the program for reducing risk factors, as outlined in the *World Health Report 2002* (WHO 2002c), clearly should be followed. However, a strong case exists for a partnership of the public health, epidemiological, and genomic sciences to develop pilot studies to define whether focusing these programs on high-risk subsets of populations will be both cost-effective and more efficient. For those many chronic diseases for which no risk factors have been defined, strategies of the same type should be established to define potential environmental factors that may be involved. Although surprises may arise along the way, such as the discovery of the infective basis for peptic ulceration, the multilayered environmental and genetic complexity of these diseases, combined with the ill-understood effects of aging, suggests that no quick or easy answers to these problems will present themselves; future planning for global health services must take this factor into consideration.

Given these uncertainties, an important place exists for the involvement and integration of the social sciences and health economics into future planning for biomedical research. Major gaps in knowledge about public perceptions and understanding of risk factors, a lack of information about the social and medical problems of aging populations, and widespread uncertainty about the most cost-effective and efficient ways of administering health care—both in developing countries and in those that have gone through the epidemiological transition and already have advanced health care systems—still exist.

In short, the emerging picture shows reasonable grounds for optimism that better and more definitive ways of preventing or curing communicable diseases will gradually become available; only the time frame is uncertain. Although there will be major improvements in management based on extensive and increasingly high-technology practice, the outlook for the prevention and definitive cure of the bulk of noncommunicable diseases is much less certain. Hence, it is vital that research in the basic biomedical sciences be directed at both the cause and the prevention of noncommunicable diseases, and that work in the fields of public health and epidemiology continues to be directed toward better use of what is known already about their prevention and management in a more cost-effective and efficient manner.

New Technologies and Developing Countries

The role of genomics and related high-technology research and practice in developing countries is discussed in detail in *Genomics and World Health 2002* (WHO 2002a). The central question addressed by the report was, given the current economic, social, and health care problems of developing countries, is it too early to be applying the rather limited clinical applications of genomic and related technology to their health care programs? The report concluded that it is not too early, and subsequent discussion has suggested that this decision was right. Where DNA technology has already proven cost-effective, it should be introduced as soon as possible (Weatherall 2003). Important examples include the common inherited disorders of hemoglobin (see chapter 34) and, in particular, the use of DNA diagnostics for communicable disease. The advantage of this approach is that it offers a technical base on which further applications can be built as they become available. It also provides the impetus to develop the training required, to initiate discussions on the many ethical issues that work of this type may involve, and to establish the appropriate regulatory bodies. The way this type of program should be organized—through North-South collaboration, local networking, and related structures, monitored by WHO—was clearly defined in the report.

For the full benefits of genomics to be made available to developing countries—and for these advances not to widen the gap in health care provision between North and South—the most pressing and potentially exciting developments from the new technologies of science and medicine will have to

be exploited by current scientific research in the industrial countries.

This need is particularly pressing in the case of the major communicable killers: malaria, tuberculosis, and AIDS. Similarly—and equally important—if developing countries are to make the best use of this new technology for their own particular disease problems, partnerships will have to be established between both academia and the pharmaceutical industries of the North and South.

Although this approach should be followed as a matter of urgency, that developing countries build up their own research capacity is equally important. *Genomics and World Health 2002* (WHO 2002a) includes some encouraging accounts of how this capacity is being achieved in Brazil, China, and India. The establishment of the Asian-Pacific International Molecular Biology Network is a good example.

It is important that work start now to apply the advances stemming from the basic biological sciences for the health of the developing world. This beginning will form a platform for the integration of future advances into health care programs for these countries. However, because of uncertainties of the time involved, more conventional public health approaches to medical care must not be neglected, and a balance should be struck between research in this area and research in the emerging biomedical sciences.

Economic Issues for Future Medical Research

The central economic issues regarding medical research in the future are how it is to be financed and how its benefits are to be used in the most cost-effective way in both industrial and developing countries. Currently, research is carried out in both private and public sectors (table 5.2). Work in the private sector is based mainly in the pharmaceutical industry and, increasingly, in the many large biotechnology companies that evolved rapidly following the genomic revolution. In the public sector, the major sites of research are universities, government research

Table 5.2 Estimated Global Health Research and Development Funding for 1998

Type of funding	Total (US$ billions)	Percentage
Public funding: high-income and transition countries	34.5	47
Private funding: pharmaceutical industry	30.5	42
Private not-for-profit funding	6.0	8
Public funding: low- and middle-income countries	2.5	3
Total	73.5	100

Source: WHO 2002b.

institutes, and centers—either within the universities or freestanding—that are funded through a variety of philanthropic sources. The input of philanthropic sources varies greatly between countries. In the United Kingdom, the Wellcome Trust provides a portion of funding for clinical and basic biomedical research that approaches that of the government, and in the United States, the Howard Hughes organization also plays a major, though proportionally less important, role in supporting medical research. Similarly, the Bill & Melinda Gates Foundation and other large international philanthropic foundations are contributing a significant amount of funding for medical research. In developing countries, such research funding as is available comes from government sources. For example, Thailand and Malaysia spend US$15.7 million and US$6.9 million each year, representing 0.9 percent and 0.6 percent of their health budgets, respectively (WHO 2002b).

As examined in the report of the WHO Commission on Macroeconomics and Health (WHO 2001), considerable discussion is taking place about how to mobilize skills and resources of the industrial countries for the benefit of the health of the developing world. However, how this international effort should be organized or, even more important, funded is still far from clear. A number of models have been proposed, including the creation of a new global institute for health research and a global fund for health research with an independent, streamlined secretariat analogous to the Global Fund to Fight AIDS, Tuberculosis, and Malaria. Recently, a number of large donations have been given—either by governments or by philanthropic bodies—to tackle some of the major health problems of the developing world. Although many of these approaches are admirable, those that involve single donations raise the critical problem of sustainability. People with experience in developing interactions between the North and South will have no doubts about the long period of sustained work that is often required for a successful outcome.

Because of the uncertainties about sustainability and the efficiency of large international bodies, it has been suggested that a virtual global network for health research be established in which the leading research agencies of the North and South take part, together with a coordinating council (Keusch and Medlin 2003). In this scheme or in a modified form (Pang 2003), both government funding agencies and philanthropic bodies would retain their autonomy and mechanisms of funding while at the same time their individual programs would be better integrated and directed toward the problems of global health.

A central problem of both private and public patterns of funding for medical research is that industrial countries have tended to focus their research on their own diseases and have, with a few exceptions, tended to ignore the broader problems of developing countries, a trend that has resulted in the well-known 10/90 gap in which more than 90 percent of the world's expenditure on health research is directed at diseases that, numerically, affect a relatively small proportion of the world's population. If the enormous potential of modern biomedical research is not to result in a widening of the gap in health care between North and South, this situation must be corrected. The governments of industrial countries may be able to encourage a more global view of research activity on the part of their pharmaceutical and biotechnology industries by various tax advantages and other mutually beneficial approaches. Progress in this direction seems likely to be slow, however. For this reason, moving quickly toward a virtual global network for research that would bring together the research agencies of the North and South holds many attractions. Although those of the North that rely on government and charitable funding may find it equally difficult to convince their governments that more of their budget should be spent on work in the developing world, they vitally need to move in this direction, possibly by turning at least some proportion of their overseas aid to this highly effective approach to developing North-South partnerships.

In short, to produce the funding required for medical research in the future and to ensure that it takes on a much more global view of its objectives, a complete change in attitude is called for on the part of the industrial countries. This transformation, in turn, will require a similar change of outlook on the part of those who educate doctors and medical scientists. The introduction of considerable sums of research monies into the international scene by governments or philanthropic bodies as single, large donations, while welcome, will not form the basis for the kind of sustainable research program that is required. Rather, the attitudes of both government funding agencies and charitable bodies in industrial countries will have to change, with a greater proportion of their funding being directed at diseases of the developing world in the future. Achieving this end will require a major program of education on the global problems of disease at every level, including governments, industry, universities, charitable organizations, and every other body that is involved in the medical research endeavor.

Issues requiring the assessment of the economic value of medical research are discussed in chapter 4.

Education

The central theme of the previous sections is that the potential fruits of the exciting developments in the biomedical sciences will be achieved only if a complete change in attitude occurs on the part of industrial countries, with the evolution of a much more global attitude to the problems of medical research and health care. Change will have to start in the universities of the industrial countries, which will need to incorporate a more global perspective in medical education so that the next generation of young people is more motivated to develop research careers that take a more international view of the problems of medical research. A major change of emphasis in education will be required and will be difficult to achieve unless those who control the university education and research programs can be convinced that funding is available for further development in these new directions (Weatherall 2003). Excellent examples of the value of the development of North-South partnerships between universities and other academic institutions do already exist.

An effective approach to increasing global funding for internationally based research is through virtual global networks involving the leading research agencies in the North and South. Hence, a similar effort will be required to educate these agencies and their governments that this approach to improving the level of health globally is cost-effective. In particular, it will be vital to persuade them that this approach may constitute an effective use of their programs of aid for developing countries. Carrying out a number of pilot studies showing the economic value of North-South partnerships in specific areas of medical research may be necessary. Indeed, a number of these partnerships have already been formed in several countries and information of this type almost certainly exists (WHO 2002a).

Of course, much broader issues involving education need to be resolved for the better exploitation of medical research. The problems of educating the public so that developing countries can partake in the advancements of the genome revolution were set out in detail in *Genomics and World Health 2002* (WHO 2002a), but a great deal of work along these lines is also required for industrial countries. People are increasingly suspicious of modern biological science and of modern high-technology medicine, a factor that, together with concerns over the pastoral skills of today's doctors, is probably playing a role in driving many communities in industrial countries toward complementary medicine (see Horton 2003). These trends undoubtedly are attributable to inadequacies of medical education and the way that science is taught in schools—reflected by the lack of scientific literacy both in the general public and in governments. If trust is to be restored between the biomedical sciences and the public, significant efforts will have to be made to improve the level of scientific literacy, and a much more open dialogue will need to be developed between scientists and the community. This requirement will be increasingly important as work on basic biomedical sciences impinges on areas such as gene therapy, stem cell research, and the collection of large DNA databases to be used for both research and therapeutic purposes in the future.

The difficulties in achieving a more global view of medical research and health care on the part of industrial countries for the future should not be underestimated. Without a major attempt to solve these difficulties, the potential of modern biomedical sciences seems certain to simply widen the gap in health care between North and South.

Ethical Issues

Few advances in scientific medicine have not raised new ethical issues for society. The genomics era has encountered many problems in this respect, and although many of the initial fears and concerns have been put to rest by sensible debate and the development of effective control bodies, new problems continue to appear (WHO 2002a). The ill-named field of therapeutic cloning is still full of unresolved issues regarding human embryo research, the creation of embryos for research purposes, and other uncertainties, but these questions should not be overemphasized at a time when most societies face even more onerous ethical issues. For example, as the size of our aging population increases, many societies may have to face the extremely difficult problem of rationing medical care. The theme recurring throughout both industrial and developing countries is how to provide an adequate level of health care equally to every income group.

Many developing countries still lack the basic structure for the application of ethical practices in research and clinical care, including the development of institutional ethics committees, governmental regulatory bodies, and independent bioethical research bodies. Every country requires a completely independent bioethics council that can debate the issues uninhibited by pressures from government, commerce, or pressure groups of any kind. Our approaches to developing a more adequate ethical framework for much of medical decision making, whether it involves preventive medicine, clinical practice, or research, constitute another neglected area that requires research input from many different disciplines.

The important question of the ethical conduct of research in the developing countries by outside agencies has been reviewed in detail recently (Nuffield Council on Bioethics 2002).

Why Do We Need Research?

It is important to appreciate that considerable public suspicion exists about both the activities and the value of biomedical research. Suspicion has been generated in part by the field's exaggerated claims over recent years, an uneasy feeling that research is venturing into areas that would best be avoided, and a lack of understanding about the complexity of many of the problems that it is attempting to solve. At the same time, many government departments that run national health care programs, the private sector (with the exception of the pharmaceutical industry), and many nongovernmental organizations set aside extremely small fractions of their overall expenditure for research. For many of those organizations, research seems irrelevant as they deal with the stresses of daily provision of programs of health care and with crisis-management scenarios that have to follow rapid change or major failures in providing health care.

One of the major challenges for the biomedical research community will be to better educate the public about its activities and to restore their faith in and support for the medical research endeavor. Educating many governments and nongovernmental organizations about the critical importance of decision making based on scientifically derived evidence will be vital. Medical care will only get more complex and expensive in the future; its problems will not be solved by short-term, politically driven activity. The need for good science, ranging from studies of molecules to communities, has never been greater.

SUMMARY

Clearly, the most important priorities for medical research are development of more effective health delivery strategies for developing countries and control of the common and intractable communicable diseases. In this context, the argument has been that much of the medical research that has been carried out in industrial countries, with its focus on noncommunicable disease and its outcomes in high-technology practice, is completely irrelevant to the needs of developing countries. This view of the medical scene, however, is short term. Although some redistribution of effort is required, every country that passes through the epidemiological transition is now encountering the major killers of industrial countries. Learning more about those killers' basic causes, prevention, and management is crucial. Although the initial costs of providing the benefits of this research are often extremely high, they tend to fall as particular forms of treatment become more widely applied. Hence, because we cannot completely rely on our current preventive measures to control these diseases, medical research must continue.

Research in basic human biology and the biomedical sciences is entering the most exciting phase of its development. However, it is difficult to anticipate when the gains of this explosion in scientific knowledge will become available for the prevention and treatment of the major killers of mankind. Thus, medical research must strike a balance between the well-tried approaches of epidemiology, public health, and clinical investigation at the bedside with the application of discoveries in the completely new fields of science that have arisen from the genome revolution.

If this balanced approach toward the future provision of health care is not to continue to worsen the gap between North and South, however, a complete change of attitude is necessary toward health care research and practice on the part of the industrial countries. A major effort will be required to educate all parties—international nongovernmental organizations, governments, universities, and the private sector—in global health problems (Weatherall 2003). Equally important will be a major change of emphasis in the universities of industrial countries toward education programs in science and medicine

to provide medical scientists of the future with a more global perspective of health and disease. If this transformation can be achieved—if it can form the basis for the establishment of networks for sustainable research programs between universities and related bodies in the North and South—much progress will be made toward distributing the benefits of biomedical research and good practice among the populations of the world. However, the great potential of advances in the biomedical sciences for global health will not come to full fruition without much closer interaction between the fields of basic and clinical research and the fields of public health, health economics, and the social sciences.

REFERENCES

Alberti, G. 2001. "Noncommunicable Diseases: Tomorrow's Pandemics." *Bulletin of the World Health Organization* 79 (10): 907.

Barker, D., ed. 2001. *Fetal Origins of Cardiovascular and Lung Disease.* New York: Marcel Dekker.

Bartram, C. R., A. deKlein, A. Hagemeijer, T. van Agthoven, A. Geurts van Kessel, D. Bootsma, and others. 1983. "Translocation of c-*Abl* Oncogene Correlates with the Presence of a Philadelphia Chromosome in Chronic Myelocytic Leukemia." *Nature* 306 (5940): 277–80.

Beeson, P. B. 1980. "Changes in Medical Therapy during the Past Half Century." *Medicine* (Baltimore) 59 (2): 79–99.

Black, D. 1980. *Inequalities in Health: Report of a Working Party, Department of Health and Society Security.* London: Her Majesty's Stationery Office.

Bumol, T. F., and A. M. Watanabe. 2001. "Genetic Information, Genomic Technologies, and the Future of Drug Discovery." *Journal of the American Medical Association* 285 (5): 551–55.

Castelli, W. P., and K. Anderson. 1986. "Population at Risk: Prevalence of High Cholesterol Levels in Hypertensive Patients in the Framingham Study." *American Journal of Medicine* 80 (Suppl. 2A): 23.

Chalmers, I. 1993. "The Cochrane Collaboration: Preparing, Maintaining, and Disseminating Systematic Reviews of the Effects of Health Care." *Annals of the New York Academy of Science* 703: 156–63; discussion 163–165.

Chen, L. C. 1996. "World Population and Health." In *2020 Vision: Health in the 21st Century.* Washington, DC: National Academy Press.

Collins, F. S., and V. A. McKusick. 2001. "Implications of the Human Genome Project for Medical Science." *Journal of the American Medical Association* 285 (5): 540–44.

Comroe, J. H. Jr., and R. D. Dripps. 1976. "Scientific Basis for the Support of Biomedical Science." *Science* 192 (4235): 105–11.

Cooter, R., and J. Pickstone. 2000. *Medicine in the Twentieth Century.* Amersterdam: Harwood.

Cowan, W. M., and E. R. Kandel. 2001. "Prospects for Neurology and Psychiatry." *Journal of the American Medical Association* 285 (5): 594–600.

Doll, R. 1985. "Preventive Medicine: The Objectives." *Ciba Foundation Symposium* 110: 3–21.

Druker, B. J., S. Tamura, E. Buchdunger, S. Ohno, G. M. Segal, S. Fanning, and others. 1996. "Effects of a Selective Inhibitor of the *Abl* tyrosine kinase on the Growth of *Bcr-Abl* Positive Cells." *Nature Medicine* 2 (5): 561–66.

Egger, M., G. Davey-Smith, and D. G. Altman. 2001. *Systematic Reviews in Health Care: Meta-Analysis in Context.* London: BMJ Publications.

Feachem, R. G. A., T. Kjellstrom, C. J. L. Murray, M. Over, and M. A. Phillips. 1992. *The Health of Adults in the Developing World.* Oxford, U.K.: Oxford University Press.

Felger, I., B. Genton, T. Smith, M. Tanner, and H. P. Beck. 2003. "Molecular Monitoring in Malaria Vaccine Trials." *Trends in Parasitology* 19 (2): 60–63.

Finch, R. G., and R. J. Williams. 1999. *Antibiotic Resistance.* London: Baillière Tindall.

Giles, J. 2003. "Biosafety Trials Darken Outlook for Transgenic Crops in Europe." *Nature* 425 (6960): 751.

Goldenberg, R. L., and A. H. Jobe. 2001. "Prospects for Research in Reproductive Health and Birth Outcomes." *Journal of the American Medical Association* 285 (5): 633–39.

Griffith, L. G., and A. J. Grodzinsky. 2001. "Advances in Biomedical Engineering." *Journal of the American Medical Association* 285 (5): 556–61.

Harris, E., and M. Tanner. 2000. "Health Technology Transfer." *British Medical Journal* 321 (7264): 817–20.

Horton, R. 2003. *Second Opinion: Doctors, Diseases and Decisions in Modern Medicine.* London: Grant Books.

Institute of Medicine. 2002. *Stem Cells and the Future of Regenerative Medicine.* Washington, DC: National Academy Press.

ISIS-2 (Second International Study of Infarct Survival) Collaborative Group. 1988. "Randomised Trial of Intravenous Streptokinase, Oral Aspirin, Both, or Neither among 17,187 Cases of Suspected Acute Myocardial Infarction: ISIS-2." *Lancet* 2 (8607): 349–60.

Joët, T., U. Eckstein-Ludwig, C. Morin, and S. Krishna. 2003. "Validation of the Hexose Transporter of *Plasmodium falciparum* as a Novel Drug Target." *Proceedings of the National Academy of Sciences of the U.S.A.* 100 (13): 7476–79.

Kaji, E. H., and J. M. Leiden. 2001. "Gene and Stem Cell Therapies." *Journal of the American Medical Association* 285 (5): 545–50.

Keusch, G. T., and C. A. Medlin. 2003. "Tapping the Power of Small Institutions." *Nature* 422 (6932): 561–62.

Klein, A., A. G. van Kessel, G. Grosveld, C. R. Bartram, A. Hagemeijer, D. Bootsma, and others. 1982. "A Cellular Oncogene Is Translocated to the Philadelphia Chromosome in Chronic Myelocytic Leukaemia." *Nature* 300 (5894): 765–67.

Land, K. M. 2003. "The Mosquito Genome: Perspectives and Possibilities." *Trends in Parasitology* 19 (3): 103–5.

Letvin, N. L., B. R. Bloom, and S. L. Hoffman. 2001. "Prospects for Vaccines to Protect against AIDS, Tuberculosis, and Malaria." *Journal of the American Medical Association* 285 (5): 606–11.

Livingston, D. M., and R. Shivdasani. 2001. "Toward Mechanism-Based Cancer Care." *Journal of the American Medical Association* 285 (5): 588–93.

Mack, M. J. 2001. "Minimally Invasive and Robotic Surgery." *Journal of the American Medical Assocation* 285 (5): 568–72.

Mattick, J. S. 2003. "Challenging the Dogma: The Hidden Layer of Non-Protein-Coding RNAs in Complex Organisms." *Bioessays* 25 (10): 930–39.

Modell, B., and V. Bulyzhenkov. 1998. "Distribution and Control of Some Genetic Disorders." *World Health Statistics Quarterly* 41: 209–18.

Niklason, L. E., and R. Langer. 2001. "Prospects for Organ and Tissue Replacement." *Journal of the American Medical Association* 285 (5): 573–76.

Noedl, H., C. Wongsrichanalai, and W. H. Wernsdorfer. 2003. "Malaria Drug-Sensitivity Testing: New Assays, New Perspectives." *Trends in Parasitology* 19 (4): 175–81.

Nossal, G. J. V. 1999. "Vaccines." In *Fundamental Immunology,* ed. W. E. Paul. Philadelphia: Lippincott-Raven.

Nowell, P. C., and D. A. Hungerford. 1960. "A Minute Chromosome in Human Chronic Granulocytic Leukemia." *Science* 132: 1497–501.

Nuffield Council on Bioethics. 2002. *The Ethics of Research Related to Healthcare in the Developing Countries.* London: Nuffield Council on Bioethics.

Olshansky, S. J., B. A. Carnes, and C. Cassel. 1990. "In Search of Methuselah: Estimating the Upper Limits to Human Longevity." *Science* 250 (4981): 634–40.

Pang, T. 2003. "Complementary Strategies for Efficient Use of Knowledge for Better Health." *Lancet* 361 (9359): 716.

Perrin, L., and A. Telenti. 1998. "HIV Treatment Failure: Testing for HIV Resistance in Clinical Practice." *Science* 280 (5371): 1871–73.

Porter, R. 1997. *The Greatest Benefit to Mankind: A Medical History of Humanity from Antiquity to the Present.* London: Harper Collins.

Roberts, L. 2004. "Polio: The Final Assault?" *Science* 303 (5666): 1960–68.

Rowley, J. D. 1973. "A New Consistent Chromosomal Abnormality in Chronic Myelogenous Leukemia Identified by Quinacrine Fluorescence and Giemsa Staining." *Nature* 243 (5405): 290–93.

Ruan, Y. J., C. L. Wei, A. L. Ee, V. B. Vega, H. Thoreau, S. T. Su, and others. 2003. "Comparative Full-Length Genome Sequence Analysis of 14 SARS Coronavirus Isolates and Common Mutations Associated with Putative Origins of Infection." *Lancet* 361 (9371): 1779–85.

Sackett, D. L., W. M. Rosenberg, J. A. Gray, R. B. Haynes, and W. S. Richardson. 1996. "Evidence Based Medicine: What It Is and What It Isn't." *British Medical Journal* 312 (7023): 71–72.

Scriver, C. R., J. L. Neal, R. Saginur, and A. Clow. 1973. "The Frequency of Genetic Disease and Congenital Malformation among Patients in a Pediatric Hospital." *Canadian Medical Association Journal* 108 (9): 1111–15.

Souhami, R. L., I. Tannock, P. Hohenberger, and J. C. Horiot, eds. 2001. *The Oxford Textbook of Oncology.* 2nd ed. Oxford, U.K.: Oxford University Press.

Tempany, C. M., and B. J. McNeil. 2001. "Advances in Biomedical Imaging." *Journal of the American Medical Association* 285 (5): 562–67.

Warrell, D. A., T. M. Cox, J. D. Firth, and E. J. Benz, eds. 2003. *Oxford Textbook of Medicine.* 4th ed. Oxford, U.K.: Oxford University Press.

Weatherall, D. J. 1995. *Science and the Quiet Art: The Role of Research in Medicine.* New York: Rockefeller University, W. W. Norton, and Oxford University Press.

———. 2003. "Genomics and Global Health: Time for a Reappraisal." *Science* 302 (5645): 597–99.

Weatherall, D. J., and J. B. Clegg. 2001a. "Inherited Haemoglobin Disorders: An Increasing Global Health Problem." *Bulletin of the World Health Organization* 79 (8): 704–12.

———. 2001b. *The Thalassaemia Syndromes.* 4th ed. Oxford, U.K.: Blackwell Scientific Publications.

———. 2002. "Genetic Variability in Response to Infection: Malaria and After." *Genes and Immunity* 3 (6): 331–37.

Webster, C. 1998. *The National Health Service: A Political History.* Oxford, U.K.: Oxford University Press.

WHO (World Health Organization). 2000. *World Health Report 2000— Health Systems: Improving Performance.* Geneva: WHO.

———. 2001. *Macroeconomics and Health: Investing in Health for Economic Development: Report of the Commission on Macroeconomics and Health.* Geneva: WHO.

———. 2002a. *Genomics and World Health 2002.* Geneva: WHO.

———. 2002b. *Global Forum for Health Research: The 10/90 Report on Health Research 2001–2002.* Geneva: WHO.

———. 2002c. *The World Health Report 2002: Reducing Risks, Promoting Healthy Life.* Geneva: WHO.

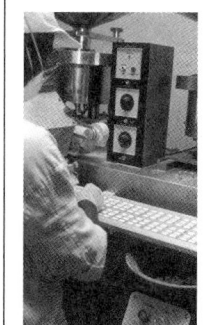

Chapter **6**

Product Development Priorities

Adel Mahmoud, Patricia M. Danzon, John H. Barton, and Roy D. Mugerwa

The overall goal of this chapter is to introduce the multistep process that leads to new product development and use and to outline the economic and institutional context for products developed specifically for major global diseases. In addition, it attempts to define the major financial efforts under way to help stimulate the process. Because product development is integrally related to intellectual property issues and to regulatory and liability concerns, these topics are also included. Data on product development for the developing countries are not systematically available. We have, therefore, used information based on analyses for developed countries and, when possible, made comparisons.

INTRODUCTION

In recent decades, scientific advances in many disciplines, particularly molecular biology, genomics, and medicinal chemistry, opened the way for developing new therapeutic agents, several vaccines, and enhanced diagnostic capabilities. The central questions for the purpose of this chapter are what drives research, discovery, and development and what institutional and financing arrangements are necessary to promote research and development (R&D) for global diseases? Medical needs and public health imperatives constitute the logical answer to the first question; however, our armamentarium for combating major global diseases suffers from certain fundamental gaps. Innovation or discovery in the health fields is the process whereby the findings of many sciences are translated from basic findings into approaches to protect health (vaccines) or reverse disease (therapeutic and diagnostic products).

Even though investigators have explored the conceptual framework for understanding how knowledge may be translated into products over the years, consensus is lacking on the specific drivers of the process or on the effects of alternative institutional arrangements.

Several features of the innovation process and its environment are essential for product development (Hilleman 2000; Nederbragt 2000; Schmid and Smith 2002). Innovation advances through a sequence of steps from discovery, through process development, to animal and human testing—a sequence with many overlapping features. Discovery may come in two ways: in a nonlinear, quantum-leap fashion that results in findings of an unexpected or unpredictable nature or in a linear fashion that builds on existing knowledge. Nonlinear processes are characteristically random despite many efforts to inject varying degrees of predictability or goal definitions (Webber and Kremer 2001). By contrast, the goal of linear innovation is defined improvement of a known process or mechanism.

Discovery

Product development is fundamentally anchored to the discovery process. In modern societies, discovery represents a societal capability that involves multiple institutions and constituents. The concept of networks of innovation has been introduced to describe one of the processes of discovery that leads to the development of pharmaceutical products or vaccines (Galambos and Sewell 1995, 272). Original scientific observations are made in organizations widely distributed across society, such as academic environments, government laboratories, biotechnology companies, or the large organizations dedicated to R&D. Because of the multiplicity of these settings and the traditions of open scientific communications, combined with the high costs of research and the importance of incentives, intellectual property issues must be taken into account.

The outcome is appreciably complex. Therefore, prescribing in a systematic way how to develop products along a planned pathway—particularly those intended for use in developing countries—is challenging. Recent decades have witnessed many attempts to develop specific drugs or vaccines to meet developing countries' needs, and the process has been difficult. Examples include pharmaceuticals to treat major global killers such as malaria and African trypanosomiasis and vaccines for most of the diarrheal diseases and respiratory infections (Nossal 2000).

Development Cycles

Discovery may set in motion a series of steps that eventually leads to the deployment of a product suitable for human use. The next step following discovery is process definition to map the steps of manufacturing and scalability to optimize the size of manufacturing. This process involves translating an idea discovered anywhere in the multiplicity of settings defined earlier, including mobilizing the energies of many sciences, to come up with a product. For instance, for a discovery in the therapeutic field to be translated into a drug, the sciences of medicinal chemistry, structural biology, and structure-function relationships are fundamental to the process. More recently, the product development process has begun using genomics and proteomics to bring about a more focused approach to defining clinical candidate products. Only then are pharmacology, toxicology, and bioavailability used in the next phase of therapeutic evaluation.

The capabilities for process definition and scalability have traditionally been concentrated in the research-based pharmaceutical industry, but several recent successful efforts in public-private partnerships (PPPs) have expanded these capabilities, such as the Medicines for Malaria Venture (MMV) and Global Alliance for TB Drug Development (GATB). Developing countries such as Brazil, India, and the Republic of Korea are now undertaking major efforts to achieve similar capabilities (Biehl 2002; Lohray 2003).

Therapeutic evaluation may begin at an in vitro or molecular level before proceeding to animal testing and the usual three phases of human assessment (Hilts 2003). The scientific disciplines of clinical research, epidemiology, and biostatistics have progressed at a significant pace in recent decades. In parallel, ethical and societal concerns about research involving human subjects and its standards, particularly across countries, cultures, and capabilities, are being extensively debated (Agre and Rapkin 2003; Barrett and Parker 2003; Emanuel and others 2004; McMillan and Conlon 2004).

The engineering aspects of product development are the next major step. Optimizing manufacturability and assessing market needs to determine the level of investment required for plant construction and operation are the two fundamental components of this phase.

One important feature of discovery and development is the length of time it takes. Estimates indicate that the average time for a new chemical entity (NCE) or vaccine to proceed from discovery through preclinical testing, human clinical trials, and regulatory approval is longer than a decade (Garber, Silvestri, and Feinberg 2004; Hilleman 1996; Rappuoli, Miller, and Falkow 2002), including the time spent on unsuccessful attempts. This timeline imposes certain pressures on how decisions are made, on the investment needed, and on competing priorities.

Development Institutions

As indicated previously, innovation and discovery occur in a multiplicity of settings. Although these settings have been concentrated in developed counties and have served the process of product development well, the challenges of developing new products for the developing world are considerable. Many countries, such as Brazil, India, and Singapore, are initiating a new wave of fundamental research institutions (Ahmad 2001; Jayaramann 2003). Their involvement in the discovery of products necessary for the health needs of developing countries is a fundamental paradigm shift. Along with the developing world's emerging biotechnology industry, a movement toward product discovery and development is under way. In addition, multiple PPPs—for example, the MMV (2002) and the GATB (2001)—are adding to the total global effort (Lyles 2003; Widdus 2001). The major feature of these new settings is their ability to focus on the immediate needs of developing countries. The challenge, however, lies in sustaining their funding and ensuring their ability to proceed from discovery to development and manufacturing, possibly with appropriate partners.

Finally, the evaluation of a product's pharmacological, biological, and toxicological properties may be carried out in developed or developing countries. Indeed, the evaluation of the safety and efficacy of products intended for developing countries should occur in those settings. Although quality control standards should be applied globally (Milstien and Belgharbi 2004), specific efforts must be directed at protecting the rights of human subjects (Agre and Rapkin 2003; Barrett and Parker 2003; Emanuel and others 2004; McMillan and Conlon 2004). In general, clinical development is heavily regulated in developed countries, and additional mechanisms exist for monitoring other aspects of product development, such as animal experimentation, use of controlled substances, and so on, but the global situation varies considerably. The time is ripe to consider the development of a global coordinated effort that involves uniform standards and reciprocity.

The analysis in the following sections focuses on the costs of developing drugs, vaccines, and diagnostics. The emphasis on drugs and vaccines reflects both the available evidence and the fact that regulatory requirements and costs are much greater for drugs and vaccines than for devices and diagnostics.

PHARMACEUTICAL PRODUCTS

The costs of developing new medicines and diagnostics reflect both the technical complexities of product development and costs related to regulatory approval, which requires clinical trials to establish product safety and efficacy. Although the relative contributions of these two components are difficult to distinguish empirically—and even conceptually—there is general consensus that increasing regulatory requirements have contributed to the rising costs of new product development in the United States. In considering the costs of new product development for diseases prevalent in low-income countries (LICs), we attempt to identify those costs that might be influenced by regulatory policy as opposed to the unavoidable costs resulting from the hard science of new product development.

R&D Costs for Drugs for Industrial Countries

The most detailed evidence on the cost of developing new drugs is from DiMasi, Hansen, and Grabowski (2003), who estimate the cost of bringing a compound to market at US$802 million in 2000 dollars. Their estimate is based on U.S. data from 10 major companies for a randomly selected sample of 68 compounds that entered human testing between 1983 and 1994 and reached approval between 1990 and 2001. The 68 compounds include 61 small molecule chemical entities, 4 recombinant proteins, 2 monoclonal antibodies, and 1 vaccine. Together, the 10 companies accounted for 42 percent of R&D by U.S. companies. The cost estimates are based on project-level data obtained from the companies for the period 1980–99. The sample was restricted to compounds that originated within these companies to avoid omitted costs of in-licensed products.

Earlier studies using similar data and methods found significantly lower R&D costs for drugs launched in the 1970s and 1980s (DiMasi and others 1991; Hansen, 1979). For the 1980s drug cohort, the estimate was US$359 million per NCE (U.S. Congress, Office of Technology Assessment 1993). Thus, the estimate for the 1990s drug cohort of US$802 million represents a significant increase over and above inflation.

Three main factors contribute to this high and rising cost of R&D. Understanding the contribution of each of these factors is important to understanding whether drug R&D costs might be lower in developing countries.

First, the inputs into pharmaceutical R&D are costly, including highly trained scientists, highly specialized capital equipment, expensive animal studies, and clinical trials involving thousands of human subjects that are often coordinated across multiple countries. Clinical trial out-of-pocket costs reflect expenditures on patients' medical treatment and monitoring, data collection, and analysis. In the study by DiMasi, Hansen, and Grobowski (2003), the average expected clinical cost, adjusted for the probability of entering each clinical phase, was US$60.6 million per compound entering human trials. In addition, the authors estimated that the out-of-pocket costs of drug discovery and preclinical development account for 30 percent of overall R&D costs, raising the total expected out-of-pocket cost to US$86.8 million per compound entering clinical trials. The average number of clinical trial patients per compound was 5,303, and the average cost per patient was US$23,500 before adjusting for the probability of entering each clinical phase.

Second, in the United States, the Food and Drug Administration (FDA) approves only roughly one in five compounds that enter human clinical trials.[1] The costs incurred for the four out of five compounds that failed must be included as costs of bringing one new compound to market. Failures occur because of safety concerns, lack of significant efficacy, and poor economic prospects. Even though the new technologies of drug discovery should eventually improve predictive accuracy for both safety and efficacy, success rates were no better in the 1990s than in the 1980s (DiMasi, Hansen, and Grabowski 2003; DiMasi and others 1991). Adjusting for failure rates raises the total out-of-pocket cost from US$86.8 million to US$403 million per approved compound.

Third, the US$802 million total cost estimate includes the opportunity cost of capital over the roughly 12-year investment period. Using an 11 percent real (net of inflation) cost of capital, DiMasi, Hansen, and Grabowski (2003) estimate the total cost of capital at US$399 million. This figure represents the return that shareholders would have received had they invested in activities that yielded immediate returns rather than in the lengthy drug discovery process. If pharmaceutical R&D is financed by—and hence must compete for—private equity capital, shareholders must be compensated for this opportunity cost. Thus, the cost of capital is appropriately included as a cost of R&D if the R&D is undertaken in commercial firms and financed by equity capital. As discussed later, if not-for-profit organizations finance R&D, the opportunity cost of capital may be lower. If we assume financing by private equity, adding the US$399 million cost of capital to the US$403 million out-of-pocket cost yields US$802 million as the capitalized cost at launch, before taxes, per approved compound. The after-tax estimate is considerably lower because, like any business expense, R&D expenses are tax deductible, plus R&D tax credits may be available in certain circumstances. However, for purposes of comparing the costs of R&D to the revenues a commercial firm would require to cover these costs, if costs are measured net of tax, then revenues must also be measured net of tax, in which case adjusting for tax makes little difference. Hereafter we use the before-tax R&D cost estimates to facilitate comparison with other estimates of R&D costs. The before-tax estimates are also most relevant to not-for-profit firms and PPPs that are not subject to taxes.

If commercial firms facing a commercial cost of capital and with no in-kind contributions (see the next section) undertake R&D, they might be able to save roughly 10 to 20 percent of their costs by conducting trials in developing countries and possibly more if they adhere to the countries' regulatory requirements, which may permit fewer and shorter trials than are normal for the FDA. Whether firms could realize those potential savings may be a matter of judgment depending on perceived liability risks. If commercial firms conduct R&D for LIC diseases in not-for-profit spinoffs, they may realize tax advantages and a lower cost of capital, which would further reduce their cost below the US$802 million estimate.

R&D Costs for Drugs for Developing Countries

Recent studies by two PPPs that focus on new product development for diseases in developing countries yield much lower cost estimates for drugs in their portfolios than those in the previous section. The GATB and the MMV estimate the costs of R&D at US$150 million (MMV 2002) and US$178 million (midpoint of the range of US$115 million to US$240 million) (GATB 2001, 101) or less than a quarter of DiMasi, Hansen, and Grabowski's (2003) estimate of US$802 million. The reasons for these large differences are instructive.

First, the GATB and MMV estimates reflect only out-of-pocket costs, with no allowance made for the opportunity cost of capital. Nevertheless, the estimates of out-of-pocket cost are less than half of the US$403 million out-of-pocket cost estimated by DiMasi, Hansen, and Grabowski (2003). This difference in out-of-pocket costs primarily reflects two factors: (a) fewer clinical trials and, hence, fewer patients in trials—namely, 1,368 patients per drug for the GATB compared with 5,303 in the DiMasi, Hansen, and Grabowski (2003) study—and (b) lower costs per patient of US$1,000 to US$3,000 for the GATB for trials run in developing countries compared with US$23,500 per patient in the DiMasi, Hansen, and Grabowski (2003) study.

Some drugs for LICs may require fewer trials, fewer patients, or both per trial because of differences in drug types and trial objectives and different regulatory requirements. For example, some of the drugs in the two PPPs' portfolios are modifications of existing drugs for which some data have been established. R&D costs for LIC drugs may also be lower to the extent that these drugs are tested for fewer indications, with less within-sample stratification by patient subgroup and less need to test for drug interactions. Clinical effects for infectious and parasitic diseases may also be greater than for chronic diseases, which permit smaller trial sizes.[2] The lower trial cost per patient for LIC drugs partly reflects the lower costs of conducting trials in developing countries, with much lower costs of medical care and personnel than in the United States. The trial duration may also be shorter because the target diseases are acute rather than chronic. To the extent that the lower out-of-pocket clinical costs in the GATB and MMV studies reflect fewer patients in trials and lower cost per patient, such savings could, in principle, apply to LIC drugs regardless of whether these drugs are developed by not-for-profit or commercial enterprises.[3]

Another factor contributing to the lower out-of-pocket costs reported by the MMV and the GATB is that these PPPs benefit from in-kind contributions of personnel, technologies, and other resources supplied by their industry and academic partners. The MMV estimates these in-kind contributions as equivalent to its own incurred costs. Thus, if these in-kind contributions are included, the full social cost for developing LIC drugs increases to US$250 million to US$300 million per compound, or only 25 to 35 percent less than the DiMasi, Hansen, and Grabowski (2003) estimate of US$403 million. However, as long as such in-kind contributions are available without charge to PPPs, the actual budget cost to PPP funders is only US$150 million to US$178 million, or less than half DiMasi, Hansen, and Grabowski's (2003) estimate.[4]

The second major determinant of R&D costs is failure rates. The GATB and MMV estimates show overall drug failure rates similar to those in DiMasi, Hansen, and Grabowski's (2003) study. Indeed, there is no obvious reason to expect significant differences in failure rates if LIC drugs face similar scientific challenges and are reviewed by the FDA or the European Medicines Evaluation Agency applying the same safety, efficacy, and risk-benefit tradeoff standards as are applied to drugs for the industrial countries. However, if the regulatory review of LIC drugs uses risk-benefit tradeoffs that reflect conditions in developing countries, then success rates might be higher, implying a lower budget cost per approved compound for LIC drugs.

Finally, the third major contributor to R&D costs is the opportunity cost of capital, which accounts for US$399 million, or almost half of DiMasi, Hansen, and Grabowski's (2003) US$802 million cost per compound. The GATB and MMV estimates do not include the cost of capital. Whether the cost of capital should be included in estimating the cost of R&D for LIC drugs depends on the circumstances and the perspective. If LIC drugs are to be developed by commercial firms that must generate a competitive return for their shareholders, then the cost estimates appropriately include a cost of capital at roughly 11 percent, as in the DiMasi, Hansen, and Grabowski (2003) study. However, if LIC drugs are developed by PPPs or other not-for-profit institutions with financing from philanthropic or governmental agencies, the opportunity cost of capital may be lower if these funders typically do not require a rate of return on their investment to compensate them for the forgone alternative uses of the funds during the investment period. For example, government investments sometimes assume a social opportunity cost of capital of about 5 percent. Using a 5 percent cost of capital for financing from philanthropic or governmental agencies implies a roughly 50 percent markup over out-of-pocket R&D costs to reflect the cost of capital rather than the roughly 100 percent estimated by DiMasi, Hansen, and Grabowski (2003), assuming the same time flow of investments.

Applying this markup to the US$150 million to US$178 million estimated out-of-pocket R&D cost for the MMV and the GATB yields a total capitalized R&D cost of roughly US$250 million for LIC drugs if they are developed by PPPs with foundation or government funding, assuming that in-kind contributions are at current levels and that trials are conducted in developing countries. Alternatively, these funders might choose to use a zero cost of capital, reflecting the importance that they attach to developing new medicines to treat currently untreatable diseases and to replace existing drugs that are increasingly ineffective because of resistance. In that case, the appropriate capitalization cost is zero, and the out-of-pocket costs of US$150 million to US$178 million are the full R&D costs per new compound for LIC diseases.

Economics of Vaccine Discovery and Development

In discussions of the economics of vaccine development, comparing the findings with those obtained for pharmaceuticals is useful. Note, however, that the two product categories are different in many fundamental and practical aspects. Pharmaceuticals are used to treat an existing clinical condition with the ultimate aim of reversing the course of disease. By contrast, vaccines are used to prevent a future threat. In addition, pharmaceuticals may be administered over a prolonged time frame and, in many chronic conditions, may be taken from the time of diagnosis for the rest of the patient's life, whereas most vaccines are administered once or a few times.

The costs of vaccine production consist of the traditional components of discovery, process development, scale-up, and manufacturing, as well as the costs pertaining to regulatory requirements, liability, and postlicensing studies (Andre 2002; Grabowski 1997). Furthermore, the economic framework for disease prevention (Kou 2002) raises many questions that are less clear than calculating the cost of treatment of a specific pathological condition in an individual or setting priorities for government budgets. Finally, the financing of vaccine purchasing and immunization programs has traditionally been separated from the totality of health care financing. Although this practice may have appeared to be advantageous at some point globally or in individual countries, the current outcome is less than satisfying in that the financing of vaccines is fragmented (Institute of Medicine 2004) and competes at a less favorable level with other budgetary priorities.

Costs of Vaccine R&D

The decision to develop a new vaccine is usually based on medical need, scientific feasibility, and market conditions. Because most currently available vaccines have been developed over relatively long periods and multiple organizations have been involved in their discovery, our cost estimates are based on historical data and on many assumptions that are probably changing rapidly (Agre and Rapkin 2003; Barrett and Parker 2003; Emanuel and others 2004; McMillan and Conlon 2004). The cost elements are similar to those for pharmaceutical R&D except for the specific regulatory procedures for vaccines, such as the completion of plant construction before phase 3 trials.

As noted earlier, estimates indicate that an NCE costs US$403 million to US$802 million in 2000 dollars (DiMasi, Hansen, and Grabowski 2003). Clarke (2002) estimates that a vaccine costs approximately US$700 million by the time the product is marketed, including not only the actual costs of products, but also such items as the cost of failures and the cost of funds (Grabowski 1997). In addition, the size of phase three clinical trials has recently escalated along with costs.

The Institute of Medicine (2004) estimates that total expenditure on vaccine R&D in 1995 was US$1.4 billion. The large pharmaceutical companies accounted for approximately 50 percent of the total (Mercer Management Consulting 1995). However, the current situation is more complex for vaccine research than for drug R&D. In 2004, only five major multinational companies were investing in vaccine R&D and production (Institute of Medicine 2004). In addition, a multitude of smaller, new biotechnology organizations in both developed and developing countries are pursuing multiple vaccine targets that are of considerable value (Nossal 2004). Since September 11, 2001, U.S. government funding for microbial threats that can be used as agents of terror has increased: Project Bioshield is devoting more than US$5 billion during the next 10 years to discovering and producing vaccines and other therapeutics (Herrera 2004). These initiatives may have spillover benefits for vaccines and therapeutics for developing countries.

Another barrier, in addition to complexity and costs that may directly or indirectly affect investment in vaccine R&D, is the condition of the vaccine market. Even though experts anticipate healthy growth in the total global vaccine market from approximately US$6 billion in 2004 to US$20 billion in 2009, the number of large private pharmaceutical companies involved in vaccine research is down to five (Mercer Management Consulting 2002). As a recent Institute of Medicine report (2004) demonstrates, other significant barriers also stand in the way of a well-functioning vaccine research and production system. These barriers include the difficulties of entering the field and of financing research, plus in the United States they include the government's role in determining pricing in relation to the government's purchase of a significant proportion of vaccines. Similar situations arise in other countries. All lead to an underappreciation of the value of vaccines and reduce the incentives for investment in future vaccine products.

As noted earlier, whether the cost of R&D for drugs or vaccines intended for use in developing countries is less than for products targeted to high-income markets is questionable. Certainly, developing vaccines for LICs requires investment from both industrial and developing countries and participation by scientists from both industrial and developing countries. In the case of vaccines, discovery similar to pharmaceuticals is a costly process. Therefore, a research infrastructure has to be supported in academic institutions and private sector and government laboratories for new ideas to emerge and to be tested. The capabilities needed to discover a new HIV or malaria vaccine are different and far more complex than those used to manufacture traditional vaccines such as whole-cell pertussis. Indeed, the technological know-how needed to discover new vaccines is embedded in the advancing edge of science.

Alternative mechanisms of financing and managing the development of new vaccines for the developing world must be identified and may require governmental, international, and philanthropic funding. Appropriate new institutions or alliances could evolve from the multiple PPPs now being pursued. The case has repeatedly been made for a massive infusion of funds and global coordination if vaccines against great killer diseases such as HIV/AIDS are to be developed (Klausner and others 2003).

Effect and Cost of Vaccination Programs

The major societal and health effect of vaccines are realized mainly when immunization programs reach a significant proportion of individuals in a society (Mahmoud 2004). The effect of vaccines in interrupting or preventing the transmission of infectious agents depends on two concepts: inducing resistance in healthy individuals before exposure and extending the umbrella of prevention to the majority of the target population to achieve herd immunity (Anderson and May 1990). When deciding to mount a vaccination program, health professionals face scientific, public health, and financial considerations. The ultimate outcome is a cost structure that has to compete against well-established budgetary constraints and comparisons. The subject of the cost-effectiveness of vaccination programs has been examined at multiple levels and in many settings (Miller and Hinman 1999). The overall conclusion derived from most quantitative techniques—for example, cost-benefit analysis, cost-effectiveness analysis, and cost utility and decision analysis—indicates that vaccination was one of the most effective health measures of the 20th century (CDC 1999).

DIAGNOSTICS

Evidence-based disease control strategies are now in place for most of the major infectious diseases affecting developing countries. Implementing these strategies depends on accurate diagnostic methods. Progress has been made in securing adequate drug supplies to treat or prevent diseases such as tuberculosis (TB), and in many instances, the most pressing need is for improved diagnostics to ensure wider and wiser use of effective therapies. Thus, an urgent need exists to develop diagnostic tests that are simple, cost-effective, and robust enough to be used in resource-constrained settings with endemic diseases.

Diagnostics Development Priorities for Developing Countries

The top priorities for developing new diagnostic methods pertain to HIV, TB, and malaria. In the field of HIV/AIDS, where the goal is to simplify the diagnosis of HIV, the need is for a noninvasive, inexpensive, and simple but highly sensitive and specific HIV test for saliva, sputum, urine, or other body secretions, as well as tests for monitoring highly active antiretroviral therapy.

In diagnosis of mycobacterium TB, the limited sensitivity of microscopy and the diagnostic challenges posed by smear-negative, extrapulmonary, and pediatric TB emphasize the need to find an alternative approach. In this context, the Gen-Probe Amplified Mycobacterium Tuberculosis Direct Test (Coll and others 2003; O'Sullivan and others 2002) and nucleic acid amplifications assays, as well as serological tests (Perkins 2000), have great potential. Diagnosing latent mycobacterium TB infection using tuberculin skin testing has major limitations, including the inability to differentiate latent TB from active TB. The QuantiFERON-TB test (Mazurek and Villarino 2003), which was approved by the FDA for detecting latent mycobacterium TB infection, and the MPB64 patch test (Perkins 2000), a mycobacterial antigen test (Nakamura and others 1998) specific to the mycobacterium TB complex, are promising and should undergo further evaluation.

For specific diagnosis of malaria, the most useful approach would be a rapid test to determine whether patients who present with fever have malaria. If this rapid test has the capability of estimating parasite density, it may help predict those at higher risk of progression to severe disease or treatment failure.

For the major noncommunicable diseases—for instance, cardiovascular diseases—portable imaging devices, such as radiographic or ultrasound machines, are becoming the new standard for diagnosis. Adaptation of these technologies to settings in developing countries is urgently needed.

Economics of Diagnostics R&D

R&D for new drugs and vaccines poses major challenges in developing countries because of financial constraints and lack of infrastructure. By contrast, both the timelines and the costs of developing diagnostics are significantly lower even though the process of developing diagnostics is in many respects similar to the development of drugs or vaccines. Whereas the costs related to clinical trials and the opportunity cost of funds are lower, the process does have additional engineering requirements. For diseases with relatively large at-risk populations, large and small biotechnology companies have been sufficiently attracted to invest in diagnostic R&D and stand to generate adequate commercial returns even for inexpensive products. For less common diseases or diagnostic indications, industry investment has been minimal, and direct R&D investment by the Special Programme for Research and Training in Tropical Diseases (TDR) (http://www.who.int/tdr) and other public sector agencies or PPPs will be needed if products are to be developed.

Diagnostics activity in the TDR's Product Research and Development Unit currently focuses on two disease areas through work carried out by the TB Diagnostics Initiative (http://www.who.int/tdr/diseases/tb/tbdi.htm) and the Sexually Transmitted Diseases Diagnostic Initiative. This work is done in partnership with academic researchers, disease control experts, public health officials from disease-endemic countries, and industry. The TDR has recently invested substantially in its capacity to support the clinical development and registration of new diagnostics and will work closely with industry, regulatory agencies, and ministries of health in industrial countries and disease-endemic countries to improve the quality and standardization of diagnostic trials and to facilitate the implementation and appropriate use of proven technologies. As an example, the mission of the TB Diagnostics Initiative is to work

closely with interested parties to stimulate interest; identify obstacles; and facilitate the development, evaluation, approval, and appropriate use of new diagnostics for TB in LICs (http://www.who.int./tdr/about/resources/contributions.htm). Current activities include research on new diagnostic targets and methodologies, product development programs to facilitate commercial and noncommercial R&D, and formal laboratory and field product evaluation trials. The Sexually Transmitted Diseases Diagnostic Initiative is a 10-year-old collaborative project established in recognition of the critical need for improved diagnostic tools for common sexually transmitted diseases. Its mission is to promote the development, evaluation, and application of diagnostic tests appropriate for use in primary health care settings in developing countries, with a focus on syphilis, chlamydia, and gonorrhea.

Cost Estimates of Diagnostics R&D

No systematic estimates of the costs of developing diagnostics are available that are comparable to the studies for pharmaceuticals. The costs of developing new diagnostics depend on the type of tool; the duration from discovery to approval; and the technicalities involved in technology acquisition, patent fees, market research, laboratory and field trials, marketing and product launch, and support costs. Table 6.1 summarizes costs related to the development of selected diagnostics for TB. Note that these are out-of-pocket costs and do not include the

Table 6.1 Costs of Developing Selected TB Diagnostics (US$)

Item	Rest of world	United States and European Union	Nucleic acid amplification United States and European Union	Screening test United States and European Union	Drug susceptibility testing United States and European Union
Location of company	Rest of world	United States and European Union	United States and European Union	United States and European Union	United States and European Union
Market research costs	10,000	100,000	50,000	500,000	500,000
Technology acquisition and patent fees		275,000	250,000	50,000	200,000
Development of prototype		3,775,000	4,000,000	4,662,000	2,825,000
Consumables used during development		1,575,000		75,000	150,000
Scale-up and validation			600,000	200,000	200,000
Total product development costs	575,000	5,625,000	4,850,000	4,987,000	3,375,000
Total costs of clinical trials (location of study sites)	180,000 (disease-endemic countries)	1,450,000 (United States and European Union)	2,000,000 (United States and European Union)	294,000 (disease-endemic countries)	
Regulatory approval costs (agencies)	100,000 (FDA, European Union)	800,000 (United States)	454,000		
Marketing and launch support costs	80,000	1,500,000	200,000		
Product support costs for one year	50,000	1,125,000	20,000		
Total	995,000	10,600,000	7,574,000	5,781,000	3,875,000

Source: http://www.who.int.tdr/about/resources/default.htm.

opportunity cost of capital (http://www.who.int./tdr/about/resources/contributions.htm).

FINANCING AND INSTITUTIONAL ARRANGEMENTS FOR NEW PRODUCT DEVELOPMENT

Research that contributes to the discovery and development of drugs, vaccines, and diagnostics occurs in public, private, and mixed settings, each with different funding mechanisms.

Public Sector

In most high-income countries (HICs), government funding from tax revenues is generally targeted to basic research—that is, research that advances understanding of underlying disease processes but is unlikely to yield commercially viable products in the near term. The research may be done in government institutions or in academic and other not-for-profit research institutions. Governments also stimulate private sector R&D through tax credits.

Private For-Profit Sector

Applied research that targets specific products is generally undertaken by the private sector using equity financing. Firms that rely on equity financing must provide a return to their investors comparable to returns on other potential investments, hereafter referred to as a competitive return. This requirement applies for multinational pharmaceutical companies, for biotechnology firms, and for firms in developing countries, unless they receive public subsidies. Start-up firms in HICs generally rely on equity capital from venture capitalists and other private investors, whereas established firms issue shares in the broadly based public equity markets but finance most of their R&D from retained earnings on existing products. The need to provide a competitive return to shareholders means that commercial firms can invest only in products that they expect will generate sufficient revenues to cover all costs, including the costs of R&D. In practice, commercial firms have focused on products with a potential market in industrial countries because of their residents' ability to pay prices sufficient to cover costs.

Differential, or "Tiered," Pricing. For global products—that is, products targeting diseases that occur in all countries, such as cardiovascular diseases—revenues generated in HICs and in the more affluent sectors of middle-income countries are sufficient to recoup the investment in R&D to the extent that, ideally, prices in LICs need to cover only the incremental or marginal costs of production for these countries.

Even with pricing at marginal cost, medicines may still be unaffordable for the poorest populations, particularly for drugs with high manufacturing costs, in which case additional subsidies may be necessary. However, the important conclusion is that for drugs for global diseases, the existence of a market in industrial countries attracts private sector investment in R&D; thus, differential (tiered) pricing provides a finance mechanism for developing new drugs that can achieve both dynamic efficiency (appropriate incentives for R&D) and static efficiency (appropriate incentives for use of existing products) (Danzon and Towse 2005).

By contrast, for drugs and vaccines that target diseases that occur predominantly in LICs, no HIC market exists in which to recoup the costs of R&D, and patents and differential pricing will not suffice to attract R&D for products that cannot expect to generate sufficient revenue to cover their development costs. In 2002, annual per capita spending on drugs alone in member states of the Organisation for Economic Co-operation and Development was US$279, while developing countries typically spent less than US$20 per capita for all health services (Sachs 2001; Troullier and others 2002). Per capita health spending on drugs by the poorest individuals, who may be the majority of patients for communicable diseases, is even lower. Thus, for products that target LIC-only diseases, even if millions of patients are in need, expected revenues are insufficient to attract private sector investment for developing new products without additional public subsidies.

For HIV/AIDS, even though the majority of the disease burden is in LICs, the markets in HICs have been sufficient to attract private sector companies to develop several drugs and to undertake considerable investment in an AIDS vaccine, albeit with little success to date. In 2001, the GATB increased the estimated size of the TB market from US$150 million to US$450 million per year, with the potential to grow to US$700 million per year (GATB 2001). This amount is within the range normally considered necessary to attract private investment. However, estimated potential revenues for antimalarials and treatments for other LIC diseases are still well below this threshold. In addition to the limited ability to pay, some developing countries still lack the health care infrastructure necessary for conducting clinical trials and for delivering medicines and vaccines effectively, which further reduces incentives for R&D investment.

Given the low potential revenues and lack of necessary infrastructure, R&D for tropical diseases and TB for the past 25 years has been far less, relative to need, than for global diseases. The number of NCEs per million disability-adjusted life years lost (a proxy for research relative to need) was 0.55 for infectious and parasitic diseases but roughly 1.25 to 1.44 for cardiovascular system diseases (Troullier and others 2002). Between 1975 and 1999, just 16 of the 1,393 NCEs registered were for tropical diseases or TB (Troullier and others 2002).[5]

Several of these products were fortuitous by-products of commercial research efforts initially intended for the oncology or veterinary market (Ridley 2003).

Multinational companies appear to be showing some signs of increasing their investment in tropical disease R&D. For example, GlaxoSmithKline, AstraZeneca, and Novartis have recently announced or established research centers devoted to tropical disease. AstraZeneca's facility in Bangalore, India, will focus on TB treatments and receive a commitment of personnel and US$40 million in investment during 2003–8. The nonprofit Novartis Institute for Tropical Diseases in Singapore is a US$122 million joint venture between Singapore and Novartis that will focus on dengue fever and TB. GlaxoSmithKline has established a research institute for TB and malaria in Spain ("Drugs for the Poor" 2003).

Orphan Drug Acts. Orphan drug acts provide additional stimulus for private sector R&D for diseases that afflict only small populations in HICs. The U.S. Orphan Drug Act grants orphan status to drugs to treat diseases that affect 200,000 or fewer patients per year in the United States. Orphan drug status provides additional R&D tax credits and seven years of market exclusivity, during which the FDA cannot approve another drug to treat the same condition unless it uses a novel mechanism of action. Such market exclusivity enhances the orphan drug's market power, enabling the developer to charge high prices that to some extent offset the low sales volumes, thereby covering the costs of R&D. The U.S. act has stimulated a sharp increase in the number of drugs developed to treat orphan conditions since its passage. The European Union recently adopted similar legislation.

The potential for orphan status in the United States and the European Union may provide some additional stimulus for commercial firms to develop drugs and vaccines for LIC diseases, but the effects are likely to be minor for several reasons. First, after one product has acquired market exclusivity, firms have few incentives to develop other products to treat the same disease. Second, the value of orphan drug status in terms of annual revenue per patient is greatest for drugs to treat chronic diseases that require daily or weekly treatment. Potential revenues for treatments for acute diseases, for which each patient needs only a short course of treatment, are likely to be smaller. Thus, though orphan drug acts may create some additional stimulus for R&D for LIC diseases, other institutional and financing mechanisms are essential. Of these, PPPs are the most promising.

"Pull" Financing Mechanisms. Since the late 1990s, organizations such as the Bill & Melinda Gates Foundation and the Rockefeller Foundation have increased their funding commitments to fight diseases in developing countries. This new funding, including funding coordinated through the Global Fund to Fight AIDS, Tuberculosis, and Malaria, is allocated primarily to paying for vaccinations and treatment. By paying for vaccines and drugs, such financing could provide additional revenues to suppliers of these products and, hence, stimulate R&D. However, for the financing of vaccines and therapeutics to serve as an effective pull mechanism for future R&D, such financing must be sustained and must pay originators enough that they can recoup the costs of R&D. Thus, purchasers such as the United Nations Children's Fund or the Global Fund face a tradeoff between paying the lowest possible prices so as to maximize their ability to supply existing medicines to current patients and paying somewhat higher prices so as to create incentives for future R&D.

Creating effective pull financing incentives for R&D is probably best done by means of explicit purchasing commitments for specific products. Some progress has been made in identifying the contractual and legal requirements of such commitments to enter into future contracts. The most promising candidates for initial implementation would be products or vaccines that are already in late stages of development or have been approved for industrial countries but for which additional purchasing commitments are needed to induce the investment necessary to undertake clinical trials and build the manufacturing capacity required to extend these products to LICs. Possible candidates are the pneumococcal vaccine and the rotavirus vaccine. For both these products, accelerated development and introduction plans have been created in the Global Alliance for Vaccines and Immunization to address the many practical issues surrounding the implementation of an advance purchase contract. When advance purchasing commitments have been successfully demonstrated on products in the late stages of development, extending this promising approach to products at earlier stages of development may be possible.

Public-Private Partnerships

In recent years, a growing number of initiatives involving partnerships between industry and government, nonprofit, and philanthropic organizations have been set up to stimulate tropical disease R&D. One of the oldest is the World Health Organization, World Bank, and United Nations Development Programme TDR, which has worked with industry, academia, and research institutions to spur R&D and has contributed to half the new drugs developed for neglected tropical diseases during the past 25 years (Ridley 2003; Troullier and others 2002) (see table 6.2 for examples of the program's initiatives). The TDR is a relatively small program, with contributions of US$30 million in 2002.

Since the late 1990s, increased government and foundation funding, particularly from the Rockefeller Foundation and the Bill & Melinda Gates Foundation, has stimulated the growth of product development PPPs, giving a "push" stimulus to R&D

Table 6.2 Selected Initiatives of the TDR

Disease	Product	Partner	Status
Uncomplicated malaria	Lapdap	GlaxoSmithKline	Dossier submitted (2002)
	Lapdap, artesunate	GlaxoSmithKline	Phase 1
	Pyronaridine, artesunate	Shin Poong	Preclinical trials
Severe malaria	Intramuscular artemether	Artecef	Registered (2000)
	Rectal artesunate	Under discussion	FDA approval letter received
Visceral leishmaniasis	Miltefosine	Zentaris	Registered (2002)
	Paromomycin	Institute for OneWorld Health	Phase 3 studies
Sleeping sickness	Intravenous eflornithine	Aventis	Registered (2001)
River blindness	Ivermectin	Merck	Registered (1989)

Source: Ridley 2003.

(Varmus and others 2004). According to the Initiative on Public-Private Partnerships for Health, about 20 PPPs were involved in product development as of 2004. Although a few focus on a specific project, most adopt a portfolio approach with multiple candidates. The latter include five targeting HIV/AIDS vaccines or microbicides; three working with malaria therapeutics or vaccines; three investigating TB therapeutics, vaccines, or diagnostics; and at least six targeting drugs for other neglected diseases (Widdus 2004).

The PPPs are heterogeneous in terms of their objectives, structure, and financing. In general, their goal is to develop products for use in developing countries with a public health rather than a commercial goal. Their sources for promising compounds include modifications of existing compounds; continued development of compounds previously abandoned because of a lack of commercial potential; and totally new initiatives coming out of academia, industry, or government laboratories. If a PPP acquires a product from another firm, the other firm typically retains patent rights in HICs and middle-income countries, and the PPP commits to noncommercial pricing in developing countries.

PPPs draw on financing from foundations and, to a lesser extent, from governments. They work closely with private industry, including large pharmaceutical and biotechnology firms, obtaining a range of in-kind contributions, including promising compounds; useful technologies; patent rights; and expertise and advice on discovery, clinical trials, manufacturing, market estimation, regulatory requirements, and so on. They operate largely as "virtual" firms, usually contracting out actual operations to other firms or to contract research or service organizations. As compounds move into human trials, PPPs must also liaise closely with disease-endemic countries regarding clinical trials, regulatory requirements, and product delivery. Thus, they face significant scientific, managerial, financing, and operational challenges.

Table 6.3 lists the leading product development PPPs and their committed funding as of early 2004. Several have received grants of US$50 million or less, with significantly larger amounts for the International AIDS Vaccine Initiative and the Malaria Vaccine Initiative. Several of the organizations rely heavily on the Bill & Melinda Gates Foundation and the Rockefeller Foundation for both their initial and continued funding (Widdus 2004). Note that the dollar funding amounts shown exclude in-kind contributions from industry and other sources, whose worth is difficult to calculate because the value to the PPPs is presumably greater than the cost to the donor.

Table 6.4 shows the product development PPPs' portfolios of products as of early 2004. The percentage of products still in preclinical development is higher for vaccines than for drugs, which may reflect the scientific challenges of developing vaccines for LIC diseases. In general, comparing funding amounts with the number of products in development across PPPs is inappropriate as an indicator of performance because the different PPPs target different problems and have received varying in-kind contributions. Also, some products are modest extensions of existing therapies, whereas others are more innovative and, hence, more risky approaches.

As table 6.3 shows, aggregate committed funding for the product development PPPs as of early 2004 was US$1.2 billion, excluding in-kind contributions. A comparison of these funding amounts to the costs per NCE suggests that current rates of investment will produce some progress, but not rapid advances. Assuming optimistically that future funding for PPPs will be US$300 million per year, that private industry will invests similar amount, and that other sources will provide US$100 million a year (all of which are probably generous estimates) would imply total investment of US$700 million per year. If this level of investment were sustained over time, it might result in two or three NCEs per year, using the conservative cost estimates of US$200 million to US$300 million per NCE. This development level would be significant progress, although it still leaves a large shortfall, given the number of diseases for which no good treatment or vaccine is available and the threat of resistance developing to existing treatments. It is

Table 6.3 Selected Endeavors by Product Development PPPs, 2004

Disease	Number of people killed annually by the disease	Number of new cases per year	PPP	Focus	Committed funds raised to date (US$ millions)
HIV/AIDS	2,800,000	5,500,000	International AIDS Vaccine Initiative	Vaccines	350
			South African AIDS Vaccine Initiative	Vaccines	45
			International Partnership for Microbicides	Microbicides	95
			Microbicides Development Programme	Microbicides	27
			Global Microbicide Project	Microbicides	64
TB	1,600,000	8,000,000	Global Alliance for TB	Drugs	42
			Aeras	Vaccines	108
			Foundation for Innovative New Diagnostics	Diagnostics	30
Malaria	1,200,000	300,000,000–500,000,000	Malaria Vaccine Initiative	Vaccines	150
			European Malaria Vaccine Initiative	Vaccines	18
			MMV	Drugs	107
Dengue fever	19,000	20,000,000	Pediatric Dengue Vaccine Initiative	Vaccines	56
Hookworm	3,000	—	Human Hookworm Vaccine Initiative	Vaccines	20
Leishmaniasis	51,000	1,000,000–1,500,000	Drugs for Neglected Diseases Initiative and Institute for OneWorld Health	Drugs	11 (Institute for OneWorld Health)
Chagas disease	14,000	16,000,000–18,000,000	Drugs for Neglected Diseases Initiative and Institute for OneWorld Health	Drugs	30 (Drugs for Neglected Diseases Initiative)
Total	5,700,000	351,000,000–353,000,000	n.a.	n.a.	1,200

Source: Sander 2004.
n.a. = not applicable; — = not available.

Table 6.4 Product Development PPPs' Portfolios, 2004

PPP	Number of products in			
	Preclinical trials	Phase 1	Phase 2	Phase 3
Aeras		2		
Drugs for Neglected Diseases Initiative[a]				3
European Malaria Vaccine Initiative				
Foundation for Innovative New Diagnostics		1	1	1
GATB[b]	10	0	1	0
Human Hookworm Vaccine Initiative	2			
International AIDS Vaccine Initiative	2	2	1	
Institute for OneWorld Health	3		1	1
International Partnership for Microbicides				
Microbicides Development Programme		1		1
MMV	14 in discovery	4	2	2
Malaria Vaccine Initiative	8	6	1	
Pediatric Dengue Vaccine Initiative				
South African AIDS Vaccine Initiative[c]	6	0		
Total	47	16	7	8
Of which drugs	26	8	5	8
Of which vaccines	19	8	2	0

Sources: Initiative on Public-Private Partnerships for Health survey, PPPs' Web sites, interviews.
a. The Drugs for Neglected Diseases Initiative has two malaria drugs in phase 3 that are partly financed by the European Union.
b. The GATB anticipates a portfolio of three phase 1 trials and expects its current phase 2 trial will enter phase 3 before 2007. Its portfolio also includes platform-related investments.
c. The South African AIDS Vaccine Initiative does not yet have any of its own products at phase 1 but is collaborating on two projects that are at this stage.

also far short of the Commission on Macroeconomics and Health's target for 2006 of US$3 billion in R&D spending for diseases in developing countries (Sachs 2001).

Industry in Developing Countries

Pharmaceutical firms in developing countries have traditionally focused on the generic sector, making use of their expertise in engineering and other skills needed for efficient drug manufacturing. More recently, the adoption of product patents has created incentives for LIC firms to invest in R&D. For example, India adopted product patents as of 2005, and several leading generic firms are already developing new products. However, assuming that these firms will focus their efforts on developing drugs for tropical diseases would be a mistake. As for-profit firms, they face similar incentives to those of commercial firms in any country, which means focusing on the global diseases that offer the greatest expected net revenues rather than diseases specific to LICs. Nonetheless, several policies might help target R&D efforts in these countries toward tropical diseases. These policies include collaboration with the product development PPPs, provision of special government funding or tax credits for products that target LIC diseases, and provision of subsidies targeting the development and scientific testing of products derived from local products and other traditional medicines.

Other Proposed Mechanisms for Increasing Affordability

In evaluating other proposals for making drugs or vaccines available in developing countries, distinguishing proposals to stimulate new product development from proposals to increase the affordability of existing drugs is critical. One proposal pertaining to affordability is that multinational companies should voluntarily license production rights to LIC producers. Experience with generic markets across countries indicates that necessary conditions for such out-licensing to reduce prices to consumers are (a) the existence of competition between multiple licensees, (b) the licensees having lower production costs than the originator firms, and (c) a mechanism that prevents middlemen and retailers from capturing any potential savings. In practice, these conditions may not be met. The more probable scenario of licensing to only one local generic manufacturer is unlikely to reduce prices to consumers.

Another proposal is that governments should purchase patent rights, paying the originator firm the estimated value of the drug (net of production costs) and then selling the product to consumers at the marginal cost of production. This proposal has several disadvantages. First, because the government would presumably have to raise taxes to pay for the patents, the tax-induced efficiency loss could offset any efficiency gain in the pharmaceutical market, so the net effect on efficiency is

unclear. Second, the presumption that patents result in suboptimal drug consumption because of monopoly pricing ignores the widespread prevalence of insurance in HICs and middle-income countries, so that, in practice, consumers face out-of-pocket prices that are already close to marginal cost. Third, and most important, is the difficulty of estimating the value of a product before its use in the market, because both positive features (additional uses) and negative features (side effects) may be discovered. In addition, distortions in the amounts paid for patent rights would distort incentives for R&D. Moreover, the proposal would reduce originator firms' incentives to invest in postlaunch improvements.

INTELLECTUAL PROPERTY

The issue of intellectual property is involved in the debate about the perceived conflict between patents and access.

The Role of Patents in Drug Development

Under a patent system, an inventor is entitled to a limited monopoly for a period of time, typically 20 years. This exclusivity may permit high prices and, consequently, an increased economic return that serves as an incentive to develop new products. The system has worked quite effectively in the pharmaceutical area, where the incentives deriving from exclusivity have resulted in important new drugs. The first generation of patients pays a higher price than subsequent generations, which provides compensation for the large research costs involved in developing a new drug. When the patent expires, the price normally falls as generic competitors enter the market.

Even though this approach has been extremely successful in the developed world, it does not generally work for products for which the main market is limited to the developing world. The total magnitude of the market in the developing world for products for HIV, malaria, TB, or less widespread diseases is likely to be too small to provide an adequate incentive for the private sector. This fact, together with the fact that patents are likely to result in higher prices, has raised important concerns in the developing world.

The Drug Access Debate

The Agreement on Trade-Related Aspects of Intellectual Property Rights (TRIPS) entered into force on January 1, 1995.[6] This agreement requires the members of the World Trade Organization (WTO), which include nearly all major trading nations, to live up to defined standards of intellectual property protection. TRIPS was part of a much broader international trade package negotiated during the Uruguay Round, one of a series of international trade negotiations that have taken place since World War II. The United States and European nations, which were the strong proponents of TRIPS, were responding to pressure from their pharmaceutical, copyright content, and trademark-based industries.

The pharmaceutical industry's concern was that a number of developing nations had made deliberate decisions to deny patent protection to pharmaceutical products and to grant protection only to processes for producing pharmaceuticals. These nations believed that inexpensive access to pharmaceutical products was so important that these products should not be patented. In its 1970 patent law, for example, India excluded pharmaceuticals from product patent protection, effectively choosing to provide low-cost pharmaceuticals for its people at the expense of eliminating incentives to create new products. This law was one of the reasons the Indian generic pharmaceutical industry was able to evolve to make and market copies of drugs that were still on patent in wealthier nations. Another concern for the pharmaceutical industry arose from the compulsory license process, a legal process available in some nations to authorize the use of a patented technology under some circumstances even over the patent holder's objection. In practice, compulsory licenses are rarely granted but are instead used as a threat to negotiate lower prices for the technology or pharmaceutical involved.

The United States was determined to change these laws and in TRIPS achieved important requirements for expanding patent protection. The most important TRIPS provision relevant to pharmaceuticals is article 27, which includes a requirement that "patents shall be available for any inventions, whether products or processes, in all fields of technology." (U.K. Commission on Intellectual Property Rights 2002). The clear intent of this language was to prohibit exclusions of pharmaceutical products as in the Indian law. Article 31 established careful procedural limitations on when a nation could grant a compulsory license. As part of the political compromise, transitional provisions gave developing nations extra time to comply with the treaty's requirements and also set up arrangements for the remaining parts of patent terms to be made available for products developed during the transition period. Because of these transitional provisions, developing nations were not generally required to provide product patents on pharmaceuticals until January 1, 2005 (a date that has since been extended to 2016 for the least developed countries).

During the years following the entry into force of TRIPS, a substantial and bitter debate over access to pharmaceutical products in developing countries focused largely on access to antiretroviral agents for HIV patients in Sub-Saharan Africa. A group of nongovernmental organizations argued that patents on these drugs in the developing world raise the prices of the products necessary to help such patients survive. The research-based pharmaceutical industry countered that many of the relevant products are not covered by patents in the nations involved and that the problem is not patents but the inadequacy of the countries' medical infrastructure.

An area of convergence has begun to emerge in relation to differential pricing: prices should be lower in developing nations than in developed nations, permitting pharmaceutical firms to recover their research expenditures in the developed world while making products available at near marginal production cost to the poor in the developing world. This differential pricing is justified because potential sales in poor nations are so small that the market provides only a minimal incentive: total sales in the poorest nations account for only about 1 percent of global pharmaceutical sales. The research-based pharmaceutical industry would prefer to achieve this differential pricing by means of a donation program or simply by charging different prices. Critics would prefer that the patent monopoly not be available to raise prices in the developing world, thereby opening up markets to local generic producers.

Movement toward agreement on differential pricing was reflected in the Doha Declaration on TRIPS agreement and public health, reached at a November 2001 WTO meeting of trade ministers. This declaration affirmed that TRIPS "should be interpreted and implemented in a manner supportive of WTO members' right to protect public health and, in particular, to promote access to medicines for all" (TRIPS, paragraph 4, 2001). It affirmed the right of nations to use the exceptions to TRIPS to address public health concerns, specifically stating that "public health crises, including those related to HIV/AIDS, tuberculosis, malaria and other epidemics, can represent a national emergency" and, thus, facilitate the right to use compulsory licensing (WTO 2003).

The Doha Declaration left an issue unresolved: the manufacture of drugs under compulsory license for nations that do not have the capability to manufacture the drugs themselves. The problem arises from the compulsory licensing article of TRIPS, which contains a provision, article 31(f), requiring that the manufacture of products under compulsory license be predominantly for the domestic market. Thus, a small Sub-Sahara African nation clearly has the right to grant a compulsory license but may have no local industry able to manufacture the product. If it asks a foreign firm to manufacture the product, that firm would be manufacturing the product primarily for export, a violation of TRIPS.

The Doha negotiators did not find a way to resolve this problem, and article 6 of the Doha Declaration called for members of the TRIPS Council (a group of national representatives) to find a solution by the end of 2002. By that time, all member countries except the United States had agreed to a procedure for waiving article 31(f). The new agreement covered products needed to address public health problems recognized in the Doha Declaration, but the United States feared that it would be expanded to a variety of other products and was unwilling to accept it. Finally, a compromise was reached in August 2003.

The United States accepted the 2002 document, provided that the General Council chairperson of the WTO made an appropriate parallel statement. The chair made the statement, which included language that the agreement would be used "in good faith to protect public health" and not be "an instrument to pursue industrial or commercial policy objectives," and recognized the need to respond to the industry's concern that products produced under this agreement would not be exported to major developed world markets (WTO 2003; see also UNAIDS 2003).

This agreement represents a step forward for access and will certainly place pressure on the research-based pharmaceutical industry to provide products in the developing world at low prices. It leaves several important problems only partly resolved, however. One is the need to prevent importation of the low-priced products into the developed world. Such imports would cut into the patent-protected market and affect incentives to develop new products. A second is political backlash. When the general public becomes aware that a product is available to the poor in a developing nation at a price far below that which patients in developed nations must pay, the political backlash for the pharmaceutical industry in the developed world may be severe.

Most important, resolving the legal problem of article 31(f) does not resolve the economic problem. It confirms that there will be no patent incentive for the development of drugs for diseases endemic to the developing nations and that public funds will be needed for this purpose. Such funds are currently inadequate.

The Research Tool Issue

Another important problem arises from the changing nature of medical research and of patenting practice. This is the research tool problem: many of the basic tools used in medical research are now themselves patented. For example, the research use of certain genetically modified mice is patented in the United States, as are the uses of many gene sequences and protein crystal coordinates. In the case of the malaria antigen merozoite surface protein 1, some 39 patent families cover various aspects of the protein (U.K. Commission on Intellectual Property Rights 2002).

Such patents can significantly complicate research and make it more expensive. Each one that might affect a particular research program requires legal analysis to determine whether it is valid and actually applies to the planned research program. If relevant, a license must be sought or the research program must be redesigned. The more patents are involved, the greater the likelihood that a patent holder will refuse to grant a license or will demand an exorbitant sum. Even though Walsh, Arora, and Cohen's (2003) study finds no cases of research programs being canceled midstream because of this problem, it finds

many cases of efforts to avoid the problem by, for example, modifying the research; conducting the research offshore in locations where the relevant patents are not in force; or, in some cases, simply ignoring the patent.

REGULATORY AND LIABILITY ISSUES

Developing and registering new products are generally lengthy and complicated processes (Abraham and Reed 2002; Baylor and McVittie 2003; FDA 2004) that are regulated both at the national level and, in some circumstances, at the international level. The role of the regulatory system extends beyond the launch of a new product to manufacturing and compliance standards and to postmarketing surveillance for clinical effects and potential untoward outcomes. For products that are intended to be deployed in global markets, manufacturers have to comply with regulatory requirements in the country of origin as well as the requirements of each country where the product may be marketed. One exception is the mutual recognition systems used currently by European Union countries (Pignatti, Boone, and Moulon 2004). The situation may be different for products intended for use only in developing countries; however, for legal and liability reasons, manufacturers in developed countries have refrained from working with two different sets of regulatory requirements.

The best example for illustrating this process is the FDA (2004). Over the years, FDA regulations have developed into a clear pathway. The process is initiated through an application by the manufacturer and a step-by-step approach toward licensing. The agency gets involved in every phase of the development process and approves in advance the experimental design, assays, and endpoints for clinical trials. After it has collected all the information, the agency examines the materials submitted and reaches a decision. The FDA process extends through regulating and approving marketing materials and postlicensing collection of efficacy data and information about possible side effects.

The FDA approval process differs somewhat for pharmaceutical products and vaccines. One of the main differences is the obligation of vaccine manufacturers to prepare materials for use in phase 3 trials in the final and approved production facility. This requirement means that the firm must invest in completing the manufacturing plant well ahead of launching a specific product, a process that can take three to six years. The regulatory process for vaccines also dictates batch release for every batch ready for deployment in the marketplace. This part of the regulatory process, although it ensures quality control, adds to costs and to the timeline.

In 1996, the European Union adopted a centralized procedure for applications and approvals through the European Medicines Evaluation Agency and through a mutual recognition process (Pignatti, Boone, and Moulon 2004). In many ways, the procedure parallels the FDA process, with several differences reflecting the fact that the European Union consists of many countries, each with a country-based process that remains as an alternative or an addition to the communitywide process. The International Conference on Harmonization of Technical Requirements for Regulation of Pharmaceuticals for Human Use was established to achieve coordination of the process of drug development between industry, Japan, the United States, and the European Union (Abraham and Reed 2002; Ohno 2002). The conference's activities have improved understanding of the regulatory process and reduced duplication.

In contrast, the absence of a unified or harmonized approach to product registration and approval at the global level adds multiple layers of complexity. National systems consist of complex processes with differing thresholds and interpretations and with changing requirements in addition to differing Global Manufacturing Program standards and enforcement. A number of recent attempts have been made to resolve the issue. First among these is the World Health Organization's effort to expand its prequalification system, to develop technical standards earlier in the approval process, and to expand the availability of reference reagents for international calibration (Milstien and Belgharbi 2004). These efforts aim at injecting a higher level of quality control and transparency into the global regulatory system. The effort may have the potential to provide a global process that transcends national borders. Such a process should provide a simplified, systematic, and disciplined system that would reduce costs and speed up market access for new products.

The issue of liability in relation to harm to individuals receiving pharmaceutical products has been extremely significant in U.S. product development. It is entirely appropriate for those developing new products to be sued if they are negligent in their research or product development, but in some cases pharmaceutical firms have been sued for side effects of drugs that may have been unforeseeable or may not even have been the result of the product. This type of liability can be a barrier to product development. Although perhaps a less serious concern since the 1993 *Daubert v. Merrell Dow Pharmaceuticals* lawsuit in the United States, a case that has been interpreted to restrict the presentation to juries of evidence determined not to be "scientific," the issue is still significant. It may also be part of the reason the U.S. vaccine industry has shrunk significantly, and it has certainly affected the direction of investment, pushing it away, for example, from products such as vaccines that are used in one or a few doses in healthy people toward products used repetitively by those who already have a chronic disease (Institute of Medicine 2004). It, thus, provides pressure directly contrary to public health priorities, which emphasize prevention and, therefore, the use of vaccines.

Whether or how this trend in the United States will affect the developing world is unclear. Europe has moved toward a liability system somewhat similar to that of the United States, but many developing nations may not have such a tort liability system. Even if they do not have such a system, groups participating in pharmaceutical development might be sued in the United States for harm occurring in the developing world. Doctrines exist that restrict such suits, but firms may fear that these doctrines are insufficiently effective. Hence, recognizing the potential costs of protecting against liability and, at the same time, ensuring that products are designed and manufactured to the highest standards will be important.

NOTES

1. The phase transition probabilities in DiMasi, Hansen, and Grabowski (2003) and the overall success probability of 0.215, conditional on entering human trials, are estimated from a larger sample of 538 investigational compounds first tested in humans between 1983 and 1994.

2. The size of trial required to estimate statistical significance depends on the magnitude of the drug effect; the extent of stratification within the total sample by patient age, condition, and so on; the required statistical confidence; and other factors.

3. DiMasi, Hansen, and Grabowski's (2003) data for average cost and average number of patients are based on actual, retrospective cost data, whereas the GATB estimates are prospective estimates (best guesses) based on prior clinical trials for tuberculosis drugs in the United States and a survey of clinical trial experts to determine administrative and data management costs.

4. The MMV estimate of in-kind contributions does not include the value of basic research conducted by universities and foundations from which it obtains its lead compounds. Similarly, commercial firms also benefit from such basic research and it is omitted from the DiMasi, Hansen, and Grabowski (2003) estimates, so comparisons are not necessarily biased by this exclusion.

5. Tropical diseases include parasitic diseases (malaria, African trypanosomiasis, Chagas disease, schistosomiasis, leishmaniasis, lymphatic filariasis, onchocerciasis, and intestinal nematode infections); leprosy; dengue fever; Japanese encephalitis; trachoma; and infectious diarrheal diseases.

6. This section is based in part on Barton (2004).

REFERENCES

Abraham, J., and T. Reed. 2002. "Progress Innovation and Regulatory Science in Drug Development: The Politics of International Standard-Setting." *Social Studies of Science* 32 (3): 337–69.

Agre, P., and B. Rapkin. 2003. "Improving Informed Consent: A Comparison of Four Consent Tools." *IRB: Ethics and Human Research* 25 (6): 1–7.

Ahmad, K. 2001. "Brazil and USA at Loggerheads over Production of Generic Antiretrovirals." *Lancet* 357: 453.

Anderson, R. M., and R. M. May. 1990. "Immunization and Herd Immunity." *Lancet* 335: 641–45.

Andre, F. E. 2002. "How the Research-Based Industry Approaches Vaccine Development and Establishes Priorities." *Developmental Biology* 110: 25–29.

Barrett, R. J., and D. B. Parker. 2003. "Rites of Consent: Negotiating Research Participation in Diverse Cultures." *Monash Bioethics Review* 22 (2): 9–26.

Baylor, N. W., and L. D. McVittie. 2003. "Changes in the Regulations for Vaccine Research and Development." In *The Jordan Report 20th Anniversary*, 45–49. Washington, DC: U.S. Department of Health and Human Services.

Biehl, J. 2002. "Biotechnology and the New Politics of Life and Death in Brazil: The AIDS Model." *Princeton Journal of Bioethics* 5: 59–74.

CDC (U.S. Centers for Disease Control and Prevention). 1999. "Achievements in Public Health 1900–1999: Impact of Vaccines Universally Recommended for Children in the United States, 1990–1998." *Morbidity and Mortality Weekly Report* 48 (12): 243–48.

Clarke, B. 2002. Presentation for the National Vaccine Advisory Committee, Washington DC.

Coll, P., M. Garrigo, C. Moreno, and N. Marti. 2003. "Routine Use of Gen-Probe Amplified Mycobacterium Tuberculosis Direct (MTD) Test for Detection of Mycobacterium Tuberculosis with Smear-Positive and Smear-Negative Specimens." *International Journal of Tuberculosis and Lung Disease* 7 (9): 886–91.

Danzon, P., and A. Towse. 2005. "Theory and Implementation of Differential Pricing for Pharmaceuticals." In *International Public Goods and Transfer of Technology under a Globalized Intellectual Property Regime*, ed. K. Maskus and J. Reichman. Cambridge, U.K.: Cambridge University Press.

DiMasi, J. A., R. W. Hansen, and H. G. Grabowski. 2003. "The Price of Innovation: New Estimates of Drug Development Costs." *Journal of Health Economics* 22: 151–85.

DiMasi, J. A., R. W. Hansen, H. G. Grabowski, and L. Lasagna. 1991. "Cost of Innovation in the Pharmaceutical Industry." *Journal of Health Economics* 10 (2): 107–42.

"Drugs for the Poor: Exotic Pursuits." 2003. *Economist*, January 30, p. 52.

Emanuel, E. T., D. Wendler, J. Killen, and C. Grady. 2004. "What Makes Clinical Research in Developing Countries Ethical? The Benchmarks of Ethical Research." *Journal of Infectious Diseases* 89: 930–37.

FDA (U.S. Food and Drug Administration). 2004. "Biological Products, Bacterial Vaccines, and Toxoids: Implementation of Efficacy Review." *Federal Register* 69: 1–23.

Galambos, L., and J. C. Sewell. 1995. *Networks of Innovation*. New York: Cambridge University Press.

Garber, D. A., G. Silvestri, and M. B. Feinberg. 2004. "Prospects for an AIDS Vaccines: Three Big Questions, No Easy Answers." *Lancet Infectious Diseases* 4: 397–414.

GATB (Global Alliance for TB Drug Development). 2001. *The Economics of TB Drug Development*. New York: GATB.

Grabowski, H. 1997. "The Effect of Pharmacoeconomics on Company Research and Development Decisions." *Pharmacoeconomics* 11: 389–97.

Hansen, R. W. 1979. "The Pharmaceutical Development Process: Estimates of Current Development Costs and Times and the Effects of Regulatory Changes." In *Issues in Pharmaceutical Economics*, ed. R. I. Chien, 151–87. Lexington, MA: Lexington Books.

Herrera, S. 2004. "U.S. Rejiggers Bioshield Bill." *Nature Biotechnology* 22: 792.

Hilleman, M. R. 1996. "Three Decades of Hepatitis Vaccinology in Historic Perspective: A Paradigm of Successful Pursuits." In *Vaccinia, Vaccination, Vaccinology: Jenner, Pasteur, and Their Successors*, ed. S. A. Plotkin and B. Fantini, 199–209. New York: Elsevier.

———. 2000. "Vaccines in Historic Evolution and Perspective: A Narrative of Vaccines Discoveries." *Vaccine* 18: 1436–47.

Hilts, P. J. 2003. *Protecting America's Health: The FDA, Business, and One Hundred Years of Regulation*. New York: Alfred A. Knopf.

Institute of Medicine. 2004. *Financing Vaccines in the 21st Century*. Washington, DC: National Academy Press.

Jayaramann, S. 2003. "Indian Biogenerics Industry Emerges." *Nature Biotechnology* 21: 1115–16.

Klausner, R. D., A. S. Fauci, L. Corey, G. J. Nabel, H. Gayle, S. Berkley, and others. 2003. "The Need for a Global HIV Vaccine Enterprise." *Science* 300: 2036–39.

Kou, U. 2002. *Guidelines for Estimating Costs of Introducing New Vaccines into the National Immunization System*. Geneva: World Health Organization, Department of Vaccines and Biologicals.

Lohray, B. B. 2003. "Medical Biotechnology in India." *Advances in Biochemical Engineering/Biotechnology* 85: 215–81.

Lyles, A. 2003. "Public-Private Partnerships at the National Institutes of Health from Discovery to Commercialization." *Clinical Therapeutics* 25 (11): 2900–2.

Mahmoud, A. 2004. "The Global Vaccination Gap" (editorial). *Science* 305: 147.

Mazurek, G. H., and M. E. Villarino. 2003. "Guidelines for Using the QuantiFERON®-TB Test for Diagnosing Latent Mycobacterium Tuberculosis Infection." *Morbidity and Mortality Weekly Report Recommendations and Reports* 52 (RR-2): 15–18.

McMillan, J. R., and C. Conlon. 2004. "The Ethics of Research Related to Health Care in Developing Countries." *Journal of Medical Ethics* 30: 204–6.

Mercer Management Consulting. 1995. "Report on the United States Vaccine Industry." Report for the Department of Health and Human Services, Washington DC.

———. 2002. "Lessons Learned: New Procurement Strategies for Vaccines." Report for the Global Alliance for Vaccines and Immunization Board, Geneva.

Miller, M. A., and A. R. Hinman. 1999. "Cost-Benefit and Cost-Effectiveness Analysis of Vaccine Policy." In *Vaccines*, 3rd ed., ed. Stanley Plotkin and Walter Orenstein, 1074–87. Philadelphia: W. B. Saunders.

Milstien, J., and L. Belgharbi. 2004. "Regulatory Pathways for Vaccines for Developing Countries." *Bulletin of the World Health Organization* 82: 128–33.

MMV (Medicines for Malaria Venture). 2002. *Annual Report 2002*. Geneva: MMV.

Nakamura, R. M., M. A. Velmonte, K. Kawajiri, C. F. Anf, R. A. Frias, M. T. Mendoza, and others. 1998. "MPB64 Mycobacterial Antigen: A New Skin Test Reagent through Patch Method for Rapid Diagnosis of Active Tuberculosis." *International Journal of Tuberculosis and Lung Disease* 2 (7): 541–46.

Nederbragt, H. 2000. "The Biomedical Disciplines and the Structure of Biomedical and Clinical Knowledge." *Theoretical Medicine and Bioethics* 21 (6): 553–66.

Nossal, G. J. V. 2000. "The Global Alliance for Vaccines and Immunization: A Millennial Challenge." *Nature Immunology* 1: 5–8.

———. 2004. "A Healthier Climate for Funding of Vaccine Research." *Nature Immunology* 5: 457–59.

Ohno, Y. 2002. "ICH Guidelines: Implementation of the 3Rs (Refinement, Reduction, and Replacement)—Incorporating Best Scientific Practices into the Regulatory Process." *Institute for Laboratory Animal Research Journal* 43 (Suppl.): 595–98.

O'Sullivan, C. E., D. R. Miller, P. S. Schneider, and G. D. Roberts. 2002. "Evaluation of Gen-Probe Amplified Mycobacterium Tuberculosis Direct Test by Using Respiratory and Nonrespiratory Specimens in a Tertiary Care Center Laboratory." *Journal of Clinical Microbiology* 40 (5): 1723–27.

Perkins, M. D. 2000. "New Diagnostic Tools for Tuberculosis." *International Journal of Tuberculosis and Lung Disease* 4 (12): S182–88.

Pignatti, E., H. Boone, and I. Moulon. 2004. "Overview of the European Regulatory Approval System." *Journal of Ambulatory Care Management* 27: 89–97.

Rappuoli, R., H. Miller, and S. Falkow. 2002. "The Intangible Value of Vaccination." *Science* 297: 937–39.

Ridley, R. 2003. "Product R&D for Neglected Diseases: 27 Years of WHO/TDR Experiences with Public-Private Partnerships." *European Molecular Biology Organization Reports* 4: S43–46.

Sachs, J. 2001. *Macroeconomics and Health: Investing in Health for Economic Development.* Geneva: World Health Organization.

Sander, A. 2004. "The Emerging Landscape of Public-Private Partnerships for Product Development." In *Combating Diseases Associated with Poverty: Financing Strategies for Product Development and the Potential Role of Public-Private Partnerships,* ed. R. Widdus and K. White, 79–80. Geneva: Initiative for Public-Private Partnerships for Health, Global Forum for Health Research.

Schmid, E. F., and D. A. Smith. 2002. "Should Scientific Innovation Be Managed?" *Drug Discovery Today* 7: 941–45.

Trouiller, P., P. Olliaro, E. Torreele, J. Orbinski, R. Laing, and N. Ford. 2002. "Drug Development for Neglected Diseases: A Deficient Market and a Public-Health Policy Failure." *Lancet* 359: 2188–94.

U.K. Commission on Intellectual Property Rights. 2002. *Integrating Intellectual Property Rights and Development Policy.* London: U.K. Commission on Intellectual Property Rights.

UNAIDS (Joint United Nations Programme on HIV/AIDS). 2003. *Accelerating Action against AIDS in Africa.* Geneva: UNAIDS.

U.S. Congress, Office of Technology Assessment. 1993. *Pharmaceutical R&D Costs, Risks, and Rewards.* OTA-H-522. Washington, DC: U.S. Government Printing Office.

Varmus, H., R. Klausner, E. Zerhouni, T. Acharya, A. S. Daar, and P. A. Singer. 2004. "Public Health: Grand Challenges in Global Health." *Science* 303: 168–69.

Walsh, J., A. Arora, and W. Cohen. 2003. "Working through the Patent Problem." *Science* 299: 1021.

Webber, D., and M. Kremer. 2001. "Perspectives on Stimulating Industrial Research and Development for Neglected Infectious Diseases." *Bulletin of the World Health Organization* 79: 735–41.

Widdus, R. 2001. "Public-Private Partnerships for Health: Their Main Targets, Their Diversity, and Their Future Direction." *Bulletin of the World Health Organization* 79: 713–20.

———. 2004. "Historical Context: Why Public-Private Partnerships for Product Development Emerged and How." In *Combating Diseases Associated with Poverty: Financing Strategies for Product Development and the Potential Role of Public-Private Partnerships,* ed. R. Widdus and K. White. Geneva: Initiative for Public-Private Partnerships for Health, Global Forum for Health Research.

WTO (World Trade Organization). 2003. "The General Council Chairperson's Statement," August 30. http://www.wto.org/english/tratop_e/trips_e/t_news_e.htm.

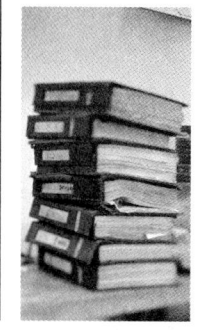

Chapter **7**

Economic Approaches to Valuing Global Health Research

David Meltzer

Health research has contributed tremendously to advancing health and welfare throughout the world. Gains in health have already been attained, and health research continues to have great potential to contribute to the well-being of persons in both low-income and high-income countries. The "10/90" reports of the Global Forum on Health Research (GFHR) have helped highlight that, although the burden of disease attributable to morbidity and mortality is greatest in developing countries, most health research has focused on the needs of developed countries and relatively little on the needs of lower-income countries (GFHR 2003). Despite the relative dearth of health research focused specifically on their most important health problems, lower-income countries have also benefited from health research, often as much from research originally motivated to serve high-income countries as from research specifically designed to address the needs of low-income countries.

In the future, health research aimed primarily at addressing the needs of affluent countries is likely to continue to produce benefits for lower-income countries, even in the absence of efforts to manage scientific research in the interest of lower-income nations. Indeed, as lower-income countries increase in income, their health problems will likely come to resemble more closely the health problems of higher-income countries. However, "trickle-down" approaches are not an efficient way of producing knowledge to advance the health and well-being of the populations of lower-income nations. Instead, a rational approach is needed that appreciates both the value of health in lower-income nations and the potential for rational scientific management to efficiently allocate resources for scientific research. The work of the GFHR and other organizations in this regard is an important step in this direction. Moreover,

recent advances in understanding about the value of improvements in health and in approaches to the value and priorities of health research provide powerful theoretical tools to address these issues.

Although the application of these principles is still in its infancy, these tools provide a valuable framework for determining the value of health research relevant to low-income countries and for maximizing the value of research that aims to promote health in those countries. In the following section, recent innovations in determining the value of health research at an aggregate level are reviewed. The conclusion is that the value of health research has been immense and is likely to increase dramatically in coming years, especially in lower-income countries. In deriving these conclusions, not only health-oriented measures of improved health, such as life years, disability-adjusted life years (DALYs), or quality-adjusted life years (QALYs), were considered, but also how increases in income may increase the value of such improvements. In a later section, recent methods that can be used to estimate the value of specific research projects are reviewed. The application of such methods promises to better identify the value of health research in specific instances, which can enhance the case for research spending to improve health in developing countries and can increase the efficiency with which available research funds are spent.

THE VALUE OF HEALTH RESEARCH

Health research can be valuable for a variety of reasons. The most obvious reason is simply the value that people place on improvements in health. Those health improvements may be reflected in increased length of life or quality of life. Other reasons that health research can be valuable include the improvements in productivity, decreases in medical care costs, and greater ability to plan for and invest in the future when health improves. Health research can also sometimes decrease costs independent of any effects on health—for example, when a lower-cost treatment can replace a higher-cost treatment of similar efficacy.

A large body of work has attempted to assess and quantify the economic value of health from these perspectives. The goal of some of this literature is a comprehensive assessment of the cost of illness (for example, Rice 1994). Such comprehensive assessments are often attempted in order to assess the cost-effectiveness of medical or public health interventions, which are frequently measured in terms of quality-adjusted life expectancy (Gold and others 1996) or DALYs (WHO 1994; World Bank 1993). Other aspects of this literature focus on single dimensions of the economic value of health. For example, Ram and Schultz (1979) performed an early analysis showing the effects of malaria eradication on productivity. Similarly, Meltzer (1992) attempted to identify the effects of mortality on investment in education, the demographic transition, and the onset of sustained economic growth. In that work, it was suggested that health can increase income because increasing life expectancy raises returns to investment in education, in turn encouraging decreases in family size and further increases in investment in the education of children and a transition to sustained human capital–based economic growth. These and other mechanisms, including shifts in the ratio of productive adults to dependents and changes in savings rates with increasing life expectancy, have been suggested to produce positive effects of health on per capita income in both the short and the long run (Bloom, Canning, and Jamison 2004).

Although some evidence suggests the importance of all these effects, recent work on the value of health in developed countries has focused primarily on the value that people place on improvements in their health. Such studies for the United States have suggested that increases in longevity over the past several decades are valued in the tens of trillions of dollars, indeed, contributing about as much to increasing welfare over the period as increases in per capita income. Subsequently, similar findings have been reported for other countries, and cross-national studies have found that the value of growth in life expectancy compared with the value of income growth has been even greater for low-income countries (Becker, Philipson, and Soares 2003). These studies have been influential in developing a broad consensus that the returns to health research are large and in producing dramatic increases in the budget for the National Institutes of Health (NIH) in the United States. The conclusions of these studies in the United States have been based on assessments of both the high value of health and the role that health research has played in improvements in health.

Although both the connection of health research to health and the valuation of health differ in important ways between lower-income and higher-income countries, these studies provide a useful framework for understanding the past and likely future value of health research in lower-income countries.

The Value of Improved Health

Several authors have contributed to the literature on the value of improvements in health: Becker, Philipson, and Soares (2003); Cutler and others (1997); Murphy and Topel (2003); and Nordhaus (2003). Although these studies differ somewhat in the analytic framework they use, the basic form of their analyses is quite similar. In essence, they all use estimates of the value of longevity on the basis of revealed preference techniques and multiply these values by the increases in longevity that have been observed to determine the value of improvements in health. Revealed preference estimates of the value of life are most commonly derived by assessing the wage premium required by workers to accept riskier jobs. This idea dates back at least to the work of Adam Smith, but the modern treatment of this issue stems primarily from the work of Thaler and Rosen (1975). For example, if the lifetime earnings of a risky mining job that has a $1/1,000$ increased risk of death compared with another mining job is US$1,000, then the statistical value of a life would be said to be US$1,000,000, since paying 1,000 workers would result in one extra death on average and require that the employer pay wages equal to 1,000 workers $\times$ US$1,000/worker = US$1,000,000.

A simple example considering the value of increases in life expectancy in the United States from 1970 to 2000 illustrates well how these sorts of estimates have been used to estimate the value of increased longevity. From 1970 to 2000, life expectancy at birth for Americans grew by a little more than 5 years, from about 75 years to about 80 years. With about 300 million Americans living during this period, this increase constitutes about 1.5 billion life years. Using a conservative revealed preference estimate of about US$4 million as the statistical value of a life (Viscusi and Aldy 2003), assuming a life expectancy of 75 to 80 years, and assuming discounting is somewhere between 0 and 3 percent annually, one gets a value of about US$50,000 to US$100,000 per life year saved. Multiplying this gain in life years and the estimate of the value of a life year, one gets a value of increased longevity over this period of about US$75 trillion to US$150 trillion, or about US$2 trillion to US$4 trillion per year. The average of these numbers translates into almost US$10,000 per person per year, which is about as large as the increase in per capita income in the United States during this period. In essence, this analysis is a simplified form of that performed by Murphy and Topel (2003).

An alternative approach to obtaining a similar number may help some readers better understand the intuition behind these effects. Over this 30-year period, the 5-year increase in life expectancy that occurred raised life expectancy by about two months (or one-sixth year) per year. With each life year valued at about US$75,000, these gains in life years are readily seen to be worth about US$10,000 per person per year.

Understanding the value of improvements in health in lower-income countries requires data both on increase in longevity and on how such increases in longevity might be valued. Data on increases in longevity are relatively easy to obtain for most countries and vary substantially across countries over time. For example, many countries that had low income in 1950, including the Arab Republic of Egypt, Mexico, and Thailand, have had an increase in life expectancy since 1950 of more than 20 years, or about three months per year, which is about 50 percent greater than the rate of growth in life expectancy in the United States. Although some countries that had low incomes in 1950 and did not experience much economic growth during this period did not increase in life expectancy over this period, the vast majority of countries with low incomes in 1950 experienced increases in life expectancy far exceeding the rate of increase in the United States and other developed countries. This fact suggests that the potential for increases in life expectancy is greater for lower-income countries than for higher-income ones, so the increase in life expectancy for lower-income countries might be expected to slow in coming years. If the rate of change in the value of health gains were determined primarily by the rate of increase in life expectancy, growth in the value of health in lower-income countries would be expected to slow in the future.

Assessing the importance of changes in life expectancy relative to changes in the value of increased life expectancy in influencing the value of health requires data on the value of increased longevity. Such data on the value of mortality reductions are limited but do exist. Viscusi and Aldy (2003) reviewed the literature on the statistical value of life across countries that vary in income. One key finding is that the statistical value of life increases with income, with an elasticity of approximately 0.5 to 0.6, so that a 100 percent increase in income leads to a 50 to 60 percent increase in the statistical value of life.

One implication of this finding is that economic growth is likely to result in increases in welfare through improved health, both because economic growth improves health and because the value of those health improvements increases as income increases. This statement can be assessed formally by analyzing change over time in the value of life (VL) = $VLY \times LY$, where VLY is the value of a life year, and LY is life expectancy. Such numbers easily show the value of health gains that have been achieved. For example, India is the poorest country for which calculations of revealed preference estimates of the statistical value of life have been done (Viscusi and Aldy 2003). This study suggests a statistical value of life of US$0.6 million, or about US$10,000 to US$20,000 per life year saved. With

gains in life expectancy of about 25 years since 1950 and a population in 2000 of about 1 billion persons, the gains in life expectancy in India alone over the period are worth about US$400 trillion, or US$8 trillion per year, equivalent to about US$800 per person per year.

Thus, as large as the US$75 trillion to US$150 trillion estimate for the health gains for the United States is, such gains are only about one-fourth as large as the gains for India. The value of the gains for India is larger for several reasons. One is just the longer period considered—30 years for the United States compared with 50 for India—although, in fact, gains in the United States were small enough between 1950 and 1970 that the longer period explains relatively little of the difference. Much larger factors are the fivefold greater increase in life expectancy in India than in the United States over the period (25 years compared with 5 years) and a population about five times as large. Thus, if health gains are valued in U.S. dollars, the value of such gains for India over this period far exceeds that for the United States. Given the 5:1 size of India and the gains in life expectancy, the ratio of those gains would be more like 25:1 than 4:1 (US$400 trillion as opposed to US$75 trillion to US$150 trillion) were it not that the statistical value of life in the United States is greater than that in India. Even if one does not feel comfortable assigning differential valuation to lives across countries, the fact that the valuation of gains in India is so much larger than the valuation of the gains in the United States using this method provides a powerful reminder of certain basics of the value of improving health in lower-income versus higher-income countries: many more people live in low-income than in high-income countries, and the potential for large increases in life expectancy is thus far greater.

Such statistics provide some insights into the value of historical improvements in health, but in terms of considering future investments, considering what can be said about the growth of the value of health in lower- versus higher-income countries in the future is useful. To do so, one finds it useful to decompose growth in the value of health into growth in life expectancy and growth in the value of longevity (growth in the value of life years). We begin with $VL = VLY \times LY$ and differentiate to obtain the finding that growth rates can be decomposed to find that $g_{VL} = g_{VLY} + g_{LY}$, so that the growth in the value of life is the sum of the growth in the value of a life year and growth in life expectancy.

To understand the meaning of this relationship, one finds it useful to consider the Viscusi and Aldy (2003) estimate of the elasticity of the value of life with respect to income. Substituting this elasticity income in the above equation, $g_{VL} = 0.5\ g_Y + g_{LY}$, where g_Y is the growth rate in per capita income. The relative magnitude of these two components is instructive. In developed countries such as the United States, where growth in life expectancy has been on the order of two months per year from a base of 75 or so years, the growth in life expectancy is $(2/12)/75 = 0.2$ percent per year. This rate is substantially smaller than the component of increased value of life related to growth in the valuation of gains in life, even with long-run real growth rates of only 2 to 3 percent, so the component attributable to growth in the value of life is $0.5 \times (2$ to 3 percent$) = 1$ to 2 percent per year. In lower-income countries in which growth in life expectancy is greater and baseline life expectancy is lower, life expectancy growth may be more important but is still not likely to exceed the effects of growth in per capita income. For example, Mali experienced dramatic growth in life expectancy of 1 percent per year (from 30 to 45 years from 1950 to 1990), but growth in per capita income in Mali from 1980 to 2000 was about 3 percent annually, translating into effects on the value of life of 1.5 percent annually. More striking perhaps is China, where growth in life expectancy from 40 to 70 years from 1950 to 1990 represented an increase of about 2 percent per year, whereas growth in per capita income (from 1980 to 2000) was about 8 percent per year (translating into effects on the value of life of about 4 percent per year). Two implications are immediately obvious:

- First, the growth in the overall value of health over the period has been large—about 2 to 6 percent annually for these initially low-income countries.
- Second, the major driver of the value of health over time has not been an increase in health per se but, instead, increases in income that produce increases in how health is valued. This finding is likely to be even more true as life expectancy increases so that continuing large increases in life expectancy become more difficult to achieve.

As noted previously, estimates such as these of the statistical value of life can understandably be criticized on the basis of associating a greater value with saving lives of wealthier persons than saving lives of poorer persons. Nevertheless, it is striking to note that in India—the only relatively low-income country for which data on the statistical value of life are available—the total value of recent health gains far exceeds even the immense gains in the United States. Data on the value of life for other low-income countries would help reinforce this finding, but the combination of the greater potential for large increases in life expectancy and for greater growth in per capita income in low-income countries in the future suggests that the total value of health gains for such countries may far exceed those of higher-income countries. Indeed, it bears emphasis that, in attempting to value health in monetary terms rather than merely health terms, such as life years or QALYs or DALYs, an important new avenue is opened by which the value of health research can increase over time even as gains in life expectancy slow with increasing life expectancy, as they have in developed countries. Despite the concern that economic approaches undervalue the health of persons with lower incomes, such

valuations clearly suggest that the potential value of health research for these countries is immense. That this discussion has focused only on the value of mortality reductions and neglected those of reductions in morbidity even further reinforces the potential gains from health research.

Not only is the magnitude of the value of these improvements in health immense in regard to how people value being healthier, but the total value of health also includes increased productivity, decreased medical care costs, and increased ability to plan for and invest in the future when health improves. Although these effects are often not easy to quantify, they may prove to be important components of the total economic value of improvements in health.

The Connection between Gains in Health and Health Research

To move from the finding that gains in health are highly valued to the finding that health research is highly valued, gains in health must be connected to health research. Making such associations is difficult even in high-income countries, but it has been done with some success. For example, Cutler and Kadiyala (2003) argue that the major recent gains in life expectancy in the United States have come from reductions in cardiovascular disease, about two-thirds of which can be tied to advances that have resulted from medical research as opposed to secular trends in nonmedical factors that promote health, such as per capita income and education. Similar calculations for lower-income countries have not been done. Nevertheless, although growth in income and education seem more likely to be important in producing increases in life expectancy for such countries, the major role of reductions in childhood infectious disease in recent gains in life expectancy suggests the great value of the research that has produced such innovations as childhood immunizations, improved sanitation, and oral rehydration therapy. Similarly, the high burden of cardiovascular disease in lower-income countries will be expected to decline in the coming years if the benefits of research can be applied in those settings.

Such conclusions speak to the value of health research as a whole for lower-income countries, and they reflect the gains that come both from research done initially to benefit higher-income countries and from research done to benefit lower-income countries. Although both of these classes of research may produce benefits for lower-income countries, discussion of their differences is in order. In the case of research done initially with the needs of high-income countries in mind, clearly some types of research benefit low-income countries more than others. For example, research that has demonstrated the power of relatively inexpensive medications to reduce mortality from cardiovascular disease (for example, aspirin in acute myocardial infarction) has much greater potential to produce large benefits for lower-income countries in the foreseeable future than does research that advances techniques for expensive acute treatments, such as cardiac catheterization. In this particular case of cardiovascular disease, estimates summarized by Cutler and Kadiyala (2003) suggest that higher-income countries have also benefited more from research that advanced such low-technology treatments than from research on high-technology treatments.

Such patterns may not be maintained across other health conditions, but they do hold out the tantalizing thought that health research initiated by high-income countries in their own interest may sometimes be directed toward work of greater value if issues of cost and generalizability to lower-income settings are reflected more greatly in decisions about research priorities. When research directed toward the needs of lower-income countries is considered, cost and feasibility must, of course, receive great attention. However, the immense reductions in mortality that have come from advances in knowledge about public health efforts—such as efficient and effective sanitation, immunization, and oral rehydration programs, all of which were developed primarily with the needs of low-income countries in mind—suggest the value of research targeted toward the needs of lower-income countries. Rigorous studies of the value of these innovations akin to those studies done to assess the value of health research for the United States are sorely needed to inform potential funders of the potential returns to such research.

METHODS OF ASSESSING THE VALUE OF HEALTH RESEARCH PROJECTS

Although the aggregate value of health research has unquestionably been large, not all health research projects are sufficiently valuable to justify their costs. Some of these latter projects are inevitable because the outcome of research is intrinsically unpredictable. However, even if one abstracts from such uncertainty by considering the expected returns from a project before one embarks on it, research projects clearly vary in their likely value relative to their cost. Such assessments are obviously difficult to make, yet they are routinely done as part of the process of deciding the allocation of research funds. These assessments have traditionally been done rather informally, even in the most closely structured settings in which research funding is sought, such as the NIH study sections in the United States that review research proposals for NIH funding.

An active discussion over the past decade has helped to identify valuable strategies for priority setting in global health research and determine their implications for research priorities in the field. The 2004 report on health research of the GFHR summarized the major contributions to this discussion (GFHR 2003). The approaches that are described date back to as early as 1990 with the work of the Commission on Health Research

for Development. They include the essential national research approach developed by the Council on Health Research for Development and approaches developed by the Ad Hoc Committee on Health Research, the Advisory Committee on Health Research, and the GFHR's own Global Forum combined matrix approach. The 2004 report compares these approaches along several dimensions that include the following:

1. Objective of priority setting
2. Focus at global or national level
3. Strategies or principles (especially relating to the process for participation by stakeholders)
4. Criteria for priority setting:
   - Burden of disease
   - Analysis of determinants of disease burden
   - Cost-effectiveness of interventions (resulting from proposed research)
   - Effect on equity and social justice
   - Ethical, political, social, and cultural acceptability
   - Probability of finding a solution
   - Scientific quality of research proposed
   - Feasibility (availability of human resources, funding, facilities)
5. Contribution to capacity strengthening.

In addition to describing the dimensions considered in these approaches to priority setting, the 2004 report also summarizes several efforts to apply these approaches in individual countries or for individual diseases or disease areas (see, for example, Remme and others 2002). The priorities identified include many of those identified in chapter 4 in this volume.

Examining these dimensions of priority setting, one finds that some are intrinsically qualitative in nature but quantitative analysis also sometimes plays an important role. For example, several approaches, including the GFHR's combined matrix approach, use DALYs to quantify the number of healthy years of life lost to the disease toward which the research is directed.

Looking forward, one may find additional quantitative approaches helpful in assessing the value of research. For example, new methods based on value-of-information (VOI) techniques have begun to be proposed to better inform such assessments. In essence, VOI techniques model the uncertainty in the outcomes of research and the value of research contingent on that uncertainty in order to assess the expected value of the research. For example, a research project that has a 5 percent chance of success that it would produce health gains worth US\$100 million and a 95 percent chance of failure, would have an expected value of $(0.05 \times US\$100 \text{ million}) + (0.95 \times US\$0) = US\$5 \text{ million}$. Although these techniques have rich roots in statistical and economic theory, they are often difficult to apply well because of the difficulty in valuing health outcomes and modeling the uncertain outcomes of research. As a result, these methods often can provide only loose bounds on the value of a research project (Meltzer 2001). Indeed, in the worst-case scenarios, in which the available information about the likely outcomes of research is essentially uninformative, VOI techniques only reproduce information on the burden and costs of illness. Nevertheless, in settings where more structure can be put into the problem, these techniques have begun to be applied successfully to specific research questions, such as the prioritization of research in Alzheimer's disease (Claxton and others 2001). In general, the more remote the connection of the research to health outcomes, the harder it is to gain meaningful information from a VOI approach. Thus VOI approaches are far better at providing information on the value of applied research than they are at providing information on the value of basic research.

For lower-income countries, this ability to illustrate the value of applied work may be especially valuable because often a technology has already been developed and the question is how best to apply it in a given setting. With the limited funds that have traditionally been available for research in lower-income countries and the high value that appears to be placed on improvements in health in these countries, VOI studies, as discussed previously, seem likely to frequently show that the benefits of research in lower-income countries far exceed the costs. It is hoped that such findings may be used to increase the pool of funds available for research in these settings. However, even if VOI techniques do not lead to increases in the total funding available for research in low-income countries, they may be helpful in informing resource allocation decisions, given available resources. In the context of a fixed research budget in which some research projects whose expected benefit exceeds their costs could still not be funded, rigorous data on the high rates of return on projects that did not make the funding line would then serve to highlight the returns to greater research in these settings. Because VOI calculations need not be complex (see box 7.1), the most important barriers to their

---

Box 7.1

Value of Information

Although VOI calculations can be quite complex (for example, Claxton and others 2001), they need not be. For a researcher seeking funding, much simpler calculations may be sufficient to build a compelling case for funding. For example, quantifying the burden of illness in life years, QALYs, or DALYs lost and converting this into a burden or cost-of-illness measure in economic terms using an estimate of the statistical value of life may even be sufficient. To take a simple example, imagine a research program in a country with a statistical value of life of US$0.6 million (for example, the estimate for India) for a disease that currently kills 1,000 people per year. If one abstracts from issues such as the age of death and how one might differentially value deaths at different ages, this would have a potential value of US$0.6 billion per year. If the research study were viewed as having a 10 percent chance of preventing 50 percent of those deaths, its expected value would be $P(\text{success}) \times$ percent efficacy $\times$ statistical value of life $= 0.1 \times 0.5 \times \text{US\$0.6 billion} = \text{US\$30 million per}$ year. Potential annual productivity gains produced by a successful treatment and annual costs of the treatment could be added to, or subtracted from, these US$0.6 billion annual benefits as well. One could go further, arguing that the research would be valuable into the future, and discount an infinite stream of those annual returns. At a discount rate (R) of 10 percent, this stream would have a value of US$20 million$/R = \text{US\$200 million}$. This result suggests that a research program costing up to this amount would be worthwhile if it could be expected to have this likelihood of success and percent efficacy. Even if those probabilities could not be reliably estimated, minimum values could be calculated at which the research program would continue to be worthwhile.

As in their use in affluent countries, such calculations are likely to suggest that health research is of great value, often being predicted to return value many times its cost even accounting for uncertainty. In the preceding example, for instance, even an immense US$100 million research program would have an expected return 20 times as large. Such results would reflect the immense value in health research but would also suggest caution: with limited research funds, not all programs whose benefits exceed their costs should be funded if more valuable projects remain unfunded. In this area, funding agencies can be helpful to the research community by highlighting how they have used calculations such as these and publicizing the ratio of research costs to returns for those projects they have been able to fund. Even when a project is not funded despite a favorable ratio of expected returns to research costs, reporting the missed opportunity will serve as a reminder to the world community of the potential of health research for lower-income countries that remains unrealized and thereby, perhaps, promote greater investment in health research to benefit the people of these countries.

useful application to research in developing countries are the lack of awareness and acceptance of these methods on the part of researchers and funders focused on these settings. Organizations concerned with international health can exercise valuable international leadership by exposing these researchers and funders to these methods and encouraging their use.

CONCLUSIONS

Improvements in health in recent decades have been of great value in both high- and low-income countries. Furthermore, future improvements in health are likely to be highly valued as the value of health increases with continuing growth in income. Health research has played a major role in the advances in health that have occurred, and the great potential value of future gains in health suggests that health research continues to merit increasing investment. New tools to prospectively assess the value of research offer the promise of even greater returns from health investment, especially for more applied research that can be closely connected to measurable benefits at the population level. Because low-income countries may often particularly benefit from applied research, these techniques to assess the value of research may be especially helpful in ensuring that the value of applied research in these settings is recognized. Providing researchers and policy makers in low- and high-income countries with the analytic tools needed to better identify and advocate for valuable opportunities for health research may be an important avenue to increasing the level and effectiveness of spending for health research.

REFERENCES

Becker, G. S., T. J. Philipson, and R. R. Soares. 2003. "The Quantity and Quality of the Life and the Evolution of World Inequality." NBER Working Paper 9765, National Bureau of Economic Research, Cambridge, MA.

Bloom, D. E., D. Canning, and D. T. Jamison. 2004. "Health, Wealth, and Welfare." *Finance and Development* 41 (1): 10–15.

Claxton, K., P. J. Neumann, S. Aranki, and M. C. Weinstein. 2001. "Bayesian Value of Information Analysis: An Application to a Policy Model of Alzheimer's Disease." *International Journal of Technology Assessment in Health Care* 17 (1): 38–55.

Cutler, D. M., and S. Kadiyala. 2003. "The Return to Biomedical Research: Treatment and Behavioral Effects." In *Measuring the Gains from Medical Research: An Economic Approach,* ed. K. M. Murphy and R. H. Topel, 110–62. Chicago: University of Chicago Press.

Cutler, D. M., E. Richardson, T. E. Keeler, and D. Staiger. 1997. "Measuring the Health of the U.S. Population." Brookings Papers on Economic Activity: Microeconomics 21782, Brookings Institution, Washington, DC.

GFHR (Global Forum for Health Research). 2003. *The 10/90 Report on Health Research 2003–2004.* Geneva: GFHR.

Gold, M. R., J. E. Siegel, L. B. Russell, and M. C. Weinstein. 1996. *Cost-Effectiveness in Health and Medicine.* New York: Oxford University Press.

Meltzer, D. 1992. "Mortality Decline, the Demographic Transition, and Economic Growth." Ph.D. dissertation, University of Chicago, Department of Economics.

———. 2001. "Addressing Uncertainty in Medical Cost-Effectiveness Analysis: Implications of Expected Utility Maximization for Methods to Perform Sensitivity Analysis and the Use of Cost-Effectiveness Analysis to Set Priorities for Medical Research." *Journal of Health Economics* 20: 109–29.

Murphy, K. M., and R. H. Topel. 2003. "The Economic Value of Medical Research." In *Measuring the Gains from Medical Research: An Economic Approach,* ed. K. M. Murphy and R. H. Topel, 41–73. Chicago: University of Chicago Press.

Nordhaus, W. D. 2003. "The Health of Nations: The Contribution of Improved Health to Living Standards." In *Measuring the Gains from Medical Research: An Economic Approach,* ed. K. M. Murphy and R. H. Topel, 9–40. Chicago: University of Chicago Press.

Ram, R., and T. W. Schultz. 1979. "Life Span, Health, Savings, and Productivity." *Economic Development and Cultural Change* 27 (April): 399–421.

Remme, J. H., E. Blas, L. Chitsulo, P. M. Desjeux, H. D. Engers, T. P. Kanyok, and others. 2002. "Strategic Emphases for Tropical Diseases Research: A TDR Perspective." *Trends in Parasitology* 18 (10): 421–26.

Rice, D. 1994. "Cost-of-Illness Studies: Fact or Fiction?" *Lancet* 344 (8936): 1519–20.

Thaler, R., and S. Rosen. 1975. "The Value of Saving a Life: Evidence from the Labor Market." In *Household Production and Consumption,* ed. N. Terleckyj, 265–68. New York: Columbia University Press.

Viscusi, W. K., and J. E. Aldy. 2003. "The Value of a Statistical Life: A Critical Review of Market Estimates throughout the World." *Journal of Risk and Uncertainty* 27 (1): 5–76.

WHO (World Health Organization). 1994. "Global Comparative Assessments in the Health Sector." In *Disease Burden, Expenditures, and Intervention Packages,* ed. C. J. L. Murray and A. D. Lopez. Geneva: WHO.

World Bank. 1993. *World Development Report: Investing in Health.* Washington, DC: World Bank.

Chapter **8**

Improving the Health of Populations: Lessons of Experience

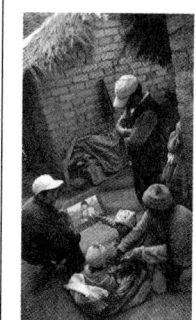

Carol Ann Medlin, Mushtaque Chowdhury, Dean T. Jamison, and Anthony R. Measham

In the past 50 years, the world has experienced enormous and unprecedented gains in the health of human populations. Progress has been especially apparent in developing countries. Average life expectancy has risen by more than 60 percent, from 40 years in 1950 to 65 years today. In 1950, roughly 28 percent of children died before their fifth birthday, but by 1990, this number had fallen to 10 percent. Furthermore, many of the world's most deadly and debilitating diseases, including leprosy, measles, poliomyelitis (polio), and many childhood illnesses, have been effectively contained in most areas and virtually eliminated in others. Smallpox, a highly contagious and deadly disease that affected more than 50 million people a year prior to 1950, has been completely eradicated.

Researchers have identified economic growth, rising incomes, and better living conditions brought about by rapid social and political transformations in many societies as major contributors to these impressive health gains. However, in recent years, the role of scientific and technological progress has emerged as a crucial, but little understood, factor underlying these gains. As Davis (1956, 306–7) observes, "It seems clear that the great reduction of mortality in underdeveloped areas since 1940 has been brought about mainly by the discovery of new methods of disease treatment applicable at reasonable cost [and] by the diffusion of these new methods."

New research has sought to validate, and indeed quantify, this basic intuition. For example, Jamison, Lau, and Wang (2005) show that technological progress (which is broadly defined as the generation or adoption of new technologies), together with education, has been a far more important contributor to declining infant mortality rates in developing

countries than income growth. Furthermore, improvements in health brought about by investments in technological progress generate an important and positive feedback loop favoring economic growth and development in these countries.

An important question that follows is what can be done to further consolidate these gains and ensure that the fruits of scientific and technology progress are placed in the hands of the people in developing countries who stand to benefit most? Because the work of the Disease Control Priorities Project (DCPP) focuses primarily on identifying the most cost-effective interventions for diseases and conditions affecting the health of populations in developing countries, this work provides the starting point for analysis. The goal is to isolate the critical factors—in particular those "actionable" through specific public policies—that have contributed to the effective deployment and scaling up of proven cost-effective technologies and services in low-income settings.

To address this question, the DCPP joined forces with the What Works Working Group of the Global Health Policy Research Network, an initiative led by the Center for Global Development in Washington, D.C., and funded by the Bill & Melinda Gates Foundation. DCPP authors were asked to identify outstanding examples of successful implementation of programs and projects geared toward the deployment of proven cost-effective interventions in their respective fields of international health and to speculate on what kinds of programmatic aspects and broader public policy decisions might have contributed to their success.

From an initial set of nominations, the What Works Working Group selected a subset of cases that conformed to strict selection criteria, researched them thoroughly, and produced a report to be widely disseminated to policy makers and leading health experts in both developed and developing countries. In parallel, the DCPP initiated a systematic review of the case materials to identify commonalities or factors that may have contributed to the deployment and scaling up of those interventions. The objective was to identify a set of specific policy levers and programmatic decisions that could facilitate the transplantation of those and other cost-effective interventions to new and different settings. This chapter presents the results of that study.

RESEARCH METHODS

The study consisted of a qualitative analysis of a set of case studies selected to help illustrate how proven, cost-effective interventions have been successfully deployed and brought to scale with dramatic results in low- and middle-income countries in Africa, Asia, and Latin America and the Caribbean. We examined evidence culled from interviews, peer-reviewed articles published in journals, and official project evaluations and attempted to organize this information in a way that would allow us to reach tentative conclusions about the most significant elements associated with the interventions' success.

The study thus followed one of Mill's (1843) five methods of experimental reasoning: the method of agreement. Such a method postulates that "if two or more instances of the phenomenon (A) . . . have only one circumstance (B) in common, the circumstance (B) in which alone all the instances agree is the cause (or effect) of the given phenomenon (A)." For this study, the phenomenon (A) is represented by success. Cases that qualified as successes had to conform to the following five criteria:

- *Scale.* All cases selected for study involved a national, regional, or global scale. Pilot projects or interventions implemented on a subnational scale were not considered.
- *Importance.* Selected cases addressed a problem of major public health significance that could be expressed, at the program's inception, in terms of disability-adjusted life years, a composite measure of mortality and morbidity caused by the disease.
- *Health impact.* Selected cases had documented evidence of a clear and measurable effect on the health of the population targeted by the intervention. Process indicators, including immunization coverage rates, were not considered an acceptable substitute for health impact data.
- *Duration.* All cases selected for study had a life span of at least five consecutive years.
- *Cost-effectiveness.* Selected cases relied on interventions that had been proven to be cost-effective at a threshold of approximately US$100 per disability-adjusted life year saved.

The unabashed focus on success meant that the study ignored potentially important information about factors that may be associated with programmatic failures or not-so-successful cases that did not meet the strict criteria described above. However, the inclusion of less-than-successful cases was not an option in light of time, resource constraints, and paucity of available documentation. Thus, a significant limitation of our study results from the lack of variance in the outcome observed. This type of selection bias is a common problem that may result from the nonrandom selection of cases in qualitative research.

Although bias cannot be eliminated without expanding the study to include unsuccessful examples, working skillfully with the presumption of bias to increase the level of confidence in the findings is possible. First, counterfactual examples, even if purely speculative (what would have happened if . . . ?), can be used to further substantiate the hypothesis that circumstance (B) has directly contributed to the observed phenomenon (A). Second, theorizing in a constructive way about what the direction of the bias might be and, therefore, minimizing its impact on the results of the study are also possible. For example, any potential bias more than likely results from overdetermining causality rather than overlooking or ignoring key factors related to success. In a related point, the study design makes discerning the relative contributions of the various factors difficult, because weights cannot be assigned easily.

Remarkably few rigorous studies of this sort attempt to track the implementation of proven, cost-effective interventions in the field. Although we have a good understanding of the efficacy of the available arsenal of interventions for treating and preventing diseases specific to low-income countries, we often know little about the range of programmatic and policy options that are needed to support these interventions in the real world. This study represents the first major contribution toward the development of a body of knowledge in that area, and the preliminary conclusions reached should be understood in that context (Collier and Brady 2004).

CASES

From an initial set of nominations received from DCPP authors as well as from other international health researchers, we selected a subset of 17 cases for study. We could not consider many cases that were nominated because of the absence of reliable data. Thus, the 17 cases selected are merely a subset of the many successes in international health that have been achieved during the past 50 years, not the full universe. Nonetheless, the cases draw from all three continents of the developing world—Africa, Asia, and Latin America and the Caribbean—and involve both communicable and noncommunicable diseases as well as curative and preventive care. Most cases are national-level programs, but a few involve regional initiatives, and one is global.

Many near misses did not make the cut. The reasons for this exclusion varied. For example, a program in Costa Rica, El Salvador, and Guatemala to promote hand washing appears to have resulted in a dramatic decline in child morbidity and mortality but did not meet the duration criterion because it was fully operational for only three years (1996–99). In another example, the evidence of a health impact was mixed: a successful schistosomiasis control program in the Arab Republic of Egypt that included treatment of blood flukes in infected individuals was later linked to high prevalence rates of hepatitis C caused by the use of improperly sterilized syringes (Frank and others 2000). Nonetheless, the most common rationale for excluding a case from this study had to do with a lack of consistent documentation and of analysis of the health impact of the program in question. Thus, a reasonable conclusion is that the true universe of cases is much larger than the subset of cases we examined.

Each case reviewed here illustrates how a discrete health intervention or combination of interventions was successfully brought to scale in a specific context. To gain insight into this process, we can distinguish between the intervention—for example, the tool or technology that has been proven to be cost-effective for the treatment or prevention of a given disease—and the programmatic characteristics and policies that contributed to the successful delivery or deployment of the intervention through specially designed programs or projects.

The following list of cases selected for review describes the programs or projects that were scaled up, identifies the specific intervention or interventions deployed, and summarizes the existing evidence about health outcomes and impact:[1]

- **Chagas disease control.** In 1991, seven countries—Argentina, Bolivia, Brazil, Chile, Paraguay, Uruguay, and later Peru—joined forces as part of an initiative for the Southern Cone countries led by the Pan American Health Organization to combat Chagas disease through a combination of surveillance activities, house-to-house spraying, and other vector control methods. *Health impact*—Disease incidence had fallen by 94 percent by 2000. By 2001, disease transmission had been halted in Chile, Uruguay, and large parts of Brazil and Paraguay. The project is ongoing.
- **Diarrheal treatment.** In Egypt, the government launched a national program in the early 1980s to promote the use by mothers of locally manufactured oral rehydration salts in a four-part strategy that included tailoring product design and branding to accommodate local preferences and customs; strengthening production and distribution channels, both public and private; training health workers; and using social marketing and a mass media campaign. *Health impact*—Between 1982 and 1987, infant and child mortality

dropped by 36 and 43 percent, respectively. Mortality attributed to diarrhea fell 82 percent among infants and 62 percent among children. The project closed in 1991.
- **Guinea worm eradication.** Twenty countries in Asia and Sub-Saharan Africa began a global campaign to eradicate guinea worm in the mid 1980s. Led by the Carter Center, the United Nations Children's Fund, the U.S. Centers for Disease Control and Prevention, and the World Health Organization, the campaign promoted improved water safety through deep-well digging, environmental control, and the use of cloth filters for drinking water; health education programs; and case management, containment, and surveillance. *Health impact*—By 1998, 9 million to 13 million cases of guinea worm had been prevented and global prevalence had dropped by 99 percent. The project is ongoing in three countries.
- **Family planning.** In Bangladesh, family planning has been promoted since the 1970s through a door-to-door outreach program conducted by young, married women who provide information about limiting family size or spacing pregnancies along with products. An extensive media campaign accompanied the outreach program. *Health impact*—Contraceptive use among married women in Bangladesh is approximately 50 percent today, compared with only 8 percent in the mid 1970s, and the average number of children per family is 3.3, down from 7 in the mid 1970s. The project is ongoing.
- **Hib vaccination.** Chile began to include the Hib vaccine as part of its national immunization program in 1996. In The Gambia, a similar initiative was introduced in 1997. *Health impact*—In Chile, the prevalence of Hib disease fell by 90 percent, and the incidence of pneumonia and other Hib-related illnesses fell by 80 percent. In The Gambia, the number of children developing Hib meningitis fell from 200 per 100,000 to 21 per 100,000 only 12 months following the introduction of the vaccine. The projects are ongoing in both countries.
- **HIV/AIDS prevention.** Thailand launched the 100 Percent Condom Program in 1991 to address the rising incidence of HIV/AIDS in the country. The program provided boxes of condoms to brothels free of charge, mandated the use of condoms by sex workers, and threatened brothels with penalties and closure for noncompliance. *Health impact*—By 1992, condom use in brothels had risen to more than 90 percent, up from 14 percent in 1989. The number of cases of new sexually transmitted infections fell from 200,000 in 1989 to 15,000 in 2001, and an estimated 200,000 new infections were averted between 1993 and 2000. The project is ongoing.
- **Health improvement of the poor using financial incentives.** In 1997, the Mexican government launched a new social welfare program designed to help lift rural families

out of poverty by providing cash payments in exchange for their participation in nutrition and supplementation programs, their use of prevention and basic health care services, and their children's school attendance. *Health impact*— After five years, the children of participating families were 12 percent less likely to experience illness than those of non-participating families, and their nutritional status had improved. Adult health indicators also improved. The project is ongoing.

- **Maternal health.** The Sri Lankan government relied on professional midwives and sustained investments in the country's health care system, including in rural areas, to improve maternal health. *Health impact*—The maternal mortality ratio fell from approximately 500 per 100,000 live births in 1950 to 60 per 100,000 in 2003. The project is ongoing.

- **Measles elimination.** In 1996, the seven southern African countries agreed to a coordinated immunization strategy, supported by improved surveillance and laboratory capacity, to eliminate measles by including the vaccine as part of routine immunization for all nine-month-old babies and organizing nationwide catch-up and follow-up campaigns for children age nine months to 14 years. *Health impact*— The number of measles cases reported annually in the region fell from 60,000 in 1996 to 117 in 2000. The number of deaths attributed to measles fell from 166 to 0 during the same period. The project is ongoing.

- **Onchocerciasis control.** The discovery of ivermectin (Mectizan) in 1978 and Merck's decision to provide it free of charge to anyone who needed it allowed early successes based on weekly aerial spraying in 11 West African countries to be further consolidated and later expanded to the other 19 endemic countries in Central and East Africa. *Health impact*—In West Africa, disease transmission has been virtually halted, and 1.5 million previously infected people are now symptom free. In Central and East Africa, the program has helped prevent an estimated 40,000 cases of blindness each year. The Onchocerciasis Control Program (OCP) ended in 2002. The African Programme for Onchocerciasis Control is ongoing.

- **Polio elimination.** In 1985, the Pan American Health Organization launched a campaign to eradicate polio from the Americas. National vaccine days were held twice a year and were targeted at children under the age of five, regardless of their immunization status, to increase coverage in countries with weak routine immunization programs. An extensive surveillance system and mop-up campaigns to address outbreaks were crucial during the campaign's final stages. *Health impact*—The last case of polio in the Americas was reported in 1991.

- **Salt fluoridation.** In Jamaica, a formal agreement between the Ministry of Health and the country's only salt producer introduced fluoridation to salt in 1987 to prevent caries.

Health impact—By 1995, the severity of caries in children between the ages of 6 and 12 had fallen by more than 80 percent. The project is ongoing.

- **Salt iodination.** China launched the National Iodine Deficiency Disorders Elimination Program in 1993. The government requires producers to iodize salt and has stepped up its monitoring and enforcement capacity to ensure compliance. *Health impact*—Total goiter rates among children between the ages of 8 and 10 years fell from 20.4 percent in 1995 to 8.8 percent in 1999. The project is ongoing.

- **Smallpox eradication.** The campaign to eradicate smallpox, led by the World Health Organization and heavily financed by the United States, was launched in the mid 1960s. Strong leadership, dedication, and commitment on the part of the international community and the timely discovery of simple, new technologies—for example, the bifurcated needle and the "ring" strategy of surveillance and containment—characterized the effort. *Health impact*—The World Health Assembly declared smallpox eradicated in May 1980.

- **Tobacco control.** Poland passed groundbreaking legislation in 1995 imposing strong warning labels on cigarette packages, banning smoking from enclosed workplaces, and prohibiting tobacco sales to minors. South Africa passed similar legislation in 1999 to strengthen a previously imposed tax of 50 percent on the retail price of cigarettes. *Health impact*—Cigarette consumption dropped 10 percent between 1990 and 1998, resulting in a 30 percent decline in lung cancer among men age 20 to 44, a nearly 7 percent decline in cardiovascular disease, and a decline in the number of babies with low birthweight. South Africa witnessed a 30 percent decline in cigarette consumption in the 1990s, especially among youths and the poor. The projects are ongoing in both countries.

- **Trachoma control.** The Moroccan National Blindness Control Program, launched in 1991, promoted the use of "SAFE" interventions (surgery, antibiotics to control the infection, facial cleanliness, and environmental improvements), with the goal of eliminating trachoma by 2005. *Health impact*—Overall prevalence rates have fallen by 75 percent since 1999, and the prevalence of active disease in children under the age of 10 has seen a 90 percent reduction since 1997. The project is ongoing.

- **Tuberculosis control.** In 1991, China launched a 10-year program in 13 of its 31 mainland provinces to apply the directly observed therapy short course (DOTS) strategy to turberculosis (TB) control. Peru, previously one of 23 high-burden countries that collectively account for 80 percent of the world's new TB cases each year, launched a similar effort the same year. *Health impact*—Within two years, China had achieved a 95 percent cure rate for new cases and a cure rate of 90 percent for those patients who had previously completed treatment unsuccessfully. The number of people with

TB declined by more than 37 percent between 1999 and 2000. The project ended in 2001, but important elements have been incorporated in the 10-year National Plan for the Prevention and Control of TB (2001–10). In Peru, disease incidence declined each year by 6 percent. The program achieved a case detection rate of 70 percent and an 85 percent cure rate. The project is ongoing.

GENERAL FINDINGS

Taken as a whole, the cases support four general findings. The first two have special relevance because they serve to disconfirm aspects of the prevailing wisdom about aid effectiveness— or at least present a serious challenge to such wisdom.

First, these cases demonstrate that a wide range of proven, cost-effective interventions exists that can and have been brought to scale in developing countries, even in extremely low-income settings with limited health infrastructure and in challenging macropolicy environments. In West Africa, aerial spraying of the blackflies' breeding sites, part of the strategy promoted by the OCP throughout the 1980s, "continued unabated through wars between member countries and coups that grounded all other aircraft" (Eckholm 1989, 20). In Sudan, despite the difficulties created by the more than 20-year civil war, and in other areas of Sub-Saharan Africa, the campaign to eradicate the guinea worm has made progress. The finding is significant in that it challenges a central tenet of the aid-effectiveness literature: that only countries with a "good" policy environment can benefit from external financial assistance (Devarajan, Dollar, and Holmgren 2001).

The aid-effectiveness literature has tended to focus on a different set of outcomes—for example, macroeconomic and structural reform—rather than on health outcomes, and this focus may partly explain the contradictory conclusions; however, an examination of whether such a conclusion is true goes well beyond the scope of this study. In any event, the cases reviewed for this study displayed a striking degree of variation in the political and economic contexts in which interventions were applied and brought to scale, and no clear pattern of association was apparent between this variation and successful outcomes in relation to health.

Second, the cases provided new evidence of the importance of the public sector to achieving successful health outcomes. This finding was a surprise, especially considering the strength of recent evidence documenting "weak links in the chain between government spending for services to improve health and actual improvements in health status" (Filmer, Hammer, and Pritchett 2000, 199). The specific roles that the public sector played in achieving these outcomes varied tremendously. In some instances, such as promoting maternal health in Sri Lanka and controlling TB in China and Peru, governments were involved in direct service provision. In other instances, the

public sector's regulatory or legislative authority was critical. Governments in Poland and South Africa passed strict laws, despite strong opposition from the tobacco industry, requiring explicit health warnings on cigarette packs, banning smoking in enclosed public places, and prohibiting tobacco media advertisements, among other things. Governments also used their authority creatively to encourage health-promoting behaviors and to discourage risky ones. In Mexico, the government provided direct cash payments to poor families in exchange for visits to health care clinics and school attendance. In Thailand, local police worked in collaboration with health officials to lend credibility to the government's threat to shut down brothels that failed to comply with the no condom, no sex policy, giving teeth to the national campaign.

Third, the cases reviewed for this study share a number of common features or attributes that appear to have contributed to the successful outcomes. Without exception, they enjoyed and managed to reap the benefits of strong leadership, effective management, realistic financing arrangements, country ownership, and openness and receptivity to learning by doing, constantly improving on strategies and processes by incorporating new research findings and technical innovation into program improvements.

For example, successful projects appeared to benefit from a strong champion who could provide the necessary leadership to bring relevant stakeholders together, encourage them to focus and coordinate their activities, and instill in them a sense of purpose and enthusiasm for their work. However, we did find that leadership came packaged in many different shapes and sizes. In Jamaica, the curiosity and persistence of a Ministry of Health dentist led to the identification of the island's only salt producer as the vehicle for fluoridation. In Mexico, President Ernesto Zedillo Ponce de León seized on the innovative proposal of a close adviser, Santiago Levy, then director-general of social security, and launched a program linking education, health, and nutrition as part of an integrated strategy to lift rural families out of poverty, and the program was not abandoned when Zedillo left office. The new Vicente Fox administration, motivated by undeniable evidence of the program's effectiveness, instead sought to expand the program into urban areas and added an educational component. In a less visible but nonetheless critical display of leadership and forward thinking, the sustained investments of the Sri Lankan government over a nearly 50-year period to build a rural health network emphasizing critical elements of maternal health have led to gains in the health of women unparalleled by countries at similar, and higher, income levels.

Strong program management was needed to ensure that plans, once conceived, were implemented effectively. Successful cases had well-delineated goals that were clearly linked to inputs, activities, outputs, and outcomes. This factor was especially evident in the case of global or regional immunization campaigns, given the many logistical challenges and the need for fluid and effective coordination of many countries and stakeholder groups, often within a highly constrained time frame. However, similar management skills are needed for health service delivery systems, especially when patient referral, tracking, and follow-up are essential components of the intervention. In China, incentive schemes to motivate physicians, extensive training and supervision of health care staff, and substantial investments in local TB dispensaries were all crucial elements in improving management capacity for large-scale rollout of the country's DOTS program, which covered a population of 573 million in 1,208 counties in 13 provinces.

A closely related requirement was having a realistic financing strategy that was compatible with a project's goals. Even when large sums of money were involved, deployment of the intervention yielded tremendous returns at a relatively low cost per disability-adjusted life year. In the case of onchocerciasis control, for which donors have invested US$560 million over a period of 28 years, transmission has been virtually halted in 20 West African countries, and nearly 600,000 cases of blindness have been averted at an annual cost of only US$1 per person. In the case of guinea worm control, in which donors have invested approximately US$88 million over a 12-year period, disease prevalence has fallen by 99 percent, and only 35,000 people remain affected, down from 3.5 million, at a cost of US$5 to US$8 per person.

Country ownership was another distinguishing feature of successful programs. A government's willingness to commit scarce funding to scaling up an intervention can be an important indication of this ownership, although not the sole predictor. Despite the extremely constrained budgets of the seven participating countries, the campaign to eliminate measles in southern Africa was almost entirely funded by their ministries of health. The Thai government covered approximately 96 percent of the cost of the 100 Percent Condom Program. In Morocco, the government bore the bulk of the costs for implementing the SAFE strategy to address blindness caused by trachoma, with contributions from the United Nations Children's Fund and the International Trachoma Initiative, an international public-private partnership.

Most of the cases we reviewed benefited from new research findings and technical innovation. Successful cases appear to display the openness and receptivity needed to make good use of new knowledge and to support ongoing research when appropriate or when gaps in knowledge prove to be a hindrance to progress. In Bangladesh, a program to treat childhood diarrhea trained mothers to make their own salt solution when the authorities determined that mass production and distribution of prepackaged oral rehydration salts was unrealistic. Control of Chagas disease in the Southern Cone of Latin America required public health officials in each country to devise and deploy environmental control strategies appropriate to local conditions and vector behavior. Finally, adoption of the ring vaccination strategy marked a crucial turning point in the global campaign to eradicate smallpox, enabling rapid containment of the disease in remote parts of the world without vaccination of every child.

In sum, a small number of features appear to be common to all the successful cases. A reasonable hypothesis suggested by the evidence is that these five attributes represent the known set of necessary, but not sufficient, conditions for successfully implementing cost-effective health interventions in the developing world.

Fourth, despite the obvious limitations of case study methods in hypothesis testing and confirmation, the evidence from the cases sheds important light on two important debates in international health policy. First, the cases suggest that much more is involved than what is currently understood about whether weak policy environments can make good use of carefully selected, strategic investments in health. As the next section indicates, different types of programmatic characteristics and policies are needed for the deployment of different types of interventions. How these characteristics interact with different policy environments—whether strong, weak, or in between—deserves further scrutiny and exploration. Second, evidence from the cases of successful government action should call into question any premature and overly general conclusions about public sector ineffectiveness in developing countries. Even though such a small sample of cases is surely insufficient to close the book on these important policy debates, it should at least encourage further study and refinement of the arguments.

INTERVENTION TYPE, PROGRAMMATIC CHARACTERISTICS, AND POLICIES

Programmatic characteristics and policies associated with successful outcomes appear to vary by intervention type. The starting point for this discussion is the intervention, technology, or tool in question. What allows for the widespread deployment of a proven, cost-effective intervention? What are the steps for converting a proven, cost-effective intervention into a fully fledged health program that has been successfully brought to scale, preferably at the national level? Is it possible to distinguish between the specific health intervention and the programmatic characteristics and public policies associated with its successful deployment?

The cases under review were grouped according to the primary type of intervention deployed by the program or project in question. The types of interventions varied in terms of their emphasis on the delivery of standardized products to a population (product-intensive interventions), the delivery of clinical services (service-intensive interventions), a personal behavior change (behavioral change interventions), the control of environmental hazards (environmental control interventions), or some combination thereof.

Further scrutiny of subgroupings of cases revealed that certain programmatic characteristics, delivery modalities, and public policy instruments also appeared to vary by intervention type. This finding appeared to substantiate the claim of the first edition of this volume (Jamison 1993, 11) that "commonalities of logistics, policy instruments, and approach" vary by intervention type and play a role in determining whether the intervention or interventions will be deployed successfully.

The typology presented here differs from the one elaborated by *World Development Report 2004: Making Services Work for Poor People* (World Bank 2004), in that the classification depends on characteristics inherent to the intervention in question. By contrast, *World Development Report 2004* identifies three classes of service delivery arrangements: individual-oriented clinical services, population-oriented outreach services, and community- and family-oriented services that support self-care. The focus is on differences in the relationship between provider and client and how these differences interact with market and public sector dynamics.[2] However, our focus was on how characteristics of the interventions themselves give rise to certain programmatic or policy imperatives that may contribute, ultimately, to successful health outcomes.

This section presents the five intervention types and explores the clusters of programmatic characteristics and policies that appear to support the successful deployment of each intervention type, based on case study analysis.

Product-Intensive Interventions

These types of interventions (box 8.1) involve the simple transfer of a standardized technology to an individual or to an entire population. They can be targeted at either prevention or cure, but the distinguishing feature is standardization. Unlike service-intensive interventions, product-intensive interventions need not be tailored to the unique health care needs of the individual receiving treatment.

To the degree that product-intensive interventions place relatively low technical demands on health care staff at the point of delivery, they may be more easily deployed in low-resource settings than other types of interventions. Compared with service-intensive interventions, they are less transaction intensive, requiring fewer interactions between providers and clients. Also, compared with behavioral-change interventions, they are less dependent on individual compliance, requiring simply that individuals make themselves available for treatment. Product-intensive interventions include mass drug administration (chemotherapy), childhood immunizations, mineral fortification, and nutritional supplementation. (These specific interventions are addressed in detail in chapters 20, 22, and 28.)

Product-intensive interventions are often, though not necessarily, linked to vertical rather than horizontal delivery modalities. According to Gonzalez (cited in Mills 1983, 1972), the vertical approach "calls for the solution of a given health problem through the application of specific measures through single-purpose machinery." By contrast, the horizontal approach "seeks to tackle . . . health problems on a wide front and on a long-term basis through the creation of a system of permanent institutions commonly known as 'general health services.'" Where health systems are weak and poorly functioning, vertical programs—in particular, mass campaigns—can be an effective means of rapidly providing coverage to a large population. However, the same approach could result in an unfortunate duplication of effort in countries where the health care system is already strong and functioning properly.

Mass Drug Administration. Of the product-intensive interventions, those that can be delivered in pill or capsule form in standardized doses, often through what is referred to as *mass drug administration,* are perhaps the least complex to deliver and, as a result, may be the least costly. Onchocerciasis, also known as river blindness, can be treated by a single dose of ivermectin administered annually to infected individuals. Lymphatic filariasis can be treated in much the same way using a two-drug combination therapy of albendazole plus either diethylcarbamazine or ivermectin administered annually in

---

Box 8.1

Product-Intensive Interventions: Illustrations from Cases

Hib vaccine

Ivermectin

Measles vaccine

Oral polio vaccine

Salt fluoridation

Salt iodination

Smallpox vaccine

Source: Authors.

single doses for four to six years (the estimated productive life span of the adult-stage parasite).

The importance of product-intensive therapies can easily be illustrated by reference to the case of onchocerciasis control in most parts of Africa. Although aerial spraying, an environmental control intervention, had been used successfully to slow disease transmission in 11 West African countries, it was not a viable option for 19 countries of East and Central Africa because of geographical differences. However, Merck scientists' discovery of ivermectin in 1978 and the company's generous commitment to provide the drug free of charge to anyone who needed it changed the parameters of what was possible. Seizing the opportunity, the African Programme for Onchocerciasis Control, an international partnership led by the World Bank, the World Health Organization, the United Nations Development Programme, and the Food and Agriculture Organization of the United Nations, was created in 1995 with the goal of eliminating onchocerciasis as a disease of public health and socioeconomic importance in East and Central Africa.

It quickly became apparent that the weak and sometimes nonfunctioning health systems of many African countries were not up to the task; thus, a new approach was tried that took advantage of the fact that the success of the intervention no longer depended on a clinic-based delivery system. Under the supervision of national public health ministries and nongovernmental organizations, community volunteers received training on organizing and managing the local ivermectin campaigns. The community-directed approach of treatment with ivermectin has been so successful that it has been considered as a possible model for delivering other types of treatments to remote areas.

Immunizations. Product-intensive interventions may vary in complexity, which has implications for their delivery or deployment. For vaccines, the need to maintain an effective cold chain adds an additional layer of complexity to the delivery system. Other pertinent factors are whether the intervention can be delivered as a single shot or iteratively, whether it can be bundled together with other products or must be delivered separately, and whether the number of distribution points is few or many. In many cases, the characteristics of the disease or condition being addressed may affect the level of complexity.

For example, the overwhelming success of the global effort to eradicate smallpox has been attributed, at least in part, to specific characteristics of the variola virus. Unlike other infectious diseases, such as malaria or yellow fever, smallpox depends solely on the human host and does not have an animal or insect carrier. Unlike polio, smallpox does not produce silent or asymptomatic infection, thereby facilitating diagnosis and surveillance of the disease (Tucker 2001). Other notable differences from other diseases have more to do with the vaccine than the virus. Tucker (2001, 64) explains that "a freeze-dried smallpox

vaccine was available that was easy to manufacture, cost only about a penny a dose, protected for several years with a single inoculation, and was relatively stable in warm climates, reducing the need for refrigeration. Whereas most vaccines took months to induce immunity, the smallpox vaccine acted with remarkable speed, providing nearly total protection within ten to twelve days." This unique set of characteristics together meant that a "surveillance-containment" approach could replace mass vaccination entirely, in effect reducing the number of distribution points required by the intervention, thereby permitting major strides in the global eradication campaign.

The more complex the intervention, the more challenging—and probably costly—it will likely be to implement. Interventions that can be delivered in a single shot or that can be easily incorporated into routine immunization (bundled) are clearly the easiest to implement. As the case of Hib vaccination in Chile illustrates, delivering the intervention was relatively straightforward after the government got past the hurdle of evaluating its cost-effectiveness relative to other interventions. The government determined that the creation of a combined diphtheria-tetanus-pertussis and Hib vaccine was worthwhile and that the vaccine could be administered as part of an already well-functioning system of routine immunization.

Some of the common complexities associated specifically with immunizations range from the need for multiple inoculations administered at regular intervals, to the need to maintain a reliable cold chain, or to the need for the large population coverage required to achieve "herd immunity"—whereby the likelihood of person-to-person transmission is drastically reduced, even among the unimmunized population. In view of these potential complexities, polio elimination in the Americas represents a remarkable achievement. The oral polio vaccine must be administered in three properly spaced doses, and coverage must be high to prevent "silent" epidemics. In the 1970s, before the campaign was launched, polio caused an estimated 15,000 cases of paralysis and 1,750 deaths each year (Musgrove 1988). However, a carefully orchestrated campaign organized around achieving and maintaining high coverage through routine immunization and national vaccination days, the prompt identification of new cases, and the aggressive control of outbreaks led to the elimination of polio from the Americas in 1991. The creation of the Inter-Agency Coordinating Committee, made up of representatives from the Pan American Health Organization, the United Nations Children's Fund, the U.S. Agency for International Development, the Inter-American Development Bank, Rotary International, and the Canadian Public Health Association, played a key role not only in generating political and financial support, but also in helping address the logistical and managerial challenges inherent to the campaign. The Inter-Agency Coordinating Committee model was so effective that it was quickly duplicated at the country level.

The technical and logistical challenges associated with measles elimination in southern Africa were no less complex. Measles is one of the most contagious of all human diseases. The measles vaccine requires 90 percent coverage to achieve herd immunity and to stop the spread of the virus. Furthermore, it often requires two doses to be effective and must be administered to infants no earlier than nine months of age, or about six months later than other recommended vaccines. If given earlier, the vaccine will fail to trigger an active immune response, because infants are passively protected by their mothers' antibodies until that age. Thus, the vaccination interval falls outside of what most routine immunizations require.

To overcome this challenge, the southern African countries adopted a strategy known as catch up, keep up, and follow up. In each country, beginning with the program's launch in 1996, the strategy involved organizing a national catch-up campaign in which mobile teams vaccinated all children, regardless of their vaccination status, between the approximate ages of 9 months and 14 years; sustained routine coverage; and ran at least one follow-up campaign several years later. The countries also strengthened their surveillance and laboratory capabilities to investigate all suspected measles cases.

Mineral Fortification. A different type of product-intensive intervention, mineral fortification, requires fewer points of delivery and is far less labor intensive. However, potential challenges include the need for a different set of technical capacities than is typical for health sector solutions; the possibility of a need for significant initial investments to modify production processes or manufacturing capabilities; and the involvement of non–health sector entities, such as private industry.

Jamaica's salt fluoridation program beautifully illustrates the simplicity of a single delivery point for an intervention. With the agreement of the island's only salt producer, Alkali Limited, in place, universal coverage was easy to achieve. All that was needed was a complementary legal and regulatory framework to oversee the process. In this case, the start-up costs were small: only US$3,000 worth or so of new equipment was needed, which the company was easily able to recoup with a slight increase in the price of salt.

In China, salt fortification with iodine was more difficult, involving a larger investment in the production process and a greater number of potential delivery points. Because salt production is licensed at the provincial level in China, implementing the change involved working with several layers of government bureaucracy; however, perhaps ironically, the system of central control eased the challenge. During a four-year period, 55 salt factories were upgraded and 112 iodination centers were established throughout the country to support the initiative. The government also introduced changes in bulk and retail packaging to help consumers more easily recognize iodized salt. The basic plan achieved nearly 90 percent coverage, but the remaining challenge is to address the numerous delivery points that function outside the national system, for instance, in areas where people live near the sea and produce their own salt.

Summary. In sum, product-intensive interventions can be extraordinarily complex even though they involve fewer transactions between providers and clients and lower technical requirements at the point of delivery than other types of interventions, particularly service-intensive interventions. However, the relative simplicity of deployment when the scientific and technical issues of development and production have been addressed may help explain why product-intensive interventions are perceived to be easier to implement than other types of interventions and why countries experiencing political and economic instability might prefer them.

Service-Intensive Interventions

Service-intensive interventions (box 8.2) include the full range of diagnostic and therapeutic health services usually provided not only in the clinic setting, but also in the home or at school. Unlike product-intensive interventions, service-intensive interventions cannot easily be standardized and may require careful—and time-consuming—monitoring and reporting on patients' progress. Thus service-intensive interventions are highly transaction intensive and typically place high technical demands on the health staff at the point of delivery. Examples range from primary care services, including essential obstetrical care, to surgical procedures, to treatment of communicable and noncommunicable diseases.

The complexity of service-intensive interventions may vary, just as in the case of product-intensive interventions. The more

---

Box 8.2

Service-Intensive Interventions: Illustrations from Cases

Bilamellar tarsal rotation procedure	Maternal health care using midwives
DOTS for TB	Primary and basic health care services

Source: Authors.

---

standardized the treatment protocol, the easier it will be to administer on a large scale. However, standardized or not, the transaction-intensive character of this type of intervention means that its successful deployment depends on the program's or project's ability to overcome potential (and likely) constraints on human resources. A related concern is the overall health system's capacity to effectively manage competing demands on these resources. In contrast to product-intensive interventions, human capacity constraints for service-intensive interventions are harder, but not impossible, to address through community mobilization or the use of volunteers, because of the need for specialized training. Chapter 71 investigates developing countries' experiences with new types of professionals in service delivery settings that have traditionally relied on physicians.

Single-Shot Surgical Services. If the intervention is relatively standardized, it can sometimes be deployed using a vertical modality in a manner similar to the more standardized, single-shot, product-intensive interventions. This was the case of the surgical procedure used in Morocco as part of the broader SAFE strategy to address trachoma. A relatively simple surgical procedure, the bilamellar tarsal rotation procedure, can be used to halt corneal damage to prevent the onset of blindness caused by repeated trachoma infections. Morocco's Ministry of Health organized mobile surgical teams of doctors and nurses to carry out the corrective surgery in small towns and communities throughout the country. In just eight years, the teams carried out more than 26,000 surgeries. The effort required the involvement of 43 physicians and 119 nurses working in 34 clinics. However, despite the relatively standardized nature of this kind of service-intensive intervention, human capacity constraints may slow progress. Compared with product-intensive interventions for which community volunteers can be recruited to assist with distribution, service-intensive interventions require a more specialized workforce. Even when nurses and other health workers with lower-level skills can substitute for more highly trained physicians, constraints on human resource capacity may persist. Morocco faces a backlog of about 15,000 cases, many of which are urgent.

Strengthened Outreach and Referral Systems. If the intervention is not easily standardized, or if it is highly transaction intensive, its successful deployment will also depend on well-developed outreach and referral systems. Outreach systems are needed to ensure that those requiring care will have access to care, and referral systems are needed to route patients requiring additional care toward specialized care and treatment facilities. However, ensuring that such systems are in place for specific programs and projects is a major challenge in countries where the health care system is already weak and under considerable strain.

The cases we reviewed relied on a variety of strategies to address this problem. Although the specific interventions varied, the strategies ranged from traditional investments in public sector provision to improve access, to supply-side incentives to address quality concerns, to demand-side incentives to strengthen the effective demand for health care services. For example, in an effort to improve maternal health even in remote areas, Sri Lanka adopted the traditional model of public sector provision, but with a twist. Instead of a physician-based solution, which would have been extremely costly, Sri Lanka relied instead on professional midwives to provide widespread access to maternal health care, building on a strong health care system that provides free health care. Midwives serve a population of 3,000 to 5,000 each and live locally. They visit pregnant women in their homes, register them for care, and encourage them to attend prenatal clinics (run by doctors). Midwives receive 18 months of training and are backed up by supervision and a well-functioning referral network. Established procedures for service delivery and supervision, along with frequent in-service training, help keep midwives current and delivering high-quality services. Health clinics are supported by a network of cottage hospitals (clinics having doctors as well as nurses assigned to them), rural hospitals, and maternity homes at the secondary level; tertiary provincial hospitals with specialist services; teaching hospitals; and specialist maternity hospitals.

China faced a similar dilemma with regard to establishing an effective system of outreach and referral to address a growing TB problem by scaling up DOTS. Although DOTS is relatively standardized as far as service interventions go (see chapter 16), the treatment protocol is highly transaction intensive, and complicated cases may require specialized treatment. DOTS is thus also highly dependent on well-developed systems of outreach and referral for its success. However, China faced a challenging situation because most village doctors who were needed to conduct patient diagnosis, treatment, and surveillance in rural areas were in private practice and had little incentive to treat patients for whom drugs were now provided free of charge. In response, the government created a financial scheme to provide incentives for these doctors to participate. For each patient enrolled in the treatment program, village doctors received US$1. They received an additional US$2 for each smear examination carried out in the county TB dispensary during a two-month period and another US$4 for each patient who completed treatment. Simultaneously, the government made significant administrative, managerial, and institutional investments. Tens of thousands of staff from TB dispensaries were trained, and supervisory systems were put into place. Furthermore, the government set up a national TB project office and a TB control center to oversee and coordinate the various levels of government involvement.

Demand-Side Incentives. Demand-side incentives can be designed to complement supply-side investments. Indeed, both skeptics and supporters of governments' ability to translate public spending into effective service provision and positive health outcomes encourage the use of demand-side incentives as a means of quality control to improve routine care (Filmer, Hammer, and Pritchett 2000). Economists consider demand-side incentives to be valuable tools for stimulating weak demand for services or for overcoming barriers to use that can artificially dampen demand. This was how at least two of the cases included in this study constructively used demand-side incentives. However, in neither case was this use an either-or proposition; that is, both demand-side and supply-side investments were relied on to generate the successful outcomes that qualified the cases for this study.

In Peru, the newly revised National Tuberculosis Control Program offered food packages, employment training, and stipends to patients to improve compliance with the drug treatment regime. Simultaneously, the program was dramatically scaled up and the number of participating health centers rose from 977 to 6,539 over the next decade. In the clinics, nurses were the medical personnel responsible for administering DOTS. In isolated rural areas, the program recruited local leaders to serve under the direction of the nursing staff to administer the treatment and follow up with patients.

Mexico's Education, Health, and Nutrition Program (originally known as PROGRESA, but now called "Oportunidades") also provides a compelling example of how a program can use demand-side incentives to stimulate demand for basic health care services. The program offers cash transfers to families in exchange for the attendance of mothers and children age five and under at nutrition monitoring clinics and to pregnant women if they agree to prenatal care visits and nutritional supplementation. The program also includes cash transfers to promote school attendance and performance. A rigorous evaluation provided evidence of the program's effect on the use of health services: after just one year of implementation, attendance at health care clinics was significantly higher in participating localities. However, the increased demand for services was also met with significant improvements in the quality of services available through public providers. Health care providers in participating localities were paid more and

received more on-the-job training, and clinics benefited from a steadier flow of pharmaceutical and other supplies.

Summary. In sum, service-intensive interventions are highly transaction intensive, especially compared with product-intensive interventions. The more standardized the intervention, the more likely that it can be delivered by means of military-like campaigns in the same manner as product-intensive interventions, although the skill level of the health workers involved will need to be higher. If complications of treatment are possible—or if the intervention cannot easily be standardized—its deployment will likely require fairly elaborate systems of outreach and referral. Although recent scholarship has strongly encouraged the use of demand-side mechanisms, particularly in an effort to address quality concerns in public sector service provision, evidence from the cases highlighted in this chapter suggests that a variety of modalities are possible and that a mix of supply- and demand-side incentives may even be desirable.

Behavioral Change Interventions

Behavioral change interventions (box 8.3) are designed to induce or encourage an individual behavior change or habit modification to achieve specific health goals. The focus is usually on prevention, but need not be exclusively so—for example, the use of oral rehydration therapy to treat childhood diarrhea. Behavioral change interventions are often linked to the uptake of a specific product, as in the case of condoms and insecticide-treated bednets. However, unlike product-intensive interventions, behavioral change interventions require active participation by the individual and cannot be passively received in the form of an injection or supplement. Also, unlike service-intensive interventions, behavioral change interventions do not depend on the involvement of a health care professional on an ongoing basis. Illustrative examples include the uptake of oral rehydration therapy for use by mothers in the home, not the clinic; face washing to prevent trachoma; and condoms to prevent HIV infection or other sexually transmitted infections.

As Jamison (2002) notes, some changes in behavioral practices associated with improved health, such as improved

---

Box 8.3

Behavioral Change Interventions: Illustrations from Cases

Stopping smoking

Using condoms to prevent HIV/AIDS

Using nylon filters to purify water

Using oral rehydration salts

Source: Authors.

---

hygiene and better nutrition, are linked to rising incomes, but the pathway for this link is not entirely clear, especially at the individual level, which makes it difficult to predict which mix of programs and policies can be used to change behavior at the population level. Information plays an important role, but the evidence suggests that its effect may be limited if it is not combined with other mechanisms to induce behavioral change.

The cases under review typically used a mix of strategies to induce behavioral change, including information, education, and communication (IEC) campaigns; regulatory policies; taxation or subsidies; and financial incentives or disincentives. The evidence is suggestive, but hardly conclusive, that a relative hierarchy exists among the available strategies and policy instruments and that some are more effective than others at altering how individuals perceive risk and weigh the costs and benefits of behavioral change. Chapter 11, for example, provides an in-depth discussion of how and when fiscal instruments may be used effectively to alter producers' and consumers' decisions in ways that encourage healthy behaviors.

Information, Education, and Communication. Recent studies have challenged the effectiveness of mass IEC campaigns (Kremer and Miguel 2003), and evidence from the cases appears to support a degree of healthy skepticism. However, IEC campaigns did appear to have an effect in the cases under review when they were accompanied by the promotion of a new technology or a product. Also, acceptability appeared to increase if the product was adapted to fit the local circumstances or cultural context. In Sub-Saharan Africa, educational campaigns to stop transmission of the guinea worm to humans have encouraged the construction and maintenance of safe water sources (through deep-well digging and the application of larvicide to contaminated ponds) and the use of cloth or nylon filters to purify drinking water, in addition to case identification and containment. The primary IEC tool was so-called worm weeks—that is, weeks of intensive health education and community mobilization.

In Egypt, in addition to nurses and physicians, mothers were a primary target of the campaign to promote the use of oral rehydration salts for the treatment of diarrhea in children, especially those under three years of age. Television was the primary educational medium and proved to be an effective strategy for reaching a broad population base, including rural, illiterate households. Appropriate product design and branding were essential. Oral rehydration salt packets were supplied in a 200-milliliter size, not the standard 1-liter packs, because mothers did not have appropriate containers at home and felt that a full liter was too much to give to a child to drink. By contrast, in Bangladesh, where few households had access to a radio, much less a television, health workers went door to door to teach mothers how to make the solution in their homes.

In these cases, the targeted population not only was aware of the health care problem, but also was eager to adopt solutions to address it. Clearly this situation does not always prevail, but a reasonable conclusion is that a relatively simple technology that addresses a recognizable, but as yet unmet, need will find a receptive audience. In Bangladesh, a mass media campaign to encourage families to have fewer children was backed up by a large cadre of female outreach workers, who went door to door in rural areas to provide information to young married women and to make family-planning commodities available to them. Market research indicates that almost all Bangladeshi women were in favor of family planning but were unable to go against their husbands' objections if they were opposed to the use of contraceptives. The fact that the campaign and the provision of contraceptive commodities addressed an unmet need among Bangladeshi women may provide a partial explanation for the rapid acceptance of the program when it was launched on a large scale.

Regulatory Policies. By contrast, other behavioral changes, such as using condoms to prevent HIV infection and other sexually transmitted infections and stopping smoking, have clearly been harder to induce, although the precise reasons for this difficulty remain elusive (see, in particular, chapters 18 and 46). Nevertheless, evidence from the cases suggests that governments can put the right mix of policies in place to either discourage high-risk behaviors or encourage health-promoting behaviors. For example, they may use regulatory policies to ensure compliance through nonfinancial means and may complement these by using fines and sanctions as an enforcement mechanism.

The Thai government's 100 Percent Condom Program is an excellent example of such a strategy. In 1991, the National AIDS Committee launched a national program to be implemented at the provincial level requiring all workers in brothels and other commercial sex establishments to refuse to have sex with any client not using a condom. The program had several components, including free distribution of condoms to health workers during regular health checks and a media campaign to raise awareness of the risks of HIV and the dangers associated with unprotected sex. What gave the program its unique character was its regulatory and enforcement component. Local governments, health authorities, and police officers were responsible for monitoring and enforcing condom use in the brothels. Those brothels that failed to comply with the strict policy would be fined or forced to shut down. The results were impressive. Condom use in brothels exceeded 90 percent in just the first year of the program, up from 14 percent in 1989. The number of new HIV infections fell by more than 80 percent, from 142,819 cases in 1991 to 25,790 cases in 2001. Furthermore, the program appears to have generated important spillover effects, or externalities, in unexpected places. For example, studies indicate that indirect sex workers—a group that cannot be reached through similar enforcement strategies—have also begun to insist that their clients use condoms.

Taxation and Subsidies. Another option for discouraging high-risk behaviors is the adoption of taxation policies. A 1997 study by the World Bank in partnership with the World Health Organization found that a price increase of 10 percent on cigarettes would lower smoking rates by about 4 percent in high-income countries and about 8 percent in low-income countries (Jha and Chaloupka 2000, 358). In South Africa, a 50 percent tax on the retail price of cigarettes contributed to a 30 percent decrease in consumption. In Poland, an increase in taxes on cigarettes from 30 to 47 percent of the retail price, in conjunction with other policies—including a ban on smoking in health care establishments, schools, enclosed spaces in the workplace, and elsewhere—contributed to a dramatic decline in smoking rates. Before the fall of communism, Poland had the highest cigarette consumption in the world, but by the end of the 1990s, there were 4 million fewer smokers compared with the previous decade, and cigarette consumption had fallen by 10 percent. These successes led to a 30 percent decrease in lung cancer among men age 20 to 44 and a 19 percent decrease among men age 45 to 64 over the same period.

The section on service-intensive investments has already discussed the remarkable power of explicit subsidies to encourage health-promoting behaviors. The Mexican case of PROGRESA offers a by now familiar example of such a strategy. Although none of the cases included in this study dealt with subsidies explicitly directed at behavioral change interventions, evidence suggests that they have a significant effect. However, as Nugent and Knaul discuss in chapter 11, poorly targeted subsidies can be costly, particularly relative to the result achieved. Much more research is needed in this area to understand the specific contexts in which subsidies can achieve their desired effects and their cost-effectiveness relative to other types of interventions.

Summary. In sum, behavioral change interventions differ from both product-intensive and environmental control interventions in that they require active participation by the individual for the intervention to be fully effective. In some cases, this requirement is also true for service-intensive interventions, but it is not as exclusively true as for behavioral change interventions. The degree to which incentives (or disincentives) are needed to induce (or discourage) behavior depends on the interaction between the usage characteristics of the intervention, the perceived risk of not using the intervention, and the perceived effectiveness of the intervention. To have an effect, policy incentives (and disincentives) must either succeed in changing the individual's risk-benefit assessment or make ignoring the policy extremely costly.

Environmental Control Interventions

As with behavioral change interventions, environmental control interventions are geared toward prevention and are used in conjunction with other treatments or alone when effective vaccines or other prophylaxes are unavailable. However, rather than focus on risk factors associated with individual behavior, environmental control interventions target risks associated with the physical environment that are largely beyond the individual's control. The *physical environment* refers to media in the natural (water, air, or soil) or man-made (housing, roads) environment. Examples of environmental control interventions include many vector control strategies, such as aerial and household spraying, water and sanitation projects, and air quality control measures. (See, in particular, chapters 41 and 43.)

Few of the cases reviewed for this study involved "pure" environmental control interventions; although in several cases environmental control measures were coupled with other types of interventions. Whenever activities involved in executing the intervention fall outside the realm of typical health care services, nonhealth government agencies will be involved, and strong political and technical leadership will be required of the ministry of health to ensure that proper attention is given to health care concerns during implementation.

Successful interventions in this category also appeared to be associated with strong multicountry partnerships, particularly in relation to vector control activities. This factor raises an interesting question concerning governments' capacity to engage in these types of partnerships. Technical capacity, although essential, is just the first hurdle, because what is ultimately required is a political and financial commitment at the highest levels in participating countries.

In the case of Chagas disease control, the Southern Cone Initiative brought together the seven countries in the endemic region under a coordinated, comprehensive, Chagas disease control strategy. This multicountry approach was led by the Pan American Health Organization, following the recognition that disease transmission from neighboring countries was threatening the health gains achieved under Brazil's national eradication plan. A central aim of the Southern Cone Initiative was to eliminate the protozoan parasite, *Trypanosoma cruzi*, in the region by coordinating technical efforts to detect and eliminate it. This coordination ensured consistent use of highly effective control measures across the region and limited any possibility of reinvasion. Infested homes throughout the region were treated with long-lasting pyrethroid insecticides and structurally improved to eliminate hiding places for the bloodsucking insects that spread the parasite. These coordinated environmental control efforts, combined with blood screening, proved to be highly successful at interrupting Chagas disease transmission in the region.

Environmental control interventions also appear to be characterized by many consecutive years of sustained activity. In some cases, this activity may take the form of ongoing maintenance of filters and distribution systems to prevent recontamination. In other cases, as in the case of vectorborne disease control in which elimination or eradication is within reach, the intervention must be sustained at least until transmission has been interrupted in humans. (The intervention may need to be sustained for much longer, or indefinitely, if the disease has an animal host.) In the case of onchocerciasis, the lifetime of the filarial load is 14 years, and vector spraying would need to be sustained for at least 14 years to cut transmission. If reinvasions or native vector population growth are allowed to take hold before the human loads die off, transmission will occur and the disease will not be effectively controlled. The OCP in West Africa has demonstrated the effectiveness of a long-term commitment to vector control in reducing the burden of onchocerciasis. Since its inception in 1974, the OCP has used aerial spraying of blackfly breeding sites to control vector populations and interrupt transmission. The original OCP area remains free of onchocerciasis transmission following the withdrawal of regular spraying after 14 years. This sustained attention proved to be highly successful in eliminating onchocerciasis transmission and infection. Even after the introduction of ivermectin drug therapy to the program, vector control has remained a key strategy for maintaining health benefits in the expansion area of the OCP.

In sum, environmental control interventions are associated with intersectoral collaboration, multicountry partnerships, sustained activity, and attentiveness to context (for example, epidemiological conditions, patterns of disease transmission, and vector behavior). These factors place special capacity requirements on governments that may differ markedly from nonenvironmental interventions. Thus, to be effective, ministries of health must be capable of advocacy and influence within the broader structures of government.

Combination or Bundled Interventions

A two-front battle involving both prevention and treatment must be waged against most diseases and conditions to achieve the desired effect on morbidity and mortality. Under such circumstances, a combination or bundling of interventions is needed, adding an additional layer of complexity to the deployment of any particular intervention. An effective malaria control strategy, for example, demands effective distribution and uptake of insecticide-treated bednets (a behavioral change intervention) and rapid treatment of malaria symptoms through strong outreach and referral systems (a service-intensive intervention). Similarly, countries have adopted a dual approach to controlling the spread of HIV/AIDS: promoting safe sex practices (a behavioral control intervention) and supporting the scale-up of antiretroviral therapy (a service-intensive intervention). In this context, global partnerships

have a critical role to play in providing technical assistance to countries in formulating policies and developing strategic plans that are tailored toward their specific needs and capabilities.

Perhaps the most successful example of bundling interventions included in our study is the Moroccan National Blindness Control Program, launched in 1991. The program was based on the development in the mid 1980s of SAFE, a comprehensive strategy to treat and prevent trachoma. The philosophy of the new strategy, which was heavily researched and promoted under the support and guidance of the Edna McConnell Clark Foundation, was to augment the traditional medical approach to the treatment of trachoma with behavioral and environmental changes. The four main interventions the strategy recommended were surgery (service-intensive intervention); antibiotics (product-intensive intervention); face washing (behavioral change intervention); and environmental activities, including water and sanitation programs (environmental control intervention).

The program consisted of a wide-ranging partnership that included five government divisions: the Ministry of Health, the Ministry of National Education, the Ministry of Employment, the Ministry of Equipment, and the National Office for Potable Water. Targets were set—Morocco's political leaders were committed to eliminating trachoma by 2005—and the institutional and policy artillery to support the initiative was quickly put in place. Mobile surgical teams were deployed to small towns and villages to perform a simple, quick, and inexpensive procedure of the eyelid to halt corneal damage in infected patients; treatment campaigns were organized to distribute the newly discovered antibiotic, azithromycin, that could be administered in a single dose; IEC campaigns were launched at the community level with the participation of the Ministry of Education to educate the population about the causes of the disease and how to prevent it; and the National Office for Potable Water has expanded water and sanitation projects in many areas of the country. By 1999, prevalence levels had dropped 75 percent, from 28 to 6.5 percent, and acute infections in children had been reduced significantly.

CONCLUSION

The accumulation of evidence presented in this study should help allay any remaining doubts about whether existing technologies and interventions, proven to be cost-effective in randomized controlled trials, can be successfully deployed to improve the lives and health of people throughout the developing world. The evidence suggests not only that it is possible, but also that it has been achieved in many parts of the world, in many different socioeconomic and political settings.

The study also found important commonalities among programs and projects that appear to have contributed to the successful deployment and rapid scale-up of cost-effective interventions. Strong leadership, effective management, realistic financing, country ownership, and application of new research findings and technical innovation all played a role in implementation and appeared to have made major contributions to the positive achievements of the cases under review.

In some respects, the study also presents a sobering view of the difficulties inherent in moving from a cost-effective intervention to a successful program or project. No single formula is available, and identification of unique characteristics and attributes that will permit the large-scale, effective deployment of many known interventions is difficult.

In addition, evidence from the case studies suggests that the programmatic characteristics and policies associated with successful outcomes vary depending on the type of intervention. Although no single formula exists, the implementation of the programs and projects structured around various types of interventions appears to depend on certain types of organizational, managerial, and financial capacities that can be anticipated and specifically targeted for strengthening before the full-scale launch of a program or project. Thus, the findings of this study may serve as pointers for future research seeking to understand the range of government capacities that are needed to support the successful deployment and scaling up of interventions in various contexts and in different parts of the world.

ACKNOWLEDGMENTS

The authors gratefully acknowledge the helpful comments and feedback from Gerald T. Keusch, Phil Musgrove, John Peabody, and members of the What Works Working Group. Thanks also to Carol Kolb for providing excellent research assistance. The basic idea for the What Works Working Group, and for the material in this chapter, came principally from Richard Klausner, and we owe him special acknowledgment.

NOTES

1. Unless otherwise indicated, the background information and health impact data presented about the 17 cases reviewed for this study are drawn from Levine and What Works Working Group (2004). All materials are available at www.cgdev.org/publication/millionssaved.

2. According to *World Development Report 2004* (World Bank 2004), because the relationship between provider and client differs, each of the three types of service arrangements will experience a different constellation of market, government, and accountability failures. The report proposes that if these failures are properly addressed and client power increases, the quality of service delivery will improve, especially among poorer groups.

REFERENCES

Collier, D., and H. E. Brady, eds. 2004. *Rethinking Social Inquiry: Diverse Tools, Shared Standards.* Lanham, MD: Rowman and Littlefield.

Davis, K. 1956. "The Amazing Decline of Mortality in Underdeveloped Areas." *American Economic Review* 46 (2): 305–18.

Devarajan, S., D. Dollar, and T. Holmgren. 2001. *Aid and Reform in Africa: Lessons from Ten Case Studies.* Washington, DC: World Bank.

Eckholm, E. 1989. "River Blindness: Conquering an Ancient Scourge." *New York Times Magazine*, January 8.

Filmer, D., J. S. Hammer, and L. H. Pritchett. 2000. "Weak Links in the Chain: A Diagnosis of Health Policy in Poor Countries." *World Bank Research Observer* 15 (2): 199–224.

Frank, C., M. K. Mohamed, G. T. Strickland, D. Lavanchy, R. R. Arthur, L. S. Magder, and others. 2000. "The Role of Parenteral Antischistosomal Therapy in the Spread of Hepatitis C Virus in Egypt." *Lancet* 355 (9207): 887–91.

Jamison, D. T. 1993. "Disease Control Priorities in Developing Countries: An Overview." In *Disease Control Priorities in Developing Countries,* ed. D. T. Jamison, W. H. Mosley, A. R. Measham, and J. L. Bobadilla, 3–34. New York: Oxford University Press.

———. 2002. "Cost-Effectiveness Analysis: Concepts and Applications." In *Oxford Textbook of Public Health,* 4th ed., ed. R. Detels, J. McEwen, R. Beaglehole, and H. Tanaka. Oxford, U.K.: Oxford University Press.

Jamison, D. T., L. J. Lau, and J. Wang. 2005. "Health's Contribution to Economic Growth in an Environment of Partially Endogenous Technical Progress." In *Health and Economic Growth: Findings and Policy Implications,* ed. G. Lopez-Casasnovas, B. Rivera, and L. Currais, 67–91. Cambridge, MA: MIT Press.

Jha, P., and F. Chaloupka. 2000. "The Economics of Global Tobacco Control." *British Medical Journal* 321: 358–61.

Kremer, M., and E. Miguel. 2003. "The Illusion of Sustainability." http://emlab.berkeley.edu/users/emiguel/miguel_illusion.pdf.

Levine, R., and the What Works Working Group with Molly Kinder. 2004. *Millions Saved: Proven Successes in Global Health.* Washington, DC: Center for Global Development.

Mill, J. S. 1843. "Of the Four Methods of Experimental Inquiry." In *A System of Logic, Raciocinative, and Inductive.* Book 3. Reprint. Toronto: University of Toronto Press, 1974.

Mills, A. 1983. "Vertical vs. Horizontal Health Programs in Africa: Idealism, Pragmatism, Resources, and Efficiency." *Social Science and Medicine* 17 (24): 1971–81.

Musgrove, P. 1988. "Is Polio Eradication in the Americas Economically Justified?" *Bulletin of the Pan American Health Organization* 22 (1): 1–16.

Tucker, J. B. 2001. *Scourge: The Once and Future Threat of Smallpox.* New York: Grove Press.

World Bank. 2004. *World Development Report 2004: Making Services Work for Poor People.* New York: Oxford University Press.

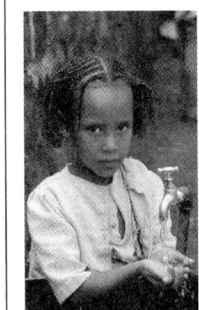

Chapter **9**

Millennium Development Goals for Health: What Will It Take to Accelerate Progress?

Adam Wagstaff, Mariam Claeson, Robert M. Hecht, Pablo Gottret, and Qiu Fang

The scale of the diseases and conditions that the Millennium Development Goals (MDGs) address is staggering:

- Almost 11 million children died before their fifth birthday in 2000 (UNICEF 2001). Less than 1 percent of these 11 million deaths (79,000) occurred in high-income countries, compared with 42 percent in Sub-Saharan Africa, 35 percent in South Asia, and 13 percent in East Asia.
- In 1998, an estimated 843 million people were considered undernourished on the basis of their food intake (FAO 2000). Of the estimated 140 million children under the age of five who were underweight, almost half (65 million) were in South Asia.
- Of the 3.1 million people who died from HIV/AIDS in 2003, almost all (99 percent) were in the developing world—74 percent in Sub-Saharan Africa alone (UNAIDS 2004). Tuberculosis and malaria together killed an equal number; most of these deaths were among the poor.
- In 1995, 515,000 women died during pregnancy or childbirth: 1,000 in the industrial world, contrasted with 252,000 in Sub-Saharan Africa (UNICEF 2001).

This burden of death and suffering is heavily concentrated in the world's poorest countries (Wagstaff and Claeson 2004). Death and disease matter in their own right, but they also act as a brake on poverty reduction. Nobel laureate Amartya Sen (2002) has described health as one of "the most important conditions of human life and a critically significant constituent of human capabilities which we have reason to value." Health also matters because it influences the living standards of both households and countries. Health expenses can easily become burdensome

for households. In Vietnam, they are estimated to have pushed 3 million people into poverty in 1993 (Wagstaff and van Doorslaer 2003).

Beyond the direct impact of ill health on households' living standards through out-of-pocket expenditures, it indirectly affects labor income through productivity and the number of hours that people can work. The effects of illness on income, which may take time to appear, are often long lasting. Malnourished children are less likely to attend school and less likely to learn when they do attend, reducing their productivity in later life. The devastating economic consequences of illness and death are evident at the macroeconomic level as well. The AIDS epidemic alone has been estimated to reduce rates of economic growth by 0.3 to 1.5 percentage points annually (Bell, Devarajan, and Gersbach 2003).

In the 1990s, the international community recognized the importance of health in development. In a period when overall official development assistance declined, development assistance to health rose in real terms. World Bank lending for health increased, with a doubling of the share of International Development Association disbursements going to health (OECD Development Assistance Committee 2000). The 1990s saw an increased global concern over the debt in the developing world, fueled in part by a perception that interest payments were constraining government health expenditures in developing countries. The enhanced Highly Indebted Poor Country Initiative, spearheaded by the International Monetary Fund and World Bank in response to the unsustainable debt burden of the poorest countries, was explicitly geared to channel freed resources into the health and other social sectors. The

Poverty Reduction Strategy Papers submitted by governments of developing countries seek debt relief or concessional (low-interest) International Development Association loans to set out their plans for fighting poverty on all fronts, including health.

The 1990s also saw the development of major new global health initiatives and partnerships, including the Joint United Nations Programme on HIV/AIDS (UNAIDS); the Global Alliance for Vaccines and Immunization; the Stop TB Partnership; the Roll Back Malaria Partnership; the Global Fund to Fight AIDS, Tuberculosis, and Malaria; and the Global Alliance for Improved Nutrition. A range of new not-for-profit organizations were set up to spur the accelerated discovery and uptake in developing countries of low-cost health technologies to address the diseases of the poor; these organizations included the International AIDS Vaccine Initiative, the Medicines for Malaria Venture, the Global Alliance for Tuberculosis, and the International Trachoma Initiative. In addition, the scale of philanthropic involvement in international health increased, with the launch of the Bill & Melinda Gates Foundation and the Packard Foundation and the continued attention to global health issues by such established entities as the Rockefeller Foundation. These initiatives brought not only new resources—funds, ideas, energy, and mechanisms—but also new challenges to harmonization in the attempt to coordinate and link global goals with local actions in the fight against disease, death, and malnutrition in the developing world.

As the 1990s closed, the international community decided that even more needed to be done. At the United Nations Millennium Summit in September 2001, heads of 147 states endorsed the MDGs, nearly half of which concern different aspects of health—directly or indirectly (box 9.1). Several other goals are indirectly related to health—for example, the goals on education and gender. Gender equality is considered important to promoting good health among children. Other health outcomes than those included in the MDGs measure progress on health—for example, targets related to noncommunicable diseases. These targets are referred to as the *MDG plus* and are included in national priority setting, especially in many middle-income countries.

THE MILLENNIUM DEVELOPMENT GOALS FOR HEALTH: PROGRESS AND PROSPECTS

Of the MDGs for which trend data are available or estimated, the fastest progress has been on malnutrition, whereas overall progress on under-five mortality and maternal mortality has been slower.

A Mixed Score at Halftime

In-depth analysis of the health-related MDGs shows a mixed score at halftime (Wagstaff and Claeson 2004):

- The number of people living in on-track countries (countries that will reach the MDGs if they maintain the rate of progress they have already achieved during the period from 1990 to the present) matters. For the malnutrition target, 77 percent of the developing world's people live in an on-track country, but in Sub-Saharan Africa only 15 percent of the people live in an on-track country.
- Different indicators show different levels of improvement. For under-five mortality, the developing world was reduced by an average of only a 2.5 percent in the 1990s, well short of the target of 4.3 percent.

Box 9.1

The Health-Related Millennium Development Goals

Goal 1—eradicating extreme poverty and hunger. This goal includes as a target the halving between 1990 and 2015 of the proportion of people who suffer from hunger, with progress to be measured in terms of the prevalence of underweight children under five years of age. The target implies an average annual rate of reduction of 2.7 percent.

Goal 4—reducing child mortality. The target is to reduce by two-thirds between 1990 and 2015 the under-five mortality rate, equivalent to an annual rate of reduction of 4.3 percent.

Goal 5—improving maternal health. The target is to reduce by three-quarters between 1990 and 2015 the maternal mortality ratio, equivalent to an annual rate of reduction of 5.4 percent.

Goal 6—combating HIV/AIDS, malaria, and other diseases. The target is to halt and begin to reverse the spread of these diseases by 2015.

Goal 7—ensuring environmental sustainability. This goal includes as a target the halving by 2015 of the proportion of people without sustainable access to safe drinking water.

Goal 8—developing a global partnership for development. This goal includes as a target the provision of access to affordable essential drugs in developing countries.

Source: United Nations Millennium Declaration, the United Nations Millennium Summit 2000.

- Regional differences are also pronounced, with Sub-Saharan Africa faring worse than other regions. In Africa, trends in reducing under-five mortality and underweight in children were barely above zero during the 1990s, and maternal mortality fell on average by just 1.6 percent a year compared with the annual target rate of 5.4 percent.
- Evidence on how the poor are faring within countries is mixed. For malnutrition, the poorest 20 percent of the population within countries appears, on average, to have been experiencing broadly similar rates of reduction to the population as a whole. However, for under-five mortality, the rate has been falling more slowly among the poor, while better-off families are seeing faster rates of progress.

Will the Second Half Go Better?

As a comparison of the child mortality experiences in the 1980s and 1990s demonstrates, past performance is not necessarily a good predictor of future performance. The fact that a country is on track on the basis of its performance in the 1990s does not guarantee that it will maintain the required annual rate of reduction of malnutrition or mortality during the second half of the MDG "window" from 2000 to 2015. Countries currently off track may possibly get on track in the second half if they can combine good policies with expanded funding for programs that address both the direct and the underlying determinants of the health-related goals.

Stimuli External to the Health Sector. The World Bank estimates that economic growth will fall somewhat in East Asia and the Pacific in 2000–15, turn from negative to positive in Europe and Central Asia as well as Sub-Saharan Africa, and increase somewhat in Latin America and the Caribbean, the Middle East and North Africa, and South Asia (Jones and others 2003). Primary education completion rates will probably grow faster in the new millennium as a result of the global education initiatives and partnerships on Education for All and the Fast-Track Initiative. However, higher rates of educational attainment among women of childbearing age will not be achieved until 2005 or so, and even then the first full round of effects on under-five mortality will not be felt until 2010.

More relevant is the fact that gender gaps in secondary education may well narrow faster in the new millennium than in the 1990s as a result of the gender MDG (Goal 3: Eliminate gender disparity in primary and secondary education by 2005 and in all levels of education no later than 2015). To achieve parity with boys by 2015 in the proportion of the population who are age 15 and have completed secondary education, girls will have to achieve a faster growth in completion rates in the new millennium than in the 1990s in most regions, especially in South Asia and in East Asia and the Pacific. If the water MDG (ensuring that households have access to safe drinking water) is to be reached, access rates will need to grow much faster in 2000–15, especially in Sub-Saharan Africa (Wagstaff and Claeson 2004). Gender equality in school and access to clean water will have a positive effect on progress toward the health MDGs. Even with economic growth and faster progress on these nonhealth goals, however, many regions will still miss many of the health targets. The picture is bleakest for under-five mortality—and for Sub-Saharan Africa.

The Goals Matter for All Countries. These goals need to be taken seriously for three main reasons:

- Faster progress is important even if targets are missed. A key message of this chapter is that progress can be accelerated in all countries through a judicious mix of spending and policy and institutional reform.
- The goals facilitate benchmarking and monitoring of results. Because the goals focus on a limited set of outcomes, monitoring and evaluating progress toward the MDGs can show what is achievable and where faster progress can be made.
- Focusing attention on national progress, as measured by distributional analysis of the MDGs, forces countries to consider how the benefits of progress are distributed among the rich and poor within each country—the poor risk being left behind even in countries making progress overall. One limitation of the MDGs and targets is that they are national averages. However, distributional analysis of MDG trends (Wagstaff and Claeson 2004) reminds us that progress needs to be for everyone, not just the better off. Progress has been uneven, with the poorer countries lagging behind the rest, and for under-five mortality, the poor within countries are lagging behind the rest of the population.

SCALING UP: DEFINING INTERVENTIONS AND REMOVING CONSTRAINTS

A lack of interventions is not the primary obstacle to faster progress toward the goals, although new interventions that can be delivered by weak health systems could greatly improve progress—for example, malaria or HIV vaccines and effective vaginal microbicides to block the spread of HIV and other sexually transmitted infections. The main obstacle is the low levels of use—especially among the poor—of existing effective interventions. For example, if use of all the proven effective preventive and treatment interventions for childhood illness were to rise from current levels to reach all, the number of under-five deaths worldwide could fall by as much as 63 percent (World Bank 2003b).

Array of Interventions, Programs, and Service Modalities

The available interventions constitute a powerful arsenal for preventing and treating the main causes of malnutrition and death (table 9.1).[1] The major diseases and conditions that the MDGs aim to prevent and control are discussed in several

Table 9.1 Effective Interventions to Reduce Illness, Deaths, and Malnutrition

MDG	Preventive interventions	Treatment interventions
Child mortality	Breastfeeding; hand washing; safe disposal of stool; latrine use; safe preparation of weaning foods; use of insecticide-treated bednets; complementary feeding; immunization; micronutrient supplementation (zinc and vitamin A); prenatal care, including steroids and tetanus toxoid; antimalarial intermittent preventive treatment in pregnancy; newborn temperature management; nevirapine and replacement feeding; antibiotics for premature rupture of membranes; clean delivery	Case management with oral rehydration therapy for diarrhea; antibiotics for dysentery, pneumonia, and sepsis; antimalarials for malaria; newborn resuscitation; breastfeeding; complementary feeding during illness; micronutrient supplementation (zinc and vitamin A)
Maternal mortality	Family planning (lifetime risk); intermittent malaria prophylaxis; use of insecticide-treated bednets; micronutrient supplementation (iron, folic acid, calcium for those who are deficient)	Antibiotics for preterm rupture of membranes, skilled attendants (especially active management of third stage of labor), basic and emergency obstetric care
Nutrition	Exclusive breastfeeding for 6 months, appropriate complementary child feeding for next 6–24 months, iron and folic acid supplementation for children, improved hygiene and sanitation, improved dietary intake of pregnant and lactating women, micronutrient supplementation for prevention of anemia and vitamin A deficiency for mothers and children, anthelmintic treatment in school-age children	Appropriate feeding of sick child and oral rehydration therapy, control and timely treatment of infectious and parasitic diseases, treatment and monitoring of severely malnourished children, high-dose treatment of clinical signs of vitamin A deficiency
HIV/AIDS	Safe sex, including condom use; unused needles for drug users; treatment of sexually transmitted infections; safe, screened blood supplies; antiretrovirals in pregnancy to prevent maternal to child transmission and after occupational exposure	Treatment of opportunistic infections, co-trimoxazole prophylaxis, highly active antiretroviral therapy, palliative care
Tuberculosis	Directly observed treatment of infectious cases to prevent transmission and emergence of drug-resistant strains and treatment of contacts, Bacillus Calmette-Guérin immunization	Directly observed treatment to cure, including early identification of tuberculosis symptomatic cases
Malaria	Use of insecticide-treated bednets, indoor residual spraying (in epidemic-prone areas), intermittent presumptive treatment of pregnant women	Rapid detection and early treatment of uncomplicated cases, treatment of complicated cases (such as cerebral malaria and severe anemia)

Source: Authors.

chapters (for example, see chapters 15, 19, 21–24, 28–31, 44, and 45). The most cost-effective interventions and programs are also discussed in several chapters (see chapters 59–62 and 65). The chapters dealing with health systems and service delivery issues and other constraints related to the health MDGs are found in the latter part of the book (see chapters 66–68, and 73).

In the case of child mortality, for example, diarrheal diseases, pneumonia, and malaria account for 52 percent of deaths worldwide (World Bank 2003b). For each of these major causes of childhood mortality, at least one proven effective preventive intervention and at least one proven effective treatment intervention exist, capable of being delivered in a low-income setting. In most cases, several proven effective interventions exist. For diarrhea—the second-leading cause of child deaths—no fewer than five proven preventive interventions and three proven treatment interventions are available.

Effective Interventions Reaching Too Few People

The high rates of malnutrition and death in the developing world have several causes. First, people do not receive the effec-

tive interventions that could save their lives or make them well nourished. In middle- and high-income countries, 90 percent of children are fully immunized, more than 90 percent of deliveries are assisted by a medically trained provider (that is, a doctor, nurse, or trained midwife, excluding traditional birth attendants), and more than 90 percent of pregnant women have at least one prenatal visit (UNICEF 2001). In South Asia, fewer than 50 percent of pregnant women receive a prenatal checkup, and only 20 percent of deliveries are assisted by a trained provider.

The story is similar for other childhood interventions—and for interventions for other goals. Condom use to prevent transmission of HIV is low in much of Sub-Saharan Africa and South Asia, and inexpensive one-time treatment with antiretroviral medicine to prevent transmission from mother to child covers only a small fraction of at-risk pregnant women in most of the developing world. In Asia, where more than 7 million people are living with HIV/AIDS, no country has yet exceeded 5 percent antiretroviral therapy coverage among those who could benefit from it (World Bank 2003c).

Just as shortfalls in coverage vary across countries, so do they vary within countries, with the poor and other deprived groups consistently lagging. These groups are less likely to receive full basic immunization coverage, to have their deliveries attended by a trained provider, and to have at least one prenatal care visit to a medically trained provider. On the positive side, the poor are often making fastest progress in coverage, reflecting in part that the better off already have high coverage rates for many interventions.

Underuse of Effective Interventions Costs Lives

The low use of effective interventions—in the developing world in general and among the poor in particular—translates into rates of mortality, morbidity, and malnutrition that are far higher than necessary. If use of all the proven effective childhood preventive and treatment interventions, for example, were to rise from their current levels to 99 percent—95 percent for breastfeeding—the number of under-five deaths worldwide could fall by as much as 63 percent (Jones and others 2003). Deaths from malaria and measles could be all but eliminated, and deaths from diarrhea, pneumonia, and HIV/AIDS could be reduced dramatically. If coverage rates of the key maternal mortality interventions were increased from current levels to 99 percent, an estimated 391,000 maternal deaths worldwide (74 percent of current maternal deaths) might be averted (Ramana 2003). One intervention stands out as especially important: access to essential obstetric care, which accounts for more than half the maternal deaths averted.

WHAT DO COUNTRIES NEED TO DO?

If the lack of interventions is not holding countries back from achieving the goals, what is? What do countries need to do to make progress toward the MDGs?

In countries with good governance, additional government health spending does reduce child mortality (Rajkumar and Swaroop 2002). Development assistance has a stronger effect in countries with strong policies and institutions than in countries with only average-quality policies and institutions—and an insignificant effect in countries where policies and institutions are weak. This assertion is also consistent with the findings of a study undertaken by the World Bank for the MDG report, *The Millennium Development Goals for Health: Rising to the Challenges* (Wagstaff and Claeson 2004). The study includes other outcomes with child mortality and uses the World Bank's Country Policy and Institutional Assessment index to measure the quality of policies and institutions.

In principle, well-governed countries with good policies and institutions could achieve the goals simply by scaling up their expenditures on existing programs in proportion to current

allocations. In practice, however, the amount of extra spending required would be difficult to attain on present trends and would even be prohibitively expensive. In the case of East Asia and the Pacific, for example, if economic growth proceeds as expected and the other relevant Millennium Development Targets are attained, the region would achieve the required rates of reduction of underweight and maternal mortality—assuming that economic growth is accompanied by the development of appropriate human resources for health—even if government health spending continues to grow at its current rate. However, the region would miss the under-five mortality target. To reach that target, a minimum of 5 percentage points would need to be added to the annual rate of growth of the government health share of gross domestic product (GDP). That would take the projected share of GDP spent on government health programs to 3.7 percent in 2015—more than twice what it would be if the 1990s pattern of growth continued (Wagstaff and Claeson 2004).

In Sub-Saharan Africa, the situation is even starker. Even if faster economic growth materializes and the other targets are achieved, the share of government health spending in GDP would need to grow nearly sixfold over the coming decade, taking the share to 12.2 percent of GDP in 2015. This percentage compares with a 2000 figure of 1.8 percent and a 2015 forecast of 2.2 percent based on the 1990s annual growth in government spending for health. In conclusion, African countries will not be able to reach the MDGs simply by multiplying their health spending along the lines of historical expenditure patterns, because the multiples required are beyond any realistic expectation of what these governments will be able to do during the next 10 years.

What Are the Implications?

Poorly governed countries cannot expect to make much progress toward the MDGs simply by scaling up their expenditures on existing programs in proportion to current allocations. Although well-governed countries could, in principle, simply scale up existing spending to reach the targets, this option is unlikely to be affordable for them or their donors.

This situation has two implications:

- First, targeting additional government spending to activities that will have the largest effect on the MDGs is important for both sets of countries.
- Second, building good policies and institutions is important for all countries: doing so increases the productivity not just of additional spending but also of existing spending commitments. What do better policies and institutions entail in the health sector? Health systems are very broad, and weak policies and institutions can arise at several points along the pathway, from government health spending to health

outcomes (Claeson and others 2001). Countries can do a number of things, with help from donors, to build stronger policies and institutions.

Improving Expenditure Allocations and Targeting

In most countries, government spending gets stuck in the cities and disproportionately accrues—in a financial sense—to people who are better off.

Geographic Targeting. Resource allocation formulas can be used to reduce government spending gaps across regions and ideally to favor geographic zones that are furthest behind. These formulas have been used, for example, as part of Bolivia's decentralization efforts since 1994 and have been associated with some large—and pro-poor—improvements in maternal and child health indicators. Targeting resources to poor regions and provinces may be most effectively implemented through nontraditional mechanisms for priority setting and implementation, such as social investment funds. In Bolivia, a recent impact evaluation concluded that such funds were responsible for a decline in under-five mortality from 88.5 to 65.6 per 1,000 live births over a five-year period (Newman and others 2002).

Changing the Allocation of Spending across Care Levels. Spending on health in developing countries is characterized by a high concentration of spending on secondary and tertiary infrastructure and personnel. Some governments have tried to scale back the share of hospital spending. Tanzania, for example, reduced the share of hospital spending from 60 percent in 2000 to 43 percent in 2002. Chapter 3 deals with the issue of how to couple expenditure reallocations across levels of care with measures to improve performance at each level of the health care system.

Targeting Specific Programs. Programs such as those delivering directly observed treatment short course (DOTS) for tuberculosis or integrated management of infant and childhood illness (IMCI) for child health are good examples of programs that may yield high returns to government spending at the margin. A recent World Bank study in India provides further support for the idea that the way government spending is allocated across programs makes a difference to its effect on the Millennium Development Indicators (World Bank 2003a). Successful public health programs—large-scale programs with a measurable health effect over at least a five-year period—are further discussed in chapter 8. All successful programs have several factors in common: technical innovation and stakeholder consensus, strong political leadership, coordination across agencies and management, effective use of information and financial resources, and participation of the beneficiary community.

Targeting Specific Population Groups. Many countries subsidize all government health services for everyone. These blanket subsidy schemes not only fail to target interventions that give rise to externalities but also fail to disproportionately benefit the poor—despite the stronger equity case for subsidizing their care and the fact that they tend to bear a disproportionate burden of malnutrition as well as child and maternal mortality. There are many proven ways to target the poor—for example, by delivering essential services in clinics or health posts that only poor families attend or by promoting and delivering services in a way that segments the market and appeals to those in low-income households.

Targeting Spending to Remove Bottlenecks. A planning and budgeting approach is to assess—for a country—the health sector impediments to faster progress, to identify ways of removing them, and to estimate both the costs of removing them and the likely effects of their removal on MDG outcomes (Soucat and others 2002). MDG analysis along these lines—referred to sometimes as *marginal budgeting for bottlenecks* (MBB)—has begun in several African countries and in some states of India (UNICEF and World Bank 2003). In Mali, key bottlenecks were identified for supporting home-based practices and delivering periodic and continual professional care. They included low access to affordable commodities and the need for community-based support for home-based care; low geographical access to preventive professional care (immunization, vitamin A supplementation, and prenatal care); shortages of qualified nurses and midwives; and an absence of effective third-party payment mechanisms for the poor for professional continuous care. Important health systems bottlenecks, such as human resources, drug availability, and health care management, are discussed in chapters 71–73.

Improving Policies toward Households as Producers and Demanders of Care

Households are at the center of any efforts to scale up; they not only demand and consume care, but they are also important producers of prevention and care. Policies to increase coverage of cost-effective interventions to reach the health MDGs, therefore, need to identify and influence the key constraints to both the production and the demand for those services at the household and community levels.

Lowering Financial Barriers. Low income is a barrier to the use of most health interventions, and economic growth is an important weapon in the war against malnutrition and mortality. However, social protection programs are also important. Successful schemes aimed at households and communities are discussed in chapter 56.

One part of the affordability equation is price. User charges for MDG interventions are to be discouraged. Why? Many of those interventions involve benefits that spill over to people who do not receive the intervention; high coverage of immunization is a classic example. However, an equity case also can be made for reducing prices facing the poor and near poor, even where no spillovers occur. Subsidies should be targeted to services with spillovers and to the poor. In practice, subsidies are often badly targeted in at least one respect if not both. Exceptions exist. In Ifakara, Tanzania, a voucher program for mosquito nets was launched successfully for pregnant women and children under five (Schellenberg and others 2001).

Some recent programs, especially in Latin America, have not only made health care affordable for the poor but have also made it profitable. Rather than simply reducing the cost of using specific interventions, these programs provide users with cash payments, which are linked to specific interventions and restricted to certain groups—often poor mothers and their children. The experience with these programs in targeting and achieving results is encouraging (Mesoamerica Nutrition Program Targeting Study Group 2002; Morris and others 2003; Palmer and others 2004).

Risk aversion coupled with the unpredictability of illness provides a motivation for pooling risks through an insurance scheme. The Arab Republic of Egypt, for example, introduced a school health insurance program for all children attending school. The program resulted in larger increases in coverage among the poor and achieved considerable effect on use and out-of-pocket expenditures (Yip and Berman 2001). However, insurance in the developing world is very limited, and those who are least able to smooth consumption without insurance are the least likely to have insurance coverage (Musgrove, Zeramdini, and Carrin 2002). Another problem is that many of the schemes are small scale, and evaluations of these schemes do not generally measure health effect or effect on equity, thus resulting in limited evidence (Palmer and others 2004).

Providing Information—Enhancing Knowledge. Lack of knowledge is a major factor behind poor health. It results in people not seeking care when needed, despite the absence of price barriers, and it also results in people—especially poor people—wasting limited resources on inappropriate care. Ignorance may also result in people not getting the maximum health gain out of inputs they have available to them and use. Many people do not know that hand washing confers much of the health benefit of piped water (see chapter 41). Not surprisingly, piped water has a much greater effect on the prevalence of diarrhea among the children of the better off and better educated. Better-educated women—especially those with a secondary education—achieve better health outcomes for themselves and their children not by using health-specific knowledge that they acquire at school, but by using general

numeracy and literacy skills learned at school to acquire health-specific knowledge later in life. Although better-educated girls will mean healthier women and healthier children in years to come, a shorter and more direct route to increasing health-specific knowledge and skills is through information dissemination, health promotion, and counseling in the health sector.

Several success stories exist. In Brazil, after health workers trained by IMCI provided information and counseling at health facilities and in the community, health knowledge among mothers improved, as did feeding practices (Santos and others 2001). After only 18 months, the nutritional status of children in the area improved as well. Social marketing and media campaigns—for example, malaria and social marketing of insecticide-treated nets (see chapter 21)—have also proved effective in some circumstances.

Reducing Time Costs Transportation systems, road infrastructure, and geography influence the demand for care delivered by formal providers through their effect on time costs, which can be substantial. In rural communities, where the roads are poor and the transportation unreliable, the time spent waiting for the transportation is also a major cost. Time costs tend to be a major issue for maternal mortality: health centers are unable to provide essential obstetric care for a complicated delivery, and women would have to travel to distant hospitals to get such services. Road rehabilitation and other transportation projects are important here, but so are subsidies linked to the use of health services. Malaysia and Sri Lanka provide free or subsidized transportation to hospitals in emergencies (Pathmanathan and others 2003). Other options for tackling inaccessibility include using outreach and establishing partnerships between government and nongovernmental organizations (NGOs), private providers, or community organizations.

Providing Access to Water and Sanitation The availability of adequate supplies of water and improved sanitation is associated with better maternal and child health outcomes, at least among the better educated, even after controlling for other influences. This result is not altogether surprising. Hand washing is easier if the household has piped water that provides readily available quantities of safe water. The safe disposal of feces is easier if the household has an improved form of sanitation. The developing world lags well behind the industrial world in both; the poorer people fare especially badly. They are less likely to be connected to a network, and the sources they rely on tend to be more costly per liter than the networked services used by the better off.

The challenge from a health perspective is to get maximum health benefits from investments in access to water and sanitation infrastructure. Efforts to work across sectors on water and health, in order to influence the health MDGs, are under way in Ethiopia, Peru, and Rwanda.

Improving Health Service Delivery

Health providers—in the public and private sectors, as well as in both formal and informal sectors—should deliver interventions of relevance to the MDGs. Many are efficient, deliver high quality services, and are responsive to their patients. Many, however, are not; many are not even there to deliver any services at all. As a result, resources—public and private—are often nonexistent, underused, or wasted.

Two things can make a difference. One is the quality of management. Better management means a clearer delineation of responsibilities and accountabilities inside organizations, a clearer link between performance and reward, and so on. Management means getting accountabilities right within an organization. The other thing that can make a difference is getting accountabilities right between the organization and the public (World Bank 2003d).

Improving Management—Increasing Accountability within Provider Organizations.

Management styles in government-funded and government-implemented health schemes have recently begun to change, focusing on performance—that is, on outputs and outcomes—rather than on inputs and processes. Good performance is rewarded, financially or in some other way. The focus is on clients and on the belief that an organization is ultimately accountable to its clients. A client-oriented strategy emphasizes customer choice and satisfaction. Business techniques enhance performance and are a standard part of strategic planning.

This new approach is evident in several countries, and elements of the approach are visible in successful nutrition and child health programs (see chapter 56). For example, in Tamil Nadu's Integrated Nutrition Program, community nutrition workers were given clearly defined duties. Information on outputs not only enabled the community to keep the workers accountable but also enabled the nutrition workers to see how their program was working. In Ceara's Programa de Agentes de Saude, which is credited with a substantial reduction in child mortality (Victora and others 2000), health agents and nurse-supervisors were assigned clear tasks and given clear responsibilities. The intended outcomes of the program were emphasized to health workers and members of the public, and the health agents were held accountable through community-based monitoring and rewarded for good performance.

Governance.

The accountability of provider organizations to the public can be improved through enhanced governance or contracting. Having community representatives participate in the governance and oversight of providers can improve the productivity and quality of public sector providers. In Burkina Faso, participation of community representatives in public primary health care clinics increased immunization coverage, the availability of essential drugs, and the percentage of women with two or more prenatal visits. In Peru, comparisons of primary health care clinics with and without community participation in governance suggested decreases in staff absenteeism and waiting times and suggested increases in perceived quality by patients (Cotlear 1999). The approach probably works best for primary care and in situations in which strong technical and advisory support is provided to community representatives who are close to the service being delivered.

Contracting.

Evidence on the effect of contracting within the public sector is mixed, and the experiences are mainly based on lessons learned from middle-income countries. In several countries in Europe and Central Asia, evidence shows a positive effect from performance-based payment, but that is not necessarily the same as contracting, which can occur without performance-related pay. The best evidence relates to the use of target payments for the attainment of a given level of coverage—for example, for immunization or cervical cytology at the primary care level (Langenbrunner 2003). In Argentina and Nicaragua, social security institutes have increased productivity by establishing capitation-based payments for an integrated package of inpatient and ambulatory services (Bitran 2001). Key influences on the success of contracts within the public sector include whether the provider has the ability to respond, whether service commitments are congruent with funding levels, whether output and key components of performance expectations are easily measurable, and how far capacity strengthening of the payer or funder is addressed.

Contracting with nonprofit organizations is most common in low-income countries (see chapter 12, which contains a longer discussion of contracting with NGOs). Most cases have had positive effects on target outcome or output variables. In Bangladesh, contracts with nonprofit organizations for planning and implementing an expanded program on immunization project were credited with a dramatic increase in immunization. In Haiti, contracting for a primary health care package also significantly increased immunization coverage (Eichler, Auxilia, and Pollock 2001). In Bangladesh, Madagascar, and Senegal, significant reductions in nutrition rates were attributed to contracting initiatives (Marek and others 1999). Only a few cases assess efficiency. Contracting with nonprofits works best when the contractors have well-functioning accountability arrangements and strong intrinsic motivation and when the government makes timely payments to the NGOs. The government needs to be capable of assessing, selecting, and managing the ongoing relationship with contractors. The methodological quality of evaluating contracting is often poor and needs to be improved. An exception is the Cambodian contracting trial that used a rigorous cluster randomized design, but the intervention groups had greater input of resources than the control communities, which may have been partly responsible for the difference in performance.

Results on contracting with for-profit private service providers are also mixed. Experience from the hospital sector warns that weak government contracting capacity often allows the provider to capture efficiency gains or to expand volume—not necessarily of cost-effective services—to generate more income. In Zimbabwe, the cost per service decreased, but the lack of volume control led to an increase in total cost (McPake and Hongoro 1995). Other adverse outcomes are possible. In Brazil, contracting with for-profit hospitals led to increases in access, but also increases in fraud (false billing) and cream-skimming to avoid costly patients (Slack and Savedoff 2001). These problems seem less pronounced in primary health care. In Peru and El Salvador, contracting with private primary health care providers increased access, choice, and consumer satisfaction (Fiedler 1996). Contracting with for-profit providers seems to work best when the government invests in the development of capacity to manage the contracting process (Mills, Bennett, and Russell 2001); when quality is at least as high in the private sector as in the public sector; and when the services involve primary care or other relatively observable services, such as diagnostic services.

Strengthening Core Public Health Functions

Vulnerable populations need to be protected from risks and damages, informed, and educated. Public health regulations need to be established and enforced. Infrastructure needs to be in place to reduce the impact of emergencies and disasters on health. All this action needs to be implemented through a public health system that is transparent and accountable. Governments in developing countries generally recognize that these public health functions are important, but they often lack the capacity and financial resources to implement them. Indeed, few low-income countries invest in these public health functions.

By employing public health professionals with core public health competencies, the government can develop and enforce standards; can monitor the health of communities and populations; and can emphasize health education, public information, health promotion, and disease prevention. Public action can help improve consumer knowledge and change attitudes so that private markets can operate effectively to meet the needs of the poor, for example, through social marketing of insecticide-treated bednets to reduce malaria transmission or of condoms for protection against HIV/AIDS.

Government-Led Monitoring and Evaluation. Integrated disease surveillance, program assessment, and collection and analysis of demographic and vital registration data are essential if governments and donors are to ascertain whether policies and programs are positively affecting health goals. Governments can use a list of intermediate indicators and proxies for the goals that can help monitor progress, test the impact of policies, and adjust programs going forward (World Bank 2001). Such indicators should be simple, easily measurable, representative, easy to understand, scientifically robust, and ethical. They need to be assessed regularly because the MDGs themselves are difficult to collect, thus entail delays, and are therefore not useful for regular monitoring of progress. Greater investments are needed in systems to monitor these intermediate indicators and to track expenditures on public health.

Although some good practices in surveillance are being developed—for example, in Brazil, China, and India—few low-income developing countries can afford to invest in the infrastructure required for strong surveillance systems. Most rely on alternative short- to medium-term solutions for data gathering, such as intermittent household surveys, health facility surveys, and simplified facility-based routine reporting. A few countries have made special efforts to improve the surveillance of a specific intervention, such as AIDS and tuberculosis treatment or childhood immunization, whereas others have attempted to monitor progress toward a specific MDG. INDEPTH (International Network of Field Sites with Continuous Demographic Evaluation of Populations and Their Health in Developing Countries), which is supported by the Rockefeller Foundation with help from other donors, coordinates a range of surveillance sites, many of them in Africa, and the Health Metrics network aims at improving the quality of surveillance data. Some governments are explicitly developing or modifying their monitoring and evaluation framework to focus on the MDGs.

Intersectoral Actions—Going Beyond the Ministry of Health. A review of the evidence base for the key determinants of the health and nutrition MDGs identifies significant potential for intersectoral synergies (Wagstaff and Claeson 2004).

Transportation Although roads and transport are vital for health services, especially for reducing maternal mortality, it is not just the physical infrastructure that matters. Also important are the availability of transportation and the affordability of its use, as shown in a study in Nigeria (Eissen, Efenne, and Sabitu 1997). Transportation and roads complement health services. A 10-year study in Rajasthan, India, found that better roads and transportation helped women reach referral facilities, but many women still died because no corresponding improvements took place at household and facility levels. Working with the transportation sector is also important for reducing HIV transmission in many settings and making progress on the HIV/AIDS-related MDG.

Hygiene Improved hygiene (use of hand washing) and sanitation (use of latrines and safe disposal of children's stools) are at least as important as drinking water quality in shaping health outcomes, specifically in reducing diarrhea and associated child mortality (Esrey and others 1991). Constructing water supply and sanitation facilities is not enough to improve health outcomes; sustained human behavior change must accompany the infrastructure investment. By collaborating with other sectors, the health sector can develop public health promotion and education strategies and implement them in partnership with agencies that plan, develop, and manage water resources. The health sector can also work with the private sector to manufacture, distribute, and promote affordable in-home water purification solutions and safe storage vessels—and advocate for water, sanitation, and hygiene interventions in strategies to reduce poverty.

Indoor Air Quality Indoor air pollution is caused by use of low-cost, traditional energy sources, such as coal and biomass for cooking and heating, the main source of energy for 3.5 billion people. Indoor air pollution is a major risk factor for pneumonia and associated deaths in children and for lung cancer in women who risk exposure during cooking (see chapter 42). Studies in China, Guatemala, and India are under way to improve access to efficient and affordable energy sources through local design, manufacturing, and dissemination of low-cost technologies, modern fuel alternatives, and renewable energy solutions. The community-based project in China was initiated by the Ministry of Health, which was troubled by the leveling off of child mortality reductions among the rural poor and was seeking ways to influence major environmental determinants of child mortality. The program combines appropriately improved stoves and ventilation with behavior-change modification; it is in an early stage of implementation, and results on outcomes are not yet available. Agricultural policies and practices influence food prices, farm incomes, diet diversity and quality, and household food security. Policies that focus on women's access to land, training, and agricultural inputs; on their roles in production; and on their income from agriculture are more likely to have a positive effect on nutrition than interventions without a focus on women, particularly if combined with other strategies, such as women's education and behavior change (Johnson-Welch 1999; Quisumbing 1995). The MDG agenda highlights the need not only to prioritize within health to achieve better health outcomes, but also to better inform priority setting in resource allocations between sectors, identifying intersectoral synergies and finding ways to maximize benefits for health.

COSTING AND FINANCING ADDITIONAL SPENDING FOR THE MDGS

Additional health spending will be required in many countries to accelerate progress toward the health goals (see chapter 12). What will it cost, and how will extra spending be financed?

Cost of Achieving the MDGs Globally

The global estimates of what it would cost to achieve the MDGs range from an additional US$20 billion to US$70 billion a year. A World Bank study (http://www.worldbank.org/html/extdr/mdgassessment.pdf) estimates that the additional official development assistance required to meet the health goals is in the range of US$20 billion to US$25 billion per year, which is roughly four times the current amount of official development assistance spending for health in 2002 (US$6.5 billion) and three times all external financing, including that of foundations and loans from multilateral sources (see chapter 13). The dramatic shortfalls in resources required to achieve the MDGs were emphasized during the 2002 Monterrey Conference on Financing for Development, which brought significant attention to issues concerning the estimation of the cost of achieving the health MDGs.

Another analysis conducted by the Commission on Macroeconomics and Health (2001) of the World Health Organization estimated that an additional US$40 billion to US$52 billion annually would be required until 2015 to scale up the coverage for malaria, tuberculosis, HIV/AIDS, childhood mortality, and maternal mortality (Kumaranayake, Kurowski, and Conteh 2001). A third study using the production frontiers approach estimated that between US$25 billion and US$70 billion of additional spending was needed to bring poorly performing countries up to the level of high performers (Preker and others 2003). A fourth study prepared by the World Bank for the Development Committee estimated at least US$30 billion annually in additional aid was needed to accelerate all the MDGs, including health (Development Committee 2003). Whatever the method of analysis, all global estimates show that reaching the MDGs will require significant additional resources compared with the current levels of funding for health.

Cost of Achieving the MDGs in Countries

Global estimates of what it costs to achieve the health MDGs are not very useful for countries wanting to plan and budget in order to reach the MDGs. The substantial range of estimates between US$20 billion and US$75 billion per year to achieve the MDGs at a global level has led to debates over the most appropriate costing method for country-specific analysis and to the development of new costing methodologies for obtaining consistent and reliable estimates to use for policy dialogue and decision making at the country levels. Some of the methods are summarized in box 9.2.

Preliminary Country Cost Estimates. Table 9.2 provides a set of preliminary country-level estimates for the cost of removing bottlenecks and accelerating progress toward the health MDGs (MBB method) and for the cost of achieving the health MDGs (Millennium Project tools) in selected countries. The estimates are presented for illustration of orders of magnitude and should not be used for intercountry comparison.

Financing Extra Health Spending

The additional resources needed to reach the MDGs are large at both country and global levels, as discussed in the previous section. The key question is how to finance the extra spending that is needed.

Encouraging Risk Pooling Rather Than Out-of-Pocket Spending. Health spending can be broken down into three categories:

- private (out-of-pocket expenditures and private insurance)
- public (financing from general revenues and social insurance contributions)
- external sources (development assistance).

Box 9.2

Estimating the Cost of Scaling Up to Achieve the MDGs

The following are the country-specific models for MDG cost analysis:

- The *MDG Needs Assessments Model* developed by the United Nations Millennium Project, (Millennium Project 2004). The Millennium Project model yields total cost estimates for full coverage of the needs of a defined population with a comprehensive set of health interventions in a given year. It uses unit cost of covering one person multiplied by the total population in need in a given year to yield the direct health cost. Additional resource requirements are added (on the basis of assumptions rather than actual inputs) for, among other items, health system improvement, salary increases for human resources, administration and management, promotion of community demand, and research and development.

- The *Marginal Budgeting for Bottlenecks Model* developed by the United Nations Children's Fund, the World Bank, and the World Health Organization (Soucat and others 2002, 2004; UNICEF and World Bank 2003). The MBB model yields additional resources required for removing a set of health system bottlenecks that are considered to hinder the delivery of health services to the population through three delivery modes: family-community, outreach, and clinical levels. The MBB method also estimates the effect on outcomes (for instance, child and maternal mortality) of increased coverage and use of the health services provided. First, a set of high-impact services are selected on the basis of a country's epidemiological needs. These services are the same as those cost-effective priority interventions identified in the relevant disease control priorities chapters. Second, health system bottlenecks hindering delivery of these services are identified. Then, strategies for

removal of bottlenecks are discussed, and the inputs are identified for improving coverage, for example, in a village. Cost estimates are based on these inputs by scaling up the cost to cover the district, province, or nation.

- Elasticity estimates through *econometric modeling* developed by the World Bank staff (Wagstaff and Claeson 2004). A few studies have used econometric techniques to analyze the effect on MDG outcomes of certain cross-sector determinants (such as economic growth, water and sanitation, education, and road infrastructure) as well as government expenditures on health. Econometric analysis has been used mostly to analyze the effect of changes in government health expenditures on outcomes using cross-sectional or panel data at a global scale. But in one particular study in India, the methodology was used to estimate the marginal costs of averting a child's death at the state level. The estimates could vary from as low as US$2.40 per child death in a low-income state to US$160 in a middle-income state in India.

- The *Maquette for Multisectoral Analysis* of MDGs is under development by the World Bank (Bourguignon and others 2004). The thesis for this new approach is that development aid is a key ingredient of a country's development process, but its effectiveness has to be assessed at the country level within each country's local implementation and macroeconomic constraints. The objective of the model is to calculate the financial needs to attain a targeted path to 2015 and determine an optimal allocation of additional funding toward different social sectors for the MDGs. This modeling framework is still at an early stage of development and will be applied later to countries. This model is anticipated to draw extensively from results of other models, such as the elasticity analysis and MBB models.

Source: Millennium Project 2003, 2004; Soucat and others 2004; Bourguignon and others 2004.

Table 9.2 Alternative Cost Estimates Using Millennium Project and Marginal Budgeting for Bottlenecks Models

Country	Model used	Cost estimate (US$ per capita per year)
Ethiopia	MBB	3.56
Madagascar (Toamasina)	MBB	2.38
Mali (one region)	MBB	3.97
Ethiopia	Millennium Project	32.00
Bangladesh	Millennium Project	20.60
Cambodia	Millennium Project	22.50
Ghana	Millennium Project	24.70
Tanzania	Millennium Project	34.70
Uganda	Millennium Project	32.10

Source: Authors.

Private spending absorbs a larger share of income in poorer countries. In low-income countries, it absorbs a larger share of GDP, on average, than domestically financed public spending. In low-income and lower-middle-income countries, it invariably means out-of-pocket expenditures rather than private insurance (Musgrove, Zeramdini, and Carrin 2002). This situation leaves many near-poor households heavily exposed to the risk of impoverishing health expenses. The risk is clearly greater the poorer the country, because poorer countries tend, on average, to have larger shares of poor people (World Bank 2000). Governments thus have a major role to play in helping shape effective risk-pooling mechanisms, in addition to increasing their own spending and targeting it to services for the poor that will have a large positive effect on the MDGs.

Getting Governments to Spend What They Can Afford

Government spending is an important part of the picture, and the issue is how much they can afford. Unlike private spending, government spending as a share of GDP is higher in richer countries. However, at any given per capita income, a surprising amount of variation occurs across countries in the share of GDP allocated to government health programs. Countries that appear able to spend similar shares of GDP on government health programs end up spending quite different amounts.

How can extra domestic resources be mobilized if countries are spending less than they can afford? Domestically financed government health spending comes from general revenues, social insurance contributions, or both. The amount of general revenues flowing into the health sector is the product of the amount of general (tax and nontax) revenues collected by the government (the *general revenue share*) and the share of general revenues allocated to the health sector (the *health share of government spending*) (Hay 2003). Low government health spending could be attributable to either share or both shares being low. In poorer countries, both shares are typically lower

than they are in richer countries. However, differences exist across countries that cannot be explained by per capita income alone.

Countries need to ascertain whether their low spending is caused by unduly low general revenues or by unduly low allocations to health and explore ways of making appropriate adjustments. Bolivia managed to raise its general revenue share consistently in the 1990s as the result of a sustained reform process begun in 1983. The health sector there has been one of the beneficiaries of this growth of tax revenues: government health spending as a share of GDP grew at an annual rate of nearly 10 percent in the 1990s.

Although raising domestic resources takes time, countries that can apparently afford to spend more out of their own resources should be encouraged to start the process. Development agencies have a role here—in providing technical support of tax reform, in helping develop government commitment to health in public expenditure allocations, and in giving financial assistance, both to ease the adjustment costs and to provide support while the gap is being closed between current and affordable spending.

Recognizing the Limits of Development Assistance. Official development assistance tends to account for a larger share of government health spending in poorer countries. Development assistance for health is especially important in Sub-Saharan Africa. Twelve countries in Sub-Saharan Africa had external funding exceeding 35 percent of total health expenditures in 2000 (World Bank 1998).

Increased development assistance is needed to achieve the MDGs. Development assistance, however, is not without its drawbacks. Many donors require that assistance be kept in parallel budgets outside the ministry of finance, which risks undermining government efforts to appropriately plan and target expenditures. Such off-budget expenditures make it difficult in some countries to properly target resources to particular interventions, geographic locations, or population groups, even though such targeting may be essential for improving the effect of expenditures on outcomes and the probability of reaching the health goals. Donors often require recipient governments to maintain separate accounts and to provide separate progress reports, thereby increasing the administrative burden on weak health ministries. Most important, donor commitments of expenditures in health are short term, whereas the needs are permanent. Thus, any external financing must at some point be substituted with additional domestic revenues or expenditure reallocations. This substitution or transition to domestic sources of funding has typically been difficult to achieve, leading to a dropoff in effort in important health programs, such as immunizations and reproductive health services.

Consensus on how to improve aid effectiveness is growing among development partners, and partners at the High Level Forum on Health MDGs (http://www.hlfhealthmdgs.org). This agenda includes supporting countries in developing more MDG-responsive Poverty Reduction Strategy Papers, tracking resource flows, strengthening monitoring and evaluation, and more effectively dealing with the human resources crisis in health. Effective monitoring can help ensure that increased external funds do not simply lead to reduced domestic financing (the *fungibility problem*) but actually boost overall spending for health. In concert with moves affecting all development assistance, donors and governments are trying to see that in the health area external funds are pooled and that ministries can use a common management and reporting format. In addition, a research agenda to support acceleration toward the health MDGs is being proposed; it needs to focus on how to translate knowledge into action and on how to remove health systems constraints to scaling up coverage of cost-effective interventions that are available but do not reach those who need them (Claeson and others 2004; Task Force on Health Systems Research 2004).

NOTE

1. *Intervention* in this chapter refers to the direct action that leads to prevention or cure.

REFERENCES

Bell, C., S. Devarajan, and H. Gersbach. 2003. *The Long-Run Economic Cost of AIDS: Theory and an Application to South Africa.* Washington, DC: World Bank.

Bitran, R. 2001. "Paying Health Providers through Capitation in Argentina, Nicaragua, and Thailand: Output, Spending, Organizational Impact, and Market Structure." USAID Partners for Health Reform Project, Washington, DC.

Bokhari, F., P. Gottret, and Y. Gai. Forthcoming. "Government Health Expenditures, Donor Funding and Health Outcomes." World Bank, Washington, DC.

Bourguignon, F., M. Bussolo, H. Lofgren, H. Timmer, and D. van der Mensbrugghe. 2004. "Towards Achieving the Millennium Development Goals in Ethiopia: An Economywide Analysis of Alternative Scenarios." World Bank, Washington, DC.

Claeson, M., C. Griffin, T. Johnston, M. McLachan, A. Soucat, A. Wagstaff, and A. Yazbeck 2001. "Poverty-Reduction and the Health-Sector." In *Poverty Reduction Strategy Sourcebook.* Washington, DC: World Bank.

Claeson, M., A. Wagstaff, E. Bos, P. Hay, and J. Baudouy. 2004. "The Case for Mobilizing New Research behind the Health Millennium Development Goals." In *Global Forum Update on Research for Health 2005,* 73–75. Geneva: Global Forum.

Commission on Macroeconomics and Health. 2001. "Macroeconomics and Health: Investing in Health for Economic Development—Report of the Commission on Macroeconomics and Health." December 20, World Health Organization, Geneva.

Cotlear, D. 1999. "Peru: Improving Health Care for the Poor." Human Development Department (Latin America and the Caribbean Human Development) Paper 57, World Bank, Washington, DC.

Development Committee. 2003. "Supporting Sound Policies with Adequate and Appropriate Financing." Discussion paper, World Bank, Washington DC.

Eichler, R. 2001. "Improving Immunization Coverage in an Innovative Primary Health Care Delivery Model: Lessons from Burkina Faso's Bottom up Planning, Oversight, and Resource Control Approach That Holds Providers Accountable for Results." Discussion paper, World Bank, Washington, DC.

Eissen, E., D. Efenne, and K. Sabitu. 1997. "Community Loan Funds and Transport Services for Obstetric Emergencies in Northern Nigeria." *International Journal of Gynecology and Obstetrics* 59 (Suppl. 2): S237–44.

Esrey, S. A., J. B. Potash, L. Roberts, and C. Shiff. 1991. "Effects of Improved Water Supply and Sanitation on Ascariasis, Diarrhea, Dracunculiasis, Hookworm Infection, Schistosomiasis, and Trachoma." *Bulletin of the World Health Organization* 69 (5): 609–21.

FAO (Food and Agriculture Organization of the United Nations). 2000. *The State of Food Security in the World.* Rome: FAO.

Fiedler, J. L. 1996. "The Privatization of Health Care in Three Latin American Social Security Systems." *Health Policy and Planning* 11 (4): 406–17.

Filmer, D., and L. Pritchett. 1999. "The Impact of Public Spending on Health: Does Money Matter?" *Social Science and Medicine* 49, pp. 1309–23.

Gwatkin, D., S. Rutstein, K. Johnson, and R. P. Pande. 2000. *Socio-economic Differences in Health, Nutrition, and Population.* Washington, DC: World Bank.

Hay, R. 2003. "The 'Fiscal Space' for Publicly Financed Health Care." Oxford Policy Institute Policy Brief, Washington, DC.

Johnson-Welch, C. 1999. "Focusing on Women Works: Research on Improving Micronutrient Status through Food-Based Interventions." International Center for Research on Women, Washington, DC.

Jones, G., R. W. Steketee, R. E. Black, Z. A. Bhutta, and S. S. Morris. 2003. "How Many Child Deaths Can We Prevent this Year?" *Lancet* 362 (9377): 65–71.

Kumaranayake, L., Christoph Kurowski, and Lesong Conteh. 2001. "Costs of Scaling Up Priority Health Interventions in Low-Income and Selected Middle-Income Countries: Methodology and Estimates." Commission for Macroeconomics and Health Working Paper WG5:19, World Health Organization, Geneva.

Langenbrunner, J. 2003. "Resource Allocation and Purchasing in ECA Region: A Review." Discussion paper, World Bank, Washington, DC.

Marek, T., I. Diallo, B. Ndiaye, and J. Rakotosalama. 1999. "Successful Contracting of Prevention Services: Fighting Malnutrition in Senegal and Madagascar." *Health Policy and Planning* 14 (4): 382–89.

McPake, B, and C. Hongoro. 1995. "Contracting Out of Clinical Services in Zimbabwe." *Social Science and Medicine* 41 (1): 13–24.

Mesoamerica Nutrition Program Targeting Study Group. 2002. "Targeting Performance of Three Large-Scale, Nutrition-Oriented Programs in Central America and Mexico." *Food and Nutrition Bulletin* 232 (2): 162–74.

Millennium Project. 2003. "Millennium Development Goal Country Case Studies: Methodology and Preliminary Results." October. United Nations, NY.

———. 2004. "Millennium Development Goals Needs Assessments: Country Case Studies of Bangladesh, Cambodia, Ghana, Tanzania, and Uganda." Unpublished working paper for the Millennium Project. United Nations, NY.

Mills, A., S. Bennett, and S. Russell. 2001. *The Challenge of Health Sector Reform: What Must Governments Do?* New York: St. Martin's Press.

Morris, S., E. Flores, P. Olinto, and J. Medina. 2003. "A Randomized Trial of Conditional Cash Transfers to Household and Peripheral Health Centres: Impact on Child Health and Demand for Health Services." Presented at Fourth International Health Economics Association World Congress, San Francisco, CA, June.

Musgrove, P., R. Zeramdini, and G. Carrin. 2002. "Basic Patterns in National Health Expenditure." *Bulletin of the World Health Organization* 80 (2): 134–42.

Newman, J., M. Pradhan, L. Rawlings, G. Ridder, R. Coa, and J. Evia. 2002. "An Impact Evaluation of Education, Health, and Water Supply Investments of the Bolivian Social Investment." *World Bank Economic Review* 6 (2): 241–74.

OECD (Organisation for Economic Co-operation and Development) Development Assistance Committee. 2000. *Recent Trends in Official Development Assistance to Health.* Paris: OECD.

Palmer, N., D. Mueller, L. Gilson, A. Mills, and A. Haines. 2004. "Health Financing to Promote Access in Low Income Settings—How Much Do We Know?" *Lancet* 364: 1365–70.

Pathmanathan, I., J. Liljestrand, J. M. Martins, L. C. Rajapaksa, C. Lissner, A. de Silva, and others. 2003. "Investing in Maternal Health: Learning from Malaysia and Sri Lanka." Health, Nutrition, and Population Department, World Bank, Washington, DC.

Preker, A. S., E. Suzuki, F. Bustero, A. Soucat, and J. Langenbrunner. 2003. "Costing the Millennium Development Goals." Background paper to *The Millennium Development Goals for Health: Rising to the Challenges,* World Bank, Washington, DC.

Quisumbing, A. R. 1995. "Gender Differences in Agricultural Productivity: A Survey of Empirical Evidence." IFPRI Discussion Paper 5. International Food Policy Research Institute, Washington, DC.

Rajkumar, A., and V. Swaroop. 2002. "Public Spending and Outcomes: Does Governance Matter?" Policy Research Working Paper 2840, World Bank, Washington, DC.

Ramana, G. 2003. Background paper for *The Millennium Development Goals for Health: Rising to the Challenges.* World Bank, Washington, DC.

Santos, I., C. G. Victora, J. Martines, H. Goncalves, D. P. Gigante, N. J. Valle, and G. Pelto. 2001. "Nutrition Counselling Increases Weight Gain among Brazilian Children." *Journal of Nutrition* 131 (11): 2966–73.

Schellenberg, J. R., S. Abdulla, R. Nathan, O. Mukasa, T. J. Marchant, N. Kikumbih, and others. 2001. "Effect of Large-Scale Social Marketing of Insecticide-Treated Nets on Child Survival in Rural Tanzania." *Lancet* 357 (9264): 1241–47.

Sen, A. 2002. "Why Health Equity?" *Health Economics* 11 (8): 659–66.

Slack, K., and W. D. Savedoff. 2001. "Public Purchaser–Private Provider Contracting for Health Services: Examples from Latin America and the Caribbean." Sustainable Development Department Technical Paper 111, Inter-American Development Bank, Washington, DC.

Soucat, A., W. Van Lerberghe, F. Diop, S. Nguyen, and R. Knippenberg. 2002. "Marginal Budgeting for Bottlenecks: A New Costing and Reallocation Practice to Buy Health Results." World Bank, Washington, DC.

———. 2004. "Marginal Budgeting for Bottlenecks: A New Costing and Resource Allocation Practice to Buy Health Results—Using Health Sector's Budget Expansion to Progress toward the Millennium Development Goals in Sub-Saharan Africa." Unpublished paper. World Bank, Washington, DC.

Task Force on Health Systems Research. 2004. "Informed Choices for Attaining the Millennium Development Goals: Towards a Cooperative Agenda for Health Systems Research." *Lancet* 364: 997–1003.

UNAIDS (United Nations Joint Programme on HIV/AIDS). 2004. *Report on the Global AIDS Epidemic.* Geneva: UNAIDS.

UNICEF (United Nations Children's Fund). 2001. *Progress since the World Summit for Children: A Statistical Review.* New York: UNICEF.

Victora, C., F. Barros, J. Vaughan, A. Silva, and E. Tomasi. 2000. "Explaining Trends in Inequities: Evidence from Brazilian Child Health Studies." *Lancet* 356 (9235):1093–38.

Wagstaff, A., and M. Claeson. 2004. *The Millennium Development Goals for Health: Rising to the Challenges.* Washington, DC: World Bank.

———. 2005. "The Millennium Development Goals for Health: Rising to the Challenges: Appendix A, pp. 169–174." World Bank. Washington, DC.

Wagstaff, A., and E. van Doorslaer. 2003. "Catastrophe and Impoverishment in Paying for Health Care: with Applications to Vietnam 1993–1998." *Health Economics* 12 (11): 921–34.

World Bank. 1998. *Assessing Aid: What Works, What Doesn't, and Why.* Oxford, U.K.: Oxford University Press.

———. 2000. *World Development Report 2000/2001: Attacking Poverty.* New York: Oxford University Press.

———. 2001. "Health, Nutrition, and Population Development Goals: Measuring Progress Using the Poverty Reduction Strategy Framework." Report of a World Bank Consultation, World Bank, Washington, DC.

———. 2003a. *Attaining the Millennium Development Goals in India: How Likely and What Will It Take?* Washington, DC: World Bank.

———. 2003b. *Global Economic Prospects and the Developing Countries.* Washington, DC: World Bank.

———. 2003c. *World Development Indicators 2003.* Washington, DC: World Bank.

———. 2003d. *World Development Report 2004: Making Services Work for Poor People.* Washington, DC: World Bank.

Yip, W., and P. Berman. 2001. "Targeted Health Insurance in a Low Income Country and Its Impact on Access and Equity in Access: Egypt's School Health Insurance." *Health Economics* 10 (3): 207–20.

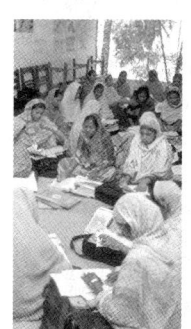

Chapter **10**

Gender Differentials in Health

Mayra Buvinić, André Médici, Elisa Fernández,
and Ana Cristina Torres

In health, more than in other social sectors, sex (biological) and gender (behavioral and social) variables are acknowledged useful parameters for research and action because biological differences between the sexes determine male-specific and female-specific diseases and because behavioral differences between the genders assign a critical role to women in relation to family health. Until recently, however, the importance of sex and gender informed work on female-specific diseases but did not carry over to diseases shared by men and women. As a result, the literature contained comparatively little about which diseases affect men and women differently, why that difference might be the case, and how to structure prevention and treatment in response to these differences. This situation has changed, however, and interest in measuring, understanding, and responding to sex and gender differentials in disease has surged, nurtured by breakthroughs in science and advances in advocacy.[1]

In line with this interest and using global burden-of-disease data for 2001, this chapter reviews worldwide gender differentials in mortality and morbidity that result in excess disease burdens for women and examines cost-effective interventions drawn from chapters 17 (on sexually transmitted infections), 26 (on maternal and perinatal conditions), 29 (on health service interventions for cancer control in developing countries), 31 (on mental disorders), 32 (on neurological disorders), 51 (on musculoskeletal disability and rehabilitation), and 57 (on contraception) to address them.

The focus on women's excess disease burden is justified to fill gaps in knowledge regarding women's health that are in part a product of male bias and male norms in clinical studies. In the past, medical research often wrongly assumed that women were biologically weaker (male bias) and extrapolated findings from trials with male subjects only (male norm) to both sexes, whereas female biology can affect the onset and progression of disease, and women's lower position in society can affect their health-seeking behaviors (Pinn 2003; Sen, George, and Ostlin 2002).

As A. K. Sen (1990) and others have indicated, gender bias results in the neglect of female children and in selective abortion and excess female mortality in China, India, and other South Asian countries, explaining the "missing" women in population counts. In addition, such bias can have intergenerational health effects, starting with maternal undernutrition and leading to fetal growth retardation, low birthweight, child undernutrition, and ailments in adult children of disadvantaged mothers (Osmania and Sen 2003).

This chapter only partially addresses women's health needs. It omits important disease conditions for women, such as lung cancer and HIV/AIDS, where men and women currently have similar disease burdens. (In the case of HIV/AIDS this balance is changing, and women's disease burden is rising over men's, especially for the 18–25 age group and for specific world regions.) It also does not cover important sources of the disease burden for women that are not measured in disability-adjusted life years (DALYs), such as burden from female genital mutilation (FGM). Last, the emphasis on disease underplays women's reproductive and other health needs.

ANTECEDENTS

The chapter's emphasis on gender differentials and inequalities in health rather than on women's absolute health conditions reflects the evolution of thinking on women and health issues.

(Annex 10.A charts these advances in the past two decades, highlighting milestones and influential publications.) In the 1960s and 1970s, the field of international women's health issues emerged from and was influenced by an interest in women's fertility behavior as a means of curbing population growth and by an interest in maternal and child health to improve child welfare, with little or no attention paid to mothers (McNamara 1981; Rosenfield and Maine 1985). Much of the work in the 1980s sought to bring a woman-centered perspective into population and maternal and child health programs. This focus included awareness of how women's lower status in society affected health delivery and health-seeking behaviors and how women's time burdens in poor households affected child health. The issues raised included the quality of care in health and family-planning programs and the nature of women's work and its impact on child survival and health (Bruce 1990; Leslie 1988). Reducing maternal mortality became a major development objective (Herz and Measham 1987).

The 1994 United Nations International Conference on Population and Development in Cairo placed women's reproductive health and rights at the center of the population and development debate, and the United Nations Women's Conference in Beijing the following year reinforced the importance of women's empowerment and of a gender perspective in health. Along with the global burden-of-disease effort, researchers estimated the loss of women's healthy years of life caused by gender violence (Heise, Pitanguy, and Germain 1994), and gender was identified as central to women's risk of and treatment for HIV/AIDS (Gupta 2000; Mann 1993). The World Health Organization analyzed how differences between women and men in access to and control over resources determine differential exposure to risk and access to the benefits of health technology and care (WHO 1998). After more than two decades almost solely devoted to maternal and reproductive health issues, attention expanded to cover a range of women's health issues unrelated to reproduction and to identify and correct gender differentials and inequities in health (Sen, George, and Ostlin 2002). These new emphases complemented renewed interest in health inequities and their reduction in the field of international health (see, for instance, Evans and others 2001).

Framework

Both sex and gender matter in health. We use the term *sex* to describe differences between men and women that are primarily biological in origin and that may be genetic or phenotypic. By contrast, we use the term *gender* to describe differences that are primarily caused by social conditions or cultural and religious beliefs and norms regarding the sexes. Structural gender inequalities that place women in a subordinate position to men underlie and contribute to gender differentials in disease (Sen, George, and Ostlin 2002). A gender perspective addresses differences between men's health and women's health that arise from this lower position and the consequent unequal power relationship between the sexes. Sex and gender can act alone, independently, or interactively in determining differentials in the burden of disease (Krieger 2003). Some women's excess health burdens, such as uterine cancer, are based almost solely on biology. At the other end of the continuum, some women's excess health burdens, such as injuries from domestic fires or domestic abuse, are solely gender based.

However, in most cases sex and gender interact to determine women's disease burdens. Two salient examples are depressive disorders and HIV/AIDS. Women are twice as likely as men to become depressed, and genetics and hormones influence the risk of depression. However, genes and sex hormones cannot entirely explain women's excess burdens, and gender factors play an important role (WHO 2000). HIV infection rates among teenage girls are 5 to 16 times higher than among teenage boys in Sub-Saharan Africa. This earlier age of HIV exposure for girls is partly explained by the greater biological efficiency of male-to-female transmission and partly by girls' lack of knowledge, opportunities, and bargaining power in sexual relations that make them prime victims of the rapid spread of the disease.

Existing knowledge about the interplay between sex and gender in determining disease is imperfect and evolving (Krieger 2003; Pinn 2003). This chapter groups women's excess health burdens from diseases into the following four broad categories:

- diseases specific to women (that is, where biology plays a major role in the disease)
- diseases related to women's average greater longevity (where both sex and gender tend to play important roles)
- diseases that result from the interaction of sex and gender
- diseases that are predominantly gender based (that is, that result from specific behavioral, social, and cultural factors associated with women's condition).

Sex and gender have a much wider influence on disease than is usually acknowledged. They influence the etiology, diagnosis, progression, prevention, treatment, and health outcomes of disease as well as health-seeking behaviors and exposure to risk. Whereas sex plays a bigger role in the etiology, onset, and progression of disease, gender and its consequences influence differential risks, symptom recognition, severity of disease, access to and quality of care, and compliance with care. In addition, poverty and social exclusion because of race and ethnicity interact with sex and gender and contribute to women's excess disease burdens in ways that are largely unexplored to date (Breen 2002).

Factors that influence gender differentials in relation to the risk of disease include (a) biological (genetic, physiological, and hormonal) differences between the sexes; (b) women's longer life expectancy; (c) nature and rate of change of women's labor force participation compared with men's participation; (d) women's differential access to social protection mechanisms (health and social insurance); (e) cultural norms, religious beliefs, and family arrangements and behaviors determining gender roles and gender hierarchy in society; (f) gender differences in educational attainment; (g) income differences between the genders resulting from the interaction of all the previous factors; and (h) interactions between race, ethnicity, income, and gender.

Women's overall underutilization of health services has been well documented. For instance, even though women in India report more illness than men, hospital records show that men receive more treatment (World Bank 1996); in Thailand, men are six times more likely than women to seek clinical treatment for malaria, a disease that affects women and men similarly (Hanson 2002); and in Brazil, the Dominican Republic, Jamaica, Paraguay, and Peru, low-income women underuse health services (Levine, Glassman, and Schneidman 2001).

Three groups of factors influence this underuse of health services. The first group is service factors, such as accessibility; affordability (money and time costs); and appropriateness or adequacy, including friendliness, of the health and social infrastructure for meeting women's needs. The second group is user factors, which include social constraints, such as restrictions on women's mobility and women's average lower incomes and greater time burdens than men's; asymmetric information about health needs and rights and the availability of services, which disproportionately affects poor women; and marital status, family roles, and work conditions affecting access and use. The third group is institutional factors, including men's decision-making power and control over health budgets and facilities, which affect local perceptions of illness and norms concerning treatment, and stigmatization and discrimination in health settings, which affect women among the poor and women of minority ethnic and racial groups.

Context

The global demographic dynamic, a product of the interplay of nature and nurture, biology and society, helps determine gender differentials in health. In 2001, the world's population, an estimated 6.2 billion, was 50.3 percent male and 49.7 percent female. The surplus male population was concentrated in the developing countries, whereas the developed countries had a higher proportion of women, primarily in the older age groups (WHO 2001).

In the developed countries, the number of women age 80 and older was more than double the number of men in the same age group. This female advantage in longevity helps shape a gender paradox in health outcomes worldwide: on average,

males live shorter but healthier lives than females. Even though more boys are born than girls, gender differences in mortality eventually change the sex balance in populations so that by age 30 or so women start outliving men, and the absolute female advantage in survivability increases with age (Kinsella and Gist 1998). Therefore, differences in life expectancy at birth by gender, using 2000 data, vary in favor of females, ranging from one year in the low-income countries of South Asia and Sub-Saharan Africa to seven years in Europe and Central Asia and nine years in the middle-income countries of Latin America and the Caribbean.

Overall, however, women have higher morbidity than men. Murray and Evans (2003) find that in relation to expected lost healthy years at birth, whereas men lose 7.8 years over their lifetimes as a result of poor health, women lose 10.2 years. In other words, women spend about 15 percent of their lives in unhealthy conditions and men spend just 12 percent. Therefore, living longer lives should not be taken to indicate better health for women. Women live less healthy lives and are saddled with higher morbidity in part because they outlive men (Verbrugge 1989). Supporting the less healthy lives assertion, women up to age 65 reported worse health status in virtually all 64 household surveys from 46 countries (Sadana and others 2000). Because of these differences in morbidity, the concept of healthy adjusted life expectancy at birth describes differences in health conditions between males and females better than the concept of life expectancy at birth.

GENDER DIFFERENTIALS IN DISEASE BURDENS

The global burden of disease for 2001 proportionally affects males slightly more than females. About 52 percent of DALY losses are attributed to males, but this proportion varies between 54.8 percent in Europe and Central Asia and 49.9 percent in South Asia. The only region where the global burden of disease affects females more than males is South Asia.

Table 10.1 shows the burden of disease by region, gender, and age group. The burden of disease during early childhood (age 0 through 4) is somewhat smaller for girls than boys; however, from age 5 through 29, females lose more DALYs than males, but only in developing countries. Larger differences favoring women appear starting at age 30 and continue until after the age of 70, when women, because of their greater longevity, lose more DALYs than men. However, when DALYs are estimated per 1,000 males and females as in table 10.1, women in the older age groups lose fewer DALYs than men both in low- and middle-income countries (LMICs) and in high-income countries (HICs).

Communicable diseases and maternal conditions contribute significantly to females' burden of disease in developing countries and add little to their burden in HICs, where

Table 10.1 DALYs by Region, Gender, and Age Group, 2001
(DALYs per 1,000 population)

Region	0–4	5–14	15–29	30–44	45–59	60–69	70–79	80+	Total
Males									
Low- and middle-income countries	754.6	75.4	137.4	194.5	349.3	600.1	799.4	950.8	271.5
East Asia and the Pacific	408.0	46.5	99.6	124.2	276.4	522.8	735.3	965.1	192.6
Europe and Central Asia	345.4	50.1	137.9	220.8	412.8	695.6	855.3	952.5	278.3
Latin America and the Caribbean	449.1	56.7	155.0	173.2	290.4	493.2	682.6	870.8	217.8
Middle East and North Africa	585.6	67.5	109.3	151.4	337.8	608.5	825.8	1,019.8	219.8
South Asia	805.2	83.0	131.9	196.0	383.0	661.7	861.7	899.6	285.1
Sub-Saharan Africa	1,480.7	142.2	248.2	532.2	609.0	778.6	1,002.5	1,194.3	528.6
High-income countries	128.2	28.6	84.4	97.0	189.6	355.7	541.5	721.5	168.2
World	698.5	70.9	131.1	178.5	315.4	540.4	721.0	856.7	256.3
Females									
Low- and middle-income countries	753.4	78.5	142.5	162.1	275.3	501.3	745.4	946.7	259.8
East Asia and the Pacific	434.9	47.1	86.2	103.4	225.7	442.9	699.5	966.8	182.1
Europe and Central Asia	303.6	39.1	87.0	117.7	223.6	423.7	663.2	909.6	212.5
Latin America and the Caribbean	395.8	51.1	101.8	120.5	222.3	423.8	604.9	827.6	179.0
Middle East and North Africa	538.0	62.7	103.6	140.6	278.3	509.2	767.6	1,069.1	203.3
South Asia	865.5	98.3	168.7	188.5	334.0	616.6	901.0	938.3	304.4
Sub-Saharan Africa	1,367.4	138.7	317.3	448.9	478.8	701.4	1,009.8	1,196.5	504.3
High-income countries	117.5	28.9	72.5	77.7	144.8	258.4	414.6	625.9	153.3
World	696.5	73.7	134.2	148.1	247.2	441.6	641.0	800.0	243.4

Source: WHO 2001.

noncommunicable diseases prevail in both women's and men's disease burden. Injuries weigh more heavily in males' than in females' burden of disease across regions. In summary, in both developed and developing countries, the overall burden of disease is higher for males than for females; however, this situation reverses in developing countries for young girls and women in their prime childbearing years. In addition, in LMICs, females are more affected than males by highly preventable communicable diseases.

WOMEN'S EXCESS DISEASE BURDENS

The 2001 global burden-of-disease data underestimate both women's and men's disease burdens because of the incompleteness of health statistics, especially in the developing world. This underestimation is probably more pronounced for women because they experience more disability—which is less well recorded than mortality—than men. This underestimation is aggravated by underreporting resulting from the stigma associated with certain diseases in women, such as sexual infections;

the prevalence of asymptomatic illness, such as sexually transmitted infections among women; the differences in health-seeking behaviors that favor males accessing formal health care, which is the main source for health statistics; and the exclusion of some conditions that affect only women, such as FGM, from global burden-of-disease estimations (Hanson 2002). Thus, the findings in the preceding section may be affected by a quality problem, and the estimates in this section are probably conservative.

Table 10.2 breaks down 11 conditions specific to women by region. In 2001, conditions specific to women accounted for 5.3 percent of women's total DALY losses, compared with 0.7 percent for two conditions (prostate cancer and benign prostate hypertrophy) specific to men.[2] Most causes of mortality or morbidity specific to women are related to maternal conditions and malignant neoplasms. The DALY losses associated with conditions specific to women are around 6 percent in both HICs and LMICs, but maternal conditions are more prevalent in LMICs, whereas neoplasms cause more DALY losses in HICs.

Table 10.2 Percentage of DALYs Resulting from Conditions Specific to Women by Region, 2001

Condition	HICs	LMICs	East Asia and the Pacific	Europe and Central Asia	Latin America and the Caribbean	Middle East and North Africa	South Asia	Sub-Saharan Africa	World
Maternal	0.5	4.0	2.0	0.8	2.5	4.1	4.9	5.7	2.8
Maternal hemorrhage	0.0	0.6	0.2	0.0	0.2	0.4	0.8	1.0	0.5
Maternal sepsis	0.1	0.8	0.5	0.2	0.7	0.7	0.9	1.1	0.7
Hypertensive disorders[a]	0.0	0.3	0.1	0.0	0.2	0.2	0.4	0.5	0.3
Obstructed labor	0.0	0.4	0.1	0.0	0.1	0.3	0.6	0.5	0.3
Abortion	0.0	0.5	0.1	0.0	0.2	0.5	0.7	0.9	0.5
Other	0.4	1.4	1.0	0.6	1.3	2.0	1.5	1.7	0.5
Neoplasms	5.5	1.7	1.8	4.1	3.1	1.4	1.5	0.8	2.2
Breast cancer[b]	3.4	0.8	1.0	2.0	1.3	0.9	0.6	0.3	1.1
Cervix uteri cancer	0.4	0.6	0.5	0.7	1.0	0.3	0.7	0.4	0.6
Corpus uteri cancer	0.8	0.1	0.1	0.7	0.5	0.1	0.0	0.0	0.2
Ovarian cancer	0.9	0.2	0.3	0.7	0.3	0.1	0.2	0.1	0.3
Chlamydia[b]	0.1	0.3	0.2	0.2	0.4	0.5	0.4	0.3	0.3
Total	6.1	6.0	4.0	5.1	6.0	6.0	6.8	6.8	5.3

Source: WHO 2001.
a. Related to maternal conditions only.
b. Even though these conditions are not specific to women, women account for more than 90 percent of the DALY losses associated with these conditions.

Table 10.3 shows the gender ratio and burden of disease of eight conditions, by region, that are more prevalent among women than among men. The selection of diseases was done using as the threshold the mean plus one standard deviation (SD) of the distribution of gender ratio scores for each disease. The diseases selected were then screened for their importance in women's disease burden, using the same criterion of the mean plus one SD in the distribution of DALY scores for women. Although some diseases, such as unipolar depressive disorders and osteoarthritis, are priorities for both HICs and LMICs, others, such as Alzheimer's disease, are more relevant in HICs, reflecting women's longer life expectancy. Conditions such as age-related vision disorders, migraine, fires, and cerebrovascular diseases have particular relevance in specific regions.

Combining gender-specific conditions and shared conditions that disproportionately affect women gives a total of 19 priority conditions for women. Taken together, these conditions represent about one-fifth of women's total DALY losses and indicate priorities for research and the search for cost-effective methods of promotion, prevention, and treatment. Note that some important contributors to females' health burdens, such as malaria and HIV/AIDS, have been omitted because females do not currently suffer disproportionately from these diseases. However, the growing feminization of the HIV/AIDS epidemic in developing countries should result in excess disease burdens for women in the near future.

We determined priority conditions affecting females in different age groups using a method that took into account both the gender ratio and the weight of specific conditions in females' total DALYs lost. The results indicate that women are affected by communicable diseases and maternal conditions until age 29 and by noncommunicable diseases after age 30, with chronic diseases having a heavy weight during the last stages of the life cycle. Conditions for which females' burden of disease is more or less double that of males at a specific stage in the life cycle are migraine at age 5 to 14, fires and panic disorder at age 15 to 29, and unipolar depressive disorders at age 60 to 69.

PRIORITY DISEASE GROUPS FOR WOMEN

Table 10.4 presents conditions with excess burdens for women divided into the four groups defined earlier.

Conditions Specific to Women

In developed countries, advances in medical technology have almost eliminated the burden of disease resulting from maternal conditions. Three types of cost-effective intervention packages for maternal conditions are the prevention of pregnancy by means of effective family-planning methods; the prevention of complications (for example, hemorrhage); and the prevention

Table 10.3 Gender Ratio and Women's Excess Burden of Disease for Top Priority Conditions by Region, 2001

Condition	World		LMICs		HICs		East Asia and the Pacific		Europe and Central Asia		Latin American and the Caribbean		Middle East and North Africa		South Asia		Sub-Saharan Africa	
	GR	BOD (percent)	GR	BOD (percent)	GR	BOD (percent)	GR	BOD (percent)	GR	BOD (percent)	GR	BOD (percent)	GR	BOD (percent)	GR	BOD (percent)	GR	BOD (percent)
Alzheimer's disease and other dementias	1.81	1.48	n.a.	n.a.	2.13	7.02	1.55	1.51	2.40	2.16	1.63	1.58	n.a.	n.a.	n.a.	n.a.	n.a.	n.a.
Osteoarthritis	1.64	1.46	1.63	1.26	1.71	3.30	1.64	2.15	1.76	2.76	n.a.	n.a.	n.a.	n.a.	n.a.	n.a.	n.a.	n.a.
Unipolar depressive disorders	1.53	4.22	1.51	3.89	1.69	7.30	n.a.	n.a.	1.73	5.15	1.72	6.94	1.44	3.86	1.56	4.33	1.54	1.17
Age-related vision disorders	n.a.	n.a.	n.a.	n.a.	n.a.	n.a.	n.a.	n.a.	1.63	2.10	n.a.	n.a.	n.a.	n.a.	n.a.	n.a.	n.a.	n.a.
Migraine	n.a.	n.a.	n.a.	n.a.	n.a.	n.a.	n.a.	n.a.	n.a.	n.a.	2.81	1.14	n.a.	n.a.	n.a.	n.a.	n.a.	n.a.
Other cardiovascular diseases	n.a.	n.a.	n.a.	n.a.	n.a.	n.a.	n.a.	n.a.	n.a.	n.a.	n.a.	n.a.	1.45	3.20	n.a.	n.a.	n.a.	n.a.
Fires	n.a.	n.a.	n.a.	n.a.	n.a.	n.a.	n.a.	n.a.	n.a.	n.a.	n.a.	n.a.	n.a.	n.a.	2.43	2.04	n.a.	n.a.
Cerebrovascular diseases	n.a.	n.a.	n.a.	n.a.	n.a.	n.a.	n.a.	n.a.	n.a.	n.a.	n.a.	n.a.	n.a.	n.a.	n.a.	n.a.	1.47	1.80

Source: WHO 2001.

n.a. = not applicable; BOD = burden of disease; GR = gender ratio.

Note: The gender ratio is the ratio of female to male DALYs.

For each world region or classification, data are shown only for those diseases that are classified as "priority" given that they meet the selection criteria according to the methodology used in this study (that is, the gender ratio was equal to or higher than the mean plus one SD of the distribution of gender ratio scores, and in a second screening, the BOD was equal to or higher than the mean plus one SD of the distribution of female DALY scores).

Table 10.4 Priority Conditions by Category, 2001

Category and condition	Gender ratio	Region where gender ratio is apparent
Conditions specific to women		
Maternal hemorrhage	n.a.	n.a.
Maternal sepsis	n.a.	n.a.
Hypertensive disorders related to maternal conditions	n.a.	n.a.
Obstructed labor	n.a.	n.a.
Abortion	n.a.	n.a.
Other maternal conditions	n.a.	n.a.
Breast cancer	244.62	World
Cervix uteri cancer	n.a.	n.a.
Corpus uteri cancer	n.a.	n.a.
Ovarian cancer	n.a.	n.a.
Chlamydia	9.76	World
Conditions associated with women's greater longevity		
Alzheimer's disease and other dementias	1.81	World
Osteoarthritis	1.64	World
Cerebrovascular diseases	1.47	Sub-Saharan Africa
Other cardiovascular diseases	1.45	Middle East and North Africa
Age-related vision disorders	1.63	Europe and Central Asia
Conditions arising from the interaction of sex and gender		
Unipolar depressive disorders	1.53	World
Migraine	2.81	Latin America and the Caribbean
Gender-based conditions		
Fires	2.43	South Asia

Source: WHO 2001.
n.a. = not applicable.

of death or disability resulting from complications through emergency obstetric care. Proven technologies also exist for screening and early detection of some neoplasms, although their implementation has been uneven. Problems pertaining to conditions in this category are not simply related to the availability of medical technologies, but also to the behavioral and social factors that influence women's exposure to risks and underuse of services as well as the economic and institutional factors that influence the availability and quality of services, especially in developing countries.

Even though the international women's health movement has promoted significant advances in the quality of care for reproductive health and maternal conditions in the past 25 years, the main challenges in relation to conditions specific to women include reaching poor and socially excluded women with basic maternal and reproductive health services; strengthening the adoption of preventive health behaviors in developing countries; extending the quality of care to other conditions specific to women, including neoplasms; and educating and empowering women to promote their own healthy behaviors.

Conditions Associated with Women's Greater Longevity

The main group of diseases with excess burdens for women associated with women's greater longevity are Alzheimer's disease; musculoskeletal disorders, such as osteoarthritis, rheumatoid arthritis, and osteoporosis; and cardiovascular diseases,[3] which together account for 12 percent of total DALY losses for women worldwide. LMICs account for about 80 percent of the DALYs resulting from these conditions, likely because of the lack of medical care during the early stages of these diseases.

Alzheimer's disease and other dementias account for 1.5 percent of total female DALYs, and this burden is almost twice as high as that for men. About 46 percent of this burden is concentrated in HICs and 54 percent in LMICs, but DALYs lost per capita are much greater in the HICs than in more densely populated LMICs. Because of population aging, during the next 50 years the number of people with Alzheimer's disease is expected to more than double, with more women affected than men (McCann and others 1997). Studies of the effects of estrogen therapy on Alzheimer's disease have been inconsistent: estrogen may increase the risk of both dementia and other diseases such as stroke in postmenopausal women (Shumaker and others 2003).

As concerns musculoskeletal disorders, osteoarthritis affects 9.6 percent of men and 18.0 percent of women age 60 or older worldwide and accounts for 1.5 percent of total female DALYs. Osteoarthritis is related to aging and is most common in overweight women over the age of 45. Demographic changes in developing countries, especially middle-income countries, indicate that osteoarthritis prevention and treatment needs will increase during the next decade. Most prevention and treatment are linked to regular exercise, healthy weight management, physical and occupational therapy, and pain management with over-the-counter medications.

Because cardiovascular diseases are generally thought of by society as "men's diseases," women tend to delay seeking treatment for cardiac-related events (Seils, Friedman, and Schulman 2001). However, cardiovascular and cerebrovascular diseases account for about 8.2 percent of total female DALYs, more than half of which is caused by cerebrovascular diseases.

In addition to age, smoking, and obesity, another risk factor that exposes women to a greater burden of cardiovascular diseases is depression, which is associated with increased morbidity and mortality from heart diseases and is highly prevalent in women (Linfante and others 2003). Also, women's symptoms of heart disease tend to be different from men's, increasing the difficulties of diagnosis (Seils, Friedman, and Schulman 2001). Finally, evidence suggests that physical activity significantly reduces the risk of cardiovascular events; however, women tend to exercise less than men (Manson and others 2002). Whether this observation can be generalized to all age groups and whether it occurs because of biological factors or social norms deserve further attention.

Conditions Arising from the Interaction of Sex and Gender

In the group of conditions resulting from the interaction of biological and social factors, unipolar depressive disorders have the most significant gender ratio and most unequal burden of disease in every region except East Asia and the Pacific. Unipolar depressive disorders account for 4.2 percent of women's global burden of disease. Even though the DALYs lost per capita are similar in LMICs and HICs, these disorders represent a higher share of women's total burden of disease in HICs (7.3 percent) than in LMICs (3.9 percent). Another important consideration is the high comorbidity between depression and other psychiatric disorders (for example, anxiety disorders). Neuropsychiatric disorders account for 11.8 percent of women's total global burden of disease and 23.5 percent in HICs.

The exact contributions of biology and society in the etiology of depression are unknown. Some believe that genetic causes account for about half of the risk for mood disorders (Zubenko and others 2002), whereas others suggest that gender roles, stressors, social relationships, and personality traits may play a larger role than hormones and neurotransmitters (Bromberger 2004). As concerns biology, aside from genetic predisposition, the fluctuation of sex hormones, especially estrogen, during women's reproductive life is believed to be an important risk factor for depression (Bromberger 2004). As concerns social factors, poverty; lack of proper nutrition and education; stressful and insecure life circumstances; and domestic and sexual violence and the concomitant feelings of loss, entrapment, and lack of control are likely at the root of depression (Bromberger 2004; WHO 2000).

Treatment for depression includes medication and psychotherapy or counseling, and instruments are available to assess the severity of depression, including prenatal and postpartum depression. In developing countries, severe depression and anxiety disorders go mostly untreated (76 to 85 percent of serious cases receive no treatment), partly because of ignorance, social barriers, and stigmatization, which may affect women's access to treatment (WHO 2004). A main challenge, therefore, is increasing women's access to treatment for depression in developing countries by creating systems that help them overcome social stigma and economic and social barriers.

In addition to treatment, prevention of depression and other mental illness needs to address women's role in society and the control they have over their lives and circumstances. According to the World Health Organization, pertinent factors are related to having sufficient autonomy to exercise some control in response to severe events, access to adequate resources to be able to make choices, and social supports (WHO 2000). The promotion of healthy behaviors, including exercise, is also crucial for prevention.

Gender-Based Conditions

The main characteristic of gender-based conditions is that they have no biological referent and can, therefore, be prevented by means of behavioral change. The role of social components in this category explains excessive health burdens for women in particular world regions. For example, women are disproportionately affected by fires in South Asia, an outcome of the violence caused by dowries. Too often women die in what are called "cooking fire accidents," whereas in reality they are murdered so that their husbands may remarry and obtain another dowry.

Another characteristic of the diseases and injuries in this category is that they are often underreported because of stigma and social pressures. As a result, the data probably underreport the true extent of the problem. FGM and domestic violence are two examples. In 2000, estimates indicated that 100 million to 140 million girls and women had undergone FGM and that more than 2 million girls were at risk. At least 28 African and Middle Eastern countries practice FGM for social, cultural, or religious reasons (WHO 2000). Unfortunately, global burden-of-disease data do not report the resulting DALYs lost. Regarding violence against women, 10 to 50 percent of women report having been physically abused by an intimate partner, and 12 to 25 percent report attempted or completed forced sex. Although men experience more absolute DALY losses from violence, women are also seriously affected. In 1998, interpersonal violence was the 10th-leading cause of death for women age 15 to 44 worldwide.

Given the complexity of these health problems, comprehensive interventions are necessary. Changes are needed in the following areas:

- legislation and law enforcement
- public policies and programs in areas such as health, education, and police and legal services
- training of service providers and creation of gender-sensitive services, especially at the community level

- education of the general public to create awareness, behavioral change, and promotion of advocacy groups
- better data collection, research, and understanding of the individual and social mechanisms sustaining these problems.

COST-EFFECTIVENESS OF INTERVENTIONS

This section summarizes the costs and health benefits of strategies to address conditions that are specific to women and conditions that affect women disproportionately. Table 10.5 presents cost-effectiveness estimates for recognized effective interventions.

Conditions Specific to Women

Conditions specific to women include the cluster of diseases related to women's maternal function plus chlamydia (which is predominantly but not exclusively a female disease) and female-specific cancers.

Maternal Conditions. The analysis developed in chapter 26 uses a model for maternal and perinatal conditions that generates 128 potential scenarios. According to the findings of this theoretical exercise, the cost per DALY averted of mother and baby packages could vary from US$77 to US$151 in Sub-Saharan Africa and from US$143 to US$278 in South Asia, depending on the complexity of the intervention.

Prenatal care prevents almost a quarter of maternal deaths, especially when backed by essential and emergency obstetric care to deal with conditions detected during the course of pregnancy care. Good prenatal care includes information, education, and communication activities and behavior-change communication to increase women's skills in relation to the identification of danger signs and potential complications and where to seek care in these cases (Dayaratna and others 2000). In Uganda, for example, integral prenatal care ranged from US$2.26 (public services) to US$6.43 (religious mission services) per pregnant woman per year (Levin and others 1999).

Another important service is supplementation with iron and folic acid. Iron deficiency accounts for 1.8 percent of women's deaths and 2.6 percent of female DALY losses. Iron and folic acid supplements administered to highly anemic pregnant women can save lives at a cost of US$13 per DALY averted (Berman and others 1991), demonstrating that this intervention is very cost-effective.

Good maternal health services can strengthen the entire health system. A health facility that is equipped to provide essential obstetric care can also treat accidents, trauma, and other medical emergencies. The costs of emergency obstetric care vary depending on the country. In Uganda, costs per

episode vary from US$73 (public hospital) to US$86 (mission hospital) (Levin and others 1999). In Bolivia, the cost of a cesarean section ranges from US$56 to US$104 (Rosenthal and Percy 1991), and the cost of a normal delivery varies from US$11 to US$16 (Dmytraczenko and others 1998).

In developing countries, 61 percent of maternal deaths occur 23 to 48 hours after delivery because of such problems as postpartum hemorrhage and hypertensive disorders or after 48 hours because of sepsis. Complications from unsafe abortions account for 13 percent of maternal deaths, though this figure is probably an underestimate because of the scarcity of data. Little information is available on costs related to postnatal care given the different kind of interventions and the severity of cases, but the literature generally agrees that emergency obstetric care can reduce costs. As concerns postabortion care, costs per case in LMICs could vary from US$4.40 to US$17.19 (Dayaratna and others 2000).

Millions of premature deaths, illnesses, and injuries could be avoided by helping women prevent unwanted pregnancies and obtain prompt treatment for reproductive health problems. The contraception costs per couple-year of protection could vary, depending on the method used, from US$6 (intrauterine device) to US$20 (condoms or injections) (Dayaratna and others 2000). A 1999 experiment by the Planned Parenthood Association of South Africa considered total health planning costs per couple-year of protection, including travel expenses to health clinics. Comparing these costs with total health planning costs in services provided by community-based doctors, the study found that the former cost US$44 per couple-year of protection and the latter cost US$42.

Chlamydia. Although not specific to women, chlamydia is nine times more prevalent among women than among men, and its consequences and treatment are much more complicated and severe for women, affecting women's and infants' health during pregnancy and the postnatal period. Chlamydia is widespread in low-income countries. Chlamydia, as well as other sexually transmitted diseases, could be prevented by using condoms, with an average cost per DALY averted in developing countries estimated at US$3.40 in noncore target groups and US$12.60 in core target groups (Mumford and others 1998). Detecting chlamydia in pregnant women could cost $4.38 per case, with treatment, at $3.82 per case, being less expensive than detection (Shultz, Schulte and Berman 1992). Chlamydia's adverse effects are trachoma (chronic conjunctivitis, endemic in Africa and Asia), reproductive tract infections, genital ulcer disease in tropical countries, and infertility. The cost of each adverse outcome averted varies from about US$85 to US$308 (Shultz, Schulte, and Berman 1992).

Neoplasms. Cancers specific to women are responsible for high levels of female morbidity and mortality, with cervical

Table 10.5 Cost-Effectiveness of Selected Interventions Aimed at Conditions Specific to Women or That Affect Women Disproportionately

Intervention	Region or country	Lower end of range	Upper end of range	Source
Maternal conditions				
Mother and baby package	LMICs	US$2 per capita	US$4 per capita	WHO 1997
Mother and baby package	LMICs	US$18 per DALY averted	US$58 per DALY averted	Raviez, Griffin, and Follmer 1995; World Bank 1993
Mother and baby package	Sub-Saharan Africa	US$77 per DALY averted	US$151 per DALY averted	Chapter 26 of this publication
Mother and baby package	South Asia	US$143 per DALY averted	US$278 per DALY averted	Chapter 26 of this publication
Integral prenatal care	Uganda	US$2.26 per pregnant woman	US$6.43 per pregnant woman	Levin and others 1999
Iron and folic acid nutritional supplementation	Low-income countries	US$13 per DALY averted in highly anemic pregnant women	n.a.	Berman and others 1991
Emergency obstetric care	Uganda	US$73 per episode	US$86 per episode	Levin and others 1999
Cesarean delivery	Bolivia	US$56 per case	US$104 per case	Rosenthal and Percy 1991
Normal delivery	Bolivia	US$11 per case	US$16 per case	Dmytraczenko and others 1998
Postabortion care (dilation and curettage)	LMICs	US$4.40 per case	US$17.19 per case	Dayaratna and others 2000
Total health-planning costs	South Africa	US$42 per couple-year of protection	US$44 per couple-year of protection	Dayaratna and others 2000
Chlamydia				
Prevention	Developing countries, 1990	US$47.98 per DALY averted (noncore target groups)	US$651.82 per DALY averted (core target groups)	Over and Piot 1993
Prevention (use of condoms)	Developing countries,	US$3.40 per DALY averted (noncore target groups)	US$12.60 per DALY averted (core target groups)	Mumford and others 1998
Detection	Various sites, 1992	US$4.38 per pregnant woman	n.a.	Shultz, Schulte, and Berman 1992
Treatment	Various sites, 1992	US$3.82 per pregnant woman	n.a.	Shultz, Schulte, and Berman 1992
Detection and treatment	Various sites, 1992	US$84.92 per adverse outcome averted in low-prevalence context (5 percent)	US$307.88 per adverse outcome averted in high-prevalence context (20 percent)	Shultz, Schulte, and Berman 1992
Neoplasms				
Detection of cervical cancer	Ecuador, 1996	US$2.95 per visit	US$3.51 per visit (laboratory costs)	Mumford and others 1998
	Honduras, 1991	US$5.60 per visit	US$12.89 per visit	Mumford and others 1998
	Zimbabwe, 1995	US$2.99 per visit	US$3.89 per visit	Mumford and others 1998
Cervical cytology screening	Vietnam, 2000	US$725 per discounted DALY averted	n.a.	Suba and others 2001
Cervical cytology screening	South Africa, 2000	US$39 per DALY averted	US$81 per DALY averted	Goldie and others 2001
Treatment of cervical cancer	Zimbabwe, 1994 Mexico, 1994	US$12.35 per visit US$52.51 per visit	US$95.82 per visit US$432.42 per visit	Mitchell, Littlefield, and Gutter 1997
Treatment of cervical cancer	Developed countries	US$2,384 to US$28,770 per DALY averted based on actual survival	n.a.	Rose and Lappas 2000
Treatment of cervical cancer	Developed countries	US$308 to US$3,712 per DALY averted based on estimated survival	n.a.	Rose and Lappas 2000
Treatment of ovarian cancer	Thailand, 1995	US$234.25 per case	US$472.27 per case	Tintara and Leetanapon 1995
Management of breast cancer	Brazil, 1995	US$1,667.88 per case	n.a.	Arredondo, Lockett, and Icaza 1995

Table 10.5 Continued

Intervention	Region or country	Lower end of range	Upper end of range	Source
Alzheimer's disease and other dementias				
Acetylcholinesterase inhibitors	Developed countries	US$13 per hour of caregiver time saved	n.a.	Marin and others 2003
	Developing countries	US$10 per hour of caregiver time saved	n.a.	Marin and others 2003
Osteoarthritis				
Celecoxib monotherapy	Sweden	US$1,394 per QALY	n.a.	Haglund and Svarvar 2000
Rofecoxib monotherapy	United Kingdom	US$2,184 per life year saved (result was sensitive to the use of gastrointestinal protective agents)	n.a.	Moore and others 2001
Different packages of drugs, including acetaminophen, naproxen, misoprostol, celecoxib, and rofecoxib	United States	US$2,001 to US$2,140 per QALY, depending on the drug combination	n.a.	Sigal 2002
Total hip arthroplasty	United States	US$6,893 per QALY for 85-year-old men	n.a.	Chang, Pellissier, and Hazen 1996
Knee replacement	Australia	US$6,000 per QALY		Sigal and others 2004

Source: Authors.

QALY = quality-adjusted life year.

Note: Costs are based in current U.S. dollars as presented in each study. Many studies do not present well-documented data regarding reference period of costs. To avoid mistakes on interpretation, we kept the costs in the currency informed by the authors.   n.a. indicates that information is not available.

cancer being one of the most important. Recommended strategies involve early detection and treatment. The following are the main strategies to prevent cervical cancer:

- screening and treatment performed during the same visit
- screening and treatment performed at two separate visits
- traditional three-visit intervention, in which a cytology sample is obtained during the first visit, a diagnostic colposcopy is performed for those who screened positive during the second visit, and treatment is provided at the third visit.

The data on costs associated with cervical cancer detection and treatment in developing countries are limited. In Honduras in 1991, costs per visit for cervical cancer detection varied from US$5.60 (small clinics) to US$12.90 (larger clinics) (Mumford and others 1998). Lower detection costs were found in Ecuador in 1996 (US$2.95 to US$3.51 per visit) and in Zimbabwe in 1995 (US$3.00 to US$3.90 per visit). Recent studies on cervical cancer screening in South Africa show that the two-visit method is more cost-effective than the traditional three-visit method, US$39 per DALY averted compared with US$81 (Goldie and others 2001). Studies in Vietnam found costs equivalent to US$725 per DALY averted with cytology screening (Suba and others 2001).

Regarding treatment of cervical cancer, Rose and Lappas's (2000) studies in developed countries find costs varying from US$2,384 to US$28,770 per DALY averted. Costs are lower in developing countries, ranging from US$52.51 to US$432.42 per visit in Mexico and from US$12.35 to US$95.82 per visit

in Zimbabwe. Differences in treatment costs are associated with the kinds of procedures used. How the results of cost-effectiveness studies for cervical cancer prevention and screening interventions in developed countries might translate to health care delivery settings in developing countries is not clear, but prevention could clearly play an important role.

Many studies of breast cancer prevention view diet as an important condition explaining the predisposition for breast cancer. Ministries of health in many developing countries invest in promotion and prevention, issuing communications and guidelines for early detection using self-testing as a cost-effective way to provide information. Few studies of the cost-effectiveness of different breast cancer treatments are available, especially in developing countries. One on the management of breast cancer in Brazil in 1995 showed extremely high costs of US$1,678 per death averted (Arredondo, Lockett, and Icaza 1995).

Conditions That Affect Women Disproportionately

Few studies on shared diseases that affect women disproportionately include gender-related considerations, especially in developing countries. Most literature on Alzheimer's disease, unipolar depressive disorders, and osteoarthritis presented in this section is based on studies in developed countries with no specific analysis of gender differences in relation to cost-effectiveness.

Alzheimer's Disease and Other Dementias. Alzheimer's disease is linked to genetic and other risk factors, including increasing age, positive family history of dementia, and lower levels of education. Treatment is based mostly on drugs, and the practical benefits of treatment translate mainly into reduced caregiver hours.

Some studies have found that interventions aimed at reducing caregiver stress, even providing low-dose antipsychotic medication, can be effective. However, the costs of undertaking such interventions have not been quantified; thus, their cost-effectiveness cannot be calculated. Institutional care for patients with any form of dementia is extremely limited in LMICs. The costs of setting up institutions for those with Alzheimer's disease and the costs of care are prohibitive. In this context, inexpensive, home-based care appears to be the only viable option for Alzheimer's disease patients in developing countries. These countries will therefore have to face the challenges of addressing families' needs in relation to financial and social support and caregiver training. Another issue is the tradeoff between women's income-earning opportunities and their traditional primary role as family caregivers.

Unipolar Depressive Disorders. Depression is among the most disabling and costly illnesses in the world, especially for women. Despite good short-term treatment outcomes, long-term outcomes remain disappointing. Costs associated with depression affect not just the sufferers themselves, but also their families and friends (time dedicated to caregiving); employers (payment for treatment and care, as well as for reduced productivity); and society (provision of mental health care financed by taxpayers). Most of these costs are difficult to obtain, but the consensus is that the indirect costs of depression are larger than the direct costs.

The treatment setting for depression is usually primary health care, with many kinds of episodic treatments combining old and new generations of antidepressants and psychosocial procedures. Averting depressive episodes results in average gains of up to 50 disability days per treated case per year. Studies of the factors influencing women's access to screening, prevention, and treatment for depression and the cost-effectiveness of treatment options should be a priority in developing countries.

Osteoarthritis. Despite clear evidence of a reduction in symptoms and delayed progression of osteoarthritis with weight reduction, no formal studies of cost-effectiveness are available. Education and exercise programs for osteoarthritis are available in developed countries, but such programs are unknown in developing countries. Studies of the effect of diet and physical exercise in preventing osteoarthritis in women are a priority not just in developed countries, but especially in developing countries with fiscally strapped health systems and growing elderly populations.

Acetaminophen is thought to be the most cost-effective initial treatment with drugs. In addition, some cost-effectiveness measures of using several kinds of medicines (acetaminophen, naproxen, misoprostol, celecoxib, and rofecoxib) under different conditions are available. Sigal (2002) shows that by using different combinations of medicines, treatment costs can vary from US$2,001 to US$2,140 per quality-adjusted life year, but these costs are prohibitive for developing countries.

Another treatment for osteoarthritis is synovial fluid replacement, but given the costs of this intervention, it is not currently recommended for developing regions. Surgical interventions for osteoarthritis, such as joint replacement, are most commonly performed in developed countries. Sigal and others (2004) review a number of interventions for osteoarthritis and suggest a cost per quality-adjusted life year of US$6,000 for knee replacements. In developing countries, however, the availability of surgical interventions is constrained by its costs and by the availability of surgeons qualified to perform the operation.

RESEARCH AGENDA

Health research and practice should give priority attention to the 19 conditions with excess burdens for women that this chapter has identified and clustered into four main groups, according to the interplay of sex and gender in their etiology, to improve women's health status worldwide. A number of cost-effective health technologies are available, but women are dying because these technologies are not available and accessible to all. Thus, a priority need is to deploy them more widely in developing countries. The research challenge is also urgent, given the unacceptably high disease burdens for women in developing countries and the rising numbers of older women worldwide. Research on sex and gender factors affecting women's disease burdens should give physicians new information that will increase their options in relation to diagnostic practices and drug approaches, not only for women, but also for men, thereby improving the provision of gender-appropriate health care for all.

Key general items in a research agenda to reduce women's excess disease burdens include the following:

· Expand and sharpen analyses of sex and gender and their interaction in the etiology, onset, progression, prevention, and treatment of diseases that women and men share, but where women face an excess health burden, and in the assessment of cost-effective interventions.
· Increase research to identify the determinants of women's underuse of health services, paying special attention to the accessibility, affordability, and appropriateness of services. Identify and analyze best practices in health service delivery that incorporate gender variables to inform training and human resource development programs for health sector providers in developing countries for both services specific to women and general services.

- Investigate how interactions between sex and gender, race, ethnicity, and poverty affect the etiology, onset, and progression of disease as well as access to and compliance with prevention and treatment. Investigate the effects of stigmatization and discrimination on service quality and use.
- Use demographic accounting methods to project and plan for the demands that women's overall greater longevity imposes on health systems and investigate cost-effective treatment options, effect of gender variables on prevention and treatment, and viable options for increasing older women's access to health and to social insurance and protection mechanisms. Investigate affordable options for family care of elderly patients that take into account the time and the physical and emotional burdens on women, the traditional family caretakers.
- Improve the methodology used for disease classification, and expand data collection efforts to address the largely unreported causes of women's disease burdens, emphasizing conditions specific to women, including FGM and other domestic-, social-, and religious-based violence against women.
- Promote research, health promotion activities, health services, and advocacy efforts that will help women adopt desirable nutrition and physical exercise practices for optimal health. Exercise is a preventive measure that can help reduce women's excess disease burdens throughout the life cycle and has numerous indirect psychological and social benefits, but it will often require changing deeply rooted cultural mores.
- Support research on the costs and effectiveness of treatments for diseases that affect both men and women but affect women disproportionately, especially in developing countries.

Research needs pertaining to specific conditions include the following:

- Carry out further testing of innovative technologies for diagnosing neoplasms specific to women and explore new options for preventing their growth and proliferation. Regarding treatment, the literature describes few best practices and cost-effective measures, especially for breast and ovarian cancer.
- Evaluate the viability of applying the results of cost-effectiveness analysis carried out in developed countries on the prevention and treatment of cancers specific to women in developing countries to help adapt viable procedures.
- Promote and study the cost-effectiveness of approaches to preventing Alzheimer's disease, osteoarthritis, and other chronic conditions related to aging.
- Compare the prevalence of Alzheimer's disease in different populations, including carrying out genetic epi-

demiology studies to assess the importance of different genetic risks.
- Expand research on the biological and behavioral determinants of depression in women, on screening alternatives, and on cost-effective prevention and treatment options adapted to specific contexts in developing countries. Explore ways to reduce the stigmatization and discrimination associated with depression in developing countries.
- Continue research to document the risks and benefits of common, but unproven, approaches of preventing and treating diseases specific to women, such as the finding that long-term hormone replacement therapy does not reduce cardiovascular disease in postmenopausal women as had long been thought but instead increases risks for cardiovascular disease and breast cancer.
- Establish a research program to document the prevalence and disease burdens associated with FGM, and seek prevention and treatment alternatives.

CONCLUSIONS

The purpose of this chapter has been to move beyond the traditional international health focus on women's diseases related to their reproductive and maternal functions and to highlight those conditions for which sex and gender considerations, if adequately incorporated into prevention and treatment, could reduce women's excess health burdens and, as a result, increase health equity. Because of the approach taken, the chapter has excluded a set of important conditions for which the gender ratio is similar or is unfavorable for men, including HIV/AIDS, injuries resulting from domestic violence, and malaria. Therefore, this chapter should not be viewed as covering all diseases and conditions important to women or all conditions that result from the interaction of sex and gender.

The chapter has two other main limitations. First, the dataset (the global burden of disease) understates certain disease burdens, especially for women, because it does not estimate disability weights for some gender-based conditions, such as FGM. Second, the information available for cost-effectiveness analysis is inadequate. Following this chapter's emphasis on the importance of sex and gender in explaining women's excess disease burdens, assuming that sex and gender considerations in prevention and treatment would affect the analysis of cost-effectiveness seemed reasonable; however, general information for assessing cost-effectiveness was deficient, and gender-related information was entirely lacking. This limitation was additional to the common limitation of cost-effectiveness analysis in terms of underestimating the value of prevention for conditions specific to women and non–health sector interventions important to women.

Annex 10.A Milestones and Influential Works in International Women's Health (1980–2003)

Year	Milestones and Influential Work	
1980		• Maternal and child health • Infant feeding practices • Women's reproductive and fertility behaviors
1984		• Child survival research (Mosley and Chen 1984) • Women's issues for child survival
1985	UN Women's Conference in Nairobi	• Gender perspective/framework (DAWN)
1987	Safe Motherhood Initiative (World Bank)	• Barber Conable speech (Conable 1986) • Herz and Measham 1987
	Reproductive Health and Dignity: Choices by Third World Women (International Women's Health Coalition)	• Germain 1987
1988	Women's Work and Child Nutrition (Leslie 1988)	• Debunks myth of incompatibility between breastfeeding and work
1989	Quality of Care for Women in Family Planning (Population Council)	• Quality of care (Bruce 1990)
1990	1990–1994: 10 Working Papers (World Bank)	• Life-stage focus: adolescents, postreproductive age, and so on • Burden focus: cervical cancer, abortion, HIV/AIDS, reproductive tract infections, violence, and so on
1992	Women's Health: Across Age and Frontier (WHO)	• Socioeconomic, cultural, and legal factors affecting women's health • Policy directions for women's nutrition
1993	Disease Control Priorities in Developing Countries (World Bank)	• Access and empowerment • Cost-effectiveness issues in women's health • Missing women in India (A. K. Sen 1990) • Sector study of women's health in India (1992)
1994	New Agenda for Women's Health and Nutrition (World Bank)	• Lifecycle approach to account for specific and cumulative effects of nutrition • Cost-effective intervention packages advocated • Women and AIDS (Mann 1993) • Stigma and lack of empowerment as risk factors
	International Conference on Population and Development, Cairo	• Agenda setting, policy making, and programming for reproductive health since the 1994 Cairo conference
1995	UN Beijing Women's Conference	• Reproductive health and rights
1996	In Her Lifetime: Female Morbidity and Mortality in Sub-Saharan Africa (Institute of Medicine)	• Burdens exclusive to, greater for, and of particular significance to women reviewed • Burdens tracked across life span
1998	Women, Aging and Health (WHO)	• Social, cultural, political, economic determinants of major health issues facing aging and postmenopausal women • Life-cycle approach
	Gender and Health: A Technical Paper (WHO)	• Role of social and cultural factors and power relations between men and women in promoting and protecting health
1999	Safe Motherhood and the World Bank	• Effect of safe motherhood on labor supply, productive capacity, community economic well-being
	Gender and HIV/AIDS (Joint United Nations Program on HIV, International Center for Research on Women)	• Gender-specific personal and societal vulnerability to HIV/AIDS
2000	Women of South East Asia: Health Profile (WHO)	• Life-cycle approach to review gender-specific and disproportionate burdens
	Improving Women's Health: Issues and Interventions (World Bank)	• Role of biological and social factors in women's exposure risk and disease progression • Life cycle approach

Year	Milestones and Influential work	
2000	2000: Investing in the Best Buys (World Bank)	• Emphasis on identifying and funding most cost-effective programs and factors that lead to program success
2002	2002: Reproductive Health Outlook: Older Women	• Health conditions and interventions for older women
	2002: International Position Paper on Women's Health and Menopause (National Institutes of Health)	• Best clinical practices to address conditions associated with menopause

Source: Adapted from an original project proposal for this volume by S. Goldie, R. Anhang, and M. Buvinić. 2004. *The Evolving Agenda for Women's Health.*

ACKNOWLEDGMENTS

The authors would like to acknowledge the useful comments of E. Barrett-Connor, Mahmoud F. Fathalla, and Philip Musgrove and the collaboration of Sue Goldie, Anthony Measham, and Sonbol A. Shahid-Salles in the preparation of this chapter.

NOTES

1. See, for instance, the documentation of efforts to understand gender differentials in infectious diseases (Altman 2004) and in unipolar depressive disorders (Gilbert 2004).

2. Males suffer the weight of some external causes in the burden of diseases more than females. For example, in 2001, mortality and morbidity caused by war and violence worldwide accounted for about 2.7 percent of males' total DALY losses and 0.6 percent of females' losses.

3. Cardiovascular diseases include cerebrovascular diseases but do not include ischemic heart disease, which affects men more than women, or coronary artery disease.

REFERENCES

Altman, L. K. 2004. "Action Urged on Diseases with Dangers for Women." *New York Times,* February 28.

Arredondo, A., L. I. Lockett, and E. de Icaza. 1995. "Cost of Diseases in Brazil: Breast Cancer, Enteritis, Cardiac Valve Disease, and Bronchopneumonia." *Revista de Saude Publica* 29 (5): 349–54.

Berman, P., J. Quinley, B. Yusuf, S. Anwar, U. Mustaini, A. Azof, and I. Iskandar. 1991. "Maternal Tetanus Immunization in Aceh Province, Sumatra: The Cost-Effectiveness of Alternative Strategies." *Social Science and Medicine* 33 (2): 185–92.

Breen, N. 2002. *Social Discrimination and Health: Gender, Race, and Class in the United States.* In *Engendering International Health,* ed. G. Sen, A. George, and P. Ostlin, 223–55. Cambridge, MA: Massachusetts Institute of Technology Press.

Bromberger, J. T. 2004. "A Psychosocial Understanding of Depression in Women: For the Primary Care Physician." *Journal of the American Medical Women's Association* 59 (3): 198–206.

Bruce, J. 1990. "Fundamental Elements of the Quality of Care: A Simple Framework." *Studies in Family Planning* 21 (2): 61–91.

Chang, R. W., J. M. Pellissier, and G. B. Hazen. 1996. "A Cost-Effectiveness Analysis of Total Hip Arthroplasty for Osteoarthritis of the Hip." *Journal of the American Medical Association* 275 (11): 858–65.

Conable, B. 1987. "Population Growth and Policies in Sub-Saharan Africa." Address to the annual meetings of World Bank and International Monetary Fund, Washington, DC. September.

Dayaratna, V., W. Winfrey, W. McGreevey, K. Hardee, J. Smith, E. Mumford, and others. 2000. *Reproductive Health Interventions: Which One Works and What Do They Cost?* Policy Project. Washington, DC: Futures Group.

Dmytraczenko, T., I. Aitken, S. E. Carrasco, J. Holley, W. Abramson, A. Valle, and M. Effen. 1998. *Evaluación del seguro de maternidad y niñez en Bolivia.* Bethesda, MD: Abt Associates.

Evans, T., M. Whitehead, F. Diderichsen, A. Bhuiya, and M. Wirth. 2001. "Challenging Inequities in Health." In *Challenging Inequities in Health: From Ethics to Action.* New York: Oxford University Press.

Germain, A. 1987. "Reproductive Health and Dignity: Choices by Third World Women." Paper commissioned for the International Conference on Better Health for Women and Children through Family Planning, Nairobi, Kenya, October 1987, by the International Women's Health Coalition, New York.

Gilbert, S. 2004. "New Clues to Women Veiled in Black." *New York Times,* March 16.

Goldie, S. J., L. Kuhn, L. Denny, A. Pollack, and T. C. Wright. 2001. "Policy Analysis of Cervical Cancer Screening Strategies in Low-Resource Settings: Clinical Benefits and Cost-Effectiveness." *Journal of the American Medical Association* 285 (24): 3107–15.

Gupta, R. G. 2000. "Approaches for Empowering Women in the HIV/AIDS Pandemic: A Gender Perspective." Paper prepared for the Expert Group Meeting on the HIV/AIDS Pandemic and Its Gender Implications, Windhoek, Namibia, November 13–17.

Haglund, U., and P. Svarvar. 2000. "The Swedish ACCES Model: Predicting the Health Economic Impact of Celecoxib in Patients with Osteoarthritis or Rheumatoid Arthritis." *Rheumatology* 39 (Suppl. 2): 51–56.

Hanson, K. 2002. "Measuring Up: Gender, Burden of Disease, and Priority Setting." In *Engendering International Health,* ed. G. Sen, A. George, and P. Ostlin, 313–45. Cambridge, MA: Massachusetts Institute of Technology Press.

Heise, L., with J. Pitanguy and A. Germain. 1994. *Violence against Women: The Hidden Health Burden.* Washington, DC: World Bank.

Herz, B., and A. R. Measham. 1987. *The Safe Motherhood Initiative: Proposals for Action.* Washington, DC: World Bank.

Kinsella, K., and Y. J. Gist. 1998. *Gender and Aging: Mortality and Health.* International Programs Center Report IB/98-2. Washington, DC: U.S Department of Commerce, Economics and Statistics Administration.

Krieger, N. 2003. "Gender, Sexes, and Health: What Are the Connections and Why Does It Matter?" *International Journal of Epidemiology* 32 (4): 652–57.

Leslie, J. 1988. "Women's Work and Child Nutrition in the Third World." *World Development* 16 (11): 1341–62.

Levin, A., T. Dmyatraczenko, F. Ssengooba, M. McEuen, F. Mirembe, M. Nakakeeto, and others. 1999. *Costs of Maternal Care Services in Masaka District, Uganda.* Bethesda, MD: Abt Associates.

Levine, R., A. Glassman, and M. Schneidman. 2001. *La Salud de la Mujer en América Latina y el Caribe.* Washington, DC: Inter-American Development Bank.

Linfante, A. H., R. Allan, S. C. Smith, and L. Mosca. 2003. "Psychosocial Factors Predict Coronary Heart Disease, but What Predicts Psychosocial Risk in Women?" *Journal of the American Medical Women's Association* 58 (4): 248–53.

Mann, J. M. 1993. "Women and AIDS: Critical Issues." Speech given at the International Center for Research on Women Meeting, New York, April 16.

Manson, J. E., P. Greenland, A. Z. LaCroix, M. L. Stefanick, C. P. Mouton, A. Oberman, and others. 2002. "Walking Compared with Vigorous Exercise for the Prevention of Cardiovascular Events in Women." *New England Journal of Medicine* 347(10): 716–25.

Marin, D., K. Amaya, R. Casciano, K. L. Puder, J. Casciano, S. Chang, and others. 2003. "Impact of Rivastigmine on Costs and on Time Spent in Caregiving for Families of Patients with Alzheimer's Disease." *International Psychogeriatrics* 15 (4): 385–98.

McCann, J., L. Hebert, D. Bennett, V. Skul, and D. Evans. 1997. "Why Alzheimer's Disease Is a Women's Health Issue." *Journal of the American Medical Women's Association* 52 (3): 132–37.

McNamara, R. 1981. "To the Massachusetts Institute of Technology: An Address of the Population Problem," April 28, 1977. In *The McNamara Years at the World Bank: Major Policy Addresses*, 415–16. Baltimore and London: John Hopkins University Press.

Mitchell, M. D., J. Littlefield, and S. Gutter. 1997. "Reproductive Health: From Policy to Practice." Draft manuscript. Management Sciences for Health, Boston, MA.

Moore, R. A., C. J. Phillips, J. M. Pellissier, and S. X. Kong. 2001. "Health Economic Comparisons of Rofecoxib versus Conventional Nonsteroidal Anti-inflammatory Drugs for Osteoarthritis in the United Kingdom." *Journal of Medical Economics* 4: 1–17.

Mosley, W. H., and L. C. Chen, eds. 1984. *Child Survival: Strategies for Research*. Cambridge, U.K.: Cambridge University Press.

Mumford, E., V. Dayaratna, W. Winfrey, J. Sine, and W. McGreevey. 1998. *Reproductive Health Costs: Literature Review*. Washington, DC: Futures Group.

Murray, C. J. L., and D. B. Evans, eds. 2003. *Health Systems Performance Assessment: Debates, Methods, and Empiricism*. Geneva: World Health Organization.

Osmania, S., and A. Sen. 2003. "The Hidden Penalties of Gender Inequality: Fetal Origins of Ill-Health." *Economics and Human Biology* 1 (1): 91–104.

Over, M., and P. Piot. 1993. "HIV Infection and Sexually Transmitted Diseases." In *Disease Control Priorities in Developing Countries*, ed. D. T. Jamison, W. H. Mosley, A. R. Measham, and J. L., Bobadilla, 455–527. New York: Oxford University Press for the World Bank.

Pinn, V. W. 2003. "Sex and Gender Factors in Medical Studies. Implications for Health and Clinical Practice." *Journal of the American Medical Association* 289 (4): 397–400.

Raviez, M., C. Griffin, and A. Follmer. 1995. "Health Policy in Eastern Africa: A Structured Approach to Resource Allocation." Unpublished report, World Bank, Washington, DC.

Rose, P. G., and P. T. Lappas. 2000. "Analysis of the Cost-Effectiveness of Concurrent Cisplatin-Based Chemoradiation in Cervical Cancer: Implications from Five Randomized Trials." *Gynecologic Oncology* 78 (1): 3–6.

Rosenfield, A., and D. Maine. 1985. "Maternal Mortality: A Neglected Tragedy—Where Is the M in MCH?" *Lancet* 2 (8446): 83–85.

Rosenthal, G., and A. Percy. 1991. "Maternal Services in Cochabamba, Bolivia: Costs, Cost-Recovery, and Changing Markets." Arlington, VA: MotherCare, John Snow.

Sadana, R., C. D. Mather, A. D. Lopez, C. J. L. Murray, and K. Iburg. 2000. "Comparative Analysis of More Than 50 Household Surveys on Health Status." Global Programme on Evidence for Health Policy Discussion Paper Series 15, World Health Organization, Geneva.

Seils, D. M., J. Y. Friedman, and K. A. Schulman. 2001. "Sex Differences in the Referral Process for Invasive Cardiac Procedures." *Journal of the American Medical Women's Association* 56 (4): 151–55.

Sen, A. K. 1990. "More Than 100 Million Women Are Missing." *New York Review of Books* 37 (20): December 20.

Sen, G., A. George, and P. Ostlin. 2002. "Engendering Health Equity: A Review of Research and Policy." In *Engendering International Health*, ed. G. Sen, A. George, and P. Ostlin, 1–33. Cambridge, MA: Massachusetts Institute of Technology Press.

Shultz K., J. Schulte, and S. Berman. 1992. "Maternal Health and Child Survival: Opportunities to Protect Both Women and Children from the Adverse Consequences of Reproductive Tract Infections." In *Reproductive Tract Infections: Global Impact and Priorities for Women's Reproductive Health*, ed. A. Germain, K. Homes, P. Piot, and J. Wasserheit, 145–82. New York: Plenum Press.

Shumaker, S., C. Legault, S. Rapp, L. Thal, R. B. Wallace, J. K. Ockene, and others. 2003. "Estrogen Plus Progestin and the Incidence of Dementia and Mild Cognitive Impairment in Postmenopausal Women." *Journal of the American Medical Association* 289 (20): 2651–62.

Sigal, L. 2002. "Cost-Effectiveness Analysis of Osteoarthritis Treatment Options." Data presented at the American College of Rheumatology 66th Annual Scientific Meeting, New Orleans, December 16.

Sigal, L., S. E. Day, A. B. Chapman, and R. H. Osbourne. 2004. "Can We Reduce Disease Burden from Osteoarthritis." *Medical Journal of Australia* 180 (5 Suppl.): S11–17.

Suba, E. J., C. H. Nguyen, B. D. Nguyen, and S. S. Raab. 2001. "De Novo Establishment and Cost-Effectiveness of Papanicolaou Cytology Screening Services in the Socialist Republic of Vietnam: Viet/American Cervical Cancer Prevention Project." *Cancer* 91 (5): 928–39.

Tintara, H., and R. Leetanapon. 1995. "Cost-Benefit Analysis of Laparoscopic Adnexectomy." *International Journal of Gynecology and Obstetrics* 50 (1): 21–25.

Verbrugge, L. M. 1989. "Gender, Aging, and Health." In *Aging and Health: Perspectives on Gender, Race, Ethnicity and Class*, ed. K. S. Markides. Newbury Park, CA: Sage.

WHO (World Health Organization). 1997. "Mother-Baby Package Costing Spreadsheet." Unpublished spreadsheet, WHO, Geneva.

———. 1998. *World Health Report 1998*. Geneva: WHO.

———. 2000. *Women's Mental Health: An Evidence Based Review*. Geneva: WHO.

———. 2001. Global Burden of Disease data. Accessible at www.fic.nih.gov/dcpp/gbd.html.

———. 2004. "Prevalence, Severity, and Unmet Need for Treatment of Mental Disorders in the World Health Organization World Mental Health Surveys." *Journal of the American Medical Association* 291 (21): 2581–90.

World Bank. 1993. *World Development Report: Investing in Health*. New York: Oxford University Press.

———. 1996. *Development in Practice: Improving Women's Health in India*. Washington, DC: World Bank.

Zubenko, G. S., H. B. Hughes III, B. S. Maher, J. S. Stiffler, W. N. Zubenko, and M. L. Marazita. 2002. "Genetic Linkage of Region Containing the CREB1 Gene to Depressive Disorders in Women from Families with Recurrent, Early-Onset, Major Depression." *American Journal of Medical Genetics* 114 (8): 980–87.

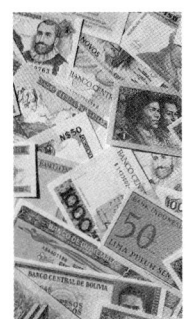

Chapter **11**

Fiscal Policies for Health Promotion and Disease Prevention

Rachel Nugent and Felicia Knaul

Governments use fiscal policy to encourage healthy behavior. The instruments of government for this purpose are taxes and subsidies, and direct provision of certain health services for free or at subsidized rates. Examples of fiscal policies for health are taxes on tobacco and alcohol, subsidies on certain foods, and tax incentives for health care purchases.

Government intervention through fiscal policy works best when public institutions and credibility are strong, the design and application of the fiscal instruments are appropriate, and consumers' and producers' responsiveness to a price signal is high. When these conditions are not present, direct provision, information and education campaigns, or legislation may be preferable in conjunction with fiscal policy.

The purpose of this chapter is to review country experiences with promoting health through fiscal policies and to examine the usefulness and success of these policies. The chapter considers both the role of fiscal policies in the production of health and the effect of these policies on the well-being of the economy—fiscal policy for health and healthy fiscal policy.[1] Little exists in the literature linking fiscal policy and health promotion except in relation to tobacco. This work contributes to filling that gap.

The chapter deals specifically with experiences at the country level with tax policies affecting some goods related to health, such as food, tobacco, alcohol, and condoms; subsidized provision of workplace promotion of healthy behavior and caregiving; and direct subsidies affecting food provision and fortification, cooking fuels, water purification and soap, condoms, bednets, vaccines, and medical research. The chapter only touches on health care provision and does not discuss its financing, either directly by governments or through insurance, because other chapters deal with those topics.

The chapter is divided into five sections:

- The first section provides a general framework through which fiscal policy options can be considered in terms of their impact on health and the health sector.
- The next section examines the experiences in developing countries of using subsidies to achieve health-related objectives (columns 1 and 2 in table 11.1).
- The third section presents examples of how taxes are used in a number of countries to promote health (column 3 in table 11.1).
- The next section discusses nonhealth goods where fiscal policies are often used and have important indirect health benefits (lower part of column 2 in table 11.1).
- The final section presents conclusions and suggestions for further research and policy development.

USE OF FISCAL POLICY FOR HEALTH IN DEVELOPING COUNTRIES

Fiscal policies come in a wide range of designs, but the main effect is either to alter the price of health-related goods or to alter the quantity available. Table 11.2 summarizes the health interventions subject to fiscal policies. The behaviors that require these interventions are divided into the following categories:

- unhealthy consumption (foods, tobacco, and alcohol), for which the most salient fiscal policies are taxes on consumers and producers, and fines

Table 11.1 Fiscal Policies for Health Promotion Covered in Chapter 11

Subsidy for or tax imposed on	Health-related products receiving direct subsidies	Subsidized provision of health	Health-related products directly taxed	Government financing of health care
Consumer	Medicine	Caregiving (partially covered)	Tobacco	Not covered
	Food		Alcohol	
	Cooking fuel		Food	
	Water purification		Imported medicine and supplies	
	Soap			
	Condoms			
	Bednets			
Producer	Vaccinations	Workplace promotion of healthy behavior (partially covered)	Fuel usage (partially covered)	
	Food additives			
	Medical research			

Source: Authors.

- health promotion and disease and accident prevention (hygiene, pollution, safety, public health, maternal and child and reproductive health, infectious disease, and healthy lifestyles), for which the most important fiscal instruments are subsidies, but which may also be affected by tax policy
- health care goods and inputs, including insurance and human resources, that may be exempted from taxation, subsidized, or guaranteed as a constitutional right
- other goods that indirectly promote health (education, housing, agriculture, energy, charitable giving, charities that provide targeted subsidies, and so on), which are often subject to their own particular tax regime or sets of subsidies that affect their production or consumption and, therefore, also affect health behavior
- research and development initiatives that can be applied to health and health care goods and are sensitive to tax exemptions and subsidies.

Fiscal interventions can have various rationales, such as macroeconomic benefits, equity, or efficiency—and promoting health may or may not be the primary goal. A fiscal policy may be designed to affect some other sphere of behavior or a good other than health—for instance, education—and the effects on health or the use of health care may be indirect. The shaded boxes in table 11.3 indicate the possible rationale behind each type of fiscal policy.

A fiscal policy should be effective, efficient, and cost-effective and should promote or maintain equity goals. An effective tax or subsidy reaches the intended target and alters health-related behavior in the desired manner. An efficient policy minimizes resource distortions and involves minimal administrative costs. A cost-effective policy has the lowest cost relative to the desired health goal.

SUBSIDIES FOR HEALTH AND HEALTH-RELATED PRODUCTS

Using examples primarily from developing countries, this section of the chapter analyzes the range of subsidies that are available to promote healthy behavior and the consumption of health-related goods. The first sections deal with consumer subsidies both to promote the consumption of health-producing goods and of health care. The second section discusses producer subsidies.

Consumer Subsidies

Governments use consumer subsidies to encourage the use of a beneficial product by lowering the price consumers pay—usually in situations where the consumers are too poor, the market prices of the good are too high, or both situations apply—to otherwise achieve a socially optimal consumption level. Examples include subsidies for staple foods, condoms, soap, insecticide-treated bednets, cooking fuels, and medicines.

Staple Foods. Ample evidence indicates that food subsidies are effective in improving nutrition; however, appropriate targeting is often a problem (Alderman 2002). Subsidies may be targeted to specific foods, specific delivery locales or geographic areas, or specific populations. Often targeting includes all three.

Food-specific subsidies, whether in the form of general subsidies, ration cards, quotas, or food stamps, increase food consumption. They will have a positive effect on health if this consumption occurs in undernourished populations that require increased caloric or nutrient intake. In some cases, food subsidy programs have had unintended macroeconomic and

Table 11.2 Use of Taxes and Subsidies to Promote Health by Type of Intervention

| Intervention | Taxes | | | | | | Tax preferences | | | Subsidies | | Rights |
	Payroll	Consumer (sales and value added tax)	Excise	Production	Input	Fines	Credits and exemptions	Director-subsidized provision	Subcontract provision	Targeted consumer subsidies	Producers	
Unhealthy consumption												
Foods												
Alcohol												
Tobacco												
Health promotion and disease and accident prevention												
Hygiene (soap)												
Pollution (for example, fuels)												
Safety (for example, seat belts)												
Public health (vaccines, clean water, supplementation, education, and information)												
Child, maternal, and reproductive health (information and education, supplementation, and medical attention)												
Infectious disease (condoms and healthy workplaces)												
Healthy lifestyles (food, exercise, and healthy workplaces)												

(Continues on the following page.)

Table 11.2 Continued

Intervention	Taxes						Tax preferences	Director-subsidized provision	Subcontract provision	Subsidies		Rights
	Payroll	Consumer (sales and value added tax)	Excise	Production	Input	Fines	Credits and exemptions	Director-subsidized provision	Subcontract provision	Targeted consumer subsidies	Producers	Rights
Health care goods												
Insurance												
Medical attention												
Medicines												
Human resources for health												
Other goods that indirectly promote health												
Personal leave												
Caregiving and family leave (maternity, paternity, and chronic illness)												
Education (for mothers or women, early childhood, or special needs)												
Housing (provision, flooring, and roofing)												
Agriculture (type of products produced or imported)												
Energy (types of fuels, heating, cars, and gasoline)												
Charitable giving												
Research and development												

Source: Authors.

Note: Shaded boxes indicate possible fiscal policies for each type of intervention.

Table 11.3 Taxes and Subsidies by Policy Rationale

Policy	Healthy behavior	Macroeconomic or fiscal benefits	Rationale Equity	Efficiency	Promotion of another good or type of behavior
Taxes					
Payroll					
Consumer (value added tax/sales)					
Levy					
Excise					
Producer					
Input					
Fines					
Subsidies					
Tax credits					
Direct provision					
Subsidized provision					
Subcontracted provision					
Targeted subsidies					
Subsidies to producers					
Rights					
Tax exemptions					

Source: Authors.

Note: The shaded boxes indicate the possible rationale behind each type of fiscal policy.

microeconomic consequences (Adams 2000; del Ninno and Dorosh 2002; Pinstrup-Anderson 1988; Siamwalla 1988). They become expensive if they are too widely available, can create incentives for black market activities, and can affect prices and volumes in agricultural and trade markets.

Indonesia switched from a general rice support system to a limited subsidy during the 1997 macroeconomic crisis. The earlier system had successfully reduced food insecurity to low levels, but higher prices increased the cost of maintaining the subsidy and led to food being smuggled out of the country (Tabor and Sawit 2001). The government targeted the new rice subsidy to the poor and issued ration cards. Within roughly a year of implementation, the subsidy was reaching an estimated 85 percent of the poor. Only about 10 percent of the subsidy appeared to be reaching nontarget population groups.

India has subsidized essential consumer goods for decades, including health-related goods such as food grains, edible oils, sugar, and fuels (S. Jha 1992). The government rationed certain goods in the belief that only the truly needy would endure waiting in lines and purchasing the poorer quality products that were involved in the subsidy schemes. This is called *self-targeting*. However, Jha shows that 40 percent of the population purchased subsidized rice in 1990, only half of whom were poor. The government recently modified the program to better target the subsidy to the poor and removed such barriers as bulk purchasing (Rao 2000).

The Arab Republic of Egypt's generalized program also illustrates the problems that beset broad food subsidy programs. The program reached its zenith in 1980, when it subsidized 20 food products and accounted for 15 percent of government expenditures (Adams 2000). The program has been scaled back to cover four staple foods and now accounts for 6 percent of government expenditures. Nevertheless, about 75 percent of the population holds ration cards entitling them to purchase the subsidized foods. The program is intended to achieve self-targeting, but the nonpoor purchase many of the subsidized foods. The program accounts for 44 percent of the total calorie supply of the poorest quintile group, but in rural areas, the rich obtain more calories from subsidized food than the poor do.

Musgrove (1993) reviews 104 supplementary feeding programs in 19 countries in Latin America and the Caribbean. The review covers a range of program sizes, from those serving 1,000 individuals to those supplying 28 million people; of types of subsidies (namely, food distribution, direct feeding, and direct payments); of levels of coverage of the targeted population, ranging from 1.9 to 100.0 percent; and of extent of coverage of the poor, varying from 5.8 to 88.0 percent. The per capita costs of reaching beneficiaries differed widely. The most common reasons for program ineffectiveness were spreading resources too thinly across beneficiaries, targeting foods with minor health benefits, choosing inappropriate beneficiaries, and encountering excessive costs in distributing resources.

These kinds of issues underscore the importance of design considerations and country conditions in creating effective and efficient food subsidy programs.

In sum, many food subsidy programs avoid the political and administrative challenges of explicit targeting by allowing universal access to the subsidies on the assumption that the needy will self-select into the programs. However, Adams (2000) shows that countries with targeted food programs—for example, Chile, Jamaica, and Peru—provide much higher income transfers to the poor than do self-targeted programs of the kind used in Egypt, Morocco, and Tunisia.

Condoms. Preliminary investigation indicates that subsidies on condoms can be effective in increasing their use in both general and high-risk populations, but whether price reduction, increased access, or education leads to greater use is not clear (Price 2001) because information campaigns about the health benefits of condoms usually accompany price subsidies. Recent surges in social-marketing schemes to distribute condoms as part of the fight against HIV/AIDS, especially in Africa, have increased condom use.[2]

Few researchers have compared HIV infection rates—or even condom use rates—before and after the introduction of a subsidy on condoms. Cohen and others (1999) conclude that in a particular jurisdiction in Louisiana, free distribution through public clinics and 1,000 small businesses in areas with high levels of HIV and other sexually transmitted diseases achieved significantly higher condom distribution than a fee-based system (77 percent use during the last sexual encounter compared with 64 percent) and that the revenues from cost recovery were insufficient to justify imposition of the fee. The dropoff in condom use during the cost-recovery period persuaded the jurisdiction to reinstate the free distribution program.

Another example suggests that promotion and information are also effective. A social-marketing effort in Turkey in the early 1990s offered condoms at a commercial price but included intensive advertising and other promotional efforts. It achieved sales well beyond original expectations and gained 41 percent of the market share (Yaser 1993).

Water Purification. The U.S. Centers for Disease Control and Prevention and the Pan American Health Organization designed the Safe Water System Initiative to improve the quality of drinking water for households that draw their water from sources outside the home. The principle underlying the initiative is to subsidize storage containers, disinfectant, and education on proper handling to avoid contamination (Quick and others 1999). Numerous countries have implemented similar initiatives, including Bangladesh, Bolivia, Burkina Faso, Kenya, and Zambia. The government provides containers and chemicals at subsidized prices, but the costs are still higher than the cost of boiling water (Quick and others 2002).

Soap. Another proven method for reducing the incidence of diarrhea and other hygiene-related diseases is hand washing, with or without soap. Whether the key factor is education or the subsidized provision of soap is unclear. Some investigators claim that small-scale programs that subsidize soap and educate households about the benefits of hand washing are self-financing because of the consequent reduction in disease (Borghi and others 2002).

Luby and others' (2001) results from Pakistan suggest that education alone may be just as effective as education accompanied by soap provision in reducing diarrheal disease. By contrast, Hoque (2003) and other researchers suggest that the cost of soap is a barrier to its widespread use among extremely poor populations and that behavioral change may be difficult to achieve without a subsidy.

Insecticide-Treated Bednets. The degree of subsidization of bednets has become a controversial issue, with some arguing for full subsidization and others for partial subsidization. Most long-term studies indicate that consumers resist purchasing bednets even at subsidized prices after they have had access to free bednets (Snow and others 1999).

A number of researchers have undertaken studies in various locations in Africa to assess the effect of selling bednets rather than providing them free to vulnerable populations (Armstrong-Schellenberg and others 2001; Kolaczinski and others 2004; Snow and others 1999). The key issue is consumers' responsiveness to changes in the prices of bednets, through either subsidies or a reduction in taxes and tariffs. Many households do not own a bednet because they cannot afford it, while other reasons are lack of information, poor access to markets, and cultural preferences (Hanson and Worrall 2002; Simon and others 2002). The evidence suggests that responsiveness to price changes alone may be modest, but in combination with removing some of the other barriers, demand for bednets could increase substantially in malaria-affected regions (Simon and others 2002).

Nigeria removed tariffs and taxes on bednet insecticide in 2001, and the 18 percent price drop resulted in an estimated 9 to 27 percent increase in purchases (Simon and others 2002). Another study that reviewed a public sector subsidy for bednets combined with private sector marketing and distribution by means of a social-marketing scheme concluded that the program was successful because 18 percent of children slept under bednets as a result; however, the low insecticide retreatment rate led the authors to conclude that subsidies were needed on both bednets and insecticide (Armstrong-Schellenberg and others 2001).

Clean Cooking Fuels. High rates of respiratory illness occur as a result of exposure to smoke and particle emissions from biomass burning in many developing countries. Fuel subsidy pro-

grams have been designed to promote the use of liquid petroleum gas, natural gas, or kerosene, which burn more cleanly and emit a low amount of smoke and particulates, but none has been efficacious or efficient (UNDP 2003).

Liquid petroleum gas subsidies have been shown to benefit middle- and higher-income families in urban areas rather than the poor (UNDP 2003). In attempting to target the poor more accurately, Côte d'Ivoire and Senegal focused subsidies on smaller liquid petroleum gas cylinders but found that poor consumers still preferred charcoal (UNDP 2003). Electricity subsidies in low-income countries are also often skewed toward the well off, who are more likely than the poor to be connected to the electricity grid (Alderman 2002).

Medicines and Medical Supplies. In relation to the direct provision of health-related goods, including drugs, supplies, and services of medical personnel, governments may subsidize and regulate drug prices, make bulk purchases from manufacturers for distribution at reduced prices, and distribute certain drugs with complete or partial subsidies to target populations. Specific interventions—for instance, antiretrovirals, vaccines, or reproductive health care—are often more heavily subsidized or may be targeted by population group or disease—for example, child and maternal health, tuberculosis, and malaria. With the exception of antiretroviral drugs, the health benefits and low costs of these medicinal interventions make them good targets for subsidization.

General Health Care. In developing countries, where informal sectors tend to be large, providing subsidized health care is an important tool for health promotion. Some countries have chosen direct provision of health goods, whereas others combine the public provision of services with subsidized health insurance for families below a certain income cutoff. Both models require identifying the families that are unable to afford health care and the types of services that are considered public goods.

One example of subsidizing the production and provision of health care is the Mexican program originally called PROGRESA and now known as Oportunidades. This program is also an example of how income transfers for other goods can affect health and how cross-subsidies can be used to strengthen the incentive effects of a fiscal policy to promote healthy behavior. The government launched the program in 1997 to provide subsidized health, nutrition, and education to poor families. By mid 2004, it was serving the majority of those living below the poverty line. Oportunidades combines a cash transfer equivalent to 20 to 30 percent of families' incomes that includes incentives for positive behaviors in relation to health, nutrition, and schooling with subsidized basic health interventions. The program is largely financed from federal budgets.

Oportunidades is successful both in terms of targeting the poorest households and in terms of achieving measurable gains in health, health care use, nutritional status and growth, school attendance, and school achievement. Gertler (2004), for example, finds significant and cumulative reduction in illness rates among children, lower prevalence of anemia, and an additional centimeter of growth in the first year of the program.

The program's success is attributable to many factors, including a rigorous longitudinal evaluation process; an integrated package of services; and the presence of financial stimuli tied to school attendance, visits to health clinics, and participation in health education initiatives. Furthermore, the program incorporates several targeting methods.

Producer Subsidies

Governments use producer subsidies to encourage production that improves health by lowering manufacturers' costs in situations in which the private market supply is inadequate to meet social needs. Examples include medical supplies, vaccines, food additives, and medical research.

Food Fortification. Governments sometimes subsidize the fortification of staple foods through the addition of selected micronutrients as a way of achieving broadly based nutrition improvements. Challenges involve maintaining a relationship between the public sector, which initiates and funds the program, and the private sector, which implements the fortification. Incentives for private providers are often needed in the form of tax exemptions, import preferences, subsidies for start-up costs, quality control, and training. Illegal markets selling nonfortified products at a lower price often arise in response (Alderman 2002; Dorosh, del Ninno, and Sahn 1996; Rao 2000).

Health Research. Government support for health research consists of the provision of direct subsidies for private sector investment, the granting of tax benefits for private research and development (R&D) investment, the establishment of property rights and a system to protect them, and the promotion of private goods by other means (OECD 2003). Despite the strong evidence from developed countries that the private sector will underinvest in R&D and that tax incentives increase R&D investment, developing countries should be cautious in applying those results to their own situations. Empirical investigations tend to conclude that producer subsidies for R&D in developing countries are not effective (Shah 1995; Zee, Stotsky, and Ley 2002). Many conditions need to be in place to realize high social returns and to minimize rent seeking and profiteering, including a strong private sector research effort that is stimulated by the public investment, the presence of appropriate targeting, a transparent and fair set of public laws and insti-

tutions to grant and monitor the tax benefits, and the ability to forgo alternative public investments.

TAXES AND TAX EXPENDITURES: DESIGN AND OUTCOMES

The following section describes various examples of the use of taxation directed at both consumers and producers. This section of the chapter also analyzes the design issues that are important in order to guarantee that these instruments contribute to achieving healthy fiscal policy.

Taxes on Consumers

Sales taxes—including excise taxes and value added taxes—and exemptions from those taxes are the most common fiscal policy tools used to influence consumers' health purchases. Examples are exempting medicines and foods from sales tax and imposing an excise tax on cigarettes and alcohol. Developed countries often use income tax incentives to provide deductions and credits for specific health care purchases. Box 11.1 discusses issues surrounding use of taxes for health.

"Sin" Taxes on Tobacco and Alcohol. A wide range of countries and local jurisdictions have taxed tobacco, with acknowledged success in reducing consumption (P. Jha 1999). The health benefits of curbing the demand for cigarettes may go beyond eliminating the health consequences of smoking and secondhand smoke if consumer expenditures are diverted from cigarettes to healthier alternatives (for example, food).

Taxes on alcohol are widespread and are used primarily to raise revenue. Governments typically impose taxes at the producer, wholesale, and retail levels that are levied as a percentage of the sale price or are based on a flat amount per unit. Harmful alcohol consumption is controlled through prohibition, government monopolization of sales, "dry" days, restrictions on hours when sales are legal, restrictions on age and locations for sales and consumption, laws against drinking and driving, limits to alcohol content, laws against the sale of certain types of alcohol, and licensing.

Alcohol taxes do contribute revenue to government coffers in developing countries, generally in higher proportions than in developed countries (WHO 2002a), but smuggling and tax evasion are common. For example, Zimbabwe raised taxes on certain beers in 1995 but repealed the increase within months when tax revenues dropped significantly (WHO 2002a). Some developing countries have lowered alcohol taxes with consequent negative results. Mauritius experienced a dramatic increase in drunk-driving arrests, alcohol-related fatalities, and hospital admissions after it reduced taxes on alcohol (WHO 2002a). In sum, alcohol taxes do reduce drinking, but the evidence that such taxes are well targeted to those most at risk of problem drinking is not strong.

Box 11.1

Using Taxes to Influence Consumption and Production Behavior

Taxes as a tool for health policy face significant implementation obstacles. First, targeting can be difficult. A close link must exist between the consumption of the product or behavior to be taxed and a specific population with a health risk. For instance, all consumers would pay a tax on "junk" food, even though it would only present a health threat to a small percentage of them. The taxed good must also be appropriately defined in relation to close substitutes; for example, taxing only certain forms of tobacco such as cigarettes, but not chewing tobacco, may increase consumption of the latter. Governments may also distinguish between locally produced goods and imported goods, often because of lobby groups. If governments place a higher tax on the good that is less harmful, this action will encourage greater consumption of the more harmful good.

Key weaknesses in using taxes for health policy include the feasibility of smuggling and the existence of large informal or illegal markets. Smuggled or contraband products that cannot be regulated or certified for quality and safety, such as alcohol or tobacco in particular, may be more harmful to health than goods that are legally produced and sold.

Any tax should be efficient in terms of both its administration and its effect on resource allocation. Tax authorities need a well-functioning system for imposing, collecting, and monitoring taxes and taxed products, and the public should perceive the system as fair and credible in order to achieve a high degree of compliance.

Finally, a tax should be cost-effective in achieving its stated goal of improving health outcomes. The net costs of imposing the tax should compare favorably with the net costs of using another policy instrument, such as regulation or direct government provision. Depending on the characteristics of the tax base, the health goal and the revenue goal may even be at odds.

Source: Authors.

Food Taxes. The issue of taxing unhealthy foods has received increasing attention in the wake of the Global Strategy on Diet, Physical Activity, and Health, which was approved by member countries of the World Health Organization (WHO 2004). The global strategy points to the rising prevalence of obesity and overweight in developing countries, along with that of nutrition-related noncommunicable diseases, and recommends that countries consider fiscal policies and other measures to reduce those problems.

Governments can use excise taxes to reduce the consumption of unhealthy foods only if tax rates are sufficient to change consumption in a way that improves health outcomes, if they tax enough harmful foods or food ingredients, and if they levy the taxes in an effective manner. Guo and others' (1999) study in China demonstrates significant potential for price changes to affect consumption. The researchers studied dietary intake in a sample of urban and rural Chinese households and show that a 10 percent increase in the price of pork potentially reduces fat consumption by 8 percent. Energy and protein intake would both drop by 2 percent. The overall effect may be different for the poor and the rich. The potentially harmful effects on the poor of increasing the price of pork would be buffered by substitutions from other food groups, such as oil, wheat flour, and coarse grains, but concerns remain that overall nutrition would worsen. These results suggest that using price changes to alter dietary intake

in a setting where overnutrition and undernutrition coexist may have mixed outcomes.

A natural experiment in Poland during the economic downturn of the 1990s suggests a beneficial role for price policy in a consumer switch from animal fats to vegetable fats with lower amounts of trans fatty acids (Zatonski, McMichael, and Powles 1998). A dramatic decline in ischemic heart disease and related circulatory system diseases during the first half of the 1990s is most easily explained by the removal of consumer subsidies from foods of animal origin, the aggressive marketing of margarines, and a general decline in food purchasing power. The major change in the food supply appeared to be a reduction in foods containing animal fats; however, no direct relationship can be conclusively attributed without further study of the Polish experience and the experiences of other countries undergoing similar transitions.

Governments may choose to address food-related health problems by taxing imports of high-fat or high-sugar food; however, such efforts conflict with rules governing international trade. Fiji, for example, tried to ban the import of mutton flaps, an extremely fatty food that was contributing to the country's obesity problem. To comply with its World Trade Organization obligations, Fiji had to ban the sale of all mutton flaps, not just imports (Evans and others 2001). One analysis suggests that the same kind of broad treatment would be necessary to grant subsidies to healthy foods, but taxing unhealthy domestic foods alone would probably not pose a problem under World Trade Organization rules (WHO 2003). Furthermore, avenues for using other regulatory and economic policies to improve the consumption of healthy foods may be acceptable under the World Trade Organization Agreement on Technical Barriers to Trade and the Agreement on Agriculture if countries can justify them as contributing to legitimate national health objectives.

Agricultural policies affect food prices, food choices, and farm incomes in addition to the food security of both rural and urban populations. Each country must assess the potential for reorienting its agricultural policies so as to produce a healthier food supply. Developing countries are generally more likely to directly subsidize food consumption than food production; however, they frequently make indirect subsidies available through the provision of cheap fuel, chemical inputs, water, and loans to the agriculture sector. These policies may be environmentally and fiscally costly and rarely contribute to improved population health.

Research is needed on individual countries' agricultural policies and food supply needs to make them more compatible (Nugent 2004). At the same time, the dynamics of food choice and the effects of price manipulation need to be better understood before tax and subsidy systems can be designed to effectively promote healthy food choices.

Sales Tax Exemptions on Healthy and Staple Foods and Medicines and Other Health Care Goods. Governments may set tax policies to ensure that certain expenditures on health-related behaviors and health goods are tax deductible or tax exempt for firms, employers, or individuals. Exemptions should apply to a limited number of goods that are easily differentiated from goods that are not exempted. Note that in countries with large informal sectors, income tax systems are weak, and fiscal policies for the deductibility of credits are unlikely to be effective.

South Africa provided value added tax exemptions for a short list of essential foods and found a varied consumption pattern by commodity, with the poor receiving most of the benefits of the maize exemption, but few of the benefits of the milk exemption (Alderman and del Ninno 1999).

Mexico imposes a 15 percent value added tax on almost all goods. Exemptions include medicines, physician's services, and some foods. Recently, a government proposal to make drug and food purchases eligible for value added tax and to channel the resulting revenues into financing programs targeted to the poor has given rise to extensive debate. Those in favor have argued that the existing subsidy is regressive because most drug and food purchases are by the wealthy (Fundación Mexicana para la Salud 2001).

Many developing countries concerned about the spread of HIV/AIDS have dropped import taxes on condoms, but others continue to impose tariffs on imports. For example, Malaysia is a major producer and imposes a 25 percent tax on imports. Brazil used to impose both an import tax and a distribution tax that amounted to a total of 45 percent of the original condom price, but it granted a permanent sales tax exemption when condom sales increased following a temporary tax holiday.

Taxes on Producers

Producer taxes are usually aimed at discouraging socially harmful products or processes. They can be imposed either on the use of certain inputs, such as more heavily polluting fuels, or on their outputs, such as emissions of air pollutants.

Theoretical and simulation models have examined the use of taxes on fuels and emissions taxes to control air pollution (World Bank 1994a, 1994b), but empirical data are lacking. Models of taxes suggest potential to induce substitution by cleaner fuels and reductions in overall energy use, but actual results will depend on the availability of fuel substitutes within countries. Data on Chilean manufacturing support the possibility of clean fuels substitution but indicate the likelihood of uneven sectoral incidence of the emissions tax. For example, bakeries were responsive to changes in relative prices, whereas metal products plants were unresponsive, and meat packers were unable to adjust their electricity demand but could reduce energy from other sources (World Bank 1994b). If this potential were realized on a global or regional basis—for example, through agreements to the Kyoto Protocol—a double benefit of reducing harmful externalities and raising significant revenues might be achieved.

FISCAL POLICY TO PROMOTE HEALTH

The fiscal policies discussed in this chapter in relation to health and health care goods can be applied to other goods and markets, such as housing and education, some of which may have important effects on health. This chapter does not provide an exhaustive discussion of the goods that indirectly promote health, but it does briefly consider some of these policies in relation to workplaces, employment leave policies, and day care. Note that policies focused on formal labor markets will not be effective in reaching large segments of the population in many countries. Policies that provide health-related services, such as day care, that are not based on formal labor market participation may have a broader effect.

Workplace Health

Governments can use tax relief and financial support to producers to encourage firm-specific actions to promote health. Many countries mandate safeguards in the workplace and levy penalties against occupational health violations. Most government actions are mandates rather than fiscal policies, but a combination of approaches may also be used.

A growing area for workplace health promotion is HIV/AIDS. Bloom and others (2004) suggest that the failure on the part of most firms to act—even if they correctly perceive the business, human, and social challenges HIV/AIDS poses—is attributable to a lack of incentives. Significant externalities (benefits to society and firms) are likely to result from promoting greater action by firms. Some private firms have begun providing HIV/AIDS prevention and treatment services to employees, families, and their communities ("Face Value: AIDS and Business" 2004). Sometimes government support is involved, but little information is available to evaluate the potential of fiscal policy.

Maternity Leave, Sick Leave, and Family Care Leave

Government policy can alter choices regarding different types of worker leave. Many countries have financial or legislative support for caregiving, although most focus on children. Rhum (1998) cites evidence that more than 100 countries—and almost all the industrial countries—have some legislation about parental leave, although in several countries it is unpaid.

Caregiving policies that allow people to take time off work to care for aged and chronically ill family members are less common than policies for child care, particularly in developing countries, but tax benefits and allowances for these types of caregiving are becoming increasingly available in the industrial countries (Brodsky, Habib, and Mizrahi 2000; Pijl 2003; Wiener 2003). Although the provision of services in kind by the government is still an important mechanism, the trend is toward empowering consumers by offering subsidies or tax deductions that allow them to choose among caregiving options. Countries tend to use a combined approach to financing that relies on payroll taxes imposed on employees and employers, general taxation, and copayments. Important issues that developing countries need to address in this respect include targeting compared with universal provision, the mechanisms to pay for or to insure care, and the extent to which long-term care should be integrated into the health care and social service systems (Brodsky, Habib, and Mizrahi 2000; WHO 2003).

Day Care and Early Childhood Education

Some countries use targeted fiscal policies, such as income tax deductions or direct provision, to increase the use and quality of early childhood education and child care services. Important health, labor market efficiency, growth, and equity arguments support subsidizing these services, particularly for low-income families, because without subsidies women may be forced to limit their work or to leave the labor market, and families

may have to use low-quality care or leave children unattended. Van der Gaag and Tan (1997) argue for public subsidies based on cost-benefit analysis of early childhood development programs. They conclude that the greatest payoff comes from targeting the most deprived families and that the private benefits are sufficient to expect better-off parents to pay.

Two large-scale, home-based day care programs targeted to poor families are Community Well-Being Homes (Hogares Comunitarios de Bienestar) run by the Colombian Institute for Family Well-Being (Instituto Colombiano de Bienestar Familiar) in Colombia (Myers 1995) and the Integrated Child Development Program in Bolivia. The former is an interesting case of a targeted cross-subsidy because the financing comes from the wealthier formal sector by means of a payroll tax, whereas the services are targeted to the poorest families. The program was 85 percent subsidized in the early 1990s. Parents paid a proportion of the caregivers' wages on a sliding-scale user fee (Young 1996). The Bolivian program includes nutrition, health, and cognitive development interventions and is one of the few early childhood programs in developing countries that has been formally evaluated (Behrman, Cheng, and Todd 2000). The evaluation shows that the program significantly increases cognitive achievement, although the results depend on age and the duration of exposure to the program.

CONCLUSIONS

A broad range of experiences cited in this chapter demonstrates that fiscal and health policies interact in a number of areas. Although substantial research has focused on tobacco and alcohol, other links—for example the promotion of health in the workplace—have been much less recognized or studied, particularly in developing countries.

The research presented in this chapter suggests that fiscal policy can be a useful tool for influencing health in developing countries. Nevertheless, budgetary limitations to withstand pressure for program expansion, leakages to unintended beneficiaries, public compliance with the tax system, and corruption among both government officials and the public are important factors to take into account in design and implementation. Table 11.4 summarizes some lessons learned on the use of fiscal policy to promote health.

Governments may find it worthwhile to examine their use of fiscal policies to identify the entire range of effects and have health ministries participate in this exercise. More generally, the chapter indicates an area for increased interaction between ministries of health and finance. Healthy fiscal policy and fiscal policy for health should be topics that are debated, agreed on, and formalized between the two areas of policy making to guarantee that those developing fiscal policy take both its economic and its health implications into account.

Table 11.4 Lessons in Using Fiscal Policy for Health Promotion

Intervention choice	Program design	Instrument design	Policy regime
• Select interventions that directly address the health objective. • Ensure that interventions are sufficient to effect the health change, but not excessive. • Choose interventions with high health returns and low costs relative to alternatives.	• Ensure that the health benefits of the desired change are apparent and significant. • Make sure that the tax base is adequate and stable and that no untaxed close substitutes are available. • Be aware that a large informal labor sector will limit the effectiveness and equity of benefit delivery. • Avoid programs whose expenses may become unsustainable because of uncontrollable factors.	• Choose the appropriate recipients for a subsidy or tax preference. • Do not spread the benefits across too large a group. • Note that targeting by demographic, geographic, or need categories is more efficient than no targeting or self-targeting. • Be aware of the price elasticities of a taxed good so that its incidence is clear.	• Ensure that policy is consistent and predictable. • Ensure that institutions carrying out a policy are open, accountable, and uncorrupted. • Consider tradeoffs between efficiency and distributional goals. • Seek non–health sector opportunities to effect health goals.

Source: Authors.

Rigorous evaluation studies are needed of most of the fiscal policy interventions discussed in this chapter. Such studies should address the health, fiscal, macroeconomic, and distributional effects of using fiscal policy to achieve health goals and should be performed in a range of countries with mixed public and private sector capacity to deliver health services. The studies should also examine the differing effects of policies in urban and rural settings and across income quintiles. Of particularly high priority are further studies of the results of subsidizing drugs, medical supplies, and hygiene interventions with or without education campaigns. Those areas may reveal new fiscal approaches for addressing the disease burden in developing countries.

DISCLAIMER AND ACKNOWLEDGMENT

The results and conclusions in this chapter are those of the authors and do not necessarily reflect the opinions of the institutions for which they work. The authors are grateful to Ana Mylena Aguilar, Hector Arreola, Ania Burczysnka, Esperanza Calleja, Marissa Courey, Monica Hurtado, Vanesa Leyva, Eugenia Rocha, Swathi Sista, and Sinaia Urrusti for excellent research assistance and to the Mexican Health Foundation's Council on Health and Competitiveness and the National Council for Science and Technology of Mexico for support for this research.

NOTES

1. The idea of healthy fiscal policy is discussed in Cook and Vlaisavljevich (1994), Joffe and Mindell (2004), and Secretaría de Salud (2001).

2. *Social marketing* is defined as the use of marketing principles to influence behavior for a socially desirable outcome. It provides a desirable product at an affordable price with adequate promotion and placement (that is, access).

REFERENCES

Adams, R. 2000. "Self-Targeted Subsidies: The Political and Distributional Impact of the Egyptian Food Subsidy System." *Economic Development and Cultural Change* 49 (1): 115–36.

Alderman, H. C. 2002. *Price and Tax Subsidization of Consumer Goods.* Social Safety Net Primer Series. Washington, DC: World Bank Institute.

Alderman, H. C., and C. del Ninno. 1999. "Poverty Issues for Zero Rating VAT in South Africa." *Journal of African Economies* 8 (2): 182–208.

Armstrong-Schellenberg, J., S. Abdulla, R. Nathan, O. Mukasa, T. J. Marchant, N. Kikumbih, and others. 2001. "Effect of Large-Scale Social Marketing of Insecticide-Treated Nets on Child Survival in Rural Tanzania." *Lancet* 357 (9264): 1241–47.

Behrman, J. R., Y. Cheng, and P. Todd. 2000. *The Impact of the Bolivian Integrated "PIDI" Preschool Program.* Philadelphia: University of Pennsylvania.

Bloom, D., L. R. Bloom, D. Steven, and M. Weston. 2004. "Business and HIV/AIDS: Who Me? A Global Review of the Business Response to HIV/AIDS." Paper prepared for the World Economic Forum's Global Health Initiative in partnership with the Harvard School of Public Health and Joint United Nations Programme on HIV/AIDS, World Economic Forum, Geneva.

Borghi, J., L. Guinness, J. Ouedraogo, and V. Curtis. 2002. "Is Hygiene Promotion Cost-Effective? A Case Study in Burkina Faso." *Tropical Medicine and International Health* 7 (11): 960–69.

Brodsky, J., J. Habib, and I. Mizrahi. 2000. *Long-Term Care in Five Developed Countries.* Geneva: World Health Organization.

Cohen, D., R. Scribner, R. Bedimo, and T. Farley. 1999. "Cost as a Barrier to Condom Use: The Evidence for Condom Subsidies in the United States." *American Journal of Public Health* 89 (4): 567–68.

Cook, E., and M. Vlaisavljevich. 1994. "Implications of Health Reform for State and Local Fiscal Policy." *National Tax Journal* 47 (3): 639–54.

del Ninno, C., and P. Dorosh. 2002. "In-Kind Transfers and Household Food Consumption: Implications for Targeted Food Programs in Bangladesh." Discussion Paper 134, International Food Policy Research Institute, Washington, DC.

Dorosh, P., C. del Ninno, and D. Sahn. 1996. "Market Liberalization and the Role of Food Aid in Mozambique." In *Economic Reform and the Poor in Africa*, ed. D. Sahn. Oxford, U.K.: Clarendon Press.

Evans, M., R. Sinclair, C. Fusimalohi, and V. Liav'a. 2001. "Globalization, Diet, and Health: An Example from Tonga." *Bulletin of the World Health Organization* 79 (9): 856–62.

"Face Value: AIDS and Business." 2004. *Economist* 373 (8404): 68.

Fundación Mexicana para la Salud. 2001. "Política Fiscal Saludable: Propuestas a Considerar sobre la Reforma Fiscal." Unpublished paper, Fundación Mexicana para la Salud, México, D.F.

Gertler, P. 2004. "Do Conditional Cash Transfers Improve Child Health? Evidence from PROGRESA's Control Randomized Experiment." *American Economic Review* 94 (2): 336–41.

Guo, X., B. Popkin, T. Mroz, and F. Zhai. 1999. "Food Price Policy Can Favorably Alter Macronutrient Intake in China." *Journal of Nutrition* 129 (5): 994–1001.

Hanson, K., and E. Worrall. 2002. *Report on the Analysis of SMITN2 End-of-Project Survey.* London: London School of Hygiene and Tropical Medicine.

Hoque, B. 2003. "Handwashing Practices and Challenges in Bangladesh." *International Journal of Environmental Health Research* 13 (Suppl. 1): S81–87.

Jha, P. 1999. *Curbing the Epidemic: Governments and the Economics of Tobacco Control.* Washington, DC: World Bank.

Jha, S. 1992. "Consumer Subsidies in India: Is Targeting Effective?" *Development and Change* 23 (4): 101–28.

Joffe, M., and Mindell, J. 2004. "A Tentative Step towards Healthy Public Policy." *Journal of Epidemiology and Community Health* 58: 966–68.

Kolaczinski, J., N. Muhammad, Q. Khan, Z. Jan, N. Rehman, T. Leslie, and others. 2004. "Subsidized Sales of Insecticide-Treated Nets in Afghan Refugee Camps Demonstrate the Feasibility of a Transition from Humanitarian Aid Towards Sustainability." *Malaria Journal* 3 (15): 1–11.

Luby, S. P., M. Agboatwalla, A. Raza, J. Sobel, E. Mintz, K. Baier, and others. 2001. "Microbiologic Effectiveness of Hand Washing with Soap in an Urban Squatter Settlement, Karachi, Pakistan." *Epidemiological Infection* 127 (2): 237–44.

Musgrove, P. 1993. "Feeding Latin America's Children." *World Bank Research Observer* 8 (1): 23–45.

Myers, R. 1995. *Early Childhood Care and Development Programs in Latin America and the Caribbean: A Review of Experience.* Washington, DC: Inter-American Development Bank. http://www.ecdgroup.com/download/gw1eccdl.pdf.

Nugent, R. 2004. "Food and Agricultural Policy in the Prevention of Non-communicable Diseases." *Food and Nutrition Bulletin* 25 (2): 200–8.

OECD (Organisation for Economic Co-operation and Development). 2003. *Tax Incentives for Research and Development: Trends and Issues.* Paris: Science Technology Industry.

Pijl, M. 2003. "The Support of Carers and Their Organizations in Some Northern and Western European Countries." In *Key Policy Issues in Long-Term Care: World Health Organization Collection on Long-Term Care*, ed. J. Brodsky, J. Habib, M. J. Hirschfeld. Geneva: World Health Organization.

Pinstrup-Anderson, P. 1988. *Food Subsidies in Developing Countries: Costs, Benefits, and Policy Options.* Washington, DC: International Food Policy Research Institute; Baltimore, MD: Johns Hopkins University Press.

Price, N. 2001. "The Performance of Social Marketing in Reaching the Poor and Vulnerable in AIDS Control Programs." *Health Policy and Planning* 16 (3): 231–39.

Quick, R., A. Kimura, A. Thevos, M. Tembo, I. Shamputa, L. Hutwanger, and E. Mintz. 2002. "Diarrhea Prevention through Household-Level Water Disinfection and Safe Storage in Zambia." *American Journal of Tropical Medicine* 66 (5): 584–89.

Quick, R., L. Venczel, E. Mintz, L. Soleto, J. Aparicio, M. Gironaz, and others. 1999. "Diarrhea Prevention in Bolivia through Point-of-Use Water Treatment and Safe Storage: A Promising New Strategy." *Epidemiology Infection* 122 (1): 83–90.

Rao, V. 2000. "Price Heterogeneity and Real Inequality: A Case Study of Poverty and Prices in Rural South India." *Review of Income and Wealth* 46 (2): 201–11.

Rhum, C. 1998. "*Parental Leave and Child Health.*" NBER Working Paper 6554, National Bureau of Economic Research, Cambridge, MA.

Secretaría de Salud. 2001. "Programa Nacional de Salud: 2001–2006—La democratización de la salud en México: Hacia un sistema universal de salud." Secretaría de Salud, México, D.F.

Shah, A., ed. 1995. *Fiscal Incentives for Investment and Innovation.* New York: Oxford University Press.

Siamwalla, A. 1988. "Some Macroeconomic Policy Implications of Consumer-Oriented Food Subsidies." In *Food Subsidies in Developing Countries: Costs, Benefits and Policy Options*, ed. P. Anderson. Baltimore: Johns Hopkins University Press, 323–30.

Simon, J., B. Larson, A. Zusman, and S. Rosen. 2002. "How Will the Reduction of Tariffs and Taxes on Insecticide-Treated Bednets Affect Household Purchases?" *Bulletin of the World Health Organization* 80 (11): 892–99.

Snow, R. W., E. McCabe, D. Mbogo, C. Molyneux, V. Mung'ala, and C. Nevill. 1999. "The Effect of Delivery Mechanisms on the Uptake of Bed Net Re-impregnation in Kilifi District, Kenya." *Health Policy and Planning* 14 (1): 18–25.

Tabor, R., and M. Sawit. 2001. "Social Protection via Rice: The OPK Rice Subsidy Program in Indonesia." *Developing Economies* 39 (3): 267–94.

UNDP (United Nations Development Programme). 2003. *World Bank Energy Sector Management Assistance Program—India: Access of the Poor to Clean Household Fuels.* New York: UNDP. http://www.worldbank.org/esmap/.

Van der Gaag, J., and J. P. Tan. 1997. *The Benefits of Early Child Development Programs: An Economic Analysis.* Washington, DC: World Bank.

WHO (World Health Organization). 2002. *Alcohol in Developing Societies: A Public Health Approach.* Geneva: WHO.

———. 2003. *Using Domestic Law in the Fight against Obesity: An Introductory Guide for the Pacific.* Geneva: WHO.

———. 2004. *Strategic Plan for Diet, Nutrition, and Physical Activity.* Geneva: World Health Assembly.

Wiener, J. 2003. "The Role of Informal Support in Long-Term Care." In *Key Policy Issues in Long-Term Care. World Health Organization Collection on Long-Term Care*, ed. J. Brodsky, J. Habib, M. J. Hirschfeld. Geneva: World Health Organization.

World Bank. 1994a. *Energy Pricing and Air Pollution: Econometric Evidence from Manufacturing in Chile and Indonesia.* Washington, DC: World Bank.

———. 1994b. *How Relative Prices Affect Fuel Use Patterns in Manufacturing: Plant-Level Experience from Chile.* Washington, DC: World Bank.

Yaser, Y. 1993. "Extensive Advertising." *Integration* 32: 32–33.

Young, M. E. 1996. *Desarrollo del Niño en la Primera Infancia: Una Inversión en el Futuro.* Washington, DC: World Bank, Human Resources Department. http://web.worldbank.org/WBSITE/EXTERNAL/TOPICS/EXTEDUCATION/EXTECD/.

Zatonski, W. A., A. J. McMichael, and J. W. Powles. 1998. "Ecological Study of Reasons for Sharp Decline in Mortality from Ischaemic Heart Disease in Poland since 1991." *British Medical Journal* 316 (7137): 1047–51.

Zee, H., J. Stotsky, and E. Ley. 2002. "Tax Incentives for Business Investment: A Primer for Policymakers in Developing Countries." *World Development* 30 (9): 1497–516.

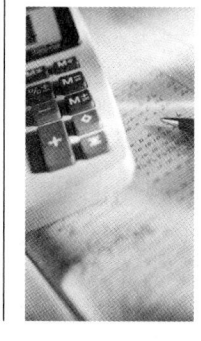

Chapter **12**

Financing Health Systems in the 21st Century

George Schieber, Cristian Baeza, Daniel Kress, and Margaret Maier

This chapter assesses health financing policy in low- and middle-income countries (LMICs). It discusses the basic functions of health financing systems and the various mechanisms for effective revenue collection, pooling of resources, and purchase of interventions (WHO 2000). It analyzes the basic financing challenges facing LMICs as a result of revenue generation and collection constraints, increasing flows of development assistance for health (DAH) coupled with donors' concerns about aid effectiveness, and the difficult economic situation facing many LMICs as a result of globalization and poor economic management.

In 2001, about US$3.059 trillion—approximately 9 percent of global gross domestic product (GDP)—was spent on health care worldwide (WHO 2004b; World Bank 2004e); however, only 12 percent of this amount was spent in LMICs, which account for 84 percent of the global population and 92 percent of the global disease burden (Mathers and others 2002). Ongoing epidemiological, demographic, and nutrition transitions will pose significant challenges for health financing systems in LMICs in the near future as the communicable disease burden lessens and the noncommunicable disease and injury burdens expand. At the same time, the current communicable disease burden in low-income countries (LICs) and in many middle-income countries (MICs), especially that caused by malaria, tuberculosis, and HIV/AIDS, poses a serious threat to public health, health systems, and economic growth.

As a result of the international focus on poverty reduction, the HIV/AIDS pandemic, and the Millennium Development Goals (MDGs), international health financing policy has evolved over the past decade from defining a basic package of cost-effective health services to figuring out how to finance and deliver those services equitably and efficiently, to recognizing the need to scale up health systems to meet basic service needs and achieve the MDGs, which will require large amounts of DAH for poor countries (see, for example, WHO 2000, 2001; World Bank 1993, 2004b).

This chapter updates and reviews the global evidence on health spending, health needs, revenue-raising capacity, organization of health financing, and trends in DAH. It discusses the key challenges that country policy makers face in ensuring access to services and financial protection while dealing with a new health policy world defined by new instruments such as sectorwide approaches (SWAps) and Poverty Reduction Strategy Papers (PRSPs). The chapter also discusses the scope and potential effects of new and relatively large global funding sources, such as the Bill & Melinda Gates Foundation; the Global Fund to Fight AIDS, Tuberculosis, and Malaria; and the Global Alliance for Vaccines and Immunization (GAVI) Vaccine Fund.

HEALTH FINANCING SYSTEMS

Health financing provides the resources and economic incentives for the operation of health systems and is a key determinant of health system performance in terms of equity, efficiency, and health outcomes.

Health Financing Functions

Health financing involves the basic functions of revenue collection, pooling of resources, and purchase of interventions.

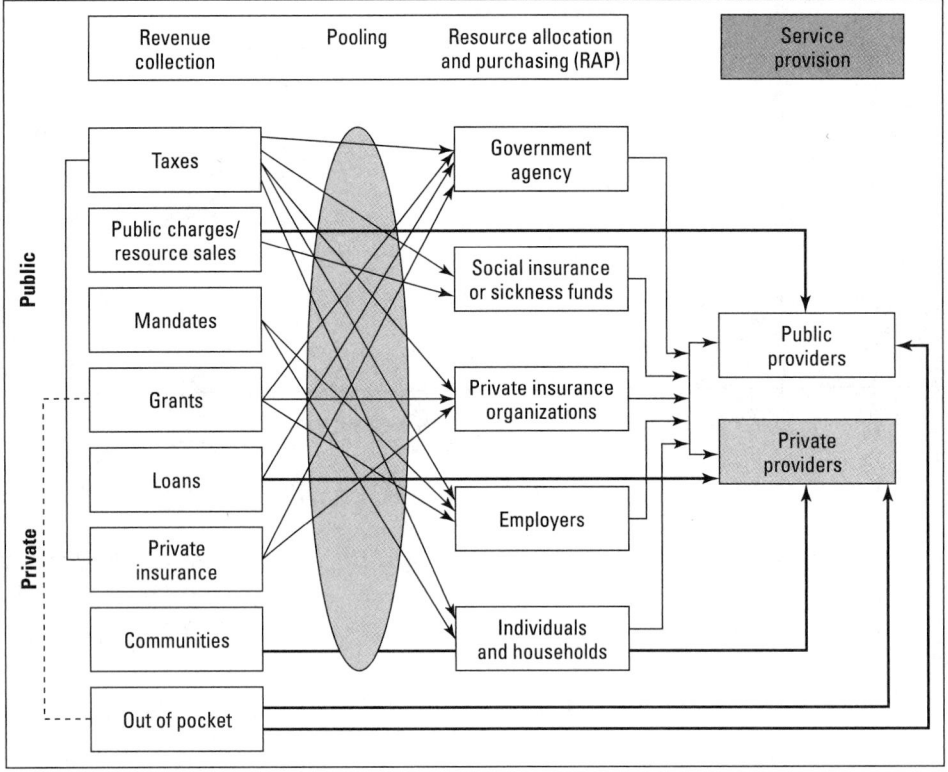

Source: Authors.

Figure 12.1 Interactions among Revenue Raising, Risk Pooling, Resource Allocation, and Service Provision

- *Revenue collection* is how health systems raise money from households, businesses, and external sources.
- *Pooling* deals with the accumulation and management of revenues so that members of the pool share collective health risks, thereby protecting individual pool members from large, unpredictable health expenditures. Prepayment allows pool members to pay for average expected costs in advance, relieves them of uncertainty, and ensures compensation should a loss occur. Pooling coupled with prepayment enables the establishment of insurance and the redistribution of health spending between high- and low-risk individuals and high- and low-income individuals.
- *Purchasing* refers to the mechanisms used to purchase services from public and private providers. Figure 12.1 illustrates these functions and their interactions.

In terms of health policy at the country level, these three financing functions translate into the following:

- raising sufficient and sustainable revenues in an efficient and equitable manner to provide individuals with both a basic package of essential services and financial protection against unpredictable catastrophic financial losses caused by illness or injury.

- managing these revenues to equitably and efficiently pool health risks; and,
- ensuring the purchase of health services in an allocatively and technically efficient manner.

These financing functions are generally embodied in the following three stylized health financing models:

- *national health service (NHS):* compulsory universal coverage, national general revenue financing, and national ownership of health sector inputs
- *social insurance:* compulsory universal coverage under a social security (publicly mandated) system financed by employee and employer contributions to nonprofit insurance funds with public and private ownership of sector inputs
- *private insurance:* employer-based or individual purchase of private health insurance and private ownership of health sector inputs.

Although these models provide a general framework for classifying health systems and financing functions, they are not useful from a micropolicy perspective because all health systems embody features of the different models. The key health policy issues are not whether a government uses general revenues or payroll taxes, but the amounts of revenues raised and the extent to which they are raised in an efficient, equitable, and sustainable manner. Similarly, nothing is intrinsically good or bad about public versus private ownership and provision. The important issue is whether the systems in place ensure access, equity, and efficiency.

Revenue Collection

Governments use a variety of financial and nonfinancial mechanisms to carry out their functions, including directly providing services; financing, regulating, and mandating service provision; and providing information (Musgrove 1996). A substantial literature is devoted to the various sources for financing health services and the economic and institutional effects of using these sources in terms of efficiency, equity, revenue-raising potential, revenue administration, and sustainability (Schieber 1997; Tait 2001; Tanzi and Zee 2000; WHO 2004b; World Bank 1993). An additional source of revenue receiving increasing attention is efficiency gains (Hensher 2001). LICs rarely use tax credits as a financing source (Tanzi and Zee 2000).

The key fiscal issue for LMICs is for their financing systems, both public and private, to mobilize enough resources to finance expenditures for basic public and personal health services without resorting to excessive public sector borrowing (and creation of excessive external debt); to raise revenues equitably and efficiently; and to conform with international standards (Tanzi and Zee 2000). Institutional constraints are particularly important, including a country's economic structure—for example, large rural populations and limited formal sector employment; ineffective tax administration; and lack of data, all of which tend to preclude LMICs from using the most efficient and equitable revenue-raising instruments (Schieber and Maeda 1997; Tait 2001). The high level of inequality in most LMICs means that governments face the difficult situation of needing to tax the politically powerful and wealthy elites to raise significant revenues in an equitable manner but of being unable to do so easily. As Tanzi and Zee (2000, 4) point out, "tax policy is often the art of the possible rather than the pursuit of the optimal."

Another area of health financing that continues to generate heated debate is user fees (that is, charges to individuals for publicly provided services). The need to significantly scale up resources to meet the MDGs in LICs has pushed the user fee issue to the forefront of this debate. Arhin-Tenkorang (2000) and Palmer and others (2004) suggest that the overall effect is negative: use decreases, particularly among the poor, and frequently, administrative costs of collecting the fees are higher than the revenue generated. Further, Kivumbi and Kintu (2002) suggest that granting waivers and exemptions for the poor is difficult, if not impossible. Given those findings, many have called for the abolition of user fees, including the United

Nations Millennium Project (2005) and the Commission for Africa (2005).

Others have argued, however, that absent resources to fund drug purchases, provide facilities with some discretionary funding, and motivate providers, use of primary health care by the poor will remain low because of both poor quality and lack of drugs, and the poor will purchase these essential services on the private market. The Bamako Initiative shows that user fees may be an important revenue source where institutions are weak, resources are limited, and the choice is between having drugs or not having them (World Bank 2003, 76–77). Furthermore, studies indicate that user fees can improve benefit incidence if user fee and waiver policies have been well designed and implemented and if providers are compensated for forgone revenues. Indeed, proponents of user fees argue that as long as the fees are set below private market levels, this "savings" may result in a net reduction in overall out-of-pocket spending for the poor (Bitrán and Giedion 2003). These diverse experiences demonstrate the difficultly involved in making blanket statements regarding user fees. As the World Bank (2003, 71) points out, "user fees, as with other public policy decisions, must balance protection of the poor, efficiency in allocation, and the ability to guarantee that services can be implemented and sustained."

Risk Pooling and Financial Protection

Preventing individuals from falling into poverty because of catastrophic medical expenses and protecting and improving the health status of individuals and populations by ensuring financial access to essential public and personal health services provide a strong basis for public intervention in financing health systems. Public intervention may be needed because of market failures in private financing and provision (for instance, information asymmetries) and instabilities in insurance markets (such as favorable risk selection by insurers and moral hazard). Indeed, in virtually all Organisation for Economic Co-operation and Development (OECD) countries except the United States, governments have decided to publicly finance or require private financing of the bulk of health services. However, given both low income levels and limits on possibilities for domestic resource mobilization in LICs and some MICs, these countries face severe challenges in publicly financing essential public and personal health services. They also often confront difficult tradeoffs with respect to financing these basic essential services and providing financial protection against the costs of catastrophic illness.

Ensuring Financial Protection. Ensuring financial protection means that no household spends so much on health that it falls into and cannot overcome poverty (ILO and STEP 2002b). Achieving adequate levels of financial protection requires maximizing prepayment for insurable health risks; achieving the largest possible pooling of health risks within a population, thereby facilitating redistribution among high- and low-risk individuals; ensuring equity through prepayment mechanisms that redistribute costs from low- to high-income individuals; and developing purchasing arrangements that promote efficient delivery of good-quality services.

Meeting those requirements depends on how health systems arrange the three key health financing functions of revenue collection, risk pooling, and purchasing. Although all health financing functions play an important role in ensuring financial protection, risk pooling and prepayment—whether through taxes or individual premiums—play the central and often the most poorly understood roles.

Risk pooling refers to the collection and management of financial resources so that large individual and unpredictable financial risks become predictable and are distributed among all members of the pool. The pooling of financial risks is at the core of traditional insurance mechanisms. Whereas pooling ensures predictability and the potential for redistribution across individual health risk categories, *prepayment* provides various options for financing those risks equitably and efficiently across high- and low-income pool members. The health financing models described earlier embody different means for creating risk pools and financing such pools through prepaid contributions.

In most LMICs, multiple public and limited private arrangements coexist, making system fragmentation the norm rather than the exception. This situation increases administrative costs; creates potential equity and risk selection problems, for example, when the wealthy are all in one pool; and limits pool sizes. Moreover, health care risks change over the life cycle of an individual or household, but because generally little correlation exists between life cycle needs and capacity to pay, subsidies are often necessary and are facilitated by risk pooling.

Risk pooling and prepayment functions are central to the creation of cross-subsidies between high-risk and low-risk (that is, a *risk subsidy*) and rich and poor (that is, an *equity subsidy*) individuals. The larger the pool, the greater the potential for spreading risks and the greater the accuracy in predicting average and total pool costs. Placing all participants in a single pool and requiring contributions according to capacity to pay rather than individual or average pool risk facilitates cross-subsidization and, depending on the level of pooled resources, can significantly increase financial protection.

However, spreading risks through insurance schemes is not enough to ensure financial protection, because it can result in low-risk, low-income individuals subsidizing high-income, high-risk individuals. Furthermore, significant portions of the population may not be able to afford insurance. For this reason, most health care systems aim not only at spreading risk, but also at ensuring equity in financing of health care services through subsidies from high- to low-income individuals. Equity subsidies are the result of such redistribution policies.

At least four alternative organizational arrangements exist for risk pooling and prepayment: ministries of health (MOHs) or NHSs, social security organizations (SSOs), voluntary private health insurance, and community-based health insurance (CBHI). Each of these is linked to distinctive instruments for revenue collection (for example, general revenues, payroll taxes, risk-rated premiums, and voluntary contributions) and for purchase of health services.

Within these organizational structures, three alternatives often coexist for generating revenues and financing equity subsidies: subsidies within a risk pool, subsidies across different risk pools, and direct public subsidies through transfers from the government. Although medical savings accounts (with or without public subsidization) are also sometimes referred to as a risk pooling mechanism, they do not pool risks over groups and, therefore, are far more limited in terms of predictability and equity subsidization. They are simply intertemporal mechanisms for smoothing health risks over an individual's or household's life cycle.

Subsidies within a risk pool, whether financed through general revenues or payroll taxes, are prerequisites for pooling risks in traditional NHSs and SSOs. The goal of collecting revenues through an income-related or general revenue–based contribution (in contrast to a risk-related contribution, as is generally the case with private insurance) is to generate subsidies from high- to low-income individuals. These systems are effective when payroll contributions are feasible, when the general revenue base is sufficient and a large proportion of the population participates in the same risk pool, or when both conditions exist. Moreover, in a system with multiple, competing, public and private insurers and a fragmented risk pool, payroll contributions may increase incentives for risk selection. In the case of a NHS or SSO, financial resources might be insufficient or inappropriate for spreading the financial risks or for creating an equity subsidy, particularly if the general revenue or payroll contribution base is regressive.

Subsidies across different risk pools involve the creation of funds, often called *solidarity* or *equalization funds,* financed by a portion of contributions to each risk pool. This mechanism is found in systems with multiple insurers in, for example, Argentina, Colombia, Germany, and the Netherlands. A key element of this mechanism's success is the implementation of adequate systems of compensation among different risk and income groups.

Finally, in many OECD countries, direct public transfers funded through general taxation are made to insurers for subsidizing health care for certain groups or for the entire population. They are also used in some LMICs, although at a limited level because of low revenue collection capacity.

In most LMICs, risk pool fragmentation significantly impedes effective risk pooling, while limited revenue-raising capacity precludes the use of broad public subsidies as the main source of finance. Therefore, targeting scarce public subsidies across different risk pooling schemes is probably the most feasible way to finance equity subsidies for the poor and those outside formal pooling arrangements. However, this method has important transaction costs. Because a significant portion of the population is excluded from the formal sector, using this mechanism for ensuring universal financial protection is limited, particularly in LICs. Even if significant subsidies are available from general taxation, the lack of insurance portability restricts its usefulness as a subsidization mechanism among risk pools because individuals may lose their coverage when they change jobs. LICs and certain MICs will be challenged both to publicly finance essential public and personal health services and to ensure financial protection through equity subsidies. Thus, LMICs should strive to achieve the best value for publicly financed health services in terms of health outcomes and equity and should try to facilitate effective risk pooling for privately financed services. Providing public financing for cost-effective interventions is one critical aspect of determining which services to finance publicly.

Distributing and Sourcing Health Expenditures. As table 12.1 shows, health spending is derived from three broad sources: public sector (expenditures financed out of general revenues and social insurance contributions), private sector (expenditures financed out of pocket and by private insurance), and external sources (grants or loans from international funding agencies). In 2001, high-income countries spent an average of 7.7 percent of their GDP on health (country weighted), MICs spent 5.8 percent, and LICs spent 4.7 percent.

Even though a clear upward trend between a country's income level and the level of public and total health spending is apparent in terms of both absolute spending and share of GDP, spending for any given income level varies a great deal, particularly at lower income levels (Musgrove, Zeramdini, and Carrin 2002). The composition of health spending also exhibits major differences. As incomes increase, both private and out-of-pocket shares of total health spending decrease. In LICs, private and out-of-pocket spending and external assistance account for the bulk of all health spending. As countries move up the income scale, public spending predominates and both out-of-pocket spending and external assistance decrease drastically.

LMICs with high levels of out-of-pocket spending have limited opportunities for risk pooling, which hinders allocative efficiency and financial protection efforts.[1] Moreover, low overall spending levels in many LICs and some MICs result in limited access to essential services and limited financial protection, particularly for the poor. As Musgrove (personal communication with G. Schieber, April 2004) indicates, if GDP is adjusted for basic subsistence needs, poor households in LICs appear to be spending a substantial share of their postsubsistence income on health, reinforcing much of the discussion that follows on the need for additional funds from external financing sources.

As also discussed by Hecht and Shah in this book (chapter 13), external funds—development assistance for health—have become an increasingly importance source of health financing in LICs, supporting some 20 percent of LIC spending. Specifically, DAH from governments, multilateral and bilateral agencies, and private foundations increased from an average of US$6.7 billion between 1997 and 1999 to US$9.3 billion in 2002. Sub-Saharan Africa received 36 percent of DAH funds in 2002, and in 13 extremely poor countries, DAH accounted for more than 30 percent of health spending (WHO 2004b).

The relationship between health expenditures and health outcomes is not always clear. Higher spending does not necessarily translate to better health outcomes. Although the evidence tenuously demonstrates a positive relationship between public spending on health and selected health indicators, it falls far short of a definitive statement (Bidani and Ravallion 1997; Filmer and Pritchett 1999; Gupta, Verhoeven, and Tiongson 2001; World Bank 1993, 2003). Health outcomes also vary across income groups, with the poor generally receiving fewer services and having worse health outcomes. As in the case of health services and health outcomes, health spending is often not pro-poor (Gwatkin and others 2003). The quality of a country's institutions also plays a key role in determining the effectiveness of health spending (Devarajan, Swaroop, and Heng-Fu 1996; Rajkumar and Swaroop 2002; Wagstaff and Claeson 2004; World Bank 1993).

Mobilizing Government Revenues. Governments of LICs have recognized the need for greater domestic investments in health. In the 2001 Abuja Declaration on HIV/AIDS, Tuberculosis, and Other Related Infectious Diseases, African leaders pledged to increase health spending to 15 percent of their government's budgets (Haines and Cassels 2004; UNECA 2001). Yet LICs' ability to raise enough revenue to meet needs and demands for publicly financed health services is highly constrained (Gupta and others 2004; Schieber and Maeda 1997). Even though revenue mobilization is directly correlated with income, wide cross-country variation in revenue mobilization within income groups is apparent. For example, Myanmar's tax revenues amounted to only 4 percent of its GDP, whereas Lesotho's were 36 percent (WHO 2002).

As table 12.2 shows, during the early 2000s, LICs collected the equivalent of about 18 percent of their GDP as revenues, whereas high-income countries collected almost 32 percent. Given projected future economic growth on the order of 4 percent for LMICs during 2006–15, they will face difficulties in mobilizing additional domestic revenues (World Bank 2004b). In other words, even though economic growth is a necessary condition for progress, it is unlikely to provide the financing

Table 12.1 Composition of Health Financing by Region and Country Income Level, 2001
(Averages)

Region and country income level	Per capita GDP (US$)	Per capita health expenditures (US$)[a]	Total health expenditures as a percentage of GDP	Public expenditures on health as a percentage of total health expenditures	Social security expenditures on health as a percentage of total public health expenditures	Private expenditures on health as a percentage of total health expenditures	Out-of-pocket expenditures on health as a percentage of total private health expenditures	Private prepaid plans as a percentage of private health expenditures	External provision for health as a percentage of total health expenditures
East Asia and the Pacific	1,387	84 (46)	5.6	59.3	11.1	40.7	83.4	3.5	11.9
Eastern Europe and Central Asia	2,053	132 (131)	5.5	67.1	42.1	32.9	94.9	3.5	2.6
Latin America and the Caribbean	3,705	237 (264)	6.4	56.2	28.5	43.8	81.5	13.7	4.0
Middle East and North Africa	2,834	102 (82)	5.6	52.7	15.6	47.3	79.1	8.1	3.1
South Asia	737	38 (21)	4.6	49.0	6.2	51.0	97.7	0.2	9.9
Sub-Saharan Africa	868	42 (29)	4.5	54.0	1.0	46.0	83.3	6.9	21.7
High-income countries	21,198	1,527 (2,860)	7.7	70.1	33.1	29.9	74.0	16.2	0.1
MICs	3,026	176 (106)	5.8	61.7	28.5	38.3	86.4	8.9	3.4
LICs	576	25 (19)	4.7	51.7	2.2	48.3	84.4	4.0	20.0

Sources: WHO 2004b; World Bank 2004e.
Note: All figures are weighted by country.
a. Per capita health expenditures include population-weighted averages (in parentheses).

Table 12.2 Average Central Government Revenues, Early 2000s

Region and country income level	Total revenue as a percentage of GDP	Tax revenue as a percentage of GDP	Social security taxes as a percentage of GDP
Americas	20.0	16.3	2.3
Asia and the Pacific	16.6	13.2	0.5
Central Europe, Baltic states, Russian Fed., and other former Soviet republics	26.7	23.4	8.1
Middle East and North Africa	26.2	17.1	0.8
Sub-Saharan Africa	19.7	15.9	0.3
Small islands (population less than 1 million)	32.0	24.5	2.8
LICs	17.7	14.5	0.7
Lower-middle-income countries	21.4	16.3	1.4
Upper-middle-income countries	26.9	21.9	4.3
High-income countries	31.9	26.5	7.2

Source: IMF 2004b.

base needed to deal with the HIV/AIDS pandemic or to achieve the health MDGs.

Trends in Health System Financing

As countries move to different stages of the income spectrum, their health financing profiles transition as well. The following discussion compares countries at different stages of the income spectrum. Given health systems' variability across time periods, countries, and income levels, the analysis provides only a snapshot. Figure 12.2 illustrates transitions in general health systems as countries move from low- to middle- to high-income status.

In LICs, almost half of health spending is private, virtually all out of pocket, and usually in the form of payments for

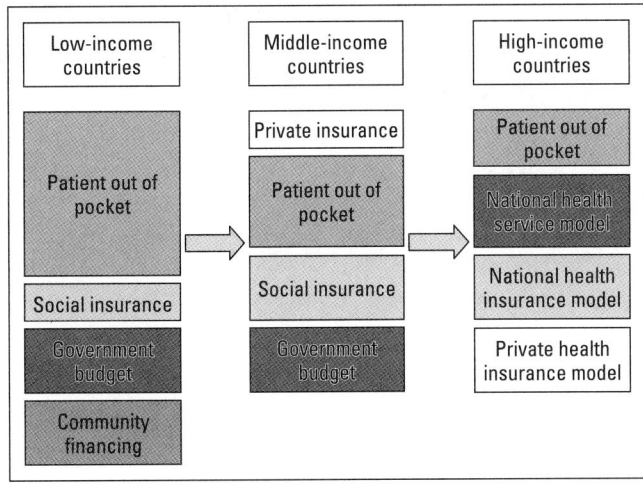

Source: Maeda 1998.

Figure 12.2 Health Care Financing System Trends by Country Income Level

privately provided health services and pharmaceuticals. The government, through the MOH, generally operates like a NHS. It provides basic public health and other services, including some tertiary-level hospital care, generally in major urban areas, to the entire population within an extremely limited budget. In general, because of the small size of formal sector employment, social insurance is limited, except perhaps for government employees. Community-based health insurance may be available to varying degrees but is unlikely to play a major role. Private health insurance, if any, is extremely limited because of people's inability to pay and institutional constraints to the industry's development, including the lack of well-developed financial markets and regulatory environments.

As countries' economies improve, government revenues tend to increase because of the expansion of the more readily taxable formal sector. Other institutions, such as financial markets, legal systems, and regulatory capabilities, are able to develop. Although private spending still accounts for some 40 percent of all health spending in MICs, the out-of-pocket share declines as private health insurance markets develop. The MOH generally continues to provide basic public health services and to serve as the insurer of last resort for the poor or for the entire population for specific chronic conditions as social health insurance mechanisms develop.

Countries move into the high-income group with improved institutions, more efficient governments, and greater revenue-raising capacity and spend a relatively small share on basic public health. With few exceptions, publicly financed universal coverage—or, in some cases, publicly mandated private coverage—becomes the goal. MOHs maintain responsibility for public health and surveillance and for the general regulatory environment but generally do not directly provide services. Risks are pooled either through a NHS, as in Italy and the

United Kingdom, or through single or multiple insurance mechanisms, as in France and Germany. The Netherlands requires wealthier individuals to be insured through a private system. Private spending declines to 30 percent, and out-of-pocket spending represents about 20 percent of total health spending. Although health financing systems are highly country specific, available information on sources of health spending and government revenues supports these stylized models.

ABSORPTION, EFFECTIVENESS, AND SUSTAINABILITY OF DONOR FUNDS

In recent years, several new dimensions have emerged in the debate on international health financing, namely the effectiveness of large increases in DAH and the enormous costs of scaling up health and other social systems to meet the MDGs. Both the donor community and recipient countries have raised concerns pertaining to countries' absorptive capacity, aid effectiveness, and sustainability.

Countries' Absorptive Capacity

Large increases in DAH channeled to LICs have raised questions about whether countries can make effective use of these new aid flows. As table 12.3 shows, absorptive capacity has macroeconomic, budgetary management, and service delivery dimensions.

Increased aid has important macroeconomic implications given its potential effect on exchange rates, inflation, balance of trade, overall competitiveness, aid dependency, domestic revenue mobilization efforts, and future recurrent costs. Most studies indicate that the macroeconomic saturation point for aid lies somewhere between 15 and 45 percent of GDP, depending on the country's policy environment (Clemens, Radelet, and Bhavnani 2004; Collier and Dollar 1999; Collier and Hoeffler 2002; Foster 2003).

Aid can have a number of negative effects. If aid flows are not included in the recipient country's budget, they can result in corruption. Aid may substitute donors' priorities for countries' priorities. A country may have insufficient human resources, physical infrastructure, or managerial capacity to use funds effectively. Resources that may already be in short supply and that are critical for effective service delivery may be diverted from other important activities. New resources may overwhelm the system, and the donors' reporting and administrative requirements may impose additional burdens on countries.

Absorptive capacity problems may also result from demand-side constraints at the individual, household, or community levels, including lack of education, limited information, travel costs, and income loss (Ensor and Cooper 2004). Conditional cash transfers are among the demand-side innovations developed to improve the use of essential public health services by the poor that have been receiving increased attention. Such programs were initially developed in Latin America as part of social safety-net programs and provide direct cash payments to poor households contingent on certain behavior, such as completing a full set of prenatal visits or attending health education classes (Rawlings 2004). Conditional cash transfers are in effect negative user fees. Even though investigators have found that such programs are quite successful in

Table 12.3 Major Constraints to Countries' Absorption of Additional External Resources

	Macroeconomic	Institutional	Physical and human	Social, cultural, and political
National government	Debt sustainability Competitiveness Dutch disease	Monetary and fiscal policy instruments Exchange rate management	Administrative, management, and planning skills Training technicians and sector specialists	Stable national political institutions Power-sharing mechanisms Social stability
Fiscal instruments and allocative mechanisms	n.a.	Public expenditure management: Budget preparation and execution Accounting and auditing	Sector management skills Connectivity and communications networks	Cultural norms Weak institutions Power-sharing mechanisms
Service delivery and local governments	n.a.	Local government institutions Private sector capacity	Accessibility Sanitation and water Roads Geography Local government skills and capacity	Cultural norms Ethnic, caste, and class relations

Source: World Bank 2004a.
n.a. = not applicable.

MICs and have the potential to improve human capital and health outcomes and reduce poverty with relatively modest administrative costs, their applicability in LICs is still unresolved.

Health sector supply and demand constraints can also hinder countries' effective employment of large increases in health resources. As Mills, Rasheed, and Tollman point out in this book (chapter 3) and elsewhere, these constraints can occur at all levels of service delivery and governances (Oliviera-Cruz, Hanson, and Mills 2003). Additional funding alone does not create sufficient conditions for overcoming structural weaknesses, particularly in the short run. If aid is targeted to specific diseases or interventions, effective use of such aid may "consume" different amounts of a country's administrative capacity. Increased public funds may supplant private spending not only by the poor, but also by the nonpoor, resulting in limited marginal effects on the poor (Filmer and Pritchett 1999).

Aid Effectiveness

Given calls for increases in aid of anywhere between US$25 billion and US$75 billion a year, the question of aid effectiveness has taken on increased importance.[2] A protracted debate has generated the following findings concerning aid (Burnside and Dollar 1997; Clemens and Radelet 2003; Clemens, Radelet, and Bhavnani 2004; Collier and Dollar 1999; Collier and Hoeffler 2002; Foster 2003; United Nations Millennium Project 2005; WHO 2001; World Bank 2004a):

- Aid has diminishing returns.
- Countries' absorptive capacity is limited.
- Aid is fungible overall and among sectors.
- Aid achieves better results in good policy environments.[3]
- Aid requires ownership by countries; for example, donor-imposed conditions rarely work.
- Aid is related to increased investment and growth.
- Debt repayments have a negative effect on economic growth.
- Aid has high transaction costs for countries.
- Aid makes governments accountable to donors as opposed to their citizens.

Serious overall and health sector–specific questions pertain to the levels, predictability, variability, fungibility, and sustainability of aid flows, and debate continues between those arguing for vertical disease–specific program assistance and those supporting broader health system reform changes (WHO 2001). As Mills, Rasheed, and Tollman show in this book (chapter 3), evidence on the effectiveness of both approaches is mixed. Aid unpredictability and uncertainty need to be addressed by aligning donors' disbursement and commitment cycles with those of recipient countries, strengthening

countries' budgetary and financial management capacity, and fostering a more transparent and predictable implementation structure (World Bank 2004a).

The effect of the composition of aid on countries' efforts to mobilize domestic resources is also critical given the strong push by heavily indebted countries, several Group of Seven (G-7) countries, and the United Nations Millennium Project for grant assistance. Gupta and others (2004) find that increases in overall aid (net loans plus grants) result in a decline in total domestic revenues; however, the effects of loans were quite different from those of grants. Each 10.0 percent increase in loans was associated with a 2.3 percent increase in domestic revenues, whereas a 10.0 percent increase in grants was associated with a 2.8 percent decrease in domestic revenues. The same study also finds higher levels of corruption result in reduced domestic revenue-raising efforts.

Fiscal Sustainability

Fiscal sustainability is an often used but rarely defined term, though it has generally been defined in terms of self-sufficiency. In its broadest context, achieving sustainability means that, over a specific period, the managing entity will generate sufficient resources to fund the full costs of a particular program, sector, or economy, including the incremental service costs associated with new investments and the servicing and repayment of external debt.

Knowles, Leighton, and Stinson (1997, 39) define *health system sustainability* as the "capacity of the health system to replace withdrawn donor funds with funds from other, usually domestic, sources" and *sustainability of an individual program* as the "capacity of the grantee to mobilize the resources to fund the recurrent costs of a project once it has terminated." However, given the enormous unmet needs in the poorest countries, coupled with stagnant economic performance, some donors are now defining sustainability on the basis of the managing entity's commitment of a stable and fixed share of program costs (Brenzel and Rajkotia 2004; Kaddar, Lydon, and Levine 2003).

In light of criticisms leveled at the International Monetary Fund (IMF) regarding its structural adjustment programs and fiscal ceilings, IMF has recently paid increased attention to fiscal sustainability. However, evaluating a country's fiscal situation and defining sustainability are not easy matters (Croce and Juan-Ramon 2003; Dunaway and N'Diaye 2004; Hemming, Kell, and Schimmelpfennig 2003; Tanzi and Zee 2000). Work is under way to develop operational indicators of debt and fiscal sustainability and to define the concept of fiscal space (Dunaway and N'Diaye 2004; Heller 2005). Understanding the details of IMF fiscal programs and ensuring stable and predictable long-term DAH are important conditions for avoiding the macroeconomic distortions discussed earlier.

HEALTH FINANCING ISSUES IN LICs

This section discusses the severe challenges LICs face in mobilizing sufficient revenues, both domestically and externally, to meet even the basic health needs of their populations.

The Needs Gap

Since the release of the 1993 World Bank *World Development Report: Investing in Health,* researchers have undertaken numerous efforts to estimate the costs of a basic package of essential health services. The Commission on Macroeconomics and Health (WHO 2001) estimated that, in 1997, the 48 poorest developing countries were spending on average US$11 per capita (US$6 per year in public funds) and that the level of spending would have to rise to US$34 per capita to ensure delivery of an essential package.[4] On the basis of these data, the Commission on Macroeconomics and Health estimated that total DAH should rise to US$27 billion in 2007 and to US$38 billion by 2015 to scale up coverage (WHO 2001).

Within the framework of the MDGs, a number of other studies have been undertaken to determine the financial resources needed to meet the goals. In this book, Wagstaff and others (chapter 9) review the estimates and methodologies from these various studies, finding that the annual cost of scaling up to meet the MDGs is between US$25 billion and US$75 billion. The United Nations Millennium Project (2005) estimates that the additional overall development assistance needed for scaling up to meet all the MDGs will be US$74 billion by 2015. All the studies indicate that most LICs will face enormous constraints in raising additional resources through domestic resource-mobilization efforts and that the international community must essentially finance most of the gap.

New Global Alliances and Funds

Recent years have witnessed a marked increase in the number of global alliances and institutions aimed at alleviating specific health sector deficiencies, a number of which owe their existence to resources made available by philanthropic organizations.[5] The GAVI Vaccine Fund and the Global Fund to Fight AIDS, Tuberculosis, and Malaria are perhaps the largest and most well known. While the GAVI Vaccine Fund is both a funder and an implementer, Roll Back Malaria is an example of an alliance that is a global partnership without a funding mechanism. Some entities like the Global Fund are purely financial vehicles with little alliance structure. The effect of these new alliances and funds is significant. Since its inception in 2000, the GAVI Vaccine Fund has raised and spent more than US$1 billion for immunization, and the Global Fund has commitments of more than US$5 billion and has signed grant agreements with more than 70 countries worth in excess of US$3 billion.

Although assessments of global initiatives and alliances are generally positive, some observers have concerns about their effects on health systems and prioritization (Travis and others 2004). Increasing concerns are being expressed about the "verticalization" of DAH and the development of separate health system "silos," each dedicated to specific diseases and activities. This strategy is especially problematic in light of the scarce human resources available for health in many LICs (Global Health Trust 2004; Joint Learning Initiative 2004).

As a result of these concerns, the G-7 countries are currently discussing a number of new, broad-based, global financing mechanisms to mobilize and facilitate the transfer of resources from developed countries to LICs, and significant progress has been made in relation to the International Finance Facility (IFF), a proposal advanced by the U.K. government. The IFF will frontload development assistance by issuing bonds on international markets that would be secured based on legally binding, long-term donor commitments. The IFF would repay bondholders using future donor payments. Depending on the number of donors involved, the IFF could raise an additional US$50 billion a year in development assistance between now and 2015. One of the many advantages of this kind of mechanism is that a portion of funding for international development is effectively taken out of the annual budgetary process in participating countries. In this way, the hope is that the revenue streams available to fund development can be rationalized, both in terms of the total volume of assistance and in terms of the stability of annual flows.

These global funds have added a major new dynamic to global health policy and a new level of influence over LICs. Large grants are approaching the World Bank's financing levels for the health sector. Moreover, such funding is often targeted to specific diseases or interventions, frequently outside the basic broadly based financing instruments required by the World Bank and the IMF. This factor raises important issues of donor coordination and harmonization of procedures and has implications for IMF fiscal ceilings.

Financing Instruments

During the past decade, a new reform instrument known as the *SWAp* has heavily influenced health financing, particularly for LICs. Concomitantly, the World Bank and the IMF have imposed a series of requirements and instruments to ensure that external assistance is targeted to the poor through PRSPs. These new policy blueprints and requirements are radically different from previous DAH mechanisms, which were largely funded on a bilateral basis through projects.

SWAps. Starting in the mid-1990s, donors and recipient countries established the SWAp to address the limitations of project-based forms of donor assistance, to ensure that overall health reform goals were met, to reduce large transaction costs for countries, and to establish genuine partnerships between donors and countries in which both had rights and responsibilities. The core elements of a SWAp follow (McLaughlin 2003, 2004):

- The government is "in the driver's seat."
- The partnership results in a shared vision and agreed-upon priorities for the sector.
- A comprehensive sector development strategy that reflects all development activities to identify gaps, overlaps, or inconsistencies.
- An expenditure framework that clarifies sectoral priorities and guides all sectoral financing and investment.
- A partnership across development assistance agencies that reduces governments' transaction costs.

SWAps explicitly recognize the need to tie health sector changes to new aid instruments, to macroeconomic and public sector management, to poverty reduction, and to achievement of the MDGs (Cassels 1997). A key aspect of this approach is to improve countries' policy-making processes, including budget and public expenditure management, by capturing all funding sources and expenditures and by putting resource allocation decisions into a medium-term budget and expenditure framework that is based on national priorities (Foster 1999). To date, SWAps are in various stages of development and implementation, and few conform fully to the specifications listed above (Institute for Health Sector Development 2003). At this point in their evolution, SWAps should be viewed as a way of coordinating development assistance and creating country ownership. They should be judged on how well they do these things compared with the previous environment characterized by multiple, stand-alone projects.

PRSPs. Starting in the mid 1990s, the World Bank and the IMF began to radically change both the focus and the tools for providing development assistance to poor countries. In response to criticisms about the ineffectiveness of previous development assistance efforts and the high level of indebtedness in some of the world's poorest countries, the two organizations focused on debt forgiveness for heavily indebted poor counties, poverty reduction, and improved economic growth. Debt forgiveness required countries to reprogram the bulk of the savings from forgiven debt into social sectors such as health and education.

In 1999, the World Bank and the IMF stipulated that all of their concessionary assistance to 81 eligible poor countries would need to be based on a Poverty Reduction Strategy Paper (IMF and World Bank 2002, 2003). This new approach was intended to the following:

- strengthen country ownership
- enhance the poverty focus of country programs

- provide a comprehensive coordination framework for the World Bank, the IMF, and other development partners
- improve public governance and accountability
- improve priority setting.

The PRSP process is country driven, involves broadly based participation, is results oriented and focused on outcomes that benefit the poor, is comprehensive in recognizing the multidimensional nature of poverty, is partnership oriented, and is based on a long-term perspective (IMF 2004a; World Bank 2004d).

The PRSP process has made poverty reduction the priority issue for development (SHC Development Consulting 2001). Because macroeconomic and sectoral strategies need to be formulated around the PRSP, health reform strategies must be included and focus on the poor. As of September 2004, about 42 LICs had developed PRSPs that are serving as the basis for World Bank and IMF financing in those countries. Extensive evaluations of PRSPs by the World Bank and the IMF, by bilateral donors, and by other development partners have painted the following mixed picture of their success (IMF 2004a; IMF and World Bank 2002, 2003; World Bank 2004d):

- PRSPs have the potential to encourage the development of country-owned, long-term strategies for poverty reduction and growth, but tensions concerning ownership among countries, the World Bank and the IMF, and other donors remain. External partners have not adapted their assistance programs to PRSP processes in a coordinated manner, and better frameworks for accountability of both countries and partners are needed.
- Country participation has improved; however, greater inclusiveness is still needed. Moreover, the process has not strengthened domestic institutional policy-making processes or accountability.
- PRSPs are an improvement over previous processes in terms of results orientation, poverty reduction focus, and long-term perspective. They have fallen short in terms of being a strategic reform road map, especially in relation to undertaking structural reforms, boosting economic growth, linking with medium-term expenditure frameworks and budgets, integrating sectoral strategies into the macroeconomic framework, assessing the social effects of macroeconomic strategies, understanding links between macroeconomics and microeconomics, integrating strategy components, and linking medium- and long-term operational targets.
- Capacity constraints have been serious impediments to effective implementation, but little attention has focused on capacity building.
- Monitoring and evaluation is still a significant weakness.

Evaluations of the health sector components of PRSPs raise many of these issues (DFID Health Systems Resource Centre 2003; WHO 2004a). As more and more partners buy into this process and as increased amounts of development assistance are funneled through PRSPs, their effectiveness will ultimately depend on country commitment, capacity, and processes; partner flexibility; and funding availability. At this stage, PRSPs still seem to be a work in progress.

Community-Based Health Insurance

As noted earlier, private and out-of-pocket spending accounts for almost half of total health spending in LICs. Given LIC governments' limited abilities to mobilize revenues, country and donor attention has turned to informal sector insurance mechanisms as a way to improve financial protection, mobilize revenues, and improve the efficiency of out-of-pocket spending. *Community-based health insurance* is an umbrella term for the various types of community financing arrangements that have emerged because of high out-of-pocket spending, uncertainty surrounding anticipated financial flows from donors, and large and unregulated private sectors. Here, CBHI refers to prepayment plans that attempt to pool risks to reduce the financial risk an individual faces because of illness (Atim and others 1998; Bennett, Creese, and Monash 1998; Bennett, Kelley, and Silvers 2004).

CBHI is found throughout the world but is particularly prevalent in Sub-Saharan Africa (Bennett, Kelley, and Silvers 2004). CBHI plans are relatively heterogeneous in terms of populations covered, services offered, regulation, management function, and objectives. The Commission on Macroeconomics and Health found that CBHI plans provided significant financial protection and extended access to a large number of rural and low-income populations (WHO 2001), but that affordability impeded access for the very poor. As a result, the commission called for increased support for CBHI and for the establishment of a cofinancing scheme that would match dollar for dollar the premiums individuals paid toward their health insurance with a government or donor dollar (WHO 2001).

One recent review of the CBHI experience found less positive results, noting "no evidence from the documents reviewed that [CBHI schemes] positively impact health status or at least the utilization of services and financial protection for their members and/or for society at large, particularly the poor" (ILO and STEP 2002a, 54). The review finds that most CBHI schemes "tend to be small organizations (70 percent covering less than 200 members) with community participation in key decisions at one point or another in their history but with limited legal or de facto ownership by the community and with significant dependence from other health subsystems or subsidies as reflected by their low market exposure" (ILO and STEP 2002a, 54).

In his assessment of CBHI, Ekman (2004, 249) notes the following:

> Overall, the evidence base is limited in scope and questionable in quality. There is strong evidence that

community-based health insurance provides some financial protection by reducing out-of-pocket spending. There is evidence of moderate strength that such schemes improve cost-recovery. There is weak or no evidence that schemes have an effect on the quality of care or the efficiency with which care is produced. In absolute terms, the effects are small and schemes serve only a limited section of the population. The main policy implication of this review is that these types of community financing arrangements are, at best, complementary to other more effective systems of health financing.

The evidence from these reviews suggests that, even though CBHI provides financial protection for those enrolled and some degree of resource mobilization, the overall effect is relatively small and schemes are less effective in reaching the very poor. Thus, CBHI is unlikely to be a panacea for substantially improving risk pooling and mobilizing resources in LICs, and for MICs, CBHI is less relevant given higher incomes and levels of formal sector employment. This finding does not suggest that CBHI should not be part of an overall solution to financing health care, but it indicates that CBHI is unlikely to play a major role.

The most critical challenge facing LICs is raising sufficient revenues to meet their basic health needs and the health MDGs. Although increased grant funding is badly needed, the large amounts of funds often targeted to a few countries and for specific diseases and interventions raise questions of country absorptive capacity, potential distortions of health systems' priorities, and interactions with IMF fiscal ceilings. Concomitantly, LICs must improve their institutions in order to increase absorptive capacity and increase the effectiveness of all official development assistance. It is also critical for the international community to reassess the entire official development assistance and DAH structure; to develop country-compatible mechanisms to reinforce promised international redistribution; and to improve the targeting, levels, predictability, and timeliness of external assistance.

HEALTH FINANCING ISSUES IN MICs

MICs benefit from higher levels of domestic funding, higher initial levels of risk pooling and prepayment, and stronger health systems than LICs. Many MICs are now focused on ensuring access and financial protection through universal health coverage. Chile, Colombia, the Republic of Korea, Mexico, Poland, and Thailand are implementing universal coverage reforms or have already done so. However, they and many other MICs still face challenges similar to those facing LICs.

Alternative Risk Pooling Arrangements

Country experience shows that the critical factors for increasing coverage—that is, the number of individuals covered and

Table 12.4 MIC Reforms and Innovations for Achieving Universal Coverage

Organizational arrangement	Reforms or innovations
Social security	Opening affiliation to self-employed and informal sector workers
	Mandating universal participation
	Providing direct public subsidies to the organization for including the poor
	Subsidizing premiums for the poor, self-employed, and workers in the informal sector
MOHs and NHSs	Separating the purchase and provision of care
	Using public and private purchasing
	Reforming provider payments
Private health insurance	Regulating voluntary health insurance
	Making private insurers eligible for mandatory social security for health
	Providing demand-side subsidies for health insurance
Integration reforms (reforms that allow synergic interaction of multiple organizational arrangements)	Using public and private purchasing
	Providing demand-side subsidies for health insurance for the poor and for high-risk groups
	Setting up risk equalization and solidarity funds
	Providing health education to stimulate demand
	Having a virtual single pool

Source: Authors.

the extensiveness of the benefit package—are increased risk pooling and prepayment and better access to equity subsidies. As discussed earlier, most MICs face fragmented risk pools (ILO and STEP 2002b). Table 12.4 presents MIC approaches to reforming risk pooling arrangements for achieving universal coverage.

Most MICs face an additional strategic decision: whether to pursue aggregation of all pools in a single organization (a single pool) or whether to allow for the existence of multiple risk pooling organizations, which would explicitly or implicitly compete for members and would be subject to the same rules regarding benefit packages, revenue collection mechanisms, and portability of benefits (that is, a virtual single pool). Colombia and Turkey have opted for the virtual single pool reform, whereas Costa Rica has chosen a single risk pool. In the OECD context, Germany and the Netherlands have virtual single pool arrangements, whereas New Zealand and the United Kingdom have single pool arrangements.

Reforms of Social Security. Because SSOs traditionally cover salaried formal sector workers from whom payroll contributions can be collected, requiring informal sector workers or self-employed workers to join is difficult. The reforms for confronting this issue range from voluntary enrollment to various types of subsidization, as detailed in table 12.4.

Country experiences are also illuminating. For instance, Chile and Mexico have opened SSOs to the informal sector and the self-employed through voluntary affiliation, yet they still face risks of adverse selection because of the voluntary nature of enrollment and the exclusion of the poorest (Bitrán and others 2000; Instituto Mexicano de Seguro Social 2003). Chile, Colombia, Costa Rica, and the Philippines have addressed exclusion either by subsidizing the SSO directly or by subsidizing premiums for the poor and informal and self-employed workers who join. The Republic of Korea and Taiwan, China, have implemented mandatory universal participation, including gradual expansion to the whole population, whereas Panama has expanded coverage to dependents of contributing members.

Some of the most important advantages underlying SSO innovations include the existence of organizational capacity and of pools of funds (or sometimes a single large fund) that allow newly enrolled individuals and groups to take advantage of the risk and income cross-subsidization mechanisms and purchasing arrangements that are already in place. This approach results in an immediate enlargement of the risk pool in contrast to creating other pooling organizations as intermediate steps for the future merging of schemes. However, SSOs usually cover only a relatively small portion of the total population, and their focus on formal sector workers and use of payroll contributions as their main revenue collection mechanisms might be an insurmountable obstacle for reaching the informal sector and the poor, particularly those in rural areas.

In countries where a SSO is well established and covers a large population, it might face problems in including informal sector workers in the absence or even the presence of public subsidies if the incentive structure is not well designed. For instance, in the case of Mexico, the SSO operates a scheme that is partially subsidized by the central government, yet the scheme still has experienced severe adverse selection and has few participants, which has also discouraged actively promoting enrollment (World Bank 2004c).

Reforms of MOHs and NHSs. MIC reform approaches for MOHs and NHSs include introducing internal markets, including separating the purchasing function from the provision of health services; using public-private purchasing; reforming provider payment systems; and decentralizing. In theory, efficiency gains in the system could be used to provide access to new enrollees, to increase the number and quality of services to all participants in the system, or to do both. Success in these areas has been limited (Baeza and Packard 2005). Effective modernization of public sector management and civil services statutes has to date been missing from most provider payment and health sector reform efforts.

Private Health Insurance Reforms in MICs. Since the 1980s, MICs have seen two main reforms related to private insurance: (a) the facilitation and promotion of voluntary health insurance, including formal recognition of competing private health insurance, and (b) the integration of regulated private insurance as one component of mandatory social security schemes for formal workers. Many MICs, such as Indonesia, Mexico, and the Philippines, now recognize and regulate voluntary private health insurance. In Chile and Colombia, private insurers participate in the provision of mandatory risk pooling for social security.

The literature provides some evidence of the potential benefits and problems resulting from the introduction of private health insurance and competition in the insurance market (Londoño and Frenk Mora 1997; Sheshinski and López-Calva 1998). However, an ample literature also deals with the equity and efficiency problems of private health insurance competition, including risk selection (insurers seeking to enroll low-risk individuals) and underservice (insurers setting barriers to the use of services, for instance, by not contracting with providers of expensive interventions or in low-income areas) (Arrow 1963; Hsiao 1994, 1995; Laffont 1990; Milgrom and Roberts 1992).

As to whether harnessing private health insurance contributes to or damages MICs' chances for achieving universal coverage, the question is whether MICs can take advantage of the benefits of introducing health insurance competition and avoid the related efficiency and equity problems. MICs must confront the feasibility of introducing specific financial, regulatory, and organizational reforms at a level of transaction costs that would not offset the benefits of competition and privatization (Baeza and Cabezas 1998; Coase 1937; Newhouse 1998; Williamson 1985).

Single Pool versus Virtual Single Pool. Most MICs must also decide whether to aggregate all pools into a single organization or to aim for a virtual single pool (Baeza and Packard 2005). The implementation of more effective and efficient cross-subsidies between groups with different income and health risks is facilitated by merging smaller pools into large pools—in some cases, national pools. Indeed, the main preliminary lessons emerging from Costa Rica, the Republic of Korea, and Taiwan (China), all of which have achieved universal coverage, suggest that the combination of a clearly defined benefit package and reforms for enlarging risk pools plays a paramount role in achieving greater inclusion through solidarity in financing and increasing access.

Yet for most MICs, the reality is that multiple pooling arrangements exist, leading to a fragmented, inefficient, and inequitable health financing situation overall. Given that developing proper regulations and incentive systems for counterbalancing such problems is complicated, both institutionally and cost-wise, fostering a virtual single pool is likely the most feasible option for these countries.

Sources of Health System Financing in MICs

As discussed earlier in this chapter, health systems use different sources of financing and revenue collection, including general taxation, payroll contributions, risk-rated premiums, and user fees. However, concern is increasing about the use of payroll contributions as a mechanism for collecting revenue. In a recent study on financial protection in Latin America, Baeza and Packard (2005) argue that to extend effective risk pooling to the informal and nonsalaried sectors and to achieve universal participation in risk pooling arrangements, policy makers need to delink health insurance financing and eligibility from labor market status or employment sector, by gradually reducing and eventually eliminating payroll contribution financing. In addition to extending protection against health shocks, this delinking might also have a positive effect on labor market mobility and formalization. This delinking can be achieved through shifting health financing toward general taxation, which is likely preferred on equity and efficiency grounds, or through risk-rating premiums as a transition if fiscal constraints do not permit full fiscal financing.

Donor Disengagement from MICs

As demonstrated both by the composition and recipients of DAH and by new health financing and policy agendas, global health financing policy is currently focused on LICs, leaving most MICs under the radar. The MDG agenda is predominantly a LIC agenda, or at least most MICs perceive it as such. Thus, the question is what to do with the MIC policy dialogue. Is the status quo tantamount to disengagement? If so, the international community is in danger of losing important financing lessons that would most likely be of great use for LICs. In addition, a more concerted effort is needed to analyze what the MDGs mean for MICs—particularly in light of their increased noncommunicable disease and injury burdens, areas that the MDGs do not address—and to invest more in the evidence base for MIC-relevant reforms. It is important to maintain broad goals, but also important to develop new MIC-specific indicators, especially for financial protection, which is at the core of poverty alleviation in MICs as well as LICs but is not explicitly reflected in the MDGs.

The PRSP process also sends a clear signal to the international community to focus on the LICs. Unfortunately, few PRSPs consider the role of the health system in ensuring financial protection and reforms of risk pooling arrangements, which are at the core of most LIC and MIC health sector financing strategies. A new approach is needed to support MICs' efforts to improve public subsidy management and health system performance to ensure financial protection. Such approaches are also critical in assisting LICs with their poverty reduction and health financing reform efforts in the future.

CONCLUSIONS

Global health financing policy is in transition. Infusions of large amounts of grant money from new financing entities have changed the players involved in shaping global health policy. Decisions made by the World Bank and the IMF in 1999 requiring PRSPs as the basis for concessionary financing have pushed LICs to develop their health policies in the context of an overall strategy framework for poverty reduction that considers intrasectoral, intersectoral, and macroeconomic tradeoffs.

Clearly, neither increased domestic resource mobilization nor future economic growth will provide the resources necessary for LICs to finance their health needs, whether defined in terms of a basic package of essential health services or whether identified within the framework of the MDGs. Increasing official development assistance is thus critical for LICs to make progress in either respect. However, the projected magnitude and speed of scaling up raises serious questions about countries' absorptive capacity, aid effectiveness, predictability, and stability and about new investments' financial sustainability at the country and donor levels. Even though empirical evidence is still lacking, concerns have arisen that new sources and increased levels of funding for disease-specific programs will lead to verticalization and could distort health systems. The donor community and countries urgently need to reform the current system of DAH, to improve institutions in developing countries, and to develop mechanisms to ensure that donors meet their DAH commitments. Finally, MIC issues need to receive greater attention.

Global health financing policy makers face the following challenges:

- The architecture for formulating, coordinating, and implementing global health financing policy at the international and country levels needs to be improved.
- The donor community needs to harmonize procedures, ensure aid predictability, and guarantee longer-term assistance.
- Donors need to meet their development assistance obligations as well as provide more assistance to help countries improve their domestic resource mobilization efforts.
- The IMF needs to improve understanding of its fiscal programs and be more flexible in reconciling fiscal constraints with increased official development assistance and DAH.
- The global community needs to improve the knowledge base in terms of good (and bad) international practice with respect to health financing. In this context, absorptive capacity constraints on both the demand and the supply sides must be removed. Better use of existing tools, including cost-effectiveness analysis, and development of new tools are needed to help poor countries realistically prioritize their financing and spending options and deal with the tradeoffs between financing essential services and providing financial protection.
- The potential for verticalization as a result of increased levels of DAH needs to be assessed rigorously and empirically, taking into account the benefits of such assistance as well as its potential distortionary effects on other programs and on health systems as a whole. By focusing limited resources on a few targeted areas, countries can achieve impressive results in terms of disease control efforts; however, many disease eradication efforts have succeeded because such efforts enhanced overall system capacity.
- The existing assistance instruments need to be objectively and fully analyzed. Examples of potential inconsistencies, such as disease-specific program grants versus PRSPs, need to be highlighted and addressed.
- The issue of financial sustainability needs to be assessed objectively and apolitically. The international donor community needs to face up to the realities of those poor countries whose economies are not sustainable in the medium term and to consider redistributional policies to assist them.
- The donor community needs to put MICs on the agenda both in terms of their economic and social development and in terms of their use as good practice examples for LICs as they transition to MIC status.

Because of the different accountabilities of the various multilateral and bilateral organizations, global funds and alliances, and private foundations, coordinating global health financing policy has become increasingly complex. Given that international redistribution of wealth is central to meeting basic needs in poor countries, the lack of an effective international mechanism to enforce agreed-on transfers of wealth is problematic. Under these circumstances, the global community must help countries prioritize on the basis of realistic expectations of promised donor assistance and harmonization.

Providing countries with advice on good practice and assisting both LICs and MICs to develop equitable and efficient institutional structures, revenue-raising mechanisms, and spending prioritizations are important areas worthy of more international focus and collaboration. Assessments of the costs and constraints in reaching the health MDGs, taking into account the large increases in marginal costs to cover the most difficult-to-reach 5 or 10 percent of the population, are important knowledge products in a resource-constrained world. Making better use of cost-effectiveness information and developing better-costing tools are necessary for assisting countries, and donors could help by providing better information on where to focus policies to remove bottlenecks to the absorption of additional resources, particularly in terms of achieving the MDGs. A needed step for assisting LIC and MIC governments is developing and disseminating evidence about effective health financing polices, both in severely resource-constrained LICs that have achieved good health outcomes and in MICs that have achieved universal coverage with good health outcomes at reasonable spending levels. Last, the donor community must harmonize its procedures, simplify aid instruments, ensure the predictability of assistance, and create a more effective global policy environment.

DISCLAIMER

The findings, interpretations, and conclusions expressed in this paper are entirely those of the authors and should not be attributed in any manner to the Bill & Melinda Gates Foundation, the RAND corporation, or to the World Bank, its affiliated organizations, the members of its Board of Directors, or the countries it represents.

NOTES

1. For a detailed analysis of country-specific and global health expenditure trends, see Musgrove, Zeramdini, and Carrin (2002).

2. In addition to aid, countries receive significant financial inflows through foreign direct investment, expatriate workers' remittances, special targeted assistance, South-South support, and so on, and these inflows must also be taken into account (World Bank 2004b).

3. Clemens, Radelet, and Bhavani's (2004) study shows that aid can be somewhat effective in countries with weaker policy environments.

4. More recent data for all LICs indicate per capita spending of US$19 if the data are population weighted and US$25 if they are country weighted. The public share is 52 percent (country weighted).

5. One of the main funding organizations is the Bill & Melinda Gates Foundation, which is investing approximately US$1.35 billion per year, with a considerable portion of that allocated to global health issues.

REFERENCES

Arhin-Tenkorang, D. 2000. "Mobilizing Resources for Health: The Case for User Fees Revisited." Working Paper 81, Center for International Development, Cambridge, MA.

Arrow, K. J. 1963. "Uncertainty and the Welfare Economics of Medical Care." *American Economic Review* 53 (5): 851–83.

Atim, C., F. Diop, J. Etté, D. Evrard, P. Marcadent, and N. Massiot. 1998. *The Contribution of Mutual Organizations to Financing, Delivery, and Access to Health Care: Synthesis and Research in Nine West and Central African Countries.* Bethesda, MD: Abt Associates, Partnerships for Health Reform Project.

Baeza, C., and M. Cabezas. 1998. "Is There a Need for Risk Adjustment in Health Insurance Competition in Latin America?" Discussion paper prepared for the World Bank, Latin America and the Caribbean Region, Human and Social Development Department, Washington, DC.

Baeza, C., and T. G. Packard. 2005. *Beyond Survival: Protecting Households from the Impoverishing Effects of Health Shocks in Latin America.* Washington, DC: World Bank.

Bennett, S., A. Creese, and R. Monash. 1998. "Health Insurance Schemes for People outside Formal Sector Employment." Discussion of Analysis, Research, and Assessment Paper 16, World Health Organization, Geneva.

Bennett, S., A. G. Kelley, and B. Silvers. 2004. *21 Questions on CBHF: An Overview of Community-Based Health Financing.* Bethesda, MD: Abt Associates, Partnerships for Health Reform Project.

Bidani, B., and M. Ravallion. 1997. "Decomposing Social Indicators Using Distributional Data." *Journal of Econometrics* 77 (1): 125–39.

Bitrán, R., and U. Giedion. 2003. "Waivers and Exemptions for Health Services in Developing Countries." Social Protection Discussion Paper 308, World Bank, Washington, DC.

Bitrán, R., J. Muñoz, P. Aguad, M. Navarrete, and G. Ubilla. 2000. "Equity in the Financing of Social Security for Health in Chile." *Health Policy* 50 (3): 171–96.

Brenzel, L., and Y. Rajkotia. 2004. "Vaccine Financing Report." Paper prepared for the World Bank Human Development Network, Health Nutrition and Population Unit, Washington, DC.

Burnside, C., and D. Dollar. 1997. "Aid, Policies, and Growth." Policy Research Working Paper 1777, World Bank, Policy Research Department, Macroeconomics and Growth Division, Washington, DC.

Cassels, A. 1997. *A Guide to Sectorwide Approaches for Health Development: Concepts, Issues, and Working Arrangements.* Geneva: World Health Organization.

Clemens, M. A., and S. Radelet. 2003. "The Millennium Challenge Account: How Much Is Too Much, How Long Is Long Enough?" Working Paper 23, Center for Global Development, Washington, DC.

Clemens, M. A., S. Radelet, and R. Bhavnani. 2004. "Counting Chickens When They Hatch: The Short-Term Effect of Aid on Growth." Working Paper 44, Center for Global Development, Washington, DC.

Coase, R. H. 1937. "The Nature of the Firm." *Economica* 4 (16): 386–405.

Collier, P., and D. Dollar. 1999. "Aid Allocation and Poverty Reduction." Unpublished manuscript, World Bank, Development Research Group, Washington, DC.

Collier, P., and A. Hoeffler. 2002. "Aid, Policy, and Growth in Post-Conflict Societies." Policy Research Working Paper 2902, World Bank, Washington, DC.

Commission for Africa. 2005. *Our Common Interest: Report of the Commission for Africa*. London: Commission for Africa. http://www.commissionforafrica.org/english/report/thereport/cfafullreport_1.pdf.

Croce, E., and V. H. Juan-Ramon. 2003. "Assessing Fiscal Sustainability: A Cross-Country Comparison." Working Paper 03/145, International Monetary Fund, Washington, DC.

Devarajan, S., V. Swaroop, and Z. Heng-Fu. 1996. "The Composition of Public Expenditures and Economic Growth." *Journal of Monetary Economics* 37 (2–3): 313–44.

DFID (Department for International Development) Health Systems Resource Centre. 2003. *A Review of Human Resource Content of PRSP and HIPC Documentation in 6 Selected African Countries*. London: DFID.

Dunaway, S., and P. N'Diaye. 2004. "An Approach to Long-Term Fiscal Policy Analysis." Working Paper 04/113, International Monetary Fund, Washington, DC.

Ekman, B. 2004. "Community-Based Health Insurance in Low-Income Countries: A Systematic Review of the Evidence." *Health Policy and Planning* 19 (5): 249–70.

Ensor, T., and S. Cooper. 2004. "Overcoming Barriers to Health Service Access: Influencing the Demand Side." *Health Policy and Planning* 19 (2): 69–79.

Filmer, D., and L. Pritchett. 1999. "The Impact of Public Spending on Health: Does Money Matter?" *Social Science and Medicine* 49 (10): 1309–23.

Foster, M. 1999. "Lessons of Experience from Sectorwide Approaches in Health." Paper prepared for the World Health Organization and the Inter-Agency Working Group on Sector-wide Approaches and Development Cooperation, Geneva.

———. 2003. *The Case for Increased Aid: Final Report to the Department for International Development*. Chelmsford, U.K.: Mick Foster Economics.

Global Health Trust. 2004. *Specific Programs and Human Resources: Addressing a Key Implementation Constraint*. Cambridge, MA: Harvard University.

Gupta, S., B. J. Clements, A. Pivovarsky, and E. R. Tiongson. 2004. "Foreign Aid and Revenue Response: Does the Composition of Aid Matter?" In *Helping Countries Develop: The Role of Fiscal Policy*, ed. S. Gupta, B. J. Clements, and G. Inchauste, 385–406. Washington, DC: International Monetary Fund.

Gupta, S., M. Verhoeven, and E. R. Tiongson. 2001. "Public Spending on Health Care and the Poor." Working Paper 01/127, International Monetary Fund, Washington, DC.

Gwatkin, D., S. Rutstein, K. Johnson, E. A. Suliman, and A. Wagstaff. 2003. *Initial Country-Level Information about Socioeconomic Differences in Health, Nutrition, and Population*. Vols. I and II. Washington, DC: World Bank.

Haines, A., and A. Cassels. 2004. "Can the Millennium Development Goals Be Attained?" *British Medical Journal* 329: 394–97.

Heller, P. 2005. "Fiscal Space-What It Is and How To Get It." *Finance and Development* 42 (2).

Hemming, R., M. Kell, and A. Schimmelpfennig. 2003. "Fiscal Vulnerability and Financial Crisis in Emerging Market Economies." Occasional Paper 218, International Monetary Fund, Washington, DC.

Hensher, M. 2001. "Financing Health Systems through Efficiency Gains." Commission on Macroeconomics and Health Working Paper Series WG3:2, World Health Organization, Geneva.

Hsiao, W. C. 1994. "'Marketization': The Illusory Magic Pill." *Health Economics* 3 (6): 351–57.

———. 1995. "Abnormal Economics in the Health Sector." *Health Policy* 32: 125–39.

ILO and STEP (International Labour Organization and Strategies and Tools against Exclusion and Poverty). 2002a. "Extending Social Protection in Health through Community Based Health Organizations." Discussion paper, ILO and STEP, Geneva.

———. 2002b. "Toward Decent Work: Social Protection for Health for All Workers and Their Families." Working paper, ILO and STEP, Geneva.

IMF (International Monetary Fund). 2004a. *Evaluation of the IMF's Role in Poverty Reduction Strategy Papers and Poverty Reduction and Growth Facility*. Washington, DC: IMF, Independent Evaluation Office.

———. 2004b. *2004 Government Finance Statistics*. Washington, DC: IMF.

IMF and World Bank. 2002. "Review of the Poverty Reduction Strategy Paper (PRSP) Approach: Early Experience with Interim PRSPs and Full PRSPs." Paper prepared for the International Development Association and the IMF, Washington, DC.

———. 2003. "Poverty Reduction Strategy Papers: Detailed Analysis and Progress to Date." Paper prepared for the International Development Association and the IMF, Washington, DC.

Institute for Health Sector Development. 2003. "Mapping of Sector-Wide Approaches in Health." Report prepared for the Swedish International Development Cooperation Authority Sectorwide Approach Seminar, San Francisco, CA, June 19.

Instituto Mexicano de Seguro Social. 2003. *Informe al Ejecutivo Federal y al Congreso de la Unión sobre la situación financiera y los riesgos del Instituto Mexicano del Seguro Social*. Mexico City: Instituto Mexicano de Seguro Social.

Joint Learning Initiative. 2004. "Human Resources for Health: Overcoming the Crisis." Harvard University Press Global Equity Initiative, Cambridge, Mass.

Kaddar, M., P. Lydon, and R. Levine. 2003. "A Critical Review of Financial Sustainability: The GAVI Experience." Discussion paper prepared for London School of Hygiene and Tropical Medicine, Workshop on the Economics of Immunization, London, October 29–30.

Kivumbi, G. W., and F. Kintu. 2002. "Exemption and Waivers from Cost Sharing: Ineffective Safety Nets in Decentralized Districts in Uganda." *Health Policy and Planning* 17 (Suppl. 1): 64–71.

Knowles, J. C., C. Leighton, and W. Stinson. 1997. *Measuring Results of Health Sector Reform for System Performance: A Handbook of Indicators*. Special Initiatives Report 1. Bethesda, MD: Abt Associates, Partnerships for Health Reform Project.

Laffont, J-J. 1990. *The Economics of Uncertainty and Information*. Cambridge, MA: Massachusetts Institute of Technology Press.

Londoño, J-L., and J. Frenk Mora. 1997. "Structured Pluralism: Toward an Innovative Model for Health System Reform in Latin America." *Health Policy* 41 (1): 1–36.

Maeda, A. 1998. "A Model for the Evolution of Health Systems." Presentation prepared for the World Bank, Washington, DC.

Mathers, C. D., C. Stein, D. M. Fat, C. Rao, M. Inoue, N. Tomijima, and others. 2002. "Global Burden of Disease 2000: Version 2 Methods and Results." Global Programme on Evidence for Health Policy Discussion Paper 50, World Health Organization, Geneva.

McLaughlin, J. 2003. "Accelerating Progress toward the Health MDGs: Important Lessons Learned from Development Assistance." Paper prepared for the World Bank, Washington, DC.

———. 2004. "The Evolution of the Sectorwide Approach (SWAp) and Explaining the Correlation between SWAps and Reform Initiatives." Paper prepared for the World Bank, Washington, D.C.

Milgrom, P., and J. Roberts. 1992. *Economics, Organization, and Management*. Englewood Cliffs, NJ: Prentice-Hall.

Musgrove, P. 1996. "Public and Private Roles in Health: Theory and Financing Patterns." Health, Nutrition, and Population Discussion Paper, World Bank, Washington, DC.

Musgrove, P., R. Zeramdini, and G. Carrin. 2002. "Basic Patterns in National Health Expenditures." *Bulletin of the World Health Organization* 80 (2): 134–46.

Newhouse, J. 1998. "Risk Adjustment: Where Are We Now?" *Inquiry* 35 (2): 122–31.

Oliviera-Cruz, V., K. Hanson, and A. Mills. 2003. "Approaches to Overcoming Constraints to Effective Health Service Delivery: A Review of the Evidence." *Journal of International Development* 15 (1): 41–65.

Palmer, N., D. H. Mueller, L. Gilson, A. Mills, and A. Haines. 2004. "Health Financing to Promote Access in Low Income Settings—How Much Do We Know?" *Lancet* 364 (9442): 1365–70.

Rajkumar, A. S., and V. Swaroop. 2002. "Public Spending and Outcomes: Does Governance Matter?" Policy Research Working Paper 2840, World Bank, Washington, DC.

Rawlings, L. 2004. "A New Approach to Social Assistance: Latin America's Experience with Conditional Cash Transfer Programs." Social Protection Discussion Paper 0146, World Bank, Washington, DC.

Schieber, G., ed. 1997. *Innovations in Health Care Financing.* Washington, DC: World Bank.

Schieber, G., and A. Maeda. 1997. "A Curmudgeon's Guide to Financing Health in Developing Countries." In *Innovations in Health Care Financing,* ed. G. Schieber, 1–40. Washington, DC: World Bank.

SHC Development Consulting. 2001. *Sector Programmes and PRSP Implementation: Chances and Challenges.* Kassel, Germany: SHC Development Consulting.

Sheshinski, E., and L. F. López-Calva. 1998. "Privatization and Its Benefits: Theory and Evidence." Consulting Assistance on Economic Reform II Discussion Paper 35, Harvard University, Cambridge, MA.

Tait, A. 2001. "Mobilization of Domestic Resources for Health through Taxation: A Summary Survey." Commission on Macroeconomics and Health Working Paper WG3:14, World Health Organization, Geneva.

Tanzi, V., and H. H. Zee. 2000. "Tax Policy for Emerging Markets: Developing Countries." Working Paper 00/35, International Monetary Fund, Washington, DC.

Travis, P., S. Bennet, A. Haines, T. Pang, Z. Q. Bhutta, A. A. Hyder, and others. 2004. "Overcoming Health Systems Constraints to Achieve the Millennium Development Goals." *Lancet* 364: 900–6.

UNECA (United Nations Economic Commission for Africa). 2001. "Abuja Declaration on HIV/AIDS, Tuberculosis, and Other Related Infectious Diseases." Paper presented at UNECA Special Summit on HIV/AIDS, Tuberculosis, and Other Related Infectious Diseases, Abuja, Nigeria, April 27. http://www.uneca.org/adf2000/Abuja%20Declaration.htm.

United Nations Millennium Project. 2005. *UN Millennium Project 2005: Investing in Development—A Practical Plan to Achieve the Millennium Development Goals.* New York: United Nations.

Wagstaff, A., and M. Claeson. 2004. *The Millennium Development Goals for Health: Rising to the Challenges.* Washington, DC: World Bank.

WHO (World Health Organization). 2000. *The World Health Report 2000: Health Systems—Improving Performance.* Geneva: WHO.

———. 2001. *Report of the Commission on Macroeconomics and Health: Investing in Health for Economic Development.* Geneva: WHO.

———. 2002. *The Report of Working Group 3 of the Commission on Macroeconomics and Health.* Geneva: WHO.

———. 2004a. *Poverty Reduction Strategy Papers: Their Significance for Health—Second Synthesis Report.* Geneva: WHO.

———. 2004b. *World Health Report 2004: Changing History.* Geneva: WHO.

Williamson, O. E. 1985. *The Economic Institutions of Capitalism.* New York: Free Press.

World Bank. 1993. *World Development Report 1993: Investing in Health.* New York: Oxford University Press.

———. 2003. *World Development Report 2004: Making Services Work for Poor People.* New York: Oxford University Press.

———. 2004a. "Aid Effectiveness and Innovative Financing Mechanisms." Report prepared for the 2004 Annual Meetings of the International Monetary Fund and the World Bank, Washington, DC, October 2–3.

———. 2004b. *Global Development Finance: Harnessing Cyclical Gains for Development.* Washington, DC: World Bank.

———. 2004c. *Poverty in Mexico: An Assessment of Conditions, Trends, and Government Strategy.* Washington, DC: World Bank.

———. 2004d. *The Poverty Reduction Strategy Initiative: An Independent Evaluation of the World Bank's Support through 2003.* Washington, DC: World Bank, Operations Evaluation Department.

———. 2004e. *2004 World Development Indicators.* Washington, DC: World Bank.

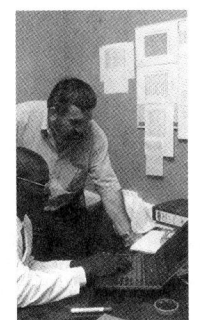

Chapter **13**

Recent Trends and Innovations
in Development Assistance for Health

Robert Hecht and Raj Shah

After nearly a decade during which levels of external development assistance for health (DAH) stagnated, an encouraging rise has occurred in the volume of such assistance. Donors and developing countries are testing and implementing innovative approaches to the use of DAH, while simultaneously seeking ways to raise the effectiveness of existing streams of aid and more traditional financing mechanisms. In short, DAH has entered a dynamic phase that holds considerable promise.

Nevertheless, it continues to suffer from a broad range of disappointments: misuse and inefficiency in the deployment of funds, gaps in essential areas that require financing support, and weaknesses in institutional and management arrangements. Substantial room for improvement exists.

This chapter documents those recent trends, analyzes the effects and assesses the performance of DAH, and points to areas that require priority attention. In the first part, we present statistics on DAH, updating the *World Development Report 1993* (World Bank 1993) and the report of the Commission on Macroeconomics and Health (CMH 2001). In the second part, we assess the performance of DAH. In the third part, we present recent innovations to underscore the current dynamic nature of such assistance. The chapter concludes with some suggestions on future directions.

TRENDS AND GAPS IN DEVELOPMENT ASSISTANCE FOR HEALTH

Despite a decline in overall official development assistance in the 1990s, DAH rose in real terms and as a proportion of official development assistance (table 13.1). New funding sources became available in 2000–2, including the Global Fund to

Fight AIDS, Tuberculosis, and Malaria and special U.S. financing for HIV/AIDS, plus rapid growth in grant awards from the Bill & Melinda Gates Foundation and in World Bank International Development Association (IDA) grants. Commitments from all external sources, including foundations, rose from an annual average of US$6.7 billion in 1997–99 to about US$9.3 billion in 2002.

Total DAH is the sum of external financing for health from several different sources: bilateral agencies as reported through the creditor reporting system of the Organisation for Economic Co-operation and Development (OECD); multilateral agencies, including the United Nations (UN) system—especially the World Health Organization (WHO), the United Nations Children's Fund, the United Nations Population Fund, and the global and regional development banks; the European Union; philanthropic organizations; and the Global Fund to Fight AIDS, Tuberculosis, and Malaria. Because no central repository of data on all the sources of DAH is currently available and comprehensive information is not published on any regular basis, painstaking and time-consuming efforts are required to assemble accurate, comparable data about all these sources.

After a long period of decline in official development assistance (grants from bilateral government channels and UN agencies plus net flows from development banks) during the 1990s, the OECD reported a real increase of 7 percent from 2001 to 2002 and a further increase of 4 percent from 2002 to 2003. Those increases took official development assistance to an all-time high, in both nominal and real terms, of US$68.5 billion. As a percentage of gross national income, this represents an increase from the all-time low of 0.22 percent recorded during most years from 1997 to 2001 to about 0.25 percent in

Table 13.1 Development Assistance for Health, Selected Years *(US$ millions)*

Source	Annual average, 1997–99	2002
Bilateral agencies	2,560	2,875
Multilateral agencies	3,402	4,649
European Commission	304	244
Global Fund to Fight AIDS, Tuberculosis, and Malaria	0	962
Bill & Melinda Gates Foundation	458	600
Total	6,724	9,330

Sources: Michaud 2003; OECD 2004a.

2003, still well below the target of 0.7 percent set by the OECD's member states in 1970. Only five countries—Denmark, Luxembourg, the Netherlands, Norway, and Sweden—currently achieve this target, and six others have now set prospective dates for its achievement—namely, Belgium (2010), Finland (2010), France (2012), Ireland (2007), Spain (2012), and the United Kingdom (2013).

Bilateral assistance for health rose from an annual average of US$2.2 billion (3.8 percent of the total) during 1997–99 to US$2.9 billion (6.8 percent) in 2002. Among the bilateral arrangements, the United States accounted for about 40 percent of the total, even though as a percentage of gross domestic product (GDP), its allocation to international development was among the lowest of all the high-income countries.

Within the UN system, DAH rose from an average of US$1.6 billion per year during 1997–99 to US$2 billion in 2002. Commitments from the development banks remained stationary at about US$1.4 billion. However, changes in accounting by the World Bank to include financing for health activities contained in projects managed by other sectors (such as urban, water and sanitation, transportation, and social development), suggest that its new commitments for health actually rose from about US$1 billion in 2001 to US$1.3 billion in 2002 and US$1.7 billion in 2003.

In the future, consensus will need to be reached on whether allocations by the multilateral development banks to projects in other sectors or to projects that are classified as multisectoral—especially broad budget support to governments, which may be specifically tied to domestic spending and policy reforms in health—should be counted as DAH. Another issue in DAH accounting involves distinguishing between allocations for health from the multilateral banks that take different forms—namely, outright grants (a recent innovation for the World Bank and the regional banks); subsidized loans for the poorest countries, which at the World Bank are IDA credits; and loans for the middle-income developing countries that reflect the actual costs of borrowing by the development banks. For example, of the US$1.7 billion in World Bank commitments for

health in 2003, about US$1 billion took the form of IDA credits, and most of the rest was in the form of loans that reflected the costs of borrowing. Because the face value of the financial commitment can be considered to be reduced by repayments in the case of subsidized and market rate loans, some argue that the net financial value of such loans, rather than their face value, should be used in calculating DAH. This calculation further complicates the task of monitoring DAH.

Despite these various cautions and qualifications, it is clear that DAH has grown in recent years. This upward trend has been driven by several factors, including (a) donors' increasing attention to the challenges presented by the Millennium Development Goals (MDGs), which are heavily centered on maternal and child health and control of communicable diseases; (b) strong global mobilization to confront the AIDS pandemic in developing countries since 1998–99, especially in Africa; and (c) donors' expanding interest in research and development (R&D) in relation to new health technologies to address the major diseases prevalent in poor countries. In contrast, external funding for health system development, human resources, and noncommunicable diseases has increased more slowly.

In terms of the areas that have benefited from the growing volume of DAH, three stand out: HIV/AIDS, immunization, and new health product development. According to Michaud (2003), in 2002 about US$900 million in DAH was for HIV/AIDS, followed by US$210 million for tuberculosis (TB), and US$160 million for malaria control. The Joint United Nations Programme on HIV/AIDS (UNAIDS) also reports a substantial rise in external financing for AIDS prevention, treatment, and social mitigation activities over the past four years (UNAIDS 2004). Most of the increase in assistance for immunization has taken place through the Global Alliance for Vaccines and Immunization (GAVI), which has amassed commitments of about US$1.3 billion to finance the expansion of existing childhood immunization programs and the accelerated introduction of hepatitis B and *Haemophilus influenzae* type B vaccines. Assistance for health technologies directed at diseases that are prevalent in the developing world has been channeled through new public-private partnerships. Examples include the International AIDS Vaccine Initiative (IAVI), the Medicines for Malaria Venture, and the International Partnership for Microbicides. Estimates indicate that the 10 largest public-private partnerships have raised more than US$1 billion over the past five years (IPPPH 2004).

In terms of the sources of the expanded volume of DAH, a small number of institutions account for much of the recent increase. Among the traditional donors, these institutions include the World Bank and the governments of Canada and the United Kingdom. At the same time, as a share of GDP, contributions from Ireland, the Netherlands, Norway, and Sweden remain high. Among nontraditional sources, the Bill &

Melinda Gates Foundation stands out as a major new player as of the late 1990s. With a focus on the development of new drugs, vaccines, and diagnostics for the developing world, the Gates Foundation's commitments for health started in 1998 and rose rapidly to some US$600 million in 2002, with annual commitments expected to approach US$1 billion in 2004 and beyond.

Development assistance for health is channeled to a large number of low- and middle-income developing countries, but the largest recipient region is Africa. In 2002, about 35 percent of all such assistance went to Africa, followed by Latin America and the Caribbean with around 14 percent, East Asia and South Asia with 11 percent each, and the Middle East with 7 percent. The remaining 22 percent was for global programs (Michaud 2003).

This growth in funding for the control of communicable diseases and new health technologies to address them is important, given the high burden of illness and premature death these diseases cause. Nevertheless, the focus on AIDS, TB, and malaria should be matched by similar increases in investments in broader health system improvements. Relatively little DAH is being channeled to address the serious problems of shortages in health workforces in poor countries and their low productivity or to deal with weaknesses in health management information systems, in supply chain logistics for drugs and commodities, and so on. Even though focused spending on AIDS, TB, and malaria will clearly touch on these weaknesses, it will not on its own go to the core of the problem or lead to sustainable solutions. For example, GAVI allocates resources to strengthen immunization infrastructure such as cold chains and to train health workers to deliver vaccinations more effectively. The Global Fund to Fight AIDS, Tuberculosis, and Malaria provides funds to prepare health workers to deliver and monitor compliance with antiretroviral treatments. Useful as those activities are, they will not address the underlying weaknesses in human resources for health in poor countries, such as low levels of pay, unattractive conditions of service, and uncertain prospects for career advancement.

The recent rise in DAH is encouraging, but it is still far short of the volume of external financing for health that is needed, according to recent estimates and political pronouncements. On a global level, estimates of what donors need to provide to help countries reach the MDGs for health have typically ranged from US$15 billion to US$35 billion per year. The Commission on Macroeconomics and Health suggested a figure of about US$30 billion a year. While preparing for the Monterrey Summit on Finance for Development, the World Bank calculated a funding gap of US$15 billion to US$25 billion a year (Devarajan, Miller, and Swanson 2002). For the United Nations General Assembly special session on AIDS in June 2001, UNAIDS suggested that spending on HIV/AIDS alone in the developing countries needed to rise to about US$9 billion annually by 2005, with about two-thirds of this amount to

come from external sources (UNAIDS 2001). At the 2004 International AIDS Conference in Bangkok, UNAIDS raised its estimate of resources needed to more than US$15 billion a year by 2010 (UNAIDS 2004).

These global calculations have been followed by more detailed costing exercises at the country level, which hold the promise of yielding more accurate and meaningful figures than the global estimates. Donors working with government specialists in developing countries have tested a variety of methods. The UN Millennium Project has used a bottom-up approach, which is based on expanded coverage of key interventions and fixed unit costs, assuming no shared costs or benefits among different interventions, omitting the possibility of private financing, and adding a rough amount for system improvements (UN Millennium Project 2004). The World Bank has followed two other approaches. One, in India, is based on observed elasticities of change in children's health and nutrition outcomes in relation to public expenditures on health, primary education, water, and so on (World Bank 2003a). Another, in Ethiopia, Mali, and other countries, is based on detailed modeling of the costs of removing bottlenecks in health service delivery to enhance the coverage, utilization, and quality of key health interventions proven to have a positive effect on maternal and child health outcomes (Soucat and others 2003; World Bank and Ministry of Health, Ethiopia 2005).

A comparison of the Millennium Project's and the World Bank's results for East Africa is interesting. The Millennium Project calculates that nearly US$30 per capita are needed in additional spending for health, whereas the World Bank calculates that about US$4 per capita are needed for Ethiopia to reduce child and maternal death rates by 30 to 40 percent by 2015. The large difference between the two sets of results suggests that more work needs to be done to move toward consensus on the best methodology for countries to use.

Part of the difference is due to technical factors. The Millennium Project approach covers all the health MDGs, whereas the bottlenecks method has focused on the MDGs pertaining to child and maternal health only. The Millennium Project also calculates costs to achieve the MDGs in their entirety, whereas the bottlenecks method addresses incremental improvements. For example, in relation to the child mortality goal, the bottlenecks analysis for Ethiopia considers a substantial decline to be from 176 to 107 deaths per 1,000 live births, but the MDG is 59 deaths per 1,000 births. In addition, the Millennium Project multiplies additional units of service by a standard cost per unit, whereas the bottlenecks method estimates the cost of system improvements and then divides this amount by the additional services rendered to derive incremental unit costs.

The two approaches also have important differences in political philosophy. The Millennium Project approach sets high targets for DAH and health spending, which are based on full achievement of the MDGs, regardless of the starting points and gaps and without addressing the feasibility of reaching the targets. The World Bank's approach is less ambitious but may be seen as more realistic and as pointing the way to implementation based on gradual improvements—improvements that countries can pursue as additional financial resources and capacity to manage them effectively are combined on the ground.

MAKING DEVELOPMENT ASSISTANCE FOR HEALTH MORE EFFECTIVE: LESSONS LEARNED

More assistance is part of the answer to helping developing countries achieve more rapidly the improved health outcomes they seek and that are enshrined in the MDGs. To this end, we need to know how effective DAH has been and what can be done to make it more effective.

Despite valid criticisms of DAH, some health programs—inspired and supported by donors—have worked at scale and contributed to more than four decades of steady improvements in health, as measured by under-five mortality and overall life expectancy. The record of public health successes in developing countries is becoming increasingly clear, as noted in a recent review of four decades of experience (Levine and What Works Working Group 2004). The success stories cover a broad spectrum of circumstances. They are found in all regions and cover both communicable and noncommunicable diseases. They have been driven by new technologies, including vaccines, drugs, and diagnostics; community- and clinic-based care; and knowledge for behavior change.

Significant gains have occurred even in the poorest countries and in those with weak institutional environments. Consider, for example, the high levels of TB case detection in the Democratic Republic of Congo and in Myanmar (Stop TB Partnership 2003), the successes in polio eradication in African countries experiencing civil wars, and the growing availability of antiretroviral therapy in Haiti.

Some of this progress can be attributed to the general effects of economic growth and improvements in education, water, and sanitation. However, specific, compelling examples of the success of DAH-backed initiatives are available. For example, programs to immunize against measles, to control river blindness and guinea worm, and to fortify salt with iodine have had sustained and widespread effects (Levine and What Works Working Group 2004). These programs have been successful at scale, have generated sustainable health improvements at the population level, and have succeeded in a broad range of institutional environments.

Recent analyses and reviews of donor-supported successes in international health have noted a set of factors that tend to contribute to positive outcomes:

- strong internal (governments) and external (donors) political leadership

- collaboration across governments, donors, and nongovernmental organizations (NGOs) in program design and implementation
- consistent, predictable funding support, even after success has been achieved
- simple and flexible technologies that can be adapted to local conditions and do not require complex skills to operate and maintain
- programmatic approaches that recognize and address the need to help build health system infrastructure, especially in human resources
- household or community participation in the design, execution, and monitoring of program activities.

Policy Environment

Development assistance for health supports a vast array of activities and services, some focused on specific diseases (polio, TB, HIV/AIDS), some on strengthening health systems (disease surveillance, nurse and midwife training), and some on particular services (reproductive and child health services). But has DAH actually changed health outcomes? Recent work from the World Bank, the Commission on Macroeconomics and Health, and others suggests that it has (Rajkumar and Swaroop 2002). However, DAH does not work as effectively in countries where the policy environment is poor, even though some carefully targeted disease control activities can confer limited benefits. With good policies and institutions (strong property rights, reduced corruption, an efficient bureaucracy), an extra 1 percent of GDP in aid is estimated to reduce infant mortality by 0.9 percent. By contrast, where policies are average, the decline is estimated at only 0.4 percent, and where policies are poor, aid is estimated to have no significant effect on infant mortality (World Bank 2004b).

The issue is not black and white: there are gradations of good policy, and as policies improve, the productivity of aid increases. For example, Bangladesh has made large strides in reducing under-five mortality in recent years, relying on NGOs to deliver many services. If Bangladesh were able to raise the quality of its governance from below average to above average, even at its same public spending levels, it would realize more rapid gains. An additional dollar of government health spending would reduce under-five mortality by 14 percent, compared with 9 percent without such improvements (World Bank 2003c).

Tradeoffs may be necessary between targeting assistance toward the neediest countries and achieving the greatest effect from DAH, but even in needy countries with weak policies, some kinds of carefully targeted assistance for health (for example, immunizations delivered by reputable NGOs) can have a positive effect. In addition, in countries with weak policies, a focus by donors on policy dialogue and technical assistance to improve the environment for DAH can set the stage for a larger infusion of financial support down the road.

Conditionality

Conditionality is making the availability of funding dependent on a government completing an agreed task, such as enacting a new health law or spending a certain share of its budget on health activities. It can work, but only if the government is committed to making such a change. Tying aid to policy changes is a common practice, but recent studies have cast doubt on the ability of such conditionality to bring about reform (World Bank 1998, 2003a). If governments are not committed to reform, conditionality will not make them reform. Donors themselves often undermine the rigor and credibility of conditions because they usually face strong internal pressures to continue disbursement of the funds anyway, even when governments do not adhere to the agreed-on conditions. On the other hand, if governments are committed to reform, conditions can help by enabling governments to commit publicly to certain reforms and persuade private investors of their seriousness. For example, the government of Uganda's commitment to decentralizing the management of basic health services and to making local authorities accountable to communities was reinforced by conditions in the Uganda poverty reduction support credit, which several donors financed. Similarly, the Chinese government's commitment to reaching the poor with TB control services was reinforced by stipulations in donor-funded TB projects that they target the country's poorest provinces and reach out to deprived households (World Bank 2003c).

Donors cannot force policies on governments, but they can help with policy design. Donors can alert governments to the reasons for reform and help nurture commitment, but at the end of the day, it is governments that have to sustain any reforms (box 13.1). Undertaking analytical work, providing training and technical assistance, disseminating ideas about policy reform and development, and stimulating debate in civil society can all be valuable activities for donors to support while a government's commitment to reform is growing.

Vietnam in the late 1980s and early 1990s is a good example. At a landmark meeting in 1986, the ruling Communist Party decided to break with the past and introduce sweeping economic reforms. In the health sector, the reforms included introducing user fees at public facilities, legalizing private medicine, deregulating the pharmaceutical industry, and opening the pharmaceuticals and medical equipment subsectors to international trade. Initially, Vietnam saw no increase in aid, but such agencies as the United Nations Development Programme and the World Bank helped facilitate the reform process by organizing international workshops for the Vietnamese to exchange ideas on policy with their neighbors.

This effort set the stage for a large inflow of donor financing, starting around 1995 and continuing to the present.

Fungibility of Development Assistance for Health

Much aid is earmarked, both across sectors and within them. One part of a development agency gives a grant to the ministry of health for a health sector reform, while another does the same for a primary education project. An agency makes a loan to the ministry of health for a TB project, while another makes a loan for a malaria control project. The donors' intent is that these activities remain tightly sealed: the funds for health sector reform are to be kept separate from the funds for the primary education project; the TB project funds are to be kept separate from the malaria control project funds. The idea is to ensure that the government makes a certain spending choice. It is based on the assumption that the choice would not be made if the government had been handed a blank check for the same amount.

The implied view of such aid is that what you see is what you get; that is, a government receives US$1 million for a water project and the net effect is US$1 million worth of extra spending on the water sector. This view has recently been challenged, with the alternative view being that aid is at least partly fungible (Burnside and Dollar 2000; World Bank 1998). Hence, as a result of the inflow of development assistance for a specific health activity, the government changes the way in which it spends the rest of its resources, both in the health sector and in terms of allocations between health and other sectors. As a result, for each dollar earmarked for a specific health project, spending on health rises by less than a dollar but by more than would have been the case had the government received an extra dollar in its overall budget. Similarly, spending for the specified purpose in the health sector rises by less than a dollar, but by more than would have been the case had the government allocated an extra dollar of its own resources to health generally.

Assessing whether aid is indeed fungible is not straightforward. The difficulty is knowing how the government would have responded had its own resources increased by the amount of the aid or had it received a blank check for the same amount. Recent research suggests that, despite considerable variation across countries, on average only 29 cents of each additional dollar of aid goes into government development programs, with the rest leaking out into nondevelopment programs such as military spending (World Bank 2004b).

One important implication of those findings is that donors should spend less time and effort trying to channel their external funding to specific programs for priority diseases and populations. Instead, a more useful exercise would be to engage in a dialogue with the government on basic changes in the overall patterns of public spending for health—that is, the total

Donors and Commitment: Nutrition in Bangladesh and Thailand

In most countries, nutrition has not become a visible issue on the national political agenda, because nutrition advocates have not succeeded in linking improved nutrition with political and economic goals or in creating popular demand to eliminate malnutrition. In Bangladesh in the early 1990s, the United Nations Children's Fund and the World Bank joined forces to present a case to the government showing how the country could not achieve its economic goals unless it reduced malnutrition. This effort persuaded the government's financial planners that funding a national nutrition program was a good investment, and the government approved a new nutrition project in 1995.

However, the issue is not just how to build initial commitment, often the main focus of organizations such as the World Bank. Commitment can be fragile, and the issue is how to broaden and maintain commitment and complement it with systematic investments in institutional capacity development. The first nutrition investment in Bangladesh was completed in 2001. Children's nutritional status and households' health-seeking behaviors improved substantially in project areas, and malnutrition rates declined. A follow-on nutrition investment was approved, but because of weak government commitment, it is struggling in the challenging policy environment in which the social sectors operate. The Ministry of Health has not assigned high priority to the program, and conflicts between the government and the NGOs involved in community activities have complicated the situation. Contradictory messages from donors and frequent changes in leadership within the government have added to the challenge.

More recently, donors and advocates for nutrition within the government have proposed that nutrition activities that build on earlier successes be included in the Health, Nutrition, and Population Sector Program, which is scheduled to be finalized and approved in early 2005.

In contrast, in Thailand, building commitment for nutrition was achieved during the 1980s and nurtured with little external support. Government-sponsored efforts through studies, workshops, and media outreach generated commitment for nutrition by building broad consensus (in the government, NGOs, and the private sector) on the benefits of nutrition—not as a welfare issue, but as a human development issue. This initial commitment was sustained by ensuring that policy statements were closely linked to national investment plans, by building strong technical and managerial capacity for nutrition in the country (often by means of external aid), and by linking those actions with a strong buy-in and demand from communities. Malnutrition rates in Thailand declined from 51 percent in the early 1980s to 18 percent in 1990 and continue to fall.

Source: Heaver 2002.

allocation and the amounts for, say, providing child health and communicable disease control services and for improving community and primary-level health delivery systems. If the government followed through on those basic changes, then donors would transfer their financial assistance to the health sector as a whole.

The finding that aid is indeed fungible has encouraged some donors to search for broader development assistance mechanisms that recognize the importance of the entire expenditure program and explicitly avoid earmarking. Such mechanisms include the Multi-Country AIDS Program in Africa, which supports national HIV/AIDS strategies; sectorwide approaches in health; and poverty reduction support credits (PRSCs) that back a broad public spending agenda.

An opposing viewpoint is that although, in general, good policies matter and the fungibility of aid tends to undermine donors' ability to earmark their funding effectively, many high-impact health services can be delivered to the population on a targeted basis even when national policies and institutions are weak—and this aid would not occur in the absence of DAH. This argument applies especially to services with simple technologies—for instance, basic childhood vaccinations that can be delivered on a single occasion through annual campaigns or disease treatment programs (such as short-course drug therapy for TB) that can be provided through tightly managed top-down efforts (Jamison 2004). The high coverage and treatment success using the directly observed short-course therapy approach for TB in the Democratic Republic of Congo in recent years, even during the civil war, can be cited as an example of how a well-protected enclave project with strong donor backing can be successful (Stop TB Partnership 2003).

Another argument against broad budget support of health sector funding or in favor of the more traditional earmarking of DAH is that it helps maintain governments' and donors' focus on implementing and monitoring specific health service interventions and on the necessary technical and managerial improvements to ensure the achievement of targets in those areas. On the basis of experience in countries such as Bangladesh, Ghana, Mozambique, and Zambia, donors are increasingly of the view that broad support to a national health sector program leads to superficial oversight of bureaucratic processes and a corresponding loss of technical focus and depth (Foster, Brown, and Conway 2000). Although a sector-wide approach is theoretically fully compatible with careful monitoring of key outputs and health outcomes and with in-depth technical improvements, in practice, achieving this mix of objectives may prove difficult.

In summary, the debate on earmarked versus broad DAH support for national health programs continues. More analysis is needed to produce clearer conclusions on the advantages and disadvantages of the two approaches.

Transaction Costs of Aid

In a single low-income country, more than 20 donors—including bilaterals, multilaterals, global programs, foundations, and large NGOs—may be involved in the health sector. The demands placed on recipient countries can be huge, and donors are starting to acknowledge this burden. They are recognizing that their individual procedures for reporting, accounting, and managing funds—which often encompass different budget structures; different ways of measuring progress toward objectives; different regulations for the procurement of goods, services, and works; and different approaches toward and cycles for disbursing funds—place heavy and unreasonable demands on recipient countries. Demands are particularly heavy in poor countries that are forced to allocate limited human resources away from service delivery to manage donor funding.

The donor community is working to harmonize and simplify its procedures to reduce these transaction costs. In the health sector, experiments are taking place in several developing countries, including Bangladesh, the Kyrgyz Republic, Mozambique, and Zambia, to determine how best to lower the costs (OECD 2004b). Some of the principles of improved donor action include the following:

- ensuring that countries, not donors, drive the coordination
- fostering strategic coherence through a poverty reduction strategy and the health, nutrition, and population analyses that feed into it
- promoting financial coherence through a medium-term expenditure framework and an agreement that all donor funding will respect the government's overall spending plans and limits
- pooling donor funds in a single account and untying aid so that the government can procure goods and services from the lowest-cost source and not just from the donor countries
- limiting the number of country coordination bodies that can bring together national and international actors involved in health.

At the same time, some of the experiments in country-level coordination of DAH reveal the difficulties of implementing the principles of better donor harmonization. In some instances, persuading donors to pool their funds and sever the links between funding and procurement has proven difficult. Some donors face pressure from their legislatures to maintain separate accounting for the use of their DAH allocations so they can claim credit for achieving progress and thus "plant flags" on individual health projects. In addition, monitoring and evaluation systems have frequently not been strong enough to yield timely and meaningful data on progress, a critical failure if disbursements are linked to performance rather than to spending on specific inputs. Multiple national coordination bodies for government, donors, and NGOs for different diseases (AIDS, TB) and services (immunization, polio eradication) also persist in many settings. In short, a number of political and technical changes are needed to ensure the successful implementation of a harmonized donor agenda at the country level in the poorest developing nations.

Unpredictability of Development Assistance for Health

Some donors have taken steps to put in place instruments for DAH that extend the length of their financial commitments. The development of multiphase funding "slices" of 3 to 5 years embedded in a 10- or 15-year program of support is one way to lengthen commitments. Nevertheless, donor financing for health is not yet as reliable or sustained as is often claimed or hoped for, even under these new, long-term arrangements. In some developing countries, cuts in DAH have been sharp. Donors' budgets are subject to the usual business and political cycles and may go up or down during their annual budgetary processes. For such countries as the Comoros and Eritrea, where the year-to-year changes in external funding can amount to as much as a fifth of all public spending for health, the fluctuations are so great that they make planning and implementing coherent national health programs nearly impossible (figure 13.1).

Further work is needed to design mechanisms for DAH that provide greater assurance of sustained financial support. The challenges are to overcome the factors that result in interruptions to long-term DAH. Those factors include changes in

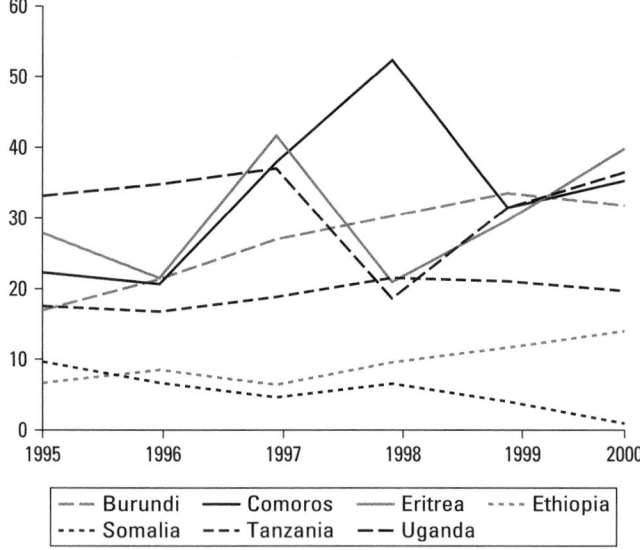

Source: World Bank 2004b.

Figure 13.1 External Financing as a Percentage of Total Health Expenditures, Selected Countries, 1995–2000

political leadership and aid agency management that lead to modifications of earlier agreements and end up reducing external funding levels or reallocating those funds to other activities.

One example of an innovative approach is the recently proposed establishment of an international finance facility. This facility would use financial commitments from governments of developed countries to tap funds in capital markets and would use those funds to frontload development assistance so as to accelerate progress toward the MDGs. The International Finance Facility for Immunization, which the United Kingdom formally announced at the World Economic Forum in January 2005 and is aiming to launch later in the year, will expand external financing for childhood vaccinations. The pilot project could be used to pledge funding against multiyear advance-purchase contracts for new vaccines (such as rotavirus vaccine) that may not reach the market for several years. Such an effort could help create a more assured market and reduce the risks for vaccine companies, thereby speeding up the introduction of these new health commodities to low-income countries (GAVI 2004b).

RECENT INNOVATIONS TO IMPROVE THE EFFECTIVENESS OF DEVELOPMENT ASSISTANCE FOR HEALTH

In recent years, donor agencies working with developing countries have been testing—and in some cases rolling out on a

large scale—a series of innovative approaches and instruments to improve the effectiveness of DAH. Those innovations include the use of broad budgetary support to countries with strong governance and institutions, the implementation of sectorwide approaches in health, the use of performance-based financing mechanisms, a shift to direct engagement with the private sector, and the implementation of programs designed to move resources expeditiously to the frontlines of the battle for improved health (that is, to communities). Evidence on the effectiveness of those innovative approaches and the conditions under which they tend to work is starting to accumulate.

Budget Support in Strong Policy Environments

In low-income settings where policies, governance, and institutions are sound, donors have increasingly sought to provide broad, untied, and flexible budget support to governments to help support a full public expenditure program aimed at raising the level of spending and the effectiveness of resource use for health. Frequently, this support has taken the form of PRSC operations, including grants and credits. The PRSC is typically built on the foundations of a national poverty reduction strategy that analyzes the links between poor health outcomes and income poverty and identifies policies that can improve the health of the general population, especially that of poor households. The policies are then used to design a medium-term public expenditure program or framework that, in turn, is backed by external funding from donors in the form of a PRSC.

This approach draws on three of the key lessons from decades of experience with DAH:

- A good policy environment improves the use of external financing.
- The fungibility of DAH makes it logical to allocate external funds to a general budget that prioritizes health rather than to narrow projects in the health sector.
- An integrated system for managing public finance for health improves national ownership of policies and programs to improve the health of the poor and raises the chances that such funding will be sustained over a long period and eventually will use domestic resources.

Plenty of examples are now available of the use of DAH for PRSCs that focus on improvements in health. The earliest health-oriented PRSCs were in Mozambique and Uganda, followed since by similar operations in Benin, Mauritania, and other low-income African countries. In Mauritania, for example, the country received a transfer of US$25 million in external financing to back a public spending plan that doubled health spending from about US$8 per capita in 2000 to US$16 per capita in 2004. The plan also emphasized increasing health investments that are designed to lower maternal and child deaths and combat communicable diseases by expanding rural health facilities, by providing higher pay and other incentives for health personnel working in rural areas, and by improving the availability of drug supplies at lower-level facilities. External financing was not earmarked for these actions in the health sector. Instead, the government committed itself to spending for these purposes from a consolidated national budget that was closely monitored by civil society, government officials, and donor representatives (World Bank 2004a). The early results from Mauritania are encouraging. Spending for health has risen, with most of the increase going to those parts of the country and for those kinds of services likely to have the largest effect on the health of the poorest households.

In middle-income countries, an analogous shift of DAH in strong policy environments has been the increasing use of single-tranche, programmatic, sector adjustment loans. These loans have emerged as a favored instrument for DAH in certain Latin American countries with sound management of public finances and internationally accepted procurement practices. Unlike the PRSCs, the programmatic sector loans have tended to target a single sector (such as health) or, occasionally, two sectors (such as health and education in the case of Brazil or health insurance and pensions in the case of Ecuador). Whereas the PRSCs have their analytical roots in poverty studies, the programmatic sector loans tend to be based on sector assessments. After the government has taken key legal, institutional, and spending actions to improve the efficiency of health spending or to target services for poor households, donor funds are transferred in a block or *tranche* to the government. In 2003, the World Bank approved four programmatic sector loans—for Brazil, Colombia, Ecuador, and Peru—totaling US$900 million (D. Cotlear, personal communication, December 12, 2003).

Another recent example is the World Bank's US$750 million Maternal and Child Insurance Program sector adjustment loan to Argentina, which followed decisions made by that government in 2003 to create a mother and child health insurance scheme for poor provinces, to increase spending for communicable diseases, and to establish a national health council to set policies on the sharing of revenues to be used for health between the central government and the provinces. The central pillar of this project, as well as the follow-on operation in 2004, is the implementation of the Maternal and Child Insurance Program. It delivers a publicly financed package of essential services to uninsured mothers and children at the provincial level. The donor funding is used in an innovative way to provide matching grants from the national to the provincial level, on the basis of a capitated payment per mother and child enrolled plus additional transfers to the province for performance. That performance is measured in terms of key health service goals (for example, coverage of vaccine programs, incidence of low birthweight, and number of prenatal consultations). In the first four months of program execution, more than 100,000 eligible women and children joined the insurance scheme.

Pooling and Donor Harmonization

As mentioned earlier, another innovation in recent years has been the use of sectorwide approaches as a way for multiple donors to pool their funds for a commonly agreed-on program and to use similar, streamlined procedures for procurement, monitoring and evaluation, and reporting. Sectorwide approaches grew out of sector investment programs for health that were launched in the early 1990s as a way to bring donors together to support broader government objectives in health.

The main features of sectorwide approaches are as follows:

a. a partnership among a broad coalition of donors, with the government taking the lead;
b. a comprehensive sector policy framework to achieve goals over the short and medium terms;
c. an agreed-on expenditure program;
d. the improvement of management systems and capacity building (Swedish International Development Cooperation Agency 2003).

The main difference between sectorwide approaches and PRSCs is that, in the former, pooled donor funding is disbursed against specific expenditure items—for example, construction of health facilities or purchase of drugs—whereas in PRSCs, donor funds are transferred to the general budget, with disbursements triggered by policy actions.

A prime example of a sectorwide approach is the Ghana health sector support program, in which 17 donor organizations have committed US$442 million over a five-year period to improve the health status of the population while focusing efforts on reducing inequalities in health. The program includes the following main spheres of action aimed at strengthening priority health interventions: developing human resources for health services, enhancing infrastructure and support services, fostering partnerships for health, improving regulation, reforming organizational arrangements, improving health sector financing, enhancing financial management systems, strengthening management information systems and performance monitoring, and linking with traditional medicine.

Performance-Based Financing

Developing countries and their international partners are increasingly adopting methods for financing health care activities that link the availability of funding to concrete, measurable results on the ground. Such performance-based financing was advocated a decade ago in the 1993 *World Development Report* (World Bank 1993) and in other policy documents in the early 1990s, although relatively little practical knowledge of this type of financing was available at the time.

Since then, much more experimentation has taken place, and the important potential—as well as the challenges—of performance-based financing for achieving national and global health goals is becoming apparent.

Performance-based financing is now being widely and actively tested at several levels of the health care system. These tests include situations in which the following occurs:

- Governments of developing countries pay health care providers in NGOs and the private sector to deliver essential health services to poor households.
- Central governments determine the transfer of funds to local governments on the basis of their performance in strengthening health services.
- Donors release funding to recipients in developing countries as and when they achieve certain key health targets.

Performance-Based Contracts with Nongovernmental Organizations. A number of governments in low-income countries are funding NGOs to deliver basic health services on a performance basis (Hecht 2004). Many of the earliest experiments are from Latin America and the Caribbean. In Haiti, for example, the government contracted NGOs to provide child health and family planning services. The government gave the NGOs an advance each year and then a quarterly sum based on a negotiated budget. At the end of the year, performance was measured against various indicators, including the extent of immunization coverage, the percentage of families using oral rehydration to treat acute diarrhea, the share of pregnant women attending prenatal care, and the average waiting times in clinics. The NGOs' performance determined the bonus they received, which could be up to 10 percent of the original negotiated budget. As a result, the Haitian NGOs made changes in their service delivery schemes and improved their performance in immunization and oral rehydration in particular (Eichler, Auxilia, and Pollack 2001). In Guatemala, the government is implementing a large performance-based program with NGOs that currently covers nearly 4 million people, mostly among the country's indigenous population (box 13.2). Similar schemes have been implemented in Argentina, El Salvador, and Nicaragua.

Box 13.2

Large-Scale Performance Contracting with Nongovernmental Organizations in Guatemala

Guatemala has successfully implemented contracting on a large scale with NGOs to deliver health services. The government started the Program to Extend Coverage of Basic Health Services in 1997, soon after the end of a long civil war. The program has continued under successive administrations. By 2000, a total of 89 NGOs were involved in providing health care to about 3.7 million people under 137 contracts.

The contracts specify a range of maternal and child health services, as well as the prevention and treatment of a number of diseases, including malaria. The NGOs are paid about US$8 per person served, mostly in cash, but also in kind in the form of such items as vaccines and medicines. Payments are released quarterly after the NGOs' performance has been checked and verified.

Performance is measured according to a series of indicators, including coverage of immunization and prenatal care, distribution of iron sulfate tablets to pregnant women and to children, and frequency of home visits by NGO outreach staff. The government has hired private firms to develop the monitoring system, which also looks at the NGOs' accounting practices.

The contracting system under the program appears to have resulted in important gains in health service delivery. Immunization rates rose from 69 percent in 1997 to 87 percent in 2001. Household surveys currently under way will be able to assess the program's effect on mothers' and children's health outcomes.

During the program's early years, the government had to overcome a number of obstacles. Government health workers resisted the scheme because they feared that contracting with NGOs was a hidden form of privatization of government health services. The NGOs were initially reluctant to get involved, because they thought that the government was demanding too much in the way of improved performance and also doubted that the government would pay them in a timely manner. Given the financial fragility of many local NGOs in Guatemala, the government had to make advance payments to the NGOs and release quarterly payments without delay to build confidence in the relationship between the public and private sectors.

Source: Hecht 2004; World Bank 2000.

More recently, countries in South Asia have begun to enter into performance-based health programs with NGOs. In Afghanistan, under a recently approved World Bank–financed project for health service rehabilitation, the government is contracting with NGOs to run health centers. NGOs that achieve specified targets will be eligible to receive additional payments of up to 10 percent of their baseline subsidies from the government.

In a similar vein, the central and state governments in India have started to reimburse NGOs and private providers on the basis of performance. The national TB program reimburses private laboratories for testing sputum samples to detect TB; it also pays NGOs and private doctors a fixed sum per infected patient who is cured using the directly observed short-course therapy approach. In one district of Kerala state where this scheme is well advanced, NGOs and private providers have helped boost coverage from some 55 percent of those infected with TB to 78 percent.

In Cambodia, government agreements and funding to NGOs to operate district health services showed impressive results compared with the standard approach, whereby the government ran district services. The NGOs operated in one of two ways: (a) on a fully contracted-out basis, with complete responsibility for service delivery, including hiring and firing staff members and setting wages and procuring and distributing essential drugs and supplies, or (b) through a pure management contract, in which the NGOs worked within the Ministry of Health system and had to strengthen the existing district structure. The NGOs that were fully contracted out raised immunization rates by 40 percentage points between 1997 and 2001, twice the rate of improvement produced by the government-run districts. The rate of growth in prenatal care in the contracted-out districts was more than triple that in the government-run districts, and the use of modern contraception methods expanded 50 percent more in the contracted-out districts (Bhushan, Keller, and Schwartz 2002).

Central Government Transfers to Local Authorities. In Brazil's Family Health Project, the central government is making per capita transfers to local municipalities on the basis of planned increases in certain services, such as safe deliveries for low-income women and poor children treated for various illnesses and monitored for their nutritional status and growth. For example, at least 40 percent of babies are to be delivered in maternity facilities managed under the government's family health program. Participating outreach workers are to provide an average of at least nine home visits to targeted low-income families each year. All doctors enrolled in the program are to undergo special training. If the municipalities reach those targets and several others, they will continue to be eligible for future financial transfers; otherwise, the level of central government support will be reduced, and remedial measures will be put in place to try to improve the targeting and effectiveness

of the activities run by the underperforming municipalities (G. M. LaForgia, personal communication, October 21, 2003).

Donor Disbursements to National Governments and Other Recipients. A number of innovative approaches are in place that make donor financing of health programs conditional on successful performance on the ground. One example is the World Bank's credit buy-down program for polio eradication (box 13.3).

GAVI has also been a pioneer in the performance-based approach to grant assistance. Through its sister organization, the Vaccine Fund, which raises and disburses funds for the alliance, GAVI provides commodity assistance to countries in the form of new and underused vaccines (hepatitis B, *Haemophilus influenzae* type B, and yellow fever, with new products for rotavirus and pneumococcus to follow); safe injection supplies; and support for strengthening national immunization systems. In addition, GAVI allocates grant funds to countries on the basis of their performance in increasing coverage rates for diptheria-pertussis-tetanus immunizations. Countries' applications to GAVI specify current coverage levels. On the basis of these data, their performance is assessed annually, and US$20 per child is given to the country for each additional child immunized with the diphtheria-pertussis-tetanus vaccine.

In 2004, GAVI made its first payment for performance verified by means of externally audited health data. Eight countries received US$15 million in performance-based payments for their achievements in increasing immunization rates to reach an additional 750,000 children. Sierra Leone, for example, qualified for these payments on the basis of its performance in raising coverage from 44 percent of children in 2000 to 62 percent in 2002, as the country emerged from civil war (GAVI 2004a).

Stronger Engagement with the Private Sector

As donors have increasingly become aware of the extent of private sector involvement in the health sector in developing countries—that is, both the share of health services delivered by private providers and the share of total health spending coming from private sources, including out-of-pocket payments—they have sought to use DAH to engage the private sector in pursuit of basic health goals.

Innovative approaches include both the transfer of development assistance to the private sector through government channels in developing countries and the provision of direct financial support to private institutions (World Bank 2003b). In the former category, social investment funds have been established in many regions as a way to channel DAH to community groups and NGOs involved in running health centers and disease control programs (Jorgensen and Domelen 2001), especially in Africa and Latin America. In a similar vein, donors

IDA Credit Buy-Downs for Polio Eradication

To ensure financing for the MDGs, governments, foundations, agencies, and development banks are all exploring new financing approaches that have the potential to increase resource flows, adjust the concessionality of funding (that is, reduce interest rates and thus increase the grant element) where appropriate, and help focus more attention on effects.

The IDA credit buy-down mechanism was recently piloted in several projects supporting polio eradication, clearly a global public good. The mechanism enhances the concessionality of IDA's assistance in priority areas, mobilizes additional resources from external partners, and focuses the attention of governments, partners, and World Bank staff on clearly defined performance objectives.

Working in partnership with the Bill & Melinda Gates Foundation, Rotary International, and the United Nations Foundation, the World Bank implemented two projects in fiscal 2003, one in Pakistan and the other in Nigeria. The partnerships will buy down a country's IDA loans on successful completion of the country's polio eradication program. Because of the generous loan terms, each grant dollar unlocks roughly US$2.50 for countries to fight polio. To fund the buy-downs, the partnership has established a trust fund with US$25 million from the Bill & Melinda Gates Foundation and US$25 million from Rotary International and the United Nations Foundation. This US$50 million investment has the potential to buy down roughly US$125 million in IDA loans. In this way, developing countries can mobilize what ultimately becomes grant funding to eradicate polio and to contribute to the global campaign to eliminate the transmission of polio.

Source: World Bank 2004d.

---

have been prime movers behind schemes to encourage governments to contract with NGOs and private hospitals and laboratories for basic services targeted to the poor, such as cataract surgery and TB case detection and treatment in India (Central TB Division 2002; World Bank 2002).

In terms of direct DAH financing to the private sector in developing countries, the most common and longstanding examples are in the social marketing of health-related personal products, such as contraceptives, kits for treating sexually transmitted infections, insecticide-impregnated bednets to prevent malaria, and point-of-use water purification kits. Donors are currently providing millions of dollars each year to subsidize the purchase of these items by poor families in developing countries. More recently, other donor engagements with the private sector have included the Global Alliance for Improved Nutrition, in which a consortium of donors that includes the Bill & Melinda Gates Foundation and the governments of Canada, the Netherlands, and the United States have pooled funds that can be used to expand the fortification of basic foods with micronutrients by private manufacturers. The Global Alliance for Improved Nutrition is helping to fortify wheat with iron in western China and in Morocco and fish sauce with vitamin A in Vietnam.

Another recent example of DAH going directly to the private sector is Avahan, the innovative AIDS prevention program that the Bill & Melinda Gates Foundation is financing in six Indian states. The program uses external financing to leverage financial and in-kind support from major Indian companies that can then be used to support a range of HIV prevention programs, such as condom promotion, peer education, and voluntary counseling and testing targeted at truck drivers, commercial sex workers, and others at high risk (Sengupta and Sinha 2004).

The other area in which donor funds are increasingly being used to stimulate private sector action and leverage private funding is through public-private partnerships for new health technologies, including vaccines, drugs, and diagnostics. Private financing, technical input, and management make sense in this area, because typically it is the private sector that has the technical knowledge and the manufacturing and distribution capacity to create and market new health products, but major scientific risks and the lack of an attractive market in poor countries are barriers to investment. The public-private partnerships aim to overcome those barriers through a combination of up-front financing for R&D (so-called push funding) and market guarantees for effective products (so-called pull financing). The 20 largest partnerships for new products have raised more than US$1.5 billion over the past decade and are beginning to see results, such as the development of new drugs for malaria and TB, promising vaccines for malaria and AIDS, and microbicides to protect against HIV infection (IPPPH 2004; Rockefeller Foundation 2004). The largest partnership, the IAVI, illustrates the innovative nature of these partnerships and the effective use of DAH (box 13.4).

Box 13.4

The International AIDS Vaccine Initiative

The International AIDS Vaccine Initiative was established in 1996 with support from the Rockefeller Foundation as an innovative way to give a boost to AIDS vaccine R&D. Optimism about AIDS vaccines in the late 1980s had given way to a series of failures and to discouragement by the end of the decade. R&D efforts were spending less than US$100 million a year. Neither governments nor private vaccine companies were investing much in research into AIDS vaccines.

IAVI's mission was defined as ensuring the development of a safe, effective, and accessible vaccine for use throughout the world. IAVI's activities were to include a combination of global advocacy, policy analysis and reform, and investments in carefully chosen R&D projects focusing on the most promising vaccine candidates.

IAVI's collaboration with the private sector has occurred at several levels. Funding for IAVI has come from six governments (Canada, Denmark, the Netherlands, Norway, the United Kingdom, and the United States); the European Union; and the World Bank, as well as from private foundations and companies. IAVI's vaccine development partnerships take many forms. They typically include an academic developer and a biotechnology company, plus researchers, laboratories, and clinical trial sites in developing countries such as India, Kenya, and Uganda. Private companies generally manufacture test lots of the AIDS vaccines and undertake bioengineering studies and enhancements to the vaccine. IAVI generally shares the risks and costs of the partnerships with the private code-

velopers, while ensuring that developing countries will have access to the vaccine at an affordable price if it turns out to be effective.

Since IAVI embarked on these vaccine development partnerships in 1999, it has spent a total of about US$200 million in this area. Five vaccine candidates are undergoing clinical trials in eight countries in Africa, Asia, Europe, and North America. IAVI is poised to spend another US$300 million in R&D during 2005–7 in an effort to accelerate the discovery, development, and licensing of a vaccine to prevent HIV infection. IAVI is also trying to stimulate expanded use of donor funding for R&D in the field of AIDS vaccines and is calling for governments to increase public financing from the current amount of around US$600 million a year to US$1.2 billion annually. At the same time, IAVI has proposed that donors create a purchase fund of several billion dollars to serve as a promise to buy large numbers of doses of an efficacious vaccine from qualified manufacturers. The U.K. government has committed itself to joining such an advance purchase fund and is urging others to join it ("Gordon Brown to Earmark" 2004).

The health and economic stakes are enormous. Without improved HIV prevention tools, an additional 100 million HIV infections are likely over the next two decades, resulting in huge economic losses. IAVI estimates that an efficacious vaccine could prevent 2 million AIDS deaths a year and generate billons of dollars in lives saved and antiretroviral treatment costs averted.

Source: IAVI 2004.

Getting Funds to the Front Line

Central government funds can easily leak as they move through the pipeline from the center to local levels. In addition, in the absence of local initiative and the right incentives, service provision can fail to reflect the views of local people. Effective DAH needs to address those impediments. It needs to channel technologies, ideas, finance, and technical assistance closer to households, health providers, and supervisory officials in ways that are consistent with national policies and are amenable to monitoring and reporting.

Development assistance for health is more likely to reach communities if they have the following:

- a decentralized system of fiduciary and technical management in the public sector

- a strong financial capacity in NGOs and private providers in cases in which the government's strategy for local development is to rely on private institutions
- a government body that is appropriately equipped and responsible for regulating the quality of public and private providers
- a balanced approach to community-driven development in health to ensure that financing for community health initiatives of the social fund type is sustainable.

Examples of DAH reaching frontline workers in an expeditious and sustainable way include block grants for districts in Uganda; social development funds in Central America; contracts with urban and rural NGOs under India's Reproductive and Child Health Program; and support to community-led initiatives under the Multi-Country AIDS Program, which financed an average of 10,000 local initiatives in each of its first four years in several African countries (World Bank 2004c).

CONCLUSIONS

Despite the promising trends in DAH over the past five to seven years, the outlook for the next few years is uncertain. What happens will depend on overall trends and innovations in development assistance, which in turn are driven by such factors as political changes and the rate of economic growth in OECD countries, and the willingness of high-income countries to honor their pledges to increase the share of GDP they devote to development.

Under most scenarios, the share of overall assistance going to health will likely continue its recent rise, given the current political focus on the global AIDS pandemic and the growing awareness of the challenges and opportunities associated with the MDGs for maternal and child health and communicable diseases.

Under a more conservative scenario, a number of factors could have a negative impact on DAH. Those factors could include an overall slowing in the rate of growth of development financing and the donor fatigue that could set in if the larger allocations for HIV/AIDS, TB, and malaria are not fully disbursed, are misused, or yield disappointing results on the ground.

Under a more optimistic scenario, DAH will continue to grow as developing countries and donors find new ways to disburse a higher volume of funds and use them effectively—for example, through subcontracts with NGOs and private health service delivery organizations. Sectorwide approaches and budget support through national poverty reduction programs may also result in expanded flows of DAH. New generations of technologies adapted to the developing world, such as more effective antimalarials, better TB diagnostics, and a vaccine to prevent HIV infection, would almost certainly attract increasing amounts of DAH.

Even under the more optimistic scenario, DAH will still face major challenges. The expected volume of financial assistance is unlikely to match the large needs of the developing world and the requirements to attain the MDGs. Countries and donors will therefore face difficult decisions in relation to priority setting and require better tools to make such allocation decisions. Cost-effectiveness analysis offers one such tool. Effective absorption of DAH will also continue to pose difficulties for countries with weak capacity. In such cases, increased use of NGOs and the private sector in general to complement public sector action may help make the information and services that poor households need to improve their health status more accessible.

Another issue is that the current architecture of development assistance does not contain a mechanism to ensure that adequate funds flow to the upstream stages of R&D on new health technologies, where the private sector lacks the market incentives to invest and where national research bodies have so far not been up to the task. The multilateral banks do not have the instruments to channel major funding to global, as opposed to national, health technology programs, and the bilateral agencies alone are not equal to this task. Even with the modest external funds allocated to the recently established public-private partnerships (such as the IAVI, the Medicines for Malaria Venture, the Global TB Drug Alliance, and the International Partnership for Microbicides), new technologies are emerging. However, they need to be reinforced with additional funding. One option would be to design a new funding facility within the multilateral banks that would allow them to allocate significant resources to global health research and product development. Another would be to use the nascent international finance facility to provide funds for global research.

To address those challenges, strong political will is the essential baseline ingredient, as recent experience with HIV/AIDS has clearly demonstrated. The United Nations and the multilateral agencies must remain firmly behind more robust DAH, as they are currently doing by means of the Millennium Project and the High-Level Forum on the Health-Related MDGs. Individual bilateral donors and foundations must continue to demonstrate their leadership. Finally, and perhaps most important, leaders and civil society organizations in poor countries need to continue to speak out for more and more effective DAH, indicating that health is their priority and that they are prepared to commit domestic resources to match the larger external flows provided through DAH.

REFERENCES

Bhushan, I., S. Keller, and B. Schwartz. 2002. *Achieving the Twin Objectives of Efficiency and Equity: Contracting for Health Services in Cambodia.* Policy Brief Series 6. Manila: Asian Development Bank.

Burnside, C., and D. Dollar. 2000. "Aid, Growth, the Incentive Regime, and Poverty Reduction." In *The World Bank: Structure and Policies,* ed. C. L. Gilbert and D. Vines, 210–27. Cambridge, U.K.: Cambridge University Press.

Central TB Division, Directorate General of Health Services, Ministry of Health and Family Welfare. 2002. *TB India 2002: RNTCP Status Report.* New Delhi: Directorate General of Health Services.

CMH (Commission on Macroeconomics and Health). 2001. *Macroeconomics and Health: Investing in Health for Economic Development—Report of the Commission on Macroeconomics and Health.* Geneva: World Health Organization.

Devarajan, S., M. J. Miller, and E. V. Swanson. 2002. "Goals for Development: History, Prospects and Costs." Discussion Paper 2819, World Bank, Washington, DC.

Eichler, R., P. Auxila, and J. Pollock. 2001. *Output-Based Health Care: Paying for Performance in Haiti.* Washington, DC: Abt Associates.

Foster, M., A. Brown, and T. Conway. 2000. *Sector-Wide Approaches for Health Development: A Review of Experience.* Geneva: World Health Organization.

GAVI (Global Alliance for Vaccines and Immunization). 2004a. *GAVI Awards for Top Performing Countries*. Geneva: GAVI.

———. 2004b. *Programmatic Aspects of the IFF Immunization Pilot*. Geneva: GAVI.

"Gordon Brown to Earmark 200 Million Pounds a Year to Fund AIDS Vaccine." 2004. *Independent* (London), December 1, p. 18.

Heaver, R. 2002. *Thailand's National Nutrition Program: Lessons in Management and Capacity Development*. Washington, DC: World Bank.

Hecht, R. 2004. "Making Health Care Accountable: The New Focus on Performance-Based Funding of Health Services." *Finance and Development* 41 (March): 16–19.

IAVI (International AIDS Vaccine Initiative). 2004. *The IAVI Strategic Plan 2005–07*. New York: IAVI.

IPPPH (Initiative for Public-Private Partnerships for Health). 2004. *Combating Diseases Associated with Poverty: Financing Strategies for Product Development and the Potential Role of Public-Private Partnerships*. Geneva: IPPPH.

Jamison, D. T. 2004. "External Finance of Immunization Programs: Time for a Change of Paradigm?" In *Vaccines: Preventing Disease and Protecting Health*, ed. C. de Quadros, 325–32. Washington, DC: Pan-American Health Organization.

Jorgensen, S., and J. V. Domelen. 2001. *Helping the Poor Manage Risks Better: The Role of Social Funds*. Washington, DC: Brookings Institution.

Levine, R., and What Works Working Group. 2004. *Millions Saved*. Washington, DC: Center for Global Development.

Michaud, C. 2003. *Development Assistance for Health: Recent Trends and Resource Allocation*. Boston: Harvard Center for Population Development.

OECD (Organisation for Economic Co-Operation and Development). 2004a. CRS Online Database on Aid Activities. http://www.oecd.org/dac/stats/idsonline.

———. 2004b. *Survey on Harmonisation and Alignment: Preliminary Edition*. Paris: OECD.

Rajkumar, A., and V. Swaroop. 2002. "Public Spending and Outcomes: Does Governance Matter?" Policy Research Working Paper 2840, World Bank, Washington, DC.

Rockefeller Foundation. 2004. *Partnering to Develop New Products for Diseases of Poverty*. New York: Rockefeller Foundation.

Sengupta, J., and J. Sinha. 2004. "Battling AIDS in India." *McKinsey Quarterly* 3. New Delhi: McKinsey.

Soucat, A., W. Van Lerberghe, F. Diop, S. Nguyen, and R. Knipperberg. 2003. *Marginal Budgeting for Bottlenecks: A New Costing and Resource Allocation Practice to Buy Health Results*. Washington, DC: World Bank.

Stop TB Partnership. 2003. *Report of the DOTS Working Group for the 22 High-Burden Countries*. Geneva: World Health Organization.

Swedish International Development Cooperation Agency. 2003. *Mapping of Sector-Wide Approaches in Health*. London: Institute for Health Sector Development.

UN (United Nations) Millennium Project. 2004. "Millennium Development Goals Needs Assessment: Case Studies of Bangladesh, Cambodia, Ghana, Tanzania, and Uganda." Working Paper, United Nations, New York.

UNAIDS (Joint United Nations Programme on HIV/AIDS). 2001. *Report on the Global HIV/AIDS Epidemic*. Geneva: UNAIDS.

———. 2004. *Global Expenditures and Requirements to Address the HIV/AIDS Pandemic*. Geneva: UNAIDS.

World Bank. 1993. *World Development Report 1993: Investing in Health*. New York: Oxford University Press.

———. 1998. *Assessing Aid: What Works, What Doesn't, and Why*. Oxford, U.K.: Oxford University Press.

———. 2000. "Large-Scale Government Contracting of NGOs to Extend Basic Health Services to Poor Populations in Guatemala." Paper prepared for the Challenge of Health Reform: Reaching the Poor, Europe and Americas Forum, San José, Costa Rica, May 24–28.

———. 2002. "India—Cataract Blindness Control Project." Implementation Completion Report 25232, World Bank, Washington, DC.

———. 2003a. *Attaining the Millennium Development Goals in India: How Likely and What Will It Take?* Washington, DC: World Bank.

———. 2003b. "Private Health: Policy and Regulatory Options for Private Participation." Private Sector and Infrastructure Network Note 264, World Bank, Washington, DC.

———. 2003c. *Progress Report and Critical Next Steps in Scaling up Education for All, Health, HIV/AIDS, and Water and Sanitation*. Washington, DC: World Bank and International Monetary Fund Development Committee.

———. 2004a. "The Mauritania Health System and Implementation of the Poverty Reduction Strategy." Africa Human Development Working Paper 39, World Bank, Washington, DC.

———. 2004b. *The Millennium Development Goals for Health: Rising to the Challenges*. Washington, DC: World Bank.

———. 2004c. *Experience in Scaling Up Support to Local Response in Multi-Country AIDS Programs (MAP) in Africa*. Washington, DC: World Bank.

———. 2004d. "Financing Modalities toward the Millennium Development Goals: Progress Note." World Bank, Washington, DC.

World Bank and Ministry of Health, Ethiopia. 2005. *Ethiopia: A Country Status Report on Health and Poverty*. Volumes I and II. Washington, DC: World Bank.

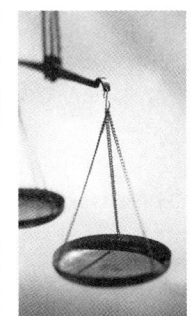

Chapter **14**

Ethical Issues in Resource Allocation, Research, and New Product Development

Dan W. Brock and Daniel Wikler

The ethical justification for developing and providing the means to reduce the burden of disease in developing countries is self-evident. Nevertheless, those who pursue these laudable ends encounter ethical dilemmas at every turn. The development of new interventions requires testing with human subjects, an activity fraught with controversy since the dawn of scientific medicine and especially problematic with poor and vulnerable participants in developing countries. Ethical dilemmas arising in setting priorities among interventions and among individuals in need of care are most acute when needs are great and resources few.

We address some of these concerns in this chapter, identifying some of the principal ethical issues that arise in the development and allocation of effective interventions for developing countries and discussing some alternative resolutions. We omit discussion of two other aspects of these ethical decisions: ensuring that the process of decision making is fair and involves the subject population (Daniels 2000; Holm 1998), and respecting legal obligations under international human rights treaties (Gruskin and Tarantola 2001).

HEALTH RESOURCE ALLOCATION

Resource allocation in health and elsewhere should satisfy two main ethical criteria. First, it should be cost-effective—limited resources for health should be allocated to maximize the health benefits for the population served. A cost-effectiveness analysis (CEA) of alternative health interventions measures their respective costs and benefits to determine their relative efficiency in the production of health. Costs are measured in monetary terms; benefits are measured in health improvements. By dividing costs by benefits, one can obtain a cost-to-effectiveness ratio for each health intervention, and interventions can be ranked by these ratios. Although a CEA is typically an economic analysis performed by health economists, it is also a measure of one ethical criterion for the evaluation of health programs. Cost-effectiveness is not merely an economic concern, because improving people's health and well-being is a moral concern, and an allocation of resources that is not cost-effective produces fewer benefits than would have been possible with a different allocation. Producing more rather than fewer benefits for people is one important ethical consideration in evaluating actions and social policies.

Second, the allocation should be equitable or just; equity is concerned with the distribution of benefits and costs to distinct individuals or groups. The maximization of benefits, which is associated with the general philosophical moral theory of utilitarianism or consequentialism, however, is routinely criticized for ignoring those considerations (Rawls 1971). Equity in health care distribution is complex and embodies several distinct moral concerns or issues that this chapter delineates (Brock 2003a). There is no generally accepted methodology comparable to CEA for determining how equitable a distribution is; nevertheless, allocations are unsatisfactory if equity considerations are ignored.

Efficiency and equity can sometimes coincide. In some of the world's poorest countries, for example, health budgets support tertiary care and travel to clinics abroad for the elite and the well connected, even as the poor are denied effective, low-cost prevention or treatment for life-threatening diseases (Birdsall and Hecht 1995). Moreover, because equity concerns the relative treatment of different individuals, CEA is largely unobjectionable when it is used only for evaluating alternative health interventions that would serve the same patients. However, considerations of equity may conflict with cost-effectiveness and so may provide moral reasons for an allocation that is not cost-effective. The discussion in this chapter accepts that CEA identifies one important ethical criterion in evaluating health care interventions—producing the most benefits possible for individuals served by those interventions—and then focuses on the other ethical criterion of ensuring equitable distribution of those benefits.

This chapter considers two types of equity issues: first, those that arise in the general construction of a CEA—that is, in determining the form of a CEA; second, those that arise in the use of the results of a CEA for resource allocation in the health sector. It is worth noting that, when applied appropriately and broadly to all social conditions and programs that significantly influence health, CEA may often support using resources to affect the so-called social determinants of health—which largely affect the incidence of disease, disability, and premature mortality—rather than using those resources on health care to treat disease. However, we shall focus largely on CEA in the evaluation of health care and public health programs.

Issues in the Construction of a Cost-Effectiveness Analysis

Cost-effectiveness analyses require decisions about which costs to include, which if any financial gains should be counted as offsetting costs, whether to include benefits beyond the effects of the intervention on health, and whether all health gains should be valued alike. None of those decisions, in our view, is exclusively a technical issue, and CEA results reflect the analysts' ethical judgments on those issues.

Evaluation of Benefits. Evaluating health benefits within a CEA involves several issues. This chapter assumes that some version of a quality-adjusted life year (QALY) is used to combine the two main benefits of health care—(a) protecting or improving health or health-related quality of life and (b) preserving life. Disability-adjusted life years (DALYs) are a variant of QALYs in that they measure the losses from disability or premature death; a CEA will determine which interventions will maximize QALYs or minimize DALYs. Calculating QALYs requires a metric evaluating the effect of different states of limitations in function on health-related quality of life, such as the Health Utilities Index (Horsman and others 2003). The Disease Control Priorities Project uses the health state valuations or disability weights of the World Health Organization (WHO). The relative value of any particular health state, typically on a scale in which "0" represents death and "1" represents full,

undiminished function (or health) is generally determined by soliciting a group of individuals' preferences for life in that state using standard gambles, time tradeoffs, visual analog scales, or person tradeoffs. In all these methods, a common issue is whose preferences to use for valuing health states. The main debate has been whether to use a randomly selected group of citizens or to use people who have the particular disability or limitation in function being evaluated.

This issue matters because a number of studies have shown that persons without disabilities generally evaluate the quality of life with a particular disability as significantly worse than do persons who have that same disability (Menzel and others 2002). If the preferences of persons without disabilities are used, their lower evaluation of quality of life with various disabilities will mean that fewer QALYs will be produced by life-saving interventions for persons with disabilities than if the preferences of persons with disabilities had been used. However, if we use the preferences of persons with disabilities, then both prevention and rehabilitation will receive less value than if the preferences of persons without disabilities had been used.

This difference in evaluations in part results from ignorance, prejudice, and stereotypes on the part of persons without disabilities about what it is like to live with various disabilities. The difference results as well from the process of adaptation to disability in which disabled persons adjust by learning new skills, cope by adjusting their expectations to their new circumstances, and accommodate by substituting new aims and activities for ones made difficult or impossible by their disabilities (Solomon and Murray 2002). They thus adopt a new valuational perspective for making health and quality-of-life evaluations. Because the adoption of this new perspective resulted from a disability, it will represent a set of values for making choices that reflects a restricted set of abilities. Nevertheless, neither the nondisabled perspective nor the adapted disabled perspective is mistaken; they are only different (Brock 1995). These differences create controversy in the literature over which perspective is correct for cost-effectiveness evaluations in health care.

A second issue is whether, in evaluating interventions that preserve or extend life, we should use life years saved (as QALYs do) or lives saved. Certainly individuals offered two interventions that would preserve their lives for different lengths of time would prefer, all other things being equal, the alternative with the longer period of survival. Moreover, when the differences are extreme—for example, extending group A's lives by a week or extending an equally numerous group B's lives by 10 years—virtually everyone would judge this difference to support giving priority to group B. This fact suggests that even the proponent of counting lives saved should require that the lives saved for a shorter period of time must still be saved for a significant period of time; what is significant will depend in part on the duration of lives saved by the alternative with which it is being compared. Some empirical studies indicate that ordinary people tend not to give much weight to differences in the duration of health benefits to different groups of persons when prioritizing between them, as long as the lesser duration benefits are viewed as significant; this attitude suggests that they favor lives saved over life years saved (Nord and others 1996). The life years saved versus lives saved controversy remains unsettled.

Should Life Years Be Age Weighted? The standard assumption in most CEAs using QALYs is that one QALY has the same social value, regardless of the age of the recipient (Gold and others 1996). Thus, equality is adopted as the weighting for QALYs achieved by recipients at different ages, and that is the approach adopted in this volume. The use of any age weighting that gives less value to benefits for the elderly than for younger persons is often charged as unjust age discrimination. Even the use of equally weighted QALYs is often charged as unjust age discrimination because, other things being equal, saving the lives of younger persons will produce more QALYs than saving the lives of older persons. The goal of lives saved, as opposed to life years saved, removes this disadvantage to the elderly from CEAs that use QALYs. However, if the relevant benefit is adding years to life, then standard CEA is neutral or impartial regarding age, in the sense that it gives the same value to a year of life extension whatever the age of its recipient.

WHO, in its burden-of-disease and resource prioritization studies that use DALYs, rejected the equal age weighting that is standard with QALYs. Instead, it gave less value to DALYs prevented for infants, young children, and the elderly, in comparison with persons in their productive adult years. WHO justified this weighting by the fact that the very young and the elderly both tend to be economically, socially, and psychologically dependent on adults during those adults' productive working and child-rearing years (Murray 1994). This justification is ethically problematic, however, because it assigns different value to meeting people's health needs on the basis of differences in the instrumental value to others of meeting their needs. This approach differentiates people solely on whether they are a means to benefiting others. The same reasoning would justify giving priority to rich over poor patients with the same medical needs because the rich are more socially productive than the poor, a practice that would be widely regarded as unjust.

Writers in this field have provided different reasons for giving greater value to QALYs for younger patients, however, that are not subject to this moral objection and that are specifically grounded in fairness. For example, Alan Williams has developed an argument to the effect that fairness requires that individuals should each receive "fair innings" of QALYs in their lives (Williams 1997). In this view, the earlier a preventable death could occur and the worse a person's past health is, the greater is the unfairness the person suffers—so the greater is

the moral urgency, grounded in fairness, of preventing the death. The younger a person is, the greater is the moral value of providing a QALY to him or her. This view leaves open to what extent the moral value of QALYs should decline with the age of the recipient. This age weighting to favor the young has been attacked by some as unjust age discrimination, but because an explicit moral justification in terms of fairness is offered for it, critics must show why that justification is unsound.

What Costs Should Count in Health Cost-Effectiveness Analyses? No controversy surrounds the inclusion in a CEA of direct costs of a health intervention program or direct health benefits to the intervention's recipients. Ethical issues do, however, arise in other aspects of the cost calculation (Brock 2003b). A full CEA of alternative health programs should take account of all the economic effects on public or private expenditures of the alternative health interventions or programs under analysis. An example is provided in the consideration of treatment for two alternative health conditions judged to have equally detrimental effects on patients' health: the first condition permits patients to continue working, and the second interferes with regular work and so has large economic costs to the patients' employers. Should the costs of treating the second be reduced by the cost savings to the employers from returning the patients to work on a regular basis? If so, the second treatment program will have a more favorable cost-effectiveness ratio than the first, even if it may be no better or worse without consideration of those economic effects. The same issue arises in many other contexts.

From the moral perspectives of both a consequentialist and a standard CEA, these indirect economic effects for others are real benefits or cost reductions and should be part of the CEA. The fundamental moral objection to giving higher priority to treating those who can be treated at lower net cost because of the economic savings to their employers is the same as that with WHO's instrumental rationale for its age weighting. One condition or group of patients gets higher priority solely because treating it or them is a means to producing economic benefits to others, thereby reducing the net social costs of their treatment. This approach violates the Kantian injunction against treating people solely as means—the first group has lower priority for treatment solely because treating that group is not a means to the economic savings to employers. It fails to give equal moral concern to the health needs of each group of patients because it discriminates against the less socially valuable patients. Conversely, at the macro level of the allocation of resources to health instead of other social goods, the WHO Commission on Macroeconomics and Health has supported increasing health investments in developing countries because such investments often more than pay for themselves in their economic and development benefits (CMH 2001). Using a "separate spheres" view, only the health benefits and health costs of alternative health interventions should determine their priority for obtaining resources, but this view remains controversial.

Another aspect of cost calculation concerns whether future health care and other costs, such as old-age payments, that will be incurred as a result of a person's life being saved should be added to the costs of treating that person now. Persons who do not die now because of a life-saving intervention will typically go on to incur future health costs that would not have been incurred had they died now. The U.S. Public Health Service Panel on cost-effectiveness recommended that inclusion of these costs be optional in CEAs (Gold and others 1996). Others have argued that, if CEA is designed to maximize lifetime utility, the future costs should be included (Meltzer 1997). These are costs that would not be incurred if the patient was not saved, but virtually no one would argue that, because of those costs, we should judge a life-saving intervention as not cost-effective and thus deserving of lower priority than interventions that do not have those effects. What does this thinking show? That we are not prepared to allocate health resources on the basis of a full CEA that accounts for all the costs incurred and saved by those interventions—that is, that some should be disregarded on ethical grounds.

Should Health Benefits and Costs Be Discounted in Cost-Effectiveness Analyses? As standard practice in CEAs, both health care costs and benefits are discounted at the same rate, for example, 3 percent or 5 percent, and the Disease Control Priorities Project applies a 3 percent discount rate to costs and benefits (Gold and others 1996). Little controversy surrounds the idea that future monetary costs and benefits should be discounted to their present value in a CEA. The same amount of money is worth more if received today than in 10 years because it can be invested at the market rate of interest if received today. For the same reason, costs that can be deferred require fewer present dollars to meet them.

The controversial issue is whether health benefits should be discounted—that is, whether the same magnitude of health benefit has progressively less social value the farther into the future it occurs. This issue is complex and has engendered an extensive literature that cannot be reviewed here, but we can at least try to focus the issue. It is appropriate to discount for the uncertainty about whether potential beneficiaries will survive to receive a future health benefit and to discount for any increased uncertainty about whether a benefit will occur because it is more distant. However, these uncertainties are reflected in the calculation of expected future benefits and do not require that future benefits be discounted. Likewise, if individuals receive a health benefit (such as regaining mobility) sooner rather than later, their total lifetime benefit may be greater, but this fact, too, is reflected in the estimation of the total benefit without discounting.

The ethical issue about discounting is whether, after taking account of such considerations, a health benefit of the same size has progressively less social value the farther into the future that it occurs. To make the issue more concrete, suppose we must decide between two programs: one will save 100 lives now, and the other, say a hepatitis vaccination program, will save 200 lives in 30 years. The vaccination program will save twice as many lives, but if we apply even a 3 percent discount rate to the future lives saved, they are equivalent to only 78 lives saved now, and we should prefer the first program. This example illustrates not only the theoretical issue, but its practical import, too, because discounting future health benefits will systematically tend to disadvantage prevention programs that must be undertaken now but whose benefits occur only at some point in the future. This reasoning applies not only to many vaccination programs, but also to most programs to change unhealthy behaviors in which the benefits generally occur at some later time.

Arguments for discounting health benefits at the same rate as costs have included consistency arguments (Weinstein and Stason 1997), avoidance of paradoxes in allocation concerning research and deferral of spending (Keeler and Cretin 1983), individual or social rates of time preference, and so forth. Those arguments cannot be reviewed here, but whether to discount health benefits is squarely an ethical question about the valuing of health benefits over time and should be explicitly addressed as such in allocating resources.

Issues in the Use of Cost-Effectiveness Analysis for Resource Allocation

It is now widely recognized that CEA alone is not a satisfactory guide to resource allocation in all cases. CEA, as customarily formulated, measures the sum of costs and benefits and largely ignores the pattern of their distribution across the affected population. In some cases, the resulting allocation will strike most observers as unfair. Health resource allocators need to take distributional issues into account along with cost-effectiveness.

Priority to the Worst Off. Justice requires a special concern for the worst off, as is reflected in aphorisms such as "you can tell the justice of a society by how it treats its least well-off members," in the well-known Difference Principle in John Rawls's theory of justice, and by the special concern for the poor within many religious traditions (Brock 2002; Rawls 1971). This concern is often understood to reflect a concern for equality—in particular, equality in outcomes or welfare between people. In the health context, it takes the form of a concern for reducing inequalities in health between persons or groups. A variety of ethical bases underpin a concern for equality in general and for equality in health in particular, and they cannot be explored here. It is important, however, to understand that concern for the worst off is different from a concern for equality, because the two can be and often are confused. Raising the position of the worst off will typically reduce inequality, but it need not always do so. Sometimes improving the position of the worst off may unavoidably improve the position of those who are better off even more and thereby increase inequality. Moreover, the concern for equality in outcomes is subject to the "leveling down" objection, in which equality is achieved by making the better-off members worse off, even when doing so in no way benefits those who are worst off. In the face of that objection, many have rejected equality in outcomes in favor of a prioritarian view, according to which benefiting people has greater moral value the worse off those people are (Parfit 1991).

A number of possible lines of reasoning support prioritarianism. For example, the worse off that people are, the greater is the relative improvement that a given size of benefit will provide them, so the more the benefit may matter to them. Alternatively, the greater the undeserved health deprivation or need that an individual suffers, the greater is the moral claim to have it alleviated or met.

However priority to the worst off is justified, an important issue is who the worst off are. In the context of resource allocation in health care, the worst off might be those who are globally worst off, those with the worst overall well-being (such as the poor), or those with the worst health (that is, the sickest). General theories of justice usually focus on people's overall well-being, often allowing a lower level in one domain of well-being to be compensated for by a higher level in another domain. However, there are both moral and pragmatic reasons for what has been called a *separate spheres view*, according to which the worst off for the purpose of health resource allocation should be considered to be those with worse health. Morally, for example, Scanlon has argued that "for differences in level to affect the relative strength of people's claims to help, these differences have to be in an aspect of welfare that the help in question will contribute to" (Scanlon 1997, 227). Pragmatically, it may generally be too difficult, costly, intrusive, and controversial, as well as too subject to mistake and abuse, to have to inquire into all aspects of people's overall levels of well-being.

Even if health allocation to the worst off should be based on levels of health, other issues remain. For example, are those with worse health those who are sickest now, at the time a health intervention would be provided for them, or those with worse health over time, taking into account past and perhaps expected future health? The latter would give special weight to meeting the health needs of those with long-term chronic diseases and disabilities. Separate spheres would still include past and future health. Should special priority also be given to those whose health is not worse now but is especially vulnerable to becoming worse?

Finally, how much priority should the worst off receive? Giving absolute priority to the worst off is implausible because it faces the bottomless pit problem—using very great amounts of resources to produce very limited or marginal gains in the health-related quality of life of the severely ill or disabled. However, there is no apparent principled basis for determining how much priority the worst off should receive.

Aggregation and Cost Differences. The aggregation problem occurs when determining at what point small benefits to a large number of persons should take priority over very large benefits to a few, because the former result in greater aggregate or total benefits (Daniels 1993; Kamm 1993). The issue can be illustrated by the initial effort to prioritize different treatment-condition pairs in the Medicaid program in the U.S. state of Oregon by what was essentially a cost-effectiveness standard. As was widely reported, capping teeth for exposed pulp was ranked just above performing appendectomies for acute appendicitis, even though appendicitis is a life-threatening condition. A variety of methodological problems affected Oregon's analysis, but this kind of result is to be expected from CEA. The Oregon Health Services Commission estimated that it was possible to provide a tooth capping for more than 100 patients for the cost of one appendectomy, so the aggregate benefits of the many tooth cappings were estimated to exceed the benefit of one appendectomy. As a consequence of results of this sort, the commission fundamentally changed its prioritization methodology to largely ignore cost differences, except in the case of roughly equally beneficial interventions. The commission essentially adopted what might be called a relative effectiveness or benefit standard (Hadorn 1991).

What Oregon's experience shows is that most people's sense of priorities is determined by a one-to-one comparison of the benefits of different interventions, in which case appendectomies are clearly a higher priority than tooth capping. That ignores the great differences in costs between different health interventions that a CEA will reflect. Is it then simply a mistake to ignore those cost differences in allocating health resources? At least two moral considerations suggest not. First, empirical studies have shown that many people ignore the cost differences because they believe that patients should not be at a disadvantage in priority for treatment simply because their condition happens to be more expensive to treat than are other patients' conditions (Nord and others 1995). Second, according to many moral theories, individuals should confront other competitors for scarce resources as individuals, and their priority for treatment should be determined by the urgency of their individual claims to treatment (Scanlon 1997).

Then again, most people and most moral theories do not reject all aggregation of different sizes and costs of health benefits in setting priorities and allocation, although there is no consensus either on when aggregation should be permitted or for what reasons. However, at a minimum, we suggest that individuals should not be denied very great health benefits—in the extreme case, life-saving interventions—merely to provide small health benefits to a large number of other persons.

Fair Chances and Best Outcomes. The thesis that resources should be targeted to interventions in which they will do the most good ascribes a higher priority to those who can be helped more easily or cheaply. This thinking, in turn, implies that some patients will lose out simply because their needs are more difficult or expensive to meet. Consider, for example, a ward with 100 patients, 50 of whom require one pill and 50 of whom require two pills to recover. The patients are otherwise similar. The clinic has 50 pills and must decide how to distribute them. To achieve the best outcome, all 50 pills should be given to the patients who need only one to recover. However, to give each patient an equal chance to recover, entitlement to treatment should be awarded randomly. Seventeen fewer cures would result.

Limited surveys indicate a sharp difference between health professionals and the general public in their responses to this conflict. Most health professionals favor distribution to one-pill patients only, and most members of the general public insist that people should not be penalized for needing two pills (Nord 1999). This division of opinion goes to the heart of CEA, which is precisely a guide to identifying the route to the best outcomes that can be hoped for with existing resources. It also creates a dilemma for those health professionals who maintain that health policy should be based on values most frequently endorsed by the population affected.

The conflict between fair chances and best outcomes arises not only from differences in the costs of treating otherwise similar groups of patients, but also when one group of patients will receive somewhat greater benefits than another at the same cost. The appeal of a fair-chances solution is greater when the difference in cost-effectiveness between the two programs is relatively small compared with the potential gain or loss to individual patients. Suppose that health program A will produce 5,000 QALYs while program B will produce 4,500 QALYs and that the effect on the health or life of each patient served is large—in the extreme, life saving. Patients who would be served by program B could complain that it is not fair that all the resources go to program A and none to B when they have nearly as pressing health needs and would be benefited by treatment nearly as much as the patients served by program A. If all cannot be treated, they might go on to argue, they deserve a fair chance to have their needs met rather than having no chance for treatment only because treating them would produce slightly less benefit than treating the patients served by program A. The small difference in benefits produced for the two groups—for example, a slightly greater life expectancy or more serious disability averted in program A—they argue, is too small to justify the tremendous difference in how the two

groups are treated. In the extreme case, some live and others die. The better outcome is produced by funding program A rather than program B, but that additional good is insufficient to justify morally the huge difference in the way the two groups of patients are treated. The conflict between fair chances and best outcomes can arise in a variety of contexts (Kamm 1993).

Preferring the most cost-effective program can also seem unfair because it compounds existing unfair inequalities. For example, screening slum-dwelling black men for hypertension targets the group with the highest incidence and greatest risk of premature death. However, it is more cost-effective to target well-to-do suburban white men, because they have more ordered lives, comply better, have personal doctors and the means to obtain medical services, are more educated, and are more likely to modify their lifestyles wisely. However, if the poor black men are not screened for this reason, it only compounds their existing unjust deprivation and, of course, is also in conflict with giving priority to the worst off.

If those who need a less cost-effective program deserve a fair chance to have their needs met, what would be a fair chance? Some argue that a fair chance is an equal chance, so some random method of selecting which program to fund should be used (Broome 1991). Others suggest proportional chances or a weighted lottery, in which the chance of each program being selected is proportional to the amount of health benefit each would produce, as a way of balancing fair chances against best outcomes (Brock 1988). Alternatively, some resources might go to each program (which is usually possible at the macro level), thereby benefiting some patients in each group—at least if their relative benefits are not strikingly dissimilar—instead of all going to the most cost-effective programs.

Another consideration supports spreading some resources to less cost-effective programs instead of devoting them all to the most cost-effective: to give all—or at least more—patients a reason to hope that their health needs will be met. This consideration may be especially important in developing countries where resource scarcity is more severe and adhering strictly to cost-effectiveness criteria could result in large numbers of patients with serious—or even life-threatening—health needs having no hope that their needs will be met.

Discrimination against Persons with Disabilities. The use of CEA in resource allocation to maximize the QALYs produced by available resources will often discriminate against persons with disabilities. Many persons with disabilities such as cystic fibrosis, HIV/AIDS, and chronic pulmonary or heart disease have reduced life expectancies or health-related quality of life as a result of their disabilities. Life-extending health care for those people will produce fewer QALYs than for people without them, all else being equal.

When health interventions are aimed at improving quality of life rather than extending life, similar discrimination can arise. The presence of disabilities can act as comorbidities, making treatment less effective or more expensive (or both) than it would otherwise be, thereby worsening its cost-effectiveness ratio relative to comparable treatment for persons without disabilities. These effects of treatment can result from a disability that exists before treatment and is unrelated to the treatment provided. So it seems that a cost-effectiveness standard for resource allocation discriminates against such persons specifically because of their disabilities. Moreover, this effect will arise not only in the case of preexisting disabilities, but also in the case of patients who become disabled as a result of treatment that is only partially effective.

Several strategies to avoid this discrimination in resource allocation have been suggested. Perhaps the most plausible, at least for the case of life-sustaining treatment, is to ignore differences in patients' posttreatment quality of life as long as each patient accepts and values that quality of life and to ignore differences in life expectancy after treatment as long as each will receive a significant gain in life extension; obviously, what counts as significant is vague and needs finer definition. Ignoring differences in life expectancy posttreatment fits with empirical evidence that individuals give little weight to duration of benefits in prioritizing between health interventions that serve different individuals.

Cutoffs for Cost per Quality-Adjusted Life Year. It is not uncommon in health care allocation to suggest the use of cutoffs tied to cost per QALY, although the cutoffs suggested vary substantially depending on the overall wealth of the country and on the amount that it spends on health care. The cutoffs can be of some value in identifying health interventions that are either good or poor buys, given the society's overall wealth and overall level of health spending. However, it is important to be clear that such cutoffs should never function as anything more than a rough initial guide in health resource allocation. The various equity considerations discussed briefly above can serve as justification for departing from or violating any cutoffs related to cost per QALY.

Responsibility for Health Needs. Some have suggested that health needs for which individuals are morally responsible should have lower priority than health needs for which individuals are not responsible (Moss and Siegler 1991). If individuals are responsible for their health needs and could have taken steps to avoid them, they have weaker claims on social resources to meet those needs than do individuals whose health needs are no fault of their own and could not have been prevented. Smoking and substance abuse are two of the most prominent examples of behaviors often cited. However, differentiating patients by whether they deserve care on the basis of whether they are responsible for their health needs does not fit

the practice or norms of medicine, which have the goal of meeting patients' medical needs.

There are strong moral reasons for considerable caution in letting health resource allocation depend on individuals' responsibility for their health needs (Wikler 2002). For that practice to be fair to those whose needs receive lower priority because of behavior, (a) the needs must have been caused by the behavior, (b) the behavior must have been voluntary, and (c) the persons must have known that the behavior would cause the health needs and that if they engaged in it their health needs resulting from it would receive lower priority. Smoking shows that these conditions are not easily satisfied. Smoking is one causal factor in much cancer and heart disease, but many smokers do not get those diseases, indicating that other factors, no doubt in part genetic differences for which individuals are not responsible, also play an important causal role. Smoking is typically begun when individuals are young adolescents, and as discussed in chapter 46, it is highly addictive, which undermines the voluntariness of continuing to smoke. Individuals in industrial countries are now generally familiar with the health risks of smoking, but this is less true among less educated populations in developing countries, where smoking is an increasing problem. No one anywhere has been informed before they smoke that, if they do, their health needs from smoking will receive lower priority for treatment than will other health needs.

Thus, it would generally be unfair to give smokers lower priority for treatment of smoking-related diseases on the grounds that they were morally responsible for those health needs, although there may be other behaviors for which individuals could more justifiably be held responsible. Moreover, attempting to make those judgments in individual cases would be extremely difficult and controversial. Given the difficulty of instituting a fair practice that allocates health resources according to people's moral responsibility for their health needs, we generally have good moral reason to preserve the egalitarian feature of the practice of medicine that looks to patients' needs for care rather than to whether they deserve care.

ETHICS IN RESEARCH AND NEW PRODUCT DEVELOPMENT

All new drugs and other medical products must be tested on human subjects before they are sold. Although participation in health research is often a valuable opportunity for participants, what happens to them is determined not only by their clinicians' therapeutic intent (if any) but also by the need to ensure that the research yields useful information. Managing the potential conflict between those motivations is often an ethically challenging task, and the issues become particularly contentious when research is conducted in developing countries.

Developing Consensus on Ethics and Human Subjects Research

The central ethical question in health research that involves human subjects is what may be asked of some individuals so that others may benefit. The question arises in any research in which human subjects are asked to participate, but is most pressing if the care that is offered to subjects provides no therapeutic benefit or if that care is compromised by the requirements of the study design. Informed consent, while in most cases a requirement for ethical justification of research involving risk, does not relieve the scientist of responsibility. The ethical question is what potential subjects may be recruited for, even if they do consent.

A rough consensus exists worldwide on the elements of research ethics and, increasingly, on the central role of the ethical review committee, or institutional review board (IRB). This consensus can be traced back to the post–World War II international determination to ensure that the kind of barbaric research practiced by Nazi scientists would not again stain the good name of medical science.[1] Three advisory documents have been particularly influential. The Nuremberg Tribunal that conducted the postwar Doctors' Trial promulgated a code of conduct for medical research that stressed the requirement of informed consent. The World Medical Association issued the first version of its Declaration of Helsinki in 1964 and has revised it several times. A further set of guidelines, issued in 1993 and revised a decade later, was published by the Geneva-based Council for International Organizations of Medical Sciences. Although they lack the force of law, these documents are widely acknowledged as international standards. Indeed, the World Medical Association's periodic revisions of the Declaration of Helsinki have become focal points for international debates over outstanding issues in research ethics.

The most elaborate codification of research ethics is the so-called Common Rule of Conduct of the U.S. Code of Federal Regulations (title 45, section 46), which derived from the work of the National Commission for the Protection of Human Subjects of Biomedical and Behavior Research of the mid 1970s. In addition to proposing rules governing many aspects of research with human subjects, the commission proposed that the IRB be given the central role in research ethics and be responsible for prior review of research proposals.[2] The IRB was a compromise, granting a measure of self-regulation to scientists and an assurance of ethical conduct to the government and the public for publicly funded investigations.

The basic elements of research ethics engender little disagreement. The research must never be brutal or inhumane, and all unnecessary risks should be eliminated. Any net risks to subjects must be justified by the prospect of potential benefits to others. Prospective participants must be told that they are in a study and must be informed of its nature and its risks and benefits. In the case of research that offers therapeutic benefit,

scientists must explore the range of reasonable therapeutic alternatives with the patient. Potential subjects must understand that their participation is completely voluntary and that they may withdraw at any time and for any reason. Because they cannot voluntarily shoulder risks, further protection must be provided to those who cannot give consent. Such people include, among others, mentally incompetent or immature participants and those involved in research (chiefly in social psychology) that requires initial deception. Consent, however, is not sufficient to ensure fairness; there should be additional safeguards against unfair distribution of the burdens and benefits of research. Finally, all research that involves potential risks should be reviewed by an IRB acting on the basis of internationally recognized ethical principles.

The global acceptance of these principles and the rapid development of capacity for ethical review attest to the perceived validity of this system of rules and procedures of ethical review. However, there has been relatively little research on how IRBs actually perform. Many IRBs in smaller institutions lack the necessary expertise to review novel or complex proposals, and their institutional setting creates a potential conflict of interest. Government investigations of the adequacy of IRBs for the tasks that are now assigned to them have often been critical (for example, Office of the Inspector General 1998, 2000). IRBs are often overworked and understaffed, resulting in ever-lengthening delays between initial submission of protocols and final approval. Regardless of the value of IRBs, predicting what will pass through them and what might provoke delay or rejection has become a significant concern for medical researchers. The system thus has costs as well as benefits, a fact that lends additional gravity to the controversies that it must resolve.

Goals of Ethical Review of Research

Although the overall purpose of ethical review is to ensure that research with human subjects is ethically defensible, the international consensus specifies several distinct goals that are sometimes in tension with each other:

- *Protection.* Ethical review committees can protect subjects by alerting investigators to unforeseen hazards and by suggesting research designs that can avoid unnecessary risk or reduce the number of subjects exposed to risk. By insisting that a clear explanation of risks and benefits be provided to potential participants, ethical review committees also help potential participants to protect themselves. Ethical review committees often take the name "Committee for the Protection of Human Subjects," reflecting a central preoccupation of research ethics today.
- *Assurance that participation is voluntary.* Some research cannot be conducted without asking some participants to

endure discomfort or pain, to delay relief from symptoms of their disease, or to risk other harm so that future patients may benefit. Permitting investigators to approach potential subjects in these cases requires an ethical judgment. In approving such a proposal, the function of the ethical review committee is not, strictly speaking, only to protect the subjects (the goal of protection would often be served more effectively by declining to do the research), but also to permit them to be enlisted in the effort to improve health care for others. Thus, a second function of ethical review is to ensure that those who agree to participate do so voluntarily and freely and that they understand what is being asked of them.

- *Equality and fairness.* Although research ethics committees have little authority to address persistent social injustices, a third concern of research ethics is that the benefits and burdens of health research be distributed fairly. This function receives relatively little attention in the literature of research ethics, despite its prominence in such well-known documents as the Belmont Report of the National Commission for the Protection of Human Subjects (1979). Many of the most notorious abuses of research subjects, including the Nazi investigations in the concentration camps, the Japanese biowarfare experiments on Chinese and other civilians, and the Tuskegee research on African Americans suffering from syphilis, were committed on subjects chosen exclusively from disadvantaged groups.

Those three goals of ethical review—protecting subjects; ensuring voluntary, informed participation; and reviewing the fairness of recruitment—are promulgated in the international guidelines and in the Common Rule (and in the regulations of other countries), but they do not always point in the same direction. For example, a research project that asks participants to endure a burden or risk—thus failing to offer full protection—can still meet the requirement of equality if the burden is equally shared.

Ethical review, thus, is not a matter of applying a checklist, but it imposes an obligation of substantial ethical judgment. A key challenge for IRBs is to earn and retain the trust of participants and of the public, a task made more difficult by the unavoidable absence of explicit criteria for approval. This problem is exacerbated by the institutional conflict of interest inherent in the placement of the IRB within the research institution, which prompts concern that the committees will downplay risks to subjects for projects that profit or benefit the institution or its influential staff members. Conversely, IRBs that are fearful of institutional embarrassment or legal sanction in the event of any harm befalling research participants might lean too far in the direction of overprotection of subjects, at the expense of important scientific research initiatives. Both concerns have been raised about the IRB system.

Current Controversies in Research Ethics

Some of the most sharply disputed issues have arisen in international collaborative research involving scientists and sponsors from wealthy countries conducting experiments in developing countries. Some of the problems are procedural. For example, U.S. agencies have insisted on the same kind of recordkeeping for IRBs in developing countries that is required of IRBs in U.S. research institutions. IRBs in developing countries may accept the same principles of accountability, but they do not have the elaborate staffs and budgets that leading IRBs rely on.

The most difficult disputes involving the ethics of research in developing countries are, however, substantive rather than procedural.

Standard of Care. The international guidelines used in navigating the ethical dilemmas of research in developing countries were created for the very different purpose of ensuring that what happened at Dachau and Auschwitz would not recur. It is not clear whether those rules usefully resolve the kinds of dilemmas that arise in, say, Uganda or Peru.

The Declaration of Helsinki, following the Nuremberg Tribunal, requires informed consent of all competent research subjects, and in section 29 states that "the benefits, risks, burdens, and effectiveness of a new method should be tested against those of the best current prophylactic, diagnostic, and therapeutic methods."

To its supporters, any departure from the letter of the Declaration of Helsinki that would permit an experiment in a poor country that would be forbidden in a rich one would constitute a double ethical standard. In their view, this clause of the Declaration of Helsinki affirms the equal importance of human lives, regardless of wealth or nationality, and stands as a safeguard against exploitation of those made vulnerable by poverty, sickness, and absence of governmental protection.

Opponents, however, argue that this position seems to rule out the possibility of testing cheap new products that may be effective, although perhaps not as effective as other products that the population could not afford. If so, it would be difficult to understand whom the single-standard-of-care position would be protecting, for surely it is better for a seriously ill person to receive a good drug, even if it is not the best, than to receive no drug at all.[3]

Both points of view deserve respect. The single-standard approach is consistent with the postwar consensus on principles of research ethics, and it offers a bright line between research that amply respects human subjects and that which might result if sponsors and scientists were tempted to roam the globe in search of human subjects who could be used as experimental material with a minimum of expense or trouble.

Opponents of the universal-standard view, however, challenge its premise. It made sense to insist on a single, universal standard when the problem was Nazi barbarity, because the prevailing standard was high and the medical criminals in the death camps denied it to the imprisoned minority—people unjustly stripped of their entitlements. In Uganda or Nepal, however, care at the highest world standard is available, if at all, to only a small elite.

A full reconciliation of those points of view may not be possible. The authors suggest that a relativized standard should be considered only when the beneficiaries will include the impoverished, sick population. Even in those cases, however, the local standard of care could be adopted in the experiment only if it met or exceeded the standard provided by other countries at similar levels of development.

Placebo Controls and Other Issues Involving Research Design. For certain purposes, scientists use a placebo control even though a proven treatment exists. Patients in these control groups thus receive care that is inferior to what they would experience in good clinical care. Until very recently, the Declaration of Helsinki flatly condemned this practice (its current language is somewhat less restrictive), but the U.S. Food and Drug Administration (FDA) accepted results of these trials in applications for approval of new drugs. The FDA's justification for this acceptance rests on two claims, one scientific and one ethical. The first is that in certain contexts (for example, for conditions such as depression, in which eligibility criteria and outcomes are subjective, to an appreciable extent, and in which symptoms fluctuate in both treated and untreated patients), active controls may produce misleading indications of equivalency, yielding seemingly positive results that may be spurious. The second is that when only placebo controls can be informative, it is sometimes justifiable to ask participants to be randomized with placebo and thereby to risk discomfort and distress (but not any appreciable risk of death or long-term impairment).

Debates over placebo controls are often joined in the context of disputes over the appropriate standard of care that arise in the case of research in developing countries, but placebo controls are controversial in trials in high-income countries, too. Placebo controls are one instance of a large category of ethical issues in research that require weighing the importance of a scientifically ideal research design against the well-being of participants. For example, a study of long-term chemotherapy to prevent the recurrence of breast cancer was halted before the designated endpoints had been reached after the study's Data Safety and Monitoring Board decided that continuing the study after a strong trend had been established favoring the chemotherapy would be unfair to the control group. It is notable that in this instance severe criticism of this decision was voiced by an organization representing women at risk for breast cancer, as well as by the editorial board of the *New York Times.* Critics of the early termination of the trial were, in effect, aligning themselves with the interests of future

beneficiaries of the research and possibly against the immediate interests of the women in the control group.

Rights of Host Communities. Ideally, research involving human subjects would be a cooperative endeavor for mutual advantage among free citizens who understand and endorse the need for research and who expect to share both in the burden of serving as research subjects and in the eventual benefit of improved health care. Societies that recruit subjects primarily from lower socioeconomic strata fall short of this ideal; those that do not offer new advances in care to all of their citizens fall even further short, raising serious questions about fairness. Furthest of all from this ideal are some instances of the increasingly common practice of recruiting research subjects among the poorest people in the poorest countries. The means for protecting human subjects in these countries are often nonexistent. Most of their citizens will be unable to afford new drugs developed by firms in industrial countries. It is not clear that these subjects participate voluntarily. Their lack of scientific education or even literacy limits their ability to understand the terms of the proposed agreement with the scientists and sponsors (particularly when consent forms, on legal advice, run to 20 dense pages), and poverty often deprives them of any alternative means of recovering their health.

Despite these potential ethical shortcomings, international collaborative research is assured of continued growth. Some of this research targets diseases affecting mainly poor people, who as a group suffer more from too little research on their populations than from too much. Even research intended to develop therapies that will be affordable only to much wealthier patients can be defended. Individual participants may receive better care than they would otherwise, and visiting scientists offer employment and technical training.

To right the perceived imbalance in what is asked of research subjects in poor countries and the value that is obtained by scientists who experiment on them, some have proposed that sponsors of research in the poorest countries compensate their hosts by offering a supplementary benefit (Glantz and others 1998). One much discussed option is access following the end of the study to any drugs or other therapies whose effectiveness is confirmed in the research. The most limited proposals would restrict this entitlement to individuals who were enrolled in the study (those who received placebo as members of a control group, for instance), and time limits (such as three years) have been proposed in the case of chronic diseases such as HIV/AIDS. More expansive community benefit proposals have called for lifetime access to the treatments by all participants, their families, other members of the local community, or even all citizens of the country. Other proposed benefits include a specified amount of technology transfer, including scientific training and the construction of clinics and laboratories, and cash payments earmarked for health care. A moderate proposal is to encourage these benefits but to require only that they be discussed and agreed on before investigations are initiated (National Bioethics Advisory Commission 2001).

These proposals are intended to restore fairness to the relationship between participants and those who benefit from research, including scientists and their sponsors and also future beneficiaries of advances in medical science. Among the potential drawbacks are the inability to specify, even roughly, how much is owed to host communities; the inability to determine whether community benefit should be required even of research funded by governments or philanthropists for the benefit of people living in the host communities; and the risk that placing these demands on proposed research projects will drive them away from these very needy sites. Some of these uncertainties may be resolved over time as a variety of approaches are attempted, particularly if they are studied and reported to officials in potential research sites.

These international collaborations would draw less scrutiny if it were clear that all subjects knew what they were getting into and participated of their own free will. Although evidence on this point is mixed, special circumstances in some countries introduce problems that will have to be addressed over the long run. Cultural differences between host populations and scientists may lead to conflicts over who has the authority to speak for the individuals invited to participate in a given study. Regulatory authorities in high-income countries have been reluctant to accept permission by a woman's husband or by a village chief on behalf of his people in lieu of individual consent. It is often unclear—particularly from the vantage point of an IRB in Europe or the United States—whether the cultural norms of the host population designate the husband or village chief as decision makers in these transactions and whether insistence on concurrent individual consent would be viewed as intrusive or insulting.

Another recurring issue is whether people enrolled in a trial of a promising therapy who are ill and very poor can rightly be viewed as volunteers. The prospect of a cure for a person who would otherwise die would seem to be irresistible, even if the treatment is not up to the standards that even less well-to-do citizens of richer countries would expect. Financial incentives, too, would predictably have a powerful effect on an individual who may always be looking for a day's wage to feed hungry children. Some IRBs limit payments to compensation for lost wages and travel expenses, but even at this level researchers are asked to change the amounts offered to avoid forcing a choice on the potential participant. As with alleged cultural differences regarding individual informed consent, IRBs operate with scant evidence on this point. It is difficult from a long distance to decide what amount of compensation undermines freedom of choice. It is also unclear whether the moral categories used in these disputes have been adequately thought through. The fact that a poor person finds an attractive offer irresistible will be viewed as evidence of coercion by some observers but nothing more than common sense by others.

Most of these controversies can be traced back to underdevelopment and the inequalities of wealth and education that prevail among and within nations today, but progress in resolving the ethical controversies that have become obstacles to badly needed health research must be made even as these disparities persist. Viewing health research in the context of development and emphasizing research that is targeted to the needs of the poor majorities in poor countries can provide a context in which trust rather than fear or suspicion is the default response in host countries. Efforts to build capacity for ethical review within the host countries, such as financial support for ethical review committees, can place the locus of decision making closer to the people who serve as subjects. Research on the effectiveness of current ethical and regulatory requirements and mechanisms might enhance the process of ethical review while reducing its bureaucratic burden. Meanwhile, the quality and appropriateness of ethical review of this research that takes place in the sponsors' countries would be enhanced by eliciting the views of officials in developing countries, clinicians, scientists, and community leaders.

NOTES

1. Because our current system of ethical review and regulation of research with human subjects derives from our resolve to prevent the recurrence of earlier abuses, it deserves mention that the standard historical account of research ethics has been seriously incomplete. While the Allies sat in judgment of the Nazi scientists at Nuremberg, abuses of similar scope and savagery practiced by Japanese biowarfare researchers on Chinese and other civilians and prisoners of war were kept secret (and their perpetrators were unpunished) following a pact with the criminal scientists to exchange data for war crimes immunity. Moreover, the Allied governments did not always honor the Nuremberg principles. In the Soviet Union, scientists attempting to develop for clandestine operations poisons that would not be identified on autopsy practiced their craft, with predictably lethal results, on hapless prisoners (Birstein 2001). Abuses in the United States, such as the Tuskegee syphilis study (Brandt 2000), have been more widely publicized, but ethical lapses in large-scale Cold War–related studies, ranging from radiation studies on urban populations (Advisory Committee on Human Radiation Experiments 1995) to surreptitious administration of mind-altering drugs such as LSD (Rockefeller Commission 1975), were state secrets.

2. In the United States, the Office of Human Research Protections, an agency of the Department of Health and Human Services, has overall responsibility for oversight of IRBs administering research using U.S. government funds. Its Web site is http://ohrp.osophs.dhhs.gov/.

3. Supporters of the single-standard view might point out that, in its current version, the Declaration of Helsinki does not require that everyone in an experiment receive the best available care, but rather that new treatments be tested against the best available care. But this defense faces further objections. In some cases, testing against the best available care (rather than against the care currently provided to the population or against placebo) will fail to provide the evidence needed to convince the ministry of health or potential donors that funds should be provided. There is a potential contradiction in any view that claims both that all patients in experiments deserve the best care and that it is ethically acceptable to test a new treatment that is not expected to be quite as good as the best currently available.

REFERENCES

Advisory Committee on Human Radiation Experiments. 1995. *Final Report*. Washington, DC: U.S. Government Printing Office.

Birdsall, N., and R. Hecht. 1995. "Swimming against the Tide: Strategies for Improving Equity in Health." Human Capital Development and Operations Policy Working Paper 55, World Bank, Washington, DC.

Birstein, V. 2001. *The Perversion of Knowledge: The True Story of Soviet Science*. Boulder, CO: Westview.

Brandt, A. 2000. "Racism and Research: The Case of the Tuskegee Syphilis Experiment." In *Tuskegee's Truths: Rethinking the Tuskegee Syphilis Study*, ed. S. M. Reverby. Chapel Hill, NC: University of North Carolina Press.

Brock, D. 1988. "Ethical Issues in Recipient Selection for Organ Transplantation." In *Organ Substitution Technology: Ethical, Legal, and Public Policy Issues*, ed. D. Mathieu. Boulder, CO, and London: Westview.

———. 1995. "Justice and the ADA: Does Prioritizing and Rationing Health Care Discriminate against the Disabled?" *Social Philosophy and Policy* 12 (2): 159–84.

———. 2002. "Priority to the Worst Off in Health Care Resource Prioritization." In *Medicine and Social Justice*, ed. M. Battin, R. Rhodes, and A. Silvers. New York: Oxford University Press.

———. 2003a. "Ethical Issues in the Use of Cost Effectiveness Analysis for the Prioritization of Health Care Resources." In *Making Choices in Health: WHO Guide to Cost-Effectiveness Analysis*, ed. T. Tan-Torres Edejer, R. Baltussen, T. Adam, R. Hutubessy, A. Acharya, D. B. Evans, and C. J. L. Murray. Geneva: World Health Organization.

———. 2003b. "Separate Spheres and Indirect Benefits." *Cost-Effectiveness and Resource Allocation* 1 (1): 4.

Broome, J. 1991. "Fairness." *Proceedings of the Aristotelian Society* 91 (1): 87–102.

CMH (Commission on Macroeconomics and Health). 2001. *Macroeconomics and Health: Investing in Health for Economic Development*. Geneva: World Health Organization.

Daniels, N. 1993. "Rationing Fairly: Programmatic Considerations." *Bioethics* 7 (2–3): 224–33.

———. 2000. "Accountability for Reasonableness." *British Medical Journal* 321: 1300–1.

Glantz, L. H., G. J. Annas, M. A. Grodin, and W. K. Mariner. 1998. "Research in Developing Countries: Taking 'Benefit' Seriously." *Hastings Center Report* 28 (6): 38–42.

Gold, M. R., J. E. Siegel, L. B. Russell, and M. C. Weinstein, eds. 1996. *Cost-Effectiveness in Health and Medicine*. New York: Oxford University Press.

Gruskin, S., and D. Tarantola. 2001. "Health and Human Rights." In *Oxford Textbook on Public Health*, ed. R. Detels and R. Beaglehole. Oxford, U.K.: Oxford University Press.

Hadorn, D. 1991. "Setting Health Care Priorities in Oregon." *Journal of the American Medical Association* 265 (17): 2218–25.

Holm, S. 1998. "Goodbye to the Simple Solutions: the Second Phase of Priority Setting in Health Care." *British Medical Journal* 317: 1000–7.

Horsman, J., W. Furlong, D. Feeny, and G. Torrance. 2003. "The Health Utilities Index (HUI®): Concepts, Measurement Properties, and Applications." *Health and Quality of Life Outcomes* 1 (1): 54.

Kamm, F. M. 1993. *Morality/Mortality. Volume One. Death and Whom to Save from It*. Oxford, U.K.: Oxford University Press.

Keeler, E. B., and S. Cretin. 1983. "Discounting of Life-Saving and Other Non-monetary Effects." *Management Science* 29 (3): 300–6.

Meltzer, D. 1997. "Accounting for Future Costs in Medical Cost-Effectiveness Analysis." *Journal of Health Economics* 16 (1): 33–64.

Menzel, P., P. Dolan, J. Richardson, and J. A. Olsen. 2002. "The Role of Adaptation to Disability and Disease in Health State Valuation: A Preliminary Normative Analysis." *Social Science and Medicine* 55 (12): 2149–58.

Moss, A. H., and M. Siegler. 1991. "Should Alcoholics Compete Equally for Liver Transplantation?" *Journal of the American Medical Association* 265 (10): 1295–98.

Murray, C. J. L. 1994. "Quantifying the Burden of Disease: The Technical Basis for Disability-Adjusted Life Years." In *Global Comparative Assessments in the Health Sector: Disease Burden, Expenditures, and Intervention Packages*, ed. C. J. L. Murray and A. D. Lopez. Geneva: World Health Organization.

National Bioethics Advisory Commission. 2001. "When Research Is Concluded—Access to the Benefits of Research by Participants, Communities, and Countries." In *Ethical and Policy Issues in International Research: Clinical Trials in Developing Countries*. Washington, DC: U.S. Government Printing Office.

National Commission for the Protection of Human Subjects of Biomedical and Behavioral Research. Office of the Secretary, U.S. Department of Health, Education, and Welfare. 1979. "The Belmont Report: Ethical Principles and Guidelines for the Protection of Human Subjects of Research." U.S. Department of Health, Education, and Welfare, Washington, DC.

Nord, E. 1999. *Cost-Value Analysis in Health Care: Making Sense out of QALYs*. Cambridge, U.K.: Cambridge University Press.

Nord, E., J. Richardson, H. Kuhse, and P. Singer. 1996. "The Significance of Age and Duration of Effect in Social Evaluation of Health Care." *Health Care Analysis* 4 (2): 103–11.

Nord, E., J. Richardson, A. Street, H. Kuhse, and P. Singer. 1995. "Who Cares about Cost? Does Economic Analysis Impose or Reflect Social Values?" *Health Policy* 34 (2): 79–94.

Office of the Inspector General, U.S. Department of Health and Human Services. 1998. *Institutional Review Boards: A Time for Reform*. Washington, DC: U.S. Government Printing Office.

———. 2000. *Protecting Human Subjects: Status of Recommendations*. Washington, DC: U.S. Government Printing Office.

Parfit, D. 1991. "Equality or Priority." Lindley Lecture. Department of Philosophy, University of Kansas, Lawrence, KS.

Rawls, J. 1971. *A Theory of Justice*. Cambridge, MA: Harvard University Press.

Rockefeller Commission (Commission on CIA Activities within the United States). 1975. *Report to the President*. Washington, DC: U.S. Government Printing Office.

Scanlon, T. M. 1997. *What We Owe to Each Other*. Cambridge, MA: Harvard University Press.

Solomon, J., and C. Murray. 2002. "A Conceptual Framework for Understanding Adaptation, Coping, and Adjustment in Health State Valuations." In *Summary Measures of Population Health*, ed. C. Murray, J. Salomon, C. Mathers, A. Lopez, and J. Lozano. Geneva: World Health Organization.

Weinstein, M., and W. B. Stason. 1997. "Foundations of Cost-Effectiveness Analysis for Health and Medical Practices." *New England Journal of Medicine* 296 (13): 716–21.

Wikler, D. 2002. "Personal and Social Responsibility for Health." *Ethics and International Affairs* 16 (2): 47–55.

Williams, A. 1997. "Intergenerational Equity: An Exploration of the 'Fair Innings' Argument." *Health Economics* 6 (2): 117–32.

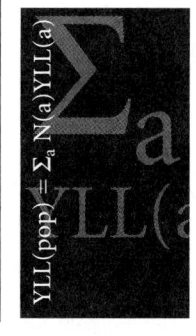

Chapter **15**

Cost-Effectiveness Analysis for Priority Setting

Philip Musgrove and Julia Fox-Rushby

The economic analyses in this volume focus on activities whose main objective is to improve health. Although the chapters vary considerably, all possess, nonetheless, a common core of definitions, assumptions, and methods of analysis. These are drawn primarily from concepts and applications in the *Oxford Textbook of Public Health* (Jamison 2002), drawing partly on the 1993 *World Development Report* (World Bank 1993). In this chapter, we summarize and explain the common features and some of the variations of economic analysis and point the reader to examples throughout the book.

First is a general discussion of cost-effectiveness analysis (CEA), which is the principal analytic tool used here. Here we explain what such analysis does and does not provide, how it is related to the concept of burden of disease, and how it can be used, along with other criteria, in setting priorities.

Because CEA is applied to specific interventions, the next section describes the several meanings of that term and the way that interventions are classified and evaluated. It is essential to understand what is being analyzed before considering in detail how the analysis is conducted.

Estimating the effectiveness of an intervention requires specifying the units in which that concept is measured. This action in turn requires choices of several parameter values, including, in the analyses reported here, the discount rate applied to future years; the disability weights that describe the severity of diseases and conditions, corresponding to the health losses that they cause; and the life expectancy at different ages, which determines how many years of healthy life can be saved by averting a death or preventing or treating a long-term health problem. We also consider briefly the nonhealth benefits that may result from a health intervention.

The subsequent section deals with the costs of interventions: first with the question of which costs to include in the analysis, and then with the conversion of costs in national currencies to equivalents in U.S. dollars for international comparisons.

Despite the common assumptions and parameter values, the economic analyses differ from chapter to chapter in how comprehensive and how exact they are, including how they deal with a variety of approximations and how the results vary from place to place or according to differences in the assumptions. This section also contains a brief description of the differences in the quality of the basic evidence and in how widely conclusions are applicable.

Estimates of the cost-effectiveness of interventions often describe what happens at the level of the individual patient or beneficiary. In the next section, we suggest two ways to consider costs and outcomes at the population level, allowing for large differences among countries in the size of population; the incidence or prevalence of a disease, condition, or risk factor; and the amount spent or available to spend on an intervention.

In the final section, we indicate how the type of analysis presented in this volume might be improved and how it can be applied to help set priorities among the large number of interventions to which limited resources can be applied.

COST-EFFECTIVENESS AND PRIORITY SETTING

The principal analytic tool throughout this volume is CEA, which compares the cost of an activity, called an *intervention*, with the known or expected health gain. The result is summarized in a cost-effectiveness ratio (CER), as explained more fully below. This ratio corresponds to the concept of (health) value for money. Favoring activities that are more cost-effective over those that are less so is consistent with the ethical view that "limited resources for health should be allocated to maximize the health benefits for the population served" (chapter 14).

Cost-effectiveness provides the clearest simple way to promote value for money in health: hence, the emphasis on it here. CEA allows comparisons throughout the health sector and not only for the same health outcome. It does not allow comparison to nonhealth outcomes unless these outcomes can be incorporated into costs, and the calculation of the CER by itself makes no pretense of monetizing the intrinsic value of health. To use CERs for choosing what to buy and what not to, decision makers must determine a maximum willingness to pay for units of health gain, unless other criteria are considered to justify buying something with relatively poor cost-effectiveness.

For risk factors, CEA requires estimating the gain in health consequent on introducing an intervention to reduce the risk of acquiring or transmitting a condition. For packages of interventions or elements of the health system, such as hospitals, effectiveness is estimated by judging how much mortality and morbidity would be reduced by providing the whole package or set of services or by operating the facility. With some exceptions, the analyses may describe but do not quantify the nonhealth benefits of an intervention. Apart from the difficulty of obtaining enough data, such quantification requires attaching values to nonhealth outcomes, which is problematic when comparisons are made over large cultural and income differences.

All comparisons are relative, with no absolute distinction between being and not being cost-effective. In assigning priorities among interventions for public funding or for other policy actions, one must also consider the magnitude of health problems to which interventions apply because that affects what is affordable. Calculations of the effect of spending US$1 million or the total cost and health gain in a population of 1 million people offer ways of looking at such choices. Equity, poverty, and risk of impoverishment from ill health may also influence priorities; so do the budgets available—and the decisions of how much to make available—for buying interventions. Finally, the effectiveness of an intervention and, therefore, the degree to which it deserves priority depend on how far it is culturally appropriate or acceptable for the population it is intended to benefit. The identical intervention, technically speaking, may lead to different degrees of use or compliance in different population groups, and information and incentives may be needed to achieve the full potential outcomes.

Cost-effectiveness is only one of at least nine criteria relevant for priority setting in health if the object is to decide how to spend public funds (Musgrove 1999). Cost matters by itself, as do the capacities of potential beneficiaries to pay for an intervention. The other criteria that may affect priorities include horizontal equity (equal treatment for people in equal circumstances); vertical equity (priority for people with worse problems); adequacy of demand; and public attitudes and wants. Two criteria—whether an intervention is a public good and whether it yields substantial externalities—are classic justifications for public intervention, because private markets could not supply them efficiently, just as in other sectors. As noted in chapter 1, the interventions analyzed in this volume are not limited to public or semipublic goods. The emphasis is on value for money—that is, whether an intervention is worth buying, not who pays for it. Nonetheless, when one is choosing which public goods to buy, several criteria become irrelevant, and cost-effectiveness can be used as the chief or even the only consideration. Cost-effectiveness can similarly determine what to include in a mandatory universal public package of health care alongside competitive voluntary insurance (Smith 2005).

Cost-effectiveness can conflict with both kinds of equity—that is, the more cost-effective of two interventions may also lead to a less equitable distribution of health benefits. Equity and cost-effectiveness are compatible when a cost-effective intervention is provided to only part of the population that would benefit from it because everyone in the group suffers from the same problem. Then expanding coverage will generally also promote horizontal equity. These equity effects are reinforced when those who are better off already benefit while the poorer and sicker population does not. Choices about vertical equity—doing more for those in greatest need—are more complicated. Doing very little for people with severe health problems—because the available interventions for those problems are not very effective at reducing their suffering—is not necessarily preferable to doing more for people with less severe problems that are more amenable to intervention. When an intervention is reaching only part of a potential beneficiary population and those not benefiting tend to have more severe illness, then expanding coverage can improve both horizontal and vertical equity. Where possible, chapters consider the equity effects of expanding or changing interventions.

Cost-Effectiveness and Disease Burden

Cost-effectiveness and disease burden are related because effectiveness is the reduction in burden caused by an intervention. This relationship holds true at the individual level. The magnitude of a health problem—the total burden in the population—is irrelevant for marginal changes in resource allocation. However, it matters for large changes from the status quo. Health interventions demand managerial capacity as well as financial and physical resources, and managerial ability may be stretched thin if it has to deal with a large number of interventions. In consequence, it may be efficient to concentrate on relatively few and somewhat less cost-effective interventions, provided they attack substantial burdens, rather than many other interventions that are more cost-effective but affect only small burdens. Moreover, even for a cost-effective intervention, high prevalence or incidence may make the cost of covering the whole potential beneficiary population prohibitive. The authors of chapter 21 indicate how expensive it would be to protect all at-risk African children from malaria with bednets, even though bednets are highly cost-effective. Conversely, an intervention that costs more per health gain may be affordable and given priority if it treats a manageable burden of disease and corresponds to a small beneficiary group. Priority turns on the available budget relative to the cost of a program; on how divisible a program is (that is, how easily it can be operated at different scales, as a technical or political matter); and on whether interventions are mutually exclusive (Karlsson and Johannesson 1996).

Because of the interaction between cost-effectiveness, disease burden, and available funds, no single threshold of maximum cost per health gain exists below which an intervention is "cost-effective." A rule of thumb, such as that any intervention is worthwhile if it costs less than two or three times income per capita, ignores this interaction and is an inadequate guide to priority setting. However, even an intervention that is considered justified by cost-effectiveness may be infeasible to deliver, for example, if the costs are monetary and come from the public budget but the benefits are nonmonetary and diffused over the population. Economic theory would suggest removing the current budget constraint by raising more revenue until the marginal social cost of the interventions plus the cost of obtaining the revenue equals the marginal social benefit. Although theoretically attractive, this escape from resource limitation may not be possible because of political reasons or because the economic cost of raising extra taxes is prohibitive.

Because so many criteria can affect priority setting and because evidence on cost-effectiveness in low- and middle-income countries is so scarce, health system policies and budgets seldom derive purely from considerations of cost versus outcomes. Even in high-income countries, where more such analyses are available, their effect has been limited, although it is growing (Gabbay and le May 2004; Glick, Polsky, and Schulman 2001; Hoffmann and others 2002; McDaid, Cookson, and ASTEC Group 2003; Sheldon and others 2004; Taylor and NICE 2002). Cost-effectiveness studies are now required by, for example, the U.S. Food and Drug Administration for labeling claims, the National Institute for Clinical Excellence before advising national policy on treatments and care in England, and the Ministry of Health in the Netherlands for new drugs (iMTA 2005).

DEFINITION AND CHARACTERISTICS OF INTERVENTIONS

The object of a CEA—the thing to which it is applied, the costs and outcomes of which are to be analyzed—is an intervention. An *intervention* is an activity using human, physical, and finan-

cial resources in a deliberate attempt to improve health by reducing the risk, duration, or severity of a health problem (Jamison 2002, table 2). The term usually refers to an activity undertaken by a health system rather than by an individual. The emphasis on a deliberate, systemic effort means that an intervention is not simply anything that improves health; for example, if more rainfall leads to higher crop yields and better nutritional status, the rain does not count as an intervention. Similarly, although breastfeeding protects infants' health, it is not itself an intervention as the word is used in this volume. In contrast, a program to encourage new mothers to breastfeed *is* an intervention (as described in chapter 27). How effective such a program is, of course, depends on how many mothers it persuades to adopt the practice when they are neither currently breastfeeding nor planning to do so.

Interventions can be directed against an injury or disease (such as trachoma), a condition associated with or deriving from a disease (such as blindness), or a risk factor that makes the disease or condition more likely (such as the lack of hygiene that leads to trachoma). An intervention may pursue primary prevention at the population level—promoting personal behavior change, controlling environmental hazards, or delivering a medical intervention such as immunization to a large population—or individual action for primary prevention, cure, acute management, chronic management, secondary prevention, rehabilitation, or palliation. Box 15.1 defines these terms, and the figure in the box illustrates how interventions may prevent ill health events or deal with their consequences. Characterizing an intervention fully also means distinguishing the level at which it is delivered (home, primary care facility, district hospital, or referral hospital); indicating whether it involves drugs, immune enhancement, surgery, or physical or psychological therapy; and determining whether it requires a physician or uses diagnostic, laboratory, or imaging procedures. Such procedures are most often evaluated relative to the interventions they screen for or lead to, because they produce no health gain by themselves (although the information they provide can be valuable for reassurance or for promoting behavioral changes).

An intervention in the everyday sense includes such activities as immunizing a child, performing a surgical procedure, or treating an infection with antibiotics. The authors of some chapters use the term only in this sense—for example, in discussing interventions that contribute to meeting the Millennium Development Goals (chapter 9). Authors of other chapters use the term in several other senses as well. It can mean modifying an existing intervention—for example, adding *Haemophilus influenzae* type B (Hib) antigen to the Expanded Program on Immunizations (EPI). Immunization against Hib is itself an intervention, but instead of analyzing it separately, one can use CEA to evaluate the additional cost of incorporating that antigen and the additional health gain that

Box 15.1

Intervention Categories, with Examples

The following figure illustrates how interventions are related to a health event; the definitions of these categories are given below.

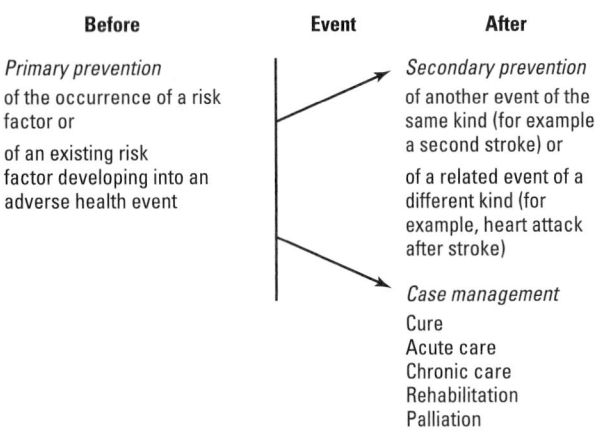

| **Before** | **Event** | **After** |

Primary prevention
of the occurrence of a risk factor or

of an existing risk factor developing into an adverse health event

Secondary prevention
of another event of the same kind (for example, a second stroke) or

of a related event of a different kind (for example, heart attack after stroke)

Case management
Cure
Acute care
Chronic care
Rehabilitation
Palliation

Interventions Related to the Occurrence of an Adverse Health Event

Population-based interventions all aim at primary prevention (as defined later), are directed to entire populations or large subgroups, and fall into three categories:

- Promoting personal behavior change (diet, exercise, smoking, sexual activity)
- Control of environmental hazards (air and water pollution, disease vectors)
- Medical interventions (immunization, mass chemoprophylaxis, large-scale screening, referral).

Personal interventions are directed to individuals and can be intended for the following:

- Primary prevention—to reduce the level of one or more risk factors, to reduce the probability of initial occurrence of disease (medication for hypertension to prevent stroke or heart attack), or to reduce the likelihood of disease when the risk factor is already present (prophylaxis for sickle cell anemia).
- Secondary prevention following the occurrence of disease—either to prevent another event of the same kind or to reduce the risk of a different but related event (medication to reduce the likelihood of a second coronary event or a first heart attack after stroke).
- Cure—to remove the cause of a condition and restore function to the status quo ante (surgery for appendicitis)
- Acute management—short-term activity to decrease the severity of acute events or the level of established risk factors, to minimize their long-term impacts (thrombolytic medication following heart attack, angioplasty to reduce stenosis in coronary arteries).
- Chronic management—continued activity to decrease the severity of chronic conditions or prevent deterioration (medication for unipolar depression, insulin for diabetes). Chronic management can include some secondary prevention.
- Rehabilitation—full or partial restoration of physical, psychological, or social function that has been damaged by a previous disease or condition (therapy following musculoskeletal injury, counseling for psychological problems).
- Palliation—to reduce pain and suffering from a condition for which no cure or rehabilitation is currently available (analgesics for headache, opiates for terminal cancer).

Source: Authors.

---

is expected to result (see chapter 20). The intervention studied is then not Hib immunization as such but the change in the full vaccination procedure. A change in the scale of an existing activity can also be considered an intervention, even if the activity itself is unchanged: that is, one can analyze the change in costs and in outcomes associated with expanding or contracting the coverage of the activity—for example, extending antiretroviral treatment for HIV and AIDS to a larger population (chapter 18) or screening more newborns for sickle cell anemia (chapter 34). In most chapters, the authors assume that expansion affects costs and outcomes linearly, so that the CER does not change. The chapters on vaccine-preventable diseases

(chapter 20) and malaria (chapter 21) provide explicit estimates of the differential costs of expanding coverage.

Adding one intervention to another to deal with the same disease or condition is also an intervention, and combinations of interventions can be analyzed to determine which is most cost-effective or how the cost-effectiveness of one intervention depends on the other activities with which it is combined. Examples include successively adding drugs for treatment of epilepsy (chapter 32) or secondary prevention of cardiovascular disease (chapter 33) or combining several quite different interventions to control tobacco addiction or alcohol (chapters 46 and 47, respectively). The analyses of community health and nutrition programs (chapter 56) and integrated management of infant and childhood illness (IMCI; chapter 63) define "the intervention" as a whole program incorporating several different activities. Generally, even less empirical evidence exists concerning combinations of interventions than for individual activities, but IMCI is an exception; it has been evaluated more thoroughly than most single interventions.

Box 15.2 includes a more detailed discussion, using a hypothetical example of three different ways to deliver immunization, of how CEA can be applied to four of the meanings of *intervention* used here: an existing intervention at its current coverage, changes in the scale of that intervention, the addition of one intervention to another when expanding coverage, and the complete shift from one intervention to a different (and more cost-effective) one.

Depending on the comparison undertaken, the result may be an average cost-effectiveness ratio (ACER) or an incremental cost-effectiveness ratio (ICER). The former compares total costs and total results, starting from zero, whereas the latter compares additional costs and additional results, starting from the current or some other level of coverage of an intervention.

Either shifting completely from one intervention to another or partially replacing one with another may reduce costs while producing more health gain. For example, if spending is high on hospitalization for acute myocardial infarction, a program using a "polypill" (several medications in a single pill) would reduce expenditures by lowering incidence (chapter 33) and would be cost saving, because less hospitalization would be needed. If the status quo is no hospitalization (as is typical at low incomes), a polypill program increases costs but may more than correspondingly increase health gains and therefore be more cost-effective. If the polypill both reduces costs and improves outcomes compared with hospitalization, it is said to dominate a hospital-only strategy. The second figure in box 15.2 illustrates the concept of dominance; table 45.4 and box 45.1 of chapter 45 provide examples of interventions that are dominated by others.

Unfortunately, reliable information on current intervention coverage, costs, and results is not always available even in high-income countries (iMTA 2005) and is extremely scarce in low- and middle-income countries. Studies showing whether an intervention is effective or cost-effective seldom cover the entire potential beneficiary population, and service provision in the private sector is often not recorded. Many chapter authors describe only the ACER of an existing or potential intervention, whereas others explicitly compare alternatives to current practice (for an example, see chapter 16).

Many of the activities analyzed here aim at promoting changes in personal behavior, by informing and persuading individuals to eat differently, to avoid smoking and excessive alcohol, to reduce the risks of sexually transmitted infections, or to practice better hygiene. Such efforts can be considered interventions in themselves, and as such are crucial for controlling HIV and AIDS (chapter 18), promoting better infant and child care (chapters 20 and 27), preventing inherited disorders (chapter 34), encouraging healthful diets and exercise (chapters 44 and 45), and avoiding addiction (chapters 46–48). But they can also be used to improve the effectiveness of other interventions by increasing awareness and demand, combating mistaken beliefs about diseases and risks, or reducing anxiety and stigma. In that sense, information, education, and communication delivered to consumers or providers or both are examples of policy instruments. They can facilitate or promote the use of such interventions as condom distribution, screening for diseases or congenital disorders, prenatal care, or immunization.

Other activities that can be classified either as interventions or as policy instruments include the following:

- *Measures to increase the quality of care,* such as some kinds of staff training or the introduction of better recordkeeping. These activities may simultaneously affect a large number of specific interventions in a health facility (chapter 70).
- *Legislation and regulation* to impose an intervention (for example, limiting the salt content of foods, chapter 45, or requiring that salt be iodized, chapter 28); to limit or prohibit an intervention that is ineffective or dangerous or to reduce unhealthful behavior such as smoking and excessive drinking (chapters 46–47); or to codify how an intervention should be delivered and determine who may provide it, as by licensing doctors, nurses, and health facilities (chapter 71).
- *Economic incentives,* which can take the form of subsidies or taxes (chapter 11) for particular items of consumption other than health goods or services, such as tobacco and alcohol (chapters 46–47) or condoms to reduce HIV transmission (chapter 18), or can be provided through protection of property rights, as for patented drugs (chapter 72).

These activities of informing, mandating, legislating, regulating, and taxing or subsidizing, which are at one remove or more from medical interventions, are also often called functions of the health system (WHO 2000, chapter 2; see also chapter 9 in this volume). Several of these instruments may be used together, such as increased taxes on tobacco or alcohol along with measures to educate consumers and to restrict the times, places, or quantities of consumption. Sometimes the instrument is needed before introducing or expanding an intervention to overcome barriers to its use or to make it cost-effective enough to be worth pursuing. Educating the affected population, for example, is crucial to screening and treatment of cancers and hemoglobin disorders. The need for a particular instrument may vary from country to country even if the

Average and Incremental Cost-Effectiveness and Intervention Choices

In the figure below, which compares three ways of delivering immunization, point *X* describes the status quo of a current intervention, delivering immunization by means of fixed facilities. At point *X*, the intervention achieves a total effect *E2* (measured as coverage or as disease reduction) at a total cost *C2*. The ratio *C2* to *E2* is the average cost-effectiveness ratio (ACER), shown by the slope of the line *O–X*. Beyond point *X*, expanding coverage becomes very costly, perhaps because the population not yet immunized is dispersed and hard to reach. (Chapter 20 includes estimates of how costs increase as immunization coverage expands but without introducing a sharp increase in costs.) Expansion to point *X1*, which increases the cost from *C2* to *C3*, yields only a small increment *E3–E2* in effect. The slope of the line *X–X1* represents the incremental cost-effectiveness ratio (ICER) of that expansion, which would raise the ACER to line *O–X1*. The line *X–X2* shows the alternative of reducing coverage, which would improve the average cost-effectiveness (to *C1/E1*) because marginal costs are rising steeply near point *X*. The ICER of the reduction in coverage is the ratio of *C2–C1* to *E2–E1*.

Raising immunization coverage at an affordable cost may require adopting the alternative of mobile vaccination teams, intervention *Y*. The hypothetical combination of fixed facilities and such teams allows increasing the effect to *E4* (complete or nearly complete immunization) at a total cost of *C4*. The ICER of the mobile teams is shown by the slope of the line *X–Y* and the resulting overall or combined ACER by the slope *O–Y*. Adopting intervention *Y* would be clearly preferable to trying to expand coverage through intervention *X* by building and staffing more fixed facilities.

An alternative even better than *Y* might subsequently be developed, represented by point *Z*—for example, community-based immunization teams that could operate either near or far from fixed facilities because they use heat-stable vaccines that do not require a cold chain. The ICER of turning to that choice, represented by the line *X–Z*, is not only more favorable than intervention *Y*, but it is even better than the current ACER, and preferable to intervention *X* at any coverage level beyond *X2*. The cost-effective choice, therefore, is not to retain intervention *X* at its current level and add *Z* beyond that point but to switch entirely from *X* (or from *X* plus *Y*, if *Y* has already been adopted) to *Z*. Because it costs less but provides a better outcome, *Z* is said to *dominate* both *X* and *Y*. The following figure illustrates dominance of one intervention by another, as well as cases in which neither of two interventions is dominant.

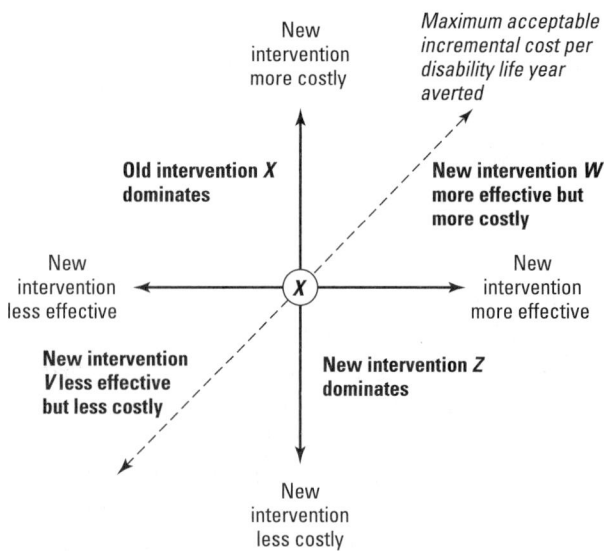

Average and Incremental Cost-Effectiveness and Intervention Choices: Comparison of Three Ways to Deliver Immunization

Comparison of Cost and of Effectiveness between Interventions: Conditions for Dominance

If intervention Z is divisible (meaning that it can be operated at any desired scale, such as $Z2$), then it is preferable to X at a cost of $C2$ because of the additional effect $E2^*$–$E2$. It can be extended all the way to $E4$, just as with intervention Y, provided only that the ICER represented by the slope X–Z is still acceptable to decision makers choosing how far to expand the intervention. That is, the cost must still appear to be justified by the increased coverage. Under either of these conditions, an obstacle to switching, or to doing so quickly, would exist only if substantial fixed costs accompanied the transition from one intervention to the other, such as recruiting or retraining staff, building health posts in communities, or setting up the system for distributing the new heat-stable vaccines.

Compared with intervention X, intervention Z is better in both dimensions (lower cost and greater effectiveness), so it is to be preferred, and is said to dominate X. However, intervention X would dominate any other treatment that is both more costly and less effective and, therefore, falls in the upper left quadrant. An intervention such as V or W may or may not be considered preferable to X (V is cheaper but also less effective, and W is more effective but also more costly). Whether either such intervention would be selected over X depends on the relation of the increased (or decreased) cost to the increased (or decreased) effectiveness. That ratio corresponds to an ICER. If a maximum acceptable, or threshold, value for the ICER is determined, as shown by the dashed diagonal line, then any intervention that falls below the dashed line would be acceptable (preferable to X), and those that fall above the dashed line would not be. Uncertainty about the estimates of cost and effectiveness means that, instead of a sharp line as in the figure, the division of preferable from nonpreferable interventions corresponds to a zone of some width that depends on the confidence intervals around the estimates. This kind of comparison can start from an existing intervention such as X in the first figure or, when there is currently no intervention, from point O in the first figure.

Source: Authors.

intervention that it facilitates is identical, because the legal, regulatory, or financial environment differs.

ESTIMATING EFFECTIVENESS IN HEALTH

Using cost-effectiveness for resource allocation requires health effects to be represented in common units in order to facilitate comparison across interventions, diseases, or conditions. All analyses start with some natural unit: cases of disease or injury, deaths, or numbers of people who quit smoking or adopt some other health-improving behavior. All interventions that avert death are alike in that regard. Preventing a child's death at a particular age, independent of the cause, means that the averted death alone is an adequate measure of outcome. However, when lives are saved at different ages—averting death from malaria at age 2 versus death from beta thalassemia at age 10–15—the outcome is no longer identical, and some measure must account for the difference in years of life saved. These cases provide another natural unit, subject to estimating how much longer a person spared death might live. The choice of life expectancy to assume for such calculations is discussed later.

The unit of time becomes a less natural and more synthetic measure if the future is discounted, as in all these analyses. *Discounting* means reducing the value of each variable in each future year by an amount that increases the further in the future that year is. The discounting procedure reflects inherent uncertainty about the future and preferences for timing of consumption, and it avoids two problems. First, outcomes that potentially generate benefits forever, such as smallpox eradication, appear to have infinite benefits if the future is not discounted and therefore seem to justify any finite cost at all. Second, it makes little sense to postpone interventions forever simply because funds to finance them could be invested today and be worth more tomorrow. Even discounting the future at the low rate of 3 percent annually has a substantial effect—that is, dividing the values for future years by successive powers of 1.03. That means dividing values for year 1 by 1.03; those for year 2 by 1.03 squared, or 1.0609; and so on. At that rate, averting an infant death saves not all the 80 calendar years of life expectancy at birth (or fewer in low-income countries) but at most 30 discounted years.

For interventions that avert mortality, analysis starts by estimating the deaths prevented, uses age at death to yield numbers of life years saved, and then discounts those years as described above. When interventions improve health by averting or reducing nonfatal disability, different disabilities must be compared in severity. As with mortality, age at the time of intervention matters for long-lasting conditions, and so does discounting. In contrast, age is irrelevant for episodes of illness or injury that are self-limited or quickly resolved by intervention, because the duration of ill health does not depend on age, and all ages are treated alike in this analysis. Discounting also makes little difference over short intervals.

Unit of Measurement of Health

The common unit of health loss or gain used here takes into account duration and severity, as well as discounting the future. The disability-adjusted life year (DALY) is a unit introduced by the World Health Organization (WHO) and the World Bank (Jamison and others 1993; Murray 1996; World Bank 1993). As previously discussed, the DALY incorporates assumptions and measurements about severity of nonfatal conditions, age at incidence or intervention, duration with and without intervention, and remaining life expectancy at that age. For interventions directed to risk factors rather than diseases, the analysis incorporates estimates of reductions in diseases that result from changes in the level of risks. Smoking cessation, for example, reduces deaths from both cardiovascular disease and cancer (chapter 46).

Published analyses, particularly in high-income countries, often use not DALYs but quality-adjusted life years (QALYs), an alternative measure of how much a year of life is worth if a person suffers one or more limitations of various kinds and degrees. QALYs can be estimated directly using a valuation method such as the *time tradeoff* (comparing and varying the time spent in one health state with time spent in another state until the quality of life is judged the same in both). Alternatively, a prescored questionnaire such as the EQ5D (a European quality of life measure) could be used. The EQ5D distinguishes three grades—no problem, an extreme problem, and total disability—on each of five dimensions of life quality—mobility, self-care, performance of usual activities, pain or discomfort, and anxiety or depression (Brooks, Rabin, and de Charro 2003). Discounting of QALYs occurs as an additional step, although some concern exists that discounting values derived from the time tradeoff approach is double discounting (Dolan and Jones-Lee 1997).

QALYs allow comparison among interventions and can easily account for comorbidity. Although the concept of DALYs averted by an intervention is similar to that of QALYs gained, no systematic formula exists for converting between DALYs and QALYs except in broad approximations (Fox-Rushby 2002). This gap is partly because DALY disability weights are specific to diseases whereas the QALY system of evaluation is not (it is based on overall health status). Authors sometimes report effectiveness results in QALYs, because they cite studies in high-income countries that often use QALYs. When some interventions are evaluated in DALYs and others in QALYs, ranking interventions according to cost-effectiveness may still be possible (see chapter 29 for examples of the use of both units).

Priority setters sometimes stop exercises in priority setting after concluding that something is or is not cost saving, without asking whether an intervention yielding a different outcome (against a different disease, for example) would be still more cost-effective. In this volume, the intent is to estimate both costs and effects, permitting all such comparisons. Knowing that one intervention achieves the same results as another at lower cost, which would be relevant if they were the only two possible interventions against a common problem, is not enough. Comparing both with another intervention with different effects may also be necessary. For example, a coronary artery bypass graft for myocardial infarction costs, on average across regions, US$37,000 per DALY gained, compared with an average of only US$409 for the polypill discussed earlier. However, both are much more expensive than saving life years for a middle-aged person by treating active tuberculosis (and thereby preventing transmission), an intervention that costs only US$15 per DALY in the absence of HIV infection, or US$102 on average where coinfection makes treatment more difficult. (In only a few cases do chapters deal explicitly with comorbidity, in part because the DALY approach considers conditions only individually.)

Parameter values for effectiveness are required in order to conduct CEA: how to value disability, compared with mortality; how to treat the future; and whether to distinguish people according to age, sex, or other characteristics. Because effectiveness is related to reduction in disease burden, nearly all these parameter choices coincide with those adopted to estimate the existing burden (see Mathers and others 2005 for a full explanation).

Because disease burden estimates discount the future at 3 percent annually, CEA in this volume does the same, for both effects and costs. This method follows the recommendations of the U.S. Public Health Service Panel on Cost-Effectiveness in Health and Medicine (Gold and others 1996) and appears appropriate whenever the benefits of an intervention begin immediately. Constant discounting (using the same percentage rate each year) undervalues interventions for which the benefits appear long after the costs have been paid. Immunization against hepatitis B can prevent liver cancer decades later (chapter 20) but, compared with the costs incurred at the moment of vaccination, appears less cost-effective if the health gain is heavily discounted during that interval. Slow discounting, with the rate falling close to zero for the more distant future, would yield a higher present value of benefits (Jamison and Jamison 2003), but given the absence of consensus on the correct form, the analyses here use constant discounting.

The limitations from a disease or condition in the absence of intervention are measured by disability weights (Mathers and others 2005), despite some controversy as to whether they adequately capture all the disability (see chapter 24 on helminthic infections). These weights range from zero for perfect health to 1.0 for death. Authors have made their own estimates whenever WHO did not provide any disability weight because the corresponding condition was not explicitly included in the burden of disease. For example, weights for anemia caused by hemoglobin disorders (chapter 34) were taken from other causes of anemia. Note that years lost to early death also are DALYs, since they include the disability weight of 1.0.

When an intervention prevents or completely cures a condition, the postintervention disability is zero. For partially successful interventions leaving residual disability, the disability weight is reduced but not eliminated. WHO has sometimes estimated weights for "treated" as opposed to "untreated" conditions (Murray and Lopez 1996, annex table 3) without specifying the intervention. This distinction is introduced for some consequences of chronic conditions: cancers not yet in the terminal stage, diabetic conditions, major psychological disorders, cataracts, various cardiovascular conditions, chronic respiratory conditions, ulcers, arthritis, cleft lip and palate, edentulism (total loss of teeth), and some burns. Chapters 31 and 33 use these values to describe intervention outcomes.

WHO burden-of-disease estimates used in the first edition of *Disease Control Priorities in Developing Countries* (Jamison and others 1993) incorporated age weights—that is, numbers attempting to describe the relative value of life at different ages. These numbers were calculated to keep the discounted integral from age 0 to 80 the same, as if no age distinction were made. The weights are zero at birth, ignoring health losses from stillbirth prior to live birth; reach a maximum at age 25; and decline almost to zero at advanced age. They are a particularly controversial element in the burden estimates (Musgrove 2000) because they value some years of life more than others, and little evidence suggests what an appropriate weight should be. In consequence, only constant age weighting (treating all years alike) is used in these analyses. Removing age weights makes no difference to an intervention that averts an infant death, but it changes the relative importance of interventions at later ages. Because life is more highly valued at advanced ages, death and disability after age 38 become more important compared with events before that age, and interventions later in life become more cost-effective. Some estimates used here therefore differ from those published previously by WHO even when all the other parameters are unchanged.

The only parameters for CEA that differ from those in the burden of disease concern life expectancy. In estimating burden, people at any age and in all regions are assumed, on the ethical criterion of valuing all lives equally, to have the same life expectancy. The only exception is that at birth males appear to have a biologically determined (not behavior-related) life expectancy of 80 years, which is shorter than the life expectancy of females by 2.5 years. However, applying these expectancies to CEA will overstate the effects of interventions when life expectancy in a population is low. Averting a death at age 5 in Sub-Saharan Africa or South Asia does not confer a high probability of living to age 80 or longer. Competing causes of death reduce the effectiveness of any single intervention, unless it affects so large a population that it actually increases life expectancy. An intervention that completely interrupted the transmission of HIV and AIDS or prevented all deaths from malaria would do that. Given the absence of evidence that any intervention actually has such a substantial effect, it is assumed in this volume that individuals face the same probability of death at each subsequent age as the existing population does.

This assumption makes interventions appear less effective when overall mortality is high than when mortality is low. For example, averting an infant death in Sub-Saharan Africa will save, on average, only 44 to 49 undiscounted life years and should not be credited with saving 80 or more. Cost-effectiveness calculations and estimates of burden of disease are inconsistent in that fully effective interventions appear able to deal with only part of the burden they aim to control. Regional rather than standard life expectancy also makes interventions in a high-mortality region appear more effective relative to outcomes where mortality is lower, when they avert deaths later in life.

Nonhealth benefits of health interventions sometimes should be taken into account, because many health interventions also yield other kinds of benefits. They often make beneficiaries mentally or physically more productive, better able to continue in and learn from school or to work and earn more. This benefit occurs particularly with interventions against non-fatal consequences, as indicated in the chapters on malnutrition (chapter 28), malaria (chapter 21), helminthic infections (chapter 24), tropical diseases (chapters 22–23), psychiatric disorders (chapter 31), and learning and developmental disorders (chapter 49). Interventions that prevent injury or restore work capacity also have such effects (chapters 39–40 and 60), as do interventions against diseases that kill in the prime of life, notably tuberculosis and AIDS (chapters 16 and 18). Nonhealth benefits also occur as time is saved when piped water is made available, as less cleaning is needed when air pollution is reduced (chapter 42), or as property damage is reduced by improved traffic safety (chapter 39).

Several chapters include discussions of the nature and, where possible, the magnitude of nonhealth benefits from health interventions. This factor is important when the health benefits, although substantial, are so costly that interventions do not appear cost-effective on health grounds alone but may be justified by large nonhealth returns. Safe water and sanitation services are the classic example (chapter 41). Because different types of benefits—health gains, increased income, time saved—cannot be compared directly, the only way of combining them into a single expression is usually to evaluate all outcomes in monetary terms. (An exception occurs when some monetary gains can be measured directly—for example, increased worker productivity from better health. Those gains can be subtracted from costs and incorporated into CEA without attributing a monetary value to the health gains.) Most chapters that account for any nonhealth benefits simply offer descriptions of them rather than incorporating them into monetary outcome indicators. Chapter 7 is an exception; it compares gains in welfare from living longer or in better health with those from higher income.

Estimating the monetary value of all benefits and adding them together for comparison with cost is what cost-benefit analysis does. Interventions are considered justified in absolute terms if the benefits exceed the costs. However, when faced with constrained budgets that cannot finance all interventions whose benefits are greater than costs, policy makers need to establish some minimum acceptable rate of return. This choice is parallel to the need to set a maximum on cost per unit of health gain when choosing according to cost-effectiveness.

Published analyses of health interventions sometimes use cost-benefit analysis, so results following that method are incorporated in some chapters here. The decision to emphasize CEA instead derives from two chief considerations. One is that, for most interventions, the health consequences seem more relevant or more important than any nonhealth outcomes. The other is that, conceptually, it is unclear what dollar value to assign to improved health, as would have to be done in most cases. Two approaches to valuing health, particularly for judging how much a life is worth, are known respectively as (a) the *value of a statistical life,* or the *human capital approach,* and (b) the *willingness-to-pay valuation,* or *contingent valuation.* The former depends on estimating earnings lost from premature death or retirement, and the latter on what people pay or indicate they would pay for care to protect or restore their health.

Both approaches reflect a society's level of income. Although they may be appropriate within a homogeneous society, if applied globally they imply that better health is worth less among poor populations than among those who are better off. Both methods are arguably more appropriate for marginal improvements (like saving travel time for commuters) than for valuing life-or-death differences, although willingness to pay is sometimes used in analyses of policies to reduce mortality. Avoiding monetary evaluation of health benefits sidesteps most of the ethical problems of valuing individual lives and requires fewer assumptions about what benefits are worth. The cost of this simplification is that occasionally substantial nonhealth benefits are not explicitly valued, so interventions may look less justified than they would be if all benefits were analyzed.

DETERMINING COSTS FOR INTERVENTIONS

Whatever outcome measures are used to evaluate an intervention, its costs must be estimated. This need raises several questions about which costs to attribute to the intervention and how some of them should be valued.

Direct and indirect costs should be distinguished, and choices should be made about which, if any, of the latter to include. In addition to the direct costs to the health system of producing an intervention, the U.S. Public Health Service guidelines (Gold and others 1996) recommend including the indirect costs to patients and their families of consuming it. This recommendation means, in particular, the value of time needed for travel, waiting, and undergoing medical tests and procedures, or the value of time used in caregiving, as well as any income forgone during treatment. Externalities, or costs imposed on third parties, such as on the school system or the environment, should also be included. The analyses in this volume generally exclude such costs and report only the direct costs of delivering interventions, partly because published analyses seldom include the various indirect costs, and they are harder to estimate. Walker and Fox-Rushby (2000) found that only 20 of 101 studies included some element of indirect costing. Valuing time according to local wages or income, for example, may underestimate how valuable time actually is to poor people. Estimating such costs, even if time is not valued in money, may show whether time or monetary costs or both account for a relatively low level of use and therefore impede expanding coverage. Applying one or more of the policy instruments discussed earlier, along with the intervention, may then be important in order for it to be cost-effective.

Including such costs also raises a question of interpretation. If an intervention appears low in cost-effectiveness because it requires much travel or waiting time, the fault may lie not with the intervention itself but with health facilities that are located too far from the beneficiary population, are understaffed, or are inefficiently managed. For this reason, cost-effectiveness is estimated assuming a functional health system that does not impose prohibitive time costs on users.

Not only the characteristics of the interventions themselves, but also the capacity to deliver interventions greatly affect cost-effectiveness across many activities. In a complete analysis, each intervention is characterized by how demanding it is of managerial or institutional capacity. This element is difficult to measure directly, but authors often provide at least an intuitive description of how easy or hard delivery of an intervention is or what factors facilitate or impede its implementation. Where capacity to deliver several interventions together is important, authors deal explicitly with the issue, as in the chapters on health facilities (chapters 64–66), resources (chapters 71–72), service management (chapter 73), and whole packages of interventions (chapters 56 and 63).

Dollar values of unit costs need to be calculated for international comparisons. The inputs used to produce an intervention—the time (and training) of human resources; drugs and supplies; and depreciation or rental value of equipment, vehicles, and buildings—are either produced in the country or imported. If the latter, they already have prices in U.S. dollars; if the former, prices in local currency must be converted to U.S. dollars for comparison with other interventions and other countries. The usual distinction between tradable and nontradable goods is that tradables move from producing to importing countries at relatively constant "world" prices. In fact, the same good may be imported at different prices to different countries or may be imported to one country but locally produced in another, so that it has both an international and a local price. This situation is increasingly true of drugs and supplies, which middle-income countries (Brazil, for example) and some low-income countries (India) now produce and sometimes export.

Prices in local currency can be converted to U.S. dollars by exchange rates or by purchasing-power parity rates (as estimated in World Bank 2003). The former may reflect under- or overvaluation of the local currency, making goods systematically cheaper or more expensive than at world prices, and they may change quickly and substantially in response to changes in a country's trade balance, indebtedness, or capital flows. Nonetheless, they represent what is actually paid for locally produced inputs at any given moment. Purchasing-power parity rates, in contrast, attempt to say what local currency is worth in purchasing power, correcting for systematic price differences. Such rates can be calculated for the country as a whole, for the health sector, or for specific inputs or combinations thereof (Wordsworth and Ludbrook 2004). This calculation means valuing local inputs at external prices, assuming they are equally productive or of equal quality in the particular country as in the countries from which purchasing-power parity rates are derived. A doctor in South Asia or Sub-Saharan Africa is treated as costing just as much as a physician in high-income countries. This approach approximates measuring the real resource cost of intervention by comparing *quantities* of inputs among countries, eliminating *price* differences as a source of cost variation. Estimates of real national income are derived this way, making poor countries usually look less poor in dollar terms than if income in local currency were valued at exchange rates.

Granted that purchasing-power parity rates are reasonable for comparing large aggregates such as income across countries, but they bear little relation to the allocation of resources and budgetary choices within a country. The cost calculations in this volume are, therefore, all based on exchange rates. Exchange rates more accurately reflect what a domestic buyer—or a foreign donor or investor—has to pay for imported versus domestic inputs and, therefore, are more relevant for choices between interventions with high or low imported content. (If exchange rates are artificially fixed, the country pays a cost for that distortion that affects all interventions to the extent that they require foreign exchange.) In general, the more an intervention is produced with local inputs, the more cost-effective it will appear when priced using exchange rates, compared with its cost at purchasing-power parity rates. For decision makers and purchasers in the country, efficiency means choosing interventions according to what they actually cost, not according to what they would cost if prices were more nearly uniform among countries. If, in local currency, physicians are paid little more than nurses are, it may make sense to employ more doctors per nurse—even if at international prices doctors would cost much more and should be replaced by nurses when possible. Of course, the staffing decision turns on the competencies of the two groups as well as on their costs; for certain health problems, more nurses might be the better choice even if they cost more.

Two other reasons besides that of efficiency in buying interventions support basing cost-effectiveness on exchange rate prices. First, authors who have used published costs (which usually involve exchange rates) rather than building up estimates from individual prices and quantities seldom break down costs into imported and domestic components. Local inputs cannot be repriced at purchasing-power parity rates or can only be repriced very approximately. Second, for readers accustomed to dealing with prices converted using exchange rates, real resource estimates may simply appear to penalize the use of local inputs by valuing them at unrealistic prices. The problem with exchange rate prices, in contrast, is that when rates change, so may the relative cost-effectiveness of interventions, as imported inputs become relatively more or less expensive. Cost-effectiveness is not static or intrinsic but depends on prices as well as on quantities and on the results of an intervention—and prices can change individually or generally, through exchange movements. Priorities sometimes need to shift because of such price changes, as well as because of technological changes that make interventions more effective, and so analyses should be kept up to date.

MORE AND LESS COMPREHENSIVE DATA AND ANALYSIS

Several authors (Drummond and others 1997; Gold and others 1996; Sloan 1995) provide similar guidance and recommendations for relatively comprehensive economic evaluation in general or for specific medical procedures. This volume aims at estimating cost-effectiveness for interventions against many different problems in all low- and middle-income regions, for which varying amounts and quality of information are available. It has therefore not always been possible to conduct as complete an analysis as would be desirable. Some degree of modeling is usually inescapable (Buxton and others 1997).

More complete analysis starts by characterizing, in each regional setting where an intervention is relevant (where the health problem causes some measurable burden and the intervention appears feasible), estimates of the quantities of inputs required (Q), the unit costs of those inputs (P), and the effectiveness or health gain (E). Authors were provided regional estimates of unit costs for the major inputs—salaries, facility costs, fuel and vehicle operation, drugs, representative equipment, diagnostic tests, and buildings (Mulligan and others 2003). The total cost of delivery is the sum of the input costs PQ, which is compared with effectiveness E and the CER calculated from the total costs and total effects of the proposed intervention or from the changes in those costs and outcomes compared with current practice.

The data on unit costs, quantities, and outcomes may all derive from published literature; what is original is how that information is combined to calculate cost-effectiveness rather than taking the ratios from existing studies. Estimates are built up using prices and physical inputs in the chapters on tuberculosis (chapter 16), vaccine-preventable diseases (chapter 20), malaria (chapter 21), cancers (chapter 29), psychiatric disorders (chapter 31), neurological disorders (chapter 32), cardiovascular disease (chapter 33), hemoglobin disorders (chapter 34), water and sanitation (chapter 41), indoor air pollution (chapter 42), tobacco (chapter 46), alcohol (chapter 47), community programs (chapter 56), family planning (chapter 57), surgery (chapter 67), emergency care (chapter 68), and complementary medicine (chapter 69). Several chapters analyze some interventions more fully and others less fully, depending on the available information.

As indicated in box 15.2, expanding or contracting the scale of an intervention may change the CER because of difficulty in reaching more of the population. The ratio may also vary because of the cost of identifying who would benefit most from the intervention—for example, whether to screen all newborns for sickle cell disease or only those of African origin (chapter 34). And expansion may change the cost-effectiveness because it would require considerable fixed investment. The costs of expanding capacity to deliver an intervention, including physical capital and training of human resources, should be amortized over a reasonable interval (10 years is the standard in this volume) and included in the total costs. Ideally, one would know the complete production function of the intervention, including the possibilities of substituting one input for another to minimize costs in response to differences in prices. However, analysis of this level of complexity is difficult to achieve, so most chapters assume fixed input proportions. Q, then, does not depend on P, and the CER varies (at most) only with coverage, prices, and outcomes. This result could be an underestimate of the true cost-effectiveness if much substitution is possible (see chapter 16 on tuberculosis).

Approximations are required when the average and incremental CERs have to be taken directly from the literature and when key parameter values are not easily available. Existing estimates of total cost or effectiveness may or may not incorporate the standard assumptions about discounting, disability weights, and life expectancy. Authors then need to judge how to adjust the available estimates for a more consistent analysis.

Local cost and outcome estimates that have not been constructed transparently from inputs and prices provide a less complete basis for secondary analysis. Where such estimates are used, information about how costs are constructed or how results vary with the scale of the intervention is usually not available, but the data may explicitly show regional differences in one or both elements, thereby permitting regionally differentiated recommendations (or may show differences so small that recommendations need not differ regionally). If costs and results refer to only one moment or are specified year by year, they can be discounted at 3 percent. Published analyses often use higher constant rates of 5, 6, or even 10 percent and may specify only total costs and outcomes rather than the respective streams through time. In that case, both costs and health gains occurring in the future are valued less, but conversion to a CER based on 3 percent discounting may be impossible and is at best only approximate. Some published analyses discount costs but not health outcomes, which makes interventions look more cost-effective when costs are spread over long intervals (for examples, see chapter 29). Imported estimates of cost and effect—that is, estimates from other regions, commonly from high-income countries—are often all that is available. Sometimes data on costs and outcomes derive from the same source; in other cases, they come from different sources and even different regions and are difficult to compare directly. More appropriate adjustments to total costs are possible with information on quantities of inputs. In the absence of data on quantities of resources used, differences in average cost can sometimes be calculated using estimates of input proportions. Such an approximation characterizes the analysis for diabetes (chapter 30), in which proportions were known in one region and assumed to be the same elsewhere and costs were estimated from regional cost ratios.

Variation of Results and Uncertainty of Estimates

Variation and uncertainty are two different aspects of cost-effectiveness estimates that also need to be accounted for in setting priorities. Because costs of inputs differ among regions, intervention costs vary even if effectiveness does not—and there are often reasons why the same intervention is more effective in one place than another. Such variation means that a single estimate of incremental or average cost-effectiveness of an intervention is not universally applicable. All estimates should ideally be local, and regional values capture only part of the real variation. For example, the average cost per DALY of chemotherapy for active or contagious tuberculosis, in the absence of HIV and AIDS, is US$15, but that figure varies from US$6 to US$31 across regions, and such wide variation is common in many chapters. Whenever the estimates of cost-effectiveness in different chapters use the same input prices, their results are comparable within a given region. Analyses that draw on published estimates for price or unit cost information are necessarily less comparable across interventions and introduce another element of variation, even in the same locale. Still more variation arises when costs or outcomes are extrapolated from one country or region to another.

Because the CER depends on many parameters and variables, of which only the discount rate and the disability weights are uniform, good analytic practice calls for sensitivity analysis to see how the ACERs and ICERs change with plausible variation in one or more parameters. Many chapters (such as chapter 26) provide such analyses, varying one value at a time, to sketch the likely range of estimates. This method is one way of dealing with uncertainty (which differs from real, known variation) about the true values of the data and seeing whether the ranking of interventions changes when those values change. Such analyses do not indicate the probability that the true CER falls in a particular interval, only under what input values it would do so. Estimating such probabilities requires knowing or assuming the statistical distributions of the parameters in question and using that information to derive confidence intervals around the point estimates. Guides to CEA recommend these approaches (Gold and others 1996), and the National Institute for Clinical Excellence requires probabilistic sensitivity analysis before approving medical treatments in the United Kingdom (NICE 2004).

Data for estimating probability distributions around mean parameter estimates are seldom available in low- and middle-income countries. Simply having available several different estimates of a parameter is inadequate for deriving a distribution, because the differences may be caused by variation in regional costs or expected life years rather than uncertainty. However, assumptions about the shape of distributions can be applied within modeling exercises to give an indication of the likely distribution of ICERs. Only a few chapters, therefore, include confidence intervals. The analyses for tuberculosis (chapter 16) and malaria (chapter 21) do, but ranges associated with most cost-effectiveness estimates (see chapter 2) reflect other causes of variation, not statistical accuracy.

Although calculations are often reported to several significant digits, such precision is not really feasible given the uncertainties in the original data: "economics is a one- or at most a two-digit science" (Morgenstern 1963). However, even crude findings can be valuable, either as guides to value for money if inaccuracies do not affect the relative order of magnitude of the results or for understanding and exploring the sources of variation and their effect on priorities as well as indicating future research needs (Claxton, Sculpher, and Drummond 2002). These issues arise, for example, when considering whether to expand the EPI or to add new antigens (chapter 20), how far to extend screening procedures (chapters 29 and 34), and when to change drugs in response to vector or parasite resistance (see chapters 21 and 23).

The quality and relevance of evidence can vary considerably, depending on whether information comes from randomized controlled trials or systematic overviews, nonrandomized studies with multivariate analyses and well-defined endpoints, or case studies or expert opinion. For these analyses, the quality of evidence also depends on geographic coverage, as distinguished in chapter 2:

- literature review of one cost-effectiveness study, in one country
- literature review of several studies in different countries in different regions
- literature review of several studies in different countries in the same region
- original analyses starting with price and quantity data in one country
- original analyses starting with price and quantity in one or more regions.

The first three categories differ in how representative published findings are; the latter two categories differ according to the data used in constructing total effects and total costs.

Besides the quality of the evidence at its source, how the results will apply to other settings matters, particularly when the data are limited to high-income countries. The more that outcomes depend on underlying biology, the more the findings will apply to low- and middle-income countries. Outcomes depending more on cultural or environmental factors are less readily transferred and require judgment and evidence as to their applicability elsewhere. Sometimes the only detailed studies refer to high-income countries, as for abuse of substances other than alcohol and tobacco (chapter 48). At the other extreme, in a few cases all or nearly all the information comes from low- and middle-income countries, and there is no need to extrapolate, as for nutritional interventions (chapter 28) and community health and nutrition programs (chapter 56).

COST-EFFECTIVENESS AND POPULATION IMPACT

An intervention CER, whether average or incremental, is based on assumptions about introduction, expansion, contraction, or modification of the activity compared with current (or sometimes "best") practice. Comparison of ratios indicates whether one intervention offers better or worse value for money than another at the individual level but says nothing about how either one affects the whole population. The analysis, therefore, includes, wherever possible, two ways of describing the latter effect. One is to consider a population of 1 million, with a typical regional age and sex structure, and to suppose that the intervention were delivered to all the potential beneficiaries. That number of people is just the prevalence or incidence of the condition times 1 million. The total cost would then be the unit cost times that number (or the cost of reaching that many people if the unit cost varies with coverage). The total health gain would be the individual effectiveness times that same number (or the overall outcome if that depends on externalities, such as the transmission of communicable disease, that are sensitive to coverage). Standardizing on a population of 1 million allows comparisons among regions and interventions in which the incidence or prevalence may vary greatly.

A second approach standardizes not on population but on expenditure: if an additional US$1 million were devoted to the resources needed for an intervention, how many people could benefit from it and how large would the health gain be? The coverage of the intervention would be US$1 million divided by the average cost, and the total gain in DALYs would be that number of people times the average effectiveness. This approach is applied in relatively few chapters because of the information requirements; its advantage is to facilitate judgments as to where increased spending would be most justified—where it would yield the largest improvement in health, reach the most people, or account for the largest share of burden from a condition. Table 1.3 in chapter 1 provides examples for some interventions to reduce child mortality, prevent or treat HIV and AIDS, reduce smoking prevalence, treat heart attack and stroke, detect and treat cervical cancer, and operate a basic surgical ward. The estimates of DALYs gained per US$1 million vary from less than 100 to more than 100,000—a thousandfold difference in value for money. Annex 26.A of chapter 26 provides both kinds of calculations, per million population, to compare the cost-effectiveness of interventions for improved maternal health in South Asia and Sub-Saharan Africa.

IMPROVEMENTS AND FURTHER APPLICATIONS

What would improve the kind of estimates and conclusions reported in this volume? Most crucially, more and better data are needed in low- and middle-income countries to reduce reliance on extrapolation from high-income countries and on expert judgments. The need for information starts, in some cases, with better estimates of incidence and prevalence, but even where the epidemiology is well known, data on coverage and outcomes of existing interventions are scarce. Evidence of what it would cost to change coverage of existing interventions or add new interventions, and with what results, is particularly scarce and depends heavily on assumptions. This situation is sometimes true even for activities that have been conducted widely for many years and have been extensively analyzed, notably the EPI (chapter 20). Analyses should when possible be conducted at the level of a country or even smaller units, to take full account of all the reasons cost-effectiveness varies from place to place

and to develop priorities on the basis of analyses appropriate to local circumstances. The methods used here are intended to help guide such efforts, and they can and should be refined through research to provide more robust help to policy.

Finally, a more concerted approach is needed for clarifying the options facing different decision makers and incorporating the results from systematic literature reviews into analytic models that compare the costs and effects of alternative interventions (Buxton and others 1997; Kuntz and Weinstein 2001). Modeling encourages explicit decision making and can deal comprehensively with the inputs and outcomes of decision options, which allows a range of uncertainties to be reflected. Thus, hypotheses about interventions can be formulated and tested statistically. Specifying models explicitly (as in chapter 16, for example) can also help identify gaps in current evidence and can capture details specific to particular populations and settings.

ACKNOWLEDGMENTS

The authors are grateful to Jo Mulligan for the estimation and explanation of input costs used in this volume; to Sonbol A. Shahid-Salles for help in drawing methodological examples from numerous chapters; to George Alleyne, Joel G. Breman, Mariam Claeson, Anthony R. Measham, and Elinor Schwartz for helpful comments; and to Dean T. Jamison and Anne Mills for overall guidance.

REFERENCES

Brooks, R., R. Rabin, and F. de Charro, eds. 2003. *The Measurement and Valuation of Health Status Using the EQ-5D: European Perspective.* (Evidence from the EuroQol BIOMED research program.) Dordrecht, Netherlands: Kluwer Academic Publishers.

Buxton, M. J., M. F. Drummond, B. A. Van Hout, R. L. Prince, T. A. Sheldon, T. Szucs, and M. Vray. 1997. "Modeling in Economic Evaluation: An Unavoidable Fact of Life." *Health Economics* 6 (3): 217–27.

Claxton, K., M. Sculpher, and M. F. Drummond. 2002. "A Rational Framework for Decision Making by the National Institute for Clinical Excellence (NICE)." *Lancet* 360 (9334): 711–15.

Dolan, P., and M. Jones-Lee. 1997. "The Time Trade-Off: A Note on the Effect of Lifetime Reallocation of Consumption and Discounting." *Journal of Health Economics* 16: 731–39.

Drummond, M. F., B. O'Brien, G. L. Stoddart, and G. W. Torrance. 1997. *Methods for the Economic Evaluation of Health Care Programmes.* Oxford, U.K.: Oxford Medical Publications.

Fox-Rushby, J. A. 2002. *Disability-Adjusted Life Years (DALYs) for Decision-Making?* London: Office of Health Economics.

Gabbay, J., and A. le May. 2004. "Evidence Based Guidelines or Collectively Constructed 'Mindlines?' Ethnographic Study of Knowledge Management in Primary Care." *British Medical Journal* 329 (7473): 1013.

Glick, H., D. Polsky, and K. Schulman. 2001. "Trial-Based Economic Evaluations: An Overview of Design and Analysis." In *Economic Evaluation in Health Care: Merging Theory with Practice*, ed. M. Drummond and A. McGuire, 113–40. Oxford, U.K.: Oxford University Press.

Gold, M. R., J. E. Siegel, L. B. Russell, and M. C. Weinstein, eds. 1996. *Cost-Effectiveness in Health and Medicine*. New York: Oxford University Press.

Hoffmann, C., B. A. Stoykova, J. Nixon, J. M. Glanville, K. Misso, and M. F. Drummond. 2002. "Do Health-Care Decision Makers Find Economic Evaluations Useful? The Findings of Focus Group Research in U.K. Health Authorities." *Value Health* 5 (2): 71–78.

iMTA (Institute for Medical Technology Assessment). 2005. *Newsletter* 3 (1): 1–3.

Jamison, D. T. 2002. "Cost-Effectiveness Analysis: Concepts and Applications." In *Oxford Textbook of Public Health*, 4th ed., ed. R. G. Detels, J. McEwen, R. Beaglehole, and H. Tanaka, 903–19. Oxford, U.K.: Oxford University Press. Also published as Disease Control Priorities Project Reprint 3.

Jamison, D. T., and J. S. Jamison. 2003. "Discounting." Disease Control Priorities Project Working Paper 4, World Bank, Washington, DC.

Jamison, D. T., W. H. Mosley, A. R. Measham, and J. L. Bobadilla, eds. 1993. *Disease Control Priorities in Developing Countries*. New York: Oxford University Press.

Karlsson, G., and M. Johannesson. 1996. "The Decision Rules of Cost-Effectiveness Analysis." *Pharmacoeconomics* 9 (2): 113–20.

Kuntz, K. M., and M. C. Weinstein. 2001. "Modelling in Economic Evaluation." In *Economic Evaluation in Health Care: Merging Theory with Practice*, ed. M. Drummond and A. McGuire, 141–71. Oxford, U.K.: Oxford University Press.

Mathers, C. D., A. Lopez, C. Stein, C. Ma Fat, C. Rao, M. Inoue, and others. 2005. "Deaths and Disease Burden by Cause: Global Burden of Disease Estimates for 2001 by World Bank Country Groups." Disease Control Priorities Project Working Paper 18, World Bank, Washington, DC.

McDaid, D., R. Cookson, and ASTEC Group. 2003. "Evaluating Health Care Interventions in the European Union." *Health Policy* 63 (2): 133–39.

Morgenstern, O. 1963. *On the Accuracy of Economic Observations*. Princeton, N.J.: Princeton University Press.

Mulligan, J., J. A. Fox-Rushby, T. Adam, B. Johns, and A. Mills. 2003. "Unit Costs of Health Care Inputs in Low and Middle Income Regions." Disease Control Priorities Project Working Paper 9, World Bank, Washington, DC.

Murray, C. J. L. 1996. "Rethinking DALYs." In *The Global Burden of Disease*, ed. C. J. L. Murray and A. D. Lopez, 1–98. Cambridge, MA: Harvard University Press.

Murray, C. J. L., and A. D. Lopez, eds. 1996. *The Global Burden of Disease*. Cambridge, MA: Harvard University Press.

Musgrove, P. 1999. "Public Spending on Health Care: How Are Different Criteria Related?" *Health Policy* 47: 207–23.

———. 2000. "A Critical Review of 'A Critical Review': The Methodology of the 1993 World Development Report, *Investing in Health*." *Health Policy and Planning* 15 (1): 110–15.

NICE (National Institute for Clinical Excellence). 2004. *Guide to the Methods of Technology Appraisal*. London: NICE. http://www.nice.org.uk.

Sheldon, T. A., N. Cullum, D. Dawson, A. Lankshear, K. Lowson, I. Watt, and others. 2004. "What's the Evidence That NICE Guidance Has Been Implemented? Results from a National Evaluation Using Time Series Analysis, Audit of Patients' Notes, and Interviews." *British Medical Journal* 329 (7473): 999.

Sloan, F. A. 1995. "Introduction." In *Valuing Health Care: Costs, Benefits, and Effectiveness of Pharmaceuticals and Other Technologies*, ed. F. A. Sloan. New York: Cambridge University Press.

Smith, P. C. 2005. "Statutory Packages of Health Care Alongside Voluntary Insurance: What Treatments Should Be Covered?" York, U.K.: Centre for Health Economics, University of York.

Taylor, R., and NICE (National Institute for Clinical Excellence). 2002. "HTA Rhyme and Reason?" *International Journal of Technology Assessment in Health Care* 18 (2): 166–70.

Walker, D., and J. A. Fox-Rushby. 2000. "Critical Review of Economic Evaluations of Communicable Disease Interventions in Developing Countries." *Health Economics* 9 (8): 681–98.

WHO (World Health Organization). 2000. *World Health Report 2000*. "Health Systems: Improving Performance." Geneva: WHO.

Wordsworth, S., and A. Ludbrook. 2004. "Comparing Costing Results in Across Country Economic Evaluations: The Use of Technology Specific Purchasing Power Parities." *Health Economics* 14 (1): 93–96.

World Bank. 1993. *World Development Report: Investing in Health*. New York: Oxford University Press.

———. 2003. *World Development Indicators*. Washington, DC: World Bank.

Part **Two**

Selecting Interventions

- Infectious Disease, Reproductive Health, and Undernutrition
- Noncommunicable Disease and Injury
- Risk Factors
- Consequences of Disease and Injury

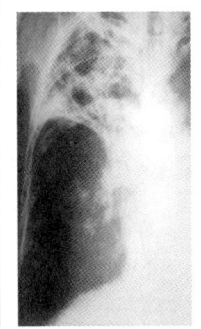

Chapter 16

Tuberculosis

Christopher Dye and Katherine Floyd

Despite the availability of drugs to cure tuberculosis (TB) since the 1940s, TB remains an important cause of death from an infectious agent, second only to the human immunodeficiency virus, or HIV (WHO 2004f). TB control is high on the international public health agenda, not only because of the enormous burden of disease, but also because short-course chemotherapy (SCC) is recognized as one of the most cost-effective of all health interventions (Jamison and others 1993). That recognition is partly attributable to an influential series of studies done in three of the poorest countries of southeastern Africa (Malawi, Mozambique, and Tanzania), which suggested that a year of healthy life could be gained for less than about US$5 (de Jonghe and others 1994; Murray and others 1991). This evidence has been central to the global promotion of the DOTS strategy, the package of measures combining best practices in the diagnosis and treatment of patients with active TB, in which direct observation of treatment during SCC is a key element (WHO 2002a, 2004c).

Although the World Health Organization (WHO) has fostered the implementation of DOTS over the past decade, four recent developments have drawn attention to a wider range of options for TB control:

- First, many more studies have investigated the costs, efficacy, and cost-effectiveness of different approaches to TB control. They are mostly studies of ways to improve the delivery of first-line drug treatment for active disease, but they include some investigations of preventive therapy (treatment of latent infection), treatment of multidrug-resistant TB (MDR-TB) using both first- and second-line drugs, and different approaches to diagnosis. They have been carried out in a variety of settings, in richer as well as poorer coun-

tries. The results have not been fully synthesized but may suggest ways to enhance DOTS.
- Second, striking increases in TB have been associated with the spread of HIV infection and drug resistance, suggesting that DOTS alone may not be enough to bring TB under control, especially in Africa and in the countries of the former Soviet Union.
- Third, there is now substantially more investment in new tools for TB control, including multimillion-dollar initiatives to develop better diagnostics, drugs, and vaccines, many of which operate under the umbrella of the Stop TB Partnership (see http://www.stoptb.org). Some of the possible products of this new research would stimulate reevaluations of the current reliance on chemotherapy, especially the development of a new high-efficacy vaccine.
- Fourth, interest in TB is renascent, not simply as the outcome of mycobacterial infection, but also as the consequence of exposure to exacerbating risks, such as tobacco smoke, air pollution, malnutrition, overcrowding, and poor access to health services. Research directed at quantifying these risks will also suggest ways to minimize them.

These developments set a big agenda for analysis. To make some inroads, this chapter presents an overview of the value for money and potential effect of the principal modes of TB control around the world. The starting point is a review of the natural history and clinical characteristics of TB and the geographical distribution of and trends in TB cases and deaths. This introduction sets the context for a discussion of the interventions that are now available to control TB and of how they have been used. We use a new method for evaluating the cost-effectiveness of infectious disease control and apply this method systematically to four groups of TB interventions as they could be implemented in six regions of the world.

The internationally agreed-on targets for TB control, embraced by the United Nations Millennium Development Goals (MDGs), are to detect 70 percent of sputum-smear-positive cases and successfully treat 85 percent of such cases by the end of 2005. The expectation is that, if these targets can be reached and maintained, incidence rates will be falling by 2015, and the TB prevalence and death rates of 1990 will be halved by 2015. Meeting these targets requires a set of interventions that are not only cost-effective but also affordable and capable of having an effect on a large scale. The final sections of the chapter discuss the absolute costs and benefits of global TB control and the potential for achieving the effect defined within the MDG framework. The main themes of the text that follows are elaborated in a series of annexes available online at http://www.fic.nih.gov/dcpp as well as at http://www.who.int/tb/publications/en/.

TUBERCULOSIS INFECTION, DISEASE, AND DEATH

Human TB is caused by infection with mycobacteria, principally *Mycobacterium tuberculosis*. Individuals with pulmonary or laryngeal TB produce airborne droplets while coughing, sneezing, or simply talking. Inhaled infectious droplets lodge in the alveoli, and bacilli are taken up there by macrophages, beginning a series of events that results in either the containment of infection or the progression to active disease (Frieden and others 2003). Following uptake by macrophages, *M. tuberculosis* replicates slowly but continuously and spreads through the lymphatic system to hilar lymph nodes. In most infected people, cell-mediated immunity, associated with a positive tuberculin test, develops two to eight weeks after infection. Activated T lymphocytes and macrophages form granulomas, which limit the further replication and spread of bacilli. Unless a later defect occurs in cell-mediated immunity, the infection remains contained within the granulomas.

The immune mechanisms are, in their details, far more complex. For example, following antigenic challenge, a suite of different T cells is responsible for the induction and suppression of protective immunity, delayed hypersensitivity, cytolysis, and the production of antibodies and memory cells. Helper T cells mature into two functionally different populations: in *M. tuberculosis* infection, the T_H1 response is associated with granuloma formation and protection, whereas the T_H2 response results in tissue-necrotizing hypersensitivity and the progression of disease. The processes that determine the balance of the two responses affect, for example, the interaction between *M. tuberculosis* and other infectious agents (Grange 2003).

When the immune response cannot suppress replication, primary infection leads to active TB (progressive primary TB).

The most common clinical manifestation is pulmonary disease, typically in the parenchyma of the middle and lower lung. In the most infectious patients, bacilli can be seen microscopically on stained sputum smears (60 to 70 percent of pulmonary cases; Marais and others 2004; Styblo 1991). Smear-negative patients may also be infectious but, per patient, contribute relatively little to transmission (Behr and others 1999; Hernandez-Garduno and others 2004). Extrapulmonary tuberculosis accounts for 10 to 30 percent of the disease but is more common among women and children (particularly lymphatic TB) and in people infected with HIV (Aaron and others 2004; Rieder 1999; Rieder, Snider, and Cauthen 1990; Shafer and Edlin 1996).

In the absence of other predisposing conditions, only about 5 percent of infected people develop progressive primary disease within five years of infection (Comstock, Livesay, and Woolpert 1974; Sutherland 1968, 1976). After five years, the annual risk of developing TB by the reactivation of latent infection is much lower($\approx 10^{-4}$ per capita per year). The risk of progressing to active disease is relatively high in infancy and lower in older children; it increases quickly during adolescence (earlier in girls) and then more slowly throughout adulthood (Comstock, Livesay, and Woolpert 1974; Nelson and Wells 2004; Sutherland, Svandova, and Radhakrishna 1982; Vynnycky and Fine 1997). Whether latent bacilli remain viable for the full life span of all infected people is unknown, but the risk of reactivation certainly persists into old age. The lifetime risk of developing TB following infection clearly depends on the prevailing transmission rate; the rule of thumb is 10 percent, but it has been calculated at 12 percent for all forms of pulmonary disease in England and Wales during the second half of the 20th century (Vynnycky and Fine 2000).

Besides the strong innate resistance to developing disease, infection is associated with an acquired immune response. This response is only partially protective (Dye and others 1998; Sutherland, Svandova, and Radhakrishna 1982; Vynnycky and Fine 1997), which helps explain why developing an effective vaccine has been difficult (few manufactured vaccines are more protective than natural immunity; Andersen 2001; Fordham von Reyn and Vuola 2002; Young and Stewart 2002). Consequently, individuals who carry a latent infection and who continue to be exposed are at risk of TB following reinfection. The importance of reinfection remains controversial, but mathematical modeling shows that the decline of TB in Europe cannot easily be explained without reinfection (Dye and others 1998; Vynnycky and Fine 1997). In addition, molecular fingerprinting has produced direct evidence that TB commonly arises from infection and reinfection in endemic areas (de Viedma and others 2002; Richardson and others 2002; van Rie and others 1999; Verver and others 2004), especially where subjects are infected with HIV (Glynn and others 2004).

The low incidence of infection and the low probability of breakdown to disease explain why TB is relatively rare. Its importance among infectious diseases is attributable not so much to the number of cases as to the high case-fatality rate among untreated or improperly treated patients. About two-thirds of untreated smear-positive patients will die within five to eight years, the majority within the first 18 months (Styblo 1991). Most of those who are still alive after eight years will have quiescent TB (self-cures, susceptible to relapse), and a few will become chronic excretors of bacilli. The case-fatality rate for untreated smear-negative cases is lower, but still of the order of 10 to 15 percent (Krebs 1930; Rieder 1999). Even among smear-positive patients receiving antituberculosis drugs, the case-fatality rate can exceed 10 percent if adherence to treatment is low or if rates of HIV infection and drug resistance are high (WHO 2004c).

Online annex 1 contains more information about factors that affect the risk to individuals of contracting infection and developing disease and the distribution of TB in populations.

EPIDEMIOLOGICAL BURDEN AND TRENDS

Surveys of the prevalence of infection and disease, assessments of the performance of surveillance systems, and death registrations yield an estimated 8.8 million new cases of TB in 2003, fewer than half of which were reported to public health authorities and WHO (online annex 2). Approximately 3.9 million cases were sputum-smear positive, the most infectious form of the disease (Corbett and others 2003; Dye and others 1999; WHO 2005). The African region has the highest estimated incidence rate (345 per 100,000 population annually), but the most populous countries of Asia harbor the largest number of cases: Bangladesh, China, India, Indonesia, and Pakistan together account for half the new cases arising each year. In terms of the total estimated number of new TB cases arising annually, about 80 percent of new cases occur in the top-ranking 22 countries.

In most countries (but not all), more cases of TB are reported among men than women. This differential is partly because women have less access to diagnostic facilities in some settings (Hudelson 1996), but the broader pattern also reflects real epidemiological differences between men and women, both in exposure to infection and in susceptibility to disease (Borgdorff and others 2000; Hamid Salim and others 2004; Radhakrishna, Frieden, and Subramani 2003). Where the transmission of *M. tuberculosis* has been stable or increasing for many years, the incidence rate is highest among young adults, and most cases are caused by recent infection or reinfection. As transmission falls, the caseload shifts to older age groups, and a higher proportion of cases comes from the reactivation of latent infection.

Globally, the TB incidence rate per capita appears to be growing slowly (online annex 2). Case numbers have been declining more or less steadily for at least two decades in Western and Central Europe, the Americas, and the Middle East. Striking increases have occurred in countries of Eastern Europe (mainly the former Soviet republics) since 1990 and in Sub-Saharan Africa since the mid 1980s, although trends in case notifications suggest that the rate of increase in both regions has slowed significantly since the mid 1990s (WHO 2005).

TB has increased in Eastern European countries because of economic decline and the general failure of TB control and other health services since 1991 (Shilova and Dye 2001). Periodic surveys indicate that more than 10 percent of new TB cases in Estonia, Latvia, and some parts of the Russian Federation are multidrug-resistant—that is, resistant to at least isoniazid and rifampicin, the two most effective anti-TB drugs (Espinal and others 2001; WHO 2004a). Drug resistance is likely to be a by-product of the events that led to TB resurgence in these countries, not the primary cause of it, for three reasons. First, resistance is generated initially by inadequate treatment caused, for example, by interruption of the treatment schedule or use of low-quality drugs. Second, resistance tends to build up over many years, and yet TB incidence increased suddenly in Eastern European countries after 1991. Third, although formal calculations have not been done, resistance rates are probably too low to attribute all of the increase in caseload to excess transmission from treatment failures.

Globally, 12 percent of new adult TB cases were infected with HIV in 2003, but there was marked variation among regions—from an estimated 33 percent in Sub-Saharan Africa to 2 percent in East Asia and the Pacific (online annex 2). HIV infection rates in TB patients have so far remained below 1 percent in Bangladesh, China, and Indonesia. The increase in TB incidence in Africa is strongly associated with the prevalence of HIV infection (Corbett and others 2002), and in populations with higher rates of HIV infection, women 15–24 years old constitute a higher proportion of TB patients (Corbett and others 2002). The rise in the number of TB cases in Africa is slowing, almost certainly because HIV infection rates are also beginning to stabilize or fall (Asamoah-Odei, Garcia Calleja, and Boerma 2004). HIV has probably had a smaller effect on TB prevalence than on incidence because HIV significantly reduces the life expectancy of TB patients (Corbett and others 2004). Where HIV infection rates are high in the general population, they are also high among TB patients; estimates for 2003 suggested that more than 50 percent of TB patients infected with HIV in Botswana, South Africa, Zambia, and Zimbabwe, among other countries.

Approximately 1.7 million people died of TB in 2003 (Corbett and others 2003), including 229,000 patients who were also infected with HIV (online annex 2). Although these are usually reported as AIDS deaths under the *International Statistical Classification of Diseases and Related Health Problems, 10th revision* (ICD-10), and by WHO, TB control programs need to know the total number of TB deaths, whatever the underlying cause.

INTERVENTIONS AGAINST TUBERCULOSIS

TB can be controlled by preventing infection, by stopping progression from infection to active disease, and by treating active disease. The principal intervention is the DOTS strategy and its variations, centered on the diagnosis and treatment of the most severe and most infectious (smear-positive) forms of TB but including treatment for smear-negative and extrapulmonary cases as well. Anti-TB drugs can also be used to treat latent *M. tuberculosis* infection and active TB in patients with HIV coinfection, and the widely used bacillus Calmette-Guérin (BCG) vaccine prevents (mainly) severe forms of TB in childhood. These biomedical interventions directed specifically against TB can be implemented in a variety of ways through medical services and public action and can be supported by other efforts to reduce environmental risk factors (online annex 1).

Vaccination

Currently, the only means of immunizing against TB is with the live attenuated vaccine BCG, although other vaccines are under development (Fruth and Young 2004; Goonetilleke and others 2003; Horwitz and others 2000; Letvin, Bloom, and Hoffman 2001; Reed and others 2003; Young and Stewart 2002). Randomized controlled trials and case-control studies have shown consistently high protective efficacy of BCG against serious forms of disease in children (73 percent [95 percent confidence limits 67–79 percent] for meningitis and 77 percent [95 percent confidence limits 58–87 percent] for miliary TB) but highly variable—and often very low—efficacy against pulmonary TB in adults (Bourdin Trunz, Fine, and Dye, forthcoming; Fine 2001; Rieder 2003). Thus, even with the high coverage now achieved, BCG is unlikely to have any substantial effect on transmission. In parts of Europe and North America that did and did not use BCG, TB declined at rates that were not measurably different (Styblo 1991). In areas of high incidence, BCG vaccination is recommended for children at birth or at first contact with health services. Vaccination is being discontinued in many low-incidence countries because the risk of infection is low and because the response to BCG confounds the interpretation of tuberculin skin tests used to track persons infected during occasional outbreaks. BCG may have substantial nonspecific effects on child mortality—that is, in reducing deaths from causes other than TB—but this possibility is still controversial (Kristensen, Aaby, and Jensen 2000).

Reported BCG vaccination coverage has increased throughout the world during the past 25 years, reaching about 100 million infants, or 86 percent of all infants, in 2002. An estimated 92 percent of children were vaccinated in Europe and 62 percent in Africa in 2002 (WHO 2001). During the past 15 years, coverage has generally been most variable among African countries and least variable in Europe and the Americas. The most complete analysis of the effect of BCG vaccination suggests that BCG given to children born in 2002 prevents about 29,700 cases of childhood meningitis and 11,500 cases of miliary TB during the first five years of life, or one case for every 3,400 and 9,300 vaccinations, respectively (Bourdin Trunz, Fine, and Dye, forthcoming).

Treatment of Latent Infection

Individuals at high risk of TB who have a positive tuberculin skin test but not active disease (for example, associates of active cases, especially children and immigrants to low-incidence countries) can be offered treatment for latent TB infection (TLTI), most commonly with the relatively safe and inexpensive drug isoniazid. Studies among those who have contacts with active cases have demonstrated that 12 months of daily isoniazid gives 30 to 100 percent protection against the development of active TB (Cohn and El-Sadr 2000; Comstock 2000). For patients who may be carrying a strain resistant to isoniazid, rifampicin daily for 4 months is an acceptable alternative (or rifabutin, if used with protease inhibitors for HIV-infected people; Cohn 2003; Menzies and others 2004). Nevertheless, TLTI is not widely used. The main reason is that compliance with long-term daily treatment tends to be poor among healthy people—a relatively high risk of TB among those who are latently infected is usually still a low risk in absolute terms. An additional reason is that the tuberculin skin test tends to be less specific when applied to individuals who have been vaccinated with BCG. Although it is sometimes possible to make separate estimates of the number of individuals in a population who have been infected and who have received BCG (Neuenschwander and others 2002), distinguishing the responses to BCG and infection is harder in any given individual.

The exceptionally high risk of TB among persons coinfected with *M. tuberculosis* and HIV is a reason for encouraging wider use of TLTI, especially in Africa. However, there are significant barriers to making TLTI effective for coinfected individuals living in areas of high transmission (in addition to those listed earlier). Although trials of TLTI with individuals infected with HIV whose tuberculin skin test was positive have averaged about 60 percent protection for up to three years (with a good deal of variability), the effects have been lost soon afterward, and little or no effect has been seen on mortality (Bucher and others 1999; Johnson and others 2001; Mwinga and others 1998; Quigley and others 2001; Whalen and others 1997; Wilkinson,

Squire, and Garner 1998). In addition, identifying *M. tuberculosis* infection is more difficult in HIV-positive individuals than in those who are HIV-negative because the former are often anergic and are, therefore, unresponsive to tuberculin. Early studies have also experienced problems with uptake and compliance. In a pilot project in Zambia, for example, only 35 percent of HIV-infected individuals identified through HIV testing and counseling services actually started TLTI, and, of those who started, only 23 percent completed at least six months of treatment (Terris-Prestholt and Kumaranayake 2003).

TLTI has been used as a component of intensive, local control campaigns, such as those carried out for North American and Greenland Eskimos, but probably had effects secondary to the prompt treatment of active disease (Comstock, Baum, and Snider 1979; Styblo 1991). At present, TLTI plays no more than an accessory role in TB control in any setting, although the number of recipients around the world has been neither directly quantified nor indirectly estimated.

Treatment of Active Disease: The DOTS Strategy

The cornerstone of TB control is the prompt treatment of active cases with SCC using first-line drugs, administered through the DOTS strategy (WHO 2002a) within targets framed by the MDGs. The DOTS strategy has five elements:

- political commitment
- diagnosis primarily by sputum-smear microscopy among patients attending health facilities
- SCC with effective case management (including direct observation of treatment)
- a regular drug supply
- systematic monitoring to evaluate the outcomes of every patient started on treatment.

Standard SCC can cure more than 90 percent of new, drug-susceptible TB cases, and high cure rates are a prerequisite for expanding case finding. Although the DOTS strategy aims primarily to provide free treatment for smear-positive patients, most DOTS programs also treat smear-negative patients, usually without a fee. DOTS can be used as the basis for more complex TB control strategies where rates of drug resistance or HIV infection are high.

Mathematical modeling and practical experience suggest that the incidence of TB will decline at 5 to 10 percent per year when 70 percent of infectious cases are detected through passive case finding and 85 percent of these cases are cured, even though that level represents a treatment success rate among all infectious cases of only 60 percent (Dye 2000; Dye and others 1998). In principle, TB incidence could be forced down more quickly, by as much as 30 percent per year, if new cases could be found soon enough to eliminate transmission. In general, the decline will be faster where a larger fraction of cases arises from recent infection (that is, in areas where transmission rates have recently been high) and slower where there is a large backlog of asymptomatic infection. As TB transmission and incidence go down, a higher proportion of cases comes from the reactivation of latent infection and the rate of decline in incidence slows. These facts explain why it should be easier to control epidemic than endemic disease: during an outbreak in an area that previously had little TB, the reservoir of latent infection will be small, and most new cases will come from recent infection.

In the control of endemic TB, largely by chemotherapy, the best results have been achieved in communities of Alaskan, Canadian, and Greenland Eskimos, where incidence was reduced at 13 to 18 percent per year from the early 1950s (Styblo 1991). Over a much wider area in Western Europe, TB declined at 7 to 10 percent per year after drugs became widely available during the 1950s, although incidence was already falling at 4 to 5 percent per year before chemotherapy (Styblo 1991). More recently, between 1994 and 2000, the incidence of pulmonary TB among Moroccan children 0 to 4 years of age fell at more than 10 percent per year, suggesting that the risk of infection was falling at least as quickly (S. Ottmani, personal communication 2005). The overall reduction in pulmonary TB was only 4 percent per year, in part because of the large reservoir of infection in adults. DOTS was launched in Peru in 1991, and high rates of case detection and cure appear to have pushed down the incidence rate of pulmonary TB by 6 percent per year (Suarez and others 2001). For epidemic TB, as a result of aggressive intervention following an outbreak in New York City, the number of MDR-TB cases fell at a rate of more than 40 percent per year (Frieden and others 1995).

Although the long-term aim of TB control is to eliminate all new cases, cutting prevalence and death rates is arguably more important. About 86 percent of the burden of TB, as measured in terms of disability-adjusted life years (DALYs) lost, is attributable to premature death rather than illness, and prevalence and mortality can be reduced faster than incidence in chemotherapy programs. Thus, the TB death rate among Alaskan Eskimos dropped at an average of 30 percent per year in the period 1950–70 and at an average of 12 percent per year throughout the Netherlands from 1950 to 1990. Indirect assessments of the effect of DOTS suggest that 70 percent of the TB deaths expected in the absence of DOTS were averted in Peru between 1991 and 2000, and more than half the TB deaths expected in the absence of DOTS are prevented each year in DOTS provinces of China (Dye and others 2000; Suarez and others 2001). There have been few direct measures of the reduction in TB prevalence over time, but surveys done in China in 1990 and 2000 showed a 32 percent (95 percent confidence limits 9–51 percent) reduction in the prevalence rate of all forms of TB in DOTS areas, as compared with the change in the prevalence rate in other parts of the country (China Tuberculosis Control Collaboration 2004; PRC Ministry of Health 2000). These findings imply that the targets of halving prevalence and death rates between 1990 and 2015 are technically feasible, at least in countries that are not burdened by high rates of HIV infection or drug resistance.

Many of the 182 national DOTS programs in existence by the end of 2003 have shown that they can achieve high cure rates: the average treatment success rate was 82 percent (that is, the percentage that were sputum-smear negative at the end of treatment plus the percentage that had completed treatment but for whom cure was not confirmed by sputum smear), not far below the 85 percent international target (WHO 2005). The outstanding deviations below that average were in Africa (73 percent) and some former Soviet republics (for example, 67 percent in Russia). Although the completion of treatment was almost a guarantee of cure before the spread of HIV and drug resistance, "completed" is an unsatisfactory way to report the outcome of treatment if cure is in doubt.

Although most TB patients probably receive some form of treatment, only 45 percent of all estimated new smear-positive cases were reported by DOTS programs to WHO in 2003. The case-detection rate in DOTS programs has been accelerating globally since 2000, but the annual increment must be still greater if the 70 percent target is to be reached by the end of 2005. Observations on the way DOTS is presently implemented suggest that a ceiling on case detection might be reached at about 50 to 60 percent (Dye and others 2003; WHO 2005). This fraction is about the same as the percentage of all cases reported annually to WHO from all sources (that is, from DOTS and non-DOTS programs). The problem is that, as DOTS programs have expanded geographically, they have not yet reached far beyond existing public health reporting systems.

ALTERNATIVE AND COMPLEMENTARY APPROACHES TO THE DIAGNOSIS AND TREATMENT OF ACTIVE DISEASE

The limitations of the DOTS strategy have stimulated numerous initiatives to improve program performance (including treatment protocols for patients carrying drug-resistant bacilli or who are infected with HIV), active case finding, collaborations within and between public and private sector health services, schemes for outpatient and community-based treatment, and integration of the management of TB and other illnesses.

Management of Drug-Resistant Disease

The higher the proportion of patients carrying drug-resistant bacilli is, the greater the need for accurate resistance testing and for the provision of alternative regimens that include at least

three drugs to which bacilli are fully susceptible. Of greatest importance is resistance to the two principal first-line drugs, isoniazid and rifampicin (that is, MDR-TB). The introduction of resistance testing, second-line drugs, longer treatment regimens (12 to 18 months), and rigorous bacteriological and clinical monitoring all increase program costs without necessarily ensuring high cure rates (equal to or greater than 85 percent). Indeed, achieving the same cure rates for MDR-TB patients as for patients carrying fully susceptible strains may not be possible. The cost-effectiveness of this component of a TB control program is therefore lower by an amount that depends on the nature of the resistance, the methods of testing and monitoring, and the choice of regimen. The higher costs and lower cure rates associated with treating drug-resistant TB are part of the argument for preventing the spread of resistance in the first place, as can be investigated with models of selection and transmission (Dye and Espinal 2001; Dye and others 2002; Dye and Williams 2000). Suarez and others (2002) have investigated the cost-effectiveness of managing drug-resistant TB in Peru, but because studies in other settings have yet to be published, an empirical overview is not yet possible. Further data will be available from studies in Estonia, the Philippines, and Russia in 2005.

Treatment of HIV Coinfection

Antiretroviral therapy for HIV-positive individuals is unlikely to prevent a large fraction of TB cases unless treatment can be given shortly after HIV infection is acquired (Sonnenberg and others 2005; Williams and Dye 2003). In general, antiretroviral therapy is likely to be most effective, not in reducing TB incidence, but in extending the life expectancy of HIV-positive patients successfully treated for TB (Friedland and others 2004). Antiretroviral therapy and DOTS are formally synergistic, because without undergoing both together, HIV-infected TB patients have a short life expectancy, typically less than five years.

Where the prevalence of HIV infection has been rising quickly, as in eastern and southern Africa, even the most energetic programs of TB chemotherapy may not be able to reverse the rise in TB incidence. However, mathematical modeling indicates that, even in the midst of a major HIV epidemic, early detection and cure are the most cost-effective ways of minimizing TB cases and deaths (Currie and others, 2005). One reason is that DOTS programs treat all TB cases, not just those linked with HIV. The alternatives—the prevention of HIV infection, TLTI, and antiretroviral therapy—are less promising strategies to control TB, at least for the coming decade, although they could be used in combination with DOTS.

Active Case Finding

The DOTS strategy is based on passive case detection for three reasons: (a) the majority of incipient TB cases develop active smear-positive, infectious disease more quickly than any reasonable interval between successive rounds of mass screening for TB symptoms or x-ray abnormalities; (b) the majority of patients severely ill with a life-threatening disease are likely to seek help quickly (Toman 1979); and (c) countries that have not yet implemented effective systems for passive case detection are not in a position to pursue cases more actively. The drawback of passive case finding is that the delays to diagnosis among symptomatic patients are often long, and health services never see some patients. To shorten delays and increase the proportion of cases detected, studies of risk can identify subpopulations in which TB tends to be relatively common. Systematic surveys of these subpopulations for active TB may be logistically feasible and affordable. The target populations include individuals infected with HIV, refugees (Marks and others 2001), contacts of active cases (Claessens and others 2002; Noertjojo and others 2002), health workers (Cuhadaroglu and others 2002), and drug users and prisoners (Nyangulu and others 1997). Despite the practical possibilities and the potential effect on transmission (Murray and Salomon 1998), active case finding is rarely done in high-burden countries, where the emphasis is still on implementing the basic DOTS strategy.

Case Finding and Treatment in the Private Sector

It is well known that many TB patients first seek treatment from private practitioners and that diagnosis and treatment in the private sector often do not meet internationally accepted standards (Uplekar, Pathania, and Raviglione 2001). A new scheme to deliver DOTS through the private sector (Public-Private Mix DOTS) operates through the provision of free drugs, by information exchange and patient referral, and with some financial support from participating governments. Two pilot projects in Hyderabad and Delhi, India, improved case-detection rates by 26 percent and 47 percent, respectively, and maintained treatment success close to the target of 85 percent (WHO 2004b). Other such projects are under way elsewhere in India as well as in Bangladesh, Indonesia, Nepal, the Philippines, and Vietnam (WHO 2004d).

Outpatient and Community-Based Treatment

Early studies of the cost-effectiveness of TB control found that full ambulatory treatment, eliminating hospitalization during the first two months (intensive phase), was cheaper and did not compromise cure rates (de Jonghe and others 1994; Murray and others 1991). Partly as a result, ambulatory treatment has become the standard of care in many high-burden countries. The natural extension, to home- and community-based treatment, has proved to be just as effective in several African settings, and even lower in cost (Adatu and others 2003; Dudley

and others 2003; Floyd and others 2003; Floyd, Wilkinson, and Gilks 1997; Moalosi and others 2003; Okello and others 2003; Sinanovic and others 2003; Vassall and others 2002; Wilkinson, Floyd, and Gilks 1997). Various schemes have been used to provide TB care in the community, in which nongovernmental organizations, volunteers (Okello and others 2003), or appointed "guardians" (Floyd and others 2003) supervise treatment, sometimes with financial incentives (Sinanovic and others 2003). Consequently, community-based care is being adopted in some countries (for example, Uganda) as standard procedure.

Integrated Management of Tuberculosis and Other Respiratory Illnesses

Surveys in nine countries found that up to one-third of patients over five years of age attending primary health centers had respiratory symptoms, of whom 5 to 10 percent were TB suspects, but only 1 to 2 percent had TB (WHO 2004e). Because TB is rare among respiratory diseases, comanaging TB with other conditions has clear advantages. The purpose of the WHO's Practical Approach to Lung Health (PAL) project is to encourage a syndromic approach to management of patients, to standardize health service delivery through the development and implementation of clinical guidelines, and to promote the necessary coordination within national health services. Preliminary investigations in the Kyrgyz Republic and Morocco suggest that PAL projects can improve the accuracy of diagnosis, encourage better practice in prescribing drugs, and strengthen primary care. However, a full analysis of costs and effects in the nine-country study remains to be done.

COST-EFFECTIVENESS OF INTERVENTIONS AGAINST TUBERCULOSIS

Some questions about investing in TB control are broad and strategic (for example, should money be spent on the control of TB rather than on the control of some other condition?); others are specific and technical (for example, which laboratory diagnostic procedures should be used?). On whatever level the question is posed, cost-effectiveness analysis (CEA) has become a prominent method for evaluating and choosing among different health interventions.

Background

Between 1980 and 2004, 32 studies of the cost-effectiveness of TB control were published from the low- and middle-income countries considered by the Disease Control Priorities Project (table 16.1; online annex 3 summarizes the 32 studies that have been published according to the country and year of publication, the question being addressed, the strategies compared, the

Table 16.1 Number of Studies on the Cost-Effectiveness of TB Control by Topic and Region, 1980–2004

Intervention	East Asia and the Pacific	Europe and Central Asia	Latin America and the Caribbean	Middle East and North Africa	South Asia	Sub-Saharan Africa	World	Total	Number that consider transmission
BCG vaccination	1	0	0	0	0	0	0	1	0
TLTI	0	0	0	0	0	3	0	3	3
Treatment of active disease: the DOTS strategy	4	2	0	1	0	2	0	9	4
Variations on DOTS: Management of drug-resistant disease	0	0	1	0	0	1	0	2	1
Treatment of HIV coinfection	0	0	0	0	0	1	0	1	0
Active case finding and diagnosis	0	1	1	0	0	4	1	7	1
Outpatient and community-based treatment	0	0	0	0	2	7	0	9	0
All interventions	5	3	2	1	2	18	1	32	9

Source: Authors.

subjects and costs considered, the effectiveness of measures used, whether or not transmission is considered, and the main results and conclusions). Almost all of these studies (28, or 88 percent) have concerned ways of finding, diagnosing, and treating patients with active TB, and most (18, or 56 percent) have been done in eight countries in Sub-Saharan Africa (Floyd 2003). Three studies (all in Sub-Saharan Africa) have investigated TLTI, and one study in Indonesia has examined BCG vaccination. The principal findings are that short-course chemotherapy for active TB is a comparatively cost-effective intervention and one of the most cost-effective of all health interventions. TB patients can be treated more cheaply and conveniently outside hospitals on an ambulatory basis, by health staff or with the help of family and community members, without compromising the success of treatment. Supplementary methods, such as standardized second-line drug treatment for MDR-TB, appear to be affordable and cost-effective in some settings.

What does not emerge from this compilation of data is a comprehensive overview of the value for money provided by current and potential interventions against TB in all major regions of the world, expressed using a common measure of effectiveness and based on a consistent approach to the evaluation of transmission. (The returns on investment in infectious disease control include the immediate benefits to individuals treated—for example, those vaccinated or given drug therapy—plus the longer-term benefits gained by preventing secondary

cases through reduced transmission.) Little work has been done in China, India, and other large countries in Asia, even though Asia carries the largest burden of TB, and only limited information is available for Europe and Central Asia, Latin America and the Caribbean, and the Middle East and North Africa. Of the 32 studies, only 10 used a measure of effectiveness that allows comparison with other diseases (table 16.2), and only 9 attempted to include an estimate of the benefits gained from reduced transmission (table 16.1). The benefits from reduced transmission are usually assessed through mathematical modeling (using computer simulations) for a given epidemiological situation, an approach that produces specific solutions for each setting rather than results that are generally applicable. In addition, although the benefits from prevented transmission are lower when TB is endemic, existing studies do not make a clear distinction between the cost-effectiveness of interventions in epidemic (outbreak) and endemic situations.

Methods

In this study, a general analytical framework was used to evaluate the total costs and total effects (defined as cases prevented, deaths averted, and DALYs gained) of the principal interventions against TB across six regions of the world (see online annexes 4–7 for further details). A dynamic infectious disease model (online annex 4) was used to derive general formulas for calculating the cost-effectiveness of interventions

Table 16.2 Number of Studies on the Cost-Effectiveness of TB Control by Effectiveness Measure and Intervention, 1980–2004

Intervention	Cases detected or cases diagnosed	Cases prevented	Cure or successful treatment rate	Deaths prevented	Years of life saved	QALYs gained	DALYs gained
BCG vaccination	0	1	0	1	0	0	0
TLTI	0	3	0	0	0	1	0
Treatment of active disease: the DOTS strategy	0	1	6	1	3	0	1
Variations on DOTS: Management of drug-resistant disease	0	0	2	2	0	0	1
Treatment of HIV coinfection	0	0	0	1	0	0	0
Active case finding and diagnosis	5	0	0	0	1	0	2
Outpatient and community-based treatment	0	0	10	0	0	1	0
All interventions	5	5	18	5	4	2	4

Source: Authors.
QALY = quality-adjusted life year.
Note: The total for all interventions is greater than the number of studies because some studies use more than one measure of effectiveness.

to control endemic (online annex 5) and epidemic (online annex 6) TB in a wide variety of settings. The formulas are approximate, but they are simple and able to provide insights into the strategies that give value for money under a wide variety of epidemiological circumstances. The model was then supplied with cost and efficacy data (online annex 7) for each of the six World Bank regions for four main groups of interventions:

- immunization with BCG (proportion of infants, *m*, assumed to be protected against severe, noninfectious childhood TB only), or a new vaccine that prevents infection and progression to pulmonary and extrapulmonary TB in children and adults
- isoniazid treatment of latent TB infection (TLTI, given at per capita rate ρ), for people infected with *M. tuberculosis*, with or without HIV coinfection and with or without the use of radiography to exclude patients with active disease
- short-course chemotherapy, delivered as a component of the DOTS strategy, for smear-positive or smear-negative pulmonary disease and extrapulmonary disease (with a combination of drugs given at per capita rate τ), and for patients infected with HIV, with or without supporting antiretroviral therapy
- treatment for MDR-TB using a standardized regimen including first- and second-line drugs or using individualized regimens of first- and second-line drugs that are tailored to each patient's drug susceptibility pattern.

Costs were considered from a health system or provider perspective. They were calculated by combining estimates of the quantities of resources required for each intervention (per patient or per person treated) with the unit prices of those resources (in 2001 U.S. dollars) using the cost categories and unit prices defined in the Disease Control Priorities costing guidelines.

COST-EFFECTIVENESS OF MANAGING ENDEMIC TUBERCULOSIS

The primary problem in global TB control is the management of disease in countries where incidence has been roughly stable for many years (that is, where TB is endemic).

Cost per Case Prevented

In monetary terms, the cost-effectiveness (*C/E*) of a new program of treatment for active infectious disease (here defined as sputum-smear positive), per case prevented, can be calculated from $C/E \approx P/\epsilon kT$, where *P* is the cost of treatment, ϵ is the efficacy of treatment, *k* is a constant determined by the mode of action of the intervention, and *T* is the duration of the intervention in years (online annex 5). The cost per case prevented is mostly in the range of US\$1,000 to US\$10,000, depending on the region of the world (figure 16.1). The exception is Europe and Central Asia, where costs are high because patients are currently treated for long periods in hospitals rather than on an

Cost per case prevented (US$)

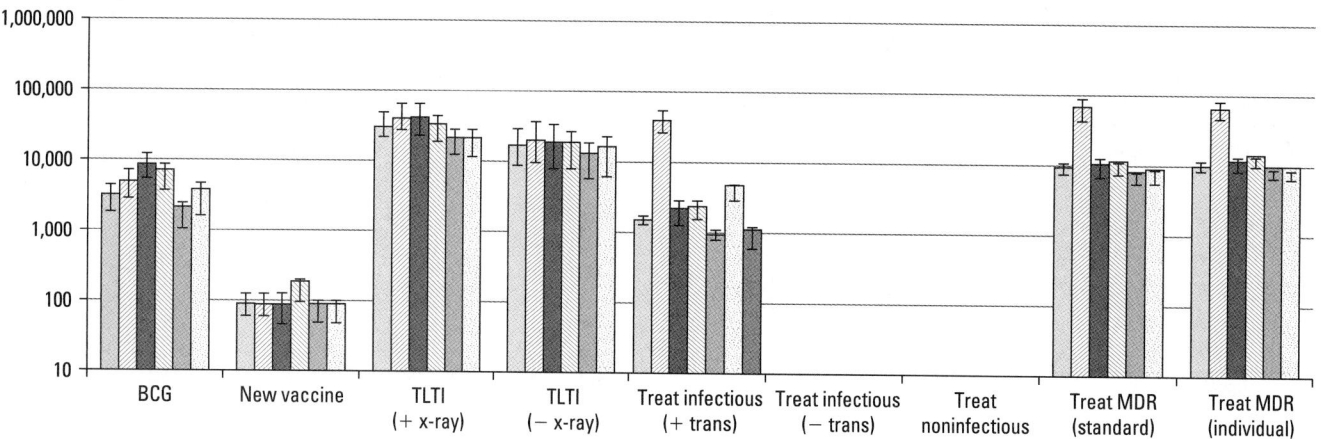

Cost per death prevented (US$)

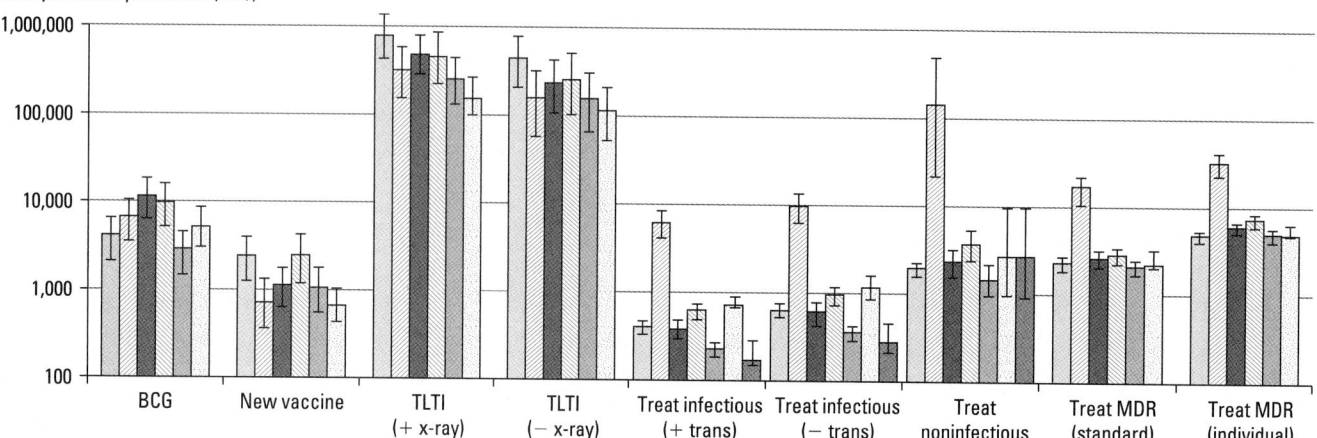

Cost per DALY gained (US$)

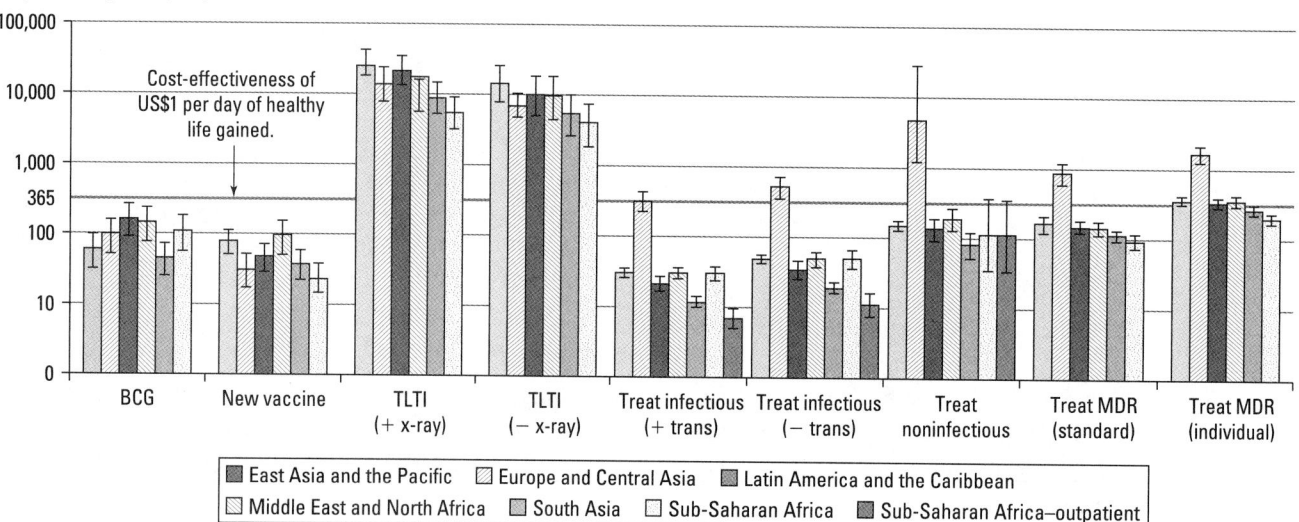

East Asia and the Pacific   Europe and Central Asia   Latin America and the Caribbean
Middle East and North Africa   South Asia   Sub-Saharan Africa   Sub-Saharan Africa–outpatient

Source: Authors.

Note: Where shown, bar 7 is for ambulatory (outpatient) treatment in Sub-Saharan Africa. The treatment of active disease saves no additional cases of TB when the effects of reducing transmission are excluded, so the cost per case prevented cannot be calculated. Cost-effectiveness of vaccination and TLTI is calculated for an initial incidence rate of 100 per 100,000 population per year. Cost-effectiveness ratios are plotted on a logarithmic scale. Error bars are 90 percent confidence limits. The horizontal gray line in the third chart marks a cost-effectiveness of US$1 per day of healthy life gained.

Figure 16.1 Cost-Effectiveness of Different Interventions against Endemic TB

ambulatory basis. These cost-effectiveness ratios (CERs) are computed from the total costs and total effects of treatment. Costs are therefore the same as the incremental costs for new programs. If costs and effects are compared with those of a previous treatment program, CERs for the treatment of active disease are often negative; that is, the program sooner or later saves money, as well as preventing TB cases. The positive CERs reported here for new treatment programs are, in this sense, upper estimates.

The cost of TLTI per active case prevented also depends on the initial incidence rate (I) and is calculated from $C/E \approx P/\epsilon kIT$ (online annex 5). The cost is substantially higher than that for the treatment of active TB: US$20,000 to US$40,000 when radiography is used to exclude patients with active disease, but it is less (US$13,000 to US$20,000) if active TB can be ruled out on the basis of symptoms and clinical examination (figure 16.1). TLTI is less cost effective than the treatment of active TB because preventive treatment would be given to latently infected individuals, most of whom were not recently infected and who are at small risk of developing active disease. In an endemic setting, there is no feasible method of identifying individuals who have recently acquired infection and who will proceed rapidly to active TB.

A new vaccine that prevents infection and, hence, the progression to pulmonary TB among people who were previously uninfected would be extremely competitive (US$90 to US$200) per case prevented if the costs were the same as those for BCG. BCG is cheap to manufacture and administer (US$1 to US$3 per dose) but less cost-effective (US$2,000 to US$8,500 per case prevented) than the treatment of active disease because it is assumed to protect against severe forms of childhood TB only and because it does not affect transmission (figure 16.1).

Cost per Death Prevented and DALY Gained

The wider benefits of treating active TB are revealed when allowing for the additional reduction in case fatality. For a 10-year program of treatment for infectious TB, the cost per death prevented is typically US$150 to US$750, and the cost per DALY gained is US$5 to US$50 for all regions except Europe and Central Asia (figure 16.1). When TB is close to the endemic equilibrium, the extra benefits gained from reducing transmission under DOTS are small: the cost per DALY gained is only 60 percent higher when transmission benefits are excluded. The treatment of noninfectious TB is less cost-effective (US$60 to US$200 per DALY gained), not primarily because transmission is unaffected, but because the case fatality of untreated smear-negative and extrapulmonary disease is relatively low. Treating infectious MDR-TB is between two and ten times more costly than treating drug-susceptible TB per death prevented (greater than US$2,000), or per DALY gained

(greater than US$90), assuming resistant bacilli are as transmissible and pathogenic as susceptible bacilli.

BCG vaccination is not much less cost-effective than the treatment of active disease (US$40 to US$170 per DALY gained; higher where the risk of infection is lower). If a new vaccine with 75 percent efficacy against pulmonary disease and other forms of TB costs the same as BCG, it would be almost as cost-effective (US$20 to US$100 per DALY gained) as the ambulatory treatment of active TB. As expected from the preceding analysis, TLTI is much more expensive than all other options (US$5,500 to US$26,000 per DALY gained) and most costly where the death rate from TB among adults is already relatively low—for example, because an effective DOTS program already exists. Although the cost-effectiveness of each intervention varies among regions, the variation among strategies is much greater, whatever the outcome measure (figure 16.1).

COST-EFFECTIVENESS OF MANAGING TUBERCULOSIS OUTBREAKS

The basic case reproduction number, R_0, is a ready-made epidemiological tool for relating effort and reward in the management of outbreaks. R_0 is the average number of secondary cases generated by a primary case introduced into a previously uninfected population (Anderson and May 1991). No country is presently free of TB, but some countries have recently suffered "epidemic" increases in incidence from previously low levels. The algebraic expression of R_0 for TB reveals how the various components of a disease's natural history and the different kinds of intervention interact with each other to influence transmission and the generation of new cases (online annex 4). For example, the cost-effectiveness of chemotherapy per $M.$ $tuberculosis$ generation is $C/E = P\sigma\tau/\epsilon R_0$, where τ is the number of TB patients treated per prevalent case per unit time, and σ is the proportion of new cases that is infectious.

The biggest resurgences of TB in recent history have been driven by the spread of HIV in Africa and are linked to the rise of drug resistance in former Soviet republics; this analysis is confined to interventions associated with these two phenomena (figure 16.2; online annex 6). Indeed, in this study, interventions related to TB with HIV are considered only in the epidemic context.

If multidrug-resistant strains of $M.$ $tuberculosis$ are assumed to have the same intrinsic transmissibility and pathogenicity as drug-susceptible strains, and given the spread of MDR-TB as an independent epidemic (Dye and Williams 2000), then treatment of MDR-TB with a standard regimen including second-line drugs is more costly per DALY gained than treatment of fully susceptible disease in Sub-Saharan Africa, but it is marginally less costly than TLTI (with an x-ray screen) over most rates of case detection and treatment (online annex 6).

Cost per case prevented (US$)

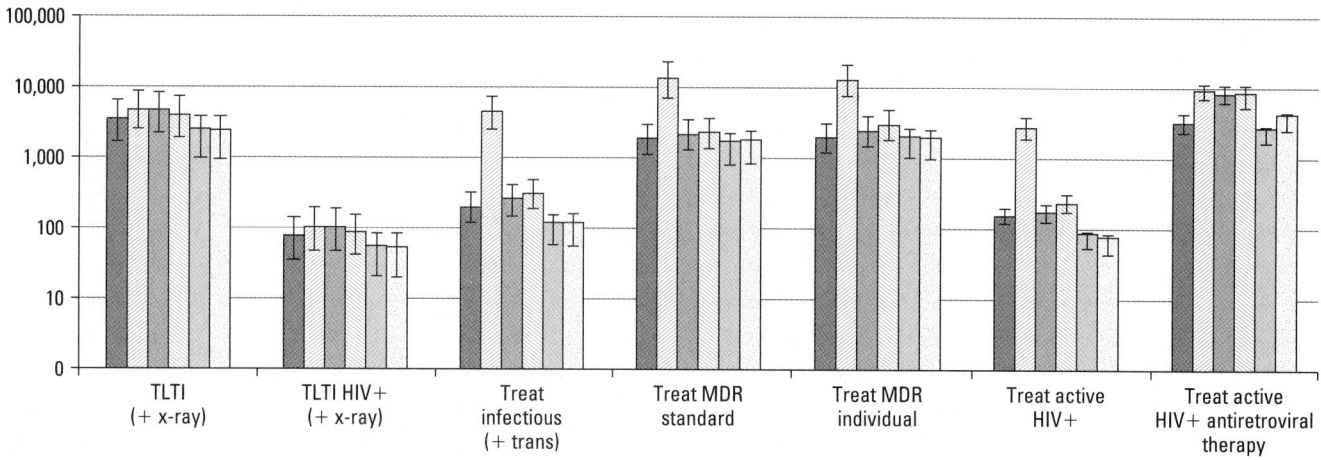

Cost per death prevented (US$)

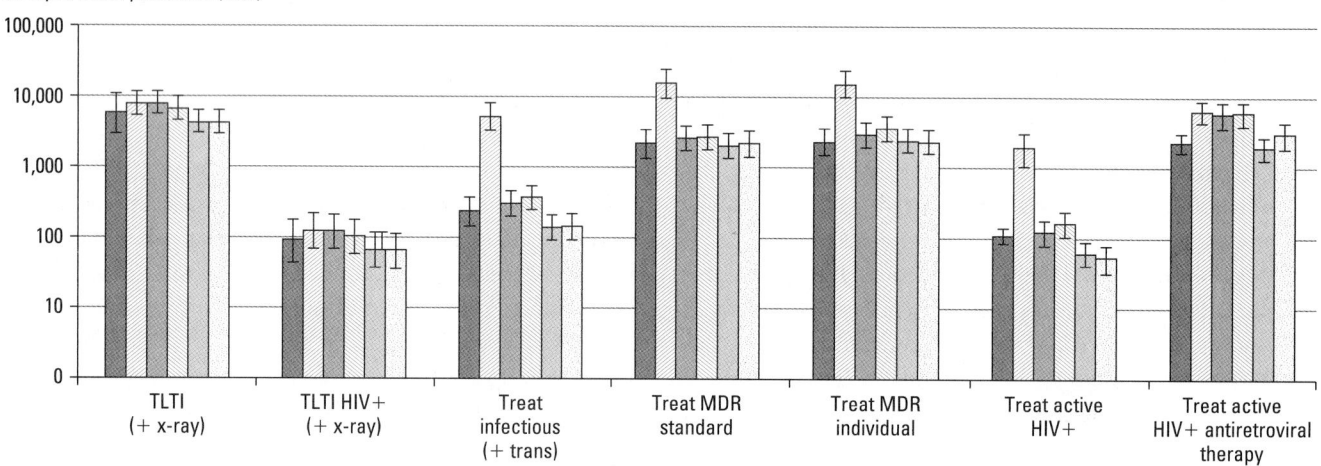

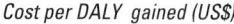
Cost per DALY gained (US$)

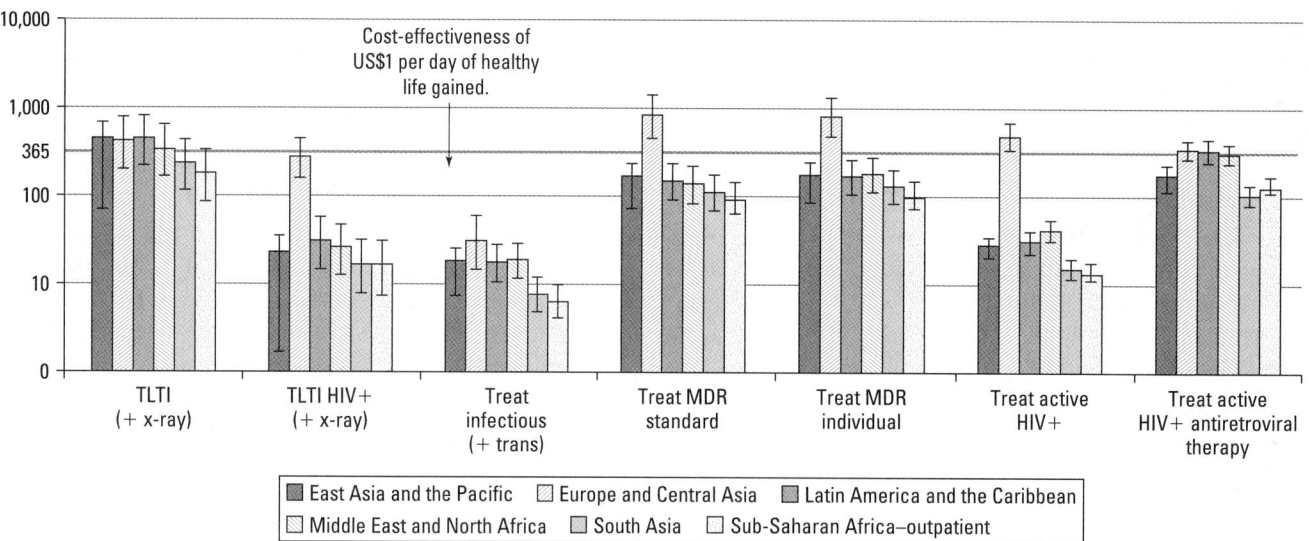

Legend:
■ East Asia and the Pacific ▨ Europe and Central Asia ▨ Latin America and the Caribbean
▨ Middle East and North Africa ▨ South Asia □ Sub-Saharan Africa–outpatient

Source: Authors.

Note: Five interventions used in the management of TB epidemics that are linked with HIV and MDR-TB (TLTI for people coinfected with TB and HIV, treatment of infectious MDR-TB with a standard or individual regimen, treatment of HIV-infected TB patients with TB drugs, treatment of HIV-infected TB patients with TB and antiretroviral drugs) are compared with two standard methods (TLTI, with active disease excluded by x-ray screen, and treatment of active infectious disease, allowing for transmission). Cost-effectiveness ratios (plotted on a logarithmic scale) vary with the treatment rate (online annex 6); for illustration here, 20 percent of eligible people are treated annually with each intervention. The horizontal gray line in the third figure marks a cost-effectiveness of US$1 per day of healthy life gained. Error bars are 90 percent confidence limits.

Figure 16.2 Cost-Effectiveness of Managing Epidemic TB

For example, at the fixed rate of treatment used to generate figure 16.2, treatment of MDR-TB with a standard regimen costs US$91 to US$846 per DALY gained, depending on the region, as compared with US$6 to US$31 for the treatment of drug-susceptible TB. The treatment of MDR-TB with regimens tailored to the resistance patterns of individual patients is more costly but also more efficacious than standardized treatment for MDR-TB and, therefore, almost equally cost-effective under this set of assumptions.

TB patients infected with HIV are more costly to treat per DALY gained than HIV-negative patients, either without antiretroviral therapy (low cost, short life expectancy) or with such therapy (high cost, long life expectancy). TLTI is a more attractive option for the management of epidemic TB than for endemic TB (compare figures 16.1 and 16.2), because during an outbreak, TLTI is directed at recent rather than remote infection. TLTI is even more cost-effective in the control of TB and HIV coinfection, because it prevents the rapid breakdown to active disease caused by immunodeficiency.

These results are indicative rather than definitive, because the calculations assume, among other things, that HIV-infected populations exist in isolation; in reality, HIV-infected people also acquire TB infection from TB patients who are not infected with HIV. Neither does this analysis address all the important questions about managing outbreaks of drug-resistant or HIV-related TB. Fuller investigations should assess, for example, the benefits to whole populations of giving antiretroviral therapy to HIV-infected individuals before they develop TB and of investing in DOTS to prevent multidrug-resistant epidemics from arising in the first place.

SUMMARY OF COST-EFFECTIVENESS ANALYSES

Box 16.1 summarizes the results of these calculations of the cost-effectiveness of managing epidemic and endemic TB. The findings are one justification for maintaining and expanding DOTS programs, on the basis of SCC for patients with active disease, as the dominant mode of TB control around the world. BCG vaccination and the treatment of MDR-TB (standard or individualized regimens) or HIV-infected TB patients (with or without supporting antiretroviral therapy) are more costly in absolute terms, but they typically cost less than US$1 per day of healthy life gained, which is less than the average economic productivity of workers in the least developed countries. TLTI appears to be relatively poor value for money, even though this analysis assumes that one course of treatment prevents active

---

Box 16.1

Cost-Effectiveness of TB Interventions: Main Findings

- The cost effectiveness of TB control depends not only on local costs but also on the local characteristics of TB epidemiology (for example, epidemic or endemic, low or high rates of HIV infection and drug resistance) and on the rate of application of any chosen intervention.
- Short-course chemotherapy for the treatment of infectious and noninfectious TB patients through the DOTS strategy is highly cost-effective for the control of either epidemic or endemic TB (US$5 to US$50 per DALY gained, for regions excluding Eastern and Central Europe). When a new treatment program is compared with a previous program, DOTS often saves money as well as preventing cases and deaths.
- Some variations on DOTS are less cost-effective but still good value for money, including the treatment of patients with MDR-TB (standard or individualized drug regimens) and with HIV infection (with or without supporting antiretroviral therapy). For these additional interventions, the cost per DALY gained is less than the annual average economic productivity per capita in the least developed countries.

- Even with relatively favorable assumptions, the treatment of latent TB infection where TB is endemic and populations are unaffected by HIV is the least cost-effective of the interventions examined here (US$5,500 to US$26,000 per DALY gained). TLTI is more cost-effective during outbreaks (US$150 to US$500 per DALY gained) and for people who are coinfected with TB and HIV (US$15 to US$300 per DALY gained).
- BCG vaccination to prevent severe forms of childhood TB is much less effective than SCC but nearly as cost-effective (US$40 to US$170 per DALY gained).
- A new vaccine that prevents pulmonary TB with high efficacy (equal to or greater than 75 percent) would be more cost-effective than BCG if the cost of immunization were the same as BCG (US$20 to US$100 per DALY gained).
- For any intervention with the potential to cut transmission (that is, excluding BCG vaccination), control of epidemic disease produces more favorable cost-effectiveness ratios than control of endemic disease, because the benefits gained from reduced transmission are greater during outbreaks.

Source: Authors.

TB for life. TLTI is more cost-effective in epidemic than in endemic settings, and it is more cost-effective when it is used to treat individuals coinfected with TB and HIV. A new, high-efficacy vaccine that prevents infection and the progression to pulmonary TB in adults, to be directed at the control of endemic TB, would be more cost-effective than BCG at the same price and almost as cost-effective as SCC.

Averted and Avertable Burden of Tuberculosis

Trends in case notifications can be used, judiciously, to assess regional and global trends in TB incidence, but no satisfactory large-scale analysis has been done of the number of cases prevented by chemotherapy (as distinct from the reductions in transmission and susceptibility associated with improved living standards). One approach to evaluating the averted and avertable burden of TB begins with the observation that 86 percent of the years of healthy life lost that are attributable to TB are from premature death, and only 14 percent are from illness. Because DALYs lost are dominated by premature death, a conservative estimate of the burden of TB alleviated can be obtained in terms of the number of deaths and associated DALYs gained, regionally and globally, since the introduction of the DOTS strategy in 1991.

Figure 16.3 is derived from recent estimates of cases and deaths and their trends by region, including those attributable to HIV coinfection (Corbett and others 2003; WHO 2004c). In the MDG baseline year, 1990, approximately 1.5 million TB deaths (28 per 100,000) occurred. BCG vaccination saved roughly 650,000 deaths from extrapulmonary TB among children between 1990 and 2003. If chemotherapy is assumed to reduce only the case-fatality rate and to have no effect on transmission and incidence, 23 million deaths (44 percent) would have been saved in non-DOTS treatment programs. The expansion to 45 percent case-detection rate under DOTS during the same period saved an estimated 2.3 million (≈5 percent) additional deaths, the largest numbers in Sub-Saharan Africa (1.1 million), East Asia and the Pacific (558,000), and South Asia (408,000). Further analysis shows that, if 70 percent of TB cases (smear positive and smear negative) can be treated under DOTS before MDG target year 2015, an estimated 1.9 million TB deaths (26 per 100,000) will occur in that year, a greater number than in 1990, but a 7 percent lower death rate per capita (Dye and others 2005).

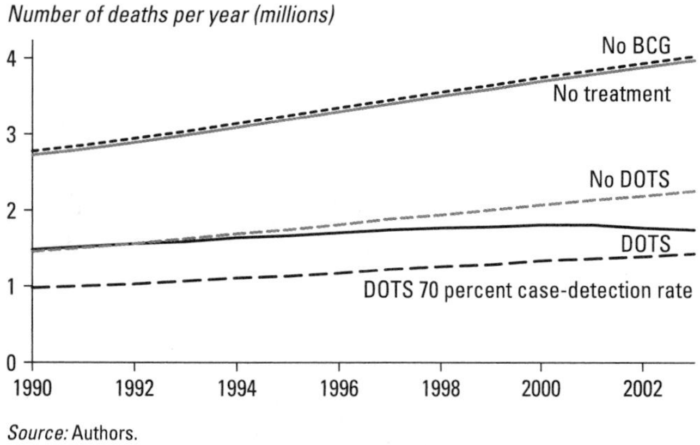

The calculations for Africa assume that treatment cures TB in the majority of HIV-infected patients even though, without antiretroviral therapy, many of these patients will die anyway. Despite these favorable assumptions, the number of TB deaths was evidently still rising in Africa in 2003, whereas it was falling in Asia, aided by the large programs of DOTS expansion in China (1991–97) and India (from 1998).

Reducing the TB death rate sufficiently to meet the MDG target requires a significant cut in incidence, as well as in case fatality. An extension of this assessment suggests that case detection must reach at least 70 percent and the TB incidence rate must fall by 5 to 6 percent annually between 2003 and 2015 (Dye and others 2005). For the world, excluding Sub-Saharan Africa and former Soviet republics, the incidence rate would have to fall at a more modest 2 percent per year.

New diagnostics, drugs, and vaccines would also help reduce the global TB burden more quickly. The most desirable of these is a vaccine that prevents pulmonary disease, whether or not vaccination subjects are already infected (a pre- or postexposure vaccine), and that confers lifetime immunity (Andersen 2001; Fordham von Reyn and Vuola 2002; McMurray 2003; Young and Stewart 2002). A new vaccine with high efficacy against pulmonary TB would almost certainly change immunization practice: mass vaccination campaigns among adults (rather than infants) would have dramatic effects, going far beyond the expectations of DOTS programs (figure 16.4; Dye 2000). A postexposure vaccine that stops progression to disease among those already infected, as well as preventing infection in others, would have greater effect than a preexposure vaccine that only prevents infection (Lietman and Blower 2000). However, such calculations are at present highly speculative, because the mode of action and efficacy of any new vaccine is unknown.

Number of deaths per year (millions)

Source: Authors.

Note: Broken and gray lines represent various hypothetical scenarios; the solid black line represents DOTS programs. The interventions are, from top to bottom: no BCG vaccination and no anti-TB treatment, no treatment, no DOTS programs, DOTS expansion from zero to 45 percent case detection over the period 1990–2003, and DOTS with 70 percent case-detection rate throughout the period 1990–2003. To make a conservative assessment of effect, the treatment of active TB is assumed to change the case-fatality rate without affecting the TB incidence rate.

Figure 16.3 Estimated Number of TB Deaths Worldwide under Various Hypothetical Scenarios and the Estimated Effect of DOTS Programs, 1990–2003

Economic Benefits of Tuberculosis Control

Preventing TB deaths brings no savings in the costs of TB control unless it is accompanied by a reduction in incidence so that fewer patients require treatment. The prompt and effective

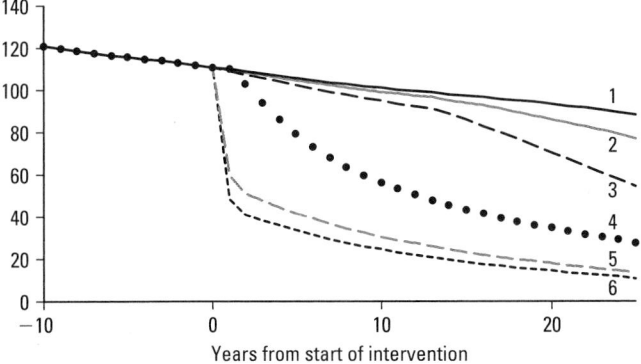

Incidence rate per 100,000 population per year

Source: Dye 2000.

Note: Lines and points show: (1) no intervention in a population where TB is already in slow decline, as in many countries in Asia and Latin America; (2) a postexposure vaccine given annually to infected infants so that 20 percent are immunized; (3) a postexposure vaccine given annually to infected infants so that 70 percent are immunized; (4) DOTS reaching 70 percent case detection and 85 percent cure by year 5 and maintained at these levels thereafter; (5) one-time mass immunization with a preexposure vaccine giving 70 percent protection to uninfected people, followed by annual vaccination of infants with the same fraction protected; and (6) one-time mass immunization with a postexposure vaccine giving 70 percent protection to uninfected people, followed by annual vaccination of infants with the same fraction protected.

Figure 16.4 Hypothetical Effect of New Vaccines on TB Incidence Rate

treatment of active disease is almost certainly reducing transmission around the world, but because the effect on incidence is necessarily slow, it has been hard to quantify in all but a few countries, notably Peru (Suarez and others 2001).

The monetary savings implied by a reduction in incidence of one-quarter (26 percent) between 2000 and 2015—which may be enough to achieve the MDG targets—could be magnified or diminished by adjustments to the DOTS strategy. On the one hand, without compromising cure rates, chemotherapy can be delivered more cheaply to outpatients than inpatients and with less reliance on x-ray diagnosis and surgical procedures. On the other hand, various additions to DOTS—contact tracing, active case finding, antiretroviral therapy for HIV-infected patients, second-line drugs for patients carrying resistant bacilli, or joint public-private schemes for the management of TB—might be desirable but more costly per year of healthy life gained. Whether the savings made by reducing incidence and improving efficiency offset the costs of DOTS add-ons will, therefore, depend on the setting.

Besides the possibility of reducing diagnostic and treatment costs, improved health and longevity yield other economic benefits, but the quantification of those benefits is always controversial. This difficulty is reflected in the limited number of cost-benefit analyses of TB control; among the few examples, one detailed study in India estimated the potential societal benefits of DOTS to be worth US$8.3 billion in 1993–94, or 4 percent of the gross domestic product (Dholakia 1996). Without attempting to extend such analyses here, we note that the preceding results also imply that large-scale treatment programs

for TB are likely to give net returns on investment or at least to appear to be good value for money in ways that go beyond the arguments from cost-effectiveness (Jack 2001).

The analysis earlier in this chapter showed that SCC typically costs up to US$30 per DALY gained for the treatment of infectious TB and up to US$200 per DALY gained for the treatment of noninfectious TB (excluding Europe and Central Asia). These figures can be compared with a recent estimate of US$1.5 billion as the annual global cost of treating 70 percent of cases with 85 percent cure (WHO 2004c). Reaching these targets would prevent approximately 2.1 million of all the TB deaths expected if no treatment were available in 2003, including 391,000 deaths prevented by DOTS (figure 16.3). Because each TB death prevented gains approximately 20 DALYs (WHO 2002b), the total cost per DALY gained would be about US$36. This rough calculation excludes any benefits in reduced transmission but includes the costs of treating smear-negative and extrapulmonary TB and is of the same order of magnitude as the results from CEA.

However the calculation is done, the cost of gaining a year of healthy life under DOTS is substantially less than the annual average productivity per capita in the low-income (gross national income [GNI] less than or equal to US$735) or least developed (GNI average US$290, http://www.worldbank.org) countries, and it is probably less than the marginal productivity of labor in the poorest communities. It is also less than twice the average annual income per capita, which has also been proposed as a benchmark for assessing whether an intervention is cost-effective (Garber and Phelps 1997). Moreover, it is less than the World Bank's definition of *absolute poverty* (living on US$1 per day or less, close to average GNI per capita for the least developed countries) and is certainly less than the monetary values that are typically placed on the value of a human life year (for example, a life was valued at US$100,000 by the 2004 Copenhagen Consensus panel, http://www.copenhagenconsensus.com). All these comparisons suggest not only that the basic DOTS strategy, and perhaps even an enhanced DOTS strategy, are cost-effective but that they also have very favorable cost-benefit ratios.

RESEARCH AND DEVELOPMENT

The preceding review and analysis suggest at least six areas for economic and epidemiological research and development:

1. *DOTS expansion.* Refinement of existing cost estimates of scaling up DOTS programs to reach and move beyond targets for case detection (70 percent) and cure (85 percent) in the poorest countries—notably in Africa—through more comprehensive planning and budgeting exercises. The analyses should include the costs of developing fully staffed

health services, with expanded and renovated infrastructure and improved management capacity where necessary, and the costs of the new initiatives that will be required to improve case detection and cure rates.

2. *Service delivery.* Assessment of the potential for health service restructuring to detect, diagnose, and treat TB patients more efficiently through syndromic management of respiratory diseases at primary health centers and through collaborations between public and private health services, between different parts of the public sector health service, and between TB and HIV/AIDS control programs.

3. *Complementary strategies.* Further investigation of the costs and effectiveness of strategies that are potentially complementary to DOTS, including active case finding and TLTI in high-risk populations, and the management of drug resistance and of patients infected with HIV.

4. *Impact and targets.* Evaluation of the actual and potential effects of the tools (mostly drugs) now being used for TB control. This research requires a better understanding of the ways human population density, age structure, migration, HIV coinfection, and drug resistance affect TB epidemiology. The analyses should check the internal consistency of international targets for the implementation and effect of chemotherapy programs, as defined by the MDGs. The analyses should also make better use of the rich body of routine surveillance data collected by all national TB control programs around the world.

5. *Risk factors.* Assessment of the reductions in TB cases and deaths that could be made by reducing exposure to environmental risk factors, notably indoor and outdoor air pollution, tobacco smoking, and malnutrition. These risk factors affect the establishment of infection, the progression to active disease, and the outcome of treatment.

6. *New diagnostics, drugs, and vaccines.* A sensitive and specific test for active TB that is cheap and simple to use at the first point of contact between patients and health services would be a major advance in diagnosis. Mycobacterial culture, which detects a higher proportion of active TB patients than sputum-smear microscopy, is a prerequisite for screening for drug resistance. However, present culture methods are slow, taking four to six weeks to obtain a result. Technology based on phage amplification and nucleic acid amplification can establish whether cultures are positive in days or hours, but this technology needs to be packaged for use in developing countries (Albert and others 2002, 2004; Johansen and others 2003; Woods 2001). The tuberculin skin test is being superseded in many developed countries by more specific methods for detecting infection (Doherty and others 2002; Pai, Riley, and Colford 2004). A test that can predict who will progress from latent to active disease, as yet hypothetical, would greatly increase the feasibility of treating latent infection.

Among a growing list of new vaccine antigens (Fruth and Young 2004), three of the most promising are now undergoing phase 1 safety trials in humans. One trial has evaluated mycobacterial antigen 85, delivered as a recombinant smallpox vaccine (Goonetilleke and others 2003). Another is testing a live attenuated BCG bacterium (rBCG30) that overexpresses antigen 85B protein and that provides guinea pigs with greater protection than BCG alone (Horwitz and others 2000). A third trial is assessing a fusion protein of two different antigens in adjuvant, referred to as Mtb72f, that is likely to be used as a booster to either BCG or rBCG30 (Reed and others 2003). Compounds that could form the basis of new drugs and new drug regimens include the nitroimidazopyran PA-824. Experiments with a mouse model of TB have shown that PA-824 has bactericidal activity similar to that of isoniazid and sterilizing activity that may rival that of rifampicin and that it is particularly active against dormant bacilli.

Among the most important recent discoveries is a diarylquinoline with a novel mode of action on the ATP synthase of *M. tuberculosis* that powerfully inhibits both drug-sensitive and drug-resistant strains of bacilli (Andries and others 2004). Alongside these laboratory studies, analytical and operational research are needed to find out what kinds of new tools will give the best returns on investment. Investigations of this kind will contribute to the introduction of new vaccines, drugs, and diagnostics and will inform the work of the Foundation for Innovative New Diagnostics (http://www.finddiagnostics.org), the Global Alliance for TB Drug Development (http://www.tballiance.org), and the AerasGlobal TB Vaccine Foundation (http://www.aeras.org).

CONCLUSIONS

After more than a decade of climbing incidence rates in Africa and former Soviet republics, the global TB epidemic appears once again to be on the threshold of decline. The spread of HIV and drug resistance, respectively, in those two regions has exacerbated the problems of TB control, but at the same time it has helped keep TB on the international public health agenda. The global incidence rate was still rising in 2003, but more slowly each year. This slowdown is not only (or even mainly) because of direct intervention through DOTS programs but because HIV epidemics are approaching peak levels in Africa and because incidence is now starting to fall again in some former Soviet republics, including Russia. Where TB incidence is already falling, prevalence and death rates should be dropping more quickly, although little evidence demonstrates this decrease yet.

The prompt diagnosis and treatment of active TB has been the mainstay of TB control and will continue to be so for the foreseeable future. Short-course chemotherapy, delivered through the DOTS strategy, is, at typically US$5 to US$350 per DALY gained, the most cost-effective among current methods for the management of TB, and in most high-burden countries, the cost is toward the lower end of this range. A comparison of the costs of treating active TB with the costs of running a previous program suggests that DOTS could actually save money in the long run. In addition, DOTS provides an operational framework for the introduction of more specialized methods in certain risk groups. The extensions to DOTS investigated here include the treatment of MDR-TB with second-line drugs, preventive therapy (TLTI) during outbreaks and for people coinfected with *M. tuberculosis* and HIV, and antiretroviral therapy for HIV-infected TB patients. Those interventions cost more than the basic DOTS strategy but are still less than a dollar for each day of healthy life gained, which provides an economic argument for their integration into enhanced DOTS programs.

Although the analyses in this chapter show that DOTS and its extensions are good value for money, they conceal various features of health systems, as yet poorly defined, that may facilitate the implementation of treatment programs. For example, if broader investment in the health sector is needed before TB control programs can work in some parts of some countries, then the full cost of DOTS could be greater. By contrast, a more integrated approach to the management of TB and other respiratory diseases in primary health facilities could lead to cost savings. Those possibilities have not yet been investigated.

The only development that could radically alter the current approach to TB control—shifting the emphasis from cure to prevention—is the discovery of a new vaccine that protects adults against infectious pulmonary disease. Whether such a vaccine would be more or less cost-effective than BCG (US$40 to US$1,600 per DALY gained) depends on price and efficacy, but the potential epidemiological effect would be far greater than that of BCG, perhaps justifying mass adult vaccination. If research and development proceed according to plan, a new vaccine of some kind could be licensed between 2010 and 2015. New drugs and diagnostics should be available earlier, shortening the delay to, and duration of, treatment.

Although cost-effectiveness studies show that DOTS is a good investment, they do not formally show that the strategy is affordable. The analytical difficulty is that CEA does not solve the practical problem of how to allocate money to TB control in combination with other interventions, or even how to combine different approaches to TB control (Tan-Torres Edejer and others 2004). Interpreted literally, CEA says that the best return on total investment is obtained by ranking interventions according to CER and then fully implementing each intervention, from smallest to largest CER, allowing for diminishing returns, until the total budget is spent. This method is unlikely to lead to a balanced health care portfolio in the poorest countries. Besides, the evidence is rarely available to carry out such a complete analysis. The results of CEA are therefore typically used more informally, along with other evidence and constraints, when a mix of health interventions is chosen.

Although this problem will recur in discussions about allocating health budgets, the case for large-scale programs of TB treatment has now been accepted in many parts of the world. That is the fruit of more than 10 years' work on burden, cost, efficacy, effectiveness, and cost-effectiveness. The governments of the less poor members of the group of 22 high-burden countries have demonstrated that they can budget for, and provide, most of the funds needed to reach target levels of case detection and cure (WHO 2004c, 2005). Some of the poorer countries among the 22 are now receiving sufficient external assistance to fill the gaps in their budgets for TB control, principally from the Global Fund to Fight AIDS, Tuberculosis, and Malaria. Consequently, the total reported budget deficit for the high-burden countries in 2005 was remarkably small—just US$119 million—and concentrated in the poorest countries (WHO 2005).

From those findings and observations arise two key questions for global TB control: If the estimated budget gap is filled, would the money be enough to ensure that enhanced DOTS programs reach 70 percent case detection and 85 percent cure—and by when? And if those targets are reached, will the effort be sufficient to achieve the MDG objectives of halving prevalence and death rates by 2015?

As yet, there are only partial answers. On the costs, it is clear that, by moving treatment out of hospitals and into the community, DOTS can often be made cheaper and more convenient for patients and health services without compromising treatment outcome. However, planning for TB control in the poorest countries is still inadequate, and budgets commonly understate the real costs of scaling up national TB control programs (WHO 2004c, 2005). Despite those weaknesses in the budgeting and funding process, the overall expenditure on TB control in high-burden countries has increased since 2000, and the injection of extra effort and money has led to a small acceleration in case finding globally. As a result, case detection under DOTS could reach 50 to 60 percent by 2005, and treatment success should be close to the target level of 85 percent.

A case-detection rate of 50 to 60 percent may not be enough. The analysis in this chapter suggests that the MDG objective of halving the death rate can be reached with 70 percent case detection globally, provided this case detection also generates a 5 to 6 percent annual reduction in the incidence rate between 2003 and 2015. The DOTS program in Peru generated a 6 to 7 percent annual reduction in the incidence rate of pulmonary TB, but that result has not yet been repeated in other high-burden countries with good control programs (for example, India, Morocco, and Vietnam). It is unlikely to be achieved in African countries that currently have high rates of HIV infection.

Although others have emphasized that the costs of infectious disease control can be related to the benefits in complex ways (Brandeau, Zaric, and Richter 2003), we advocate the use of a powerful new method of carrying out CEA, which is based on the observation that mathematical models can be used to generate simple (albeit approximate) and general formulas that relate reward to effort in the management of both epidemic (based on R_0) and endemic (based on dynamics in the vicinity of equilibrium) TB. The results are similar to those obtained by using more complex simulations in specific settings, and they are accurate enough to offer a choice between interventions (Currie and others, 2005). The generality of the method exposes more clearly the reasons some interventions are comparatively cost-effective and indicates the range of conditions under which specific cost-effectiveness results apply. The scope for using this approach for other infectious diseases remains to be explored, but it should be readily applicable in the evaluation of new approaches to TB control, whether through vaccination, drug treatment, the reduction of environmental risks, or improved service delivery.

ACKNOWLEDGMENTS

The authors wish to thank Uli Fruth, Kreena Govender, Ulla Griffiths, Mehran Hosseini, Anne Mills, Mark Perkins, Catherine Watt, Diana Weil, and Brian Williams for help of various kinds during the preparation of this chapter.

REFERENCES

Aaron, L., D. Saadoun, I. Calatroni, O. Launay, N. Memain, V. Vincent, and others. 2004. "Tuberculosis in HIV-Infected Patients: A Comprehensive Review." *Clinical Microbiology and Infection* 10: 388–98.

Adatu, F., R. Odeke, M. Mugenyi, G. Gargioni, E. McCray, E. Schneider, and D. Maher. 2003. "Implementation of the DOTS Strategy for Tuberculosis Control in Rural Kiboga District, Uganda, Offering Patients the Option of Treatment Supervision in the Community, 1998–1999." *International Journal of Tuberculosis and Lung Disease* 7: S63–71.

Albert, H., A. Heydenrych, R. Brookes, R. J. Mole, B. Harley, E. Subotsky, and others. 2002. "Performance of a Rapid Phage-Based Test, FASTPlaqueTBTM, to Diagnose Pulmonary Tuberculosis from Sputum Specimens in South Africa." *International Journal of Tuberculosis and Lung Disease* 6 (6): 529–37.

Albert, H., A. Trollip, T. Seaman, and R. J. Mole. 2004. "Simple, Phage-Based (FASTPlaque) Technology to Determine Rifampicin Resistance of *Mycobacterium tuberculosis* Directly from Sputum." *International Journal of Tuberculosis and Lung Disease* 8: 1114–19.

Andersen, P. 2001. "TB Vaccines: Progress and Problems." *Trends in Immunology* 22: 160–68.

Anderson, R. M., and R. M. May. 1991. *Infectious Diseases of Humans: Dynamics and Control.* Oxford, U.K.: Oxford University Press.

Andries, K., P. Verhasselt, J. Guillemont, H. W. Gohlmann, J. M. Neefs, H. Winkler, and others. 2004. "A Diarylquinoline Drug Active on the ATP Synthase of Mycobacterium Tuberculosis." *Science* 307: 223–27.

Asamoah-Odei, E., J. M. Garcia Calleja, and J. T. Boerma. 2004. "HIV Prevalence and Trends in Sub-Saharan Africa: No Decline and Large Subregional Differences." *Lancet* 364: 35–40.

Behr, M. A, S. A. Warren, H. Salamon, P. C. Hopewell, A. Ponce de Leon, C. L. Daley, and P. M. Small. 1999. "Transmission of *Mycobacterium tuberculosis* from Patients Smear-Negative for Acid-Fast Bacilli." *Lancet* 353: 444–49.

Borgdorff, M. W., N. J. Nagelkerke, C. Dye, and P. Nunn. 2000. "Gender and Tuberculosis: A Comparison of Prevalence Surveys with Notification Data to Explore Sex Differences in Case Detection." *International Journal of Tuberculosis and Lung Disease* 4: 123–32.

Bourdin Trunz, B., P. E. M. Fine, and C. Dye. Forthcoming. Global Impact of BCG Vaccination on Childhood Tuberculous Meningitis and Miliary Tuberculosis.

Brandeau, M. L., G. S. Zaric, and A. Richter. 2003. "Resource Allocation for Control of Infectious Diseases in Multiple Independent Populations: Beyond Cost-Effectiveness Analysis." *Journal of Health Economics* 22: 575–98.

Bucher, H. C., L. E. Griffith, G. H. Guyatt, P. Sudre, M. Naef, P. Sendi, and M. Battegay. 1999. "Isoniazid Prophylaxis for Tuberculosis in HIV Infection: A Meta-Analysis of Randomized Controlled Trials." *AIDS* 13: 501–7.

China Tuberculosis Control Collaboration. 2004. "The Effect of Tuberculosis Control in China." *Lancet* 364: 417–22.

Claessens, N. J. M., F. F. Gausi, S. Meijnen, M. M. Weismuller, F. M. Salaniponi, and A. D. Harries. 2002. "High Frequency of Tuberculosis in Households of Index TB Patients." *International Journal of Tuberculosis and Lung Disease* 6: 266–69.

Cohn, D. L. 2003. "Treatment of Latent Tuberculosis Infection." *Seminars in Respiratory Infections* 18: 249–62.

Cohn, D. L., and W. M. El-Sadr. 2000. "Treatment of Latent Tuberculosis Infection." In *Tuberculosis: A Comprehensive International Approach*, ed. L. B. Reichman and E. S. Hershfield, 471–502. New York: Marcel Dekker.

Comstock, G. W. 2000. "How Much Isoniazid Is Needed for Prevention of Tuberculosis among Immunocompetent Adults? In Reply." *International Journal of Tuberculosis and Lung Disease* 4: 485–86.

Comstock, G. W., C. Baum, and D. E. Snider. 1979. "Isoniazid Prophylaxis among Alaskan Eskimos: A Final Report of the Bethel Isoniazid Studies." *American Review of Respiratory Disease* 119: 827–30.

Comstock, G. W., V. T. Livesay, and S. F. Woolpert. 1974. "The Prognosis of a Positive Tuberculin Reaction in Childhood and Adolescence." *American Journal of Epidemiology* 99: 131–38.

Corbett, E. L., S. Charalambous, V. M. Moloi, K. Fielding, A. D. Grant, C. Dye, and others. 2004. "Human Immunodeficiency Virus and the Prevalence of Undiagnosed Tuberculosis in African Gold Miners." *American Journal of Respiratory Critical Care Medicine* 170: 673–79.

Corbett, E. L., R. W. Steketee, F. O. ter Kuile, A. S. Latif, A. Kamali, and R. J. Hayes. 2002. "HIV-1/AIDS and the Control of Other Infectious Diseases in Africa." *Lancet* 359: 2177–87.

Corbett E. L., C. J. Watt, N. Walker, D. Maher, B. G. Williams, M. C. Raviglione, and C. Dye. 2003. "The Growing Burden of Tuberculosis: Global Trends and Interactions with the HIV Epidemic." *Archives of Internal Medicine* 163: 1009–21.

Cuhadaroglu, C., M. Erelel, L. Tabak, and Z. Kilicaslan. 2002. "Increased Risk of Tuberculosis in Health Care Workers: A Retrospective Survey at a Teaching Hospital in Istanbul, Turkey." *BioMed Central Infectious Diseases* 2: 14.

Currie, C. S. M., K. Floyd, B. G. Williams, and C. Dye. 2005. "Cost Affordability and Cost-Effectiveness of Strategies to Control Tuberculosis in Countries with High HIV, Prevalence." *BMC Public Health* 5 (1): 130.

de Jonghe, E., C. J. Murray, H. J. Chum, D. S. Nyangulu, A. Salomao, and K. Styblo. 1994. "Cost-Effectiveness of Chemotherapy for Sputum Smear-Positive Pulmonary Tuberculosis in Malawi, Mozambique and Tanzania." *International Journal of Health Planning and Management* 9: 151–81.

de Viedma, D. G., M. Marin, S. Hernangomez, M. Diaz, M. J. R. Serrano, L. Alcala, and E. Bouza. 2002. "Reinfection Plays a Role in a Population Whose Clinical/Epidemiological Characteristics Do Not Favor Reinfection." *Archives of Internal Medicine* 162: 1873–79.

Dholakia, R. 1996. *The Potential Economic Benefits of the DOTS Strategy against TB in India.* Geneva: World Health Organization.

Doherty, T. M., A. Demissie, J. Olobo, D. Wolday, S. Britton, T. Eguale, and others. 2002. "Immune Responses to the *Mycobacterium tuberculosis*–Specific Antigen ESAT-6 Signal Subclinical Infection among Contacts of Tuberculosis Patients." *Journal of Clinical Microbiology* 40 (2): 704–6.

Dudley, L., V. Azevedo, R. Grant, J. H. Schoeman, L. Dikweni, and D. Maher. 2003. "Evaluation of Community Contribution to Tuberculosis Control in Cape Town, South Africa." *International Journal of Tuberculosis and Lung Disease* 7 (Suppl. 1): S48–55.

Dye, C. 2000. "Tuberculosis 2000–2010: Control, but Not Elimination." *International Journal of Tuberculosis and Lung Disease* 4 (Suppl. 2): S146–52.

Dye, C., and M. A. Espinal. 2001. "Will Tuberculosis Become Resistant to All Antibiotics?" *Proceedings of the Royal Society of London, Series B, Biological Sciences* 268: 45–52.

Dye, C., G. P. Garnett, K. Sleeman, and B. G. Williams. 1998. "Prospects for Worldwide Tuberculosis Control under the WHO DOTS Strategy." *Lancet* 352: 1886–91.

Dye, C., S. Scheele, P. Dolin, V. Pathania, and M. C. Raviglione. 1999. "Global Burden of Tuberculosis: Estimated Incidence, Prevalence, and Mortality by Country." *Journal of the American Medical Association* 282: 677–86.

Dye, C., C. J. Watt, D. M. Bleed, S. M. Hosseini, and M. C. Raviglione. 2005. "The Evolution of Tuberculosis Control, and Prospects for Reducing Incidence, Prevalence and Deaths Globally." *Journal of the American Medical Association* 293: 2767–75.

Dye, C., C. J. Watt, D. M. Bleed, and B. G. Williams. 2003. "What Is the Limit to Case Detection under the DOTS Strategy for Tuberculosis Control?" *Tuberculosis* 83: 35–43.

Dye, C., and B. G. Williams. 2000. "Criteria for the Control of Drug-Resistant Tuberculosis." *Proceedings of the National Academy of Sciences USA* 97: 8180–85.

Dye, C., B. G. Williams, M. A. Espinal, and M. C. Raviglione. 2002. "Erasing the World's Slow Stain: Strategies to Beat Multidrug-Resistant Tuberculosis." *Science* 295: 2042–46.

Dye, C., F. Zhao, S. Scheele, and B. G. Williams. 2000. "Evaluating the Impact of Tuberculosis Control: Number of Deaths Prevented by Short-Course Chemotherapy in China." *International Journal of Epidemiology* 29: 558–64.

Espinal, M. A., A. Laszlo, L. Simonsen, F. Boulahbal, S. J. Kim, A. Reniero, and others. 2001. "Global Trends in Resistance to Antituberculosis Drugs." *New England Journal of Medicine* 344: 1294–1303.

Fine, P. E. M. 2001. "BCG Vaccines and Vaccination." In *Tuberculosis: A Comprehensive International Approach*, ed. L. B. Reichman, and E. S. Hershfield, 503–24. New York: Marcel Dekker.

Floyd, K. 2003. "Costs and Effectiveness: The Impact of Economic Studies on TB Control." *Tuberculosis* (Edinburgh) 83: 187–200.

Floyd, K., J. Skeva, T. Nyirenda, F. Gausi, and F. Salaniponi. 2003. "Cost and Cost-Effectiveness of Increased Community and Primary Care Facility Involvement in Tuberculosis Care in Lilongwe District, Malawi." *International Journal of Tuberculosis and Lung Disease* 7 (Suppl. 1): S29–37.

Floyd, K., D. Wilkinson, and C. Gilks. 1997. "Comparison of Cost Effectiveness of Directly Observed Treatment (DOT) and Conventionally Delivered Treatment for Tuberculosis: Experience from Rural South Africa." *British Medical Journal* 315 (7): 1407–11.

Fordham von Reyn, C., and J. M. Vuola. 2002. "New Vaccines for the Prevention of Tuberculosis. *Clinical Infectious Diseases* 35: 465–74.

Frieden, T. R., P. I. Fujiwara, R. M. Washko, and M. A. Hamburg. 1995. "Tuberculosis in New York City—Turning the Tide." *New England Journal of Medicine* 333: 229–33.

Frieden, T., T. R. Sterling, S. S. Munsiff, C. J. Watt, and C. Dye. 2003. "Tuberculosis." *Lancet* 362: 887–99.

Friedland, G., S. Abdool Karim, Q. Abdool Karim, U. Lalloo, C. Jack, N. Gandhi, and W. El Sadr. 2004. "Utility of Tuberculosis Directly Observed Therapy Programs as Sites for Access to and Provision of Antiretroviral Therapy in Resource-Limited Countries." *Clinical Infectious Diseases* 38 (Suppl. 5): S421–28.

Fruth, U., and D. Young. 2004. "Prospects for New TB Vaccines: Stop TB Working Group on TB Vaccine Development." *International Journal of Tuberculosis and Lung Disease* 8: 151–55.

Garber, A. M., and C. E. Phelps. 1997. "Economic Foundations of Cost-Effectiveness Analysis." *Journal of Health Economics* 16: 1–31.

Glynn, J. R., M. D. Yates, A. C. Crampin, B. M. Ngwira, F. D. Mwaungulu, G. F. Black, and others. 2004. "DNA Fingerprint Changes in Tuberculosis: Reinfection, Evolution, or Laboratory Error?" *Journal of Infectious Diseases* 190: 1158–66.

Goonetilleke, N. P., H. McShane, C. M. Hannan, R. J. Anderson, R. H. Brookes, and A. V. Hill. 2003. "Enhanced Immunogenicity and Protective Efficacy against *Mycobacterium tuberculosis* of Bacilli Calmette-Guérin Vaccine Using Mucosal Administration and Boosting with a Recombinant Modified Vaccinia Virus Ankara." *Journal of Immunology* 171: 1602–9.

Grange, J. 2003. "Immunophysiology and Immunopathology." In *Clinical Tuberculosis*, 3rd ed., ed. P. D. O. Davies, 88–104. London: Arnold.

Hamid Salim, M. A., E. Declercq, A. Van Deun, and K. A. R. Saki. 2004. "Gender Differences in Tuberculosis: A Prevalence Survey Done in Bangladesh." *International Journal of Tuberculosis and Lung Disease* 8: 952–57.

Hernandez-Garduno, E., V. Cook, D. Kunimoto, R. K. Elwood, W. A. Black, and J. M. FitzGerald. 2004. "Transmission of Tuberculosis from Smear Negative Patients: A Molecular Epidemiology Study." *Thorax* 59: 286–90.

Horwitz, M. A., G. Harth, B. J. Dillon, and S. Maslesa-Galic. 2000. "Recombinant Bacillus Calmette-Guérin (BCG) Vaccines Expressing the *Mycobacterium tuberculosis* 30-kDA Major Secretory Protein Induce Greater Protective Immunity against Tuberculosis Than Conventional BCG Vaccines in a Highly Susceptible Animal Model." *Proceedings of the National Academy of Sciences USA* 97: 13853–58.

Hudelson, P. 1996. "Gender Differentials in Tuberculosis: The Role of Socio-Economic and Cultural Factors." *Tubercle and Lung Disease* 77: 391–400.

Jack, W. 2001. "The Public Economics of Tuberculosis Control." *Health Policy* 57: 79–96.

Jamison, D. T., W. H. Mosley, A. R. Meashem, and J. L. Bobadilla. 1993. *Disease Control Priorities in Developing Countries.* New York: Oxford University Press.

Johansen, I. S., B. Lundgren, A. Sosnovskaja, and V. Ø. Thomsen. 2003. "Direct Detection of Multidrug-Resistant *Mycobacterium tuberculosis* in Clinical Specimens in Low- and High-Incidence Countries by Line Probe Assay." *Journal of Clinical Microbiology* 41 (9): 4454–56.

Johnson, J. L., A. Okwera, D. L. Hom, H. Mayanja, C. Mutuluuza Kityo, P. Nsubuga, and others. 2001. "Duration of Efficacy of Treatment of Latent Tuberculosis Infection in HIV-Infected Adults." *AIDS* 15: 2137–47.

Krebs, W. 1930. "Die Fälle von Lungentuberkulose in der aargauischen Heilstätte Barmelweid aus den Jahren 1912–1927." *Beiträge zur Klinik der Tuberkulose* 74: 345–79.

Kristensen, I., P. Aaby, and H. Jensen. 2000. "Routine Vaccinations and Child Survival: Follow Up Study in Guinea-Bissau, West Africa." *British Medical Journal* 321: 1435–38.

Letvin, N. L., B. R. Bloom, and S. L. Hoffman. 2001. "Prospects for Vaccines to Protect against AIDS, Tuberculosis, and Malaria." *Journal of the American Medical Association* 285: 606–11.

Lietman, T., and S. M. Blower. 2000. "Potential Impact of Tuberculosis Vaccines as Epidemic Control Agents." *Clinical Infectious Diseases* 30 (Suppl. 3): S316–22.

Marais B. J., R. P. Gie, H. S. Schaaf, A. C. Hesseling, C. C. Obihara, L. J. Nelson, and others. 2004. "The Clinical Epidemiology of Childhood Pulmonary Tuberculosis: A Critical Review of Literature from the Pre-Chemotherapy Era." *International Journal of Tuberculosis and Lung Disease* 8: 278–85.

Marks, G. B., J. Bai, G. J. Stewart, S. E. Simpson, and E. A. Sullivan. 2001. "Effectiveness of Postmigration Screening in Controlling Tuberculosis among Refugees: A Historical Cohort Study, 1984–1998." *American Journal of Public Health* 91: 1797–99.

McMurray, D. N. 2003. "Recent Progress in the Development and Testing of Vaccines against Human Tuberculosis." *International Journal of Parasitology* 33: 547–54.

Menzies, D., M. J. Dion, B. Rabinovitch, S. Mannix, P. Brassard, and K. Schwartzman. 2004. "Treatment Completion and Costs of a Randomized Trial of Rifampin for 4 Months versus Isoniazid for 9 Months." *American Journal of Respiratory and Critical Care Medicine* 170: 445–49.

Moalosi, G., K. Floyd, J. Phatshwane, T. Moeti, N. Binkin, and T. Kenyon. 2003. "Cost-Effectiveness of Home-Based Care versus Hospital Care for Chronically Ill Tuberculosis Patients, Francistown, Botswana." *International Journal of Tuberculosis and Lung Disease* 7 (Suppl. 1): S80–85.

Murray, C. J. L., E. de Jonghe, H. J. Chum, D. S. Nyangulu, A. Salomao, and K. Styblo. 1991. "Cost Effectiveness of Chemotherapy for Pulmonary Tuberculosis in Three Sub-Saharan African Countries." *Lancet* 338: 1305–8.

Murray, C. J. L., and J. A. Salomon. 1998. "Modeling the Impact of Global Tuberculosis Control Strategies." *Proceedings of the National Academy of Sciences USA* 95: 13881–86.

Mwinga, A., M. Hosp, P. Godfrey-Faussett, M. Quigley, P. Mwaba, B. N. Mugala, and others. 1998. "Twice Weekly Tuberculosis Preventive Therapy in HIV Infection in Zambia." *AIDS* 12: 2447–57.

Nelson, L. J., and C. D. Wells. 2004. "Global Epidemiology of Childhood Tuberculosis." *International Journal of Tuberculosis and Lung Disease* 8: 636–47.

Neuenschwander, B. E., M. Zwahlen, S. J. Kim, E. G. Lee, and H. L. Rieder. 2002. "Determination of the Prevalence of Infection with *Mycobacterium tuberculosis* among Persons Vaccinated against Bacillus Calmette-Guérin in South Korea." *American Journal of Epidemiology* 155: 654–63.

Noertjojo, K., C. M. Tam, S. L. Chan, J. Tan, and M. Chan-Yeung. 2002. "Contact Examination for Tuberculosis in Hong Kong Is Useful." *International Journal of Tuberculosis and Lung Disease* 6: 19–24.

Nyangulu, D. S., A. D. Harries, C. Kang'ombe, A. E. Yadidi, K. Chokani, T. Cullinan, and others. 1997. "Tuberculosis in a Prison Population in Malawi." *Lancet* 350: 1284–87.

Okello, D., K. Floyd, F. Adatu, R. Odeke, and G. Gargloni. 2003. "Cost and Cost-Effectiveness of Community-Based Care in Rural Uganda." *International Journal of Tuberculosis and Lung Disease* 7 (Suppl. 1): S72–79.

Pai, M., L. W. Riley, and J. M. Colford Jr. 2004. "Interferon-gamma Assays in the Immunodiagnosis of Tuberculosis: A Systematic Review." *Lancet Infectious Diseases* 4 (12): 761–76.

PRC (People's Republic of China) Ministry of Health. 2000. *Report on Nationwide Random Survey for the Epidemiology of Tuberculosis in 2000.* Beijing: PRC Ministry of Health.

Quigley, M. A., A. Mwinga, M. Hosp, I. Lisse, D. Fuchs, J. D. H. Porter, and P. Godfrey-Faussett. 2001. "Long-Term Effect of Preventive Therapy for Tuberculosis in a Cohort of HIV-Infected Zambian Adults." *AIDS* 15: 215–22.

Radhakrishna, S., T. R. Frieden, and R. Subramani. 2003. "Association of Initial Tuberculin Sensitivity, Age, and Sex with the Incidence of Tuberculosis in South India: A 15-Year Follow-Up." *International Journal of Tuberculosis and Lung Disease* 7: 1083–91.

Reed, S. G., M. R. Alderson, W. Dalemans, Y. Lobet, and Y. A. W. Skeiky. 2003. "Prospects for a Better Vaccine against Tuberculosis." *Tuberculosis* 83: 213–19.

Richardson, M., N. M. Carroll, E. Engelke, G. D. Van Der Spuy, F. Salker, Z. Munch, and others. 2002. "Multiple Mycobacterium Tuberculosis Strains in Early Cultures from Patients in a High-Incidence Community Setting." *Journal of Clinical Microbiology* 40: 2750–54.

Rieder, H. L. 1999. "Epidemiologic Basis of Tuberculosis Control." Paris: International Union against Tuberculosis and Lung Disease.

———. 2003. "BCG Vaccines." In *Clinical Tuberculosis,* 3rd ed., ed. P. D. O. Davies, 337–53. London: Arnold.

Rieder, H. L., D. E. Snider Jr., and G. M. Cauthen. 1990. "Extrapulmonary Tuberculosis in the United States." *American Review of Respiratory Disease* 141: 347–51.

Shafer, R. W., and B. R. Edlin. 1996. "Tuberculosis in Patients Infected with Human Immunodeficiency Virus: Perspective on the Past Decade." *Clinical Infectious Diseases* 22: 683–704.

Shilova, M. V., and C. Dye. 2001. "The Resurgence of Tuberculosis in Russia." *Philosophical Transactions of the Royal Society of London, Series B, Biological Sciences* 356: 1069–75.

Sinanovic, E., K. Floyd, L. Dudley, V. Azevedo, R. Grant, and D. Maher. 2003. "Cost and Cost-Effectiveness of Community-Based Care for Tuberculosis in Cape Town, South Africa." *International Journal of Tuberculosis and Lung Disease* 7 (Suppl. 1): S56–62.

Sonnenberg, P., J. R. Glynn, K. Fielding, J. Murray, P. Godfrey-Faussett, and S. Shearer. 2005. "How Soon after Infection with HIV Does the Risk of Tuberculosis Start to Increase? A Retrospective Cohort Study in South African Gold Miners." *Journal of Infectious Diseases* 191: 150–58.

Styblo, K. 1991. *Epidemiology of Tuberculosis.* 2nd ed. The Hague: Royal Netherlands Tuberculosis Association.

Suarez, P. G., K. Floyd, J. Portocarrero, E. Alarcon, E. Rapiti, G. Ramos, and others. 2002. "Feasibility and Cost-Effectiveness of Standardised Second-Line Drug Treatment for Chronic Tuberculosis Patients: A National Cohort Study in Peru." *Lancet* 359: 1980–89.

Suarez, P. G., C. J. Watt, E. Alarcon, J. Portocarrero, D. Zavala, R. Canales, and others. 2001. "The Dynamics of Tuberculosis in Response to 10 Years of Intensive Control Effort in Peru." *Journal of Infectious Diseases* 184: 473–78.

Sutherland, I. 1968. "The Ten-Year Incidence of Clinical Tuberculosis Following 'Conversion' in 2,550 Individuals Aged 14 to 19 Years." Unpublished progress report of the Tuberculosis Surveillance and Research Unit, KNCV, The Hague, Netherlands.

———. 1976. "Recent Studies in the Epidemiology of Tuberculosis, Based on the Risk of Being Infected with Tubercle Bacilli." *Advances in Tuberculosis Research* 19: 1–63.

Sutherland, I., E. Svandova, and S. Radhakrishna. 1982. "The Development of Clinical Tuberculosis Following Infection with Tubercle Bacilli: 1. A Theoretical Model for the Development of Clinical Tuberculosis Following Infection, Linking from Data on the Risk of Tuberculosis Infection and the Incidence of Clinical Tuberculosis in the Netherlands." *Tubercle* 63: 255–68.

Tan-Torres Edejer, T., R. Baltussen, T. Adam, R. Hutubessy, A. Acharya, D. B. Evans, and C. J. L. Murray, eds. 2004. *WHO Guide to Cost-Effectiveness Analysis.* Geneva: World Health Organization.

Terris-Prestholt, F., and L. Kumaranayake. 2003. "Cost Analysis of the Zambian ProTEST Project: A Package to Reduce the Impact of Tuberculosis and Other HIV-Related Diseases." Unpublished report, London School of Hygiene and Tropical Medicine.

Toman, K. 1979. *Tuberculosis Case-Finding and Chemotherapy. Questions and Answers.* Geneva: World Health Organization.

Uplekar, M., V. Pathania, and M. Raviglione. 2001. "Private Practitioners and Public Health: Weak Links in Tuberculosis Control." *Lancet* 358: 912–16.

van Rie, A., R. Warren, M. Richardson, T. C. Victor, R. P. Gie, D. A. Enarson, and others. 1999. "Exogenous Reinfection as a Cause of Recurrent Tuberculosis after Curative Treatment." *New England Journal of Medicine* 341: 1174–79.

Vassall, A., S. Bagdadi, H. Bashour, H. Zaher, and P. V. Maaren. 2002. "Cost-Effectiveness of Different Treatment Strategies for Tuberculosis in Egypt and Syria." *International Journal of Tuberculosis and Lung Disease* 6: 1083–90.

Verver, S., R. M. Warren, Z. Munch, E. Vynnycky, P. D. van Helden, M. Richardson, and others. 2004. "Transmission of Tuberculosis in a High Incidence Urban Community in South Africa." *International Journal of Epidemiology* 33: 351–57.

Vynnycky, E., and P. E. M. Fine. 1997. "The Natural History of Tuberculosis: The Implications of Age-Dependent Risks of Disease and the Role of Reinfection." *Epidemiology and Infection* 119: 183–201.

———. 2000. "Life Time Risks, Incubation Period, and Serial Interval of Tuberculosis." *American Journal of Epidemiology* 152: 247–63.

Whalen, C. C., J. L. Johnson, A. Okwera, D. L. Hom, R. Huebner, P. Mugyenyi, and others. 1997. "A Trial of Three Regimens to Prevent Tuberculosis in Ugandan Adults Infected with the Human Immunodeficiency Virus." *New England Journal of Medicine* 337: 801–8.

WHO (World Health Organization). 2001. *Vaccine Preventable Diseases: Monitoring System—2001 Global Summary.* Geneva: WHO, Department of Vaccines and Biologicals.

———. 2002a. *An Expanded DOTS Framework for Effective Tuberculosis Control.* Geneva: WHO.

———. 2002b. *The World Health Report: Reducing Risks, Promoting Healthy Life.* Geneva: WHO.

———. 2004a. *Anti-Tuberculosis Drug Resistance in the World.* Report 3. Geneva: WHO.

———. 2004b. *Cost and Cost-Effectiveness of Public-Private Mix DOTS: Evidence from Two Pilot Projects in India.* Geneva: WHO.

———. 2004c. *Global Tuberculosis Control: Surveillance, Planning, Financing.* Geneva: WHO.

———. 2004d. *Public-Private Mix for DOTS: Global Progress.* Geneva: WHO.

———. 2004e. *Respiratory Care in Primary Care Services—A Survey in 9 Countries.* Geneva: WHO.

———. 2004f. *World Health Report 2004: Changing History.* Geneva: WHO.

———. 2005. *Global Tuberculosis Control: Surveillance, Planning, Financing.* Geneva: WHO.

Wilkinson, D., K. Floyd, and C. F. Gilks. 1997. "Costs and Cost-Effectiveness of Alternative Tuberculosis Management Strategies in South Africa—Implications for Policy." *South African Medical Journal* 87 (4): 451–55.

Wilkinson, D., S. B. Squire, and P. Garner. 1998. "Effect of Preventive Treatment for Tuberculosis in Adults Infected with HIV: Systematic Review of Randomised Placebo Controlled Trials." *British Medical Journal* 317: 625–29.

Williams, B. G., and C. Dye. 2003. "Antiretroviral Drugs for Tuberculosis Control in the Era of HIV/AIDS." *Science* 301: 1535–37.

Woods, G. L. 2001. "Molecular Techniques in Mycobacterial Detection." *Archives of Pathology and Laboratory Medicine* 125 (1): 122–26.

Young, D. B., and G. R. Stewart. 2002. "Tuberculosis Vaccines." *British Medical Bulletin* 62: 73–86.

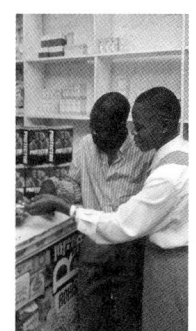

Chapter **17**

Sexually Transmitted Infections

Sevgi O. Aral and Mead Over, with Lisa Manhart
and King K. Holmes

Sexually transmitted infections (STIs) are responsible for an enormous burden of morbidity and mortality in many developing countries because of their effects on reproductive and child health (Wasserheit 1989) and their role in facilitating the transmission of HIV infection (Laga, Diallo, and Buvé 1994).

INTRODUCTION

Largely because of the HIV epidemic, interest in STIs has increased over the past two decades. During that time, the epidemiology of STIs has changed in developing countries, partly as a result of modifications in STI case management approaches and partly because of behavioral changes in response to the HIV epidemic. At the same time, advances in STI prevention have enhanced understanding of the intricacies of STI transmission dynamics and the role of interventions in the control of STIs. However, what has not changed is as significant as what has changed: the epidemiology of STIs still differs substantially in the industrial countries and the developing world. The sociocultural and economic contexts in developing countries influence the epidemiology of STIs and help make them an important public health priority.

Incidence and prevalence rates of STIs are generally high in both urban and rural populations and vary considerably across areas. Because diagnosis and treatment of STIs are often delayed, inadequate, or both, rates of STI complications are also high in developing countries. Those complications include pelvic inflammatory disease, ectopic pregnancy, and chronic abdominal pain in women; adverse pregnancy outcomes, including abortion, intrauterine death, and premature delivery;

neonatal and infant infections and blindness in infants; infertility in both men and women; urethral strictures in men; genital malignancies, such as cancer of the cervix uteri, vulva, vagina, penis, and anus; arthritis secondary to gonorrhea and chlamydia; liver failure and liver cancer secondary to hepatitis B or human T cell lymphotropic virus type I; and central nervous system disease secondary to syphilis (Holmes and Aral 1991; Meheus, Schulz, and Cates 1990; van Dam, Dallabetta, and Piot 1999). Thus, STI sequelae affect mostly women and children.

In developing countries, high levels of STIs and high rates of complications and sequelae result largely from inadequacies in health service provision and health care seeking (Aral and Wasserheit 1999). STI care is provided by a large variety of health care providers, many of whom are poorly trained in STI case management, and the quality of care they provide is often less than desirable (Moses and others 1994; WHO 1991). Health care seeking for STIs is frequently inadequate, particularly among women (van Dam 1995), because of the low levels of awareness regarding sexual health, the stigmatization associated with genital symptoms, and the asymptomatic nature of many STIs. A study in Nairobi, Kenya, found that 42 percent of patients had been symptomatic for more than a week before coming to a clinic and that 23 percent had been symptomatic for more than two weeks (Moses and others 1994).

Setting up good-quality STI services is considerably more difficult in resource-poor settings than elsewhere. Variables that affect the duration of infectiousness include adequacy of health workers' training, attitudes of health workers toward such marginalized groups as sex workers, patient loads at health centers, availability of drugs and clinic supplies, and costs of care (Moses and others 2002). Thus, improvements pertaining to all these factors would greatly improve STI-related services, help reduce the duration of infectiousness, and decrease the incidence of STIs (Aral 2002a). However, in many countries in the developing world, worsened economic conditions and the increasing burden of HIV/AIDS have negatively affected these variables. For example, in South Africa, the ratio of hospital beds to population declined from 6.5 per 1,000 in 1976 to 2.3 in 1996; during 1999, approximately 300 professionally trained nurses left the country each month; and student enrollments in nursing school declined from 12,282 in 1996 to 10,398 in 1999 (Aral 2002a).

Sexual behaviors also contribute to the STI burden in developing countries. These behaviors are heavily influenced by the sociocultural, economic, and political contexts, which in the past two decades have deteriorated at an accelerated rate in many areas. Societal change has included rising levels of inequality within countries, growing inequality between countries, increased levels of globalization, increased proportions of people who live in cultures they were not born in, and a larger proportion of the world's population living in postconflict societies (Aral 2002a). One effect of these changes is an increase in multipartner sexual activity, which in turn increases the rate at which infected and susceptible individuals are sexually exposed to each other and consequently the rate at which STIs spread.

Changes in STI Epidemiology, Management, and Prevention since 1993

Since 1993, STI epidemiology and management have evolved interactively, particularly in developing countries. Technological advances in diagnosis, screening, and treatment; evaluation and widespread implementation of new case-management algorithms; and changes in risk behaviors in response to the AIDS epidemic have all influenced the dynamic typology of STIs (Wasserheit and Aral 1996).

The introduction of nucleic acid amplification tests, which have improved the sensitivity and expanded the repertoire of usable specimens, has heralded a new era in STI diagnosis. The use of urine and vaginal swabs in diagnosis has enabled providers to supply diagnostic and screening services outside traditional clinical facilities and has greatly enhanced the coverage of outreach activities (Schachter 2001). Unfortunately, many of these tests are currently too expensive for routine use in developing countries. Single-dose oral azithromycin has improved the treatment of several bacterial STIs (Lau and Qureshi 2002), but quinolones are apparently becoming ineffective for gonorrhea in some locations (Donovan 2004).

A major recent advance in STI prevention is the early success of a prophylactic, monovalent human papillomavirus (HPV) type 16 vaccine (Koutsky and others 2002); HPV vaccines may be able to help prevent genital and anal cancers in the foreseeable future. Researchers are evaluating multivalent vaccines for preventing moderate to severe cervical dysplasia as well. Other advances include easier episodic treatment of genital herpes (Strand and others 2002) and the use of suppressive therapy to reduce the transmission of genital herpes to regular partners (Corey and others 2004). In a related development, a prophylactic vaccine against herpes simplex virus type 2 (HSV-2) has shown limited efficacy in that it has proved partly effective for HSV-seronegative women, but not for men or herpes simplex virus type 1 (HSV-1) seropositive women (Stanberry and others 2002). Prevention successes of the recent past include STI sequelae, such as pelvic inflammatory disease and cervical cancer. A randomized controlled trial showed that selective screening of women for *Chlamydia trachomatis* significantly reduced the incidence of pelvic inflammatory disease (Scholes and others 1996).

Widespread implementation of syndromic management as an approach to STI case management has apparently had a considerable effect on the epidemiology of STIs, particularly in resource-poor settings (King Holmes and Michael Alary, personal communication, May 15, 2003).

In some developing countries, including Cambodia, the Dominican Republic, and Thailand, sexual risk behaviors have been changing over the past decade. In Uganda, for example, the age of sexual debut has increased, the frequency of sex with casual partners has decreased, and the use of condoms has increased (Stoneburner and Low-Beer 2004). During the 1990s, demographic and health surveys in 29 developing countries asked individuals if they had done anything to avoid AIDS (Low-Beer and Stoneburner 2003): almost 80 percent of men and 50 percent of women surveyed reported that they had. Specific behavior changes reported included increased monogamy, reduced number of partners, avoidance of sex workers, and increased condom use.

By contrast, in developed countries, recent years have seen behavior changes in the opposite direction; for example, in many European countries and in the United States, risk behaviors among men who have sex with men have increased significantly (CDC 2004; L. Doherty and others 2002). In addition, Grémy and Beltzer (2004) report declines in condom use among heterosexual adult populations in Europe. Investigators attribute increases in risk behaviors to the introduction and availability of antiretroviral therapy for HIV infection and the difficulties in sustaining preventive behaviors in the long term, referred to as *prevention fatigue*. Some researchers speculate that the widespread introduction of antiretroviral therapy in developing countries may have a similar disinhibitory effect on sexual behaviors and that changes in sexual behavior may offset the beneficial effect of antiretroviral therapy (Blower and others 2001; Blower and Farmer 2003; Blower and Volberding 2002; Over and others 2004).

Advances in STI prevention in recent decades have enhanced understanding of transmission dynamics and the role of interventions. Investigators have articulated the following five emergent insights about STI epidemiology and prevention over the past two decades:

- Populations consist of many diverse subpopulations, and each population-level epidemic trajectory consists of many distinct subpopulation epidemic trajectories (Pisani and others 2003). The epidemic trajectories of specific STIs differ depending on when and where the infection was introduced; the natural history and transmissibility of the infection; the structure of sexual networks; the demographic, economic, social, and epidemiological context; and the state of the health system (Aral and others 2005).
- Temporal dimensions are important in relation to STI epidemiology (Aral and Blanchard 2002). At the individual level, concurrency of partnerships and gaps between partnerships are risk factors for the acquisition and transmission of STIs (Adimora and others 2002; Agrawal, Gillespie, and Foxman 2001; Kraut and Aral 2001). At the population level, investigators have described the evolution of STI epidemics through sometimes predictable phases, characterized by changing patterns in the distribution and transmission of STI pathogens within and between subpopulations (UNAIDS and WHO 2000; Wasserheit and Aral 1996).
- Sexual networks are important in the transmission dynamics of STIs at the population level, and position in a sexual network is important in the transmission and acquisition of STIs at the individual level (Morris 2004).
- Trajectories whereby STI epidemics evolve differ for different types of population-pathogen interactions (Aral 2002a; Blanchard 2002; Garnett 2002). Whereas highly infectious, short-duration bacterial STIs—for instance, gonorrhea—depend on the presence of core groups marked by multiple sex partnerships of short duration for their spread, less infectious, long-duration viral STIs—for example, HSV—depend on the presence of multiple partnerships of longer duration.
- Interactions among sexually transmitted pathogens affect STI epidemic trajectories at the population level (Wasserheit 1991). The inconsistent findings of three landmark randomized community trials evaluating the effect of STI treatment on HIV transmission (Grosskurth and others 1995; Kamali and others 2003; Wawer and others 1999) can be accounted for by the complex, multifactorial, multilevel, and phase-specific nature of STI epidemics (Orroth 2003).

Epidemiology and Control

The epidemiology of STI pathogens, the local prevention and care infrastructure, and the cultural and sociopolitical context vary considerably within and across developing countries. At the same time, health care delivery for STIs varies by type of institution and location, although inadequate resources are universal in the developing world, as are recordkeeping, data management, and data analysis. The limited data that are available suggest that STIs are a major public health burden in the developing world. Although the prevalence and incidence of bacterial STIs have apparently declined because of expanded syndromic management, changes in sexual behavior, and death of high-risk populations, the prevalence and incidence of viral STIs seem to have increased over the past decade.

Syndromic Management. Health systems can use three different approaches to manage patients presenting with symptoms suggestive of an STI. First, etiology-based management relies on identifying causative micro-organisms or detecting specific antibodies. It requires costly and often technically complex laboratory diagnosis, trained personnel, quality assurance programs, and infrastructure. Second, clinical diagnosis–based management is rapid, inexpensive, and requires less infrastructure than etiology-based management; however, clinical diagnosis is often inaccurate, may miss multiple infections, and may result in undertreatment or overtreatment. Third, syndromic management, which is based on the recognition of a constellation of clinical signs and symptoms, is inexpensive, can be standardized, and can be used by both physicians and paramedical personnel, though it often results in some overtreatment. Nevertheless, syndromic management has been recommended as a realistic approach for managing symptomatic patients in developing countries (Over and Piot 1993). Implementation issues associated with the syndromic management approach involve inadequate local evaluation of treatment algorithms because of a lack of local data, inconsistencies in implementation, and inadequate monitoring (Dallabetta, Gerbase, and Holmes 1998; Hawkes and Santhya 2002; WHO 2001b).

Limitations of the syndromic management approach include the inability to directly target the subclinical STI pool, the variability of STI symptoms and signs, the potential for wasting antibiotics, the risk of promoting drug resistance, and the unintended consequence of decreasing the skill levels of health care providers (Dallabetta Gerbase, and Holmes 1998; Donovan 2004). Moreover, syndromic management tends to undermine STI surveillance efforts because cases are managed and treated in the absence of a specific clinical or laboratory diagnosis (O'Farrell 2002).

Role of Core Groups and Bridge Populations. Core groups—that is, groups of individuals who have large numbers of sex partners who themselves have large numbers of sex partners—play an important role in the spread and persistence of STIs and are characterized by a high prevalence of STIs. Examples of core groups include sex workers, drug users, truck drivers, and bar girls. Because a case treated or prevented in a core group member tends to prevent that person from infecting several others, interventions that target core groups tend to be more effective and more cost-effective than interventions that target the general population (Ainsworth and Over 1997; Over 1999; Over and Piot 1993). In situations in which a high prevalence of STIs is concentrated in core groups, so-called bridge populations (individuals who have sexual links with members of both high- and low-prevalence subpopulations) may play an important role in disseminating infection from core groups to the general population (Aral 2000; Aral and others 1999; Gorbach and others 2000; Morris and others 1996).

Several variables influence the relative importance of core groups in the spread of STIs, including the characteristics of the specific pathogen, such as its transmissibility and duration of infectiousness; the phase of a particular epidemic; and the duration of sexual partnerships among those involved in multipartner sexual activity (Aral 2002a, 2002b; Blanchard 2002; Garnett 2002; Wasserheit and Aral 1996). The role of core groups in STI dissemination tends to be greater during the initial and later phases of epidemics, when infection is highly concentrated in small, high-risk subpopulations, than during the middle phases of epidemics, when infection tends to be widely spread across subpopulations. The importance of core groups appears to be greater in populations in which most people are involved in sexual activity with a single partner and only a small minority of people engage in short-term sexual partnerships with a large number of sex partners (Laumann and Youm 1999).

Antibiotic Use and Drug Resistance. Antibiotic use is unregulated in many developing countries, and antibiotics are frequently misused and overused, which results in drug resistance. Resistance to antimicrobial drugs is increasing mortality and morbidity from infectious diseases (Hart and Kariuki 1998). STIs are among the most frequently occurring infections worldwide, with more than 76 percent estimated to occur in the developing world (WHO 2001a). *Neisseria gonorrhoeae* has shown great versatility in developing resistance to antimicrobial drugs, including sulfonamides, penicillins, and tetracycline. Fluoroquinolones such as ciprofloxacin and ofloxacin have proved highly effective in treating gonorrhea, but after widespread and often inappropriate use of fluoroquinolones, resistant *N. gonorrhoeae* has emerged. In some areas, such resistance leaves third-generation cephalosporins as the only predictably effective antibiotic treatment for gonorrhea.

STIs and HIV/AIDS. Because HIV is a sexually transmitted infection, people who are infected with another STI also tend to be at increased risk of HIV infection and vice versa. However, beyond this correlation resulting from common risk behaviors, STIs and HIV may facilitate each other's transmission.

BACTERIAL AND VIRAL STIs AND THEIR SEQUELAE

Both bacterial and viral STIs are widespread in developing countries; recently, incidence of bacterial STIs has declined while that of viral STIs has been increasing.

Natural History of Bacterial STIs and Their Sequelae

Chancroid is a genital ulcer disease caused by *Haemophilus ducreyi*. Its incidence has declined greatly in both developed and developing countries. This decline has been associated with the provision of STI diagnostic and therapeutic services to sex workers (Steen 2001) and with improved syndromic management of genital ulcers. Like other genital ulcer diseases, chancroid is associated with increased acquisition and transmission of HIV (Donovan 2004).

Syphilis is a genital ulcer disease caused by *Treponema pallidum*. In 1999, the World Health Organization (WHO) estimated the global prevalence of syphilis at 12 million (WHO 2001a), with high prevalence rates in South and Southeast Asia and Sub-Saharan Africa. Those most likely to be affected are populations in developing countries and disadvantaged subpopulations in developed countries. Since 1999, syphilis outbreaks have reemerged in many developed countries among men who have sex with men (CDC 2004; L. Doherty and others 2002). Among heterosexuals, sexual contact with sex workers is an important risk factor. If untreated, syphilis during pregnancy may lead to stillbirth and congenital syphilis (Genc and Ledger 2000).

Gonorrhea is a discharge disease caused by *N. gonorrhoeae*. In 1999, WHO estimated its global prevalence at 62.4 million (WHO 2001a). Like syphilis, its prevalence is high in South and Southeast Asia and Sub-Saharan Africa, in many developing countries elsewhere, and among high-risk groups and disadvantaged subpopulations in developed countries. Community surveys reveal a substantial pool of asymptomatic gonococcal infections (Chandeying and others 2000; Turner and others 2002). Following the emergence of AIDS, gonorrhea cases declined among men having sex with men, sex workers, and the general population in the developed world and among sex workers in many developing countries (Donovan 2004).

In most populations tested, infection with *Chlamydia trachomatis* is the most common bacterial STI. In 1999, WHO estimated the global prevalence of chlamydial infection to be 92 million (WHO 2001a). Chlamydial infection is common in most countries, especially among young people. Key risk factors are being younger than 25 and having a new sex partner. Many women with uncomplicated infection are asymptomatic or have mild symptoms. Like untreated gonococcal infection, untreated chlamydial infection can cause pelvic inflammatory disease, chronic pelvic pain, and ectopic pregnancy. Chlamydial infection is an important acquired cause of infertility in women (Simms and Stephenson 2000). Roughly half of men with urethral chlamydial infection develop symptomatic urethritis, chlamydial infection is the most common cause of epididymitis in young men, and both men and women may develop chlamydial conjunctivitis or reactive arthritis (Stamm 1999). Research also suggests that chlamydial infection in men may be associated with reduced fecundity among couples (Idahl and others 2004). In addition, chlamydial infection can affect neonates: many delivered vaginally become infected, developing conjunctivitis or, less often, chlamydia pneumonia (Donovan 2004). The role of *C. trachomatis* in preterm births and in cervical cancer awaits further clarification through research (Samoff and others 2004; Wallin and others 2002).

In the absence of control programs, the prevalence of *Trichomonas vaginalis* varies greatly across countries, ranging from less than 1 percent among urban women to more than 20 percent in underserved populations in the same country (Brown and Brown 2000), and may increase with age. WHO estimated the global prevalence of *T. vaginalis* at 174 million in 1999. The introduction of nucleic acid amplification tests highlighted the poor sensitivity of microscopy in the detection of *T. vaginalis*. Even though most infected people are asymptomatic, *T. vaginalis* can cause vaginitis with vaginal discharge in women and urethritis in men. *T. vaginalis* has been associated with preterm birth and may promote the sexual transmission of HIV (Laga and others 1993). However, a randomized controlled trial did not show that screening and treatment for *T. vaginalis* to prevent preterm birth were effective (Klebanoff and others 2001).

Like *T. vaginalis,* bacterial vaginosis and vulvovaginal candidiasis cause vaginal symptoms in women, are extremely prevalent in developing countries, and in one or more studies have been associated with HIV acquisition or HIV genital shedding by women (Donovan 2004). Although often referred to as reproductive tract infections rather than STIs, they are managed in conjunction with STIs, and bacterial vaginosis is associated with some of the same risk factors as other STIs.

Viral STIs and Their Sequelae

Both HSV-1 and HSV-2 infect the genital and anal areas, but HSV-2 causes the most clinical recurrences in the genital tract. Symptoms are mild in most of those infected and tend to go unrecognized and undiagnosed (Corey 2000; Scoular 2002). Genital herpes establishes a lifelong infection that in some people is associated with significant morbidity. Complications of

HSV-2 include severe primary disease, meningitis, hepatitis, erythema multiforme, and neonatal herpes (Donovan 2004). Infected neonates may die or develop severe neurological sequelae despite antiviral therapy. In contrast to bacterial STIs, HSV-2 may be transmitted to sex partners many years after initial infection and during periods when the infected individual may be asymptomatic. Infection with HSV-2 is now one of the most common STIs worldwide and is the most frequent cause of genital ulcers in almost all areas; however, this observation may be related to better diagnostic technologies rather than a genuine alteration in the spectrum of genital ulcer disease (Corey and Handsfield 2000). Improved control of chancroid and syphilis as well as actual increases in the sexual transmission of HSV-2 in areas with advanced HIV epidemics, where HIV-related immunosuppression causes more frequent and more severe HSV-2 disease, may also play a role. Estimates indicate that 10 to 30 percent of adults worldwide are infected with HSV-2 (Brugha and others 1997). Prevalence increases with age and is higher in women and high-risk populations.

HPV types are grouped into low-risk (nononcogenic) and high-risk (oncogenic) types. Low-risk types, including types 6 and 11, cause benign anogenital warts, whereas high-risk types, including HPV 16, 18, 31, and 45, occasionally lead to genital and anal squamous cell cancers. The introduction of nucleic acid amplification tests revealed that genital and anal HPV infection is common even among relatively sexually inexperienced individuals (Giuliano and others 2002; Stone and others 2002). Investigators believe that most adults become infected with HPV but that only a few develop warts or genital or anal cancer. Infection with a high-risk HPV type is implicated in nearly all cases of invasive cervical cancer (Walboomers and others 1999) and with vaginal, vulvar, and anal cancers.

In developed countries, hepatitis B virus is spread predominantly by sexual and injecting drug-use transmission. Indeed, the first three trials of hepatitis B vaccine successfully demonstrated prevention of sexual transmission of hepatitis B virus in men who have sex with men (Manhart and Holmes 2005). In developing countries, hepatitis B is more often acquired perinatally or during childhood, but a rise in seroincidence in adolescence and young adulthood in some countries probably reflects sexual or injecting drug-use transmission. Hepatitis B virus causes acute hepatitis and in some people causes chronic hepatitis that can lead to cirrhosis and liver cancer.

Human T cell lymphotropic virus type I (and perhaps in more cases type II) is, like hepatitis B virus, transmitted perinatally and sexually. In some high-risk populations, for example, female sex workers in Latin America, human T cell lymphotropic virus type I infection is substantially more common than HIV infection. This infection causes a serious form of spastic paralysis or human T cell lymphotropic-associated myelopathy, as well as T cell lymphoma or leukemia.

Coinfection with Sexually Transmitted Pathogens

The epidemiology and natural history of coinfection with more than one sexually transmitted pathogen may have important intervention and economic implications. Coverage by clinical services, outreach, access, partner management, and treatment may be different with coinfection than with independent infections. Although coinfections with HIV and other STIs have received a great deal of attention in recent years, researchers have not focused on overlaps among non-HIV STIs in a similar systematic manner. A number of biological mechanisms may lead to coinfection with STIs: infection with one pathogen may increase the probability of acquiring or transmitting another pathogen; infection with one pathogen may increase or decrease the frequency, the severity, or both of symptoms associated with another sexually transmitted pathogen; and presence of one STI may affect the natural history of another STI. High-risk behaviors and networks often lead to coinfection.

Empirical data on coinfection are limited. Most studies have been conducted in developed countries and have focused on co-occurrences of chlamydial and gonococcal infection. Earlier studies of coinfection assessed the proportion of gonorrhea cases with concurrent chlamydial infection in a variety of clinical settings. Reported levels of coinfection were 4 to 64 percent among attendees at STI clinics, 46 percent among prenatal clinic attendees, and 4 to 25 percent at primary health care facilities (Creighton and others 2003). The proportion of those with chlamydia who also have gonorrhea has been assessed less well, and estimates have ranged between 3 and 4 percent (Creighton and others 2003).

Sexual Behavior and Sexual Health Care

Unprotected sex with an infected partner is the most important risk factor for acquiring an STI. This risk is influenced by the behaviors of the individual and the probability that the partner is infected, which is determined by the prevalence and distribution of infection in the population as well as the partner's behaviors. Current approaches to STI epidemiology recognize at least three distinct components of transmission dynamics at the population level: likelihood of sexual exposure between infected and uninfected individuals, transmissibility of infection upon exposure between an infected and an uninfected person, and duration of infection among those infected (Aral and Holmes 1999; Over and Piot 1993). The first of these components is entirely behavioral, and behavior plays an important role in the last two—for example, condom use, sexual practices, and health care–seeking behaviors.

Demographic and Social Risk Markers. The prevalence and incidence of STIs vary across societies and subpopulations defined by age, gender, race and ethnicity, and socioeconomic status (Fenton, Johnson, and Nicoll 1997). In all societies, adolescents and young people are at greater risk for acquiring most STIs. Women tend to have a higher prevalence and incidence of all STIs (except for men who have sex with men) and suffer more of the serious complications, such as pelvic inflammatory disease, ectopic pregnancy, infertility, and chronic abdominal pain. For many STIs, the probability of transmission from an infected man to a susceptible woman is higher than from an infected woman to a susceptible man. Social and behavioral patterns also increase women's vulnerability to STIs; for instance, many men have concurrent sex partnerships, which increase their risk for transmitting infection to their female sex partners. In addition, many young women have sex with older male partners, who expose them to the higher STI prevalence rates in older age groups.

In most societies, minority racial ethnic groups have higher STI rates than other groups. Both in the United Kingdom (Fenton, Johnson, and Nicoll 1997) and in the United States (Laumann and Youm 1999), assortative sexual mixing and higher rates of sexual mixing with members of core groups emerge as determinants of ethnicity differentials in STI rates. The prevalence of concurrent partnerships is also higher among racial ethnic minorities (Kraut-Becher and Aral 2003). The relative inadequacy of STI health services and of health care–seeking behaviors among minority racial ethnic groups may also contribute to their higher prevalence of STIs (Aral and Wasserheit 1999).

Socioeconomic status differentials in STI prevalence and incidence are similar to ethnicity differentials. However, the multicollinearity between the two factors makes delineating the independent contributions of either variable to differentials in STI prevalence and incidence difficult.

Behavioral Risk Factors for Exposure to Infected Sex Partners. Most sexual behaviors of individuals are associated with exposure to sex partners infected with sexually transmitted pathogens and, consequently, with acquisition of STI. These behavioral factors include number of sex partners over the individual's lifetime, over the past year, and over a short term (Fenton and others 2001; Laumann and Youm 1999); frequency or number of sexual encounters (Garnett and Rottingen 2001); having sex with members of groups with high STI prevalence, such as core groups and sex workers (Fenton and others 2001; Laumann and Youm 1999) or older age groups (Service and Blower 1996); and position in a sexual network (I. A. Doherty and others 2005). Some sexual behaviors of individuals are associated with transmission of STIs, and for those infected the behaviors increase the probability that people will transmit their infections to susceptible sex partners. These behaviors include having concurrent partnerships (Koumans and others 2001; Kraut-Becher and Aral 2003; Morris and Kretzchmar 1995) and having short gaps between sex partners in serial monogamous partnerships (Kraut-Becher and Aral 2003).

Sex partners' behaviors are also critical determinants of exposure to infection. Investigators use many behavioral and epidemiological indicators to assess partners' risk of having infection, including existence and number of new sex partners; presence of concurrent partnerships; gap between sex partners; partners' number of partners; and risk status of partners' partners—for example, if they have sex with sex workers or men who have sex with men (Aral 2002b).

Behavioral Risk Factors Associated with STI Acquisition and Transmission on Exposure to Infected Partners. Certain behaviors influence the likelihood of an infected person's transmitting infection to a susceptible partner, including condom use, sexual practices such as anal intercourse, vaginal douching, and use of drying agents in the vagina (Bailey, Plummer, and Moses 2001; Donovan 2000a, 2000b). The probability of transmission varies depending on the pathogen and is much higher for bacterial STIs, such as gonorrhea, syphilis, and chlamydia, than for other STIs, such as HIV infection. Thus, preventive behaviors such as condom use may be more effective in preventing the latter than the former (National Institute for Allergy and Infectious Diseases 2001). In addition, the probability of both acquisition and transmission is significantly affected by such nonbehavioral cofactors as circumcision status (Aral and Holmes 1999).

Overall, oral sex and anal sex tend to be practiced less often in the developing world than in the developed world (Vos 1994). Insertion of herbs to tighten or dry the vagina and other practices of vaginal clearing and wiping are widespread (Brown and Brown 2000). Condom use is increasing in some countries—for example, India, Thailand, and Uganda—especially during high-risk encounters.

Behaviors Associated with the Duration of Infectiousness. The duration of infectiousness is an important component of transmission dynamics. Because effective treatment curtails the duration of curable STIs, the speed with which infected individuals seek treatment and the speed and effectiveness with which health care providers supply effective treatment together determine duration. To the extent that suppressive therapies truncate the period of infectiousness of viral STIs, as they do for HSV-2 and HIV infection, duration is also important in the transmission dynamics of incurable viral STIs.

Behaviors that can reduce the average duration of infectiousness include timely and appropriate health care seeking, effective participation in risk assessment, and compliance with therapy and prevention recommendations on the part of those infected and at risk (Aral and Wasserheit 1999). Health care seeking depends on perceived seriousness and causality of symptoms, availability and accessibility of health care, costs (including opportunity costs) of treatment, perceived and actual quality of care, and beliefs about the appropriate provider to consult. The proportion of those infected seeking care is highly variable, and delays in seeking treatment can be substantial. In many places, the proportion of people seeking timely care from appropriately trained providers is limited (Hawkes and Santhya 2002; Moses and others 2002; Rekart 2002).

Behaviors on the part of health care providers that ensure timely and accurate diagnosis, appropriate treatment, and nonjudgmental attitudes toward those infected would also help reduce the duration of infectiousness of STIs. However, establishing effective, accessible, affordable, and decentralized services is difficult (Over 2004; World Bank 2003). The major barriers Moses and others (2002) identified in Nairobi reflect the situation in many developing countries. Those barriers include inadequate basic training and inefficient deployment of health workers; attitudes of health workers toward marginalized groups (for instance, female sex workers); high patient loads at health centers; lack of supportive supervision; inadequate referral systems; chronic shortages of supplies and drugs; and inadequate recording of health information. User fees can be a substantial additional barrier, though they may contribute to the sustainability of the treatment program and improve the provider's incentives.

Behavioral Interactions. Both at the individual and the population levels, people's risk behaviors respond to changing circumstances. In many developing countries where HIV incidence has been high, people have adopted compensatory behavior changes, such as delayed age of sexual debut, reduced number of sex partners, and increased use of condoms (Shelton and others 2004; Stoneburner and Low-Beer 2004), especially with high-risk partners (Peterman and others 2000). Some people now seek health care when they suspect they have been exposed to an STI.

At the same time, risk behaviors can overlap: people who initiate sexual activity early in life tend to have many partners, and people who engage in risky sex tend to also use drugs and alcohol. A history of sexual abuse or of being an abuser is also positively associated with high-risk sexual behaviors and drug use (Aral 2004). The adoption of preventive behaviors raises the possibility that people will compensate by changing other behaviors in response; for example, many believe that the widespread adoption of antiviral therapy or condom use may lead to increases in the numbers of sex partners (Blower and others 2001; Blower and Farmer 2003; Over and others 2004). Although constructing mathematical models to explore the effects of such changes in behavior is helpful, empirical research in varied contexts is urgently needed to identify the variables that determine patterns of interaction among risky and preventive behaviors. Two such variables may be individual autonomy and awareness of the epidemiological context.

Societal Determinants of STIs. Sexual networks and patterns of sexual partnership formation and dissolution constitute a major mechanism through which the political economy and the sociolegal system influence the rate of spread of STIs in a population. Sexual networks that are highly critical to the rate of spread of STIs include those involving sex work; exchange of sex for drugs, gifts, or material needs; and anonymous sex. The frequency of sex in exchange for money or other goods appears to be highly sensitive to changes in the political economy and the sociolegal system. Internal conflicts, war, economic crises, and social collapse are accompanied by the establishment of major sex markets or the expansion of existing ones. For example, following the collapse of the former Soviet Union, the number and size of commercial sex and sex-drug networks expanded significantly (Aral and St. Lawrence 2002; Aral and others 2005). The availability and use of condoms also influence the rate of spread of STIs.

Many developing countries continuously face political conflict, war, economic deterioration, mass migration, and increasing inequality plus the effect of globalization. In addition, in most developing societies, gender power relationships are marked by great inequality. Those contextual factors lead to sexual networks and sexual mixing patterns that are highly conducive to the spread of STIs. Sexual partnerships are often not stable, and in the long-term absence of a spouse, both men and women (but especially men) have other partners.

In addition, as economic needs rise, the number of women who exchange sex for material needs increases. Wilson and others (1989) estimate that approximately 10 percent of the female population in Bulawayo, Zimbabwe, had engaged in full- or part-time sex work at some time in their lives, whereas Aral and St. Lawrence's (2002) estimates for Saratov, Russian Federation, are closer to 25 percent. As the supply of sex workers increases, the demand for their services often increases in parallel. Economic need also affects sexual mixing patterns. In most developing countries, young girls commonly have "sugar daddies"—that is, older, often married men who provide them with material goods in return for sex while also exposing them to chronic STIs typical of relatively older cohorts (Gregson and others 2002).

Gender inequalities put women in a highly vulnerable position in many ways. For example, Decosas and Padian (2002) find that, among women attending family-planning and primary health care clinics in Zimbabwe, 17 percent had at some time received a gift in exchange for sex, 22 percent had been forced to have sex with a steady partner, 5 percent had been forced to have sex with a nonsteady partner, 35 percent were certain their steady partner had other partners, 27 percent said their partners had STI symptoms, 24 percent said their partner was intoxicated during sexual intercourse more than half the time, and only 10 percent had used a condom in the previous three months.

Income and Inequality. A cross-country database (George Schmid, personal communication, September 15, 2004) enables us to analyze the association between national STI prevalence rates and two important economic variables: gross national income per capita and the degree of income inequality as measured by the Gini coefficient.[1] As table 17.1 shows, these two variables explain 45 percent of the variation in STI prevalence in low-risk groups and 16 percent of STI prevalence in high-risk groups. Figure 17.1 illustrates the relationship between each of these two economic variables and STI prevalence.

Poor countries' higher prevalence rates of STIs are unsurprising and could be explained by the fact that people in richer countries are likely to seek and find care for STIs more quickly. More notable is that income inequality is such a strong predictor of STI prevalence even after controlling for gross national income per capita. Furthermore, income inequality is a strong predictor of STI prevalence among high-risk groups, where income per capita performs less well. A possible explanation for this finding is that greater inequality creates more active markets for commercial and casual sex as higher-income men negotiate for the sexual services of lower-income sex workers (Aral 2002b; Over 1998).

Table 17.1 Cross-Country Regressions of Average STI Prevalence on Per Capita Income and the Gini Coefficient of Inequality for Low- and High-Risk Groups, Selected Countries

Category	Average prevalence of STIs in low-risk groups	Average prevalence of STIs in high-risk groups
Gross national income purchasing power parity per capita, log, 19–2001	−0.862**	−0.194+
Gini index, 1990s	7.731**	2.73*
Dummy for syphilis	0.093	−0.051
Dummy for chlamydia	1.992**	0.308
Dummy for herpes	3.611**	1.507**
Constant	−0.515	−1.751
R^2	0.45	0.16
Number of countries	204	147

Source: Authors' calculations from Schmid and others 2004.

Note: * = probability of less than 0.05 percent; ** = probability of less than 0.01 percent. Positive numbers indicate a probability of 0.1 to 0.2 percent. Both regressions pool data across these STIs: syphilis, chlamydia, and herpes. The coefficients of the dummies show that the estimated prevalence rates are significantly higher for herpes than for the other diseases. Among low-risk groups, the prevalence of chlamydia is higher than that of syphilis. Standard errors (not shown) are estimated using the White correction for heteroskedasticity under the assumption that the observations for a single country are comparable to a cluster of data. Other explanatory variables that were unsuccessful in explaining a significant proportion of the variance included percentage of the population foreign born, percentage of the population that is Muslim, male-to-female literacy gap, urban male-to-female population ratio, and military personnel per 1,000 urban population.

a. Gross national income per capita

Average national prevalence of STIs among low-risk groups
(deviations from mean)

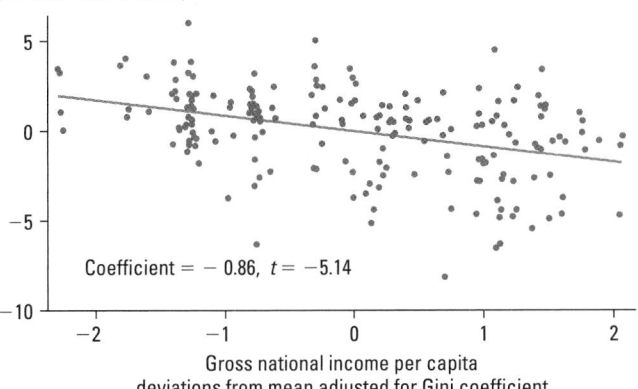

Coefficient = −0.86, t = −5.14

Gross national income per capita
deviations from mean adjusted for Gini coefficient

b. Income inequality

Average national prevalence of STIs among low-risk groups
(deviations from mean)

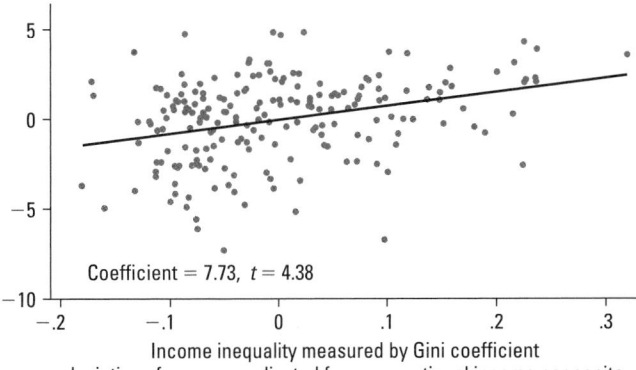

Coefficient = 7.73, t = 4.38

Income inequality measured by Gini coefficient
deviations from mean adjusted for gross national income per capita

Source: Authors' calculations based on personal communication with George Schmid
(April 5, 2004).

Figure 17.1 Association between Per Capita Income and Income
Inequality with STI Prevalence for Low-Risk Groups, Selected
Countries

BURDEN OF STIs AND BENEFITS OF CONTROL

On the basis of an independent analysis of cross-country data
on STI prevalence, we believe that WHO may have underestimated the burden of STIs relative to that of HIV and other diseases (www.fic.nih.gov/dcpp/gbd.html). Adjusting the WHO
estimates on the basis of our calculations increases the estimate
of years of life lost burden by about 18.1 percent and the overall estimate of disability-adjusted life years (DALYs) lost by
about 8.2 percent.

DALYs Gained from Effectively Preventing or Treating STIs

In the first edition of this volume, chapter 20 presented estimates of the so-called static and dynamic burdens of preventing or curing a single case of an STI and of HIV (Over and Piot
1993). We reproduce those estimates in table 17.2 for four of
the STIs.[2] The static benefit column estimates the average
number of DALYs saved for a single person by curing or preventing his or her own case of each disease. These estimates
are based on specific assumptions regarding the distribution of
incidence, case-fatality rates, and severity across age ranges.
Although updating these estimates to 2004 and varying them
by region would ideally be possible, we have not found any
more recent data. If the person who is cured of an STI ceases to
be sexually active, the static benefit would be the only benefit of
curing or preventing his or her case; however, most individuals
who have contracted an STI remain sexually active and are
therefore likely to communicate that STI to others. An STI
prevented or cured in a sexually active person will prevent
additional cases in that person's sex partners, in the sex partners' partners, and so on. Thus, the dynamic benefit columns
indicate the magnitude of those additional benefits.

The key finding is that preventing or curing a case of any
of the STIs in a core group member generates approximately

Table 17.2 Discounted DALYs Saved Per Case Prevented or Cured

STI	Static benefits	Dynamic benefits		Total benefits	
		Member of noncore group	Member of core group	Member of noncore group	Member of core group
Chancroid	0.2	0.2	1.6	0.4	1.8
Chlamydia	1.1	4.4	43.0	5.5	44.1
Gonorrhea	0.9	3.6	36.4	4.5	37.3
Syphilis	3.8	16.0	157.0	19.8	160.8
For comparison					
HIV without ulcers	19.5	35.1	340.1	54.6	359.6
HIV with ulcers	19.5	39.2	410.7	58.7	430.2

Source: Over and Piot 1993, table 20-16, appendix 20B.

10 times the dynamic benefits of the same intervention in a person in a noncore group. This result is driven by the assumption that a member of a noncore group has a new sexual contact every 50 days, or about seven new contacts per year, whereas a member of a core group has 10 times as many contacts. Within this model, the results are proportional to the frequency of partner change, so that the dynamic benefits of curing or preventing a case in a sex worker who has two partners a day would be approximately 10 times as great as for a member of the core group in table 17.2. The implication is that preventing or curing a case of syphilis in a sex worker can result in up to 1,600 DALYs of benefit, a health effect that is likely to be competitive with any discussed in the other chapters in this volume.

Impact of STIs on HIV

The preceding discussion does not address the possibility that STI infections increase HIV transmission. On this point the evidence is mixed, with a study in Mwanza, Tanzania (Grosskurth and others 1995), demonstrating a statistically significant 40 percent reduction in HIV incidence attributable to an STI intervention, while two studies (Kamali and others 2003; Wawer and others 1999) in Uganda failed to show any such effect. Recent reanalyses (Orroth 2003) of the data from these studies suggest that the effect of an STI intervention on an HIV epidemic will vary depending on the sexual activity and resulting prevalence of STIs among those being treated.

None of the randomized controlled trials of the effect of STI treatment on HIV prevention exclusively targeted the most sexually active people in the community. In Mwanza, Tanzania, and Masaka, Uganda, treatment was provided to those who sought it at health care clinics. In Rakai, Uganda, treatment was given to all adults in all households, regardless of whether the individual complained of STI symptoms. Data on the prevalence of HIV infection in the three communities suggest that the HIV and STI epidemics were both at an earlier stage in Mwanza and were therefore more concentrated among those more sexually active. Thus, the people who became symptomatic and sought treatment were among the most sexually active people in Mwanza, and treating them would therefore have had a greater effect on HIV incidence than would treating an average person in the two Ugandan sites. Conversely, in the more generalized epidemics in Uganda, a larger proportion of new infections occurred within stable HIV-1 serodiscordant couples.

An alternative, less rigorous way to test for the effect of STI prevalence on HIV infection is to study the cross-sectional correlation in ecological data. In a replication of an earlier study (Over 1998), we have attempted to explain urban HIV prevalence in a cross-country sample by the prevalence of syphilis and gonorrhea seven years earlier after controlling for six other potentially confounding variables. The results of these cross-

country regressions are presented in table 17.3.[3] Columns (1) and (2) of table 17.3 present the results of regressions estimated on the subsets of countries for which data are available on all eight explanatory variables and on the dependent variable (2002 urban HIV prevalence). Their specifications differ only by the replacement of the prevalence of syphilis as an explanatory variable in column (1) with the prevalence of gonorrhea in column (2). Columns (3) and (4) repeat the same two regressions by replacing missing values of the two prevalence rates with estimates that are based on a regression of these rates on the other variables in the regression. This procedure expands the samples dramatically from 56 and 38 to 181 and 180, respectively.[4]

In interpreting these regressions, note first that all four specifications explain more than half of the variance in 2002 urban HIV prevalence, a remarkably good fit for cross-sectional regressions. In all these specifications, the lagged value of an STI prevalence is a statistically significant predictor of HIV prevalence approximately seven years later. The coefficient for gonorrhea is larger than the coefficient for syphilis and is more statistically significant in the augmented sample, though less so in the basic sample.

After the age of the epidemic is controlled for, several other variables contribute to explaining the variation in HIV prevalence. These variables include national income per capita (richer countries have lower infection rates), the percentage of the population that is Muslim (a higher percentage is associated with lower infection rates), and the ratio of males to females in the sexually active age range (higher ratios are associated with higher infection rates).

The major difference between the regressions using the augmented sample and those using the basic sample is in the statistical significance of the estimated coefficient of income inequality as measured by the Gini coefficient. When the sample is expanded to take advantage of the available data, the coefficient stabilizes at about 5.3 and is statistically significant at the 0.01 probability value, suggesting that an increased degree of income inequality is associated with increased HIV infection even after controlling for STI prevalence. This result lends support to the idea that income inequality is just as important as poverty in setting the stage for HIV transmission.

As with the results of any ecological or cross-sectional analysis, questions of attribution and interpretation arise. Is the statistically significant coefficient of syphilis or gonorrhea capturing a biological effect of an STI on increasing the transmission probability during sexual intercourse? Or is the coefficient instead simply reflecting the fact that greater sexual activity spreads all STIs, including gonorrhea, syphilis, and HIV? Is the coefficient of the percentage of the population that is Muslim capturing differential sexual activity or the prevalence of male circumcision, which is increasingly recognized as biologically protective? A biological interpretation of both the STI and the Muslim coefficients is suggested by the fact that the variable

Table 17.3 Multiple Regression of circa 2002 Urban HIV Prevalence on circa 1995 STI Prevalence and Other Socioeconomic Variables

Category	(1) Basic sample with syphilis	(2) Basic sample with gonorrhea	(3) Augmented sample with syphilis	(4) Augmented sample with gonorrhea
Age of epidemic (urban low) in 2002[a]	0.177 (4.07)***	0.131 (2.00)*	0.12 (2.90)***	0.08 (1.70)*
Per capita national income, median 1996–2001	−1.344 (2.82)***	−1.177 (2.30)**	−0.929 (3.63)***	−0.949 (4.45)***
Income equality, Gini index, 1990s	0.125 (0.04)	3.186 (0.83)	5.349 (2.77)***	5.258 (2.79)***
Percentage of the population that is Muslim, 1999	−0.026 (4.05)***	−0.031 (3.50)***	−0.015 (3.45)***	−0.02 (4.10)***
Urban male-to-female ratio for those age 20–39, 1999	6.178 (2.03)**	6.199 (1.40)	3.27 (1.29)	3.038 (1.19)
Urban high-risk population dummy (1 if yes, 0 is no)	1.17 (2.83)***	0.564 (0.85)	0.894 (2.64)***	0.37 (0.71)
Logit syphilis in low-risk group, 1995[b]	0.31 (2.46)**		0.233 (1.78)*	
Logit gonorrhea in low-risk group, 1995[b]		0.502 (1.92)*		0.479 (1.86)*
Constant	0.297 (0.05)	−0.791 (0.11)	−2.117 (0.63)	0.054 (0.02)
Number of observations	56	38	181	180
Number of countries	40	29	101	100
R^2	0.57	0.56	0.5	0.51

Source: Authors' calculations. Syphilis and gonorrhea prevalence in 1995 (George Schmid, personal communication, April 5, 2004). HIV prevalence circa 2002 is from the urban low-risk tables in the U.S. Bureau of Census database on HIV prevalence. Other variables are from World Bank data.
* = significant at 10 percent; ** = significant at 5 percent; *** = significant at 1 percent.
Note: The figures in parentheses are robust *t*-statistics.
a. *Age of epidemic* is defined as the number of years since the first case of HIV/AIDS was reported.
b. The logarithm of the ratio of the prevalence to 1 minus the prevalence of the given STI for the low risk population in 1995.

urban male-to-female ratio is probably already capturing much of the variation in the most risky sexual behavior: the practice of prostitution.

Increasing the availability of treatment for STIs and for HIV infection reduces the prevalence of the former and increases the prevalence of the latter. Thus, this statistical relationship between STI prevalence and HIV prevalence, even if once valid, will no longer obtain. Under current conditions, estimating the effect of a change in the prevalence rate of an STI on the incidence rate of HIV would be more relevant.

If we assume that in 2002 the HIV epidemic was approaching equilibrium in many urban settings and that prior to antiretroviral treatment the median duration of the illness was about 10 years, the prevalence of HIV infection is approximately equal to 10 times the incidence rate. Thus, a 10 percentage point increase in the prevalence of syphilis or gonorrhea is estimated to increase the incidence of HIV by 0.27 percentage points for syphilis and 0.57 for gonorrhea. For comparisons,

the Mwanza trial found that a reduction in the prevalence of male urethritis of 0.6 percent was associated with a decrease of 0.7 percent in the incidence of HIV (Grosskurth and others 1995). Thus, the present study suggests an effect about one-fourth as strong as that of the Mwanza study.

EFFECTIVENESS OF THE PRINCIPAL INTERVENTIONS

Unlike HIV interventions, STI interventions benefit from a large body of rigorous evaluations. STI interventions that have been rigorously evaluated for effectiveness can be organized by intervention level (that is, individual, group, or community); by the outcomes measured; and by the intervention modality used (for example, behavior change, vaccination, topical microbicide use, screening, or treatment). Prevention outcomes may measure the prevention of acquisition, of transmission, and of complications of STIs (Manhart and Holmes 2005). This section reviews the interventions for which the strongest evidence exists.

Individual-Level Interventions

A large number of STI interventions that have been rigorously evaluated are individual-level interventions.

Preventing Acquisition. The following have been the main means of preventing STI acquisition:

- *Behavior change.* Counseling on risk reduction was the most frequently used behavior-change approach. Most studies showed a reduction in risk behaviors as a result of counseling, and some showed decreases in STI outcomes (Kamb and others 1998).
- *Antimicrobial prophylaxis.* Two studies (Harrison and others 1979; Kaul and others 2004) showed reductions in the incidence of gonococcal, chlamydial, or trichomonal infections following antimicrobial prophylaxis.
- *Vaccines and passive immunization.* A yeast-derived HPV type 16 vaccine was 100 percent efficacious in preventing persistent HPV-16 infection in young college women (Koutsky and others 2002), and a bivalent HPV type 16 and type 18 vaccine was also highly efficacious in preventing those infections. An HSV-2 glycoprotein D-adjuvant vaccine among those with no serological evidence of prior HSV-1 infection partially protected women, but not men, from experiencing genital herpes disease, with 73 percent efficacy for such women in one trial and 74 percent in another (Stanberry and others 2002).
- *Microbicides.* To date, studies have not identified any efficacious topical microbicides.
- *Male circumcision.* Even though cross-sectional evidence suggesting that male circumcision decreases the risk of acquiring chancroid and HIV is strong, outcome data are not yet available from ongoing randomized trials in Kenya, South Africa, and Uganda.

Preventing Transmission. All individual-level interventions aimed at preventing transmission have involved curative or suppressive therapy. Giving tinidazole to male partners of females treated for vaginal trichomoniasis infections significantly reduced recurrences in the females; administering valacyclovir to positive members of HSV-2 serodiscordant couples reduced the incidence of symptomatic genital herpes and HSV-2 seroconversion in the uninfected partners; patient-delivered therapy to partners of women with chlamydial infection demonstrated a nonsignificant trend toward reduced risk of reinfection with *C. trachomatis*; and expedited partner therapy (usually patient delivered) significantly reduced persistent

or recurrent gonococcal or chlamydial infection in the index patient (Golden and others 2005).

Preventing Complications. Risk-based screening for *C. trachomatis* infection resulted in a 56 percent reduction in the subsequent risk of incident pelvic inflammatory disease (Scholes and others 1996). Several trials have shown that antiviral suppression decreases clinical and virological recurrences of genital herpes (Corey and Handsfield 2000).

Group-Level Interventions

Studies of behavior-change methods in small-group settings to reduce the acquisition of STIs had mixed outcomes. Behavior-change approaches resulted in significant reduction in incident STIs; antimicrobial prophylaxis and provision of female condoms did not.

Community-Level Interventions

Four community-level randomized trials have sought to reduce the prevalence and transmission of STIs by shortening the duration of infectiousness within the general population (Manhart and Holmes 2005).

The "Mema Kwa Vigara" study in Mwanza, Tanzania, randomized 20 communities to intervention and control communities. The intervention consisted of school-based sexual and reproductive health education, enhanced reproductive health services for youths, condom distribution, and community activities. Knowledge and reported behaviors improved; however, no differences were apparent between the intervention and control communities in relation to HIV or HSV-2 seroincidence, incidence of other STIs, or pregnancy outcomes (Hayes and others 2003).

A second study in Mwanza, Tanzania, randomized communities to intervention and control conditions. The intervention consisted of syndromic treatment of STIs. The results showed a 40 percent reduction in HIV incidence and reductions in symptomatic urethritis in men and prevalence of syphilis seroreactivity; the prevalence of gonorrheal or chlamydial infection in prenatal women did not change (Grosskurth and others 1995; Mayaud and others 1997).

In a community randomized trial in Masaka, Uganda, one community received information, education, and communication; a second community received information, education, and communication plus syndromic management of STIs; and the control received community development assistance. The results showed no differences in HIV-1 incidence. The incidence of HSV-2 seroconversion declined in the community receiving information, education, and communication only; the incidence of syphilis and of gonorrhea decreased in the community receiving information, education, and communication plus

STI syndromic management; and condom use increased in all three communities (Kamali and others 2003).

In Rakai, Uganda, a community randomized trial evaluated the efficacy of repeated mass treatment of STIs. Relative to control communities, in intervention communities the prevalence of *T. vaginalis* in women was reduced significantly, but no significant reduction was apparent in prevalence of gonorrhea, chlamydial infection, new syphilis seroreactivity, and bacterial vaginosis; in HIV incidence; or in history of urethral or vaginal discharge or genital ulcer disease (Wawer and others 1999). A subanalysis of pregnant participants showed a reduction in the prevalence of several STIs in women tested near delivery and in potentially STI-related pregnancy, puerperal, and neonatal morbidity (Gray and others 2001).

Conclusions on Interventions

The review of STI intervention research suggests several, perhaps counterintuitive, insights:

- First, most evidence is on individual-level interventions aimed at reducing STI acquisition, even though individual-level interventions may be costly and difficult to sustain.
- Second, behavior change is the most commonly evaluated modality, followed by treatment.
- Third, theory-based behavioral interventions failed to show an effect as often as behavioral interventions not based on theory.
- Fourth, behavioral interventions delivered in small group settings were as effective as those delivered to individuals (Manhart and Holmes 2005).
- Fifth, the effect of a particular behavior change on STI risk depended on the type of STI; however, the number of partners may be more predictive of risk for highly infectious STIs than for HIV, and unprotected sex acts may be more predictive of risk for HIV than for highly infectious STIs (Semaan and others 2002). Thus, behavioral interventions may have different effects on STIs of differing infectiousness.
- Finally, the number of intervention trials that demonstrate declines in risk behaviors combined with either no effect on STIs or increases in STIs is increasing. This observation calls into question the use of behavioral outcome measures as indicators of biomedical outcomes (Aral and Peterman 2002).

INTERVENTION COSTS AND COST-EFFECTIVENESS

Widespread implementation of effective interventions depends on cost and cost-effectiveness considerations.

Organization of STI Control Activities in Poor Countries

In poor countries, patients can typically obtain treatment for an STI in a public sector health care facility. Many countries have publicly funded, stand-alone STI clinics, but the typical pattern is for health care personnel to provide care for STIs as part of their regular practice in general outpatient clinics. Despite the availability of such publicly funded care, or perhaps because of concerns about anonymity, many STI patients in poor countries avoid public facilities in favor of traditional healers and private pharmacies. A recent study of the cost-effectiveness of delivering STI treatment through trained pharmacists in Peruvian cities included reports of the popularity of self-treatment in Brazil, Cameroon, Ghana, Nepal, South Africa, Thailand, Vietnam, and Zambia (Adams and others 2003). After reviewing this literature, Adams and others selected the point estimate of 0.4 as their best guess for the proportion of STI patients seeking treatment from a pharmacy in Lima.

Determinants of the Costs of Interventions

We adopt a government perspective in analyzing the costs and cost-effectiveness of interventions. Thus, we define the costs of an activity as the total budgetary expenditure attributable to that activity—that is, the total budget for buildings, equipment, personnel, and supplies, with adjustments made when buildings are used for multiple purposes.

We define the unit costs of an activity as the total budgetary expenditure during a stated time period divided by the number of units of output during that same period. Because the same activity can have several outputs, this definition necessarily entails some ambiguity. For example, an intermediate output of the delivery of STI treatment services is the patient treated, whereas a more final output is the patient cured. An even more complete measure of output would include the secondary infections averted as a result of the cure.

One of the reasons that many economists prefer cost-benefit analysis to cost-effectiveness analysis is that the former attaches a dollar value to each of the outputs of an activity and then aggregates across the outputs to construct a summary measure of the total benefit of the activity. However, this simple result hides many arbitrary assumptions that are required to value the separate outputs. One of the most arbitrary of these assumptions is the assignment of a dollar value to a healthy life year. So instead we present costs and cost-effectiveness denominated in the outputs for which we have data. We then go as far as we can toward aggregation by adopting the conventions of the healthy life year and the disability-adjusted healthy life year.

Kumaranayake and others' (2004) background study for this chapter reviews the literature on the unit costs of STI treatment. They identify 35 studies on this topic that provide a total of 77 unit cost estimates. These are grouped in table 17.4 by the disease or syndrome being treated and by the output that was

Table 17.4 Average Estimated Costs per Unit of Output, by Disease or Syndrome and Type of Output
(2001 US$)

Disease or syndrome	Treatment	Cure	Average
Syphilis	36.04	n.a.	36.04
	(5.91)	n.a.	(5.91)
Urethral discharge	14.29	89.07	29.25
	(20.68)	(0)	(37.94)
Genital ulcer	23.16	100.60	48.97
	(21.73)	(83.74)	(59.56)
Venereal disease	25.47	82.65	31.83
	(18.56)	(111.55)	(37.12)
Pelvic inflammatory disease	7.12	n.a.	7.12
	(3.09)	n.a.	(3.09)
Vaginal discharge	48.23	102.92	81.04
	(0)	(89.63)	(70.10)
Total	24.05	96.10	39.49
	(19.04)	(73.44)	(47.23)

Source: Authors' calculations based on a literature review done as a background study for this chapter by Kumaranayake and others 2004.
n.a. = not applicable.
Note: The figures in parentheses are standard deviations. The 42 observations in the table are individual unit cost estimates distributed across separate studies.

costed. Of the 46 estimates of the unit cost of treatment, only 33 could be interpreted as, or converted to, 2001 U.S. dollars, and the same applied to 9 of the 10 estimates of the unit cost of a cure. Table 17.4 summarizes the results of these studies by the disease or syndrome that occasioned the treatment.

The most notable thing about the summary statistics is their variability: the cost per unit of output can vary by a factor of 100 or more. Even though the mean dollar cost per cure could plausibly be almost four times that of treatment alone, the standard errors are so large as to make the difference statistically insignificant.

The same point—that is, that unit costs vary enormously from one site to another—is made by the preliminary results of a study by Dandona and others (2005). The cost per case treated in the study varies by a factor of 10 across the 14 sites. Furthermore, the two sites that treat the fewest and the most cases per year also display the highest costs, a finding that suggests the existence of both economies and diseconomies of scale.

The variables that determine the costs—and therefore the cost-effectiveness—of STI treatment include the following:

- delivery by the public or private sector
- economies of scale
- economies of scope
- prevalence and incidence
- epidemic phase
- transmission efficiency
- health system characteristics

- population composition and concentration
- resource combinations and input prices
- incentives to providers for high quality and quantity of service delivery
- willingness to pay for treatment as a function of price, income, and distance
- stigmatization
- disutility of condom use.

SCALING UP CONTROL STRATEGIES

Throughout the history of STI control, tension has been apparent between those who support prioritizing resources for the small proportion of people with the most sexual contacts and those who advocate spreading prevention, screening, and treatment resources more thinly over the entire population. Opponents of prioritization argue that most of the people who practice the riskiest behavior are hard to find and that attempts to find them would expose those individuals to stigmatization and repressive measures.

A group of researchers at the University of North Carolina has developed and applied a novel approach to STI interventions that has demonstrated in several countries that finding the people who practice the riskiest sexual behavior without targeting them as individuals is possible (Weir and others 2003). As an example of this approach, consider its application to Madagascar, a country where risky sexual behavior had previously been thought to be too common to be identified or to be distinguished from less risky behavior.

In May 2003, the Malagasy Steering Committee, which consisted of representatives of the Ministry of Health, local government officials, and other knowledgeable experts, selected five towns judged to be at high risk for STIs for a pilot study. The Priorities for Local AIDS Control Effort (PLACE) method applied in these towns was, first, to interview adults at random on the streets of the city to find out where people go to meet and socialize and, second, to visit and collect data on these locations and the people who frequent them.

In each of the five cities, the informants tended to agree on the most frequented sites. They identified between 70 and 267 unique socialization sites of various types, ranging from bars and restaurants to beaches and brothels. Interviews with people frequenting the sites revealed them to be much more sexually active than the average Malagasy adult. According to the 1997 demographic and health survey, 13 percent of women outside the capital city, Antananarivo, had two or more sexual partners in the previous year. In contrast, the percentage of women at the socialization sites who had had more than two partners ranged from 46 to 68 percent. According to the demographic and health survey, only about 3 percent of women outside Antananarivo had four or more partners in the previous year, but the percentage of women at the study sites having this many partners was 10 times larger. The men interviewed at these sites were even more sexually active than the women.

The pilot study also investigated whether information on or products for prevention of STIs, HIV, or both were available at the socialization sites. In the five towns, the proportion of sites where condoms were available on the day of the visit varied from 27 to 54 percent. These percentages are not negligible and are undoubtedly much higher than they were 10 years ago, and the availability of condoms at so many of these sites is a tribute to the success of the condom social-marketing campaign. However, the statistics also indicate substantial room for improvement, for example, by distributing condoms in 100 percent of identified socialization sites. The feasibility of such a program is enhanced by information from the PLACE study that more than 80 percent of the owners or managers of these sites expressed their willingness to host STI and HIV prevention programs, and more than half were willing to sell condoms.

Researchers have carried out similar PLACE studies in Burkina Faso, Ghana, South Africa, and elsewhere. Unfortunately, in none of these countries has this extensive risk mapping been followed by the implementation of prevention programs at all the identified locations. Until such programs are implemented and evaluated, no African country will be able to claim that it has scaled up the most effective type of STI prevention to population levels.

RESEARCH AND DEVELOPMENT AGENDA

Priorities for global STI research include the following:

- The development and evaluation of therapeutic (drug treatment or vaccines), behavioral, and structural interventions to prevent or reduce STIs and their sequelae. Given the spread of drug-resistant strains of gonorrhea and other STIs, new pharmaceutical products and new combination therapies are needed to prevent and treat STIs.
- The development and evaluation of mechanisms to accurately quantify the disease burden in order to prioritize activities.
- The development and evaluation of inexpensive and practical rapid diagnostic tests to permit early detection and treatment of STIs.
- The conducting of studies to evaluate effective prevention modalities for persons at highest risk for STIs.
- The undertaking of health services research to gain an understanding of practical and cost-effective STI prevention strategies or systems that ideally can be integrated into existing public health infrastructure. When an individual is treated for an STI, this treatment has both positive and neg-

ative spillover effects (externalities). The right combination of patient and provider incentives needs to be found that will maximize the beneficial spillovers while minimizing the harmful ones.
- The implementation of studies in support of global elimination programs.

Because of the clandestine nature of most sexual behavior, STIs are probably massively underreported, which in turn leads to an underestimation of their importance. New survey and measurement tools have been developed. They now need to be applied to populations in poor countries to improve these estimates.

In addition, randomized controlled trials need to be conducted in different settings to test the hypothesis that treating or preventing STIs in high-risk individuals has beneficial spillover effects by preventing infections among low-risk individuals. An improved understanding of the determinants of high-risk sexual behavior and the role that such behavior can sometimes play in helping women to escape from poverty and helping men to cope with it is also needed, as is a better understanding of the full range of benefits of effective STI interventions for high-risk individuals and their dependents.

As concerns disease modeling and surveillance, further improvements are needed in understanding the implications for interventions of different kinds of local, regional, and international sex networks.

Tools

Because of the difficulty of persuading patients to adhere to a course of medication for the prescribed period, single-dose therapy would be valuable. Rapid, point-of-care diagnostics are also a high priority, so that drugs can be targeted at pathogens more accurately. New approaches for treating chronic STIs should be incorporated into prevention strategies, and blister packs of antibiotics that can be sold over the counter for syndromic management of STIs should be available.

Vaccines would be particularly valuable, both for preventing and for potentially treating chronic viral STIs and chlamydial infection, which is often asymptomatic but is responsible for considerable morbidity.

Diagnostics tests that could be used at home or at social meeting spots may help people decide whether to engage in risky sex. Packages of diagnostic tests that change color when the contents expire would also be useful.

Intervention Methods

Syndromic management algorithms have now existed for more than a decade. However, treatment algorithms are sensitive to changes in the relative prices of pharmaceuticals and diagnostic reagents, in the prevalence of the various STIs, in pathogens' resistance, and so on. Thus, every country needs some ability to respond to local changes by developing or modifying algorithms as needed.

As concerns intervention packaging, many policy makers continue to believe that the most sexually active people are hard to find. This belief hampers efforts to target these people with STI prevention programs. The PLACE methods developed at the University of North Carolina offer an opportunity to correct that impression and should be packaged with other urban public health functions. Packaging sex education into school curricula is a challenge in most of the world. As enrollment rates for poor children, especially girls, rise, the presence of a strong, culturally appropriate, sex education curriculum will lay the foundation for strong STI prevention and treatment campaigns.

As this chapter has argued, the determinants of the unit costs of STI treatment and prevention are largely unknown. We recommend health services and operations research to study the determinants of the unit costs of STI prevention and treatment services. The purpose of this research would be to learn not only how to deliver care in the most cost-effective ways, but also how to build systems that achieve that technological frontier in a high percentage of public and private facilities and pass those cost savings on to the government and to patients. Given the beneficial spillover effects from effective STI prevention and treatment among those who are most sexually active, research is needed to learn how the PLACE approach to targeting can be implemented most cost-effectively in different cultural contexts.

Finally, improved understanding of the best way to design an STI treatment system, including the rewards and penalties that best motivate providers (to be polite, discrete, prompt, efficient, and accurate in following best practice, evidence-based treatment protocols) and patients (to seek and then to adhere to treatment) is a priority. Improved data on the costs of each STI intervention at the pilot stage and after scaling up to the national level are also necessary.

CONCLUSIONS

Regarding the cost-effectiveness of STI control, the position this chapter takes is "it depends." The health benefit in terms of numbers of disability-adjusted, discounted, healthy life years saved by curing or preventing a case of syphilis varies from 3 years in a person who has ceased all sexual activity to as many as 161 years in a sex worker with two partners a day. The cost of treating that prostitute for syphilis varies from US$5 to US$100. Thus, the cost per DALY of syphilis treatment can range from 100/3 or US$33 per DALY to 5/161 or less than US$0.05 per DALY.

As we learn more about the complexities of delivering STI treatment services and take into account the diversity of risk behavior, the ease with which STI interventions can be ascribed a simple cost-effectiveness ratio has declined. If no easy way to summarize experience to date with a simple cost-effectiveness ratio is available, how should we analyze economic investments in STI treatment? We believe that the way forward is a better understanding of why STI treatment and other health services vary so much in terms of their efficiency and effectiveness from one setting to another. By studying the determinants of this variation, we should gain an improved understanding of the full costs of high-quality STI service delivery and its place in the health sector investment picture.

ACKNOWLEDGMENTS

The authors would like to acknowledge Becca Feldman, Patricia Jackson, Dilip Parajuli, and Melanie Ross for their outstanding support in the preparation of this chapter.

NOTES

1. The Gini coefficient is a measure of inequality that here we apply to income. If income is distributed equally in the population, the coefficient is equal to 0, and if a few individuals hold almost all the wealth, the coefficient is close to 1.

2. Given that WHO has expended enormous efforts to estimate discounted years of life lost, disability years lost, and DALYs lost as a result of STIs, the simplest and most direct approach for computing the DALY benefits of preventing or curing an STI in a single patient would be to use WHO's years of life lost, disability years lost, or DALY per case assumptions. Alternatively, one could simply divide WHO's aggregate values of these indicators by the incidence rate of each disease in each region to obtain the estimated burden per incident case. Unfortunately, neither the case-specific burden numbers nor the incidence rates that correspond to the DALY aggregates are available from WHO.

3. In contemporaneous data, STIs can either affect or be affected by HIV prevalence. To focus on the effects of an STI on HIV infection, we lag infection by an STI by seven years. Though partially correcting for simultaneity bias, this strategy does not allow us to identify whether lagged STI prevalence is directly affecting HIV infection or only serving as a proxy for the risky sexual behavior that drives both epidemics.

4. The samples include two measures of HIV prevalence (low- and high-risk groups) for some countries. These measures enable us to expand the sample used in the column (1) regression from 40 countries to 56 separate observations. Equations are estimated with Stata's cluster option to correct the standard errors of the coefficients for the correlation between the errors on separate observations from the same country. The variable urban high-risk dummy is used to shift the intercept coefficient for the high-risk sample in comparison with the low-risk one.

REFERENCES

Adams, E. J., P. J. Garcia, G. P. Garnett, W. J. Edmunds, and K. K. Holmes. 2003. "The Cost-Effectiveness of Syndromic Management in Pharmacies in Lima, Peru." *Sexually Transmitted Diseases* 30 (5): 379–87.

Adimora, A. A., V. J. Schoenbach, D. M. Bonas, F. E. Martinson, K. H. Donaldson, and T. R. Stancil. 2002. "Concurrent Sexual Partnerships among Women in the United States." *Epidemiology* 13 (3): 320–27.

Agrawal, D., B. Gillespie, and B. Foxman. 2001. "Sexual Behavior across the Lifespan: Results from a Random-Digit Dialing Survey of Women Aged 60–94." *International Journal of STD and AIDS* 12 (Suppl. 2): 186.

Ainsworth, M., and M. Over. 1997. *Confronting AIDS: Public Priorities in a Global Epidemic.* New York: Oxford University Press.

Aral, S. O. 2000. "Behavioral Aspects of Sexually Transmitted Diseases: Core Groups and Bridge Populations." *Sexually Transmitted Diseases* 27 (6): 327–28.

———. 2002a. "Determinants of STD Epidemics: Implications for Phase Appropriate Intervention Strategies." *Sexually Transmitted Infections* 78 (Suppl. 1): i3–13.

———. 2002b. "Understanding Racial-Ethnic and Societal Differentials in STI: Do We Need to Move beyond Behavioral Epidemiology?" *Sexually Transmitted Infections* 78 (1): 2–3.

———. 2004. "Editorial Response: Mental Health—A Powerful Predictor of Sexual Health?" *Sexually Transmitted Diseases* 31 (1): 13–14.

Aral, S. O., and J. F. Blanchard. 2002. "Phase Specific Approaches to the Epidemiology and Prevention of Sexually Transmitted Diseases." *Sexually Transmitted Infections* 78 (Suppl. 1): i1–2.

Aral, S. O., and K. K. Holmes. 1999. "Social and Behavioral Determinants of the Epidemiology of STDs: Industrialized and Developing Countries." In *Sexually Transmitted Diseases,* 3rd ed., ed. K. K. Holmes, P. F. Sparling, P.-A. Mardh, S. M. Lemon, W. E. Stamm, P. Piot, and J. N. Wasserheit, 139–76. New York: McGraw Hill.

Aral, S. O., J. P. Hughes, B. Stoner, W. Whittington, H. H. Handsfield, R. M. Anderson, and others. 1999. "Sexual Mixing Patterns in the Spread of Gonococcal and Chlamydial Infections." *American Journal of Public Health* 89 (6): 825–33.

Aral, S. O., and T. A. Peterman. 2002. "A Stratified Approach to Untangling the Behavioral/Biomedical Outcomes Conundrum." *Sexually Transmitted Diseases* 29 (9): 530–32.

Aral, S. O., and J. S. St. Lawrence. 2002. "The Ecology of Sex Work and Drug Use in Saratov Oblast, Russia." *Sexually Transmitted Diseases* 29 (12): 798–805.

Aral, S. O., J. S. St. Lawrence, R. Dyatlov, and A. Kozlov. 2005. "Commercial Sex Work, Drug Use, and Sexually Transmitted Infections in St. Petersburg, Russia." *Social Science and Medicine* 60 (10): 2181–90.

Aral, S. O., and J. N. Wasserheit. 1999. "STD-Related Health Care Seeking and Health Service Delivery." In *Sexually Transmitted Diseases,* 3rd ed., ed. K. K. Holmes, P. F. Sparling, P.-A. Mardh, S. M. Lemon, W. E. Stamm, P. Piot, and J. N. Wasserheit, 1295–306. New York: McGraw Hill.

Bailey, R. C., F. A. Plummer, and S. Moses. 2001. "Male Circumcision and HIV Prevention: Current Knowledge and Future Research Directions." *Lancet Infectious Diseases* 1 (4): 223–31.

Blanchard, J. F. 2002. "Populations, Pathogens, and Epidemic Phases: Closing the Gap between Theory and Practice in the Prevention of Sexually Transmitted Diseases." *Sexually Transmitted Infections* 78 (Suppl. 1): i183–88.

Blower, S. M., A. N. Aschenbach, H. B. Gershengorn, and J. O. Kahn. 2001. "Predicting the Unpredictable: Transmission of Drug-Resistant HIV." *Nature Medicine* 7 (9): 1016–20.

Blower, S. M., and P. Farmer. 2003. "Predicting the Public Health Impact of Antiretrovirals: Preventing HIV in Developing Countries." *AIDScience.* http://www.aidscience.org/Articles/AIDScience033.asp.

Blower, S. M., and P. Volberding. 2002. "What Can Modeling Tell Us about the Threat of Antiviral Drug Resistance?" *Current Opinion in Infectious Diseases* 15 (6): 609–14.

Brown, J. E., and R. C. Brown. 2000. "Traditional Intravaginal Practices and the Heterosexual Transmission of Disease: A Review." *Sexually Transmitted Diseases* 27 (4): 183–87.

Brugha, R., K. Keersmaekers, A. Renton, and A. Meheus. 1997. "Genital Herpes Infection: A Review." *International Journal of Epidemiology* 26 (4): 698–709.

CDC (U.S. Centers for Disease Control and Prevention). 2004. "Increases in Fluoroquinolone-Resistant *Neisseria gonorrhoeae* among Men Who Have Sex with Men: United States 2003 and Revised Recommendations for Gonorrhea Treatment 2004." *Morbidity and Mortality Weekly Review* 53 (16): 335–38.

Chandeying, V., S. Skov, P. Duramad, B. Makepeace, M. Ward, and P. Khunigij. 2000. "The Prevalence of Urethral Infections amongst Asymptomatic Young Men in Hat Yai, Southern Thailand." *International Journal of STD and AIDS* 11 (6): 402–5.

Corey, L. 2000. "Herpes Simplex Type 2 Infection in the Developing World: Is It Time to Address this Disease?" *Sexually Transmitted Diseases* 27 (1): 30–31.

Corey, L., and H. H. Handsfield. 2000. "Genital Herpes and Public Health: Addressing a Global Problem." *Journal of the American Medical Association* 283 (6): 791–94.

Corey, L., A. Wald, R. Patel, S. L. Sacks, S. K. Tyring, T. Warren, and others. 2004. "Once-Daily Valacyclovir to Reduce the Risk of Transmission of Genital Herpes." *New England Journal of Medicine* 350 (1): 11–20.

Creighton, S., M. Tenant-Flowers, C. B. Taylor, R. Miller, and N. Low. 2003. "Co-infection with Gonorrhoea and Chlamydia: How Much Is There and What Does It Mean?" *International Journal of STD and AIDS* 14 (2): 109–13.

Dallabetta, G. A., A. C. Gerbase, and K. K. Holmes. 1998. "Problems, Solutions, and Challenges in Syndromic Management of Sexually Transmitted Diseases." *Sexually Transmitted Infections* 74 (Suppl. 1): S1–11.

Dandona, L., P. Sisodia, Y. K. Ramesh, S. G. Kumar, A. A. Kumar, M. C. Rao, and others. 2005. "Cost and Efficiency of HIV Voluntary Counselling and Testing Centres in Andhra Pradesh, India." *National Medical Journal of India* 18 (1): 26–31.

Decosas, J., and N. Padian. 2002. "The Profile and Context of the Epidemics of Sexually Transmitted Infections Including HIV in Zimbabwe." *Sexually Transmitted Infections* 78 (Suppl. 1): i40–46.

Doherty, I. A., N. S. Padian, C. Marlow, and S. O. Aral. 2005. "Determinants and Consequences of Sexual Networks as They Affect the Spread of Sexually Transmitted Infections." *Journal of Infectious Diseases* 191 (Suppl. 1): S42–54.

Doherty, L., K. A. Fenton, J. Jones, T. C. Paine, S. P. Higgins, D. Williams, and A. Palfreeman. 2002. "Syphilis: Old Problem, New Strategy." *British Medical Journal* 325 (7356): 153–56.

Donovan, B. 2000a. "The Repertoire of Human Efforts to Avoid Sexually Transmissible Diseases: Past and Present. Part 1—Strategies Used before or Instead of Sex." *Sexually Transmitted Infections* 76 (1): 7–12.

———. 2000b. "The Repertoire of Human Efforts to Avoid Sexually Transmissible Diseases: Past and Present. Part 2—Strategies Used during or after Sex." *Sexually Transmitted Infections* 76 (2): 88–93.

———. 2004. "Sexually Transmissible Infections Other Than HIV." *Lancet* 363 (9408): 545–56.

Fenton, K. A., A. M. Johnson, and A. Nicoll. 1997. "Race, Ethnicity, and Sexual Health." *British Medical Journal* 314 (7096): 1703–4.

Fenton, K. A., C. Korovessis, A. M. Johnson, A. McCadden, S. McManus, K. Wellings, and others. 2001. "Sexual Behaviour in Britain: Reported Sexually Transmitted Infections and Prevalent Genital Chlamydia Trachomatis Infection." *Lancet* 358 (9296): 1851–54.

Garnett, G. P. 2002. "The Geographical and Temporal Evolution of Sexually Transmitted Disease Epidemics." *Sexually Transmitted Infections* 78 (Suppl. 1): i14–19.

Garnett, G. P., and J. A. Rottingen. 2001. "Measuring the Risk of HIV Transmission." *AIDS* 15 (5): 641–43.

Genc, M., and W. J. Ledger. 2000. "Syphilis in Pregnancy." *Sexually Transmitted Infections* 76 (2): 73–79.

Giuliano, A. R., R. Harris, R. L. Sedjo, S. Baldwin, D. Roe, M. R. Papenfuss, and others. 2002. "Incidence, Prevalence, and Clearance of Type-Specific Human Papillomavirus Infections: The Young Women's Health Study." *Journal of Infectious Diseases* 186 (4): 462–69.

Golden, M. R., W. L. Whittington, H. H. Handsfield, J. P. Hughes, W. E. Stamm, M. Hogben, and others. 2005. "Effect of Expedited Treatment of Sex Partners on Recurrent or Persistent Gonorrhea or Chlamydial Infection." *New England Journal of Medicine* 352 (7): 676–85.

Gorbach, P. M., H. Sopheab, T. Phalla, H. B. Leng, S. Mills, A. Bennett, and others. 2000. "Sexual Bridging by Cambodian Men: Potential Importance for General Population Spread of STD/HIV Epidemics." *Sexually Transmitted Diseases* 27 (6): 320–26.

Gray, R. H., F. Wabwire-Mangen, G. Kigozi, N. K. Sewankambo, D. Serwadda, L. H. Moulton, and others. 2001. "Randomized Trial of Presumptive Sexually Transmitted Disease Therapy during Pregnancy in Rakai, Uganda." *American Journal of Obstetrics and Gynecology* 185 (5): 1209–17.

Gregson, S., C. A. Nyamukapa, G. P. Garnett, P. R. Mason, T. Zhuwau, M. Carael, and others. 2002. "Sexual Mixing Patterns and Sex-Differentials in Teenage Exposure to HIV Infection in Rural Zimbabwe." *Lancet* 359 (9321): 1896–903.

Grémy, I., and N. Beltzer. 2004. "HIV Risk and Condom Use in the Adult Heterosexual Population in France between 1992 and 2001: Return to the Starting Point?" *AIDS* 18 (5): 805–9.

Grosskurth, H., F. Mosha, J. Todd, E. Mwijarubi, A. Klokke, K. Senkoro, and others. 1995. "Impact of Improved Treatment of Sexually Transmitted Diseases on HIV Infection in Rural Tanzania: Randomized Controlled Trial." *Lancet* 346 (8974): 530–36.

Harrison W. O., R. R. Hooper, P. J. Wiesner, A. F. Campbell, W. W. Karney, G. H. Reynolds, and others. 1979 "A Trial of Minocycline Given after Exposure to Prevent Gonorrhea." *New England Journal of Medicine* 300 (19): 1074–78.

Hart, C. A., and S. Kariuki. 1998. "Antimicrobial Resistance in Developing Countries." *British Medical Journal* 317 (7159): 647–50.

Hawkes, S., and K. G. Santhya. 2002. "Diverse Realities: Sexually Transmitted Infections and HIV in India." *Sexually Transmitted Diseases* 78 (Suppl. 1): i31–39.

Hayes, R., J. Chagalucha, H. Grosskurth, A. Obasi, J. Todd, B. Cleophas-Mazige, and others. 2003. "Mema Kwa Vijana, a Randomized Controlled Trial of an Adolescent Sexual and Reproductive Health Intervention Programme in Rural Mwanza, Tanzania: 1. Rationale and Trial Design" (Abstract 0695). Paper presented at the 15th Biennial Congress of the International Society of Sexually Transmitted Diseases Research, Ottawa, July 27–30.

Holmes, K. K., and S. O. Aral. 1991. "Behavioral Interventions in Developing Countries." In *Research Issues in Human Behavior and STD in the AIDS Era*, ed. J. N. Wasserheit, S. O. Aral, and K. K. Holmes, 318–44. Washington, DC: American Society of Microbiology Publications.

Idahl, A., J. Boman, U. Kumlin, and J. I. Olofsson. 2004. "Demonstration of *Chlamydia trachomatis* IgG Antibodies in the Male Partner of the Infertile Couple Is Correlated with a Reduced Likelihood of Achieving Pregnancy." *Human Reproduction* 19 (5): 1121–26.

Kamali, A., M. Quigley, J. Nakiyingi, J. Kinsman, J. Kengeya-Kayondo, R. Gopal, and others. 2003. "Syndromic Management of Sexually-Transmitted Infections and Behaviour Change Interventions on Transmission of HIV-1 in Rural Uganda: A Community Randomized Trial." *Lancet* 361 (9358): 645–52.

Kamb, M. L., M. Fishbein, J. M. Douglas Jr., F. Rhodes, J. Rogers, G. Bolan, and others. 1998. "Efficacy of Risk-Reduction Counseling to Prevent Human Immunodeficiency Virus and Sexually Transmitted Diseases: A Randomized Controlled Trial." *Journal of the American Medical Association* 280 (13): 1161–67.

Kaul, R., J. Kimani, N. J. Nagelkerke, K. Fonck, E. N. Ngugi, F. Keli, and others. 2004 "Monthly Antibiotic Chemoprophylaxis and Incidence of Sexually Transmitted Infections and HIV-1 Infection in Kenyan Sex Workers: A Randomized Controlled Trial." *Journal of the American Medical Association* 291 (21): 2555–62.

Klebanoff, M. A., J. C. Carey, J. C. Hauth, S. L. Hillier, R. P. Nugent, E. A. Thom, and others. 2001. "Failure of Metronidazole to Prevent Preterm Delivery among Pregnant Women with Asymptomatic *Trichomonas vaginalis* Infection." *New England Journal of Medicine* 345 (7): 487–93.

Koumans, E. H., T. A. Farley, J. J. Gibson, C. Langley, M. W. Ross, M. McFarlane, and others. 2001. "Characteristics of Persons with Syphilis in Areas of Persisting Syphilis in the United States: Sustained Transmission Associated with Concurrent Partnerships." *Sexually Transmitted Diseases* 28 (9): 497–503.

Koutsky, L. A., K. A. Ault, C. M. Wheeler, D. R. Brown, E. Barr, F. B. Alvarez, and others. 2002. "A Controlled Trial of a Human Papillomavirus Type 16 Vaccine." *New England Journal of Medicine* 347 (21): 1645–51.

Kraut, J., and S. O. Aral. 2001. "Patterns of Age Mixing Are Associated with STDs in the USA." *International Journal of STD and AIDS* 12 (Suppl. 2): 188.

Kraut-Becher, J. R., and S. O. Aral. 2003. "Gap Length: An Important Factor in Sexually Transmitted Disease Transmission." *Sexually Transmitted Diseases* 30 (3): 221–25.

Kumaranayake, L., P. Vickerman, D. Walker, S. Samoshkin, V. Romantzov, Z. Emelyanova, and others. 2004. "The Cost-Effectiveness of HIV Preventive Measures among Injecting Drug Users in Svetlogorsk, Belarus." *Addiction* 99 (12): 1565–76.

Laga, M., M. O. Diallo, and A. Buvé. 1994. "Interrelationship of STD and HIV: Where Are We Now?" *AIDS* 8 (Suppl.): S119–24.

Laga, M., A. Manoka, M. Kivuvu, B. Malele, M. Tuliza, N. Nzila, and others. 1993. "Non-ulcerative Sexually Transmitted Diseases as Risk Factors for HIV-1 Transmission in Women: Results from a Cohort Study." *AIDS* 7 (1): 95–102.

Lau, C. Y., and A. K. Qureshi. 2002. "Azithromycin versus Doxycycline for Genital Chlamydial Infections: A Meta-Analysis of Randomized Clinical Trials." *Sexually Transmitted Diseases* 29 (9): 497–502.

Laumann, E. O., and Y. Youm. 1999. "Racial-Ethnic Group Differences in the Prevalence of Sexually Transmitted Diseases in the United States: A Network Explanation." *Sexually Transmitted Diseases* 26 (5): 250–61.

Low-Beer, D., and R. L. Stoneburner. 2003. "Behaviour and Communication Change in Reducing HIV: Is Uganda Unique?" *African Journal of AIDS Research* 2: 9–21.

Manhart, L., and K. K. Holmes. 2005. "Randomized Controlled Trials of Individual-Level, Population-Level, and Multilevel Interventions for Preventing Sexually Transmitted Infections: What Has Worked?" *Journal of Infectious Diseases* 191 (Suppl. 1): S7–24.

Mayaud, P., F. Mosha, J. Todd, R. Balira, J. Mgara, B. West, and others. 1997. "Improved Treatment Services Significantly Reduce the Prevalence of Sexually Transmitted Diseases in Rural Tanzania: Results of a Randomized Controlled Trial." *AIDS* 11 (15): 1873–80.

Meheus, A., K. F. Schulz, and W. Cates Jr. 1990. "Development of Prevention and Control Programs for Sexually Transmitted Diseases in Developing Countries." In *Sexually Transmitted Diseases*, 2nd ed., ed. K. K. Holmes, P.-A. Mardh, and P. F. Sparling, 1041–46. New York: McGraw-Hill.

Morris, M., ed. 2004. *Network Epidemiology: A Handbook for Survey Design and Data Collection.* Oxford, U.K.: Oxford University Press.

Morris, M., and M. Kretzchmar. 1995. "Concurrent Partnerships and Transmission of Dynamics in Networks." *Social Networks* 17: 299–318.

Morris, M., C. Podhisita, M. J. Wawer, and M. S. Handcock. 1996. "Bridge Populations in the Spread of HIV/AIDS in Thailand." *AIDS* 10 (11): 1265–71.

Moses, S., E. N. Ngugi, J. E. Bradley, E. K. Njeru, G. Eldridge, E. Muia, and others. 1994. "Health Care–Seeking Behavior Related to the Transmission of Sexually Transmitted Diseases in Kenya." *American Journal of Public Health* 84 (12): 1947–51.

Moses, S., E. N. Ngugi, A. Costigan, C. Kariuki, I. Maclean, R. C. Brunham, and others. 2002. "Response of a Sexually Transmitted Infection Epidemic to a Treatment and Prevention Program in Nairobi, Kenya." *Sexually Transmitted Infections* 78 (Suppl. 1): i114–20.

National Institute for Allergy and Infectious Diseases. 2001. *Scientific Evidence on Condom Effectiveness for Sexually Transmitted Disease Prevention.* Workshop report. Bethesda, MD: National Institute for Allergy and Infectious Diseases.

O'Farrell, N. 2002. "Donovanosis." *Sexually Transmitted Infections* 78 (6): 452–57.

Orroth, A. K. 2003. "Investigations of the Proportion of HIV Infections Attributable to Sexually Transmitted Diseases in Sub-Saharan Africa Based on Data from the Mwanza and Rakai Trials." Ph.D. thesis, Faculty of Medicine, University of London.

Over, M. 1998. "The Effects of Societal Variables on Urban Rates of HIV Infection in Developing Countries: An Exploratory Analysis." In *Confronting AIDS: Evidence from the Developing World,* ed. M. Ainsworth, L. Fransen, and M. Over, 40–51. Brussels: European Commission.

———. 1999. "The Public Interest in a Private Disease: An Economic Perspective on the Government Role in STD and HIV Control." In *Sexually Transmitted Diseases,* 3rd ed., ed. K. K. Holmes, P. F. Sparling, P.-A. Mardh, S. M. Lemon, W. E. Stamm, P. Piot, and J. N. Wasserheit, 3–15. New York: McGraw-Hill.

———. 2004. "Impact of the HIV/AIDS Epidemic on the Health Sectors of Developing Countries." In *The Macroeconomics of HIV/AIDS,* ed. M. Haacker. Washington, DC: International Monetary Fund.

Over, M., P. Heywood, J. Gold, I. Gupta, S. Hira, and E. Marseille. 2004. *HIV/AIDS Treatment and Prevention in India: Modeling the Costs and Consequences.* Washington, DC: World Bank.

Over, M., and P. Piot. 1993. "HIV Infection and Sexually Transmitted Diseases." In *Disease Control Priorities in Developing Countries,* ed. D. T. Jamison, W. H. Mosley, A. R. Measham, and J. L. Bobadilla, 455–527. New York: Oxford University Press.

Peterman, T. A., L. S. Lin, D. R. Newman, M. L. Kamb, G. Bolan, J. Zenilman, and others. 2000. "Does Measured Behavior Reflect STD Risk? An Analysis of Data from a Randomized Controlled Behavioral Intervention Study: Project RESPECT Study Group." *Sexually Transmitted Diseases* 27 (8): 446–51.

Pisani, E., G. P. Garnett, N. C. Grassly, T. Brown, J. Stover, C. Hankins, and others. 2003. "Back to Basics in HIV Prevention: Focus on Exposure." *British Medical Journal* 326 (7403): 1384–87.

Rekart, M. L. 2002. "Sex in the City: Sexual Behavior, Societal Change, and STDs in Saigon." *Sexually Transmitted Infections* 78 (Suppl. 1): i47–54.

Samoff, E., E. Koumans, L. Markowitz, and others. 2004. "An Assessment of Factors Associated with Type-Specific Human Papillomavirus Persistence in an Adolescent Clinic Population Using Generalized Estimating Equations—Atlanta, Georgia, 1999–2003." Oral presentation at the Epidemic Intelligence Service National Conference, Atlanta, Georgia, April 19.

Schachter, J. 2001. "NAATs to Diagnose *Chlamydia trachomatis* Genital Infection: A Promise Still Unfulfilled." *Expert Review of Molecular Diagnostics* 1 (2): 137–44.

Schmid, G. P., A. Buve, P. Mugyenyi, G. P. Garnett, R. J. Hayes, B. G. Williams, and others. 2004. "Transmission of HIV-1 Infection in Sub-Saharan Africa and Effect of Elimination of Unsafe Injections." *Lancet* 363 (9407): 482–88.

Scholes D., A. Stergachis, F. E. Heidrich, H. Andrilla, K. K. Holmes, and W. E. Stamm. 1996. "Prevention of Pelvic Inflammatory Disease by Screening for Cervical Chlamydial Infection." *New England Journal of Medicine* 334 (21): 1362–66.

Scoular, A. 2002. "Using the Evidence Base on Genital Herpes: Optimizing the Use of Diagnostic Tests and Information Provision." *Sexually Transmitted Infections* 78 (3): 160–65.

Semaan, S., L. Kay, D. Strouse, E. Sogolow, P. D. Mullen, M. S. Neumann, and others. 2002. "A Profile of U.S.-Based Trials of Behavioral and Social Interventions of HIV Risk Reduction." *Journal of Acquired Immune Deficiency Syndrome* 30 (Suppl. 1): S30–50.

Service, S. K., and S. M. Blower. 1996. "Linked HIV Epidemics in San Francisco" (letter). *Journal of Acquired Immune Deficiency Syndromes and Human Retrovirology* 11 (3): 311–13.

Shelton, J. D., D. T. Halperin, V. Nantulya, M. Potts, H. D. Gayle, and K. K. Holmes. 2004. "Partner Reduction Is Crucial for Balanced 'ABC' Approach to HIV Prevention." *British Medical Journal* 328 (7444): 891–93.

Simms, I., and J. M. Stephenson. 2000. "Pelvic Inflammatory Disease Epidemiology: What Do We Know and What Do We Need to Know?" *Sexually Transmitted Infections* 76 (2): 80–87.

Stamm, W. E. 1999. "*Chlamydia trachomatis* Infections of the Adult." In *Sexually Transmitted Diseases,* 3rd ed., ed. K. K. Holmes, P. F. Sparling, P.-A. Mardh, S. M. Lemon, W. E. Stamm, P. Piot, and J. N. Wasserheit, 407–22. New York: McGraw-Hill.

Stanberry, L. R., S. L. Spruance, A. L. Cunningham, D. I. Bernstein, A. Mindel, S. Sacks, and others. 2002. "Glycoprotein-D-Adjuvant Vaccine to Prevent Genital Herpes." *New England Journal of Medicine* 347 (21): 1652–61.

Steen, R. 2001. "Eradicating Chancroid." *Bulletin of the World Health Organization* 79 (9): 818–26.

Stone, K. M., K. L. Karem, M. R. Sternberg, G. M. McQuillan, A. D. Poon, E. R. Unger, and others. 2002. "Seroprevalence of Human Papillomavirus Type 16 in the United States." *Journal of Infectious Diseases* 186 (10): 1369–402.

Stoneburner, R. L., and D. Low-Beer. 2004. "Population-Level HIV Declines and Behavioral Risk Avoidance in Uganda." *Science* 304 (5671): 714–18.

Strand, A., R. Patel, H. C. Wulf, K. M. Coates, and International Valacyclovir HSV Study Group. 2002. "Aborted Genital Herpes Simplex Virus Lesions: Findings from a Randomized Controlled Study." *Sexually Transmitted Infections* 78 (6): 435–39.

Turner, C. F., S. M. Rogers, H. G. Miller, W. C. Miller, J. N. Gribble, J. R. Chromy, and others. 2002. "Untreated Gonococcal and Chlamydial Infection in a Probability Sample of Adults." *Journal of the American Medical Association* 287 (6): 726–33.

UNAIDS and WHO (Joint United Nations Programme on HIV/AIDS and World Health Organization). 2000. *Guidelines for Second Generation HIV Surveillance.* WHO/CDS/EDC/2000.5, UNAIDS/00.03E. Geneva: Working Group on Global HIV/AIDS and STI Surveillance.

van Dam, C. J. 1995. "HIV, STD, and Their Current Impact on Reproductive Health: The Need for Control of Sexually Transmitted Diseases." *International Journal of Gynecology and Obstetrics* 50 (Suppl. 2): S121–29.

van Dam, C. J., G. Dallabetta, and P. Piot. 1999. "Prevention and Control of Sexually Transmitted Diseases in Developing Countries." In *Sexually Transmitted Diseases,* 3rd ed., ed. K. K. Holmes, P. F. Sparling, P.-A. Mardh, S. M. Lemon, W. E. Stamm, P. Piot, and J. N. Wasserheit, 1381–90. New York: McGraw-Hill.

Vos, T. 1994. "Attitudes to Sex and Sexual Behavior in Rural Matabeleland, Zimbabwe." *AIDS Care* 6 (2): 193–203.

Walboomers, J. M. M., M. V. Jacobs, M. M. Manos, F. X. Bosch, J. A. Kummer, K. V. Shah, and others. 1999. "Human Papillomavirus Is a Necessary Cause of Invasive Cervical Cancer Worldwide." *Journal of Pathology* 189 (1): 12–19.

Wallin K. L., F. Wiklund, T. Luostarinen, T. Angstrom, T. Anttila, and F. Bergman. 2002. "A Population-Based Prospective Study of Chlamydia Trachomatis Infection and Cervical Carcinoma." *International Journal of Cancer* 101 (4): 371–74.

Wasserheit, J. N. 1989. "The Significance and Scope of Reproductive Tract Infections among Third World Women." *International Journal of Gynecology and Obstetrics* 3 (Suppl.): 145–68.

———. 1991. "Epidemiological Synergy: Interrelationships between HIV Infection and Other STDs." In *AIDS and Women's Health: Science for Policy and Action,* ed. L. Chen, J. Sepulveda, and S. Segal, 47–72. New York: Plenum Press.

Wasserheit, J. N., and S. O. Aral. 1996. "The Dynamic Topology of Sexually Transmitted Disease Epidemics: Implications for Prevention Strategies." *Journal of Infectious Diseases* 174 (Suppl. 2): S201–13.

Wawer, M. J., N. K. Sewankambo, D. Serwadda, T. C. Quinn, L. A. Paxton, N. Kiwanuka, and others. 1999. "Control of Sexually Transmitted Diseases for AIDS Prevention in Uganda: A Randomized Community Trial—Rakai Project Study Group." *Lancet* 353 (9152): 525–35.

Weir, S., C. Pailman, X. Mahlalela, N. Coetzee, F. Meidany, and J. T. Boerma. 2003. "From People to Places: Focusing AIDS Prevention Where It Matters Most." *AIDS* 17 (6): 895–903.

WHO (World Health Organization). 1991. *Management of Patients with Sexually Transmitted Disease: Report of a WHO Study Group.* Technical Report Series 810. Geneva: WHO.

———. 2001a. *Global Prevalence and Incidence of Selected Curable Sexually Transmitted Infections: Overview and Estimates.* Geneva: WHO.

———. 2001b. *Guidelines for the Management of Sexually Transmitted Infections.* Geneva: WHO.

Wilson, D., P. Chiroro, S. Lavelle, and C. Mutero. 1989. "Sex Worker, Client Sex Behaviour, and Condom Use in Harare, Zimbabwe." *AIDS Care* 1 (3): 269–80.

World Bank. 2003. *World Development Report 2004: Making Services Work for Poor People.* New York: Oxford University Press.

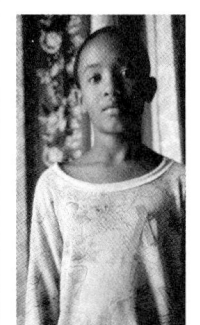

Chapter **18**

HIV/AIDS Prevention and Treatment

Stefano Bertozzi, Nancy S. Padian, Jeny Wegbreit, Lisa M. DeMaria, Becca Feldman, Helene Gayle, Julian Gold, Robert Grant, and Michael T. Isbell

Although global commitment to control the HIV/AIDS pandemic has increased significantly in recent years, the virus continues to spread with alarming and increasing speed. By the end of 2005, an estimated 40 million people worldwide were living with HIV infection or disease, a notable rise from the 35 million infected with HIV in 2001 (UNAIDS 2005). In 2005, close to 5 million new HIV infections and 3 million AIDS deaths occurred, more of both than in any previous year. Sub-Saharan Africa remains the region most affected by HIV/AIDS; however, the virus is now spreading rapidly in Asia and parts of Eastern Europe.

Despite the rapid spread of HIV, several countries have achieved important success in curbing its transmission. The extraordinary potential of HIV prevention is exemplified by such diverse efforts as Thailand's 100 percent condom program, Uganda's remarkable decrease in HIV prevalence, and the community-based syndromic management of sexually transmitted infections (STIs) in Mwanza, Tanzania. Box 18.1 describes characteristics common to these programs.

Successes also include the development and effective use of highly sensitive and specific HIV screening tests, which have virtually eliminated infection from the blood supply in the developed world and in most parts of the developing world (WHO 2002a). In addition, the administration of a short course of nevirapine to mothers during labor and to newborns postpartum reduces the risk of mother-to-child transmission (MTCT) by as much as 47 percent (Guay and others 1999). However, recent data suggest that such short-term successes may be at the expense of resistance and viral failure once treatment is introduced after delivery (Eshleman and others 2001).

Enormous advances in HIV/AIDS treatment regimens have fundamentally altered the natural history of the disease and sharply reduced HIV-related morbidity and mortality in countries where such treatments are accessible. The advent of antiretroviral drugs in the late 1980s began a revolution in the management of HIV, which can be seen as analogous to the use of penicillin for treating bacterial infections in the 1940s. The most notable advance on the treatment front is the use of combination antiretroviral therapy, which is far more effective than monotherapy (zidovudine or AZT), the standard of care when the first edition of this volume was published. Recent declines in the price of combination antiretroviral therapy in developing countries from US$15,000 per year to less than US$150 in some countries have prompted numerous developing countries to introduce antiretroviral therapy through the public sector. These declines also pose difficult questions regarding the optimal allocation of limited resources for HIV/AIDS, as well as the potential impact on already strained health care infrastructures.

OBSTACLES TO HIV CONTROL

Obstacles to effective HIV control include lack of prevention and care coverage and lack of rigorous evaluations. Both are discussed below.

Lack of Coverage and Access to Prevention Services

Notwithstanding these treatment strides, global efforts have not proved sufficient to control the spread of the pandemic or to extend the lives of the majority of those infected. The desired level of success has not yet been achieved for several reasons.

Most people who could benefit from available control strategies, including treatment, do not have access to them. Modelers commissioned by the World Health Organization (WHO) and the Joint United Nations Programme on HIV/AIDS (UNAIDS) determined that existing interventions could prevent 63 percent of all infections projected to occur between 2002 and 2010 (Stover and others 2002). Nonetheless, a 2003 survey of coverage revealed that fewer than one in five people at high risk of infection had access to the most basic prevention services, including condoms, AIDS education, MTCT prevention, voluntary counseling and testing (VCT), and harm reduction programs (Global HIV Prevention Working Group 2003). WHO and UNAIDS estimate that only about 7 percent of the nearly 6 million people in need of treatment receive it and that the number of people who require antiretroviral therapy increases by 8,000 each day (UNAIDS 2004).

Current coverage shortfalls, combined with the relentless expansion of the epidemic, underscore the acute need for rapid scale-up of prevention and treatment interventions—an imperative that the international community has acknowledged but that remains to be realized after more than 15 years. However, the activities of the Global Fund to Fight AIDS, Tuberculosis, and Malaria and the U.S. President's Emergency Plan for AIDS Relief (a five-year, US$15 billion initiative) suggest a growing commitment to tackle these issues. The latter aims to provide antiretroviral drugs for 2 million HIV-infected people, to prevent 7 million new infections, to provide care for 10 million individuals, and to develop health system capacity in Vietnam and in Africa and the Caribbean. Even though 15 countries are currently slated to receive support from the President's Emergency Plan, many of the countries most affected by HIV/AIDS— including Lesotho, Malawi, Swaziland, and Zimbabwe—are not included in the list of beneficiary countries.

Because antiretroviral therapy has historically been unavailable in most developing countries, national programs have lacked the means to undertake a comprehensive approach to HIV/AIDS (notable exceptions are Argentina, Brazil, and Mexico, which provide universal coverage for antiretroviral therapy). As discussed in chapter 8, control of the pandemic demands a two-front battle that emphasizes both prevention and care. Even though the prospect of greater access to treatment increases the feasibility of integrating prevention and care in resource-limited settings, it also raises new questions regarding the selection of optimal prevention programs to pair with treatment programs.

Lack of Rigorous Evaluations

In addition to poor coverage of key interventions, perhaps the greatest challenge to effective global control is the lack of reliable evidence to guide the selection of interventions for specific areas or populations. In the same way that global policy makers are increasingly recognizing the need for rigorous evaluation of development programs to ensure their success and eliminate waste, the need for reliable scientific evaluations of AIDS control programs is equally paramount for the same reasons. There are simply not enough resources to do everything everywhere; choices must be made and priorities set. In the HIV/AIDS field, this information deficit is especially pronounced with respect to HIV prevention in general and prevention implemented on a population level in particular. Currently, the allocation of resources for HIV/AIDS prevention is seldom evidence based, primarily because of a lack of data on both the effectiveness and the cost of interventions (Feachem 2004).

Few evaluations have collected data specifically on HIV infection as an outcome (Fleming and DeMets 1996). In the case of care and treatment, success and failure are more readily and rapidly apparent, leading to a substantial degree of auto-correction of ineffective policies. In contrast, with respect to HIV prevention, it is unlikely that those infections that might have occurred in the absence of a prevention program would be monitored, thus reducing the meaningfulness of the auto-feedback cycle for prevention. This underscores the importance of proactive, rigorous evaluation to differentiate success from failure in a timely manner. Sound evidence on the effectiveness of HIV prevention measures is especially important in light of the tendency of many governments and international aid agencies to avoid programs that address sexual behaviors, drug use, and highly stigmatized and vulnerable populations.

In addition, prevention studies have rarely incorporated the well-defined control or comparison groups necessary to identify contextual factors that are essential for appropriately tailoring interventions to the diverse regional settings and the myriad of microenvironments in which HIV transmission occurs (Grassly and others 2001). Contextual data are similarly critical for developing strategies to combat HIV/AIDS-related stigma and restrictive social and gender norms, which often frustrate attempts to address sexual and addictive behaviors associated with HIV transmission. Even where national efforts have succeeded in curbing the spread of the epidemic, as in Senegal and Uganda, evidence often does not clearly indicate the specific, well-defined, contextual features that account for success.

The lack of both contextual data and sound evidence regarding the effectiveness of HIV interventions hinders policy makers' ability to tailor HIV interventions to the nature and stage of national epidemics, something that the authors argue is necessary to address HIV/AIDS effectively. In the absence of such data, HIV/AIDS expenditures undoubtedly incorporate an unacceptable degree of waste, people are unnecessarily becoming infected with HIV, and HIV-infected individuals are dying prematurely.

Why has this type of research not been more forthcoming? In part it is because, by definition, such research is less innovative scientifically and also typically less experimental than research to develop new interventions. It is handicapped both in competing for traditional research funding and in receiving academic recognition. The only way to redress the imbalance is through specific earmarking of significant research funds.

ACTION UNDER UNCERTAINTY

Even though the current deficit in evaluation research is glaring, the magnitude and seriousness of the global pandemic means that action is nevertheless required. Moreover, despite such gaps in knowledge, we can still improve control strategies by tailoring interventions to the nature and scope of the epidemic. Summarized below is what is known with regard to the burden of disease, the determinants of transmission, and the effectiveness and cost-effectiveness of existing prevention interventions.

Burden of Disease

As a result of large-scale implementation of data collection methods for surveillance worldwide and enhanced methods for validating and interpreting HIV-related data, the HIV/AIDS epidemic is probably one of the best documented epidemics in history. An increasing number of data sources contribute to reasonably accurate estimates and a more nuanced understanding of the epidemic's trends. Unfortunately, this relatively accurate picture of where the epidemic is and has been is not matched by similarly convincing maps of the factors that explain its spread.

Although no single country has been spared the virus, the epidemic has affected certain regions of the world disproportionately, and Sub-Saharan Africa remains by far the hardest hit region (table 18.1). With only 10 percent of the world's population, it accounts for more than 75 percent of all HIV infections worldwide and more than 75 percent of AIDS-related deaths estimated for 2003. Asia and the Pacific, with several large and populous countries, account for 7.4 million infections, or 19.5 percent of the current burden of disease. Prevention and treatment efforts in Sub-Saharan Africa and Asia—regions that together represent 85 percent of all current infections—have dictated, and will continue to dictate, global trends in the burden of HIV- and AIDS-related mortality.

Between 1997 and 2001, the percentage of women living with HIV/AIDS increased from 41 to 50 percent. This trend is most apparent in Sub-Saharan Africa, where women represent 57 percent of adults living with HIV and 75 percent of HIV-infected young people. Even though women account for a smaller share of infections in Asia (28 percent), the disease burden among women and girls is likely to rise as the epidemic becomes generalized. More detailed information about the global burden of HIV/AIDS, regional differences, and trends over time is available in the UNAIDS (2005) report on the global AIDS epidemic.

Determinants of Infection

HIV transmission predominantly occurs through three mechanisms: sexual transmission, exposure to infected blood or blood products, or perinatal transmission (including breast-feeding). The likelihood of transmission is heavily affected by social, cultural, and environmental factors that often differ markedly between and within regions and countries. There is also some indication that molecular, viral, immunological, or other host factors might influence the likelihood of HIV transmission. For a more detailed discussion of sexual behaviors and the contextual determinants of infection, see chapter 17.

Table 18.1 Deaths and Disability-Adjusted Life Years Attributed to AIDS by Region, Age, and Gender, 2001

Region	Number (thousands)			
	Total	Both sexes, age 0–14	Both sexes, age 15+	Percentage female
Deaths				
World	2,576	439	2,133	46
High-income countries	22	0	21	23
Low- and middle-income countries	2,554	439	2,111	46
Sub-Saharan Africa	2,058	408	1,651	51
East Asia and the Pacific	107	5	100	25
Europe and Central Asia	28	0	27	14
Latin America and the Caribbean	83	8	73	36
Middle East and North Africa	4	0	2	25
Southeast Asia	272	18	255	23
Disability-adjusted life years				
World	71,460	13,586	57,875	47
High-income countries	665	7	660	23
Low- and middle-income countries	70,795	13,579	57,215	47
Sub-Saharan Africa	56,820	12,526	44,294	52
East Asia and the Pacific	3,121	195	2,927	25
Europe and Central Asia	982	25	957	18
Latin America and the Caribbean	2,354	260	2,092	36
Middle East and North Africa	105	20	84	39
Southeast Asia	7,413	553	6,861	25

Source: Mathers and others 2006.

Table 18.2 Estimated HIV Transmission Risk per Exposure

Type of exposure	Estimated risk HIV transmission per exposure
Receptive anal intercourse	≤ 3.0 percent (1/125 to 1/31) (DeGruttola and others 1989)
Receptive vaginal intercourse	≤ 0.1 percent (1/2,000 to 1/667) (Mastro and others 1994; Wiley, Herschkorn, and Padian 1989)
Insertive vaginal or anal intercourse	≤ 0.1 percent (1/3,333 to 1/1,111) (Nagachinta and others 1997; Peterman and others 1988)
Needlestick injury	= 0.3 percent (1/313) (Henderson and others 1990)
Use of contaminated injecting drug equipment	= 0.6 percent (1/149) (Kaplan and Heimer 1992)
Mucous membrane	= 0.1 percent (1/1,111) (Ippolito, Puro, and De Carli 1993)

Source: Authors.

Sexual Transmission. Worldwide, sexual intercourse is the predominant mode of transmission, accounting for approximately 80 percent of infections (Askew and Berer 2003). Sexual intercourse accounts for more than 90 percent of infections in Sub-Saharan Africa. Although many people who know they are infected reduce their risk behaviors, studies in developed countries suggest that a substantial percentage nevertheless continue to engage in unprotected sex (Marks, Burris, and Peterman 1999). The risk of sexual transmission is determined by behaviors that influence the likelihood of exposure to an infected individual and by infectivity in the event of exposure. This also includes factors related to the infectiousness of the infected partner and the susceptibility of the uninfected partner.

Infectivity The per contact infectivity of HIV from sexual transmission varies depending on sexual activity (Royce and others 1997). Anal intercourse carries a higher transmission probability than penile-vaginal intercourse, and male-to-female transmission is more likely than female-to-male transmission. Data on infectivity by transmission mode are shown in table 18.2.

Biological Mediators of Infectivity Untreated STIs increase the risk of sexual HIV transmission several-fold (Institute of Medicine 1997). Numerous epidemiological studies have supported the association of genital ulcers in general and of genital herpes (herpes simplex virus 2, or HSV-2) in particular with HIV infection (Hook and others 1992). Not only does the biological interaction between HSV-2 and HIV enhance the transmission and acquisition of HIV, but HIV infection is also associated with more frequent reactivation of HSV-2. The presence of herpetic ulcers and lesions allows an entry point for HIV in the uninfected individual, and the presence of high copy numbers of HIV ribonucleic acid (RNA) in HSV-2 lesions in HIV-infected individuals underscores the importance for HIV prevention of controlling HSV-2 infections (Mbopi Keou and others 1999).

Vaginal infections are also emerging as important risk factors for HIV. For example, infection with trichomonas increases the risk for HIV seroconversion (Buve 2002). In addition, higher trichomonas rates have been detected in regions of Sub-Saharan Africa that have higher HIV rates, and investigators working throughout Sub-Saharan Africa report similar results, with odds ratios from 1.5 to 56.8 (Gregson and others 2001). In addition, studies have shown an increased risk of HIV acquisition in patients who have bacterial vaginosis (Martin and others 1999).

Circumcision also affects HIV transmission. In a meta-analysis of 27 studies (Weiss, Quigley, and Hayes 2000), uncircumcised men were almost twice as likely to be infected with HIV as those who were circumcised. Studies that controlled adequately for other risks and studies that separately assessed risk in high-risk populations, such as STI clinic attendees or truck drivers, found an even stronger protective effect of circumcision. Similarly, an ecological study comparing two high-prevalence Sub-Saharan African cities with two low-prevalence cities found that circumcised individuals were substantially less likely to be infected with HIV (Auvert and others 2001). Two recent studies conducted in Kenya and India (Donnelly 2004; Reynolds and others 2004) found that uncircumcised men had an HIV rate 7 to 11 times greater than circumcised men. More recently, results from a randomized controlled trial conducted in South Africa indicated that the risk of HIV acquisition was reduced by more than 60 percent of men randomized for circumcision (controlling for sexual behavior, including condom use and health seeking behavior) in a community where more than 30 percent of the women were infected (Auvert and others 2005).

Before circumcision among adult males becomes a widespread policy recommendation, results are still pending in two similar trials. Obviously one issue is the acceptability of such a procedure as well as the fact that some increase in high risk sexual activity was noted among the men who were circumcised, although this did not offset the results of the intervention.

The risk of sexual transmission is also strongly correlated with the plasma level of virus in the infected individual (Quinn and others 2000); thus, infectivity varies over the natural progression of the disease. Individuals are most infectious subsequent to infection and again during the late stage of the disease. Antiretroviral therapy significantly reduces the level of virus, often to the point that standard tests cannot detect HIV in the patient's blood (Palella and others 1998). Available data suggest that viral load reductions induced by antiretroviral therapy will lower infectiousness. Studies have shown a close relationship between the amount of viral suppression and the risk of vertical transmission (Garcia and others 1999). Quinn and others (2002) show that the risk of sexual transmission between couples in Africa was strongly related to the level of viral load in the infected partner.

Exposure to Infected Blood or Blood Products. Injection drug use and blood transfusion are two mechanisms of HIV exposure to infected blood. Determinants of each are discussed below.

Injection Because of the efficiency of HIV transmission through needle sharing, the introduction of HIV into an urban network of injecting drugs users can quickly lead to extraordinarily high HIV prevalence in this population. Sharing of injection equipment and frequency of injection are both important correlates of HIV infection (Chaisson and others 1989). Attendance at shooting galleries, where sharing with anonymous injecting partners is likely to occur, is also an independent risk factor across many studies (Vlahov and others 1990). Injecting cocaine (associated with "booting" or "kicking," where blood is drawn into the syringe and then injected) and having a number of needle-sharing partners are also associated with HIV infection (Anthony and others 1991).

Blood Transfusion The probability of becoming infected through an HIV-contaminated transfusion is estimated at more than 90 percent (UNAIDS 1997), and the amount of HIV in a single contaminated blood transfusion is so large that individuals infected in this manner may rapidly develop AIDS. Currently, between 5 and 10 percent of HIV infections worldwide are transmitted through the transfusion of contaminated blood products (WHO 2002a). Setting up and maintaining a safe blood supply will virtually eliminate HIV transmission through transfusions.

Perinatal Transmission. Perinatal HIV transmission includes both vertical transmission and transmission during breastfeeding. Determinants of each are discussed below.

Vertical Transmission Perhaps the most compelling evidence of the significance of viral load and transmission risk has been documented with respect to MTCT. Maternal viral load, as quantified by RNA polymerase chain reaction, is associated with increased risk in each mode of vertical transmission. A recent randomized clinical trial in Kenya found that maternal plasma HIV RNA levels higher than 43,000 copies per milliliter were associated with a fourfold increase in vertical transmission (John and others 2001).

Independent of HIV RNA levels in maternal plasma, additional risk factors include cervical HIV deoxyribonucleic acid (DNA), vaginal HIV DNA, and cervical or vaginal ulcers. Chorioamnionitis has also been documented as a risk factor for MTCT among African mothers (Ladner and others 1998), as has exposure to maternal blood during labor and delivery. Newell (2003) estimates that for every hour an infant is exposed to ruptured membranes, the risk of transmission increases by 2 percent.

Breastfeeding Transmission through breastfeeding is likely associated with an elevated viral load in the breast milk, which in turn is associated with maternal plasma viral load and CD4 T cell levels. Mastitis has also been associated with increased risk of vertical transmission. Meta-analyses suggest that the cumulative probability of HIV infection increases from 0.6 percent at age 6 months to 9.2 percent at age 3 (Read 2003). A study in Malawi, however, indicates that most transmission occurs in the early breastfeeding months, with an incidence per month of 0.7 percent at age 1 to 5 months, 0.6 percent at age 6 to 11 months, and 0.3 percent at age 12 to 17 months (Miotti and others 1999). In one study, infants who were breastfed in combination with receiving other supplementary foods were twice as likely to be infected at age 6 months than infants fed exclusively on breast milk or on formula (Coutsoudis and others 2001). The hypothesis is that antigens and bacterial contaminants present in supplemental fluids and foods consumed by infants who are not exclusively breastfed may cause inflammation and microtrauma to the infant's intestinal gut, thereby facilitating viral transmission. Another hypothesis is that mixed feeding increases the risk of subclinical or clinical mastitis in the mother, which could increase milk viral load (Semba and others 1999).

Decisions about breastfeeding are further complicated by recent data indicating possible increased mortality among breastfeeding mothers (Nduati and others 2001) and by the stigma associated with not breastfeeding in countries where abstaining from breastfeeding is tantamount to disclosing a woman's HIV status.

Effectiveness and Cost-Effectiveness of Prevention Interventions

Below we discuss the need for ongoing surveillance and contextual data to determine the effectiveness of HIV interventions and how best to implement those interventions. We then discuss the existing effectiveness and cost-effectiveness data.

Essential Background Data for Any Intervention. Because the prioritization of prevention strategies for any epidemic requires accurately identifying the epidemiological profile (discussed below), maintaining a sound and reliable public health surveillance system is a prerequisite for an effective prevention response. An understanding of HIV and STI prevalence and trends, as well as the prevalence and distribution of behaviors that contribute to the epidemic's spread, should be supplemented by national monitoring systems that track sources and uses of funding to promote greater accountability. In addition, data are needed to identify and characterize key contextual issues that affect the selection of interventions.

Although surveillance is essential for an optimally strategic public health response, its utility depends on the degree to which the information it yields is effectively deployed. As noted below, countries with concentrated epidemics should prioritize interventions that are targeted to the populations at highest risk. In Latin America, however, where information on national AIDS funding is strongest, the proportion of limited prevention resources that is not targeted to the populations at highest risk of infection varies from less than 5 percent to more than 50 percent (Saavedra 2000). This range strongly suggests that resource allocation is frequently not based on available epidemiological and effectiveness data.

Table 18.3 summarizes information about the effectiveness of the interventions discussed below.

Cost-Effectiveness Estimates for Prevention Interventions. How countries spend funds and which interventions they prioritize should be guided by estimates of the relative cost-effectiveness of such interventions. Unfortunately, reliable estimates of cost-effectiveness are largely lacking, for a number of reasons. The main reason is that HIV prevention interventions are difficult to force into a typology that clearly distinguishes one intervention from another. For example, the counseling component of VCT has a strong information-sharing element that overlaps with (a) information, education, and communication (IEC) through the media; (b) peer interventions; and (c) the counseling component of STI treatment. Similarly, the psychological support offered through counseling is comparable to support provided through support groups or to interventions designed to increase social support. Such overlap and duplication among components of different interventions complicate efforts to estimate both the effectiveness and the cost-effectiveness of different interventions.

Several authors have recently reviewed estimates of cost-effectiveness for the prevention interventions described here (Creese and others 2002; Jha and others 2001; Marseille and others 2002; Walker 2003). These reviews address a number of

Table 18.3 Effectiveness of HIV Interventions

Intervention	Outcome	Effect	Citations
School-based education	Sexual debut	The number of students reporting early sexual debut was significantly lower in the intervention group in both studies.	Hayes and others 2003; Stanton and others 1998
	Multiple sex partners	The number of students reporting multiple sex partners was significantly lower in the intervention group in both studies.	Fawole and others 1999; Hayes and others 2003
	Condom use	Condom use was significantly higher in the intervention group in three of the four studies and nonsignificantly higher in one study.	Fawole and others 1999; Harvey, Stuart, and Swan 2000; Hayes and others 2003; Stanton and others 1998
	HIV incidence	The study found no significant differences in HIV incidence.	Hayes and others 2003
	STI prevalence and incidence	The study found no significant differences in STI prevalence and incidence.	Hayes and others 2003
Abstinence education	Condom use	The study found no significant differences in condom use.	Jemmott, Jemmott, and Fong 1998
	Early sexual debut	The study found no significant differences in early sexual debut.	Meekers 2000
VCT[a]	Condom use	Condom use was significantly higher in the intervention group in six of the seven studies and unchanged in one study.	Bentley and others 1998; Bhave and others 1995; Deschamps and others 1996; Jackson and others 1997; Kamenga and others 1991; Levine and others 1998; Voluntary HIV-1 Counseling and Testing Efficacy Study Group 2000
	Unprotected intercourse	Unprotected intercourse was significantly lower in the intervention group in both studies.	Deschamps and others 1996; Voluntary HIV-1 Counseling and Testing Efficacy Study Group 2000
	HIV incidence	HIV incidence was significantly lower in the intervention group in one of the studies and nonsignificantly lower in the other study.	Bhave and others 1995; Celentano and others 2000
	STI prevalence and incidence	STI prevalence and incidence were significantly lower in the intervention group in all three studies.	Celentano and others 2000; Jackson and others 1997; Levine and others 1998
Peer-based programs	Condom use	Condom use was significantly higher in the intervention group in all four studies.	Kelly and others 1997; Norr and others 2004; Sikkema and others 2000; Stanton and others 1996
	Unprotected intercourse	Unprotected intercourse was significantly lower in the intervention group in all four studies.	Basu and others 2004; Kegeles, Hays, and Coates 1996; Kelly and others 1997; Sikkema and others 2000
	Communication about condoms with partner	Communication was significantly higher in the intervention group.	Lauby and others 2000
	HIV incidence	HIV incidence was significantly lower in the intervention group in both studies.	Ghys and others 2002; Katzenstein and others 1998
	STI prevalence and incidence	STI prevalence and incidence were significantly lower in the intervention group.	Ghys and others 2002
Condom promotion and distribution and IEC[a]	Condom use	Condom use was significantly higher in the intervention group in 10 of the 11 studies and unchanged in 1 study.	Bentley and others 1998; Bhave and others 1995; Egger and others 2000; Ford and others 1996; Jackson and others 1997; Jemmott, Jemmott, and Fong 1998; Kagimu and others 1998; Laga and others 1994; Levine and others 1998; Ngugi and others 1988; Pauw and others 1996

(Continues on the following page.)

Table 18.3. Continued

Intervention	Outcome	Effect	Citations
	HIV incidence	HIV incidence was significantly lower in the intervention group in two out of three studies and nonsignificantly lower in one study.	Bhave and others 1995; Celentano and others 2000; Laga and others 1994
	STI prevalence and incidence	STI prevalence and incidence were significantly lower in the intervention group in all four studies.	Bhave and others 1995; Celentano and others 2000; Jackson and others 1997; Laga and others 1994; Levine and others 1998
Condom social marketing	Condom use	Condom use was significantly higher in the intervention group in one study; no significant differences were found in the other study.	Agha, Karlyn, and Meekers 2001; Meekers 2000
	Early sexual debut	The study found no significant differences in early sexual debut.	Meekers 2000
STI treatment[a]	HIV incidence	HIV incidence was significantly lower in the intervention group in two of the studies, but the other two studies found no significant differences.	Grosskurth and others 1995; Kamali and others 2003; Laga and others 1994; Wawer and others 1999
	STI prevalence and incidence	The prevalence and incidence of STIs were significantly lower in the intervention group in all six studies.	Jackson and others 1997; Kamali and others 2003; Laga and others 1994; Mayaud and others 1997; Wawer and others 1999
Antiretroviral therapy to reduce MTCT	Mother-to-infant transmission[b]	Significant reduction in mother-to-infant HIV transmission in the intervention group was found in all eight studies, with a range of 33 to 67 percent reduction in transmission.	Ayouba and others 2003; Connor and others 1994; Dabis and others 1999; Guay and others 1999; Jackson and others 2003; PETRA Study Team 2002; Shaffer and others 1999; Wiktor and others 1999
MTCT feeding substitutions	Mother-to-infant transmission	Use of breast milk substitutes prevented 44 percent of infant infections and was associated with significantly improved HIV-1-free survival.	Nduati and others 2000
Harm reduction in injecting drug users	HIV incidence	Significant reduction in HIV incidence in the intervention group was found in both studies.	Des Jarlais and Friedman 1996; Hurley, Jolley, and Kaldor 1997
	Reuse or sharing of syringes	Significant reduction in needle sharing in the intervention group was found in all three studies; correlation between needle exchange program attendance and lower needle sharing was found in one study.	Jenkins and others 2001; Ksobiech 2003; Peak and others 1995; Vlahov and others 1997
Drug substitution for injecting drug users	Drug use	This meta-analysis found significantly lower rates of drug use.	Metzger, Navaline, and Woody 1998
Blood safety	HIV infections averted	HIV screening was associated with a reduction in HIV infections by both studies.	Foster and Buve 1995; Laleman and others 1992
	Units of HIV-positive blood averted	HIV screening was associated with a reduction in units of HIV-positive blood.	Jacobs and Mercer 1999
Universal precautions	Blood volume transferred in needlestick injury	Glove material reduced the transferred blood volume by 46 to 86 percent.	Mast, Woolwine, and Gerberding 1993
Antiretroviral therapy for prevention, postexposure prophylaxis	HIV seroconversion	The study found a significant relationship between seroconversion and not having received antiretroviral therapy.	Cardo and others 1997
Behavior change for those HIV positive	Condom use	Condom use was significantly higher in the intervention group.	Kalichman and others 2001
	Unprotected intercourse	Unprotected intercourse was significantly lower in the intervention group.	Kalichman and others 2001

Source: Authors.

a. Studies examined may have included educational components, condom promotion and distribution components, HIV testing and counseling, or STI treatment.

b. The types of MTCT antiretroviral therapy varied in theses studies.

Table 18.4 Cost-Effectiveness of Interventions by Epidemic Profile

| Intervention | Epidemic profile (2001 US$) | | | | UNAIDS estimate of need for 2007 | |
	Low-level epidemic (Middle East and North Africa)	Concentrated epidemic (East Asia and the Pacific, Europe and Central Asia, Latin America and the Caribbean, South Asia)	Generalized low-level epidemic (Sub-Saharan Africa)	Generalized high-level epidemic (Sub-Saharan Africa)	2003 US$ millions	Percentage of all prevention needs
Surveillance	No CE studies found	No CE studies found	No CE studies found	No CE studies found	—	—
IEC	No CE studies found	No CE studies found	No CE studies found	No CE studies found	129	1
School-based education	No CE studies found	India (E/D/no STIs) US$1,350 per HIV infection US$68 per DALY (World Bank 1999)	No CE studies found	No CE studies found	100	1
Abstinence education	No CE studies found	No CE studies found	No CE studies found	No CE studies found	—	—
VCT	No CE studies found	India US$196 per HIV infection US$10 per DALY (World Bank 1999)	Chad (M/S/no STIs) US$891 to US$5,213 per HIV infection US$45 to US$261 per DALY (Hutton, Wyss, and N'Diekhor 2003) Kenya and Tanzania (M/S/STI) US$270 to US$376 per HIV infection US$14 to US$19 per DALY (Sweat and others 2000)	No CE studies found	2,175	22

(Continues on the following page.)

Table 18.4 Continued

Intervention	Epidemic profile (2001 US$)				UNAIDS estimate of need for 2007	
	Low-level epidemic (Middle East and North Africa)	Concentrated epidemic (East Asia and the Pacific, Europe and Central Asia, Latin America and the Caribbean, South Asia)	Generalized low-level epidemic (Sub-Saharan Africa)	Generalized high-level epidemic (Sub-Saharan Africa)	2003 US$ millions	Percentage of all prevention needs
Peer-based programs	No CE studies found	United States (E/S/no STIs) US$71,113 per HIV infection, US$3,556 per DALY (Pinkerton and others 1998) United States (E/D/no STIs) US$14,934 to US$18,719 per HIV infection US$747 to US$936 per DALY (Kahn and others 2001) India (sex workers) US$52 per HIV infection US$3 per DALY (World Bank 1999) India (high-risk men) US$303 per HIV infection US$15 per DALY (World Bank 1999)	Chad (sex workers) US$6 to US$30 per HIV infection US$0 to US$2 per DALY (Hutton, Wyss, and N'Diekhor 2003) Chad (high-risk men) US$24 to US$1,476 per HIV infection US$1 to US$74 per DALY (Hutton, Wyss, and N'Diekhor 2003) Chad (youths) US$129 to infinity per HIV infection US$6 to infinity per DALY (Hutton, Wyss, and N'Diekhor 2003) Cameroon (E/D/STIs) US$67 to US$137 per HIV infection US$3 to US$7 per DALY (Kumaranayake and others 1998)	No CE studies found	3,696	37
Condom promotion and distribution and IEC	No CE studies found	No CE studies found	No CE studies found	South Africa (female condom) (M/D/STI) US$378 to US$4,094 per HIV infection US$19 to US$205 per DALY (Marseille and others 2001)	1,093	11

Intervention						
Condom social marketing	No CE studies found	No CE studies found	Chad US$77 per HIV infection US$4 per DALY (Hutton, Wyss, and N'Diekhor 2003)	No CE studies found	198	2
STI treatment	No CE studies found	No CE studies found	Chad US$1,675 per HIV infection US$84 per DALY (Hutton, Wyss, and N'Diekhor 2003) Tanzania (E/S/STI) US$326 per HIV infection US$16 per DALY (Gilson and others 1997) Kenya (E/D/STI) US$11 to US$16 per HIV infection US$1 per DALY (Moses and others 1991)	South Africa (E/STI) US$2,093 per HIV infection US$105 per DALY (Vickerman and others forthcoming)	783	8
Antiretroviral therapy to reduce MTCT	No CE studies found	Mexico (M) US$39,230 to US$42,528 per HIV infection US$2,124 to US$2,303 per DALY (Rely and others 2003) India $2,527 per HIV infection $126 per DALY (World Bank 1999)	Zambia (E) US$848 per HIV infection US$34 per DALY (Stringer and others 2003) Chad (AZT) US$924 to US$4,044 per HIV infection US$37 to US$162 per DALY (Hutton, Wyss, and N'Diekhor 2003) Chad (breastfeeding advice) US$1,241 to US$4,382 per HIV infection US$50 to US$175 per DALY (Hutton, Wyss, and N'Diekhor 2003)	South Africa (M) US$1,650 to US$3,844 per HIV infection US$66 to US$154 per DALY (Wilkinson, Floyd, and Gilks 1998) Sub-Saharan Africa (M) US$5,279 to US$11,444 per HIV infection US$211 to US$458 per DALY (Marseille, Kahn, and Saba 1998) Sub-Saharan Africa (nevirapine) (M) US$142 to US$306 per HIV infection US$6 to US$12 per DALY (Marseille and others 1999)	320	3

(Continues on the following page.)

Table 18.4 Continued

Intervention	Epidemic profile (2001 US$)				UNAIDS estimate of need for 2007	
	Low-level epidemic (Middle East and North Africa)	Concentrated epidemic (East Asia and the Pacific, Europe and Central Asia, Latin America and the Caribbean, South Asia)	Generalized low-level epidemic (Sub-Saharan Africa)	Generalized high-level epidemic (Sub-Saharan Africa)	2003 US$ millions	Percentage of all prevention needs
MTCT, feeding substitution	No CE studies found	No CE studies found	No CE studies found	No CE studies found	—	—
Harm reduction for injecting drug users	No CE studies found	Belarus (E) US$353 per HIV infection US$18 per DALY (Kumaranayake and others 2004) Russia (E) US$564 per HIV infection US$28 per DALY (Bobrik 2004)	No CE studies found	No CE studies found	241	2
Drug substitution for injecting drug users	No CE studies found	No CE studies found	No CE studies found	No CE studies found	—	—
Blood safety	0.01–1 percent HIV prevalence (M/D/STIs) US$374 to US$45,173 per HIV infection US$19 to US$2,259 per DALY (Over and Piot 1996)		Chad US$75 to US$151 per HIV infection US$4 to US$8 per DALY (Hutton, Wyss, and N'Diekhor 2003) Zambia (E/D/STI) US$215 to US$262 per HIV infection US$11 to US$13 per DALY (Watts, Goodman, and Kumaranayake 2000) Zambia (E) US$41 per HIV infection US$2 per DALY (Foster and Buve 1995)	Zimbabwe (E) US$166 to US$1,010 per HIV infection US$8 to US$51 per DALY (McFarland and others 1995) 1–40 percent HIV prevalence US$9 to US$1,806 per HIV infection US$0.45 to $90 per DALY (Over and Piot 1996)	230	2

	Middle East (M)	Southeast Asia	Africa		
Sterile injection	US$393 per DALY (Dziekan and others 2003)	Southeast Asia US$143 to US$593 per DALY; Americas US$1,851 to US$56,642 per DALY; Western Pacific US$953 per DALY (Dziekan and others 2003)	US$91 to US$230 per DALY (Dziekan and others 2003)	94	1
Universal precautions	No CE studies found	No CE studies found	No CE studies found	663	7
Antiretroviral therapy for prevention and postexposure prophylaxis	No CE studies found	United States (E/S/no STIs) US$76,584 per HIV infection US$3,829 per DALY (Pinkerton, Holtgrave, and Bloom 1998)	No CE studies found	1	<1
Vaccines	No CE studies found	No CE studies found	No CE studies found	—	—
Behavior change for those who are HIV+	No CE studies found	No CE studies found	No CE studies found	112	1

Source: Authors.

— = not available.

CE = cost-effectiveness.

Note: The authors have categorized each of the studies. The first time each study is mentioned, it is identified by whether it was modeled (M) or empirical (E); whether it calculated primary HIV infections averted (S, for static) or if it also showed secondary infections averted (D, for dynamic); and where appropriate, we indicate if the study also looked at the impact on STIs. The cost-effectiveness of these interventions will differ depending on the population to which they are targeted, (that is, mass interventions versus targeted interventions). In addition, the cost-effectiveness of each intervention may vary greatly by study, because each cost-effectiveness study is not uniform. No cost-effectiveness studies of male condom promotion were found, because condom promotion, distribution, and IEC are generally part of a larger program with many components and studies did not distinguish between the costs of individual components of such programs.

Comprehensive Sex Education Versus Abstinence-Only Education

The available data on sex education suggest the following:

- Sex education, including condom promotion, does not encourage or increase sexual activity (Kirby 2001).
- Sex education reduces risk and positively affects sexual behaviors. In general, sex education programs increase knowledge about AIDS and related issues, increase intention to use condoms, and increase condom use among sexually active youths (Kim and others 1997).

- Abstinence-only education is not effective in promoting healthy sexual behaviors. Programs that promote both postponement of intercourse and contraceptive use were more effective in changing behaviors than those that stressed abstinence alone. None of the abstinence-only programs that have been evaluated demonstrated an overall positive effect on sexual behavior, nor did they affect contraceptive use among sexually active participants (Kirby 1997).

Source: Authors.

methodological issues that will not be repeated here. The reviews agree that the availability of cost and cost-effectiveness analyses for HIV/AIDS prevention strategies is limited and that the need for such knowledge for planning and decision-making purposes is urgent.

Table 18.4 summarizes available cost-effectiveness estimates for the four UNAIDS epidemic profiles that are described later in table 18.5. The estimates of cost per disability-adjusted life year (DALY) saved assume a uniform 20 DALYs lost per infected adult (Murray and Lopez 1996) and 25 DALYs lost per infected child (Marseille and others 1999) and do not account for the increasing proportion of people living with HIV/AIDS in developing countries who will have access to antiretroviral therapy over the coming years.

General Interventions Relevant for All Modes of Transmission

The following are general interventions not specifically targeting the mode of transmission:

- *Information, education, and communication.* This intervention includes education on HIV/AIDS and condom use through pamphlets, brochures, and other promotional materials in classroom or clinic settings or through the radio, television, or press. In general, discerning the effectiveness of IEC alone is difficult, because IEC is often included in condom promotion and distribution interventions. Here we consider the effectiveness of IEC in concert with condom promotion and distribution. Of all available prevention interventions, providing information and education about HIV/AIDS is perhaps the most difficult to assess for cost-effectiveness. Numerous studies have shown that information alone is typically insufficient to change risk behavior. Accurate information, however, is indisputably the basis for informed policy discourse—a vital ingredient in the fight against fear-based stigma and discrimination. In

the absence of studies to guide the level of investment in IEC, the only reasonable alternative seems to be to implement IEC on the basis of data derived from relative levels of knowledge and understanding in the population. For example, if only 25 percent of the sexually active population were able to describe how HIV is transmitted and prevented, clearly more IEC would be needed, but if 75 percent of the population understood the basic facts about HIV/AIDS, the need for additional funding would be diminished.

- *School-based sex education.* School-based sex education programs, an aspect of IEC, provide information to young people and reinforce healthy norms in a school setting (Peersman and Levy 1998). Limited data have shown differences in students who have been exposed to school-based sex education (summarized in table 18.3). Box 18.2 reviews the effectiveness of abstinence-only education and comprehensive sex education, subsets of school-based sex education. In light of more recent controlled studies that have not shown an effect on condom use, STIs, or HIV infection, any cost-effectiveness estimate is extremely speculative.
- *Voluntary counseling and testing.* This intervention enables people to know their HIV status and provides counseling support to help them cope with the outcome. Knowledge of serostatus may lead individuals to avoid engaging in risky behaviors (Sweat and others 2000). Cost-effectiveness estimates of VCT vary widely, and as with many other prevention interventions, these estimates are extremely sensitive to the prevalence of HIV in the population that is seeking testing.
- *Peer-based programs.* Peer interventions use influential members of a targeted community to disseminate information or teach specific skills. Such interventions have generally been found to be effective in reducing unsafe behaviors. Work on the cost-effectiveness of peer-based interventions in developing countries has been minimal. In Chad, Hutton, Wyss, and N'Diekhor (2003) reviewed data on 12 prevention

interventions and integrated them into a comparative analysis. Their findings suggest that peer education for sex workers is likely to be highly cost-effective and to entail one-fifth the cost of the next most favorable intervention, blood safety. However, the estimated cost-effectiveness for the same intervention directed toward young people and high-risk men is 33- to 36-fold lower.

Interventions to Prevent Sexual Transmission Below we discuss the effectiveness and cost-effectiveness of interventions that target sexual transmission of HIV:

- *Condom promotion, distribution, and social marketing.* Condom promotion, distribution, and social marketing vary by epidemic profile. The evidence on condom promotion and distribution programs indicates that such programs result in significantly higher condom use and significantly lower STI incidence (see table 18.3). Given the central role that condom promotion, distribution, and social marketing has played in HIV prevention programs, the lack of data on the relative cost-effectiveness of such programs 20 years into their implementation is striking. It is beyond dispute that the use of a condom by sexual partners who are HIV-discordant is extraordinarily cost-effective, given the low cost and high effectiveness of the condom in preventing HIV transmission. Information on the relative costs and effectiveness of different approaches to increasing condom use by serodiscordant sexual partners is not available, with the shortage of information being far more acute for effectiveness than for costs. In the absence of empirical evidence, decision makers are reduced to formulating policy on the basis of theory and common sense. Even inefficient use of condoms by seroconcordant couples is likely to be highly cost-effective because of the reduction in other STIs, cervical cancer, and unwanted pregnancies. However, more reliable information on

strategies to optimize the effectiveness and cost-effectiveness of condom programs is urgently needed.
- *STI screening and treatment.* The latest analyses suggest that STI control may be most effective as an HIV prevention strategy when initiated earlier in the course of national epidemics and when sexual risk behaviors are high (Orroth and others 2003). In most developing countries, the greatest benefits from treating STIs almost certainly accrue from averting the morbidity and mortality caused directly by STIs rather than indirectly because of reduced HIV transmission. Estimates of the cost-effectiveness of STI treatment purely as a way to reduce HIV transmission vary widely.

Prevention of Mother-to-Child Transmission The existing data on the effectiveness and cost-effectiveness of HIV interventions target MTCT in order of decreasing cost-effectiveness as follows:

- *Avoidance of unwanted pregnancies among infected mothers.* One of the most effective strategies to reduce HIV among infants is to provide better contraception services. See box 18.3 for details.
- *Use of antiretroviral therapy.* Evidence indicates that the provision of antiretroviral drugs to infected mothers significantly reduces vertical transmission (see table 18.4). The provision of antiretroviral therapy to prevent MTCT is highly cost-effective, to the point of being cost-saving for women who already know that they are infected. When screening of women is involved, cost-effectiveness declines as HIV prevalence falls, because of the larger number of women who must be screened to identify an HIV-positive woman (Rely and others 2003).
- *Feeding substitution.* Whereas in high-income countries the health community recommends complete avoidance of breastfeeding for HIV-infected mothers to prevent postnatal

---

Box 18.3

Preventing Mother-to-Child Transmission: Antiretroviral Therapy or Contraception?

The differential effect of contraceptive delivery versus antiretroviral therapy in preventing HIV can be shown by comparing the provision of effective contraception and of nevirapine to a population of 1,000 HIV-infected women. In the absence of an intervention, approximately 150 infants would be infected with HIV during delivery (Cates 2004). If nevirapine were available, the number of infected infants would be reduced to 82 (the expected 47 percent decline). If effective contraceptive services were

available, this number would be reduced to 49. If both strategies were adopted, the number of infected infants would be further reduced to 25.

The greatest difference between providing antiretroviral therapy and providing contraception is the number of infants orphaned in the future because their mothers die of HIV infection. Three models all come to this conclusion (Reynolds and others 2004; Stover and others forthcoming; Sweat and others 2004).

Source: Authors.

HIV transmission, in developing countries the feasibility of this approach is often limited by such factors as cost, sustainability, lack of safe water, health, and child spacing and by sociocultural factors (Coutsoudis 2002). Prolonged breastfeeding more than doubles the likelihood of MTCT (Nduati and others 2000). Because evidence indicates that mixed feeding (breast milk and formula or other substance) has a higher risk of transmission than exclusive breastfeeding (Coutsoudis and others 1999), mothers should be counseled on the superiority of early weaning over mixed feeding. Even fewer data are available on the cost-effectiveness of feeding substitution.

Prevention of Bloodborne Transmission Below we discuss the effectiveness and cost-effectiveness of harm reduction for injecting drug users, implementation of blood safety practices, and provision of sterile injections:

- *Harm reduction for injecting drug users.* Harm reduction involves a combination of health promotion strategies for users, including needle and syringe exchange programs, ready access to effective drug treatment and substitution, and provision of counseling and condoms. Brazil, which has reduced the incidence of HIV and kept HIV prevalence from reaching projected levels, has relied on strong official support for harm reduction as a cornerstone of its national prevention program (Mesquita and others 2003). A limited number of studies have shown significant reductions in HIV incidence among those exposed to needle exchange programs, and several studies have shown significant reductions in needle sharing (see table 18.3). Methadone maintenance is both safe and effective as a treatment for drug addiction (National Consensus Development Panel on Effective Medical Treatment of Opiate Addiction 1998) and may help reduce the risk of HIV transmission by enabling individuals to avoid the drug-using behaviors that can lead to HIV infection (Metzger, Navaline, and Woody 1998; Needle and others 1998). However, the effect of drug treatment modalities on the rate of HIV transmission is currently limited by laws in many countries that prohibit or restrict the use of methadone maintenance or other drug substitution strategies. The evidence supporting the cost-effectiveness of needle exchange programs in high-income countries is strong. However, little has been published in relation to developing countries, partly because these programs have not been as widely implemented as hoped. Given the low cost of syringes, the extremely high efficiency of HIV transmission by this route, and the demonstrated effectiveness of harm reduction programs in changing syringe-sharing behavior, needle exchange programs should be one of the most cost-effective interventions.
- *Implementation of blood safety practices.* Transmission of HIV can be virtually eliminated in health care settings through a blood safety program that ensures (a) a national blood transfusion service; (b) the recruitment of voluntary, low-risk donors; (c) the screening of all donated blood for HIV; and (d) the reduction of unnecessary and inappropriate transfusions (UNAIDS 1997). Available evidence indicates that HIV screening is effective in reducing HIV infections (see table 18.4). Blood screening for HIV is costly but has been shown to be cost-effective in numerous studies in developing countries (see table 18.3) (Foster and Buve 1995; Hutton, Wyss, and N'Diekhor 2003; Watts, Goodman, and Kumaranayake 2000). The evidence appears to support the WHO and UNAIDS recommendations that all countries, regardless of the nature of the epidemic in the country, should implement a comprehensive blood safety program.
- *Universal precautions.* A critical component of standard infection control in health care settings is a prohibition on reusing needles and syringes. A controversy has recently arisen among researchers who contend that HIV infections have been significantly misclassified because of the undercounting of cases that result from unsafe injection practices by misattributing such cases to heterosexual transmission (Gisselquist and others 2003). However, after much investigation, WHO and the U.S. Department of Health and Human Services concluded that even though transmission caused by unsafe injections may have been underreported, it nevertheless does not account for an appreciable amount of HIV transmission (WHO and UNAIDS 2003). Cost-effectiveness analyses indicate that a combined policy strategy of single-use syringes and interventions to minimize injection use could reduce injection-related infections by as much as 96.5 percent, or 8.86 million DALYs between 2000 and 2030, at an average cost of US$102 per DALY. Additional cost-effectiveness studies are needed to guide decisions regarding the optimal choice of technology in this area.

To prevent bloodborne transmission of HIV and other diseases, health care workers, emergency personnel, and others who might experience occupational exposure to blood or body fluids are advised to take universal precautions. This approach, which treats all bodily fluids as potentially infectious, includes the use of gloves, gowns, and goggles; the proper disposal of waste; and the use of sterile injection and other infection control practices (CDC 1989). Studies have demonstrated that the use of protective gear, such as gloves, reduces the likelihood of blood exposure in health care settings.

Although the cost-effectiveness of implementing universal precautions increases as HIV prevalence increases, universal precautions are unlikely to be cost-effective in resource-limited settings especially where HIV prevalence is low. Postexposure prophylaxis with antiretroviral agents is considered the standard of care after occupational needlestick exposure to blood from an HIV-infected person.

Cost-effectiveness analyses of postexposure prophylaxis have been conducted only in high-income countries and have concluded that this intervention is not cost-effective (Low-Beer and others 2000; Pinkerton, Holtgrave, and Bloom 1998).

PREVENTION IN THEORY AND PRACTICE: USING EPIDEMIC PROFILES AND CONTEXTUAL FACTORS TO INFORM PREVENTION GUIDELINES

Prevention studies and national experiences over the past 20 years strongly suggest that prevention strategies are likely to be most effective when they are carefully tailored to the nature and stage of the epidemic in a specific country or community. UNAIDS has developed epidemiological categories for characterizing individual epidemics on the basis of prevalence of infection in particular subpopulations and in the general population (table 18.5).

As a complement to the guidance provided by the epidemic profile, Grassly and others (2001) recommend assessing the prevalence of other STIs; estimating the extent of mixing between high- and low-risk groups (for example, men who have sex with men who have sexual contact with female partners); and estimating the prevalence of high-risk sexual behaviors in the population (such as lack of condom use with casual partners). They also cite two other critical contextual factors: the capacity of the health service and the social, economic, and legislative context, including social norms and attitudes about sexual and drug use behaviors and the acceptance of breastfeeding. Contextual factors that may play a role in the success of interventions include the status of women, the stigmatization of high-risk groups, and the presence of armed conflict and social upheaval. Together, the epidemic profile and the context in which the epidemic occurs suggest various prevention strategies.

General Prevention Guidelines by Type of Epidemic

Generally, it is more important to change the behavior of people who have high levels of risk behavior than it is to change that of

people with lower levels of risk behavior. However, the difference in the effectiveness between the two falls as epidemics become more generalized, and as the average and maximum size of the connected components (number of people linked to each other directly or through others by their sexual or injecting risk behavior). Thus, in heavily affected countries, or those where the virus has the potential to spread rapidly, prevention interventions are likely to become extremely cost-effective even when targeted at individuals with relatively low levels of risk behavior. Consequently, countries with low-level and concentrated epidemics should emphasize interventions that target individuals at especially high risk of becoming infected or of transmitting the virus, whereas countries with generalized epidemics should also invest heavily in interventions that target entire populations or population subgroups. Thus, any determination of the likely effectiveness and cost-effectiveness of specific interventions in particular circumstances requires an accurate understanding of the stage and nature of the national epidemic.

The countrywide successes discussed in boxes 18.4 and 18.5 highlight population-level interventions that modify social norms as well as highlighting legislative and economic factors. Other examples include instituting government regulation of brothels and interventions to change social norms among sex workers in Thailand, implementing national sex education and blood safety programs in Senegal in concert with creating a national registry of sex workers, and mandating involvement by women in politics in Uganda.

Low-Level Epidemic. Providing widespread VCT, screening for STIs, universal precautions, and postexposure prophylaxis may not be cost-effective in a low-level epidemic. In this setting, such as in the Middle East and North Africa, HIV/AIDS control strategies should emphasize the following:

- surveillance and individual-level interventions that target key populations
- IEC, including limited education through the mass media and sex education in schools

Table 18.5 Epidemic Profiles

Extent of HIV infection	Highest prevalence in a key population[a] (percent)	Prevalence in the general population (percent)	WHO region
Low level	< 5	< 1	Middle East and North Africa
Concentrated[b]	> 5	< 1	East Asia and the Pacific, Europe and Central Asia, Latin America and the Caribbean, South Asia
Generalized low level	≥ 5	1–10	Sub-Saharan Africa
Generalized high level	≥ 5	≥ 10	Sub-Saharan Africa

Source: Adapted from UNAIDS 2004.

a. Key populations include sex workers, men who have sex with men, and drug injecting users.

b. We consider three types of concentrated epidemics depending on the key population most affected: sex workers, men who have sex with men, or drug injecting users.

Thailand's 100 Percent Condom Program

Thailand's HIV prevalence, fueled primarily by high rates of commercial sex work and low levels of condom use, began to rise rapidly in the late 1980s. Beginning in 1989, the Thai government initiated a nationwide condom distribution and education campaign focusing on commercial sex workers and their clients to ensure 100 percent condom use in all commercial sex encounters. Elements thought to contribute to the program's success include

- government-mandated 100 percent condom use in commercial sex establishments
- mass condom promotion advertising campaign
- education in commercial sex workplaces

- government-distributed condoms
- STI testing and treatment
- surveillance and tracking of infections to points of origin
- strong political and financial commitment
- active involvement of provincial and local governments.

Despite this unprecedented success, evidence indicates that enforcement of the 100 Percent Condom Program is not as strong today as when it was initially implemented. A recent study in Bangkok found that 89 percent of sex workers used condoms, a decline from 96 percent in 2000 (UNDP 2004).

Source: Authors.

Uganda HIV/AIDS Prevention Program

Like many countries in Sub-Saharan Africa, Uganda experienced a rapid increase in HIV incidence and a generalization of the epidemic in the late 1980s and early 1990s. By 1991, overall HIV prevalence was 21 percent (Low-Beer and Stoneburner 2003); however, the trajectory of Uganda's epidemic has differed markedly from that of its neighbors. By 2001, overall HIV prevalence had fallen to 5 percent, with dramatic decreases in incidence among key populations, such as soldiers, pregnant women, and young women (USAID 2002). Critical components of Uganda's HIV prevention program include

- having strong political support, especially from President Yoweri Museveni

- implementing interventions to empower women and girls
- having a strong focus on youths
- engaging in active efforts to fight stigma and discrimination
- emphasizing open communication about HIV/AIDS
- engaging the religious leadership and faith-based organizations
- creating Africa's first confidential VCT interventions
- emphasizing STI control and prevention.

Source: Authors.

- prevention programs for people living with HIV/AIDS and harm reduction for injecting drug users
- VCT that is available to key populations with the highest levels of risk behavior and infection rates
- MTCT prevention to mothers known to be infected with HIV
- screening all blood for transfusions and providing sterile injections
- addressing market inefficiencies in condom procurement and distribution—including strategies such as bulk purchases and incentives

- responding to community attitudes toward sexual activity, as they may dictate people's response to sex education materials.

Concentrated Epidemic. In a concentrated epidemic, as in countries in East Asia and the Pacific, Europe and Central Asia, Latin America and the Caribbean, and South Asia, prevention priorities should include the following:

- ongoing surveillance
- subsidized VCT and promotion of VCT among key populations

- HIV screening of pregnant women, guided by individuals' risk profiles
- peer-based programs for key populations to educate individuals at risk, promote safer behaviors, and distribute condoms
- harm reduction for injecting drug users, including needle exchange and drug substitution programs
- STI screening and treatment for key risk groups
- targeted distribution and promotion of condoms to key populations with condom distribution linked to VCT and STI care.

In addition, contextual factors, such as government acceptance of needle exchange programs, incarceration of drug users, and harassment of sex workers, will likely have a major impact on the effectiveness of prevention efforts. Because HIV/AIDS is typically concentrated in socially or economically marginalized populations in countries with concentrated epidemics, attention to socioeconomic factors and to the stigmatization of key populations will also be vital to an effective response.

Generalized Low-Level Epidemic. In a generalized low-level epidemic, such as in some countries in Sub-Saharan Africa (for example, Tanzania), the emphasis on targeted interventions must be maintained or even strengthened. Interventions for broader populations must also be aggressively implemented. These prevention priorities should include the following:

- maintaining surveillance of STIs, risk behaviors, and HIV infections in the entire population, with a particular focus on young people
- extending mass media IEC beyond basic education
- providing routine voluntary and confidential HIV testing and STI screening and promoting treatment beyond key populations
- providing subsidized and social marketing of condoms and strengthened distribution to ensure universal access
- offering HIV screening to all pregnant women
- broadening peer approaches and targeted IEC to include all populations with higher rates of STIs and risk behavior.

Contextual factors remain critical to the success of prevention efforts in generalized low-level epidemics, but population-level factors now have greater priority. The most important is likely to be the status of women, especially with regard to their ability to control their sexual interactions, to negotiate VCT, to be protected from abuse, and to have property rights following the death of a spouse.

Generalized High-Level Epidemic. In a generalized high-level epidemic, such as in some countries in Sub-Saharan Africa (for instance, Botswana and Zimbabwe), an attack on all fronts is required. Prevention efforts should focus on broadly based,

population-level interventions that can mobilize an entire society so as to address prevention and care at all levels. Prevention should include the following:

- mapping and maintaining surveillance of risk behaviors, STIs, and HIV infection
- offering routine, universal HIV testing and STI screening and universal promotion of treatment
- promoting condom use and distributing condoms free in all possible venues
- providing VCT for couples seeking to have children
- counseling pregnant women and new mothers to make informed and appropriate choices for breastfeeding.
- implementing individual-level approaches to innovative mass strategies with accompanying evaluations of effectiveness
- using the mass media as a tool for mobilizing society and changing social norms
- using other venues to reach large numbers of people efficiently for a range of interventions—workplaces, transit venues, political rallies, schools and universities, and military camps
- establishing official institutional policies to provide for harm reduction among injecting drug users.

In a generalized high-level epidemic, contextual factors—such as poverty and the fragility of the health care infrastructure—will dramatically affect service provision at every level. The status of women, an important factor in all epidemics, becomes an overriding concern in this setting, requiring priority action to radically alter gender norms and reduce the economic, social, legal, and physical vulnerability of girls and women.

PREVENTION-CARE SYNERGY

In addition to the benefits antiretroviral therapy has for the individual being treated (Komanduri and others 1998; Ledergerber and others 2001), it almost certainly has other effects on populations where therapy is widely available. Effective antiretroviral therapy appears to decrease the infectiousness of treated individuals. Chemoprophylaxis in exposed, uninfected people may reduce transmission. In addition, availability of treatment may destigmatize the disease and make prevention programs more effective (Castro and Farmer 2005).

However, these benefits in relation to reduced transmission may be offset by a "disinhibition" of risk behavior that is associated with greater availability of antiretroviral therapy, by the spread of drug-resistant HIV, or by increases in the incidence of exposure to partners with HIV infection because of increased survival. These sometimes opposing effects of offering therapy may differ to such a degree that the net effects of widespread therapy on transmission rates may vary among risk groups and across geographic regions.

Table 18.6 Effect of Antiretroviral Therapy on Transmission Dynamics

Area or behavior affected	Treatment effects expected to decrease transmission	Treatment effects expected to increase transmission
Viral load	Decreased infectiousness of the treated partner is substantial even with monotherapy (Musicco and others 1994). Transmission after exposure to individuals with a viral load of less than 1,500 copies per milliliter is extremely rare (Quinn and others 2000). No cases of sexual transmission from a partner with undetectable viremia have been reported.	As survival increases, the incidence of exposure to partners with HIV infection may increase (Hammer and others 1997).
Prophylaxis	Decreased susceptibility may occur during postexposure prophylaxis (Cardo and others 1997).	None.
Drug resistance	Impaired fitness and decreased viral load during drug-resistant viremia (Deeks and others 2000) appear to allow persistent decreases in infectiousness even after drug resistance has occurred (Leigh Brown and others 2003).	Impaired virological responses to therapy in the person who is infected by a resistant virus may partially offset the beneficial effect on infectiousness (Little and others 2002; Grant, Kahn, and others 2002). However, primary infection with a resistant virus may also be associated with slower progression of the disease (Grant, Hecht, and others 2002).
Risk behavior	Treatment may provide incentives for HIV testing and counseling, which has been associated with decreased risk behavior and HIV incidence. The availability of treatment may reduce stigma directly, and also indirectly by increasing the visibility of people living with HIV/AIDS. Risk reduction counseling during treatment programs may reduce risk behavior.	Decreased fear of HIV and disinhibition of risk behavior are possibilities (Katz and others 2002). Risk behavior by people who are sick and who recover their health status may increase (Stolte and others 2001).
Sexual networks	Decreased fear of HIV may foster more informed risk behavior, including increased use of testing and more thoughtful partner selection, including serosorting and sorting by risk level (McConnell and Grant 2003).	Decreased fear of HIV may disinhibit risk behavior, reduce serosorting, and increase mixing between higher- and lower-risk groups in the population.
Epidemiological	The effective prevalence of infectious people will decrease because of treatment effects on infectiousness or increased serosorting.	Treatment-induced reduction in mortality may increase the prevalence of infection, although many being treated will be less infectious or better informed regarding risk reduction strategies. A rebound of viral load with treatment failure may mean that treatment postpones transmission rather than reducing it.

Source: Authors.

Table 18.6 reviews the information available on the population effects of antiretroviral therapy and makes suppositions about potential effects for those areas for which data and research are lacking. The information in the table suggests that widespread therapy using currently available combination regimens will provide a net benefit in relation to the transmission of HIV. However, because confidence in this prediction is not high, the population consequences of therapy programs must be evaluated and monitored with active surveillance of prescribing patterns, sexual risk behavior, STI prevalence, HIV incidence and prevalence, and prevalence of primary drug resistance and sexual networks of risk behavior.

CARE AND TREATMENT

This section reviews evidence of the cost-effectiveness of HIV/AIDS care and treatment interventions in resource-limited settings. Until relatively recently, the majority of HIV clinical care in resource-limited countries was confined to managing the terminal stage of infection, including extremely late diagnosis of opportunistic infections and cancers, use of basic palliative symptom management, and short-term hospitalization just before death. Few people were aware of their HIV status until the onset of severe HIV-associated illness, and most did not seek help from the health care system until they were already terminally ill.

The advent of primary prophylaxis and treatment for opportunistic infections, including tuberculosis, prolonged survival to a limited extent but did nothing to restore immune function. Such restoration was not possible until the advent of antiretroviral therapy. Because clinical intervention in HIV is so recent in resource-limited settings, few cost-effectiveness studies are available. Those that are available on the treatment of and prophylaxis for opportunistic infections were largely conducted before the availability of antiretroviral therapy and therefore need to be reestimated to be relevant for decision making today. Fortunately, because the determinants of biological responses are better conserved across countries and cultural settings than the determinants of behavior, effectiveness data from high-income countries can help inform decisions about treatment in resource-limited settings.

Unlike drugs for many other high-burden health conditions in developing countries, antiretroviral therapy for HIV and drugs for some of its associated opportunistic infections depend on medications that are still under patent protection. Nevertheless, generic drug makers in India and Thailand have produced a range of effective antiretroviral therapies that combine multiple drugs into single tablets and reduce the pill burden to one tablet twice daily. These companies have made it possible for prices to drop dramatically for some antiretroviral therapy combinations—to less than US$250 per year, compared with more than US$4,000 for the same combinations (from the original manufacturers) in high-income countries. In response to this threat, some multinational pharmaceutical companies have introduced a system of price differentiation among countries depending on their per capita income and HIV/AIDS burden.

In addition, the World Trade Organization's Agreement on Trade-Related Aspects of Intellectual Property Rights (TRIPS) includes a provision that permits compulsory licensing of pharmaceutical products in cases of national emergency and other circumstances of extreme emergency, which is clearly the case for HIV/AIDS in much of the developing world. A 2003 World Trade Organization decision also made it easier for low- and middle-income countries (LMICs) to import cheaper generics made under compulsory licensing if the countries are unable to manufacture the medicines themselves (WTO 2003). As a result, some countries, including Brazil, India, and Thailand, have begun to produce generic versions of antiretroviral drugs to be sold at greatly reduced prices. The TRIPS provision has also improved developing countries' bargaining power with large pharmaceutical companies, to the point that some countries have been able to secure drugs from the original manufacturers at substantially reduced prices. As a result, the relative cost-effectiveness of different drug combinations has been in rapid flux, increasing the importance of updating recommendations frequently.

Diagnostic HIV Testing

A positive HIV test can be confirmed within one month of infection. Infection is diagnosed in two ways: by a biological test that detects the presence of HIV antibodies or by diagnosis of an opportunistic infection that is a clear sign of HIV disease. The most widely used biological test in high-income countries, conducted in a laboratory on a blood sample, is called an ELISA (enzyme-linked immunosorbent assay). Obtaining a result may take several days. Rapid tests that can provide results in 20 minutes are being used more widely as their costs fall. When the prior probability of infection is low and resources are

abundant, following up an initially positive ELISA with a second ELISA—and even a Western blot test if the second ELISA is positive—may be appropriate (this is typically done in high-income countries).

However, in a high-prevalence environment where the prior probability is high and resources are scarce, such an approach is almost certainly not cost-effective. Each additional confirmatory test decreases the number of false positive results, thereby averting the costs associated with such a result. The costs of averting a false positive result range from US$425 with a single confirmatory rapid test or ELISA to more than US$500,000 for a confirmatory Western blot test following two positive ELISAs as the prevalence of HIV in patients who are clinically suspected of being infected is varied from 5 to 50 percent (these calculations are based on assumptions in John Snow, Inc. 2003 and WHO 2004). These results suggest that LMICs should not use a second confirmatory test unless the prevalence among patients is extremely low.

Palliative Care

Palliative care has traditionally focused on patients in the terminal stages of disease. More recent definitions of palliative care, including WHO's definition, have been broadened to encompass quality-of-life issues of patients and their families throughout the course of a life-threatening illness (WHO 2002b). The control of pain and other symptoms is the crux of any palliative care model, but the WHO model also addresses patients' and their families' psychological, social, and spiritual problems. Under this definition, in many developing countries, most people living with HIV/AIDS are not receiving the minimum standard of palliative care. Of the 5 million people living with HIV/AIDS in South Africa, one of the wealthiest countries in Sub-Saharan Africa, Carlisle (2003) estimates that only 250,000 have access to palliative care services. In the face of a growing epidemic of historic dimensions, the provision of comprehensive palliative care represents a critical, but neglected, global priority.

Health care professionals have promoted community home-based care as an affordable way to expand the coverage of palliative care (Hansen and others 1998), but the great heterogeneity among home-based care programs complicates comparisons. Most programs for which data are available are community-based outreach programs administered by local clinics or hospitals. These programs can consist of simple home visits to provide basic care for AIDS patients or may be comprehensive schemes that provide care, palliative medications, meals, psychosocial support and counseling, and links to primary and secondary health care.

Studies indicate that home-based care has considerable potential to deal cost-effectively with the palliative care needs of HIV/AIDS patients (Ramsay 2003; UNAIDS 2001; Uys and Hensher 2002; Wenk, Bertolino, and Pussetto 2000). Although a Zimbabwe study found that home visits were associated with extensive travel time and costs (Hansen and others 1998), little research has examined the extent to which home-based care can be used to substitute for hospitalization, nor is evidence available to determine the most cost-effective combination of palliative care strategies. Most people living with HIV/AIDS do incur some end-of-life costs in the formal health care sector. In one South African study, primary care clinic and hospital costs accounted for 39 and 18 percent, respectively, of the costs of care in the last year of life, whereas community home-based care accounted for 42 percent (Uys and Hensher 2002).

Higginson and others' (2003) meta-analysis concludes that overall evidence demonstrates a positive effect of home-based palliative care, especially its effect on pain management and symptom control. Available data do not permit estimating a cost per DALY of community-based palliative care programs, but a review of available studies suggests that palliative care provided by health professionals in the home is unlikely to be cost-effective in low-income countries. However, low-cost, community-based models have been developed that require minimal external resources and function almost like care cooperatives among affected households. These models are likely to be highly cost-effective.

Symptom-Based Care. Pain management is extremely important in HIV and is addressed in chapter 52. Diarrhea, nausea, vomiting, and skin problems are all symptoms that are targeted for treatment in palliative care. Oral rehydration for diarrheal treatment costs pennies per episode. Nausea and vomiting are prevalent in people with AIDS and can lead to anorexia and weight loss (UNAIDS 2000). Treating nausea costs an estimated US$1.75 per episode (Willbond and others 2001), and continuous treatment of nausea and vomiting in end-stage patients costs about US$2 per day (World Bank 1997).

Approximately 90 percent of people with HIV suffer from some form of skin condition. These conditions include infections, drug reactions, scabies, pressure sores, and cancers. Skin often becomes dry in the middle and late stages of AIDS because of dehydration caused by persistent diarrhea, vomiting, and malabsorption. The cost of treating an episode of skin rash is estimated to be US$2 (UNAIDS 2000). No estimates are available on the benefits of providing such care in terms of DALYs, especially to terminally ill patients.

Psychosocial Support. Psychosocial support is an integral component of the multidisciplinary management strategies that care providers regard as essential for people with HIV (Murphy and others 2004). Support for patients and families can have a positive effect on adherence to therapies and can contribute to the critical aim of integrating prevention with treatment and care.

Psychosocial support and counseling has a positive effect on the quality of life of people living with HIV/AIDS. Cook's (2004) study of U.S. women demonstrated that the use of mental health services was associated with reduced mortality and that AIDS-related deaths were more likely among women who had symptoms of chronic depression. While results have not been replicated in resource-constrained countries, an assessment of clinic-based psychosocial support and counseling services in northern Thailand showed that 50% of PLWHA became more positive about their lives and 40% stated that they learned how to live with the disease (Tsunekawa and others 2004). Although few data are available on the costs of various strategies, interventions for psychosocial support appear to be cost-effective—especially where innovative solutions, such as group counseling sessions, are implemented. Although studies indicate an improved quality of life for these patients, little information is available on the cost of the interventions. Additional evaluation research is needed to guide decisions about how much to invest in psychosocial support.

Nutrition Programs and Food Security. Strong evidence indicates that malnutrition and AIDS work in tandem at both the individual and the societal levels. Infection with HIV increases the risk of malnutrition in the individual, while malnutrition worsens the impact of HIV and AIDS. Similarly, HIV/AIDS can both cause and be worsened by food insecurity. This reciprocity must be considered when planning specific program responses.

Protein deficiency is a well-known cause of cell-mediated immunodeficiency (Vanek 1953). HIV-infected individuals need to consume more energy than uninfected individuals: as much as 10 percent greater consumption for asymptomatic individuals and 20 to 30 percent more for symptomatic individuals. Malnutrition alters the susceptibility of individuals to HIV infection and their vulnerability to its various sequelae, increases the risk of HIV transmission from mothers to babies, and accelerates the progression of HIV infection (Gillespie, Haddad, and Jackson 2001).

Small studies of adults with AIDS, including those on antiretroviral therapy, have shown that daily micronutrient supplementation increases bodyweight, reduces HIV RNA levels, improves CD4 counts, and reduces the incidence of opportunistic infections. Fawzi and others' (2004) large trial among pregnant women infected with HIV in Tanzania demonstrates that multivitamin supplements (a) decrease the risk of progression to WHO stage 4 (progression from HIV to AIDS, the most advanced level of HIV infection) or death from AIDS-related causes and (b) reduce many HIV-related symptoms. The multivitamins used in the trial cost US$15 per person per year (Fawzi and others 2004).

The World Food Program guidelines prioritize three nutrition interventions for people living with HIV/AIDS: counseling on specific behaviors, prescribed or targeted nutrition supplements, and links with food-based interventions and programs. The guidelines cite three types of nutrition supplements: food rations to manage mild weight loss and nutrition-related side effects of antiretroviral therapy and to address nutritional needs in food-secure areas; micronutrient supplements for specific HIV-positive risk groups; and therapeutic foods for addressing moderate and severe malnutrition in HIV-positive adults and children. Cost-effectiveness data in support of these recommendations are not available, but the low costs of supplementation, coupled with the likely benefits to other malnourished household members, suggest that such interventions will be highly cost-effective.

Infection with HIV/AIDS can severely undermine an individual's food security, affecting the availability, stability, access to, and use of essential foods. The epidemic is stunting progress in rural development and causing significant increases in rural poverty and destitution in the countries most affected by the epidemic (Bonnard 2002). Thus, interventions must consider the epidemic's impact on the broader community and not solely on people living with the disease. Care-related household and community-level interventions include school feeding with special take-home rations for families caring for orphans, food for training programs that promote income-generating activities, and food for work to support homestead production

activities (Van Liere 2002). Chapter 56 estimates that sustained community nutrition programs would *save* US\$200 to US\$250 per DALY. Such programs targeted at communities at especially high risk are likely to be even more cost-effective (World Food Programme 2001).

Treatment of Opportunistic Infections and Secondary Prophylaxis

Even as the availability of antiretroviral therapy increases in many developing countries, appropriate diagnosis and management of life-threatening opportunistic infections, including HIV-associated cancers, remain the most important aspects of the care of patients with HIV disease. Opportunistic infections usually begin five to seven years after infection (Munoz, Sabin, and Phillips 1997) and occur progressively as uncontrolled HIV replication destroys the immune system (Colebunders and Latif 1991). Figure 18.1 describes the cascade of infections that occur as the immune system is depleted. Opportunistic infections are typically caused by organisms that exist in the environment of the body (on the skin, in the lungs and gastrointestinal system) and remain latent until HIV has impaired the immune system.

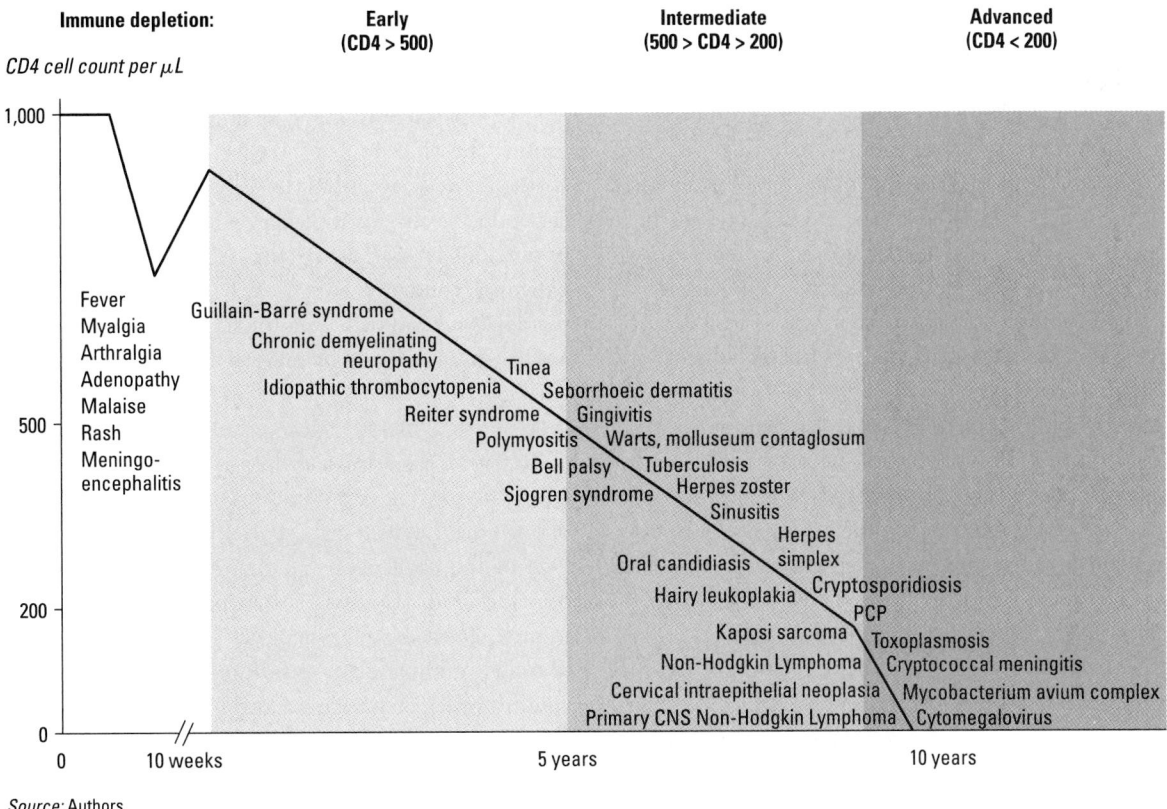

Source: Authors.

Figure 18.1 Cascade of Infections and Cancers That Develop as Immune Function Is Depleted

The epidemiology of opportunistic infections is complex; it is related to the severity of individual immune depletion and shows considerable intercountry variation. Each infection has its unique clinical expression, requiring specific diagnostic techniques and treatment. Many opportunistic infections can be prevented by judicious use of chemoprophylaxis, ranging from the low-cost (cotrimoxazole to prevent *Pneumocystis jiroveci* pneumonia [PCP] at less than US$20 per year) to the extremely expensive (ganciclovir to prevent cytomegalovirus at more than US$10,000 per year) (Schneider and others 1995; Spector and others 1996). In high-income countries, antiretroviral therapy has so effectively controlled viral replication that the process of HIV-related immune destruction has been slowed or halted, leading to marked declines in the incidence of opportunistic infections and a dramatic reduction in their resultant high death toll (McNaghten and others 1999). Unfortunately, the emerging problem of poor adherence to drug regimes is now making HIV resistance to antiretroviral therapy more prevalent in high-income countries, triggering a resurgence of opportunistic infections.

More than 20 infections and cancers have been associated with severe immune depletion. The most common pathogens and cancers include bacteria such as *Mycobacteria tuberculosis* and *avium;* protozoa such as *Cryptosporidium, Strongyloides,* and *Toxoplasma;* fungi such as *Candida,* PCP, *Cryptococcus, Aspergillis,* and *Penicillium* (the latter largely restricted to South and Southeast Asia); viruses such as cytomegalovirus, herpes simplex, and herpes zoster; and cancers such as Kaposi sarcoma and non-Hodgkin lymphoma.

The range of complications arising from continued HIV infection varies from country to country, reflecting the differences in infectious agents that populations have encountered earlier in life or are exposed to when immunosuppressed. In high-income countries, the most common opportunistic infections are PCP, esophageal candidiasis, cytomegalovirus retinitis, cryptococcal meningitis, toxoplasma encephalopathy, cryptosporidium diarrhea, and human herpes virus–8 and Kaposi sarcoma (Bacellar and others 1994; Hoover and others 1993; Lanjewar and others 1996; Selik, Starcher, and Curran 1987). In resource-limited countries, because of the higher background prevalence of infectious agents, it is more common to encounter tuberculosis, cryptococcal meningitis, toxoplasma encephalopathy, infectious diarrhea, and nonspecific wasting (slim disease) (Hira and others 1998; Hira, Dore, and Sirisanthana 1998a; Sengupta, Lal, and Srinivas 1994).

The time from HIV infection to manifestation of the first AIDS-defining illness varies within populations. In high-income countries, reports on the natural history of untreated HIV infection suggest that AIDS occurs between 7 and 10 years after infection (Alcabes and others 1993; Lui and others 1988). The time can be as short as 24 months (Anzala and others

1995) in some individuals, whereas some long-term survivors remain disease free for longer than 15 years (Easterbrook 1994). In developing countries, disease progression, though not as well studied, appears to be more rapid (Morgan and others 1997). Once an AIDS-defining illness occurs, the average time to death seems to be similar across countries, reported at approximately 12 to 18 months in Uganda and the United States (Carre and others 1994).

The time from presentation with an AIDS-defining opportunistic infection to death depends on the type of infection, the availability of care, and the patient's adherence to prescribed prophylaxis and treatment. Even as access to antiretroviral therapy increases, prophylaxis for opportunistic infections remains one of the most important ongoing and successful care strategies for patients with advanced HIV disease. In high-income countries, the widespread use of such simple interventions as cotrimoxazole for PCP prophylaxis has had a significant effect in delaying the onset of PCP, the most common initial AIDS-defining event, thus positively influencing survival (Hoover and others 1993). However, prophylaxis for opportunistic infections appears to be underused in LMICs.

Prevention of PCP or any other opportunistic infection does not halt the relentless erosion of the immune system and provides only a short-term prolongation of life (Morgan and others 1997). The only way to halt or delay the progression of HIV disease is to interrupt viral replication.

Role of Antiretroviral Therapy in Relation to Opportunistic Infections. Antiretroviral therapy is effective in reducing viral load and partially enabling immune restoration, thereby preventing the onset and recurrence of opportunistic infections. If taken strictly according to directions, antiretroviral therapy can induce a sustained recovery of CD4 cell reactivity against opportunistic pathogens in severely immunosuppressed patients (Li and others 1998). The effectiveness of antiretroviral therapy is determined by its ability to rapidly reduce viral load and to sustain low levels of viral activity. This viral activity is what has an independent effect on increasing or decreasing susceptibility to opportunistic infections (Kaplan and others 2001).

Initiating antiretroviral therapy can also have detrimental effects by causing complications from latent or undiagnosed opportunistic infections, especially in resource-poor settings. One of the challenges in initiating antiretroviral therapy in resource-limited settings is that patients tend to present late in their illness, usually when they have an opportunistic infection that prompts them to seek medical care, or in the case of countries with lax pharmaceutical policy, when they buy antiretroviral therapy from a private pharmacy. It is well documented that initiating antiretroviral therapy in severely immunosuppressed patients can result in illnesses associated with reconstitution of the immune system (Shelburne and others 2005). These illnesses can occur with all presenting opportunistic infections and may be more serious than the infection itself. The major problem with care of patients in this situation is that they may believe the illness is a side effect of their antiretroviral therapy and refrain from medicating. Training clinicians to recognize and treat immune reconstitution disease is therefore essential.

Management of Opportunistic Infections. The three components of effective management of oppportunistic infections are diagnosis, treatment, and secondary prophylaxis. As immune function continues to deteriorate, secondary prophylaxis is required to prevent recurrence of the treated infection. Some of the most common infections, such as PCP, can be diagnosed with a reasonable degree of confidence by clinical history and treated empirically (Kaplan, Masur, and Holmes 2002). Less frequently occurring infections often require sophisticated diagnostic equipment and skilled clinicians to confirm a diagnosis from a wide range of pathogenic possibilities before starting complex and expensive treatment. For example, toxoplasmosis can be accurately diagnosed only by a lumbar puncture and CT brain scan (and in some cases an MRI), and cryptosporidium diagnosis requires specialized laboratory techniques.

The full spectrum of options for treating opportunistic infections in developing countries has not been systematically evaluated for cost-effectiveness. Because of the effect of antiretroviral therapy on both the efficacy of treatment of individual infections and on life expectancy (and therefore on potential DALYs gained from treating a life-threatening infection), the limited economic evaluations conducted are already out of date. In particular, chronic infections such as *Mycobacterium avium* complex and cytomegalovirus may be more effectively treated over the medium term by reversing immunosuppression with antiretroviral therapy than by directly treating the infectious agent. Other treatment regimens for opportunistic infections that were marginally cost-effective before antiretroviral therapy may now become substantially more cost-effective if the patient can begin the therapy following treatment of the infection, thereby extending life expectancy. Table 18.7 shows the cost-effectiveness of care and treatment options for opportunistic infections and antiretroviral therapy.

In most resource-limited settings, few specialized diagnostic facilities are available for opportunistic infections. Clinicians have little training in the diagnosis and management of complex opportunistic infections, and laboratory backup is either nonexistent or so expensive that end users cannot afford it. The spectrum of opportunistic infections in LMICs is such that most require highly technical facilities for confirmation of diagnosis. Consider *M. tuberculosis*, the most prevalent such infection in Thailand. The rate of latent tuberculosis becoming clinically active in the presence of HIV increases from a lifetime risk of 10 percent in the general population to an annual risk of 10 percent for those coinfected with HIV (Pape and others 1993). Hence, after five years, about 40 percent of HIV-infected people with latent tuberculosis will have developed active disease.

Primary Prophylaxis for Opportunistic Infections

Before the advent of antiretroviral therapy, the use of prophylaxis to decrease the risk of acquiring opportunistic infections was the only intervention available to delay the onset of life-threatening infections (Kitahata and others 1996). With the development of antiretroviral therapy in the 1990s, the prevalence of many opportunistic infections has been greatly reduced, and the use of prophylaxis has decreased correspondingly (Palella and others 2003). Nevertheless, prophylaxis for opportunistic infections remains necessary in patients who lack access to antiretroviral therapy, in extremely immunosuppressed patients until the therapy takes effect, in patients who do not wish to or who cannot take antiretroviral therapy, in patients for whom such therapy fails, and in the small group of patients who are unable to recover sufficient CD4 cells despite good inhibition of viral replication (Berenguer and others 2004). Note that extensive clinical research is still being carried out in relation to the withdrawal of secondary prophylaxis following immune restoration with antiretroviral therapy.

Treatment of HIV Infection with Antiretroviral Therapy

Combination therapy with multiple antiretroviral drugs is associated with prolonged survival. Whereas monotherapies are associated with one year or less of additional survival, the survival benefit conferred by combination therapy appears to be sustainable for extended periods (Palella and others 2003). Long-term toxicities related to treatment may include atherosclerosis, lipodystrophy, hepatic failure, and cardiac failure. Researchers are still evaluating the effects of these toxicities on HIV/AIDS mortality.

Cost-Effectiveness Considerations in the Choice and Initiation of Antiretroviral Therapy. WHO has issued global guidelines for scaling up antiretroviral therapy access; the guidelines promote a combination of stavudine, lamivudine, and nevirapine (as a fixed-dose formulation) as initial therapy. A number of clinical trials have produced results outlining differential efficacy for a number of antiretroviral therapy combinations, which provide guidance in the selection of appropriate drugs for treating HIV (Yeni and others 2004). The preferred first-line medications in developing countries are dictated by these considerations, in addition to pricing and patent concerns.

Table 18.7 Cost-Effectiveness of Care and Treatment for HIV/AIDS

Intervention	Source	Cost-effectiveness (2001 US$/DALY)	
		Before or when initiating antiretroviral therapy	**Failed or no antiretroviral therapy**
HIV testing and diagnosis			
Confirmatory ELISA, Western blot	No cost-effectiveness studies found in developing countries	—	—
Palliative care			
Pain alleviation	Chapter 52	420/year of pain-free life added	420/year of pain-free life added
Symptom-based care	No cost-effectiveness studies found in developing countries	—	—
Nutrition interventions	Chapter 56	200–250 for HIV-negative individuals	200–250 for HIV-negative individuals
End-of-life care	No cost-effectiveness studies found in developing countries	—	—
Treatment of opportunistic infections, per episode			
Oral candidias	Modeling estimates based on efficacy trials reported from HIVInsite (CHI, 2005) and drug costs (UNICEF and others 2004)	0.5–157	1–394
Esophageal candidiasis		0.4–55	1–165
Histoplasmosis		12–77	81–539
Kaposi's sarcoma		6,236–63,700	12,460–127,400
Cryptococcal meningitis		3–86	21–546
Penicilliosis		11–72	76–483
Mycobacterium avium complex		31–51	87–320
Cytomegalovirus		586–995	4,875–5,120
PCP		0.4–5	3–35
Toxoplasmosis		5–44	31–291
Herpes simplex virus		3–32	7–80
Tuberculosis	Chapter 16	200–370	50–450
	South Africa (Floyd, Wilkinson, and Gilks 1997); Malawi, Mozambique, Tanzania (Murray and others 1991); Uganda (Saunderson 1995)	Short-course ambulatory: 2–16 Short-course hospital: 3–8 Community-based directly observed therapy: 14–22	Short-course ambulatory: 2–16 Short-course hospital: 3–8 Community-based directly observed therapy: 14–22
Opportunistic infection prophylaxis			
PCP	Modeling estimates based on efficacy trials reported from HIVInsite (CHI, 2005) and drug costs: (UNICEF and others 2004)	29–1487	590–29,817
Toxoplasmosis		14–412	252–8,265
Mycobacterium avium complex		786–3,604	2,247–18,020
Cytomegalovirus		151,855–972,955	976,209–4.5 million
Tuberculosis preventive therapy	Uganda (Bell, Rose, and Sacks 1999); Chapter 16	15–300 (Isoniazid, Rifampicin plus pyrazinamide, Isoniazid plus rifampicin)	15–300 (Isoniazid, Rifampicin plus pyrazinamide, Isoniazid plus rifampicin)
Early detection and screening for opportunistic infections			
HPV screening and treatment	South Africa (Goldie and others 2001)	Direct visual inspection using acetic acid: < 4/years of life saved	Direct visual inspection using acetic acid: < 4/years of life saved
Antiretroviral therapy			
First-line antiretroviral therapy	Sub-Saharan Africa (Marseille, Hofmann, and Kahn 2002)	350	350
Second-line (and subsequent) antiretroviral therapy	India (Over and others 2004)	492/patient year[a]	492/patient year[a]
	No cost-effectiveness studies found in developing countries	—	—
Adherence interventions	No cost-effectiveness studies found in developing countries	—	—
Monitoring response to antiretroviral therapy	No cost-effectiveness studies found in developing countries	—	—

Source: Authors.

— = not available.

a. Antiretroviral therapy for the poorest HIV positive adults. The estimates include the cost of drugs, clinic visits, and laboratory tests for physician monitoring of treatment and assumes 50 percent condom use in the general population.

Antiretroviral Drugs

Current antiretroviral drugs can be divided into three classes:

- *Nucleoside analogue reverse transcriptase inhibitors* (NRTIs) were the first type of drug available to treat HIV infection in 1987. When HIV infects a cell, it copies its own genetic code into the cell's DNA, and the cell is then programmed to create new copies of HIV. To reproduce, HIV must first convert its RNA into DNA using the enzyme reverse transcriptase. Nucleoside analogue reverse transcriptase inhibitors act like false building blocks and compete with the cell's nucleosides, thereby preventing DNA synthesis. This inhibits reverse transcriptase, which prevents HIV from infecting cells and duplicating itself.

- *Nonnucleoside reverse transcriptase inhibitors* (NNRTIs) started to be approved in 1997. Like nucleoside analogue reverse transcriptase inhibitors, nonnucleosides also interfere with HIV's ability to infect cells by targeting reverse transcriptase. In contrast to nucleoside analogue reverse transcriptase inhibitors, nonnucleosides bind directly to the enzyme. This blocks the binding site of the reverse transcriptase and inhibits the binding of nucleotides.

- *Protease inhibitors* (PIs) were first approved in 1995. PIs interfere with viral replication by binding to the viral protease enzyme and preventing it from processing viral proteins into their functional forms and thereby rendering the resulting viral particles noninfectious (Peiperl, Coffey, and Volberding 2005).

Source: Authors.

In recent years, the most volatile parameter in cost-effectiveness analyses for HIV/AIDS has been the prices of antiretroviral drugs, which have dropped by about two orders of magnitude for some LMICs. Price reductions have not been consistent across countries, nor have they necessarily been larger for the poorest countries. This variability in pricing greatly complicates the establishment of national guidelines regarding which regimens to prescribe under which circumstances, because the ranking of regimens varies among and within countries as relative prices change. Box 18.6 discusses the three classes of drugs used in antiretroviral therapy.

Because of their higher manufacturing costs and their more recent introduction into the market, protease inhibitors are more expensive than either nucleoside reverse transcriptase inhibitors or nonnucleoside reverse transcriptase inhibitors. They are also more difficult to manufacture, making them less attractive to generic manufacturers. Although the difference is less marked, nucleoside reverse transcriptase inhibitors tend to cost less than nonnucleoside reverse transcriptase inhibitors.

Ranking different antiretroviral therapy regimens by their cost-effectiveness is more complex than doing so for most therapeutic situations, because a high proportion of patients will develop resistance to or intolerance of initial therapy and will need to stop their initial regimen and then initiate a second (and perhaps a subsequent) regimen, if available. One U.S. cohort study suggests that for 50 percent of patients the prescribed protease inhibitor–based regimen fails within a year (Deeks and others 1999). As a result, the cost-effectiveness of a regimen is a function not only of its effectiveness in isolation, but also of its impact on the effectiveness of future regimens. Thus, the comparative cost-effectiveness of different sequences of regimens needs to be considered.

The effectiveness of antiretrovirals depends on not only the benefits conferred but also the associated side effects, the toxicity level of the drugs, and patients' adherence to the drug regimen. The ability of care providers to detect incipient toxicity at an early stage also influences the magnitude of side effects and toxicities. In low-income settings with limited laboratory capacity, a greater proportion of side effects will not be detected until they become severe. As a result, the relative cost-effectiveness profiles will change depending on the availability of toxicity monitoring.

Initiating antiretroviral therapy has a proven benefit for patients with a CD4 count of fewer than 350 cells per cubic millimeter (Palella and others 2003). In patients with a higher CD4 count, the benefits of antiretroviral therapy are believed to be outweighed by the toxicities that may accrue from continued drug exposure (Mallal and others 2000). Concerted research efforts are needed to gauge both the average costs of care and the survival benefits of identifying patients and initiating antiretroviral therapy while their immune function is still competent, compared with the costs and survival benefits associated with starting care late, on presentation of an opportunistic infection—as is currently the norm in LMICs.

Drug Resistance. Drug resistance occurs as the virus evolves to escape the inhibitory effects of antiretroviral drugs. The capacity of HIV to mutate is extraordinary, as the wide diversity of HIV variants that occurs worldwide demonstrates. Viral diversification is driven by low-fidelity enzymes (which have a high rate of mutation) that carry out replication of the viral genome.

Drug resistance resulting from being infected by a drug-resistant HIV strain is known as primary drug resistance. Secondary drug resistance develops as a consequence of treatment. Primary HIV drug resistance to nucleoside reverse transcriptase inhibitors, nonnucleoside reverse transcriptase inhibitors, and protease inhibitors has been reported (Salomon and others 2000; Wegner and others 2000). The first reports of transmission of drug resistance have typically occurred within a few years of a drug's introduction into clinical practice. The proportion of newly infected people who acquire drug-resistant HIV has implications for the choice of first-line regimen. Primary resistance in recently infected individuals in high-income countries is stable or has been in decline since 2000, following a rise between 1996 and 1999. Almost nothing is known regarding primary drug resistance among those recently infected in low-income countries, although this question will become more important with the increased availability of antiretroviral therapy in resource-limited settings.

Drug resistance is associated with increases in plasma viral RNA levels and attenuation of the responses of CD4 counts to therapy. Nonetheless, clinical and epidemiological observations suggest that drug resistance does not completely offset the benefits of therapy (Deeks and others 1999; Ledergerber and others 1999). Individuals with drug-resistant HIV typically have plasma viral RNA levels that remain 3- to 10-fold lower than pretreatment levels. Furthermore, patients with drug resistance experience more rapid immunological decline and disease progression if they discontinue their drugs (Nijhuis, Deeks, and Boucher 2001).

Importance of Adherence to Prescribed Therapy. With certain drugs, resistance can develop in as little as two weeks if therapy is suboptimal (which can be less than 90 percent adherence). Conversely, patients who adhere to therapy can obtain continued viral suppression for many years without the need for second- or third-line options. Research has shown that drug adherence is one of the most important predictors of continued treatment response (Mannheimer and others 2002). Patients in resource-limited countries are likely to be subjected to a number of influences that challenge their ability to adhere to the prescribed therapy, including limited education and the consequent poorer understanding of their disease state, unstable housing and financial circumstances, a limited number of treatment options, and clinicians with limited antiretroviral therapy treatment experience (Kitahata and others 1996). Those factors, in addition to the toxicity of the therapy, influence adherence and future disease progression rates (Duran and others 2001) and lead to an increase in drug resistance. Thus, poorly coordinated scale-up of antiretroviral therapy in some developing countries has the potential to jeopardize both the duration of clinical benefit for the first wave of patients who receive substandard care and future response rates as the prevalence of drug resistance increases (Harries and others 2001).

Studies in India, Mexico, Senegal, and Uganda point to poor adherence (which for some classes of drugs can be adherence of less than 95 percent), inadequate doses and regimens, and poor monitoring as factors that contribute to more rapid development of antiretroviral therapy resistance (Oyugi and Bangsberg 2004, Laniece and others 2004, Bautista and others 2003, Liechty and Bangsberg 2003). By contrast, experiences in Haiti and Uganda suggest that it is possible to achieve adherence rates in developing countries equal to or better than those observed in high-income countries (Farmer and others 2001; Mitty and others 2002).

Second-Line and Subsequent Therapies. Studies from high-income countries have unequivocally demonstrated that the probability that an antiretroviral therapy regimen will achieve viral suppression diminishes with each subsequent regimen (Deeks and others 1999). Similarly, the mean duration of viral suppression for those who achieve suppression is also lower for subsequent regimens (Deeks and others 1999). This finding is entirely expected because failing a previous regimen is associated with lower adherence, higher toxicity, or side effects and increased resistance, all of which increase the probability of similar problems occurring with subsequent regimens. Thus, the expected survival benefit per month of antiretroviral therapy declines with each change of regimen. In contrast, the monthly cost of therapy rises as a patient moves from first-line to more expensive protease inhibitor–based second-line and subsequent therapies. Given this steadily declining cost-effectiveness, wealthier countries are likely to offer a greater number of regimen changes than poorer countries.

Laboratory Monitoring of Immune Function to Guide Therapy

Laboratory monitoring determines when antiretroviral therapy should be initiated and when it should be changed because of toxicity, lack of efficacy, or resistance. The optimal frequency and precision of monitoring depends on numerous factors, principally the following:

- the expected rate of change of variables of interest
- the expected frequency of events, such as development of resistance, adherence failure, and side effects
- the relative cost of monitoring versus the cost of providing ineffective treatment
- the magnitude of the secondary effects of monitoring (motivating prevention, motivating adherence).

WHO has suggested a pragmatic approach to monitoring, with inexpensive, easy-to-measure parameters (bodyweight or body mass index, body temperature, hemoglobin, liver enzymes, and clinical symptoms) for monitoring in low-income countries. More specialized markers—namely, CD4 count, viral load, and resistance genotyping—would be restricted to sentinel sites and tertiary care services (Gutierrez and others 2004), at least initially.

The large price reductions for antiretroviral drugs are only now starting to be mirrored in the costs of monitoring tests as new technologies are introduced, collective bargaining is undertaken, and international pressure mounts on diagnostic manufacturers to provide more favorable pricing for LMICs. Commercial cytometric CD4 measurements are now available to some developing countries at less than US$5 per test (R. Göhde, personal communication, 2004). Viral load testing is still significantly more expensive, but even those prices have dropped to US$20 following negotiations on behalf of low-income countries by the William Jefferson Clinton Foundation. Even when the potential savings become an operational reality in developing countries, the costs of laboratory monitoring will still represent an important proportion of the costs of providing antiretroviral therapy.

Monitoring to Guide Initiation of Antiretroviral Therapy. If laboratory monitoring is performed, its optimal frequency must be determined. The closer patients get to an antiretroviral therapy threshold, the more often they must be tested to detect a CD4 decline that falls within a specific CD4 range. As use of antiretroviral therapy expands in LMICs and as the costs of drugs fall relative to the costs of laboratory monitoring, collecting empirical data and constructing models to compare different monitoring strategies is becoming increasingly urgent.

In the absence of capacity to perform CD4 counts, several studies suggest that total lymphocyte count can be used as a proxy because of the correlation between the two counts (Badri and Wood 2003). Research has also shown that falling body mass index is highly predictive of disease progression (Pistone and others 2002). In light of those findings, the cost-effectiveness of CD4 monitoring in developing countries must be considered in terms of its incremental improvement over total lymphocyte

monitoring or body mass index monitoring rather than being compared with no monitoring at all.

Testing for Primary Resistance. Testing for resistance in individual patients is still costly, because of both the cost of the diagnostic kit and the sophisticated laboratory capacity required to perform the tests. Because primary resistance is far less prevalent in LMICs than in high-income countries, no serious consideration is being given at this time to initiating individual resistance testing in the developing world. However, the choice of optimal first-line and subsequent treatment strategies should be guided by information about the prevalence of primary resistance to different antiretroviral drugs in a particular country, which indicates that population-level monitoring of the prevalence of resistance among antiretroviral-naive people living with HIV/AIDS is important.

Monitoring Response to Therapy. Ideally, therapeutic failure should be detected as soon as possible to permit the implementation of clinical strategies to address toxicity, drug resistance, or poor adherence. Therapeutic failure leads to rising viral load and falling immune competence and to the subsequent development of opportunistic infections. Unfortunately, earlier detection comes at a price: testing for increases in viral load, which can be detected soonest, is more expensive than CD4 testing, which in turn is more expensive than the less sensitive monitoring of total lymphocyte count, which is more expensive than monitoring body mass index or waiting until clinical signs of failure appear. Where facilities for detecting early failure are absent, first-line therapy should be replaced by a completely new combination at failure, usually a protease inhibitor–based combination.

Monitoring Toxicity. Available antiretroviral drugs have significant toxicity. Such toxicity is often insidious, progressing unnoticed until the patient's health has been seriously impaired. Examples include zidovudine-associated anemia, nevirapine-associated impaired liver function, and didanosine-associated pancreatitis. Fortunately, the most commonly encountered serious toxicities can be detected either on clinical examination or with inexpensive laboratory tests. Data on the relative cost-effectiveness of different toxicity monitoring regimens are unavailable. Current guidelines identify what monitoring should be conducted in conjunction with specific antiretroviral drugs, depending on whether laboratory capacity is available (WHO 2004).

Unfortunately, in the absence of a quantitative analysis of the costs of monitoring and the benefits associated with early detection of toxicity, it is difficult to provide guidance on the minimum laboratory capacity that should accompany the delivery of specific treatment combinations. Clearly, extremely low-cost monitoring tests are warranted for toxicities that occur frequently. The preeminent example is anemia monitoring for patients receiving zidovudine. Hemoglobin levels can be monitored for less than US$0.02 per test, which is almost certainly cost-effective given that the incidence of anemia with zidovudine therapy is approximately 10 percent in advanced-stage patients and that anemia frequently progresses to life-threatening levels if not detected.

RESEARCH AGENDA

As in many other areas of public health in developing countries, a profound tension exists between (a) the need for research to discover new technologies and interventions for both prevention and care and (b) the need for research to learn how to effectively apply the technologies that are currently available. The most important barrier to control is lack of

---

Box 18.7

Interventions in the Pipeline or in Trial

The following interventions are currently being developed or evaluated:

- *Microbicides.* Most microbicide products are currently in preclinical development; however, 18 products are being evaluated in clinical research studies, most in small phase 1 safety and acceptability trials. Three phase 3 effectiveness trials are currently under way.
- *Diaphragms.* The safety and effectiveness of the diaphragm and Replens gel in preventing HIV and STIs among women are being tested in an ongoing phase 3 randomized controlled trial in South Africa and Zimbabwe. Two trials, in the Dominican Republic and Madagascar, are planned to test the diaphragm's effectiveness against bacterial STIs. Several other trials in Sub-Saharan Africa are planned to test the acceptability and safety of the diaphragms plus microbicides.
- *Circumcision.* Two randomized controlled trials are under way in Kenya and Uganda to examine whether circumcision confers protection among adult men.
- *Community-based VCT.* Project Accept is a community-based VCT trial in 32 communities in South Africa, Tanzania, and Zimbabwe and 14 communities in Thailand. Communities are randomized to receive either a community-based VCT intervention or a standard clinic-based VCT. The community-based VCT intervention has three major strategies: to make VCT more available in community settings, to engage the community through outreach, and to provide posttest support.
- *HSV-2 treatment.* One study in six countries will determine the efficacy of twice-daily acyclovir in reducing susceptibility to HIV infection among high-risk, HIV-negative, HSV-2 seropositive women and men who have sex with men. A companion study will also be conducted to assess whether acyclovir reduces HIV infectiousness in individuals infected with both HSV-2 and HIV.
- *Tenofovir for preexposure use.* Studies are now enrolling participants at three West African sites and will soon begin in Botswana, Malawi, Thailand, and the United States.
- *Antiretroviral therapy to prevent sexual transmission.* A phase 3, randomized, controlled, multisite trial to assess whether antiretroviral therapy can prevent sexual transmission of HIV in serodiscordant couples will begin in Brazil, India, Malawi, Thailand, and Zimbabwe.
- *Vaccines.* Although preliminary results from a phase 3 clinical trial in Thailand found that AIDSVAX failed to protect against infection, several other vaccines are being developed. Merck and GlaxoSmithKline have unveiled sizable vaccine programs and moved products into human testing. An International AIDS Vaccine Initiative U.K.-Kenya team is in the midst of intermediate human trials of DNA/MVA (modified vaccinia virus Ankara), and Aventis Pasteur is taking ALVAC-AIDSVAX into the final phase of trials. The South African AIDS Vaccine Initiative is preparing for the country's first trials, India's prime minister has pledged national resources for vaccines, and the European Union is broadening its vaccine research for HIV.
- *Behavior change programs for people with HIV.* In recent years, a growing number of public health experts have proposed implementing prevention interventions that target people with HIV (De Cock, Marum, and Mbori-Ngacha 2003; Janssen and others 2001), although evidence on the most effective strategies to encourage safer behavior among people with HIV is lacking.

Source: Authors.

---

knowledge about how best to implement packages of existing interventions at the appropriate scale to maximize the effect of prevention and care interventions and to protect the human rights of those affected by the epidemic. Accurate surveillance data are needed on risk behaviors, and effectiveness research is needed to discern what interventions work where and how they do so. Unfortunately, few rigorous evaluations of new or existing interventions have been conducted using large prospective cohorts, with the result that, for many interventions, convincing data on effectiveness are not available. Finally, research on policy or structural interventions, which by definition must be conducted on a population level, is also insufficient. These interventions include the development and testing of such policy tools as changing the tax structure, regulating the sex industry, and guaranteeing property rights and access to credit for women.

Box 18.7 lists new prevention interventions in the pipeline. Although numerous promising interventions are listed, results for most of these strategies are at best years away. Centuries hence, when future generations study the history of our time and the epidemic that killed 50 million or perhaps many more, the most difficult question to answer may well be "why did they invest so little for so long in developing a vaccine?" Creating such knowledge is about as close as one can get to a pure international public good, and the lack of global cooperation in adequately funding such research is an indictment of global commitment to multilateral cooperation. However, given both the uncertainty about whether developing an effective vaccine is possible and the long delay until a new vaccine can be widely applied, vaccine development efforts must be accompanied by the development of other new biomedical and behavioral prevention technologies.

In contrast, research on care and treatment has been far more successful than research on prevention, and innovation in new therapies continues apace. The ability of HIV to rapidly evolve resistance to antiretroviral drugs, combined with the existence of an important market in high- and middle-income countries, appears to ensure continued investment in new drug development. In addition, because treatment generally has important commercial returns, HIV therapies, unlike behavioral interventions, have benefited the most from private sector investment. The paradox is that research on the behavioral aspects of adherence to drug regimens would improve the effectiveness of antiretroviral therapy, and thereby benefit both commercial and public interests.

The greatest research challenges in relation to care and treatment in developing countries do not revolve around new drug development. They revolve around how to adapt care and treatment strategies to low-income, low-technology, low–human resource capacity settings in ways that maximize adherence; minimize toxicity, monitoring, and costs; and maximize the prolongation of high-quality life from antiretroviral therapy—all without damaging existing and often fragile health care infrastructure that must also address other health concerns. Although simplified regimens, such as delivering multiple drugs in a single tablet and fewer doses per day, are desirable everywhere, they are especially important in low-resource settings. Similarly, low-technology, low-cost monitoring tests for antiretroviral therapy toxicity and for immunological and virological responses to treatment are especially needed in low-income countries, which otherwise must centralize testing—an especially difficult prospect when transport and communications systems are poorly developed.

CONCLUSION

Despite the glaring deficits in AIDS research, the magnitude and seriousness of the global pandemic calls for action in the absence of definitive data. The appropriate mix and distribution of prevention and treatment interventions depends on the stage of the epidemic in a given country and the context in which it occurs. In the absence of firm data to guide program objectives, national strategies may not accurately reflect the priorities dictated by the particular epidemic profile, resulting in highly inefficient investments in HIV/AIDS prevention and care. This waste undoubtedly exacerbates funding shortfalls and results in unnecessary HIV infections and premature deaths. The lack of good data—and thus the ability to tailor responses to epidemics—may be somewhat understandable when the burden of disease is minimal and the resources dedicated to it are similarly small. Neither is the case for HIV/AIDS.

ACKNOWLEDGMENTS

We are deeply indebted to Andrew Beggs, Susan Foster, James Kahn, Lilani Kumaranayake, Elliot Marseille, Fern Terris-Prestholt, Seema Vyas, and Charlotte Watts for their background papers that have informed this chapter. We also owe thanks to Sevgi Aral, Geoffrey Garnett, Robin Jackson, Marie Laga, Meg Newman, Mead Over, and David Vlahov for their work on several sections of this chapter. Finally, we would like to thank Martin Gross and Phillip Machingura for their invaluable contributions throughout this chapter.

NOTE

1. See http://www.hivinsite.org/global?page=cr-00-04 for a compilation of international guidelines.

BIBLIOGRAPHY

Agha, S., A. Karlyn, and D. Meekers. 2001. "The Promotion of Condom Use in Non-Regular Sexual Partnerships in Urban Mozambique." *Health Policy and Planning* 16 (2): 144–51.

Alcabes, P., A. Munoz, D. Vlahov, and G. H. Friedland. 1993. "Incubation Period of Human Immunodeficiency Virus." *Epidemiologic Reviews* 15 (2): 303–18.

Anthony, J. C., D. Vlahov, K. E. Nelson, S. Cohn, J. Astemborski, and L. Solomon. 1991. "New Evidence on Intravenous Cocaine Use and the Risk of Infection with Human Immunodeficiency Virus Type 1." *American Journal of Epidemiology* 134: 1175–89.

Anzala, O. A., N. J. Nagelkerke, J. Bwayo, D. Holton, S. Moses, and E. Ngugi. 1995. "Rapid Progression to Disease in African Sex Workers with Human Immunodeficiency Virus Type 1 Infection." *Journal of Infectious Diseases* 171 (3): 686–89.

Askew, I., and M. Berer. 2003. "The Contribution of Sexual and Reproductive Health Services to the Fight against HIV/AIDS: A Review." *Reproductive Health Matters* 11 (22): 51–73.

Auvert, B., A. Buve, E. Lagarde, M. Kahindo, J. Chege, N. Rutenberg, and others. 2001. "Male Circumcision and HIV Infection in Four Cities in Sub-Saharan Africa." *AIDS* 15 (Suppl. 4): S31–40.

Auvert, B., A. Puren, D. Taljaard, E. Lagarde, R. Sitta, and J. Tambekou. 2005. "Impact of Male Circumcision on the Female-to-Male Transmission of HIV." Paper presented at the 3rd IAS Conference on HIV Pathegenosis and Treatment. Rio de Janeiro, July 24–27.

Ayouba, A., G. Tene, P. Cunin, Y. Foupouapouognigni, E. Menu, A. Kfutwah, and others. 2003. "Low Rate of Mother-to-Child Transmission of HIV-1 after Nevirapine Intervention in a Pilot Public Health Program in Yaounde, Cameroon." *Journal of Acquired Immune Deficiency Syndrome* 34 (3): 274–80.

Bacellar, H., A. Munoz, E. N. Miller, B. A. Cohen, D. Besley, O. A. Selnes, and others. 1994. "Incidence of Clinical AIDS Conditions in a Cohort of Homosexual Men with CD4+ Cell Counts <100/mm3: Multicenter AIDS Cohort Study." *Journal of Infectious Diseases* 170 (5): 1284–87.

Badri, M., and R. Wood. 2003. "Usefulness of Total Lymphocyte Count in Monitoring Highly Active Antiretroviral Therapy in Resource-Limited Settings." *AIDS* 17 (4): 541–45.

Basu, I., S. Jana, M. J. Rotheram-Borus, D. Swendeman, S. J. Lee, P. Newman, and R. Weiss. 2004. "HIV Prevention among Sex Workers in India." *Journal of Acquired Immune Deficiency Syndrome* 36 (3): 845–52.

Bautista, S., T. Dmytraczenko, G. Kombe, and S. Bertozzi. 2003. Costing of HIV/AIDS Treatment in Mexico. In *Technical Report No. 020.* Edited by Project PHRplus. Bethesda, MD: Abt Associates, Inc.

Bell, J. C., D. N. Rose, and H. S. Sacks. 1999. "Tuberculosis Preventive Therapy for HIV-Infected People in Sub-Saharan Africa Is Cost-Effective." *AIDS* 13 (12): 1549–56.

Bentley, M. E., K. Spratt, M. E. Shepherd, R. R. Gangakhedkar, S. Thilikavathi, R. C. Bollinger, and S. M. Mehendale. 1998. "HIV Testing and Counseling among Men Attending Sexually Transmitted Disease Clinics in Pune, India: Changes in Condom Use and Sexual Behavior over Time." *AIDS* 12 (14): 1869–77.

Berenguer, J., F. Laguna, J. Lopez-Aldeguer, S. Moreno, J. R. Arribas, J. Arrizabalaga, and others. 2004. "Prevention of Opportunistic Infections in Adult and Adolescent Patients with HIV Infection: GESIDA/National AIDS Plan Guidelines, 2004." *Enfermedades Infecciosas y Microbiologia Clinica* 22 (3): 160–76.

Bertozzi, S. M., N. S. Padian, J. Wegbreit, B. Feldman, L. DeMaria, H. Gayle, and others. Forthcoming. "HIV/AIDS Prevention and Treatment." Disease Control Priorities Project Working Paper 39, Bethesda, MD. http://www.fic.nih.gov/dcpp/wps.html.

Bhave, G., C. P. Lindan, E. S. Hudes, S. Desai, U. Wagle, S. P. Tripathi, and J. S. Mandel. 1995. "Impact of an Intervention on HIV, Sexually Transmitted Diseases, and Condom Use among Sex Workers in Bombay, India." *AIDS* 9 (Suppl. 1): S21–30.

Bobrik, A. 2004. "HIV Prevention among IDUs in Russia: A Cost-Effectiveness Analysis." Paper presented at the 14th International Conference on the Reduction of Drug-Related Harm, April, Chiang Mai, Thailand.

Bonnard, P. 2002. "HIV/AIDS Mitigation Using What We Already Know." Technical Note 5, Food and Nutrition Technical Assistance (FANTA) Project, Washington, DC.

Buve, A. 2002. "HIV Epidemics in Africa: What Explains the Variations in HIV Prevalence?" *International Union of Biochemistry and Molecular Biology Life* 53 (4–5): 193–95.

Cardo, D. M., D. H. Culver, C. A. Ciesielski, P. U. Srivastava, R. Marcus, D. Abiteboul, and others. 1997. "A Case-Control Study of HIV Seroconversion in Health Care Workers after Percutaneous Exposure." Centers for Disease Control and Prevention Needlestick Surveillance Group. *New England Journal of Medicine* 337 (21): 1485–90.

Carlisle, D. 2003. "Africans Are Dying of AIDS without Pain Relief." *British Medical Journal* 327 (7423): 1069.

Carre, N., C. Deveau, F. Belanger, F. Boufassa, A. Persoz, C. Jadand, and others. 1994. "Effect of Age and Exposure Group on the Onset of AIDS in Heterosexual and Homosexual HIV-infected Patients: SEROCO Study Group." *AIDS* 8 (6): 797–802.

Castro, A., and P. Farmer. 2005. "Understanding and Addressing AIDS-Related Stigma: From Anthropological Theory to Clinical Practice in Haiti." *American Journal of Public Health* 95 (1): 53–59.

Cates, W. 2004. "A Funny Thing Happened on the Way to FHI." *Sexually Transmitted Diseases* 31 (1): 3–7.

CDC (U.S. Centers for Disease Control and Prevention). 1989. *Guidelines for the Prevention of HIV and Hepatitis B.* Atlanta: CDC.

Celentano, D. D., K. C. Bond, C. M. Lyles, S. Eiumtrakul, V. F. Go, C. Beyrer, and others. 2000. "Preventive Intervention to Reduce Sexually Transmitted Infections: A Field Trial in the Royal Thai Army." *Archives of Internal Medicine* 160 (4): 535–40.

Chaisson, R. E., P. Bacchetti, D. Osmond, B. Brodie, M. A. Sande, and A. R. Moss. 1989. "Cocaine Use and HIV Infection in Intravenous Drug Users in San Francisco." *Journal of the American Medical Association* 261 (4): 561–65.

CHI (Center for HIV Information). 2005. "HIV Insite." University of California, San Francisco. http://hivinsite.org.

Colebunders, R. L., and A. S. Latif. 1991. "Natural History and Clinical Presentation of HIV-1 Infection in Adults." *AIDS* 5 (Suppl. 1): S103–12.

Connor, E. M., R. S. Sperling, R. Gelber, P. Kiselev, G. Scott, M. J. O'Sullivan, and others. 1994. "Reduction of Maternal-Infant Transmission of Human Immunodeficiency Virus Type 1 with Zidovudine Treatment." Pediatric AIDS Clinical Trials Group Protocol 076 Study Group. *New England Journal of Medicine* 331 (18): 1173–80.

Cook, J. A., D. Grey, J. Burke, M. H. Cohen, A. C. Gurtman, J. L. Richardson, and others. 2004. "Depressive Symptoms and AIDS-Related Mortality among a Multisite Cohort of HIV-Positive Women." *American Journal of Public Health* 94 (7): 1133–40.

Coutsoudis, A. 2002. "Breastfeeding and HIV Transmission." In *Public Health Issues in Infant and Child Nutrition*, vol. 48, ed. R. E. Black and K. F. Michaelsen. Nestle Nutrition Workshop Series. Philadelphia: Lippincott Williams & Wilkins.

Coutsoudis, A., K. Pillay, L. Kuhn, E. Spooner, W. Y. Tsai, and H. M. Coovadia. 2001. "Method of Feeding and Transmission of HIV-1 from Mothers to Children by 15 Months of Age: Prospective Cohort Study from Durban, South Africa." *AIDS* 15 (3): 379–87.

Coutsoudis, A., K. Pillay, E. Spooner, L. Kuhn, and H. M. Coovadia. 1999. "Influence of Infant-Feeding Patterns on Early Mother-to-Child Transmission of HIV-1 in Durban, South Africa: A Prospective Cohort Study." South African Vitamin A Study Group. *Lancet* 354 (9177): 471–76.

Creese, A., K. Floyd, A. Alban, and L. Guinness. 2002. "Cost-Effectiveness of HIV/AIDS Interventions in Africa: A Systematic Review of the Evidence." *Lancet* 359 (9318): 1635–43.

Dabis, F., P. Msellati, N. Meda, C. Welffens-Ekra, B. You, O. Manigart, and others. 1999. "6-Month Efficacy, Tolerance, and Acceptability of a Short Regimen of Oral Zidovudine to Reduce Vertical Transmission of HIV in Breastfed Children in Côte d'Ivoire and Burkina Faso: A Double-Blind Placebo-Controlled Multicentre Trial." DITRAME Study Group. *Lancet* 353 (9155): 786–92.

De Cock, K. M., E. Marum, and D. Mbori-Ngacha. 2003. "A Serostatus-Based Approach to HIV/AIDS Prevention and Care in Africa." *Lancet* 362 (9398): 1847–49.

Deeks, S. G., J. D. Barbour, J. N. Martin, M. S. Swanson, and R. M. Grant. 2000. "Sustained CD4+ T Cell Response after Virologic Failure of Protease Inhibitor–Based Regimens in Patients with Human Immunodeficiency Virus Infection." *Journal of Infectious Diseases* 181 (3): 946–53.

Deeks, S. G., F. M. Hecht, M. Swanson, T. Elbeik, R. Loftus, P. T. Cohen, and others. 1999. "HIV RNA and CD4 Cell Count Response to Protease Inhibitor Therapy in an Urban AIDS Clinic: Response to Both Initial and Salvage Therapy." *AIDS* 13 (6): F35–43.

DeGruttola, V., G. R. Seage, K. H. Mayer, C. R. Horsburgh. 1989. "Infectiousness of HIV between Male Homosexual Partners." *Journal of Clinical Epidemiology* 42 (9): 849–56.

Des Jarlais, D. C., and S. R. Friedman. 1996. "HIV Epidemiology and Interventions among Injecting Drug Users." *International Journal of Sexually Transmitted Diseases and AIDS* 7 (Suppl. 2): 57–61.

Deschamps, M. M., J. W. Pape, A. Hafner, and W. D. Johnson. 1996. "Heterosexual Transmission of HIV in Haiti." *Annals of Internal Medicine* 125 (4): 324–30.

Donnelly, J. 2004. "Circumcised Men Less Likely to Get AIDS." *Boston Globe*, November 16.

Duran, S., M. Saves, B. Spire, V. Cailleton, A. Sobel, P. Carrieri, and others. 2001. "Failure to Maintain Long-Term Adherence to Highly Active Antiretroviral Therapy: The Role of Lipodystrophy." *AIDS* 15 (18): 2441–44.

Dziekan, G., D. Chisholm, B. Johns, J. Rovira, and Y. J. Hutin. 2003. "The Cost-Effectiveness of Policies for the Safe and Appropriate Use of Injection in Healthcare Settings." *Bulletin of the World Health Organization* 81 (4): 277–85.

Easterbrook, P. J. 1994. "Non-Progression in HIV Infection." *AIDS* 8 (8): 1179–82.

Egger, M., J. Pauw, A. Lopatatzidis, D. Medrano, F. Paccaud, and G. D. Smith. 2000. "Promotion of Condom Use in a High-Risk Setting in Nicaragua: A Randomised Controlled Trial." *Lancet* 355 (9221): 2101–05.

Eshleman, S. H., M. Mracna, L. A. Guay, M. Deseyve, S. Cunningham, M. Mirochnick, and others. 2001. "Selection and Fading of Resistance Mutations in Women and Infants Receiving Nevirapine to Prevent HIV-1 Vertical Transmission (HIVNET 012)." *AIDS* 15 (15): 1951–57.

Farmer, P., F. Leandre, J. Mukherjee, R. Gupta, L. Tarter, and J. Y. Kim. 2001. "Community-Based Treatment of Advanced HIV Disease: Introducing DOT-HAART (Directly Observed Therapy with Highly Active Antiretroviral Therapy)." *Bulletin of the World Health Organization* 79 (12): 1145–51.

Fawole, I. O., M. C. Asuzu, S. O. Oduntan, and W. R. Brieger. 1999. "A School-Based AIDS Education Programme for Secondary School Students in Nigeria: A Review of Effectiveness." *Health Education Resources* 14 (5): 675–83.

Fawzi, W., G. Msamanga, G. Antelman, C. Xu, E. Hertzmark, D. Spiegelman, and others. 2004. "Effect of Prenatal Vitamin Supplementation on Lower-Genital Levels of HIV Type 1 and Interleukin Type 1 Beta at 36 Weeks of Gestation." *Clinical Infectious Diseases* 38 (5): 716–22.

Feachem, R. G. 2004. "The Research Imperative: Fighting AIDS, TB, and Malaria." *Tropical Medicine and International Health* 9 (11): 1139–41.

Fleming, T. R., and D. L. DeMets. 1996. "Surrogate End Points in Clinical Trials: Are We Being Misled?" *Annals of Internal Medicine* 125: 605–13.

Floyd, K., D. Wilkinson, and C. Gilks. 1997. "Comparison of Cost Effectiveness of Directly Observed Treatment (DOT) and Conventionally Delivered Treatment for Tuberculosis: Experience from Rural South Africa." *British Medical Journal* 315 (7120): 1407–11.

Ford, K., D. N. Wirawan, P. Fajans, P. Meliawan, K. MacDonald, and L. Thorpe. 1996. "Behavioral Interventions for Reduction of Sexually Transmitted Disease/HIV Transmission among Female Commercial Sex Workers and Clients in Bali, Indonesia." *AIDS* 10 (2): 213–22.

Foster, S., and A. Buve. 1995. "Benefits of HIV Screening of Blood Transfusions in Zambia." *Lancet* 346 (8969): 225–27.

Garcia, P. M., L. A. Kalish, J. Pitt, H. Minkoff, T. C. Quinn, S. K. Burchett, and others. 1999. "Maternal Levels of Plasma Human Immunodeficiency Virus Type 1 RNA and the Risk of Perinatal Transmission. Women and Infants Transmission Study Group." *New England Journal of Medicine* 341 (6): 394–402.

Ghys, P. D., M. O. Diallo, V. Ettiegne-Traore, K. Kale, O. Tawil, M. Carael, and others. 2002. "Increase in Condom Use and Decline in HIV and Sexually Transmitted Diseases among Female Sex Workers in Abidjan, Côte d'Ivoire, 1991–1998." *AIDS* 16 (2): 251–58.

Gillespie, S., L. Haddad, and R. Jackson. 2001. "HIV/AIDS Food and Nutrition Security: Impacts and Actions." Paper prepared for the 29th Session of the ACC/SCN Symposium on Nutrition and HIV/AIDS.

Gilson, L., R. Mkanje, H. Grosskurth, F. Mosha, J. Picard, A. Gavyole, and others. 1997. "Cost-Effectiveness of Improved Treatment Services for Sexually Transmitted Diseases in Preventing HIV-1 Infection in Mwanza Region, Tanzania." *Lancet* 350 (9094): 1805–9.

Gisselquist, D., J. J. Potterat, R. Rothenberg, E. M. Drucker, S. Brody, D. Brewe, and others. 2003. "Examining the Hypothesis That Sexual Transmission Drives Africa's HIV Epidemic." *AIDScience* 3 (10). http://www.aidscience.org/Articles/AIDScience032.asp.

Global HIV Prevention Working Group. 2003. *Access to HIV Prevention—Closing the Gap*. Menlo Park, CA: Kaiser Family Foundation.

Göhde, R. 2004. Personal Communication. HIV/AIDS Project Coordinator, Müster, Germany.

Goldie, S. J., L. Kuhn, L. Denny, A. Pollack, and T. C. Wright. 2001. "Policy Analysis of Cervical Cancer Screening Strategies in Low-Resource Settings: Clinical Benefits and Cost-Effectiveness. *Journal of the American Medical Association* 285 (24): 3107–15.

Grant, R. M., F. M. Hecht, M. Warmerdam, L. Liu, T. Liegler, C. J. Petropoulos, and others. 2002. "Time Trends in Primary HIV-1 Drug Resistance among Recently Infected Persons." *Journal of the American Medical Association* 288 (2): 181–88.

Grant, R. M., J. Kahn, M. Warmerdam, L. Liu, C. J. Petropoulos, N. S. Hellman, and F. Hecht. 2002. "Transmission and Transmissibility of Drug Resistant HIV-1 (368-M)." Paper presented at 9th Conference on Retroviruses and Opportunistic Infections, Seattle, February 24–28.

Grassly, N. C., G. P. Garnett, B. Schwartlander, S. Gregson, and R. M. Anderson. 2001. "The Effectiveness of HIV Prevention and the Epidemiological Context." *Bulletin of the World Health Organization* 79 (12): 1121–32.

Gregson, S., P. R. Mason, G. P. Garnett, T. Zhuwau, C. A. Nyamukapa, R. M. Anderson, and S. K. Chandiwana. 2001. "A Rural HIV Epidemic in Zimbabwe? Findings from a Population-Based Survey."

International Journal of Sexually Transmitted Diseases and AIDS 12 (3): 189–96.

Grosskurth, H., F. Mosha, J. Todd, E. Mwijarubi, A. Klokke, K. Senkoro, and others. 1995. "Impact of Improved Treatment of Sexually Transmitted Diseases on HIV Infection in Rural Tanzania: Randomised Controlled Trial." *Lancet* 346 (8974): 530–36.

Guay, L. A., P. Musoke, T. Fleming, D. Bagenda, M. Allen, C. Nakabiito, and others. 1999. "Intrapartum and Neonatal Single-Dose Nevirapine Compared with Zidovudine for Prevention of Mother-to-Child Transmission of HIV-1 in Kampala, Uganda: HIVNET 012 Randomised Trial." *Lancet* 354 (9181): 795–802.

Gutierrez, J. P., B. Johns, T. Adam, S. M. Bertozzi, T. T. Edejer, R. Greener, and others. 2004. "Achieving the WHO/UNAIDS Antiretroviral Treatment 3 by 5 Goal: What Will It Cost?" *Lancet* 364 (9428): 63–64.

Hammer, S. M., K. E. Squires, M. D. Hughes, J. M. Grimes, L. M. Demeter, J. S. Currier, and others. 1997. "A Controlled Trial of Two Nucleoside Analogues Plus Indinavir in Persons with Human Immunodeficiency Virus Infection and CD4 Cell Counts of 200 Per Cubic Millimeter or Less." *New England Journal of Medicine* 337 (11): 725–33.

Hansen, K., G. Woelk, H. Jackson, R. Kerkhoven, N. Manjonjori, P. Maramba, and others. 1998. "The Cost of Home-Based Care for HIV/AIDS Patients in Zimbabwe." *AIDS Care* 10 (6): 751–59.

Harries, A. D., D. S. Nyangulu, N. J. Hargreaves, O. Kaluwa, and F. M. Salaniponi. 2001. "Preventing Antiretroviral Anarchy in Sub-Saharan Africa." *Lancet* 358 (9279): 410–14.

Harvey, B., J. Stuart, and T. Swan. 2000. "Evaluation of a Drama-in-Education Programme to Increase AIDS Awareness in South African High Schools: A Randomized Community Intervention Trial." *International Journal of Sexually Transmitted Diseases and AIDS* 11 (2): 105–11.

Hayes, R., J. Chagalucha, H. Grosskurth, A. Obasi, J. Todd, B. Cleophas-Mazigr, and others. 2003. "Mema Kwa Vijana: A Randomised Controlled Trial of an Adolescents Sexual and Reproductive Health Intervention Programme in Rural Mwanza, Tanzania: 2 Intervention and Process Indicators." Paper presented at the International Society of Sexually Transmitted Diseases Research Congress, Ottawa, July 27–30.

Henderson, D. K., B. J. Fahey, M. Will, J. M. Schmitt, K. Carey, D. E. Koziol, and others. 1990. "Risk for Occupational Transmission of Human Immunodeficiency Virus Type 1 (HIV-1) Associated with Clinical Exposures: A Prospective Evaluation." *Annals of Internal Medicine* 113 (1): 740–46.

Higginson, I. J., I. G. Findlay, D. M. Goodwin, K. Hood, A. G. Edwards, A. Cook, and others. 2003. "Is There Evidence That Palliative Care Teams Alter End-of-Life Experiences of Patients and Their Caregivers?" *Journal of Pain and Symptom Management* 25 (2): 150–168.

Hira, S. K., G. J. Dore, and T. Sirisanthana. 1998. "Clinical Spectrum of HIV/AIDS in the Asia-Pacific Region." *AIDS* 12 (Suppl. B): S145–54.

Hira, S. K., H. L. Dupont, D. N. Lanjewar, and Y. N. Dholakia. 1998. "Severe Weight Loss: The Predominant Clinical Presentation of Tuberculosis in Patients with HIV Infection in India." *National Medical Journal of India* 11 (6): 256–58.

Hook, E. W., R. O. Cannon, A. J. Nahmias, F. F. Lee, C. H. Campbell, D. Glasser, and others. 1992. "Herpes Simplex Virus Infection as a Risk Factor for Human Immunodeficiency Virus Infection in Heterosexuals." *Journal of Infectious Diseases* 165 (2): 251–55.

Hoover, D. R., A. J. Saah, H. Bacellar, J. Phair, R. Detels, R. Anderson, and others. 1993. "Clinical Manifestations of AIDS in the Era of Pneumocystis Prophylaxis: Multicenter AIDS Cohort Study." *New England Journal of Medicine* 329 (26): 1922–26.

Hurley, S. F., D. J. Jolley, and J. M. Kaldor. 1997. "Effectiveness of Needle-Exchange Programmes for Prevention of HIV Infection." *Lancet* 349 (9068): 1797–800.

Hutton, G., K. Wyss, and Y. N'Diekhor. 2003. "Prioritization of Prevention Activities to Combat the Spread of HIV/AIDS in Resource-Constrained Settings: A Cost-Effectiveness Analysis from Chad, Central Africa." *International Journal of Health Planning and Management* 18 (2): 117–36.

Ippolito, G., V. Puro, and G. De Carli. 1993. "The Risk of Occupational Human Immunodeficiency Virus Infection in Health Care Workers: Italian Multicenter Study." Italian Study Group on Occupational Risk of HIV Infection. *Annals of Internal Medicine* 153 (12): 1451–58.

Institute of Medicine, ed. 1997. *The Hidden Epidemic: Confronting Sexually Transmitted Diseases.* Washington, DC: National Academy Press.

Jackson, D. J., J. P. Rakwar, B. A. Richardson, K. Mandaliya, B. H. Chohan, J. J. Bwayo, and others. 1997. "Decreased Incidence of Sexually Transmitted Diseases among Trucking Company Workers in Kenya: Results of a Behavioural Risk-Reduction Programme." *AIDS* 11 (7): 903–09.

Jackson, J. B., P. Musoke, T. Fleming, L. A. Guay, D. Bagenda, M. Allen, and others. 2003. "Intrapartum and Neonatal Single-Dose Nevirapine Compared with Zidovudine for Prevention of Mother-to-Child Transmission of HIV-1 in Kampala, Uganda: 18-Month Follow-up of the HIVNET 012 Randomised Trial." *Lancet* 362 (9387): 859–68.

Jacobs, B., and A. Mercer. 1999. "Feasibility of Hospital-Based Blood Banking: A Tanzanian Case Study." *Health Policy and Planning* 14 (4): 354–62.

Janssen, R. S., D. R. Holtgrave, R. O. Valdiserri, M. Shepherd, H. D. Gayle, and K. M. De Cock. 2001. "The Serostatus Approach to Fighting the HIV Epidemic: Prevention Strategies for Infected Individuals." *American Journal of Public Health* 91 (7): 1019–24.

Jemmott, J. B., L. S. Jemmott, and G. T. Fong. 1998. "Abstinence and Safer Sex: HIV Risk-Reduction for African American Adolescents." *Journal of the American Medical Association* 279 (19): 1529–36.

Jenkins, C., H. Rahman, T. Saidel, S. Jana, and A. M. Hussain. 2001. "Measuring the Impact of Needle Exchange Programs among Injecting Drug Users through the National Behavioural Surveillance in Bangladesh." *AIDS Education and Prevention* 13 (5): 452–61.

Jha, P., L. M. E. Vaz, F. Plummer, N. Nagelkerke, B. Willbond, E. Ngugi, and others. 2001. "The Evidence Base for Interventions to Prevent HIV Infection in Low- and Middle-Income Countries." Commission on Macroeconomics and Health Working Paper. WG5: 2. Commission on Macroeconomics and Health, Geneva, Switzerland.

John, G. C., R. W. Nduati, D. A. Mbori-Ngacha, B. A. Richardson, D. Panteleeff, A. Mwatha, and others. 2001. "Correlates of Mother-to-Child Human Immunodeficiency Virus Type 1 (HIV-1) Transmission: Association with Maternal Plasma HIV-1 RNA Load, Genital HIV-1 DNA Shedding, and Breast Infections." *Journal of Infectious Diseases* 183 (2): 206–12.

John Snow Inc. 2003. Fact Sheets for Diagnostic Tests. http://deliver.jsi.com/2002/archives/hivaids/test_kits/index.cfm.

Kagimu, M., E. Marum, F. Wabwire-Mangen, N. Nakyanjo, Y. Walakira, and J. Hogle. 1998. "Evaluation of the Effectiveness of AIDS Health Education Interventions in the Muslim Community in Uganda." *AIDS Education and Prevention* 10 (3): 215–28.

Kahn, J. G., S. M. Kegeles, R. Hays, and N. Beltzer. 2001. "Cost-Effectiveness of the Mpowerment Project, a Community-Level Intervention for Young Gay Men." *Journal of Acquired Immune Deficiency Syndrome* 27 (5): 482–91.

Kalichman, S. C., D. Rompa, M. Cage, K. DiFonzo, D. Simpson, J. Austin, and others. 2001. "Effectiveness of an Intervention to Reduce HIV Transmission Risks in HIV-Positive People." *American Journal of Preventive Medicine* 21 (2): 84–92.

Kamali, A., M. Quigley, J. Nakiyingi, J. Kinsman, J. Kengeya-Kayondo, R. Gopal, and others. 2003. "Syndromic Management of Sexually Transmitted Infections and Behaviour Change Interventions on

Transmission of HIV-1 in Rural Uganda: A Community Randomised Trial." *Lancet* 361 (9358): 645–52.

Kamenga, M., R. W. Ryder, M. Jingu, N. Mbuyi, L. Mbu, F. Behets, and others. 1991. "Evidence of Marked Sexual Behavior Change Associated with Low HIV-1 Seroconversion in 149 Married Couples with Discordant HIV-1 Serostatus: Experience at an HIV Counselling Center in Zaire." *AIDS* 5 (1): 61–67.

Kaplan, E. H., and R. Heimer. 1992. "A Model-Based Estimate of HIV Infectivity via Needle-Sharing." *Journal of Acquired Immune Deficiency Syndrome* 5 (11): 1116–18.

Kaplan, J. E., D. L. Hanson, J. L. Jones, and M. S. Dworkin. 2001. "Viral Load as an Independent Risk Factor for Opportunistic Infections in HIV-Infected Adults and Adolescents." *AIDS* 15 (14): 1831–36.

Kaplan, J. E., H. Masur, and K. K. Holmes. 2002. "Guidelines for Preventing Opportunistic Infections among HIV-Infected Persons—2002: Recommendations of the U.S. Public Health Service and the Infectious Diseases Society of America." *Morbidity and Mortality Weekly Report* 51 (RR-8): 1–52.

Katz, M. H., S. K. Schwarcz, T. A. Kellogg, J. D. Klausner, J. W. Dilley, S. Gibson, and others. 2002. "Impact of Highly Active Antiretroviral Treatment on HIV Seroincidence among Men Who Have Sex with Men: San Francisco." *American Journal of Public Health* 92 (3): 388–94.

Katzenstein, D. A., W. McFarland, M. Mbizvo, A. S. Latif, R. Machekano, J. Parsonnet, and others. 1998. "Peer Education among Factory Workers in Zimbabwe: Providing a Sustainable HIV Prevention Intervention." Paper presented at the 12th International Conference on AIDS, Geneva, June 28–July 3.

Kegeles, S. M., R. B. Hays, and T. J. Coates. 1996. "The Mpowerment Project: A Community-Level HIV Prevention Intervention for Young Gay Men." *American Journal of Public Health* 86 (8): 1129–36.

Kelly, J. A., D. A. Murphy, K. J. Sikkema, T. L. McAuliffe, R. A. Roffman, L. J. Solomon, and others. 1997. "Randomised, Controlled, Community-Level HIV-Prevention Intervention for Sexual-Risk Behaviour among Homosexual Men in U.S. Cities: Community HIV Prevention Research Collaborative." *Lancet* 350 (9090): 1500–5.

Kim, N., B. Stanton, X. Li, K. Dickersin, and J. Galbraith. 1997. "Effectiveness of the 40 Adolescent AIDS-Risk Reduction Interventions: A Quantitative Review." *Journal of Adolescent Health* 20 (3): 204–15.

Kirby, D. 1997. *No Easy Answers: Research Findings on Programs to Reduce Teen Pregnancy*. Washington, DC: National Campaign to Prevent Teen Pregnancy.

———. 2001. *Emerging Answers: Research Findings on Programs to Reduce Teen Pregnancy*. Washington, DC: National Campaign to Prevent Teen Pregnancy.

Kitahata, M. M., T. D. Koepsell, R. A. Deyo, C. L. Maxwell, W. T. Dodge, and E. H. Wagner. 1996. "Physicians' Experience with the Acquired Immunodeficiency Syndrome as a Factor in Patients' Survival." *New England Journal of Medicine* 334: 701–6.

Komanduri, K. V., M. N. Viswanathan, E. D. Wieder, D. K. Schmidt, B. M. Bredt, M. A. Jacobson, and others. 1998. "Restoration of Cytomegalovirus-Specific CD4+ T-Lymphocyte Responses after Ganciclovir and Highly Active Antiretroviral Therapy in Individuals Infected with HIV-1." *Nature Medicine* 4 (8): 953–56.

Ksobiech, K. 2003. "A Meta-Analysis of Needle Sharing, Lending, and Borrowing Behaviors of Needle Exchange Program Attenders." *AIDS Education and Prevention* 15 (3): 257–68.

Kumaranayake, L., P. Mangtani, A. Boupda-Duate, J. C. Foumena Abada, C. Cheta, Z. Njoumemi, and C. Watts. 1998. "Cost-Effectiveness of an HIV/AIDS Peer Education Programme among Commercial Sex Workers (CSW): Results from Cameroon [abstract no. 33592]." Paper presented at the World AIDS Conference, Geneva, June 28–July 3.

Kumaranayake, L., P. Vickerman, D. Walker, S. Samoshkin, V. Romantzov, Z. Emelyanova, and others. 2004. "The Cost-Effectiveness of HIV

Preventive Measures among Injecting Drug Users in Svetlogorsk, Belarus." *Addiction* 99 (12): 1565–76.

Ladner, J., V. Leroy, P. Hoffman, M. Nyiraziraje, A. De Clercq, P. Van de Perre, and F. Dabis. 1998. "Chorioamnionitis and Pregnancy Outcome in HIV-Infected African Women: Pregnancy and HIV Study Group." *Journal of Acquired Immune Deficiency Syndrome and Human Retrovirology* 18 (3): 293–98.

Laga, M., M. Alary, N. Nzila, A. T. Manoka, M. Tuliza, F. Behets, and others. 1994. "Condom Promotion, Sexually Transmitted Diseases Treatment, and Declining Incidence of HIV-1 Infection in Female Zairian Sex Workers." *Lancet* 344 (8917): 246–48.

Laleman, G., K. Magazani, J. H. Perriens, N. Badibanga, N. Kapila, M. Konde, and others. 1992. "Prevention of Blood-borne HIV Transmission Using a Decentralized Approach in Shaba, Zaire." *AIDS* 6 (11): 1353–58.

Laniece, I., K. Diop, A. Desclaux, K. Sow, B. Ciss, B. Ndiaye, and I. Ndoye. 2004. "Determinants of long-term adherence to antiretroviral drugs among adults followed over four years in Dakar, Senegal." Abstract presented at the XV International AIDS Conference, July 11–16, Bangkok, Thailand.

Lanjewar, D. N., B. S. Anand, R. Genta, M. B. Maheshwari, M. A. Ansari, S. K. Hira, and others. 1996. "Major Differences in the Spectrum of Gastrointestinal Infections Associated with AIDS in India versus the West: An Autopsy Study." *Clinical Infectious Disease* 23 (3): 482–85.

Lauby, J. L., P. J. Smith, M. Stark, B. Person, and J. Adams. 2000. "A Community-Level HIV Prevention Intervention for Inner-City Women: Results of the Women and Infants Demonstration Projects." *American Journal of Public Health* 90 (2): 216–22.

Ledergerber, B., M. Egger, M. Opravil, A. Telenti, B. Hirschel, M. Battegay, and others. 1999. "Clinical Progression and Virological Failure on Highly Active Antiretroviral Therapy in HIV-1 Patients: A Prospective Cohort Study." Swiss HIV Cohort Study. *Lancet* 353 (9156): 863–68.

Ledergerber, B., A. Mocroft, P. Reiss, H. Furrer, O. Kirk, M. Bickel, and others. 2001. "Discontinuation of Secondary Prophylaxis against *Pneumocystis carinii* Pneumonia in Patients with HIV Infection Who Have a Response to Antiretroviral Therapy: Eight European Study Groups." *New England Journal of Medicine* 344 (3): 168–74.

Leigh Brown, A. J., S. D. Frost, W. C. Mathews, K. Dawson, N. S. Hellmann, E. S. Daar, and others. 2003. "Transmission Fitness of Drug-Resistant Human Immunodeficiency Virus and the Prevalence of Resistance in the Antiretroviral-Treated Population." *Journal of Infectious Diseases* 187 (4): 683–86.

Levine, W. C., R. Revollo, V. Kaune, J. Vega, F. Tinajeros, M. Garnica, and others. 1998. "Decline in Sexually Transmitted Disease Prevalence in Female Bolivian Sex Workers: Impact of an HIV Prevention Project." *AIDS* 12 (14): 1899–906.

Li, T. S., R. Tubiana, C. Katlama, V. Calvez, H. Ait Mohand, and B. Autran. 1998. "Long-Lasting Recovery in CD4 T-Cell Function and Viral-Load Reduction after Highly Active Antiretroviral Therapy in Advanced HIV-1 Disease." *Lancet* 351 (9117): 1682–86.

Liechty, C. A., and D. R. Bangsberg. 2003. "Doubts about DOT: antiretroviral therapy for resource-poor countries." *AIDS* 17 (9): 1383–1387.

Little, S. J., S. Holte, J. P. Routy, E. S. Daar, M. Markowitz, A. C. Collier, and others. 2002. "Antiretroviral-Drug Resistance among Patients Recently Infected with HIV." *New England Journal of Medicine* 347 (6): 385–94.

Low-Beer, D., and R. Stoneburner. 2003. "Behavior and Communication Change in Reducing HIV: Is Uganda Unique?" *African Journal of AIDS Research* 2 (1): 9–21.

Low-Beer, S., A. E. Weber, K. Bartholomew, M. Landolt, D. Oram, J. S. Montaner, and others. 2000. "A Reality Check: The Cost of Making Post-Exposure Prophylaxis Available to Gay and Bisexual Men at High Sexual Risk." *AIDS* 14 (3): 325–26.

Lui, K. J., W. W. Darrow, and G. W. Rutherford III. 1988. "A Model-Based Estimate of the Mean Incubation Period for AIDS in Homosexual Men." *Science* 240 (4857): 1333–35.

Mallal, S. A., M. John, C. B. Moore, I. R. James, and E. J. McKinnon. 2000. "Contribution of Nucleoside Analogue Reverse Transcriptase Inhibitors to Subcutaneous Fat Wasting in Patients with HIV Infection." *AIDS* 14 (10): 1309–16.

Mannheimer, S., G. Friedland, J. Matts, C. Child, and M. Chesney. 2002. "The Consistency of Adherence to Antiretroviral Therapy Predicts Biologic Outcomes for Human Immunodeficiency Virus-Infected Persons in Clinical Trials." *Clinical Infectious Diseases* 34 (8): 1115–21.

Marks, G., S. Burris, and T. A. Peterman. 1999. "Reducing Sexual Transmission of HIV from Those Who Know They Are Infected: The Need for Personal and Collective Responsibility." *AIDS* 13 (3): 297–306.

Marseille, E., P. B. Hofmann, and J. G. Kahn. 2002. "HIV Prevention before HAART in Sub-Saharan Africa." *Lancet* 359 (9320): 1851–56.

Marseille, E., J. G. Kahn, K. Billinghurst, and J. Saba. 2001. "Cost-Effectiveness of the Female Condom in Preventing HIV and STDs in Commercial Sex Workers in Rural South Africa." *Social Science and Medicine* 52 (1): 135–48.

Marseille, E., J. G. Kahn, F. Mmiro, L. Guay, P. Musoke, M. G. Fowler, and others. 1999. "Cost-Effectiveness of Single-Dose Nevirapine Regimen for Mothers and Babies to Decrease Vertical HIV-1 Transmission in Sub-Saharan Africa." *Lancet* 354 (9181): 803–9.

Marseille, E., J. G. Kahn, and J. Saba. 1998. "Cost-Effectiveness of Antiviral Drug Therapy to Reduce Mother-to-Child HIV Transmission in Sub-Saharan Africa." *AIDS* 12 (8): 939–48.

Marseille, E., S. F. Morin, C. Collins, T. Summers, T. J. Coates, and J. G. Kahn. 2002. "Cost-Effectiveness of HIV Prevention in Developing Countries." In *HIV InSite Knowledge Base*. http://hivinsite.ucsf.edu/InSite?page=kb-08-01-04.

Martin, H. L., B. A. Richardson, P. M. Nyange, L. Lavreys, S. L. Hillier, B. Chohan, and others. 1999. "Vaginal Lactobacilli, Microbial Flora, and Risk of Human Immunodeficiency Virus Type 1 and Sexually Transmitted Disease Acquisition." *Journal of Infectious Diseases* 180 (6): 1863–68.

Mast, S. T., J. D. Woolwine, and J. L. Gerberding. 1993. "Efficacy of Gloves in Reducing Blood Volumes Transferred during Simulated Needlestick Injury." *Journal of Infectious Diseases* 168 (6): 1589–92.

Mastro T. D., G. A. Satten, T. Nopkesorn, S. Sangkharomya, and I. M. Longini. 1994. "Probability of Female-to-Male Transmission of HIV-1 in Thailand." *Lancet* 343 (8891): 204–7.

Mathers, C. D., A. Lopez, C. Stein, D. Ma Fat, C. Rao, M. Inoue, and others. 2006. "The Burden of Disease and Mortality by Condition: Data, Methods and Results for the Year 2001." In the *Global Burden of Disease in 2001*, ed. A. Lopez, C. Mathers, M. Ezzati, D. Jamison, and C. J. L. Murray. New York: Oxford University Press.

Mayaud, P., F. Mosha, J. Todd, R. Balira, J. Mgara, B. West, and others. 1997. "Improved Treatment Services Significantly Reduce the Prevalence of Sexually Transmitted Diseases in Rural Tanzania: Results of a Randomized Controlled Trial." *AIDS* 11 (15): 1873–80.

Mbopi Keou, F. X., G. Gresenguet, P. Mayaud, H. A. Weiss, R. Gopal, D. W. Brown, and others. 1999. "Genital Herpes Simplex Virus Type 2 Shedding Is Increased in HIV-Infected Women in Africa." *AIDS* 13: 536–37.

McConnell, J., and R. Grant. 2003. "Sorting out Serosorting Using Social Network Methods. Paper presented at the 10th Conference on Retroviruses and Opportunistic Infections, Boston, February 10–14.

McFarland, W., J. G. Kahn, D. A. Katzenstein, D. Mvere, and R. Shamu. 1995. "Deferral of Blood Donors with Risk Factors for HIV Infection Saves Lives and Money in Zimbabwe." *Journal of Acquired Immune Deficiency Syndrome and Human Retrovirology* 9 (2): 183–192.

McNaghten, A. D., D. L. Hanson, J. L. Jones, M. S. Dworkin, and J. W. Ward. (1999). "Effects of Antiretroviral Therapy and Opportunistic Illness Primary Chemoprophylaxis on Survival after AIDS Diagnosis: Adult/Adolescent Spectrum of Disease Group." *AIDS* 13 (13): 1687–95.

Meekers, D. 2000. "The Effectiveness of Targeted Social Marketing to Promote Adolescent Reproductive Health: The Case of Soweto, South Africa." *Journal of HIV/AIDS Prevention and Education for Adolescents and Children* 3 (4): 73–92.

Mesquita, F., D. Doneda, D. Gandolfi, M. I. Nemes, T. Andrade, R. Bueno, and others. 2003. "Brazilian Response to the Human Immunodeficiency Virus/Acquired Immunodeficiency Syndrome Epidemic among Injection Drug Users." *Clinical Infectious Diseases* 37 (Suppl. 5): S382–85.

Metzger, D. S., H. Navaline, and G. E. Woody. 1998. "Drug Abuse Treatment as AIDS Prevention." *Public Health Reports* 113 (Suppl. 1): 97–106.

Miotti, P. G., T. E. Taha, N. I. Kumwenda, R. Broadhead, L. A. Mtimavalye, L. Van der Hoeven, and others. 1999. "HIV Transmission through Breastfeeding: A Study in Malawi." *Journal of the American Medical Association* 282 (8): 744–49.

Mitty, J. A., V. E. Stone, M. Sands, G. Macalino, and T. Flanigan. 2002. "Directly Observed Therapy for the Treatment of People with Human Immunodeficiency Virus Infection: A Work in Progress." *Clinical Infectious Disease* 34 (7): 984–90.

Morgan, D., G. H. Maude, S. S. Malamba, M. J. Okongo, H. U. Wagner, D. W. Mulder, and others. 1997. "HIV-1 Disease Progression and AIDS-Defining Disorders in Rural Uganda." *Lancet* 350 (9073): 245–50.

Moses, S., F. A. Plummer, E. N. Ngugi, N. J. Nagelkerke, A. O. Anzala, and J. O. Ndinya-Achola. 1991. "Controlling HIV in Africa: Effectiveness and Cost of an Intervention in a High-Frequency STD Transmitter Core Group." *AIDS* 5 (4): 407–11.

Munoz, A., C. A. Sabin, and A. N. Phillips. 1997. "The Incubation Period of AIDS." *AIDS* 11 (Suppl. A): S69–76.

Murphy, D. A., W. D. Marelich, D. Hoffman, and W. N. Steers. 2004. "Predictors of Antiretroviral Adherence." *AIDS Care* 16 (4): 471–84.

Murray, C. J., E. DeJonghe, H. J. Chum, D. S. Nyangulu, A. Salomao, and K. Styblo. 1991. "Cost-Effectiveness of Chemotherapy for Pulmonary Tuberculosis in Three Sub-Saharan African Countries." *Lancet* 338 (8778): 1305–8.

Murray, C. J., and A. D. Lopez. 1996. *The Global Burden of Disease: A Comprehensive Assessment of Mortality and Disability from Diseases, Injuries, and Risk Factors in 1990 and Projected to 2020*. Boston: Harvard University Press.

Musicco, M., A. Lazzarin, A. Nicolosi, M. Gasparini, P. Costigliola, C. Arici, and others. 1994. "Antiretroviral Treatment of Men Infected with Human Immunodeficiency Virus Type 1 Reduces the Incidence of Heterosexual Transmission." Italian Study Group on HIV Heterosexual Transmission. *Archives of Internal Medicine* 154 (17): 1971–76.

Nagachinta, T., A. Duerr, V. Suriyanon, N. Nantachit, S. Rugpao, C. Wanapirak, and others. 1997. "Risk Factors for HIV-1 Transmission from HIV-Seropositive Male Blood Donors to Their Regular Female Partners in Northern Thailand." *AIDS* 11 (14): 1765–72.

National Consensus Development Panel on Effective Medical Treatment of Opiate Addiction. 1998. "Effective Medical Treatment of Opiate Addiction." *Journal of the American Medical Association* 280: 1936–43.

Nduati, R., G. John, D. Mbori-Ngacha, B. Richardson, J. Overbaugh, A. Mwatha, and others. 2000. "Effect of Breastfeeding and Formula Feeding on Transmission of HIV-1: A Randomized Clinical Trial." *Journal of the American Medical Association* 283 (9): 1167–74.

Nduati, R., B. A. Richardson, G. John, D. Mbori-Ngacha, A. Mwatha, J. Ndinya-Achola, and others. 2001. "Effect of Breastfeeding on

Mortality among HIV-1 Infected Women: A Randomised Trial." *Lancet* 357 (9269): 1651–55.

Needle, R. H., S. L. Coyle, J. Normand, E. Lambert, and H. Cesari. 1998. "HIV Prevention with Drug-Using Populations—Current Status and Future Prospects: Introduction and Overview." *Public Health Reports* 113 (Suppl. 1): 4–18.

Newell, M. L. 2003. "Antenatal and Perinatal Strategies to Prevent Mother-to-Child Transmission of HIV Infection." *Transactions of the Royal Society of Tropical Medicine and Hygiene* 97 (1): 22–24.

Ngugi, E. N., F. A. Plummer, J. N. Simonsen, D. W. Cameron, M. Bosire, P. Waiyaki, and others. 1988. "Prevention of Transmission of Human Immunodeficiency Virus in Africa: Effectiveness of Condom Promotion and Health Education among Prostitutes." *Lancet* 2 (8616): 887–90.

Nijhuis, M., S. Deeks, and C. Boucher. 2001. "Implications of Anti-retroviral Resistance on Viral Fitness." *Current Opinions in Infectious Diseases* 14 (1): 23–28.

Norr, K. F., J. L. Norr, B. J. McElmurry, S. Tlou, and M. R. Moeti. 2004. "Impact of Peer Group Education on HIV Prevention among Women in Botswana." *Health Care for Women International* 25 (3): 210–26.

Orroth, K. K., E. L. Korenromp, R. G. White, A. Gavyole, R. H. Gray, and L. Muhangi. 2003. "Higher-Risk Behaviour and Rates of Sexually Transmitted Diseases in Mwanza Compared to Uganda May Help Explain HIV Prevention Trial Outcomes." *AIDS* 17 (18): 2653–60.

Over, M., P. Heywood, J. Gold, I. Gupta, S. K. Hira, and E. Marseille. 2004. *HIV/AIDS Treatment and Prevention in India: Modeling the Cost and Consequences.* Health, Nutrition, and Population Series. Washington, DC: World Bank.

Over, M., and P. Piot. 1996. "Human Immunodeficiency Virus Infection and Other Sexually Transmitted Diseases in Developing Countries: Public Health Importance and Priorities for Resource Allocation." *Journal of Infectious Diseases* 174 (Suppl. 2): S162–75.

Oyugi, J., and D. Bangsberg. 2004 "Treatment outcomes and adherence to generic Triomune® and Maxivir® therapy in Kampala, Uganda." XV International AIDS Conference. Bangkok, Thailand, July 10–16.

Palella, F. J., K. M. Delaney, A. C. Moorman, M. O. Loveless, J. Fuhrer, G. A. Satten, and others. 1998. "Declining Morbidity and Mortality among Patients with Advanced Human Immunodeficiency Virus Infection." HIV Outpatient Study Investigators. *New England Journal of Medicine* 338 (13): 853–60.

Palella, F. J., M. Deloria-Knoll, J. S. Chmiel, A. C. Moorman, K. C. Wood, A. E. Greenberg, and others. 2003. "Survival Benefit of Initiating Antiretroviral Therapy in HIV-Infected Persons in Different CD4+ Cell Strata." *Annals of Internal Medicine* 138 (8): 620–26.

Pape, J. W., S. S. Jean, J. L. Ho, A. Hafner, and W. D. Johnson. 1993. "Effect of Isoniazid Prophylaxis on Incidence of Active Tuberculosis and Progression of HIV Infection." *Lancet* 342 (8866): 268–72.

Pauw, J., J. Ferrie, R. Rivera-Villegas, J. Medrano-Martinez, A. Gorter, and M. Egger. 1996. "A Controlled HIV/AIDS-Related Health Education Programme in Managua, Nicaragua." *AIDS* 10 (5): 537–44.

Peak, A., S. Rana, S. H. Maharjan, D. Jolley, and N. Crofts. 1995. "Declining Risk for HIV among Injecting Drug Users in Kathmandu, Nepal: The Impact of a Harm-Reduction Programme." *AIDS* 9 (9): 1067–70.

Peersman, G., and J. Levy. 1998. "Focus and Effectiveness of HIV-Prevention Efforts for Young People." *AIDS* 12 (Suppl. A): S191–96.

Peipert, L., and Coffey, S. "About the Antiretroviral Drug Profiles." In HIV InSite Knowledge Base, ed. L. Peipert, S. Coffey, P. Volberding. http://hivinsite.ucsf.edu.

Peterman, T. A., R. L. Stoneburner, J. R. Allen, H. W. Jaffe, and J. W. Curran. 1988. "Risk of Human Immunodeficiency Virus Transmission from Heterosexual Adults with Transfusion-Associated Infections." *Journal of the American Medical Association* 259 (1): 55–58.

PETRA Study Team. 2002. "Efficacy of Three Short-Course Regimens of Zidovudine and Lamivudine in Preventing Early and Late Transmission of HIV-1 from Mother to Child in Tanzania, South Africa, and Uganda: A Randomised, Double-Blind, Placebo-Controlled Trial." *Lancet* 359 (9313): 1178–86.

Pinkerton, S. D., D. R. Holtgrave, and F. R. Bloom. 1998. "Cost-Effectiveness of Post-Exposure Prophylaxis Following Sexual Exposure to HIV." *AIDS* 12 (9): 1067–78.

Pinkerton, S. D., D. R. Holtgrave, W. J. DiFranceisco, L. Y. Stevenson, and J. A. Kelly. 1998. "Cost-Effectiveness of a Community-Level HIV Risk Reduction Intervention." *American Journal of Public Health* 88 (8): 1239–42.

Pistone, T., S. Kony, M. A. Faye-Niang, C. T. Ndour, P. M. Gueye, D. Henzel, and others. 2002. "A Simple Clinical and Paraclinical Score Predictive of CD4 Cell Counts below 400/mm3 in HIV-Infected Adults in Dakar University Hospital, Senegal." *Transactions of the Royal Society of Tropical Medicine and Hygiene* 96 (2): 167–72.

Quinn, T. C., M. J. Wawer, N. Sewankambo, D. Serwadda, C. Li, F. Wabwire-Mangen, and others. 2000. "Viral Load and Heterosexual Transmission of Human Immunodeficiency Virus Type 1" Rakai Project Study Group. *New England Journal of Medicine* 342 (13): 921–29.

Ramsay, S. 2003. "Leading the Way in African Home-Based Palliative Care." *Lancet* 362 (9398): 1812–13.

Read, J. S. 2003. "Human Milk, Breastfeeding, and Transmission of Human Immunodeficiency Virus Type 1 in the United States." American Academy of Pediatrics Committee on Pediatric AIDS. *Pediatrics* 112 (5): 1196–205.

Rely, K., S. Bertozzi, C. Avila-Figueroa, and M. T. Guijarro. 2003. "Cost-Effectiveness of Strategies to Reduce Mother-to-Child HIV Transmission in Mexico, a Low-Prevalence Setting." *Health Policy and Planning* 18 (3): 290–98.

Reynolds, H. W., B. Janowitz, R. Homan, and L. Johnson. 2004. "Cost-Effectiveness of Two Interventions to Avert HIV-Positive Births." Poster presentation at the XV International AIDS Conference, Bangkok, Thailand, July 11–16, 2004.

Reynolds, S. J., M. E. Shepherd, A. R. Risbud, R. R. Gangakhedkar, R. S. Brookmeyer, A. D. Divekar, and others. 2004. "Male Circumcision and Risk of HIV-1 and Other Sexually Transmitted Infections in India." *Lancet* 363 (9414): 1039–40.

Royce, R. A., A. Sena, W. Cates, and M. S. Cohen. 1997. "Sexual Transmission of HIV." *New England Journal of Medicine* 336 (15): 1072–78.

Saavedra, J. 2000. "Economy and AIDS in Latin America." In *AIDS in Latin America: A Multidisciplinary Vision,* ed. by J. A. Izazola. Mexico City: FUNSALUD.

Salomon, H., M. A. Wainberg, B. Brenner, Y. Quan, D. Rouleau, P. Cote, and others. 2000. "Prevalence of HIV-1 Resistant to Antiretroviral Drugs in 81 Individuals Newly Infected by Sexual Contact or Injecting Drug Use." Investigators of the Quebec Primary Infection Study. *AIDS* 14 (2): F17–23.

Saunderson, P. R. 1995. "An Economic Evaluation of Alternative Programme Designs for Tuberculosis Control in Rural Uganda." *Social Science and Medicine* 40 (9): 1203–12.

Schneider, M. M., T. L. Nielsen, S. Nelsing, A. I. Hoepelman, J. K. Eeftinck Schattenkerk, Y. van der Graaf, and others. 1995. "Efficacy and Toxicity of Two Doses of Trimethoprim-Sulfamethoxazole as Primary Prophylaxis against *Pneumocystis carinii* Pneumonia in Patients with Human Immunodeficiency Virus: Dutch AIDS Treatment Group." *Journal of Infectious Diseases* 171 (6): 1632–36.

Selik, R. M., E. T. Starcher, and J. W. Curran. 1987. "Opportunistic Diseases Reported in AIDS Patients: Frequencies, Associations, and Trends." *AIDS* 1 (3): 175–82.

Semba, R. D., N. Kumwenda, D. R. Hoover, T. E. Taha, T. C. Quinn, L. Mtimavalye, and others. 1999. "Human Immunodeficiency Virus

Load in Breast Milk, Mastitis, and Mother-to-Child Transmission of Human Immunodeficiency Virus Type 1." *Journal of Infectious Diseases* 180 (1): 93–98.

Sengupta, D., S. Lal, and Srinivas. 1994. "Opportunistic Infection in AIDS." *Journal of the Indian Medical Association* 92 (1): 24–26.

Shaffer, N., R. Chuachoowong, P. A. Mock, C. Bhadrakom, W. Siriwasin, N. L. Young, and others. 1999. "Short-Course Zidovudine for Perinatal HIV-1 Transmission in Bangkok, Thailand: A Randomised Controlled Trial." Bangkok Collaborative Perinatal HIV Transmission Study Group. *Lancet* 353 (9155): 773–80.

Shelburne, S. A., F. Visnegarwala, J. Darcourt, E. A. Graviss, T. P. Giordano, A. C. White Jr., and others. 2005. "Incidence and Risk Factors for Immune Reconstitution Inflammatory Syndrome during Highly Active Antiretroviral Therapy." *AIDS* 19 (4): 399–406.

Sikkema, K. J., J. A. Kelly, R. A. Winett, L. J. Solomon, V. A. Cargill, R. A. Roffman, and others. 2000. "Outcomes of a Randomized Community-Level HIV Prevention Intervention for Women Living in 18 Low-Income Housing Developments." *American Journal of Public Health* 90 (1): 57–63.

Spector, S. A., G. F. McKinley, J. P. Lalezari, T. Samo, R. Andruczk, S. Follansbee, and others. 1996. "Oral Ganciclovir for the Prevention of Cytomegalovirus Disease in Persons with AIDS: Roche Cooperative Oral Ganciclovir Study Group." *New England Journal of Medicine* 334 (23): 1491–97.

Stanton, B. F., X. Li, J. Kahihuata, A. M. Fitzgerald, S. Neumbo, G. Kanduuombe, and others. 1998. "Increased Protected Sex and Abstinence among Namibian Youth Following a HIV Risk-Reduction Intervention: A Randomized, Longitudinal Study." *AIDS* 12 (18): 2473–80.

Stanton, B. F., X. Li, I. Ricardo, J. Galbraith, S. Feigelman, and L. Kaljee. 1996. "A Randomized, Controlled Effectiveness Trial of an AIDS Prevention Program for Low-Income African-American Youths." *Archives of Pediatric Adolescent Medicine* 150 (4): 363–72.

Stolte, I. G., N. H. Dukers, J. B. de Wit, J. S. Fennema, and R. A. Coutinho. 2001. "Increase in Sexually Transmitted Infections among Homosexual Men in Amsterdam in Relation to HAART." *Sexually Transmitted Infections* 77 (3): 184–86.

Stover, J., N. Fuchs, D. Halperin, A. Gibbons, and D. Gillespie. 2003. "Costs and Benefits of Adding Family Planning to Services to Prevent Mother-to-Child Transmission of HIV (PMTCT)." Unpublished paper. The Futures Group.

Stover, J., N. Walker, G. P. Garnett, J. A. Salomon, K. A. Stanecki, P. D. Ghys, and others. 2002. "Can We Reverse the HIV/AIDS Pandemic with an Expanded Response?" *Lancet* 360 (9326): 73–77.

Stringer, E. M., M. Sinkala, J. S. Stringer, E. Mzyece, I. Makuka, R. L. Goldenberg, and others. 2003. "Prevention of Mother-to-Child Transmission of HIV in Africa: Successes and Challenges in Scaling Up a Nevirapine-Based Program in Lusaka, Zambia." *AIDS* 17 (9): 1377–82.

Sweat, M. D., S. Gregorich, G. Sangiwa, C. Furlonge, D. Balmer, C. Kamenga, and others. 2000. "Cost-Effectiveness of Voluntary HIV-1 Counseling and Testing in Reducing Sexual Transmission of HIV-1 in Kenya and Tanzania." *Lancet* 356 (9224): 113–21.

Sweat, M. D., K. R. O'Reilly, G. P. Schmid, J. Denison, and I. de Zoysa. 2004. "Cost-Effectiveness of Nevirapine to Prevent Mother-to-Child HIV Transmission in Eight African Countries." *AIDS* 18 (12): 1661–71.

Tsunekawa, K., S. Moolphate, H. Yanai, N. Yamada, S. Summanapan, and J. Ngamvithayapong. 2004. "Care for People Living with HIV/AIDS: An Assessment of Day Care Centers in Northern Thailand." *AIDS Patient Care and Sexually Transmitted Diseases* 18 (5): 305–14.

UNAIDS (Joint United Nations Programme on HIV/AIDS). 1997. *Blood Safety and AIDS: UNAIDS Point of View*. Geneva: UNAIDS.

———. 2000. *AIDS: Palliative Care*. UNAIDS Technical Update. Geneva: UNAIDS.

———. 2001. *Eight Case Studies of Home and Community Care for and by People with HIV/AIDS*. Geneva: UNAIDS.

———. 2004. *AIDS Epidemic Update: December 2004*. Geneva: UNAIDS.

———. 2005. AIDS Epidemic Update. December 2005. Geneva: UNAIDS.

UNDP (United Nations Development Programme). 2004. *Thailand's Response to HIV/AIDS: Progress and Challenges*. Bangkok: UNDP.

UNICEF (United Nations Children's Fund), UNAIDS (Joint United Nations Programme on HIV/AIDS), WHO (World Health Organization), and Médécins sans Frontières. 2004. *Sources and Prices of Selected Medicines and Diagnostics for People Living with HIV/AIDS*. Geneva: WHO.

USAID (United States Agency for International Development). 2002. *What Happened in Uganda?* Washington, DC: USAID.

Uys, L., and M. Hensher. 2002. "The Cost of Home-Based Terminal Care for People with AIDS in South Africa." *South African Medical Journal* 92 (8): 624–28.

Van Liere, M. 2002. "HIV/AIDS and Food Security in Sub-Saharan Africa." Paper presented at the Seventh Annual Economic Community of West African States Nutrition Forum. Banjul, The Gambia, September 2–6.

Vanek, J., O. Jírovec, and J. Lukes. 1953. "Interstitial Plasma Cell Pneumonia in Infants." *Annals of Paediatrics* 180: 1–21.

Vickerman, P., F. Terris-Prestholt, S. Delany, L. Kumaranayake, H. Rees, and W. Watts. Forthcoming. "Are Targeted HIV Prevention Activities Still Cost-Effective in High Prevalence Settings? Results from an STI Treatment Intervention for Sex Workers in Hillbrow, South Africa." *Sexually Transmitted Diseases*.

Vlahov, D., B. Junge, R. Brookmeyer, S. Cohn, E. Riley, H. Armenian, and others. 1997. "Reductions in High-Risk Drug Use Behaviors among Participants in the Baltimore Needle Exchange Program." *Journal of Acquired Immune Deficiency Syndrome and Human Retrovirology* 16 (5): 400–6.

Vlahov, D., A. Munoz, J. C. Anthony, S. Cohn, D. D. Celentano, and K. E. Nelson. 1990. "Association of Drug Injection Patterns with Antibody to Human Immunodeficiency Virus Type 1 among Intravenous Drug Users in Baltimore, Maryland." *American Journal of Epidemiology* 132 (5): 847–56.

Voluntary HIV-1 Counseling and Testing Efficacy Study Group. 2000. "Efficacy of Voluntary HIV-1 Counseling and Testing in Individuals and Couples in Kenya, Tanzania, and Trinidad: A Randomized Trial." *Lancet* 356: 103–12.

Walker, D. 2003. "Cost and Cost-Effectiveness of HIV/AIDS Prevention Strategies in Developing Countries: Is There an Evidence Base?" *Health Policy and Planning* 18 (1): 4–17.

Watts, C., H. Goodman, and L. Kumaranayake. 2000. "Improving the Efficiency and Impact of Blood Transfusion Services in the Context of Increasing HIV Prevalence." Health Policy Unit, London.

Wawer, M. J., N. K. Sewankambo, D. Serwadda, T. C. Quinn, L. A. Paxton, N. Kiwanuka, and others. 1999. "Control of Sexually Transmitted Diseases for AIDS Prevention in Uganda: A Randomised Community Trial." Rakai Project Study Group. *Lancet* 353 (9152): 525–35.

Wegner, S. A., S. K. Brodine, J. R. Mascola, S. A. Tasker, R. A. Shaffer, M. J. Starkey, and others. 2000. "Prevalence of Genotypic and Phenotypic Resistance to Anti-Retroviral Drugs in a Cohort of Therapy-Naive HIV-1 Infected U.S. Military Personnel." *AIDS* 14 (8): 1009–15.

Weiss, H. A., M. A. Quigley, and R. J. Hayes. 2000. "Male Circumcision and Risk of HIV Infection in Sub-Saharan Africa: A Systematic Review and Meta-Analysis." *AIDS* 14 (15): 2361–70.

Wenk, R., M. Bertolino, and J. Pussetto. 2000. "Direct Medical Costs of an Argentinean Domiciliary Palliative Care Model." *Journal of Pain and Symptom Management* 20 (3): 162–65.

WHO (World Health Organization). 2002a. "Blood Safety: Aide-Memoire for National Blood Programmes." WHO, Geneva.

———. 2002b. "Definition of Palliative Care." WHO, Geneva.

———. 2004. "Scaling Up Antiretroviral Therapy in Resource-Limited Settings: Treatment Guidelines for a Public Health Approach." WHO, Geneva.

WHO (World Health Organization) and UNAIDS (Joint United Nations Programme on HIV/AIDS). 2003. "Expert Group Stresses That Unsafe Sex Is Primary Mode of HIV Transmission in Africa." Press release, Geneva, March 14.

Wiktor, S. Z., E. Ekpini, J. M. Karon, J. Nkengasong, C. Maurice, S. T. Severin, and others. 1999. "Short-Course Oral Zidovudine for Prevention of Mother-to-Child Transmission of HIV-1 in Abidjan, Côte d'Ivoire: A Randomised Trial." *Lancet* 353 (9155): 781–85.

Wiley, J. A., S. J. Herschkorn, and N. S. Padian. 1989. "Heterogeneity in the Probability of HIV Transmission per Sexual Contact: The Case of Male-to-Female Transmission in Penile-Vaginal Intercourse." *Statistics in Medicine* 8 (1): 93–102.

Wilkinson, D., K. Floyd, and C. F. Gilks. 1998. "Antiretroviral Drugs as a Public Health Intervention for Pregnant HIV-Infected Women in Rural South Africa: An Issue of Cost-Effectiveness and Capacity." *AIDS* 12 (13): 1675–82.

Willbond, B., P. Thottingal, J. Kimani, L. M. E. Vaz, and F. A. Plummer. 2001. "The Evidence Base for Interventions in the Care and Management of AIDS in Low and Middle Income Countries." Commission on Macroeconomics and Health Working Paper Series, Paper WG5: 29. Commission on Macroeconomics and Health, Geneva.

World Bank. 1997. *Confronting AIDS: Public Priorities in a Global Epidemic.* New York: Oxford University Press.

———. 1999. "Project Appraisal Document on a Proposed Credit in the Amount of SDR 140.82 Million to India for Second National HIV/AIDS Control Project." World Bank, Washington, DC.

World Food Programme. 2001. *Food Security and HIV/AIDS: WFP Executive Board Third Regular Session.* Rome: WFP.

WTO (World Trade Organization). 2003. "Decision Removes Final Patent Obstacle to Cheap Drug Imports." Press release, August 30.

Yeni, P. G., S. M. Hammer, M. S. Hirsch, M. S. Saag, M. Schechter, C. C. Carpenter, and others. 2004. "Treatment for Adult HIV Infection: 2004 Recommendations of the International AIDS Society–USA Panel." *Journal of the American Medical Association* 292 (2): 251–65.

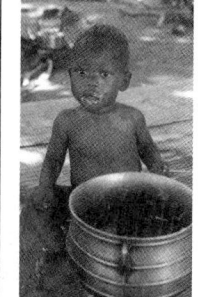

Chapter **19**

Diarrheal Diseases

Gerald T. Keusch, Olivier Fontaine, Alok Bhargava, Cynthia Boschi-Pinto, Zulfiqar A. Bhutta, Eduardo Gotuzzo, Juan Rivera, Jeffrey Chow, Sonbol A. Shahid-Salles, and Ramanan Laxminarayan

Diarrheal diseases remain a leading cause of preventable death, especially among children under five in developing countries. This chapter reviews and prioritizes a number of available interventions.

The normal intestinal tract regulates the absorption and secretion of electrolytes and water to meet the body's physiological needs. More than 98 percent of the 10 liters per day of fluid entering the adult intestines are reabsorbed (Keusch 2001). The remaining stool water, related primarily to the indigestible fiber content, determines the consistency of normal feces from dry, hard pellets to mushy, bulky stools, varying from person to person, day to day, and stool to stool. This variation complicates the definition of *diarrhea,* which by convention is present when three or more stools are passed in 24 hours that are sufficiently liquid to take the shape of the container in which they are placed. The frequent passage of formed stool is not diarrhea (Black and Lanata 2002). Although young nursing infants tend to have five or more motions per day, mothers know when the stooling pattern changes and their children have diarrhea (Ronsmans, Bennish, and Wierzba 1988). The interval between two episodes is also arbitrarily defined as at least 48 hours of normal stools. These definitions enable epidemiologists to count incidence, relapses, and new infections.

TRANSMISSION

Diarrhea is caused by infectious organisms, including viruses, bacteria, protozoa, and helminths, that are transmitted from the stool of one individual to the mouth of another, termed *fecal-oral transmission.* Some are well known, others are recently discovered or emerging new agents, and presumably many remain to be identified. They differ in the route from the stool to the mouth and in the number of organisms needed to cause infection and illness. Among bacteria, the ability to survive stomach acid is an important determinant of the inoculum size required to cause illness. For example, *Shigella* bacteria are resistant to low pH, and a few thousand organisms suffice, which are readily transferred by direct person-to-person contact or through contamination of inanimate objects, such as a cup. In contrast, bacteria readily killed by acid, such as *Vibrio cholerae,* require millions of organisms to cause illness, and therefore must first multiply in food or water to an infectious dose. Some pathogens, such as rotavirus, display a sharp host species preference, and others have a broad host range. Among *Salmonella* bacteria, certain bio-serotypes are adapted to infect animals and pose no threat to humans, and others are adapted to humans and do not infect animals. The majority, however, are not adapted to a specific host and can infect either humans or domestic animals, thus facilitating transmission of these organisms to humans. Less than a dozen of the more than 2,500 individual *Salmonella* cause the majority of human infections, reflecting the requirement for genes that encode essential virulence factors.

The ability to identify virulence genes and their products has led to new molecular approaches to epidemiology and diagnosis, and undoubtedly will lead to new measures to prevent and treat diarrhea. Molecular methods also allow the separation of organisms that otherwise appear to be identical. Nonpathogenic *Escherichia coli* in normal stool cannot be separated from diarrhea-causing *E. coli* by standard methods; however, identification of virulence genes or factors distinguishes five groups of *E. coli* that cause illnesses ranging from cholera-like watery diarrhea to neonatal diarrhea, persistent diarrhea, and bloody diarrhea (Nataro and Kaper 1998).

LABORATORY DIAGNOSIS

Etiologic diagnosis of diarrhea is valuable for public health interventions and case management. Microbiological culture and microscopy remain the standard, despite their limited sensitivity. Their effectiveness is further reduced by antibiotic use, and patients with severe illness are more likely both to be cultured and to have taken antibiotics. Even when cultures are positive, the delay in laboratory identification limits their cost-effectiveness for managing individual patients. The information is always epidemiologically and clinically important; however, during epidemics, culturing every patient is unnecessary when the causative organism is known. Antimicrobial resistance data are essential to guide initial antibiotic choices.

New rapid tests to detect inflammatory mediators or white or red blood cells in stool offer the promise of distinguishing between secretory and inflammatory disease and optimizing case management (Huicho and others 1996). High background levels, probably from frequent infections, limits the use of such tests in developing countries, where they would be most useful (Gill and others 2003).

Simple microscopy for protozoa or helminths can be quick and effective when the proper sample is obtained and a well-trained technician is available to examine a fresh specimen, but these prerequisites are often not available in developing countries. Newer immunological and nucleic acid–based tests to detect pathogen-specific factors hold great promise for all diarrhea agents, but they are too expensive or require specialized instrumentation and trained technicians. For the foreseeable future, then, syndromic diagnosis will be the norm.

SYNDROMIC DIAGNOSIS

Three major diarrhea syndromes exist. They are acute watery diarrhea, which results in varying degrees of dehydration; persistent diarrhea, which lasts 14 days or longer, manifested by malabsorption, nutrient losses, and wasting; and bloody diarrhea, which is a sign of the intestinal damage caused by inflammation. The three are physiologically different and require specific management. Syndromic diagnosis provides important clues to optimal management and is both programmatically and epidemiologically relevant.

Acute watery diarrhea can be rapidly dehydrating, with stool losses of 250 milliliters per kilogram per day or more, a quantity that quickly exceeds total plasma and interstitial fluid volumes and is incompatible with life unless fluid therapy can keep up with losses. Such dramatic dehydration is usually due to rotavirus, enterotoxigenic *E. coli*, or *V. cholerae* (the cause of cholera), and it is most dangerous in the very young.

Persistent diarrhea is typically associated with malnutrition, either preceding or resulting from the illness itself (Ochoa, Salazar-Lindo, and Cleary 2004). Even though persistent diarrhea accounts for a small percentage of the total number of diarrhea episodes, it is associated with a disproportionately increased risk of death. In India, persistent diarrhea accounted for 5 percent of episodes but 14 percent of deaths, and a mortality rate three times higher than briefer episodes (Bhan and others 1989). In Pakistan, persistent diarrhea accounted for 8 to 18 percent of episodes but 54 percent of deaths (Khan and others 1993). In Bangladesh, persistent diarrhea associated with malnutrition was responsible for nearly half of diarrhea deaths, and the relative risk for death among infants with persistent diarrhea and severe malnutrition was 17 times greater than for those with mild malnutrition (Fauveau and others 1992). Persistent diarrhea occurs more often during an episode of bloody diarrhea than an episode of watery diarrhea, and the mortality rate when bloody diarrhea progresses to persistent diarrhea is 10 times greater than for bloody diarrhea without persistent diarrhea. HIV infection is another risk factor for persistent diarrhea in both adults and children (Keusch and others 1992). Management focuses on overcoming the nutritional alterations initiated by persistent diarrhea.

Bloody diarrhea, defined as diarrhea with visible or microscopic blood in the stool, is associated with intestinal damage and nutritional deterioration, often with secondary sepsis. Some dehydration—rarely severe—is common, as is fever. Clinicians often use the term *bloody diarrhea* interchangeably with dysentery; however, dysentery is a syndrome consisting of the frequent passage of characteristic, small-volume, bloody mucoid stools; abdominal cramps; and tenesmus, a severe pain that accompanies straining to pass stool. Those features show the severity of the inflammation. Agents that cause bloody diarrhea or dysentery can also provoke a form of diarrhea that clinically is not bloody diarrhea, although mucosal damage and inflammation are present, and fecal blood and white blood cells are usually detectable by microscopy. The release of host-derived cytokines causes fever, altering host metabolism and leading to the breakdown of body stores of protein, carbohydrate, and fat and the loss of nitrogen and other nutrients. Those losses must be replenished during convalescence, which takes much longer than the illness does to develop. For these reasons, bloody diarrhea calls for management strategies that are markedly different than those for watery or persistent diarrhea. New bouts of infection that occur before complete restoration of nutrient stores can initiate a downward spiral of nutritional status terminating in fatal protein-energy malnutrition (Keusch 2003).

DIARRHEA, ENVIRONMENT, AND POVERTY

Diarrheal disease affects rich and poor, old and young, and those in developed and developing countries alike, yet a strong relationship exists between poverty, an unhygienic environment, and the number and severity of diarrheal episodes—especially for children under five.

Poverty is associated with poor housing, crowding, dirt floors, lack of access to sufficient clean water or to sanitary disposal of fecal waste, cohabitation with domestic animals that may carry human pathogens, and a lack of refrigerated storage for food—all of which increase the frequency of diarrhea. Poverty also restricts the ability to provide age-appropriate, nutritionally balanced diets or to modify diets when diarrhea develops so as to mitigate and repair nutrient losses. The impact is exacerbated by the lack of adequate, available, and affordable medical care. Thus, the young suffer from an apparently never-ending sequence of infections, rarely receive appropriate preventive care, and too often encounter the health care system when they are already severely ill.

Although the presence of blood in the stool is a recognized danger signal, prompting more urgent care seeking, even these patients either are not treated early or receive poor medical care. Ironically, the poor spend considerable amounts on inappropriate care and useless drugs purchased from local shops and untrained practitioners. If antibiotics are properly prescribed, poverty often limits the purchase of a full course of treatment or leads to cessation of treatment as soon as symptoms improve, even though the infection has not been cured.

PUBLIC HEALTH SIGNIFICANCE OF DIARRHEAL ILLNESSES

Continuing surveillance and longitudinal studies allow tracking of current levels and trends in diarrhea incidence and mortality and provide the basis for future projections and for evaluations of different control strategies.

Morbidity

Comparisons over time of the global burden of diarrheal diseases have revealed secular trends and demonstrated the impact of public health interventions (Bern and others 1992; Kosek, Bern, and Guerrant 2003; Snyder and Merson 1982). The long-term consequences of diarrhea are only now being systematically assessed and are not reflected in earlier studies.

Reviews in 1992 (Bern and others) and 2003 (Kosek, Bern, and Guerrant) are similar in many ways—for example, assessing morbidity at least twice weekly—but differ significantly in the use of different sources for data on children under five and in the inclusion of studies differing in design and data

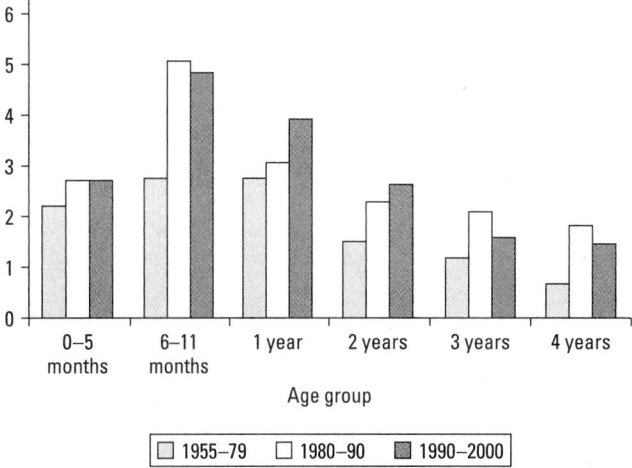

Number of episodes per person per year

Figure 19.1 Median Age-Specific Incidences for Diarrheal Episodes per Child per Year from Three Reviews of Prospective Studies in Developing Areas, 1955–2000

Source: Authors.

collection protocols (and only the later study includes data from China). Remarkably, the estimated median incidence of diarrheal disease in children under five in developing countries has not changed much since the early 1990s (figure 19.1): 3.2 episodes per child per year in 2003 (Parashar and others 2003) compared with 3.5 episodes per child per year in 1993 (Jamison and others 1993). However, many fewer surveys were available for the most recent review (31 in 20 countries) compared with the 1993 consensus (276 in 60 countries), reflecting diminished support for the systematic collection of incidence data. Incidence rates in Sub-Saharan Africa and Latin America are clearly greater than in Asia or the Western Pacific, while subject to greater data limitations from individual countries. Incidence continues to show a peak in infants age 6 to 11 months, dropping steadily thereafter.

The seemingly lower estimates of diarrheal incidence before 1980 (Snyder and Merson 1982) are likely due to methodological differences. These estimates are not precise or directly comparable; the trends are most relevant. The persistently high rates of diarrhea throughout the 1990s despite intensive efforts at control, particularly among children age 6 to 24 months, is of particular concern. Early childhood diarrhea during periods of critical postnatal development may have long-term effects on linear growth and on physical and cognitive functions.

Data on the incidence of shigellosis, the principal cause of bloody diarrhea in developing countries, are even more limited. Kotloff and others' (1999) review of studies on *Shigella* infection estimates that more than 113 million episodes occur every year in children under five in developing countries, or 0.2 episodes of bloody diarrhea per year caused by *Shigella* species.

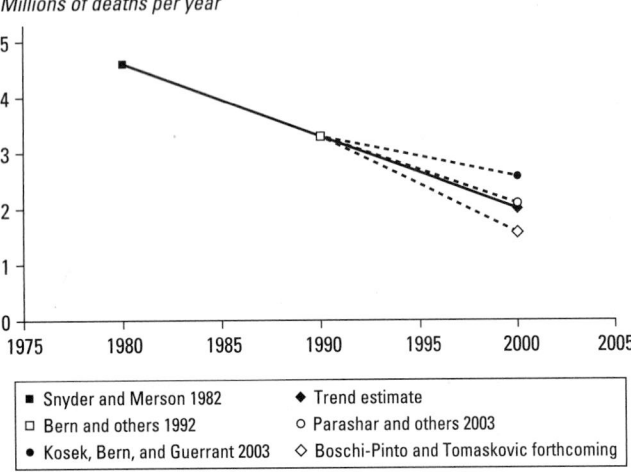

Source: Authors.

Figure 19.2 Estimates of Diarrhea Mortality, 1975–2000

Mortality

Bern and others (1992); Kosek, Bern, and Guerrant (2003); and Snyder and Merson (1982) also estimate diarrheal mortality using data from longitudinal studies with active surveillance in place (figure 19.2). The estimate before 1980 was 4.6 million deaths per year. This estimate dropped to 3.3 million per year between 1980 and 1990 and to 2.6 million per year between 1990 and 2000. Two other studies (Parashar and others 2003; Boschi-Pinto and Tomaskovic forthcoming) report even lower figures for 1990–2000: 2.1 million and 1.6 million deaths per year, respectively. Methodological variations (inclusion of studies with different designs and data collection methods and inclusion of data from China, different sources for estimating the number of children under five, and different strategies for calculating mortality for this age group) may account for some of the striking differences. However, the end of the 20th century witnessed significant reductions in diarrheal deaths in children under five.

This steady decline in diarrheal mortality, despite the lack of significant changes in incidence, is most likely due to modern case management (introduced since the 1980s) and to the improved nutrition of infants and children. Major recommendations include the following:

- counseling mothers to begin suitable home-prepared rehydration fluids immediately on the onset of diarrhea
- treating mild to moderate dehydration early with oral rehydration solution (ORS), reserving intravenous electrolytes for severe dehydration
- continuing breastfeeding and complementary foods during diarrhea and increasing intake afterward
- limiting antibiotic use to cases of bloody diarrhea or dysentery and avoiding antidiarrheal and antimotility drugs

- advising mothers to increase fluids and continue feeding during future episodes.

Victora and others' (2000) review provides evidence that this strategy, and especially oral rehydration therapy (ORT), has influenced the outcome of dehydrating diarrhea. Data from 99 national surveys carried out in the mid 1990s and compiled by the United Nations Children's Fund (UNICEF) increasingly show that diarrhea patients are appropriately managed in most parts of the world, with overall use rates of ORS or recommended home fluids reaching 49 percent. Country case studies in Brazil, the Arab Republic of Egypt, Mexico, and the Philippines showed a dramatic reduction of diarrhea mortality as ORT use rates increased from close to zero in the early 1980s to 35 percent in Brazil, 50 percent in Egypt, 81 percent in Mexico, and 33 percent in the Philippines in the early 1990s. Hospital admissions for diarrhea also plummeted (Victora and others 2000). As mortality attributable to acute dehydration decreased, the proportionate mortality associated with persistent diarrhea increased. Data from Brazil and Egypt suggest that even relatively low ORT use rates can positively affect mortality, because ORT use tends to be much higher for severe illness (Victora and others 2000).

Worldwide mortality caused by *Shigella* infection is estimated to be 600,000 deaths per year among children under five, or a quarter to a third of all diarrhea-related mortality in this age group (Kotloff and others 1999). Because mortality caused by bloody diarrhea is not tracked separately, it is difficult to assess the impact of standard case management recommendations, and disease-specific trends cannot be tracked. In the past few years, however, data from the International Centre for Diarrheal Disease Research, in Bangladesh, have shown a marked decrease in the rate of hospitalization caused by *Shigella*, especially *S. dysenteriae* type 1, the most severe form of shigellosis. Some investigators have suggested that this decrease may be because *Shigella* infections are now in the low part of a 10-year cycle (Legros 2004). The observed change could also be explained by better case management with more efficacious antimicrobials. More comprehensive, syndrome-specific surveillance data will be required if rational control priorities are to be set, because the options for dehydrating and bloody diarrheal diseases differ substantially.

Despite national data that indicate a significant decline in mortality (Baltazar, Nadera, and Victora 2002; Miller and Hirschhorn 1995), diarrheal diseases remain among the five top preventable killers of children under five in developing countries and among the top two in many.

Long-Term Consequences

The long-term consequences of diarrheal diseases remain poorly studied, and analyses of global trends have not considered them. Niehaus and others (2002) recently evaluated the long-term consequences of acute diarrheal disease on psychomotor and cognitive development in young children. Following a cohort of 47 children in a poor urban community in northeastern Brazil, they correlated the number of diarrheal episodes in the first two years of life with measures of cognitive function obtained four to seven years later. They found a significant inverse correlation (average decrease of 5.6 percent) between episodes of early diarrheal disease and overall intellectual capacity and concentration, even when controlling for maternal education or helminth infection, which are known to be independent predictors of malnutrition and cognitive defects. Test scores were also 25 to 65 percent lower in children with an earlier history of persistent diarrhea.

Recent evidence suggests that genetic factors may also be involved in the developmental response to repeated diarrhea (Oria and others 2005). Better and more sensitive assessment tools are needed to define the relationships between diarrheal diseases and developmental disorders and to calculate individual and societal costs and the cost-effectiveness of interventions. In addition, early childhood malnutrition resulting from any cause reduces physical fitness and work productivity in adults (Dobbing 1990).

PREVENTIVE STRATEGIES

Strategies for controlling diarrheal diseases have remained substantially unchanged since the 1993 edition of this volume (Martinez, Phillips, and Feachem 1993). The World Health Organization (WHO 2004) recently reevaluated these interventions to determine the extent to which they have been effectively implemented and their effect.

Promotion of Exclusive Breastfeeding

Exclusive breastfeeding means no other food or drink, not even water, is permitted, except for supplements of vitamins and minerals or necessary medicines. The optimal duration of exclusive breastfeeding is six months (WHO 2001). A meta-analysis of three observational studies in developing countries shows that breastfed children under age 6 months are 6.1 times less likely to die of diarrhea than infants who are not breastfed (WHO Collaborative Study Team 2000). Exclusive breastfeeding protects very young infants from diarrheal disease in two ways: first, breast milk contains both immune (specific) and nonimmune (nonspecific) antimicrobial factors; second, exclusive breastfeeding eliminates the intake of potentially contaminated food and water. Breast milk also provides all the nutrients most infants need up to age 6 months. When exclusive breastfeeding is continued during diarrhea, it also diminishes the adverse impact on nutritional status.

Those data underpin the global campaign to promote exclusive breastfeeding for the first six months of life by increasing both the initiation and the duration of exclusive breastfeeding. The strategies include the following:

- hospital policies and actions to encourage breastfeeding and discourage bottle feeding
- counseling and education provided by peers or health workers
- mass media and community education
- mothers' support groups.

Interventions focused on hospital practices apply where most women deliver in such facilities. Such interventions have shown up to a 43 percent increase in exclusive breastfeeding with good institutional policies and retraining of health staff (Westphal and others 1995). Interventions focused on education and counseling increase exclusive breastfeeding by 4 to 64 percent (Sikorski and others 2002). Peer-counseled women are less likely to stop exclusive breastfeeding than are those who receive either professional support or no support, and their infants are 1.9 to 2.9 times less likely to have diarrhea (Barros and others 1995; Haider and others 1996). No large-scale peer counseling programs exist; therefore, feasibility is unknown. Community-based mother's support groups are sustainable, but they have low coverage and are biased toward women who are already motivated to breastfeed (Bhandari and others 2003). Mass media can be effective where media coverage is high, where production skills are good, and where it addresses barriers to breastfeeding instead of just proclaiming its benefits. We found no studies that examined the relationship between breastfeeding promotion and diarrheal disease mortality; however, estimates suggest such promotion could decrease all-cause mortality in children under five by 13 percent (Jones and others 2003).

Maternal HIV infection has put a new wrinkle in the "breast is best" dogma because of the risk of transmission of infection to the infant (De Cock and others 2000). There is a trade-off, however, between the risk of mortality associated with replacement feeding and the risk of HIV infection, especially where safe replacement feeding is difficult. For women who are HIV-negative or whose status is unknown, WHO currently recommends exclusive breastfeeding for at least six months (WHO 2000). The best option for HIV-positive women is acceptable, affordable, sustainable, and safe replacement feeding. If this option is not possible, there are four alternatives: (a) heat-treated breast milk, (b) HIV-negative wet nurses, (c) uncontaminated donor milk, or (d) exclusive breastfeeding for six months and rapid discontinuation thereafter (WHO 2003).

A danger of promoting replacement feeding is that uninfected women or women with unknown HIV status will adopt the practice. Even in high-prevalence communities, the best option for women with unknown status for the overall health of their children appears to be exclusive breastfeeding for six months. In Coutsoudis and others' (1999) cohort study in South Africa, the risk of mother-to-infant transmission of HIV after three months of exclusive breastfeeding was similar to that with no breastfeeding and significantly lower than that with mixed feeding. Providing antiretroviral therapy to the mother should significantly extend the period of safe breastfeeding for the initially HIV-negative infants of HIV-positive mothers.

Improved Complementary Feeding Practices

Ideally, complementary foods should be introduced at age 6 months, and breastfeeding should continue for up to two years or even longer to increase birth intervals (WHO 2003). There is a strong inverse association between appropriate, safe complementary feeding and mortality in children age 6 to 11 months. Malnutrition is an independent risk predictor for the frequency and severity of diarrheal illness. There is a vicious cycle in which sequential diarrheal disease leads to increasing nutritional deterioration, impaired immune function, and greater susceptibility to infection. The cycle may be broken by interventions to decrease infection incidence to reduce malnutrition (Keusch and Scrimshaw 1986) or improving nutritional status to reduce the burden of infection (Victora and others 1999).

Improved feeding practices to prevent or treat malnutrition could save as many as 800,000 lives per year (Jones and others 2003). Pediatricians have long been aware of an increase in diarrhea incidence during weaning from exclusive breast milk feeding. Microbial contamination of complementary foods (Mondal and others 1996) and nutritionally inadequate diets during and after diarrhea episodes (Badruddin and others 1991) increase the risk. Contamination of complementary foods can potentially be reduced by educating caregivers on hygienic practices (Guptill and others 1993), improving home food storage (English and others 1997), fermenting foods to reduce pathogen multiplication (Kimmons and others 1999), or ingesting nonpathogenic probiotic microorganisms that colonize the gut and help resist pathogens (Allen and others 2004). These interventions have not been evaluated at scale in communities, and effectiveness trials are lacking.

We could not find any reports on the effects of complementary feeding interventions on mortality. Five efficacy trials to improve the intake of complementary foods noted a net increase in energy intake of between 65 and 300 kilocalories a day and improvements of 0.25 to 0.46 standard deviations in weight-for-age and 0.04 to 0.35 standard deviations in height-for-age (Caulfield, Huffman, and Piwoz 1999). By extrapolation, this increment in growth should translate into a 2 to 13 percent reduction in deaths associated with malnutrition (Black and others 1995).

Brown, Dewey, and Allen (1998) reviewed experiences with large-scale complementary feeding interventions in 14 countries. They demonstrate that it is possible to provide nutritionally improved complementary foods in diverse cultural settings and that poor mothers are willing to prepare new foods their children will eat. However, caregivers face considerable time and resource constraints in providing such foods, especially during episodes of illness. A pilot study in Brazil that implemented nutritional counseling through the Integrated Management of Childhood Illness Program reported significant weight gain in children age one year or more, but not in younger children (Santos and others 2001).

Unfortified complementary foods do not meet all essential micronutrient requirements. Although improvements in vitamin A status do not significantly reduce the incidence of diarrhea and other common childhood illnesses, vitamin A supplementation can reduce the frequency of severe diarrhea (Barreto and others 1994) and mortality (Ross and others 1995). Chapter 28 describes interventions to promote vitamin A intake. Zinc supplementation also reduces the incidence of diarrhea.

Rotavirus Immunization

Almost all infants acquire rotavirus diarrhea early in life, and rotavirus accounts for at least one-third of severe and potentially fatal watery diarrhea episodes—primarily in developing countries, where an estimated 440,000 vaccine-preventable rotavirus deaths per year occur (Parashar and others 2003), compared with about a dozen in a developed country such as France (Fourquet and others 2003). An effective rotavirus vaccine would have a major effect on diarrhea mortality in developing countries.

In 1998, a quadrivalent Rhesus rotavirus–derived vaccine that reduced the frequency of severely dehydrating rotavirus—but not the overall incidence of rotavirus infections—was licensed in the United States (Glass and others 1999). It was cost-effective, even at US$100 for a full course of immunization, when direct economic losses resulting from health care expenses and indirect costs of lost productivity and wages for the caretakers were considered (Tucker and others 1998). The strategy was clear: use the high-priced vaccine routinely in industrial countries to subsidize its use in developing countries. However, postmarketing surveillance detected an apparent increase in a relatively rare event, intussusception, a condition in which the intestine telescopes on itself, causing a potentially serious obstruction (CDC 1999a). The relationship was strongest with the first dose of vaccine given with the first or second dose of diphtheria-pertussis-tetanus vaccine (Peter and others 2002), although this was counterbalanced by a decrease in the incidence of intussusception in older children (Murphy and others 2003).

The overall reduced incidence in immunized infants compared with nonimmunized infants in these studies suggested that the vaccine may actually protect against later adverse events. Nonetheless, the ensuing controversy led to a reversal of the recommendation for universal immunization in the United States and withdrawal of the vaccine from the market, precluding the possibility of its deployment in developing countries (CDC 1999b). Because very young infants are less prone to develop intussusception, initial immunization at birth might have been entirely safe.

Despite this setback, efforts to produce an effective and safe rotavirus vaccine continue. The Rhesus vaccine has been relicensed to another manufacturer, and new vaccines derived from human or bovine rotavirus are undergoing field trials in developing countries (Dennehy 2005). A monovalent human rotavirus vaccine was introduced in Mexico in 2005. The entry of both China and India into rotavirus vaccine development and their potential for manufacturing quality vaccines at low cost will make it easier to deploy an effective vaccine where it is really needed.

Cholera Immunization

Endemic cholera is primarily a pediatric disease, although adult morbidity and mortality are significant, especially during epidemics. The lethality of cholera is due to the physiological consequences of rapid and profound dehydration. Oral rehydration therapy has dramatically improved survival and reduced the cost of treatment. Wherever parenteral and oral rehydration is readily available, even in epidemic situations, a cholera mortality rate above 1 percent indicates failure of the public health system to provide appropriate case management.

A vaccine would further reduce the morbidity and mortality associated with cholera in endemic areas; however, developing an effective, safe vaccine has proven difficult. The most immunogenic and protective vaccines tested thus far are administered orally. Two such vaccines have been licensed: an attenuated live vaccine and a heat-killed vaccine combined with recombinant cholera toxin B subunit, which functions as an immunoadjuvant (Graves and others 2000; Ryan and Calderwood 2000). Many developing countries can produce the killed vaccine, especially without cholera toxin B. Current oral cholera vaccines appear to be safe and offer reasonable protection for a limited period; however, the main users have been individual travelers from industrial countries who may be exposed to the risk of cholera while traveling in endemic areas.

The use of oral cholera vaccine in mass vaccination campaigns as an adjunct to good case management, disposal of fecal waste, and access to safe water during humanitarian disasters has recently been reviewed (WHO 1999). Analysis of an outbreak in Micronesia suggested that a single dose was useful in limiting the spread of cholera (Calain and others 2004). But because ORT is so inexpensive and useful in preventing death, immunization is not a high priority. Only Vietnam routinely deploys cholera vaccine.

Operational information on the costs, logistics, and availability of vaccines for use by global programs and on the vulnerable populations in high-risk settings who would benefit from cholera vaccine remains limited. Although scientific interest in a cholera vaccine remains high, its public health priority is less than that of a vaccine for rotavirus or *Shigella*.

Measles Immunization

Measles is known to predispose to diarrheal disease secondary to measles-induced immunodeficiency. Feachem and Koblinsky (1983) estimate that measles vaccine given to 45 to 90 percent of infants would prevent 44 to 64 percent of measles cases, 0.6 to 3.8 percent of diarrheal episodes, and 6 to 26 percent of diarrheal deaths among children under five. Global measles immunization coverage is now approaching 80 percent, and the disease has been eliminated from the Americas, raising hopes for global elimination in the near future (GAVI 2005), with a predictable reduction in diarrhea as well.

Improved Water and Sanitary Facilities and Promotion of Personal and Domestic Hygiene

Human feces are the primary source of diarrheal pathogens. Poor sanitation, lack of access to clean water, and inadequate personal hygiene are responsible for an estimated 90 percent of childhood diarrhea (WHO 1997). Promotion of hand washing reduces diarrhea incidence by an average of 33 percent (Huttly, Morris, and Pisani 1997); it works best when it is part of a package of behavior change interventions. Effects on mortality have not been demonstrated. However, the required behavior change is complex, and significant resources are needed. Antiseptic soaps are more costly than plain hand soap and confer little advantage. Washing hands after defecating or handling children's feces and before handling food is recommended, but it entails an average of 32 hand washes a day and consumes 20 liters of water (Graef, Elder, and Booth 1993). If soap is too costly, ash or mud can be used, but access to water remains essential (Esrey 1996).

Six rigorous observational studies demonstrated a median reduction of 55 percent in all-cause child mortality associated with improved access to sanitation facilities (Esrey, Feachem, and Hughes 1985). The greatest effect of improving sanitation systems will be in areas of high population density and wherever the entire community, rather than single households, adopts the intervention. Current technology can be costly and difficult to maintain, and in some settings it is simply not feasible.

CASE MANAGEMENT

Two recent advances in managing diarrheal disease—(a) newly formulated ORS containing lower concentrations of glucose and salts and (b) zinc supplementation—used in combination with promotion of exclusive breastfeeding, general nutritional support, and selective and appropriate use of antibiotics, can further reduce the number of diarrheal deaths among children. Families and communities are key to achieving case management goals by making these recommendations routine practice in homes and health facilities.

New Oral Rehydration Solutions

For more than 25 years, UNICEF and WHO have recommended a single formulation of glucose-based ORS considered optimal for cholera, irrespective of cause or age group affected. This formulation has proven effective and without significant adverse effects (Ruxin 1994), but because watery stools persist and duration of diarrhea is not reduced, mothers' and health workers' acceptance of current ORSs has been suboptimal.

During the past 20 years, efforts to improve ORS to treat dehydration from all types of diarrhea and reduce stool output or duration have continued—for example, by reducing the sodium content in line with sodium losses for noncholera diarrhea. Compared with standard ORS, lower sodium and glucose ORS reduces stool output, vomiting, and the need for intravenous fluids (Hanh, Kim, and Garner 2001). If household use increases, new ORS can reduce childhood deaths from noncholera diarrhea (Duggan and others 2004), and it appears to be as effective as standard ORS for children or adults with cholera. A WHO expert group now recommends that ORS containing 75 milliequivalents of sodium and 75 millimoles of glucose per liter (total osmolarity, 245 milliosmoles per liter) be used everywhere (WHO and UNICEF 2004).

Zinc Supplementation

A review of all relevant clinical trials indicates that zinc supplements given during an episode of acute diarrhea reduce both duration and severity and could prevent 300,000 deaths in children each year (Black 2003). WHO and UNICEF now recommend that all children with acute diarrhea be given zinc in some form for 10 to 14 days during and after diarrhea (10 milligrams per day for infants younger than 6 months and 20 milligrams per day for those older than 6 months) (WHO and UNICEF 2004).

Pilot studies in Brazil, Egypt, Ethiopia, India, Mali, Pakistan, and the Philippines that include zinc routinely in the management of acute diarrhea not only show an improvement over ORS alone but also suggest two important new effects: (a) use rates of ORS increase, and (b) use rates of antidiarrheals and

antimicrobials decrease significantly (Baqui and others 2004). Large community-based studies are being implemented to corroborate these potentially important findings.

Management of Bloody Diarrhea

The primary treatment for shigellosis, the most common and severe cause of bloody diarrhea, is antimicrobials. The choice of effective, safe, and inexpensive oral drugs for use in developing countries has, however, become problematic because of the increasing prevalence of antimicrobial drug resistance (Salam 1998). Tetracycline, ampicillin, and the fixed-ratio combination of trimethoprim and sulfmethoxazole, once used as first-line treatment, are no longer reliably effective. When epidemic dysentery caused by multidrug-resistant *S. dysenteriae* type 1 appeared in Africa and Asia in the 1980s and 1990s, nalidixic acid was pressed into use (Salam and Bennish 1988). Nalidixic acid is a drug used primarily for urinary tract infections, but it is also effective against *Shigella*. Clinical responses were initially excellent, but with continued use, resistance to nalidixic acid has been increasing in many parts of the world (Dutta and others 2003).

A number of other drugs have been tested and shown effective, including ceftriaxone, azithromycin, pivmecillinam, and some new generation 5-fluoroquinolones, such as ciprofloxacin (Salam 1998). Because of its effectiveness, safety, ease of administration by the oral route, short course, and low cost (US$0.10 for a three-day course for a 15-kilogram child), ciprofloxacin is the current drug of choice for shigellosis (Zimbasa Dysentery Study Group 2002). However, ciprofloxacin-resistant strains are already appearing (Pazhani and others 2004), and it is only a matter of time before resistance becomes widespread, especially if the drug is readily available and indiscriminately used. Because of these concerns, development of a vaccine for *Shigella* is critical. The Diseases of the Most Impoverished initiative, supported by the Bill & Melinda Gates Foundation (Nossal 2003), which promotes vaccine development for *Shigella*, cholera, and typhoid, is a significant advance since the previous edition of this volume.

COST-EFFECTIVENESS OF INTERVENTIONS

Cost-effectiveness ratios of diarrheal disease interventions were calculated by World Bank region in terms of disability-adjusted life years (DALYs) averted for a model population of 1 million, following the standardized guidelines of the Disease Control Priorities Project for economic analyses (see chapter 15). Europe and Central Asia were excluded because data were lacking owing to the low prevalence of disease. Input variables included (a) region-specific diarrhea morbidity rates adapted from Kosek, Bern, and Guerrant (2003); (b) region-specific underlying mortality rates and age structures provided by the Disease Control Priorities Project; (c) median intervention effectiveness rates (that is, percentage of diarrheal morbidity reduction and percentage of diarrheal mortality reduction); and (d) median per capita intervention costs gathered from the literature and from personal communications (table 19.1).

Because approximately 90 percent of all cases in the developing world occur in children under five, the analysis focused on this age group alone. Uniform intervention effectiveness rates were assumed for all regions because region-specific information was not available. Regional variations in cost-effectiveness were due to regional variations in the prevalence of diarrheal disease, in the diarrhea-attributable morbidity and mortality, and in the intervention cost, where region-specific information was available.

Disability-adjusted life years are averted through the avoidance of cotemporaneous disability and mortality attributable to diarrhea. We did not consider long-term developmental and cognitive effects of childhood diarrhea or the external benefits of interventions unrelated to diarrhea (for instance, benefits of measles immunization unrelated to diarrhea or other health benefits of improved public water and sanitation). Therefore, our estimates err on the conservative side.

We explored two general categories of interventions: early interventions that take place within the first year of life—breastfeeding promotion and immunizations for rotavirus (with the prototype Rhesus reassortant tetravalent vaccine), cholera (with live oral vaccine), and measles—and other interventions that treat an entire cohort of children under five simultaneously (improved water and sanitation). For early interventions, cost-effectiveness ratios were calculated by considering the cost of treating all newborns in a single year and the benefits (DALYs averted) from those treatments that occur over the first five years of life. These benefits include avoided mortality that allows individuals to live to the expected life expectancy for the region. Other interventions included ORT and improved water and sanitation infrastructure. Because a single year of these interventions yields only cotemporaneous benefits—because effectively treated individuals do not necessarily live to life expectancy given that they are likely to be reinfected the next year—we calculated cost-effectiveness of a five-year intervention. Analysis of a five-year intervention enabled us to consider the case in which an entire cohort of children age zero to four avoids early childhood diarrheal mortality because of the intervention and receives the benefit of living to life expectancy.

Disability and deaths averted for those benefiting from improved water and sanitation were calculated from only the fraction of the model populations currently without access. For each region, the proportion of rural and urban children age zero to four currently without access to improved water and sanitation was calculated using region-specific information from *World Bank Development Indicators* (World Bank 2002)

for 2000. Infrastructure improvements for rural and urban populations were considered separately because of differences in infrastructure type and cost, although the same effectiveness rates were used for both.

The per child treatment costs and effectiveness rates used are presented in table 19.1. Cost per treatment of ORT varied widely depending on the type and method of ORT implemented. Oral rehydration therapy can be as inexpensive as US\$0.02 per child treated—the cost of a home remedy with sugar and salt. However, treatment can become substantially more expensive if commercially manufactured ORS is used or if there are substantial personnel or infrastructure costs (Martinez, Phillips, and Feachem 1993). Finally, our analysis considered only long-run marginal costs (which vary with the number of individuals treated) and did not include fixed costs of initiating a program where none currently exists.

Figure 19.3 shows the cost-effectiveness of all interventions over the first five years of life. Two interventions administered during the first year of life—breastfeeding promotion (US\$930 per DALY) and measles immunization (US\$981 per DALY)—were the most cost-effective. ORT (US\$1,062 per DALY) and water and sanitation in rural areas (US\$1,974 per DALY) were the next most cost-effective, but only if they were implemented continuously for five years, thereby allowing an entire cohort of effectively treated children age zero to four to survive past the age at which they are most at risk for diarrheal infection, disability, and mortality. Rotavirus immunization (US\$2,478 per DALY), cholera immunization (US\$2,945 per DALY), and water and sanitation in urban areas (US\$6,396 per DALY) were the least cost-effective.

Among the early interventions, breastfeeding promotion was less effective than other interventions but also less expensive than rotavirus and measles vaccination (table 19.1). Cholera vaccination was less expensive than breastfeeding promotion, but it was also many times less effective because of the significantly higher prevalence of diarrhea that is not related to cholera—making cholera vaccination the least cost-effective of the early interventions considered. Oral rehydration therapy and water and sanitation interventions were more effective than breastfeeding and vaccination interventions in reducing morbidity and mortality caused by diarrhea, but they were also more expensive. However, our analysis for water and sanitation did not consider the benefits of this intervention other than those related to health, and the high cost-effectiveness ratio is more a limitation of our methodology than of the intervention itself.

The high cost-effectiveness ratio for ORT is attributable to the high variation in reported treatment costs, which may inflate the median cost used in this analysis (table 19.2). Given the range of reported treatment costs (table 19.1), the cost-effectiveness ratio of ORT could be as low as US\$4 per DALY or as high as US\$2,124 per DALY in low- and middle-income countries. High variation in reported treatment costs results in

Table 19.1 Cost and Effectiveness Values Used to Calculate Cost-Effectiveness Ratios for Select Interventions for Diarrhea for Children under Age Five

Model regions	Sources	Source regions or countries	Median cost/child (2001 US$)	Cost/child range (2001 US$)	Median diarrhea morbidity reduction (percent)	Morbidity reduction range (percent)	Median diarrhea mortality reduction (percent)	Mortality reduction range (percent)
Breastfeeding promotion								
Costs								
LMICs, EAP, MENA, SA, SSA	Horton and others 1996; Martinez, Phillips, and Feachem 1993	LMICs, Brazil, Honduras, Mexico	8.98	0.46–17.50				
LAC	Horton and others 1996	Brazil, Honduras, Mexico	1.86	0.46–3.26				
Effectiveness (age 0 to 5)								
All	Feachem and Koblinsky 1984	LMICs			4.5	1–8	10.5	4–17
Rotavirus immunization with RRV-TV								
Costs								
LMICs, EAP, LAC, MENA, SSA	Martinez, Phillips, and Feachem 1993; Narula, Tiwari, and Puliyeh 2004	LMICs, India	53.80	3.33–104.30				
SA	Narula, Tiwari, and Puliyeh 2004	India	104.30	—				
Effectiveness (age 0 to 5)								
All	Parashar and others 1998[a]	Brazil, Peru, R. B. de Venezuela			8.54	—	24.1	—
Cholera immunization with live oral vaccine								
Costs								
LMICs, EAP, MENA, SA, SSA	Cookson and others 1997; Martinez, Phillips, and Feachem 1993	LMICs, Argentina	3.65	1.70–5.60				
LAC	Cookson and others 1997	Argentina	1.70	—				
Effectiveness (age 0 to 5)								
All	de Zoysa and Feachem 1985	Bangladesh			0.095	0.06–0.13	1.5	1–2

Measles immunization

Costs

LMICs, LAC, MENA, SA	Duke 1999; Feachem and Koblinsky 1983; Phillips, Feachem, and Mills 1987; Martinez, Phillips, and Feachem 1993; Shann 2000	LMICs, Côte d'Ivoire, Ghana, Indonesia, Papua New Guinea, Zambia	13.26	0.52–26.00		
EAP	Duke 1999; Phillips, Feachem, and Mills 1987; Shann 2000	Indonesia, Papua New Guinea	1.62	0.52–1.10		
SSA	Feachem and Koblinsky 1983; Phillips, Feachem, and Mills 1987	Côte d'Ivoire, Ghana, Zambia	15.00	4.00–26.00		

Effectiveness (age 0 to 5)

All	Feachem and Koblinsky 1983	LMICs	2.2	0.6–3.8	16	6.4–25.6

Water supply and sanitation improvement

Costs (rural)

All	Esrey, Feachem, and Hughes 1985	LMICs	25.00	—		

Costs (urban)

All	Esrey, Feachem, and Hughes 1985	LMICs	81.00	—		

Effectiveness (age 0 to 5)

All	Esrey, Feachem, and Hughes 1985; Esrey and others 1991	LMICs	24	22–26	65	—

(Continues on the following page.)

Table 19.1 Continued

Model regions	Sources	Source regions or countries	Median cost/child (2001 US$)	Cost/child range (2001 US$)	Median diarrhea morbidity reduction (percent)	Morbidity reduction range (percent)	Median diarrhea mortality reduction (percent)	Mortality reduction range (percent)
Oral rehydration therapy								
Costs								
LMICs	Horton and Claquin 1983; Islam, Mahalanabis, and Majid 1994; Qualls and Robertson 1989; Shepard, Brenzel, and Nemeth 1986; WHO and UNICEF 2001	Bangladesh, Arab Rep. of Egypt, The Gambia, Honduras, Indonesia, Malawi, Swaziland, Turkey	5.50	0.02–11.00				
EAP	Shepard, Brenzel, and Nemeth 1986	Indonesia	0.71	0.02–1.40				
LAC	Shepard, Brenzel, and Nemeth 1986	Honduras	2.59	0.02–5.16				
MENA	Shepard, Brenzel, and Nemeth 1986	Arab Rep. of Egypt	4.89	0.02–9.75				
SA	Horton and Claquin 1983; Islam, Mahalanabis, and Majid 1994	Bangladesh	2.91	0.02–5.80				
SSA	Shepard, Brenzel, and Nemeth 1986; Qualls and Robertson 1989	The Gambia, Malawi, Swaziland	5.51	0.02–11.00				
Effectiveness (age 0 to 5)								
All	Boschi-Pinto and Tomaskovic forthcoming	LMICs			0	—	95	—

Source: Authors.

LMICs = low- and middle-income countries; EAP = East Asia and the Pacific; LAC = Latin America and the Caribbean; MENA = Middle East and North Africa; SA = South Asia; SSA = Sub-Saharan Africa; — = not available.

a. Effectiveness calculated based on vaccine efficacy reported in Parashar and others (1998) and under the assumption that rotavirus infection is responsible for 20 percent of all diarrheal morbidity and severe infection is responsible for 33.3 percent of all diarrheal mortality.

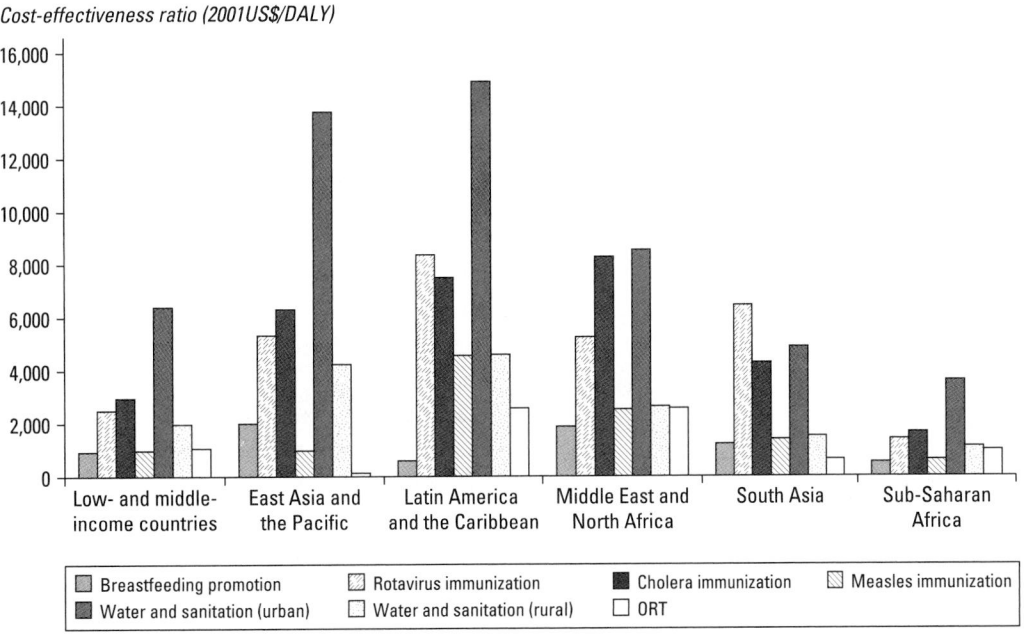

Cost-effectiveness ratio (2001US$/DALY)

Legend:
- Breastfeeding promotion
- Water and sanitation (urban)
- Rotavirus immunization
- Water and sanitation (rural)
- Cholera immunization
- ORT
- Measles immunization

Source: Authors.

Figure 19.3 Cost-Effectiveness: Intervention at Birth through Age 5 with Benefits that Occur over Five Years (age 0–4)

Table 19.2 Cost-Effectiveness Ratios of Oral Rehydration Therapy Interventions Based on Minimum, Median, and Maximum per Capita Costs (2001 US$/DALY)

Region	Minimum cost	Median cost	Maximum cost
Low- and middle-income countries	4	1,062	2,124
East Asia and the Pacific	4	132	260
Latin America and the Caribbean	20	2,570	5,120
Middle East and North Africa	10	2,564	5,113
South Asia	4	642	1,279
Sub-Saharan Africa	4	988	1,972

Source: Authors.

high variation in cost-effectiveness for the other regions as well. There remains little doubt, however, about the effect of widespread use of ORT on diarrhea morbidity and mortality and about the associated direct and indirect cost savings for treatment and hospitalization.

RESEARCH AGENDA

Good evidence now supports the view that promoting ORT in conjunction with other key interventions, preventive as well as curative, has had a large role in the marked reduction in deaths of children caused by diarrhea (Victora and others 2000).

Preventive strategies—such as breastfeeding, improving complementary feeding and using micronutrient supplementation or fortification, and increasing coverage with the full set of Expanded Programme on Immunization vaccines (especially measles vaccine)—are all useful and effective (GAVI 2005). Failure to separately track the full impact of bloody diarrhea—especially *Shigella* infection—on morbidity and mortality or to effectively implement good clinical management (including guidelines for and control over the use of antibiotics) has contributed to the continuing burden of bloody diarrhea and dysentery worldwide and the alarming increase in antibiotic resistance. The challenges for the next decade will be to increase or ensure universal appropriate implementation of these interventions in developing countries and to avoid a situation in which they compete for funding and staff time. Delivery of good-quality services is essential, and much remains to be learned through research before this requirement can be met.

Other interventions, such as vaccines against rotavirus, *Shigella,* or cholera, are either not yet available or not ready for universal administration. Progress toward the development of these vaccines, with the highest priority for the first two, is encouraging, but further investments in research and development will be required before large-scale implementation of these interventions can be considered. The cost of these vaccines will remain a major constraint for poor people, who cannot pay for the costs of development and ensure reasonable profits for industry. However, increased public investment in fundamental and applied research, vaccine purchase schemes, and development of low-cost, high-quality manufacturing capacity in developing countries may change the prevailing dynamics. By creating public-private partnerships for vaccine development, organized as targeted product development programs, the public sector, private foundations, and industry are taking steps toward these goals.

Because of the fecal-oral transmission of enteric pathogens, improving the supply of safe water and the ability to safely dispose of fecal waste are the best ways to reduce the burden of morbidity and mortality. However, major investments and critical improvements in water and sanitary waste disposal on the necessary scale are unlikely to occur in the next decade or two. Local low-tech solutions can be useful, and enhanced efforts to find ways to improve water cleanliness at the point of use and to build simple latrines that will be used consistently are needed (chapter 41). However, in the face of HIV and the attention being given to tuberculosis and malaria, coordinated efforts to build safe water and sanitation capacity at the local level, one village at a time, that are sufficient to significantly influence the burden of illness are unlikely—even though many more infants and children die each year of preventable and treatable diarrhea than of HIV/AIDS.

The cycle of research, followed by implementation, followed by research has enabled the development of improved tools to manage diarrheal diseases—tools that have the potential to further drive down diarrhea mortality. The challenge is to achieve high coverage and good practice with ORT and correct diarrhea case management, including antimicrobial and nutrition interventions. Interventions to integrate health care through programmatic initiatives such as the Integrated Management of Childhood Illness program, critically evaluated elsewhere in this book (chapter 63), could be essential to ensure this high coverage. Some concern remains that in low-resource settings such targeted vertical programs may be abandoned, to the detriment of the goals for disease burden reduction that they were established to achieve.

The challenge posed by the case management of bloody diarrhea is a different matter. Until a vaccine is available, the keystone for managing bloody diarrhea will continue to be the early use of effective antimicrobial agents. That is made difficult by increasing drug resistance, aided by the widespread indiscriminate and inappropriate use of antimicrobials, and the increasingly difficult task of finding a safe, inexpensive, and effective oral agent and then ensuring that the drug is given in a clinically optimal manner. From a technical perspective, the development of a vaccine against *Shigella* infections is still in its infancy and in need of greater investment. For both watery and bloody diarrhea, the challenge of developing drugs to normalize the pathophysiology caused by the infection remains a scientific challenge and a distant hope.

CONCLUSIONS

Existing interventions to prevent or treat diarrheal diseases have proven their efficacy in reducing mortality, but a major challenge for the next 10 years will be to scale up these interventions to achieve universal utilization coverage. The United Nations Millennium Development Goal to reduce the mortality rate among children under five by two-thirds by 2015 will be easier to attain if the scale-up goals are reached. New products and tools could significantly improve the efficacy of these interventions—for example, rapid specific diagnostics, new treatment strategies based on reversing the pathophysiology of the infection, simple and effective ways to produce clean water and control human waste, and vaccines to prevent illness. However, these products and tools will not become widely available in time to influence the achievement of the Millennium Development Goals. Continued investment in diarrheal disease research across the spectrum of basic, social and behavioral, and applied investigations is, therefore, essential, including expanded behavioral research to understand how parents assess risk and how actionable health messages can be presented in different cultures and settings.

REFERENCES

Allen, S. J., B. Okoko, E. Martinez, G. Gregorio, and L. F. Dans. 2004. "Probiotics for Treating Infectious Diarrhea." Cochrane Database Systematic Reviews (2): CD003048.

Badruddin, S., A. Islam, K. H. Hendricks, Z. A. Bhutta, S. A. Shaikh, J. D. Snyder, and A. M. Molla. 1991. "Dietary Risk Factors Associated with Acute and Persistent Diarrhea in Karachi, Pakistan." *American Journal of Clinical Nutrition* 51: 745–49.

Baltazar, J. C., D. P. Nadera, and C. G. Victora. 2002. "Evaluation of the National Control of Diarrhoeal Diseases Programme in the Philippines, 1980–93." *Bulletin of the World Health Organization* 80: 637–43.

Baqui, A. H., R. E. Black, S. El Arifeen, M. Yunus, K. Zaman, N. Begum, and others. 2004. "Zinc Therapy for Diarrhoea Increased the Use of Oral Rehydration Therapy and Reduced the Use of Antibiotics in Bangladeshi Children." *Journal of Health, Population, and Nutrition* 22 (4): 440–42.

Barreto, M. L., L. M. P. Santos, A. M. O. Assis, M. P. N. Araujo, G. G. Farenzena, P. A. B. Santos, and R. L. Fiaccone. 1994. "Effect of Vitamin A Supplementation on Diarrhoea and Acute Lower Respiratory-Tract Infections in Young Children in Brazil." *Lancet* 344: 228–31.

Barros, F. C., T. C. Semer, S. Tonioli Filho, E. Tomasi, and C. G. Victora. 1995. "The Impact of Lactation Centers on Breastfeeding Patterns, Morbidity, and Growth: A Birth Cohort Study." *Acta Paediatrica* 84: 1221–26.

Bern, C., J. Martines, I. de Zoysa, and R. I. Glass. 1992. "The Magnitude of the Problem of Diarrhoeal Disease: A Ten-Year Update." *Bulletin of the World Health Organization* 70: 705–14.

Bhan, M. K., N. Bhandari, S. Sazawal, J. Clemens, and P. Raj. 1989. "Descriptive Epidemiology of Persistent Diarrhoea among Young Children in Rural North India." *Bulletin of the World Health Organization* 67: 281–88.

Bhandari, N., R. Bahl, S. Mazumdar, J. Martines, R. E. Black, and M. K. Bhan. 2003. "Infant Feeding Study Group: Effect of Community-Based Promotion of Exclusive Breastfeeding on Diarrhoeal Illness and Growth: A Cluster Randomised Controlled Trial." *Lancet* 361: 1418–23.

Black, M. M., H. Dubowitz, J. Hutcheson, J. Berenson-Howard, and R. H. Starr, Jr. 1995. "A Randomized Clinical Trial of Home Intervention for Children with Failure to Thrive." *Pediatrics* 95: 807–14.

Black, R. E. 2003. "Zinc Deficiency, Infectious Disease, and Mortality in the Developing World." *Journal of Nutrition* 133 (Suppl. 1): 1485S–89S.

Black, R. E., and C. F. Lanata. 2002. "Epidemiology of Diarrheal Diseases in Developing Countries." In *Infections of the Gastrointestinal Tract*, 2nd ed., ed. M. J. Blaser, P. D. Smith, J. I. Ravdin, H. B. Greenberg, and R. L. Guerrant, 11–29. Philadelphia: Lippincott, Williams, and Wilkins.

Boschi-Pinto, C., and L. Tomaskovic. Forthcoming. "Deaths from Diarrhoeal Diseases among Children under Five Years of Age in the Developing World: A Review." *Bulletin of the World Health Organization*.

Brown, K., K. Dewey, and L. Allen. 1998. *Complementary Feeding of Young Children in Developing Countries: A Review of Current Scientific Knowledge*. WHO/NUT/98.1. Geneva: World Health Organization.

Calain, P., J. P. Chaine, E. Johnson, M. L. Hawley, M. J. O'Leary, H. Oshitani, and C. L. Chaignat. 2004. "Can Oral Cholera Vaccination Play a Role in Controlling a Cholera Outbreak?" *Vaccine* 22: 2444–51.

Caulfield, L. E., S. L. Huffman, and E. G. Piwoz. 1999. "Interventions to Improve Intake of Complementary Foods by Infants 6 to 12 Months of Age in Developing Countries: Impact on Growth and on the Prevalence of Malnutrition and Potential Contribution to Child Survival." *Food and Nutrition Bulletin* 20:183–200.

CDC (U.S. Centers for Disease Control and Prevention). 1999a. "Intussusception among Recipients of Rotavirus Vaccine: United States, 1998–1999." *Morbidity and Mortality Weekly Reports* 48: 577–81.

———. 1999b. "Suspension of Rotavirus Vaccine after Reports of Intussusceptions: United States, 1999." *Morbidity and Mortality Weekly Reports* 53 (34): 786–89.

Cookson, S. T., D. Stamboulian, J. Demonte, L. Quero, C. M. De Arquiza, A. Aleman, and others. 1997. "A Cost-Benefit Analysis of Programmatic Use of CVD 103-Hgr Live Oral Cholera Vaccine in a High-Risk Population." *International Journal of Epidemiology* 26: 212–19.

Coutsoudis, A., K. Pillay, E. Spooner, L. Kuhn, and H. M. Coovadia. 1999. "Influence of Infant-Feeding Patterns on Early Mother-to-Child Transmission of HIV-1 in Durban, South Africa: A Prospective Cohort Study." *Lancet* 354: 471–76.

De Cock, K. M., M. G. Fowler, E. Mercier, I. de Vincenzi, J. Saba, E. Hoff, and others. 2000. "Prevention of Mother-to-Child HIV Transmission in Resource-Poor Countries: Translating Research into Policy and Practice." *Journal of the American Medical Association* 283: 1175–82.

Dennehy, P. H. 2005. "Rotavirus Vaccines: An Update." *Current Opinion in Pediatrics* 17: 88–92.

de Zoysa, I., and R. G. Feachem. 1985. "Interventions for the Control of Diarrhoeal Diseases among Young Children: Rotavirus and Cholera Immunization." *Bulletin of the World Health Organization* 63: 569–83.

Dobbing, J. 1990. "Early Nutrition and Later Achievement." *Proceedings of the Nutrition Society* 49: 103–18.

Duggan, C., O. Fontaine, N. F. Pierce, R. I. Glass, D. Mahalanabis, N. H. Alam, and others. 2004. "Scientific Rationale for a Change in the Composition of Oral Rehydration Solution." *Journal of the American Medical Association* 291: 2628–31.

Duke, T. 1999. "Haemophilus influenzae Type B Vaccine in Papua New Guinea: What Can We Expect, and How Should We Determine Priority for Child Health Interventions?" *Papua and New Guinea Medical Journal* 42: 1–4.

Dutta, S., D. Dutta, P. Dutta, S. Matsushita, S. K. Bhattacharya, and S. Yoshida. 2003. "*Shigella dysenteriae* Serotype 1, Kolkata, India." *Emerging Infectious Diseases* 9: 1471–74.

English, R. M., J. C. Badcock, T. Giay, T. Ngu, A. M. Waters, and S. A. Bennett. 1997. "Effect of Nutrition Improvement Project on Morbidity from Infectious Diseases in Preschool Children in Vietnam: Comparison with Control Commune." *British Medical Journal* 315: 1122–25.

Esrey, S. A. 1996. "Water, Waste, and Well-Being: A Multicountry Study." *American Journal of Epidemiology* 143: 608–23.

Esrey, S. A., R. Feachem, and J. M. Hughes. 1985. "Interventions for the Control of Diarrhoeal Diseases among Young Children: Improving Water Supplies and Excreta Disposal Facilities." *Bulletin of the World Health Organization* 63: 757–72.

Esrey, S. A., J. B. Potash, L. Roberts, and C. Shiff. 1991. "Effects of Improved Water Supply and Sanitation on Ascariasis, Diarrhoea, Dracunculiasis, Hookworm Infection, Schistosomiasis, and Trachoma." *Bulletin of the World Health Organization* 69: 609–21.

Fauveau, V., F. J. Henry, A. Briend, M. Yunus, and J. Chakraborty. 1992. "Persistent Diarrhea as a Cause of Childhood Mortality in Rural Bangladesh." *Acta Paediatrica Supplement* 381: 12–14.

Feachem, R. G. A., and M. A. Koblinsky. 1983. "Interventions for the Control of Diarrhoeal Diseases among Young Children: Measles Immunization." *Bulletin of the World Health Organization* 61: 641–52.

———. 1984. "Interventions for the Control of Diarrhoeal Diseases among Young Children: Promotion of Breast-Feeding." *Bulletin of the World Health Organization* 62: 271–91.

Fourquet, F., J. C. Desenclos, C. Maurage, and S. Baron. 2003. "Acute Gastroenteritis in Children in France: Estimates of Disease Burden through National Hospital Discharge Data." *Archives of Pediatrics* 10: 861–68.

GAVI (Global Alliance for Vaccines and Immunization). 2005. "Outcomes: Most Recent Data on the Impact of Support from GAVI/The Vaccine Fund and the Work of GAVI Partners." http://www.vaccinealliance.org/General_Information/About_alliance/progupdate.php.

Gill, C., J. Lau, S. L. Gorbach, and D. H. Hamer. 2003. "Diagnostic Accuracy of Stool Assays for Inflammatory Bacterial Gastroenteritis in Developed and Resource-Poor Countries." *Clinical Infectious Diseases* 37: 365–75.

Glass, R. I., J. S. Bresee, U. D. Parashar, R. C. Holman, and J. R. Gentsch. 1999. "First Rotavirus Vaccine License: Is There Really a Need?" *Acta Paediatrica Supplement* 88: 2–8.

Graeff, J. A., J. P. Elder, and E. M. Booth. 1993. *Communication for Health and Behavior Change: A Developing Country Perspective*. San Francisco, CA: Jossey Bass.

Graves, P., J. Deeks, V. Demicheli, M. Pratt, and T. Jefferson. 2000. "Vaccines for Preventing Cholera." *Cochrane Database Systematic Reviews* (4): CD000974.

Guptill, K. S., S. A. Esrey, G. A. Oni, and K. H. Brown. 1993. "Evaluation of a Face-to-Face Weaning Food Intervention in Kwara State, Nigeria: Knowledge, Trial, and Adoption of a Home-Prepared Weaning Food." *Social Science and Medicine* 36: 665–72.

Haider, R., A. Islam, J. Hamadani, N. J. Amin, I. Kabir, M. A. Malek, and others. 1996. "Breastfeeding Counselling in a Diarrhoeal Hospital." *Bulletin of the World Health Organization* 74: 173–79.

Hanh, S. K., Y. J. Kim, and P. Garner. 2001. "Reduced Osmolarity Oral Rehydrations Solution for Treating Dehydration Due to Diarrhoea in Children: A Systematic Review." *British Medical Journal* 323: 81–85.

Horton, S., and P. Claquin. 1983. "Cost-Effectiveness and User Characteristics of Clinic-Based Services for the Treatment of Diarrhea: A Case Study in Bangladesh." *Social Science and Medicine* 17: 721–29.

Horton, S., T. Sanghvi, M. Phillips, J. Fielder, R. Perez-Escamilla, C. Lutter, and others. 1996. "Breastfeeding Promotion and Priority Setting in Health." *Health Policy and Planning* 11: 156–68.

Huicho, L., M. Campos, J. Rivera, and R. L. Guerrant. 1996. "Fecal Screening Tests in the Approach to Acute Infectious Diarrhea: A Scientific Overview." *Pediatric Infectious Disease* 15: 486–94.

Huttly, S. R., S. S. Morris, and V. Pisani. 1997. "Prevention of Diarrhoea in Young Children in Developing Countries." *Bulletin of the World Health Organization* 75: 163–74.

Islam, M. A., D. Mahalanabis, and N. Majid. 1994. "Use of Rice-Based Oral Rehydration Solution in a Large Diarrhea Treatment Centre in Bangladesh: In-House Production, Use, and Relative Cost." *Journal of Tropical Medicine and Hygiene* 97: 341–46.

Jamison, D. T., H. W. Mosley, A. R. Measham, and J. L. Bobadilla. 1993. *Disease Control Priorities in Developing Countries*. Oxford, U.K.: Oxford University Press.

Jones, G., R. W. Steketee, R. E. Black, Z. A. Bhutta, S. S. Morris, and the Bellagio Child Survival Study Group. 2003. "How Many Child Deaths Can We Prevent This Year?" *Lancet* 362: 65–71.

Keusch, G. T. 2001. "Toxin-Associated Gastrointestinal Disease: A Clinical Overview." In *Molecular Medical Microbiology*, ed. M. Sussman, 1083–88. New York: Academic Press.

———. 2003. "The History of Nutrition: Malnutrition, Infection, and Immunity." *Journal of Nutrition* 133: 336S–40S.

Keusch, G. T., and N. S. Scrimshaw. 1986. "Selective Primary Health Care: Strategies for Control of Disease in the Developing World—XXIII. The Control of Infection to Reduce the Prevalence of Infantile and Childhood Malnutrition." *Reviews of Infectious Diseases* 8: 273–87.

Keusch, G. T., D. M. Thea, M. Kamenga, K. Kakanda, M. Mbala, and F. Davachi. 1992. "Persistent Diarrhea Associated with AIDS." *Acta Paediatrica Scandinavica* 381 (Suppl.): 45–48.

Khan, S. R., F. Jalil, S. Zaman, B. S. Lindblad, and J. Karlberg. 1993. "Early Child Health in Lahore, Pakistan: X—Mortality." *Acta Paediatrica Supplement* 390: 109–17.

Kimmons, J. E., K. H. Brown, A. Lartey, E. Collison, P. P. Mensah, and K. G. Dewey. 1999. "The Effects of Fermentation and/or Vacuum Flask Storage on the Presence of Coliforms in Complementary Foods Prepared for Ghanaian Children." *International Journal of Food Science and Nutrition* 50: 195–201.

Kosek, M., C. Bern, and R. L. Guerrant. 2003. "The Global Burden of Diarrhoeal Disease, as Estimated from Studies Published between 1992 and 2000." *Bulletin of the World Health Organization* 81: 197–204.

Kotloff, K. L., J. P. Winickoff, B. Ivanoff, J. D. Clemens, D. L. Swerdlow, P. J. Sansonetti, and others. 1999. "Global Burden of Shigella Infections: Implications for Vaccine Development and Implementation of Control Strategies." *Bulletin of the World Health Organizaton* 77: 651–66.

Legros, D. 2004. "Shigellosis: Report of a Workshop." *Journal of Health, Population and Nutrition* 22: 445–49.

Martinez, J., M. Phillips, and R. G. A. Feachem. 1993. "Diarrheal Diseases." In *Disease Control Priorities in Developing Countries*, ed. D. Jamison, W. H. Moseley, A. R. Measham, and J. S. Bobadilla, 91–115. Oxford, U.K.: Oxford University Press.

Miller, P., and N. Hirschhorn. 1995. "The Effect of a National Control of Diarrheal Diseases Program on Mortality: The Case of Egypt." *Social Science and Medicine* 40: S1–30.

Mondal, S. K., P. G. Gupta, D. N. Gupta, S. Ghosh, S. N. Sikder, K. Rajendran, and others. 1996. "Occurrence of Diarrheal Diseases in Relation to Infant Feeding Practices in a Rural Community in West Bengal, India." *Acta Paediatrica* 85: 1159–62.

Murphy, B. R., D. M. Morens, L. Simonsen, R. M. Chanock, J. R. La Montagne, and A. Z. Kapikian. 2003. "Reappraisal of the Association of Intussusception with the Licensed Live Rotavirus Vaccine Challenges Initial Conclusions." *Journal of Infectious Diseases* 187 (8): 1301–8.

Narula, D., L. Tiwari, and J. M. Puliyeh. 2004. "Rotavirus Vaccines." *Lancet* 364: 245–46.

Nataro, J., and J. B. Kaper. 1998. "Diarrheagenic Escherichia coli." *Clinical Microbiological Reviews* 11: 142–201.

Niehaus, M. D., S. R. Moore, P. D. Patrick, L. L. Derr, B. Lorntz, A. A. Lima, and R. L. Guerrant. 2002. "Early Childhood Diarrhea Is Associated with Diminished Cognitive Function 4 to 7 Years Later in Children in a Northeast Brazilian Shantytown." *American Journal of Tropical Medicine and Hygiene* 66: 590–93.

Nossal, G. J. 2003. "Gates, GAVI, the Glorious Global Funds, and More: All You Ever Wanted to Know." *Immunology and Cell Biology* 81: 20–22.

Ochoa, T. J., E. Salazar-Lindo, and T. G. Cleary. 2004. "Management of Children with Infection-Associated Persistent Diarrhea." *Seminars in Pediatric Infectious Diseases* 15: 229–36.

Oria, R. B., P. D. Patrick, H. Zhang, B. Lorntz, C. M. de Castro Costa, G. A. Brito, and others. 2005. "APOE4 Protects Cognitive Development in Children with Heavy Diarrhea Burdens in Northeast Brazil." *Pediatric Research* 57: 310–16.

Parashar, U. D., J. S. Bresee, J. R. Gentsch, and R. I. Glass. 1998. "Rotavirus." *Emerging Infectious Diseases* 4: 561–70.

Parashar, U. D., E. G. Hummelman, J. S. Bresee, M. A. Miller, and R. I. Glass. 2003. "Global Illness and Deaths Caused by Rotavirus Disease in Children." *Emerging Infectious Diseases* 9: 565–72.

Pazhani, G. P., B. Sarkar, T. Ramamurthy, S. K. Bhattacharya, Y. Takeda, and S. K. Niyogi. 2004. "Clonal Multidrug-Resistant Shigella Dysenteriae Type 1 Strains Associated with Epidemic and Sporadic Dysenteries in Eastern India." *Antimicrobial Agents and Chemotherapy* 48: 681–84.

Peter, G., M. G. Myers, the National Vaccine Advisory Committee, and the National Vaccine Program Office. 2002. "Intussusception, Rotavirus, and Oral Vaccines: Summary of a Workshop." *Pediatrics* 110: e67.

Phillips, M. A., R. G. A. Feachem, and A. Mills. 1987. *Options for Diarrhoeal Disease Control: The Cost and Cost-Effectiveness of Selected Interventions for the Prevention of Diarrhea*. London: Evaluation and Planning Centre for Health Care.

Qualls, N., and R. Robertson. 1989. "Potential Uses of Cost Analyses in Child Survival Programs: Evidence from Africa." *Health Policy and Planning* 4: 50–61.

Ronsmans, C., M. L. Bennish, and T. Wierzba. 1988. "Diagnosis and Management of Dysentery by Community Health Workers." *Lancet* 8610: 552–55.

Ross, D. A., B. R. Kirkwood, F. N. Binka, P. Arthur, N. Dollimore, S. S. Morris, and others. 1995. "Child Morbidity and Mortality Following Vitamin A Supplementation in Ghana: Time since Dosing, Number of Doses, and Time of Year." *American Journal of Public Health* 85:1246–51.

Ruxin, J. N. 1994. "Magic Bullet: The History of Oral Rehydration Therapy." *Medical History* 38: 363–97.

Ryan, E. T., and S. B. Calderwood. 2000. "Cholera Vaccines." *Clinical Infectious Diseases* 31: 561–65.

Salam, M. A. 1998. "Antimicrobial Therapy for Shigellosis: Issues on Antimicrobial Resistance." *Japanese Journal of Medical Science and Biology* 51 (Suppl.): S43–62.

Salam, M. A., and M. L. Bennish. 1988. "Therapy for Shigellosis: I. Randomized, Double-Blind Trial of Nalidixic Acid in Childhood Shigellosis." *Journal of Pediatrics* 113: 901–7.

Santos, I., C. G. Victora, J. Martines, H. Goncalves, D. P. Gigante, N. J. Valle, and G. Pelto. 2001. "Nutrition Counseling Increases Weight Gain among Brazilian Children." *Journal of Nutrition* 131: 2866–73.

Shann, F. 2000. "Immunization: Dramatic New Evidence." *Papua and New Guinea Medical Journal* 43: 24–29.

Shepard, D. S., L. E. Brenzel, and K. T. Nemeth. 1986. "Cost-Effectiveness of Oral Rehydration Therapy for Diarrheal Diseases." Technical Note 86–26, Population, Health and Nutrition Department, World Bank, Washington, DC.

Sikorski, J., M. J. Renfrew, S. Pindoria, and A. Wade. 2002. "Support for Breastfeeding Mothers." Cochrane Database of Systematic Reviews (1): CD001141.

Snyder, J. D., and M. H. Merson. 1982. "The Magnitude of the Global Problem of Acute Diarrhoeal Disease: A Review of Active Surveillance Data." *Bulletin of the World Health Organization* 60: 604–13.

Tucker, A. W., A. C. Haddix, J. S. Bresee, R. C. Holman, U. D. Parashar, and R. I. Glass. 1998. "Cost-Effectiveness Analysis of a Rotavirus Immunization Program for the United States." *Journal of the American Medical Association* 279: 1371–76.

Victora, C. G., J. Bryce, O. Fontaine, and R. Monasch. 2000. "Reducing Deaths from Diarrhoea through Oral Rehydration Therapy." *Bulletin of the World Health Organization* 78: 1246–55.

Victora, C. G., B. R. Kirkwood, A. Ashworth, R. E. Black, S. Rogers, S. Sazawal, and H. Campbell. 1999. "Potential Interventions for the Prevention of Childhood Pneumonia in Developing Countries: Improving Nutrition." *American Journal of Clinical Nutrition* 70: 309–20.

Westphal, M. F., J. A. Taddei, S. I. Venancio, and C. M. Bogus. 1995. "Breastfeeding Training for Health Professionals and Resultant Institutional Changes." *Bulletin of the World Health Organization* 73: 461–68.

WHO (World Health Organization). 1997. *Health and Environment in Sustainable Development Five Years after the Health Summit.* WHO/EHG/97.8. Geneva: WHO.

———. 1999. "Potential Use of Oral Cholera Vaccines in Emergency Situations." WHO/CDS/CSR/EDC/99.4. Report of a WHO meeting, Geneva, May 12–13.

———. 2000. "New Data on the Prevention of Mother-to-Child Transmission of HIV and Their Policy Implications." Report of a WHO technical consultation on behalf of a United Nations Population Fund, United Nations Children's Fund, and Joint United Nations Programme on HIV/AIDS interagency task team on mother-to-child transmission of HIV, Geneva, October 11–13.

———. 2001. "The Optimal Duration of Exclusive Breastfeeding: Results of a WHO Systematic Review." http://www.who.int/inf-pr-2001/en/note2001-07.html.

———. 2003. *HIV and Infant Feeding—Framework for Priority Action.* Geneva: WHO.

———. 2004. *Family and Community Practices That Promote Child Survival, Growth, and Development—A Review of Evidence.* Geneva: WHO.

WHO Collaborative Study Team. 2000. "Effect of Breastfeeding on Infant and Child Mortality Due to Infectious Diseases in Less Developed Countries: A Pooled Analysis." *Lancet* 355: 1104.

WHO and UNICEF (United Nations Children's Fund). 2001. "Reduced Osmolarity Oral Rehydration Salts (ORS) Formulation." WHO/FCH/CAH/01.22. Report from a meeting of experts jointly organized by the United Nations Children's Fund and the World Health Organization, Geneva.

———. 2004. *Joint Statement: Clinical Management of Acute Diarrhoea.* WHO/FCH/CAH/04.7. Geneva: WHO; New York: UNICEF.

World Bank. 2002. *World Development Indicators.* CD-ROM. Washington, DC: World Bank.

Zimbasa (Zimbabwe, Bangladesh, South Africa) Dysentery Study Group. 2002. "Multicenter, Randomized, Double Blind Clinical Trial of Short Course versus Standard Course Oral Ciprofloxacin for Shigella Dysenteriae Type 1 Dysentery in Children." *Pediatric Infectious Disease Journal* 21: 1136–41.

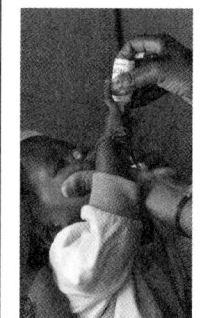

Chapter **20**

Vaccine-Preventable Diseases

Logan Brenzel, Lara J. Wolfson, Julia Fox-Rushby, Mark Miller, and Neal A. Halsey

Vaccination against childhood communicable diseases through the Expanded Program on Immunization (EPI) is one of the most cost-effective public health interventions available (UNICEF 2002; World Bank 1993). By reducing mortality and morbidity, vaccination can contribute substantially to achieving the Millennium Development Goal of reducing the mortality rate among children under five by two-thirds between 1990 and 2015. Accelerated research into the development of new vaccines has been made possible in part by innovative public-private partnerships, such as the Global Alliance for Vaccines and Immunization (GAVI). GAVI focuses on expanding access by immunization programs in developing countries to new and underused vaccines, such as those for hepatitis B and *Haemophilus influenzae* type B (Hib). These newer, more expensive vaccines are challenging previous notions of the cost-effectiveness of immunization. Analyses of their costs and cost-effectiveness are particularly important because of the need to determine the level of resources required in the future to improve immunization programs, to cover the costs of new vaccines, and to allocate scarce public and external resources available for immunization in the most optimal manner.

This chapter analyzes the costs and cost-effectiveness of scaling up the EPI and introducing selected new vaccines into the program. It also summarizes the epidemiology of diseases preventable through immunization and estimates the disease burden with and without immunization programs. In addition, the chapter discusses the organization, delivery, and financing of immunization programs and highlights future prospects and areas for further study.

Several areas overlap with other chapters. For example, the vaccines that prevent measles, tuberculosis, diphtheria,

pertussis, Hib, and *Neisseria meningitis* prevent respiratory diseases. Some vaccines, such as those against measles and pertussis, prevent diseases that cause or contribute to malnutrition. Chapter 16 provides an in-depth review of tuberculosis and a discussion of the potential impact of bacillus Calmette-Guérin (BCG) vaccines. This chapter also does not discuss some new vaccines, including conjugate *Streptococcus pneumoniae*, influenza, typhoid fever, and rotavirus, because other chapters deal with those diseases and vaccines. Vaccines to prevent mumps and varicella that are routinely used in some developed countries are not included in most vaccination programs in developing countries. Other interventions that can reduce the burden of vaccine-preventable diseases and are not covered in this chapter include clean umbilical cord care to reduce the incidence of neonatal tetanus, vitamin A therapy to reduce the case-fatality rate (CFR) from measles, and intensive clinical care that can reduce the mortality associated with most of the vaccine-preventable diseases.

CAUSES AND EPIDEMIOLOGY OF DISEASES PREVENTED BY VACCINES USED IN NATIONAL IMMUNIZATION PROGRAMS

The epidemiology and burden of vaccine-preventable diseases vary by country and region partly because of differences in vaccine uptake. Numerous other factors that contribute to the disease burden include geography, seasonal patterns, crowding, nutritional status, travel to and from other countries, and possibly genetic differences in populations that affect disease severity. Table 20.1 summarizes the features of selected vaccines

Table 20.1 Selected Vaccine-Preventable Diseases and Vaccines

Category	Tuberculosis	Diphtheria	Tetanus	Pertussis	Poliomyelitis	Measles[a]	Rubella	Hib	Hepatitis B	Yellow fever	Meningococcal disease	Japanese encephalitis
Causative agent	Mycobacterium tuberculosis	Toxin-producing bacterium (Corynebacterium diphtheriae)	Toxin-producing bacterium (Clostridium tetani)	Bacterium (Bordetella pertussis)	Virus (serotypes 1, 2, and 3)	Virus	Virus	Bacterium (Haemophilus influenzae type B)	Virus	Virus	Neisseria meningitis groups A, B, C, Y, W135	Virus
Reservoir	Humans (some bovine)	Humans	Animal intestines; soil	Humans	Humans	Humans	Humans	Humans	Humans	Monkeys and humans	Humans	Birds and mammals
Spread	Airborne droplet nuclei from sputum-positive persons	Close respiratory or cutaneous contact	Spores enter the body through wounds or the umbilical cord stump	Close respiratory contact	Fecal-oral; close respiratory contact	Close respiratory contact and aerosolized droplets	Close respiratory contact and aerosolized droplets	Close respiratory contact	Blood, perinatal, household, occupational, or sexual transmission	Bites by infected mosquitoes	Close respiratory contact	Bites by infected mosquitoes
Transmission period	As long as sputum acid-fast bacilli are positive	Usually under two weeks; some chronic carriers	No person-to-person transmission	Usually under three weeks (starts before cough is apparent)	A few days before and after acute symptoms	Four days before rash until two days afterward	A few days before to seven days after rash; up to one year of age in congenitally infected	Chronic carriage for months	Up to lifelong chronic carriage and transmission	Infected individuals can transmit the disease when bitten by a mosquito vector during the viremic phase (the first three or four days of illness)	Chronic carriage for months	Unknown, rare cases for several months
Subclinical infection	Common but not important in transmission	Common	No	Mild illness common: may not be diagnosed	More than 100 subclinical infections for each paralytic case	May occur in children under one, but relative importance is minimal	Common	Common	Common, especially in infants	Common	Common	Common
Duration of natural immunity	Not known; reactivation of old infection commonly causes disease	Lasting protective immunity not produced by infection; second attack possible	Lasting protective immunity not produced by infection; second attack possible	Incomplete and waning protection	Lifelong type-specific immunity	Lifelong	Lifelong	Uncertain; no protection against carriage and those previously infected may develop some disease (epiglottitis)	If develops, lifelong	Lifelong	Uncertain; no protection against carriage	Lifelong

	Tuberculosis	Diphtheria	Tetanus	Pertussis	Poliomyelitis	Measles	Rubella	Hepatitis B	Haemophilus influenzae type b	Yellow fever	Meningococcal meningitis	Japanese encephalitis
Risk factors for infection (for unvaccinated individuals)	High population densities in regions with historically poor control; low socioeconomic status; poor access to care; immunodeficiency; malnutrition; alcoholism; diabetes	Crowding; low socioeconomic status	Wound contaminated by soil; umbilical cord; agricultural work	Young age; crowding	Poor environmental hygiene and sanitation	Highly transmissible agent with nearly 100 percent infectivity except for isolated populations; crowding, low socioeconomic status	Highly transmissible; crowding; low socioeconomic status	Carrier mother, sibling, or sex partner; multiple sex partners; intravenous drug use; unsafe injection practices	Failure to breastfeed; crowding; low socioeconomic status; immune deficiency, including HIV	Young age; forest workers; season (late rainy season, early dry season)	Crowding; respiratory viral infections, especially influenza	Young age; forest workers; season
Case-fatality rate[b]	See chapter 16	2 to 20 percent	25 to 90 percent	Up to 10 percent in infants and children	2 to 10 percent	0.05 to 10.0 percent	Less than 0.1 percent	Acute, more than 1 percent; chronic, 25 percent (delayed)	Meningitis, 5 to 90 percent; pneumonia 5 to 25 percent	10 to 40 percent	Untreated 90 to 100 percent; treated 5 to 20 percent	5 to 30 percent
Vaccine (number of doses); route	BCG attenuated Mycobacterium bovis (1); intradermal	Diphtheria toxoid (three to five primary including booster doses in most countries); intramuscular	Tetanus toxoid (three to five in children, including booster doses in many countries; five for women of childbearing age; adult boosters for injury prevention); intramuscular	Killed whole-cell or acellular pertussis (three to five, including booster doses in most countries); intramuscular	Live (OPV) (three to four primary plus campaigns)[c] killed (IPV) (three to four)	Measles (two); subcutaneous	Rubella (one or two); subcutaneous	Hepatitis B surface antigen (three to four); intramuscular	Capsular polysaccharide linked to protein Hib (three to five); intramuscular	Yellow fever attenuated live virus (1 plus boosters); subcutaneous	Vaccines for A, C, Y, W135 only; unconjugated polysaccharides given subcutaneously or intramuscularly; one dose with repeat three to five years later for high-risk persons; conjugated: for C only or A, C, Y, + W135, one dose given intramuscularly	Live attenuated (two, China only); killed (two); booster commonly used but of uncertain value
Vaccine efficacy	0 to 80 percent for pulmonary tuberculosis; 75 to 86 percent for meningitis and miliary tuberculosis	More than 87 percent	More than 95 percent (more than 80 percent after two doses) in infants	70 to 90 percent	OPV: more than 95 percent in industrial countries; 72 to 98 percent in developing countries; lower protection against type 3 than 1 and 2; IPV: more than 95 percent	95 percent at 12 months of age; 85 percent at 9 months of age from one dose, more than 98 percent from two doses	95 percent (at 12 months and up)	75 to 95 percent; efficacy against chronic infection in infants born to carrier mothers; more than 95 percent for exposure at older ages	More than 95 percent for invasive disease	90 to 98 percent	Unconjugated polysaccharides: poor efficacy under two years of age; conjugated polysaccharides: approximately 95 percent and up serogroup specific	Live attenuated: 90 percent (after one dose at one year); 94 to 100 percent (after two doses one to two months apart); inactivated: 80 percent (declining to 55 percent after one year; no decrease in another study)

(Continues on the following page.)

Table 20.1 Continued

Category	Tuberculosis	Diphtheria	Tetanus	Pertussis	Poliomyelitis	Measles[a]	Rubella	Hib	Hepatitis B	Yellow fever	Meningococcal disease	Japanese encephalitis
Duration of immunity after primary series	Unknown; some evidence that immunity wanes with time	Variable: probably around five years; longer in presence of natural boosting or booster doses	10 years or more	Unknown; wanes with time	Presumed lifelong for both OPV and IPV, but unknown	Lifelong in most; rare cases of waning immunity after one dose, not two	Lifelong in most; presumed rare cases of waning immunity after one dose, not two	Unknown, but lasts for at least three years beyond period of greatest exposure	More than 15 years; further follow-up is continuing	For at least 10 years and possibly for life	Unconjugated wanes rapidly for children under five, more than three to five years for older children; conjugated uncertain	Unknown, may be lifelong
Schedule	Given at or near birth in populations at high risk	Three-dose schedule recommended at 6, 10, and 14 weeks in developing countries for DTP vaccine; other schedules in common use; booster doses at 18 months and four to six years also suggested	Normally given as DTP vaccine to children; unimmunized pregnant women should be given two doses of tetanus toxoid or tetanus-reduced diphtheria toxoid, and a total of five doses is required to provide protection through all childbearing years	Usually given in childhood as combination vaccine (DTP)	OPV: four doses (birth, 6, 10, and 14 weeks) in polio-endemic countries; birth dose may be omitted elsewhere with fourth dose given later; supplemental doses (up to 10) given in national campaigns for eradication; IPV: three to four doses: 2, 4, 6 to 18 months, and four to six years	First dose at 9 or 12 to 15 months]; a second opportunity to receive a dose of measles vaccine (either through routine [18 months or four to six years] or supplemental immunization activities) should be provided for all children	First dose at 12 to 15 months; when given, a second dose with measles vaccine	Three or four doses; usually given during the same visit as for DTP	Several schedules: at birth, 6, and 14 weeks; with first three doses of DTP, birth dose needed if mother is a carrier and recommended if perinatal transmission of hepatitis B is frequent; four doses total can be given although only three are required	One dose at 9 to 12 months with measles in countries where yellow fever poses a risk	Unconjugated: one dose at two years or older and second dose three to five years later for high risk; conjugate C: three doses at two, three, and four or two, four, and six months for infants; one dose for older children and adults; conjugate A, C, Y, W135 currently only approved for one dose at 11 years or older	Live: one year and two years; killed: days 0, 7, and 30 followed by booster two years later and then every three years

Status as of the end of 2001	158 countries using BCG; 85 percent coverage	All countries; 78 percent coverage	Childhood: all countries; 78 percent coverage	All countries; 78 percent coverage	All countries; 79 percent routine, plus supplemental coverage	Routine first dose all countries, 77 percent coverage; second opportunity, 164 out of 192 countries	110 countries in 2003	89 countries; global coverage less than 18 percent	147 countries; global coverage 42 percent	29 of 43 countries at risk using vaccine; 30 percent coverage in target population	European countries, Canada (and United States in 2005)	Southeast Asia
Comments	Reasons for varying efficacy are multifactorial, including differences in vaccines	Recent trends to lower antibody levels in adults without booster doses because of waning immunity and less natural boosting	Five doses in adults provide protection for more than 20 years	Variability in whole cell vaccines; acellular vaccines used in some developed countries	Primary series gives incomplete protection in developing countries	Lower efficacy when maternal antibody present	Lower efficacy when maternal antibody present	None	Efficacy lower if injected into fat	None	None	None

Sources: WHO 2002, 2004.

DTP = diphtheria-tetanus-pertussis; IPV = inactivated polio vaccine; OPV = oral polio vaccine.

a. Measles vaccine is given as measles, measles-rubella, or measles-mumps-rubella vaccine. The latter two vaccines are routinely used in industrial countries and are increasingly being adopted in other countries. The World Health Organization recommends that the combination measles-rubella or measles-mumps-rubella vaccines be introduced only after careful evaluation of public health priorities within each country and following the establishment of an adequate program for measles control as demonstrated by high coverage rates as part of a well-functioning childhood immunization program.

b. Note that variations in case-fatality rates are related to access to care, type of care administered, setting, age at onset of disease, and other factors. The ranges presented in this table reflect both uncertainty as to actual case-fatality rates and the variability of populations.

c. As of 2003, an injected IPV is given alone or in combination with OPV in 31 countries. IPV is currently not recommended for routine use in developing countries because of its relatively high cost and uncertain efficacy when given at 6, 10, and 14 weeks. The usual recommended IPV schedule is 2, 4, and 6 to 18 months. Routine use of OPV is expected to cease following polio eradication. Stockpiles of monovalent OPV for each of the three virus types are under development to protect against vaccine-associated paralytic poliomyelitis and outbreaks of circulating vaccine-derived polioviruses.

in use in childhood immunization programs throughout the world.

Burden of Vaccine-Preventable Diseases

A number of vaccine-preventable diseases are not reportable events in many countries. The estimates of the burden of disease by the World Health Organization (WHO) are based on a combination of often incomplete vital registration data, mortality survey data, and mathematical models using numerous assumptions. Most models of vaccine-preventable diseases are derived from the susceptible fraction of the population (calculated from natural immunity from presumed historical infections in regions without previous vaccination and historical immunization coverage rates), infectivity rates of disease, sequelae of diseases, and estimates of local CFRs. The degree of accuracy of these models is only as good as the data supporting the assumptions. The disease burden is most appropriately represented by a range of values reflecting uncertainty. In this chapter, we estimate the burden of disease as the number of deaths and DALYs per World Bank region in 2001. The following description draws in part on discussion of methods for burden of disease calculations reflected in the Global Immunization and Vision Strategy of WHO and the United Nations Children's Fund (UNICEF) (Wolfson and Lydon 2005).

Diphtheria

Diphtheria is caused by a toxin-producing strain of the bacterium *Corynebacterium diphtheriae,* which is transmitted by means of respiratory droplets. The 2001 WHO estimates of diphtheria mortality are extrapolations from reported deaths in countries with full or partial vital registration systems.

Before the widespread use of immunization, more than 5 percent of people living in temperate climates suffered from clinical diphtheria at some point during their lifetimes (Griffith 1979). Rates exceeding 100 cases per 100,000 population were seen in Europe during World War II (Galazka, Robertson, and Oblapenko 1995). The CFRs from respiratory tract diphtheria have been 2 to 20 percent, with an average of 10 percent for patients receiving good medical care (Feigin, Stechenberg, and Hertel 2004). To estimate diphtheria deaths in the absence of vaccination and to project future deaths with and without vaccination, we assumed an average incidence rate of 15 per 100,000 and CFRs of 2.5 percent in developed countries, 5.0 percent in Europe and Central Asia, and 10.0 percent elsewhere (Birmingham and Stein 2003; Galazka and Robertson forthcoming).

Tetanus

Clostridium tetani is maintained in nature and is found in all countries. Spores remain viable for many years in soil and dust,

especially in areas contaminated by animal feces (Cherry and Harrison 2004). The organism is usually transmitted through burns, cuts, and other penetrating injuries. Neonatal tetanus is the most common presentation in developing countries. The portal of entry is usually the umbilical stump but has been associated with circumcision and other surgical procedures (Birmingham and others 2004; Stanfield and Galazka 1984). Children born to women who do not have protective levels of tetanus antibody are susceptible to neonatal tetanus.

The estimated burden of neonatal tetanus assumes that in areas with low rates of skilled delivery, all births not protected by the immunization of pregnant women are subject to a preimmunization era neonatal tetanus mortality rate expressed as deaths per 1,000 live births (Birmingham and others 2004; Griffiths and others 2004). In other areas, we assume that births not protected through immunization or skilled delivery are subject to an incidence and CFR equal to 25 percent of the preimmunization era neonatal tetanus mortality rate.[1]

CFRs are directly associated with the quality of medical care available. With the availability of secondary and tertiary care, CFRs have declined to 25 percent or less (Cherry and Harrison 2004; Wassilak and others 2004). The CFRs used to derive cases from estimated deaths range from 40 percent in developed countries to 80 percent in the poorest developing countries. We estimate the tetanus burden other than for neonates by applying an estimated age distribution of total tetanus to the estimated neonatal tetanus deaths (Galazka and others forthcoming) and region-specific CFRs, which indicate a range of from 27 percent among children age one to four in developed countries to 65 percent among those age 80 or older in developing countries.

Pertussis

Bordetella pertussis is transmitted through respiratory excretions and occurs throughout the world. Most pertussis in developing countries occurs in school-age children. In developed countries, mild or asymptomatic infections in adults are believed to be common sources of transmission to very young infants (Edwards and Decker 2004). Clinical manifestations include an initial 7 to 10 days of rhinorrhea progressing to a cough that becomes paroxysmal or spasmodic, usually associated with profuse rhinorrhea (Cherry and Heininger 2004). Clinical pneumonia is seen in approximately 10 percent of infants.

Our estimates for the burden of pertussis followed the model described in Crowcroft and others (2003). We estimated that the proportion of susceptible children becoming infected in countries with vaccination coverage of less than 70 percent over the previous five years was 30 percent by age 1, 80 percent by age 5, and 100 percent by age 15. For countries with coverage of more than 70 percent in the past five years, we assumed that 10 percent of susceptible children were infected by age 1, 60 percent by age 5, and 100 percent by age 15. A vaccine efficacy of 80 percent was assumed for preventing infection and 95 percent for preventing deaths. The CFR was 0.20 percent in infants, 0.04 percent in children age one to four, and 0 percent in those older than five in low-mortality countries; and 3.7 percent among infants, 1 percent among children age one to four, and 0 percent in those older than five in high-mortality countries.

Poliomyelitis

Before the availability of polio vaccines, as many as 90 percent of children in the developing world were infected with all three types of the polio virus in the first two or three years of life (Sutter and Kew 2004). In developed countries, transmission occurred primarily in school-age children and more than 90 percent of infections were asymptomatic; 4 to 8 percent of children had nonspecific febrile illness and less than 1 percent developed acute flaccid paralysis (Sutter and Kew 2004).

Children with residual paralysis require rehabilitation. Surgical intervention is necessary if contractures develop because of the lack of rehabilitative services following the acute illness. These children are at increased risk of premature death because of late onset postpolio muscle atrophy (postpolio syndrome), which occurs 20 to 40 or more years after acute illness.

Disease burden estimates are based on actual active surveillance. The estimated 1,000 deaths a year caused by polio reflect past infections and current deaths. Following Robertson (1993), we obtained the number of cases and deaths in the absence of immunization by applying an incidence rate of 1 per 1,000 population under age five and CFRs of from 2.5 percent in developed countries to 10.0 percent in Sub-Saharan Africa. To determine current cases, we applied an estimate of notification efficiency to reported cases.

Measles

Measles is an acute respiratory viral infection. Children born to immune mothers are protected against clinical measles from passively acquired maternal antibodies until they are five to nine months of age. More than 90 percent of infections are associated with clinical disease (Krugman 1963). Complications include pneumonia, diarrhea, encephalitis, and blindness, especially in children with vitamin A deficiency. In recent years, CFRs have been estimated at 3 percent in many developing countries, but historically they have been as high as 30 percent in some community-based studies (Aaby 1988; Aaby and Clements 1989; Moss, Clements, and Halsey 2003; Perry and Halsey 2004).

For a disease such as measles in which infection is almost universal in the absence of immunity, small changes in the CFR result in large changes in estimates of total mortality. Increased complication and mortality rates occur in children who are younger than five, vitamin A deficient, or infected with HIV or who have acquired measles from a household contact (Perry and Halsey 2004). Declines in CFRs in the past two decades are associated with the tendency of the disease to infect older children, decreased crowding, and improved nutritional status in many developing countries (Perry and Halsey 2004). At the same time, recent studies indicate CFRs of 0.4 to 9.7 percent in Sub-Saharan African countries with low immunization coverage (Perry forthcoming).

Considerable controversy is associated with the number of deaths resulting from measles, because of difficulty in accurately specifying the cause of death in children afflicted with measles and in separating complications of measles from those of other conditions. In addition, CFRs, which have decreased rapidly in many countries, vary significantly. The natural history model used in this chapter is based on Stein and others (2003), modified to account for the effect of supplementary immunization activities.

We derived estimates of the burden of disease in countries with high-quality surveillance data and high sustained coverage of measles vaccine by adjusting the number of reported cases by a reporting efficiency factor ranging from 5 to 40 percent. In estimating the future burden of disease, the averted burden of disease, and the burden in countries without both adequate surveillance and sustained high coverage, we assumed that the average number of cases per year is equal to the number of children in the current birth cohort who are not protected by either routine or supplemental vaccination. WHO (2005a) estimates that in 2001, 611,000 deaths (approximately 5 percent of all childhood mortality) were attributable to measles.

An alternative proportional mortality approach, which is based on retrospective verbal autopsy studies in 18 countries to derive the proportional causes of child deaths in 42 high-mortality countries, also has appeared in the literature (Morris, Black, and Tomaskovic 2003). This model suggests that measles may have accounted for approximately 3 percent of all childhood deaths in 2000.

In countries with a high disease burden, the true number of measles deaths may be somewhere between the proportional mortality and natural history estimates. WHO (2005b) uses a hybrid method that estimates that measles was responsible for an average of 4 percent of mortality among children under five between 2000 and 2003, or approximately 400,000 deaths per year. If the actual number of deaths in 2001 was 400,000, then the cost per death averted will be lower than what has been estimated for this chapter, and the effect of increasing coverage will be overestimated because fewer deaths could be prevented.

Both of the approaches described have strengths and limitations. We adopt the natural history approach for this analysis because the chapter includes deaths at all ages and the model can adapt to recent changes in CFRs and coverage rates.

However, the natural history method is sensitive to the accuracy of parameter inputs such as CFRs and may underestimate the effect of herd immunity. Further modeling efforts would need to incorporate sensitivity testing around a range of parameter estimates.

In the absence of vaccination, the measles virus would infect almost 100 percent of the population, including most of the 688 million children under five in the developing world. Using the methods described here, approximately 125 million cases and 1.8 million to 2.0 million deaths per year would be expected in the absence of vaccination.

Haemophilus influenzae Type b (Hib)

Hib is transmitted through the respiratory tract and causes meningitis, pneumonia, septic arthritis, skin infections, epiglottitis, osteomyelitis, and sepsis. Deaths caused by Hib occur primarily from meningitis and pneumonia. In developed countries, approximately half of diagnosed invasive infections are meningitis (Wenger and Ward 2004). In developing countries, a larger proportion of identified cases is meningitis resulting from underdiagnosis of other clinical syndromes (Martin and others 2004; Peltola 2000). Intervention studies have demonstrated significant reductions in pneumonia in vaccinated compared with unvaccinated children (Levine and others 1998; Mulholland and others 1997). Although infections occur throughout the world, the incidence of Hib disease may be lower in some Asian countries than in Africa and the Americas (Gessner and others 2005).

We derived estimates of Hib disease burden from incidence rates and CFRs for meningitis and pneumonia. We derived country-specific estimates of the incidence of Hib meningitis from the literature on incidence in the prevaccine era (Bennett and others 2002). For countries without meningitis incidence data, we used the average incidence in countries with similar epidemiological profiles. Regional averages ranged from 219 cases per 100,000 to 3 per 100,000 population in children under one, and 1 to 15 per 100,000 population in children age one to four. The CFR for meningitis is nearly 100 percent in the absence of intensive antibiotic therapy, but it can be reduced to 5 to 8 percent when appropriate therapy is available (Swartz 2004). We derived CFRs in a manner similar to that used for incidence rates and adjusted them on the basis of country-specific data on access to care. Regional means ranged from 3 to 32 percent.

Estimating the burden of Hib pneumonia is much more complex. A rapid assessment method assumes five pneumonia cases for every meningitis case (WHO 2001). An alternative approach assumes that Hib is responsible for a fixed proportion (about 20 percent) of acute lower respiratory infection deaths in the absence of immunization (Peltola 2000). We derived pneumonia CFRs from a literature review of lower respiratory infections in children (Bennett and others 2002), with average CFRs ranging from 1 percent among infants in developed countries to 12 percent in Sub-Saharan Africa.

Hepatitis B

In many developed countries, most transmission of hepatitis B occurs during or after adolescence, coinciding with the onset of sexual activity and of drug abuse involving unsafe reuse of needles and syringes (McQuillan and others 1999). In many African countries, transmission occurs primarily in early childhood through mucosal contact with infectious body fluids and unsafe injection practices (Margolis, Alter, and Hadler 1997). Some Asian countries have a high rate of chronic carrier states, and the primary mode of transmission is mothers to infants (Beasley 1988; Mast and others 2004). The rate of symptomatic disease is only about 1 percent in infancy and 10 percent in early childhood, but it increases to 30 to 40 percent in adults. Serosurveys for carrier states of hepatitis B are available for almost all nations (WHO 1996).

Models of hepatitis B disease burden are based on estimated ratios between infected and carriage states at various ages or estimates of the percentage of carriers that progress to hepatoma, fulminant hepatitis, or cirrhosis at later stages of life (Miller and McCann 2000). The model we used for estimating hepatitis B mortality estimates the age- and sex-specific progression of hepatitis B surface antigen infection to disease incorporating competing mortality, particularly because individuals infected with HIV are more likely to perish from HIV before the full mortality impact from hepatitis B infection (Gay and others 2001; Griffiths, Hutton, and Pascoal 2005).

Whereas most vaccine-preventable diseases that result in death occur at an early age shortly after the age of vaccination, deaths from hepatitis B occur many years into the future. Countries that introduce hepatitis B vaccines today will not reap most of the benefits for many years. In the absence of vaccination, we estimated approximately 1.4 million future deaths attributable to hepatitis B for the 2001 birth cohort after accounting for competing mortality. Global vaccination of 35 percent would prevent more than 500,000 of those future deaths. Discounting the value of future hepatitis B deaths to their equivalent value in the present to make the burden of disease prevented equivalent to that of other vaccine-preventable diseases results in approximately 87,000 deaths averted.

Yellow Fever

Yellow fever virus is transmitted by mosquitoes, primarily *Aedes eqypti*, with a three- to six-day incubation period. Patients present with intense headache, fever, chills, and myalgia, among other symptoms. Although once much more widespread, yellow fever is now limited to West and Central Africa, the northern half of South America, and Panama. In approximately

15 to 20 percent of yellow fever patients, severe disease occurs, with liver and kidney failure and cardiovascular collapse. The CFR varies, with increased severity in older adults (Monath 2004). The average CFR in patients in Africa with jaundice is 20 percent (Monath and others 1980; Nasidi and others 1989).

On the basis of surveillance data adjusted for underreporting, WHO (1992) estimates the global burden of yellow fever at 200,000 cases and 30,000 deaths in 1990. Most cases and deaths occur in 33 African countries, where 1 in 80 cases is assumed to be reported. In South American countries, 1 in 10 cases is assumed to be reported. We use the implied incidence rate and a CFR of 15 percent to project future mortality. Between 1990 and 2001, some improvement in routine coverage of yellow fever vaccine occurred, but the overall burden of yellow fever is unlikely to have declined.

ESTIMATES OF THE CURRENT BURDEN OF VACCINE-PREVENTABLE DISEASES AND OF THE BURDEN AVERTED BY VACCINATION

Table 20.2 provides WHO estimates of deaths from selected vaccine-preventable diseases for 2001, taking immunization coverage rates into account. The greatest burden of disease is in Sub-Saharan Africa, which accounts for 58 percent of pertussis deaths, 41 percent of tetanus deaths, 59 percent of measles deaths, and 80 percent of yellow fever deaths. East Asia and the Pacific has the greatest burden from hepatitis B, with 62 percent of deaths worldwide. South Asia also experienced a high disease burden, particularly for tetanus and measles.

Table 20.2 also shows the extent of mortality in the absence of immunization and the estimated number of deaths averted by vaccination. In 2001, vaccination averted up to 52 percent of yellow fever deaths, 61 percent of measles deaths, 69 percent of tetanus deaths, 78 percent of pertussis deaths, 94 percent of diphtheria deaths, and 98 percent of polio deaths that would have occurred in the absence of vaccination. These results demonstrate the significant effect that vaccination programs have had on worldwide disease burden. The figures also show that vaccination programs have been less successful in reducing the disease burden in Sub-Saharan Africa, where coverage rates are lower.

Table 20.3 reports WHO estimates of disability-adjusted life years (DALYs) lost from vaccine-preventable diseases by region for 2001, demonstrating the high burden of disease worldwide from disability associated with sequelae of hepatitis B (liver cancer and cirrhosis), pertussis, and tetanus.[2]

EXPANDED PROGRAM ON IMMUNIZATION

WHO initiated the EPI in 1974 to provide countries with guidance and support to improve vaccine delivery and to help make vaccines available for all children (Hadler and others 2004;

Turk 1982; WHO 1974). A standard immunization schedule was established in 1984 on the basis of a review of immunological data for the original EPI vaccines: BCG, diphtheria-tetanus-pertussis (DTP), oral polio, and measles vaccines (Halsey and Galazka 1985).

Today, national immunization programs in developing countries are responsible for improving access to the traditional EPI antigens and introducing new vaccines. In 2002, the EPI introduced the Reaching Every District strategy, which focused on achieving an 80 percent coverage rate of DTP3 in 80 percent of districts and using immunization contacts to deliver other high-priority child health interventions. In addition to delivering vaccinations, national immunization programs are concerned with the quality and safety of immunization through the adoption of safe injection technologies (autodisabled syringes, storage boxes, and incinerators) and proper cold chain and vaccine stock maintenance.

In most developing countries, immunizations are provided through a system of fixed facilities at different levels of the health system. Immunization campaigns are discrete, time-limited efforts at national or subnational levels that usually focus on specific antigens (for example, polio). Mobile strategies rely on the use of specialized vehicles to transport health professionals and vaccines to deliver services to remote or migrating populations. Outreach is a strategy by which staff members from a health facility travel to villages and surrounding areas to administer vaccines. Extended outreach refers to more targeted and intensive efforts.

In 1999, the major international development partners involved in immunization (for example, WHO, UNICEF, the World Bank, and bilateral donors) joined the Bill & Melinda Gates and Rockefeller Foundations, the vaccine industry, and nongovernmental organizations to create GAVI (http://www.vaccinealliance.org) to increase access to new and underused vaccines in the world's poorest countries, improve access to basic immunization services, and accelerate research and development pertaining to new vaccines and delivery technology. Through the Vaccine Fund, GAVI raised more than US$1.3 billion to strengthen immunization systems, introduce new vaccines, and support safe injection practices. More than US$3 billion has been pledged for the next 10 years. Between 2000 and 2003, an additional 4 million children were vaccinated with DTP3, 42 million with hepatitis B, nearly 5 million with Hib, and more than 3 million with yellow fever vaccine.

COSTS AND COST-EFFECTIVENESS OF EXISTING VACCINATION PROGRAMS

Brenzel and Claquin (1994) and GAVI (2004) estimate the cost per fully immunized child (FIC) for the traditional six EPI antigens as approximately US$20.[3] We evaluated the cost per

Table 20.2 Estimated Number of Deaths in the Absence of Vaccination, Deaths from Vaccine-Preventable Diseases, and Deaths Averted by Vaccination, All Ages, by Region and Vaccine, 2001
(thousands)

Disease	Total	High income	East Asia and the Pacific	Europe and Central Asia	Latin America and the Caribbean	Middle East and North Africa	South Asia	Sub-Saharan Africa
Diphtheria								
If no vaccination	78	3	28	4	8	5	21	10
Estimated deaths	5	<1	1	<1	<1	<1	3	1
Deaths averted	73	3	27	4	8	5	18	9
Pertussis								
If no vaccination	1,343	7	377	4	138	93	428	296
Estimated deaths	301	<1	3	<1	6	8	108	176
Deaths averted	1,042	7	374	4	132	85	320	120
Tetanus								
If no vaccination	936	<1	110	<1	20	23	543	239
Estimated deaths	293	<1	27	<1	1	4	140	121
Deaths averted	643	<1	83	<1	19	19	403	118
Poliomyelitis								
If no vaccination	52	1	15	1	3	4	17	11
Estimated deaths[a]	<1	<1	<1	0	0	0	0	0
Deaths averted	51	n.a.	15	1	3	4	17	11
Measles								
If no vaccination	2,000	6	301	36	6	55	567	1,025
Estimated deaths[b]	676	<1	77	4	<1	7	239	348
Deaths averted	1,237	5	229	28	6	40	351	578
Hib								
If no vaccination	468	<1	28	2	9	14	199	216
Estimated deaths	463	<1	28	2	5	14	199	215
Deaths averted	5	<1	<1	<1	4	<1	<1	1
Hepatitis B								
If no vaccination	600	34	370	36	11	17	75	58
Estimated deaths	600	34	370	36	11	17	75	58
Deaths averted[c]	<1	<1	<1	<1	<1	<1	<1	<1
Yellow fever								
If no vaccination	63	n.a.	n.a.	n.a.	8	n.a.	n.a.	54
Estimated deaths	30	n.a.	n.a.	n.a.	6	n.a.	n.a.	24
Deaths averted	33	n.a.	n.a.	n.a.	2	n.a.	n.a.	30

Source: Mathers and others 2006 and authors' calculations.
n.a. = not available.
Note: Totals may not add due to rounding.
a. Primarily deaths at older ages caused by delayed effect of poliomyelitis in childhood.
b. See text for discussion of uncertainty regarding measles estimates. The values shown here are an updated version of the 2001 estimates.
c. Deaths averted to date from the use of the hepatitis B vaccine in infant immunization programs are minimal, largely because of the long time period (20 to 40 years) to see mortality effects.

Table 20.3 DALYs Lost from Vaccine-Preventable Diseases, All Ages By Region, 2001 *(thousands)*

Disease	Total	High income	East Asia and the Pacific	Europe and Central Asia	Latin America and the Caribbean	Middle East and North Africa	South Asia	Sub-Saharan Africa
Diphtheria	164	<1	18	2	8	1	90	45
Tetanus	8,342	5	762	2	17	110	3,965	3,481
Pertussis	11,542	139	584	81	366	326	3,930	6,116
Poliomyelitis	145	8	49	2	6	8	55	17
Measles	23,129	23	2,318	236	13	470	6,527	13,539
Hepatitis B[a]								
Acute hepatitis B	2,169	86	675	79	95	111	585	536
Liver cancer	9,168	1,223	5,925	379	277	138	464	762
Cirrhosis of the liver	15,780	2,146	3,890	2,084	1,513	686	4,249	1,212
Meningitis[b]	5,607	131	1,071	403	591	328	2,142	941
Lower respiratory infections[c]	85,920	2,314	10,827	2,111	3,043	2,974	34,196	30,455

Source: Mathers and others 2006 and Authors' calculations.

Note: Totals may not add due to rounding.

a. Includes all DALYs attributable to the three conditions. Hepatitis B is the underlying cause of only a portion of the liver cancer and cirrhosis of the liver DALYs.

b. Includes all DALYs attributable to meningitis, including Hib, *S. pneumococcus*, and *N. meningitides*.

c. Includes all DALYs attributable to lower respiratory infections, including Hib and *S. pneumococcus*.

FIC for the childhood EPI cluster antigens by World Bank region on the basis of published and unpublished data. These studies used a standard costing approach that estimated the costs of labor, vaccines, supplies, transportation, communication, training, maintenance, and overhead and included the annualized value of equipment, vehicles, and building space (Khaleghian 2001; USAID, Asia–Near East Region 1988; WHO 1988). The number of FICs in these studies was measured using community-based sample surveys (Henderson and Sundaresen 1982).

Our literature review found 102 estimates of total and unit immunization program costs from 27 countries between 1979 and 2003 for different immunization delivery strategies (Berman and others 1991;1 Beutels 1998, 2001; Brenzel 2005; Brenzel and Claquin 1994; Brinsmead, Hill, and Walker 2004; Creese 1986; Creese and Domínguez-Ugá 1987; Domínguez-Ugá 1988; Edmunds and others 2000; Griffiths and others 2004; Levin and others 2001; Pegurri, Fox-Rushby, and Walker 2005; Robertson and others 1992; Soucat and others 1997; Steinglass, Brenzel, and Percy 1993). All costs were converted to 2001 U.S. dollar equivalents. Because total and unit costs are related to population size, table 20.4 reports population-weighted results only. National immunization program refers to total national costs for all strategies.

The population-weighted mean cost per FIC for all regions and all strategies is approximately US$17, with a range of US$3 to US$31. The lowest mean population-weighted cost per FIC

was for extended outreach services (US$5.81), perhaps because the strategy is a more targeted approach. Routine facility-based strategies had lower average costs (US$13.65 per FIC) than campaigns (US$26.82 per FIC) or mobile strategies (US$25.84 per FIC). Higher unit costs associated with these strategies are possibly attributable to a different mix of inputs as well as greater expenses for per diems, fuel, and social mobilization. The results also vary by World Bank region, with East Asia and the Pacific (US$13.25) and Sub-Saharan Africa (US$14.21) having lower estimates of cost per FIC than Europe and Central Asia (US$24.12) and the Middle East and North Africa (US$22.15).

The findings of our analysis are generally supported by the literature (Creese 1986; Brenzel and Claquin 1994; Khaleghian 2001), which has shown that variation in the cost per FIC is related to the mix of delivery strategies, the prices of key inputs such as vaccines, and the overall scale of programs. In addition, an analysis of 13 national financial sustainability plans for immunization reveals a wide range in the cost per FIC by region and strategy.[4]

Recurrent costs are the lion's share of total immunization costs (80 percent for fixed facility strategy and 92 percent for campaigns), which has implications for the need for continuous and predictable program financing. Labor costs account for the largest share (roughly 30 to 46 percent of total cost) for all strategies except extended outreach. Vaccine costs range from 8 percent for mobile strategies to 29 percent for extended

Table 20.4 Estimates of the Population-Weighted Annual Cost for the Traditional Vaccines per FIC, by Immunization Strategy and Region, 2001
(2001 US$)

Strategy	East Asia and the Pacific (*n* = 4)	Europe and Central Asia (*n* = 1)	Latin America and the Caribbean (*n* = 1)	Middle East and North Africa (*n* = 1)	South Asia (*n* = 10)	Sub-Saharan Africa (*n* = 15)	All regions (*n* = 32)
National immunization program	—	—	18.10	22.15	24.82 (23–27) *n* = 2	21.05 (17–26) *n* = 2	23.52 (17–27) *n* = 6
Fixed facility	20.00 (18–22) *n* = 2	24.12	—	—	13.79 (6–24) *n* = 7	6.31 (3–31) *n* = 6	13.65 (3–31) *n* = 16
Campaign	—	—	—	—	—	26.82 (13–28) *n* = 3	26.82 (13–28) *n* = 3
Mobile	—	—	—	—	—	25.84 *n* = 1	25.84 *n* = 1
Outreach	6.50 (4–9) *n* = 2	—	—	—	7.11 *n* = 1	—	7.10 (4–9) *n* = 3
Extended outreach	—	—	—	—	—	5.81 (5.8–13) *n* = 3	5.81 (5.8–13) *n* = 3
Mean for all strategies	13.25 (4–22)	24.12	18.10	22.15	17.11 (6–27)	14.21 (3–31)	16.91 (3–31)

Source: Authors' calculations for the traditional vaccines based on the literature.

— = not available.

Note: Mean values are used in the analysis. Ranges for estimates are reported in parentheses. Europe and Central Asia, Latin America and the Caribbean, and the Middle East and North Africa are limited to one observation for each region, which may not be indicative of the cost per FIC in each region. However, in lieu of using region-specific estimates, the overall average (US$13.65) would be applied, which may underestimate the cost per FIC in these more developed regions, where higher unit costs for delivery of health services would be expected.

outreach strategies. Transportation costs account for the second-largest share of EPI costs for mobile strategies, while building costs account for a greater share of fixed facility strategies.

Using data from table 20.4 on costs per FIC and multiplying by the size of the population covered, we estimate US$1.17 billion for the total cost of immunization programs in developing countries in 2001, with a range of US$717 million to US$1.48 billion. At US$20 per FIC, the cost of the six traditional vaccines in developing countries would have amounted to US$1.57 billion in 2001. Table 20.5 shows that the estimated cost per death averted ranges from US$205 in South Asia and Sub-Saharan Africa to US$3,540 in Europe and Central Asia. These results suggest that the cost per death averted rises with coverage rates. Europe and Central Asia, Latin America and the Caribbean, and the Middle East and North Africa had higher coverage rates in 2001, resulting in fewer deaths that could be averted. The table also shows that the cost per DALY from the traditional EPI vaccines ranges from US$7 to US$438, depending on region, mix of strategy, and levels of scale.

Our analysis highlights the variation in cost per FIC by region and strategy and demonstrates the value of more disaggregated results for making policy decisions. However, given the limited sample of estimates available for the regions and strategies, the results should be used as an indicative guide for policy making and not as a substitute for country-specific cost-effectiveness evaluations of strategies. In addition, our estimates do not take into account household costs, such as time spent seeking services, and other social costs. Our estimates also do not consider the direct and indirect costs of acute illnesses prevented by vaccination or the costs of long-term complications from disease and of adverse events associated with vaccination (though the latter are unlikely to have a significant impact on costs because rates of serious complications are extremely low). Furthermore, the analysis focuses on FICs and underemphasizes the benefits of partial immunization. Future economic evaluations of immunization program alternatives could consider these factors as a critical step in determining the allocation of scarce resources among high-priority health interventions.

Table 20.5 Average Cost per FIC, Total Immunization Cost, Cost per Death Averted and Cost per DALY for the Traditional Immunization Program by Region

Strategy	East Asia and the Pacific	Europe and Central Asia	Latin America and the Caribbean	Middle East and North Africa	South Asia	Sub-Saharan Africa
Cost/FIC (2001 US$) (from table 20.4)	13.25	24.12	18.10	22.15	17.11	14.21
Percentage of FIC	78.22	93.72	86.36	90.90	58.86	50.20
Estimated total immunization cost (2001 US$ millions)	316	131	174	152	227	172
Estimated deaths averted (thousands, from table 20.2)	728	37	174	153	1,109	867
Estimated cost/death averted (2001 US$)	434	3,540	1,030	993	205	205
Estimated cost/DALY (2001 US$)	85	395	438	166	16	7

Source: Authors' calculations.

Note: DALY estimates are the sum total for diphtheria, pertussis, tetanus, polio, and measles from table 20.3.

COST-EFFECTIVENESS OF INCREASING IMMUNIZATION COVERAGE FOR THE TRADITIONAL EPI

WHO (2004) estimates that in 2001, 30 million children were inadequately immunized with DTP. Achieving higher coverage rates by improving access for remote populations, accelerating immunization delivery strategies, and introducing new vaccines will mean increasing the level of investment (Batt, Fox-Rushby, and Castillo-Riquelme 2004).

We estimated the costs of scaling up EPI coverage for a hypothetical population of 1 million in each region between 2002 and 2011. Costs were reported in 2001 dollars, and a 3 percent discount rate was applied. Brenzel (2005) provides details on the methods. The costs of scaling up coverage are based on vaccine and delivery costs per dose. We derived vaccine costs from the unit price of each vaccine (provided by WHO, UNICEF, and the Vaccine Fund); wastage rates for vaccines and injection supplies by strategy; the required injection supplies; and the number of doses per FIC. A 2 percent adjustment was made for inflation. We used data on the cost per FIC generated earlier to derive delivery costs per dose by strategy and region by subtracting the costs of vaccines, injection supplies, and fixed costs.

Fixed costs were excluded from the scaling-up exercise because they were assumed to remain constant during the projection period.

- First, the largest projected coverage increase of 9 percentage points (figure 20.1) may not require additional infrastructure investments.
- Second, how and to what extent fixed costs would change by region is uncertain, and a conservative approach would be to exclude them.
- Third, because most immunization costs are recurrent costs, the analysis focuses on these.

Percentage of FICs

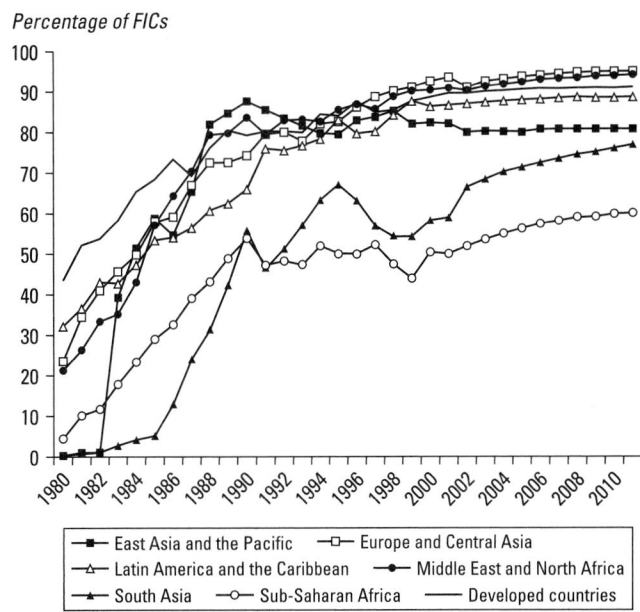

Source: Authors' estimation.

Figure 20.1 Coverage of FICs Projected to 2011

- Finally, because the scale factor is derived from the unit costs of a health center visit, the assumption of constant fixed costs in the short run appears reasonable.

Previous studies have found that the main cost drivers of immunization costs are the mix of strategies and the scale of immunization programs (Brenzel and Claquin 1994; Domínguez-Ugá 1988; Robertson and others 1992; Soucat and others 1997). Countries are unlikely to achieve 90 percent or more coverage relying on fixed facilities alone because of limited population access. We estimate the proportion of FICs obtained for each strategy by region.[5] The best mix of strategies for increasing coverage will vary by country depending on the dispersion of the population, the access to health facilities, the vaccines being delivered, and the effectiveness of various strategies in reaching target populations. Estimates are also adjusted for the level of scale by a factor derived from the unit cost per health center contact by coverage level (Mulligan and others 2003), and details are provided in Brenzel (2005).

The total additional cost of reaching higher coverage levels was divided by the number of deaths averted. Coverage projections for 2002–11 were based on statistical modeling of official WHO and UNICEF estimates for the period between 1995 and 2002 for all developing countries. The model relates coverage in future years to that in the previous year, with the relationship between past and future coverage differing for each region and economic status combination.

Figure 20.1 shows historical and projected coverage rates by region. The figure shows that coverage increased in all the regions during the late 1980s under universal childhood immunization. After 1990, when funding for universal childhood immunization waned, the figure indicates the subsequent stagnation and, in some cases, the declines in coverage rates. For the scaling-up period, we project that the coverage of FICs will increase from 78 to 79 percent in East Asia and the Pacific, from 92 to 95 percent in Europe and Central Asia, from 88 to 90 percent in Latin America and the Caribbean, from 91 to 95 percent in the Middle East and North Africa, from 70 to 79 percent in South Asia, and from 52 to 61 percent in Sub-Saharan Africa. The projections show that three of the six regions are expected to achieve 90 percent FIC by 2011. East Asia and the Pacific, South Asia, and Sub-Saharan Africa will require additional intensive efforts to achieve higher coverage rates.

Table 20.6 reports the results of the scaling-up analysis for the traditional EPI vaccines, for tetanus toxoid vaccination for women of reproductive age, and for selected new vaccines. The discounted incremental cost per child vaccinated with the traditional EPI vaccines ranges from US$10.89 in Latin America and the Caribbean to US$12.84 in the Middle East and North Africa. The number of discounted deaths averted because of full immunization depends on incremental coverage rates and varies from 747 in Europe and Central Asia to 14,584 in Sub-Saharan Africa, resulting in regional variations in the discounted incremental cost per death averted from US$169 in Sub-Saharan Africa to US$1,754 in Europe and Central Asia.[6]

DALYs were estimated indirectly based on the ratio of deaths to DALYs for each disease in 2001. This ratio is applied to the hypothetical population in each World Bank region over the projection period. Calculated this way, the number of DALYs averted will not account for changes in the average age of infection that ordinarily results from expanding immunization coverage. This method over-estimates the number of DALYs and thus under-estimates the cost/DALY. Cost-effectiveness ratios should be treated as indicative only. The cost/DALY ranges from $2 to $20 for scaling up traditional immunizations.

For tetanus toxoid immunization, the additional discounted cost per person vaccinated ranges from US$3.28 to US$4.06. The cost per death averted varies from US$271 to more than US$190,000. The results of this analysis fall within the range of estimates reported in the literature (Berman and others 1991; Steinglass, Brenzel, and Percy 1993). Differences in coverage levels and in protection against neonatal tetanus through skilled delivery contribute to the variation in results across regions.

The analysis shows both an increase in costs and potential benefits from scaling up immunization programs. In practice, the costs and benefits related to scaling up in any one region will be highly dependent on a few countries or subnational areas within countries. Aggregate country- or region-level data do not reveal the efficiency that could best be obtained by targeting immunization efforts on specific countries or geographic areas rather than making diffuse investments across regions. For instance, Miller and others (1998) show that India and Nigeria contribute the most to estimates of global measles deaths; therefore, reducing transmission in those countries would contribute the most to reducing the global disease burden caused by measles.

Despite its importance for policy, empirical and country-specific evidence on how immunization program costs change as coverage increases is lacking. Because scaling up immunization coverage will require more intensive efforts to find unvaccinated children, an extra cost for vaccinating each additional child is generally expected. Nevertheless, most cost-effectiveness studies assume constant returns to scale (Elbasha and Messonnier 2004; Karlsson and Johannesson 1998) even when emerging evidence suggests that the cost of vaccinating each additional child may rise with the size of delivery unit (Valdmanis, Walker, and Fox-Rushby 2003). Box 20.1, which focuses on scaling up traditional immunization coverage, and box 20.2, which focuses on new antigens, summarize the results of two studies that shed more light on this subject.

COSTS AND COST-EFFECTIVENESS OF ADDING NEW ANTIGENS TO THE CURRENT IMMUNIZATION SCHEDULE

We also estimated the additional costs per person vaccinated and cost per death averted of introducing new and underused vaccines into the traditional EPI in a hypothetical population of 1 million in each region between 2002 and 2011. The new vaccines considered protect against hepatitis B, yellow fever, Hib, measles, rubella, Japanese encephalitis, and meningococcal A, as well as inactivated polio vaccine (IPV). For comparison purposes, we assumed that new vaccines were introduced in 2002.

The additional cost of combination vaccines is net of the original cost of DTP vaccination to avoid duplication. The

Table 20.6 Average Cost per Person Vaccinated and per Death Averted for Scaling Up Immunization Coverage and Adding in Selected New Vaccines in a Hypothetical Population of 1 million for 2002–11
(2001 US$, current vaccine prices)

	East Asia and the Pacific	Europe and Central Asia	Latin America and the Caribbean	Middle East and North Africa	South Asia	Sub-Saharan Africa
Traditional EPI (mix of strategies)						
Incremental discounted cost/person vaccinated	12.03	11.54	10.89	12.84	11.58	11.16
Incremental discounted deaths averted	3,165	747	2,552	4,576	7,584	14,584
Incremental discounted cost/death averted	478	1,754	791	698	274	169
Tetanus toxoid (mix of strategies)						
Incremental discounted cost/person vaccinated	4.06	3.34	3.28	3.34	3.98	3.88
Incremental discounted deaths averted	343	2	200	465	2,815	2,412
Incremental discounted cost/death averted	1,541	>190,000	3,117	1,880	271	394
Second opportunity for measles (fixed facility)						
Incremental discounted cost/person vaccinated	1.08	1.05	0.98	1.19	1.04	1.00
Incremental discounted deaths averted	1,138	599	95	1,304	2,509	9,646
Incremental discounted cost/death averted	119	199	1,906	228	74	23
DTP-hepatitis B and Hib (pentavalent) vaccine (mix of strategies)						
Incremental discounted cost/person vaccinated	15.14	14.61	15.69	16.23	15.24	11.68
Incremental discounted deaths averted	47	19	116	274	192	1,796
Incremental discounted cost/death averted	>40,000	>85,000	>25,000	>14,000	>14,000	1,433
Yellow fever (campaigns)						
Incremental discounted cost/person vaccinated	n.a.	n.a.	1.43	n.a.	n.a.	1.42
Incremental discounted deaths averted	n.a.	n.a.	94	n.a.	n.a.	376
Incremental discounted cost/death averted	n.a.	n.a.	2,810	n.a.	n.a.	834
Incremental discounted cost/person vaccinated (mix of strategies)						
Hepatitis B monovalent (birth dose)	2.26	2.15	2.36	2.37	2.24	2.02
DTP-hepatitis B (tetravalent)	7.85	7.57	7.34	8.03	7.55	7.26
Rubella (campaigns)	1.20	1.19	1.20	1.07	1.19	1.19
Meningococcal A (fixed facilities)	n.a.	n.a.	n.a.	2.73	n.a.	2.33
Japanese encephalitis (fixed facilities)	4.56	n.a.	n.a.	n.a.	4.37	n.a.
Injectable polio vaccine (monovalent)	7.12	6.72	6.42	7.32	6.85	6.60
Injectable polio vaccine (combination with DTP)	13.88	14.84	14.62	15.28	14.77	14.19

Source: Authors' calculations.
Note: n.a. refers to not applicable when a specific disease is not prevalent in a specific region.

delivery cost per FIC was apportioned to individual antigens on the basis of the share of number of doses per FIC for that antigen (Brenzel 2005). Cost estimates are based on the number of doses required for full immunity (that is, hepatitis B, Hib, and IPV vaccines require three doses for full immunity, and meningococcal A requires two doses for full immunity). Results are reported in table 20.6.

The analysis also assumes that an additional visit to a health facility is required for new doses (depending on timing in the EPI schedule). Combination vaccines may be more cost-efficient because of potential savings in supplies, syringes, and health workers' time, in addition to the overall health benefits of reducing the number of required injections. However, if the combination vaccine does not reduce the number of visits a child would ordinarily need to make to a health facility, any cost savings may be subsumed by the higher costs of increasing coverage.

The discounted incremental cost per person ranges from less than US$1 to US$16.23, depending on the unit price of

Marginal Costs of Immunization Services in India

A study in Tamil Nadu evaluated immunization costs and coverage using a longitudinal panel dataset of immunization program costs (Brenzel 1995). Data were collected from a stratified, random sample of facilities between 1989 and 1991 for the North Arcot District Polio Control Program.[a] The sample included 120 observations of 59 different health centers: 17 followed for three years (29 percent), 27 followed for two years (46 percent), and 15 with a single observation (25 percent). Total immunization costs included the cost of labor, vaccines, injection supplies, transportation, and overhead and the value of equipment, vehicles, and buildings.

During this period, coverage rates for FICs increased from 5 to 77 percent. The table shows that the cost per dose and the cost per FIC increased during this period.[b] Changes in the cost per dose were highly statistically significant, whereas no statistical differences were apparent in the cost per FIC during the study period.

Comparison of Total Facility Immunization Costs, Immunization Activity, and Unit Costs by Year, North Arcot District Polio Control Program, 1989–91
(2001 US$)

Indicator	Year 1	Year 2	Year 3	Overall
Total costs	996	1,337	980	1,104
Variable costs	697	1,260	917	958
Cost/dose	1.09	1.98	1.33	1.47
Cost/FIC	13.11	27.92	17.07	19.37

Source: Brenzel (1995).

a. The program was a joint effort by the Indian Council for Medical Research, the Centre for Advanced Research in Virology at the Christian Medical Centre and Hospital in Vellore, and the governments of Tamil Nadu and India.

b. Higher costs in the second year reflect a change in the organization of the primary health care system in 1990 to improve access to basic services.

The study used data from the health facility sample to explain the determinants of immunization costs, which were modeled as a function of outputs, input prices, and other production-related variables that influence the cost function with respect to outputs. A random effects estimation was performed on the analysis sample relating the natural logarithm of health facility costs to the type of polio vaccine in use, estimated target population, and size of geographical area serviced by the health facility and natural logarithms of the number of FICs per facility, the number of hours spent by a village health nurse on immunization services per facility, and the number of small pieces of equipment used for immunization service delivery.

The analysis revealed a significant association between facility cost and the number of FICs, the hours worked by village health nurses, the area served, and the type of polio vaccine. When calculated using mean values, the marginal cost per FIC was Rs 24.43 (US$1.30) lower than the associated average cost per FIC of Rs 183 (US$9.80), implying that the average cost curve lies above the marginal cost curve for the sample of health facilities in India. A declining relationship is apparent between costs and coverage for this sample of facilities, calling into question assumptions of constant returns to scale. The results suggest that, in India, average cost-effectiveness ratios would overestimate total resource needs. Using a single-point estimate of average unit costs to determine the use of scarce public health resources will result in suboptimal resource allocations.

vaccine, the type of vaccine, the delivery strategy, and the coverage levels. The results lead to several conclusions:

- First, the additional incremental cost per person vaccinated is relatively small for some new vaccines.
- Second, because fixed costs are excluded, the results represent conservative estimates of additional costs.
- Third, because of price uncertainty, cost variations are greatest for newer vaccines, such as the DTP-IPV combination.

The second opportunity for measles has the lowest cost per death averted, ranging from US$23 to US$1,906 for fixed

facility strategies, and from US$65 to US$1,363 for campaigns These results are consistent with the literature. Foster, McFarland, and John (1993) find an incremental cost per death averted ranging from US$335 to US$552 in urban areas and from US$327 to US$706 in rural areas. The Africa Measles Partnership (2004) estimates a cost per death averted of US$131 to US$393 in the African context, but these figures include the costs of infrastructure.

In the hypothetical populations, the incremental cost per death averted for the pentavalent vaccine ranged from US$1,433 to more than US$85,000, depending mostly on the number of potential deaths that could be averted. Although a

An Immunization Costing Study of Adding New Vaccines to the EPI in Peru

Data were collected from 19 government health facilities in three districts in Peru, including five hospitals and 14 health centers (Walker and others 2004). Total annual costs per center included vaccines, supplies, personnel, cold chain, overhead, and shared inputs. The average cost per dose for traditional EPI antigens plus yellow fever varied from US$1.50 to US$3.20 per dose as shown in the table, with vaccines and personnel accounting for the bulk of costs.

At 2,000 doses, the marginal cost of delivering one more dose is US$1.08, increasing to US$5.33 for 12,000 doses. Average and marginal costs are equal (US$1.18) when 5,000 doses are provided per site. When an outlier delivering many vaccines at a high cost was removed, cost-minimizing output rose to 6,000 doses at US$1.11.

Although each vaccination facility is likely to be associated with different average and marginal costs, considering vaccine provision across a range of providers is relevant, because targets for vaccination can be set by site. Information about marginal costs can help determine what the most efficient size for vaccination facilities is in the long run and how to minimize costs across different size units in the short run, given targets (see figure).

When hepatitis B, Hib, and the pentavalent vaccine (DTP-hepatitis B-Hib) are added to the delivery schedule, the total annual additional cost increases to US$4,121, US$11,886, and US$25,261, respectively, with an average

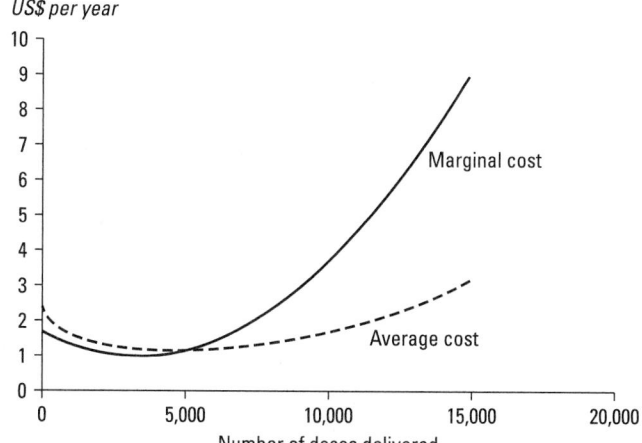

US$ per year

Source: Authors' calculations.

Marginal and Average Vaccination in Sample Facilities in Peru
(2001 US$)

incremental cost per dose of vaccine of US$0.20, US$4.14, and US$4.24, respectively. Adding these new vaccines increased the total cost of providing 5,100 doses from US$5,840 to US$9,415 and changed the minimum average cost from US$1.18 per dose to US$1.68. Therefore, the addition of new vaccines shifts both average and marginal costs upward.

Mean Cost per Dose by Type of Facility, Selected Districts in Peru
(2001 US$)

Cost items	Health post	Health center	Rural hospital	Provincial hospital	Department hospital (Ayacucho)	National hospital
Recurrent items						
Vaccines	0.59	0.87	1.39	1.03	0.60	0.31
Syringes	0.04	0.05	0.07	0.04	0.05	0.03
Personnel	0.46	0.28	1.17	0.33	0.76	0.29
Other	0.05	0.03	0.03	0.04	0.03	0.13
Capital items	0.01	0.02	0.09	0.01	0.03	0.02
Direct costs	1.15	1.25	2.75	1.45	1.47	0.78
Indirect costs	0.33	0.26	0.41	0.30	0.45	1.19
Average cost	1.48	1.51	3.17	1.79	1.92	1.98

Source: Walker and others (2004).
Note: Totals may not sum exactly because of rounding.

wide range of results was found, these estimates are supported by the literature. Miller (1998) estimated between US$3,127 and US$3.2 million per life saved for Hib vaccine. Brinsmead, Hill, and Walker's (2004) systematic review of the literature on the cost-effectiveness of Hib vaccine finds wide variations in results because of methodological differences and epidemiological and health system characteristics. The discounted incremental cost of introducing the pentavalent (DTP–hepatitis B–Hib) vaccine is roughly equal to the total mean cost of the traditional vaccine package estimated earlier. This finding implies that introducing this combination vaccine may double the financial requirements, an implication that is supported by data from national financial sustainability plans for immunization (Lydon 2004).

The incremental discounted cost per person vaccinated with a birth dose of hepatitis B is approximately US$2, and that for the tetravalent vaccine was between US$7 and US$8. The 10-year time period for our analysis is too short to accumulate deaths averted resulting from hepatitis B vaccination because deaths from liver cancer occur at older ages. Beutels's (1998, 2001) reviews of studies of the cost-effectiveness of introducing hepatitis B vaccine indicate that results vary depending on assumptions of endemicity and the methodology used, with a cost per death averted ranging from US$3,500 to US$271,800.

Rubella vaccination had a low additional cost per person vaccinated, at slightly more than US$1. Golden and Shapiro (1984) found that vaccinating all prepubertal children with rubella vaccine had the highest benefit-cost ratio (ranging from US$1.70 to US$1.96). Most benefits were future cost savings from long-term institutional care. When rubella was delivered in combination with measles and mumps, the benefit-cost ratios varied from US$4.70 to US$38.80 (Hinman and others 2002).

The additional cost per person vaccinated with one dose of Japanese encephalitis vaccine was between US$4.37 and US$4.56. A study in Thailand using two doses showed a cost per child ranging from US$2.31 to US$4.20, depending on the mode of delivery (Siraprapasiri, Sawaddiwudhipong, and Rojanasuphot 1997). Ding and others (2003) estimate a cost per case averted of US$258 and a cost per DALY averted of US$16.80 for a five-dose inactivated Japanese encephalitis vaccine.

Our analysis suggests an additional discounted cost per person vaccinated for injectable polio vaccine of between US$6.60 and US$7.32, depending on coverage levels and mix of delivery strategy. The additional discounted unit cost of the combination DTP-IPV vaccine was higher, ranging from US$13.88 to US$15.28. These results are also sensitive to the current prices of the vaccine, which will probably decline in coming years. Brenzel (1995) finds that in India the cost per case prevented for the combination DTP-polio vaccine was much lower than for oral polio vaccine (OPV), primarily because the combination vaccine was associated with a greater reduction in the number of polio cases. Miller and others (1996) suggest that

introducing IPV into routine vaccination in the United States would cost an additional US$15 million to US$28 million depending on the type of schedule adopted, resulting in a cost per vaccine-associated paralytic poliomyelitis case prevented of approximately US$3 million. Sangrugee, Caceres, and Cochi (2004) found that the least costly option would be for programs to stop providing OPV after postpolio eradication and certification and that optionally introducing IPV with universal IPV had the highest costs and the lowest expected number of vaccine-associated paralytic poliomyelitis cases. If the unit price of IPV fell to US$0.47, switching to IPV from OPV would be economically worthwhile.

FINANCIAL SUSTAINABILITY OF IMMUNIZATION PROGRAMS

Even though research has demonstrated that vaccination against childhood diseases is one of the most cost-effective health interventions, governments in many developing countries are considering how to meet the financing requirements of immunization programs, particularly as new vaccines are introduced and programs are scaled up. GAVI is working with countries to prepare for the transition from grant funding and to secure the overall financial sustainability of national programs. Approximately 55 countries have prepared national financial sustainability plans for immunization. These plans help countries evaluate the current and future costs and financing of national immunization programs and identify strategies to address future funding gaps (GAVI 2004; http://www.who.int/immunization_financing/en).

According to a recent analysis of financial sustainability plans, specific costs for immunization programs represent an average of 2 percent of total health spending and 6 percent of government health spending and are equivalent to less than 0.2 percent of gross domestic product on average. However, this profile changes after new and more expensive vaccines are introduced. In some countries, program-specific costs for immunization can reach as high as 20 percent of government health spending with introduction of combination vaccines (Lydon 2004). This share is related to the current unit price of the vaccine, which is expected to decline.

Governments and their development partners are challenged to find ways to finance and sustain immunization programs. In countries that are implementing reforms to achieve greater transparency and fiscal discipline through sectorwide approaches and medium-term expenditure frameworks, the additional financing requirements are compounded by the need to operate within a fixed budget for the health sector, so that increased funding needs for one program may necessitate budget cuts for others. This example illustrates the potential tradeoffs that exist at the country level, which create both opportunities for more open policy dialogue in relation to priority setting for the use of scarce public funds and risks that the cost of new vaccines may not be readily integrated into national plans and budgets. Because of the financial implications of reaching higher coverage levels and simultaneously introducing new vaccines, policy makers will not only have to weigh the cost-worthiness of alternative investments but also have to understand their long-term budgetary implications.

IMPROVING THE COSTS AND COST-EFFECTIVENESS OF IMMUNIZATION PROGRAMS

The cost-effectiveness of immunization programs could be improved by either reducing costs or improving programs' health benefits. Programs could reduce costs by using a more efficient mix of delivery strategies, reducing vaccine wastage, and using lower-cost inputs while maintaining the same quality of service. Reductions in the price of vaccines in the near future will also reduce costs. Innovations in vaccine technology may result in more widespread use of vaccine vial monitors, and increased use of heat-stable vaccines could potentially reduce the cost of the cold chain, although these innovations may themselves add to costs. The number of children and adults immunized can be increased by creating additional demand for vaccination; reducing missed opportunities; and reducing the dropout rate between the first and third doses of DTP, hepatitis B, and other vaccines. Finally, changes in the EPI schedule could affect total costs by reducing the number of doses required to achieve immunity and thereby reducing the number of visits, resulting in savings in the costs of labor, supplies, transport, and perhaps overhead.

The EPI schedule was established in 1984 based on a review of immune responses to diphtheria, tetanus, pertussis, polio, and measles vaccines starting at different ages and with varying intervals between doses (Halsey and Galazka 1985). The EPI schedule administers three doses of DTP at the shortest possible intervals to complete the immunization series as early in life as possible. However, if the primary series could be reduced to two doses with a booster dose at 12 to 15 months of age, the cost savings from reduced visits and one fewer dose of DTP in countries that administer a fourth dose of DTP would be considerable. Additional serological studies would be needed to compare the existing EPI schedule with the theoretical schedule before a new schedule could be adopted. Also, other vaccines to be introduced into immunization programs would need to be revaluated in this schedule. Two doses of IPV administered beginning at two months of age induce protective levels of antibodies between 95 and 100 percent for each of the three polio types (Halsey and others 1997; Plotkin and Vidor 2004).

Some countries with a low incidence of tuberculosis (such as those of Eastern Europe) are considering the discontinuation of routine BCG vaccination, given the low risk of acquiring tuberculosis in early childhood. If the BCG were not administered during the first month of life, program costs would be reduced by the value of one visit and by the costs associated with vaccine purchase, shipping, storage, and administration.

RESEARCH AGENDA

Private and public sector investment in research and development pertaining to new vaccines and improved use of existing vaccines is considerable. Most research and development is focusing on vaccines likely to have the greatest effect in the developed world and the best financial return; however, by means of public-private partnerships for product development, foundations have stepped in to support vaccine research and development for diseases for which the greatest burden occurs in developing countries.

New vaccines are being developed that could be incorporated into EPI schedules, including vaccines that protect against rotavirus, *S. pneumoniae*, malaria, cervical cancer associated with human papilloma virus, HIV/AIDS, and dengue. New and improved vaccines are also being developed to protect against meningococcal infections in infancy and Japanese encephalitis (NIH 2000). WHO recently created the Initiative for Vaccine Research Department to facilitate global coordination of research and development efforts for these and other vaccines.

In compiling data for this chapter, we noted a number of key gaps in knowledge that could usefully drive a research agenda and contribute to more evidence-based policy making in the future (Fox-Rushby and others 2004). First, little is currently known about how and why delivery costs change with increasing numbers of vaccinations and at higher coverage rates and whether economies of scale can be achieved. Little is known about the relative cost-effectiveness of different strategies to increase coverage given different baseline coverage rates. This issue relates to other questions of the optimal timing for introducing new vaccines and of how decisions should vary given different epidemiological and economic settings. Future research should therefore consider the extent to which cost-effectiveness analyses need to be repeated for every country or context or whether (and how) estimating and validating relationships across countries and accounting for uncertainty in estimates of costs and effects are possible.

Second, more attention needs to be given to measuring effect. For example, even though the coverage of single antigens required to reach particular levels of FICs should be accounted for, economic evaluations need to move beyond such indicators of output to measuring effect on the quantity and quality of life. In evaluating different schedules, methodological research needs to focus on how to incorporate the combined effects of multiple vaccinations in this respect. Remarkably few studies have considered the effect on nonhealth benefits, such as economic growth and welfare. The larger the package of vaccinations considered, the more important this question becomes.

CONCLUSIONS

This chapter confirms that vaccination of children and women with the traditional EPI vaccines is a highly cost-effective public health intervention, although cost-effectiveness ratios vary by region, delivery strategy, and level of scale. Overall, vaccination has had a significant effect on reducing mortality and morbidity from childhood diseases and will be a priority intervention for achieving the child health Millennium Development Goals. Improving and sustaining measles control are among the most cost-effective interventions in high-mortality regions.

Establishing and maintaining high immunization coverage rates in many of the poorest developing countries have proven challenging for those with high population growth rates, limited infrastructure and resources, and fluctuating demand for services. According to historical coverage rate trends, Europe and Central Asia, Latin America and the Caribbean, and the Middle East and North Africa are expected to achieve 90 percent coverage of FIC by 2011, with East Asia and the Pacific, South Asia, and Sub-Saharan Africa lagging behind.

Increasing and sustaining higher immunization coverage rates will require further efforts so that disease control can be maintained, particularly when a perception exists at the community level that vaccine-preventable diseases are no longer a major public health issue. At higher coverage rates, further disease burden reductions will be smaller, which will affect relative cost-effectiveness. Targeted approaches in countries or at subnational levels could potentially yield high returns, especially in those areas with poor control of vaccine-preventable diseases.

Our analysis shows that the cost per FIC will increase as countries scale up immunization coverage and introduce new vaccines. Adding more antigens to traditional EPIs has been successfully accomplished in many countries, especially for Hib and hepatitis B vaccines. Although many of the new vaccines under consideration are more expensive than those for the original six targeted EPI diseases, they may still be relatively cost-effective compared with other interventions and with treatment costs. Our analysis shows a wide range of cost-effectiveness estimates depending on the type of vaccine, vaccine prices, coverage levels, and delivery strategy, with the additional incremental cost per person being relatively small for some new vaccines. Declines in unit prices of new vaccines also will affect cost-effectiveness results.

Financing and sustaining immunization programs are challenges that governments in developing countries and their development partners will face. The financial implications of reaching higher coverage levels and the simultaneous desire to introduce new vaccines will require policy makers to consider both the relative cost-effectiveness of interventions and the long-term budgetary implications.

Although global and regional estimates of cost-effectiveness of interventions are useful guides, further analytical work will be needed to evaluate the relative benefits (deaths and cases averted and DALYs) and costs (delivery and treatment) of vaccines for different delivery strategies and higher coverage rates, particularly at the country level.

ACKNOWLEDGMENTS

The authors thank Tina Proveaux for editorial and technical assistance and Howard Barnum, Mariam Claeson, Felicity Cutts, Tony Measham, and Philip Musgrove for reviewing drafts of the manuscript. Santiago Cornejo and Ravi Cheerukupalli provided valuable inputs.

NOTES

1. For our analysis, the preimmunization era neonatal tetanus mortality rate per 1,000 live births is used: developed countries, 0.1; East Asia and the Pacific, 4.7; Europe and Central Asia, 0.4; Latin America and the Caribbean, 4.4; Middle East and North Africa, 4.7; South Asia, 15.3; and Sub-Saharan Africa, 10.2.

2. Because disease classification does not have a one-to-one correspondence with those prevented by vaccine, according to table 20.3 is based on estimates of the proportion of these illnesses that may be preventable by specific vaccines. For example, some meningitis and acute lower respiratory infections are caused by Hib or *S. pneumoniae*, and some cirrhosis is caused by hepatitis B.

3. A *fully immunized child* is a standard term that refers to a child who has received one dose of BCG vaccine, three doses each of oral polio vaccine and DTP vaccines, and one dose of measles vaccine. The number of FICs does not include children who have been partially immunized, so this measure underestimates the total effect on the disease burden. However, the number of FICs is representative of the effectiveness of the delivery system in providing access to immunization services to children. The authors are aware that fully vaccinating a child does not correspond to full immunity.

4. The mean population-weighted cost per FIC for the financial sustainability plans for immunization was US$21.06. The plans use DTP3 coverage as a proxy for FICs rather than coverage measured through population-based surveys (http://www.who.int/immunization_financing/en).

5. Assumptions about the relative distribution of FICs by strategy and region were based loosely on such factors as the proportion of the population with access to health services for fixed facilities and the likelihood of active mobile strategies.

6. A proxy for the total number of deaths averted is the sum of the individual deaths averted for each antigen in the traditional EPI. This figure may overestimate the actual number of deaths averted by fully immunizing children and therefore underestimate the cost per death averted. However, the values estimated by region appear to support previously reported estimates, and direct estimation of deaths averted was impossible given data and model limitations.

REFERENCES

Aaby, P. 1988. "Malnutrition and Overcrowding/Intensive Exposure in Severe Measles Infection: Review of Community Studies." *Reviews of Infectious Diseases* 10: 478–91.

Aaby, P., and C. J. Clements. 1989. "Measles Immunization Research: A Review." *Bulletin of the World Health Organization* 67: 443–48.

Africa Measles Partnership. 2004. "Measles Investment Case." Board of the Global Alliance for Vaccines and Immunization. http://www.vaccinealliance.org/resources/Measles_Investment_Case_FINAL_w_addendum.pdf.

Batt, K., J. Fox-Rushby, and M. Castillo-Riquelme. 2004. "The Costs, Effect, and Cost-Effectiveness of Strategies to Increase Coverage of Routine Immunizations in Low- and Middle-Income Countries: Systematic Review of the Grey Literature." *Bulletin of the World Health Organization* 82: 689–96.

Beasley, R. P. 1988. "Hepatitis B Virus: The Major Etiology of Hepatocellular Carcinoma." *Cancer* 61: 1942–56.

Bennett, J. V., A. E. Platonov, M. P. E. Slack, P. Mala, A. H. Burton, and S. E. Robertson. 2002. *Haemophilus influenzae Type B (Hib) Meningitis in the Pre-vaccine Era: A Global Review of Incidence, Age Distributions, and Case-Fatality Rates*. WHO/V&B/02.18. Geneva: World Health Organization. http://www.who.int/vaccines-documents/DocsPDF02/www696.pdf.

Berman, P., J. Quinley, B. Yusuf, S. Anwar, U. Mustaini, A. Azof, and B. Iskandar. 1991. "Maternal Tetanus Immunization in Aceh Province, Sumatra: The Cost-Effectiveness of Alternative Strategies." *Social Science and Medicine* 33: 185–92.

Beutels, P. 1998. "Economic Evaluations Applied to HB Vaccination: General Observations." *Vaccine* 16: S84–92.

———. 2001. "Economic Evaluations of Hepatitis B Immunization: A Global Review of Recent Studies (1994–2000)." *Health Economics* 10: 751–74.

Birmingham, M., and C. Stein. 2003. "The Burden of Vaccine-Preventable Diseases." In *The Vaccine Book*, ed. B. R. Bloom and P.-H. Lambert, 1–21. San Diego, CA: Elsevier.

Birmingham, M., L. Wolfson, M. Kurian, U. Griffiths, F. Gasse, and J. Vandelaer. 2004. "Estimating the Burden of Neonatal Tetanus." Unpublished manuscript.

Brenzel, L. 1995. "Final Report on the Longitudinal Cost-Effectiveness Study of the North Arcot District Polio Control Program (NADPCP)." Resources for Child Health Project, U.S. Agency for International Development, Arlington, VA.

———. 2005. "Methods Used to Estimate the Costs of Scaling Up Immunization Services for the Vaccine Preventable Disease Chapter, Disease Control Priorities Project." World Bank, Washington, DC.

Brenzel, L., and P. Claquin. 1994. "Immunization Programs and Their Costs." *Social Science and Medicine* 39: 527–36.

Brinsmead, R., S. Hill, and D. Walker. 2004. "Are Economic Evaluations of Vaccines Useful to Decision Makers? Case Study of *Haemophilus Influenzae* Type B Vaccines." *Pediatric Infectious Disease Journal* 23: 32–37.

Cherry, J. D., and R. E. Harrison. 2004. "Tetanus." In *Textbook of Pediatric Infectious Diseases*, ed. R. D. Feigin, J. D. Cherry, G. J. Demmler, and S. L. Kaplan, 1766–76. Philadelphia: Elsevier.

Cherry, J. D., and U. Heininger. 2004. "Pertussis and Other *Bordetella* Infections." In *Textbook of Pediatric Infectious Diseases*, ed. R. D. Feigin, J. D. Cherry, G. J. Demmler, and S. L. Kaplan, 1588–1608. Philadelphia: Elsevier.

Creese, A. L. 1986. "Cost-Effectiveness of Potential Immunization Interventions against Diarrheal Disease." *Social Science and Medicine* 23: 231–40.

Creese, A. L., and M. A. Domínguez-Ugá. 1987. "Cost-Effectiveness of Immunization Programs in Colombia." *Pan American Health Organization Bulletin* 21: 377–94.

Crowcroft, N. S., C. Stein, P. Duclos, and M. Birmingham. 2003. "How Best to Estimate the Global Burden of Pertussis?" *Lancet Infectious Diseases* 3: 413–18.

Ding, D., P. E. Kilgore, J. D. Clemens, L. Wei, and X. Zhi-Yi. 2003. "Cost-Effectiveness of Routine Immunization to Control Japanese Encephalitis in Shanghai, China." *Bulletin of the World Health Organization* 81: 334–42.

Domínguez-Ugá, M. A. 1988. "Economic Analysis of the Vaccination Strategies Adopted in Brazil in 1982." *Bulletin of the World Health Organization* 22: 250–68.

Edmunds, D. J., A. Dejene, Y. Mekkonen, M. Haile, W. Alemnu, and D. J. Nokes. 2000. "The Cost of Integrating Hepatitis B Virus Vaccine into National Immunization Programs: A Case Study from Addis Ababa." *Health Policy and Planning* 15: 408–16.

Edwards, K. M., and M. D. Decker. 2004. "Pertussis Vaccine." In *Vaccines*, ed. S. A. Plotkin and W. A. Orenstein, 471–528. Philadelphia: Saunders.

Elbasha, E. H., and M. L. Messonnier. 2004. "Cost-Effectiveness Analysis and Health Care Resource Allocation: Decision Rules under Variable Returns to Scale." *Health Economics* 13: 21–35.

Feigin, R. D., B. W. Stechenberg, and P. Hertel. 2004. "Diphtheria." In *Textbook of Pediatric Infectious Diseases*, ed. R. D. Feigin, J. D. Cherry, G. J. Demmler, and S. L. Kaplan, 1305–13. Philadelphia: Elsevier.

Foster, S. O., D. A. McFarland, and A. M. John. 1993. "Measles." In *Disease Control Priorities in Developing Countries*, ed. D. T. Jamison, W. H. Mosley, A. R. Measham, and J. L. Bobadilla, 161–87. New York: Oxford University Press and World Bank. http://www.fic.nih.gov/dcpp/dcp1/dcp1-ch8.pdf.

Fox-Rushby, J. A., M. Kaddar, R. Levine, and L. Brenzel. 2004. "The Economics of Vaccination in Low- and Middle-Income Countries." *Bulletin of the World Health Organization* 82: 640.

Galazka, A., M. Birmingham, M. Kurian, and F. Gasse. Forthcoming. "Tetanus." In *The Global Epidemiology of Infectious Disease*, ed. C. J. L. Murray and A. D. Lopez. Cambridge, MA: Harvard University Press.

Galazka, A. M., and S. E. Robertson. Forthcoming. "Diphtheria." In *The Global Epidemiology of Infectious Disease*, ed. C. J. L. Murray and A. D. Lopez, Cambridge, MA: Harvard University Press.

Galazka, A. M., S. E. Robertson, and G. P. Oblapenko. 1995. "Resurgence of Diphtheria." *European Journal of Epidemiology* 11: 95–105.

GAVI (Global Alliance for Vaccines and Immunization). 2004. "Guidelines for Preparing a National Immunization Financial Sustainability Plan." Geneva, GAVI. http://www.who.int/immunization_financing/tools/en/FSP_Guidelines_April%202004_En.pdf.

Gay, N. J., W. J. Edmunds, E. Bah, and C. B. Nelson. 2001. *Estimating the Global Burden of Hepatitis B*. Geneva: World Health Organization.

Gessner, B. D., A. Sutanto, M. Linehan, I. G. G. Djelantik, T. Fletcher, K. Ingerani, and others. 2005. "The Incidence of Vaccine-Preventable *Haemophilus influenzae* Type B Pneumonia and Meningitis in Indonesian Children Using a Hamlet-Randomized Vaccine Probe Design." *Lancet* 365 (9453): 43–52.

Golden, M., and G. L. Shapiro. 1984. "Cost-Benefit Analysis of Alternative Programs of Vaccination against Rubella in Israel." *Public Health* 98: 179–90.

Griffith, A. H. 1979. "The Role of Immunization in the Control of Diphtheria." *Developments in Biological Standards* 43: 3–13.

Griffiths, U. K., G. Hutton, and E. D. Pascoal. 2005. "The Cost-Effectiveness of Introducing Hepatitis B Vaccine into Infant Immunization Services in Mozambique." *Health Policy Plan* 20 (1): 50–59.

Griffiths, U. K., L. J. Wolfson, A. Quddus, M. Younus, and R. A. Hafiz. 2004. "Incremental Cost-Effectiveness of Supplementary Immunization

Activities to Prevent Neo-natal Tetanus in Pakistan." *Bulletin of the World Health Organization* 82: 643–51.

Hadler, S. C., S. L. Cochi, J. Bilous, and F. T. Cutts. 2004. "Vaccination Programs in Developing Countries." In *Vaccines*, ed. S. A. Plotkin and W. A. Orenstein, 1407–42. Philadelphia: Saunders.

Halsey, N. A., M. Blatter, G. Bader, M. L. Thoms, F. F. Willingham, J. C. O'Donovan, and others. 1997. "Inactivated Poliovirus Vaccine Alone or Sequential Inactivated and Oral Poliovirus Vaccine in Two-, Four-, and Six-Month-Old Infants with Combination *Haemophilus influenzae* Type B/Hepatitis B Vaccine." *Pediatric Infectious Disease Journal* 16: 675–79.

Halsey, N., and A. Galazka. 1985. "The Efficacy of DPT and Oral Poliomyelitis Immunization Schedules Initiated from Birth to 12 Weeks of Age." *Bulletin of the World Health Organization* 63 (6): 1151–69.

Henderson, R. H., and T. Sundaresan. 1982. "Cluster Sampling to Assess Immunization Coverage: A Review of Experience with a Simplified Sampling Method." *Bulletin of the World Health Organization* 60: 253–60.

Hinman, A. R., B. Irons, M. Lewis, and K. Kandola. 2002. "Economic Analyses of Rubella and Rubella Vaccines: A Global Review." *Bulletin of the World Health Organization* 80: 264–70.

Karlsson, G., and M. Johannesson. 1998. "Cost-Effectiveness Analysis and Capital Costs." *Social Science and Medicine* 46: 1183–91.

Khaleghian, P. 2001. "Immunization Financing and Sustainability: A Review of the Literature." Special Initiatives Report 40. Bethesda, MD: Partnerships for Health Reform Project, Abt Associates.

Krugman, S. 1963. "Measles and Poliomyelitis Vaccines." *New York State Journal of Medicine* 63: 2973–77.

Levin, A., S. England, J. Jorissen, B. Garshong, and J. Teprey. 2001. *Case Study on the Costs and Financing of Immunization Services in Ghana*. Report by PHR plus. Bethesda, MD: Abt Associates.

Levine, M. M., R. Lagos, O. S. Levine, I. Heitmann, N. Enriquez, M. E. Pinto, and others. 1998. "Epidemiology of Invasive Pneumococcal Infections in Infants and Young Children in Metropolitan Santiago, Chile, a Newly Industrializing Country." *Pediatric Infectious Disease Journal* 17: 287–93.

Lydon, P. 2004. "Financial Sustainability Plan Analysis: A Look across 22 GAVI Countries." World Health Organization, Geneva.

Margolis, H. S., M. J. Alter, and S. C. Hadler. 1997. "Viral Hepatitis." In *Viral Infections of Humans: Epidemiology and Control*, ed. A. S. Evans and R. A. Kaslow, 363–418. New York: Plenum.

Martin, M., J. M. Casellas, S. A. Madhi, T. J. Urquhart, S. D. Delport, F. Ferrero, and others. 2004. "Impact of *Haemophilus influenzae* Type B Conjugate Vaccine in South Africa and Argentina." *Pediatric Infectious Disease Journal* 23: 842–47.

Mast, E., F. Mahoney, M. A. Kane, and H. S. Margolis. 2004. "Hepatitis B Vaccine." In *Vaccines*, ed. S. A. Plotkin and W. A. Orenstein, 299–338. Philadelphia: Saunders.

Mathers, C. D., A. D. Lopez, and C. J. L. Murray. 2006. "The Burden of Disease and Mortality by Condition: Data, Methods, and Results for the Year 2001." In *Global Burden of Disease and Risk Factors*. ed. Alan D. Lopez, Colin D. Mathers, Majid Ezzati, Dean T. Jamison, and Christopher J. L. Murray. New York: Oxford University Press.

McQuillan, G. M., P. J. Coleman, D. Kruszon-Moran, L. A. Moyer, S. B. Lambert, and H. S. Margolis. 1999. "Prevalence of Hepatitis B Virus Infection in the United States: The National Health and Nutrition Examination Surveys, 1976 through 1994." *American Journal of Public Health* 89: 14–18.

Miller, M. A. 1998. "An Assessment of the Value of *Haemophilus influenzae* Type B Conjugate Vaccine in Asia." *Pediatric Infectious Disease Journal* 17: S152–59.

Miller, M. A., and L. McCann. 2000. "Policy Analysis of the Use of Hepatitis B, *Haemophilus influenzae* Type B-, *Streptococcus pneumoniae*-Conjugate, and Rotavirus Vaccines in National Immunization Schedules." *Health Economics* 9: 19–35.

Miller, M. A., S. C. Redd, S. Hadler, and A. Hinman. 1998. "A Model to Estimate the Potential Economic Benefits of Measles Eradication for the United States." *Vaccine* 20: 1917–22.

Miller, M. A., R. W. Sutter, P. M. Strebel, and S. C. Hadler. 1996. "Cost-Effectiveness of Incorporating Inactivated Poliovirus Vaccine into the Routine Childhood Immunization Schedule." *Journal of the American Medical Association* 276: 967–71.

Monath, T. P. 2004. "Yellow Fever Vaccine." In *Vaccines*, ed. S. A. Plotkin and W. A. Orenstein, 1095–176. Philadelphia: Saunders.

Monath T. P., R. B. Craven, A. Adjukiewicz, M. Germain, D. B. Francy, L. Ferrara, and others. 1980. "Yellow Fever in The Gambia, 1978–79: Epidemiologic Aspects with Observations on the Occurrence of Orungo Virus Infections." *American Journal of Tropical Medicine and Hygiene* 29: 912–28.

Morris, S. S., R. E. Black, and L. Tomaskovic. 2003. "Predicting the Distribution of Under-Five Deaths by Cause in Countries without Adequate Vital Registration Systems." *International Journal of Epidemiology* 32: 1041–51.

Moss, W. J., C. J. Clements, and N. A. Halsey. 2003. "Immunization of Children at Risk of Infection with Human Immunodeficiency Virus." *Bulletin of the World Health Organization* 81: 61–70.

Mulholland, K., S. Hilton, R. Adegbola, S. Usen, A. Oparaugo, C. Omosigho, and others. 1997. "Randomised Trial of *Haemophilus influenzae* Type B Tetanus Protein Conjugate Vaccine [Corrected] for Prevention of Pneumonia and Meningitis in Gambian Infants." *Lancet* 349: 1191–97.

Mulligan, J.-A., J. A. Fox-Rushby, T. Adam, B. Johns, and A. Mills. 2003. "Unit Costs of Health Care Inputs in Low- and Middle-Income Regions." Disease Control Priorities Project Working Paper 9. DCPP, National Institutes of Health, Bethesda, MD. http://www.fic.nih.gov/dcpp/wpb9.pdf.

Nasidi, A., T. P. Monath, K. DeCock, O. Tomori, R. Cordellier, O. D. Olaleye, and others. 1989. "Urban Yellow Fever Epidemic in Western Nigeria, 1987." *Transactions of the Royal Society of Tropical Medicine and Hygiene* 83: 401–6.

NIH (National Institutes of Health). 2000. "Jordan Report 20th Anniversary: Accelerated Development of Vaccines." http://www.niaid.nih.gov/dmid/vaccines/jordan20/. NIH, Bethesda.

Pegurri, E., Fox-Rushby, J., and Walker, D. 2005. "The Effects and Costs of Expanding Coverage of Immunization Services in Developing Countries: A Systematic Literature Review." *Vaccine* 23: 1624–35.

Peltola, H. 2000. "Worldwide *Haemophilus influenzae* Type B Disease at the Beginning of the 21st Century: Global Analysis of the Disease Burden 25 Years after the Use of the Polysaccharide Vaccine and a Decade after the Advent of Conjugates." *Clinical Microbiology Reviews* 13: 302–17.

Perry, R. T. Forthcoming.

Perry, R. T., and N. A. Halsey. 2004. "The Clinical Significance of Measles: A Review." *Journal of Infectious Diseases* 189 (Suppl. 1): S4–16.

Plotkin, S. A., and E. Vidor. 2004. "Poliovirus Vaccine: Inactivated." In *Vaccines*, ed. S. A. Plotkin and W. A. Orenstein, 625–50. Philadelphia: Saunders.

Robertson, R. L., A. J. Hall, P. E. Crivelli, Y. Lowe, H. M. Inskip, and S. K. Snow. 1992. "Cost-Effectiveness of Immunizations: The Gambia Revisited." *Health Policy and Planning* 7: 111–22.

Robertson, S. E. 1993. *The Immunological Basis for Immunization Series Module 6: Poliomyelitis*. WHO/EPI/GEN/93.16. Geneva: World Health Organization.

Sangrugee N, V. Caceres, and S. Cochi. 2004. "Cost Analysis of Post-polio Certification Immunization Policies." *Bulletin of the World Health Organization* 82: 9–15.

Siraprapasiri T., W. Sawaddiwudhipong, and S. Rojanasuphot. 1997. "Cost-Benefit Analysis of Japanese Encephalitis Vaccination Program in Thailand." *Southeast Asian Journal of Tropical Medicine and Public Health* 28: 143–48.

Soucat, A., D. Levy-Bruhl, X. De Bethune, P. Gbedonou, J.-P. Lamarque, O. Bangoura, and others. 1997. "Affordability, Cost-Effectiveness, and Efficiency of Primary Health Care: The Bamako Initiative Experience in Benin and Guinea." *International Journal of Health Planning and Management* 12: S81–108.

Stanfield, J. P., and A. Galazka. 1984. "Neonatal Tetanus in the World Today." *Bulletin of the World Health Organization* 62: 647–69.

Stein, C. E., M. Birmingham, M. Kurian, P. Duclos, and P. Strebel. 2003. "The Global Burden of Measles in the Year 2000: A Model That Uses Country-Specific Indicators." *Journal of Infectious Diseases* 187 (Suppl. 1): S8–15.

Steinglass, R., L. Brenzel, and A. Percy. 1993. "Tetanus." In *Disease Control Priorities in Developing Countries*, ed. D. T. Jamison, W. H. Mosley, A. R. Measham, and J. L. Bobadilla, 189–220. New York: Oxford University Press and World Bank.

Sutter, R. W., and O. M. Kew. 2004. "Poliovirus Vaccine: Live." In *Vaccines*, ed. S. A. Plotkin and W. A. Orenstein, 651–706. Philadelphia: Saunders.

Swartz, M. N. 2004. "Bacterial Meningitis: A View of the Past 90 Years." *New England Journal of Medicine* 351: 1826–28.

Turk, D. C. 1982. "Clinical Importance of *Haemophilus influenzae*: 1981." In *Haemophilus influenzae*, ed. S. H. Sell and P. G. Wright, 3–9. New York: Elsevier.

UNICEF (United Nations Children's Fund). 2002. *State of the World's Vaccines and Immunization.* New York: United Nations.

USAID (U.S. Agency for International Development), Asia–Near East Region. 1988. "Resources for Child Health Project." Asia-Near East Bureau Guidance for Costing of Health Services Delivery Projects, Arlington, VA.

Valdmanis, V., D. Walker, and J. Fox-Rushby. 2003. "Are Vaccination Sites in Bangladesh Scale Efficient?" *International Journal of Technology Assessment in Health Care* 19: 692–97.

Walker, D., N. R. Mosqueira, M. E. Penny, C. F. Lanata, A. D. Clark, C. F. B. Sanderson, and J. Fox-Rushby. 2004. "Variation in the Costs of Delivering Routine Immunization Services in Peru." *Bulletin of the World Health Organization* 82: 676–82.

Wassilak, S, G. F. Trudy, V. Murphy, M. H. Roper, and W. A. Orenstein. 2004. "Tetanus Toxoid." In *Vaccines*, ed. S. A. Plotkin and W. A. Orenstein, 745–82. Philadelphia: Saunders.

Wenger, J. D., and J. Ward. 2004. "*Haemophilus influenzae* Vaccine." In *Vaccines*, ed. S. A. Plotkin and W. A. Orenstein, 229–68. Philadelphia: Saunders.

WHO (World Health Organization). 1974. *Handbook of Resolutions.* Vol. 1, 1.8. World Health Assembly, Fourteenth plenary meeting, 23 May 1974. Geneva: WHO.

———. 1988. *EPICost.* Geneva: WHO.

———. 1992. *Global Health Situation and Projections: Estimates.* WHO/HST/92.1. Geneva: WHO. whqlibdoc.who.int/hq/1992/WHO_HST_92.1.pdf.

———. 1996. "HBsAG Endemicity." http://wwwstage/vaccines-surveillance/graphics/htmls/hepbprev.htm. WHO, Geneva.

———. 2001. *Estimating the Local Burden of Haemophilus influenzae Type b (Hib) Disease Preventable by Vaccination: A Rapid Assessment Tool.* WHO/V&B/01.27. Geneva: WHO.

———. 2002. *Core Information for the Development of Immunization Policy, 2002 Update.* WHO/V&B/02.28. Geneva: WHO. http://www.who.int/vaccines-documents/DocsPDF02/www557.pdf.

———. 2004. "Progress toward Global Immunization Goals, 2001." http://www.who.int/vaccines/. WHO, Geneva.

———. 2005a. "Progress in Reducing Global Measles Deaths: 1999–2003." *Weekly Epidemiological Record* 80 (9): 78–81.

———. 2005b. *World Health Report 2005: Make Every Mother and Child Count.* Geneva: WHO.

Wolfson, L., and P. Lydon. 2005. "Methodology for Estimating Baseline and Future Levels of Costing (and Impact) for the Global Immunization Vision and Strategy 2005–2015, Draft 1.1." World Health Organization, Geneva.

World Bank. 1993. *Investing in Health: World Development Report, 1993.* New York: Oxford University Press.

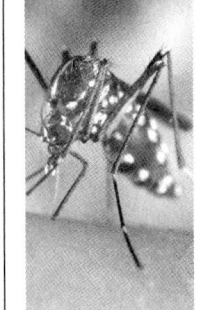

Chapter **21**

Conquering Malaria

Joel G. Breman, Anne Mills, Robert W. Snow, Jo-Ann Mulligan,
Christian Lengeler, Kamini Mendis, Brian Sharp, Chantal Morel,
Paola Marchesini, Nicholas J. White, Richard W. Steketee, and
Ogobara K. Doumbo

Malaria is the most important of the parasitic diseases of humans, with 107 countries and territories having areas at risk of transmission containing close to 50 percent of the world's population (Hay and others 2004; WHO 2005). More than 3 billion people live in malarious areas and the disease causes between 1 million and 3 million deaths each year (Breman, Alilio, and Mills 2004; Snow and others 2003). Recent estimates of the global falciparum malaria morbidity burden have increased the number to 515 million cases, with Africa suffering the vast majority of this toll (Snow and others 2005). In addition, almost 5 billion clinical episodes resembling malaria occur in endemic areas annually, with more than 90 percent of this burden occurring in Africa (Breman 2001; Breman, Alilio, and Mills 2004; Carter and Mendis 2002; Snow and others 1999, 2003; Snow, Trape, and Marsh 2001).

The disease has resurged in many parts of the tropics, and nonmalarious countries face continual danger from importation. Contributing to this resurgence are the increasing problems of *Plasmodium falciparum* resistance to drugs and of the *Anopheles* vectors' resistance to insecticides. The recent findings that insecticide-treated nets (ITNs) are extremely cost-effective in preventing malaria and overall deaths and that intermittent preventive therapy (IPT) (treatment doses given during periods of vulnerability) is effective for protecting pregnant women and their fetuses, along with the discovery of new drugs (artemisinins) and their use in combination with other antimalarials and promising vaccine trials, have given great impetus to the battle against this scourge (Alonso and others 2004; Armstrong-Schellenberg and others 2001; Lengeler 2004; Newman and others 2003; Yeung and others 2004).

CAUSES, EPIDEMIOLOGY, MANIFESTATIONS, AND DIAGNOSIS

Four species of the genus *Plasmodium* cause malarial infections in humans: *P. falciparum*, *P. vivax*, *P. ovale*, and *P. malariae*. Virtually all deaths are caused by falciparum malaria. Human infection begins when the malaria vector, a female anopheline mosquito, inoculates plasmodial sporozoites from its salivary gland into humans during a blood meal. The sporozoites mature in the liver and are released into the bloodstream as merozoites. These invade red blood cells, causing malaria fevers. Some forms of the parasites (gametocytes) are ingested by anopheline mosquitoes during feeding and develop into sporozoites, restarting the cycle.

P. falciparum predominates in Haiti, Papua New Guinea, and Sub-Saharan Africa, while *P. vivax* is more common in Central America and the Indian subcontinent and causes more than 80 million clinical episodes of illness yearly (Mendis and others 2001). The prevalence of these two species is approximately equal in the Indian subcontinent, eastern Asia, Oceania, and South America. *P. malariae* is found in most endemic areas, especially throughout Sub-Saharan Africa, but is much less common than the other species. *P. ovale* is unusual outside Africa, and where it is found accounts for less than 1 percent of isolates.

While more than 40 anophelines can transmit malaria, the most effective are those such as *Anopheles gambiae*, which are long-lived, occur in high densities in tropical climates, breed readily, and bite humans in preference to other animals. The entomological inoculation rate (EIR)—that is, the number of sporozoite-positive mosquito bites per person per year—is the most useful measure of malarial transmission and varies from less than 1 in some parts of Latin America and Southeast Asia to more than 300 in parts of tropical Africa.

The epidemiology of malaria may vary considerably within relatively small geographic areas. In tropical Africa or coastal Papua New Guinea, with *P. falciparum* transmission, more than one human bite per infected mosquito can occur per day and people are infected repeatedly throughout their lives. In such areas, morbidity and mortality during early childhood are considerable. For survivors, some immunity against disease develops in these areas, and by adulthood, most malarial infections are asymptomatic. This situation, with frequent, intense, year-round transmission, is termed *stable malaria*. In areas where transmission is low, erratic, or focal, full protective immunity is not acquired and symptomatic disease may occur at all ages. This situation is termed *unstable malaria*. An epidemic or complex emergency can develop when changes in environmental, economic, or social conditions occur, such as heavy rains following drought or migrations of refugees or workers from a nonmalarious to an endemic region. A breakdown in malaria control and prevention services intensifies epidemic conditions. Epidemics occur most often in areas with unstable malaria, such as Ethiopia, northern India, Madagascar, Sri Lanka, and southern Africa. Many other African countries situated in the Sahelian and Sub-Saharan areas are susceptible to epidemics (Djimdé and others 2004; Worrall, Rietveld, and Delacollette 2004). Public health specialists have only recently begun to appreciate the considerable contribution of urban malaria, with up to 28 percent of the burden in Africa occurring in rapidly growing urban centers (Keiser and others 2004).

The determinants of malaria and of risk factors for patients and communities relate to intrinsic (human, parasite, and vector) and extrinsic (environmental, control, and socioeconomic) factors (figure 21.1)(Breman 2001). Both humoral and cellular immunity are necessary for protection.

Anemia may be quite common among young children living in areas with stable transmission, particularly where the parasite is resistant to chloroquine, sulfadoxine-pyrimethamine (SP), or other drugs. Correctly and promptly treated, uncomplicated falciparum malaria has a mortality rate of approximately 0.1 percent (Sudre and others 1992). Once vital organ dysfunction occurs or the proportion of erythrocytes infected increases to more than 3 percent, mortality rises steeply. Coma is a characteristic and ominous feature of falciparum malaria, and despite treatment it is associated with death rates of some 20 percent among adults and 15 percent among children. Convulsions, usually generalized and often repeated, occur in up to 50 percent of children with cerebral malaria (CM) (Mung'Ala-Odera, Snow, and Newton 2004). Whereas less than 3 percent of adults suffer neurological sequelae, roughly 10 to 15 percent of children surviving CM—especially those with hypoglycemia, severe malarial anemia (SMA), repeated

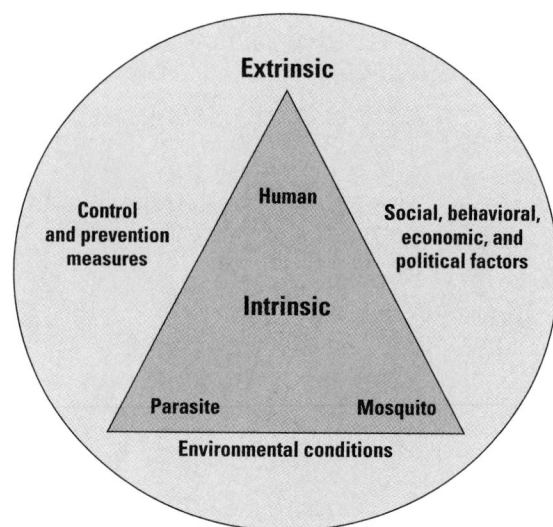

Source: Breman 2001.

Figure 21.1 Determinants of the Malaria Burden: Intrinsic and Extrinsic Factors

seizures, and deep coma—have some residual neurological deficit when they regain consciousness. Protein-calorie undernutrition and micronutrient deficiencies, particularly zinc and vitamin A, contribute substantially to the malaria burden (Caulfield, Richard, and Black 2004).

In areas with intense and stable transmission, falciparum malaria in primigravid and secundigravid women is associated with low birthweight (average reduction of about 170 grams) and consequently with increased infant and childhood mortality (Steketee and others 2001). HIV infection predisposes all pregnant women to more frequent and severe malaria, and the reverse may also be true (Ter Kuile and others 2004). *P. vivax* malaria in pregnancy is also associated with a reduction in birthweight (average reduction of some 100 grams), and this effect is greater in multigravid than in primigravid women (Nosten and others 1999).

The confirmatory diagnosis of clinical malaria rests on the microscopic demonstration of asexual forms of the parasite in stained peripheral blood smears. Newer diagnostic tests using antigen and nucleic acid detection methods are being evaluated. These tests are promising, but their limitations in relation to species sensitivity (except for *P. falciparum*), parasite quantitation, field feasibility, and costs necessitate further development and evaluation (Warhurst and Williams 2004).

BURDEN OF DISEASE

In 2001, the World Health Organization (WHO) ranked malaria as the eighth-highest contributor to the global disease burden as reflected in disability-adjusted life years (DALYs), and the

Table 21.1 Deaths and DALYs from Deaths Attributable to All Causes and to Malaria by WHO Region, 2000

Region	Population	Deaths, 2000 All causes Thousands	Deaths, 2000 All causes Percent	Deaths, 2000 Malaria Thousands	Deaths, 2000 Malaria Percent	Malaria deaths as a percentage of all deaths	DALYs from deaths, 2000 All causes Thousands	DALYs from deaths, 2000 All causes Percent	DALYs from deaths, 2000 Malaria Thousands	DALYs from deaths, 2000 Malaria Percent	Malaria DALYs as a percentage of all DALYs
World	6,122,211	56,554	100.0	1,124	100.0	2.00	1,467,257	100.0	42,279	100.0	2.90
Africa	655,476	10,681	18.9	963	85.7	9.00	357,884	24.4	36,012	85.2	10.10
Americas	837,967	5,911	10.5	1	<0.1	0.02	145,217	9.9	108	0.2	0.07
Eastern Mediterranean	493,091	4,156	7.3	55	4.9	1.30	136,221	9.3	2,050	4.8	1.50
Europe	874,178	9,703	17.2	<1	<0.1	<0.010	151,223	10.3	20	0.04	0.01
Southeast Asia	1,559,810	14,467	25.6	95	8.5	0.70	418,844	28.5	3,680	8.7	0.90
Western Pacific	1,701,689	11,636	20.6	10	0.9	<0.09	257,868	17.6	409	1.0	0.20

Source: Breman, Alilio, and Mills 2004; WHO 2002b.
Percentages may not add up to 100 percent because of rounding.

second highest in Africa (WHO 2002a). The DALYs attributable to malaria were estimated largely from the effects of *P. falciparum* infection as a direct cause of death and the much smaller contributions of short-duration, self-limiting, or treated mild febrile events, including malaria-specific mild anemia and neurological disability following CM (Murray and Lopez 1996, 1997). The estimate assumes that each illness event or death can be attributed only to a single cause that can be measured reliably. Table 21.1 shows deaths and DALYs from deaths attributable to malaria and to all causes by WHO region (WHO 2002a). It does not include the considerable toll caused by the burden of malaria-related moderate and severe anemia, low birthweight, and comorbid events (Snow and others 2003). Sub-Saharan African children under four represent 82 percent of all malaria-related deaths and DALYs. Malaria accounts for 2.0 percent of global deaths and 2.9 percent of global DALYs. In the African region of WHO, 9.0 percent of deaths and 10.1 percent of DALYs are attributable to malaria.

Recent analysis of falciparum malaria morbidity concludes that 515 (interquartile range 298 to 659) million cases occur yearly (table 21.2). This figure is 92 percent higher than the 278 million malaria cases estimated by WHO for 1998, which also includes those attributable to *P. vivax*, and 200 percent higher than previous estimates for areas outside of Africa (Snow and others 2005). While the malaria incidence globally is 236 episodes per 1,000 persons per year in all endemic areas, it ranges from about 400 to 2,000 (median 830) episodes per 1,000 persons per year in areas with intense, stable (hyperendemic and holoendemic) transmission; these areas represent 38 percent of all falciparum-endemic areas.

Background

Recent estimates of malaria deaths have varied from 0.5 million to 3.0 million per year (Breman 2001; Breman, Alilio, and

Table 21.2 Population at Risk for Falciparum Malaria, Cases and Attack Rates by World Health Organization Region, 2002*

Region	Population at risk in millions (percent)	Cases in millions (IQR) (percent)	Falciparum attack rate (1,000 persons at risk per year)
World	2,211 (100)	515 (100) [298–659]	236
Africa	521 (24)	365 (71) [216–374]	701
Americas	55 (3)	4 (1) [2–8]	73
Eastern Mediterranean	176 (8)	12 (2) [5–25]	68
Europe	4 (<1)	<1 (<1) [<1–1]	157
Southeast Asia	1,314 (59)	119 (23) [66–224]	91
Western Pacific	142 (6)	15 (3) [9–26]	106

Source: Modified from Snow and others 2005.
IQR = interquartile range, urban-adjusted.

Mills 2004; Snow and others 2003). Of the 10.6 million yearly deaths in children younger than 5 years 8 percent are ascribed to malaria (Bryce and others 2005). In 1998, an empirical analysis of malaria mortality undertaken on behalf of WHO used malaria risk maps to capture measures of disability, morbidity, and mortality associated with *P. falciparum* prevalence rates among African populations and yielded an estimate of about 1 million (Korenromp and others 2003; Snow and Marsh 2002; Snow and others 2003; Snow, Trape, and Marsh 2001). Each malarious country must now measure its own burden and progress toward decreasing that burden (WHO 2005).

Geographic and climate-driven (mainly rainfall) models of suitability for malaria transmission characterize the diversity of malaria transmission across the African continent (Craig, Snow, and le Sueur 1999; Snow and others 1999). Four distinct areas can be identified:

- class 1, no transmission (northern and parts of southern Africa)
- class 2, marginal risk (mainly in some areas of southern Africa and in high-altitude [>1500 meters] settings)
- class 3, seasonal transmission with epidemic potential (along the Sahara fringe and in highlands)
- class 4, stable and unstable malarious areas (most areas south of the Sahara to southern Africa and below an altitude of around 1,500 meters).

Direct Consequences of *P. falciparum* Infection

Two major syndromes, CM and moderate (hemoglobin less than 11 grams per deciliter) and severe (hemoglobin less than 8 grams per deciliter) malarial anemia, contribute directly and significantly to malaria mortality (tables 21.3 and 21.4). The differences in numbers derive from the different methods of calculating the burden. Children presenting with an acute febrile disease, peripheral parasitemia, and low hemoglobin concentrations account for the majority of inpatient admissions in

Table 21.4 Deaths from Malaria in Children Under Five, Africa, 2001

Cause of malaria-related death	Number of malaria deaths
Cerebral malaria	110,000
Severe malarial anemia	190,000–974,000
Respiratory distress	110,000
Hypoglycemia	153,000–267,000
Low birthweight	62,000–363,000
Total deaths from malaria	625,000–1,824,000
All-cause deaths[a]	962,000–2,806,000

Sources: Breman, Alilio, and Mills 2004; Murphy and Breman 2001.
a. Children under five represent 65 percent of all deaths in Africa as per Snow and others (2003).

Table 21.3 Malaria-Related Mortality and Morbidity, Africa, 2000

Condition	Number (range)	Percentage affected by age in years		
		0–4	5–14	≥15
Mortality and Morbidity				
Malaria-specific mortality	1,144,572[a] (702,957–1,605,448)	65	19	16
Maternal mortality (anemia)	5,300	n.a.	n.a.	100
Infant mortality (pregnancy related)	71,000–190,000	100	n.a.	n.a.
Fatal adverse events from malaria drugs	2,300	100	Unknown	Unknown
HIV from blood transfusion necessitated by malaria	5,300–8,500	100		—
Epilepsy-related mortality after cerebral malaria	Unknown	Unknown	Unknown	Unknown
Malaria-related anemia, undernutrition, and HIV mortality	Unknown	Unknown	Unknown	Unknown
Episodes of malaria (thousands)	213,549 (134,322–324,617)	51	35	14
Illness days from malaria (thousands)	803,699 (494,416–1,298,872)	69	21	10
Neurocognitive sequelae after CM				
Hemiparesis	360–400		100	Unknown
Quadriparesis	770–860		100	Unknown
Hearing impairment	650–730		100	Unknown
Visual impairment	300–330		100	Unknown
Behavioral difficulties	1,540–1,720		100	Unknown
Language deficits	7,000–7,800		100	Unknown
Epilepsy	2,700–3,000		100	Unknown
Effects on cognition	Unknown	Unknown	Unknown	Unknown

Source: Breman, Alilio, and Mills 2004; Snow and others 2003.
n.a. = not applicable.
— = not available.
Note: Figures in parentheses are interquartile ranges.
a. WHO (2002b) reports 1,124,000 deaths from malaria.

areas with stable transmission. The arbitrary definition of 5 grams of hemoglobin per deciliter is prognostic for a fatal outcome and proves useful clinically as a criterion for transfusion. Lactic acidosis commonly coexists with hypoglycemia and is (with coma, repeated convulsions, shock, and hyperparasitemia) an important predictor of death from severe malaria (White and Breman 2005; WHO 2000b).

The vast majority of deaths in developing countries occur outside the formal health service, and in Africa, most government civil registration systems are incomplete (Breman 2001; Greenberg and others 1989). Newer demographic and disease-tracking systems are being used globally and should help rectify the woefully inadequate vital statistics available for malaria and other diseases (INDEPTH 2002).

Health personnel usually attribute causes of death during demographic surveillance system surveys through a verbal autopsy interview with relatives of the deceased about the symptoms and signs associated with the terminal illness. Both the specificity and the sensitivity of verbal autopsy vary considerably depending on the background spectrum of other common diseases, such as acute respiratory infection, gastroenteritis, and meningitis, which share common clinical features with malaria (Korenromp and others 2003).

In malarious Africa, some 30 to 60 percent of outpatients with fever may have parasitemia. Monthly surveillance of households will detect a quarter of the medical events that are detected through weekly surveillance, and weekly contacts with cohorts identify approximately 75 percent of events detected through daily surveillance (Snow, Menon, and Greenwood 1989). Given the predominance of fevers, malaria case management in Africa and other endemic areas usually centers on presumptive diagnosis.

Estimates of the frequency of fever among children suggest one episode every 40 days. If we assume that the perceived frequency of fever in Africa is similar across all transmission areas (and possibly all ages), African countries would witness approximately 4.9 billion febrile events each year. Estimates indicate that in areas of stable malaria risk, a minimum of 2.7 billion exposures to antimalarial treatment will occur each year for parasitemic persons, or 4.93 per person per year (Snow and others 2003). While these diagnostic, patient management, and drug delivery assumptions are debatable, they indicate the magnitude of the challenges malaria presents.

The case-fatality rates of CM are high, even with optimal management. Murphy and Breman (2001) report a mean case-fatality rate of 19.2 percent and Snow and others (2003) cite a figure of 17.5 percent. Those who succumb at home without optimal treatment will have higher case-fatality rates.

Studies of neurological sequelae after severe malaria indicated that 3 to 28 percent of survivors suffered from such sequelae, including prolonged coma and seizures (Mung' Ala-Odera, Snow, and Newton 2004). CM is associated with hemipare-

sis, quadriparesis, hearing and visual impairments, speech and language difficulties, behavioral problems, epilepsy, and other problems (table 21.3). The incidence of neurocognitive sequelae following severe malaria is only a fraction of the true residual burden, and the impact of milder illness is unknown.

Studies of children presenting to hospital with malaria and hemoglobin of less than or equal to 5 grams per deciliter indicate a median transfusion rate of 80.1 percent. Thus, 275,400 to 442,290 surviving SMA admissions, newborn through 14 years, will be exposed to blood transfusion each year in Sub-Saharan Africa. As a result, each year 5,300 to 8,500 children, age birth through 14 years, living in stable endemic areas of Africa are likely to acquire HIV infection because of exposure to blood transfusion to manage SMA (Colebunders and others 1991; Savarit and others 1992).

Indirect and Comorbid Risks

The DALY model of malaria does not sufficiently take it into account as an indirect cause of broader morbid risks. Some consider anemia to be caused indirectly unless linked to acute, high-density parasitemia. Similarly, low birthweight may also be indirectly attributable to malaria, and a child's later undernutrition and growth retardation linked to malaria infection enhances the severity of other concomitant or comorbid infectious diseases through immune suppression. Thus, malaria infection contributes to broad causes of mortality beyond the direct fatal consequences of infection and is probably underestimated (Breman, Alilio, and Mills 2004; Snow and others 2003).

In Africa, pregnant women experience few malaria-specific fever episodes but have an increased risk of anemia and placental sequestration of the parasite. Maternal clinical manifestations are more apparent in areas with less intense transmission, particularly in Asia. Estimates indicate that in Sub-Saharan Africa, malaria-associated anemia is responsible for 3.7 percent of maternal mortality, or approximately 5,300 maternal deaths annually.

Prematurity and intrauterine growth retardation resulting in low birthweight associated with maternal malaria account for 3 to 8 percent of infant mortality in Africa (Steketee and others 1996, 2001). Assuming an infant mortality rate of 105 per 1,000 live births, Snow and others (2003) calculate that in 2000, 71,000 to 190,000 infant deaths were attributable to malaria in pregnancy (table 21.3). Other studies indicate that malaria-associated low birthweight accounted for 62,000 to 363,000 infant deaths (Murphy and Breman 2001).

Anemia among African children is caused by a combination of nutritional deficiencies and iron loss through helminth infection, red cell destruction, decreased red cell production as a result of infectious diseases, and genetically determined hemoglobinopathies. Chronic or repeated infections, often associated with parasite resistance to drugs, are more likely to involve bone marrow suppression (Menendez, Fleming, and Alonso 2000).

Murphy and Breman (2001) estimate that 190,000 to 974,000 deaths per year in Sub-Saharan Africa are attributable to SMA. Children residing in areas where the prevalence of *P. falciparum* was more than 25 percent had a 75 percent prevalence of anemia. By modeling the relationship between anemia and parasite prevalence, Snow and others (2004) found that mild anemia rose 6 percent for every 10 percent increase in the prevalence of infection. Reducing the incidence of new infections through ITNs or the prevalence of blood-stage infections through chemoprophylaxis or IPT for children halved the risk of anemia.

Caulfield, Richard, and Black (2004) report that iron, zinc, and protein-calorie deficits are responsible for a considerable amount of malaria-related mortality and morbidity and indicate that 57.3 percent of deaths of underweight children under five are attributable to nutritional deficiencies. One striking feature of the global distribution of anthropometric markers of undernutrition is its congruence with the distribution of endemic malaria. Improved growth among young children has more recently been demonstrated in The Gambia and Kenya in a comparison of those protected and unprotected by ITNs (Ter Kuile and others 2003).

Early during the HIV epidemic, Greenberg and others (1988) and Greenberg (1992) demonstrated that malaria-associated anemia treated with unscreened blood transfusions contributed to HIV transmission. At the same time, two longitudinal cohort studies in Kenya and Uganda and one hospital-based case-control study in Uganda demonstrated that HIV infection approximately doubles the risk of malaria parasitemia and clinical malaria in nonpregnant adults and that increased HIV immunosuppression is associated with higher-density parasitemias (French and others 2001; Whitworth and others 2000). In pregnant women, the presence of HIV increases the rate and intensity of parasitemia and frequency of anemia (Ter Kuile and others 2004). The increasing incidence of HIV-associated febrile illnesses may lead to increased use of antimalarials. Some believe that the recommended use of trimethoprim-sulfamethoxazole for prophylaxis of bacterial pneumonia and other infections in HIV/AIDS patients may contribute to SP resistance and that monitoring is required. Yet, evaluation of trimethoprim-sulfamethoxazole for malaria prophylaxis in Mali did not show any increases in parasite resistance mutations specific for these drugs (Thera and others 2005).

Malaria accounts for 13 to 15 percent of medical reasons for absenteeism from school, but little information is available on the performance of parasitized schoolchildren (Holding and Kitsao-Wekulo 2004). A randomized placebo control study of chloroquine prophylaxis in Sri Lankan schoolchildren demonstrated an improvement in mathematics and language scores by those who received chloroquine but found no difference in absenteeism (Fernando and others 2003) As noted earlier, malaria may result in low birthweight, and low birthweight can lead to a range of persistent impaired outcomes, predominantly behavioral difficulties, cerebral palsy, mental retardation, blindness, and deafness. The recently launched studies of intermittent preventive treatments during infancy (IPTi) should provide a more precise means of examining the benefits of IPTi and consequences on learning and performance of infection early in life (Holding and Kitsao-Wekulo 2004; Rosen and Breman 2004; Schellenberg and others 2005).

INTERVENTIONS AND THEIR EFFECTIVENESS

Malaria will be conquered only by full coverage, access to, and use of antimalarial services by priority groups; rapid, accurate diagnosis; prompt and effective patient management (diagnosis, treatment, counseling and education, referral); judicious use of insecticides to kill and repel the mosquito vector, including the use of ITNs; and control of epidemics. Eliminating malaria from most endemic areas remains a distant, huge, but surmountable challenge because of the widespread *Anopheles* breeding sites; the large number of infected people; the use of ineffective antimalarial drugs; and the inadequacies of resources, infrastructure, and control programs. The Roll Back Malaria Partnership, which began in 1998, aims to halve the burden of malaria by 2010 and has developed strategies and targets for 2005 (box 21.1). While ambitious, the initiative is making substantial progress by means of effective and efficient deployment of currently available interventions (WHO 2003, 2005). Indeed, Brazil, Eritrea, India, and Vietnam are reporting recent successes in reducing the malaria burden (Barat 2005). Despite the enormous investment in developing a malaria vaccine administered by means of a simple schedule and recent promising results in the laboratory and in field trials in Africa, no effective, long-lasting vaccine is likely to be available for general use in the near future (Alonso and others 2004; Ballou and others 2004).

Drug Use

Proper use of drugs is essential. Early diagnosis and effective treatment of patients lends credibility to the malaria program, strengthens confidence in the health care system by families and communities, and raises the esprit of clinicians and public health workers.

Early Diagnosis and Treatment. Early diagnosis and effective treatment can cure infection, prevent further morbidity and progression to severe disease and death, and arrest transmission. This intervention requires timely and accurate diagnosis; use of efficacious drugs; education of patients and their families about the disease, home management, and prevention; and referral to higher levels of the health system. The following are critical to the effectiveness of this intervention:

- *Timeliness.* A febrile malaria attack warrants early treatment. If left untreated, a proportion of *P. falciparum* malaria infections, perhaps 1 in 250 (and to a far lesser extent infections with other malaria species) will progress to severe disease within a few hours to a few days (Greenwood and others 2005). The globally agreed goal is that diagnosis and effective treatment should be provided within 24 hours of the onset of symptoms and signs.

- *Diagnosis and effective drug treatment.* An accurate diagnosis of malaria is based on detection of the parasite and, if laboratory diagnosis is not feasible, on clinical grounds. Health workers must monitor the therapeutic efficacy of drugs closely and change treatment policies when parasite resistance to chloroquine (figure 21.2), SP, and other drugs emerges (Baird 2005; Laxminarayan and others 2006; WHO 2002a). Concerns include unreliable and inaccurate microscopy and the disadvantages of alternative tests plus the widespread distribution and use of substandard and counterfeit drugs. The recommended treatments for malaria in areas with resistance to single drugs are combination treatments, preferably artemisinin combination therapy (ACT) (WHO 2001a, 2001b, 2003a, 2005). While ACT is a welcome, life-saving approach, more information on the cost-effectiveness of this new strategy is needed (Arrow, Panosian, and Gellband 2004; Yeung and others 2004). Baird (2005) reports that ACT costs range from US$2.00 (artesunate-amodiaquine, three doses in 48 hours) to US$9.12 (artemether-lumefantrine, six doses in 48 hours) per adult treatment; WHO has obtained the latter drug for US$2.40 per adult treatment for qualified purchasers, meaning those from low-income malarious countries.

- *Location of clinical management.* Effective management of patients requires skilled and well-equipped personnel at all levels of the health system. The two strategies for delivering antimalarials effectively are through health facilities and in or near the home when access to health facilities is limited. Given the pervasiveness of malaria infections, more information on the most effective and efficient ways to promote home treatment is urgently needed.

Evidence for the effectiveness of early diagnosis and treatment is available from two different epidemiological conditions

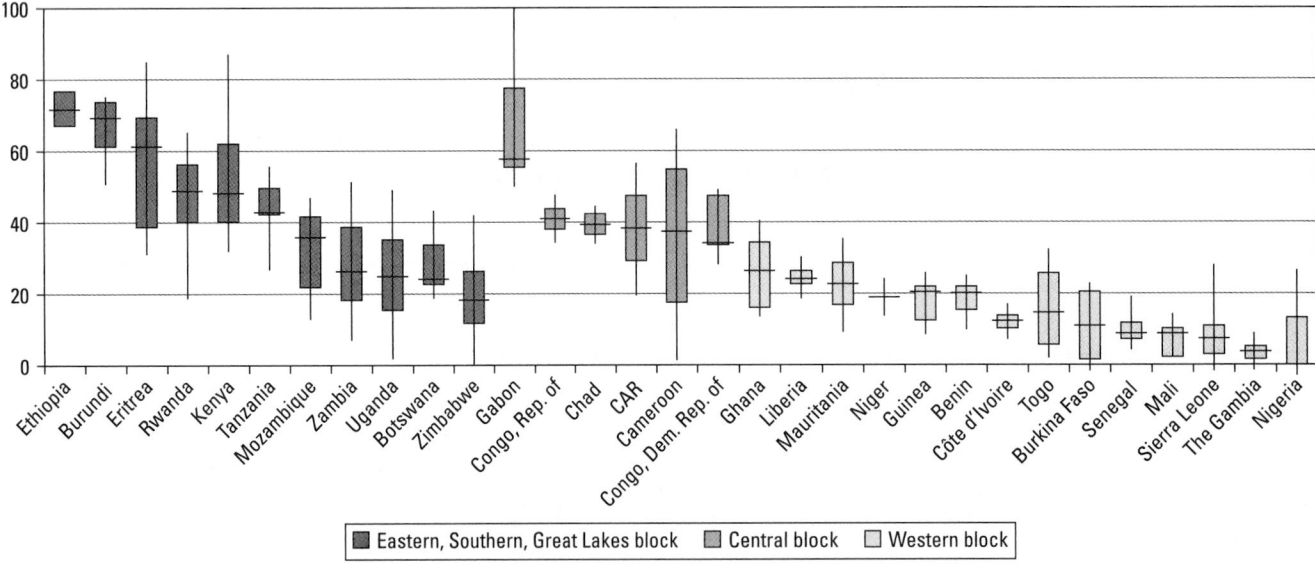

Eastern, Southern, Great Lakes block ■   Central block ■   Western block □

Source: WHO 2005.

Note: WHO has established 126 sentinel sites in 36 African countries that monitor the efficacy of locally used antimalarial drugs by following patients in clinics. The box indicates the 25th–75th percentile, the vertical line the lower and upper values, and where the lines cross the median.

Figure 21.2 Chloroquine Treatment Failure in Africa, 1997–2002

and health systems. In areas of low to moderate transmission, for example, southern Africa, the Americas, and Southeast Asia, where health care systems are relatively effective, the two major consequences of prompt and effective intervention are reduction of the period of infectivity of infected persons, and thus reduced transmission and incidence, and a lowered case-fatality rate and overall mortality. In Vietnam and the KwaZulu-Natal province of South Africa, *P. falciparum* malaria incidence and mortality rates fell when effective treatment policies (artesunate and ACT) replaced failing monotherapies (Hung and others 2002). The effective drug policies were implemented in conjunction with enhanced vector control; thus, effective treatment alone does not account for the fall in malaria incidence and mortality.

In areas with stable, high transmission of *P. falciparum* malaria—for instance, Papua New Guinea and Sub-Saharan Africa—where access to treatment is poor, little is known about the impact of early and effective treatment on malaria transmission. With a high EIR (10 to 1,000), a reduction in transmission intensity is unlikely to affect the incidence of disease until low EIRs (less than 10) are reached.

IPT in Pregnancy and Infancy. IPT is recommended in pregnancy in areas with high and stable transmission of *P. falciparum* malaria; IPT usually consists of two curative doses of antimalarial treatment. The recommended drug is SP given during the second and third trimesters of pregnancy during prenatal care visits. IPT in infancy involves giving infants treatment doses during vaccination or well-baby visits to health clinics.

In primigravid and secundigravid women, the incidence of severe maternal anemia, the incidence and density of placental parasitemia, and the incidence of low birthweight were 25 to 95 percent lower when mothers were given IPT than when they were not (Kayentao and others 2005; Steketee and others 2001). While initial studies indicate that IPT in infancy reduces anemia and febrile episodes, more research is needed. SP is becoming ineffective for IPT, and health experts are suggesting ACT as a replacement (White 2005).

Chemoprophylaxis. Chemoprophylaxis is advised by travel medicine specialists for nonresidents of endemic areas who are exposed to malaria for short periods. WHO does not recommend chemoprophylaxis for permanent residents of endemic areas because of low feasibility and compliance and high costs relative to the public health benefits (WHO 1996, 2000a, 2000b). The choice of chemoprophylaxis will depend on the drug-sensitivity profile, tolerance, side effects, costs, regimen, and compliance by patients (Baird 2005; Kain, Shanks, and Keystone 2001; White and Breman 2005). The effectiveness of chemoprophylaxis will depend mainly on patient compliance and parasite susceptibility.

Supervision and Policy Change. In relation to drug use, all control activities must be supervised and evaluated rigorously to ensure high-quality care for patients and program effectiveness and efficiency (Bryce and others 1994; Jha, Bangoura, and Ranson 1998). Studies in 37 countries indicate the need for a treatment policy change to ACT (WHO 2002a). Several countries in Africa, Asia, and South America are now implementing ACT as the first-line treatment for uncomplicated malaria (WHO 2005). Many countries are also trying to improve the time lag before treatment. More than 83 percent of the population in the three malarious provinces in South Africa is within 10 kilometers of a health facility (Sharp and le Sueur 1996). In Burkina Faso, Ethiopia, and Uganda, where access to clinics was poor and difficult, mothers and community health workers were empowered to dispense treatment, which resulted in major reductions in mortality and morbidity in children (Kidane and Morrow 2000; Pagnoni and others 1997; Sirima and others 2003).

Insecticide-Treated Nets

The use of ITNs (bednets, curtains, and other materials) to provide personal protection by killing or repelling mosquitoes is one of the major strategies of malaria control (RBM 2002). Pyrethroids are recommended for the periodic treatment or re-treatment of the protective materials.

The effectiveness of ITNs depends on their acceptability by the population at risk and their affordability. It is contingent on the habits, biology, and susceptibility of the mosquito vector; the compliance of the human population; and the concentration of insecticide on or in the fiber, which has to be maintained by regular re-treatment or by incorporating the insecticide in the fiber for long duration.

Over 20 studies in Africa and Asia have demonstrated more than 50 percent protective efficacy for individual users of ITNs in reducing malaria episodes, 29 percent protection against severe malarial disease, and substantial protection against anemia (Lengeler 2004). Most importantly, the use of ITNs reduced child mortality by 18 percent in five sites in Sub-Saharan Africa (Lengeler 2004).

Lengeler's (2004) review demonstrates the efficacy of ITNs in both stable and unstable transmission areas. Widespread use of ITNs resulted in an overall reduction in mortality of 19 percent, protected against anemia, and had a substantial impact on mild disease episodes. One large-scale rural study in Tanzania found that ITNs and untreated nets reduced mortality of children one month to four years, with protective efficacies of 27 and 19 percent, respectively (Armstrong-Schellenberg and others 2001). Re-treating ITNs semiannually or just before the annual peak in transmission is essential for effective vector control and is proving a major logistical and financial challenge. Fortunately, new types of nets with a long-lasting insecticidal property are now available, and re-treatment will soon cease to be an issue. The salutary impact of large-scale ITN programs has been demonstrated in China (Tang 2000), Tanzania (Abdulla and others 2001; Armstrong-Schellenberg and others 2001; WHO 2005), and Vietnam (Hung and others 2002). More operational experience is

required to inform national initiatives to scale up ITN use (Lengeler and Sharp 2003); yet, recent encouraging reports show that Eritrea, Malawi, Togo, Zambia, and other countries in Africa are already scaling up nationally with high coverage.

Vector Control

The reduction of *Anopheles* breeding and biting of humans involves different methods of insecticide and repellent application, environmental management, and behavioral change of populations at risk.

Indoor Residual Spraying of Dwellings with Insecticide. Indoor residual spraying (IRS) is the application of long-lasting insecticides (up to six months) on the walls of dwellings. Insecticides repel mosquitoes from entering houses or impart a lethal dose of the insecticide on the female mosquito when it rests on a sprayed surface, thereby preventing subsequent transmission. IRS is most effective against indoor-biting (endophilic) mosquito vectors. Vector susceptibility and post-feeding behavior are the main criteria to be considered when choosing an insecticide: organophosphates, carbamates, and pyrethroids are the main compounds used although some countris still rely on organochlorines (dichlorodiphenyl-trichloroethane, or DDT).

The effectiveness of this intervention depends on cost, toxicity, acceptability of the insecticide, its residual effects, and local political and international partnership commitment. Malaria incidence decreased sharply following the use of IRS in large-scale programs in many parts of Africa, the Americas, Asia, and Europe (Lengeler and Sharp 2003).

In southern Africa, more than 13 million people in six countries are protected from malaria (WHO 2002c). Control was initiated through the use of IRS and supported by engineering approaches, larviciding, prompt diagnosis, and effective treatment. Examples of successful and sustained malaria elimination using IRS with effective drug treatment are available from Cyprus, Greece, Portugal, Spain, and the former Yugoslavia and its successor states (Curtis and Mnzava 2000). The most successful malaria control efforts were linked closely to research and took place in many parts of Asia, where the notable example is the near eradication of malaria from Sri Lanka in the early 1960s, and in Central and South America from the late 1950s to early 1970s (Alilio, Bygbjerg, and Breman 2004; Carter and Mendis 2002; Gilles 2002).

Larviciding and Fogging. Larviciding is the application of chemical insecticides, including those of biological origin and insect growth regulators, to breeding sites. These may be applied to all mosquito breeding sites or targeted to the breeding sites of specific vectors. Recommended compounds, formulations, and dosages for larviciding are available through the WHO Pesticides Evaluation Scheme. Fogging or space spraying with insecticides requires specialized equipment, because the particle size of the insecticide determines its suspension qualities in the air, the number of droplets, and the penetration of space. The insecticide is not effective for as long as with IRS or ITNs, and application must occur during periods of peak target mosquito activity, generally at night.

Larviciding is not generally indicated for large-scale vector control in rural endemic areas because of the difficulty of locating all breeding sites, their often temporary nature, and the required frequency of application. Thus, larviciding is usually limited to urban areas, refugee camps, and industrial and development projects. Despite its impact on mosquito density and its contribution to reducing transmission, larviciding is not as effective as IRS and ITNs in reducing mosquito longevity (Najera and Zaim 2002).

Civil Engineering. Draining and filling larval breeding sites is one of the oldest methods of mosquito control and must be targeted to the breeding sites of locally important malaria vectors. Civil engineering strategies can require costly heavy equipment and materials and are useful for eliminating permanent breeding sites in urban areas, which are increasing globally, and at development project sites where earth removal has occurred.

Home Repellents and Insecticide Use

Commercially available mosquito repellents are applied directly on the skin or clothing as aerosols, lotions, or creams and contain active ingredients that protect the individual from mosquito bites. Commercially available mosquito coils containing pyrethroids can be burnt to repel mosquitoes, and electrically heated dispensers serve a similar function. Some communities in endemic regions use smoke, burning herbs, or plants to deter mosquitoes from entering the home.

N,N-diethyl-meta-toluamide (DEET) is the most widely used and effective ingredient in commercially available repellents (Curtis and others 1991). While several studies have shown that mosquito coils are effective at repelling mosquitoes, they are not as effective as ITNs (Charlwood and Jolly 1984).

Health Education and Counseling

Health education is the provision of information via newspapers, radio, or television, and health counseling is interactive, is individual, and involves the transfer of skills. The provision of information to households on ways to prevent malaria is needed in all endemic communities. It should cover the importance of early treatment and where to access it, the use of referral services, and the significance of full compliance with treatment and other interventions. The necessary information can be provided by community and voluntary health workers.

These persons are an extension of the health system and work under the direct supervision of health facility staff or nongovernmental organizations and in conformity with standards and norms established by the national government (Gilles 2002). Such information can help to increase the standard of patient care and prevention programs by promoting citizen and community advocacy and demand for control.

ECONOMICS OF MALARIA CONTROL INTERVENTIONS

Goodman, Coleman, and Mills's (2000) study represents the most thorough attempt to compare the cost-effectiveness of a wide range of malaria control interventions. They find that in a very low-income country, the cost-effectiveness range per DALY averted was US$19 to US$85 for ITNs (nets plus insecticide), US$32 to US$58 for residual spraying (two rounds per year), US$3 to US$12 for chemoprophylaxis for children (assuming an existing delivery system), US$4 to US$29 for IPT for pregnant women, and US$1 to US$8 for case-management improvements. Goodman, Coleman, and Mills (2000) find that even though some interventions are relatively cheap, achieving high coverage may require a level of expenditure currently out of reach for many African countries and that overcoming operational barriers to achieving widespread coverage is likely to require substantial assistance from external donors.

Analysis

The following analysis incorporates new knowledge on the effects of interventions and on their costs for a low-income, Sub-Saharan African population living in an area of high, stable transmission. The modeling draws on a wide range of sources on the costs and effects of each intervention, extrapolated across settings and operational conditions. The approach allows for changing cost-effectiveness over time, for example, as resistance to antimalarial drugs or insecticides increases. To address problems of uncertainty in relation to many of the parameters, we used probabilistic sensitivity analysis, which allows for multivariate uncertainty by assigning ranges rather than point estimates to input variables. We assumed that cost and effectiveness input variables follow uniform triangular or normal continuous probability distributions (Mulligan, Morel, and Mills 2005).

We consider the cost-effectiveness of a limited subset of interventions: ITNs, IRS, IPT during pregnancy, and patient management with a change of the first-line drug. We include costs to the provider and the community and incremental out-of-pocket expenses for households, but because of major valuation and measurement problems, we do not include the indirect costs of patients' time to seek care and of the lost productivity resulting from morbidity. We consider only gross costs for all interventions except patient management, given the uncertainty inherent in estimating savings.

Insecticide-Treated Nets. We based our analysis of ITNs on the delivery mechanism used in the WHO Special Programme for Research and Training in Tropical Diseases (WHO/TDR) trials, where householders, community health workers, and program staff worked together to treat the nets. In relation to insecticide, we considered permethrin and deltamethrin. Deltamethrin is effective for a year; thus, re-treatment is annual. Permethrin lasts for six months; thus, we assumed two treatments per year if the transmission season is longer than six months. The activities undertaken were the training of staff and community health workers, a campaign to inform the community about the intervention, the procurement and transport of the insecticide and nets, and the initial treatment and the re-treatment of the nets. We calculated cost-effectiveness for each intervention for two scenarios: one whereby nets were distributed to households and the second whereby treatment was arranged for existing nets. We drew estimates of the effectiveness of ITNS from a recent meta-analysis of WHO/TDR-sponsored trials conducted in Sub-Saharan Africa (Lengeler 2004). We adjusted the key parameter and effectiveness estimates to account for the proportion of children sleeping and not sleeping under a recently treated net.

With one treatment per year using deltamethrin, the mean cost per DALY averted was US$11 (90 percent range of US$5 to US$21). With one treatment of permethrin per year the cost-effectiveness ratio (CER) increased slightly to a mean of US$12 (90 percent range of US$6 to US$20). Two treatments of permethrin per year increased the mean CER to US$17 (90 percent range of US$9 to US$31). Even if net coverage is low and nets have to be distributed and treated, the intervention remains an extremely attractive use of resources. Moreover, the model includes health benefits only for children under five. If we included benefits for other household members, the CERs would be lower.

Insecticide Residual Spraying. We considered four insecticides for our analysis of the cost-effectiveness of IRS: DDT; malathion; and two pyrethroids, deltamethrin and lambda-cyhalothrin. We used the results of the Cochrane Review meta-analysis of ITN trials conducted in Africa to approximate the results of spraying on morbidity and mortality and adjusted effectiveness estimates to account for noncompliance (Lengeler 2004).

We found little difference between the CERs for the four insecticides when one round of spraying was done per year: they ranged from US$5 to US$18. With two rounds per year, costs increased, but we assumed that effectiveness remained the same, so all the CERs approximately doubled to US$11 to

US$34. These results should be interpreted with caution because of uncertainty in relation to the estimates of effectiveness in children under five. The model was based on one round of spraying per year in areas of seasonal transmission and two rounds per year in areas of high, intense (perennial) transmission. Effectiveness will depend on the length of the transmission seasons and on the insecticide. DDT lasts for six months or more, lambda-cyhalothrin for three to six months, and malathion and deltamethrin for only two to three months (Lengeler 2004; Lengeler and Sharp 2003).

IPT during Pregnancy. We analyzed the cost-effectiveness of IPT assuming that primigravid women are given two or three doses of SP at a prenatal clinic. We analyzed benefits to the child by decreased mortality and benefits to the mother resulting from changes in the incidence of severe anemia. We estimated the effect of IPT on the neonatal mortality rate as a function of increased birthweight based on the Cochrane meta-analysis of malaria prevention in pregnancy (Gülmezoglu and Garner 1998). The model allowed for level of drug resistance, probability of initial attendance at a prenatal clinic, probability of returning for a second visit, probability of returning for a third visit, and compliance with the drug regimen. We estimated both incremental and average costs.

The incremental CER for IPT in pregnancy using SP had a 90 percent range from US$9 to US$21 with a mean of US$13. Average total cost-effectiveness had a mean of US$24 (90 percent range of US$16 to US$35).

Change in First-Line Drug. We analyzed the cost-effectiveness of changing first-line therapies to SP and to ACT using a patient-management model with a decision-tree framework in which a patient presents with uncomplicated malaria at an outpatient facility and progresses to full recovery, recovery with neurological sequelae, or death. Three potential drug policy changes were considered (see table 21.5). For current drug policies we assumed either chloroquine or SP as the first-line drug, with SP or amodiaquine as a second-line drug and quinine as the third-line drug. We then examined the cost-effectiveness of policy switches to either SP or ACT as first-line drug (with amodiaquine as second line and quinine as third line).

Amodiaquine was chosen as the second-line drug in the new drug policy because, like chloroquine and SP, it is relatively cheap. Low compliance, adverse effects, and potential cross-resistance between amodiaquine and chloroquine excluded it from first-line selection. We omitted other potential drugs to limit the scope of analysis.

We used commonly found levels of drug resistance to create likely ranges. When used as second-line treatment, we assumed that a drug faced half the level of resistance than when it was used as a first-line drug. We estimated the growth rate of resistance to each drug based on its expected current location along

Table 21.5 Change in First-Line Drug

Scenario	Current drug policy			New drug policy		
	First-line drug	Second-line drug	Third-line drug	First-line drug	Second-line drug	Third-line drug
A	Chloroquine	SP	Quinine	SP	Amodiaquine	Quinine
B	Chloroquine	SP	Quinine	ACT	Amodiaquine	Quinine
C	SP	Amodiaquine	Quinine	ACT	Amodiaquine	Quinine

Source: Authors.

Resistance to current drug (percent)

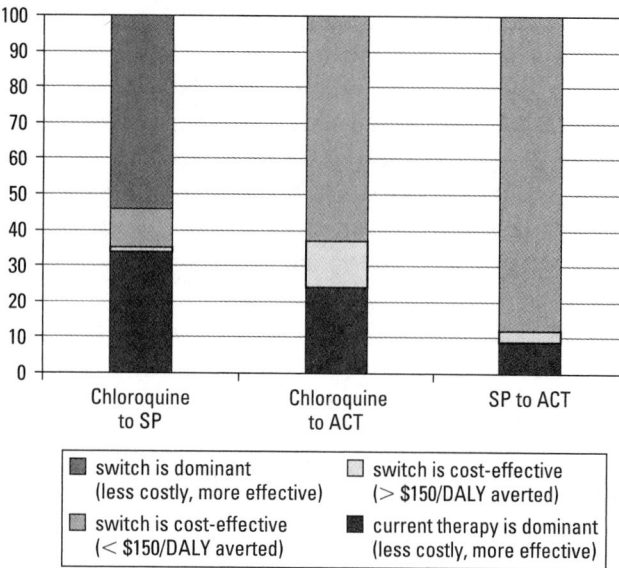

Figure 21.3 Cost-Effectiveness of Switching the First-Line Drug

a sigmoid growth curve. We assessed compliance with each drug based on the length and complexity of each regimen. We gave the widest range (20 to 70 percent) to compliance with ACT, which usually requires a three-day treatment, to account for the different lengths of regimen and variety of formulations.

Figure 21.3 shows that a switch from chloroquine to SP is cost-effective (less than $150 per DALY averted) when chloroquine resistance is above 35 percent. Switching from chloroquine to ACT becomes cost-effective as chloroquine resistance reaches around 37 percent. Switching from SP to ACT becomes cost-effective as SP resistance reaches 12 percent. This low threshold is due to the high growth rate of resistance to SP when it is used as a first-line therapy.

Results and Interpretation. Table 21.6 presents the average CERs for the interventions reviewed. All interventions can be considered attractive using a cutoff of US$150 per DALY averted. For the childhood preventive interventions, the level of existing infrastructure is a key factor in influencing cost-effectiveness. ITNs are an even better use of resources if

Table 21.6 CERs for ITNs, IRS, and IPT (2001 US$)

Intervention	Mean cost per DALY averted	90 percent range
ITNs (net + insecticide treatment)		
Deltamethrin	11	5–21
Permethrin (1 treatment)	12	6–20
Permethrin (2 treatments)	17	9–31
ITNs (without provision of nets)		
Deltamethrin	5	2–7
Permethrin (1 treatment)	6	3–9
Permethrin (2 treatments)	11	6–17
IRS (1 round)		
Melathion	12	8–18
DDT	9	5–13
Deltamethrin	10	6–14
Lambda-cyhalothrin	10	6–14
IRS (2 rounds)		
Malathion	24	15–34
DDT	17	11–24
Deltamethrin	18	12–27
Lambda-cyhalothrin	19	12–28
IPT		
Incremental costs	13	9–21
Average costs	24	16–35

Source: Authors' calculations.

net coverage is already high, and IPT is even more cost-effective if prenatal care coverage is good. However, even if levels of infrastructure are poor, these interventions are still attractive based on cost-effectiveness criteria.

Curtis and Mnzava's (2000) review comparing worldwide trials of ITNs and IRS for malaria control suggests that they were of equivalent effectiveness. Lengeler and Sharp (2003 21,) also conclude that choosing between IRS and ITNs is "largely a matter of operational feasibility and availability of local resources, rather than one of malaria epidemiology or cost-effectiveness." DDT is the cheapest insecticide but is seldom used because of concerns about its environmental impact. An updated systematic review of the health effects of IRS as well as a full economic comparison between spraying with DDT and other insecticides and ITNs is urgently required. Such reviews should include the environmental benefits of reducing DDT levels and the costs of alternative interventions.

As effective patient management, IPT, and other approaches toward drug use become more widespread, drug resistance will increase, which will affect cost-effectiveness. In terms of first-line treatment, while a switch from chloroquine to SP is unlikely to be costly, cost-effectiveness depends on the initial level of severe resistance to each drug. A switch from chloroquine to ACT is likely to be costly but more effective, given that resistance to ACT is essentially nonexistent and the growth rate of resistance to ACT is likely to be low (Yeung and others 2004). Given the high growth rate of resistance to SP, switching to ACT becomes cost-effective when SP resistance surpasses 12 percent, a relatively low threshold. A switch from chloroquine to ACT appears to be highly cost-effective at all initial levels of chloroquine resistance above 37 percent. Recent studies indicate the remarkable effectiveness of the ACT artemether-lumefantrine in East African areas of chloroquine, amodiaquine, and SP resistance (Mutabingwa and others 2005; Piola and others 2005); it is expected that the availability of ACTs will increase and the costs will decrease in the near future.

Affordability and Scaling Up

Cost-effectiveness analyses can identify which interventions are the most efficient to implement, but information is also needed on affordability. Some interventions are cheap, such as prevention in pregnancy. Achievement of high coverage with an intervention to prevent childhood malaria (for example, ITNs) has a high total cost, which needs to be borne in part by external funding. For example, full coverage of children (assuming 22 percent of the population is under five years of age) would cost US$2.81 million per 1 million persons of the general population covered (assuming the provision of nets plus two rounds of permethrin). The same coverage with IRS would cost about US$4.01 million using deltamethrin (two rounds).

In addition to the difficulties of financial feasibility, the implementation of ITN interventions poses operational and logistical challenges. A number of strategic approaches are available for national ITN upscaling (RBM 2002). The main ones are social marketing (for example, in Malawi and Kenya), assisted commercial sector development (Senegal, Mali, Tanzania), and totally free distribution (Togo). An important feature of all the approaches is that their cost per net distributed decreases significantly as the scale of the undertaking increases, so it is hard to use available estimates to project cost in national programs.

Independent of the main ITN distribution strategy, a number of countries are implementing additional actions targeted at the main high-risk groups. For example, a national voucher scheme is currently being implemented in Tanzania to provide every pregnant woman in the country with a free ITN, and a net is being distributed to children at the time of measles vaccination in Togo.

Re-treatment of ITNs on a large-scale remains a formidable operational issue, and free distribution of insecticide in the way it is done in Vietnam and China is probably the best way forward. This should occur while waiting the availability of long-lasting insecticidal nets that do not require retreatment.

Curtis and Maxwell (2002) point to the successful experience of Vietnam, where ITNs now protect 10 million people and the public health service provides free insecticide. This approach in Africa would require a substantial commitment by donors and governments given that most African governments spend only around US$4 per capita per year on health (World Bank 2003). Eritrea, with 65 percent ITN coverage, and other African countries are beginning to make great strides in getting ITNs to their populations (Barat 2006; WHO 2005; World Bank 2005).

The move toward ACT poses the most difficult questions in relation to the long-term affordability of malaria control interventions. After scale-up, estimates indicate that the additional annual costs of ACT versus current failing drugs range from US$300 million to US$500 million globally (Arrow, Panosian, and Gellband 2004), with the precise amount depending on the extent to which all fevers are treated. This figure does not include drugs for nonmalarial fevers in endemic areas and the costs for the substantial health system strengthening required to make the most effective use of ACT. These include the costs of improved drug regulation, pharmacovigilance, diagnostics, and implementation of different drug policies for different population groups. The introduction of ACT has permanently changed the economic landscape of malaria control. Innovative funding solutions at the global level are required to ensure that effective drugs are made available to the most vulnerable groups. The Global Fund to Fight AIDS, Tuberculosis, and Malaria is providing the major leadership and resources for securing ACTs and other commodities, and many other agencies and organizations are joining coalitions to combat malaria through control, research, training, funding, and advocacy activities (Breman, Alilio, and Mills 2004; Feacham 2004: http://www. theglobalfund.org/en).

Economic Benefits of Malaria Control

Given the substantial total costs of several malaria control interventions, the case for introducing them can be strengthened by evidence on non-health-related benefits, especially evidence of income gains or prevention of income losses. Three different approaches to measuring such benefits are assessing the direct and indirect costs of malaria, studying the relationship between malaria and the output of agricultural or industrial activities, and exploring the macroeconomic impact of malaria. Only the third approach sheds much light on the benefits of control as opposed to the burden of the disease in the absence of control. This point is important, because in places facing the most severe malaria problems, direct information on the economic benefits of control is largely unavailable.

Direct and Indirect Costs of Malaria. The standard approach has been to view the two key determinants of the economic costs of malaria as the direct costs of expenditure on prevention and treatment and the indirect costs of productive labor time lost because of malaria morbidity and mortality, and to estimate the total economic impact by adding the direct and indirect costs (Mills 1992). Households use a range of preventive measures (mosquito coils, aerosol sprays, bednets, and mosquito repellents) to differing degrees. A review of evidence for Sub-Saharan Africa found that monthly per capita household expenditures ranged from US$0.05 per person in rural Malawi to US$2.10 in urban Cameroon, equivalent to US$0.24 and US$15 per household in 1999 U.S. dollars (Chima, Goodman, and Mills 2003). The costs of treatment for malaria include out-of-pocket expenditures for consultation fees, drugs, transport, and subsistence at a distant health facility. For Sub-Saharan Africa, these costs ranged between US$0.41 and US$3.88 per person, equivalent to between US$1.88 and US$26 per household per year. Household expenditure on treatment is usually highly regressive, consuming a much larger proportion of income in the poorest households.

Computations of public expenditures on malaria prevention and treatment are imprecise because most fall within general health service expenditures. About 20 to 40 percent of outpatient visits in malarious Africa are for fever, and suspected malaria among inpatients ranges from 0.5 to 50.0 percent of admissions. Kirigia and others (1998) found that inpatient treatment for pediatric malaria absorbed 15 percent of the annual recurrent costs of inpatient care in one Kenyan hospital and 9 percent in another. Ettling and Shepard (1991) estimated that Rwanda's Ministry of Health spent 19 percent of its operating budget on malaria treatment. Because of the dominance of out-of-pocket spending by households, public expenditures on malaria generally account for a minority of total malaria expenditure.

The methods used to measure and value time lost and a day's work vary considerably between studies; the average time lost per episode for a sick adult and for an adult caring for sick children ranged from one to five days. The average indirect cost per episode ranged from US$0.68 for children under 10 years of age in Malawi to US$23 per adult episode in Ethiopia. Authors have concluded that aggregate productivity losses can be significant for households and for the economy as a whole. In Malawi, the indirect costs of malaria were equiv-

alent to 2.6 percent of annual household income (Ettling and others 1994), and Russell (2004) reports that malaria generally consumes less than 10 percent of family income. Leighton and Foster (1993) estimate that the total annual value of malaria-related production losses was 2 to 6 percent of gross domestic product in Kenya and 1 to 5 percent in Nigeria. The productivity consequences of mortality have received relatively little attention.

The direct and indirect cost approach involves two methodological problems. First, calculations are based mainly on days of illness and neglect mortality, debility (usually from anemia), and neurological and other long-term sequelae. Second, households' coping strategies are likely to reduce the immediate impact of illness, although in the long term they may impose costs through the sale of assets such as livestock, which jeopardizes a household's asset base.

Relationship between Malaria and Output. With the exception of a study of cotton production in Côte d'Ivoire, where the prevalence of parasitemia above a cutoff density had a major impact on labor efficiency (Audibert, Mathonnat, and Henry 2003), studies have not succeeded in identifying impacts on output. One possibility is that the risk of malaria may discourage the planting of crops that require intensive cultivation, the settlement and cultivation of fertile land, or the development of tourism and industry in suitable locations, but good evidence is lacking.

Macroeconomic Impact of Malaria. Recent empirical cross-country comparisons of economic growth indicate that eliminating malaria would have a strong positive impact on economic development. Gallup and Sachs (2001) use cross-country regression analysis to relate the growth in gross domestic product per capita between 1965 and 1990 to initial income levels, initial human capital stock, policy variables, geographical variables, and a malaria index calculated as the product of the fraction of land area with endemic malaria in 1965 and the fraction of malaria cases that were due to *P. falciparum* in 1990. Their results suggest that countries with a substantial amount of malaria grew 1.3 percent per year less than countries with little or no malaria between 1965 and 1990 (controlling for other influences on growth) and that a 10 percent reduction in malaria was associated with 0.3 percent higher growth per year. McCarthy, Wolf, and Wu (2000) employ a similar approach to explore the impact of malaria on average per capita growth rates during three five-year periods. They find a significant negative association between malaria and economic growth, although the estimated impact differed sharply across countries. The impact was smaller than that found by Gallup and Sachs (2001), exceeding 0.25 percent per year in only a quarter of the sample countries and averaging 0.55 percent for those in Sub-Saharan Africa.

Benefit-Cost Ratios

Mills and Shillcutt 2004 related the evidence on the macroeconomic benefits of malaria control to information on the costs of reducing malaria to calculate a benefit-cost ratio (Mills and Shillcutt 2004). Depending on the assumptions, the benefit-cost ratio ranged between 1.9 and 4.7 (using a 3 percent discount rate). In terms of economic growth alone malaria control is extremely cost beneficial.

RESEARCH PRIORITIES

Current interventions to combat malaria remain inadequate for achieving the increased levels of successful patient management and prevention to which all malarious countries aspire and for which ambitious targets have been set (box 21.1). Greatly increased support for malaria research and for developing institutional capacity must occur to make advances and to bring them to populations in need. The WHO Scientific Working Group on Malaria and others have identified four major areas of research as follows (Remme and others 2002; WHO 1996, 2003c).

Patient Management

Patient management, including treatment, should address the following:

- evaluation of treatment effectiveness and of access to treatment for uncomplicated malaria in children and during pregnancy, with an emphasis on home management and evaluation of alternative delivery systems
- investigation of the pathogenesis of malaria, in particular anemia and immune response mechanisms
- evaluation of new approaches, for example, rectal drug administration, for managing severe illness
- evaluation of ACT, including delivery approaches via the public and private sectors
- development of new drugs with novel targets; the Medicines for Malaria Ventura (MMV) is spearheading this activity.

Prevention Research

Prevention research should focus on the following:

- new approaches to drug-based malaria prevention, including IPT in children and during pregnancy
- strategies for scaling up the use of ITNs.

Innovative Approaches

Innovative approaches should use new technologies, including recent advances in sequencing the DNA of *P. falciparum* and *A. gambiae,* to achieve the following:

- discover and develop drugs, diagnostics, vaccines, insecticides, and antiparasite effector molecules using genomics

- carry out strategic and basic research on vector-parasite-host interactions
- assess mechanisms for addressing drug and insecticide resistance
- develop and carry out field evaluations of transgenic methods for interrupting malaria transmission.

Policy Research

Social, economic, and policy research should focus on the following:

- developing and applying a common methodology for measuring socioeconomic status
- carrying out policy and operational research on the impact, viability, sustainability, and optimal balance of public-private partnerships
- investigating ethical, legal, and social issues pertaining to new malaria-related tools.

Capacity strengthening for research and operations (including clinical trials) is urgently needed. This strengthening will result in the ability to better evaluate new drugs and vaccines and existing malaria control tools (ITNs, IPT) and to tackle the scaling up of malaria strategies.

A classification of research priorities by time frame includes the three-year, five-year, and ten-year targeting.

Three-year completion targeting includes the following:

- apply to the U.S. Food and Drug Administration (FDA) with evidence for two separate fixed-dose artemisinin combinations at a target adult treatment price of US$1.00, or US$0.60 or less for children; two combinations are necessary, as one may fail in testing or have other unforeseen problems
- evaluate the two best candidate ACT drugs for IPT in pregnant women and in infancy and early childhood (IPTi)
- launch studies to reach an evidence-based conclusion on the costs and benefits of long-lasting ITNs versus IRS in Sub-Saharan Africa and other endemic areas
- carry out operational studies to determine the best methods of deploying ACT through the public and private sectors so that first-level patient management can occur at the home and at the village levels; this involves studying packaging and distribution networks, assessing adherence, and addressing how to deploy and supervise use of artesunate rectal suppositories
- conduct economic reviews and predictive modeling to make an economic case for increased international investment in malaria control, including collecting detailed data from several scaled-up, national, fully supported control programs employing the best available strategies and interventions

- conduct in Africa and other endemic continents a maximum number of FDA-compliant phase I and phase II malaria vaccine trials to select candidates for clinical trials.

The five-year completion target is as follows:

- develop and deploy more sensitive, specific, and predictive diagnostic tests that are inexpensive and practical
- carry out operational studies on how to deploy diagnostics in areas of low, intermediate, and high transmission.

The ten-year completion target has these focuses:

- develop an inexpensive, safe, and synthetic trioxane antimalarial drug
- develop another new drug with a target and resistance mechanism that is unrelated to existing drugs
- carry out basic insecticide research to develop new approaches to both personal protection and residual house spraying
- launch successful phase III and phase IV field testing of malaria vaccines to prevent clinical illness and transmission with licensure by regulatory bodies
- use genomic, proteomic, and bioinformatic tools to better understand the pathogenesis of malaria, to design new drugs and vaccine candidates for training scientists, and to transfer technologies
- train a critical mass of leaders in science and operations to carry out the required research in support of control.

CONCLUSION

Given the heavy burden of malaria, the need to use existing strategies and interventions in scaled-up programs more effectively and to deploy them more widely is urgent and merits the highest priority, especially in Africa. While existing tools can be improved, newer tools are required. The history of malaria research and control shows that they are synergistic. Integrating research and control activities has resulted in success in several areas of the world, and will result in vanquishing malaria early in the 21st century.

REFERENCES

Abdulla, S., J. A. Schellenberg, R. Nathan, O. Mukasa, T. Marchant, T. Smith, and others. 2001. "Impact on Malaria Morbidity of a Programme Supplying Insecticide Treated Nets in Children Age under Two Years in Tanzania: Community Cross-Sectional Study." *British Medical Journal* 322: 270–73.

Alilio, M. S., I. Bygbjerg, and J. G. Breman. 2004. "Are Multilateral Malaria Research and Control Programs the Most Successful? Lessons from the Past 100 Years." *American Journal of Tropical Medicine and Hygiene* 70 (Suppl. 2): 268–78.

Alonso, P. L., J. Sacarlal, J. J. Aponte, A. Leach, E. Macete, J. Milman, and others. 2004. "Efficacy of the RTS,S/AS02A Vaccine against *Plasmodium falciparum* Infection and Disease in Young African Children: Randomised Controlled Trial." *Lancet* 364: 1411–20.

Armstrong-Schellenberg, J. R., S. Abdulla, R. Nathan, O. Mukasa, T. J. Marchant, N. Kikumbih, and others. 2001. "Effect of Large-Scale Social Marketing of Insecticide-Treated Nets on Child Survival in Rural Tanzania." *Lancet* 357: 1241–47.

Arrow, K. J., C. B. Panosian, and H. Gellband, eds. 2004. *Saving Lives, Buying Time: Economics of Malaria Drugs in an Age of Resistance.* Washington, DC: National Academy Press for Institute of Medicine.

Audibert, M., J. Mathonnat, and M. C. Henry. 2003. "Malaria and Property Accumulation in Rice Production Systems in the Savannah Zone of Côte d'Ivoire." *Tropical Medicine and International Health* 8 (5): 471–83.

Baird, J. K. 2005. "Effectiveness of Antimalarial Drugs." *New England Journal of Medicine* 352: 1565–77.

Ballou, R., M. Arevalo-Herrera, D. Carucci, T. L. Richie, G. Corradin, C. Diggs, and others. 2004. "Update on the Clinical Development of Candidate Malaria Vaccines." *American Journal of Tropical Medicine and Hygiene* 71 (Suppl. 2): 239–47.

Barat, L. M. 2006. "Four Malaria Success Stories: How Malaria Burden Was Successfully Reduced in Brazil, Eritrea, India, and Vietnam." *American Journal of Tropical Medicine and Hygiene* 74 (1): 12–16.

Breman, J. G. 2001. "The Ears of the Hippopotamus: Manifestations, Determinants, and Estimates of the Malaria Burden." *American Journal of Tropical Medicine and Hygiene* 64 (Suppl. 1–2): 1–11.

Breman, J. G., M. S. Alilio, and A. Mills. 2004. "Conquering the Intolerable Burden of Malaria: What's New, What's Needed: A Summary." *American Journal of Tropical Medicine and Hygiene* 71 (Suppl. 2): 1–15.

Bryce, J., C. Boschi-Pinto, K. Shibuya, R. E. Black, and the WHO Child Health Epidemiology Reference Group. 2005. "WHO Estimates of the Causes of Deaths of Children." *Lancet* 365 (9465): 1114–6.

Bryce, J., J. B. Roungou, P. Nguyen-Dinh, J. F. Naimoli, and J. G. Breman. 1994. "Evaluation of National Malaria Control Programmes in Africa." *Bulletin of the World Health Organization* 72 (3): 371–81.

Carter, R., and K. Mendis. 2002. "Evolutionary and Historical Aspects of the Burden of Malaria." *Clinical Microbiological Reviews* 15 (4): 564–94.

Caulfield, L., S. A. Richard, and R. Black. 2004. "Undernutrition as an Underlying Cause of Malaria Morbidity and Mortality." *American Journal of Tropical Medicine and Hygiene* 71 (Suppl. 2): 55–63.

Charlwood, D., and D. Jolly. 1984. "The Coil Works against Mosquitoes in Papua, New Guinea." *Transactions of the Royal Society of Tropical Medicine and Hygiene* 78: 678.

Chima, R., C. Goodman, and A. Mills. 2003. "The Economic Impact of Malaria in Africa: A Critical Review of the Evidence." *Health Policy* 63 (1): 17–36.

Colebunders, R., R. Ryder, H. Francis, W. Nekwei, Y. Bahwe, I. Lebughe, and others. 1991. "Seroconversion Rate, Mortality, and Clinical Manifestations Associated with the Receipt of a Human Immunodeficiency Virus-Infected Blood Transfusion in Kinshasa, Zaire." *Journal of Infectious Diseases* 164 (3): 450–56.

Craig, M. H., R. W. Snow, and D. le Sueur. 1999. "A Climate-Based Distribution Model of Malaria Transmission in Sub-Saharan Africa." *Parasitology Today* 15: 105–11.

Curtis, C. F., J. D. Lines, B. Lu, and A. Renz. 1991. "Natural and Synthetic Repellents." In *Control of Disease Vectors in the Community*, ed. C. F. Curtis, 75–92. London: Wolfe.

Curtis, C. F., and C. Maxwell. 2002. "Free Insecticide for Nets Is Cost-Effective." *Trends in Parasitology* 18: 204–5.

Curtis, C. F., and A. E. P. Mnzava. 2000. "Comparison of House Spraying and Insecticide-Treated Nets for Malaria Control." *Bulletin of the World Health Organization* 78 (12): 1389–1401.

Djimdé, A. A., A. Dolo, A. Quattara, S. Diakité, C. V. Plowe, and O. K. Doumbo. 2004. "Molecular Diagnosis of Resistance to Antimalarial Drugs during Epidemics and in War Zones." *Journal of Infectious Diseases* 190 (4): 853–55.

Ettling, M. B., D. A. McFarland, L. J. Schultz, and L. Chitsulo. 1994. "Economic Impact of Malaria in Malawian Households." *Tropical Medicine and Parasitology* 45: 74–79.

Ettling, M. B., and D. S. Shepard. 1991. "Economic Cost of Malaria in Rwanda." *Tropical Medicine and Parasitology* 42 (3): 214–18.

Feacham, R. G. A. 2004. "The Research Imperative: Fighting AIDS, TB, and Malaria." *Tropical Medicine and International Health* 9 (11): 1139–41.

Fernando, D., R. Wickremasinghe, K. N. Mendis, and A. R. Wickremasinghe. 2003. "Cognitive Performance at School Entry of Children Living in Malaria-Endemic Areas of Sri Lanka." *Transactions of the Royal Society of Tropical Medicine and Hygiene* 97 (3): 161–65.

French, N., J. Nakiyingi, E. Lugada, C. Watera, J. A. Whitworth, and C. F. Gilks. 2001. "Increasing Rates of Malarial Fever with Deteriorating Immune Status in HIV-1 Infected Ugandan Adults." *AIDS* 15 (7): 899–906.

Gallup, J. L., and J. D. Sachs. 2001. "The Economic Burden of Malaria." *American Journal of Tropical Medicine and Hygiene* 64 (Suppl. 1): 85–96.

Gilles, H. M., ed. 2002. "Historical Outline." In *Essential Malariology,* 4th ed., ed. D. A. Warrell and H. M. Gilles, 1–7. New York: Arnold.

Goodman, C., P. Coleman, and A. Mills. 2000. *Economic Analysis of Malaria Control in Sub-Saharan Africa.* Geneva: Global Forum for Health Research.

Greenberg, A. E. 1992. "HIV and Malaria." In *AIDS in the World,* ed. J. M. Mann, D. J. Tarantola, and T. W. Netter, 143–48. Cambridge, MA: Harvard University Press.

Greenberg, A. E., P. Nguyen-Dinh, J. M. Mann, N. Kabote, R. L. Colebunders, H. Francis, and others. 1988. "The Association Between Malaria, Blood Transfusions, and HIV Seropositivity in a Pediatric Population in Kinshasa, Zaire." *Journal of the American Medical Association* 259: 545–49.

Greenberg, A. E., M. Ntumbanzondo, N. Ntula, L. Mawa, J. Howell, and F. Davachi. 1989. "Hospital-Based Surveillance of Malaria-Related Paediatric Morbidity and Mortality in Kinshasa, Zaire." *Bulletin of the World Health Organization* 67 (2): 189–96.

Greenwood, B. M., K. Bojang, C. J. M. Whitty, and G. A. T. Targett. 2005. "Malaria." *Lancet* 365 (9469): 1487–98.

Gülmezoglu, A. M., and P. Garner. 1998. "Malaria in Pregnancy in Endemic Areas (Cochrane Review)." *Cochrane Library* 3, Oxford, Update Software.

Hay, S. I., D. J. Rogers, J. F. Toomer, and R. W. Snow. 2004. "Annual *Plasmodium falciparum* Entomological Inoculation Rates (EIR) across Africa: Literature Survey, Internet Access, and Review." *Transactions of the Royal Society of Tropical Medicine and Hygiene* 94: 113–27.

Holding, P. A., and P. K. Kitsao-Wekulo. 2004. "Describing the Burden of Malaria on Child Development: What Should We Be Measuring and How Should We Be Measuring It?" *American Journal of Tropical Medicine and Hygiene* 71 (Suppl. 2): 71–79.

Hung, I. Q., P. J. Vries, P. T. Giao, N. V. Nam, T. Q. Binh, M. T. Chong, and others. 2002. "Control of Malaria: A Successful Experience from Viet Nam." *Bulletin of the World Health Organization* 80 (8): 660–66.

INDEPTH (International Network of Field Sites with Continuous Demographic Evaluation of Populations and Their Health in Developing Countries). 2002. *Population, Health, and Survival at INDEPTH Sites.* Vol. 1 of *Population and Health in Developing Countries.* Ottawa: International Development Research Centre.

Jha, P., O. Bangoura, and R. Ranson. 1998. "The Cost-Effectiveness of Forty Health Interventions in Guinea." *Health Policy and Planning* 13 (3): 249–62.

Kain, K. C., G. D. Shanks, and J. S. Keystone. 2001. "Malaria Chemoprophylaxis in the Age of Drug Resistance: I. Currently Recommended Drug Regimens." *Clinical Infectious Diseases* 33 (2): 226–34.

Kayentao, K., M. Kodio, R. D. Newman, H. Maiga, D. Doumtabe, A. Ongoiba, and others. 2005. "Comparison of Intermittent Preventive Treatment with Chemoprophylaxis for the Prevention of Malaria during Pregnancy in Mali." *Journal of Infectious Diseases* 191 (1): 109–16.

Keiser, J., J. Utzinger, M. Caldas de Castro, T. A. Smith, M. Tanner, and B. H. Singer. 2004. "Urbanization in Sub-Saharan Africa and Malaria Control." *American Journal of Tropical Medicine and Hygiene* 71 (Suppl. 2): 118–27.

Kidane, G., and R. H. Morrow. 2000. "Teaching Mothers to Provide Home Treatment of Malaria in Tigray, Ethiopia: A Randomised Trial." *Lancet* 356 (9229): 550–55.

Kirigia, J. M., R. W. Snow, J. Fox-Rushby, and A. Mills. 1998. "The Cost of Treating Pediatric Malaria Admissions and the Potential Impact of Insecticide-Treated Mosquito Nets on Hospital Expenditure." *Tropical Medicine and International Health* 3: 145–50.

Korenromp, E. L., B. G. Williams, E. Gouws, C. Dye, and R. W. Snow. 2003. "Measuring Trends in Childhood Malaria Mortality in Africa: A New Assessment of Progress toward Targets Based on Verbal Autopsy." *Lancet Infectious Diseases* 3: 349–58.

Laxminarayan, R., Z. Bhutta, A. Duse, P. Jenkins, T. O'Brien, I. N. Okeke, A. Pablo-Mendez, K. P. Klugman. 2006. "Drug Resistance." In D. T. Jamison, J. G. Breman, A. Measham, and others, *Disease Control Priorities in Developing Countries,* eds. 2nd. ed. New York: Oxford University Press, ch. 55.

Leighton, C., and R. Foster. 1993. "Economic Impacts of Malaria in Kenya and Nigeria." Abt Associates, Health Financing and Sustainability Project, Bethesda, Maryland.

Lengeler, C. 2004. "Insecticide-Treated Bed Nets and Curtains for Preventing Malaria." Cochrane Database Systematic Reviews (2) CD000363.

Lengeler, C., and B. Sharp. 2003. "Indoor Residual Spraying and Insecticide-Treated Nets." In *Reducing Malaria's Burden. Evidence of Effectiveness for Decision Makers.* Washington DC: Global Health Council, 17–24. http://www.globalhealth.org

McCarthy, F. D., H. Wolf, and Y. Wu. 2000. "The Growth Costs of Malaria." In NBER Working Paper 7541, National Bureau of Economic Research, Cambridge, MA.

Mendis, K., B. J. Sina, P. Marchesini, and R. Carter. 2001. "The Neglected Burden of *Plasmodium vivax* Malaria." *American Journal of Tropical Medicine and Hygiene* 64 (Suppl. 1): 97–105.

Menendez, C., A. F. Fleming, and P. L. Alonso. 2000. "Malaria-Related Anemia." *Parasitology Today* 16: 469–76.

Mills, A. 1992. "The Economic Evaluation of Malaria Control Technologies: The Case of Nepal." *Social Science and Medicine* 34: 965–72.

Mills, A., and S. Shillcutt. 2004. "The Challenge of Communicable Disease." In *Global Crises, Global Solutions,* ed. B. Lomborg. Cambridge, U.K.: Cambridge University Press.

Mulligan, J., C. Morel, and A. Mills. 2005. "Cost-Effectiveness of Malaria Control Interventions." Disease Control Priorities Project Background Paper, Disease Control Priorities Project, Bethesda, MD.

Mung'Ala-Odera, V., R. W. Snow, and C. R. J. C. Newton. 2004. "The Burden of the Neurocognitive Impairment Associated with Falciparum Malaria in Sub-Saharan Africa." *American Journal of Tropical Medicine and Hygiene* 71 (Suppl. 2): 64–70.

Murphy, S. C., and J. G. Breman. 2001. "Gaps in the Childhood Malaria Burden in Africa: Cerebral Malaria, Neurologic Sequelae, Anemia, Respiratory Distress, Hypoglycemia, and Complications of Pregnancy." *American Journal of Tropical Medicine and Hygiene* 64 (Suppl. 1): 57–56.

Murray, C. J. L., and A. D. Lopez. 1996. *The Global Burden of Disease: A Comprehensive Assessment of Mortality and Disability from Diseases, Injuries, and Risk Factors in 1990 and Projected to 2020.* Cambridge, MA: Harvard University Press.

————. 1997. "Mortality by Cause for Eight Regions of the World: Global Burden of Disease Study." *Lancet* 349: 1269–76.

Mutabingwa, T. K., D. Anthony, A. Heller, R. Hallett, J. Ahmed, C. Drakeley, and others. 2005. "Amodiaquine Aone, Amodiaquine+Sulfadoxine-Pyrimethamine, Amodiaquine+Artesunate, and Artemether-Lumefantrine for Outpatient Treatment of Malaria in Tanzanian Children: a Four-Armed Randomized Effectiveness Trial." *Lancet* 365 (9469): 1474–80.

Najera, J. A., and M. Zaim. 2002. *Malaria Vector Control: Decision Making Criteria and Procedures for Judicious Use of Insecticides.* WHO/CDS/WHOPES/2002.5. Geneva: World Health Organization.

Newman, R. D., M. E. Parise, L. Slutsker, B. Nahlen, and R. W. Steketee. 2003. "Safety, Efficacy, and Determinants of Effectiveness of Antimalarial Drugs during Pregnancy: Implications for Prevention Programs in *Plasmodium falciparum*–Endemic Sub-Saharan Africa." *Tropical Medicine and International Health* 6: 488–506.

Nosten, F., R. McGready, J. A. Simpson, K. L. Thwai, S. Balkan, T. Cho, and others. 1999. "Effects of *Plasmodium vivax* Malaria in Pregnancy." *Lancet* 354 (9178): 546–49.

Pagnoni, F., N. Convelbo, J. Tiendrebeogo, S. Cousens, and F. Esposito. 1997. "A Community-Based Programme to Provide Prompt and Adequate Treatment of Presumptive Malaria in Children." *Transactions of the Royal Society of Tropical Medicine and Hygiene* 91 (5): 512–17.

Piola, P., C. Fagg, F. Bajunirwe, S. Biraro, F. Grandesso, E. Ruzagira, and others. 2005. "Supervised Versus Unsupervised Intake of Six-Dose Artemether-Lumefantrine for Treatment of Acute, Uncomplicated *Plasmodium falciparum* Malaria in Mbarara, Uganda: A Randomized Trial." *Lancet* 365 (9469): 1467–73.

RBM (Roll Back Malaria). 2002. *Scaling-up Insecticide-Treated Netting Programmes in Africa: A Strategic Framework for Coordinated National Action.* Geneva: WHO/CDS/RBM/2002.

Remme, J. H., E. Blas, L. Chitsulo, P. M. Desjeux, H. D. Engers, T. P. Kanyok, and others. 2002. "Strategic Emphasis for Tropical Diseases Research: A TDR Perspective." *Trends in Parasitology* 18 (10): 421–26.

Rosen, J. B., and J. G. Breman. 2004. "Malaria Intermittent Preventive Treatment in Infants (ITPi), Chemoprophylaxis, and Childhood Vaccinations." *Lancet* 363 (9418): 1386–88.

Russell, S. 2004. "The Economic Burden of Illness for Households in Developing Countries: Catastrophic or Manageable? A Review of Studies Focusing on Malaria, TB, and HIV/AIDS." *American Journal of Tropical Medicine and Hygiene* 71 (Suppl. 2): 147–55.

Savarit, D., K. M. De Cock, R. Shutz, S. Konate, E. Lackritz, and A. Bondurand. 1992. "Risk of HIV Infection from Transfusion with Blood Negative for HIV Antibodies in a West African City." *British Medical Journal* 305 (6852): 498–502.

Schellenberg, D. S., C. Menendez, J. J. Aponte, E. Kahigwa, M. Tanner, H. Mshinda, and P. Alonso. 2005. "Intermittent Preventive Treatment for Tanzanian Infants: Follow-up to Age 2 Years of a Randomized Placebo-Controlled Trial." *Lancet* 365 (9469): 1481–83.

Sharp, B. L., and D. le Sueur. 1996. "Malaria in South Africa—The Past, the Present, and Selected Implications for the Future." *South African Medical Journal* 86 (1): 83–89.

Sirima, S. B., A. Konaté, A. B. Tiono, N. Convelho, S. Cousins, and F. Pagnoni. 2003. "Early Treatment of Childhood Fevers with Pre-packaged Antimalarial Drugs in the Home Reduces Severe Malaria Morbidity in Burkina Faso." *Tropical Medicine and International Health* 8 (2): 1–7.

Snow, R. W., M. H. Craig, U. Deichmann, and K. Marsh. 1999. "Estimating Mortality, Morbidity, and Disability Due to Malaria among Africa's Non-pregnant Population." *Bulletin of the World Health Organization* 77: 624–40.

Snow, R. W., M. H. Craig, C. R. J. C. Newton, and R. W. Steketee. 2003. "The Public Health Burden of *Plasmodium falciparum* Malaria in Africa: Deriving the Numbers." Working Paper 11, Disease Control Priorities Project, Bethesda, MD.

Snow, R. W., C. A. Guerra, A. M. Noor, H. Y. Myint, and S. I. Hay. 2005. "The Global Distribution of Clinical Episodes of *Plasmodium falciparum* Malaria." *Nature* 434: 214–17.

Snow, R. W., E. Korenromp, C. Drakely, and E. Gouws. 2004. "Pediatric Mortality in Africa: *Plasmodium falciparum* Malaria as a Cause or Risk?" *American Journal of Tropical Medicine and Hygiene* 70 (Suppl. 2): 16–24.

Snow, R. W., and K. Marsh. 2002. "The Consequences of Reducing *Plasmodium falciparum* Transmission in Africa." *Advances in Parasitology* 52: 235–64.

Snow, R. W., A. Menon, and B. M. Greenwood. 1989. "Measuring Morbidity from Malaria." *Annals of Tropical Medicine and Parasitology* 83: 321–23.

Snow, R. W., J. F. Trape, and K. Marsh. 2001. "The Past, Present, and Future of Childhood Malaria Mortality in Africa." *Trends in Parasitology* 17: 593–97.

Steketee, R. W., B. L. Nahlen, M. E. Parise, and C. Menendez. 2001. "The Burden of Malaria in Pregnancy in Malaria-Endemic Areas." *American Journal of Tropical Medicine and Hygiene* 64 (Suppl.): 28–35.

Steketee, R. W., J. J. Wirima, A. W. Hightower, L. Slutsker, D. L. Heymann, and J. G. Breman. 1996. "The Effect of Malaria and Malaria Prevention in Pregnancy on Offspring Birthweight, Prematurity, and Intrauterine Growth Retardation in Rural Malawi." *American Journal of Tropical Medicine and Hygiene* 55 (Suppl.): 33–41.

Sudre, P., J. G. Breman, D. McFarland, and J. P. Koplan. 1992. "Treatment of Chloroquine Resistant Malaria in African Children: A Cost-Effectiveness Analysis." *International Journal of Epidemiology* 21: 146–54.

Tang, L. 2000. "Progress in Malaria Control in China." *Chinese Medical Journal* 113 (1): 89–92.

Ter Kuile, F. O., M. Parise, F. Verhoef, V. Udhayakumar, R. D. Newman, A. M. Van Eijk, and others. 2004. "The Burden of Co-infection with Human Immunodeficiency Virus Type 1 and Malaria in Pregnant Women in Sub-Saharan Africa." *American Journal of Tropical Medicine and Hygiene* 70 (Suppl. 2): 41–54.

Ter Kuile, F. O., D. J. Terlouw, S. K. Kariuki, P. A. Phillips-Howard, L. B. Mirel, W. A. Hawley, and others. 2003. "Impact of Permethrin-Treated Bednets on Malaria, Anemia, and Growth in Infants in an Area of Intense Perennial Malaria Transmission in Western Kenya." *American Journal of Tropical Medicine and Hygiene* 68 (Suppl. 4): 68–77.

Thera, M. A., P. S. Sehdev, D. Coulibaly, K. Traore, M. N. Garba, and others. 2005. "Impact of Trimethoprim-Sulfamethoxa-Infectious Diseases." *Journal of Infections Diseases* 192 (10): 1823–29.

Warhurst, D. C., and J. E. Williams. 2004. "Laboratory Procedures for Diagnosis of Malaria." In *Malaria: A Hematological Perspective,* ed. S. H. Abdalla and G. Pasvol, 1–27, London: Imperial College Press.

White, N. J. 2005. "Intermittent Presumptive Treatment for Malaria." *PLoS Medicine* 2 (1): 63.

White, N. J., and J. G. Breman. 2005. "Malaria and Babesiosis: Diseases Caused by Red Blood Cell Parasites." In *Harrison's Principles of Internal Medicine,* 16th ed., ed. D. Kasper, E. Braunwald, A. S. Fauci, S. L. Hauser, D. L. Longo, and J. L. Jameson, 1218–33. McGraw-Hill: New York.

Whitworth, J., D. Morgan, M. Quigley, A. Smith, B. Mayania, H. Eotu, and others. 2000. "Effect of HIV-1 and Increasing Immunosuppression on Malaria Parasitaemia and Clinical Episodes in Adults in Rural Uganda: A Cohort Study." *Lancet* 356 (9235): 1051–56.

WHO (World Health Organization). 1996. *Investing in Health Research and Development: Report of the Ad Hoc Committee on Health Research Relating to Future Intervention Options.* TDR/Gen/96.1. Geneva: WHO.

————. 2000a. *Twentieth Report of the WHO Expert Committee on Malaria.* Technical Report Series 892. Geneva: WHO.

————. 2000b. "Severe and Complicated Malaria." *Transactions of the Royal Society of Tropical Medicine and Hygiene* 95 (Suppl.): 51–90.

————. 2001a. *Antimalarial Drug Combination Therapy. Report of a WHO Technical Consultation 4–5 April, 2001.* WHO/CDS/RBM/2001.35. Geneva: WHO.

————. 2001b. "The Use of Antimalarial Drugs." Report of a WHO Informal Consultation, WHO, Geneva.

————. 2002a. *Monitoring Antimalarial Drug Resistance.* WHO/CDS/CSR/EPH/2002.1 WHO/CDS/RBM/2002.39. Geneva: WHO.

————. 2002b. *World Health Report 2002: Reducing Risks, Promoting Healthy Life.* Geneva: WHO.

————. 2002c. *South African Malaria Control Programme. Roll Back Malaria in Southern Africa. Baseline Survey 2001.* Harare, Zimbabwe: WHO.

————. 2003a. *Access to Antimalarial Medicines: Improving the Affordability and Financing of Artemisinin-Based Combination Therapies.* Geneva: WHO.

————. 2003b. *The Africa Malaria Report 2003.* Geneva: WHO; New York: United Nations Children's Fund.

————. 2003c. *The Scientific Working Group on Malaria Research.* TWR/SWG/03.03. Geneva: WHO.

————. 2005. *The World Malaria Report 2005: Roll Back Malaria.* Geneva: WHO.

World Bank. 2003. *2003 World Development Indicators.* Washington, DC: World Bank.

————. 2005. *Rolling Back Malaria, Global Strategy and Booster Program.* Washington, DC: World Bank.

Worrall, E., A. Rietveld, and C. Delacollette. 2004. "The Burden of Malaria Epidemics and Cost-Effectiveness of Interventions in Epidemic Situations in Africa." *American Journal of Tropical Medicine and Hygiene* 71 (Suppl. 2): 136–40.

Yeung, S., W. Pongtavornpinyo, I. M. Hastings, A. J. Mills, and N. J. White. 2004. "Antimalarial Drug Resistance, Artemisinin-Based Combination Therapy (ACT), and the Contribution of Modeling to Elucidating Policy Choices." *American Journal of Tropical Medicine and Hygiene* 71 (Suppl. 2): 179–86.

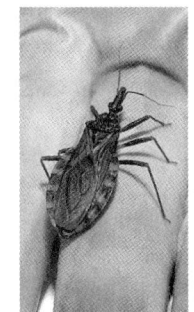

Chapter **22**

Tropical Diseases Targeted for Elimination: Chagas Disease, Lymphatic Filariasis, Onchocerciasis, and Leprosy

Jan H. F. Remme, Piet Feenstra, P. R. Lever, André Médici, Carlos Morel, Mounkaila Noma, K. D. Ramaiah, Frank Richards, A. Seketeli, Gabriel Schmunis, W. H. van Brakel, and Anna Vassall

Tropical diseases are infectious diseases that are found predominantly in the tropics, where ecological and socioeconomic conditions facilitate their propagation. Climatic, social, and economic factors create environmental conditions that facilitate transmission, and the lack of resources prevents affected populations from obtaining effective prevention and adequate care. Tropical diseases are diseases of the poor, and investments in control and research to develop more effective intervention tools and strategies have been minimal (Gwatkin, Guillot, and Heuveline 1999; Remme and others 2002). For some, however, effective intervention methods have been developed, and successful control has been achieved.

This chapter focuses on four tropical diseases—Chagas disease, lymphatic filariasis (LF), onchocerciasis, and leprosy—for which effective means of control are available. All four diseases are targeted for elimination as a public health problem. Control strategies are being implemented at scale and have already achieved a major reduction in the burden of disease, and the causative agent has even been eliminated in some previously endemic areas. Those successes have not come easily, and much remains to be done to ensure complete and sustained control of the diseases.

DISEASE CHARACTERISTICS AND TRANSMISSION

Chagas disease, LF, onchocerciasis, and leprosy are all parasitic infections, but their causative agents, modes of transmission, and geographic distribution differ. Chagas disease is caused by infection with a protozoan, leprosy by a mycobacterium, and LF and onchocerciasis by filarial nematodes. Three are vector-borne diseases, but leprosy is transmitted directly from person to person. Chagas disease occurs only in the Americas, onchocerciasis is found predominantly in Africa, and LF and leprosy occur in all tropical regions.

Chagas Disease

Chagas disease—also known as American trypanosomiasis—is a zoonotic disease caused by the protozoan hemoflagellate *Trypanosoma cruzi* that is mainly transmitted by large, blood-sucking, reduviid bugs of the subfamily *Triatominae* (known as *kissing bugs*). Infection with this blood parasite has been recorded in more than 150 species of 24 families of domestic and wild mammals as well as in humans. In the vertebrate host, *T. cruzi* usually infects macrophage, muscle, and nerve cells.

Human infection with *T. cruzi* most commonly originates through contact of broken skin or mucosa with the excretion of infected insect vectors. The incubation period ranges from 7 to 15 days, leading to the acute phase of infection—characterized by patent parasitemia—which may last up to four weeks. The acute phase may be without obvious symptoms. Romaña's sign—that is, uniocular, bipalpebral edema with regional lymphadenopathy—is diagnostic of the acute infection but occurs in less than 5 percent of infections.

If a recent infection is untreated, the individual will remain infected for life. After an asymptomatic period of 10 years or more, some 10 to 40 percent of those infected will develop cardiac or digestive complications that are characteristic of the chronic stage of the disease. In chagasic myocardiopathy the most common symptoms are dyspnea and arrhythmias. Electrocardiographic alterations can occur, such as right bundle branch block, left anterior hemiblock, or both, which may require a pacemaker implant. Apical aneurisms are also typical of advanced chagasic cardiopathy, which may rupture on excessive exercise, leading to sudden death. Chagas disease can also involve intestinal complications characterized by severe dilatations of parts of the digestive tract known as megasyndromes. Megaesophagus and megacolon are the most common. Symptoms of megaesophagus are dysphagia and odinophagia and subsequent malnutrition. Chagasic megacolon is characterized by constipation and meteorism. As a result of colon distension and contractions, abdominal pain is frequent, and fecalomas are a complication.

More than 120 species of *Triatominae* and three transmission cycles are recognized. The domestic cycle, responsible for maintaining infection in humans, occurs mostly in rural or periurban areas where houses have adobe walls and thatched roofs. Humans, dogs, cats, and in some countries guinea pigs are the main parasite reservoirs in this cycle. The vector lives and multiplies in cracks in the walls, holes in the roof, under and behind furniture and pictures, and so on. The sylvatic cycle involves sylvatic triatomine bugs that become infected and in turn infect rodents, marsupials, and other wild animals. The third is the peridomestic cycle in which mammals participate (domestic rodents, marsupials, livestock, cats, dogs) by moving freely in and out of human dwellings, and sylvatic bugs are attracted to lights in houses and to food. This peridomestic cycle acts as a link between the domestic and sylvatic cycles. Occasionally, infected sylvatic species of *Triatominae* fly into houses and contribute to transmission either by feeding and defecating on the people or their domestic animals or (indirectly) by contaminating food and drink in which the parasites can survive. In the Amazon region, cases of acute Chagas disease have been associated with sylvatic *Triatominae* contaminating sugarcane or fruit juice.

Transmission by blood transfusion is the second-most common way of acquiring *T. cruzi* infection. The true incidence of infection through blood transfusion is unknown, because most cases are not recognized. In transfusionally acquired *T. cruzi* infection, the incubation period is 30 or more days, and the most common symptoms are fever, general lymph node enlargement, and splenomegaly (Schmunis and others 2001).

Transplacental transmission of *T. cruzi* can occur, and estimates indicate that 5 percent of newborns born to chagasic mothers will become infected. Less common routes of transmission are by transplantation with an infected organ or,

more rarely, through contaminated food or infection in the laboratory (WHO 2002a).

Lymphatic Filariasis

LF is caused by species of nematode parasites—*Wuchereria bancrofti, Brugia malayi,* and *Brugia timori*—and is transmitted by mosquitoes (WHO 2002c). The adult filarial parasites live in the lymphatics of humans. After mating, each female worm produces several thousand offspring, microfilariae, during its lifetime. The microfilariae are found in humans' internal organs and appear in peripheral blood at times that coincide with the vector's biting activity. The biting mosquito ingests the microfilariae along with the blood meal, and they develop into infective-stage larvae in 10 to 12 days. When an infective mosquito bites a human, the infective-stage larvae are transmitted to the human host and develop into the adult stage in about one year. The adult parasites live 5 to 10 years, of which the fecund life span is 4 to 6 years. Several hundreds to thousands of infective mosquito bites are necessary to establish infection.

Of the three parasite species, *W. bancrofti* accounts for nearly 90 percent of LF infections worldwide. *B. malayi* is prevalent only in some parts of South and Southeast Asia, and *B. timori* is found only in Indonesia. Several species of *Culex, Anopheles, Aedes,* and *Mansonia* mosquitoes are involved in the transmission of LF. *C. quinquefasciatus* is the major vector in Africa, Asia, and South America and transmits nocturnally periodic *W. bancrofti.* Among anophelines, *An. gambiae* and *An. funestus* play a significant role in Africa. Several *Aedes* species, particularly *Ae. polynesiensis,* are the major vectors in the South Pacific islands, where diurnally subperiodic *W. bancrofti* is common. *B. malayi* is primarily transmitted by *Mansonia* and *Anopheles* species.

Infected people can harbor microfilaremia without overt clinical manifestations. The disease process is determined primarily by living adult worms, inflammatory responses caused by the death of adult worms, and secondary bacterial infections. The inflammatory response begins with the death of or damage to adult worms, which leads to host reaction and acute filarial lymphangitis. A heavy worm burden and the presence of worms in the scrotal area precipitate the development of hydrocele, chyluria, chylocele, and lymph scrotum. Lymphatic dysfunction caused by dilatation of the lymphatic vessels makes the patient more prone to repeated secondary bacterial infection, which precipitates lymphedema and elephantiasis. Microfilariae play an important role in the pathogenesis of tropical pulmonary eosinophilia (Dreyer and others 2000).

Onchocerciasis

Onchocerciasis is an infection with the filarial parasite *Onchocerca volvulus.* The main complications are severe eye disease that can lead to blindness and severe skin disease with unsightly lesions and intense itching (WHO 1995a). *O. volvulus* is transmitted by vector blackflies of the genus *Simulium*, whose larvae and pupae develop in rapidly flowing, well-oxygenated streams and rivers. As a result, onchocerciasis is often known as *river blindness*. The most important vectors are members of the *S. damnosum* complex in Africa and the Middle East and *S. neavei* in parts of East Africa. Of the many vectors in the Americas, the most important are *S. ochraceum, S. metallicum, S. oyapockense, S. guianense,* and *S. exiguum.*

When taking a blood meal, infected *Simulium* vectors deposit one or more infective (third-stage) *O. volvulus* larvae, which reach adulthood in the human host after about a year but may live as long as 14 years. The adult worms typically entwine in nodules where they mate, producing microfilariae that migrate into the skin, eyes, and other organs. These microfilariae are unable to develop into adult worms without first being ingested in the blood meal of a blackfly vector. The microfilariae transform in the vector over a period of 6 to 12 days to produce the third-stage larvae that are infective to humans.

The thousands of microfilariae that do not succeed in reaching a blackfly vector die in the human body, provoking inflammatory reactions in tissues. Inflammation in the eyes leads to irreversible ocular lesions, resulting first in impaired vision and finally in total blindness (WHO 1995a). The death of microfilariae in the skin gives rise to intense itching, dermatitis, depigmentation, and atrophy of the skin (Murdoch and others 2002). A less common complication is lymphadenitis, which may lead to hanging groin and elephantiasis of the genitals, and increasing evidence indicates that onchocerciasis is a risk factor for epilepsy and hyposexual dwarfism in certain areas (Boussinesq and others 2002). The greater is the body load of adult worms and microfilariae, the greater is the risk of developing skin and eye disease.

The disease pattern of onchocerciasis—in particular the severity of ocular disease—varies considerably between geographic zones. Onchocercal blindness can be extensive in hyperendemic communities of the West African savannas, whereas in forest villages with a comparable intensity of infection, the skin manifestations tend to be the main complications of the disease (Dadzie and others 1989; Murdoch and others 2002). These differences may reflect the existence of different vector-parasite complexes, with strains of *O. volvulus* that differ in pathogenicity (Zimmerman and others 1992). The vector-parasite complex in the West African savanna is responsible for the most severe form of ocular onchocerciasis in the world: in the most affected villages, more than 10 percent of the population may be blind because of onchocerciasis.

Leprosy

Leprosy is caused by *Mycobacterium leprae*, a gram-positive, strongly acid-fast bacterium. *M. leprae* is an obligate, intracellular parasite that resides predominantly in macrophages. It is the only bacterium that infects peripheral nerves, showing a preference for Schwann cells, particularly of unmyelinated fibers.

The disease spectrum of leprosy ranges from a single self-healing, hypopigmented macule to a generalized illness causing widespread peripheral nerve damage and affecting even bones and internal organs. Skin lesions may be well- or ill-defined hypopigmented macules, plaques, or nodules that are localized or distributed over the whole skin. They may be hypaesthetic, anesthetic, hyperaesthetic, or have normal sensibility. Nerve lesions occur in dermal nerves as well as in superficial sensory nerves and mixed nerve trunks. One or more nerves may be enlarged on palpation. Signs such as clawing of fingers and toes, "absorption" of digits caused by repeated injury, and dry skin are secondary to impairment of motor, sensory, and autonomic nerve function.

A diagnosis of leprosy is based on finding at least one of three so-called cardinal signs (ILA 2002):

- diminished sensibility in a typical macule or plaque in the skin
- palpable enlargement of one or more peripheral nerve trunks at specific sites
- demonstration of acid-fast mycobacteria in a slit skin smear.

Currently, patients are classified based on clinical signs only, but skin smear results are taken into account when available. Patients who have more than five skin lesions or who have a positive skin smear are classified as *multibacillary;* others are classified as *paucibacillary.*

The skin signs of leprosy are relatively harmless, but complications of the disease may lead to severe consequences, such as blindness, infertility, disfigurement, and severe sensory and motor disability. Reactions—that is, episodes of acute inflammation caused by hypersensitivity to bacterial antigens—can be particularly severe. Patients can develop nerve damage without any obvious sign of these reactions, but after neuropathy has become irreversible, it may lead to secondary impairments, such as wounds, contractures, and shortening of digits. As a result of visible impairments or activity limitations—or simply because of the diagnosis of leprosy—many people experience psychosocial problems (van Brakel 2000).

The exact mode of transmission of *M. leprae* is still not fully understood, but the respiratory tract seems to play an important role. The primary reservoir of infection is the human host. Untreated multibacillary leprosy patients are able to shed large amounts of *M. leprae* from the nose, and household and social contacts of such patients are at a higher risk of developing leprosy than the general population (van Beers, Hatta, and Klatser 1999). *M. leprae*–specific DNA sequences have been isolated from the noses of apparently healthy individuals, and widespread seropositivity against *M. leprae*–specific antigens has been demonstrated in endemic areas, although the role of these individuals in transmitting leprosy is not fully understood. Effective antileprosy treatment usually renders a patient noninfectious within a few days.

DISEASE BURDEN

Information on the number of people infected is often difficult to obtain for tropical diseases. Many infected people may be without obvious symptoms, those with symptoms may not seek care at public health facilities, and those who do may not be reported. Routine health information systems provide little information on the number of people infected in the population. Surveys are more informative but are rarely done. A better picture emerges only when control programs need to map the distribution of the disease as a basis for targeting large-scale interventions. Hence, the apparent paradox is that intensification of disease control may result in a significant initial increase in estimates of the burden of disease through better epidemiological data.

Chagas Disease

Chagas disease is an important public health problem in 17 countries in Latin America. Estimates from the 1980s indicated that some 16 million to 18 million individuals were infected (WHO 1991), and in the 1990s, a series of multinational control initiatives was launched that was designed to interrupt transmission by eliminating domestic insect vectors and improving the serological screening of blood donors. As a result, estimates of the number of infected people were revised to 9.8 million in 2001 (Schmunis 2000). The estimated burden of disease in terms of disability-adjusted life years (DALYs) declined from 2.7 million in 1990 (World Bank 1993) to 586,000 in 2001 (Mathers, Murray, and Lopez 2006). Because of migration, *T. cruzi*–infected individuals can be found outside Latin America (for example, in Spain or the United States).

Estimates from the 1980s suggested that 5 million people in the Americas had symptoms of Chagas disease (WHO 1991). These estimates decreased to 1.2 million to 2.8 million in the 1990s. The World Health Organization (WHO) attributed 45,000 yearly deaths to Chagas disease (WHO 1991). WHO decreased its mortality estimates to 13,000 in 2001 (WHO 2002d).

In all affected countries, Chagas disease has been responsible for a high burden of disease and significant direct and indirect costs. Reports from Brazil in the late 1980s suggested that the aggregate costs for pacemakers and intestinal surgeries for Chagas disease were US$250 million per year, excluding the costs of consultations, care, and supportive treatment for chronic chagasic patients, which amounted to US$1,000 per

year per patient, and disability awards, which in one state accounted for US$399,600 (Dias 1987; Schofield and Dias 1991). In Bolivia, in 1992, aggregate treatment costs were estimated at US$21 million. In Chile, in 1997, aggregate treatment costs for Chagas disease were estimated at US$14 million to US$19 million (Schenone 1998), and in Uruguay, in 1996, costs were estimated at US$15 million (Salvatella and Vignolo 1996).

Lymphatic Filariasis

LF is endemic in 83 countries, with 1.1 billion people living in known endemic areas. In 1992, the WHO Expert Committee estimated that 78 million people were infected (WHO 2002c). This estimate was later revised to 119 million, and current estimates indicate that LF is responsible for the loss of 4.6 million DALYs per year. Many endemic areas lack reliable data on the prevalence of LF, and estimates of the number infected may increase when more precise data become available from epidemiological mapping. Nationwide mapping in four neighboring countries in West Africa showed that LF was endemic in a much wider area than expected, and the findings resulted in a dramatic increase in the estimated number infected (Gyapong and others 2002).

Epidemiological trends have varied widely among different regions in recent decades. LF was controlled or eliminated from several islands in the Pacific, and China has seen a dramatic reduction in infection levels. Unfortunately, in India and Africa, the most endemic areas of the world, recent decades have witnessed little change (WHO 2002c).

The acute form of the disease is common and causes severe hardship in endemic communities. Infected individuals suffer from one to eight acute episodes per year, and during each episode, affected patients are bedridden for three to five days.

Morbidity caused by chronic LF is mostly lifelong, and the disease is considered the second leading cause of disability in the world (WHO 1995b). Patients affected by elephantiasis or hydrocele are often victims of societal discrimination, and the disease impairs their educational and employment opportunities, marriage prospects, and sexual life. Case-control studies in India revealed that affected individuals are 27 percent less productive than their uninfected counterparts (Ramu and others 1996). The patients work less and often switch to lighter jobs, leading to a loss of more than 1 billion person-days per year in India alone (Ramaiah and others 2000), which translates into an annual economic loss equivalent to 0.63 percent of gross national product.

Onchocerciasis

More than 99 percent of those infected with *O. volvulus* reside in 30 endemic countries in Africa, with the remainder living in the Republic of Yemen and six countries of the Americas.

In 1995, the WHO Expert Committee on Onchocerciasis estimated that 17.7 million people were infected, of whom about 270,000 were blind and another 500,000 were severely visually impaired (WHO 1995a). However, more recent information from rapid epidemiological mapping of onchocerciasis (Noma and others 2002) by the African Programme for Onchocerciasis Control (APOC) indicates that the number of those infected is twice as high and that some 37 million people were infected in 1995. This revised estimate corresponds to an estimated 1.99 million DALYs lost because of onchocerciasis in 1995.

Using the most recent rapid epidemiological mapping data and the latest APOC data on treatment coverage and assuming that four rounds of ivermectin treatment will reduce the prevalence of troublesome itching by 85 percent and the burden of visual impairment and blindness by 35 percent give a DALY estimate of 1.49 million DALYS lost for 2003 (see table 22.1).

In addition to the burden of blindness and severe itching, onchocerciasis has important socioeconomic consequences. In the West African savanna, fear of blindness has resulted in the depopulation of fertile river valleys, severely affecting agricultural production. It was this socioeconomic impact, and not just the health impact, that led to the creation of the Onchocerciasis Control Program (OCP) in West Africa in 1975 (Remme 2004b).

Even though the importance of onchocercal blindness has long been recognized, only in 1995 did research demonstrate that the public health importance of onchocercal skin disease was even greater. Troublesome itching associated with dermal onchocerciasis makes working, studying, or interacting socially difficult (Murdoch and others 2002; Vlassoff and others 2000). Onchocercal itching now accounts for 60 percent of DALYs lost (Remme 2004a). Other skin manifestations, such as reactive skin lesions, are not included in the DALY estimates, even though they are highly prevalent and have major psychosocial and economic impacts. Onchocercal skin disease also diminishes people's income-generating capacity, and the school dropout rate is twice as high among children from households in which the head of household is affected by onchocercal skin disease (Benton 1998).

Leprosy

In May 2001, 10 years after the World Health Assembly had adopted a resolution to eliminate leprosy by the end of the millennium, the target—a prevalence rate of less than 1 per 10,000—had been achieved at the global level. The number of cases registered for treatment worldwide fell from 5.4 million in 1985 to 460,000 by the end of 2003 (WHO 2004a); however, this trend should not be taken at face value because the reduction is attributable mainly to such factors as the shortening of treatment duration for multibacillary patients and the cleaning up of patient registers.

Leprosy is reported from all regions of the world, but the burden of disease, which is estimated at 192,000 DALYs, is concentrated in a few countries. During 2003, 513,798 new cases were detected, of which more than 80 percent were in Brazil, India, Madagascar, Mozambique, Nepal, and Tanzania (WHO 2004a). India alone accounted for about 75 percent of the new cases. Case detection has remained remarkably stable over the past decade. Trends in case detection rates should be analyzed in conjunction with the proportion of new patients with grade 2 impairment (an indicator of the delay between onset of the disease and diagnosis) and the proportion of children among new cases (an indicator of recent transmission).

Virtually all published data on leprosy-related disability concern impairments. In 1997, WHO estimated the global prevalence of patients with visible impairments (disability grade 2) as 2 million. A similar number may have sensory impairment without deformity. Sensory and motor impairment that are already present at diagnosis are important risk factors for developing additional impairment and disability. Evidence indicates that sensory impairment itself causes significant functional disability.

The prevalence of activity limitations among people affected by leprosy is unknown. Van Brakel and Anderson's (1998) survey in Nepal finds that among those with any impairment, about 20 percent had limitations in relation to one or more indoor activities and up to 34 percent had significant limitations in relation to common outdoor activities. Even less is known about the prevalence of restrictions on social and economic participation. Surveys are urgently needed to assess the extent of patients with leprosy-related disabilities who require intervention.

Two difficulties affect the validity of DALY estimates for leprosy. The first is the lack of data, particularly on the burden of functional and psychosocial disability caused by leprosy. The second is that the effect of leprosy often goes well beyond the affected individual; the psychosocial consequences may affect the whole family. People without any visible signs of leprosy may be stigmatized simply because they are known to be a leprosy patient. Even after completing treatment, people may remain stigmatized.

Summary of DALY Estimates

Table 22.1 summarizes the DALY estimates for each of the four diseases by World Bank region. The high estimate for LF reflects not only its wider distribution and the larger number of people affected, but also the reduction in the burden for the other three diseases as a result of control efforts. For those diseases for which there has been significant progress toward elimination, public health officials should remain aware of the

Table 22.1 DALYs Lost, by Disease and World Bank Region
(thousands)

Disease (date of information)	East Asia and the Pacific	Europe and Central Asia	Latin America and the Caribbean	Middle East and North Africa	South Asia	Sub-Saharan Africa	High-income countries	Total
Chagas disease (2001)	0	1	583	0	0	0	1	585
LF (2001)	373	1	9	4	2,412	1,656	212	4,667
Onchocerciasis (2003)	0	0	2	0.4	0	481	0	484
Onchocerciasis (latest APOC data)	0	0	2	0.4	0	1,487	0	1,490
Leprosy (2001)	34	0	18	2	113	24	1	192

Source: Mathers, Lopez, and Murray 2006; WHO 2004b; authors' calculations.

burden of disease that is currently averted but that might return if control were not to be sustained before transmission has been completely eliminated.

INTERVENTIONS AND THEIR EFFECTIVENESS

For each of the four diseases in this chapter, effective interventions are available.

Chagas Disease

The primary approaches to control of Chagas disease are halting transmission and providing adequate treatment for those infected. The two most important routes of transmission are insect vectors and blood transfusion from infected donors; thus, control programs focus on eliminating domestic vector populations and improving the serological screening of blood donors.

Vector Control. *Triatoma infestans* lives only inside houses and in the peridomestic area. Work during the late 1940s suggested that spraying houses with residual insecticides could eliminate vectors' domestic populations. The effect and sustainability of such vector control programs can be enhanced when they are combined with improved housing and when communities are well informed and closely involved in vector surveillance activities.

Argentina and Brazil initiated programs for nationwide vector control in the 1960s, and Chile and Uruguay did so in the 1970s. These programs were strengthened in 1991 by the Southern Cone Initiative, a multinational effort to eliminate infestation by *T. infestans* launched by the ministries of health of Argentina, Bolivia, Brazil, Chile, Paraguay, and Uruguay and coordinated by the WHO Regional Office for the Americas. Similar regional initiatives for Central America and the Andean

Pact regions, targeted primarily against *Rhodnius prolixus,* followed in 1997.

The results in the Southern Cone region have been impressive, with vast areas now free of domestic infestation with *T. infestans* and other vector species. In Argentina, seroprevalence rates among men age 18 to 20 drafted for military service decreased from 5.8 percent in 1981 to 1.2 percent in 1993. The number of cases of Chagasic cardiomyopathy, when compared with the number expected in the absence of control, indicates a decrease of 81 percent in the population up to 18 years of age. In 2001, a WHO commission certified that 4 of the 18 endemic provinces were free of vectorial transmission. In Brazil, domestic infestation rates decreased by 98.3 percent between 1991 and 2000. Of the 11 Brazilian states that were originally endemic for *T. infestans,* 9 have been certified as free of vectorial transmission. In Chile, house infestation rates decreased from 28.80 percent in 1982 to less than 0.01 percent in 1999, when the country was certified free of vectorial transmission. Uruguay also achieved a dramatic reduction in house infestation rates, from 5.7 percent in 1983 to 0.3 percent in 1997, when it too was certified as free of vectorial transmission. Bolivia and Paraguay have not yet eliminated transmission, but thousands of houses have been sprayed since 1991.

Blood Transfusion Control. The purpose of screening for *T. cruzi* in blood banks is to eliminate all units of potentially infected blood. Argentina and Brazil require screening to be done using two serological tests to reduce the risk of false negatives; however, the cost-benefit ratio of the two-test approach may be questionable in countries where prevalence is low and the reagents used for diagnosis are highly sensitive.

In 1993, the national coverage of blood donor screening was analyzed in four Central American and six South American countries (Schmunis and others 1998). At that time, only Honduras, Uruguay, and República Bolivariana de Venezuela screened 100 percent of donors, and even in those countries infected transfusions were possible because of the lack of sensitivity of the reagents used. Since then, the sensitivity and specificity of serological tests have improved, and more countries have passed legislation requiring the screening of all blood donors. By 2001, seven endemic countries were screening 100 percent of blood donors for *T. cruzi*, four were screening more than 99 percent of donors, and two were screening about 90 percent; but four countries were still screening fewer than 25 percent of donors. In countries with a high number of immigrants from Latin America, such as Spain and the United States, thousands of individuals are potentially infected, and screening of blood donors for *T. cruzi* infection may be indicated in these countries.

Treatment. If untreated, most individuals infected with *T. cruzi* will remain infected for life. Spontaneous cure is rare. Only two drugs, nifurtimox and benznidazole, are effective for treating *T. cruzi*. Both are highly effective for acute infections and can be used in cases of congenital Chagas disease. Their effectiveness for treating chronic cases remains unclear, but increasing evidence indicates that they are effective in clearing parasitemia when administered to young cases, which may impede the development of chronic lesions. Both drugs may cause serious side effects and should be administered under medical supervision.

Lymphatic Filariasis

In recent years, new control tools and strategies have become available for LF (Ottesen and others 1997), and the World Health Assembly has adopted a resolution on the global elimination of LF. The Global Programme for the Elimination of Lymphatic Filariasis was launched in 2000 with the primary goals of interrupting transmission and preventing suffering and disability caused by the disease (Ottesen 2000).

The core strategy for interrupting transmission is annual mass drug administration (MDA) to treat the entire at-risk population for a period long enough to ensure that levels of blood microfilariae remain below those necessary to sustain transmission. Two annual, single-dose, two-drug regimens are recommended for MDA: ivermectin plus albendazole in African countries that are coendemic for onchocerciasis, and diethylcarbamazine plus albendazole for all other endemic countries. Where feasible, diethylcarbamazine-fortified salt as the only source of domestic salt for a period of at least six months would be an alternative strategy to MDA.

The principal strategy for alleviating suffering and decreasing the disability caused by LF focuses on decreasing secondary bacterial and fungal infection of limbs or genitals whose lymphatic function has already been compromised by filarial infection. Operationally, a regimen of meticulous local hygiene of affected areas and the creation of hope and understanding among patients and their communities are the principal strategic approaches (Dreyer, Dreyer, and Noroes 2002).

Mass Treatment. It is not yet known how many years of MDA are needed to eliminate LF transmission, but empirical evidence on the effect of MDA on transmission is progressively becoming available. In *Anopheles*-transmitted *W. bancrofti* in Papua New Guinea, four rounds of MDA with diethylcarbamazine or diethylcarbamazine plus ivermectin that reached about 88 percent of the target population reduced the annual transmission potential (the estimated number of infective-stage larvae inoculated per person per year) by 97 percent and 84 percent in low- and high-transmission areas, respectively. In India, where *W. bancrofti* is transmitted by *C. quinquefasciatus*, six rounds of MDA that reached 54 to 75 percent of the target population reduced the annual transmission potential by 95 and 80 percent in diethylcarbamazine- and ivermectin-treated villages, respectively (Ramaiah and others 2003). Modeling studies indicate that the required duration of treatment will depend largely on the treatment coverage achieved and the extent of systematic noncompliance to treatment—that is, noncompliance by the same individuals during successive treatment rounds (Stolk and others 2003). The physiology of the vectors also plays a role, because with *Culex*-transmitted LF, the critical microfilariae density required to interrupt transmission is thought to be lower than in areas where *Anopheles* is the vector.

The addition of albendazole to the two established antifilarial drugs—diethylcarbamazine and ivermectin—is based on clinical trials indicating that the combination therapy is as good as or better than single-drug therapy and that albendazole may enhance the macrofilaricidal action of diethylcarbamazine. Albendazole is also effective and safe against intestinal helminth infections, and its inclusion may enhance compliance with MDA. However, clinical trials have not yet been conclusive, and more robust evidence on the advantages of combination therapy is needed (Addiss and others 2004; Gyapong and others 2005). Community trials are ongoing in India and Africa, and preliminary results of a trial in south India suggest that the combination of diethylcarbamazine and albendazole may indeed achieve greater reduction in the prevalence of antigenemia than diethylcarbamazine alone (Rajendran and others 2002). A study in Nigeria showed that the addition of albendazole to ivermectin had an additive effect on reducing LF mosquito infection rates. (Richards and others 2005).

Vector Control. Vector control has sometimes been extremely effective against LF. In the Solomon Islands, 9 to 10 years of vector control virtually eliminated LF. In India, five years of integrated vector control in an urban area reduced the overall prevalence of microfilariae by 28 percent and the prevalence in children by 92 percent. Studies suggest that 11 to 12 years of effective vector control may eliminate LF (Ramaiah, Das, and Dhanda 1994). Vector control combined with chemotherapy produced the best results. The introduction of polystyrene beads in vector breeding habitats and treatment with diethylcarbamazine reduced the annual infective biting rate in Tanzania by 99.7 percent (Maxwell and others 1990). In India, vector control combined with single-dose treatment with diethylcarbamazine plus ivermectin reduced the annual transmission potential by 96 percent, compared with 60 percent using chemotherapy alone (Reuben and others 2001).

Such results, along with the limitations of MDA for completely eliminating microfilariae in some situations, have reactivated the debate on the role of vector control in LF elimination (Burkot and Ichimori 2002). However, few endemic countries have an adequate vector control infrastructure.

In some African countries, the same vector species transmit both LF and malaria. In such situations, the effect of malaria control measures, particularly insecticide-treated bednets, on LF vector densities and transmission needs further evaluation. A review of the role and feasibility of community-based vector control strategies and large-scale application of biological control agents is also needed.

Morbidity Management. The second objective of the Global Programme for the Elimination of Lymphatic Filariasis is to decrease the disability caused by LF. Simple and cheap methods have been developed for managing lymphedema, using water and soap occasionally supplemented with antibiotics. Studies in India, Africa, and the Americas have shown that such methods can significantly improve the quality of life of those affected, but implementation of this strategy has greatly lagged behind the MDA campaigns.

Onchocerciasis

Onchocerciasis control is based on vector control and large-scale ivermectin treatment.

Vector Control. Vector control used to be the only feasible intervention when available drugs were too toxic for large-scale use. Following success with vector control in Kenya, where the application of larvicides resulted in local elimination of the vector *S. neavei,* and in selected locations in West Africa, where the application of larvicides effectively stopped local vector breeding but could not prevent reinvasion of infective vectors from elsewhere, vector control was considered feasible in the West African savanna if carried out on a large scale. In 1975, the OCP started large-scale vector control operations using helicopters for weekly spraying of larvicides over the vector breeding sites in river rapids (Molyneux 1995). The operation ultimately covered some 50,000 kilometers of rivers over a geographic area of 1,235,000 square kilometers. The OCP's strategy was to maintain vector control for at least 14 years to interrupt transmission and eliminate the parasite reservoir. Despite initial problems with reinvasion by infective flies, the strategy proved effective, eliminating onchocerciasis as a public health problem throughout the OCP area. The OCP was successfully concluded in 2002, but concerns remain about the possible recrudescence of onchocerciasis through reinvasion by infected blackflies or migration of infected persons into OCP areas. The OCP countries, therefore, need to maintain effective surveillance to identify any recurrences of infection (Richards and others 2001).

Treatment with Ivermectin. In 1987, Merck & Co., the manufacturer of ivermectin, agreed to donate the drug for onchocerciasis control for as long as needed (Peters and Phillips 2004). Clinical and community trials involving more than 70,000 people showed that annual ivermectin treatment was safe, prevented ocular and dermal morbidity, and significantly reduced transmission; however, ivermectin is a microfilaricide and does not kill the adult worms, and long-term treatment is needed to sustain suppression of the microfilarial load (Remme 2004b). Additional research is needed to determine the extent to which repeated treatments reduce the reproductive capacity of the adult worm population over time.

The introduction of ivermectin allowed the OCP to achieve its objective in 12 years instead of 14 by combining vector control with ivermectin treatment, but most important, it also provided an opportunity to control onchocerciasis in endemic areas outside the OCP where vector control was not feasible. This ability led to the creation of two other regional programs for controlling onchocerciasis in endemic areas of Africa and the Americas: APOC (Remme 1995) and the Onchocerciasis Elimination Program for the Americas (OEPA) (Richards and others 2001).

The World Bank and WHO launched APOC in 1995 to serve 19 onchocerciasis-endemic countries outside the OCP. APOC's principal strategy is to establish annual ivermectin distribution in highly endemic areas to prevent eye and skin morbidity. In partnership with ministries of health and nongovernmental organizations, APOC currently provides more than 35 million ivermectin treatments per year and aims to reach 65 million treatments per year before its scheduled termination in 2010. APOC uses an approach referred to as *community-directed treatment with ivermectin,* whereby local communities rather than health services direct the treatment process (Amazigo and others 2002). A community decides collectively whether it wants ivermectin treatment, how it will collect ivermectin tablets from the medical supply entity, when and how the tablets will be distributed, who will be responsible for distribution and recordkeeping, and how the community will monitor the process. Health workers provide only the necessary training and supervision. To date, communities have responded enthusiastically to this approach (Seketeli and others 2002), and interest is now growing in exploring this strategy for interventions against other diseases (Homeida and others 2002).

In the Americas, *O. volvulus* transmission occurs only in a few small areas in six endemic countries. Accordingly, OEPA's strategy is based on intense ivermectin treatment twice a year that should allow eventual cessation of ivermectin delivery without the risk of recrudescence (Richards and others 2001). OEPA was launched in 1992 and is currently reaching more than 85 percent of its intended target population.

Leprosy

The objectives of leprosy control are to interrupt transmission, to cure patients, to prevent the development of associated deformities, and to rehabilitate those patients already afflicted with deformities. The strategy involves early case detection and the provision of adequate chemotherapy and comprehensive patient care (ILA 2002).

Multidrug Therapy. Dapsone therapy for leprosy was introduced in the late 1940s and successfully used as monotherapy for two decades. In the 1970s, resistance to dapsone emerged, and WHO introduced multidrug therapy (MDT) in 1982. Paucibacillary patients were to be given a six-month regimen of daily dapsone and supervised monthly rifampicin. Multibacillary patients were to be treated with a three-drug regimen for two years or, where feasible, until the skin smear had become negative. This regimen followed the paucibacillary regimen, adding a smaller daily dose of clofazimine and a larger supervised dose once a month.

These regimens have had good results, with a relapse incidence of less than 0.1 percent per year (ILA 2002). No multidrug-resistant leprosy has been reported so far, and reports of rifampicin-resistant *M. leprae* have been few. In 1998, the standard multibacillary MDT regimen was shortened to 12 months. Long-term relapse rates for the 12-month regimen are not yet available.

Public health specialists expected that wide application of MDT together with earlier diagnosis resulting from the upgrading of leprosy services would have a considerable effect on transmission; however, by 2002, clear evidence of a reduction in transmission had not been seen.

Immunoprophylaxis and Chemoprophylaxis. Several randomized trials have shown that vaccination with the bacillus Calmette-Guérin (BCG) vaccine reduces the risk of developing leprosy (Fine and Smith 1996), with the level of protection varying from 20 to 80 percent. Chemoprophylaxis based on dapsone or intramuscular acedapsone conferred overall protection against leprosy of about 60 percent (Smith and Smith 2000). Two large trials are currently under way in Bangladesh and Indonesia to investigate the efficacy of one or two doses of rifampicin in preventing leprosy, with preliminary results from the Indonesian trial indicating a significant protective effect.

Prevention of Disabilities. As concerns primary prevention, leprosy-related disability is preventable, but when peripheral neuropathy has become established, it is irreversible and leads to lifelong morbidity and disability (Bekri and others 1998; Meima and others 1999). Early case detection and treatment are therefore likely to be the most effective interventions in relation to preventing disability. When detected and treated in time with corticosteroids, primary impairments may be reversible, but because many patients present late, some 11 to 51 percent do not recover or get worse.

In relation to secondary prevention, the main strategy is self-care to prevent worsening of impairments in people who already have irreversible neural impairment or secondary impairments such as wounds and contractures. The role of health care workers is to educate patients so that they can be responsible for the daily management of the effects of nerve function impairment. An essential part of secondary prevention is the use of protective footwear by people with anesthetic feet. Several studies have shown that the use of locally acceptable, appropriate footwear is a cost-effective intervention for those with a loss of plantar sensation (ILA 2002). Reconstructive surgery, protective footwear for people with insensitive feet, and assistive devices to correct or prevent activity limitations are also used in secondary prevention.

As concerns tertiary prevention, the stigma attached to leprosy often prevents patients from participating in normal community activities. Strategies include counseling of those affected and their families, neighbors, and communities; vocational training; and advocacy work.

Rehabilitation. Impairments often lead to activity limitations and restrictions on social participation, which can be prevented by correcting the underlying impairment if it is not yet irreversible. After impairment is established, activity limitations can still be minimized with the help of reconstructive surgery or appropriate assistive devices, such as orthoses, grip aids, calipers, or prostheses. A large but unknown percentage of people succeed in overcoming activity limitations by themselves. Some require rehabilitation interventions, such as physical or occupational therapy, reconstructive surgery, or temporary socioeconomic assistance.

Intervention Effectiveness

For all four diseases covered in this chapter, interventions are available that are effective under routine control conditions. The feasibility of eliminating these diseases as public health problems from most endemic areas is therefore not in doubt; however, questions remain about the effectiveness and sustainability of control under specific conditions and about the feasibility of eliminating the parasites and transmission. The vector control strategy for Chagas disease worked well in the Southern Cone countries, but the sylvatic reservoir of *T. cruzi* remains unaffected, and continued surveillance will be essential. Vector control is more challenging in the Andean and Central American countries, where some of the vectors are not domiciliated. For LF, the number of years of MDA and the treatment coverage required to interrupt transmission remain unknown, just as the epidemiological conditions and the number of rounds of ivermectin treatment required to achieve the same for onchocerciasis are not yet known. For leprosy, the key questions remain how much effect MDT has on transmission and when the incidence of new cases can be expected to decline significantly. Hence, the sustainability of control remains a critical issue.

The control programs for three of the diseases depend on drug donations. To date, the pharmaceutical companies donating the drugs and the donors supporting drug distribution have shown impressive commitment to the programs, but if their commitment were to lapse, the control programs would collapse and the diseases would return as public health problems. Another risk is drug resistance. The control programs rely on just a few drugs, and even though drug resistance is not currently apparent, if it were to emerge, the essential tools for control would be lost. Hence, although elimination is in sight, the battle has not yet been won, and research to develop new and improved interventions and strategies for these tropical diseases remains important.

COSTS AND COST-EFFECTIVENESS OF INTERVENTIONS

The published information on cost-effectiveness of interventions for the four diseases is incomplete, and this section provides some new data on the cost per DALY averted that is not available in the literature.

Chagas Disease

For the Southern Cone countries, investment in the control of Chagas disease since 1991 has been about US$320 million, well within the original estimates of US$190 million to US$350 million (Schofield and Dias 1991). Initial predictions of cost-effectiveness suggested an internal rate of return (IRR) for the initiative of about 14 percent, but point studies during the course of the interventions suggest actual IRRs of about 30 percent for Brazil (Akhavan 1998) and more than 60 percent for the province of Salta, Argentina (Basombrio and others 1998).

Brazil had an estimated 2 million infected individuals in 1995. Annual follow-up of the 1.6 million asymptomatic cases would have cost US$98 million. Diagnosis of megasyndromes for 6 percent of infected individuals at an average cost of US$141 each would add US$16.9 million, and corrective surgery for 3 percent of the latter would add US$60 million. Cardiac pacemakers for 5 percent of infected individuals at US$3,000 each would add another US$30 million, so that the partial direct costs for medical attention in Brazil in 1995–96 would have been US$205 million.

In Argentina, the costs for medical attention in 1992 were US$435 for acute cases, US$122 per patient for asymptomatic cases, US$336 for moderate cardiopathy, and US$1,135 for severe cardiopathy. Given that Argentina had 2 million infected individuals, and assuming that 85 percent of them would have been asymptomatic, 9 percent would have had mild cardiopathy, 4 percent would have had moderate cardiopathy, and 2 percent would have had severe cardiopathy, then total expenditures for medical attention would have amounted to US$457 million.

In Chile, aggregate treatment costs were estimated at US$37 million in 1991. New estimates in 1997 using the government payment schedule and an estimate of 142,000 people infected, including 26,545 with myocardiopathy of which 9,652 were severe cases, resulted in an estimated cost of US$14 million to US$19 million. In Uruguay, annual costs for treatment were estimated at US$15 million for 1996.

These treatment costs are significantly higher than the costs of vector control, which for 1996 were US$13 million in Argentina, US$28 million in Brazil, US$650,000 in Chile, and US$4,000 in Uruguay. Akhavan's (1998) study in Brazil estimates a cost of US$260 per DALY prevented, and Robles's (1997) study in Bolivia indicated a cost of US$362 to prevent one year of life lost.

Data on the cost-effectiveness of treating those infected are sparse; however, Robles's (1997) study in Bolivia estimates the costs of treating infected children under the age of five, coming up with a cost of US$3,009 per death averted or about US$100 per DALY averted.

Lymphatic Filariasis

The most widely used interventions for LF control are MDA, vector control, and administration of diethylcarbamazine-fortified salt. We estimate the cost-effectiveness of those strategies in terms of DALYs averted from studies in India on the costs and effectiveness of control and for different scenarios for the minimum duration of control required to achieve sustained interruption of transmission. These scenarios assume that all three strategies are implemented in areas with similar levels of endemicity of *Culex*-transmitted Bancroftian filariasis and that the available cost data for India apply.

We consider three scenarios (table 22.2). *Elim1* is an optimistic elimination scenario under which sustained interruption of transmission is achieved after a relatively short period

Table 22.2 Costs per DALY Averted for LF

Scenario	Mass drug administration			Vector control			Diethylcarbamazine-fortified salt		
	Elim1	Elim2	Control	Elim1	Elim2	Control	Elim1	Elim2	Control
Duration (years)	6	10	30	10	5	30	2	4	30
Costs of control operations per capita (US$)	0.35	0.65	2.22	2.92	6.64	22.74	0.09	0.29	3.56
Cost per DALY averted (US$)	4.40	8.10	29.00	47.50	84.30	302.50	1.10	3.62	46.48

Source: Authors' calculations.

of intervention (six annual rounds of MDA, 10 years of vector control, and 2 years of diethylcarbamazine-fortified salt). *Elim2* is a conservative elimination scenario under which sustained interruption is achieved only after a longer period of intervention (10 years of MDA, 15 years of vector control, and 4 years of diethylcarbamazine-fortified salt). *Control* is a scenario under which transmission is brought to low levels but not interrupted and where control efforts will have to continue.

Because of the slow dynamics of filariasis transmission and disease, the prevalence of the chronic disease manifestations (lymphedema and hydrocele) on which the DALY estimates are based will not fully reflect the effect of control for many years. We have therefore tried to predict the trend in chronic disease over a 30-year period. Recent findings from a longitudinal study (Ramaiah and others 2003) of the effect of MDA in Pondicherry, India, showed that the prevalence of hydrocele and lymphedema had declined by 58 percent after seven annual treatment rounds with diethylcarbamazine. We assumed that from the seventh year of intervention, any further reduction in disease prevalence was attributable exclusively to reduced incidence as a result of reduced transmission, and that 30 years after the initiation of the intervention, the prevalence of disease would have fallen by 90 percent. We assumed that the effect of diethylcarbamazine-fortified salt was similar to that of MDA, whereas for vector control we assumed that prevalence would decline with a delay of seven years.

The predicted costs per DALY averted (table 22.3) indicate that MDA and diethylcarbamazine-fortified salt are extremely cost-effective. Elimination with MDA costs about US$4 to US$8 per DALY averted, and even if transmission were not interrupted and MDA would have to be continued for 30 years (control scenario), the cost would be still only be around US$29 per DALY averted. Diethylcarbamazine-fortified salt would be the cheapest intervention, but governments rarely favor it, and compliance can be difficult to ensure. Vector control is at least 10 times more expensive in terms of DALYs averted, but it offers additional benefits in terms of malaria and dengue control and significant relief from mosquito nuisance.

The effect of MDA on hydrocele and lymphedema is not yet well established and the results of the Indian trial on which

the previous calculations are based may be too optimistic. However, even under much less favorable assumptions that the prevalence of hydrocele and lymphedema declines by 20 percent after 7 years of MDA and by 75 percent after 30 years, the estimated cost per DALY averted would be only 50 percent higher than those given in table 22.3, and the interventions would still be very cost-effective.

The prevention of chronic disease also has direct economic benefits (Ramaiah and Das 2004). The cost of preventing one case of chronic disease through six rounds of MDA in India has been estimated at US$8.41. The economic benefits include savings of 58.24 working days per year per case, yielding wages of US$39.39 and treatment costs of US$1.44. On average, chronic patients lose 11 years of productive life; thus, the average economic benefits total US$449.13 per chronic case averted. This figure gives a benefit-cost ratio of 52.6, perhaps one of the highest for any disease control program.

Onchocerciasis

Investment in onchocerciasis control has included about US$570 million provided by donors to the OCP during 1975–2002, US$140 million provided and earmarked for APOC for 1996–2010, and US$10 million for OEPA for 1991–2003. The African onchocerciasis control programs are considered highly cost-effective. No cost-benefit analysis has yet been published for OEPA.

The OCP has been highly successful. More than 40 million people in the program's 11 countries are now considered free from infection and eye lesions, more than 1.5 million people are no longer infected, and more than 200,000 cases of blindness have been prevented. Sixteen million children born since the program began are free of onchocerciasis. The socioeconomic effect has also been dramatic: 25 million hectares of fertile land in the river valleys were made available for resettlement and agriculture. A cost-benefit analysis of the OCP has estimated the net present value for the OCP over a 39-year project horizon from 1974 to 2002 as US$485 million (Kim and Benton 1995). This figure corresponds to an IRR of 20 percent, resulting mainly from increased labor because of prevention of blindness (25 percent of benefits) and increased land use (75 percent of benefits).

A similar cost-benefit analysis for APOC also considered benefits in terms of additional labor resulting from blindness prevention (Benton 1998). It did not consider land use because depopulation of river valleys is rarely seen in APOC countries, where the forest type of onchocerciasis predominates. Nevertheless, the estimated IRR for APOC remained almost as high as that for the OCP (17 percent), because the cost is lower but the number of people served is far greater.

The estimated rates of return for the OCP and APOC did not include the effects of control on onchocercal skin disease. Hence, these rates underestimate the benefits, because troublesome itching accounts for more than 50 percent of the DALYs attributable to onchocerciasis. The cost of ivermectin, which is donated by Merck, was not included in our analyses.

To estimate the approximate cost per DALY averted, we considered the burden of disease and treatment with ivermectin in APOC countries. Using the latest epidemiological mapping data, we estimate that, in 1995, 34.6 million people were infected in APOC countries and that 1.86 million DALYs were lost. Currently more than 44 percent of those infected are covered by community-directed treatment with ivermectin, and expectations are that treatment will be expanded to cover most of the remainder before the end of APOC in 2010. Information from areas where ivermectin treatment has been in effect for more than 15 years shows that the prevalence and intensity of onchocerciasis infection have fallen to low levels (Borsboom and others 2003), and computer simulations predict that the disease could not become a public health problem again for at least another 10 to 20 years if treatment were halted (Remme, Alley, and Plaisier 1995). We therefore estimate that 15 years of ivermectin treatment at 65 percent coverage will prevent at least 25 years of onchocercal disease. If we assume that 70 percent of endemic communities will ultimately be covered by community-directed treatment with ivermectin and that 80 percent of those communities will maintain annual treatment at 65 percent coverage for at least 15 years, at least 26 million DALYs would be prevented over a 25-year period.

The predicted cost of community-directed treatment with ivermectin in APOC countries is US$145 million by the international donor community plus US$64 million by ministries of health and collaborating nongovernmental organizations, giving a total of US$209 million. Therefore we estimate that the cost of community-directed treatment is approximately US$7 per DALY averted.

The ultimate cost-benefit of onchocerciasis control will depend on how long effective control programs will need to be maintained to keep the disease under control. National governments and ministries of health should plan to invest in ivermectin distribution and in surveillance activities for the foreseeable future. Thus, a case must continually be made with

national decision makers that if investments do not continue, recrudescence of infection is likely. One strategy for sustaining national investment is to show that ivermectin distribution systems can be made polyfunctional. Treatment programs based on MDA for intestinal parasites, schistosomiasis, and LF and on vitamin A distribution can be integrated with ivermectin distribution programs and thereby further improve cost-benefit ratios. The use of community-directed treatment with ivermectin is also envisaged as a way of strengthening peripheral and district health systems (Homeida and others 2002).

Leprosy

Costs associated with leprosy control include case detection, treatment, prevention of disability, and rehabilitation. We calculate the incremental health service cost to arrive at the average cost of curing a patient with leprosy. Our estimates are based on the limited published cost data available, program expenditure data, and expert opinion, although costs are likely to differ substantially by country.

As case-detection rates decrease, the average cost of detecting one case increases. The previous edition of this volume estimated a cost of US$2 per case detected based on a case-detection rate of about 300 per 100,000; however, case-detection rates are now considerably lower in most countries (Dharmshaktu and others 1999; Ganapati and others 2001; Smith 1999). Many leprosy control programs now rely on voluntary case finding supported by information, education, and communication activities to raise or maintain people's awareness of the early signs and symptoms of leprosy. We estimate the cost of this approach to be about US$1 per case detected. Nevertheless, if active methods are still used in areas where case-detection rates are low, the cost of case detection may be as high as US$108.

The costs of diagnosing and treating leprosy have fallen in the past decade, and diagnosis by clinical examination only is now recommended. We therefore exclude the cost of skin smears. In addition, a shortening of the treatment regimen has lowered drug costs to about US$12 for a multibacillary case and US$1 for a paucibacillary case. Globally, almost 40 percent of leprosy cases are classified as multibacillary cases, with the remaining 60 percent being paucibacillary cases. Thus, we estimate the average drug cost as US$5.40 per case.

The cost of treatment, however, is more than the cost of drugs alone. WHO guidelines recommend that a multibacillary case receive supervised treatment for 12 months and that a paucibacillary patient receive treatment for 6 months. Using cost data from Ethiopia and Pakistan, we estimate these treatment costs at US$20 to US$30 in low-income countries. Data from studies of tuberculosis interventions show that community-supervised treatment may reduce costs by up to 50 percent (Khan and others 2002), and this approach is being advocated as part of "flexible MDT delivery" (ILA 2002) and "accompanied MDT" (WHO 2002b). Reducing the nondrug costs of treating leprosy to about US$10 to US$20 per patient may, therefore, be possible. We thus estimate the costs of treating a case of leprosy with MDT to be between US$15.40 and US$35.40 per case, depending on the strategy used.

About 10 to 20 percent of new leprosy cases are likely to suffer a reaction during or after MDT. We estimate treatment of those reactions to cost US$25 per patient. Of these patients, 1 percent may develop severe complications requiring hospitalization, at an estimated cost of US$480 per patient. In addition, 10 percent of new cases will develop neural or secondary impairments and may require footwear and education about wound management. We estimate the lifetime cost of protective footwear at US$300 per patient (Seboka, Saunderson, and Currie 1998) and education at US$10 per patient. In 1 percent of cases, reconstructive surgery may be required at about US$455 per patient. We therefore estimate the average incremental cost of interventions for prevention of disability to be US$44.15 per new case of disability. Because about 3 percent of new patients will need rehabilitation, we estimate the average cost at under US$1 for each new case of leprosy detected (Jagannathan and others 1993). However, a backlog of old cases exists. Although data in this area are weak, up to a third of the 4 million people living with leprosy globally (2 million with grade 1 disability and 2 million with grade 2 disability) could require rehabilitation.

Few data are available on the program costs associated with leprosy. A review of expenditure in Asia found that up to 40 percent of the total costs could be classified as programmatic costs, although this amount may now be less because leprosy programs have increasingly been integrated into general health services. Data from Indonesia demonstrate that program costs can be reduced by up to 35 percent by integrating them with tuberculosis programs (Plag 1995). We therefore estimate the average cost of finding, treating, and preventing disabilities and rehabilitating a new case of leprosy at US$76 to US$264.

In practice, many leprosy programs will also be providing disability prevention and rehabilitation interventions to a large backlog of patients, so the average cost per new case will be higher than here. Programs that face a high proportion of multibacillary cases and cases presenting with high levels of disability are also likely to have higher costs.

Assuming a cure rate of around 85 percent, we estimate the costs of curing one patient of leprosy to be about US$93 per new case. Using data from India (25 percent of those with leprosy will self-cure, an average age of onset of 27, a disability weighting of 0.152, and a life expectancy at age 25 to 29 of 44.75), we estimate the cost per DALY of detecting and treating a new case of leprosy to be US$38.

In addition, assuming a 90 percent success rate, we calculate a cost per DALY of US$7 for patients needing treatment for

Table 22.3 Cost-Effectiveness Estimates for the Main Interventions for Each Disease

Intervention	Cost per DALY averted (US$)	Internal rate of return (percent)
Chagas disease		
Vector control	260	30–60
Treatment (children under five)	100	—
LF		
MDA	4–29	—
Diethylcarbamazine-fortified salt	1–46	—
Vector control	48–303	—
Onchocerciasis		
MDA	7	17 (APOC)
Vector control	—	20 (OCP)
Leprosy		
Case detection and treatment	38	—
Prevention of disability	1–110	—

Source: Authors' calculations.
MDA = mass drug administration, — = not available.

reactions and ulcers, US$75 for those needing footwear and self-care education, and US$110 for those needing reconstructive surgery. These estimates provide only a broad indication because data on the effectiveness of these interventions are scarce, and the application of the disability weight of 0.152 to all interventions may overestimate their benefits.

Data on the economic effect of leprosy at the national level are not available. However, leprosy affects those who are economically active, with a peak in incidence at 10 to 20 years of age and again at 30 to 50 years of age. Studies of the impact of leprosy on productivity show that deformity from leprosy can reduce the probability of obtaining employment and can reduce household income and expenditure on food (Diffey and others 2000; Kopparty 1995). In addition, leprosy can have a significant social impact because participation in the community may be restricted. This impact continues well beyond the actual treatment period because leprosy-related impairments have a tendency to get worse over time even after the infection has been arrested.

Summary

Available information indicates that interventions for the four diseases are highly cost-effective and that the benefit-cost ratio of control is high (table 22.3).

RESEARCH NEEDS AND PRIORITIES

Because the diseases in this chapter are targeted for elimination as public health problems, it is sometimes assumed that research for these diseases is no longer necessary and that all

Table 22.4 Control Strategies, Major Challenges, and Research Needs for Each Disease

Disease	Principal control strategy	Major problems and challenges	Major research needs
Chagas disease	Interruption of transmission through domestic vector control and improved blood transfusion	Control of nondomiciliated vectors Sustained vector control Millions of those infected still at risk of disease	Strategies for surveillance of nondomiciliated vectors Better drugs and diagnostics
LF	Interruption of transmission through periodic mass treatment Disability alleviation by local hygiene measures	Need for high treatment coverage Unknowns in elimination strategy Limited effect of current drugs	Strategies for high treatment coverage Evidence base for elimination strategies Drug that kills or sterilizes adult worms
Onchocerciasis	Periodic mass treatment to eliminate the disease as a public health problem	Need to sustain high coverage for decades Risk of ivermectin resistance Eradication not possible with current tools	Strategies for sustained high treatment coverage Feasibility of elimination with ivermectin Drug that kills or sterilizes adult worms
Leprosy	Case finding and multidrug treatment Rehabilitation and prevention of disability	Incomplete MDT coverage Need to integrate and sustain control Impact on transmission not known	Integration and sustainability of control Improved diagnosis of infection Prevention and management of nerve damage

Source: Remme and others 2002.

available resources should be allocated to elimination efforts. However, research remains critical to address questions pertaining to how to achieve elimination with currently available tools and especially to how to optimize implementation in different epidemiological, sociocultural, and health system settings. Epidemiological questions on the required intervention coverage, frequency, and duration need to be answered to guide elimination strategies, and research on the risk, prevention, and control of recrudescence is crucial to ensure sustained success.

The Special Programme for Research and Training in Tropical Diseases, a joint project of the United Nations Children's Fund, United Nations Development Programme, World Bank, and WHO, recently undertook a systematic analysis of research needs for each of the 10 tropical diseases in its portfolio (Remme and others 2002). This analysis involved assessing the burden of disease and recent epidemiological trends, reviewing current control strategies, and identifying the major problems and challenges for disease control and the research needed to address these challenges. Table 22.4 summarizes the results of this analysis for the four diseases discussed in this chapter.

Chagas disease has two main research priorities. The first is the development of new vector control strategies that will allow the successful elimination campaign used in the Southern Cone countries to be extended to the Central American and Andean countries, where the vectors are often not domiciliated. The second is the development of effective and affordable treatment for the millions of people already infected and the prevention of chronic complications.

For onchocerciasis and LF, the main research priorities are similar: implementation research to improve MDA; epidemiological research to determine if, when, and with what treatment coverage the parasite reservoir can be locally eliminated for different vector-parasite complexes; and research to develop a macrofilaricide and improved diagnostics that would facilitate elimination.

For leprosy, the research needs were further reviewed during a Scientific Working Group (Special Programme for Research and Training in Tropical Diseases 2003). The meeting arrived at a clear consensus of three top priorities for leprosy research: implementation research on sustainable and integrated residual leprosy control activities, improved diagnosis of infection, and improved approaches for preventing and managing nerve damage.

These are the current main priorities for research in support of elimination. Eradication is not currently anticipated for any of the diseases; thus, research on better tools and strategies that will allow a permanent solution for these infectious diseases is also needed. Furthermore, currently available control tools may be lost because of factors such as resistance, and research to develop replacement tools is essential now.

CONCLUSION

Tropical diseases are often viewed as neglected, because the investments made to fight them appear negligible compared with the massive amounts expended globally on the health problems of developed countries. Tropical diseases are truly diseases of the poor, but despite the limited resources available for research and control, simple and effective interventions have been developed and delivered to populations in need for the four tropical diseases discussed in this chapter. Thus, experience with these four diseases sends a powerful message: success is possible, even for neglected tropical diseases of poor populations in developing countries. Elimination of these diseases as public health problems can be achieved, and investments in tropical disease research and control can make a significant contribution to poverty reduction.

An important reason for the success was that the interventions were extremely cost-effective. The available cost-effectiveness data, though limited, show convincingly that intervention against these diseases is a good investment, and the argument for investment gets better when other economic benefits, not reflected in DALYs, are taken into account, such as increased food production when fertile land along river valleys became available for agriculture after the control of onchocerciasis in West Africa and increased labor productivity after effective filariasis control in India.

The pharmaceutical industry also played a major role through large drug donations, and the creation of intercountry control programs provided effective mechanisms for implementing interventions, technical support, and coordination. Another reason for the success was a focused research program that ensured the development of interventions based on simple and sustainable approaches that use cheap and "appropriate" technology and that are potentially multifunctional.

Chagas disease, LF, onchocerciasis, and leprosy are now on target for elimination as public health problems from large parts of the world. However, these diseases cannot be eradicated using current tools, and much remains to be done to expand and sustain the control efforts and undertake the necessary research to improve the control efforts as well as to develop more definite solutions. It will be essential, therefore, that donors and ministries of health not abandon these programs because of their success.

REFERENCES

Addiss, D., J. Critchley, H. Ejere, P. Garner, H. Gelband, and C. Gamble. 2004. "Albendazole for Lymphatic Filariasis." Cochrane Database of Systematic Reviews (1) CD003753.

Akhavan, D. 1998. *Análise de custo-efetividade do programa de controle da doença de Chagas no Brasil.* Brasília: Pan American Health Organization.

Amazigo, U. V., M. Obono, K. Y. Dadzie, J. Remme, J. Jiya, R. Ndyomugyenyi, and others. 2002. "Monitoring Community-Directed Treatment Programs for Sustainability: Lessons from the African Programme for Onchocerciasis Control (APOC)." *Annals of Tropical Medicine and Parasitology* 96 (Suppl. 1): S75–92.

Basombrio, M. A., C. J. Schofield, C. L. Rojas, and E. C. del Rey. 1998. "A Cost-Benefit Analysis of Chagas Disease Control in North-western

Argentina." *Transactions of the Royal Society of Tropical Medicine and Hygiene* 92 (2): 137–43.

Bekri, W., S. Gebre, A. Mengiste, P. R. Saunderson, and S. Zewge. 1998. "Delay in Presentation and Start of Treatment in Leprosy Patients: A Case-Control Study of Disabled and Non-Disabled Patients in Three Different Settings in Ethiopia." *International Journal of Leprosy and Other Mycobacterial Diseases* 66 (1): 1–9.

Benton, B. 1998. "Economic Impact of Onchocerciasis Control through the African Programme for Onchocerciasis Control: An Overview." *Annals of Tropical Medicine and Parasitology* 92 (Suppl. 1): S33–39.

Borsboom, G. J. J. M., B. A. Boatin, N. J. D. Nagelkerke, H. Agoua, K. L. B. Akpoboua, E. W. S. Alley, and others. 2003. "Impact of Ivermectin on Onchocerciasis Transmission: Assessing the Empirical Evidence That Repeated Ivermectin Mass Treatments May Lead to Elimination/Eradication in West-Africa." *Filaria Journal* 2 (1): 8.

Boussinesq, M., S. D. Pion, Demanga-Ngangue, and J. Kamgno. 2002. "Relationship between Onchocerciasis and Epilepsy: A Matched Case-Control Study in the Mbam Valley, Republic of Cameroon." *Transactions of the Royal Society of Tropical Medicine and Hygiene* 96 (5): 537–41.

Burkot, T., and K. Ichimori. 2002. "The PacELF Program: Will Mass Drug Administration Be Enough?" *Trends in Parasitology* 18 (3): 109–15.

Dadzie, K. Y., J. Remme, A. Rolland, and B. Thylefors. 1989. "Ocular Onchocerciasis and Intensity of Infection in the Community: II. West African Rainforest Foci of the Vector *Simulium yahense*." *Tropical Medicine and Parasitology* 40 (3): 348–54.

Dharmshaktu, N. S., B. N. Barkakaty, P. K. Patnaik, and M. A. Arif. 1999. "Progress towards Elimination of Leprosy as a Public Health Problem in India and Role of Modified Leprosy Elimination Campaign." *Leprosy Review* 70 (4): 430–39.

Dias, J. C. 1987. "Control of Chagas' Disease in Brazil." *Parasitology Today* 3 (11): 336–41.

Diffey, B., M. Vaz, M. J. Soares, A. J. Jacob, and L. S. Piers. 2000. "The Effect of Leprosy-Induced Deformity on the Nutritional Status of Index Cases and Their Household Members in Rural South India: A Socioeconomic Perspective." *European Journal of Clinical Nutrition* 54 (8): 643–49.

Dreyer, G., P. Dreyer, and J. Noroes. 2002. "Recommendations for the Treatment of *Bancroftian filariasis* in Symptomless and Diseased Patients." *Revista da Sociedade Brasileira de Medicina Tropical* 35 (1): 43–50.

Dreyer, G., J. Noroes, J. Figueredo-Silva, and W. F. Piessens. 2000. "Pathogenesis of Lymphatic Disease in *Bancroftian filariasis*: A Clinical Perspective." *Parasitology Today* 16 (12): 544–48.

Fine, P. E., and P. G. Smith. 1996. "Vaccination against Leprosy: The View from 1996." *Leprosy Review* 67 (4): 249–52.

Ganapati, R., C. R. Revankar, V. V. Pai, S. Kingsley, and S. N. Prasad. 2001. "Can Cost of Leprosy Case Detection in Urban Areas Be Further Reduced?" *International Journal of Leprosy and Other Mycobacterial Diseases* 69 (4): 349–51.

Gwatkin, D. R., M. Guillot, and P. Heuveline. 1999. "The Burden of Disease among the Global Poor." *Lancet* 354 (9178): 586–89.

Gyapong, J. O., D. Kyelem, I. Kleinschmidt, and others. 2002. "The Use of Spatial Analysis in Mapping the Distribution of *Bancroftian filariasis* in Four West African Countries." *Annals of Tropical Medicine and Parasitology* 96 (7): 695–705.

Gyapong, J. O., V. Kumaraswami, G. Biswas, and E. A. Ottesen. 2005. "Treatment Strategies Underpinning the Global Programme to Eliminate Lymphatic Filariasis." *Expert Opinion on Pharmacotherapy* 6 (2): 179–200.

Homeida, M., E. Braide, E. Elhassan, U. V. Amazigo, B. Liese, B. Benton, and others. 2002. "APOC's Strategy of Community-Directed

Treatment with Ivermectin (CDTI) and Its Potential for Providing Additional Health Services to the Poorest Populations: African Programme for Onchocerciasis Control." *Annals of Tropical Medicine and Parasitology* 96 (Suppl. 1): S93–104.

ILA (International Leprosy Association). 2002. "Report of the International Leprosy Association Technical Forum, Paris, France, 22–28 February 2002." *International Journal of Leprosy and Other Mycobacterial Diseases* 70 (Suppl. 1): S1–62.

Jagannathan, S. A., V. Ramamurthy, S. J. Jeyaraj, and S. Regina. 1993. "A Pilot Project on Community Based Rehabilitation in South India: A Preliminary Report." *Indian Journal of Leprosy* 65 (3): 315–22.

Khan, M. A., J. D. Walley, S. N. Witter, A. Imran, and N. Safdar. 2002. "Costs and Cost-Effectiveness of Different DOT Strategies for the Treatment of Tuberculosis in Pakistan: Directly Observed Treatment." *Health Policy and Planning* 17 (2): 178–86.

Kim, A., and B. Benton. 1995. *Cost-Benefit Analysis of the Onchocerciasis Control Programme (OCP)*. Washington, DC: World Bank.

Kopparty, S. N. 1995. "Problems, Acceptance, and Social Inequality: A Study of the Deformed Leprosy Patients and their Families." *Leprosy Review* 66 (3): 239–49.

Mathers, C. D., A. Lopez, and C. J. L. Murray. 2006. "The Burden of Disease and Mortality by Condition: Data, Methods, and Results for the Year 2001." In *Global Burden of Disease and Risk Factors*, ed. A. Lopez, C. Mathers, M. Ezzati, D. Jamison, and C. Murray. New York: Oxford University Press.

Maxwell, C. A., C. F. Curtis, H. Haji, S. Kisumku, A. I. Thalib, and S. A. Yahya. 1990. "Control of *Bancroftian filariasis* by Integrating Therapy with Vector Control Using Polystyrene Beads in Wet Pit Latrines." *Transactions of the Royal Society of Tropical Medicine and Hygiene* 84 (5): 709–14.

Meima, A., P. R. Saunderson, S. Gebre, K. Desta, G. J. van Oortmarssen, and J. D. Habbema. 1999. "Factors Associated with Impairments in New Leprosy Patients: The AMFES Cohort." *Leprosy Review* 70 (2): 189–203.

Molyneux, D. H. 1995. "Onchocerciasis Control in West Africa: Current Status and Future of the Onchocerciasis Control Programme." *Parasitology Today* 11: 399–402.

Murdoch, M. E., M. C. Asuzu, M. Hagan, W. H. Makunde, P. Ngoumou, K. F. Ogbuagu, and others. 2002. "Onchocerciasis: The Clinical and Epidemiological Burden of Skin Disease in Africa." *Annals of Tropical Medicine and Parasitology* 96 (3): 283–96.

Noma, M., B. E. Nwoke, I. Nutall, P. A. Tambala, P. Enyong, A. Namsenmo, and others. 2002. "Rapid Epidemiological Mapping of Onchocerciasis (REMO): Its Application by the African Programme for Onchocerciasis Control (APOC)." *Annals of Tropical Medicine and Parasitology* 96 (Suppl. 1): S29–39.

Ottesen, E. A. 2000. "The Global Programme to Eliminate Lymphatic Filariasis." *Tropical Medicine and International Health* 5 (9): 591–94.

Ottesen, E. A., B. O. Duke, M. Karam, and K. Behbehani. 1997. "Strategies and Tools for the Control/Elimination of Lymphatic Filariasis." *Bulletin of the World Health Organization* 75 (6): 491–503.

Peters, D. H., and T. Phillips. 2004. "Mectizan Donation Program: Evaluation of a Public-Private Partnership." *Tropical Medicine and International Health* 9 (4): A4–15.

Plag, I. 1995. *Guidelines for Cost Analysis in Leprosy Control Programmes*. Amsterdam: Royal Tropical Institute.

Rajendran, R., I. P. Sunish, T. R. Mani, A. Munirathinam, S. M. Abdullah, D. J. Augustin, and K. Satyanarayana. 2002. "The Influence of the Mass Administration of Diethylcarbamazine, Alone or with Albendazole, on the Prevalence of Filarial Antigenaemia." *Annals of Tropical Medicine and Parasitology* 96 (6): 595–602.

Ramaiah, K. D., and P. K. Das. 2004. "Mass Drug Administration to Eliminate Lymphatic Filariasis in India." *Trends in Parasitology* 20 (11): 499–502.

Ramaiah, K. D., P. K. Das, and V. Dhanda. 1994. "Estimation of Permissible Levels of Transmission of *Bancroftian filariasis* Based on Some Entomological and Parasitological Results of a Five-Year Vector Control Program." *Acta Tropica* 56 (1): 89–96.

Ramaiah, K. D., P. K. Das, E. Michael, and H. Guyatt. 2000. "The Economic Burden of Lymphatic Filariasis in India." *Parasitology Today* 16 (6): 251–53.

Ramaiah, K. D., P. K. Das, P. Vanamail, and S. P. Pani. 2003. "The Impact of Six Rounds of Single-Dose Mass Administration of Diethylcarbamazine or Ivermectin on the Transmission of *Wuchereria bancrofti* by *Culex quinquefasciatus* and Its Implications for Lymphatic Filariasis Elimination Programs." *Tropical Medicine and International Health* 8 (12): 1082–92.

Ramu, K., K. D. Ramaiah, H. Guyatt, and D. Evans. 1996. "Impact of Lymphatic Filariasis on the Productivity of Male Weavers in a South Indian Village." *Transactions of the Royal Society of Tropical Medicine and Hygiene* 90 (6): 669–70.

Remme, J. H. F. 1995. "The African Programme for Onchocerciasis Control: Preparing to Launch." *Parasitology Today* 11: 403–6.

———. 2004a. "The Global Burden of Onchocerciasis in 1990." In *Global Burden of Disease 1990*. Geneva: World Health Organization. http://www3.who.int/whosis/burden/gbd2000docs/Onchocerciasis%201990.pdf.

———. 2004b. "Research for Control: The Onchocerciasis Experience." *Tropical Medicine and International Health* 9 (2): 243–54.

Remme, J. H. F., E. S. Alley, and A. P. Plaisier. 1995. "Estimation and Prediction in Tropical Disease Control: The Example of Onchocerciasis." In *Epidemic Models: Their Structure and Relation to Data*, ed. D. Mollison, 372–92. Cambridge, U.K.: Cambridge University Press.

Remme, J. H., F. Blas, L. Chitsulo, P. M. Desjeux, H. D. Engers, T. P. Kanyok, and others. 2002. "Strategic Emphases for Tropical Diseases Research: A TDR Perspective." *Trends in Parasitology* 18 (10): 421–26.

Reuben, R., R. Rajendran, I. P. Sunish, T. R. Mani, S. C. Tewari, J. Hiriyan, and others. 2001. "Annual Single-Dose Diethylcarbamazine plus Ivermectin for Control of *Bancroftian filariasis*: Comparative Efficacy with and without Vector Control." *Annals of Tropical Medicine and Parasitology* 95 (4): 361–78.

Richards, F. O., B. Boatin, M. Sauerbrey, and A. Seketeli. 2001. "Control of Onchocerciasis Today: Status and Challenges." *Trends in Parasitology* 17 (12): 558–63.

Richards F. O., D. Pam, A. Kal, G. Gerlong, J. Oneyka, Y. Sambo, and others. 2005 "Significant Decrease in the Prevalence of *Wuchereria bancrofti* Infection in Anopheline Mosquitoes Following the Addition of Albendazole to Annual, Ivermectin-Based, Mass Treatments in Nigeria." *Annals of Tropical Medicine and Parasitology* 99 (2): 155–64.

Robles, M. C. 1997. *Analisis costo-efectividad de las intervenciones de salud en Bolivia*. La Paz: Unidad de Análisis de Políticas Sociales.

Salvatella, A. R., and W. Vignolo. 1996. "Una aproximación a los costos de internación por cardiopatia Chagasica en Uruguay." *Revista da Sociedade Brasileira de Medicina Tropical* 29 (Suppl.): 114–18.

Schenone, H. 1998. "Human Infection by *Trypanosoma Cruzi* in Chile: Epidemiology Estimates and Costs of Care and Treatment of the Chagasic Patient." *Boletin Chileno de Parasitologia*. 53 (1–2): 23–26.

Schmunis, G. A. 2000. "A tripanossomiase Americana e seu impacto na saude publica das Americas." In *Trypanosoma cruzi e doença de Chagas*, 2nd ed., ed. Z. Brener, Z. Andrade, and M. Barral-Neto, 1–15. Rio de Janeiro: Guanabara-Koogan.

Schmunis, G. A., F. Zicker, J. R. Cruz, and P. Cuchi. 2001. "Safety of Blood Supply for Infectious Diseases in Latin American Countries, 1994–1997." *American Journal of Tropical Medicine and Hygiene* 65 (6): 924–30.

Schmunis, G. A., F. Zicker, F. Pinheiro, and D. Brandling-Bennett. 1998. "Risk of Transfusion-Transmitted Infectious Diseases in Latin America." *Emerging Infectious Diseases* 4: 5–11.

Schofield, C. J., and J. C. Dias. 1991. "A Cost-Benefit Analysis of Chagas' Disease Control." *Memórias do Instituto Oswaldo Cruz* 86 (3): 285–95.

Seboka, G., P. Saunderson, and H. Currie. 1998. "Footwear for Farmers Affected by Leprosy." *Leprosy Review* 69 (2): 182–83.

Seketeli, A., G. Adeoye, A. Eyamba, E. Nnoruka, P. Drameh, U. V. Amazigo, and others. 2002. "The Achievements and Challenges of the African Programme for Onchocerciasis Control (APOC)." *Annals of Tropical Medicine and Parasitology* 96 (Suppl. 1): 15–28.

Smith, C. M., and W. C. Smith. 2000. "Chemoprophylaxis Is Effective in the Prevention of Leprosy in Endemic Countries: A Systematic Review and Meta-Analysis. MILEP2 Study Group—Mucosal Immunology of Leprosy." *Journal of Infection* 41 (2): 137–42.

Smith, W. C. 1999. "Future Scope and Expectations: Why, When, and How LECs Should Continue." *Leprosy Review* 70 (4): 498–505.

Special Programme for Research and Training in Tropical Diseases. 2003. *Report of the Scientific Working Group Meeting on Leprosy.* Geneva: World Health Organization.

Stolk, W. A., S. Swaminathan, G. J. van Oortmarssen, P. K. Das, and J. D. Habbema. 2003. "Prospects for Elimination of Bancroftian Filariasis by Mass Drug Treatment in Pondicherry, India: A Simulation Study." *Journal of Infectious Diseases* 188 (9): 1371–81.

van Beers, S. M., M. Hatta, and P. R. Klatser. 1999. "Patient Contact Is the Major Determinant in Incident Leprosy: Implications for Future Control." *International Journal of Leprosy and Other Mycobacterial Diseases* 67 (2): 119–28.

van Brakel, W. H. 2000. "Peripheral Neuropathy in Leprosy and Its Consequences." *Leprosy Review* 71 (Suppl.): S146–53.

van Brakel, W. H., and A. M. Anderson. 1998. "A Survey of Problems in Activities of Daily Living among Persons Affected by Leprosy." *Asia Pacific Disability and Rehabilitation Journal* 9 (2): 62–67.

Vlassoff, C., M. Weiss, E. B. Ovuga, C. Eneanya, P. T. Nwel, S. S. Babalola, and others. 2000. "Gender and the Stigma of Onchocercal Skin Disease in Africa." *Social Science and Medicine* 50 (10): 1353–68.

WHO (World Health Organization). 1991. *Control of Chagas' Disease: Report of a WHO Expert Committee.* Technical Report 811. Geneva: WHO.

———. 1995a. *Onchocerciasis and Its Control: Report of a WHO Expert Committee on Onchocerciasis Control.* Technical Report 852. Geneva: WHO.

———. 1995b. *World Health Report 1995: Bridging the Gaps.* Geneva: WHO.

———. 2002a. *Control of Chagas Disease: Second Report of the WHO Expert Committee.* Technical Report 109. Geneva: WHO.

———. 2002b. *The Final Push Strategy to Eliminate Leprosy as a Public Health Problem: Questions and Answers.* Geneva: WHO.

———. 2002c. *Lymphatic Filariasis: The Disease and Its Control.* Technical Report 71. Geneva: WHO.

———. 2002d. *The World Health Report 2002: Reducing Risks, Promoting Healthy Life.* Technical Report 248. Geneva: WHO.

———. 2004a. *World Health Organization: Leprosy Elimination Project Status Report 2003.* Geneva: WHO.

———. 2004b. *World Health Report 2004: Changing History.* Geneva: WHO.

World Bank. 1993. *World Development Report 1993: Investing in Health.* New York: Oxford University Press.

Zimmerman, P. A., K. Y. Dadzie, G. De Sole, J. Remme, E. S. Alley, and T. R. Unnasch. 1992. "*Onchocerca volvulus* DNA Probe Classification Correlates with Epidemiologic Patterns of Blindness." *Journal of Infectious Diseases* 165 (5): 964–68.

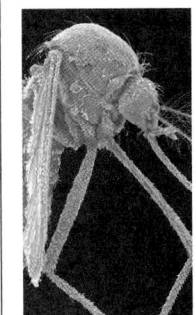

Chapter **23**

Tropical Diseases Lacking Adequate Control Measures: Dengue, Leishmaniasis, and African Trypanosomiasis

Pierre Cattand, Phillippe Desjeux, M. G. Guzmán, Jean Jannin,
A. Kroeger, André Médici, Philip Musgrove, Mike B. Nathan,
Alexandra Shaw, and C. J. Schofield

Dengue, leishmaniasis, and African trypanosomiasis (sleeping sickness) are serious diseases that the World Health Organization (WHO) characterizes as lacking effective control measures. They are transmitted by insect vectors and can result in epidemic outbreaks. Specific treatment is unavailable for dengue, although good supportive treatment can drastically reduce mortality. For the leishmaniases and for sleeping sickness, treatment relies largely on antiquated drugs based on antimony and arsenic, respectively. Sustained control of the insect vectors is difficult for dengue and leishmaniasis because their high reproductive potential allows the vector populations to recover quickly after intervention wherever adequate breeding conditions exist. By contrast, tsetse flies, the vectors for sleeping sickness, have a much lower reproductive potential and could be eliminated over large areas, given adequate organization and surveillance. Through the African Union, African nations are developing a large-scale initiative for areawide elimination of tsetse flies, partly because of sleeping sickness, but also because of their importance as vectors of animal trypanosomiasis, which poses a serious constraint to livestock development and agriculture.

DISEASE CHARACTERISTICS AND TRANSMISSION

Dengue

Dengue is a mosquitoborne viral disease with a high capacity for epidemic outbreaks. Infection can be asymptomatic or can present with symptoms ranging from mild, self-limiting, febrile illness to severe, life-threatening disease. Two clinical pictures are recognized: (a) dengue fever (DF) and (b) dengue hemorrhagic fever (DHF) or dengue shock syndrome (DSS).

The four dengue serotypes, known as dengue 1, 2, 3, and 4, constitute a complex of the flaviviridae transmitted by *Aedes* mosquitoes, particularly *Ae. aegypti*. Infection by any of the four serotypes induces lifelong immunity against reinfection by the same serotype, but only partial and transient protection against the others. Sequential infection by different serotypes seems to be the main trigger for DHF/DSS.

Disease Manifestations. The incubation period is four to six days. Infants and young children usually develop fever, sometimes accompanied by a rash. Older children and adults may develop either a mild febrile syndrome or classic DF with fever, headache, myalgias, arthralgia, nausea, vomiting, and rash. Skin bleeding, petechiae, or ecchymosis are observed in some patients. Bleeding from the nose, gums, and gastrointestinal tract; hematuria; or hypermenorrhea can accompany the clinical picture. Leukopenia is common and thrombocytopenia is sometimes observed. DF can be incapacitating, but the prognosis is favorable and the case-fatality rate is low.

By contrast, DHF/DSS can be life threatening. It is characterized by high fever, bleeding, thrombocytopenia, and hemoconcentration (Nimmanitya 1993; PAHO 1994). Plasma leakage differentiates DHF/DSS from classic DF. Severity is classified as mild (grades I and II) or severe (grades III and IV), with the main difference being shock in the latter. In some epidemics, hepatomegaly has been prominent. As with DF, DHF generally begins with a sudden temperature rise accompanied by facial flush and other nonspecific manifestations, such as anorexia, vomiting, headache, and muscle or joint pains. The most common hemorrhagic manifestation is a positive tourniquet test, although petechiae, ecchymosis, epistaxis, and gingival or gastrointestinal bleeding may also be observed. After three or four days, when the temperature returns to normal or below, the patient's condition can suddenly deteriorate with signs of circulatory disturbance. The patient may sweat, be restless, have cool extremities, and show changes in pulse rate and blood pressure. Many recover spontaneously or after brief fluid therapy, but some proceed to shock with typical signs of circulatory failure. Initially patients may be lethargic but become restless and rapidly enter a critical stage of shock. Some patients evolve to severe circulatory failure (DSS), presenting a rapid and weak pulse, a narrow pulse pressure or hypotension, cold and clammy skin, and an altered mental state. DSS is fatal in 5 to 10 percent of cases if fluid management is inadequate or delayed.

Transmission and Epidemiological Trends. The dengue virus is transmitted from humans to humans by *Aedes* mosquitoes, of which the most important is *Ae. aegypti* (Bennett and others 2002; Gubler 1979; Tardieux and others 1990). Female mosquitoes ingest the virus while feeding on viremic individuals, and after an 8- to 12-day incubation period they can transmit the virus to other humans during blood feeding (Watts and others 1987). Thereafter, the female mosquito remains infective for life. Transmission of the virus from infected females to their progeny has been documented, but its epidemiological significance is not well understood (Hull and others 1984; Rosen and others 1983).

Although believed to be of African origin, *Ae. aegypti* is now established throughout the tropics and subtropics, exploiting almost any water-filled container as larval habitat. *Ae. aegypti* is also the urban vector of yellow fever. *Ae. albopictus* also transmits dengue and is an important secondary vector in parts of Southeast Asia and the Pacific. This species is of Asian origin but has spread to parts of Africa, the Americas, and Europe by depositing egg masses in used car tires, which are traded around the world.

Major epidemics of denguelike illness were documented in the 18th and 19th centuries in Africa, the Americas, and Asia, and clinical descriptions of illness compatible with dengue in China date from about 265. During 1900–50, dengue epidemics occurred in Australia, China, Greece, India, Japan, Malaysia, Thailand, and Vietnam and in the Caribbean (Gubler and Kuno 1997). DHF was first recognized in the 1950s, although a similar hemorrhagic fever was reported in Philadelphia in 1780, in Australia in 1897, and in Greece in 1928. Dengue is now endemic in Africa, the Americas, the Eastern Mediterranean, Southeast Asia, and the Western Pacific. According to WHO, it occurs in more than 100 countries and an estimated 2.5 billion people are at risk.

The increase in dengue epidemics can be attributed to rising levels of urbanization, which promote contact between humans and *Ae. aegypti;* inadequate domestic water supplies; and increasing international travel, migration, and trade, which help disseminate vectors and the virus. Epidemiological changes in the Americas since the 1970s illustrate this process. During the 1940s through the 1960s, the *Ae. aegypti* control program was successful in most of the region, with several countries declaring complete eradication. However, after some years, reinfestation with *Ae. aegypti* was apparent, and by 1995 it had returned to most of the previously infested countries. Reinvasion by the vector was followed by increased circulation of the virus, and the region evolved from nonendemic to hypoendemic (sporadic epidemics caused by a single serotype) to hyperendemic (simultaneous circulation of multiple serotypes resulting in frequent epidemics). DHF became a major public health problem. Before 1981, 5 countries in the region reported only a few cases of DHF, but by 2002, 21 countries reported more than 14,000 cases and 250 deaths (Gubler 2002; Guzmán and Kouri 2002, 2003; Guzmán and others 2002).

Leishmaniasis

Leishmaniasis (or the leishmaniases) refers to infections caused by protozoan parasites of the genus *Leishmania* transmitted by female sandflies (*Phlebotominae*). More than 20 *Leishmania* species are pathogenic to humans, and more than 30 species of sandflies are proven vectors. The disease tends to be focal in distribution. In anthroponotic foci, sandflies transmit parasites from human to human, and in zoonotic foci, sandflies transmit the parasites between mammal hosts and from them to humans.

Disease Manifestations. The different species of *Leishmania* cause illness of differing severity. Visceral leishmaniasis (VL), caused by species of the *L. donovani* complex, is usually fatal if untreated. Mucocutaneous leishmaniasis, caused by the *L. braziliensis* complex, is highly disfiguring and mutilating, and it can be fatal because of secondary complications. Cutaneous leishmaniasis (CL), caused by the *L. major, L. donovani,* and *L. braziliensis* complexes, may be a simple, self-limiting skin ulcer, but it can be disabling when numerous lesions occur. Diffuse cutaneous leishmaniasis, caused by the *L. mexicana* and *L. aethiopica* complexes, is longer lasting because of deficient immune responses.

Epidemiological Trends. Leishmaniasis is found in 88 countries worldwide. VL occurs in 62 of those countries, with most of the estimated 500,000 annual cases occurring in poorer rural and suburban areas of Bangladesh, Brazil, India, Nepal, and

Sudan. Mucocutaneous leishmaniasis is mainly limited to South and Central America, whereas most of the estimated 1 million to 1.5 million annual CL cases occur in the Middle East (Afghanistan, Algeria, the Islamic Republic of Iran, Saudi Arabia, and the Syrian Arab Republic) and in Brazil and Peru (Desjeux 1996). Reliable data on incidence and prevalence are scarce because only 33 endemic countries provide official notification of infection.

Leishmaniasis transmission is increasing in several areas. For example, the number of cases of CL in Kabul, Afghanistan, increased from 14,200 in 1994 to 65,000 in 2002, and the number of cases of VL in northeastern Brazil increased from 1,840 in 1998 to 6,000 in 2002. Such increases reflect the following environmental, land-use, and behavioral changes that increase exposure to the sandflies:

- Rural-urban migration seems to have contributed to urbanizing VL in Brazil, whereas in East Africa, VL seems to be more closely associated with migrations of seasonal workers and refugees. Transborder migrations between Bangladesh, India, and Nepal are also a risk factor for VL.
- New settlements in high-risk endemic areas, such as those established by people migrating from high plateaus to tropical plains in some Andean countries, increase their exposure to vectors.
- Development in areas of zoonotic transmission, such as road building, mining, oil prospecting, forestry, and ecotourism, and military activity increase risks for those involved (Desjeux 2001).
- Deteriorating social and economic conditions in the poorer suburbs of some cities may contribute to increasing transmission, especially of VL.

Leishmaniasis can be an opportunistic infection in people with HIV/AIDS, and coinfections have been reported in 34 countries (Desjeux and Alvar 2003). Malnutrition or HIV/AIDS coinfection can also increase disease severity by impairing the immune response.

African Trypanosomiasis

African trypanosomiasis is caused by parasites transmitted by tsetse flies (*Glossinidae*). The most important are forms of *Trypanosoma brucei* that infect humans and livestock, and *T. congolense* and *T. vivax* that infect only livestock. Human infection causes severe disease known as sleeping sickness, which is acute in the case of infection with *T. brucei rhodesiense* but more chronic with *T.b. gambiense*. Both forms lead to central nervous involvement and are fatal without appropriate treatment.

Disease Manifestations. Parasites are transmitted by the bite of infected tsetse flies. They multiply locally in extracellular spaces,

producing a characteristic lesion or chancre. The parasites circulate in blood and lymph, resulting in waves of parasitemia with episodes of fever, often accompanied by chills, rigor, malaise, prostration, and weight loss. These symptoms may occur within days of development of the chancre and constitute the hemolymphatic early stage. Febrile episodes become less severe as the disease progresses, and after a variable period the parasites invade the central nervous system and cerebrospinal fluid, leading to the late stage, with meningoencephalitis typically accompanied by severe and protracted headache, apathy, sleep disorders, irritability, and antisocial behavior.

The clinical features of late-stage sleeping sickness can resemble AIDS. With *T.b. rhodesiense*, meningoencephalitis typically occurs within weeks of initial infection, whereas with *T.b. gambiense*, this syndrome occurs later, sometimes after several years. Untreated disease causes relentless deterioration in cerebral function, with patients becoming increasingly difficult to rouse and passing into coma and death. Infection does not seem to confer immunity, so reinfection can occur after treatment.

Transmission and Vectors. Male and female tsetse flies are obligate bloodsuckers and can transmit trypanosomes, which undergo cyclical development in the infected flies. With *T.b. gambiense*, the main reservoir host is people, so tsetse flies mainly transmit from person to person, although increasing evidence suggests that pigs and some other animals are also important reservoirs. With *T.b. rhodesiense*, the main reservoir hosts are cattle and related animals, so transmission occurs mainly from animals to humans, although transmission from human to human also occurs (Okoth 1986). Mechanical (Frézil 1983), sexual (Rochas and others 2004), and transplacental (De Raadt 1985; Libala, Wery, and Ruppol 1978; Traub and others 1978) transmission have been described but are believed to be insignificant.

Thirty-one species and subspecies of *Glossina* are recognized. All probably can transmit trypanosomes, but only eight are known vectors for human infection. Animal trypanosomiasis can be found wherever wild tsetse flies occur, but human trypanosomiasis is usually associated with historic foci with strong epidemic potential. Most *T.b. gambiense* transmission is attributed to *G. palpalis* species occupying riverine and forest habitats in West and Central Africa, whereas *T.b. rhodesiense* transmission is mainly attributed to *G. morsitans* species in East African savannas. *G. fusca* species, although important vectors of animal trypanosomiasis, are considered insignificant for human forms.

Tsetse flies have an unusual life cycle. An inseminated female nurtures the egg and larva in her uterus, depositing the mature larva on the ground, where it burrows and pupates. Thus, each female produces only one offspring at a time. She produces up to 12 during her two- to three-month adult life span. The intrinsic population growth rate is low. Even small increases in average daily mortality rates can cause population decline, even to extinction.

Epidemiological Trends. Tsetse flies occur in parts of 37 countries in Sub-Saharan Africa. Animal trypanosomiasis is widespread throughout this region, but human disease is focused in areas of 20 countries. Over the entire tsetse-fly belt, WHO estimates that 60 million people are at risk of infection, with a standing prevalence of about 300,000 infections. Of these, probably fewer than 15 percent are diagnosed and treated (Cattand, Jannin, and Lucas 2001). For *T.b. rhodesiense*, epidemiological work in Uganda estimated that for every individual correctly diagnosed and treated, a further 12 cases are undiagnosed and unreported (Odiit 2003). The incidence of sleeping sickness has been increasing steadily since the 1970s, with epidemics in several areas, particularly the Democratic Republic of Congo (DRC) and northern Angola. In 1998–99, some 45,000 new cases were reported each year, representing a 10-fold increase since the 1960s. Most current epidemics are due to *T.b. gambiense*, although major epidemics of *T.b. rhodesiense* occurred in Uganda in 1978, 1980, and 1988.

The apparent increase is largely attributable to a decline in tsetse and trypanosomiasis control operations, which are influenced both by changing political priorities and by civil unrest and war. In the DRC, some 10,000 cases were diagnosed annually during the 1980s, but after four years with little or no control, the number of reported cases rose to 30,000 per year. In Angola, cases rose sixfold following the interruption of control operations because of war. Transmission is also occurring in new locations. In 1999, urban and periurban transmission was reported in Kinshasa, DRC, and in Luanda, Angola, and a new focus was reported in Soroti, Uganda, where an epidemic of *T.b. rhodesiense* disease followed the introduction of infected cattle (Fèvre and others 2001).

DISEASE BURDEN

All three diseases affect substantial populations. Globally, WHO estimates that 500,000 cases of DHF occur annually. Assuming that DHF cases constitute 6 percent of all clinical dengue cases (that is, all other cases are classical DF) implies a total of almost 8 million new infections per year. For leishmaniasis, current estimates suggest an overall prevalence of 12 million people infected in an at-risk population of 350 million, suggesting more than 2 million new infections each year. The prevalence of sleeping sickness is estimated at 300,000 people, with 60 million people considered to be at risk. Uncertainty about the true number of cases makes all these estimates approximate, particularly because incidence is increasing. In terms of disability-adjusted life years (DALYs) lost to these diseases (table 23.1), a dengue or trypanosomiasis death accounts for 27 to 28 DALYs lost. Leishmaniasis kills less often than trypanosomiasis, but each death is responsible for a loss of 34 DALYs.

Dengue

In hyperendemic areas of Southeast Asia, where multiple virus serotypes are circulating, DF and DHF are mainly childhood diseases and in some countries are leading causes of pediatric hospitalization and death, particularly in Cambodia, Myanmar, and Vietnam. Worldwide, 80 to 90 percent of deaths occur before age 15. In recent years in the Americas, DHF in adults in endemic form has been reported frequently (Diaz and others 1988; Guzmán and others 1999; Harris and others 2000; Zagne and others 1994). In some countries, the disease is more frequent among females, and in Cuba, significantly more severe cases occur among Caucasians than among those of African descent (Kouri, Guzmán, and Bravo 1987). Dengue causes relatively few deaths, estimated at 19,000 in 2001, corresponding to a case-fatality rate of 3.8 percent for DHF. Nonetheless, it can cause a substantial burden: in Puerto Rico during 1984–94, the

Table 23.1 Number of Deaths and DALYS Caused by Dengue, Leishmaniasis, and African Trypanosomiasis, by World Bank Region, 2001
(thousands)

Region	Dengue		Leishmaniasis		African trypanosomiasis		Total	
	Deaths	DALYs	Deaths	DALYs	Deaths	DALYs	Deaths	DALYs
East Asia and the Pacific	8	217	2	48	0	0	10	265
Europe and Central Asia	0	0	0	6	0	0	0	6
Latin America and the Caribbean	2	59	0	37	0	0	2	96
Middle East and North Africa	0	8	1	48	1	22	2	78
South Asia	9	240	40	1,306	0	0	49	1,546
Sub-Saharan Africa	0	4	8	312	48	1,310	56	1,626
Total	19	528	51	1,757	49	1,332	119	3,617

DALY loss per million population was similar to that for the entire Latin America and Caribbean region from malaria, tuberculosis, intestinal helminths, and the childhood disease cluster (Meltzer and others 1998).

Economic Impact. Studies in Thailand estimated the economic impact of dengue as equivalent to US$12.6 million in 1994, of which patients and their families incurred 45 percent (Okanurak, Sornmani, and Indaratna 1997). Kouri and others (1989) estimate the cost of the 1981 DHF epidemic in Cuba at US$103 million, constituting US$41 million in medical care, US$5 million in social security disability payments, US$14 million in lost production, and US$43 million for vector control. For Southeast Asia, Shepard and others (2004) estimate individual treatment costs of US$139 for DHF and US$4.29 for DF (including health clinic visits, hospitalization, medications, travel expenses, and parents' time seeking treatment for their children). This estimate implies annual costs in the region of US$105 million—US$69.5 million for DHF and US$35.5 million for DF. Extrapolating from current trends (on the basis of cases reported to WHO since 1960), this figure will increase to an average of US$118 million each year through the first decade of the 21st century. Using the Thailand study to add the value of productive work lost doubles this figure to US$236 million. Thus, during the next decade, Southeast Asian economies could lose a total of US$2.36 billion because of DF and DHF. Additional economic losses are expected because of the impact of dengue outbreaks on tourism.

Social Impact. During the transmission season, parents familiar with DHF are anxious about their children's survival and the financial consequences of emergency medical care. In Cambodia, even relatively modest out-of-pocket health expenditures can lead to debt and poverty (Van Damme and others 2004). The psychological burden is poorly understood and warrants further study.

Even though dengue affects all strata of society, it may selectively affect the poorest. Most larval habitats in dengue-endemic communities are artificial: water storage containers, flower vases, discarded food containers, used tires, and habitats created by poor design of roof gutters and drains. Local vector ecology is largely determined by community social and cultural practices and infrastructure, and increasing urbanization typically attracts the poor to periurban settlements with deficient water supplies. Studies in the República Bolivariana de Venezuela (Barrera, Avila, and Gonzalez-Teller 1993; Barrera and others 1995) and in Thailand (Nagao and others 2003) have shown higher *Ae. aegypti* infestations where water distribution systems are deficient or unreliable. Along the border between Mexico and the United States, Reiter and others (2003) attribute the low dengue seroprevalence reported in Laredo, Texas, to factors such as air conditioning that limited human-vector contact, whereas in contiguous Nuevo Laredo on the Mexican side, where per capita income was one-seventh of that in Laredo, seroprevalence was much higher despite lower vector densities.

In countries with weak or unprepared health services, epidemics of dengue can be extremely disruptive and health services can be rapidly overwhelmed. Frequently, governments declare states of emergency to mobilize additional resources against dengue outbreaks, sometimes deploying the army to eliminate or apply larvicides to larval habitats. These responses are often launched at or after the peak of the epidemic, and the decline in transmission is unjustifiably attributed to the intervention rather than to the natural epidemic decline.

Leishmaniasis

In 2001, leishmaniasis killed an estimated 51,000 people, including 40,000 in South Asia and 8,000 in Sub-Saharan Africa, representing 0.3 percent and less than 0.1 percent, respectively, of all deaths (table 23.1). Nearly all deaths occurred at ages 5 to 29. Males were more affected than females, especially in Sub-Saharan Africa, where the ratio was three to one.

Economic Impact. Treatment for leishmaniasis is expensive, especially for VL. For many countries, the cost of treating all leishmaniasis patients would far exceed their total health budgets. For a WHO-recommended course of pentavalent antimonials, current drug costs per patient are US$150 for sodium stibogluconate, US$120 for meglumine antimoniate, and US$30 for generic sodium stibogluconate. Cases not responding to antimonials may require second-line, more toxic drugs, such as amphotericin B at a cost of US$60 or pentamidine at a cost of US$70. Less toxic amphotericin in liposomes is effective, but costs US$1,500 per patient. The first oral drug for VL, miltefosine, currently costs US$120 per patient.

In addition to drug costs, the additional costs of drug delivery can be high, especially for patients in remote areas. Patients often live far from a treatment center, and the expense of hospitalization may lead to interrupted treatment, facilitating resistance and requiring additional therapy. Without treatment, severe leishmaniasis can become chronic and debilitating, incapacitating patients and making them unable to work and vulnerable to poverty, malnutrition, and secondary infections.

Social Impact. Even self-limiting CL can leave disfiguring scars, which have associated stigma and may affect marriage prospects. CL can be disabling when lesions are numerous, and the most severe form, recidivans leishmaniasis, is difficult to treat, long-lasting, and disfiguring. In individuals with a defective cell-mediated immune response, the disseminated lesions of diffuse cutaneous leishmaniasis resemble those of leprosy. They do not heal spontaneously and frequently recur after treatment. Diffuse cutaneous leishmaniasis is recognized as a special public health problem, both clinically and because of its severe emotional consequences.

The lesions of mucocutaneous leishmaniasis can cause extensive destruction and distortion of oronasal and pharyngeal cavities, leading to mutilation of the face. Patients may be shunned and, in severe cases, even incarcerated. Although mainly associated with *L. braziliensis* and *L. guyanensis* in the Americas, mucocutaneous leishmaniasis has been reported in Africa, Asia, and Europe as a complication of *L. donovani* and *L. major* infections and, in immunosuppressed patients, of *L. infantum*.

Untreated VL is usually fatal. Even after recovery, patients may develop a chronic form of CL that usually requires prolonged and expensive therapy.

African Trypanosomiasis

WHO estimates the number of deaths caused by sleeping sickness as 48,000 in 2001 (table 23.1), although current estimates are in the range of 50,000 to 100,000 per year. Men are affected at nearly twice the rate of women. In relation to mortality, of all parasitic diseases in Sub-Saharan Africa, trypanosomiasis ranks behind only malaria. As concerns DALYs, the health burden is similar to that of schistosomiasis. In Sudan, 33 DALYs on average are lost because of each premature death from sleeping sickness (McFarland 2003). In Uganda, 23 DALYs were lost per death, but only 0.21 DALYs per successfully treated individual (Odiit and others 2004). Underreporting makes deriving estimates for the whole continent difficult: 100,000 deaths per year would imply more than 2 million DALYs lost, compared with the WHO estimate of 1.31 million (830,000 for males and 480,000 for females) (table 23.1).

Economic Impact. Information on age at death indicates that sleeping sickness mainly affects economically active adults. Data from Uganda show nearly 25 percent of cases occurring in those age 20 to 29 and more than 60 percent in those age 10 to 39 (Odiit 2003). Thus, when people become ill, their families not only become burdened with the care of seriously ill individuals but also often lose their breadwinners. Poor diagnostic support in many areas means that families often invest in a number of treatments that have no effect on the disease. In a *T.b. rhodesiense* area of Uganda, Odiit and others (2004) find that some patients made up to seven visits to health facilities before being correctly diagnosed, with just under three-quarters initially being diagnosed with malaria. For the 11 of 12 who were never diagnosed or were told that they had a different fatal disease, the costs to and burdens on their families can only be imagined.

In addition to the economic losses caused by interruption of their work, sleeping sickness patients face direct financial costs. Even though WHO now provides specific first-line drugs at no cost in excess of delivery and administration, hospitalization and treatment are expensive. In the DRC, Gouteux and others (1987) estimate that total costs are equivalent to at least 25 percent of a year's income from agriculture.

Social Impact. The importance of sleeping sickness lies not only in the number of new cases reported, but also in its potential for epidemic outbreaks causing thousands of deaths: during recent epidemics in the DRC, in some villages up to 70 percent of the population became infected. Because of the severity of the disease, one case can affect all family members, placing a burden on the whole community, reducing the labor force, interrupting agricultural activities, and jeopardizing food security. Although untreated trypanosomiasis is lethal, treated patients often remain incapacitated, perpetuating the cycle of poverty, malnutrition, and disease. DALYs do not take into account the psychosocial impact and the "minor" disabilities. In adults, loss of memory and ability to concentrate is common. Such disabilities are often accompanied by reading and writing difficulties and occasionally by extreme incoherence. These disabilities greatly affect everyday life, particularly for those school-age children who, even after successful treatment, do not recover fully and cannot pursue their studies (Frézil 1983).

Burden of Animal Trypanosomiasis. Animal trypanosomiasis constrains agricultural production—in particular, the use of draft power. Cattle infected with *T.b. brucei*, *T. vivax*, or *T. congolense* quickly succumb to a wasting form of anemia. In many areas with a high tsetse challenge, such as Central Africa, cattle are few or not present at all. Elsewhere, countries invest an estimated total of US$30 million to US$50 million per year in some 35 million doses of veterinary trypanocides to prevent the disease in livestock (Geerts and Holmes 1998). About 60 percent of the cattle at risk are not treated, and the disease is thought to kill about 1 million a year. Current drugs are more than 40 years old, and drug resistance is increasing, as are problems of drug availability and accessibility, counterfeit drugs, and drug mismanagement (Geerts and Holmes 1998). Constraints on draft power mean that farmers can till only small plots, making subsistence farmers extremely vulnerable to food shortages. Milk yields are lower in infected cows, and animal trypanosomiasis lowers fertility and increases mortality, thereby constraining the overall growth rate of the number of livestock (Swallow 2000). Kristjanson and others (1999) estimate annual direct losses of US$1.3 billion per year as a result of lowered production of milk and meat, with aggregate agricultural losses attributable to trypanosomiasis estimated at US$4.5 billion per year.

MANAGEMENT AND CONTROL STRATEGIES

Dengue

Patient Management and Treatment. Classic dengue fever is generally self-limiting. No specific treatment is available, but supportive treatment must be given, including fluid replacement when necessary. Early recognition of DHF cases—indicated by intense, continuous abdominal pain; persistent vomiting; and restlessness or lethargy—and early supportive treatment are of utmost importance to reduce case-fatality rates (Martinez 1992). For differential diagnosis, a wide spectrum of viral and bacterial infections should be considered, especially leptospirosis, malaria, yellow fever, chikungunya virus, rubella, and influenza.

Vector Control. Although good patient management can be effective for individual cases, currently no alternative to vector control is available for the prevention of dengue. Most endemic countries have a vector control component in their programs; however, the application of vector control measures is frequently insufficient, ineffective, or both and is currently failing to reduce the public health burden to an acceptable level.

Most *Aedes* control programs rely on the application of larvicides and adulticidal insecticide space sprays (Zaim and Jambulingham 2004). Because *Ae. aegypti* characteristically breeds in water that does not contain high levels of organic pollutants, control measures typically must be applied to water stored for household purposes, including drinking water. WHO currently approves five insecticides for application to potable water (FAO 1999; WHO 1991). Since the early 1970s, the organophosphate temephos has been the most widely used, but increasing levels of resistance to this insecticide are reducing the duration of effectiveness of treatments in some countries (Brengues and others 2003; Lima and others 2003; Rodriguez and others 2001). An additional challenge is the growing objection among householders, particularly in Latin America, to the application of chemicals to drinking water.

Biological control agents, including larvivorous fish and copepods, have had a demonstrable role in integrated control of *Ae. aegypti,* but operational difficulties—particularly a lack of facilities and of expertise in mass rearing and the need for repeated introduction of these agents into some container habitats—have largely precluded their widespread use. One encouraging exception is Vietnam, where indigenous species of predatory copepods are increasingly used to control semipermanent larval habitats of *Ae. aegypti* (Kay and others 2002; Nam and others 2000). However, some communities have strong cultural objections to the introduction of live animals into household water storage containers—for example, in Thailand, where bathing with water that contains small fish or other creatures is widely regarded as unacceptable.

Environmental management is generally considered the core component of dengue prevention and control, including cleanup campaigns, regular emptying and cleaning of containers, installation of water supply systems, solid waste management, and urban planning. However, huge investments in infrastructure are needed to increase access to safe and reliable water supplies, to provide solid waste management services, and to dispose of liquid waste. In addition to overall health gains, such provision would have a major effect on vector ecology, although the relationship is not invariably an inverse one. Cost-recovery mechanisms, such as the introduction of metered water, may encourage household collection and storage of roof catchment rainwater that can be harvested at no cost. Although unproven, the installation of community water services in rural townships and villages may be contributing to the rural spread of dengue in Southeast Asia and elsewhere.

At the household and community levels, where most vector control efforts are centered, increasing attention is given to such activities as covering or frequently cleaning water storage vessels, removing discarded food and beverage containers, and storing or disposing of used tires in such a way that they do not collect rainwater. Such tasks would seem to be simple and well suited to engagement by communities, but with a few exceptions, achievements to date have been unspectacular. Nevertheless, such community-based interventions are widely seen as the most promising way of achieving sustainable control through behavior change (Parks and Lloyd 2004).

Leishmaniasis

Leishmaniasis control is based primarily on finding and treating cases, combined where feasible with vector control and, in some zoonotic foci, control of animal reservoirs.

Diagnosis and Treatment. For VL, serological diagnosis is usually based on the enzyme-linked immunosorbent assay (ELISA), indirect fluorescent antibody tests, and direct agglutination tests, including a new direct agglutination test kit using lyophilized antigen, which avoids the need for refrigeration (Schallig and others 2001). A dipstick test based on a highly specific recombinant antigen is also available, together with a latex agglutination test that can be used to detect antigens in urine (Attar and others 2001; Sundar and others 1998). Parasitological diagnosis relies on microscopy of aspirates of the spleen, bone marrow, and lymph nodes.

Specific treatment includes the first-line drugs, which are pentavalent antimonials (sodium stibogluconate and meglumine antimoniate), and the second-line drugs, which are amphotericin B and AmBisome (amphotericin B in liposomes). Miltefosine for VL was registered in India in 2002, and aminosidine (paromomycin) has just completed phase 3 clinical trials and follow-up. For CL, parasitological diagnosis is made from skin smears followed by treatment with pentavalent antimonials. Treatment is given locally if lesions are few and relatively small, or systemically if lesions are more numerous. For mucocutaneous leishmaniasis, diagnosis relies on serology because patients generally develop a strong humoral response.

Vector and Reservoir Control. In foci of peridomestic or intradomestic transmission, vector control can be carried out by indoor residual spraying using pyrethroid insecticides. Individual protection using pyrethroid-impregnated bednets is also used in some areas. In zoonotic foci of VL, control has also included culling stray dogs—and pet dogs if found to be infected—although this practice is often poorly accepted by communities and is probably of limited effectiveness. Trials with insecticide-treated dog collars are showing some promise as an alternative way to reduce the peridomestic reservoir of infection (Mazloumi Gavgani and others 2002). For zoonotic CL, rodent reservoirs can be controlled using poisoned bait and environmental management, including physical destruction of rodents' burrows.

African Trypanosomiasis

For human trypanosomiasis, control consists primarily of active and passive case finding and treatment, occasionally associated with vector control operations. Dissemination of sleeping sickness can be prevented by regular surveillance of the population at risk, including diagnosis and treatment; control of the tsetse-fly population can affect the transmission of sleeping sickness as well as of animal trypanosomiasis. In *T.b. rhodesiense* foci, where cattle are reservoirs of the disease, treating cattle with trypanocides is being investigated as an additional approach to controlling outbreaks.

Case Finding and Treatment. No single clinical sign is regarded as pathognomonic for sleeping sickness. Tests have been developed to detect antibodies, circulating antigens, or trypanosomal DNA, but all require parasitological confirmation. For mass screening, infection can be confirmed by the card agglutination trypanosomiasis test, which is easy to perform and relatively inexpensive. Parasitological confirmation is by microscopy of lymph node aspirates and of thin or thick blood films. Concentration methods increase sensitivity. The most sensitive is the miniature anion exchange centrifugation technique. The capillary tube centrifugation technique is less sensitive but is commonly used in the field because of its ease and rapidity of use and its low cost.

Determining the stage of disease is essential, because early- and late-stage infections require different treatments. The criteria for late-stage infection are based on cerebrospinal fluid analysis.

Sleeping sickness is fatal if untreated. No vaccination exists. Specific drugs are currently available free through WHO. Pentamidine is used to treat early-stage *T.b. gambiense* infection, and suramine is used for early-stage *T.b. rhodesiense*. The organoarsenical compound melarsoprol (Arsobal) is used for the late stages of both. Eflornithine has been introduced to treat late-stage *T.b. gambiense* but is difficult to administer. Nifurtimox, although not yet registered for the treatment of sleeping sickness, has been used on compassionate grounds to treat patients unresponsive to melarsoprol.

Vector Control. A wide range of techniques for tsetse control is available (Maudlin, Holmes, and Miles 2004). Most current approaches exploit the acute susceptibility of tsetse flies to biodegradable pyrethroid insecticides. Spraying can be applied from the ground to known fly resting sites or at ultra-low volume from the air. Spraying is carried out sequentially to kill all flies initially present and thereafter to kill each generation of newly emerging flies. The sequential aerosol technique uses extremely low levels of insecticide and has been effective in Botswana, Somalia, South Africa, and Zambia. It is also useful against epidemic outbreaks of sleeping sickness, where a rapid cessation in contact between humans and tsetse flies is needed.

Tsetse flies can also be controlled using traps and targets. Targets are combinations of cloth and netting baited with an odor attractant and impregnated with a pyrethroid insecticide. Traps work on the same principle, but the fly is encouraged to enter a net or plastic chamber where it remains trapped. Live bait techniques are also used. Cattle are treated with a veterinary formulation of pyrethroid insecticides applied as sprays or pour-ons, which kill both tsetse flies and ticks. This technique has been successfully used in Burkina Faso, Ethiopia, Kenya, Tanzania, Zambia, and Zimbabwe (Kuzoe and Schofield 2005).

The sterile insect technique involves mass release of sterilized male tsetse flies, which compete with local males to mate with females. Because female tsetse flies generally mate only once, the result is infertile offspring and a decline of the wild tsetse population. This technique is expensive, because it requires large-scale rearing of flies, and it is only recommended for use once the wild tsetse population has been suppressed to low levels using other techniques. A combination of insecticide spraying and trap deployment followed by the sterile insect technique has been successfully used to eliminate *G. austeni* from Zanzibar (Vreysen and others 2000).

Degrees of resistance to trypanosome infection are found in the N'dama, Dwarf, and Savannah Shorthorn breeds in West Africa and, to a lesser extent, in some Orma Boran breeds in East Africa. However, even though these cattle show tolerance, can control parasitemia, and resist development of anemia, they can ultimately succumb to the disease.

COSTS AND COST-EFFECTIVENESS OF INTERVENTIONS

Dengue

Few studies are available on the cost-effectiveness of vector control for reducing dengue transmission. One of the difficulties is that the level of vector population control needed to reduce transmission is influenced by the human population's past exposure to the circulating virus serotype. A direct relationship is apparent between seroprevalence rates and levels of vector abundance needed for epidemic transmission. Thus, the paradox is that, as herd immunity declines over time in response to effective vector control, progressively lower vector densities can maintain the same level of transmission.

Modeling of the dynamics of dengue transmission is helping to improve understanding of the interrelationships between virus, vector, and host (Ferguson, Donnelly, and Anderson 1999; Focks and others 1995; Newton and Reiter 1992; Shepard 2001), but the absence of epidemiologically defined target levels for vector control has hindered calculations of cost-effectiveness. According to Shepard and others (2004), average annual costs for dengue vector control per 1,000 population were US$15 in 1998 in Indonesia, US$81 in 1994 and US$188 in 1998 in Thailand, US$240 in 2002 in Malaysia, and US$2,400 in 2000 in Singapore. In 1997, spending on dengue control in 14 Latin American countries ranged from US$20 to US$3,560 per 1,000 population, with a median of US$260. For 17 Caribbean islands in 1990, the corresponding expenditures ranged from US$140 to US$8,490, with a median of US$1,340 (Nathan 1993). By contrast, McConnell and Gubler's (2003) study in Puerto Rico concludes that larval control programs that achieve a 50 percent reduction in dengue transmission and cost less than US$2.50 per person would be cost-effective in that setting. From research based on analytical models (Shepard 2001) and primary data from Singapore, we estimate the cost of using environmental management for control at US$3,139 per DALY averted and the cost of using insecticides at US$1,992 per DALY averted.

Dengue case management depends on the severity of the illness. Despite the lack of information about cost-effective interventions to treat dengue cases, Shepard (2001) estimates an average cost of US$587 per DALY averted by appropriate case management. Were a dengue vaccine to become available, the Shepard model estimates that immunization would cost US$3,040 per DALY averted.

Leishmaniasis

Case Finding and Treatment. For leishmaniasis, diagnosis represents a small proportion of the cost of case finding and treatment, with diagnostic tests becoming available at approximately US$1.50 for the dipstick, US$3.00 for the direct agglutination test using freeze-dried antigen, and US$1.50 for the urine latex agglutination text. These tests can be used in the field. A study in Nepal (Pokhrel 1999) comparing outreach case detection using serology (the dipstick) with parasitological diagnosis at health centers (bone marrow aspirate) concluded that the median cost per VL case detected was US$25 in the outreach program, compared with US$145 at health centers (of which more than 50 percent was due to absence from work). Treatment costs increased these figures to US$131 and US$200 per patient, respectively.

In India, an examination of the costs of drugs and hospitalization and of the evolution of the disease under treatment (cure, relapse, failure, intolerance) indicated that the final cost of successful treatment depends largely on the basic drug cost, which averaged US$86 per patient successfully treated with miltefosine (using reduced pricing because of the large number of patients), US$467 for treatment with amphotericin B, and US$1,613 for treatment with AmBisome. Given current estimates of about 100,000 cases of VL each year in the state of Bihar, India, the estimated total cost of treatment using miltefosine as a first-line drug and amphotericin B as a second-line drug would be about US$11 million, or approximately US$110 per patient (personal communication with P. Olliaro and S. Sundar on treatment options for kalaazar [visceral leishmaniasis], 2003). By contrast, analysis of humanitarian relief interventions by Médecins sans Frontières–Holland that combined case finding with treatment after a VL epidemic in southern Sudan indicated total costs of US$394 per patient, or an average cost of US$595 per life saved (Griekspoor, Sondorp, and Vos 1999). Thus, the average cost per DALY averted was US$18.40.

Vector Control. Vector control is rarely carried out as a specific approach to leishmaniasis control, and cost-effectiveness estimates are not available. In general, domestic and peridomestic sandfly vectors are more susceptible to indoor residual spraying than are other domestic vectors, such as anopheline mosquitoes or triatomine bugs, so that transient suppression of sandfly populations is seen as an additional benefit of malaria or Chagas disease vector control in areas where these vectors coincide. However, insecticide-treated bednets, which are becoming widely deployed against malaria transmission, may also become cost-effective for reducing leishmaniasis in areas of domestic transmission. In Yenice, Turkey, the use of impregnated bednets reduced the incidence of CL from 1.90 percent to 0.04 percent between 2000 and 2001 (Alten and others 2003).

African Trypanosomiasis

Case Finding and Treatment. WHO (1986, 1998) has analyzed the costs of *T.b. gambiense* control by means of case finding and treatment based on practice in Côte d'Ivoire and

Uganda. This work and other studies indicate that, at current prices, the cost of active detection using the card agglutination trypanosomiasis test with parasitological confirmation varies around US$1 per person screened or slightly more for mobile teams. However, mobile teams are more effective in screening a high proportion of the population and are also more successful in ensuring that a high proportion of patients receive treatment. Unit costs are currently US$0.33 per person for the card agglutination trypanosomiasis test and US$2.20 for the miniature anion exchange centrifugation technique. Less sensitive parasitological techniques, such as examination of lymph node aspirate or blood smears, cost only a few cents but may miss a third to half of patients.

By contrast, treatment is expensive despite the availability of free drugs. Treatment of early-stage disease incurs costs of more than US$100 per person, rising to more than US$250 for late-stage treatment with melarsoprol and about US$700 with eflornithine (WHO 1998). The long hospitalization period is a major component of costs during the second stage, although work undertaken by Burri and others (2000) on a shorter melarsoprol regimen offers opportunities for reducing these costs.

Despite the costs and the risk of complications, treating sleeping sickness patients in the second stage of the disease is cost-effective. In Uganda, costs were less than US$10 per DALY averted for melarsoprol treatment and less than US$20 per person for eflornithine (Politi and others 1995). Similarly, in southern Sudan, the cost per DALY averted ranged from US$4 to US$22 (Trowbridge and others 2001). Shaw and Cattand (2001) considered the costs of case finding and treatment for *T.b. gambiense* infection for three delivery options and a wide range of prevalences. Given the limited information available on DALYs gained or on the effect on transmission of reducing the size of the human reservoir, they estimate that under different scenarios the costs per DALY averted tend to converge. For most assumptions, the cost per DALY averted fell below a US$25 threshold at prevalences of 0.5 to 1.0 percent but rose sharply at low prevalences, which explains the reluctance of control programs to invest in screening operations when prevalence is less than 0.2 percent. With better quantitative understanding of the effects of screening and removing patients from the reservoir in preventing future epidemics, investigators could demonstrate that even at low prevalences screening for sleeping sickness is highly cost-effective.

Vector Control. Several countries have undertaken community-based programs to trap tsetse flies, notably Côte d'Ivoire, where costs came to US$2.30 per person protected per year (Laveissière and others 1994), and Uganda, which achieved a cost of US$0.50 per person protected per year (Lancien and Obayi 1993). Vector control costs have been studied in more detail in the context of livestock disease (Maudlin, Holmes, and Miles 2004). These costs vary according to the technique used and the environmental context, often ignoring overheads for organizing and planning. With that caveat in mind, the figures per square kilometer cited for local tsetse-fly eradication range from about US$250 to US$550 at current prices for aerial spraying (based on experience in Somalia, South Africa, Zambia, and Zimbabwe); US$250 to US$400 per square kilometer for ground spraying; and US$200 to US$400 per square kilometer for targets. However, the cost of traps and targets falls to US$25 to US$60 per square kilometer for control or suppression operations alone. Projects treating cattle with insecticides have been implemented at costs of US$50 to US$60 per square kilometer. Use of the sterile insect technique is much more expensive because it relies on prior suppression of fly populations using another technique. The overall costs of the experimental eradication of *G. austeni* from Zanzibar using the sterile insect and other techniques were about US$3,000 per square kilometer, although the International Atomic Energy Agency (IAEA) envisages that the cost of the sterile insect technique component could be reduced to less than US$800 per square kilometer as the technology is developed and applied on a sufficiently large scale (Dr. Udo Feldmann, IAEA, Vienna, personal communication).

PROBLEMS AND CHALLENGES FOR DISEASE CONTROL

Dengue

Potential for Vaccine Development. The occurrence of DHF in children and adults with previous dengue antibodies, acquired passively or actively, has been the most important challenge for the development of a dengue vaccine. Lack of a suitable animal model, insufficient knowledge of disease pathogenesis, and limited research funding have also had a negative influence. Researchers generally agree that a dengue vaccine must confer long-lasting protection against the four dengue serotypes. Currently, they are following different strategies in the development of several vaccine candidates. Some vaccines are currently undergoing human clinical trials—for example, live attenuated dengue and yellow fever chimeric vaccines. The conventional live attenuated vaccines are entering phase 3 trials, while the chimeric vaccines are presently in phase 1 and phase 2 trials. Others are in the preclinical phase of development. To accelerate the development of a dengue vaccine, a new initiative—the pediatric dengue vaccine initiative—has been launched, with the major objective of mobilizing resources to accelerate the development of a safe and effective pediatric dengue vaccine (Almond and others 2002; Halstead and Deen 2002; Pang 2003).

Vector Control. Without a vaccine, vector control remains the only available strategy against dengue. Selective, integrated vector control with community and intersectoral participation, active disease surveillance based on a strong health information system, emergency preparedness, capacity building and training, and vector control research constitute the major elements of WHO's global strategy for dengue prevention and control. Since the eradication era, few examples of successful dengue prevention and control on a national scale are available. Exceptions include Cuba and Singapore, both island states. Cuba, with approximately 11 million inhabitants, has been able to interrupt dengue transmission. Despite being in an endemic area, the country has maintained low vector densities and has successfully controlled epidemics in recent years (Arias 2002). Critical factors contributing to this achievement are the strong dengue surveillance system, which integrates environmental, entomological, epidemiological, clinical, and virological surveillance in conjunction with the public health infrastructure, and a strong vector control program, along with good intersectoral coordination, active community involvement, and strong political commitment.

A limited array of tools is available for vector control interventions, any one of which can control at least part of the vector population or provide personal protection. However, approaches are converging, at least at the policy level, toward application of vector control tools through social or community mobilization. Consensus is growing that community-based approaches are desirable and necessary, and many believe that only through such approaches can a degree of sustainability be accomplished in relation to dengue vector control. Even though few such interventions have expanded beyond the pilot stage, the decentralization of budgetary and operational responsibilities for program delivery appears to offer opportunities for strengthening and expanding this integrated vector management approach.

Increasing levels of resistance of *Ae. aegypti* to temephos imply shorter intervals between treatments. This situation is already a reality in some countries, including Brazil and several Caribbean islands (Carvalho and da Silva 1999; Rawlins 1998). Resistance of adult mosquitoes to malathion and to pyrethroids has been reported in the Americas and in Asia (WHO 1992) and is likely to reduce the efficacy of space spraying. Given the peridomestic ecology of *Ae. aegypti* in most regions and the widespread use of pyrethroids for public health purposes and in household insecticide products, the rate of development of pyrethroid resistance is likely to accelerate. At the same time, few new insecticide products are becoming available in the public health market because of the costs involved in development and registration compared with the returns on investment from the relatively small commercial market. The high cost of re-registration of existing products is also contributing to the withdrawal of some insecticides from the market.

New Risk Factors. Environmental changes, particularly those related to climate, directly affect the incidence and prevalence of vectorborne diseases. However, social factors, such as lifestyles and population density, particularly in the case of dengue, are also important. Using an empirical model of the effect of population and climate change on the global distribution of dengue fever, Hales and others (2002) conclude that predicted changes in humidity will increase the areas with a climate suitable for dengue transmission.

The world is also becoming increasingly urbanized: during 2000–25, Asia's urban population is expected to double, and that of Latin America and the Caribbean is expected to increase by almost 50 percent. The resulting high human population densities, coupled with lifestyles that increasingly contribute to the proliferation of larval habitats and infrastructural deficiencies in relation to water supply and sanitation, are such that effective delivery of vector control on the scale needed is beyond the reach of many governments. The increasing global trend in international travel also facilitates the dissemination of virus serotypes and strains between vulnerable populations.

Genetic variability is another element to be considered. The genetic diversity of the viruses is increasing, with some genotypes associated with severe disease (Cologna and Rico-Hesse 2003; Leitmeyer and others 1999; Rico-Hesse and others 1997). Recombination has been demonstrated in all four serotypes, but the implications in terms of pathogenesis are unknown. In addition to recombination, mutations, gene flow, and other factors could further influence the genetic diversity and selection of virulent strains (Holmes and Burch 2000). At the same time, in addition to initial observations of the higher risk of DHF in Caucasian than in those of African descent, a few reports associate some human leukocyte antigen alleles with disease severity (Bravo, Guzmán, and Kouri 1987; LaFleur and others 2002; Loke and others 2001; Paradoa, Trujillo, and Basanta 1987; Stephens and others 2002). The sequence of infecting viruses and, more recently, the longer interval between primary and secondary infection as a risk factor for DHF, add a new perspective to the problem (Guzmán and others 2002; Nisalak and others 2003).

Leishmaniasis

Because the primary control strategy against leishmaniasis is based on case finding and treatment, the priority for control is developing and implementing improved diagnostic methods and better treatments that are more amenable to field use. A parallel requirement is for the development of more cost-effective drug delivery systems, especially ones that take advantage of new oral drugs, such as miltefosine, and the planned registration and local production of aminosidine in India.

Improved Diagnostics and Treatment. Even though the new serological tests, such as the dipstick, lyophilized direct agglutination test kit, and latex agglutination urine test, represent major improvements, they are not yet widely used in endemic countries. Moreover, they are indirect tests that cannot provide direct parasitological confirmation of infection or of cure immediately following treatment. Current parasitological tests tend to be highly invasive and can be costly to perform; therefore, simple molecular-based tests would be an advantage.

For leishmaniasis treatment, development of the oral VL drug, miltefosine, represents a substantial improvement, but it remains expensive and with a long treatment regimen and cannot be administered to pregnant women because of the risk of teratogenicity. Further clinical evaluation is required to establish the possibility of shorter treatment regimes and the potential of combination therapy to inhibit the development and spread of drug resistance. Another oral drug, sitamaquine, is currently under development and will require similar clinical and implementation studies. Clinical trials of aminosidine (paromomycin) are proceeding, and use of this drug against VL may become widespread. An improved understanding of disease pathogenesis would be helpful in refining the criteria for cure and in improving patients' prognosis.

Vaccine Development. The leishmaniases offer substantial opportunities for vaccine development, and a crude vaccine against CL has been widely used in parts of the Middle East. Trials of a second-generation vaccine that includes three *Leishmania* antigens are currently in progress.

Vector Control. Control of domestic and peridomestic sandfly vectors will probably continue as an additional benefit accruing to programs against other insect vectors using indoor residual spraying or insecticide-treated bednets. However, in areas where dogs are among the main reservoir hosts, increased use of insecticide-treated dog collars would merit further appraisal. Such collars not only would reduce the likelihood of new infections in dogs, but also could reduce the risk of transmission from dogs to humans.

African Trypanosomiasis

Improved Diagnostics. Serological diagnosis is reliable for verifying infection; however, most district hospitals or peripheral health units have neither the facilities nor the necessary expertise to perform and read serological tests. In the past, serological diagnosis, based on indirect fluorescent antibody tests and ELISA, was restricted to central-level facilities or specialized mobile teams. The card agglutination trypanosomiasis test has substantially simplified the use of serology but requires specifically equipped health units with a cold chain.

Parasitological diagnosis, such as the miniature anion exchange centrifugation test, is more expensive and complicated to use in field surveys despite the development of a simplified sterile kit version. Molecular diagnostics are not yet developed to a level appropriate for widespread field use.

Treatment. Despite the availability of drugs free of charge from WHO, treatment is hampered by the length of hospitalization required and by the toxicity of currently available drugs. In addition, inability to use the same drug in the early and late stages of the disease complicates the treatment protocol. The existing late-stage drug, melarsoprol, is unsafe, its secondary reactions are numerous, and the occurrence of a lethal encephalopathic syndrome in 5 to 10 percent of treated cases means that patients on melarsoprol must be hospitalized. A new oral drug for the early stage, soon to be registered, must be introduced in the field, which will take several years.

Drug resistance is well established in animal trypanosomes. For *T. congolense, T. vivax,* and *T. evansi,* resistance to all available drugs has been reported, along with trypanosome populations with multiple drug resistance (Geerts and Holmes 1998). Much less information is available on human pathogenic trypanosomes. The resurgence of human African trypanosomiasis in recent years has been accompanied by increasing reports of treatment failure using melarsoprol. As early as 1960, *T.b. rhodesiense* patients in Uganda were reported to have relapsed after two or more courses of melarsoprol, and in 1977, a 40 percent melarsoprol relapse rate was reported in the DRC.

Relapses after treatment with early-stage drugs remain rare. Whether relapses after melarsoprol treatment reflect parasite drug resistance or host factors is unknown. Furthermore, even though increasing rates of melarsoprol failure have been observed in several countries, the magnitude and geographic distribution of the problem have not been determined. Analyses of existing data are complicated by the lack of a standard treatment regimen and the range of clinical and laboratory criteria used to define a relapse.

Vector Control. Even though available techniques to control tsetse flies can be highly effective (Maudlin, Holmes, and Miles 2004), all are constrained by the difficulties of applying them on a large enough scale for long enough to achieve sustainable results. Insecticide spraying is efficient but is difficult to sustain because of logistical constraints and high costs. Targets and traps are effective, but their deployment is difficult to sustain for long periods, and implementation through community participation requires constant motivation and supervision to remain effective. To address these problems, the African Union has launched the Pan African Initiative (PATTEC), which focuses on identifying regions where elimination of the tsetse fly may be feasible using currently available techniques. This initiative is designed as part of a poverty reduction strategy that aims at eliminating the problem of tsetseborne animal trypanosomiasis, but in several areas it will also reduce the risk of human infections.

SUMMARY

For dengue, leishmaniasis, and African trypanosomiasis, the longstanding problem is the lack of adequate specific treatment. For dengue, no specific treatment is available. For the leishmaniases and African trypanosomiases, specific treatment has long depended on antiquated drugs that would be considered far too toxic for introduction under modern registration systems. Even though progress is being made, especially in relation to the development of new oral drugs for leishmaniasis, in purely pragmatic terms what is currently available will probably represent almost the entire therapeutic arsenal for the coming decades. Even without toxicological problems, the development and registration of a new candidate drug will, given current requirements, take at least a decade.

Although basic research will continue (table 23.2), the current challenge is to make better use of what is already available. Dengue can be prevented with available vector control tools and strategies designed to reduce the risk of transmission. This method requires a sustainable surveillance system capable of providing early warning and predictions based on experience of factors predisposing to new epidemic outbreaks. To a large extent, it becomes a management exercise that accepts that some dengue transmission will occur but aims at preempting epidemic outbreaks rather than instigating emergency measures after an outbreak is in full crudescence. Moreover, because preemptive measures and emergency responses are competing strategies, analyses of their relative cost-effectiveness would be appropriate.

Case finding and treatment for the leishmaniases and African trypanosomiases depend on the effectiveness of the diagnostic and treatment packages. Such packages are available, and research is required into the most cost-effective means for large-scale implementation. Again, the management exercise is to accept that some transmission will occur but to be aware that cases can be found and treated with minimal losses to healthy life. As with dengue, predictive surveillance will help focus attention on those areas where outbreaks seem most likely, and rapid, accurate diagnostics are crucial both to avoid the waste and danger of mistreatment and to minimize delays in administering the specific treatment required. But should such approaches rely on health centers, on mobile teams, or on some combination of the two? To what degree can the specialist diagnosis and treatment teams be integrated into more general approaches to health care? And, most crucially, how is the epidemiological surveillance to be organized: disease and vector notification, geographic information system mapping, analysis, and prediction?

For the leishmaniases, vector control seems unlikely to become a major component of disease control except where sandfly distribution overlaps with that of other vectors or where use of personal protection measures can be more widely encouraged. For dengue, vector control is a major component,

Table 23.2 Control Strategies, Major Challenges, and Research Needs of Each Disease

Disease	Principal control strategy	Major problems and challenges	Major research needs
Dengue	Interruption of transmission through vector control	Lifestyles that provide abundant artificial larval habitats	Vector control thresholds to interrupt transmission
	Patient management and supportive treatment	Urban water infrastructure and management	Behavioral changes conducive to dengue prevention
		Sustainable vector control	Pathogenesis and disease prognosis
		Early diagnosis and treatment	Vaccine development
		Vaccine development	
Leishmaniasis	Case detection and treatment	Rapid field diagnosis	Molecular-based field diagnostic kits
		Deployment of oral drugs for treatment	Effective, safe, oral drug treatments, including combination therapy
		Vaccine development	Diagnosis and treatment strategies
African trypanosomiasis	Case detection and treatment	Rapid field diagnosis, including determination of stage of infection	Molecular-based field diagnostic kits
	Interruption of transmission through vector control	Safer drug treatment regimens	Effective, safe, oral drug treatments
		Sustainable large-scale vector control	Vector population genetics to determine areas amenable to vector population elimination

Source: Authors.

but unless *Aedes* eradication appears again on the agenda, predicting the levels of control required in specific situations will require much greater understanding of transmission dynamics. Significant resources have been wasted on emergency dengue vector control, which has subsequently been seen to have had little more than a palliative effect, whereas sustained suppression of vector populations may require changes in urban water management and in human behavior that exceed the usual remit of health specialists.

For African trypanosomiasis, however, the prospects for sustainable vector control are more promising. The vector's low reproductive rate, combined with its extreme sensitivity to ultra-low doses of biodegradable insecticides, put tsetse flies among the most promising candidates for large-scale elimination. Campaigns against tsetse flies during the past century were invariably successful until they were discontinued and the controlled areas became reinvaded. Thus, the operational issue is to design large-scale international programs that can successively eliminate tsetse populations and prevent reinvasion of controlled areas, as contemplated by the African Union's Pan African Initiative.

In essence, all three diseases face parallel needs involving some marginal improvements to existing control techniques, but, most important, they require a management exercise that acknowledges the long-term need for surveillance, adequate reporting, case finding, and treatment. The primary challenges seem to reside less in the domain of new tools and more in the deployment of what is already available.

REFERENCES

Almond, J., J. Clemens, H. Engers, S. B. Halstead, H. B. Khiem, A. Pablos-Mendez, and others. 2002. "Accelerating the Development and Introduction of a Dengue Vaccine for Poor Children, 5–8 December 2001, Ho Chi Minh City, Vietnam." *Vaccine* 20: 3043–46.

Alten, B., S. Çağlar, S. Kaynaş, and F. M. Şimşek. 2003. "Evaluation of Protective Efficacy of K-OTAB Impregnated Bednets for Cutaneous Leishmaniasis Control in Southeast Anatolia, Turkey." *Journal of Vector Ecology* 28 (1): 53–64.

Arias, J. 2002. "El Dengue en Cuba." *Revista Panamericana de Salud Pública* 11: 221–22.

Attar, A. J., M. L. Chance, S. El-Safi, J. Carney, A. Azazy, M. El-Hadi, and others. 2001. "Latex Agglutination Test for the Detection of Urinary Antigens in Visceral Leishmaniasis." *Acta Tropica* 78 (1): 11–16.

Barrera, R., J. Avila, and S. Gonzalez-Teller. 1993. "Unreliable Supply of Potable Water and Elevated *Aedes aegypti* Larval Indices: A Causal Relationship?" *Journal of the American Mosquito Control Association* 9: 189–95.

Barrera, R., J. C. Navarro, J. D. Mora, D. Dominguez, and J. Gonzalez. 1995. "Public Service Deficiencies and *Aedes aegypti* Breeding Sites in Venezuela." *Bulletin of the Pan American Health Organization* 29: 193–205.

Bennett, K. E., K. E. Olson, M. de Lourdes Munoz, I. Fernandez-Salas, J. A. Farfan-Ale, S. Higgs, and others. 2002. "Variation in Vector Competence for Dengue 2 Virus among 24 Collections of *Aedes aegypti*

from Mexico and the United States." *American Journal of Tropical Medicine and Hygiene* 67: 85–92.

Bravo, J. R., M. G. Guzmán, and G. P. Kouri. 1987. "Why Dengue Haemorrhagic Fever in Cuba? 1: Individual Risk Factors for Dengue Haemorrhagic Fever/Dengue Shock Syndrome (DHF/DSS)." *Transactions of the Royal Society of Tropical Medicine and Hygiene* 81: 816–20.

Brengues, C., N. J. Hawkes, F. Chandre, L. McCarroll, S. Duchon, P. Guillet, and others. 2003. "Pyrethroid and DDT Cross-Resistance in *Aedes aegypti* Is Correlated with Novel Mutations in the Voltage-Gated Sodium Channel Gene." *Medical and Veterinary Entomology* 17: 87–94.

Burri, C., S. Nkunku, A. Merolle, T. Smith, J. Blum, and R. Brun. 2000. "Efficacy of New, Concise Schedule for Melarsoprol in Treatment of Sleeping Sickness Caused by *Trypanosoma brucei gambiense*: A Randomised Trial." *Lancet* 355: 1419–25.

Carvalho, A. de F., and I. G. da Silva. 1999. "Atividade larvicida do temephos a 1% sobre o *Aedes aegypti* (Lin., 1762), em diferentes criadouros artificiais." *Revista de Patologia Tropical* 28: 211–32.

Cattand, P., J. Jannin, and P. Lucas. 2001. "Sleeping Sickness Surveillance: An Essential Step towards Elimination." *Tropical Medicine and International Health* 6: 348–61.

Cologna, R., and R. Rico-Hesse. 2003. "American Genotype Structures Decrease Dengue Virus Output from Human Monocytes and Dendritic Cells." *Journal of Virology* 77: 3929–38.

Cref, B. J., T. C. Jones, R. Badar, D. Sampaio, R. Teixeira, and W. D. J. Johnson. 1987. "Malnutrition as a Risk Factor for Severe Visceral Leishmaniasis." *Journal of Infectious Diseases* 156: 1030–33.

De Raadt, P. 1985. "Trypanosomes et leishmanioses congénitales." *Archives Françaises de Pédiatrie* 42: 925–27.

Desjeux, P. 1996. "Leishmaniasis: Public Health Aspects and Control." *Clinics in Dermatology* 14: 417–23.

———. 2001. "The Increase in Risk Factors for the Leishmaniases Worldwide." *Transactions of the Royal Society of Tropical Medicine and Hygiene* 95: 239–43.

Desjeux, P., and J. Alvar. 2003. "Leishmania/HIV Co-infections: Epidemiology in Europe." *Annals of Tropical Medicine and Parasitology* 97 (Suppl. 1): S3–15.

Diaz, A., G. Kouri, M. G. Guzmán, L. Lobaina, J. Bravo, A. Ruiz, and others. 1988. "Description of the Clinical Picture of Dengue Hemorrhagic Fever/Dengue Shock Syndrome (DHF/DSS) in Adults." *Bulletin of the Pan American Health Organization* 22: 133–44.

FAO (Food and Agriculture Organization of the United Nations). 1999. *Pesticide Residues in Food, 1999: Report of the Joint Meeting of the FAO Panel of Experts on Pesticide Residues in Food and the Environment and the WHO Core Assessment Group on Pesticide Residues.* Paper 153. Rome: FAO Plant Production and Protection.

Ferguson, N. M., C. A. Donnelly, and R. M. Anderson. 1999. "Transmission Dynamics and Epidemiology of Dengue: Insights from Age-Stratified Sero-Prevalence Surveys." *Philosophical Transactions of the Royal Society of London, Series B, Biological Sciences* 354: 757–68.

Fèvre, E. M., P. G. Coleman, M. Odiit, S. C. Welburn, and M. E. J. Woolhouse. 2001. "The Origins of a New *Trypanosoma brucei rhodesiense* Sleeping Sickness Outbreak in Eastern Uganda." *Lancet* 358: 625–28.

Focks, D. A., E. Daniels, D. G. Haile, and J. E. Keesling. 1995. "A Simulation Model of the Epidemiology of Urban Dengue Fever: Literature Analysis, Model Development, Preliminary Validation, and Samples of Simulation Results." *American Journal of Tropical Medicine and Hygiene* 53: 489–506.

Frézil, J. L. 1983. *La trypanosomiase humaine en République Populaire du Congo.* Travaux et documents de l'ORSTOM 155, Paris, ORSTOM.

Geerts, S., and P. H. Holmes. 1998. *Drug Management and Parasite Resistance in Bovine Trypanosomiasis in Africa.* Programme against African Trypanosomiasis Technical and Scientific Series 1. Rome: Food and Agriculture Organization of the United Nations.

Gouteux, J. P., P. Bansimba, F. Noireau, and J. L. Frezil. 1987. "Le coût du traitement individuel de la trypanosomiase à *T. b. gambiense* dans le foyer du niari (Congo)." *Médecine Tropicale* 47: 61–63.

Griekspoor, A., E. Sondorp, and T. Vos. 1999. "Cost-Effectiveness Analysis of Humanitarian Relief Interventions: Visceral Leishmaniasis Treatment in the Sudan." *Health Policy and Planning* 14: 70–76.

Gubler, D. J. 1979. "Variation in Susceptibility to Oral Infection with Dengue Viruses among Geographic Strains of *Aedes aegypti.*" *American Journal of Tropical Medicine and Hygiene* 28: 1045–52.

———. 2002. "Epidemic Dengue/Dengue Hemorrhagic Fever as a Public Health, Social, and Economic Problem in the 21st Century." *Trends in Microbiology* 2: 100–3.

Gubler, D. J., and G. Kuno, eds. 1997. *Dengue and Dengue Hemorrhagic Fever.* New York: CAB International.

Guzmán, M. G., M. Alvarez, R. Rodriguez, D. Rosario, S. Vazquez, L. Valdes, and others. 1999. "Fatal Dengue Hemorrhagic Fever in Cuba, 1997." *International Journal of Infectious Diseases* 3: 130–35.

Guzmán, M. G., and G. Kouri. 2002. "Dengue: An Update." *Lancet Infectious Disease* 2: 33–42.

———. 2003. "Dengue and Dengue Hemorrhagic Fever in the Americas: Lessons and Challenges." *Journal of Clinical Virology* 27: 1–13.

Guzmán, M. G., G. Kouri, L. Valdes, J. Bravo, S. Vazquez, and S. B. Halstead. 2002. "Enhanced Severity of Secondary Dengue-2 Infections: Death Rates in 1981 and 1997 Cuban Outbreaks." *Pan American Journal of Public Health* 11: 223–27.

Hales, S., N. de Wet, J. Maindonald, and A. Woodward. 2002. "Potential Effect of Population and Climate Changes on Global Distribution of Dengue Fever: An Empirical Model." *Lancet* 360: 830–34.

Halstead, S. B., and J. Deen. 2002. "The Future of Dengue Vaccines." *Lancet* 360: 1243–45.

Harris, E., E. Videa, E. Perez, E. Sandoval, Y. Tellez, M. A. Perez, and others. 2000. "Clinical, Epidemiologic, and Virologic Features of Dengue in the 1998 Epidemic in Nicaragua." *American Journal of Tropical Medicine and Hygiene* 63: 5–11.

Holmes, E. C., and S. S. Burch. 2000. "The Causes and Consequences of Genetic Variation in Dengue Virus." *Trends in Microbiology* 8: 74–77.

Hull, B., E. Tikasingh, M. de Souza, and R. Martinez. 1984. "Natural Transovarial Transmission of Dengue 4 Virus in *Aedes aegypti* in Trinidad." *American Journal of Tropical Medicine and Hygiene* 33: 1248–50.

Kay, B. H., V. S. Nam, T. V. Tien, N. T. Yen, T. V. Phong, V. T. Diep, and others. 2002. "Control of *Aedes* Vectors of Dengue in Three Provinces of Vietnam by Use of *Mesocyclops* (Copepoda) and Community-Based Methods Validated by Entomologic, Clinical, and Serological Surveillance." *American Journal of Tropical Medicine and Hygiene* 66: 40–48.

Kouri, G. P., M. G. Guzmán, and J. R. Bravo. 1987. "Why Dengue Haemorrhagic Fever in Cuba? 2: An Integral Analysis." *Transactions of the Royal Society of Tropical Medicine and Hygiene* 81: 821–23.

Kouri, G. P., M. G. Guzmán, J. R. Bravo, and C. Triana. 1989. "Dengue Haemorrhagic Fever/Dengue Shock Syndrome: Lessons from the Cuban Epidemic." *Bulletin of the World Health Organization* 67: 375–80.

Kristjanson, P. M., B. M. Swallow, G. J. Rowlands, R. L. Kruska, and P. N. de Leeuw. 1999. "Measuring the Costs of African Animal Trypanosomosis: The Potential Benefits of Control and Returns to Research." *Agricultural Systems* 59: 79–98.

LaFleur, C., J. Granados, G. Vargas-Alarcon, J. Ruiz-Morales, C. Villareal-Garza, L. Higuera, and others. 2002. "HLA-DR Antigen Frequencies in Mexican Patients with Dengue Virus Infection: HLA-DR4 as a Possible Genetic Resistance Factor for Dengue Hemorrhagic Fever." *Human Immunology* 63: 1039–44.

Lancien, J., and H. Obayi. 1993. "La lutte contre les vecteurs de la maladie du sommeil." *Bulletin de la Société Française de Parasitiologie* 11: 107–17.

Laveissière, C., O. Grébuat, J. J. Lemasson, A. H. Meda, D. Couret, F. Doua, and others. 1994. *Les communautés rurales et la lutte contre la maladie du sommeil en forêt de Côte d'Ivoire.* OCCGE-WHO/TRY/94.1. Geneva: World Health Organization.

Leitmeyer, K. C., D. W. Vaughn, D. M. Watts, R. Salas, I. Villalobos, C. Ramos, and R. Rico-Hesse. 1999. "Dengue Virus Structural Differences That Correlate with Pathogenesis." *Journal of Virology* 73: 4738–47.

Libala, K., M. Wery, and J. F. Ruppol. 1978. "Congenital Transmission of *Trypanosoma gambiense.*" *Annales de la Société Belge de Médecine Tropicale* 58: 65–66.

Lima, J. B., M. P. Da-Cunha, R. C. Da Silva, A. K. Galardo, S. Soares Sda, I. A. Braga, and others. 2003. "Resistance of *Aedes aegypti* to Organophosphates in Several Municipalities in the State of Rio de Janeiro and Espírito Santo, Brazil." *American Journal of Tropical Medicine and Hygiene* 68: 329–33.

Loke, H., D. B. Betchell, C. X. T. Phuong, M. Dung, J. Schneider, N. J. White, and others. 2001. "Strong HLA Class I-Restricted T Cell Responses in Dengue Hemorrhagic Fever: A Double-Edged Sword?" *Journal of Infectious Disease* 184: 1369–73.

Martinez, E. 1992. *Dengue hemorrágico en criancas.* Havana: Editorial José Marti.

Maudlin, I., P. H. Holmes, and M. A. Miles, eds. 2004. *The Trypanosomiases.* Wallingford, U.K.: CABI Publishing.

Mazloumi Gavgani, A. S., M. H. Hodjati, H. Mohite, and C. R. Davies. 2002. "Effect of Insecticide-Impregnated Dog Collars on Incidence of Zoonotic Visceral Leishmaniasis in Iranian Children: A Matched-Cluster Randomised Trial." *Lancet* 360: 374–79.

McConnell, J. K., and D. J. Gubler. 2003. "Guidelines on the Cost-Effectiveness of Larval Control Programs to Reduce Dengue Transmission in Puerto Rico." *Pan American Journal of Public Health* 14: 9–16.

Meltzer, M. I., J. G. Rigau-Pérez, G. G. Clark, P. Reiter, and D. J. Gubler. 1998. "Using Disability-Adjusted Life Years to Assess the Economic Impact of Dengue in Puerto Rico: 1984–1994." *American Journal of Tropical Medicine and Hygiene* 59: 265–71.

Nagao, Y., U. Thavara, P. Chitnumsup, A. Tawatsin, C. Chansang, and D. Campbell-Lendrum. 2003. "Climatic and Social Risk Factors for *Aedes* Infestation in Rural Thailand." *Tropical Medicine and International Health* 8: 650–59.

Nam, V. S., N. T. Yen, M. Holynska, J. W. Reid, and B. H. Kay. 2000. "National Progress in Dengue Vector Control in Vietnam: Survey for *Mesocyclops* (Copepoda), Micronecta (Corixidae), and Fish as Biological Control Agents." *American Journal of Tropical Medicine and Hygiene* 62: 5–10.

Nathan, M. B. 1993. "Critical Review of *Aedes aegypti* Control Programs in the Caribbean and Selected Neighboring Countries." *Journal of the American Mosquito Control Association* 9: 1–7.

Newton, E. A. C., and P. Reiter. 1992. "A Model of the Transmission of Dengue Fever with an Evaluation of the Impact of Ultra-Low Volume (ULV) Insecticide Applications on Dengue Epidemics." *American Journal of Tropical Medicine and Hygiene* 47: 709–20.

Nimmanitya, S. 1993. *Clinical Manifestations of Dengue/Dengue Haemorrhagic Fever.* Regional Publication, SEARO 22. New Delhi: World Health Organization, Regional Office for Southeast Asia.

Nisalak, A., T. P. Endy, S. Nimmanitya, S. Kalayanrooj, U. Thiyakorn, R. M. Scott, and others. 2003. "Serotype-Specific Dengue Virus Circulation and Dengue Disease in Bangkok, Thailand, from 1973 to 1999." *American Journal of Tropical Medicine and Hygiene* 68: 191–202.

Odiit, M. 2003. "The Epidemiology of *Trypanosoma brucei rhodesiense* in Eastern Uganda." Ph.D. thesis, University of Edinburgh, Scotland.

Odiit, M., A. Shaw, S. C. Welburn, E. M. Fevre, P. G. Coleman, and J. J. McDermott. 2004. "Assessing the Patterns of Health-Seeking Behavior and Awareness among Sleeping-Sickness Patients in Eastern Uganda." *Annals of Tropical Medicine and Parasitology* 98: 339–48.

Okanurak, K., S. Sornmani, and K. Indaratna. 1997. "The Cost of Dengue Hemorrhagic Fever in Thailand." *Southeast Asian Journal of Tropical Medicine and Public Health* 28: 711–17.

Okoth, J. O. 1986. "Peridomestic Breeding Sites of *Glossina fuscipes fuscipes* Newst. in Busoga, Uganda, and Epidemiological Implications for Trypanosomiasis." *Acta Tropica* 43: 283–86.

PAHO (Pan American Health Organization). 1994. *Dengue and Dengue Hemorrhagic Fever in the Americas: Guidelines for Prevention and Control.* PAHO Scientific Publication 548. Washington, DC: PAHO.

Pang, T. 2003. "Vaccines for the Prevention of Neglected Diseases: Dengue Fever." *Current Opinions in Biotechnology* 14: 332–36.

Paradoa, M. L., Y. Trujillo, and P. Basanta. 1987. "Association of Dengue Hemorrhagic Fever with the HLA System." *Haematologia* 20: 83–87.

Parks, W., and L. Lloyd. 2004. *Planning Social Mobilization and Communication for Dengue Fever Prevention and Control: A Step-by-Step Guide.* WHO/CDS/WMC/2004.2. Geneva: World Health Organization.

Pokhrel, S. 1999. "Cost-Effectiveness of Early Case Detection for Visceral Leishmaniasis in Nepal," M.Sc. thesis, Chulalongkorn University, Thailand.

Politi, C., G. Carrin, D. Evans, F. A. S. Kuzoe, and P. D. Cattand. 1995. "Cost-Effectiveness Analysis of Alternative Treatments of African Gambiense Trypanosomiasis in Uganda." *Health Economics* 4: 273–87.

Rawlins, S. C. 1998. "Spatial Distribution of Insecticide Resistance in Caribbean Populations of *Aedes aegypti* and Its Significance." *Pan American Journal of Public Health* 4: 243–51.

Reiter, P., S. Lathrop, M. Bunning, B. Biggerstaff, D. Singer, T. Tiwari, and others. 2003. "Texas Lifestyle Limits Transmission of Dengue Virus." *Emerging Infectious Diseases* 9: 86–89.

Rico-Hesse, R., L. M. Harrison, R. A. Salas, D. Tovar, A. Nisalak, C. Ramos, and others. 1997. "Origins of Dengue Type 2 Viruses Associated with Increased Pathogenicity in the Americas." *Virology* 230: 244–51.

Rochas, G., A. Martins, G. Gama, F. Brandão, and J. Atougia. 2004. "Possible Cases of Sexual and Congenital Transmission of Sleeping Sickness." *Lancet* 363: 247.

Rodriguez, M. M., J. Bisset, D. M. de Fernandez, L. Lauzan, and A. Soca. 2001. "Detection of Insecticide Resistance in *Aedes aegypti* (Diptera: Culicidae) from Cuba and Venezuela." *Journal of Medical Entomology* 38: 623–28.

Rosen, L., D. A. Shroyer, R. B. Tesh, J. E. Freier, and J. C. Lien. 1983. "Transovarial Transmission of Dengue Viruses by Mosquitoes: *Aedes albopictus* and *Aedes aegypti.*" *American Journal of Tropical Medicine and Hygiene* 32: 1108–19.

Schallig, H. D. F. H., G. J. Schoone, C. C. M. Kroon, A. Hailu, F. Chappuis, and H. Veeken. 2001. "Development and Application of Simple Diagnostic Tools for Visceral Leishmaniasis." *Medical Microbiology and Immunology* 190: 69–71.

Shaw, A. P. M., and P. Cattand. 2001. "Analytical Tools for Planning Cost-Effective Surveillance in Gambiense Sleeping Sickness." *Médecine Tropicale* 61: 412–21.

Shepard, D. S. 2001. "Modeling in CE Analysis." Brandeis University, Heller School, Schneider Institute for Health Policy. http://www.sihp.brandeis.edu/Shepard/module-10-8-01.ppt.

Shepard, D. S., J. A. Suaya, S. Halstead, M. B. Nathan, D. J. Gubler, R. T. Mahoney, and others. 2004. "Cost-Effectiveness of a Pediatric Dengue Vaccine." *Vaccine* 22: 1275–80.

Stephens, H. A. F., R. Klaythong, M. Sirikong, D. W. Vaughn, S. Green, S. Kalayanarooj, and others. 2002. "HLA-A and B Allele Associations with Secondary Dengue Virus Infections Correlate with Disease Severity and the Infecting Viral Serotype in Ethnic Thais." *Tissue Antigens* 60: 309–18.

Swallow, B. M. 2000. *Impacts of Trypanosomiasis on African Agriculture.* Programme against African Trypanosomiasis Technical and Scientific Series 2. Rome: Food and Agriculture Organization of the United Nations.

Tardieux, I., O. Poupel, L. Lapchin, and F. Rodhain. 1990. "Variation among Strains of *Aedes aegypti* in Susceptibility to Oral Infection with Dengue Virus Type 2." *American Journal of Tropical Medicine and Hygiene* 43: 308–13.

Traub, N., P. Hira, C. Chintu, and C. Mhango. 1978. "Congenital Trypanosomiasis: Report of a Case Due to *Trypanosoma brucei rhodesiense.*" *East African Medical Journal* 55: 477–81.

Trowbridge, M., D. McFarland, M. Richer, M. Adeoye, and A. Moore. 2001. "Cost-Effectiveness of Programs for Sleeping Sickness Control: American Society of Tropical Medicine and Hygiene, 49th Annual Meeting, Houston, TX, 2000, Abstract 417." *American Journal of Tropical Medicine and Hygiene* 62 (Suppl. 3): 312.

Van Damme, W., L.Van Leemput, I. Por, W. Hardeman, and B. Meessen. 2004. "Out-of-Pocket Health Expenditure and Debt in Poor Households: Evidence from Cambodia." *Tropical Medicine and International Health* 9: 273–80.

Vreysen, M. J. B., K. M. Saleh, M. Y. Ali, M. A. Abdullah, Z. R. Zhu, K. G. Juma, and others. 2000. "*Glossina austeni* (Diptera: Glossinidae) Eradicated on the Island of Unguja, Zanzibar, Using the Sterile Insect Technique." *Journal of Economic Entomology* 93: 123–35.

Watts, D. M., D. S. Burke, B. A. Harrison, R. E. Whitmire, and A. Nisalak. 1987. "Effect of Temperature on the Vector Efficiency of *Aedes aegypti* for Dengue 2 Virus." *American Journal of Tropical Medicine and Hygiene* 36: 143–52.

WHO (World Health Organization). 1986. *Epidemiology and Control of African Trypanosomiasis.* Report of a WHO Expert Committee. Technical Report Series 739. Geneva: WHO.

———. 1991. *Safe Use of Pesticides.* Fourteenth Report of the WHO Expert Committee on Vector Biology and Control. Technical Report Series 813. Geneva: WHO.

———. 1992. *Vector Resistance to Pesticides.* Fifteenth Report of the WHO Expert Committee on Vector Biology and Control. Technical Report Series 818. Geneva: WHO.

———. 1998. *African Trypanosomiasis: Control and Surveillance.* Report of a WHO Expert Committee. Technical Report Series 881. Geneva: WHO.

Zagne, S. M. O., V. G. F. Alves, R. M. R. Nogueira, M. P. Miagostovich, E. Lampe, and W. Tavares. 1994. "Dengue Hemorrhagic Fever in the State of Rio de Janeiro, Brazil: A Study of 56 Confirmed Cases." *Transactions of the Royal Society of Tropical Medicine and Hygiene* 88: 677–79.

Zaim, M., and P. Jambulingham. 2004. *Global Insecticide Use for Vector-Borne Disease Control.* 2nd ed. WHO/CDS/WHOPES/GCDPP/2004.9. Geneva: World Health Organization.

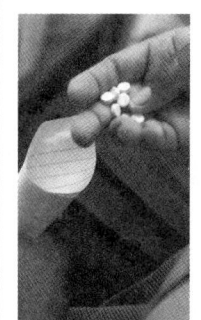

Chapter **24**

Helminth Infections: Soil-Transmitted Helminth Infections and Schistosomiasis

Peter J. Hotez, Donald A. P. Bundy, Kathleen Beegle, Simon Brooker, Lesley Drake, Nilanthi de Silva, Antonio Montresor, Dirk Engels, Matthew Jukes, Lester Chitsulo, Jeffrey Chow, Ramanan Laxminarayan, Catherine M. Michaud, Jeff Bethony, Rodrigo Correa-Oliveira, Xiao Shu-Hua, Alan Fenwick, and Lorenzo Savioli

Helminth infections caused by soil-transmitted helminths (STHs) and schistosomes are among the most prevalent afflictions of humans who live in areas of poverty in the developing world. The morbidity caused by STHs and schistosomes is most commonly associated with infections of heavy intensity. Approximately 300 million people with heavy helminth infections suffer from severe morbidity that results in more than 150,000 deaths annually (Crompton 1999; Montresor and others 2002). In addition to their health effects, helminth infections also impair physical and mental growth in childhood, thwart educational advancement, and hinder economic development. Because of the geographic overlap of these afflictions and their impact on children and adolescents, the World Health Organization (WHO); the World Bank; and other United Nations agencies and bilaterals; and civil society are working to integrate STH and schistosome control through a program of periodic school-based, targeted anthelmintic drug treatments.

CAUSES AND CHARACTERISTICS OF HELMINTH INFECTIONS

Emphasis is placed on the four most common STH infections and the three most common schistosome infections. Together, these infections account for most of the global helminth disease burden.

Soil-Transmitted Helminths

The four most common STHs are roundworm (*Ascaris lumbricoides*), whipworm (*Trichuris trichiura*), and the anthropophilic hookworms (*Necator americanus* and *Ancylostoma duodenale*). Recent estimates suggest that *A. lumbricoides* infects 1.221 billion people, *T. trichiura* 795 million, and hookworms 740 million (de Silva and others 2003) (table 24.1). The greatest numbers of STH infections occur in the Americas, China and East Asia, and Sub-Saharan Africa. *Strongyloides stercoralis* is also a common STH in some of these regions, although detailed information on the prevalence of strongyloidiasis is lacking because of the difficulties in diagnosing human infection. The life cycles of *Ascaris*, *Trichuris*, and hookworm follow a general pattern. The adult parasite stages inhabit the gastrointestinal tract (*Ascaris* and hookworm in the small intestine; *Trichuris* in the colon), reproduce sexually, and produce eggs, which are passed in human feces and deposited in the external environment.

STH infections rarely cause death. Instead, the burden of disease is related less to mortality than to the chronic and insidious effects on the hosts' health and nutritional status (Stephenson, Latham, and Ottesen 2000; Stoltzfus and others 1997). Hookworms have long been recognized as an important cause of intestinal blood loss leading to iron deficiency and protein malnutrition. The iron deficiency anemia that accompanies moderate and heavy hookworm burdens is sometimes referred to as *hookworm disease* (Hotez and others 2004). When host

Table 24.1 Global Prevalence and Distribution of Helminth Infections

Helminth infections	Total cases	Major geographic areas
STH infections	≥ 2 billion	
Ascariasis	1.221 billion	Sub-Saharan Africa, India, China and East Asia
Trichuriasis	795 million	Sub-Saharan Africa, India, China and East Asia
Hookworm	740 million	Sub-Saharan Africa, Americas, China and East Asia
Schistosomiasis	187 million	
S. haematobium	119 million	Sub-Saharan Africa
S. mansoni	67 million	Sub-Saharan Africa, Americas
S. japonicum	1 million	China and East Asia

Source: de Silva and others 2003.

iron stores are depleted, the extent of iron deficiency anemia is linearly related to the intensity of hookworm infection (Stoltzfus and others 1997). Because of their underlying poor iron status, children, women of reproductive age, and pregnant women are frequently the ones most susceptible to developing hookworm anemia (Brooker, Bethony, and Hotez 2004). Iron deficiency anemia during pregnancy has been linked to adverse maternal-fetal consequences, including prematurity, low birthweight, and impaired lactation (WHO 2002).

Chronic STH infections resulting from *Ascaris*, *Trichuris*, and hookworm can dramatically affect physical and mental development in children (WHO 2002). Studies have also shown that the growth and physical fitness deficits caused by chronic STH infections are sometimes reversible following treatment with anthelmintic drugs (Stephenson, Latham, and Ottesen 2000). The effects on growth are most pronounced in children with the heaviest infections, but light infections may also contribute to growth deficits if the nutritional status of the community is poor (Stephenson, Latham, and Ottesen 2000).

Schistosomiasis

Five major species of parasitic trematodes of the family Schistosomatidae—*Schistosoma haematobium*, *S. intercalatum*, *S. japonicum*, *S. mansoni*, and *S. mekongi*—infect humans. These parasites have a complex, indirect life cycle involving an intermediate snail host. Disease is caused primarily by schistosome eggs, which are deposited by adult worms in the blood vessels surrounding the bladder or intestines. Urinary schistosomiasis, in which the bladder is affected, is caused by infection with *S. haematobium,* which occurs mainly in Africa. Intestinal schistosomiasis results from infection with *S. mansoni,* which occurs in the Middle East, South America, and Africa, and from

infection with *S. japonicum,* which occurs in parts of China and the Philippines (Ross and others 2002). Two other schistosome species are known to cause intestinal schistosomiasis in restricted geographical areas: *S. intercalatum,* found in Central Africa, and *S. mekongi,* found in Cambodia and the Lao People's Democratic Republic. Schistosomiasis is estimated to affect 187 million people worldwide (table 24.1).

A serious acute illness accompanied by fever and lymphadenopathy, known as Katayama Syndrome, can result from heavy schistosome infections. Chronic disease is mostly due to perforation of blood vessels and entrapment of eggs by host tissues. The host's reaction to entrapped eggs results in granuloma formation. *S. haematobium* causes bladder wall pathology, leading to ulcer formation, hematuria, and dysuria. Granulomatous changes and ulcers of the bladder wall and ureter can lead to bladder obstruction, dilatation, secondary urinary tract infections and subsequent bladder calcification, renal failure, lesions of the female and male genital tracts, and hydronephrosis. *S. haematobium* is also associated with increased risk of bladder cancer. The morbidity commonly associated with *S. mansoni* infection includes lesions of the liver, portal vein, and spleen, leading to periportal fibrosis, portal hypertension, hepatosplenomegaly, splenomegaly, and ascites. Schistosomiasis also causes chronic growth faltering and can contribute to anemia (Ross and others 2002).

EPIDEMIOLOGY OF STH INFECTIONS AND SCHISTOSOMIASIS

The most striking epidemiological features of human helminth infections are aggregated distributions in human communities, predisposition of individuals to heavy (or light) infection, rapid reinfection following chemotherapy, and age-intensity profiles that are typically convex (with the exception of hookworm).

For all the major human STH and schistosome infections studied to date, worm burdens exhibit a highly aggregated (overdispersed) distribution so that most individuals harbor just a few worms in their intestines, although a few hosts harbor disproportionately large worm burdens (Anderson and May 1991). As a rule, 20 percent of the host population harbors approximately 80 percent of the worm population. This overdispersion has many consequences, both with regard to the population biology of the helminths and the public health consequence for the host, because heavily infected individuals are simultaneously at highest risk of disease and the major source of environmental contamination. One feature that may help explain overdispersion is that individuals tend to be predisposed to heavy (or light) infections. Predisposition has been demonstrated for all four major STHs and the schistosomes. The underlying cause of such predisposition remains poorly understood. However, a combination of heterogeneity in exposure to infection or differences in susceptibility to infection and the ability to mount effective immunity (genetic and nutritional factors) is likely to be important.

People of all ages rapidly reacquire infection following treatment, but in schistosomiasis, older people reacquire infection at slower rates than younger ones (Kabatereine and others 1999). The rate of reinfection is specific to certain species of helminths and depends on the life expectancy of that species (short-lived helminths reinfect more rapidly), on the intensity of transmission within a given community, and on the treatment efficacy and coverage. The basic reproductive rate (R_o) describes the transmission potential of a parasite (and thus its ability to reinfect the host). It defines the average number of female offspring produced during the life span of the parasite that survive to reproductive maturity in the absence of density dependence. R_o is determined by parasite immigration and death rates as well as by host density (and, in schistosomiasis, also snail density). A parasite will fail to become established unless R_o is greater than unity (Anderson and May 1991). Adult worms usually survive between one and four years, whereas eggs can sometimes remain viable for several more years in the environment. Therefore, reinfection rates will remain high until adults are removed with chemotherapy and until infective stages, through time, become uninfective. In reality, density-dependent processes regulate parasite populations; at endemic equilibrium, the effective reproductive ratio equals unity (that is, each female replaces herself). Control programs rely on reducing the effective reproductive ratio long enough for the parasite population to be driven to local elimination. Theoretically, R_o provides useful insights, and it is helpful to think of control programs attempting to break the transmission cycle by reducing R_o to less than unity. Therefore, estimates can be made about how long and how many rounds of chemotherapy are required to treat intestinal helminths. For example, A. lumbricoides with an R_o of three and a life expectancy of one year will need to be treated annually with a drug that is 95 percent efficacious and with coverage of more than 91 percent of the population. Where R_o is five—that is, in areas where transmission is higher—treatment must be given more frequently than once a year (Anderson and May 1991).

The age-dependent patterns of infection prevalence are generally similar among the major helminth species, exhibiting a rise in childhood to a relatively stable asymptote in adulthood (figure 24.1). Maximum prevalence of A. lumbricoides and T. trichiura is usually attained before five years of age, and the maximum prevalence of hookworm and schistosome infections is usually attained in adolescence or in early adulthood. The nonlinear relationship between prevalence and intensity has the consequence that the observed age-prevalence profiles provide little indication of the underlying profiles of age intensity (age in relation to worm burden). Because intensity is

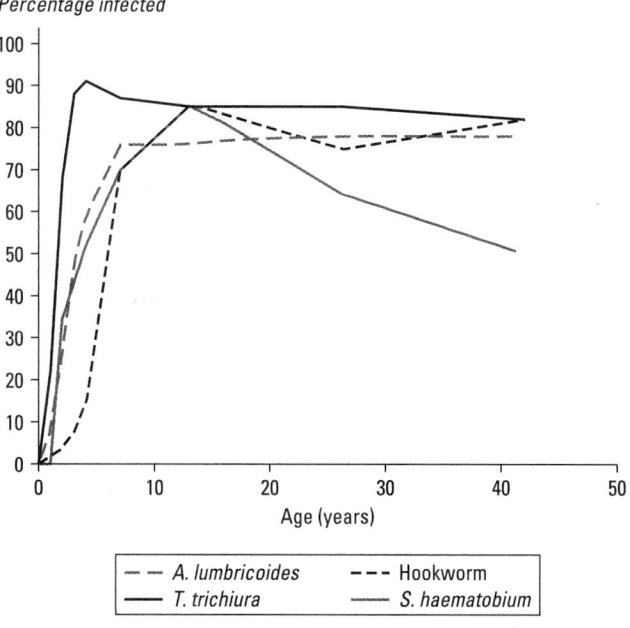

a. Prevalence

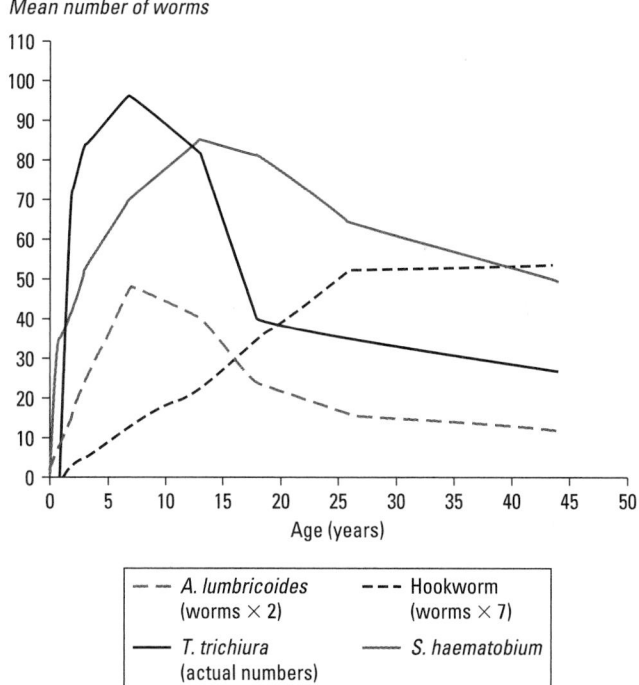

b. Intensity

Source: Bundy 1995; reproduced and modified from Hotez, Arora, and others 2005.

Figure 24.1 Age-Associated Prevalence and Intensity Profiles of STH and Schistosome Infections: Typical Age Profiles of Prevalence and Intensity of STH Infections and Schistosomiasis

linked to morbidity, the age-intensity profiles provide a clearer understanding of which populations are vulnerable to the different helminths (figure 24.1). For A. lumbricoides and T. trichiura infections, the age-intensity profiles are typically convex in form, with the highest intensities in children 5 to

15 years of age (Bundy 1995). For schistosomiasis, a convex pattern is also observed, with a similar peak but with a plateau in adolescents and young adults 15 to 29 years of age (Kabatereine and others 1999). In contrast, the age-intensity profile for hookworm exhibits considerable variation, although intensity typically increases with age until adulthood and then plateaus (Brooker, Bethony, and Hotez 2004). In East Asia it is also common to find the highest intensities among the elderly. However, more generally, children and young adults are at higher risk of both harboring higher levels of infection (thus greater levels of morbidity) and becoming reinfected more quickly. Both may occur at vital stages in a child's intellectual and physical development.

Risk Factors

Both host-specific and environmental factors have been identified that may affect the risk of acquiring or harboring heavy-intensity helminth infections.

Genetics. No genes that control for human helminth infection have yet been identified. However, recent genome scans have identified a locus possibly responsible for controlling *S. mansoni* infection intensity on chromosome 5q31-33 and loci controlling *A. lumbricoides* intensity on chromosomes 1 and 13. There is also evidence for genetic control of pathology attributable to *S. mansoni*, with linkage reported to a region containing the gene for the interferon gamma receptor 1 subunit (Quinnell 2003).

Behavior, Household Clustering, and Occupation. Specific occupations, household clustering, and behaviors influence the prevalence and intensity of helminth infections (Bethony and others 2001), particularly for hookworm, in which the highest intensities occur among adults (Brooker, Bethony, and Hotez 2004). Engagement in agricultural pursuits, for example, remains a common denominator for hookworm infection. Behavioral and occupational factors, through their effect on water contact, interact with environmental factors to produce variation in the epidemiology of schistosomiasis.

Poverty, Sanitation, and Urbanization. STH and schistosomiasis depend for transmission on environments contaminated with egg-carrying feces. Consequently, helminths are intimately associated with poverty, poor sanitation, and lack of clean water. The provision of safe water and improved sanitation are essential for the control of helminth infection. Although the STH and schistosome infections are neglected diseases that occur predominantly in rural areas, the social and environmental conditions in many unplanned slums and squatter settlements of developing countries are ideal for the persistence of *A. lumbricoides* (Crompton and Savioli 1993). Schistosomiasis transmission can also occur in urban areas.

Climate, Water, and Season. Adequate warmth and moisture are key features for each of the STHs. Wetter areas exhibit increased transmission, and in some endemic areas, both STH and schistosome infections exhibit marked seasonality (Brooker and Michael 2000). Recent use of geographical information systems and remote sensing has identified the distributional limits of STH and schistosomes on the basis of temperature and rainfall patterns (Brooker and Michael 2000). For schistosomiasis, specific snail intermediate hosts prefer certain types of aquatic environments. Construction of dams is known to extend the range of snail habitats, thereby promoting the reemergence of schistosomiasis.

BURDEN OF THE DISEASE

The revised estimates in 2003 (de Silva and others 2003) use the methodology developed by Chan and others (1994) and build on recent applications of geographical information systems to derive updated atlases of helminth infections. To reflect recent changes in the epidemiology of infection, de Silva and others used data from only 1990 onward. These data confirm that STH infections are the most prevalent infections of humans and that a large proportion of the population in developing countries is at risk. Of the 187 million cases of schistosomiasis estimated to occur worldwide, most are caused by *S. haematobium* in Sub-Saharan Africa (table 24.1).

WHO (2002) estimates that 27,000 people die annually from STH infections and schistosomiasis (case fatality rate of 0.0014 percent). Many investigators, however, believe that this figure is an underestimate. Crompton (1999) estimated that 155,000 deaths annually occur from these infections (case fatality rate of 0.08 percent), whereas Van der Werf and others (2003), using the limited data available from Africa, estimated the schistosomiasis mortality alone at 280,000 per year (case fatality rate of 0.014 percent) because of nonfunctioning kidneys (from *S. haematobium*) and hematemesis (from *S. mansoni*). Therefore, the difference between estimates for helminth-associated mortality is more than 10-fold.

Because it is uncommon for STHs and schistosomes to kill their human host, citing mortality figures provides only a small window on their health impact. Instead, measurements of disease burden using disability-adjusted life years (DALYs) and similar tools portray a more accurate picture for helminthic disease burden. WHO estimates the global burden of disease from STH infections and schistosomiasis on the basis of the enormous number of infected individuals, together with an associated low disability weight (Van der Werf and others 2003). However, because an estimated 2 billion people are infected with STHs and schistosomes, even minor adjustments to the disability weights produce enormous variations in DALYs or other measurements of disease burden. This helps to explain why, for instance, in 1990 the disease burden for the STH infections and schistosomiasis was almost 18 million DALYs, whereas the 2001 estimate was only 4.7 million DALYs. In the intervening 11 years, the DALYs were as low as 2.6 million. Such disparities are substantial when one considers that the 1990 estimate ranks helminths close to major disease entities such as tuberculosis, measles, and malaria, whereas the lowest estimate during the 1990s ranks helminth infections on a par with gonorrhea, otitis media, and iodine deficiency. The Disease Control Priorities Project helminth working group has determined that the WHO global burden of disease estimates are low because they do not incorporate the full clinical spectrum of helminth-associated morbidity and chronic disability, including anemia, chronic pain, diarrhea, exercise intolerance, and undernutrition (King, Dickman, and Tisch 2005). However, for this chapter, the average disability weights estimated by WHO are used throughout. Some of the specific controversies are described below.

A. Lumbricoides and T. Trichiura infections

Because the most significant physical and intellectual growth disturbances occur as a consequence of moderate and heavy worm burdens, the age-associated epidemiology of *A. lumbricoides* and *T. trichiura* infections has focused attention on infected school-age children in developing countries (Bundy 1995). In a revised estimate of the probable number of ascariasis infections worldwide and a better categorization of the morbidity, de Silva, Chan, and Bundy (1997) indicated that 59 million of the 1.2 billion people infected (including 51 million children less than 15 years of age) were at risk of faltering growth, decreased physical fitness, or both as a result of infection. They estimated that about 1.5 million children would never make up the deficit in growth, even if treated. In addition to these chronic, insidious effects, they estimated that about 11.5 million individuals (almost all of them children) were at risk of more acute clinical illness. Their figures also indicated that at least 10,500 deaths annually were directly attributable to one of the serious complications of ascariasis; children account for more than 90 percent of those deaths. The actual threshold at which *A. lumbricoides* and *T. trichiura* worm burdens result in childhood morbidity is controversial because of the nonlinear relationship between intensity and pathogenesis and the difficulties of measuring and attributing morbidity in underserved populations suffering from other underlying conditions (Bundy 1995).

Hookworm Infection

Hookworm infection causes more DALYs lost than any other helminthiasis with the exception of lymphatic filariasis. Even these DALY measurements may still underestimate the true disease burden of iron deficiency anemia and protein malnutrition resulting from hookworm disease. Iron deficiency anemia alone results in approximately 12 million DALYs lost annually, making it the world's most important nutrition problem. Data on the epidemiology of iron deficiency anemia in East Africa and elsewhere point to the important contribution of hookworms to this condition (Stoltzfus and others 1997). In Tanzania, where hosts' iron stores are often depleted, there is a correlation between the number of adult hookworms in the intestine and the amount of host blood loss (Stoltzfus and others 1997). However, it is unclear whether current disability weights effectively incorporate the full contribution of hookworm to severe iron deficiency anemia among iron-depleted populations or whether they take host protein losses and malnutrition into account. There is increasing interest in the importance of hookworm anemia in preschool children, especially in Africa (Brooker, Bethony, and Hotez 2004), where infants and preschool children are particularly vulnerable to the developmental and behavioral deficits caused by iron deficiency anemia (Stephenson, Latham, and Ottesen 2000). Closer assessment of the impact of hookworm on another important iron-deficient population—namely, women of reproductive age—could also significantly increase current DALY estimates. Approximately 44 million of these women harbor hookworms (Bundy, Chan, and Savioli 1995). In addition, severe anemia in pregnancy is associated with neonatal prematurity, reduced birthweight, and impaired lactation (Christian, Khatry, and West 2004).

Schistosomes

Scientists and public health workers disagree on the current assessments of both morbidity and mortality attributable to schistosomiasis. Several investigators have now initiated a process to recalculate the burden of disease attributable to schistosomiasis, focusing much more on the clinical course of the different types of schistosomiasis and chronic sequelae (King, Dickman, and Tisch 2005; Michaud, Gordon, and Reich 2003). Through a comprehensive literature review combined with mathematical modeling, Van der Werf and others (2003) estimate that urinary schistosomiasis in Africa results in approximately 18 million cases of bladder wall pathology and 20 million cases of hydronephrosis, and African intestinal schistosomiasis results in approximately 8.5 million cases of hepatomegaly. Mortality in Africa attributable to urinary and intestinal schistosomiasis was extrapolated from these figures using a limited number of studies reporting case fatality rates for nonfunctioning kidney and hematemesis. From these extrapolations, Fenwick and others (2003) conclude that in Africa the mortality attributable to urinary schistosomiasis could be as high as 150,000 per year, and the number dying as a result of intestinal schistosomiasis could be as high as 130,000 per year.

COST-EFFECTIVENESS ANALYSIS OF INTERVENTIONS

Classifying Interventions

The three major interventions are anthelmintic drug treatment, sanitation, and health education.

Anthelmintic Drug Treatment. Anthelmintic drug treatment ("deworming") is aimed at reducing morbidity by decreasing the worm burden. Repeated chemotherapy at regular intervals (periodic deworming) in high-risk groups can ensure that the levels of infection are kept below those associated with morbidity (figure 24.2) and will frequently result in immediate improvement in child health and development. Anthelmintic drug treatment can prevent the development of irreversible consequences of schistosomiasis in adulthood. For ascariasis and trichuriasis, for which intensity peaks among school-age children, frequent and periodic deworming may reduce transmission over time. Obstacles that diminish the effectiveness of periodic deworming are the low efficacy of single-dose mebendazole and albendazole for the treatment of hookworm and trichuriasis, respectively (Adams and others 2004; Albonico and others 1994); high rates of posttreatment reinfection for STHs in areas of high endemicity (Albonico and others 1995); and diminished efficacy with frequent and repeated use (Albonico and others 2003), possibly because of anthelmintic resistance (see the section "Research and Development").

Improved Sanitation. Improved sanitation is aimed at controlling transmission by reducing soil and water contamina-

tion. Sanitation is the only definitive intervention to eliminate STH infections, but to be effective it should cover a high percentage of the population. Therefore, because of the high costs involved, implementing this strategy is difficult where resources are limited (Asaolu and Ofoezie 2003). Moreover, when used as the primary means of control, it can take years or even decades for sanitation to be effective (Brooker, Bethony, and Hotez 2004).

Health Education. Health education is aimed at reducing transmission and reinfection by encouraging healthy behaviors. For STH infections and schistosomiasis, the aim is to reduce contamination of soil and water by promoting the use of latrines and hygienic behavior. Without a change in defecation habits, periodic deworming cannot attain a stable reduction in transmission. Health education can be provided simply and economically and presents no contraindications or risks. Furthermore, its benefits go beyond the control of helminth infections. In this perspective, it is reasonable to include this component in all helminth control programs.

Other Control Measures. In specific epidemiological conditions, environmental or chemical control of snails can be useful tools for reducing the transmission of schistosomiasis. Research to develop new tools for control is in progress, including vaccine development programs for hookworm infection and schistosomiasis (see "Research and Development").

Choosing Interventions

Periodic deworming stands out as the most cost-effective means to reduce the morbidity of STH and schistosome infections.

Periodic Anthelmintic Therapy. Periodic anthelmintic therapy, or periodic deworming, represents the main measure in areas where infections are intensely transmitted, resources for disease control are limited, and funding for sanitation is lacking. Drug treatment can be administered in the community using different strategies:

- *Universal treatment.* The entire community is treated, irrespective of age, sex, infection status, and other characteristics.
- *Targeted treatment.* Treatment targets population groups, which may be defined by age, sex, or other social characteristics, irrespective of the infectious status.
- *Selective treatment.* Treatment targets individual-level application of anthelmintic drugs, which is selected on the basis of either diagnosis or a suspicion of current infection.

Recommended drugs for use in public health interventions to control STH infection are the benzimidazole anthelmintics

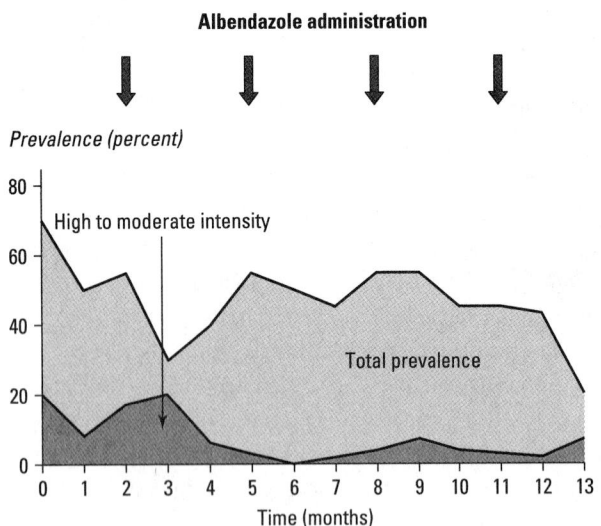

Albendazole administration

Prevalence (percent)

Source: Albonico and others, forthcoming.

Figure 24.2 Predicted Effect on *Ascaris* and *Trichuris* Prevalence Following Frequent and Periodic Dewormings with Benzimidazole Anthelmintics

(BZAs), albendazole (single dose: 400 mg, reduced to 200 mg for children between 12 and 24 months), or mebendazole (single dose: 500 mg), as well as levamisole or pyrantel pamoate (WHO 2002). Praziquantel (PZQ) (single dose: 40–60 mg/kg) is the major drug used for the treatment of schistosomiasis. However, therapy with oxamniquine has been the cornerstone for treatment of *S. mansoni* infection in South American national control programs over the past 20 years. The efficacy of oxamniquine and PZQ is comparable, although that of PZQ is slightly better. The BZAs and PZQ are inexpensive; they have undergone extensive safety testing and have been used by millions of individuals with only a few minor side effects. Drugs that do not need dosage according to weight, such as BZAs (in school-age children), are considered easier to use for population-based interventions; however, the use of proxy indicators—for example, substituting height for weight—has proved a successful implementation strategy for PZQ (Hall and others 1999).

Distribution Strategy and Frequency of Treatment. The selection of the distribution strategy and the frequency of treatment is based on epidemiological data. The recommended strategy for helminth control is a population-based approach, in which individuals in targeted communities are treated irrespective of their infection status (WHO 2002). This strategy is justified for several reasons, including the simplicity and safety of delivering treatment. Individual diagnosis is difficult and expensive and offers no safety benefit.

The intrinsic transmission potential of the parasite species determines the frequency of treatment (see "Epidemiology of STH Infections and Schistosomiasis," earlier in this chapter). To control morbidity in areas of intense transmission (prevalence greater than 70 percent and more than 10 percent of moderate- and heavy-intensity infection), WHO (2002) recommends treatment two or three times a year for STH infections. In areas with a lower intensity of transmission (prevalence between 40 and 60 percent and less than 10 percent of moderate- and heavy-intensity infection), intervention once a year is recommended (WHO 2002).

School-Age Children as a High-Risk Population. School-age children typically have the highest intensity of worm infection of any age group, and chronic infection negatively affects all aspects of children's health, nutrition, cognitive development, learning, and educational access and achievement (World Bank 2003). Regular deworming can cost-effectively reverse and prevent much of this morbidity. Furthermore, schools offer a readily available, extensive, and sustained infrastructure with a skilled workforce that is in close contact with the community. With support from the local health system, teachers can deliver the drugs safely. Teachers need only a few hours of training to understand the rationale for deworming and to learn how to give out the pills and keep a record of their distribution. School-

based deworming also has major externalities for untreated children and the whole community. By reducing transmission in the community of *Ascaris* and *Trichuris* infections, deworming substantially improves the health and school participation of both treated and untreated children, both in treatment schools and in neighboring schools (Bundy and others 1990; Miguel and Kremer 2003).

These observations provided a basis for the adoption of resolution 54.19 at the 2001 World Health Assembly, which urged member states to ensure access to essential drugs for STH and schistosome infections in endemic areas for the treatment of clinical cases and groups at high risk for morbidity (box 24.1). To achieve this goal, WHO has developed a broad partnership that promotes the incorporation of deworming into existing institutions and programs, for both the education sectors and the health sectors. The Partnership for Parasite Control was launched in 2001 with the aim of mobilizing resources and promoting synergy among public and private efforts for the control of soil-transmitted helminths and schistosomiasis at global and national levels. School-based deworming has its full effect when delivered within an integrated school health program that includes elements of the Focusing Resources on Effective School Health (FRESH) framework.

Other At-Risk Populations. Not only school-age children can benefit from treatment. Preschool children (one to five years of age) are vulnerable to the developmental and behavioral deficits caused by iron deficiency anemia, and recent analyses by Brooker, Bethony, and Hotez (2004) indicate that hookworm is an important contributor to anemia in that age group (see "Estimating Intervention Effectiveness"). Women of reproductive age (15 to 49 years of age) are particularly susceptible to iron deficiency anemia because of iron loss during menstruation and because of increased needs during pregnancy (Bundy, Chan, and Savioli 1995). In certain circumstances, male worker populations can also be at increased risk (Guyatt 2000).

Estimating Intervention Effectiveness

The evidence base for the health and educational effect of periodic deworming has accumulated significantly over the past decade.

STH Infections. All the anthelmintic drugs mentioned above substantially reduce the number of adult worms in the gastrointestinal tract. This effect is also reflected in reduced fecal egg counts. In some cases, however, the efficacy of single-dose mebendazole or albendazole on hookworm and *Trichuris* infections is low (Adams and others 2004; Albonico and others 1994). Moreover, pyrantel pamoate has little effect on *T. trichiura*.

The 54th World Health Assembly

The 54th World Health Assembly, which met in May 2001, urged member states to ensure access to essential drugs for schistosomiasis and STH infections in endemic areas for the treatment of clinical cases and groups at high risk for morbidity. The helminth infections of concern are the major schistosomes and STHs outlined in the text. The World Health Assembly determined that simple and sustainable control measures can relieve a generally underestimated and unnecessary disease burden in high-transmission areas. The following minimal targets, aimed at reducing morbidity by 80 percent, can be achieved by all countries in which such disease is endemic as an integral part of the primary health care system: (a) access to adequate diagnosis and essential anthelmintic drugs in all health services in all endemic areas, even at peripheral levels, for the treatment of symptomatic cases and of children, women, and other groups at high risk of morbidity; (b) regular administration of chemotherapy to at least 75 percent of all school-age children at risk for morbidity by 2010; and (c) sustained, community-based efforts to improve sanitation, clean water supplies, and health education.

Source: WHO 2002.

Overall, however, anthelmintic treatment significantly improves physical and cognitive outcomes in the following ways:

- *Preschool children.* Periodic distribution of anthelmintics has a positive effect on motor and language development and reduces malnutrition in very young children (Stoltzfus and others 2004).
- *School-age children.* Treating school-age children has a considerable effect on their nutritional status (Stoltzfus and others 2004), anemia, physical fitness, appetite, growth (Stephenson, Latham, and Ottesen 2000), and intellectual development (Drake and others 2000).
- *Women of reproductive age.* Studies of pregnant women conducted by Christian, Khatry, and West (2004) in Nepal indicate that albendazole treatment improves maternal hemoglobin as well as birth-weight and child survival.

Schistosomiasis. As with STH infections, anthelmintic chemotherapy for schistosomiasis has an important effect on child development, growth, and physical fitness (WHO 2002). Richter (2003) recently summarized details of the effect of PZQ on organ pathology. In *S. haematobium* infections, reversal of urinary tract pathology can be seen six months after a cure. In *S. mansoni* and *S. japonicum* infections, much of the intestinal pathology regresses after chemotherapy. However, more than one PZQ treatment is usually necessary to reverse hepatic pathology, especially in areas of intense transmission. Early intervention with PZQ is preferable to reverse organ pathology.

Intervention Costs

Several studies have evaluated the costs of school-based periodic deworming in several different settings, whereas comparable studies on other interventions are still lacking.

Periodic Deworming. The advantage of periodic deworming lies in its simplicity (one tablet per child) and safety. Teachers and other personnel without medical training can easily apply the simple measures, which can be incorporated without difficulty in existing health and nonhealth activities that reach the high-risk group. Several organizations, including nongovernmental organizations, include an STH and schistosome infection-control package within their routine activities and, with very limited budgets, relieve the burden of helminth infections in the population covered. The costs of albendazole and PZQ are available through the International Drug Price Indicator Guide (http://www.msh.org). Delivery systems for deworming have often depended on vertical programs, in which mobile teams visit schools or communities to carry out treatment (WHO 2002). Estimated costs for this approach are outlined in table 24.2. For STH infections in Tanzania, Nigeria, and Montserrat, the costs range from US$0.21 to US$0.51 per treatment. However, by training teachers and other school officials to administer anthelmintic drugs, the system could achieve low-cost delivery by "piggy-backing" on existing programs in the educational sector (WHO 2002). Specific examples of such programs conducted in Ghana and Tanzania are summarized in the section "Implementation of Control Strategies: Lessons of Experience," later in this chapter. It was found that delivery of school-based targeted anthelmintic treatment could cost as little as US$0.03 per child, which may be as low as one-tenth of the estimated costs for vertical delivery (WHO 2002). Thus, at current drug prices, the total cost (drug plus delivery) of a single treatment with albendazole or mebendazole may be as low as US$0.05, and that of a combined treatment with PZQ may be as low as US$0.25 per child (WHO 2002).

Table 24.2 Recent Examples of Delivery Costs for a Single Mass Treatment

Strategy	Drug	Country	Delivery cost per treatment US$	Percentage of total cost
Mobile team	Albendazole	Montserrat	0.51	67
	Albendazole	Bangladesh	—	42
	Levamisole	Nigeria	0.32	81
	PZQ	Tanzania	0.21	24
School-based	Albendazole	Ghana	0.04	17
	Albendazole	Tanzania	0.03	13
Out-of-school children		Arab Rep. of Egypt	0.16–0.21	40–47

Source: Guyatt 2003.
— = not available.

Integrating drug distribution through the school system rather than using mobile teams, along with a marked decline in the price of BZAs and PZQ, has resulted in a 10-fold reduction in delivery costs. However, those costs are artificially low because they do not include the external costs for the coordinating center responsible for supporting those approaches (Guyatt 2003). It has been estimated, for instance, that mass albendazole treatment of school-age children in Kenya could cost more than US$3 million each year, equivalent to some 4 percent of current national public expenditure on health care (Guyatt 2003). This analysis has not been evaluated against actual operations, however, and current estimates from the parasite control authorities in Kenya suggest that the actual cost is likely to be far less. Large-scale chemotherapy programs for helminth control continue to rely heavily on donor support, suggesting that some affected countries may be unable to support the costs of deworming.

Monitoring of control programs is an important part of the managerial process, and it should be carried out at minimum cost so as not to divert resources from the intervention (Brooker and others 2004). It is recommended that, at the planning stage, approximately 5 to 10 percent of the program budget be reserved for monitoring activities (Montresor and others 2002).

Improved Sanitation. When sanitation improvements are made alongside deworming, the results obtained last longer. However, the investment needed to reach the level required to interfere with STH transmission could be high. To correctly evaluate the advantage of such investments, one must take into account the consequences for other health indicators and for economic development. An efficient sanitation infrastructure removes the underlying cause of most poverty-related communicable diseases and can boost the economic development of a country. The resources needed to improve hygienic standards can be huge and require the cooperation of several sectors of society (Asaolu and Ofoezie 2003). Currently, these are qualitative judgments, and no cost-effectiveness analysis (CEA) estimates exist for sanitation in this context.

Health Education and Communication. Measures to increase the health awareness of the population are included as an essential component of any population-based activity aimed at controlling morbidity attributable to helminth infections. However, the effectiveness of those activities in reducing transmission of infection varies according to different reports. In some cases, health education can decrease costs, increase levels of knowledge, and decrease reinfection rates (Lansdown and others 2002). Health education efforts can build trust and engage communities, aspects that are crucial to the success of public health initiatives. No CEA estimates exist for health education in this context.

Linking Costs and Effects of Interventions

Interventions to reduce morbidity from helminth infections fall into two categories: targeting the transmission mechanisms and treating individuals directly. The former encompasses improvements in infrastructure, including water supply and sanitation, and health education. The latter entails the periodic drug treatment of the population. Substantial improvements through prevention may be a long-term outcome of economic growth in general, because wealthier households have improved sanitation facilities and practices, but those improvements are not an option in the short term without large investments in infrastructure. As shown in the previous section, deworming options dominate on both effectiveness and cost-effectiveness criteria. Costs continue to fall as drug costs decrease. With better data and detailed mapping of disease distribution within communities, targeting individuals at high risk becomes more feasible, thus improving the cost-effectiveness of control programs (Michaud, Gordon, and Reich 2003).

The High Cost-Effectiveness of Mass Treatment for Helminth Infection

The combination of low-cost treatment and high prevalence rates suggests that the cost per DALY averted from treating helminth infections will be quite low. Following the consistent framework described in mass treatment of school-age children for both STH infections and schistosomiasis proves to be extremely cost-effective. In fact, benefit-cost ratios would be even higher if the analyses incorporated the additional benefits associated with externalities for the untreated. For a population of 1 million people in low- and middle-income countries, if treatment is limited to school-age children treated 1.1 times per year with albendazole and then reinfected, the cost per DALY averted is estimated at US$3.41 for STH infections. That is, if spending were capped at US$1 million, total DALYs would be reduced by nearly 300,000. The estimate of cost per DALY is higher for schistosomiasis relative to STH infections because of higher drug costs and lower disability weights. Depending on whether generics or original formulations are used, the cost per DALY averted ranges from US$3.36 to US$6.92. However, in combination, treatment with both albendazole and PZQ proves to be extremely cost effective, in the range of US$8 to US$19 per DALY averted.

Source: Authors.

Evidence from existing programs that narrow the intervention to school-age children (a high-risk group) shows that the treatment costs of chemotherapy for helminth infections are quite low—well below US$1 per school-age child. This finding is in part due to the accessibility of the target group and the cost savings of incorporating delivery into existing school and health programs. Moreover, as discussed in the following sections, the economic benefits of targeting this group may be substantial. Still other targeted groups may also have low cost per treatment when treatment is merged into existing programs. For example, interventions through prenatal care programs for pregnant women may be cost-effective. Likewise, evidence on costs of treatment through existing integrated management of infant and childhood illness (IMCI) programs for small children and health campaigns (such as vaccination and micronutrient programs) find low cost per case treated (Montresor and others 2002).

Several factors can potentially alter the ranking of interventions in regard to cost-effectiveness, although there are no existing studies to evaluate this. Previous analysis may underestimate the effectiveness and overestimate the cost-benefit ratios of mass treatment of school-age children if the externalities of treatment are not considered (Miguel and Kremer 2003). The cost-effectiveness of school-based deworming programs will change as the programs are extended to cover children who are not enrolled in school. Such program extensions are likely to have greater costs because they entail additional staff and outreach efforts per case treated. However, the effectiveness of mass treatment of school-age children (both enrolled and not enrolled) may be greater. Children who are not enrolled in school come from households with lower income levels. Lower income, which leads to poorer sanitation conditions, is associated with greater incidence and intensity of infections. Expanding mass treatment to children not enrolled in school will result in treating populations that have higher incidence and intensity, thus raising effectiveness (box 24.2).

Distributional and Equity Consequences

Interventions to control helminth infections can have equity implications in several dimensions. Programs designed to target communities with high prevalence or high intensity of helminth infection focus on areas with lower income, as described in the sections on the causes, characteristics, and epidemiology of such infections. Although no studies undertake benefit-incidence analysis of public spending on such health services, this targeting implies that state subsidies on deworming services will be of most benefit to lower-income groups. With the increasing availability of poverty maps, empirical evaluation of the equity implications of deworming will be feasible.

AVERTED, AVERTABLE, AND NONAVERTABLE BURDEN

In the short run, deworming can avert helminth infections. In the long run, it is assumed that as income levels grow and infrastructure improves, the number of infections averted by reducing transmission will increase. However, given the slow rate of poverty reduction in the 1990s for the poorest regions, such as Sub-Saharan Africa, waiting for economic development to lead to a reduction in infections is only, at best, a slow-paced solution for the majority of the infected population. It is more likely that most averted infections will depend on periodic deworming. Thus, the question remains as to what portion of existing infections is potentially avertable through recommended interventions and what portion is currently averted with existing programs. For schistosomiasis, successful programs in several countries, including Brazil, China, and the Arab Republic of Egypt, and the issues related to the sustainability of these successes have been described (see "Implementation of Control Strategies: Lessons of Experience" later in this chapter). However, the number of averted schistosomiasis infections in Sub-Saharan Africa is likely to be small, because few serious attempts at widespread control have been made in recent years, and not much of the burden of STH and schistosome infections is currently averted through private treatment. In part, the low number of averted infections may be due to the lack of information on the part of infected individuals, the insidious nature of the condition, and the lack of drugs in the public or private health delivery system.

ECONOMIC BENEFITS OF INTERVENTION

The characteristics of helminth infections make a compelling case for public sector intervention if based only on the evidence related to the intervention's effect on health. From an economic perspective, the public sector has several reasons to become involved in improving health outcomes. First, other benefits may be gained, in addition to the benefit for the treated individual. Second, some forms of intervention are almost pure public goods; that is, no one can be excluded from using the goods or services the interventions deliver, and the private sector is thus unlikely to deliver them. Finally, preventive measures, such as information on the value of washing hands, may not be delivered through the private sector. The lack of knowledge about infections and subclinical symptoms may make individuals less likely to seek treatment. In analyzing the gains of interventions for worm control, one should account for the burden of helminth infections, which extends well beyond the health impacts and DALYs. The economic implications may be quite large.

The negative correlation between helminth infections and income level is clearly demonstrated both within and between countries (de Silva and others 2003). However, causality cannot be inferred from this established relationship; poverty promotes higher worm burdens, yet poor health induced by helminths can lead to lower income. There may also be opportunity costs to uninfected household members residing with infected persons. Few studies have been designed to evaluate, either directly or indirectly, the magnitude of the effect of deworming on economic productivity. The indirect evidence at the micro level suggests that helminth infection has a significant impact on adult productivity and, subsequently, on earnings. More direct evidence for children shows that helminth infection has long-term implications for educational attainment and economic status.

Studies are increasingly documenting a causal impact of adult health (broadly defined) on labor force participation, wages, and productivity in developing countries (Thomas and Strauss 1997). Moreover, helminth infection is known to affect some of the health conditions related to productivity—namely, iron deficiency anemia and wasting. Guyatt (2000) reviews numerous studies relating these conditions to physical fitness and productivity; Haas and Brownlie (2001) review studies on the effect of iron supplementation on work. The studies generally show productivity gains linked to better health along the various health dimensions studied. However, although some evidence points to the indirect impact of STHs on income earnings, these relationships have not been adequately studied, either directly or indirectly.

More compelling links between helminth infection and economic well-being may exist for children. The strong association between worm burden and poor health outcomes for children suggests that infections may affect school enrollment, attendance, grade repetition, and grade attainment. In turn, the potential impact on educational outcomes has implications for the assessment of the economic benefits of intervention. Numerous studies have demonstrated the benefits of schooling, showing that the return on education is quite high. Increased education is associated with, among other things, higher worker productivity and generally higher productivity in nonmarket production activities, including greater farmer efficiency and productivity (Psacharopoulos and Patrinos 2002).

Although observational studies show that lower levels of learning and schooling are linked to helminth infection (World Bank 2003), establishing a causal relationship requires adequately controlling for all unobserved or confounding factors. Miguel and Kremer (2003) note that several methodological issues hamper many existing randomized treatment-control evaluations. First, externalities associated with interventions can lead to underestimating impacts among the untreated population. Second, sample selection and attrition issues can affect the validity of findings, although the direction of this effect is ambiguous. Third, existing studies typically evaluate the impact of deworming on cognitive skills, likely the culmination of several years of health and education investments, as assessed by tests administered to treated and untreated children. Although studies find an effect on cognitive skills for those with the heaviest worm burden, they do not focus on other important education outcomes, which are likely to be more affected in the short run by health improvements, such as school enrollment and school attendance.

The study by Miguel and Kremer (2003) in Kenya attempts to address those shortcomings through improved study design and analytical methods. In addition to providing health gains, deworming reduced total primary school absenteeism by at least one-quarter in the first two years of the project. The gains were largest for the youngest children, who suffered from more

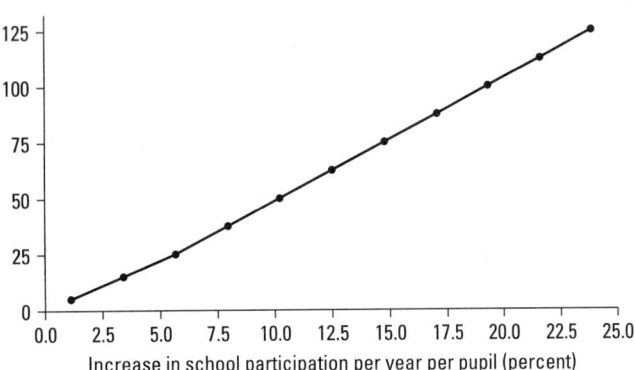

Net presented value of discounted wages (US$)

Note: Assumptions are as follows: a 7 percent return to an additional year of school; wage gains earned over 40 years in the workforce, discounted at 5 percent per year with no wage growth; and annual wage earnings of US$400 per year, which is below the estimated agricultural and nonagricultural annual wages for low-income countries in the World Bank (2003).

Figure 24.3 Returns to School Participation

intense worm infections. Externalities would cause a substantial underestimation of this effect. In terms of cost-effectiveness as an *educational* intervention, deworming proved to be far more effective at improving school attendance than other educational interventions implemented in a study in Kenya. Deworming offers a high rate of return, increasing the net present value of discounted wages by more than US$30 per treated child compared with per treatment costs of under US$1. For realistic estimates of returns to schooling, these results show in general that the net present discounted value of lifetime earnings is high compared with the costs of treatment even for small gains in school participation (figure 24.3).

Bleakley (2003) examined the effect of a hookworm control program undertaken about 1910 in the southern part of the United States. Hookworm infection was estimated to cause a 23 percent drop in the probability of school attendance, and children with greater exposure to the hookworm eradication campaign were more likely to be literate. Moreover, the long-term follow-up of affected cohorts showed that hookworm infection in childhood led to significantly lower wages in adulthood.

Helminth infections in preschool-age children can have consequences for subsequent schooling, such as delaying primary school enrollment and school attainment, thereby affecting future labor market outcomes. Bobonis, Miguel, and Sharma (2003) conducted a study of preschool-age children, using iron supplementation and deworming drugs administered to children two to six years of age. Preliminary results indicate that, in addition to the weight gain associated with treatment, average preschool participation rates increased sharply by 6.3 percentage points among assisted children older than two, reducing preschool absenteeism by roughly one-fifth.

Beyond the current impacts on schooling and implications for cognition, helminth infection in children can have long-term implications for economic outcomes in adulthood through its effect on physical growth. Height has been shown to affect wage-earning capacity as well as participation in the labor force for men and women (Thomas and Strauss 1997). This relationship may be strongest in settings where infection rates are highest—that is, low-income areas, where physical endurance yields high returns in the labor market.

IMPLEMENTATION OF CONTROL STRATEGIES: LESSONS OF EXPERIENCE

Two case studies illustrate the profound health effects of periodic deworming.

Case Study Number 1: Periodic Deworming in Ghana and Tanzania

The Partnership for Child Development (PCD) undertook an evaluation of the use of schools in Ghana and Tanzania for the delivery of health interventions, including research into the processes, costs, and benefits (PCD 1999). The effort also involved operations research and evaluation of programs with regard to health and education outcomes and people's perceptions of the programs (Hall and others 1999). The results demonstrated the following:

- Simple interventions, such as deworming, have the potential to improve children's health and educational achievement, especially for those worst affected and most disadvantaged.
- The delivery of school-based health services is efficient and cost-effective and is supported by the key stakeholders involved. Implementers of the school health programs in the education and health sectors and the community are positive regarding the teacher's role in health provision, as long as the health interventions are simple, safe, familiar, and effective and are seen as responding to local needs.
- The provision of health services through schools need not require long and complex training, nor significantly add to the workload of teachers or administrators.
- Delivery through the existing education sector could occur effectively without any additional infrastructure, as long as the existing educational system is adequately functional.

The results of the evaluation of these programs also highlighted the need for deworming to be carried out in the context of a wider framework of school health, which includes core activities such as effective and nondiscriminatory school health policies, provision of safe water and sanitation, and effective health education (http://www.freshschools.org and http://www.schoolsandhealth.org).

Case Study Number 2: Schistosomiasis Control in Egypt

In 1937, the prevalence of schistosomiasis in rural areas was about 50 percent, almost every boy had blood in his urine by the age of 12, and bladder cancer was the commonest cancer in Egypt. Molluscicides, from copper sulfate to niclosamide, have been used to try to kill the host snails, and drugs from antimony-based compounds, through niridazole, metrifonate, and PZQ, have been used to treat the millions of infected Egyptians. Finally, after a 14-year control campaign using PZQ, the prevalence of schistosomiasis has been reduced to below 10 percent. With infection intensities now low, the serious health consequences of schistosomiasis have disappeared. The program was started in 1988, when using loans from the African Development Bank and the World Bank, Egypt invested heavily in the purchase of PZQ, encouraging local production, to control morbidity caused by schistosomiasis. Since the drug was first made available in 1988, some 45 million doses have been dispensed. A television campaign has encouraged people to submit samples for diagnosis and to receive free treatment if their diagnoses are positive. Since 1997, a mass chemotherapy campaign was used to target populations in high-prevalence villages and children in selected governorates where prevalence was greater than 20 percent. In addition, molluscicides have been applied in canals around high-prevalence villages. The widespread use of PZQ has given dramatic results. Morbidity, including hematuria, has almost disappeared, and bladder cancer is on the decline.

RESEARCH AND DEVELOPMENT

Among the important tasks to be done to control helminth infections are collection of better data on helminth disease burden, research on the health and economic effects (and safety) of periodic deworming, monitoring of the emergence of anthelmintic drug resistance, and development of new tools to supplement or complement existing control strategies.

Health and Economic Impact

Overall, better estimates of disease burden are needed (Michaud, Gordon, and Reich 2003), especially with respect to obtaining a consistent and agreed-on estimate for the DALYs attributed to helminth infections. In a systematic review of randomized deworming trials, Dickson and others (2000) conclude that, although data support the effects of deworming on weight gain, there are inconsistencies among trials and insufficient evidence as to whether such interventions improve cogni-

tive performance. Plausible mechanisms by which helminths suppress growth in childhood and exert negative impacts on intelligence, cognition, and school performance are largely unstudied and unknown. In addition, some reports have questioned whether albendazole itself could adversely affect growth (Forrester and others 1998). Those issues require clarification as widespread deworming programs become more common. The impact of helminths on populations other than schoolchildren, including preschool-age children, women of childbearing age, and adult workers, appears to be substantial. However, those populations are understudied. Also unclear is the impact of childhood STH and schistosome infections on productivity in adulthood. The effect of chemotherapy on many of the manifestations of schistosomiasis has not been assessed systematically. It has been postulated that PZQ treatment of schistosomiasis promotes partial immunity by destroying worms in the vasculature and releasing parasite antigens (Colley and Secor 2004). In contrast, the frequent and periodic treatment of STH infections (Albonico and others 1995) do not appear to promote natural protective immunity.

The role of helminths and coinfections also warrants further exploration. Some studies suggest that HIV-1 infection may promote susceptibility to schistosomiasis (Secor, Karanja, and Colley 2004), and human T-cell lymphotropic virus-1 (HTLV-1) infection may promote susceptibility to strongyloidiasis. In addition, emerging evidence indicates that STH and schistosome infections may promote susceptibility to other infectious agents, possibly including HIV/AIDS and malaria (Fincham, Markus, and Adams 2003). This phenomenon, if verified in an epidemiologic study, would further increase helminth-associated DALY estimates.

Anthelmintic Drug Resistance and New Drug Development

A concern about the feasibility of sustainable control with BZAs is the possible emergence of drug resistance among human STHs. BZA resistance occurs because of the spread of point mutations in nematode-tubulin alleles. This phenomenon has already resulted in widespread BZA drug resistance among STHs of ruminant livestock. There is still no direct evidence for BZA resistance among human STHs, although such resistance could account for an observed failure of mebendazole for human hookworm in southern Mali, as well as a diminished efficacy against hookworm in Zanzibar following frequent and periodic use of mebendazole (Albonico and others 2003). PZQ resistance must also be considered, especially as it begins to be widely used in Sub-Saharan Africa (Hagan and others 2004). Should PZQ resistance develop, there will be new demands for antischistosomal drugs. Recently, the artemisins have shown activity against schistosomulae and were successful in protecting against *S. japonicum* in China (Hagan and others 2004).

Anthelmintic Vaccines

The high rates of reinfection that can occur following treatment with anthelmintic drugs and concern about emerging drug resistance have prompted the search for alternative control tools. For most helminth infections, reduction in adult worm burden has been considered the "gold standard" for vaccine development. For schistosomiasis, however, a vaccine that targets parasite fecundity and egg viability, thereby reducing pathology and transmission, would also represent an important breakthrough. A 28-kDa glutathione S-transferase (GST) has shown promise as a protective antigen for *S. haematobium* infection (Capron and others 2005). The *S. haematobium* vaccine project based on GST has successfully passed phase 1 testing; the research group, which is based at the Pasteur Institute, is embarking on phase 2 clinical trials in Senegal and Niger. Additional schistosomiasis vaccines are also undergoing early-stage development. Efforts are also under way by the Human Hookworm Vaccine Initiative to develop and test a first-generation recombinant hookworm vaccine (Brooker and others 2005; Hotez, Bethony, and others 2005). The first vaccine manufactured under current good manufacturing practices and tested for quality control and toxicity is the *Na*-ASP-2 hookworm vaccine, which was developed from research demonstrating human correlates of immunity and partial protection data in vaccinated laboratory animals. Phase 1 human trials for evaluating the safety and immunogenicity of the *Na*-ASP-2 hookworm vaccine are in progress. Additional research is needed to determine how an anthelmintic vaccine can be incorporated into existing control programs, as well how it would be used for at-risk populations not currently targeted for periodic deworming in schools.

CONCLUSIONS: PROMISES AND PITFALLS

Fulfilling the mandate of World Health Assembly resolution 54.19 will require the regular treatment of hundreds of millions of children over decades. The obstacles in this undertaking are formidable, and success will depend on the ability of countries to identify or create reliable and sustained infrastructures for this purpose. A focus on using preexisting school systems may be key to achieving this goal. The treatment of schoolchildren for *A. lumbricoides*, *T. trichiura*, and schistosome infections achieves large externalities that reduce infection in other vulnerable age groups. However, the different epidemiology of hookworm raises concerns about the risks to preschool children and women of reproductive age who remain untreated. Providing regular treatment to these populations appears to be a less cost-effective option, largely because of the absence of a preexisting infrastructure. This situation presents a strong argument for developing a hookworm vaccine that could be used to protect these vulnerable groups. It has yet to be seen whether the emergence of BZA drug resistance is a genuine concern that could derail global deworming efforts in much the same way that resistance to DDT and chloroquine has affected the ambitions for global malaria control. It is possible that the specific dynamics of helminth populations will provide sufficient genetic flow to maintain susceptibility in much the same way that insecticides remain the effective staple of global agribusiness. Until new technologies become available, anthelmintic chemotherapy for school-age children remains the most practical and substantive means to control STH and schistosome infections in the developing world.

REFERENCES

Adams, V. J., C. J. Lombard, M. A. Dhansay, M. B. Markus, and J. E. Fincham. 2004. "Efficacy of Albendazole against the Whipworm *Trichuris Trichiura*—A Randomized, Controlled Trial." *South African Medical Journal* 94: 972–76.

Albonico, M., Q. Bickle, M. Ramsan, A. Montresor, L. Savioli, and M. Taylor. 2003. "Efficacy of Mebendazole and Levamisole Alone or in Combination against Intestinal Nematode Infections after Repeated Targeted Mebendazole Treatment in Zanzibar." *Bulletin of the World Health Organization* 81: 343–52.

Albonico, M., A. Montresor, D. W. Crompton, and L. Savioli. Forthcoming. "Intervention for the Control of Soil-Transmitted Helminthiasis." *Advances in Parasitology.*

Albonico, M., E. Renganathan, A. Bosman, U. M. Kisumku, K. S. Alawi, and L. Savioli. 1994. "Efficacy of a Single Dose of Mebendazole on Prevalence and Intensity of Soil-Transmitted Nematodes in Zanzibar." *Tropical and Geographic Medicine* 46: 142–46.

Albonico, M., P. G. Smith, E. Ercole, A. Hall, H. M. Chwaya, K. S. Alawi, and L. Savioli. 1995. "Rate of Reinfection with Intestinal Nematodes after Treatment of Children with Mebendazole or Albendazole in a Highly Endemic Area." *Transactions of the Royal Society of Tropical Medicine and Hygiene* 89: 538–41.

Anderson, R. M., and R. M. May. 1991. *Infectious Diseases of Humans.* Oxford, U.K.: Oxford University Press.

Asaolu, S. O., and I. E. Ofoezie. 2003. "The Role of Health Education and Sanitation in the Control of Helminth Infections." *Acta Tropica* 86: 283–94.

Bethony, J., J. T. Williams, H. Kloos, J. Blangero, L. Alves-Fraga, G. Buck, and others. 2001. "Exposure to *Schistosoma mansoni* Infection in a Rural Area in Brazil: II. Household Risk Factors." *Tropical Medicine and International Health* 6: 136–45.

Bleakley, H. 2003. "Disease and Development: Evidence from Hookworm Eradication in the American South." *Journal of the European Economic Association* 1: 376–86.

Bobonis, G., E. Miguel, C. Sharma. 2003. "Iron Deficiency Anemia and School Participation." University of California–Berkeley. http://emlab.berkeley.edu/users/emiguel/miguel_anemia.pdf.

Brooker, S., J. Bethony, and P. J. Hotez. 2004. "Human Hookworm Infection in the 21st Century." *Advances in Parasitology* 58: 197–288.

Brooker, S., J. M. Bethony, L. Rodrigues, N. Alexander, S. Geiger, and P. J. Hotez. 2005. "Epidemiological, Immunological and Practical Considerations in Developing and Evaluating a Human Hookworm Vaccine." *Expert Review of Vaccines* 4: 35–50.

Brooker, S., and E. Michael. 2000. "The Potential of Geographical Information Systems and Remote Sensing in the Epidemiology and Control of Human Helminth Infections." *Advances in Parasitology* 47: 245–87.

Brooker, S., S. Whawell, N. B. Kabatereine, A. Fenwick, and R. M. Anderson. 2004. "Evaluating the Epidemiological Impact of National Control Programmes for Helminths." *Trends in Parasitology* 11: 537–45.

Bundy, D. A. 1995. "Epidemiology and Transmission of Intestinal Helminths." In *Enteric Infection 2, Intestinal Helminths,* ed. M. J. G. Farthing, G. T. Keusch, and D. Wakelin, 5–24. London: Chapman & Hall Medical.

Bundy, D. A., M. S. Chan, and L. Savioli. 1995. "Hookworm Infection in Pregnancy." *Transactions of the Royal Society of Tropical Medicine and Hygiene* 89: 521–22.

Bundy, D. A., M. S. Wong, L. L. Lewis, and J. Horton. 1990. "Control of Geohelminths by Delivery of Targeted Chemotherapy through Schools." *Transactions of the Royal Society of Tropical Medicine and Hygiene* 84: 115–20.

Capron, A., G. Riveau, M. Capron, and F. Trottein. 2005. "Schistosomes: The Road from Host-Parasite Interactions to Vaccines in Clinical Trials." *Trends in Parasitology* 21: 143–49.

Chan, M. S., G. F. Medley, D. Jamison, and D. A. Bundy. 1994. "The Evaluation of Potential Global Morbidity Attributable to Intestinal Nematode Infections." *Parasitology* 109: 373–87.

Christian, P., S. K. Khatry, and K. P. West. 2004. "Antenatal Anthelmintic Treatment, Birthweight, and Infant Survival in Rural Nepal." *Lancet* 364: 981–83.

Colley, D. G., and E. W. Secor. 2004. "Immunoregulation and World Health Assembly Resolution 54.19: Why Does Treatment Control Morbidity?" *Parasitology International* 53: 143–50.

Crompton, D. W. 1999. "How Much Helminthiasis Is There in the World?" *Journal of Parasitology* 85: 397–403.

———. 2001. "Ascaris and Ascariasis." *Advances in Parasitology* 48: 285–375.

Crompton, D. W., and L. Savioli. 1993. "Intestinal Parasitic Infections and Urbanization." *Bulletin of the World Health Organization* 71: 1–7.

de Silva, N. R., S. Brooker, P. J. Hotez, A. Montresor, D. Engles, and L. Savioli. 2003. "Soil-Transmitted Helminth Infections: Updating the Global Picture." *Trends in Parasitology* 19: 547–51.

de Silva, N. R., M. S. Chan, and D. A. P. Bundy. 1997. "Morbidity and Mortality Due to Ascariasis: Re-estimation and Sensitivity Analysis of Global Numbers at Risk." *Tropical Medicine and International Health* 2: 519–28.

Dickson, R., S. Awasthi, P. Williamson, C. Demellweek, and P. Garner. 2000. "Effects of Treatment for Intestinal Helminth Infection on Growth and Cognitive Performance in Children: Systematic Review of Randomised Trials." *British Medical Journal* 320: 1697–701.

Drake, L. J., M. C. H. Jukes, R. J. Sternberg, and D. A. P. Bundy. 2000. "Geohelminth Infections (Ascariasis, Trichuriasis, and Hookworm): Cognitive and Developmental Impacts." *Seminars in Pediatric Infectious Diseases* 11: 245–51.

Fenwick, A., L. Savioli, D. Engels, N. R. Bergquist, and M. H. Todd. 2003. "Drugs for the Control of Parasitic Diseases: Current Status and Development in Schistosomiasis." *Trends in Parasitology* 19: 509–15.

Fincham, J. E., M. B. Markus, and V. J. Adams. 2003. "Could Control of Soil-Transmitted Helminthic Infection Influence the HIV/AIDS Pandemic?" *Acta Tropica* 86: 315–33.

Forrester, J. E., J. C. Bailar III, S. A. Esrey, M. V. Jose, B. T. Castillejos, and G. Ocamp. 1998. "Randomised Trial of Albendazole and Pyrantel in Symptomless Trichuriasis in Children." *Lancet* 353: 1103–8.

Guyatt, H. L. 2000. "Do Intestinal Nematodes Affect Productivity in Adulthood?" *Parasitology Today* 16: 153–58.

———. 2003. "The Cost of Delivering and Sustaining a Control Programme for Schistosomiasis and Soil-Transmitted Helminthiasis." *Acta Tropica* 86: 267–74.

Haas, J. D., and T. Brownlie. 2001. "Iron Deficiency and Reduced Work Capacity: A Critical Review of the Research to Determine a Causal Relationship." *Journal of Nutrition* 131 (Suppl.): 676S–88S.

Hagan, P., C. C. Appleton, G. C. Coles, J. R. Kusel, and L. A. Tchuem-Tchuente. 2004. "Schistosomiasis Control: Keep Taking the Tablets." *Trends in Parasitology* 20: 92–97.

Hall, A., C. Nokes, S. T. Wen, S. Adjei, C. Kihamia, L. Mwanri, and others. 1999. "Alternatives to Bodyweight for Estimating the Dose of Praziquantel Needed to Treat Schistosomiasis." *Transactions of the Royal Society of Tropical Medicine and Hygiene* 93: 652–58.

Hotez, P. J., S. Arora, J. Bethony, M. E. Bottazzi, A. Loukas, R. Correa-Oliveira, and S. Brooker. 2005. "Helminth Infections of Children: Prospects for Control." In *Hot Topics in Infection and Immunity in Children,* ed. A. J. Pollard and A. Finn. New York: Springer.

Hotez, P. J., J. Bethony, M. E. Bottazzi, S. Brooker, and P. Buss. 2005. "Hookworm—'The Great Infection of Mankind.'" *Public Library of Science Medicine* 2: e67.

Hotez, P. J., S. Brooker, J. M. Bethony, M. E. Bottazzi, A. Loukas, and S. H. Xiao. 2004. "Current Concepts: Hookworm Infection." *New England Journal of Medicine* 351: 799–807.

Kabatereine, N. B., B. J. Vennervald, J. H. Ouma, J. Kemijumbi, A. E. Butterworth, D. W. Dunne, and A. J. Fulford. 1999. "Adult Resistance to Schistosomiasis Mansoni: Age-Dependence to Reinfection Remains Constant in Communities with Diverse Exposure Patterns." *Parasitology* 118: 101–5.

King, C. H., K. Dickman, and D. J. Tisch. 2005. "Reassessment of the Cost of Chronic Helmintic Infection: A Meta-analysis of Disability-Related Outcomes in Endemic Schistosomiasis." *Lancet* 365: 1561–69.

Lansdown, R., A. Ledward, A. Hall, W. Issac, E. Yona, J. Matulu, and others. 2002. "Schistosomiasis, Helminth Infection, and Health Education in Tanzania: Achieving Behaviour Change in Primary Schools." *Health Education Research* 17: 425–33.

Michaud, C. M., W. S. Gordon, and M. R. Reich. 2003. "The Global Burden of Disease Due to Schistosomiasis." Disease Control Priorities Project Working Paper 19. http://www.fic.nih.gov/dcpp/wps/wp19.pdf.

Miguel, E. A., and M. Kremer. 2003. "Worms: Identifying Impacts on Education and Health in the Presence of Treatment Externalities." *Econometrica* 72 (1): 159–217.

Montresor, A., D. W. T. Crompton, T. W. Gyorkos, and L. Savioli. 2002. *Helminth Control in School-Age Children: A Guide for Managers of Control Programmes.* Geneva: World Health Organization.

PCD (Partnership for Child Development). 1999. "The Cost of Large-Scale School Health Programmes Which Deliver Anthelmintics to Children in Ghana and Tanzania." *Acta Tropica* 73 (2): 183–204.

Psacharopoulos, G., and H. Patrinos. 2002. "Returns to Investment in Education: A Further Update." Working Paper 2881, World Bank, Washington, DC.

Quinnell, R. J. 2003. "Genetics of Susceptibility to Human Helminth Infection." *International Journal of Parasitology* 33: 1219–31.

Richter, J. 2003. "The Impact of Chemotherapy on Morbidity Due to Schistosomiasis." *Acta Tropica* 86: 161–83.

Ross, A. G., P. B. Bartley, A. C. Sleigh, G. R. Olds, Y. Li, G. M. Williams, and D. P. McManus. 2002. "Schistosomiasis." *New England Journal of Medicine* 346: 1212–20.

Secor, W. E., D. M. Karanja, and D. G. Colley. 2004. "Interactions between Schistosomiasis and Human Immunodeficiency Virus in Western Kenya." *Memorias do Instituto Oswaldo Cruz* 99 (5 Suppl. 1): 93–95.

Stephenson, L. S., M. C. Latham, and E. A. Ottesen. 2000. "Malnutrition and Parasitic Helminth Infections." *Parasitology* 121 (Suppl.): S23–28.

Stoltzfus, R. J., H. M. Chwaya, A. Montresor, J. M. Tielsch, J. K. Jape, M. Albonico, and L. Savioli. 2004. "Low Dose Daily Iron Supplementation Improves Iron Status and Appetite but Not Anemia, Whereas Quarterly Anthelmintic Treatment Improves Growth, Appetite, and Anemia in Zanzibari Preschool Children." *Journal of Nutrition* 134: 348–56.

Stoltzfus, R. J., M. L. Dreyfuss, H. M. Chwaya, and M. Albonico. 1997. "Hookworm Control as a Strategy to Prevent Iron Deficiency Anemia." *Nutrition Reviews* 55: 223–32.

Thomas, D., and J. Strauss. 1997. "Health and Wages: Evidence on Men and Women in Urban Brazil." *Journal of Econometrics* 77: 159–85.

Van der Werf, M. J., S. J. de Vlas, S. Brooker, C. W. Looman, N. J. Nagelkerke, J. D. Habbema, and D. Engels. 2003. "Quantification of Clinical Morbidity Associated with Schistosome Infection in Sub-Saharan Africa." *Acta Tropica* 86: 125–39.

WHO (World Health Organization). 2002. *Prevention and Control of Schistosomiasis and Soil-Transmitted Helminthiasis.* WHO Technical Series Report 912. Geneva: WHO.

World Bank. 2003. *School Deworming at a Glance.* Public Health at a Glance Series. http://www.worldbank.org/hnp.

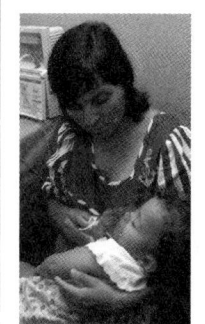

Chapter **25**

Acute Respiratory Infections in Children

Eric A. F. Simoes, Thomas Cherian, Jeffrey Chow, Sonbol Shahid-Salles, Ramanan Laxminarayan, and T. Jacob John

Acute respiratory infections (ARIs) are classified as upper respiratory tract infections (URIs) or lower respiratory tract infections (LRIs). The upper respiratory tract consists of the airways from the nostrils to the vocal cords in the larynx, including the paranasal sinuses and the middle ear. The lower respiratory tract covers the continuation of the airways from the trachea and bronchi to the bronchioles and the alveoli. ARIs are not confined to the respiratory tract and have systemic effects because of possible extension of infection or microbial toxins, inflammation, and reduced lung function. Diphtheria, pertussis (whooping cough), and measles are vaccine-preventable diseases that may have a respiratory tract component but also affect other systems; they are discussed in chapter 20.

Except during the neonatal period, ARIs are the most common causes of both illness and mortality in children under five, who average three to six episodes of ARIs annually regardless of where they live or what their economic situation is (Kamath and others 1969; Monto and Ullman 1974). However, the proportion of mild to severe disease varies between high- and low-income countries, and because of differences in specific etiologies and risk factors, the severity of LRIs in children under five is worse in developing countries, resulting in a higher case-fatality rate. Although medical care can to some extent mitigate both severity and fatality, many severe LRIs do not respond to therapy, largely because of the lack of highly effective antiviral drugs. Some 10.8 million children die each year (Black, Morris, and Bryce 2003). Estimates indicate that in 2000, 1.9 million of them died because of ARIs, 70 percent of them in Africa and Southeast Asia (Williams and others 2002). The World Health Organization (WHO) estimates that 2 million children under five die of pneumonia each year (Bryce and others 2005).

CAUSES OF ARIs AND THE BURDEN OF DISEASE

ARIs in children take a heavy toll on life, especially where medical care is not available or is not sought.

Upper Respiratory Tract Infections

URIs are the most common infectious diseases. They include rhinitis (common cold), sinusitis, ear infections, acute pharyngitis or tonsillopharyngitis, epiglottitis, and laryngitis—of which ear infections and pharyngitis cause the more severe complications (deafness and acute rheumatic fever, respectively). The vast majority of URIs have a viral etiology. Rhinoviruses account for 25 to 30 percent of URIs; respiratory syncytial viruses (RSVs), parainfluenza and influenza viruses, human metapneumovirus, and adenoviruses for 25 to 35 percent; corona viruses for 10 percent; and unidentified viruses for the remainder (Denny 1995). Because most URIs are self-limiting, their complications are more important than the infections. Acute viral infections predispose children to bacterial infections of the sinuses and middle ear (Berman 1995a), and aspiration of infected secretions and cells can result in LRIs.

Acute Pharyngitis. Acute pharyngitis is caused by viruses in more than 70 percent of cases in young children. Mild pharyngeal redness and swelling and tonsil enlargement are typical. Streptococcal infection is rare in children under five and more common in older children. In countries with crowded living conditions and populations that may have a genetic predisposition, poststreptococcal sequelae such as acute rheumatic fever and carditis are common in school-age children but may also occur in those under five. Acute pharyngitis in conjunction with the development of a membrane on the throat is nearly always caused by *Corynebacterium diphtheriae* in developing countries. However, with the almost universal vaccination of infants with the DTP (diphtheria-tetanus-pertussis) vaccine, diphtheria is rare.

Acute Ear Infection. Acute ear infection occurs with up to 30 percent of URIs. In developing countries with inadequate medical care, it may lead to perforated eardrums and chronic ear discharge in later childhood and ultimately to hearing impairment or deafness (Berman 1995b). Chronic ear infection following repeated episodes of acute ear infection is common in developing countries, affecting 2 to 6 percent of school-age children. The associated hearing loss may be disabling and may affect learning. Repeated ear infections may lead to mastoiditis, which in turn may spread infection to the meninges. Mastoiditis and other complications of URIs account for nearly 5 percent of all ARI deaths worldwide (Williams and others 2002).

Lower Respiratory Tract Infections

The common LRIs in children are pneumonia and bronchiolitis. The respiratory rate is a valuable clinical sign for diagnosing acute LRI in children who are coughing and breathing rapidly. The presence of lower chest wall indrawing identifies more severe disease (E. Mulholland and others 1992; Shann, Hart, and Thomas 1984).

Currently, the most common causes of viral LRIs are RSVs. They tend to be highly seasonal, unlike parainfluenza viruses, the next most common cause of viral LRIs. The epidemiology of influenza viruses in children in developing countries deserves urgent investigation because safe and effective vaccines are available. Before the effective use of measles vaccine, the measles virus was the most important viral cause of respiratory tract–related morbidity and mortality in children in developing countries.

Pneumonia. Both bacteria and viruses can cause pneumonia. Bacterial pneumonia is often caused by *Streptococcus pneumoniae* (pneumococcus) or *Haemophilus influenzae,* mostly type b (Hib), and occasionally by *Staphylococcus aureus* or other streptococci. Just 8 to 12 of the many types of pneumococcus cause most cases of bacterial pneumonia, although the specific types may vary between adults and children and between geographic locations. Other pathogens, such as *Mycoplasma pneumoniae* and *Chlamydia pneumoniae,* cause atypical pneumonias. Their role as a cause of severe disease in children under five in developing countries is unclear.

The burden of LRIs caused by Hib or *S. pneumoniae* is difficult to determine because current techniques to establish bacterial etiology lack sensitivity and specificity. The results of pharyngeal cultures do not always reveal the pathogen that is the cause of the LRI. Bacterial cultures of lung aspirate specimens are often considered the gold standard, but they are not practical for field application. Vuori-Holopainen and Peltola's (2001) review of several studies indicates that *S. pneumoniae* and Hib account for 13 to 34 percent and 1.4 to 42.0 percent of bacterial pneumonia, respectively, whereas studies by Adegbola and others (1994), Shann, Gratten, and others (1984), and Wall and others (1986) suggest that Hib accounts for 5 to 11 percent of pneumonia cases.

Reduced levels of clinical or radiological pneumonia in clinical trials of a nine-valent pneumococcal conjugate vaccine provide an estimate of the vaccine-preventable disease burden (*valency* indicates the number of serotypes against which the vaccine provides protection; *conjugate* refers to conjugation of polysaccharides to a protein backbone). In a study in The Gambia, 37 percent of radiological pneumonia was prevented, reflecting the amount of disease caused by *S. pneumoniae,* and mortality was reduced by 16 percent (Cutts and others 2005).

Upper respiratory tract colonization with potentially pathogenic organisms and aspiration of the contaminated secretions have been implicated in the pathogenesis of bacterial pneumonia in young children. Infection of the upper respiratory tract with influenza virus or RSVs has been shown to increase the binding of both *H. influenzae* (Jiang and others 1999) and *S. pneumoniae* (Hament and others 2004; McCullers and Bartmess 2003) to lining cells in the nasopharynx. This finding may explain why increased rates of pneumococcal pneumonia parallel influenza and RSV epidemics. A study in South Africa showed that vaccination with a nine-valent pneumococcal conjugate vaccine reduced the incidence of virus-associated pneumonia causing hospitalization by 31 percent, suggesting that pneumococcus plays an important role in the pathogenesis of virus-associated pneumonia (Madhi, Petersen, Madhi, Wasas, and others 2000).

Entry of bacteria from the gut with spread through the bloodstream to the lungs has also been proposed for the pathogenesis of Gram-negative organisms (Fiddian-Green and Baker 1991), but such bacteria are uncommon etiological agents of pneumonia in immune-competent children. However, in neonates and young infants, Gram-negative pneumonia is not uncommon (Quiambao forthcoming).

Viruses are responsible for 40 to 50 percent of infection in infants and children hospitalized for pneumonia in developing countries (Hortal and others 1990; John and others 1991; Tupasi and others 1990). Measles virus, RSVs, parainfluenza viruses, influenza type A virus, and adenoviruses are the most important causes of viral pneumonia. Differentiating between viral and bacterial pneumonias radiographically is difficult, partly because the lesions look similar and partly because bacterial superinfection occurs with influenza, measles, and RSV infections (Ghafoor and others 1990).

In developing countries, the case-fatality rate in children with viral pneumonia ranges from 1.0 to 7.3 percent (John and others 1991; Stensballe, Devasundaram, and Simoes 2003), with bacterial pneumonia from 10 to 14 percent and with mixed viral and bacterial infections from 16 to 18 percent (Ghafoor and others 1990; Shann 1986).

Bronchiolitis. Bronchiolitis occurs predominantly in the first year of life and with decreasing frequency in the second and third years. The clinical features are rapid breathing and lower chest wall indrawing, fever in one-third of cases, and wheezing (Cherian and others 1990). Inflammatory obstruction of the small airways, which leads to hyperinflation of the lungs, and collapse of segments of the lung occur. Because the signs and symptoms are also characteristic of pneumonia, health workers may find differentiating between bronchiolitis and pneumonia difficult. Two features that may help are a definition of the seasonality of RSVs in the locality and the skill to detect wheezing. RSVs are the main cause of bronchiolitis worldwide and can cause up to 70 or 80 percent of LRIs during high season (Simoes 1999; Stensballe, Devasundaram, and Simoes 2003). The recently discovered human metapneumovirus also causes bronchiolitis (Van den Hoogen and others 2001) that is indistinguishable from RSV disease. Other viruses that cause bronchiolitis include parainfluenza virus type 3 and influenza viruses.

Influenza. Even though influenza viruses usually cause URIs in adults, they are increasingly being recognized as an important cause of LRIs in children and perhaps the second most important cause after RSVs of hospitalization of children with an ARI (Neuzil and others 2002). Although influenza is considered infrequent in developing countries, its epidemiology remains to be investigated thoroughly. The potential burden of influenza as a cause of death in children is unknown. Influenza virus type A may cause seasonal outbreaks, and type B may cause sporadic infection. Recently, avian influenza virus has caused infection, disease, and death in small numbers of individuals, including children, in a few Asian countries. Its potential for emergence in human outbreaks or a pandemic is unknown, but it could have devastating consequences in developing countries (Peiris and others 2004) and could pose a threat to health worldwide. New strains of type A viruses will almost certainly arise through mutation, as occurred in the case of the Asian and Hong Kong pandemics in the 1950s and 1960s.

HIV Infection and Pediatric LRIs

Worldwide, 3.2 million children are living with HIV/AIDS, 85 percent of them in Sub-Saharan Africa (UNAIDS 2002). In southern Africa, HIV-related LRIs account for 30 to 40 percent of pediatric admissions and have a case-fatality rate of 15 to 34 percent, much higher than the 5 to 10 percent for children not infected with HIV (Bobat and others 1999; Madhi, Petersen, Madhi, Khoosal, and others 2000; Nathoo and others 1993; Zwi, Pettifor, and Soderlund 1999). *Pneumocystis jiroveci* and cytomegalovirus are important opportunistic infections in more than 50 percent of HIV-infected infants (Jeena, Coovadia, and Chrystal 1996; Lucas and others 1996). Gram-negative bacteria are also important in more than 70 percent of HIV-infected malnourished children (Ikeogu, Wolf, and Mathe 1997). Patient studies have confirmed the frequent association of these bacteria but added *S. pneumoniae* and *S. aureus* as important pathogens (Gilks 1993; Goel and others 1999). The first South African report on the overall burden of invasive pneumococcal disease reported a 41.7-fold increase in HIV-infected children compared with uninfected children (Farley and others 1994).

INTERVENTIONS

Interventions to control ARIs can be divided into four basic categories: immunization against specific pathogens, early diagnosis and treatment of disease, improvements in nutrition, and safer environments (John 1994). The first two fall within the purview of the health system, whereas the last two fall under public health and require multisectoral involvement.

Vaccinations

Widespread use of vaccines against measles, diphtheria, pertussis, Hib, pneumococcus, and influenza has the potential to substantially reduce the incidence of ARIs in children in developing countries. The effects of measles, diphtheria, and pertussis vaccines are discussed in chapter 20. The limited data on influenza in developing countries do not permit detailed analysis of the potential benefits of that vaccine. This chapter, therefore, focuses on the potential effects of Hib and pneumococcal vaccines on LRIs.

Hib Vaccine. Currently three Hib conjugate vaccines are available for use in infants and young children. The efficacy of Hib vaccine in preventing invasive disease (mainly meningitis, but also pneumonia), has been well documented in several studies in industrialized countries (Black and others 1992; Booy and others 1994; Eskola and others 1990; Fritzell and Plotkin 1992; Heath 1998; Lagos and others 1996; Santosham and others 1991) and in one study in The Gambia (K. Mulholland and others 1997). All studies showed protective efficacy greater than 90 percent against laboratory-confirmed invasive disease, irrespective of the choice of vaccine. Consequently, all industrialized countries include Hib vaccine in their national immunization programs, resulting in the virtual elimination of invasive Hib disease because of immunity in those vaccinated and a herd effect in those not vaccinated. Available data from a few developing countries show a similar herd effect (Adegbola and others 1999; Wenger and others 1999).

The initial promise and consequent general perception was that Hib vaccine was to protect against meningitis, but in developing countries the vaccine is likely to have a greater effect on preventing LRIs. The easily measured effect is on invasive disease, including bacteraemic pneumonia. The vaccine probably has an effect on nonbacteremic pneumonia, but this effect is difficult to quantify because of the lack of an adequate method for establishing bacterial etiology. In Bangladesh, Brazil, Chile, and The Gambia, Hib vaccine has been associated with a reduction of 20 to 30 percent in those hospitalized with radiographically confirmed pneumonia (de Andrade and others 2004; Levine and others 1999; K. Mulholland and others 1997; WHO 2004a). However, results of a large study in Lombok, Indonesia, were inconclusive with regard to the effect of Hib vaccine on pneumonia (Gessner and others 2005).

Pneumococcal Vaccines. Two kinds of vaccines are currently available against pneumococci: a 23-valent polysaccharide vaccine (23-PSV), which is more appropriate for adults than children, and a 7-valent protein-conjugated polysaccharide vaccine (7-PCV). A 9-valent vaccine (9-PCV) has undergone clinical trials in The Gambia and South Africa, and an 11-valent vaccine (11-PCV) is being tried in the Philippines.

Studies of the efficacy of the polysaccharide vaccine in preventing ARIs or ear infection in children in industrialized countries have shown conflicting results. Whereas some studies of this vaccine show no significant efficacy (Douglas and Miles 1984; Sloyer, Ploussard, and Howie 1981), studies from Finland show a generally protective effect against the serotypes contained in a 14-PSV (Douglas and Miles 1984; Karma and others 1980; Makela and others 1980). The efficacy was more marked in children over two years of age than in younger children. The only studies evaluating the effect of the polysaccharide vaccine in children in developing countries are a series of three trials conducted in Papua New Guinea (Douglas and Miles 1984; Lehmann and others 1991; Riley and others 1981; Riley, Lehmann, and Alpers 1991). The analysis of the pooled data from these trials showed a 59 percent reduction in LRI mortality in children under five at the time of the vaccination and a 50 percent reduction in children under two. On the basis of these and other studies, the investigators concluded that the vaccine had an effect on severe pneumonia. The greater-than-expected efficacy in these trials was attributed to the greater contribution of the more immunogenic adult serotypes in pneumonia in Papua New Guinea (Douglas and Miles 1984; Riley, Lehmann, and Alpers 1991). On account of the poor immunogenicity of the antigens in the 23-PSV against prevalent pediatric serotypes, attention is now directed at more

immunogenic conjugate vaccines (Mulholland 1998; Obaro 1998; Temple 1991).

The 7-PCV and 9-PCV have been evaluated for efficacy against invasive pneumococcal disease in four trials, which demonstrated a vaccine efficiency ranging from 71.0 to 97.4 percent (58 to 65 percent for HIV-positive children, among whom rates of pneumococcal disease are 40 times higher than in HIV-negative children) (Black and others 2000; Cutts and others 2005; Klugman and others 2003; O'Brien and others 2003).

In the United States, the 7-PCV was included in routine vaccinations of infants and children under two in 2000. By 2001 the incidence of all invasive pneumococcal disease in this age group had declined by 69 percent and disease caused by the serotypes included in the vaccine and related serotypes had declined by 78 percent (Whitney and others 2003). Similar reductions were confirmed in a study in northern California (Black and others 2001). A slight increase in rates of invasive disease caused by serotypes of pneumococcus not included in the vaccine was observed, but it was not large enough to offset the substantial reduction in disease brought about by the vaccine. The studies also found a significant reduction in invasive pneumococcal disease in unvaccinated older age groups, especially adults age 20 to 39 and age 65 and older, suggesting that giving the vaccine to young children exerted a considerable herd effect in the community. Such an advantage is likely to occur even where the prevalence of adult HIV disease is high and pneumococcal disease may be recurrent and life threatening.

The effect of the vaccine on pneumococcal pneumonia as such is difficult to define given the problems of establishing the bacterial etiology of pneumonia. Three studies have evaluated the effect of the vaccine on radiographic pneumonia (irrespective of the etiological agent) and have shown a 20.5 to 37.0 percent reduction in radiographically confirmed pneumonia (9.0 percent for HIV-positive individuals) (Black and others 2000; Cutts and others 2005; Klugman and others 2003).

Several field trials have evaluated the efficacy of PCV against ear infection. Even though the vaccine resulted in a significant reduction in culture-confirmed pneumococcal otitis, no net reduction of ear infection was apparent among vaccinated children, probably because of an increase in the rates of otitis caused by types of pneumococci not covered by the vaccine, *H. influenzae* and *Moraxella catarrhalis* (Eskola and others 2001; Kilpi and others 2003). However, a trial in northern California showed that the vaccine had a protective effect against frequent ear infection and reduced the need for tympanostomy tube placement (Fireman and others 2003). Thus, a vaccine for ear infection may be beneficial in developing countries with high rates of chronic otitis and conductive hearing loss and should be evaluated by means of clinical trials.

The most striking public health benefit of a vaccine in developing countries would be a demonstrable reduction in mortality. Although the primary outcome in The Gambia trial was initially child mortality, it was changed to radiological pneumonia. Nevertheless, the trial showed a 16 percent (95 percent confidence level, 3 to 38) reduction in mortality. This trial was conducted in a rural area in eastern Gambia where access to round-the-clock curative care, including case management, is difficult to provide. This trial demonstrates that immunization delivered through outreach programs will have substantial health and economic benefits in such populations. One additional study evaluating the effect of an 11-PCV on radiological pneumonia is ongoing in the Philippines; results are expected in the second half of 2005.

Case Management

The simplification and systematization of case management for early diagnosis and treatment of ARIs have enabled significant reductions in mortality in developing countries, where access to pediatricians is limited. WHO clinical guidelines for ARI case management (WHO 1991) use two key clinical signs: *respiratory rate*, to distinguish children with pneumonia from those without, and *lower chest wall indrawing*, to identify severe pneumonia requiring referral and hospital admission. Children with audible stridor when calm and at rest or such danger signs of severe disease as inability to feed also require referral. Children without these signs are classified as having an ARI but not pneumonia. Children showing only rapid breathing are treated for pneumonia with outpatient antibiotic therapy. Children who have a cough for more than 30 days are referred for further assessment of tuberculosis and other chronic infections.

Pneumonia Diagnosis Based on Rapid Breathing. The initial guidelines for detecting pneumonia based on rapid breathing were developed in Papua New Guinea during the 1970s. In a study of 200 consecutive pediatric outpatients and 50 consecutive admissions (Shann, Hart, and Thomas 1984), 72 percent of children with audible crackles in the lungs had a respiratory rate of 50 or more breaths per minute, whereas only 19 percent of children without crackles breathed at such a rapid rate. Therefore, the initial WHO guidelines used a threshold of 50 breaths per minute, at or above which a child with a cough was regarded as having pneumonia.

The major concern was the relatively low sensitivity of this approach, which could miss 25 to 40 percent of cases of pneumonia. A study in Vellore, India, found that sensitivity could be improved by lowering the threshold to 40 for children age 1 to 4, while keeping the 50 breaths per minute cutoff for infants age 2 months through 11 months (Cherian and others 1988). Subsequent studies showed that when these thresholds were used, sensitivity improved from 62 to 79 percent in the Philippines and from 65 to 77 percent in Swaziland, but at the same time, the specificity fell from 92 to 77 percent in the Philippines and 92 to 80 percent in Swaziland (Mulholland and

others 1992). On the basis of these and other data (Campbell, Byass, and others 1989; Kolstad and others 1997; Perkins and others 1997; Redd 1994; Simoes and others 1997; Weber and others 1997), WHO recommends a respiratory rate cutoff of 50 breaths per minute for infants age 2 through 11 months and 40 breaths per minute for children age 12 months to 5 years.

Rapid breathing, as defined by WHO, detects about 85 percent of children with pneumonia, and more than 80 percent of children with potentially fatal pneumonia are probably successfully identified and treated using the WHO diagnostic criteria. Antibiotic treatment of children with rapid breathing has been shown to reduce mortality (Sazawal and Black 2003). The problem of the low specificity of the rapid breathing criterion is that some 70 to 80 percent of children who may not need antibiotics will receive them. Nevertheless, for primary care workers for whom diagnostic simplicity is essential, rapid breathing is clearly the most useful clinical sign.

Pneumonia Diagnosis Based on Chest Wall Indrawing. Children are admitted to hospital with severe pneumonia when health workers believe that oxygen or parenteral antibiotics (antibiotics administered by other than oral means) are needed or when they lack confidence in mothers' ability to cope. The rationale of parenteral antibiotics is to achieve higher levels of antibiotics and to overcome concerns about the absorption of oral drugs in ill children.

The Papua New Guinea study (Shann, Hart, and Thomas 1984) used chest wall indrawing as the main indicator of severity, but studies from different parts of the world show large differences in the rates of indrawing because of variable definitions. Restriction of the term to lower chest wall indrawing, defined as inward movement of the bony structures of the chest wall with inspiration, has provided a better indicator of the severity of pneumonia and one that can be taught to health workers. It is more specific than intercostal indrawing, which frequently occurs in bronchiolitis.

In a study in The Gambia (Campbell, Byass, and others 1989), a cohort of 500 children from birth to four years old was visited at home weekly for one year. During this time, 222 episodes of LRI (rapid breathing, any chest wall indrawing, nasal flaring, wheezing, stridor, or danger signs) were referred to the clinic. Chest indrawing was present in 62 percent of these cases, many with intercostal indrawing. If all children with any chest indrawing were hospitalized, the numbers would overwhelm pediatric inpatient facilities.

Studies in the Philippines and Swaziland (E. Mulholland and others 1992) found that lower chest wall indrawing was more specific than intercostal indrawing for a diagnosis of severe pneumonia requiring hospital admission. In the Vellore study (Cherian and others 1988), lower chest wall indrawing correctly predicted 79 percent of children with an LRI who were hospitalized by a pediatrician.

Antimicrobial Options for Oral Treatment of Pneumonia. The choice of an antimicrobial drug for treatment is based on the well-established finding that most childhood bacterial pneumonias are caused by *S. pneumoniae* or *H. influenzae*. A single injection of benzathine penicillin, although long lasting, does not provide adequate penicillin levels to eliminate *H. influenzae*. WHO has technical documents to help assess the relevant factors in selecting first- and second-line antimicrobials and comparisons of different antimicrobials in relation to their antibacterial activity, treatment efficacy, and toxicity (WHO 1990).

The emergence of antimicrobial resistance in *S. pneumoniae* and *H. influenzae* is a serious concern. In some settings, in vitro tests show that more than 50 percent of respiratory isolates of both bacteria are resistant to co-trimoxazole, and penicillin resistance to *S. pneumoniae* is gradually becoming a problem worldwide.

In pneumonia, unlike in meningitis, in vitro resistance of the pathogen does not always translate into treatment failure. Reports from Spain and South Africa suggest that pneumonia caused by penicillin-resistant *S. pneumoniae* can be successfully treated with sufficiently high doses of penicillin. Amoxicillin is concentrated in tissues and in macrophages, and drug levels are directly correlated with oral dosages. Therefore, higher doses than in the past—given twice a day—are now being used to successfully treat ear infections caused by penicillin-resistant *S. pneumoniae*. Amoxicillin is clearly better than penicillin for such infections. The situation with co-trimoxazole is less clear (Strauss and others 1998), and in the face of high rates of co-trimoxazole resistance, amoxicillin may be superior for children with severe pneumonia.

Intramuscular Antibiotics for Treatment of Severe Pneumonia. Even though chloramphenicol is active against both *S. pneumoniae* and *H. influenzae,* its oral absorption is erratic in extremely sick children. Thus, the WHO guidelines recommend giving intramuscular chloramphenicol at half the daily dose before urgent referral of severe pneumonia cases. An additional rationale is that extremely sick children may have sepsis or meningitis that are difficult to rule out and must be treated immediately. Although intravenous chloramphenicol is superior to intramuscular chloramphenicol, the procedure can delay urgently needed treatment and adds to its cost.

Investigators have questioned the adequacy and safety of intramuscular chloramphenicol. Although early studies suggested that adult blood levels after intramuscular administration were significantly less than those achieved after intravenous administration, the intramuscular route gained wide acceptance following clinical reports that confirmed its efficacy. Local complications of intramuscular chloramphenicol succinate are rare, unlike the earlier intramuscular preparations. Although concerns about aplastic anemia following chloramphenicol are common, this complication is extremely rare in young children. There is no evidence that intramuscular chloramphenicol succinate is more likely to produce side effects than other forms and routes of chloramphenicol.

Hypoxemia Diagnosis Based on WHO Criteria. The ARI case-management and integrated management of infant and childhood illness (IMCI) strategies depend on accurate referral of sick children to a hospital and correct inpatient management of LRI with oxygen or antibiotics. Hypoxemia (deficiency of oxygen in the blood) in children with LRI is a good predictor of mortality, the case-fatality rate being 1.2 to 4.6 times higher in hypoxemic LRI than nonhypoxemic LRI (Duke, Mgone, and Frank 2001; Onyango and others 1993), and oxygen reduces mortality. Thus, it is important to detect hypoxemia as early as possible in children with LRI to avert death. Although diagnoses of acute LRIs are achieved very easily by recognizing tachypnoea, and although severe LRI is associated with chest wall indrawing, the clinical recognition of hypoxemia is more problematic. Different sets of clinical rules have been studied to predict the presence of hypoxemia in children with LRI (Cherian and others 1988; Onyango and others 1993; Usen and others 1999). Although some clinical tools have a high sensitivity for detecting hypoxemia, a good number of hypoxemic children would still be missed using these criteria. Pulse oximetry is the best tool to quickly detect hypoxemia in sick children. However, pulse oximeters are expensive and have recurring costs for replacing probes, for which reasons they are not available in most district or even referral hospitals in developing countries.

Treatment Guidelines. Current recommendations are for co-trimoxazole twice a day for five days for pneumonia and intramuscular penicillin or chloramphenicol for children with severe pneumonia. The problems of increasing resistance to co-trimoxazole and unnecessary referrals of children with any chest wall indrawing have led to studies exploring alternatives to the antibiotics currently used in ARI case management. One study indicated that amoxicillin and co-trimoxazole are equally effective for nonsevere pneumonia (Catchup Study Group 2002), though amoxicillin costs twice as much as co-trimoxazole. With respect to the duration of antibiotic treatment, studies in Bangladesh, India, and Indonesia indicate that three days of oral co-trimoxazole or amoxicillin are as effective as five days of either drug in children with nonsevere pneumonia (Agarwal and others 2004; Kartasasmita 2003). In a multicenter study of intramuscular penicillin versus oral amoxicillin in children with severe pneumonia, Addo-Yobo and others (2004) find similar cure rates. Because patients were treated with oxygen when needed for hypoxemia and were switched to other antibiotics if the treatment failed, this regimen is not appropriate for treating severe pneumonia in an outpatient setting.

WHO recommends administering oxygen, if there is ample supply, to children with signs and symptoms of severe pneumonia and, where supply is limited, to children with any of the following signs: inability to feed and drink, cyanosis, respiratory rate greater than or equal to 70 breaths per minute, or severe chest wall retractions (WHO 1993). Oxygen should be administered at a rate of 0.5 liter per minute for children younger than 2 months and 1 liter per minute for older children. Because oxygen is expensive and supply is scarce, especially in remote rural areas in developing countries, WHO recommends simple clinical signs to detect and treat hypoxemia. Despite those recommendations, a study of 21 first-level facilities and district hospitals in seven developing countries found that more than 50 percent of hospitalized children with LRI were inappropriately treated with antibiotics or oxygen (Nolan and others 2001)—and in several, oxygen was in short supply. Clearly, providing oxygen to hypoxemic babies is lifesaving, though no randomized trials have been done to prove it.

Prevention and Treatment of Pneumonia in HIV-Positive Children. Current recommendations of a WHO panel for managing pneumonia in HIV-positive children and for prophylaxis of *Pneumocystis jiroveci* are as follows (WHO 2003):

- *Nonsevere pneumonia up to age 5 years.* Oral co-trimoxazole should remain the first-line antibiotic, but oral amoxicillin should be used if it is affordable or if the child has been on co-trimoxazole prophylaxis.
- *Severe or very severe pneumonia.* Normal WHO case-management guidelines should be used for children up to 2 months old. For children from 2 to 11 months, injectable antibiotics and therapy for *Pneumocystis jiroveci* pneumonia are recommended, as is starting *Pneumocystis jiroveci* pneumonia prophylaxis on recovery. For children age 12 to 59 months, the treatment consists of injectable antibiotics and therapy for *Pneumocystis jiroveci* pneumonia. *Pneumocystis jiroveci* pneumonia prophylaxis should be given for 15 months to children born to HIV-infected mothers; however, this recommendation has seldom been implemented.

COST-EFFECTIVENESS OF INTERVENTIONS

Pneumonia is responsible for about a fifth of the estimated 10.6 million deaths per year of children under five. Where primary health care is weak, reducing mortality through public health measures is a high priority. As noted earlier, the available interventions are primary prevention by vaccination and secondary prevention by early case detection and management.

The cost-effectiveness of Hib vaccines is discussed in chapter 20. We did not attempt an analysis of the cost-effectiveness of pneumococcal vaccines, because global and regional estimates of the pneumococcal pneumonia burden are currently being developed and will not be available until later in 2005. In addition, current vaccine prices are relatively stable in developed countries, but the prices for low- and middle-income countries are expected to be substantially lower when vaccines are purchased through a global tender.

We evaluate case-management intervention strategies for LRIs in children under five. Health workers who implement case management diagnose LRIs on the basis of fast breathing, lower chest wall indrawing, or selected danger signs in children with respiratory symptoms. Because this method does not distinguish between pneumonia and bronchiolitis, nor between bacterial and viral pneumonia, we group these conditions into the general category of "clinical pneumonia" (Rudan and others 2004). This approach assumes that a high proportion of clinical pneumonia is of bacterial origin and that health workers can considerably reduce case fatality through breathing rate diagnosis and timely administration of antibiotics (Sazawal and Black 2003). We calculated treatment costs by World Bank region using standardized input costs provided by the volume editors and costs published in the *International Drug Price Indicator Guide* (Management Sciences for Health 2005) and other literature (table 25.1). The analysis addresses four categories of case management, which are distinguished by the severity of the infection and the point of treatment:

- nonsevere pneumonia treated by a community health worker
- nonsevere pneumonia treated at a health facility
- severe pneumonia treated at a hospital
- very severe pneumonia treated at a hospital.

Information about these categories of case management and their outcomes is drawn from a report on the methodology and assumptions used to estimate the costs of scaling up selected health interventions aimed at children (WHO and Child Adolescent Health forthcoming). We assumed a total of three follow-up visits for each patient treated by a community health worker rather than the twice-daily follow-ups for 10 days recommended by the report. We also assumed that all severe pneumonia patients receive an x-ray examination, rather than just 20 percent as suggested by the report. Moreover, we assumed a five-hour workday for a community health worker, the minimum workday required for community health workers under the Child Health and Survival initiative of the U.S. Agency for International Development (Bhattacharyya and others 2001).

Table 25.2 presents region-specific estimates of average treatment costs per episode for the four case-management strategies. Because we considered the prices of tradable commodities such as drugs and oxygen to be constant across

Table 25.1 Inputs for Case Management of Pneumonia in Low- and Middle-Income Countries

Condition and intervention	Cost per unit (2001 US$)	Quantity	Percentage of patients
Nonsevere pneumonia at the community level			
Oral amoxicillin (15 mg/kg)	0.03/dose	3 doses/day for 3 days	100
Acetaminophen (100-mg tablet)	0.001/dose	6 doses	100
Community health worker hour[a]	1.83/hour	1 initial 1-hour visit and 3 follow-up visits	100
Nonsevere pneumonia at the facility level			
Oral amoxicillin (15 mg/kg)	0.03/dose	3 doses/day for 3 days	100
Acetaminophen (100-mg tablet)	0.001/dose	6 doses	100
Oral salbutamol (2-mg tablet)	0.003/dose	3 doses/day for 4 days	10
Outpatient health facility visit[a]	1.72/visit	1 visit	100
Severe pneumonia at the hospital level			
Oral amoxicillin (15 mg/kg)	0.03/dose	3 doses/day for 5 days	100
Nebulized salbutamol (2.5 mg)	0.13/dose	6 doses/day for 4 days	50
Injectable ampicillin (50 mg/kg)	0.21/dose	4 doses/day for 3 days	100
X-ray[a]	9.21/test	1 test	100
Oxygen (1 liter/minute)[b]	20/day	3.5 days	50
Inpatient hospital care[a]	10.8/day	3 days	100
Very severe pneumonia at the hospital level			
Oral amoxicillin (15 mg/kg)	0.03/dose	3 doses/day for 5 days	100
Nebulized salbutamol (2.5 mg)	0.13/dose	6 doses/day for 4 days	50
Injectable ampicillin (50 mg/kg)	0.21/dose	4 doses/day for 5 days	100
Injectable gentamicin (2.5 mg/kg)	0.14/dose	1 dose/day for 10 days	100
Oral prednisolone (1 mg/kg)	0.02/dose	1 dose/day for 3 days	5
X-ray[a]	9.21/test	1 test	100
Oxygen (1 liter/minute)[b]	20/day	5 days	100
Inpatient hospital care[a]	10.8/day	5 days	100

Source: Management Sciences for Health 2005.
Note: We assumed that the average patient weighs 12.5 kilograms.
a. Provided by the volume editors. Input costs vary by region.
b. Median costs obtained from Dobson 1991; Pederson and Nyrop 1991; Schneider 2001; WHO 1993.

Table 25.2 Average per Episode Treatment Costs of Case-Management Interventions for Acute Lower Respiratory Infection *(2001 US$)*

Region	Nonsevere, community level	Nonsevere, facility level	Severe, hospital level	Very severe, hospital level
Low- and middle-income countries	8	2	82	172
East Asia and the Pacific	6	2	75	160
Latin America and the Caribbean	13	4	134	256
Middle East and North Africa	22	3	113	223
South Asia	5	2	66	148
Sub-Saharan Africa	7	2	64	145

Source: Authors' calculations.

regions, regional variations were due to differences in hospital and health worker costs. Latin America and the Caribbean and the Middle East and North Africa had the highest treatment costs.

We calculated region-specific cost-effectiveness ratios (CERs) for a model population of 1 million in each region, following the standardized guidelines for economic analyses (see chapter 15 for details). Input variables included the treatment costs detailed in tables 25.1 and 25.2, region-specific LRI morbidity rates, adapted from Rudan and others (2004), region-specific mortality rates and age structures provided by the volume editors, and region-specific urban to rural population ratios (World Bank 2002). The Europe and Central Asia region was excluded from this analysis because of a lack of incidence information. In the absence of region-specific information, we assumed uniform intervention effectiveness rates.

Disability-adjusted life years are averted through reduced duration of illness and decreased mortality with treatment. We assumed an average illness duration of 8.5 days for those not treated and of 6.0 days for those treated. We used a case-fatality reduction of 36.0 percent on account of treatment (Sazawal and Black 2003) and a diagnosis specificity of 78.5 percent for patients diagnosed based on breath rate alone. The disability weight cotemporaneous with infection was 0.28. We did not consider disabilities caused by chronic sequelae of LRIs because it is unclear whether childhood LRI causes long-term impaired lung function or whether children who develop impaired lung function are more prone to infection (von Mutius 2001).

Because a single year of these interventions yields only cotemporaneous benefits—because effectively treated individuals do not necessarily live to life expectancy given that they are likely to be infected again the following year—we calculated the cost-effectiveness of a five-year intervention. This time period enabled us to consider the case in which an entire cohort of newborns to four-year-olds avoids early childhood clinical pneumonia mortality because of the intervention and receives the benefit of living to life expectancy. Finally, this analysis considered only long-run marginal costs, which vary with the number of individuals treated, and did not include the fixed costs of initiating a program where none currently exists.

Table 25.3 presents the region-specific CERs of the four case-management categories as well as the CER for providing all four categories to a population of 1 million people. Among all low- and middle-income countries, treatment of nonsevere clinical pneumonia was more cost-effective at the facility level

than at the community level, and of all four case-management categories, treatment of very severe clinical pneumonia at the hospital level was the least cost-effective. Treatment of non-severe clinical pneumonia at the facility level was more cost-effective than treatment by a community health worker because of the lower cost of a single visit to a health facility than of multiple visits by a health worker. The CER of providing all levels of treatment to all low- and middle-income countries was estimated at US$398 per disability-adjusted life year.

Because we assumed that effectiveness rates were constant, regional variations in the CER for each case-management category were due only to variations in the intervention costs, and the relative cost-effectiveness rankings for the strategies was the same for all the regions. Variation in the CERs for providing all categories of care was also due to region-specific urban to rural population ratios. We assumed that all patients in urban areas seek treatment at the facility level or higher, whereas 80 percent of nonseverely ill patients in rural areas receive treatment at the community level and the remainder seek treatment at the facility level.

IMPLEMENTATION OF ARI CONTROL STRATEGIES: LESSONS OF EXPERIENCE

The lessons of ARI prevention and control strategies that have been implemented by national programs include the vaccination and case-management strategies discussed below.

Vaccine Strategies

Hib vaccine was introduced into the routine infant immunization schedule in North America and Western Europe in the early 1990s. With the establishment of the Global Alliance for Vaccines and Immunization (GAVI) and the Vaccine Fund, progress is being made in introducing it in developing countries, although major hurdles remain. By 2002, only 84 of the 193 WHO member nations had introduced Hib vaccine. Five

Table 25.3 CERs of Case-Management Interventions for Pneumonia
(2001US$/disability-adjusted life year)

Region	Nonsevere, community level	Nonsevere, facility level	Severe, hospital level	Very severe, hospital level	Provision of all four interventions
Low- and middle-income countries	208	50	2,916	6,144	398
East Asia and the Pacific	439	91	6,511	13,945	900
Latin America and the Caribbean	547	424	14,719	28,106	1,941
Middle East and North Africa	733	180	6,810	13,438	1,060
South Asia	140	28	1,931	4,318	264
Sub-Saharan Africa	139	24	1,486	3,376	218

Source: Authors' calculations.

countries have since been approved for support from GAVI for Hib vaccine introduction in 2004–5.

The United States added 7-PCV to the infant immunization program in 2000. Several other industrialized countries have plans to introduce the vaccine into their national immunization programs in 2005, whereas others recommend the use of the vaccine only in selected high-risk groups. In some of these last countries, the definition of *high risk* is quite broad and includes a sizable proportion of all infants. The currently licensed 7-PCV lacks certain serotypes important in developing countries, but the 9-PCV and 11-PCV would cover almost 80 percent of serotypes that cause serious disease worldwide.

Despite the success of Hib vaccine in industrial countries and the generally appreciated importance of LRIs as a cause of childhood mortality, as a result of a number of interlinked factors, uptake in developing countries has been slow. Sustained use of the vaccine is threatened in a few of the countries that have introduced the vaccine. First, the magnitude of disease and death caused by Hib is not recognized in these countries, partly because of their underuse of bacteriological diagnosis (a result of the lack of facilities and resources). Second, because the coverage achieved with traditional Expanded Program on Immunization vaccines remains low in many countries, adding more vaccines has not been identified as a priority. Third, developing countries did not initiate efforts to establish the utility of the vaccine until after the vaccine had been licensed and used routinely for several years in industrialized countries. Consequently, Hib vaccination has been perceived as an intervention for rich countries. As a result of all these factors, actual demand for the vaccine has remained low, even when support has been available through GAVI and the Vaccine Fund.

In 2004, the GAVI board commissioned a Hib task force to explore how best to support national efforts to make evidence-based decisions about introducing the Hib vaccine. On the basis of the task force's recommendations, the GAVI board approved establishment of the Hib Initiative to support those countries wishing either to sustain established Hib vaccination or to explore whether introducing Hib vaccine should be a priority for their health systems. A consortium consisting of the Johns Hopkins Bloomberg School of Public Health, the London School of Hygiene and Tropical Medicine, the Centers for Disease Control and Prevention, and the WHO has been selected to lead this effort.

Case-Management Strategies

Sazawal and Black's (2003) meta-analysis of community-based trials of the ARI case-management strategy includes 10 studies that assessed its effects on mortality, 7 with a concurrent control group. The meta-analysis found an all-cause mortality reduction of 27 percent among neonates, 20 percent among infants, and 24 percent among children age one to four. LRI-specific mortality was reduced by 42, 36, and 36 percent, respectively. These data clearly show that relatively simplified, but standardized, ARI case management can have a significant effect on mortality, not only from pneumonia, but also from other causes in children from birth to age four. Currently, the ARI case-management strategy has been incorporated into the IMCI strategy, which is now implemented in more than 80 countries (see chapter 63).

Despite the huge loss of life to pneumonia each year, the promise inherent in simplified case management has not been successfully realized globally. One main reason is the underuse of health facilities in countries or communities in which many children die from ARIs. In Bangladesh, for example, 92 percent of sick children are not taken to appropriate health facilities (WHO 2002). In Bolivia, 62 percent of children who died had not been taken to a health care provider when ill (Aguilar and others 1998). In Guinea, 61 percent of sick children who died had not been taken to a health care provider (Schumacher and others 2002). Schellenberg and others' (2003) study in Tanzania shows that children of poorer families are less likely to receive antibiotics for pneumonia than children of better-off families and that only 41 percent of sick children are taken to a health facility. Thus, studies consistently confirm that sick children, especially from poor families, do not attend health facilities.

A number of countries have established large-scale, sustainable programs for treatment at the community level:

- The Gambia has a national program for community-level management of pneumonia (WHO 2004b).
- In the Siaya district of Kenya, a nongovernmental organization efficiently provides treatment by community health workers for pneumonia and other childhood diseases (WHO 2004b).
- In Honduras, ARI management has been incorporated in the National Integrated Community Child Care Program, whereby community volunteers conduct growth monitoring, provide health education, and treat pneumonia and diarrhea in more than 1,800 communities (WHO 2004b).
- In Bangladesh, the Bangladesh Rural Advancement Committee and the government introduced an ARI control program covering 10 subdistricts, using volunteer community health workers. Each worker is responsible for treating childhood pneumonia in some 100 to 120 households after a three-day training program.
- In Nepal during 1986–89, a community-based program for management of ARIs and diarrheal disease was tested in two districts and showed substantial reductions in LRI mortality (Pandey and others 1989, 1991). As a result, the program was integrated into Nepal's health services and is being implemented in 17 of the country's 75 districts by female community health volunteers trained to detect and treat pneumonia.

- In Pakistan, the Lady Health Worker Program employs approximately 70,000 women, who work in communities providing education and management of childhood pneumonia to more than 30 million people (WHO 2004b).

RESEARCH AND DEVELOPMENT AGENDA

The research and development agenda outlined below summarizes the priorities that have been established by advisory groups to the Initiative for Vaccine Research (vaccine intervention strategies) and the WHO Division of the Child and Adolescent Health (case-management strategies).

Vaccine Intervention Strategies

The GAVI task force on Hib immunization made a number of recommendations that vary depending on the country. Countries that have introduced Hib vaccine should focus on documenting its effect and should use the data to inform national authorities, development partners, and other agencies involved in public health to ensure sustained support to such vaccination programs. Countries eligible for GAVI support that have not yet introduced Hib vaccines are often hindered by a lack of local data and a lack of awareness of regional data. They can address these issues through subregional meetings at which country experts can pool data and review information from other countries. In addition, most of the countries need to carry out economic analyses that are based on a standardized instrument. Finally, all countries that face a high Hib disease burden need to develop laboratory facilities so that they can establish the incidence of Hib meningitis at selected sites. Countries in which the disease burden remains unclear may have limited capacity to document the occurrence of Hib disease using protocols that are based on surveillance for meningitis invasive disease. They will need to explore the possibilities of using alternative methods for measuring disease burden, including the use of vaccine-probe studies.

On the basis of experience with introducing Hib and hepatitis B vaccines, GAVI took a proactive approach and in 2003 established an initiative based at the Johns Hopkins School of Public Health in Baltimore to implement an accelerated development and introduction program for pneumococcal vaccines (the PneumoADIP; see http://www.preventpneumonia.org). The program's intent is to establish and communicate the value of pneumococcal vaccines and to support their delivery. Establishing the value of the vaccine involves developing local evidence about the burden of disease and the vaccines' potential effect on public health. This effort can be accomplished through enhanced disease surveillance and relevant clinical trials in a selected number of lead countries. Once established, the evidence base will be communicated to decision makers and key opinion leaders to ensure that data-driven decisions are made. Once the cost-effectiveness of routine vaccination is established, delivery systems will have to be established, and countries will need financial support so that the vaccines can be introduced into their immunization programs. These activities are being initiated before the launch of vaccine formulations designed for use in developing countries, so as to inform capacity planning, product availability, and pricing.

Case-Management Strategies

In 2003, WHO's Division of Child and Adolescent Health convened a meeting to review data and evidence from recent ARI case-management studies and to suggest the following revisions to case-management guidelines and future research priorities:

- Nonsevere pneumonia:
  — Improve the specificity of clinical diagnostic criteria.
  — Reassess WHO's current recommended criteria for detecting and managing treatment failure, given the high rates of therapy failure.
  — Reanalyze data from short-course therapy studies to better identify determinants of treatment failure.
  — Carry out placebo-controlled trials among children presenting with wheezing and pneumonia in selected settings that have a high prevalence of wheezing to determine whether such children need antibiotics.
- Severe pneumonia: In a randomized clinical trial in a controlled environment, Addo-Yobo and others (2004) showed that oral amoxicillin is as effective as parenteral penicillin or ampicillin; however, the following actions need to be undertaken before it can be recommended on a general basis:
  — Analyze data on exclusions from the trial.
  — Identify predictors that may help distinguish children who require hospitalization and who subsequently deteriorate.
  — Reassess WHO's current recommended treatment failure criteria for severe pneumonia, given the overall high rates of therapy failure.
  — Conduct descriptive studies in a public health setting in several centers worldwide, to evaluate the clinical outcomes of oral amoxicillin in children age 2 to 59 months who present with lower chest wall indrawing.
  — Document the effectiveness of WHO's treatment guidelines for managing children with pneumonia and HIV infection.
- LRI deaths:
  — To help develop more effective interventions to reduce LRI mortality, study the epidemiology of LRI deaths in various regions in detail, using routine and advanced laboratory techniques.
- Oxygen therapy:
  — Carry out studies to show the effectiveness of oxygen for managing severe respiratory infections.

— Collect baseline information about the availability and delivery of oxygen and its use in hospital settings in low-income countries.

— Explore the utility of pulse oximetry for optimizing oxygen therapy in various clinical settings.

— Undertake studies to improve the specificity of clinical signs in the overlapping signs and symptoms of malaria and pneumonia.

— Study rapid diagnostic tests for malaria to assess their effectiveness in differentiating between malaria and pneumonia.

— Examine the effect of widespread use of co-trimoxazole on sulfadoxine-pyrimethamine resistance to *Plasmodium falciparum*.

• Etiology: Data on the etiology of pneumonia in children are somewhat out of date, and new etiological studies are needed that use modern technology to identify pathogens.

CONCLUSIONS: PROMISES AND PITFALLS

The evidence clearly shows that the WHO case-management approach and the wider use of available vaccines will reduce ARI mortality among young children by half to two-thirds. The systematic application of simplified case management alone, the cost of which is low enough to be affordable by almost any developing country, will reduce ARI mortality by at least one-third. The urgent need is to translate this information into actual implementation.

The case-management strategy has to be applied and prospectively evaluated so that emerging problems of antimicrobial resistance, reduced efficacy of current treatment with the recommended antimicrobials, or emergence of unexpected pathogens can be detected early and remedial steps can be taken rapidly. If community-level action by health workers is supplemented by the introduction of the IMCI strategy at all levels of primary care, then both applying and evaluating this strategy will be easier. Such synergy may also help in gathering information that will help further fine-tune clinical signs, so that even village health workers can better distinguish bronchiolitis and wheezing from bacterial pneumonia. The criticism that the case-management steps may result in overuse of antimicrobials should be countered by documenting their current overuse and incorrect use by doctors and other health workers. Although there is a resurgent interest in basing interventions at the community level, our analysis suggests that doing so may not be cost-effective. Indeed, ARI case management at the first-level facility may still be the most cost-effective when coupled with better care-seeking behavior interventions.

The international medical community is only beginning to appreciate the potential benefits of Hib and pneumococcal vaccines. They are currently expensive compared with Expanded Program on Immunization vaccines, but the price of Hib vaccine may fall with the entry of more manufacturers into the market in the next few years. Nevertheless, convincing evidence of the vaccines' cost-effectiveness is required to facilitate national decisions on introducing the vaccine and using it sustainedly. In low-income countries, positive cost-benefit and cost-effectiveness ratios alone appear to be insufficient to enable the introduction of these vaccines into national immunization programs.

REFERENCES

Addo-Yobo, E., N. Chisaka, M. Hassan, P. Hibberd, J. M. Lozano, P. Jeena, and others. 2004. "Oral Amoxicillin versus Injectable Penicillin for Severe Pneumonia in Children Aged 3 to 59 Months: A Randomised Multicentre Equivalency Study." *Lancet* 364 (9440): 1141–48.

Adegbola, R. A., A. G. Falade, B. E. Sam, M. Aidoo, I. Baldeh, D. Hazlett, and others. 1994. "The Etiology of Pneumonia in Malnourished and Well-Nourished Gambian Children." *Pediatric Infectious Disease Journal* 13 (11): 975–82.

Adegbola, R. A., S. O. Usen, M. Weber, N. Lloyd-Evans, K. Jobe, K. Mulholland, and others. 1999. "*Haemophilus influenzae* Type B Meningitis in The Gambia after Introduction of a Conjugate Vaccine." *Lancet* 354 (9184): 1091–92.

Agarwal, G., S. Awasthi, S. K. Kabra, A. Kaul, S. Singhi, and S. D. Walter (ISCAP Study Group). 2004. "Three-Day versus Five-Day Treatment with Amoxicillin for Non-Severe Pneumonia in Young Children: A Multicentre Randomised Controlled Trial." *British Medical Journal* 328: 791. http://bmj.bmjjournals.com/cgi/content/full/328/7443/791.

Aguilar, A. M., R. Alvarado, D. Cordero, P. Kelly, A. Zamora, and R. Salgado. 1998. *Mortality Survey in Bolivia: The Final Report—Investigating and Identifying the Causes of Death for Children under Five.* Vienna, VA: Basic Support for Institutionalizing Child Survival Project.

Berman, S. 1995a. "Otitis Media in Children" *New England Journal of Medicine* 332 (23): 1560–65.

———. 1995b. "Otitis Media in Developing Countries." *Pediatrics* 96 (1, part 1): 126–31.

Bhattacharyya, K., P. Winch, K. LeBan, and M. Tien. 2001. "Community Health Worker Incentives and Disincentives: How They Affect Motivation, Retention, and Sustainability." Basic Support for Institutionalizing Child Survival Project for the U.S. Agency for International Development, Arlington, VA.

Black, R. E., S. S. Morris, and J. Bryce. 2003. "Where and Why Are 10 Million Children Dying Every Year?" *Lancet* 361 (9376): 2226–34.

Black, S. B., H. R. Shinefield, B. Fireman, E. Lewis, P. Ray, J. R. Hansen, and others (Northern California Kaiser Permanente Vaccine Study Center Group). 2000. "Efficacy, Safety, and Immunogenicity of Heptavalent Pneumococcal Conjugate Vaccine in Children." *Pediatric Infectious Disease Journal* 19 (3): 187–95.

Black, S. B., H. R. Shinefield, B. Fireman, and R. Hiatt. 1992. "Safety, Immunogenicity, and Efficacy in Infancy of Oligosaccharide Conjugate *Haemophilus influenzae* Type B Vaccine in a United States Population: Possible Implications for Optimal Use." *Journal of Infectious Diseases* 165 (Suppl. 43): S139–43.

Black, S. B., H. R. Shinefield, J. Hansen, L. Elvin, D. Laufer, and F. Malinoski. 2001. "Postlicensure Evaluation of the Effectiveness of Seven-Valent Pneumococcal Conjugate Vaccine." *Pediatric Infectious Disease Journal* 20 (12): 1105–7.

Bobat, R., H. M. Coovadia, D. Moodley, and A. Coutsoudis. 1999. "Mortality in a Cohort of Children Born to HIV–1 Infected Women from Durban, South Africa." *South African Medical Journal* 89 (6): 646–48.

Booy, R., S. Hodgson, L. Carpenter, R. T. Mayon-White, M. P. Slack, J. A. Macfarlane, and others. 1994. "Efficacy of *Haemophilus influenzae* Type B Conjugate Vaccine PRP-T." *Lancet* 344 (8919): 362–66.

Bryce, J., C. Boschi-Pinto, K. Shibuya, R. E. Black, and the WHO Child Health Epidemiology Reference Group. 2005. "WHO Estimates of the Causes of Death in Children." *Lancet* 365: 1147–52.

Campbell, H., J. R. M. Armstrong, and P. Byass. 1989. "Indoor Air Pollution in Developing Countries and Acute Respiratory Infection in Children." *Lancet* 1 (8645): 1012.

Campbell, H., P. Byass, A. C. Lamont, I. M. Forgie, K. P. O'Neill, N. Lloyd-Eans, and B. M. Greenwood. 1989. "Assessment of Clinical Criteria for Identification of Severe Acute Lower Respiratory Tract Infections in Children." *Lancet* 1 (8633): 297–99.

Catchup Study Group. 2002. "Clinical Efficacy of Co-Trimoxazole versus Amoxicillin Twice Daily for Treatment of Pneumonia: A Randomized Controlled Clinical Trial in Pakistan." *Archives of Disease in Childhood* 86: 113–18.

Cherian, T., T. J. John, E. A. Simoes, M. C. Steinhoff, and M. John. 1988. "Evaluation of Simple Clinical Signs for the Diagnosis of Acute Lower Respiratory Tract Infection." *Lancet* 2: 125–28.

Cherian, T., E. A. Simoes, M. C. Steinhoff, K. Chitra, M. John, P. Raghupathy, and others. 1990. "Bronchiolitis in Tropical South India." *American Journal of Diseases of Children* 144 (9): 1026–30.

Cutts, F. T., S. M. A. Zaman, G. Enwere, S. Jaffar, O. S. Levine, J. B. Okoko, and others. 2005. "Efficacy of Nine-Valent Pneumococcal Conjugate Vaccine against Pneumonia and Invasive Pneumococcal Disease in The Gambia: Randomised, Double-Blind, Placebo-Controlled Trial." *Lancet* 365 (9465): 1139–46.

de Andrade, A. L., J. G. de Andrade, C. M. Martelli, S. A. Silva, R. M. de Oliveira, M. S. Costa, and others. 2004. "Effectiveness of *Haemophilus influenzae* B Conjugate Vaccine on Childhood Pneumonia: A Case-Control Study in Brazil." *International Journal of Epidemiology* 33 (1): 173–81.

Denny, F. W. Jr. 1995. "The Clinical Impact of Human Respiratory Virus Infections." *American Journal of Respiratory and Critical Care Medicine* 152 (4, part 2): S4–12.

Dobson, M. 1991. "Oxygen Concentrators Offer Cost Savings for Developing Countries: A Study Based on New Guinea." *Anaesthesia* 146: 217–19.

Douglas, R. M., and H. B. Miles. 1984. "Vaccination against *Streptococcus pneumoniae* in Childhood: Lack of Demonstrable Benefit in Young Australian Children." *Journal of Infectious Diseases* 149 (6): 861–69.

Duke T, J. Mgone, and D. Frank. 2001. "Hypoxaemia in children with severe pneumonia in Papua New Guinea." *International Journal of Tuberculosis and Lung Disease* 5: 511–19.

Eskola, J., H. Kayhty, A. K. Takala, H. Peltola, P. R. Ronnberg, E. Kela, and others. 1990. "A Randomized, Prospective Field Trial of a Conjugate Vaccine in the Protection of Infants and Young Children against Invasive *Haemophilus influenzae* Type B Disease." *New England Journal of Medicine* 323 (20): 1381–87.

Eskola, J., T. Kilpi, A. Palmu, J. Jokinen, J. Haapakoski, E. Herva, and others. 2001. "Efficacy of a Pneumococcal Conjugate Vaccine against Acute Otitis Media." *New England Journal of Medicine* 344 (6): 403–9.

Farley, J. J., J. C. King, P. Nair, S. E. Hines, R. L. Tressier, and P. E. Vink. 1994. "Invasive Pneumococcal Disease among Infected and Uninfected Children of Mothers with Human Immunodeficiency Virus Infection." *Journal of Pediatrics* 124: 853–58.

Fiddian-Green, R. G., and S. Baker. 1991. "Nosocomial Pneumonia in the Critically Ill: Product of Aspiration or Translocation?" *Critical Care Medicine* 19: 763–69.

Fireman, B., S. B. Black, H. R. Shinefield, J. Lee, E. Lewis, and P. Ray. 2003. "Impact of the Pneumococcal Conjugate Vaccine on Otitis Media." *Pediatric Infectious Disease Journal* 22 (1): 10–16.

Fritzell, B., and S. Plotkin. 1992. "Efficacy and Safety of a *Haemophilus influenzae* Type B Capsular Polysaccharide-Tetanus Protein Conjugate Vaccine." *Journal of Pediatrics* 121 (3): 355–62.

Gessner B. D., A. Sutanto, M. Linehan, I. G. Djelantik, T. Fletcher, I. K. Gerudug, and others. 2005. "Incidences of Vaccine-Preventable Haemophilus Influenzae Type B Pneumonia and Meningitis in Indonesian Children: Hamlet-Randomised Vaccine-Probe Trial." *Lancet* 365 (9453): 43–52.

Ghafoor, A., N. K. Nomani, Z. Ishaq, S. Z. Zaidi, F. Anwar, M. I. Burney, and others. 1990. "Diagnoses of Acute Lower Respiratory Tract Infections in Children in Rawalpindi and Islamabad, Pakistan." *Reviews of Infectious Diseases* 12 (Suppl. 8): S907–14.

Gilks, C. F. 1993. "Pneumococcal Disease and HIV Infection." *Annals of Internal Medicine* 118: 393–94.

Goel, A., L. Bamford, D. Hanslo, and G. Hussey. 1999. "Primary Staphylococcal Pneumonia in Young Children: A Review of 100 Cases." *Journal of Tropical Pediatrics* 45 (4): 233–36.

Hament, J. M., P. C. Aerts, A. Fleer, H. Van Dijk, T. Harmsen, J. L. Kimpen, and T. F. Wolfs. 2004. "Enhanced Adherence of *Streptococcus pneumoniae* to Human Epithelial Cells Infected with Respiratory Syncytial Virus." *Pediatric Research* 55 (6): 972–78.

Heath, P. T. 1998. "*Haemophilus influenzae* Type B Conjugate Vaccines: A Review of Efficacy Data." *Pediatric Infectious Disease Journal* 17 (9 Suppl.): S117–22.

Hortal, M., C. Mogdasy, J. C. Russi, C. Deleon, and A. Suarez. 1990. "Microbial Agents Associated with Pneumonia in Children from Uruguay." *Reviews of Infectious Diseases* 12 (Suppl. 8): S915–22.

Ikeogu, M. O., B. Wolf, and S. Mathe. 1997. "Pulmonary Manifestations in HIV Seropositive and Malnourished Children in Zimbabwe." *Archives of Disease in Childhood* 76: 124–28.

Jeena, P. M., H. M. Coovadia, and V. Chrystal. 1996. "*Pneumocystis carinii* and *cytomegalo* Virus Infections in Severely Ill HIV-Infected African Infants." *Annals of Tropical Paediatrics* 16: 361–68.

Jiang, Z., N. Nagata, E. Molina, L. O. Bakaletz, H. Hawkins, and J. A. Patel. 1999. "Fimbria-Mediated Enhanced Attachment of Nontypeable *Haemophilus influenzae* to Respiratory Syncytial Virus-Infected Respiratory Epithelial Cells." *Infection and Immunity* 67: 187–92.

John, T. J. 1994. "Who Determines National Health Policies?" In *Vaccination and World Health: Fourth Annual Public Health Forum of the London School of Hygiene and Tropical Medicine*, ed. F. T. Cutts and P. G. Smith, 205–11. Chichester, U.K.: John Wiley.

John, T. J., T. Cherian, M. C. Steinhoff, E. A. Simoes, and M. John. 1991. "Etiology of Acute Respiratory Infections in Children in Tropical Southern India." *Reviews of Infectious Diseases* 13 (Suppl. 6): S463–69.

Kamath, K. R., R. A. Feldman, P. S. S. Rao, and J. K. Webb. 1969. "Infection and Disease in a Group of South Indian Families." *American Journal of Epidemiology* 89: 375–83.

Karma, P., J. Luotonen, M. Timonen, S. Pontynen, J. Pukander, E. Herva, and others. 1980. "Efficacy of Pneumococcal Vaccination against Recurrent Otitis Media: Preliminary Results of a Field Trial in Finland." *Annals of Otology, Rhinology, and Laryngology* Suppl. 89 (3, part 2): 357–62.

Kartasasmita, C. 2003. "Three versus Five Days Oral Cotrimoxazole for Nonsevere Pneumonia." Paper presented at the World Health Organization Consultative Meeting on Reviewing Current Research and Management of Acute Respiratory Infections, Geneva, September 29–October 1.

Kilpi, T., H. Ahman, J. Jokinen, K. S. Lankinen, A. Palmu, H. Savolainen, and others. 2003. "Protective Efficacy of a Second Pneumococcal Conjugate Vaccine against Pneumococcal Acute Otitis Media in Infants and Children: Randomized, Controlled Trial of a Seven-Valent Pneumococcal Polysaccharide-Meningococcal Outer Membrane Protein Complex Conjugate Vaccine in 1,666 Children." *Clinical Infectious Diseases* 37 (9): 1155–64.

Klugman, K. P., S. A. Madhi, R. E. Huebner, R. Kohberger, N. Mbelle, N. Pierce, and others. 2003. "A Trial of a 9-Valent Pneumococcal Conjugate Vaccine in Children with and Those without HIV Infection." *New England Journal of Medicine* 349 (14): 1341–48.

Kolstad, P. R., G. Burnham, H. D. Kalter, N. Kenya-Mugisha, and R. E. Black. 1997. "The Integrated Management of Childhood Illness in Western Uganda." *Bulletin of the World Health Organization* 75 (Suppl. 1): 77–85.

Lagos, R., I. Horwitz, J. Toro, O. San Martin, P. Abrego, C. Bustamante, and others. 1996. "Large Scale, Postlicensure, Selective Vaccination of Chilean Infants with PRP-T Conjugate Vaccine: Practicality and Effectiveness in Preventing Invasive *Haemophilus influenzae* Type B Infections." *Pediatric Infectious Disease Journal* 15: 216–22.

Lehmann, D., T. F. Marshall, I. D. Riley, and M. P. Alpers. 1991. "Effect of Pneumococcal Vaccine on Morbidity from Acute Lower Respiratory Tract Infections in Papua New Guinean Children." *Annals of Tropical Paediatrics* 11 (3): 247–57.

Levine, O. S., R. Lagos, A. Munoz, J. Villaroel, A. M. Alvarez, P. Abrego, and others. 1999. "Defining the Burden of Pneumonia in Children Preventable by Vaccination against *Haemophilus influenzae* Type B." *Pediatric Infectious Disease Journal* 18 (12): 1060–64.

Lucas, S. B., C. S. Peacock, A. Hounnou, K. Brattegaard, K. Koffi, M. Honde, and others. 1996. "Disease in Children Infected with HIV in Abidjan, Côte d'Ivoire." *British Medical Journal* 312: 335–38.

Madhi, S. A., K. P. Klugman, and the Vaccine Trialist Group. 2004. "A Role for *Streptococcus pneumoniae* in Virus-Associated Pneumonia." *Nature Medicine* 10 (8): 811–13.

Madhi, S. A., K. Petersen, A. Madhi, M. Khoosal, and K. P. Klugman. 2000. "Increased Disease Burden and Antibiotic Resistance of Bacteria Causing Severe Community Acquired Lower Respiratory Tract Infections in Human Immunodeficiency Virus 1 Infected Children." *Clinical Infectious Diseases* 31: 170–76.

Madhi, S. A., K. Petersen, A. Madhi, A. Wasas, and K. P. Klugman. 2000. "Impact of Human Immunodeficiency Virus Type 1 on the Disease Spectrum of *Streptococcus pneumoniae* in South African Children." *Pediatric Infectious Disease Journal* 19 (12): 1141–47.

Makela, P. H., M. Sibakov, E. Herva, J. Henrichsen, J. Luotonen, M. Timonen, and others. 1980. "Pneumococcal Vaccine and Otitis Media." *Lancet* 2 (8194): 547–51.

Management Sciences for Health. 2005. *International Drug Price Indicator Guide.* Cambridge, MA: Management Sciences for Health.

McCullers, J. A., and K. C. Bartmess. 2003. "Role of Neuraminidase in Lethal Synergism between Influenza Virus and *Streptococcus pneumoniae.*" *Journal of Infectious Diseases* 187: 1000–9.

Monto, A. S., and B. M. Ullman. 1974. "Acute Respiratory Illness in an American Community: The Tecumseh Study." *Journal of the American Medical Association* 227 (2): 164–69.

Mulholland, E. K., E. A. Simoes, M. O. Castales, E. J. McGrath, E. M. Manalac, and S. Gove. 1992. "Standardized Diagnosis of Pneumonia in Developing Countries." *Pediatric Infectious Disease Journal* 11: 77–81.

Mulholland, K., S. Hilton, R. Adegbola, S. Usen, A. Oparaugo, C. Omosigho, and others. 1997. "Randomised Trial of *Haemophilus influenzae* Type-B Tetanus Protein Conjugate Vaccine for Prevention of Pneumonia and Meningitis in Gambian Infants." *Lancet* 349 (9060): 1191–97.

Mulholland, K., S. Usen, R. Adegbola, and M. Weber. 1998. "Use of Pneumococcal Polysaccharide Vaccine in Children." *Lancet* 352 (9127): 575–76.

Nathoo, K. J., F. K. Nkrumah, D. Ndlovu, D. Nhembe, J. Pirie, and H. Kowo. 1993. "Acute Lower Respiratory Tract Infection in Hospitalized Children in Zimbabwe." *Annals of Tropical Paediatrics* 13: 253–61.

Neuzil, K. M., Y. Zhu, M. R. Griffin, K. M. Edwards, J. M. Thompson, S. J. Tollefson, and P. F. Wright. 2002. "Burden of Interpandemic Influenza in Children Younger Than 5 Years: A 25-Year Prospective Study." *Journal of Infectious Diseases* 185: 147–52.

Nolan T., P. Angos, A. J. Cunha, L. Muhe, S. Qazi, E. A. Simoes, and others. 2001. "Quality of Hospital Care for Seriously Ill Children in Less-Developed Countries." *Lancet* 357 (9250): 106–10.

Obaro, S., A. Leach, and K. W. McAdam. 1998. "Use of Pneumococcal Polysaccharide Vaccine in Children," *Lancet* 352 (9127): 575.

O'Brien, K. L., L. H. Moulton, R. Reid, R. Weatherholtz, J. Oski, L. Brown, and others. 2003. "Efficacy and Safety of Seven-Valent Conjugate Pneumococcal Vaccine in American Indian Children: Group Randomised Trial." *Lancet* 362 (9381): 355–61.

Onyango F. E., M. C. Steinhoff, E. M. Wafula, S. Wariua, J. Musia, and J. Kitonyi. 1993. "Hypoxaemia in Young Kenyan Children with Acute Lower Respiratory Infection." *British Medical Journal* 306 (6878): 612–15.

Pandey, M. R., N. M. Daulaire, E. S. Starbuck, R. M. Houston, and K. McPherson. 1991. "Reduction in Total Under-Five Mortality in Western Nepal through Community-Based Antimicrobial Treatment of Pneumonia." *Lancet* 338 (8773): 993–97.

Pandey, M. R., P. R. Sharma, B. B. Gubhaju, G. M. Shakya, R. P. Neupane, A. Gautam, and others. 1989. "Impact of a Pilot Acute Respiratory Infection (ARI) Control Programme in a Rural Community of the Hill Region of Nepal." *Annals of Tropical Paediatrics* 9 (4): 212–20.

Pederson, J., and M. Nyrop. 1991. "Anaesthetic Equipment for a Developing Country." *British Journal of Anaesthesia* 66: 264–70.

Peiris, J. S., W. C. Yu, C. W. Leung, C. Y. Cheung, W. F. Ng, J. M. Nicholls, and others. 2004. "Re-emergence of Fatal Human Influenza A Subtype H5N1 Disease." *Lancet* 363 (9409): 617–19.

Perkins, B. A., J. R. Zucker, J. Otineo, H. S. Jafari, L. Paxton, S. C. Redd, and others. 1997. "Evaluation of an Algorithm for Integrated Management of Childhood Illness in an Area of Kenya with High Malaria Transmission." *Bulletin of the World Health Organization* 75 (Suppl. 1): 33–42.

Quiambao, B. P., E. A. Simoes, E. Abucejo-Ladesma, L. S. Gozum, S. P. Lupisan, L. T. Sombrero, and P. J. Ruutu (ARIVAC Consortium). Forthcoming. "Serious Community Acquired Pediatric Infections in Rural Asia (Bohol Island, Philippines)." *Pediatric Infectious Disease Journal.*

Redd, S. 1994. "Diagnosis and Management of Acute Respiratory Infections in Lesotho." *Health Policy and Management* 5: 255–60.

Riley, I. D., F. A. Everingham, D. E. Smith, and R. M. Douglas. 1981. "Immunization with a Polyvalent Pneumococcal Vaccine: Effect of Respiratory Mortality in Children Living in the New Guinea Highlands." *Archives of Disease in Childhood* 56 (5): 354–57.

Riley, I. D., D. Lehmann, and M. P. Alpers. 1991. "Pneumococcal Vaccine Trials in Papua New Guinea: Relationships between Epidemiology of Pneumococcal Infection and Efficacy of Vaccine." *Reviews of Infectious Diseases* 13 (Suppl. 6): S535–41.

Rudan, I., L. Tomaskovic, C. Boschi-Pinto, and H. Campbell (WHO Child Health Epidemiology Reference Group). 2004. "Global Estimate of the Incidence of Clinical Pneumonia among Children under Five Years of Age." *Bulletin of the World Health Organization* 82 (12): 895–903.

Santosham, M., M. Wolff, R. Reid, M. Hohenboken, M. Bateman, J. Goepp, and others. 1991. "The Efficacy in Navajo Infants of a Conjugate Vaccine Consisting of *Haemophilus influenzae* Type B Polysaccharide and *Neisseria meningitidis* Outer-Membrane Protein Complex." *New England Journal of Medicine* 324 (25): 1767–72.

Sazawal, S., and R. E. Black. 2003. "Pneumonia Case Management Trials Group: Effect of Pneumonia Case Management on Mortality in

Neonates, Infants, and Preschool Children—A Meta-analysis of Community-Based Trials." *Lancet Infectious Diseases* 3: 547–56.

Schellenberg, J. A., C. G. Victora, A. Mushi, D. de Savigny, D. Schellenberg, H. Mshinda, and others. 2003. "Inequities among the Very Poor: Health Care for Children in Rural Southern Tanzania." *Lancet* 361 (9357): 561–66.

Schneider, G. 2001. "Oxygen Supply in Rural Africa: A Personal Experience." *International Journal of Tuberculosis and Lung Disease* 5 (6): 524–26.

Schumacher, R., E. Swedberg, M. O. Diallo, D. R. Keita, H. Kalter, and O. Pasha. 2002. *Mortality Study in Guinea: Investigating the Causes of Death in Children under Five*. Arlington, VA: Save the Children and the Basic Support for Institutionalizing Child Survival Project.

Shann, F. 1986. "Etiology of Severe Pneumonia in Children in Developing Countries." *Pediatric Infectious Disease* 5 (2): 247–52.

Shann, F., M. Gratten, S. Germer, V. Linnemann, D. Hazlett, and R. Payne. 1984. "Aetiology of Pneumonia in Children in Goroka Hospital, Papua New Guinea." *Lancet* 2 (8402): 537–41.

Shann, F., K. Hart, and D. Thomas. 1984. "Acute Lower Respiratory Tract Infections in Children: Possible Criteria for Selection of Patients for Antibiotic Therapy and Hospital Admission." *Bulletin of the World Health Organization* 62: 749–51.

Simoes, E. A. 1999. "Respiratory Syncytial Virus Infection." *Lancet* 354 (9181): 847–52.

Simoes, E. A., T. Desta, T. Tessema, T. Gerbresellassie, M. Dagnew, and S. Gove. 1997. "Performance of Health Workers after Training in Integrated Management of Childhood Illness in Gondar, Ethiopia." *Bulletin of the World Health Organization* 75 (Suppl. 1): 43–53.

Sloyer, J. L. J., J. H. Ploussard, and V. M. Howie. 1981. "Efficacy of Pneumococcal Polysaccharide Vaccine in Preventing Acute Otitis Media in Infants in Huntsville, Alabama." *Reviews of Infectious Diseases* 3 (Suppl.): S119–23.

Stensballe, L. G., J. K. Devasundaram, and E. A. Simoes. 2003. "Respiratory Syncytial Virus Epidemics: The Ups and Downs of a Seasonal Virus." *Pediatric Infectious Disease Journal* 22 (2 Suppl.): S21–32.

Strauss, W. L., S. A. Qazi, Z. Kundi, N. K. Nomani, and B. Schwartz (Co-trimoxazole Study Group). 1998. "Antimicrobial Resistance and Clinical Effectiveness of Co-trimoxazole versus Amoxycillin for Pneumonia among Children in Pakistan: Randomised Controlled Trial." *Lancet* 352: 270–74.

Temple, K., B. Greenwood, H. Inskip, A. Hall, M. Koskela, and M. Leinonen. 1991. "Antibody Response to Pneumococcal Capsular Polysaccharide Vaccine in African Children." *Pediatric Infectious Disease Journal* 10 (5): 386–90.

Tupasi, T. E., M. G. Lucero, D. M. Magdangal, N. V. Mangubat, M. E. Sunico, C. U. Torres, and others. 1990. "Etiology of Acute Lower Respiratory Tract Infection in Children from Alabang, Metro Manila." *Reviews of Infectious Diseases* 12 (Suppl. 8): S929–39.

UNAIDS (Joint United Nations Programme on HIV/AIDS). 2002. *AIDS Epidemic Update*. Geneva: UNAIDS.

Usen S., M. Weber, K. Mulholland, S. Jaffar, A. Oparaugo, C. Omosigho, and others. 1999. "Clinical Predictors of Hypoxaemia in Gambian Children with Acute Lower Respiratory Tract Infection: Prospective Cohort Study." *British Medical Journal* 318 (7176): 86–91.

Van den Hoogen, B. G., J. C. de Jong, J. Groen, T. Kuiken, R. de Groot, R. A. Fouchier, and A. D. Osterhaus. 2001. "A Newly Discovered Human Pneumovirus Isolated from Young Children with Respiratory Tract Disease." *Nature Medicine* 7: 719–24.

von Mutius, E. 2001. "Pediatric Origins of Adult Lung Disease." *Thorax* 56: 153–57.

Vuori-Holopainen, E., and H. Peltola. 2001. "Reappraisal of Lung Tap: Review of an Old Method for Better Etiologic Diagnosis of Childhood Pneumonia." *Clinical Infectious Diseases* 32 (5): 715–26.

Wall, R. A., P. T. Corrah, D. C. Mabey, and B. M. Greenwood. 1986. "The Etiology of Lobar Pneumonia in The Gambia." *Bulletin of the World Health Organization* 64 (4): 553–58.

Weber, M. W., E. K. Mulholland, S. Jaffar, H. Troedsson, S. Gove, and B. M. Greenwood. 1997. "Evaluation of an Algorithm for the Integrated Management of Childhood Illness in an Area with Seasonal Malaria in The Gambia." *Bulletin of the World Health Organization* 75 (Suppl. 1): 25–32.

Wenger, J. D., J. DiFabio, J. M. Landaverde, O. S. Levine, and T. Gaafar. 1999. "Introduction of Hib Conjugate Vaccines in the Non-industrialized World: Experience in Four 'Newly Adopting' Countries." *Vaccine* 18 (7–8): 736–42.

Wenger, J. D., and M. M. Levine, eds. 1997. *Epidemiological Impact of Conjugate Vaccine on Invasive Disease Caused by* Haemophilus influenzae *Type B*. New York: Marcel Dekker.

Whitney, C. G., M. M. Farley, J. Hadler, L. H. Harrison, N. M. Bennett, R. Lynfield, and others. 2003. "Decline in Invasive Pneumococcal Disease after the Introduction of Protein-Polysaccharide Conjugate Vaccine." *New England Journal of Medicine* 348 (18): 1737–46.

WHO (World Health Organization). 1990. "Antibiotics in the Treatment of Acute Respiratory Infections in Young Children." Unpublished document WHO/ARI/90.10, available on request from the Division of Child Health and Development, formerly the Division of Diarrhoeal and Acute Respiratory Disease Control, WHO, Geneva.

———. 1991. "Management of the Young Child with an Acute Respiratory Infection. Supervisory Skills Training Module." Unpublished document, available on request from the WHO Division of Child Health and Development, formerly the Division of Diarrhoeal and Acute Respiratory Disease Control, WHO, Geneva.

———. 1993. "Oxygen Therapy for Acute Respiratory Infections in Young Children in Developing Countries." Geneva, WHO. http://www.who.int/child-adolescent-health/New_Publications/CHILD_HEALTH/WHO_ARI_93.28.htm.

———. 2002. *The Multicountry Evaluation of IMCI Effectiveness, Cost and Impact (MCE): Progress Report, May 2001–April 2002.* WHO/FCH/CAH/02.16. Geneva: Division of Child and Adolescent Health and Development, WHO.

———. 2003. *Consultative Meeting on Management of Children with Pneumonia and HIV Infection, 30–31 Jan. 2003, Harare, Zimbabwe.* WHO/FCH/CAH/03.4. Geneva: WHO.

———. 2004a. "Review Panel on *Haemophilus influenzae* Type B (Hib) Disease Burden in Bangladesh, Indonesia, and Other Asian Countries, Bangkok, 28–29 January 2004." *Weekly Epidemiological Record* 79 (18): 173–75.

———. 2004b. "WHO/UNICEF Joint Statement: Management of Pneumonia in Community Settings." WHO/FCH/CAG/04.06. WHO, Geneva.

WHO (World Health Organization) and Child Adolescent Health. Forthcoming. *Report on the Methodology and Assumptions Used to Estimate Costs of Scaling Up Selected Child Health Interventions to 95% in Order to Reduce Under-Five Mortality.* Geneva: WHO.

Williams, B. G., E. Gouws, C. Boschi-Pinto, J. Bryce, and C. Dye. 2002. "Estimates of Worldwide Distribution of Child Deaths from Acute Respiratory Infections." *Lancet Infectious Diseases* 2: 25–32.

World Bank. 2002. *World Development Indicators.* CD-ROM. Washington, DC: World Bank.

Zwi, K. J., J. M. Pettifor, and N. Soderlund. 1999. "Paediatric Hospital Admissions at a South African Urban Regional Hospital: The Impact of HIV, 1992–1997." *Annals of Tropical Paediatrics* 19: 135–42.

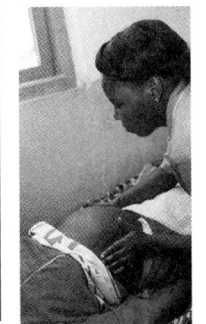

Chapter **26**

Maternal and Perinatal Conditions

Wendy J. Graham, John Cairns, Sohinee Bhattacharya, Colin H. W. Bullough, Zahidul Quayyum, and Khama Rogo

The Millennium Declaration includes two goals directly relevant to maternal and perinatal conditions: reducing child mortality and improving maternal health. The fact that two out of the eight Millennium Development Goals (MDGs) are exclusively targeted at mothers and children is testament to the significant proportion of the global burden of disease they suffer and to the huge inequities within and between countries in the magnitude of their burden. Achieving these goals is inextricably linked at the biological, intervention, and service delivery levels (Bale and others 2003).

Maternal and child health services have long been seen as inseparable partners, although over the past 20 years the relative emphasis within each, particularly at a policy level, has varied (De Brouwere and Van Lerberghe 2001). The launch of the Safe Motherhood Initiative in the late 1980s, for example, brought heightened attention to maternal mortality, whereas the International Conference on Population and Development (ICPD) broadened the focus to reproductive health and, more recently, to reproductive rights (Germain 2000). Those shifts can be linked with international programmatic responses and terminology—with the preventive emphasis of, for instance, prenatal care being lowered as a priority relative to the treatment focus of emergency obstetric care. For the child, integrated management of childhood illnesses has brought renewed emphasis to maintaining a balance between preventive and curative care. The particular needs of the newborn, however, have only started to receive significant attention in the past three or four years (Foege 2001).

Although health experts agree that the single clinical interventions needed to avert much of the burden of maternal and perinatal death and disability are known, they also accept that these interventions require a functioning health system to have an effect at the population scale. Levels of maternal and perinatal mortality are thus regarded as sensitive indicators of the entire health system (Goodburn and Campbell 2001), and they can therefore be used to monitor progress in health gains more generally. What is also clear is that maternal mortality and the neonatal component of child mortality continue to represent two of the most serious challenges to the attainment of the MDGs, particularly in South Asia and Sub-Saharan Africa.

An estimated 210 million women become pregnant each year, and close to 60 million of these pregnancies end with the death of the mother ($\approx$500,000) or the baby or as abortions. This chapter focuses on the adverse events of pregnancy and childbirth and on the intervention strategies to eliminate and ameliorate this burden.

EPIDEMIOLOGY OF MATERNAL AND PERINATAL CONDITIONS

Much has been written about the lack of reliable data on maternal and perinatal conditions in developing countries (AbouZahr 2003; Graham 2002; Save the Children 2001). Weak routine information systems, inadequate vital registration, and reliance on periodic household surveys as the main source of population-based data are all familiar obstacles to improving public health in poor countries (Godlee and others 2004). Recognizing the implications of these obstacles for prioritizing health needs and interventions is important and is now endorsed by a global movement toward evidence-based decision making for policy and practice (Evans and Stansfield 2003).

However, there has been much less appreciation of the consequences for evaluations of effectiveness—and thus cost-effectiveness—of the weaknesses in current outcomes measurement and in routine data collection. Those weaknesses also affect the monitoring of progress toward the MDGs. Initiatives for improved health surveillance are thus urgently needed (CMH 2002). For the vast majority of the world's population, the magnitude of adverse maternal and perinatal outcomes is not known reliably. It is impossible to determine whether many of the patterns apparently observed, especially at a cause-specific level, are real or are artifacts of the measurement process.

Definitions

The terms *maternal* and *perinatal* encompass a continuum of health states—from the most positive (complete physical, mental, and social well-being) to the most negative—and a huge number of clinical conditions. This chapter focuses on eight major conditions, hereafter referred to as the *focus conditions,* which are estimated to account for about 75 percent of maternal deaths and more than 60 percent of perinatal deaths. For the mother, these conditions are hemorrhage, sepsis, hypertensive disorders of pregnancy, obstructed labor, and unsafe abortion. For the baby, they are low birthweight, birth asphyxia, and infection (table 26.1).

We define *maternal conditions* as encompassing events occurring from conception to 42 days postpartum (WHO 1992a). The chapters on women's health, family planning, adolescent health, and surgery address the longer-term sequelae of pregnancy and childbirth; the preconception period; pregnancy at an early age; and specific interventions, such as repair of obstetric fistulas. Within the period from conception to 42 days postpartum, two broad categories of conditions can be distinguished: those arising specifically from pregnancy and parturition (*direct obstetric conditions*), and those aggravated by or aggravating to pregnancy (*indirect obstetric conditions*). Because the latter conditions, such as malaria, HIV/AIDS, or anemia, are not exclusive to pregnant or parturient women, they are not dealt with here but in the relevant disease-specific chapters.

Regarding perinatal conditions, we focus on those for which interventions can be directed to the baby through the mother during pregnancy or delivery. Our discussion is complemented by the discussion in chapter 27, which concentrates on the neonate, including special care of the small baby and emergency care of the sick newborn.

Formal definitions of perinatal conditions tend to vary by data source. Taken literally, they refer to conditions that arise in the perinatal period (Murray and Lopez 1998), which are not the same as events that occur in the perinatal period—that is, from 28 weeks of gestation to the end of the seventh day of life. For example, death resulting from conditions that arise in the perinatal period can happen at any age, although it tends to take place during the neonatal period (up to 28 days of life). By contrast, perinatal deaths include both stillborn babies and those who are born alive but die before the end of the seventh day. Early neonatal deaths only include live births.

Nature and Characteristics

Pregnancy and childbirth are not inherently pathological. Maintaining an effective balance, however, between preserving normality and ensuring a state of readiness to deal with abnormality represents a fundamental challenge to health systems and a tension in safe motherhood programming. Although this balance between prevention and treatment is not peculiar to maternal and perinatal conditions (or complications), the following additional characteristics are relevant to assessing the burden as well as the effectiveness of interventions:

- The principle of "first, do no harm" has particular significance in this area, because many preventive practices related to pregnancy and childbirth can readily become harmful in unskilled hands—for example, inappropriately early induction of labor or poor forceps technique. The iatrogenic burden of maternal and perinatal conditions is rarely factored into assessments of intervention effectiveness.
- The lives of two individuals, mother and baby, are potentially at stake (Stoll and Measham 2001); however, interventions will not necessarily benefit both equally, and indeed, some will be in direct conflict.
- A large number of maternal and perinatal conditions present clinically not as single entities but as complexes, such as hemorrhage and sepsis or preterm delivery and birth asphyxia. For the mother, the situation may be further complicated by the role of underlying conditions, such as HIV/AIDS underlying puerperal sepsis.
- The most extreme negative outcome, death of both the mother and the baby, is highly concentrated around the time of delivery, from the onset of labor or abortion to 48 hours postpartum or postabortion. Estimates indicate that about two-thirds of maternal deaths occur within this time window (AbouZahr 1998), and the proportion for perinatal deaths appears to be even higher (Bale and others 2003). For the mother, however, a growing number of studies highlight the contribution of direct and indirect causes of deaths, including violence, when a one-year postpartum reference period is used (Etard, Kodio, and Traore 1999; Hoj and others 2003).
- The initial clinical presentation of some conditions can be severe, with rapid escalation to a life-threatening state, and these conditions often require surgical intervention.
- A distinct clinical feature of some maternal conditions is their unpredictability (AbouZahr 1998). This fact has had a

Table 26.1 Maternal and Perinatal Focus Conditions and Risk Factors for These Conditions

Condition	Definition or complications and sequelae	Case fatality rate[a] (percent)	Average duration until death if condition fatal	Timing of presentation	Risk factors for condition — Distal or proximate	Risk factors for condition — Direct, physiological	Risk factors for death from condition — Distal or proximate	Risk factors for death from condition — Direct, physiological
Maternal								
Hemorrhage	*Definition* Antepartum hemorrhage: bleeding from the genital tract during the last 3 months of pregnancy	Not available	12 hours	28 weeks of gestation up to delivery	Primigravidity Grand multiparity (greater than 4) Fibroids Anemia	Placental abnormalities (including placenta previa; abruption; placenta accreta, percreta, increta; other adhesions) Polyhydramnios Multiple gestation Previous third-stage complication Previous cesarean section Preeclampsia, eclampsia Intrauterine death Hepatitis Induced labor Prolonged labor Precipitate labor Forceps delivery Cesarean section Chorioamnionitis Disseminated intravascular coagulation	Remote location Anemia Coagulopathies	Lack of blood transfusion Badly managed third stage of labor Delay or absence of oxytocic treatment
	Primary postpartum hemorrhage: excessive bleeding (more than 500 milliliters) from the genital tract following delivery	1.0[b]	2 hours	Delivery to 24 hours after delivery				
Sepsis	*Definition* Infection of the genital tract or extragenital infections following childbirth	1.3	6 days	Delivery to 6 weeks postpartum	Immunosuppression Anemia Sexually transmitted infections Inadequate prenatal care	Prolonged labor Obstructed labor Premature rupture of membranes Frequent pelvic examinations Intrauterine death Foreign body insertion (for example, herbs) Episiotomy Instrumental delivery	Delivery by untrained personnel Immunosuppression Anemia Lack of knowledge about warning signs Lack of postnatal care Cultural practices	Misdiagnosis Inappropriate use of antibiotics Lack of access to intravenous antibiotics

(Continues on the following page.)

Table 26.1 Continued

Condition	Definition or complications and sequelae	Case fatality rate[a] (percent)	Average duration until death if condition fatal	Timing of presentation	Risk factors for condition — Distal or proximate	Risk factors for condition — Direct, physiological	Risk factors for death from condition — Distal or proximate	Risk factors for death from condition — Direct, physiological
						Cesarean section; Unhygienic delivery conditions; Retained products of conception		
Hypertensive disorders of pregnancy	*Definition* Raised blood pressure with proteinuria	1.7	2 days (eclampsia)	28 weeks of gestation to 2 days postpartum	Extremes of maternal age; Primigravidity; Genetic predisposition; Racial or geographical predisposition; Diabetes and chronic hypertension; Lack of prenatal care	Multiple gestations; Molar pregnancy; Previous history of pregnancy-induced hypertension or chronic hypertension	Cultural practices; Lack of knowledge; Lack of prenatal care	Appearance of complications, such as cardiovascular and cerebral complications, hemolysis, elevated liver enzyme, low platelets syndrome; Disseminated intravascular coagulation; Eclampsia
Obstructed labor	*Definition* Labor in which progress is arrested by mechanical factors	0.7	3 days	During labor	Malnutrition; Rickets in childhood; Bony deformity of pelvis; Achondroplasia; Short stature; Primigravidity; Grand multiparity; Adolescent pregnancy	Cephalopelvic disproportion; Malpresentation, position	Lack of access to cesarean delivery; Lack of access to instrumental delivery and symphysiotomy; Scarred uterus; Inappropriate use of oxytocin	Uterine rupture; Hemorrhage; Sepsis; Exhaustion, dehydration
Unsafe abortion	*Definition* Procedure for terminating an unintended pregnancy carried out by people lacking the necessary skills or in an environment that does not conform to minimal medical standards or both	0.3	6 hours to 6 days	After first missed period to 22 weeks of gestation or fetal weight of less than 500 grams	Unwanted pregnancy; Adolescence; Unmarried status; Absence of legal abortion services; Lack of access to contraception; Lack of access to safe abortion services; Sexually transmitted infections	Absence of aseptic technique; Foreign body insertion; Poisoning from abortifacients	Sociocultural factors; Lack of access to safe termination services; Lack of access to postabortion care	Perforated uterus; Poisoning from abortifacients; Peritonitis; Septic shock; Acute renal failure; Hepatorenal failure; Bowel injury, perforation; Hemorrhagic shock; Peritonitis

Perinatal[c]

Condition	Complications or sequelae				Risk factors			Resulting complications
Low birthweight (less than 2,500 grams)[d]	*Complications or sequelae* Respiratory insufficiency in preterm infants with lung immaturity presenting as respiratory distress syndrome because of surfactant deficiency Neonatal cerebral injury caused by periventricular hemorrhage mediated by perinatal stress such as hypotension or trauma Severe physiological jaundice of preterm infant Difficulties in establishing spontaneous feeding and inability to tolerate feeds resulting from prematurity Failure of closure of the ductus arteriosus, frequently seen in preterm babies with lung disease Hypoglycemia and other metabolic disorders related to prematurity	50 80 50 20 70 2	5 days 3 days 1–5 days 1–14 days 3 days to months 7 days	Less than 24 hours 1–4 days 2–5 days First day 3–14 days Birth	Extremes of maternal age Race, ethnicity Low socioeconomic status Unmarried status Lack of education Parity (0 or greater than 4) Smoking, alcohol use Maternal malnutrition Maternal diabetes or hypertension Genetic factors Rubella, other viral infection Poor obstetric history Diethylstilboestrol, other toxic exposure High altitude Absent or inadequate prenatal care	Multiple pregnancy Short interpregnancy interval First or second trimester bleeding Placenta previa Preeclampsia Anemia Hyperemesis Isoimmunization Fetal abnormalities Cervical incompetence Oligohydramnios or polyhydramnios	Lack of adequate neonatal care facility Lack of knowledge and understanding	Birth asphyxia Intraventricular hemorrhage Central nervous system injury Respiratory infection Respiratory distress syndrome Necrotizing enterocolitis Cholestatic liver disease Other infections Sudden infant death syndrome Neonatal coagulopathy
Birth asphyxia (excluding birth trauma)	*Complications or sequelae* Absent or depressed breathing at birth Neonatal encephalopathy: clinically evident disturbance in neurological behavior, commonly with early neonatal seizures in term babies, resulting from an event causing hypoxia during delivery	20 30	20 minutes 3 days to life	Birth (5 minutes) Birth to first 12 hours	Drugs taken during labor, including anesthesia Maternal diabetes Maternal hypertension Preeclampsia Any other severe illness	Prolonged or obstructed labor Abruptio placentae Placental infarct, insufficiency Postmaturity Prematurity or low birthweight Multiple pregnancies Placenta previa or separation Cord prolapse	Badly conducted labor Lack of fetal monitoring Lack of partograph Lack of neonatal resuscitation facilities	Central nervous system injury Neonatal encephalopathy (seizures and recurrent apnea)

(Continues on the following page.)

Table 26.1 Continued

Condition	Definition or complications and sequelae	Case fatality rate[a] (percent)	Average duration until death if condition fatal	Timing of presentation	Risk factors for condition		Risk factors for death from condition	
					Distal or proximate	Direct, physiological	Distal or proximate	Direct, physiological
Infection	*Complications or sequelae* Neonatal sepsis of early onset resulting from intrauterine or intrapartum infection	30–40	5 days	First 3 days	Lack of adequate prenatal care	Premature rupture of membranes	Congenital HIV infection	Preterm delivery
	Neonatal sepsis of late onset resulting from nosocomial infection or lack of immunity to commensal bacteria	15	5 days	After 3 days	Maternal infection	Preterm delivery	Lack of adequate neonatal care	Septic shock
					Lack of maternal immunization	Birth asphyxia		Respiratory failure
					Unhygienic cultural practices	Unhygienic delivery and cord care		Hepatorenal failure
								Coagulopathies
	Tetanus neonatorum, commonly resulting from unhygienic cutting of the cord or care of the cord stump	80	3–7 days	3–14 days				
	Congenital syphilis resulting from transplacental infection with *Treponema pallidum* after 18 weeks gestation	30	5 days	Birth onward				
	HIV infection transmitted either intrapartum or postpartum			Direct effects mainly after neonatal period				

Source: Maternal conditions: Chamberlain 1995; case fatality rates: AbouZahr 2003; mechanical factors of obstructed labor: WHO 1994; unsafe abortion: WHO 1992b; low birthweight: Bale and others 2003, p. 324, Robertson 1993; infections: Robertson 1993; risk factors: Calder and Dunlop 1992, Murray and Lopez 1998. Case fatality rates: Robertson 1993, Yasmin and others 2001; birth asphyxia: Bale and others 2003, p. 324, Robertson 1993; infections: Robertson 1993; risk factors: Calder and Dunlop 1992, Murray and Lopez 1998.

a. Case fatality rates assume that no intensive care is available, because this is the norm in South Asia and Sub-Saharan Africa.
b. Case fatality for severe pph (blood loss ≥ 1000 ml).
c. Excludes stillbirths.
d. Includes preterm deliveries and small for gestational age.

profound effect on the prioritization of interventions in safe motherhood, and it is an area in urgent need of further research. The situation is confused by the alternative endpoints, such as death or disability, and by the extent to which there are clear and predictable risk factors. Table 26.1 summarizes some of these key characteristics as they relate to the eight focus conditions.

Causes and Conceptual Frameworks

One of the most frequently quoted figures in safe motherhood is that 88 to 98 percent of maternal deaths are avoidable with moderate levels of health care (WHO 1986). This advocacy statement simplifies the multiple pathways leading to death and, thus, the multiple opportunities for primary and secondary prevention. In part, this simplicity is a further reflection of the grouping together of clinical conditions that in reality are distinctly different in terms of prevalence, case fatality, and scope for intervention, such as eclampsia and puerperal sepsis or congenital anomalies and birth asphyxia. The multiple endpoints and conditions, for both the mother and the fetus or newborn, have implications for what is regarded as an antecedent (a cause, a determinant, or a risk factor)[1] and what is regarded as a consequence (an outcome or a sequela).

A large number of conceptual frameworks depict pathways to adverse maternal and perinatal outcomes (Bale and others 2003; McCarthy and Maine 1992). Several identify three levels of contributory factors, which are also found in causal models for general health outcomes (WHO 2002): (a) distal, (b) proximal or intermediate, and (c) physiological or direct. Table 26.1 highlights the risk factors for the focus maternal and perinatal conditions. The distal determinants emphasize that maternal and perinatal well-being is not just a medical issue. Improvements throughout the health sector must be complemented by attention to wider social, economic, and cultural factors as well as to reproductive rights (CMH 2002). Many conceptual frameworks also differentiate between the timing of interventions: before pregnancy, during pregnancy, during labor and delivery, or during the postpartum period. Similarly, a further distinction can be made in terms of the timing of the outcome, although from a programmatic perspective, such a temporal focus may lead to fragmented care for women and their babies.

Levels, Trends, and Differentials

The latest regional estimates of maternal mortality are for 2000–1 (table 26.2), with most of the figures for the developing world produced by modeling (WHO 2004b). More than 99 percent of annual maternal deaths occur in the developing world. At a national level, the magnitude of the differential in terms of lifetime risk is almost 500-fold between the highest figure for a

developing country (1 in 6) and the lowest estimate for a developed country (1 in 29,800) (WHO 2004b). This differential is often cited as the largest discrepancy between the developing and developed world of all public health statistics, reflecting major differences both in obstetric risk, as measured by the maternal mortality ratio, and in levels of fertility, as reflected in the total fertility rate.

In terms of medical causes of maternal mortality, even greater caution is needed regarding the reliability of any patterns observed, because of their dependence on whether the data are health service based or population based and on coding conventions. Figure 26.1a shows the percentage distribution among direct causes at a crude global level. Direct causes account for about 80 percent of all maternal deaths, with indirect causes responsible for the remainder. Of the direct causes, hemorrhage is generally regarded as the most common and may be underestimated, because health facilities are unaware of many such deaths, given the short interval between onset and death (see table 26.1). In terms of indirect causes, the pattern varies enormously between different parts of the world, primarily according to the prevalence of HIV/AIDS, malaria, and tuberculosis.

The published data on severe maternal morbidity are weaker still. A recent World Health Organization (WHO) systematic review indicates how prevalence figures vary hugely according to the criteria used to identify cases (Say, Pattinson, and Gulmezoglu 2004). Using disease-specific criteria, WHO found that prevalence ranged from 0.80 to 8.23 percent. Using organ system criteria, WHO found that the range was 0.38 to 1.09 percent. Finally, using management-based criteria, WHO found that the range was 0.01 to 2.99 percent. Estimates suggest that for every maternal death, at least 16 or 17 other women suffer a life-threatening complication during pregnancy or childbirth (Gay and others 2003) and at least 30 women are left with long-term disabilities, such as an obstetric fistula (UNFPA 2003). These estimates must be regarded as crude approximations, most originating from small-scale studies and most in urgent need of updating and verification. Given the varying case fatality rates shown in table 26.1, the fact that the distributional pattern for morbidity (figure 26.1b) does not completely mirror the one for mortality is not surprising.

As concerns mortality in babies, an estimated 5.7 million perinatal deaths occur each year, 47 percent as stillbirths and 53 percent in the first week of life (J. Zupan, personal communication, August 25, 2004). Many of those deaths are linked directly with complications experienced by the mothers, and several studies have shown that the survival prospects for a baby whose mother dies are generally poor—less than 1 percent in one study in Bangladesh (Koenig, Fauveau, and Wojtyniak 1991). In 2004, neonatal deaths represented 36 percent of all deaths of children under five in developing

Table 26.2 Estimates of Maternal Mortality by Region, 2000–1

Region	Maternal mortality ratio (maternal deaths per 100,000 live births), 2000	Number of maternal deaths as modeled by WHO, 2000	Estimated number of maternal deaths, 2001	Lifetime risk of maternal death (1 in number shown)	Range of uncertainty of maternal mortality ratio estimates		Total fertility rate
					Lower estimate	Upper estimate	
Central and Eastern Europe, Commonwealth of Independent States, Baltic states, Europe, and Central Asia	64	3,400	3,000	770	29	100	1.6
East Asia and the Pacific	110	37,000	37,000	360	44	210	2.0
Eastern and Southern Africa	980	123,000	—	15	490	1,500	5.5
Latin America and the Caribbean	190	22,000	16,000	160	110	280	2.6
Middle East and North Africa	220	21,000	15,000	100	85	380	3.7
South Asia	560	205,000	199,000	43	370	760	3.5
Sub-Saharan Africa	940	240,000	237,000	16	400	1,500	5.7
Western and Central Africa	900	118,000	—	16	310	1,600	5.9
High-income countries	13	1,300	1,000	4,000	8	17	1.6
Low- and middle-income countries	440	527,000	507,000	61	230	680	3.0
Low-income countries	890	236,000	—	17	410	1,400	5.4
World	400	529,000	508,000	74	210	620	2.7

Source: WHO 2004b, 2004d; UN 2002.

— = not available.

Note: The regions are those used by the United Nations Children's Fund.

countries, with about 1 million of these 3.94 million neonatal deaths occurring in the first week of life (Jamison and others 2004). Table 26.3 presents modeled estimates for early neonatal deaths in 2001. The data on the magnitude and patterns of stillbirths remain particularly poor.

Given weak sources of information, the dearth of reliable trends data is hardly surprising. At a global level, a major difficulty arises from the need to use models to estimate maternal mortality. As the basic methodology for the models has changed over time, the data are not appropriate for trend assessment. AbouZahr and Wardlaw (2001) provide patchy support for downward trends in some parts of the world, mostly on the basis of civil registration data and mostly restricted to countries with maternal mortality ratios of less than 100 per 100,000 live births—thus notably excluding South Asia and Sub-Saharan Africa. Even where declines appear to have occurred, they did so prior to 1990. Countries with sustained falls since then, such as Argentina and China, cannot be regarded as representative of all developing countries. Cause-specific trend data are extremely rare, often gathered through small-scale hospital-based studies

or special inquiries (see, for example, Pattinson 2002). Recent WHO (2004c) statistics on unsafe abortion show an apparent decrease in incidence in all world regions, although the risk of death remains high at 50 per 100,000 live births, and in parts of Sub-Saharan Africa the risk is as high as 140 per 100,000 live births (Rogo, Bohmer, and Ombaka 1999). These adverse events, however, are often also the most seriously underreported, as elaborated further in chapter 57.

The availability of reliable trends data for perinatal mortality is even more problematic. A demand for population-based estimates for newborn mortality is comparatively recent; thus, there has been insufficient time to accumulate multiple data points. Demographic and health surveys (DHSs) are a key source for tracking trends in infant and child mortality. Several DHSs now have data that can be disaggregated to show neonatal deaths, but only a few have information on stillbirths, and the quality of that information is still being assessed. Information from WHO suggests that early neonatal death rates fell slightly, from 28 per 1,000 live births around 1980 to about 25 per 1,000 in 2000, for low- and middle-income countries,

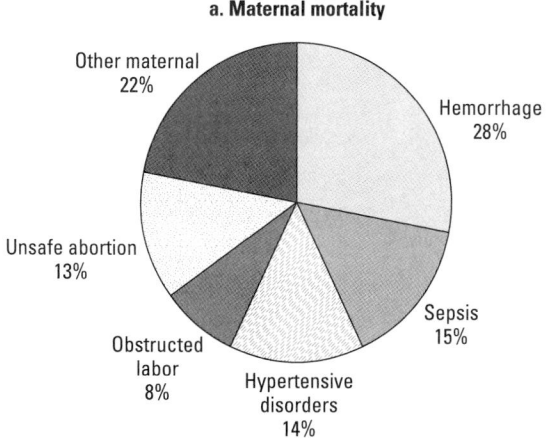

a. Maternal mortality

Other maternal 22%

Hemorrhage 28%

Unsafe abortion 13%

Sepsis 15%

Obstructed labor 8%

Hypertensive disorders 14%

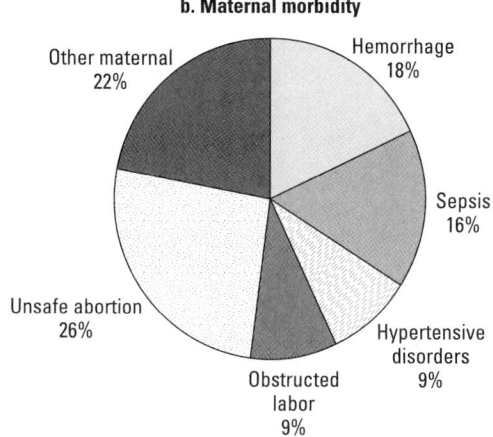

b. Maternal morbidity

Other maternal 22%

Hemorrhage 18%

Unsafe abortion 26%

Sepsis 16%

Hypertensive disorders 9%

Obstructed labor 9%

Source: Mortality: WHO 2004d; Morbidity: Murray and Lopez 1998.

Note: Nonobstetric (indirect) causes of death and morbidity, such as tuberculosis and malaria, have been excluded.

Figure 26.1 Medical Causes of Direct Maternal Mortality and Morbidity *(percentage distribution)*

and the equivalent trend for stillbirths is suggested to be a drop from 36 per 1,000 deliveries to 22 per 1,000 deliveries (J. Zupan, personal communication, August 25, 2004).

Two types of differentials are particularly relevant: geographic (or regional) and socioeconomic. Table 26.2 indicates the wide variation in the magnitude of maternal mortality across regions, and a similar difference can be seen between countries. In terms of absolute numbers of deaths, just 13 countries account for 70 percent of the global total (WHO 2004b).[2] Caution is again needed, because the poorest countries also have the weakest information systems and, therefore, have estimates derived solely from modeling. One regression model (WHO 2004b), for example, uses independent variables, such as the percentage of deliveries with health professionals present and the proportion of deaths of women of reproductive age that are maternal deaths. Those variables are themselves subject to error and likely to be least reliable where information systems are weakest. Geographic differences in maternal mortality within countries are poorly documented, although remote populations are often assumed to suffer the highest levels because of poor access to emergency obstetric care. Although this assumption seems logical, few reliable data are available to confirm or refute it, and the possibility of high levels of mortality in urban areas linked to unsafe abortion (Thonneau and others 2002) makes the topic of geographic differentials a priority for research.

Until recently, socioeconomic differentials in mortality have tended to be inferred from utilization patterns for prenatal care and health professionals at delivery. The DHSs continue to provide the main data sources in this regard, for both international and national analyses, and they demonstrate huge differences between wealth quintiles. A relevant recent development, however, is the familial technique, which can be used to examine socioeconomic differences in maternal mortality using existing survey data (Graham and others 2004). Because

Table 26.3 Early Neonatal Deaths by Gender and Cause, 2001 *(thousands)*

Cause	World[a]			South Asia			Sub-Saharan Africa[a]		
	All	Male	Female	All	Male	Female	All	Male	Female
Perinatal conditions[b]	2,522	1,400	1,123	1,086	596	489	573	332	241
Low birthweight[c]	1,301	710	591	757	406	351	243	141	102
Birth asphyxia (including birth trauma)	739	432	307	192	122	70	240	139	101
Other perinatal conditions[d]	482	258	225	137	68	68	90	52	38

Source: WHO 2004d.

a. Excludes the island of Mayotte.

b. Excludes stillbirths, congenital malformations, neonatal tetanus, congenital syphilis, acquired infections (respiratory and sepsis), and diarrhea.

c. Includes preterm deliveries and small for gestational age.

d. Includes all conditions originating in the perinatal period (P00–P96 codes in perinatal chapter of WHO 1992a), apart from low birthweight and asphyxia.

Table 26.4 DALYs for Perinatal and Maternal Conditions by Gender, Selected Regions, 2001 *(thousands)*

Condition	World[a]			South Asia			Sub-Saharan Africa[a]		
	All	Male	Female	All	Male	Female	All	Male	Female
Maternal	26,789	n.a.	26,789	10,069	n.a.	10,069	9,743	n.a.	9,743
Hemorrhage	3,928	n.a.	3,928	1,718	n.a.	1,718	1,643	n.a.	1,643
Sepsis	5,348	n.a.	5,348	1,857	n.a.	1,857	1,843	n.a.	1,843
Hypertensive disorders of pregnancy	1,895	n.a.	1,895	742	n.a.	742	842	n.a.	842
Obstructed labor	2,506	n.a.	2,506	1,185	n.a.	1,185	919	n.a.	919
Unsafe abortion	3,507	n.a.	3,507	1,467	n.a.	1,467	1,557	n.a.	1,557
Perinatal[b]	90,505	49,384	41,117	37,721	20,442	17,279	20,046	11,351	8,697
Low birthweight[c]	43,073	23,241	19,832	25,015	13,292	11,723	7,891	4,501	3,391
Birth asphyxia (including birth trauma)	31,972	17,945	14,025	8,283	4,957	3,326	9,256	5,195	4,062
Other perinatal conditions[d]	15,460	8,198	7,260	4,423	2,193	2,230	2,899	1,655	1,244

Source: WHO 2004d.
n.a. = not applicable.
a. Excludes the island of Mayotte.
b. Excludes stillbirths, congenital malformations, neonatal tetanus, congenital syphilis, acquired infections (respiratory and sepsis), and diarrhea.
c. Includes preterm deliveries and small for gestational age.
d. Includes all conditions originating in the perinatal period (P00–P96 codes in perinatal chapter of WHO 1992a) apart from low birthweight and asphyxia.

maternal health and health care are clearly associated with still-births and early neonatal deaths, the same differentiating factors are likely to apply to perinatal outcomes. Indeed, data from many DHSs show large gaps between rich and poor in relation to neonatal mortality, with the greatest average disparity being found in Latin American and the Caribbean (http://www.worldbank.org/poverty/health/).

Attributable Burden

The estimation of maternal and perinatal conditions as part of international assessments of the burden of disease has long been controversial, and much has been written about the problems and potential distortions of priorities (AbouZahr 1998; Sadana 2001). Some of those criticisms relate to methods of valuation based on disability-adjusted life years (DALYs), especially in relation to discounting and the omission of stillbirths, and others to the inaccuracies and selectivity of the base data on the incidence of complications, on case fatalities, and on disabilities. Table 26.4 presents DALYs for South Asia and Sub-Saharan Africa for the focus conditions for 2001. Those two regions together account for 74 percent of the global burden of maternal conditions and 64 percent of the global burden of perinatal conditions.

The significance of the burden of maternal and perinatal conditions is clear from two recent global assessments (CMH 2002; WHO 2002). The approaches the two initiatives adopted have led to different conclusions about public health priorities.

The former focused on avoidable mortality resulting primarily from direct obstetric conditions, whereas the latter considered population risk assessments and highlighted the contribution of indirect obstetric problems—especially micronutrient deficiencies—and the role for preventive strategies. Clearly, the choice between different measures of burden has a crucial influence both on the strategic approach to achieving health gains and on the prioritization of interventions.

INTERVENTIONS

Given the scope and nature of the burden of maternal and perinatal conditions, no quick fix is available and, thus, no single intervention warrants exclusive attention. Rather, clusters or packages of interventions need to be considered, and this understanding has long been reflected in maternity services throughout the world (Milne and others 2004). Even though these clusters can be characterized or differentiated solely on the basis of content—namely, the component interventions—in practice, the health system or implementation context is also a defining factor.

Levels and Types of Interventions

Box 26.1 presents one example of a comprehensive strategy for safe motherhood. It illustrates the range of programmatic

Components of a Comprehensive Safe Motherhood Strategy

The following are part of a comprehensive safe motherhood strategy:

- community education on safe motherhood and newborn care
- evidence-based prenatal care and counseling
  — nutritional advice
  — iron and folate supplements (multivitamins and micronutrients)
  — iodization of edible oils and salt and vitamin A in areas of endemic deficiency
  — blood pressure screening

— screening and treatment for syphilis
— antiretrovirals, where voluntary counseling and testing undertaken, and breastfeeding advice
— tetanus toxoid immunization
— treatment of urinary tract infections
- skilled assistance at delivery
- care of obstetric complications and emergencies
- postpartum care
- safe abortion and postabortion services
- family-planning information and services
- adolescent reproductive health education and services

Source: Dayaratna and others 2000.

issues raised by maternal and perinatal conditions:

- the scope for both primary and secondary prevention
- the difference between the individual receiving specific interventions (here, the mother) and the beneficiary (the baby)
- the multiple effects of single (component) interventions on different outcomes
- the multiple benefits to the same outcome of different interventions
- the short- and long-term time frames for interventions and outcomes
- the balance between supply-side and demand-side interventions
- the role for interventions outside the health sector.

Three main pathways are available for averting adverse outcomes: preventing pregnancy, preventing complications, and preventing death or disability from complications. The first pathway is the only truly primary preventive strategy. It requires intervention to avert the occurrence or mistiming of pregnancy by means of effective family-planning methods, as discussed in chapter 57. This preventive approach is relevant for those women who are able to and wish to avoid or delay pregnancy, but it has a limited role for those not in this position, estimated at between 15 and 57 percent of women age 15 to 29 (WHO 2002). As concerns the primary prevention of complications, comparatively limited reliable evidence is available on the true size of the avoidable fraction for many conditions at a population level. The emphasis in this preventive pathway is on maintaining normality and on managing mild complications—and thus on good quality of care. Finally,

maternal death and disability may be avoided by effective, timely, and appropriate clinical interventions, often referred to as *emergency obstetric care.*

Given this complexity and the multiple approaches used to address maternal and perinatal conditions, no perfect framework for categorizing interventions exists. We, therefore, cluster the alternative intervention pathways on the basis of the following three parameters:

- level of care—home, primary, and secondary
- time period—pregnancy, labor and delivery, and postpartum
- strategic approach—population-based versus personal interventions.

Quality of Evidence

Pregnancy and childbirth have been the subjects of medical investigation for centuries and, indeed, are among the oldest clinical specialties. As a consequence, a substantial body of opinion exists on the signs, symptoms, etiology, prognosis, natural history, and management and treatment options for many maternal and perinatal complications, particularly in developed countries. Much of it can be regarded as conventional wisdom acquired through practice. In contrast, a comparatively small proportion of interventions can be regarded as based on evidence, by contemporary scientific standards, and arrived at through the conduct of robust research. Thus, in specification of the content of intervention clusters, a built-in tension exists between using the best available knowledge and using only evidence that passes minimum quality criteria. Equally important is recognizing the fundamental distinction between knowing what is effective at an individual case-management level, for which an evidence base exists for maternal and perinatal conditions, and demonstrating effectiveness at the aggregate levels of composite strategies and entire countries or regions, for which robust evidence is extremely limited (Graham 2002).

Population-Based Interventions

The primary aim of population-based interventions is to reduce the risks leading to adverse outcomes at the population level rather than at the individual level (WHO 2002). Population-based interventions are essentially preventive and seek to promote healthy behaviors, thereby reducing incidence in the entire population. In the case of maternal and perinatal conditions, such an approach could be adopted for two major risk factors: lack of contraception and maternal undernutrition. The grade of evidence for these population-based interventions is primarily level C for the former, but a mixture of A and B for the latter.[3]

Fertility Behavior Change. Fertility behavior is ultimately the primary exposure factor for both maternal and perinatal conditions. Investigators have shown that the frequency (number and spacing), the timing with regard to age, and the desirability of pregnancy are associated with increased risks, although some dispute remains about the effect of birth intervals. Researchers have also investigated the influence of those factors on perinatal conditions, finding clear associations with old or young maternal age, short interpregnancy intervals, and high or first birth order, with many of those variables also being interrelated (Bale and others 2003).

Lack of effective use of contraception may result in unwanted or mistimed pregnancies. Unintended pregnancies are known to be associated with adverse maternal outcomes, including unsafe abortion. Contraceptive behavior is clearly determined by a host of socioeconomic, cultural, religious, and medical factors (Hussain, Fikree, and Berendes 2000; Marston and Cleland 2003; Mwageni, Ankomah, and Powell 2001), which also have a bearing on intervention options. Most of the options on the demand side focus on information, education, and communication; those on the supply side focus on client-friendly services. At a macro level, those intervention options have been credited with the substantial increase in contraceptive use in developing countries over the past 40 years, which, in turn, is seen as a contributor to the overall fall in the total fertility rate from 6 to 3 (Cleland and Ali 2004). Nevertheless, a significant unmet need for contraception persists in many developing countries, with high levels of unsafe abortion as a proxy indicator of that need.

As regards evidence of the effectiveness of family planning in explicitly reducing maternal mortality or disability, no primary sources are available, but there are a variety of modeled estimates, such as Prata and others (2004), Walsh and others (1993), and Winikoff and Sullivan (1987). Model estimates vary enormously in terms of the size of the effect, depending primarily on assumptions about the proportion of maternal deaths caused by unsafe abortion. Investigators estimate the potential gain from the avoidance of unintended or mistimed pregnancies to be a 20 percent decrease in maternal deaths in developing countries (Donnay 2000; Kurjak and Bekavac 2001; UNICEF 1999).

Nutritional Interventions. Maternal undernutrition encompasses two main dimensions: underweight and micronutrient deficiencies (principally iron and vitamin A). Unlike many of the direct maternal complications, which are acute at onset and of relatively short duration, these nutritional problems are chronic and long term and, indeed, are intergenerational (Tomkins 2001). The physiological mechanisms by which undernutrition exerts an influence on outcomes in the mother and baby are not entirely understood, but a large body of epidemiological evidence supports associations with, for example, fetal growth or length of pregnancy (Villar and others 2002). Those findings have originated mostly from populations with either severe levels of undernutrition or significant cofactors, such as malaria and other infections.

Considerable uncertainty surrounds the issue of timing potential interventions, with conflicting opinions about making targeted interventions during pregnancy; addressing undernutrition among girl children or adolescents, and applying strategies for women of reproductive age, including periconceptual women (Gay and others 2003; Rush 2000). Further debate relates to the use of supplements versus food fortification. A systematic review by Villar and others (2002) of randomized controlled trials to prevent or treat adverse maternal outcomes and preterm delivery concludes that limited evidence supports large-scale interventions with multivitamins, minerals, or protein-energy supplementation, but that iron and folic acid are effective against anemia. Rouse (2003) emphasizes the potential cost-effectiveness of vitamin A or beta-carotene supplementation in reducing maternal mortality if the findings of West and others (1999) from Nepal are replicable elsewhere.

Personal Interventions

When we consider interventions directed at individuals rather than whole populations, the need for a continuum of care for mother and baby in terms of time (before and after delivery), place (linking home and health services through an effective referral chain), and person (the provider of care) is important. A variety of conceptual frameworks emphasize this continuum and the dangers of fragmentation. Care to prevent or treat the vast majority of maternal and perinatal conditions can be provided at home, at the primary level (clinic or health center), and at the secondary level (district hospital),[4] with the district or equivalent regarded as the essential planning unit for service delivery (WHO 1994). This system is comparable to the "close-to-client" health system that the Commission on Macroeconomics and Health (CMH 2002) has proposed, whereby trained staff members other than doctors provide much of the care, with an emphasis on primary prevention and management of acute conditions.

Home-Based Care. Two topical interventions that fall into the category of home-based care are (a) information, education, and communication and birth preparedness and (b) male involvement (for home-based newborn care, see chapter 27). Evidence in this cluster of interventions falls predominantly into the level C category.

Birth Preparedness Many descriptive studies indicate that women, relatives, and other members of the community frequently do not recognize danger signs in pregnancy, childbirth, or the puerperium, and that lack of recognition can have serious consequences for mother and baby (Gay and others 2003). Health education interventions at prenatal clinics appear to be less successful at raising awareness and increasing the use of emergency obstetric care than the use of pictorial cards (Khanum and others 2000) or community education (Bailey, Szaszdi, and Schieber 1995).

Birth preparedness includes planning for the place and the attendant at delivery, as well as arranging for rapid transfer to a health center or hospital, when needed, and sometimes identifying a compatible blood donor in the case of hemorrhage (Portela and Santarelli 2003). Initiatives to promote birth preparedness can clearly be home or community based, but studies have emphasized the importance of linkages with prenatal care so as to include appropriate recommendations for intrapartum care (Shehu, Ikeh, and Kuna 1997). In circumstances in which prenatal services are of poor quality or are underused, traditional birth attendants or relatives are often the only source of information; thus, initiatives need to reach those individuals too.

Male Involvement Many studies have observed positive benefits from the involvement of male partners in care-seeking behavior related to pregnancy and delivery (Gay and others 2003). That involvement is now advocated as an essential element of WHO's Making Pregnancy Safer Initiative (WHO 2003). Models and mechanisms for achieving this involvement have not been robustly evaluated, and considerable controversy concerns those that are based on behavioral and social cognitive theories that presume lack of knowledge as the root problem (Portela and Santarelli 2003; Raju and Leonard 2000).

Primary-Level Care. Primary-level care is widely regarded as the crucial entry point to maternity services—and also to care before and after pregnancy. The focus here is essentially preventive, but with the capacity to detect problems, to manage mild complications appropriately, and to stabilize and then refer cases that require higher-level care. Although the name used for primary care facilities varies from country to country, we employ the commonly used term *health center*. In terms of functionality in relation to maternal and perinatal care, the health center should provide prenatal, delivery (including management of complicated abortion), and postpartum care (including family planning and postabortion counseling), as well as care of the newborn.

The management of complicated cases is usually discussed at two levels: basic emergency obstetric care (BEmOC) and comprehensive emergency obstetric care (CEmOC), the distinction being made on the basis of the number of signal or essential clinical functions performed.[5] This distinction forms the basis of a set of process indicators that the United Nations (UN) has endorsed for program monitoring (UNFPA 2003). The capacity of health centers to provide BEmOC depends on the availability of supplies, drugs, infrastructure, and skilled providers. Some of the signal functions may not always be performed by midwives or nurses, sometimes because of the regulation of roles by the government or professional bodies. For this reason, a further distinction can be made between full BEmOC, which comprises six functions, some of which may require a doctor, and obstetric first aid, which includes two signal functions universally performed by midwives and nurses: the administration of antibiotics or oxytocics, intravenously or intramuscularly.

Routine Prenatal Care The literature available on routine prenatal care is extensive, and there is a long history of assessing the component interventions (Hall, MacIntyre, and Porter 1985; Rooney 1992). In safe motherhood programs, prenatal care provides one of the rare examples of robust assessment of an intervention package (Villar and others 2001). As Bale and others (2003) note, even though many of the component clinical interventions are effective in terms of perinatal outcomes (Bergsjo and Villar 1997), reliable evidence of an effect on maternal mortality in developing countries is not available (McDonagh 1996). However, where early detection is followed by appropriate treatment, prenatal care does seem to reduce adverse outcomes from specific maternal conditions, including hypertensive disorders of pregnancy, urinary tract infections, and breech presentations (Carroli, Rooney, and Villar 2001; Villar and Bergsjo 1997). Conversely, the limited effectiveness of prenatal risk screening at a population level is now widely acknowledged (Graham 1998). The poor predictive value of many screening tools for maternal complications reinforces the importance of access to emergency obstetric care for all women who develop a need for it and underlies calls for skilled attendance at all deliveries. Many health experts, however, do accept screening and treatment for syphilis and immunization with tetanus toxoid as important prenatal interventions (Bale and others 2003). Similarly, the prevention and treatment of anemia and of malaria, with prophylaxis or bednets, are widely regarded as essential elements of routine prenatal care. Nutritional supplementation, however, remains more controversial.

Prenatal care has been assessed not only in terms of content, but also in relation to alternative models of the number and timing of visits (Munjanja, Lindmark, and Nystrom 1996). Strong evidence exists on the cost-effectiveness of a targeted, four-visit schedule (Villar and others 2001) that includes an educational element on the recognition of danger signs and the use of skilled attendance at delivery.

The principal sources of international data on levels, trends, and differentials in prenatal care coverage are the DHSs. The latest statistics show comparatively high coverage levels when measured in terms of one or more visits—levels average 71 percent for Sub-Saharan Africa—but comparatively little improvement between 1990 and 2000. Within countries, wide socioeconomic differentials in uptake are apparent.

Delivery Care As indicated earlier, the risks of adverse outcomes in mother and baby are usually highest during the intrapartum period. Even though health experts have long appreciated this fact, prioritization of this element of safe motherhood is comparatively recent. Much has been written both on this shift in emphasis and on the underlying rationale, as well as on what skilled attendance at delivery should comprise (De Brouwere and Van Lerberghe 2001). Investigators have suggested a variety of conceptual models for defining content, with varying degrees of emphasis on the attendant and on the enabling environment (Bell and others 2003). All these models recognize that skilled attendance encompasses both normal and complicated deliveries, with the focus on the former and on the management of mild complications at the primary level, as is consistent with BEmOC, and with referral to CEmOC at the secondary level when necessary.

Key unresolved issues at the primary level relate to the skills and scope of work of the attendant, especially in relation to being a multipurpose health worker, and to the potential role of nonprofessionals, such as auxiliaries and trained traditional birth attendants (Buttiens, Marchal, and De Brouwere 2004). Work by Koblinsky and Campbell (2003) has helped to inform this debate by proposing four basic models of delivery care that vary according to configurations of place of delivery and attendant. Evidence on the effectiveness of the alternative models at a population level is lacking, and support for skilled attendance at delivery is, thus, based primarily on historical and contemporary ecological analysis (De Brouwere and Van Lerberghe 2001). Conversely, high-grade

evidence supports a number of clinical interventions, such as active management of the third stage of labor, as well as essential newborn care.

Once again, the principal sources of data on levels and trends in coverage of skilled attendants at delivery are the DHSs. The data, however, are based on women's self-reports of who attended their deliveries, include only live births, and have major definitional uncertainties. Some countries, for example, use terms such as *supervised deliveries* and include as attendants both auxiliaries and trained traditional birth attendants (see Bell, Curtis, and Alayon 2003 for a critique of these data). A global analysis of trends in deliveries by skilled attendants showed wide variations in progress across different regions, with the latest figures for Sub-Saharan Africa, Asia, and Latin America and the Caribbean for 1990–2003 being 48, 59, and 82 percent, respectively (AbouZahr and Wardlaw 2001; WHO 2004a). The proportion of deliveries with health professionals present (doctors, midwives, nurses) is one of the proxy indicators for the MDG on maternal health (Graham and Hussein 2004). It demonstrates not only major differentials between countries, but also wide variation in uptake across socioeconomic groups within countries (De Brouwere and Van Lerberghe 2001). Although skilled attendants do not necessarily operate only in fixed health facilities such as health centers, the DHS data show low levels of professional attendance in the community. Promoting skilled attendance is thus essentially advocating for institutionalizing deliveries.

Postpartum Care Primary care services continue to neglect the postpartum period despite significant morbidity among mothers and babies during this time. Routine performance of postnatal checks is not widespread, and most contacts with services after delivery tend to focus on educational messages on, for example, danger signs, breastfeeding, nutrition, and lifestyle.

Postabortion Care One significant area of service delivery that does not fit well with descriptive frameworks based on prenatal, intrapartum, and postpartum care is the management of complicated abortions. Unsafe abortion accounts for a significant proportion of the burden of maternal conditions, but it is still treated as the poor relation in the debate on intervention strategies (De Brouwere and Van Lerberghe 2001). In particular, with the prioritization in recent years of skilled attendance at delivery, both the service base for and the provider of postabortion care have become less well defined (Dayaratna and others 2000). This crucial element of obstetric care falls into BEmOC in the case of mild complications and CEmOC for more serious cases, but whether it is regarded as part of prenatal, delivery, or postnatal services appears to vary from setting to setting. Moreover, postabortion care illustrates the dangers of the fragmentation of broader reproductive health care, because primary prevention and counseling after treatment for complications tend to fall within the remit of family-planning services, whereas emergency care at the primary level is usually provided as part of maternity services and at the secondary level may fall within obstetrics or gynecology services.

Secondary-Level Care. Secondary-level care is hospital-based care, generally at the district level, including CEmOC. As a center for referral, this level of care needs to be linked to the primary level through an effective chain of communications (Murray and others 2001). The focus at the district hospital is on secondary prevention, with the ability to manage the principal maternal and perinatal conditions discussed earlier; thus, district hospitals must be able to provide surgical interventions and the requisite backup, such as blood banks (Kusiako, Ronsmans, and Van der Paul 2000). In many countries, however, the district hospital is also the local provider of preventive services, including prenatal and normal delivery care; as such, it is responsible for attending to a wide mix of uncomplicated and complicated cases.

Although no high-grade evidence of the effectiveness of CEmOC is available, many health experts agree that maternal mortality cannot be significantly reduced in the absence of such care (Bale and others 2003). The issue thus becomes one of the cost-effectiveness of other strategies, given the presence of CEmOC. The UN agencies have endorsed the threshold of one CEmOC facility per 500,000 people. Data indicating the attainment of this ratio—and, indeed, the percentage of met need for CEmOC—are not widely available. Similarly, reliable information on geographic or socioeconomic differentials in access to CEmOC is extremely limited.

Policy Considerations and Approaches

The health of mothers and babies is a human right and needs to be underpinned by policies and laws that increase access to information and good-quality, affordable health services (Germain 2000). A positive policy environment is crucial for promoting maternal health and reducing the burden of maternal and perinatal conditions. Such policy considerations need to go beyond the health sector to include related issues, such as transportation, nutrition, girls' access to education, and gender biases in the control of economic resources. Through a human rights–based approach, programs can be fashioned to ensure that every woman has the right to make informed decisions about her own health and has access to quality services before, during, and after childbirth (Freedman 2001).

The ICPD marked a dramatic shift not only by putting the concepts of rights and choice center stage, but also by introducing the reproductive health paradigm. The first decade of the ICPD plan of action was marked by major improvements in policies related to maternal health in most of the 179 signatory countries. However, as observed at the ICPD + 10 Conference, many promised changes remain at the level of policy pronouncement and have not yet been implemented. The stagnation is most notable in relation to maternal mortality and the HIV pandemic, especially in Sub-Saharan Africa. The failure to fully implement the ICPD consensus can be attributed to lack of political will, inadequate funding for programs to further reproductive health, and weak health systems. It is too early to judge the effect of the MDG proclamation (Johansson and Stewart 2002), although it could well suffer the same fate unless special attention is given to maternal and child health in the context of sectorwide approaches and Poverty Reduction Strategy Papers (UNFPA 2003). Some suspect that both these modalities may not give reproductive health the focus and attention it requires, because competing needs may crowd it out. Others argue, however, that sectorwide approaches can be a boon for maternal health because they offer a more effective platform for addressing ailing health systems (Goodburn and Campbell 2001).

Whether at the national or international level, advocacy for maternal and perinatal health should focus on the following seven key message areas:

- magnitude of the problem
- factors influencing maternal and perinatal outcomes
- functions of maternal health programs and which interventions work
- consequences of not addressing maternal and perinatal health
- costs of improving maternal and perinatal health
- responsibilities at each level of the health system and beyond
- policy and legal impediments to implementing comprehensive safe motherhood and newborn health programs.

Major advocacy networks, such as the Partnership for Safe Motherhood and Newborn Health, the White Ribbon Alliance, and the Healthy Newborn Partnership, seek to promote maternal and newborn health at the global level. Their purpose is to create awareness by changing the language of discourse, building international political commitment, developing global guidelines, and improving access to technical information for providers and program managers.

COST-EFFECTIVENESS OF SELECTED INTERVENTION PACKAGES

Cost-effectiveness analysis (CEA) faces several major challenges with respect to evaluating the prevention and treatment of maternal and perinatal conditions. First is the sheer range of conditions and potential interventions. The breadth of the clinical area implies the need to make tough choices with respect to which packages of interventions to compare. A second and related challenge is the lack both of reliable data on the burden of conditions and of high-grade evidence on the effectiveness and costs of packages. As a result, we can assess only the relative cost-effectiveness of different packages of interventions by means of modeling. Thus, the third set of challenges is associated with modeling, which makes the analysis vulnerable to all the usual criticisms of the modeling of cost-effectiveness—in particular, uncertainty about the direction of any bias introduced and the difficulty of establishing the validity of the model (Sheldon 1996). Finally, there are the related issues of the appropriateness to maternal and perinatal conditions of standard outcome measures used in the model—in particular, DALYs, which exclude stillbirths and indirect maternal conditions (AbouZahr 1999; De Brouwere and Van Lerberghe 2001).

Selected Intervention Packages

For some of the reasons mentioned in the previous subsection, researchers have made few attempts to model packages of interventions for maternal and perinatal conditions, and many of those attempts do not specify content in sufficient detail to replicate the package. Our approach is to define content by beginning with a literature search of best practices in preventing and managing the focus maternal and perinatal conditions, acknowledging that, by excluding conditions that impose a lesser burden, we ignore interventions that might be highly effective and cost-effective. We then grouped those interventions that are considered effective and that are either being or likely to be implemented on a substantial scale into packages of care, bearing in mind previous CEA work, such as the WHO mother-baby package (WHO 1994). Expert panels then reviewed the component interventions and the packages and assisted with identifying resource requirements. Given the complementary CEA elsewhere in this volume on interventions relevant to maternal and perinatal conditions such as family planning, we focus on care during pregnancy, postpregnancy care, and care immediately postdelivery—in other words, on clusters or packages of interventions typically referred to as *prenatal care, delivery* or *intrapartum care,* and *emergency obstetric care.* Table 26.5 outlines the content of those packages.

When one considers the intervention packages, contextual factors are clearly crucial. Given the particularly high burden in South Asia and Sub-Saharan Africa, we chose those two regions as the specific health system scenarios for this chapter. Those regions are also characterized by high levels of poverty and encompass some of the most heavily indebted countries in the world.

Comparison of Alternative Intervention Package Scenarios. Following the approach of generalized CEA (Hutubessy and

others 2003), we evaluated intervention packages with respect to a counterfactual (base scenario), varying the content and coverage. We also performed sensitivity analyses to examine the effects of changing the values of key variables for costs, effectiveness, or both. Each intervention package scenario specifies different dimensions of prenatal and intrapartum care provided at primary and secondary care facilities. As regards the assumed pathways through which women with normal or complicated pregnancies may or may not access care, the crucial entry point in our model is prenatal care. That choice influences the detection and treatment of mild and severe complications during the antepartum period at both the primary and the secondary levels, as well as the proportion of women delivering with a health professional present and with improved access to emergency care for intrapartum or abortion-related complications. In our CEA model, these effects are achieved primarily through two types of interventions:

- improvements in the quality of care, incorporating the technical content or the proportion of women in receipt of the care needed (that is, met need)
- increases in the coverage of care—namely, the proportion of women accessing care.

Routine prenatal care can be characterized in terms of whether it is a basic or an enhanced package—in other words, its technical content (table 26.5)—and by the percentage of women accessing the package—in other words, its coverage. Delivery at a primary-level health center is viewed as having a single quality dimension in terms of content—namely, whether BEmOC is available for women who develop mild complications, including complicated abortion (table 26.5). BEmOC is assumed to require the presence of a doctor at the health center; otherwise, only obstetric first aid is presumed to be available, covering just the two signal functions described earlier.

A percentage of women with severe complications who access primary care will go on to secondary care. This percentage is assumed to be 20 or 50 percent of complicated cases attending primary care. Our model makes no provision for women who access secondary care directly in the event of a serious complication, although it does allow for those who were attending the hospital as their local provider of primary care. Of those women who access the secondary care facility from the primary level, a proportion will receive the CEmOC that they need (assumed to vary between 50 and 90 percent of complicated cases that reach secondary care). This figure reflects such issues as staff skills and motivation and the availability of drugs and equipment. For the other quality-of-care element—namely, the technical content of CEmOC—we consider two levels: with (enhanced package) and without (base package) selected interventions for high-risk babies (table 26.5).

Table 26.5 Care Packages at the Primary and Secondary Levels

Level of care and condition	Content	Base package	Enhanced package
Routine prenatal care at the primary level[a]	Clinical examination, including for severe anemia, height and weight, blood pressure	√	√
	Obstetric examination for gestational age estimation and uterine height, fetal heart, detection of malpresentation and position, and referral	√	√
	Gynecological examination	√	√
	Urine test (multiple dipstick)	√	√
	Laboratory tests: hemoglobin, blood type and rhesus status, syphilis and other symptomatic testing for sexually transmitted diseases	√	√
	Advice on emergencies, delivery, lactation, and contraception	√	√
	Education about clean delivery, warning signs, and premature rupture of membranes	√	√
	Iron and folic acid supplementation	√	√
	Multivitamin supplementation	—	√
	Tetanus toxoid immunization	√	√
	HIV voluntary testing and counseling	—	√
	Antimalarial chemoprophylaxis in endemic areas	—	√
	Screening and treatment for syphilis	√	√
	Balanced protein-energy supplementation for all women	—	√
Delivery care at the primary level[b]	Clean delivery technique, clean cord cutting, clean delivery of baby and placenta	√	√
	Active management of the third stage of labor, including oxytocics	√	√
	Episiotomy in appropriate cases	√	√
	Recognition and first-line management of delivery complications (for example, obstructed labor, early detection of cephalopelvic disproportion, malposition and malpresentation, previous cesarean delivery, postpartum hemorrhage, and preeclampsia or eclampsia) and referral	√	√
	Intravenous fluid	√	√
	Intravenous uterotonics, if bleeding occurs	√	√
	Partograph	√	√
	Essential newborn care	√	√
	Intravenous antibiotics	√	√
	Magnesium sulfate	—	√
	Forceps or vacuum extraction	—	√
	Manual removal of placenta	—	√
	Removal of retained products of conception	—	√
	Corticosteroids for preterm labor	—	√
	Antiretrovirals for prevention of mother-to-child transmission of HIV	—	√
	Antibiotics for premature rupture of membranes	—	√
CEmOC package at the secondary level[c]			
Postpartum hemorrhage	Recognition of high-risk cases and arrangements for delivery in a facility	√	√
	Grouping of blood	√	√
	Iron and folate supplementation	√	√
	Blood transfusion	√	√
	Uterotonic drugs, oxytocics	√	√
	Bimanual compression of uterus	√	√
	Manual removal of placenta	√	√
	Uterine packing or balloon tamponade	√	√
	Fluid replacement	√	√
	Hysterectomy	√	√
	Removal of products of conception	√	√
	Secondary postpartum hemorrhage management (antibiotics, uterotonics, removal of products of conception, and fluid and blood replacement)	√	√

(Continues on the following page.)

Table 26.5 Continued

Level of care and condition	Content	Base package	Enhanced package
Antepartum hemorrhage	Early detection of major placenta previa and abruption	√	√
	Grouping and saving blood	√	√
	Iron and folate supplementation	√	√
	Cesarean section for major-degree placenta previa, abruption with a live baby	√	√
	Blood and fluid replacement	√	√
	Oxytocics	√	√
Sepsis	Antibiotics for premature rupture of membranes, cesarean section	√	√
	Fluid and blood transfusion	√	√
	Intravenous antibiotics	√	√
	Evacuation of products of conception	√	√
	Drainage of abscess	√	√
	Treatment of shock with fluids or blood, nitroglycerine	√	√
Pregnancy-induced hypertension	Early detection and management of preeclampsia	√	√
	Calcium supplementation in high-risk cases	√	√
	Aspirin to prevent preeclampsia	√	√
	Antioxidants to prevent preeclampsia	√	√
	Intravenous magnesium sulfate	√	√
	Antihypertensive drugs to reduce blood pressure	√	√
	Immediate delivery if more than 36 weeks	√	√
	Magnesium sulfate and antihypertensives for postpartum eclampsia	√	√
Obstructed labor	Partograph	√	√
	Cesarean section	√	√
	Symphysiotomy	√	√
	Destructive operation	√	√
	Antibiotics	√	√
	Fluid and blood transfusion	√	√
	Hysterectomy	√	√
Abortion	Evacuation of retained products of conception	√	√
	Intravenous antibiotics	√	√
	Fluid or blood transfusion	√	√
	Postabortion contraceptive advice	√	√
Ectopic pregnancy	Proof puncture (culdocentesis)	—	—
	Laparotomy and salpingectomy	—	—
	Blood transfusion (autotransfusion)	√	√
High-risk infant	Forceps or vacuum extraction[d]	√	√
	Corticosteroids for preterm labor	—	√
	Antiretrovirals for prevention of mother-to-child transmission of HIV	—	√
	Antibiotics for premature rupture of membranes	—	√

Source: Authors.

— = not available.

a. The base package includes the four-visit schedule recommended by WHO (Villar and others 2001).

b. The base package includes the provision of obstetric first aid (intravenous or intramuscular antibiotics and oxytocics). The enhanced package includes the availability of a doctor, and thus the full range of BEmOC (UNFPA 2003). In some settings, experienced midwives or clinical officers may perform all six BEmOC functions.

c. At the hospital level, prenatal or delivery care will also be provided for normal, uncomplicated cases and, thus, also includes all care listed in the first two panels of the table.

d. Forceps or vacuum delivery can also be used for several other conditions, such as prolonged labor (not obstructed), fetal distress, preterm birth, aftercoming head of breech, and preeclampsia to speed up delivery.

The base case for our CEA model assumes the following:

- basic technical content for the prenatal care package
- prenatal care coverage for 50 percent of pregnancies
- only obstetric first aid (two signal functions) available in health centers
- 20 percent of women with severe complications accessing secondary care
- 50 percent of those severe cases receiving the CEmOC that they need.

The different assumptions regarding quality of care and coverage can be combined in many different ways, yielding a large number of potential packages and a larger number of potential comparisons between those and the base package. However, not all possible scenarios are meaningful. For example, because the base prenatal care package does not screen for HIV, matching that package with enhanced delivery care that provides antiretrovirals to reduce vertical transmission would be inappropriate. We identified six packages for comparison with the base case, representing a range of safe motherhood strategies and focusing on prenatal and delivery care. Table 26.6 summarizes these alternatives and indicates their essential characteristics from a safe motherhood perspective.

Resource Use and Costs

We adopted an ingredients approach (Creese and Parker 1994) to identify resource use. For this type of bottom-up costing, we prepared lists for primary- and secondary-level care facilities of types of personnel, drugs, supplies (medical and nonmedical), medical and surgical equipment relevant for the interventions, and capital items (vehicles, buildings, building space). For most of the scenarios, our identification of resources was based on the WHO mother-baby package costing tool (WHO 1999), with necessary modifications because of the content of care packages indicated in table 26.5. We estimated the costs for clinical personnel on the basis of salaries for different grades according to the guidelines provided by the volume editors for the two selected regions. The time required by different staff members for each care intervention and the changes in time and personnel because of varying content and coverage of packages were informed by expert panel reviews, and we then calculated the costs. We valued the other nontraded inputs using information primarily provided by WHO-CHOICE (2004).

Cost-Effectiveness Ratios

The CEA involves a number of fixed and variable assumptions (see annex 26.A). The most important assumptions concern the reducible burden of these conditions, the effectiveness of the interventions, and the availability of appropriate human resources. We have assumed that increases in care can be achieved without major capital investments and that human resources are not in short supply; therefore, more could be used (with given wage rates) as required for increased activity and enhanced coverage.

Table 26.7 summarizes the findings of the CEA in terms of incremental cost-effectiveness ratios (ICERs) for the six primary comparisons between the base scenario and alternative intervention packages for a population of 1 million. Table 26.8 gives details of total costs, deaths averted, life years saved, and DALYs averted. Table 26.9 shows the findings of the sensitivity analysis in terms of how the ICERs change when different assumptions (see annex 26.A) are made with respect to effectiveness, met need, and inpatient costs.

In interpreting the results, note that they are point estimates. Even though they are based on the best information currently available, all the inputs into the model are subject to some degree of uncertainty. Without access to robust data on individual costs and effects or without specifying distributions for each variable, it is impossible to identify confidence limits for the estimated ICERs. Thus, we do not know, for example, whether the difference in the incremental cost per DALY averted for Sub-Saharan Africa between increased coverage at the primary level (US$92) and improved quality of CEmOC (US$151) reflects a genuine difference in cost-effectiveness or whether there are overlapping confidence intervals (table 26.7).

With those important caveats in mind, at first sight the results for South Asia and Sub-Saharan Africa appear quite different. For each intervention package, regardless of the specific assumptions made, the cost per DALY averted is always lower in Sub-Saharan Africa. The higher costs of care in Sub-Saharan Africa (see annex 26.A) are thus more than compensated for by the higher effectiveness, which is a result of the region's greater burden. However, some important similarities are apparent between South Asia and Sub-Saharan Africa. Leaving aside options 3b and 5b (the options without nutritional supplements), the results for both regions show a consistent pattern. Improvements in the overall quality of care, especially at the primary level through the provision of BEmOC (option 3a), together with increased overall coverage (option 5a), are the most cost-effective intervention packages—and both include nutritional supplements. They are followed by increased coverage at the primary level (option 2). Improved quality of CEmOC (option 4) is the least cost-effective option. Removing nutritional supplements from the packages makes relatively little difference in Sub-Saharan Africa, slightly increasing cost-effectiveness, but in South Asia, options 3b and 5b become less cost-effective with the nutritional supplements removed. The explanation lies in the ICERs of nutritional supplements as such, which are US$48 or US$45 in South Asia and US$118 or US$110 in Sub-Saharan Africa, depending on whether the

Table 26.6 Comparisons Undertaken for CEA

Abbreviated description of package	Option number	Primary level		Secondary level			Interpretation	Safe motherhood strategy	Resource implications
		Coverage	Quality of care: technical content	Coverage^a	Quality of care: Percentage receiving care needed	Quality of care: technical content			
Routine maternity care	Base	50 percent of pregnant women attend prenatal care; 50 percent of pregnant women have professional intrapartum care[b]	See first two panels of table 26.5	20 percent of complicated cases at the primary level referred to the secondary level	50 percent of those reaching the secondary level receive the CEmOC needed	See table 26.5[c]	Basic package of prenatal and delivery care	Content of package essentially the same as WHO mother-baby package, plus magnesium sulfate and active management of labor	Costs typical of WHO mother-baby package
Increased primary-level coverage	2	70 percent prenatal care; 70 percent delivery care	No change from base	No change from base	No change from base	No change from base	Benefit from increasing coverage	Information, education, and communication for increasing uptake of prenatal and delivery care	Costs of information, education, and communication; increased personnel; drugs
Improved overall quality of care with nutritional supplements	3a	No change from base	Enhanced prenatal and delivery care (BEmOC)	No change from base	70 percent	Enhanced CEmOC (adds interventions for high-risk babies)	Benefit from enhancing quality (content and receipt of care needed) at the primary and secondary levels	Provision of BEmOC at the primary level	Costs of doctors and equipment at the primary level, training for BEmOC and CEmOC, costs of BPS
Improved overall quality of care without nutritional supplements	3b	No change from base	Enhanced prenatal and delivery care (BEmOC) without BPS	No change from base	70 percent	Enhanced CEmOC (adds interventions for high-risk babies)	As for 3a without BPS	As for 3a	As for 3a without costs of BPS

Improved quality of CEmOC	4	No change from base	No change from base	No change from base	No change from base	80 percent	No change from base	Benefit from increased percentage of women with severe complications receiving the CEmOC needed	Improved quality of CEmOC	Cost of additional personnel time and drugs
Improved overall quality of care and coverage with nutritional supplements	5a	70 percent prenatal care; 70 percent delivery care	Enhanced prenatal and delivery care (BEmOC)	50 percent	90 percent	Enhanced CEmOC (adds interventions for high-risk babies)	Benefit from improved quality (technical content and percentage receiving care needed) and coverage at the primary and secondary levels	Comprehensive package: improved coverage and content with BPS	Costs of providing and running ambulances, costs of additional personnel and drugs, training for BEmOC and CEmOC, costs of BPS
Improved overall quality of care and coverage without nutritional supplements	5b	70 percent prenatal care; 70 percent delivery care	Enhanced prenatal and delivery care (BEmOC) without BPS	50 percent	90 percent	Enhanced CEmOC (adds interventions for high-risk babies)	Benefit from improved quality and coverage at the primary and secondary levels without BPS	Improved coverage and content without BPS	As for 5a without the costs of BPS

Source: Authors.

BPS = balanced protein-energy supplementation.

a. Defined in terms of the percentage of complicated cases at the primary level referred to and reaching the secondary level.

b. Includes obstetric first aid for complicated cases, including abortion and postpartum complications.

c. The secondary level will also provide some prenatal and delivery care for normal cases, as defined in the first two panels of table 26.5 for the base package at the primary level.

Table 26.7 ICERs per Million Population, South Asia and Sub-Saharan Africa
(U.S. dollars)

Option number	Alternative compared with the base package	Incremental cost per death averted		Incremental cost per life-year saved		Incremental cost per DALY averted	
		South Asia	Sub-Saharan Africa	South Asia	Sub-Saharan Africa	South Asia	Sub-Saharan Africa
2	Increased primary-level coverage	6,129	3,337	217	119	148	92
3a	Improved overall quality of care with nutritional supplements	5,017	2,729	165	90	142	83
3b	Improved overall quality of care without nutritional supplements	8,975	2,538	296	84	240	77
4	Improved quality of CEmOC	10,532	5,089	372	195	255	151
5a	Improved overall quality of care and coverage with nutritional supplements	5,297	2,915	177	98	144	86
5b	Improved overall quality of care and coverage without nutritional supplements	7,944	2,865	269	96	203	84

Source: Authors' calculations.

Table 26.8 Costs and Effectiveness of Intervention Packages per Million Population, South Asia and Sub-Saharan Africa

Option number	Intervention package	Total costs (US$)	Number of deaths averted	Number of life years saved	Number of DALYs averted	Percentage of DALYs averted that are maternal
South Asia						
1	Routine maternity care	408,976	79	2,240	3,273	50
2	Increased primary-level coverage	603,071	111	3,136	4,582	50
3a	Improved overall quality of care with nutritional supplements	829,505	163	4,793	6,225	26
3b	Improved overall quality of care without nutritional supplements	757,433	118	3,415	4,727	35
4	Improved quality of CEmOC	420,918	80	2,272	3,320	50
5a	Improved overall quality of care and coverage with nutritional supplements	1,287,354	245	7,201	9,354	26
5b	Improved overall quality of care and coverage without nutritional supplements	1,186,123	177	5,131	7,103	35
Sub-Saharan Africa						
1	Routine maternity care	602,646	192	5,406	6,969	47
2	Increased primary-level coverage	859,027	269	7,568	9,757	47
3a	Improved overall quality of care with nutritional supplements	1,164,833	398	11,652	13,753	24
3b	Improved overall quality of care without nutritional supplements	1,049,209	368	10,733	12,770	26
4	Improved quality of CEmOC	617,724	195	5,483	7,069	47
5a	Improved overall quality of care and coverage with nutritional supplements	1,785,971	597	17,508	20,664	24
5b	Improved overall quality of care and coverage without nutritional supplements	1,633,956	552	16,127	19,188	26

Source: Authors' calculations.

Table 26.9 Sensitivity Analysis Results, South Asia and Sub-Saharan Africa
(incremental cost per DALY averted, US$)

Option number	Alternative compared with base package	Best estimate	Effectiveness assumption		Met need assumption		Inpatient cost assumption	
			High	Low	High	Low	High	Low
South Asia								
2	Increased primary-level coverage	148	113	163	147	150	213	109
3a	Improved overall quality of care with nutritional supplements	142	100	163	143	144	142	143
3b	Improved overall quality of care without nutritional supplements	240	180	326	241	242	240	240
4	Improved quality of CEmOC	255	193	311	373	260	446	204
5a	Improved overall quality of care and coverage with nutritional supplements	144	104	164	144	149	152	136
5b	Improved overall quality of care and coverage without nutritional supplements	203	153	250	203	210	227	189
Sub-Saharan Africa								
2	Increased primary-level coverage	92	70	104	91	93	191	84
3a	Improved overall quality of care with nutritional supplements	83	64	90	83	84	83	83
3b	Improved overall quality of care without nutritional supplements	77	61	85	77	78	77	77
4	Improved quality of CEmOC	151	114	166	228	151	326	130
5a	Improved overall quality of care and coverage with nutritional supplements	86	66	94	86	89	123	82
5b	Improved overall quality of care and coverage without nutritional supplements	84	66	93	84	87	123	79

Source: Authors' calculations.

comparison is with or without increased coverage (options 5a and 3a, respectively). This difference reflects the high burden from low birthweight in South Asia and, thus, the gain from nutritional supplements.

Comparing the content of the three most cost-effective intervention packages (3a, 5a, and 2) suggests that much can be achieved through improvements at the primary care level. Improved quality in relation to managing complications—in other words, the provision of BEmOC—and increases in coverage (a combination of options 3a and 2) at the primary level are likely to have even lower ICERs than those shown in table 26.7. This finding is consistent with the Commission on Macroeconomics and Health's emphasis on close-to-client services (CMH 2002), and it is highlighted further in chapter 53. As noted earlier, given the importance of prompt intervention in the event of obstetric complications, the effectiveness of intervention packages that may reduce delays by bringing services closer to communities is hardly surprising.

The benefits from option 2 were achieved essentially by increasing prenatal care coverage from 50 to 70 percent, because our model assumes that those women taking advantage of professional delivery are those who have also had prenatal contact. Prenatal care is, thus, a crucial entry point to the health system. Small changes in prenatal care coverage (20 per-

cent) lead to larger numbers of women also benefiting from the rest of the care package in terms of obstetric first aid and CEmOC.

This issue is important for safe motherhood and newborn health, because the role of prenatal care has been subject to intense debate about its benefits relative to resource use (De Brouwere and Van Lerberghe 2001; Maine and Rosenfield 1999). Much of this discussion has focused on the lack of evidence on the direct contribution of prenatal care to reducing maternal mortality (McDonagh 1996; Rooney 1992), which, in turn, is explained partly by the poor performance of at-risk screening tools. However, differentiating the contribution to the prevention of maternal deaths of the prenatal care component alone is difficult. Ultimately, life-saving interventions depend on the functioning of the entire health system, including an effective referral network.

Our model also made assumptions about women's willingness and capacity to respond to referral to higher levels of care in case of complications. This willingness and capacity depend on many factors and are undoubtedly also driven by communities' perceptions of quality of care. As noted earlier, coverage rates of prenatal care are already high in many Sub-Saharan African countries, but significant socioeconomic differentials are apparent within countries. Our model does not address this equity dimension but, given the recent work showing higher risks of maternal death among the poorest groups (Graham and others 2004), targeting disadvantaged women for improvements in uptake might be worth considering (Gwatkin and Deveshwar-Bahl 2002; De Brouwere and Van Lerberghe 2001).

Whereas option 2, increased primary-level coverage, relates predominantly to the demand side of the health system (Williams 1987), the most cost-effective packages (3a and 5a) focus on the supply side, particularly at the health center level. The latter packages are particularly relevant to the baby, including screening of the HIV status of the mother and treatment with antiretrovirals at the time of delivery to reduce the risk of mother-to-child transmission, as well as provision of antimalarials. As a consequence, these options have a particularly marked effect on the burden from perinatal conditions, accounting for two-thirds to three-fourths of the total DALYs averted (table 26.8). Note that these cost-effective options include a doctor at the health center level to provide all six BEmOC functions. In some situations, highly skilled midwives will be able to act in this capacity, which would reduce costs and further increase cost-effectiveness.

The most comprehensive packages in our model provide for improved quality of care and coverage at both the primary and the secondary levels (options 5a and 5b). Costing US$1.79 and US$1.63 per capita, respectively, in Sub-Saharan Africa (as calculated from the total costs of these packages shown in table 26.8, and divided by the base of 1 million people), these are also the most expensive packages. Not surprisingly, therefore, these two options avert much higher numbers of DALYs, with the package that includes nutritional supplementation averting nearly three times as many DALYs as the base package (table 26.8). In CEA, generally the most comprehensive packages—that is, those that result in the greatest gain in quality and coverage and, thus, cost the most—are often not cost-effective, and yet our analysis found otherwise. This finding may partly be explained by the linear assumptions about effectiveness in the model and the assumption that the marginal cost of care is constant. Such a finding also stresses both the importance of a well-functioning health system (rather than an excessive focus on one element) and the absence of any quick fix. Moreover, we did not model these more comprehensive options as perfect but unrealistic scenarios. We also still allowed for 30 percent of pregnant women not attending prenatal care, 50 percent of severe complications at a primary level not reaching CEmOC, and 10 percent of those reaching secondary care not receiving the emergency treatment they need.

Finally, a note of caution is warranted on the interpretation of the CEA results. First, our model has necessarily used a number of assumptions for which data are extremely limited, and it remains fairly crude, having been subject to only a limited sensitivity analysis. Second, many comparisons are possible from our model, but we have selected only six. Thus, we may not have identified even more cost-effective intervention packages, such as a combination of options 3a and 2.

ECONOMIC BENEFITS OF INTERVENTION

A narrow definition of the economic benefits of safe motherhood interventions would focus primarily on the impact of maternal mortality and morbidity on household investment and consumption. Investment in this context refers not so much to financial investment as to investment in improving housing conditions, agricultural productivity, education, and so on. The key elements to capture include the loss of productivity and the disruption of planned investment and consumption. In addition to the loss of a woman's own productivity, consequent effects are likely on the productivity of other household members—effects that may be particularly long lived in the case of young children whose health and education suffer because of their mother's death. The household will also be worse off because it will have diverted resources from preferred consumption and investment activities in response to the health crisis. Thus, recognizing the dynamic consequences of maternal death and disability and selecting an appropriate time horizon for the analysis are important.

The potential benefits to individual households arising from investments in safe motherhood are relatively clear, although challenges in quantifying and valuing them remain. The benefits may, however, be more widely spread in that improvements in safe motherhood may reduce poverty, which in turn may stimulate economic development. Increased economic development may then feed back into further improvements in maternal health, generating a virtuous cycle. The mechanisms whereby changes in maternal health affect other parts of the economy may be identified by a close examination of the influence of maternal health on productivity and educational attainment.

A number of links may exist between safe motherhood and the performance of the health care system; therefore, strategies to improve safe motherhood may be a means of achieving wider health service improvements (Goodburn and Campbell 2001). Jowett (2000, 213) notes that "to improve a facility's capacity to respond to obstetric emergencies, it is necessary to have the skills and supplies to deal with trauma, give blood transfusions and anesthesia, and have a functional operating theatre." Thus, initiatives in safe motherhood could be an entry point for wider health sector reform and improvement.

LESSONS FOR IMPLEMENTATION

The findings from the CEA indicate potential health gains and the reduced burden that may be achieved by implementing selected packages of interventions. Such implementation assumes, first, that decision makers accept the evidence and are willing and able to act and, second, that an enabling health system environment exists within which the requisite scale and quality of care can be effectively delivered. These factors are not peculiar to safe motherhood, but they undoubtedly help explain the significant gap between evidence and action that many argue is one of the main obstacles to progress (Godlee and others 2004; Villar and others 2001). The gains from bridging this gap would be significant: the MDGs for child survival and maternal health might become more than mere rhetoric for poor regions if intervention packages of the scope and nature described here were implemented. The most cost-effective of the packages averted nearly 50 percent more direct maternal deaths than the base package. This gain would be encouraging, but the prospects for achieving it by 2015 are weak (Johansson and Stewart 2002).

At the macro level, a supportive policy environment clearly is crucial, as noted earlier. At the micro level, an enabling health system implies a reduction in the disequilibrium between the demand and supply sides (Williams 1987), with particular attention to three interrelated issues: access, quality, and finance. The CEA reported in this chapter emphasizes the potential benefits to mother and baby of improved access to care, particularly the importance of entry to the health system through primary-level services. The increases in coverage could be achieved by a variety of mechanisms but clearly require both demand- and supply-side interventions.

On the supply side, this chapter has shown that improved quality of care at both the primary and the secondary levels encompassing technical, infrastructural, and human resource dimensions (Pittrof, Campbell, and Filippi 2002) is a particularly cost-effective option. The widespread call for all women to deliver with skilled attendance immediately raises major questions about quality of care and capacity, because much of the developing world faces an acute shortage, as well as an unequal geographic distribution, of health professionals.

Our CEA assumes that redistributing human resources within countries will accommodate the increased uptake of care by women, although the most effective mechanisms for achieving this goal, such as incentives, use of nonphysicians, and increased private sector involvement, have not yet been established (De Brouwere and Van Lerberghe 2001). What is clear, however, is the importance of the interplay between supply and demand, with the supply of quality care stimulating demand for care and vice versa. Quality care includes an effective referral system (Murray and others 2001) to ensure the required match between the various levels of care different women and their babies need at different times (De Brouwere and Van Lerberghe 2001). Such systems require not only financial resources to support transportation, communications, and feedback mechanisms, but also structured fee and exemption strategies to reduce both inappropriate self-referral

to hospitals and financial barriers to access on the part of the poor.

The financing of prenatal and delivery care services at an adequate and sustainable level is a subject of much debate and uncertainty, given the difficulty of distinguishing these elements from broader health expenditure categories (De Brouwere and Van Lerberghe 2001). Given the low level of overall per capita expenditure on health in developing countries—estimated at US$13 in 2002 for the poorest 49 countries (Bale and others 2003)—attaining our base intervention package (costing approximately US$0.41 per capita in South Asia and US$0.60 in Sub-Saharan Africa) does not sound unrealistic at current resource levels (see table 26.8, and divide by base population of 1 million people).

The effects of health sector reforms, particularly decentralization of management and budget holding, appear to be mixed in terms of increasing resource flows into maternity services, with both apparent positive benefits, as in Bolivia (De Brouwere and Van Lerberghe 2001), and negative effects through the exacerbation of inequities (Russell and Gilson 1997). Effective management decisions on finance, access, and quality require information, an essential ingredient for stimulating action. To allocate scarce resources where they are likely to achieve the greatest gain, countries need information to assess the burden of ill health, evaluate the performance of current intervention strategies, identify the scope for improvement and implement changes, and close the loop by evaluating effects and cost-effectiveness (Lawn, McCarthy, and Ross 2001).

Even though the challenges that the poorest countries face today clearly differ in many respects from those that developed or transition countries experienced in the past, six historical lessons provide particularly relevant insights. First, examples abound of supportive policy contexts and individual champions of progress in addressing maternal and newborn health, such as those reported by De Brouwere and Van Lerberghe (2001). Second, historical data on the uptake of prenatal care demonstrate that community-based providers and advocates played a crucial role. Third, the role of various professionals and professional bodies has not always been positive, particularly as regards the "war" between advocates for home and institutional deliveries (Koblinsky and Campbell 2003). Moreover, good historical evidence indicates that excessive rates of forceps deliveries and other interventions were significant contributors to maternal mortality in countries such as the United Kingdom and the United States (Buekens 2001). Fourth, primary-level care depends on an effective referral system being in place to maintain the confidence of both women and providers (Loudon 1997). Fifth, to reduce the burden of maternal and perinatal conditions, the system of health care financing must facilitate access for the poorest groups and guarantee service quality (De Brouwere and Van Lerberghe 2001). Finally, the role of population-based information on births and maternal deaths was crucial in ensuring that actions were locally relevant (Sorenson and others 1998), in demonstrating progress, and thus in stimulating further action. This crucial role is particularly apparent in the literature on several European countries in the past century (Graham 2002; De Brouwere and Van Lerberghe 2001).

RESEARCH AND DEVELOPMENT NEEDS

The priorities for research and development arising from this chapter need to be put in the context of wider requirements for safe motherhood and newborn health that have been well articulated elsewhere (see, for example, Bale and others 2003). The general heading under which the specific needs emerging from this chapter can be grouped is evidence-based decision making, which has five crucial requirements:

- recognizing the weakness of current approaches to allocating scarce health care resources in poor countries
- making efforts to improve the scope and quality of data on the burden from maternal and perinatal conditions
- carrying out robust evaluation of the costs and effectiveness of intervention strategies
- using reliable evidence to inform the decision-making process
- implementing prioritized strategies and robust, continuous assessment of their performance.

Within those major areas, specific topics relevant to the CEA undertaken here include the following:

- *Ascertaining the burden of maternal and perinatal conditions.* Greater clarity and consensus are needed on the scope of this important burden category and the implications of significant current exclusions, such as indirect maternal conditions and stillbirths. Practical assessment tools are needed to enable meta-analysis and other modeling approaches to systematically factor in data constraints. Huge gaps in knowledge exist with regard to the levels and consequences of maternal morbidity (Say, Pattinson, and Gulmezoglu 2004), the contribution of iatrogenic factors, the unpredictability of maternal complications, and the levels of mortality. Most of those gaps require significant developments in relation to available measurement tools and in poor countries' capacity to use them as part of routine health surveillance. These improvements not only are needed to inform future CEA but also have wider implications for global health monitoring.
- *Implementing change.* In addition to evidence on the content of intervention strategies, assessments of how to implement changes are urgently needed. A limitation of our analysis is that, even though the model may be a reasonable representation of the resource and health consequences of different intervention packages, the way to achieve the required

change, such as a particular increase in the uptake of prenatal care, may not be known. Thus, the ICERs may be too low, in that they do not fully capture the costs of the intervention.
- *Estimating cost-effectiveness.* More sophisticated economic models need to be developed to facilitate the evaluation of a wider range of safe motherhood strategies, particularly as better primary evidence becomes available from other studies and initiatives using a variety of outcome measures (Cairns, McNamee, and Hernandez 2003). Similarly, probabilistic sensitivity analysis would be a valuable development that would permit fuller exploration of the uncertainties regarding the model's parameters.

CONCLUSIONS

In 2001, maternal and perinatal conditions represented the single largest contributor to the global burden of disease, at nearly 6 percent of total DALYs (Mathers and others 2004). Reducing that burden is widely stated as a priority at both national and international levels, but the track record of translating the rhetoric into action on a sufficiently large and equitable scale to make a difference at the population level remains disappointing. The literature abounds with examples of this disappointment (see, for example, Maine and Rosenfield 1999; Weil and Fernandez 1999). Many reasons account for the limited progress, especially in the poorest regions of the world, and researchers offer many interpretations of the bottlenecks. Lack of evidence on the size of the burden and on the effectiveness of alternative intervention strategies figures prominently in these interpretations.

The modeling in this chapter is, therefore, based on imperfect knowledge and needs to be supplemented with data from primary evaluations. The findings do, however, provide some tentative insights into programmatic options that may represent the optimal use of resources in South Asia and Sub-Saharan Africa. In this context, three issues deserve emphasis. First, for intervention packages to achieve the degree of cost-effectiveness shown here, improvements are needed across health systems, and both the supply and the demand sides need to be addressed. Second, crucial entry points to this system can be achieved at the primary level, particularly through prenatal care. The effect of increasing the volume of women in contact with these services is likely to manifest itself in an increased proportion of deliveries with skilled attendance and of deliveries in which women obtain access to emergency obstetric care. Finally, the quality of these services is crucial, and even with only 50 percent uptake of care, benefits can still be achieved in terms of overall DALYs averted and of reduced maternal and perinatal mortality.

Initiatives to improve the quality of care, particularly at a primary level, thus appear to be cost-effective options for the poorest regions of the world. Overall those findings appear to lend support to a safe motherhood and newborn health strategy that is close to the client and boosts community confidence in health systems.

ANNEX 26.A: CEA MODEL ASSUMPTIONS

We assumed that there are four primary-level health facilities (health centers) and one secondary-level care facility (district hospital) for every 500,000 people. We estimated the numbers of pregnancies and births from the crude birth rate for each region. We assumed that pregnant mothers attending for routine prenatal care are equally distributed between the five facilities and that each facility provides similar routine prenatal and delivery care. Routine prenatal care is assumed to comprise four visits—except for mothers with complications, who make six visits. Mothers with complications are referred to the district hospital after their first visit if they cannot be treated at the health center. We assumed that complications such as anemia and sexually transmitted diseases are treated without referral to secondary care, as are preeclampsia and incomplete abortion, if a doctor is present at the facility. The average number of bed days is assumed to be three days for normal deliveries and six days for cesarean section and other complications. Table 26.A1 shows the U.S. dollar costs per inpatient bed day used in the main analysis and in the sensitivity analysis.

We assumed the existence of excess capacity, so that an increase in prenatal care coverage from 50 to 70 percent would not require an increase in the number or capacity of existing health care facilities, and the increased costs would mostly be increases in variable costs. For increased coverage of prenatal care, we assumed a need for increased expenditure on education, information, and communication. Enhanced prenatal care and comprehensive emergency obstetric care are assumed to require additional expenditures on training, assumed to be 10 percent of total personnel costs. We assumed that the additional costs of basic emergency obstetric care compared with obstetric first aid are largely due to providing doctors at each health center. We also assumed that 8 percent of mothers require cesarean section as a result of either maternal or perinatal complications. About 2 percent of mothers are assumed to require treatment for preterm delivery, and 1 percent for premature rupture of membranes.

In practice, the proportion of women with serious complications receiving comprehensive emergency obstetric care varies widely, from 3 percent in Cameroon to 75 percent in Sri Lanka (Averting Maternal Death and Disability Working Group on Indicators 2003). The scenarios considered in this chapter assume that either 20 or 50 percent of women with serious complications reach secondary care, and that 50, 70, 80, or 90 percent of those women receive the elements of comprehensive emergency obstetric care that they need, depending on which intervention package is being considered. For the sensitivity analysis, we used low values of 30, 50, 60, and 70 percent and high values of 70, 80, 90, and 95 percent. We assumed that ambulances are available, so that when the proportion of mothers with severe complications reaching secondary care is increased, the additional costs are only the additional driver time and the increased costs of running and maintaining the vehicle.

The prevalence and incidence of different maternal conditions are taken from the WHO mother-baby package (WHO 1994). World Health Organization estimates of the burden of different maternal and perinatal conditions (WHO 2004d) have been applied to a population of 1 million, with a particular crude birth rate to generate an estimate of the potential number of deaths that could be avoided, the years of life that could be saved, and the DALYs that could be averted. The assumptions regarding the effectiveness of the interventions with respect to maternal and perinatal conditions were based primarily on the WHO's mother-baby package and a review of the literature; they are shown in table 26.A2. We assumed that each intervention has the same effect on the number of deaths, years of life saved, and DALYs. The effectiveness of interventions is assumed to be additive.

ACKNOWLEDGMENTS

We would like to thank the many individuals who helped prepare this chapter. In particular, we acknowledge the expert input regarding perinatal conditions from Joy Lawn and Jelka

Table 26.A1 Costs Per Inpatient Bed Day, South Asia and Sub-Saharan Africa
(U.S. dollars)

Cost of inpatient bed day	South Asia		Sub-Saharan Africa	
	Primary level	Secondary level	Primary level	Secondary level
Best estimate	6.51	8.50	6.17	8.05
Low	2.64	3.45	1.92	2.51
High	14.52	18.94	41.79	54.52

Source: DCPP2: Guidelines for Authors.

Table 26.A2 Assumed Effectiveness of Interventions
(percentage of DALYs, deaths, and years of life lost averted)

Condition	Best estimate	Low	High
Maternal			
Hemorrhage	85	80	90
Sepsis	75	70	90
Hypertensive disorders of pregnancy (including eclampsia)	76	71	95
Obstructed labor	80	75	95
Unsafe abortion	75	70	90
Perinatal			
Low birthweight			
In context without nutritional supplements[a]	8	3	14
In context with nutritional supplements[a]	28	23	44
Birth asphyxia (including birth trauma)			
In context without enhanced delivery care package[a]	40	35	60
In context with enhanced delivery care package[a]	70	65	90
Infections, including tetanus	60	55	80
Sepsis (newborn)	40	35	60
HIV/AIDS	60	55	80

Source: expert panels; WHO 1994, 2004d; Steketee and others 2001; Prendiville, Elbourne, and Chalmers 1998; Eclampsia Trial Collaborative Group 1995.
Note: Two extra interventions added to WHO mother-baby package: active management of the third stage of labor and magnesium sulfate for hypertensive disorders of pregnancy.
a. See table 26.6.

Zupan. Thanks are also given to our colleagues at the University of Aberdeen, particularly Joyce Boor, Julia Hussein, Emma Pitchforth, Nara Tagiyeva-Milne, and Karen Witten. We acknowledge and thank our colleagues Paul McNamee and Rodolpho Hernandez from the Health Economics Research Unit at the University of Aberdeen for their thorough review of the cost-effectiveness analysis. Thanks also to our expert panel members: Deanna Ashley, Gary Darmstadt, Catherine Hauptfleisch, Jilly Ireland, Joy Lawn, Cecil Klufio, Elizabeth Molyneux, Ashalata Shetty, Sribala Sripad, Vijay Kumar Tandle, Sumesh Thomas, and Jelka Zupan.

NOTES

1. *Antecedent* is here defined as a factor that changes the probability of an adverse outcome or sequela, either positively (protecting) or, more usually, negatively (aggravating). A risk factor may be a leading contributor to the global burden because of high prevalence in the population or because of a large increase in the probability of adverse outcomes (WHO 2002).

2. Afghanistan, Angola, Bangladesh, China, the Democratic Republic of Congo, Ethiopia, India, Indonesia, Kenya, Nigeria, Pakistan, Tanzania, and Uganda.

3. We use a simple three-way distinction for levels of evidence. *Level A* refers to evidence from randomized clinical trials or systematic overviews of trials; *level B* relates to nonrandomized studies, often with multivariate

analyses; and *level C* is assigned to case series, case studies, or expert opinion.

4. This chapter does not deal with tertiary and specialist levels of care or with rehabilitative care or care for chronic conditions.

5. The six functions of BEmOC are (a) administering antibiotics intravenously or intramuscularly, (b) administering oxytocics intravenously or intramuscularly, (c) manually removing the placenta, (d) administering anticonvulsants intravenously or intramuscularly, (e) carrying out instrumental delivery, and (f) removing retained products of conception. The two additional functions in CEmOC are blood transfusion and cesarean section. For a facility to be regarded as a BEmOC or CEmOC site, respectively, it must perform all six or all eight functions regularly and must be assessed every three to six months (UNFPA 2003).

REFERENCES

AbouZahr, C. 1998. "Maternal Mortality Overview." In *Health Dimensions of Sex and Reproduction,* ed. C. J. Murray and A. D. Lopez, 111–64. Geneva: World Health Organization.

———. 1999. "Disability-Adjusted Life Years and Reproductive Health: A Critical Analysis." *Reproductive Health Matters* 7 (14): 118–29.

———. 2003. "Global Burden of Maternal Death and Disability." *British Medical Bulletin* 67: 1–11.

AbouZahr, C., and T. Wardlaw. 2001. "Maternal Mortality at the End of a Decade: Signs of Progress?" *Bulletin of the World Health Organization* 79 (6): 561–68.

Averting Maternal Death and Disability Working Group on Indicators. 2003. "Program Note: Using UN Process Indicators to Assess Needs in Emergency Obstetric Services: Morocco, Nicaragua, and Sri Lanka." *International Journal of Gynaecology and Obstetrics* 80: 222–30.

Bailey, P., J. Szaszdi, and B. Schieber. 1995. "Analysis of the Vital Events Reporting System of the Maternal and Neonatal Health Project: Quetzaltenango, Guatemala." MotherCare Technical Working Paper 3, John Snow, Arlington, VA.

Bale, J., B. Stoll, A. Mack, and A. Lucas, eds. 2003. *Improving Birth Outcomes: Meeting the Challenges in the Developing World.* Washington, DC: National Academy of Sciences and Institute of Medicine.

Bell, J., S. L. Curtis, and S. Alayon. 2003. "Trends in Delivery Care in Six Countries." Department of Homeland Security Analytical Studies 7, Opinion Research Corporation and Macro International Research Partnership for Skilled Attendance for Everyone (SAFE), Calverton, MD.

Bell, J., J. Hussein, B. Jentsch, G. Scotland, C. Bullough, and W. J. Graham. 2003. "Improving Skilled Attendance at Delivery: A Preliminary Report of the SAFE Strategy Development Tool." *Birth* 30 (4): 227–34.

Bergsjo, P., and J. Villar. 1997. "Scientific Basis for the Content of Routine Antenatal Care: II. Power to Eliminate or Alleviate Adverse Newborn Outcomes; Some Special Conditions and Examinations." *Acta Obstetrica et Gynecologica Scandinavica* 76 (1): 15–25.

Buekens, P. 2001. "Is Estimating Maternal Mortality Useful?" *Bulletin of the World Health Organization* 79 (3): 179.

Buttiens, H., B. Marchal, and V. De Brouwere. 2004. "Skilled Attendance at Childbirth: Let Us Go beyond the Rhetorics." *Tropical Medicine and International Health* 9 (6): 653–54.

Cairns, J., P. McNamee, and R. Hernandez. 2003. "Measurement and Valuation of Economic Outcomes." Economic Outcomes Work Program, Draft Concept Paper, IMMPACT (Initiative for Maternal Mortality Programme Assessment), Dugald Baird Centre, University of Aberdeen, Scotland.

Calder, A. A., and W. Dunlop, eds. 1992. *High Risk Pregnancy.* Oxford, U.K.: Butterworth-Heinemann.

Carroli, G., C. Rooney, and J. Villar. 2001. "How Effective Is Antenatal Care in Preventing Maternal Mortality and Serious Morbidity? An Overview of the Evidence." *Paediatric and Perinatal Epidemiology* 15 (Suppl. 1): 1–42.

Chamberlain, G., ed. 1995. *Turnbull's Obstetrics*. 2nd ed. London: Churchill Livingstone.

Cleland, J., and M. Ali. 2004. "Reproductive Consequences of Contraceptive Failure in 19 Developing Countries." *Obstetrics and Gynecology* 104 (2): 314–20.

CMH (Commission on Macroeconomics and Health). 2002. *Improving the Health Outcomes of the Poor*. Report of Working Group 5 of the Commission on Macroeconomics and Health. Geneva: World Health Organization.

Creese, A., and D. Parker. 1994. *Cost Analysis in Primary Care: A Training Manual for Programme Managers*. Geneva: World Health Organization.

Dayaratna, V., W. Winfrey, W. McGreevey, K. Hardee, K. Smith, E. Mumford, and others. 2000. *Reproductive Health Interventions: Which Ones Work and What Do They Cost?* Washington, DC: Policy Project.

De Brouwere, V., and W. Van Lerberghe, eds. 2001. *Safe Motherhood Strategies: A Review of the Evidence*. Vol. 17 of Studies in Health Services Organisations and Policy. Antwerp, Belgium: ITG Press.

Donnay, F. 2000. "Maternal Survival in Developing Countries: What Has Been Done; What Can Be Achieved in the Next Decade." *International Journal of Gynecology and Obstetrics* 70 (1): 89–97.

Eclampsia Trial Collaborative Group. 1995. "Which Anticonvulsant for Women with Eclampsia? Evidence from the Collaborative Eclampsia Trial." *Lancet* 345 (8963): 1455–63.

Etard, J. F., B. Kodio, and S. Traore. 1999. "Assessment of Maternal Mortality and Late Maternal Mortality among a Cohort of Pregnant Women in Bamako, Mali." *British Journal of Obstetrics and Gynaecology* 106 (1): 60–65.

Evans, T., and S. Stansfield. 2003. "Health Information in the New Millennium: A Gathering Storm?" *Bulletin of the World Health Organization* 81 (12): 856.

Foege, W. 2001. "Managing Newborn Health in the Global Community." *American Journal of Public Health* 91 (10): 1563–64.

Freedman, L. P. 2001. "Using Human Rights in Maternal Mortality Programs: From Analysis to Strategy." *International Journal of Gynecology and Obstetrics* 75 (1): 51–60.

Gay, J., K. Hardee, N. Judice, K. Agarwal, K. Flemming, A. Hairston, and others. 2003. *What Works: A Policy and Program Guide to the Evidence on Family Planning, Safe Motherhood, and STI/HIV/AIDS Interventions*. Safe Motherhood Module 1. Washington, DC: Policy Project.

Germain, A. 2000. "Population and Reproductive Health: Where Do We Go Next?" *American Journal of Public Health* 90 (12): 1845–47.

Godlee, F., N. Pakenham-Walsh, D. Ncayiyana, B. Cohen, and A. Packer. 2004. "Can We Achieve Health Information for All by 2015?" *Lancet* 364 (9430): 295–300.

Goodburn, E., and O. Campbell. 2001. "Reducing Maternal Mortality in the Developing World: Sector-Wide Approaches May Be the Key." *British Medical Journal* 322 (7291): 917–20.

Graham, W. J. 1998. "Every Pregnancy Faces Risks." *Planned Parenthood Challenges* 1: 13–14.

———. 2002. "Now or Never: The Case for Measuring Maternal Mortality." *Lancet* 359 (9307): 701–04.

Graham, W. J., A. E. Fitzmaurice, J. S. Bell, and J. A. Cairns. 2004. "The Familial Technique for Linking Maternal Death and Poverty." *Lancet* 363 (9402): 23–27.

Graham, W. J., and J. Hussein. 2004. "The Right to Count." *Lancet* 363 (9402): 67–68.

Gwatkin, D., and G. Deveshwar-Bahl. 2002. "Socioeconomic Inequalities in Use of Safe Motherhood Services in Developing Countries." Paper presented at the Inter-Agency Safe Motherhood Meeting, London, February 6.

Hall, M., S. MacIntyre, and M. Porter. 1985. *Antenatal Care Assessed*. Aberdeen, Scotland: Aberdeen University Press.

Hoj, L., D. da Silva, K. Hedegaard, A. Sandstrom, and P. Aaby. 2003. "Maternal Mortality: Only 42 Days?" *British Journal of Obstetrics and Gynaecology* 110 (11): 995–1000.

Hussain, R., F. F. Fikree, and H. W. Berendes. 2000. "The Role of Son Preference in Reproductive Behaviour in Pakistan." *Bulletin of the World Health Organization* 78 (3): 379–88.

Hutubessy, R. C., R. M. Baltussen, T. Tan-Torres Edejer, and D. Evans. 2003. "Generalised Cost-Effectiveness Analysis: An Aid to Decision Making in Health." In Making Choices in Health: WHO *Guide to Cost-Effectiveness Analysis*, ed. T. Tan-Torres Edejer, R. M. Baltussen, T. Adam, R. Hutubessy, A. Acharya, D. B. Evan, and C. J. L. Murray, 277–88. Geneva: World Health Organization.

Jamison, D. T., J. S. Jamison, J. Lawn, S. Shahid-Salles, and J. Zupan. 2004. "Incorporating Deaths Near the Time of Birth into Estimates of the Global Burden of Disease." Working Paper 26, Disease Control Priorities Project, Bethesda, MD.

Johansson, C., and D. Stewart. 2002. "The Millennium Development Goals: Commitments and Prospects." Working Paper 1, Human Development Report Office Working Papers and Notes, United Nations Development Programme, New York.

Jowett, M. 2000. "Safe Motherhood Interventions in Low-Income Countries: An Economic Justification and Evidence of Cost Effectiveness." *Health Policy* 53 (3): 201–28.

Khanum, P. A., M. A. Quaiyum, A. Islam, and S. Ahmed. 2000. "Complication of Pregnancy and Childbirth: Knowledge and Practices of Women in Rural Bangladesh." Working Paper 131, International Centre for Diarrhoeal Disease Research, Dhaka.

Koblinsky, M. A., and O. Campbell, eds. 2003. *Reducing Maternal Mortality: Learning from Bolivia, China, Egypt, Honduras, Indonesia, Jamaica, and Zimbabwe*. Washington, DC: World Bank.

Koenig, M. A., V. Fauveau, and B. Wojtyniak. 1991. "Mortality Reductions from Health Interventions: The Case of Immunization in Bangladesh." *Population and Development Review* 17 (1): 87–104.

Kurjak, A., and I. Bekavac. 2001. "Perinatal Problems in Developing Countries: Lessons Learned and Future Challenges." *Journal of Perinatal Medicine* 29 (3): 179–87.

Kusiako, T., C. Ronsmans, and L. Van der Paul. 2000. "Perinatal Mortality Attributable to Complications of Childbirth in Matlab, Bangladesh." *Bulletin of the World Health Organization* 78 (5): 621–27.

Lawn, J. E., B. J. McCarthy, and S. R. Ross. 2001. *The Healthy Newborn: A Reference Manual for Program Managers*. Atlanta, GA: Centers for Disease Control and Prevention and CARE. http://www.cdc.gov/reproductivehealth/health_newborn.htm.

Loudon, I. 1997. "Midwives and the Quality of Maternal Care." In *Midwives, Society and Childbirth: Debates and Controversies in the Modern Period*, ed. H. Marland and A. M. Rafferty, 180–200. London and New York: Routledge.

Maine, D., and A. Rosenfield. 1999. "The Safe Motherhood Initiative: Why Has It Stalled?" *American Journal of Public Health* 89 (4): 480–82.

Marston, C., and J. Cleland. 2003. "Do Unintended Pregnancies Carried to Term Lead to Adverse Outcomes for Mother and Child? An Assessment in Five Developing Countries." *Population Studies* 57 (1): 77–94.

Mathers, C. D., A. Lopez, C. Stein, D. Ma Fat, C. Rao, M. Inoue, and others. 2004. "Deaths and Disease Burden by Cause: Global Burden of Disease Estimates for 2001 by World Bank Country Groups." Working Paper 18, Disease Control Priorities Project, Bethesda, MD.

McCarthy, J., and D. Maine. 1992. "A Framework for Analyzing the Determinants of Maternal Mortality." *Studies in Family Planning* 23 (1): 23–33.

McDonagh, M. 1996. "Is Antenatal Care Effective in Reducing Maternal Morbidity and Mortality?" *Health Policy and Planning* 11 (1): 1–15.

Milne, L., G. Scotland, N. Tagiyeva-Milne, and J. Hussein. 2004. "Safe Motherhood Program Evaluation: Theory and Practice." *Journal of Midwifery and Women's Health* 49 (4): 338–44.

Munjanja, S. P., G. Lindmark, and L. Nystrom. 1996. "Randomised Controlled Trial of a Reduced-Visits Programme of Antenatal Care in Harare, Zimbabwe." *Lancet* (North American ed.) 348 (9024): 364–69.

Murray, C. J. L., and A. D. Lopez, eds. 1998. *Health Dimensions of Sex and Reproduction.* In Vol. 3 of *Global Burden of Disease and Injury.* Cambridge, MA: Harvard University Press.

Murray, S. F., S. Davies, P. Kumwenda, and A. Yusuf. 2001. "Tools for Monitoring the Effectiveness of District Maternity Referral Systems." *Health Policy and Planning* 16 (4): 353–61.

Mwageni, E., A. Ankomah, and R. Powell. 2001. "Sex Preference and Contraceptive Behaviour among Men in Mbeya Region, Tanzania." *Journal of Family Planning and Reproductive Health Care* 27 (2): 85–89.

Pattinson, B. 2002. *Saving Mothers: Second Report on Confidential Enquiries into Maternal Deaths in South Africa, 1999–2001.* Pretoria: Department of Health.

Pittrof, R., O. Campbell, and V. Filippi. 2002. "What Is Quality in Maternity Care? An International Perspective." *Acta Obstetrica et Gynecologica Scandinavica* 81 (4): 277–83.

Portela, A., and C. Santarelli. 2003. "Empowerment of Women, Men, Families, and Communities: True Partners for Improving Maternal and Newborn Health." *British Medical Bulletin* 67 (1): 59–72.

Prata, N., F. Greig, J. Walsh, and M. Potts. 2004. "Setting Priorities for Safe Motherhood Interventions in Resource Scarce Settings." Paper submitted to the Population Association of America, 2004 Annual Meeting, School of Public Health, University of California–Berkeley, April 1–3.

Prendiville, W. J., D. Elbourne, and I. Chalmers. 1988. "The Effects of Routine Oxytocics Administration in the Management of the Third Stage of Labour: An Overview of the Evidence from Controlled Trials." *British Journal of Obstetrics and Gynaecology* 95 (1): 3–16.

Raju, S., and A. Leonard. 2000. *Men as Supportive Partners in Reproductive Health: Moving from Rhetoric to Reality.* New Delhi: Population Council South and East Asia Regional Office.

Robertson, N. R. C. 1993. *A Manual of Normal Neonatal Care.* London: Arnold.

Rogo, K., L. Bohmer, and C. Ombaka. 1999. "Developing Community-Based Strategies to Decrease Maternal Morbidity and Mortality Due to Unsafe Abortion: Pre-intervention Report." *East African Medical Journal* 76 (11 Suppl.): S1–71.

Rooney, C. 1992. *Antenatal Care and Maternal Health: How Effective Is It? A Review of the Evidence.* WHO/MSM/92.4. Geneva: World Health Organization.

Rouse, D. J. 2003. "Potential Cost-Effectiveness of Nutrition Interventions to Prevent Adverse Pregnancy Outcomes in the Developing World." *Journal of Nutrition* 133 (Suppl.): 1640S–44S.

Rush, D. 2000. "Nutrition and Maternal Mortality in the Developing World." *American Journal of Clinical Nutrition* 72 (Suppl.): 212–40.

Russell, S., and L. Gilson. 1997. "User Fee Policies to Promote Health Service Access for the Poor: A Wolf in Sheep's Clothing." *International Journal of Health Services* 27 (2): 359–79.

Sadana, R. 2001. "Quantifying Reproductive Health and Illness." Ph.D. dissertation, Harvard School of Public Health, Boston, MA.

Save the Children. 2001. *State of the World's Newborns: Saving Newborn Lives.* Washington, DC: Save the Children.

Say, L., R. Pattinson, and M. Gulmezoglu. 2004. "WHO Systematic Review of Maternal Morbidity and Mortality: The Prevalence of Severe Acute Maternal Morbidity (Near Miss)." *Reproductive Health* 1: 3. http://www.reproductive-health-journal.com/content/1/1/3.

Shehu, D., A. T. Ikeh, and M. J. Kuna. 1997. "Mobilizing Transport for Obstetric Emergencies in Northwestern Nigeria." *International Journal of Gynecology and Obstetrics* 59 (2): 173–80.

Sheldon, T. A. 1996. "Problems of Using Modeling in the Economic Evaluation of Health Care." *Health Economics* 5: 1–11.

Sorensen, G., K. Emmons, H. K. Hunt, and D. Johnston. 1998. "Implications of the Results of Community Intervention Trials." *Annual Review of Public Health* 19: 379–416.

Steketee, R. W., B. L. Nahlen, M. E. Parise, and C. Mendez. 2001. "The Burden of Malaria in Pregnancy in Malaria-Endemic Area." *American Journal of Tropical Medicine and Hygiene* 64 (1.2 Suppl.): 28–35.

Stoll, B. J., and A. R. Measham. 2001. "Children Can't Wait: Improving the Future for the World's Poorest Infants." *Journal of Pediatrics* 139 (5): 729–33.

Thonneau, P., N. Goyaux, S. Goufodji, and J. Sundby. 2002. "Abortion and Maternal Mortality in Africa." *New England Journal of Medicine* 347 (24): 1984–85.

Tomkins, A. 2001. "Nutrition and Maternal Morbidity and Mortality." *British Journal of Nutrition* 85 (2): 93–99.

UN (United Nations). 2002. *UN Population Division Population Estimates and Projections,* 2000 rev.

UNFPA (United Nations Population Fund). 2003. *Maternal Mortality Update 2002: A Focus on Emergency Obstetric Care.* New York: UNFPA.

UNICEF (United Nations Children's Fund). 1999. "World Summit for Children Goals: End of Decade Indicators for Monitoring Progress." Executive Directive EXD/1999-03, New York.

Villar, J., H. Ba'aqeel, G. Piaggio, P. Lumbiganon, J. M. Belizan, U. Farnot, and others. 2001. "WHO Antenatal Care Randomized Trial for the Evaluation of a New Model of Routine Antenatal Care." *Lancet* (North American ed.) 357 (9268): 1551–64.

Villar, J., and P. Bergsjo. 1997. "Scientific Basis for the Content of Routine Antenatal Care I." *Acta Obstetrica et Gynecologica Scandinavica* 76 (1): 1–14.

Villar, J., M. Merialdi, A. M. Gulmezoglu, E. Abalos, G. Carroli, R. Kulier, and M. de Oni. 2002. "Nutritional Interventions during Pregnancy for the Prevention or Treatment of Maternal Morbidity and Preterm Delivery: An Overview of Randomized Controlled Trials." *Journal of Nutrition* 133 (5): 1606S–25S.

Walsh, J., A. Fiefer, A. Measham, and P. Gertler. 1993. "Maternal and Perinatal Health." In *Disease Control Priorities in Developing Countries,* ed. D. Jamison, H. Mosley, A. Measham, and J. Bobadilla, 363–90. Oxford, U.K.: Oxford Publications.

Weil, O., and H. Fernandez. 1999. "Is Safe Motherhood an Orphan Initiative?" *Lancet* 354 (9182): 940–43.

West, K. P. Jr., J. Katz, S. K. Khatry, S. C. LeClerq, E. K. Pradhan, S. R. Shrestha, and others. 1999. "Double Blind, Cluster Randomised Trial of Low Dose Supplementation with Vitamin A or Beta Carotene on Mortality Related to Pregnancy in Nepal." *British Medical Journal* 318 (7183): 570–75.

WHO (World Health Organization). 1986. "Maternal Mortality: Helping Women off the Road to Death." *World Health Organization Chronicle* 40: 175–183.

———. 1992a. *International Classification of Diseases and Related Health Problems,* 10th rev. Geneva: WHO.

———. 1992b. *The Prevention and Management of Unsafe Abortion.* WHO/MSM/92.5. Report of a Technical Working Group. Geneva: WHO.

———. 1994. *Mother-Baby Package.* WHO/FHE/MSM/94.11. Geneva: WHO.

———. 1999. *Mother-Baby Package Costing Spreadsheet.* WHO/FCH/RHR/99.17. Geneva: WHO.

———. 2002. *Reducing Risks, Promoting Healthy Life: The World Health Report 2002.* Geneva: WHO.

———. 2003. *Making Pregnancy Safer: Global Action for Skilled Attendants for Pregnant Women.* WHO/RHR/02.17. Geneva: WHO.

———. 2004a. "Global Monitoring and Evaluation, Proportion of Births Attended by Skilled Health Personnel: Global, Regional, and Subregional Estimates." Geneva, WHO, Department of Reproductive Health and Research. http://www.who.int/reproductive-health/global_monitoring/data_regions.html.

———. 2004b. *Maternal Mortality in 2000: Estimates Developed by WHO, UNICEF, UNFPA.* Geneva: WHO.

———. 2004c. *Unsafe Abortion: Global and Regional Estimates of the Incidence of Unsafe Abortion and Associated Mortality in 2000.* 4th ed. Geneva: WHO.

———. 2004d. *Global Burden of Disease for the Year 2001 by World Bank Region, for Use in Disease Control Priorities in Developing Countries,* 2nd ed. Bethesda, MD: National Institutes of Health. http://www.fic.nih.gov/dcpp/gbd.html.

WHO-CHOICE (Choosing Interventions That Are Cost Effective). 2004. "Choosing Interventions That Are Cost Effective." Geneva. http://www3.who.int/whosis/menu.cfm?path=whosis,cea&language=english.

Williams, A. 1987. "Health Economics: The Cheerful Face of the Dismal Science?" In *Health and Economics,* ed. A. Williams. 1–11. Basingstoke and London: Macmillan.

Winikoff, B., and M. Sullivan. 1987. "Assessing the Role of Family Planning in Reducing Maternal Mortality." *Studies in Family Planning* 18 (3): 128–43.

Yasmin, S., D. Osrin, E. Paul, and A. Costello. 2001. "Neonatal Mortality of Low Birth-Weight Infants in Bangladesh." *Bulletin of the World Health Organization* 79 (7): 608–14.

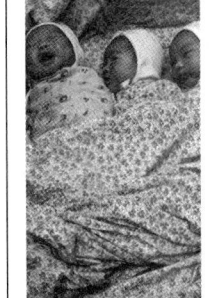

Chapter **27**

Newborn Survival

Joy E. Lawn, Jelka Zupan, Geneviève Begkoyian,
and Rudolf Knippenberg

The second half of the 20th century witnessed impressive reductions in the risk of under-five child mortality, which was halved between 1960 and 1990. The greatest reduction was for children after the first month of life, with relatively little decrease in the neonatal period (the first 28 days of life). Neonatal deaths, estimated at approximately 4 million annually, now account for 38 percent of the world's deaths of children under five. The fourth Millennium Development Goal (MDG) aspires to a global target, by 2015, of reducing the under-five mortality rate by two-thirds, which implies approximately 30 deaths per 1,000 live births for children under five. Currently, there are an estimated 30 deaths per 1,000 live births in the neonatal period alone. Thus, the fourth MDG cannot be achieved without substantial reduction in neonatal deaths (Lawn, Cousens, and Zupan 2005).

Addressing neonatal mortality requires links within the continuum of care from maternal health through pregnancy, childbirth, and early neonatal care, and into child health programs. Such services can be delivered through a combination of care at the family-community level, outreach, and clinical care (figure 27.1). Yet neither child survival nor safe motherhood programs have adequately addressed newborn deaths. The first week of life, when 75 percent of neonatal and 50 percent of maternal deaths occur, is associated with low health care coverage, particularly in poor communities. Investing in maternal, neonatal, and child health (MNCH) services will improve the survival of newborns and reduce stillbirths and maternal and child deaths. The first weeks of life are also a time of behavioral transition, representing an opportunity to promote healthy behaviors that have benefit beyond the neonatal period.

This chapter provides an overview of neonatal deaths, presenting the epidemiology as a basis for program priorities and summarizing the evidence for interventions within a health systems framework, providing cost and impact estimates for packages that are feasible for universal scale-up. The focus of the chapter is restricted to interventions during the neonatal period. The priority interventions identified here are largely well known, yet global coverage is extremely low. The chapter concludes with a discussion of implementation in country programs with examples of scaling up, highlighting gaps in knowledge.

NEONATAL DEATHS

One reason neonatal survival has received little attention relative to the huge number of deaths is the invisibility of those deaths. Most deaths during the neonatal period occur at home and are often unregistered even in transition countries (Lumbiganon and others 1990). Social invisibility is linked to an expectation of high mortality; many traditional societies do not name newborns for up to six weeks. Data presented here are derived from full-coverage vital registration for 72 countries, which cover less than 4 percent of all neonatal deaths; demographic and health surveys, which cover 75 percent of global neonatal deaths; and statistical modeling, for the 20 percent of neonatal deaths in countries without data (WHO forthcoming). Population-based data on neonatal morbidity or long-term disability in low- and middle-income countries (LMICs) are scarce. The World Health Organization (WHO) has estimated that three conditions (birth asphyxia, prematurity,

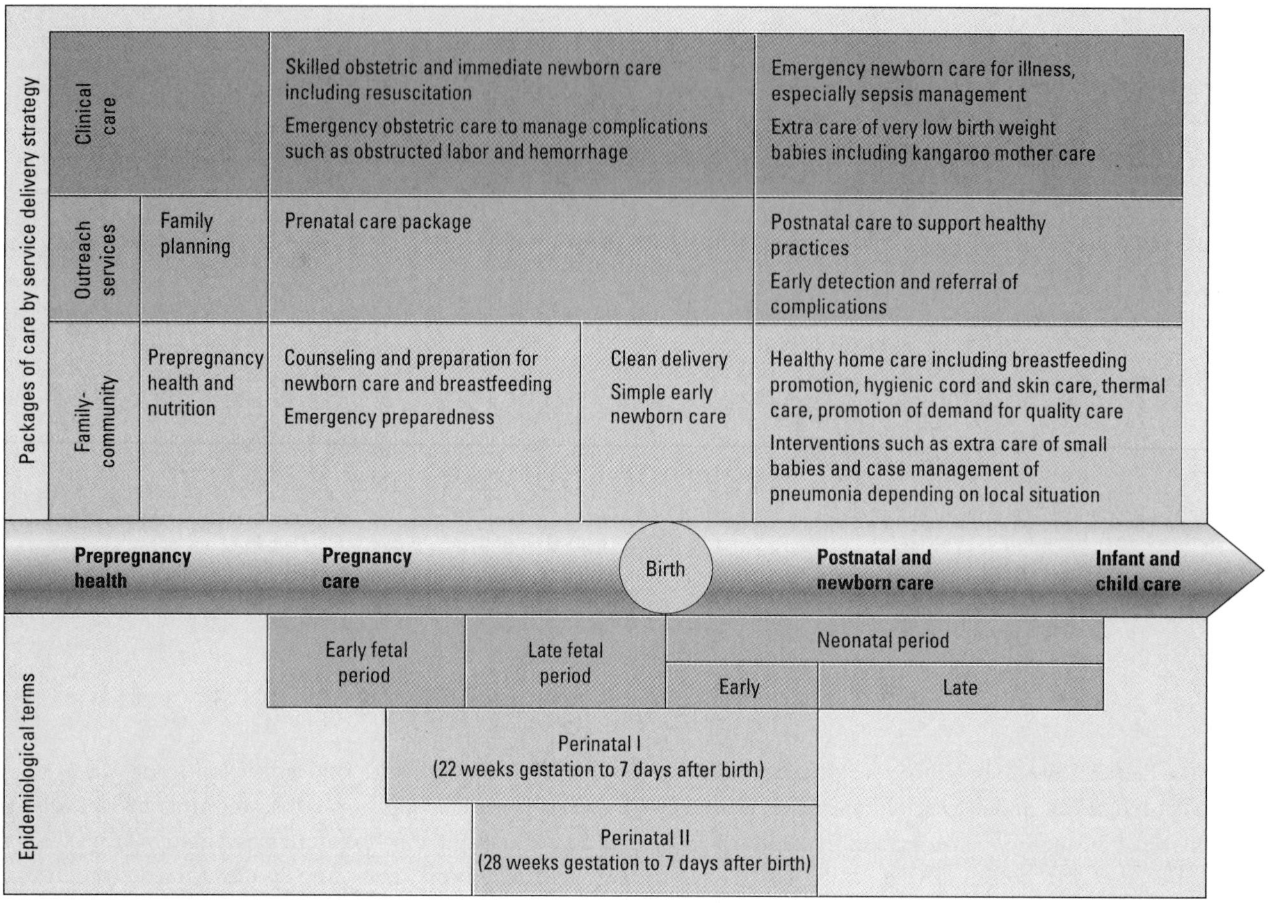

Figure 27.1 The Continuum of Care for Mothers, Newborns, and Children, Showing Epidemiological Terms around the Time of Birth and Packages of Care Relevant to Newborn Health, According to Service Delivery Level

Note: International Classification of Diseases version 10 recommends perinatal I for national data collection. The World Health Organization recommends perinatal II for international comparisons of data.

and "other perinatal causes"), collectively termed *perinatal causes,* contribute to 6.3 percent of global disability-adjusted life years (WHO 2003a). Although these causes represent only part of the neonatal burden, the WHO estimate is more than triple that of HIV, yet receives remarkably little attention.

Where Do Newborns Die?

Only 1 percent of neonatal deaths occur in high-income countries. These countries have average neonatal mortality rate (NMR) of 4 per 1,000 live births, whereas in LMICs the average NMR is 33 per 1,000 live births, with a range of 2 to 70 (table 27.1). The highest number of neonatal deaths occur in South Asia because of the large populations of this region. The six countries with the highest numbers of neonatal deaths in 2000 include the populous nations of India (1.09 million neonatal deaths annually), China (416,000), Pakistan (298,000), Nigeria (247,000), Bangladesh (153,000), and Ethiopia (147,000). Of the 20 countries with the highest NMRs, 80 percent are in Sub-Saharan Africa. The highest rates occur in countries there that have experienced recent civil unrest, such as Liberia (65 per 1,000 live births), Sierra Leone

(60 per 1,000 live births), Mozambique (55 per 1,000 live births), and Ethiopia (52 per 1,000 live births).

When Do Newborns Die?

Each year 3 million newborns die during their first seven days of life, accounting for 75 percent of all neonatal deaths. At least 1 million babies die during their first 24 hours of life (Lawn, Cousens, and Zupan 2005). If mortality rates during the first five years of life are adjusted to rates per week, the risk in the first week of life is massively higher than during any other time of life: 24 per 1,000 in the first week compared with 3 per week for the rest of the first month and only 0.12 per week after the first year of life. Yet the first week is the very period in the continuum of care when services are most likely to be lacking, particularly in poor communities, where most deaths occur.

Time Trends in Neonatal Mortality

As shown in figure 27.2, the disparity in NMRs between LMICs and high-income countries is increasing over time, especially during the early neonatal period, which saw an almost 60 percent reduction in high-income countries between 1983 and

Table 27.1 NMRs and Neonatal Deaths by Region for 2000, and Variation in NMR by Income Quintile and by Region

| Region | NMR per 1,000 live births (range across countries) | Median NMR by income quintile by region | | Number (percentage) of neonatal deaths (thousands) | Percentage of deaths during the neonatal period among children under five |
		Poorest quintile	Richest quintile		
World	30	—	—	3,998 (100)	38
High-income countries	4 (1–11)	—	—	42 (1)	63
Low- and middle-income countries	33 (2–70)	—	—	3,956 (99)	38
Region					
Africa	44 (9–70)	48	34	1,128 (28)	24
Americas	12 (4–34)	35	18	195 (5)	48
Eastern Mediterranean	40 (4–63)	38	28	603 (15)	40
Europe	11 (2–38)	—	—	116 (3)	49
South Asia	38 (11–43)	50	28	1,442 (36)	50
Western Pacific	19 (1–40)	28	17	514 (13)	56

Source: Authors' calculations, based on NMRs and under-five mortality, WHO and UNICEF estimates; NMR by income quintile based on analysis of demographic and health survey data for 50 countries, 1995–2002.
— = not available.

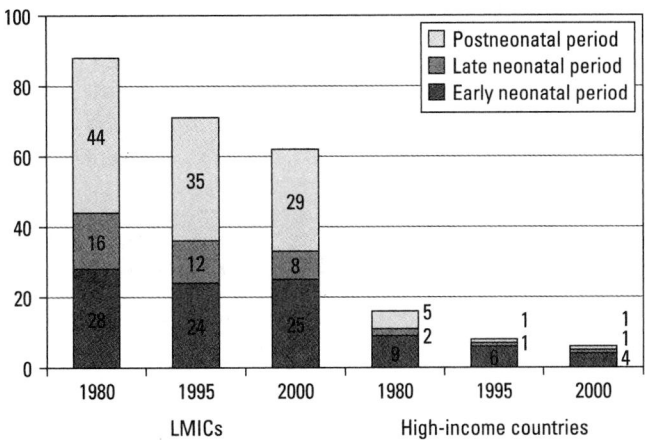

Source: Authors' calculations, based on UNICEF, various years; WHO 1998c; and WHO forthcoming.

Figure 27.2 Trends in Early and Late Neonatal and Postneonatal Mortality, by Country Income Levels

2000, compared with about a 15 percent reduction in LMICs. There has been no measurable decline in the regional average NMR for sub-Saharan Africa. However some regions have made significant progress in reducing NMRs, particularly Latin America and the Western Pacific. Some low-income countries such as Bangladesh, Indonesia, and Sri Lanka have achieved NMR reductions of 40 to 50 percent. In South Asia and Sub-Saharan Africa, the decline in late neonatal deaths was influenced by the halving of neonatal tetanus deaths that occurred during the 1990s as a result of increased tetanus toxoid protection and clean delivery practices. By 2000, two-thirds of LMICs had eliminated neonatal tetanus and an additional 22 countries were nearing this goal.

Historical data also show more rapid reductions in postneonatal mortality, steady reductions in late neonatal mortality, and slower reductions in early neonatal deaths. In England, the NMR fell from more than 30 per 1,000 live births in 1940 to 10 per 1,000 in 1975. This fall occurred before intensive care, which was introduced only when the NMR had fallen below 15 per 1,000. The greatest reduction of NMR coincided with the introduction of free prenatal care, high coverage of skilled childbirth care, and the availability of antibiotics. Although the number of postneonatal and late neonatal deaths is amenable to public health interventions (such as immunization and improved hygiene and nutrition), larger reduction of early neonatal deaths and of maternal deaths requires a system that provides effective clinical care—particularly during childbirth, which is more challenging.

Direct Causes of Neonatal Death

Fewer than 3 percent of the world's neonatal deaths occur in countries that have vital registration data that are reliable enough to use in cause-of-death analysis. Population-based information in high-mortality settings often depends on verbal autopsy tools of variable quality. The Child Health Epidemiology Reference Group undertook an extensive exercise to derive global estimates for program-relevant causes of neonatal death, including preterm birth, asphyxia, sepsis/pneumonia, neonatal tetanus, diarrhea, and other causes, with the latter including specific but less prevalent causes such as jaundice. For low-mortality countries, vital registration data from 45 countries with full vital registration coverage (cumulative sample size of 96,797) were included. For high-mortality countries, studies were identified through extensive systematic searches, and a meta-analysis was performed after applying inclusion criteria and using standard case definitions (56 studies, cumulative sample size of 13,685). Models were developed to simultaneously estimate the seven selected causes of death by country (Lawn, Cousens, and Wilczynska forthcoming).

Three causes of death—infections (pneumonia, diarrhea, and tetanus) (36 percent), preterm birth (28 percent), and asphyxia (23 percent)—account for the majority of neonatal deaths. Causes of death vary between the early and late neonatal periods, with deaths caused by preterm birth, asphyxia, and congenital defects occurring predominantly during the first week of life and infection being the major cause of neonatal deaths thereafter. Neonatal tetanus, a totally preventable condition, still accounts for more than a quarter of a million deaths, even after the second global elimination deadline has passed. Most neonatal tetanus deaths occur in 20 countries in South Asia and Sub-Saharan Africa, all of which have very high NMRs. Variation in causes of neonatal death is seen between and within countries, closely associated with the NMR level. Where the NMR is high (more than 45 per 1,000 live births), more than half of neonatal deaths are due to infections; where the NMR is low, prematurity and congenital abnormalities are the major causes of death (Lawn, Cousens, and Zupan 2005). Hence, information regarding the local epidemiology is important in prioritizing interventions.

Indirect Causes of Neonatal Death

An estimated 20 million low birthweight (LBW) infants (that is, weighing less than 2,500 grams), are born each year—25 percent of them in South Asia (Blanc and Wardlow 2005). Although globally only 16 percent of newborns have LBW, 60 to 80 percent of neonatal deaths occur in LBW infants (Lawn, Cousens, and Wilczynska forthcoming). LBW is due to short gestation (preterm birth), intrauterine growth restriction (IUGR), or both. Globally, almost one-third of neonatal deaths are directly attributable to preterm birth. In contrast, an analysis of vital registration data for 45 countries and of five population-based studies suggests that a maximum of 1 to 2 percent of neonatal deaths are directly attributable to IUGR in full-term neonates (Lawn, Cousens, and Wilczynska forthcoming). Prematurity and full-term IUGR are also indirect causes or risk factors for neonatal deaths, particularly deaths resulting from infection. The relative risk among preterm infants is much higher than for full-term IUGR infants (Yasmin and others 2001). Complex technology is not necessary to avoid most deaths in moderately preterm newborns. Extra attention to warmth and feeding and to prevention or early treatment of infections is crucial (Lawn, McCarthy, and Ross 2001).

Maternal health and health care are important determinants of neonatal survival. Neonatal outcomes are affected by female health throughout the life cycle, from child, through adolescence, and into pregnancy (Pojda and Kelley 2000). In general, intrapartum risk factors are associated with greater increases in risk of neonatal death than factors identified during pregnancy, which are in turn associated with greater increases in risk than prepregnancy factors (Lawn, Cousens, and Zupan 2005). Obstructed labor and malpresentation present the highest risk and require skilled intervention. The mother's death substantially increases the risk of death for her child. Greenwood and others (1987) report that of mothers who died in labor ($N = 8$), all the babies died within one year.

Delays in access to care for severely ill young infants are common. Peterson and others (2004), in a study in Uganda, find that almost 80 percent of the caregivers of severely ill young infants did not comply with recommended referrals to a health facility. The reason given in 90 percent of the cases was lack of money, underscoring the need for pro-poor financing mechanisms and promotion of community demand for care. This recalls the "three delays" model for maternal deaths, which outlines delays in recognition of illness and in access to care and provision of care once at a health facility (Thaddeus and Maine 1994).

Poverty is the root cause of many maternal and neonatal deaths, either because it increases the prevalence of risk factors such as maternal infections or because it reduces access to care. An analysis of 50 demographic and health surveys between 1995 and 2002 reveals that, within regions, the poorest quintiles have an NMR that is, on average, 20 to 50 percent higher than that for the highest income quintile (table 27.1). Deliberate programmatic focus is required to ensure that care reaches poor families.

Applying Lessons from Epidemiology to Programs

There are almost 4 million neonatal deaths annually. Given that the proportion of child deaths that occur during the neonatal period (currently 38 percent) will increase over time, the MDG for child survival cannot be met without a significant reduction in the NMR. Most neonatal deaths are in Sub-Saharan Africa and South Asia and are due to preventable causes. Historical data demonstrate that the NMR can be reduced to 15 per 1,000 without intensive care.

Priority should be given to two main gaps in the provision of care. The first is the continuum of care by time. The period through pregnancy and childbirth into infancy contains a gap at childbirth and during the first week of life, when most neonatal deaths—and also most maternal deaths—occur. Addressing this gap will involve strengthening safe motherhood and child survival services and institutionalizing links at the subnational, national, and global levels. The second gap is between levels of care (figure 27.1)—particularly with the family-community level, since poor and rural communities account for the majority of neonatal and maternal deaths. Approaches are needed to better link homes and health care, supplying care closer to such communities, increasing demand for skilled care, and empowering communities, including poor communities, to make healthful decisions.

INTERVENTIONS

We undertook literature searches and categorized interventions by time period (during pregnancy, and intrapartum and post-natal or neonatal periods) (table 27.2). We focus on interventions delivered during the neonatal period that are likely to reduce neonatal deaths, as opposed to those delivered during the neonatal period that yield later benefits (for example, prevention of mother to child transmission of HIV). Although rigorous evaluation of evidence is vital, evidence is not available for some well-established interventions. In the case of neonatal resuscitation, for example, a randomized controlled trial is impossible for ethical reasons, yet the intervention is a corner-stone of neonatal care in high-income settings. Some important practices, such as cleanliness, have undergone little rigorous evaluation but are obviously beneficial (Bhutta and others 2005). On the basis of level of evidence and feasibility of implementation, we grouped interventions into three categories:

- Universally applicable interventions are selected on the basis of mortality impact, cost, and feasibility. Some of these interventions are feasible only after skilled care is available. Other interventions are feasible immediately, even in the absence of skilled care. A particular example is improved family care practices. Interventions may apply to different newborns as follows:
  — essential newborn care for all babies at all levels
  — extra newborn care for babies with specific risk factors, such as LBW
  — emergency newborn care for babies who are ill, particularly those with infections.
- Additional interventions should apply where neonatal mortality is lower and capacity is greater. These interventions are more complex, requiring more skilled staff members and additional commodities, and therefore cost more for less reduction in mortality. Universal scaling up cannot be recommended at present, but these interventions become important for further reduction of mortality and disabilities after universal care packages are in place.
- Situational interventions are necessary because of locally prevalent risk factors, such as HIV or malaria.

The packages of newborn care selected for universal scale-up are summarized in table 27.3 and discussed in the following subsections, starting with family-community interventions and followed by essential, extra, and emergency newborn care packages.

Family-Community Care of the Newborn

Family care of the newborn is important for all newborns. It includes promoting positive behaviors such as breastfeeding and demand for health care throughout the neonatal period

and afterward (WHO 2003c). Cleanliness (for example, cord care and hand washing), warmth provision, and exclusive breastfeeding reduce neonatal illnesses, especially infection. Implementation of this package will depend on the setting, the coverage of facility delivery, and the availability of community workers or other channels but is feasible even in poorly developed health systems (Knippenberg and others 2005). The role and value of the mother are central.

Although much has been written to describe traditional newborn care practices, few studies assess behavior change. An exception is the study by Meegan and others (2001) of the Masai in Kenya, where behavioral messages about cord care practices were associated with the virtual elimination of neonatal tetanus—with no increase in tetanus toxoid immunizations. The Warmi Project in rural Bolivia demonstrated that raising community awareness of maternal, fetal, and neonatal health issues through women's community groups increased family-planning coverage, attendance at prenatal and postnatal services, and the presence of trained traditional birth assistants at childbirth, resulting in a 62 percent reduction of perinatal mortality (O'Rourke, Howard-Grabman, and Seoane 1998). A cluster randomized trial in rural Nepal, where 90 percent of women deliver at home, also used female facilitators working with women's groups. Comparing the 12 intervention villages with their paired villages showed a 30 percent reduction in the NMR (mainly late NMRs) mediated through increased health seeking and improved home behaviors (such as doubling the rates of practices such as hand washing and use of clean delivery kits) and strengthening of the health system (Manandhar and others 2004).

A family-community package promoting good home care of the newborn—particularly cleanliness, warmth, and exclusive breastfeeding—would have an expected reduction in the NMR of 10 to 40 percent, varying with the baseline NMR and the potential for accessing care. The effect might be greater if the package successfully addressed harmful local practices. The effect of early care seeking for illness will depend on the capacity of the primary and referral health care levels to manage neonatal illness. Thus, community-level interventions with no supply-side strengthening will have only a limited effect. Many questions remain about how best to work with families and communities, given widely differing cultures and behaviors and the varying capacities of existing community health workers (Darmstadt and others 2005), and about the wider application of demand subsidies.

Essential Newborn Care at the Time of Birth

WHO (2003d) defines essential newborn care as the care of the newborn at birth, including cleaning, drying, and warming the infant; initiating exclusive breastfeeding early; and caring for the cord. Essential care of the newborn is necessary for all

Table 27.2 Interventions to Reduce Fetal and Neonatal Mortality by Timing of Intervention and by Scalability of Intervention

Period	Interventions for universal coverage (priority interventions for high-mortality settings)	Additional interventions (where the health care system has additional capacity and the NMR is lower; for example, transition countries)	Situational interventions (where specific conditions are prevalent)
Prepregnancy	Family planning [B]: • delay age of first pregnancy to after 18 • space births by two to three years • provide opportunity for women to reduce births to their desired number and to avoid pregnancy after age 45 Prevention, identification, and management of sexually transmitted diseases [A] Micronutrient deficiency prevention strategies • iodination of salt [B]	Rubella immunization either of girls only or of all population if regular coverage can be maintained at more than 80 percent of the population [A] Periconceptual or preconceptual provision of folate [A] Information counseling and support for • smoking [RF A] • alcohol and drug abuse [RF A] • women experiencing violence [RF A]	HIV prevalent: • primary prevention strategies [B] • voluntary counseling and testing and option of antiretroviral therapy [A] High prevalence of recessive conditions (such as sickle cell disease) or high rates of consanguineous marriages: offer genetics counseling [RF A]
During pregnancy • Essential for all pregnancies	Four-visit prenatal care package, including • two tetanus immunizations [A] • iron and folate supplements [B] • syphilis screening and treatment [A] • identification and referral of multiple pregnancy, abnormal lie, preeclampsia [B] • birth planning and emergency preparedness [C] • prenatal counseling and preparation for breastfeeding [C]	Identification and treatment of bacteriuria [A] Information counseling and support for • smoking cessation [RF A] • alcohol and drug abuse [RF A] • healthy diet and avoidance of unhelpful dietary taboos [C] • women experiencing violence [RF A]	HIV prevalent: • primary prevention strategies [B] • voluntary counseling and testing and option of antiretroviral therapy [A]
• Extra care for those at risk of complications	Extra prenatal care (more frequent visits, more skilled caregiver) if • multiple pregnancy or abnormal lie (breech or transverse) [RF A] • pregnancy-induced hypertension or preeclampsia [RF A] • diabetes [RF A] • severe anemia [RF A] • previous fetal or neonatal death [RF A]	External cephalic version for breech presentation at 36 weeks [A] Fetal growth monitoring [A]	Malaria endemic: • intermittent presumptive treatment monthly after 20 weeks [A] • insecticide-treated bednets [B based on effect on LBW, not on NMR] Hookworm infestation prevalent: • presumptive treatment with mebendazole [B]
• Emergency for those with complications (first referral level and above)	Management of emergencies, including • preeclampsia or eclampsia [A] • bleeding in pregnancy [A*] • uterine infection [RF A]	In utero transfer of high-risk pregnancies [B]	Iodine deficiency prevalent: • iodine supplementation [B] Famine: • targeted food supplementation [B] Group B streptococcus prevalent: • screening and treatment [A]
Birth • Essential	Skilled care in labor, including • monitoring progress of labor (partograph), maternal and fetal well-being [A] • infection control [A*] ***Newborn resuscitation*** if required [A*]	Supportive companion in labor [A]	Mother HIV positive: • antiretroviral therapy [A]

Table 27.2 Continued

Period	Interventions for universal coverage (priority interventions for high-mortality settings)	Additional interventions (where the health care system has additional capacity and the NMR is lower; for example, transition countries)	Situational interventions (where specific conditions are prevalent)
• Extra care	Extra care if • preterm (<37 weeks) or prolonged (>18 hours) rupture of membranes or evidence of chorioamnionitis; give antibiotics to woman [A] • failure to progress in labor including instrumental vaginal delivery (vacuum) if required [RF A] ***Newborn resuscitation*** if required [A*]	Tocolytics in preterm labor and transfer to higher-level care if available [A] If preterm labor, then give prenatal steroid injection to mother [A]	Maternity waiting home if limited access to emergency obstetric care, high-risk condition identified, and culturally acceptable [B]
• Emergency	Emergency obstetric care for acute intrapartum emergencies: [A*] • obstructed labor and fetal distress • bleeding, infections, or eclampsia ***Neonatal resuscitation*** if required [A*]		
Postnatal and newborn • Essential	***Essential newborn care for all newborns,*** including • early and exclusive breastfeeding [B] • warmth provision and avoidance of bathing during first 24 hours [C] • infection control, including cord care and hygiene [B] • postpartum vitamin A provided to mother [B] • eye antimicrobial provided to prevent ophthalmia [A] • information and counseling for home care and emergency preparedness [C]	Trained breastfeeding counselors undertaking home visits [A] Vitamin K (cost-effective as prophylaxis for all babies in transition countries) [B] Routine newborn screening programs for sickle cell disease, glucose 6 phosphate dehydrogenase deficiency [B]	Hepatitis B prevalent: • give hepatitis B immunization early [A] Mother HIV positive: • provide counseling and support for feeding choices [C]
• Extra care	***Extra care for small babies*** (preterm or term IUGR) and multiple births, severe congenital abnormalities: • extra attention to warmth, feeding support, and early identification and management of complications [B] • kangaroo mother care [A: morbidity not mortality data] • vitamin K injection [B]	Provide special or intensive care for preterm babies [A]	Mother with tuberculosis: • keep baby with mother and give izoniazid prophylaxis Mother with syphilis: • treat the baby even if asymptomatic [A*]
• Emergency	***Emergency care*** providing specific and supportive care according to evidence-based guidelines for the following: • severe infections [A] • neonatal encephalopathy (following acute intrapartum insult) • severe jaundice or bleeding [A*] • neonatal tetanus	Provide special care for sick and small babies using skilled nurses and a higher nurse-to-patient ratio [B]	

Source: Authors, based on extensive literature review. References detailed on http://www.fic.nih.gov/dcpp/.

Note: A = rigorous meta-analysis or at least one good randomized controlled trial exists, RF A = evidence regarding risk is strong, B = well-conducted clinical studies exist but no randomized controlled trial done, C = some descriptive evidence and expert committee consensus exists, A* = unethical to test rigorously and widely practiced as standard (for example, blood transfusion, neonatal resuscitation). **Bold** text signifies priority packages or interventions considered in detail in this chapter.

Table 27.3 Packages for Universal Scale-up of Newborn Care

Intervention package	Contents	Number of target population per year (millions)	Implementation strategy	Estimated current coverage (percent) South Asia	Estimated current coverage (percent) Sub-Saharan Africa	Reduction in all-cause NMR (percent)	Comments on evidence
Family-community care of the newborn at home after birth	Healthy home care practices (exclusive breastfeeding, warmth protection, clean cord care, care seeking for emergencies); if birth outside a facility, then clean delivery kit.	All newborn infants: World 130 South Asia and Sub-Saharan Africa 63	Women's groups and community health workers doing postnatal visits, with links to the formal health care system, including support for referral. If appropriate, extra care of moderately small babies at home and community-based management of acute respiratory infections.	36	28	10–40	Mortality reduction based on studies in high NMR settings with weak health systems. Extra care of LBW infants and community management of acute respiratory infections not included in range shown.
Essential newborn care at the time of birth	Immediate drying, warmth, early breastfeeding, hygiene maintenance, and infection prevention	All newborn infants: World 130 South Asia and Sub-Saharan Africa 63	Skilled attendant, or if no skilled attendant available, some simple postnatal practices are feasible at home with other cadres of workers.	11	14	20–30	Based on conservative combining of single interventions (for example, breastfeeding) in the package.
Neonatal resuscitation	Resuscitation after birth if required	Newborns not breathing at birth: World 6.5 South Asia and Sub-Saharan Africa 3.2	Skilled attendant.	3	3	10–25	Limited studies, mainly from lower NMR settings with high percentage of asphyxia deaths, so range from studies was reduced.
Extra care of small newborns	Extra support for warmth (kangaroo mother care), feeding, and illness identification and management	LBW neonates: World 20.0 South Asia and Sub-Saharan Africa 10.7	Facility-based care for severely preterm babies. Community-based care is effective for moderately preterm babies.	<10	<10	20–40	Most studies are nonrandomized controlled trials at the community level in settings with extremely high LBW rates. Effect depends on baseline NMR and LBW rates.
Emergency care of ill newborns	Management of ill infants, especially those with neonatal infections	Neonates with illnesses: World 13.0 South Asia and Sub-Saharan Africa 6.3	Facility-based care with antibiotics and supportive care. Community-based management with oral antibiotics for acute respiratory infections.	<20	<20	20–50	Meta-analysis of effect on the NMR of oral antibiotic management of acute respiratory infections in the community in high-mortality settings.
Neonatal packages plus MCH package	Neonatal packages as above, in addition to family planning, prenatal care, and comprehensive obstetric care packages	All newborn infants: World 130 South Asia and Sub-Saharan Africa 63	Supply of care throughout pregnancy, childbirth, and postnatal period with increased demand and improved referral systems.	<5	<5	—	No study data identified. Marginal budgeting for bottlenecks tool suggests 58 percent in South Asia and 71 percent in Sub-Saharan Africa.

Source: Local data or Darmstadt and others 2005; Knippenberg and others 2005; Lawn, Cousens, and Zupan 2005.
Note: The range of reduction of all-cause NMRs given for each package is independent of the others; hence, the total is greater than 100 percent.

infants and is ideally provided by a skilled attendant, but in the absence of skilled care, many of the tasks can be carried out at home by alternative cadres of workers. WHO's essential care package includes resuscitation, which we consider separately because the skill level required is more complex.

Clean care of the umbilical cord (clean blade and tie) is important in reducing the incidence of neonatal tetanus and umbilical sepsis, but evidence for topical treatment of the cord remains unclear (Zupan and Garner 2000). Hand washing is important at all levels of care. Hypothermia is an important and preventable contributor to morbidity and mortality, especially in preterm babies. The so-called warm chain involves ensuring that childbirth takes place in a warmed room, drying the newborn, encouraging skin-to-skin contact between the newborn and the mother, and avoiding bathing for at least 12 hours (Lawn, McCarthy, and Ross 2001). In hospitals in LMICs, many newborns are hypothermic, and staff knowledge and practices could be improved (Dragovich and others 1997).

The effects of exclusive breastfeeding have been intensively studied, and the positive effect on infant mortality is unequivocal, although studies often do not specify the effect on neonatal mortality and morbidity. The WHO collaborative trial found the risk of mortality in nonbreastfed neonates to be 2.5 to 7.0 times greater than for breastfed neonates (WHO Collaborative Group 2000). The practice of keeping well babies close to their mothers and allowing feeding on demand increases breastfeeding rates, reducing both hypothermia and nosocomial infections (WHO 1998b). Unfortunately, as exemplified by the low proportion of hospitals that are certified as baby friendly, this practice is poorly implemented. Supportive policy, such as the International Code of Marketing of Breastmilk Substitutes, is also important at the national level.

The effect of essential newborn care has not been formally tested as a package, although exclusive breastfeeding, cleanliness, infection control measures, and hypothermia avoidance all individually reduce neonatal mortality and morbidity.

Nevertheless, only 11 percent of babies in South Asia and 14 percent in Sub-Saharan Africa are exclusively breastfed to three months. The Bellagio group estimated a 15 percent reduction in the NMR through 99 percent coverage of exclusive breastfeeding and an 11 percent impact reduction through clean delivery (Jones and others 2003). Conservatively, an essential newborn care package may result in a 10 to 25 percent reduction in the NMR, but field trials of a combined package are still required. No economic assessments were identified.

Newborn Resuscitation

Approximately 5 to 10 percent of newborns do not breathe spontaneously and require stimulation. About half of those have difficulty initiating breathing, requiring resuscitation (WHO 1998a). The major reasons for failure to breathe include preterm birth and acute intrapartum events resulting in hypoxic brain injury. Basic resuscitation using a self-inflating bag and air is effective for the majority of these newborns, although some may be too premature or have already experienced severe hypoxic brain injury and die despite resuscitation.

Monitoring labor and providing effective obstetric care can reduce the need for resuscitation (Dujardin, Sene, and Ndiaye 1992), but resuscitation may be required even with good obstetric care. Therefore, every skilled attendant should be competent in newborn resuscitation (box 27.1).

For most babies who do not breathe at birth, ventilation with a self-inflating bag and mask is lifesaving, and the time to first breath differs little between use of a self-inflating bag and mask and use of endotracheal intubation. Evidence is growing that most newborns can be successfully resuscitated without the use of oxygen (Saugstad 2001), although a small proportion of infants require such advanced resuscitation techniques as endotracheal intubation, oxygen, chest compression, or drugs. Such advanced resuscitation is appropriate only in institutions that provide ventilation. In the 1980s, the high cost of a self-inflating

---

Box 27.1

Institutionalizing a Neonatal Resuscitation Program in a Chinese Province

A hospital-based study from China reports baseline surveillance of 1,722 newborns followed by a two-year prospective assessment of 4,751 newborns, while instituting standardized resuscitation guidelines. Previous traditional resuscitation involved infusing central stimulants plus vitamin C and 50 percent glucose; wiping the baby with alcohol; and pressing the philtrum. Health professionals recognized that asphyxia was the leading cause of

neonatal death and the second leading cause of infant death nationally. They also recognized that child survival goals could not be met unless asphyxia was addressed. They developed and implemented an evidence-based neonatal resuscitation program, training staff in using the new guidelines. The early NMR fell significantly—by 66 percent, to 3.4 per 1,000.

Source: Zhu and others 1997.

bag and mask led to the development of a prototype mouth-to-mask device operated by blowing expired air. A study by Massawe and others (1996) in two teaching hospitals, one in Tanzania and the other in India, found that resuscitators using this device could maintain a maximum of only 20 breaths per minute, one-third of the recommended rate. Low-cost (less than US$5) versions of the bag and mask are now available, and it is the recommended device for resuscitation.

Although small-scale studies show that nonprofessional cadres can learn the technique of resuscitation (Bang and others 1999; Kumar 1995), a significant effect on mortality has not been demonstrated, and the feasibility of maintaining competency and the cost-effectiveness of training such cadres have yet to be ascertained. If traditional birth assistants attend, say, 20 deliveries a year, they would encounter a baby requiring resuscitation an average of only once a year, so the effect would be lower, and the cost per life saved higher, compared with a facility-based midwife who does 200 or more deliveries a year. Thus, more research is required before home resuscitation by traditional birth assistants can become a widespread policy. In the meantime, it should be ensured that where skilled attendants exist, they have the skills and equipment to perform neonatal resuscitation.

Because a randomized controlled trial would be considered unethical, the studies identified apply a before-and-after comparison. No cost assessments were identified. Achieving wider coverage of resuscitation is a challenge, especially for the 47 percent of the world's babies born at home.

Extra Care for Small Babies

Because 60 to 80 percent of neonatal deaths occur in LBW babies, targeting this group for additional preventive and early curative care is a logical approach to mortality reduction. Addressing deaths among severely preterm infants (fewer than 32 weeks of gestation) is more complex, but most preterm infants are moderately preterm (33.0 to 36.9 weeks). Excess mortality from acquired infections and other complications can largely be prevented or managed without intensive care.

A number of community-based studies have undertaken simplified identification of small babies and provided extra care at home, especially feeding (including the use of a dropper or cup feeding if required), warmth promotion, and cord cleanliness. The reported NMR reductions range from 25 percent (Pratinidhi and others 1986) to 42 percent (Daga and others 1988). Datta (1985) applied a comprehensive approach, including weighing all babies and providing extra home support to LBW infants through feeding counseling and early recognition of and referral for illness, alongside strengthening of local health systems. Compared with a control area, the NMR was reduced by more than 30 percent, with the greatest reduction among the group of 1,500- to 2,500-gram babies. In Bang and others' (1999) study, 90 percent of neonatal deaths were in LBW

infants, and all LBW babies were targeted for increased home visits. Special sleeping bags were provided for warmth, and support was given for breastfeeding and early treatment of possible infections. The NMR fell by 87 percent in the moderately preterm group (35 to 37 weeks) (Bang and others 1999).

So-called kangaroo mother care involves continuous skin-to-skin contact between mother and baby to provide thermal stability and promote exclusive breastfeeding for clinically stable preterm infants. The published evidence relates to facility-based care with or without kangaroo mother care after discharge. Mortality impact data for kangaroo mother care are lacking, but a review by Conde-Agudelo, Diaz-Rossello, and Belizan (2000) that included three randomized controlled trials found that serious morbidity was reduced by about 60 percent at the six-month follow-up visit. Although cost has not been formally evaluated, it must be considerably less than for incubator care. The lack of assessments of kangaroo mother care at community level is a research gap.

A few studies in health facilities in LMICs have reported increased survival of LBW infants with improved care. One from Papua New Guinea demonstrated a 56 percent reduction in the NMR with the introduction of standards for care and of basic technology (Duke, Willie, and Mgone 2000). Data from Ghana showed a 28 percent reduction in mortality for LBW infants with support for breastfeeding, attention to warmth, and early management of infections and jaundice using standard protocols (Lawn, McCarthy, and Ross 2001).

The reported effect for extra care of LBW babies in the community varies between 20 and 40 percent, excluding Bang and others' (1999) study because additional interventions were involved. Given the high LBW prevalence in these studies, the effect may be less in other settings with a lower LBW prevalence. Data from facilities that do not offer intensive care suggest a similar or slightly larger effect. Cost-effectiveness assessments were not identified.

Emergency Care for Ill Newborns

For many of the world's 4 million neonatal deaths, the immediate cause is a neonatal illness presenting as an emergency either soon after birth (such as complications of preterm birth and asphyxia) or later (because of neonatal tetanus or community-acquired infections). Other important but less prevalent conditions include jaundice and hemorrhagic disease of the newborn. Long-term disability follows many neonatal conditions, but it is poorly documented. Many serious neonatal problems present with similar signs: inability to feed, breathing difficulty, and temperature instability. All those conditions have high fatality rates, particularly neonatal tetanus (Institute of Medicine 2003) and neonatal encephalopathy (Ellis and others 1999), and preventive interventions may be the most realistic option in those conditions. Early phototherapy for jaundice reduces both mortality and chronic disability subsequent to kernicteris and is feasible in facilities (WHO 2003b). We focus on the clinical neonatal management of infection, which is the most prevalent neonatal illness and the most feasible to scale up.

A meta-analysis of community-based trials of case management of pneumonia in Africa and Asia yields a summary estimate for NMR reduction of 27 percent (Sazawal and Black 2003). The antibiotic regime used was mainly oral co-trimoxazole, although two studies included injectable penicillins. Bang and others' (1999) study in rural India reports a 62 percent reduction in the NMR with a home-based package for neonatal sepsis that included injectable gentamicin, although this reduction may be related to a number of simultaneously introduced interventions in addition to the gentamicin.

The effect of emergency care on neonatal sepsis can be assumed to be similar to the range in Sazawal and Black's (2003) meta-analysis: 20 to 60 percent. Published cost data were not identified apart from the Bang and others (1999) study, which indicated a cost of US$5.30 per neonate treated. This cost estimate includes the time of community health workers and the cost of equipment and drugs, but not associated supervision or system costs.

MARGINAL IMPACT AND COST OF SCALING UP UNIVERSAL NEONATAL PACKAGES

Because newborn health depends on services in the continuum of care for mother, newborn, and child, a vertical program would be duplicative, expensive, and inappropriate (Tinker and others 2005). Hence costing and impact estimates will be based on marginal additions of neonatal-specific packages to existing maternal and child health (MCH) services (table 27.4). This scenario reflects the reality in many South Asian and Sub-Saharan African contexts, where MCH services exist but do not yet include newborn interventions. We will cost packages, because packages are more cost-effective than single interventions, and the emphasis is on the packages described for universal scale-up (table 27.3). The benefits take into account only neonatal deaths averted, whereas many of the interventions will also reduce maternal deaths, stillbirths, and childhood morbidity and disability—and therefore the benefits underestimate gains for both the fourth and the fifth MDGs.

Costing and impact simulations are provided using the "marginal budgeting for bottlenecks" tool, a prioritization tool developed by the United Nations Children's Fund (UNICEF), the World Bank, and WHO. The inputs for the analysis presented here are as follows:

- *Baseline epidemiology* uses NMRs from the latest demographic and health surveys by country or state and recent local relevant demographic data, such as crude birth rates.
- *Cause-specific neonatal mortality estimates* by country are from the Child Health Epidemiology Reference Group's

neonatal estimates by country (Lawn, Cousens, and Wilczynska forthcoming).

- *Baseline coverage estimates* for the neonatal packages presented in table 27.3 are taken from local data, if available (for example, exclusive breastfeeding prevalence), or drawn from coverage estimates in the *Lancet* newborn series (Darmstadt and others 2005; Knippenberg and others 2005; Lawn, Cousens, and Zupan 2005).
- *Impact estimates* for neonatal mortality are from the literature, as presented in this chapter. The range uses the 95 percent confidence interval, rounded to the nearest 5 percent where available (table 27.3). If the data were from an efficacy trial or a before-and-after trial, the range in the literature was reduced to reflect the expected effectiveness, based on expert opinion. Cause-specific mortality was used to allow combinations of effects across packages, and the assumptions applied were aligned with those used in the *Lancet* neonatal series (Darmstadt and others 2005)—although the packages here differ, because this chapter is restricted to the neonatal period. The assumptions for cause-specific impact are detailed at http://www.fic.nih.gov/dcpp. The effect for outcomes other than neonatal ones was based on data in the marginal budgeting for bottlenecks tool, primarily from the *Lancet* Bellagio series (Jones and others 2003) and Cochrane reviews. Effects are combined in a residual manner; for example, deaths averted by preventive strategies are removed from the pool before curative approaches are applied, and hence the total effect is less than the sum of the effects. Years of life lost were calculated using local average life expectancy discounted at 3 percent per year. This measure equates to the fatal outcome component of disability-adjusted life years, as described in chapter 15.
- *Specific costs of adding the intervention packages* are calculated on the basis of the cadre of worker, additional personnel time, in-service training, supervision, performance incentives, travel and subsistence costs for referral care, drugs, and equipment. Demand promotion and community mobilization are included. The costs of time, training, and incentives are based on national salary levels, using real country data or World Bank databases. The costs of commodities are based on the UNICEF supply system (http://www.supply.unicef.dk/Catalogue/). The cost of strengthening health systems, including improving management and logistics, constructing new facilities, and deploying and training new cadres of workers, is included in the comprehensive MCH package.

Table 27.4 presents the estimated NMR effects and per capita costs, in selected Indian states and Sub-Saharan African countries, of strengthening health systems to increase coverage with existing MCH packages (without neonatal care after birth). It then presents the additional specific costs of including

Table 27.4 Estimated Marginal Effect and Cost of Adding Neonatal Packages to Existing MCH Packages for Three Scenarios in Selected Indian States and Sub-Saharan African Countries

| Package | NMR reduction 2004–15 (range of lower and upper efficacy, percent) | | | | Cost per capita (US$) | | | | Additional cost per neonatal YLL averted for 20 percent increase in coverage for lower and upper efficacy ranges (US$) | |
| | India[a] | | Sub-Saharan Africa[b] | | India[a] | | Sub-Saharan Africa[b] | | India[a] | Sub-Saharan Africa[b] |
	Scenario 1	Scenario 2	Scenario 1	Scenario 2	Scenario 1	Scenario 2	Scenario 1	Scenario 2		
MCH package (no neonatal care after birth)[c]	12–12	27–27	11–11	24–24	2.00	4.80	2.40	5.10	480	506
Marginal impact or cost of adding neonatal packages to the MCH package										
Family-community package[d]	3–8	5–15	2–6	6–14	0.30	0.60	0.23	0.37	100–257	100–270
Clinical packages[e]	0–9	0–22	1–9	3–22	0.04	0.10	0.11	0.23	11–265	25–360
Total impact or cost with combined MCH and neonatal-specific packages	13–26	27–58	11–23	24–46	2.40	5.50	2.80	5.70	244–516 (average 380)	282–583 (average 432)

Source: Estimates by authors, using the "marginal budgeting for bottlenecks" tool as detailed in the text.

YLL = years of life lost. YLL includes neonatal fatal outcomes only and is based on local life expectancy discounted at 3 percent per year.

Scenario 1: increasing coverage by 20 percent.

Scenario 2: meeting fourth MDG, necessitating about 45–60 percent NMR reduction, depending on the percentage of under-five mortality that is neonatal.

Note: No specific neonatal outreach package is shown, because this is in prenatal care as part of the MCH package or home postnatal visits in the family-community package

a. Five states in India are represented: Gujarat, Madhya Pradesh, Orissa, Rajasthan, and West Bengal.

b. Five countries in Sub-Saharan Africa are represented: Benin, Ethiopia, Madagascar, Mali, and Rwanda.

c. The MCH package consists of family planning, prenatal and obstetric care, and child health services (comprehensive integrated management of infant and childhood illness including prevention and community activities) and includes system strengthening costs.

d. Includes interventions listed in table 27.3 under family-community package plus extra care of moderately small babies at home and community-based management of acute respiratory infections.

e. Includes clinical care packages listed in table 27.3 (essential newborn care, neonatal resuscitation, extra care of small newborns, and emergency care of ill newborns).

neonatal packages at the family-community level and in clinical services and, finally, the combined costs for comprehensive MNCH. Results are shown for two coverage scenarios:

- *Scenario 1:* increasing coverage of the interventions by 20 percent from the baseline
- *Scenario 2:* increasing coverage to the level required to meet the fourth MDG, necessitating about a 45 to 60 percent reduction in NMR, depending on the baseline percentage of under-five mortality that is neonatal.

Table 27.4 shows that the addition of neonatal packages will reduce neonatal deaths at an average cost of about US$0.50 per capita per year for up to a 15 percent reduction in NMR at the family-community level and about US$0.20 per capita for a 22 percent NMR reduction at the clinical care level. Although the cost per capita is low for clinical care, the cost per case treated is higher, and the lag time to scale up is longer. The family-community neonatal package in India is estimated to cost US$100 to US$257 per year of life saved (table 27.4), which corresponds to about US$2,800 to US$7,800 per death averted. That is similar to the results of US$3,442 per neonatal death averted or US$111 per life year saved in a community participatory package in Nepal (US$4,397 and US$142, respectively, with health system strengthening) (Manandhar and others 2004).

The comprehensive MNCH package (the MCH package plus integrated neonatal packages) is more expensive than the neonatal packages alone: US$2.40 to US$2.80 per capita and per year for a 20 percent increase in coverage, and US$5.50 to US$5.70 to achieve the mortality reduction necessary to meet the fourth MDG (including the health system strengthening and demand-side approaches required). However, the effect of the MNCH packages on the NMR is more than double that of the neonatal packages alone—for example, a reduction of up to 58 percent in NMRs in Africa, compared with up to 22 percent using interventions in the neonatal period only. This finding emphasizes the advantages of a comprehensive approach across the continuum of care. Hence, the average cost per year of life saved is still low at US$380 (India) and US$432 (Sub-Saharan Africa) for a 20 percent increase in coverage, including costs of system strengthening. If the coverage of the MCH plus neonatal packages were to reach 90 percent, those packages would avert up to 71 percent of neonatal deaths in the African countries and up to 76 percent in the Indian states.

In settings where the current coverage of skilled care is low, opportunities exist to start with family care and extra care of LBW babies while building toward more challenging clinical packages. Some clinical care packages—such as simple extra care of the small baby or the provision of oral antibiotics for pneumonia later in the neonatal period—can be adapted for delivery through community health systems. Varying the cadres of worker involved or the level of health system at which

the package is delivered may reduce the cost of the package, but it also necessitates extra supervision and attention to links with the formal health system. Box 27.2 describes the projected effect and cost of various packages in Ethiopia for a 12-year program to improve maternal and child survival targeted at achieving the fourth MDG by 2015. Outreach services such as prenatal care alone have an effect of about 10 percent on NMRs, but when they are combined with a family package using community health promoters, an additional 30 percent reduction in the NMR is projected in Ethiopia.

Outreach and family care options are more feasible initially. Yet if commitment toward moving to strengthen the clinical care system is lacking, the potential reduction in NMRs over time from those options is limited, and the cost per death averted is higher. Although the estimated cost (averaged over 12 years, with gradually increasing amounts) is low, the input is higher than the current government and donor health expenditure of the countries examined. Thus, spending in India would have to be doubled, and in some African countries probably tripled. Considerable new funding is required at the national and international levels, as well as more efficient allocation and absorption of existing funds (Martines and others 2005).

IMPLEMENTATION

Effective interventions exist and are low cost, especially when added to existing programs, but current coverage is low, especially for the poor, who have the highest mortality risk. Approximately 53 percent of women worldwide deliver with a skilled attendant: fewer than 30 percent in the poorest countries and more than 98 percent in the richest countries. In Sub-Saharan Africa, average coverage with skilled care has increased at only 0.2 percent per year in the past decade; without faster progress, coverage of skilled attendance will still be less than 50 percent in 2015. Analysis in 50 low-income countries showed that the richest 20 percent of women were, on average, almost five times as likely to use a skilled attendant as the poorest 20 percent (Knippenberg and others 2005). Hence, coverage is low, progress is slow, and inequity is high.

Each country or decision-making unit starts with a different epidemiology and varying coverage and capacity in its health system. No single recipe for strengthening newborn care in health systems is available. Scaling up MNCH care will involve systematic steps to assess local situations and opportunities, improve care within current constraints, and overcome supply and demand constraints—especially for the poor. No country or program can achieve multiple new interventions at once, and scaling up human resources takes time. Therefore, phasing approaches is essential not only to allow faster approaches to reach the poor soon, but also to allow consistent strengthening of the health system (Knippenberg and others 2005).

Steps to Increase Coverage of Key MNCH Interventions in Ethiopia

Ethiopia is one of the poorest countries in the world, with gross national income of US$100 (in 2000), less than half the average for Sub-Saharan Africa. Neonatal deaths of some 135,000 a year account for 29 percent of child deaths. According to a 2000 demographics and health survey, coverage of care is extremely low: only 6 percent of women deliver with a skilled attendant present and only 8 percent receive postnatal care within 48 hours of delivery. The poor and those in rural areas have even lower coverage. Health professionals are in short supply. At the same time, obstetric services may be unused even when accessible because of issues of affordability and acceptability (most health workers are male).

In 2004, the government and major stakeholders held a national partnership conference to develop a national plan for scaling up child survival interventions. The government decided on a health extension package that would deploy two female health extension workers to each *kebele* (commune of 5,000 inhabitants). Those workers are mainly responsible for MNCH interventions, such as immunization, micronutrient supplementation, and family planning, but they also have other public health and some clinical responsibilities. In addition, one primary

school graduate per 50 families will be trained to promote healthy family behaviors.

Estimates based on the marginal budgeting for bottlenecks tool suggest that, during the first eight years, progressive scaling up of the health extension and health promoters packages, together with some upgrading of clinical services, will cost an additional US$4 per person per year. That effort could result in a 30 percent reduction in the NMR, attributable mostly to improved behaviors, such as clean delivery and exclusive breastfeeding, and to increased demand for care. Increased coverage with family planning and tetanus toxoid vaccination through the health extension package accounts for about 10 percent of the NMR reduction. By the end of the 12-year period, an additional 30 percent reduction in NMR is expected from strengthening clinical services. A comprehensive package of family-based, outreach, and clinical services is projected to reduce the NMR by nearly 50 percent, associated with a 25 percent reduction in the maternal mortality ratio—as compared with a less than 5 percent reduction in the maternal mortality ratio with family and outreach care alone. The incremental annual cost of almost US$10 per person is more than three times current public spending on health of US$2.70.

Source: Knippenberg and others 2005.

Step 1: Assess the Situation and Advocate for Action for Newborn Health

Careful examination of local data is required (Lawn, McCarthy, and Ross 2001). Newborn health should be included in general health sector and public sector planning—for instance, for education and transportation. When governments set mortality reduction targets for children under five, they should consider setting simultaneous targets for reducing NMRs (Martines and others 2005). The level of participation—involving multiple stakeholders, including women and communities—and the political will to implement and finance such plans are also crucial to success. Reaching every pregnant woman and every newborn with effective care involves everyone: the family and community provide home care and advocate for access to preventive and curative care; the health system supplies care during normal pregnancy, childbirth, and postnatal care, along with emergency obstetric and young infant care services if required; and the government and global policy makers provide supportive policy and resources, in particular to ensure that there are enough health care providers, such as

midwives. National champions can be effective in promoting progress. Global partnerships may also play a role in facilitating broad national plans and promoting donor convergence in implementation (Tinker and others 2005).

The government of Nepal recently held a series of stakeholder meetings and developed a plan for a national newborn health strategy. Representatives from such diverse backgrounds as neonatology, safe motherhood programs, and community mobilization efforts met over a five-month period to create an operational plan for newborn care through 2017 (Khadka, Moore, and Vikery 2003).

Step 2: Achieve Optimal Newborn Care within the Constraints of the Current Health System

Because situations vary even within countries, data-driven prioritization and good leadership are crucial to using resources well (Lawn, McCarthy, and Ross 2001). Program areas related to newborn health include safe motherhood, child survival, immunization, family planning, and nutrition, along with management of sexually transmitted diseases, prevention of

Adding Newborns to IMCI in India

An estimated 1.1 million neonatal deaths occur annually in India—approximately 28 percent of the world's total. Between 1960 and 1990, India achieved a 50 percent reduction in infant mortality, but in the 1990s, the decline in the infant mortality rate slowed, partially because of the increasing proportion of infant deaths during the neonatal period. The government looked for ways to add to existing programs and to increase coverage of services, especially given that most neonatal deaths occur in the first few days of life in home settings.

Two major adaptations have been made to the standard IMCI approach:

- Integrated management of neonatal illness was introduced into the global generic guidelines for IMCI, which do not cover illness in the first week of life.
- Focus on outreach services and family care, taking the program into communities to achieve higher coverage, is being promoted through a variety of strategies, namely:
  — three home visits in 10 days for normal weight babies, with a further three in the subsequent three

weeks if the infant is LBW, to provide essential newborn care, extra care of the LBW infant, and early identification and referral for sepsis
  — improved coordination between auxiliary nurse-midwives and community health workers to assist with the integration of health and nutrition services at household levels.

The marginal cost of adding N (for neonatal) into IMCI in relation to clinical care is estimated at less than US$0.10 per person, given the existence of traditional IMCI programs. Training the health and nutrition workers (2 per 1,000 population) and providing home visits is estimated to cost US$0.22 per person. In 2002, the government began to test the integrated management package in 50 districts of United Nations Children's Fund areas of programming. This initiative has prompted policy makers to scale up implementation throughout the country during the 2005–10 phase of its Reproductive and Child Health Program.

Source: Adapted from K. Suresh, M. Babille, and V. K. Paul, personal communication, April 2004.

maternal-child transmission of HIV, and prevention of malaria during pregnancy. The reality is that such interventions have not reached most women and children and that existing services fail to coordinate along the continuum of care. This situation results in gaps in service and missed opportunities. In Africa, for example, the regional average for prenatal care coverage is 64 percent, yet coverage of tetanus toxoid immunization is 42 percent (Knippenberg and others 2005). Syphilis treatment is another opportunity that frequently is missed during prenatal care (Gloyd, Chai, and Mercer 2001). Including the newborn in transport and funding programs that currently address only maternal emergencies may be of little marginal cost for significant benefit. In India, where integrated management of infant and childhood illness (IMCI) is being scaled up, the marginal cost of adding selected neonatal conditions to the clinical care component of IMCI is low, estimated at less than US$0.10 per capita (box 27.3).

In many settings in South Asia and Sub-Saharan Africa, even where midwives are in place they do not have the skills required for newborn care. Competency-based training in neonatal resuscitation is a rarity and must be incorporated into preservice as well as in-service training (box 27.1). India's National Neonatology Forum identified birth asphyxia as a leading

cause of neonatal deaths and launched the Neonatal Resuscitation Program, developing a course with standard guidelines and certification of competency (Deorari and others 2001). Between 1990 and 1992, more than 12,000 physicians and nurses were trained. The effect of the program was evaluated in 14 teaching hospitals in India. Changes in resuscitation practices were noted, and asphyxia-related mortality fell significantly. The prevalence of survivors with disabilities was not assessed.

An alternative model of skill strengthening has been tested in South Africa, where significant improvements in knowledge and skills have been documented as a result of the Perinatal Education Programme, a distance-run self-taught course (Woods and Theron 1995). More than 30,000 midwives in South Africa have passed the examinations, and the program's manuals are used in many undergraduate medical and nursing schools.

Numerous publications have detailed suboptimal hospital management of women in labor or newborns, variously reported as contributing to 10 to 75 percent of all perinatal deaths (Lawn and Darmstadt forthcoming). Thus, there is scope for improving outcomes and client satisfaction in virtually all settings. For example, in much of Sub-Saharan Africa, a

South Africa and the Perinatal Problem Identification Programme: Locally Owned Data for Decision Making

Care for pregnant women and newborns in South Africa ranges from unattended childbirth in rural mud huts to advanced obstetric and intensive neonatal care. National perinatal mortality is estimated at 40 per 1,000 live births, with regional and racial disparities. During the 1990s, growing awareness of the importance and preventability of newborn deaths resulted in the development of the Perinatal Problem Identification Programme. Under the program, basic data are entered into a computer program that calculates perinatal mortality, supporting the identification of avoidable factors to aid the prioritization of actions to address key problems. More than 44 sites across the country use the Perinatal Problem Identification Programme, covering almost 80,000 births annually, or approximately 10 percent of deliveries, with 3,045 perinatal deaths (2000). Avoidable factors were identified in 83 percent of deaths, with half of these being patient related, such as a delayed response to complications. A

further 14 percent of avoidable factors were administrative and, in particular, were related to transportation and lack of staff members. About 25 percent of the avoidable factors involving health workers pertained to intrapartum care, especially poor monitoring (not using the partograph) and inadequate response to problems identified during labor. Half of the cesarean sections were delayed by an hour or more.

The program identified the following national priorities to reduce perinatal deaths:

- reducing intrapartum asphyxia, especially in rural areas—for instance, using maternity waiting homes and addressing transport delays
- improving intrapartum management by means of protocols (partograph and effective monitoring), competency-based training, and ongoing audit
- implementing syphilis screening and treatment more effectively.

Source: Authors, based on data from Pattinson 2002.

---

significant proportion of women deliver in facilities that collect data that could be used to identify achievable improvements in care (box 27.4).

Step 3: Phase the Systematic Scaling-Up of Newborn Care

Although some resource-poor countries have succeeded in building functional systems (box 27.5), the process, especially for clinical care, takes time. Professional care during childbirth and childhood illnesses is the ideal, but significant costs are involved in increasing the numbers of professionals and retaining them, especially in rural posts. Even maintaining current staff presents challenges, given low pay and high frustration. To markedly increase coverage requires new commitment now to a massive expansion in the number of midwives and to innovative approaches to retain staff, especially in hard-to-serve areas. Supply constraints must be systematically identified and targeted—notably, human resources, accessibility to facilities, financial barriers, and supply of commodities and drugs (Knippenberg and others 2005). Demand-side strategies are also important, including consideration of subsidies for preventive care or transport for emergency care.

In the meantime, most neonatal deaths continue to occur in underserved and poor communities that will wait the longest for access to skilled care. Each year, 60 million women deliver without skilled care present. There is a moral imperative to

reach those women now. Feasible strategies to reduce NMRs exist (for example, efforts to improve family behaviors, tetanus toxoid immunization campaigns, and community-based management of acute respiratory infections) and have been demonstrated in poorly developed health care systems. Interim strategies are available, such as linking a group of traditional birth attendants with skilled attendants (Koblinsky, Campbell, and Heichelheim 1999) or medical assistants to perform cesarean sections. Policy conflicts between skilled and community approaches are not helpful. Both approaches are required. With phased program planning, community services can be used now while professional care is being strengthened. The community services can then promote demand for skilled care (Knippenberg and others 2005).

Step 4: Monitor Coverage and Measure Effect and Cost

In most high-mortality countries, NMRs are measured only intermittently (typically every five years through demographic and health surveys). Tracking of coverage indicators, and especially equity of coverage, is important for managing program decision making. Information is lacking, and the information that is available is often not used to improve care. Governments must be encouraged to report funding, coverage, and outcomes related to national plans for maternal, neonatal, and child survival. Donors should also be accountable for reporting funding flows and ensuring that commitments are kept (Martines and others 2005).

RESEARCH PRIORITIES

The overwhelming priority in newborn health research remains how to reach underserved populations. This effort involves demonstrating the effect, cost, and scaling up process for packages of interventions. The processes of adapting effective packages to different settings using various cadres of health workers and of identifying indicators of successful implementation that are replicable are all basic to scaling up yet have been little studied. Costing of newborn health interventions is a major gap. Virtually no published examinations of the marginal benefits and costs of adding neonatal interventions to existing programs aimed at safe motherhood, IMCI, HIV/AIDS, malaria, and sexually transmitted diseases are available. A demonstration of such synergies will help influence policy makers to incorporate neonatal issues into these and other programs. Testing innovative approaches to protect poor families from user costs is also important.

Given that preterm birth accounts for almost 30 percent of neonatal deaths and contributes indirectly to many more deaths, reducing the incidence of preterm birth and decreasing deaths among preterm infants are important areas for study. Low-tech extra care of small babies has the potential to reduce deaths significantly, but the effectiveness of various home and facility packages, including the potential of emollients for preventing infections, needs to be tested. A large industry is developing high-tech devices for newborn care to address the 2 percent of neonatal deaths in rich countries. Yet there is little investment in the development and testing of low-cost, simple, robust devices in the settings where most fetal and neonatal deaths occur.

Understanding is lacking of the effects of maternal infections, particularly of synergies between HIV, malaria, and sexually transmitted diseases (Ticconi and others 2003) as well as the potential synergy between maternal infections and apparent asphyxial injury to neonates (Peebles and Wyatt 2002).

Incidence and intervention data regarding neonatal morbidity and disability at the population level are entirely lacking in LMICs. Improved tools for assessing cause-specific mortality and morbidity outcomes are required to advance answers to many of these questions (Lawn, Cousens, and Wilczynska forthcoming).

CONCLUSIONS

Reductions in neonatal mortality are necessary to meet the fourth MDG. High-impact, low-cost, feasible interventions are available. They could avert approximately 70 percent of the world's 4 million neonatal deaths, according to analysis presented here, an estimate similar to the estimates in the *Lancet* neonatal series (Darmstadt and others 2005). Large gains in neonatal survival are linked to other health gains, such as reduced childhood morbidity and disability, prevention of stillbirths, and improved maternal survival, thus contributing also to the achievement of the fifth MDG.

The success of some low-income countries is encouraging, but in South Asia and Sub-Saharan Africa, coverage is generally low, progress is slow, and inequity is high. While countries continue to move toward a more comprehensive health care system, simpler approaches at family-community level and through outreach services can save many lives now, even in the poorest settings. Well-known interventions, such as neonatal resuscitation and case management of infections, can be added to other programs, particularly safe motherhood and IMCI programs, at low marginal cost. However, to reach the MDGs, skilled care is required. Scaling up coverage to ensure professional midwives reach those in underserved areas will require major new investment to generate and retain more skilled staff members, along with the necessary supportive infrastructure. This investment will involve increased spending, which—as shown here—may double current national health expenditures per capita in Asia and triple them in many African countries. Even if poor countries spend more and spend better, outside funding will be required.

Current investment in MNCH by most national governments and international donors is utterly inadequate compared with investment in conditions that have higher profiles yet lower mortality rates. The deaths of 10,000 newborns each day are unconscionable when most could be saved now at relatively low cost if the political will to do so existed.

ACKNOWLEDGMENTS

The following individuals are gratefully acknowledged for reviewing this chapter: Gary Darmstadt, Affette Mccaw-Binns, Barbara Stoll, and Anne Tinker. We thank Saving Newborn Lives, especially Julia Ruben, for editing assistance.

Joy E. Lawn was supported by the Bill & Melinda Gates Foundation through a grant to Save the Children/USA for the Saving Newborn Lives initiative.

REFERENCES

Bang, A. T., R. A. Bang, S. B. Baitule, M. H. Reddy, and M. D. Deshmukh. 1999. "Effect of Home-Based Neonatal Care and Management of Sepsis on Neonatal Mortality: Field Trial in Rural India." *Lancet* 354 (9194): 1955–61.

Bhutta, Z., G. L. Darmstadt, B. Hasan, and R. Haws. 2005. "Community-Based Interventions for Improving Perinatal and Neonatal Outcomes in Developing Countries: A Review of the Evidence." *Pediatrics* 115 (2): 520–603.

Blanc, A., and T. Wardlow. 2005. "Monitoring Low Birth Weight: An Evaluation of International Estimates and an Updated Estimation Procedure." *Bulletin of the World Health Organization* 83 (3): 178–85.

Conde-Agudelo, A., J. L. Diaz-Rossello, and J. M. Belizan. 2000. "Kangaroo Mother Care to Reduce Morbidity and Mortality in Low Birthweight Infants." *Cochrane Database of Systematic Reviews* (2) CD00277 [PMID:].

Daga, S. R., A. S. Daga, S. Patole, S. Kadam, and Y. Mukadam. 1988. "Foot Length Measurement from Foot Print for Identifying a Newborn at Risk." *Journal of Tropical Pediatrics* 34 (1): 16–19.

Darmstadt, G. L., Z. A. Bhutta, S. N. Cousens, T. Adam, L. de Bernis, and N. Walker. 2005. "Evidence-Based, Cost-Effective Interventions That Matter: How Many Newborns Can We Save and at What Cost?" *Lancet* 365 (9463): 977–88.

Datta, N. 1985. "A Study of Health Problems of Low Birth Weight Babies in a Rural Community and the Feasibility of Intervention Package Likely to Improve Their Health Status." Ph.D. dissertation, Postgraduate Institute of Medical Education and Research, Chandrigarh, India.

Deorari, A. K., V. K. Paul, M. Singh, and D. Vidyasagar. 2001. "Impact of Education and Training on Neonatal Resuscitation Practices in 14 Teaching Hospitals in India." *Annals of Tropical Paediatrics* 21 (1): 29–33.

Dragovich, D., G. Tamburlini, A. Alisjahbana, R. Kambarami, J. Karagulova, O. Lincetto, and others. 1997. "Thermal Control of the Newborn: Knowledge and Practice of Health Professionals in Seven Countries." *Acta Paediatrica* 86 (6): 645–50.

Dujardin, B., H. Sene, and F. Ndiaye. 1992. "Value of the Alert and Action Lines on the Partogram." *Lancet* 339 (8805): 1336–38.

Duke, T., L. Willie, and J. M. Mgone. 2000. "The Effect of Introduction of Minimal Standards of Neonatal Care on In-Hospital Mortality." *Papua New Guinea Medical Journal* 43 (1–2): 127–36.

Ellis, M., N. Manandhar, P. S. Shrestha, L. Shrestha, D. S. Manandhar, and A. M. Costello. 1999. "Outcome at One Year of Neonatal Encephalopathy in Kathmandu, Nepal." *Developmental Medicine and Child Neurology* 41 (10): 689–95.

Gloyd, S., S. Chai, and M. A. Mercer. 2001. "Antenatal Syphilis in Sub-Saharan Africa: Missed Opportunities for Mortality Reduction." *Health Policy and Planning* 16 (1): 29–34.

Greenwood, A. M., B. M. Greenwood, A. K. Bradley, K. Williams, F. C. Shenton, S. Tulloch, and others. 1987. "A Prospective Survey of the Outcome of Pregnancy in a Rural Area of The Gambia." *Bulletin of the World Health Organization* 65 (5): 635–43.

Institute of Medicine. 2003. *Improving Birth Outcomes: Meeting the Challenge of the Developing World.* Washington, DC: National Institutes of Science.

Jamison, D. T., S. Shahid-Salles, J. S. Jamison, J. Lawn, and J. Zupan. 2006. "Incorporating Deaths Near the Time of Birth into Estimates of the Global Burden of Disease." In *Global Burden of Disease and Risk Factors*, eds. Alan Lopez, Colin Mathers, Majid Ezzati, Dean Jamison, and Christopher Murray. New York: Oxford University Press.

Jones, G., R. W. Steketee, R. E. Black, Z. A Bhutta, and S. S. Morris. 2003. "How Many Child Deaths Can We Prevent this Year?" *Lancet* 362 (9377): 65–71.

Khadka, N., J. Moore, and C. Vikery. 2003. "Nepal's Neonatal Health Strategy: A Policy Framework for Program Development." In *Shaping Policy for Maternal and Neonatal Health: A Compendium of Case Studies*, ed. S. Crump, 47–52. Washington, DC: JHPIEGO. http://www.mnh.jhpiego.org/resources/shapepolicy.asp.

Knippenberg, R., J. E. Lawn, G. L. Darmstadt, G. Bekyorian, H. Fogstadt, N. Waleign, and V. Paul. 2005. "Systematically Scaling Up Newborn Care in Countries." Neonatal Series Paper 3. *Lancet* 365: 1087–98.

Koblinsky, M. A., ed. 2003. *Reducing Maternal Mortality: Learning from Bolivia, China, Egypt, Honduras, Indonesia, Jamaica, and Zimbabwe.* Washington, DC: World Bank. http://www-wds.worldbank.org/servlet/WDSContentServer/WDSP/IB/2003/06/06/000094946_030528 0402518/Rendered/PDF/multi0page.pdf.

Koblinsky, M. A., O. Campbell, and J. Heichelheim. 1999. "Organizing Delivery Care: What Works for Safe Motherhood?" *Bulletin of the World Health Organization* 77 (5): 399–406.

Kumar, R. 1995. "Birth Asphyxia in a Rural Community of North India." *Journal of Tropical Pediatrics* 41 (1): 5–7.

Lawn, J. E., S. N. Cousens, and K. Wilczynska. Forthcoming. *Estimating the Cause of Death for 4 Million Neonates in the Year 2000.*

Lawn, J. E., S. N. Cousens, and J. Zupan. 2005. "Four Million Neonatal Deaths: When? Where? Why?" Neonatal Series Paper 1. *Lancet* 365 (9462): 891–900.

Lawn, J. E., and G. L. Darmstadt. Forthcoming. "A Review of Strategies to Address Birth Asphyxia Especially for the Poor." *Journal of Perinatology* (Suppl.).

Lawn, J. E., B. McCarthy, and S. R. Ross. 2001. *The Healthy Newborn: A Reference Guide for Program Managers.* Atlanta: Centers for Disease

Control and Prevention and CARE. http://www.cdc.gov/reproductive-health/health_newborn.htm.

Lumbiganon, P., M. Panamonta, M. Laopaiboon, S. Pothinam, and N. Patithat. 1990. "Why Are Thai Official Perinatal and Infant Mortality Rates So Low?" *International Journal of Epidemiology* 19 (4): 997–1000.

Manandhar, D. S., D. Osrin, B. P. Shrestha, N. Mesko, J. Morrison, K. M. Tumbahangphe, and others. 2004. "Effect of a Participatory Intervention with Women's Groups on Birth Outcomes in Nepal: Cluster-Randomised Controlled Trial." *Lancet* 364 (9438): 970–79.

Martines, J., V. K. Paul, Z. A. Bhutta, M. Koblinsky, A. Soucat, N. Walker, and others. 2005. "Increasing Newborn Survival: A Call to Action." *Lancet* 365 (9465): 1189–97.

Massawe, A., C. Kilewo, S. Irani, R. J. Verma, A. B. Chakrapam, T. Ribbe, and others. 1996. "Assessment of Mouth-to-Mask Ventilation in Resuscitation of Asphyctic Newborn Babies: A Pilot Study." *Tropical Medicine and International Health* 1 (6): 865–73.

Mathers C. D., C. J. L. Murray, and A. D. Lopez. 2006. "The Burden of Disease and Mortality by Condition: Data, Methods and Results for the Year 2001." In *Global Burden of Disease and Risk Factors*, eds. Alan Lopez, Colin Mathers, Majid Ezzati, Dean Jamison, and Christopher Murray. New York: Oxford University Press.

Meegan, M. E., R. M. Conroy, S. O. Lengeny, K. Renhault, and J. Nyangole. 2001. "Effect on Neonatal Tetanus Mortality after a Culturally-Based Health Promotion Programme." *Lancet* 358 (9284): 640–41.

O'Rourke, K., L. Howard-Grabman, and G. Seoane. 1998. "Impact of Community Organization of Women on Perinatal Outcomes in Rural Bolivia." *Revista Panamericana de Salud Pública* 3: 9–14.

Pattinson, R. C., ed. 2002. *Saving Babies 2001: Second Perinatal Care Survey of South Africa*. Pretoria: MRC Unit for Maternal and Infant Health Care Strategies.

Peebles, D. M., and J. S. Wyatt. 2002. "Synergy between Antenatal Exposure to Infection and Intrapartum Events in Causation of Perinatal Brain Injury at Term." *British Journal of Obstetrics and Gynaecology* 109 (7): 737–39.

Peterson, S., J. Nsungwa-Sabiiti, W. Were, X. Nsabagasani, G. Magumba, J. Nambooze, and G. Mukasa. 2004. "Coping with Paediatric Referral—Ugandan Parents' Experience." *Lancet* 363 (9425): 1955–56.

Pojda, J., and L. M. Kelley, eds. 2000. *Low Birth Weight: Report of a Meeting in Dhaka, Bangladesh, 14–17 June 1999*. Nutrition Policy Paper 18. Geneva: United Nations Subcommittee on Nutrition.

Pratinidhi, A., U. Shah, A. Shrotri, and N. Bodhani. 1986. "Risk-Approach Strategy in Neonatal Care." *Bulletin of the World Health Organization* 64: 291–97.

Saugstad, O. D. 2001. "Resuscitation of Newborn Infants with Room Air or Oxygen." *Seminars in Neonatology* 6 (3): 233–39.

Sazawal, S., and R. E. Black. 2003. "Effect of Pneumonia Case Management on Mortality in Neonates, Infants, and Preschool Children: A Meta-analysis of Community-Based Trials." *Lancet Infectious Diseases* 3 (9): 547–56.

Thaddeus, S., and D. Maine. 1994. "Too Far to Walk: Maternal Mortality in Context." *Social Science and Medicine* 38 (8): 1091–110.

Ticconi, C., M. Mapfumo, M. Dorrucci, N. Naha, E. Tarira, A. Pietropolli, and others. 2003. "Effect of Maternal HIV and Malaria Infection on Pregnancy and Perinatal Outcome in Zimbabwe." *Journal of Acquired Immune Deficiency Syndrome* 34 (3): 289–94.

Tinker A., P. ten Hoope-Bender, S. Azfar, F. Bustreo, and R. Bell. 2005. "A Continuum of Care to Save Newborn Lives." *Lancet* 365 (9462): 822–52.

WHO (World Health Organization). 1998a. *Basic Newborn Resuscitation: Practical Guide*. WHO/RHT/MSM/98.1, 1–32. Geneva: WHO.

———. 1998b. *Evidence for the Ten Steps to Successful Breastfeeding*. WHO/CHD/98.9, 1–118. Geneva: WHO.

———. 2003a. *Global Burden of Disease, 2000*. Version c. Geneva: WHO.

———. 2003b. *Pregnancy, Childbirth, Postpartum, and Newborn Care: A Guide for Essential Practice*. Geneva: WHO.

———. 2003c. *Working with Individuals, Families, and Communities*. Geneva: WHO.

———. Forthcoming. *Neonatal and Perinatal Mortality, Estimates for 2000*. Geneva: WHO.

WHO (World Health Organization) Collaborative Group. 2000. "Effect of Breastfeeding on Infant and Child Mortality Due to Infectious Diseases in Less Developed Countries: A Pooled Analysis." *Lancet* 355: 451–55.

Woods, D. L., and G. B. Theron. 1995. "The Impact of the Perinatal Education Programme on Cognitive Knowledge in Midwives." *South African Medical Journal* 85 (3): 150–53.

Yasmin, S., D. Osrin, E. Paul, and A. Costello. 2001. "Neonatal Mortality of Low-Birth-Weight Infants in Bangladesh." *Bulletin of the World Health Organization* 79 (7): 608–14.

Zhu, X. Y., H. Q. Fang, S. P. Zeng, Y. M. Li, H. L. Lin, and S. Z. Shi. 1997. "The Impact of the Neonatal Resuscitation Program Guidelines (NRPG) on the Neonatal Mortality in a Hospital in Zhuhai, China." *Singapore Medical Journal* 38 (11): 485–87.

Zupan, J., and P. Garner. 2000. "Topical Umbilical Cord Care at Birth." *Cochrane Database of Systematic Reviews* (3) CD001057 [DOI:10.1002/14651858].

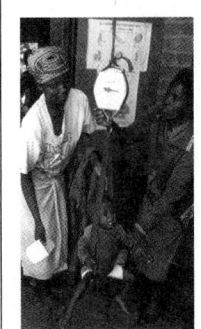

Chapter **28**

Stunting, Wasting, and Micronutrient Deficiency Disorders

Laura E. Caulfield, Stephanie A. Richard, Juan A. Rivera, Philip Musgrove, and Robert E. Black

Undernutrition and micronutrient deficiencies contribute substantially to the global burden of disease (Ezzati and others 2002). Impoverished communities experience high rates of undernutrition and increased exposure to infectious diseases caused by crowding and inadequate sanitation. Women of reproductive age and children experience devastating health consequences as a result of limited resources, cultural influences, and biological vulnerabilities. Undernutrition and infectious diseases exist in a baleful synergy: undernutrition reduces immunological capacity to defend against diseases, and diseases deplete and deprive the body of essential nutrients. Undernutrition and infectious diseases further exacerbate poverty through lost wages, increased health care costs, and—most insidiously—impaired intellectual development that can significantly reduce earning potential. Health experts have recently recognized the long-term effects of early undernutrition and inadequate infant feeding for obesity and chronic diseases, including diabetes and cardiovascular diseases. This chapter summarizes the problems of undernutrition and vitamin A, iron, zinc, and iodine deficiencies in young children and current programmatic efforts to prevent and treat them.

NATURE, CAUSES, AND BURDEN OF UNDERNUTRITION

The following section describes the magnitude, distribution, and etiology of growth faltering and specific micronutrient deficiencies in young children.

Growth Faltering

Because nutritional inputs are necessary for children's growth, undernutrition is generally characterized by comparing the weights or heights (or lengths) of children at a specific age and sex with the distribution of observed weights or heights in a reference population of presumed healthy children of the same age and sex and then calculating z-scores, that is, the difference between a child's weight or height and the median value at that age and sex in the reference population, divided by the standard deviation (SD) of the reference population. A child whose height-for-age is less than -2 SD is considered stunted, because the chances of the child's height being normal are less than 3 percent. A child whose weight-for-age is less than -2 SD is considered underweight, and one whose weight-for-height is less than -2 SD is deemed wasted. *Stunting* results from chronic undernutrition, which retards linear growth, whereas *wasting* results from inadequate nutrition over a shorter period, and *underweight* encompasses both stunting and wasting. Typically, growth faltering begins at about six months of age, as children transition to foods that are often inadequate in quantity and quality, and increased exposure to the environment increases their likelihood of illness.

Although knowledge about the prevalence of stunting and wasting is preferred, information about underweight is more available globally. The high correlation between stunting and underweight and the low prevalence of wasting mean that the prevalence of underweight directly describes the magnitude of the problem of growth faltering and stunting in young children. About 130 million children under the age of five are underweight, with the highest prevalences in South Asia and Sub-Saharan Africa (table 28.1). The prevalence of stunting, underweight, and wasting is decreasing in most areas of the world; however, in most of Africa, stunting is increasing.

Childhood malnutrition diminishes adult intellectual ability and work capacity, causing economic hardships for individuals and their families. Malnourished women tend to deliver premature or small babies who are more likely to die or suffer from suboptimal growth and development (Allen and Gillespie 2001). Poor early nutrition leads to poor school readiness and performance, resulting in fewer years of schooling, reduced productivity, and earlier childbearing. Thus, poverty, undernutrition, and ill-health are passed on from generation to generation. Undernutrition impedes economic progress in all developing countries.

Undernutrition raises the likelihood that a child will become sick and will then die from the disease. Morbidity and mortality are highest among those most severely malnourished; however, given the high prevalence of mild to moderate underweight, the mildly or moderately underweight individuals experience

the greatest total burden of disease (Fishman and others 2004). Children whose weight-for-age is less than −1 SD are also at increased risk of death, and undernutrition is responsible for 44 to 60 percent of the mortality caused by measles, malaria, pneumonia, and diarrhea. Overall, eliminating malnutrition would prevent 53 percent of deaths in young children, with most of those deaths occurring in South Asia and Sub-Saharan Africa (table 28.2).

Morbidity attributable to undernutrition depends on the nature of the illness. Susceptibility to a highly infectious disease such as measles is unlikely to be affected by nutritional status: all individuals are equally likely to become infected if they are unvaccinated and naive. However, 5 to 16 percent of pneumonia, diarrhea, and malaria morbidity is attributable to moderate to severe underweight (Fishman and others 2004). As table 28.3 shows, the number of disability-adjusted life years (DALYs) attributable to undernutrition is high and, as with mortality, is concentrated in South Asia and Sub-Saharan Africa. The tremendous costs associated with the care and treatment of childhood diseases that could be partially

Table 28.1 Estimated Prevalence of Selected Nutritional Deficiencies in Children Ages Birth through Four, by Region *(percent)*

Region	Weight-for-age less than −2 SD	Weight-for-age −2 SD through less than −1 SD	Vitamin A deficiency	Iron deficiency anemia	Zinc deficiency
East Asia and the Pacific	18	29	11	40	7
Eastern Europe and Central Asia	6	21	<1	22	10
Latin America and the Caribbean	6	23	15	46	33
Middle East and North Africa	21	35	18	63	46
South Asia	46	44	40	76	79
Sub-Saharan Africa	32	38	32	60	50
High-income countries	2	14	0	7	5

Sources: Underweight: Fishman and others 2004; vitamin A: Rice, West, and Black 2004; iron: Stoltzfus, Mullany, and Black 2004; zinc: Caulfield and Black 2004.

Table 28.2 Estimated Deaths of Children Ages Birth through Four Attributable to Selected Nutritional Deficiencies by Region *(thousands)*

Region	Weight-for-age less than −1 SD[a]	Vitamin A deficiency	Iron deficiency anemia[b]	Zinc deficiency
East Asia and the Pacific	125	11	18	15
Eastern Europe and Central Asia	14	0	3	4
Latin America and the Caribbean	22	6	10	15
Middle East and North Africa	305	70	10	94
South Asia	870	157	66	252
Sub-Saharan Africa	1,334	383	21	400
High-income countries	0	0	6	0

Sources: Underweight: Fishman and others 2004; vitamin A: Rice, West, and Black 2004; iron: Stoltzfus, Mullany, and Black 2004; zinc: Caulfield and Black 2004.
a. In high-income countries, the percentage of children at each weight-for-age criterion are those expected in a healthy population.
b. Considers only deaths directly attributable to iron deficiency anemia in children. Does not include perinatal deaths attributable to maternal iron deficiency anemia.

Table 28.3 Estimated DALYs Lost by Children Ages Birth through Four Attributable to Selected Nutritional Deficiencies by Region *(thousands)*

Region	Weight-for-age less than −1 SD	Vitamin A deficiency	Iron deficiency anemia[a]	Zinc deficiency	Iodine deficiency
East Asia and the Pacific	5,777	994	241	1,004	66
Eastern Europe and Central Asia	489	1	66	149	409
Latin America and the Caribbean	725	218	109	587	83
Middle East and North Africa	10,308	2,403	109	3,290	381
South Asia	27,879	4,761	704	8,510	366
Sub-Saharan Africa	45,131	13,552	596	14,094	748
High-income countries	0	0	40	2	2

Sources: Underweight: Fishman and others 2004; vitamin A: Rice, West, and Black 2004; iron: Stoltzfus, Mullany, and Black 2004; zinc: Caulfield and Black 2004.
a. Only considers DALYs directly attributable to iron deficiency anemia. Not included are DALYs due to perinatal deaths attributable to maternal iron deficiency anemia.

prevented through improvements in child nutrition have not been quantified.

Evidence is accumulating that early malnutrition increases the risk of numerous chronic diseases later (Caballero 2001; Gluckman and Hanson 2004). Associations of early undernutrition with diabetes, hypertension, renal disease, and cardiovascular disease mean that child undernutrition also leads to high adult health care costs.

Vitamin A Deficiency

Vitamin A deficiency (VAD) is a common cause of preventable blindness and a risk factor for increased severity of infectious disease and mortality (Rice, West, and Black 2004). One of the first symptoms of marginal VAD is night blindness. If VAD worsens, additional symptoms of xerophthalmia arise, eventually resulting in blindness. A child who becomes blind from VAD has only a 50 percent chance of surviving the year. Even if children survive, blindness severely diminishes their economic potential. VAD may cause anemia in some regions, but it does not appear to impair children's growth (Ramakrishnan and others 2004).

Increased mortality is associated with VAD, most likely because of the detrimental effects on the immune system, which result in increased severity of illness (Sommer and West 1996). According to Rice, West, and Black (2004), VAD is responsible for almost 630,000 deaths each year from infectious disease (table 28.2), accounting for 20 to 24 percent of the mortality from measles, diarrhea, and malaria (Rice, West, and Black 2004). Attributable fractions are highest where VAD is prevalent and mortality is high. Linking morbidity with VAD is far more difficult. Vitamin A supplementation decreases the severity of diarrhea and complications from measles, but in some trials, supplementation has been associated with increased lower respiratory infections.

VAD results from inadequate intakes of vitamin A because of low intakes of animal foods; inadequate intakes of nonanimal sources of carotenoids that are converted to vitamin A; and

inadequate intakes of fat, which facilitates the absorption of carotenoids. Dietary sources of preformed vitamin A include liver, milk, and egg yolks. Dark green leafy vegetables such as spinach, as well as yellow and orange noncitrus fruits (mangoes, apricots, papayas) and vegetables (pumpkins, squash, carrots), are common sources of carotenoids (vitamin A precursors), which are generally less bioavailable than preformed vitamin A but tend to be more affordable.

Table 28.1 shows recent estimates of the prevalence of VAD in young children (Rice, West, and Black 2004). Of those affected, 250,000 to 500,000 each year will lose their sight as a result. The overall prevalence of VAD is decreasing markedly because of increased awareness of VAD as a public health problem and increased measles immunization and vitamin A supplementation or fortification programs. However, the prevalence of VAD is increasing or is unknown in some regions because of political instability, high rates of infectious disease, and increasing poverty.

Iron Deficiency

More than 2 billion people, mostly women and young children, are thought to be iron deficient (Stoltzfus and Dreyfuss 1998). Iron is found in all plant foods but is more plentiful and bioavailable in meat. Deficiency results from insufficient absorption of iron or excess loss. Absorption is tightly regulated in the intestines, depending on the iron status of the individual, the type of iron, and other nutritional factors. Once iron is absorbed, it is well conserved. Iron is depleted primarily through blood loss, including from parasitic infections such as schistosomiasis and hookworm.

Mainly found in hemoglobin, iron is essential for the binding and transport of oxygen, as well as for the regulation of cell growth and differentiation (Beard 2001). Iron deficiency is the primary cause of anemia, although vitamin A deficiency, folate deficiency, malaria, and HIV also result in anemia. Iron deficiency anemia is most prevalent in South Asia and Sub-Saharan

Africa, but it is not limited to developing countries (table 28.1). Iron deficiency results in neurological impairment, which may not be fully reversible (Grantham-McGregor and Ani 1999). Finally, iron deficiency is known to decrease immune function, but some investigators have also hypothesized that deficiency protects against infectious disease or that iron supplementation increases infectious disease (Caulfield, Richard, and Black 2004). Iron deficiency and anemia do not appear to contribute to growth faltering (Ramakrishnan and others 2004).

Stoltzfus, Mullany, and Black (2004) find that iron deficiency anemia was an underlying factor in 841,000 deaths per year resulting from maternal and perinatal causes, and it directly causes the deaths of 134,000 young children annually (table 28.2). Worldwide, iron deficiency is a substantial contributor to DALY losses (table 28.3).

Iodine Deficiency

Iodine is necessary for the thyroid hormones that regulate growth, development, and metabolism and is essential to prevent goiter and cretinism. Inadequate intake can result in impaired intellectual development and physical growth. A range of impairments resulting from iodine deficiency are referred to as iodine deficiency disorders (IDD) (Hetzel 1983) and can include fetal loss, stillbirth, congenital anomalies, and hearing impairment. The vast majority of deficient individuals experience mild mental retardation. This decrease in mental ability and work capacity may have significant economic consequences. Iodine deficiency has not, however, been associated with the incidence or severity of infectious disease, and studies implicating deficiency as an underlying cause of mortality are limited. Because of this, few child deaths can be attributed to iodine deficiency, but the directly attributable DALY losses remain considerable (table 28.3).

The prevalence of iodine deficiency is often estimated from the prevalence of palpable goiter, but this method is not sensitive to milder expressions of deficiency. Iodine deficiency is thought to be a public health problem in a community if goiter is detected in more than 5 percent of the school-age population. A prevalence greater than 30 percent means that the deficiency is severe. According to World Health Organization (WHO) estimates, goiter rates among school-age children exceed 5 percent in 130 countries, putting 2,225,000 people at risk of IDD. A high prevalence of IDD occurs in Eastern Europe and Central Asia, the Eastern Mediterranean and North Africa, South Asia, and Sub-Saharan Africa (WHO 1999). Iodized salt programs are decreasing iodine deficiency in many regions; however, this reduction is offset by apparent increases in other regions, where public health officials are now aware of the problem because of increased surveillance.

Switzerland and the United States embarked on iodine fortification programs in earnest in the early 1920s. Success resulted in enthusiastic political and financial support for increased global coverage, and control of IDD through salt iodation represents a great achievement in international public health. Nevertheless, significant numbers of people remain at risk.

Zinc Deficiency

Zinc is ubiquitous within the body and is vital to protein synthesis, cellular growth, and cellular differentiation. Studies in children have demonstrated important roles for zinc in relation to immune function, growth, and development (Brown and others 2002; Shankar and Prasad 1998).

Zinc deficiency results from inadequate intakes and, to some extent, increased losses. Only animal flesh, particularly oysters and shellfish, is a good source of zinc, and fiber and phytates inhibit absorption. Thus, as with iron deficiency, populations consuming a primarily plant-based diet are susceptible. Deficiency can also result from losses during diarrheal illness.

Consensus is currently lacking on how to measure zinc deficiency in individuals. The International Zinc Nutrition Consultative Group recommended using serum or plasma zinc concentrations to identify the risk of deficiency at the population level. In addition, the group used information on absorbable zinc in the food supplies of 176 countries to estimate the proportion of each national population at risk of inadequate intake (table 28.1). This information was used to calculate the burden of disease (table 28.2) associated with zinc deficiency in young children. Prevalence is not expected to decrease unless the implementation of zinc-related interventions increases substantially (Caulfield and Black 2004).

The health consequences of severe zinc deficiency have been elucidated over the past 40 years, whereas the health risks of mild to moderate deficiency have been described only recently. Clinical presentations of severe deficiency include growth retardation, impaired immune function, skin disorders, hypogonadism, anorexia, and cognitive dysfunction. Mild to moderate deficiency increases susceptibility to infection, and the benefits of zinc supplementation on the immune system are well documented (Shankar and Prasad 1998). Zinc can prevent and palliate diarrhea and pneumonia (Zinc Investigators' Collaborative Group and others 1999, 2000) and also may reduce malaria morbidity in young children (Caulfield, Richard, and Black 2004). Improvements in growth have been demonstrated (Brown and others 2002), which may operate directly or indirectly through increased immune function and decreased infectious disease.

Zinc deficiency is estimated to be responsible for about 800,000 deaths annually from diarrhea, pneumonia, and malaria in children under five (table 28.2). Sub-Saharan Africa, the Eastern Mediterranean, and South Asia bear the heaviest attributable burden of pneumonia and diarrhea, with Sub-Saharan Africa accounting for nearly the entire attributable malaria burden.

INTERVENTIONS

Clearly, growth faltering and micronutrient deficiency disorders are prevalent, have deleterious consequences for children's health and development, and are primary contributors to the global burden of disease. Economic development is not the only path to solving childhood undernutrition. Improvements in family income may not translate into increased food intakes because the income elasticity for caloric intake is relatively low. The effects on micronutrient deficiencies might be greater if the food sources of those nutrients (meat, seafood, eggs, fortified food products) were more sensitive to income increases and if children had access to those foods. Price subsidies may reduce undernutrition in young children if targeted to foods consumed by them; the potential contribution of price subsidies to family nutrition is discussed elsewhere (see chapter 11). This chapter focuses on specific public health measures that are intended to address the problems directly. Progress has been made in some areas, but the current magnitude of the problems and of the associated disease burden underscore the need for more investment in nutritional interventions.

Growth Faltering and Childhood Stunting

Infants and young children falter in their growth because of inadequate dietary intakes and recurrent infectious diseases, which reduce appetite, increase metabolic requirements, and increase nutrient loss. Even though this problem is understood, progress to reduce malnutrition has been slow. Over time, thinking on how to reduce growth faltering and childhood stunting has shifted. Whereas previous efforts focused almost exclusively on identifying and rehabilitating severely malnourished children, current efforts emphasize prevention through combined nutritional and disease prevention and treatment interventions.

Initially, these efforts to prevent undernutrition focused on diseases rather than on improved child feeding practices as such. However, according to Becker, Black, and Brown (1991), despite the devastating effects of illness on nutritional status, improving dietary intakes is more effective than disease prevention efforts in reducing undernutrition. Because of dramatic reductions in appetite during illness, efforts to improve dietary intakes initially focused on maintaining energy intakes despite anorexia and on increasing intakes during recuperation, when appetite may be normal or high. More recent interventions aim at feeding healthy children optimal diets, which includes paying attention to dietary quality. Finally, some have argued that, for nutritional advice to be effective, it needs to be provided alongside growth monitoring and promotion; however, it is increasingly recognized that messages for prevention are largely universal and that integrated growth monitoring and promotion are not the only model for service delivery.

Promotion of Optimal Feeding of Infants and Young Children. Much of the early focus on optimal feeding was on breastfeeding, which should be immediate and exclusive until six months of age. At that time nutritious and safe foods should be added to a diet that is still based on breast milk until early in the second year of life. A consensus has been reached that six months is the recommended duration of exclusive breastfeeding (WHO 2002) and that the total duration is a decision left to the mother.

Multiple approaches exist to promote the initiation of breastfeeding and to prolong exclusive breastfeeding—health education; professional support; lay support; health sector changes (for example, infant friendly hospitals); and media campaigns—through health facilities and community programs. A recent Cochrane review estimates the potential effectiveness of these approaches (Sikorski and others 2002). Women who received any form of support for breastfeeding were 22 percent less likely to stop exclusive breastfeeding, and women who received lay support, in particular, were 34 percent less likely to stop exclusive breastfeeding. Substantial evidence indicates that interventions can be effective in prolonging breastfeeding and exclusive breastfeeding and that operational research is needed for program implementation and sustainability. If such programs were fully successful, they would reduce deaths in children under five by 13 percent (Jones and others 2003).

Complementary feeding is the process of introducing other foods and liquids into the child's diet when breast milk alone is no longer sufficient to meet nutritional requirements. According to Brown, Dewey, and Allen (1998), complementary feeding practices are suboptimal from several perspectives:

- Complementary foods are introduced too early or too late.
- Foods are served too infrequently or in insufficient amounts, or their consistency or energy density is inappropriate.
- The micronutrient content of foods is inadequate to meet the child's needs, or other factors in the diet impair the absorption of foods.
- Microbial contamination may occur.

In addition, because children often do not eat all the food offered to them, interaction between the caregiver and the child, along with other psychosocial aspects of care during feeding, requires attention. The amount of complementary food a child needs depends on breast milk intake. Guidelines are available for determining energy and nutrient intakes from complementary foods, given breast milk intakes (Dewey and Brown 2003).

Several reviews of the multiple approaches to improving infant and young child feeding practices are available (Allen and Gillespie 2001; Caulfield, Huffman, and Piwoz 1999; Dewey 2002; Hill, Kirkwood, and Edmond 2004; Swindale and others 2004). Caulfield, Huffman, and Piwoz (1999) review

16 programs in 14 countries to improve dietary intakes of infants 6 to 12 months of age. The programs were designed to promote exclusive breastfeeding and appropriate feeding during illness up to age three, and the content and approaches reflected current thinking regarding nutrition and behavior change. The approaches employed included using the mass media to reach both caregivers and the population as a whole to change cultural norms about complementary feeding and using one-on-one or small group interactions with community health workers to provide individualized information and support.

Most of the projects achieved good coverage (50 to 70 percent), with rates varying depending on the communication strategy. They resulted in large shifts in maternal knowledge and attitudes and changes in infant feeding practices. In the few programs assessing dietary intakes, intakes improved by 70 to 165 kilocalories per day. Differences in nutritional status at 12 months indicated weight-for-age and height-for-age gains of 0.24 to 0.87 SD. Even with a 50 percent overestimation of the effects, the effect of such programs could translate into tangible reductions in malnutrition and attributable mortality. In addition, these calculations do not consider the cumulative reduction in malnutrition from programs that benefit children's growth into the second and third years of life. Jones and others (2003) use the results of the analysis, along with knowledge of the relationship between underweight and child mortality, to estimate that programs to promote complementary feeding could reduce by 6 percent the deaths of children under five in developing countries.

Many programs provide supplemental food to participants either to provide them an incentive for participating in other activities (to offset time costs and increase consumer demand for preventive services) or to rehabilitate severely malnourished children. Although the latter approach is traditionally considered for supplemental food programs, the former approach is more common. Indeed, India's Integrated Child Development Services Program, the world's largest supplemental food program, plans to shift from rehabilitation to the use of supplemental food as a "magnet" for providing other integrated child development services (Kapil 2002). No consensus exists on when or how to include supplemental food to reduce undernutrition, and inefficient targeting is frequently a key constraint to effectiveness. Swindale and others' (2004) review of the effectiveness of food-assisted child survival programs concludes that such programs are reducing malnutrition by 2.0 to 2.5 percent per year.

Despite evidence of the effectiveness of nutritional interventions in improving feeding practices and preventing undernutrition, few programs take a comprehensive approach toward optimizing infant feeding, perhaps because of a lack of consensus on the key components of a comprehensive strategy. In 2002, participants at a WHO consultation developed 10 guiding principles for optimal feeding of the breastfed child (PAHO and WHO 2003). These principles, outlined in box 28.1, build on lessons from previous programmatic efforts such as those reviewed here and provide a basis for designing comprehensive programs to reduce malnutrition. The international public health community faces the challenge of implementing and evaluating these approaches.

Disease Control and Prevention. Interventions to prevent or decrease malnutrition or infectious disease are expected to decrease child mortality, and interventions that accomplish both will have the greatest effect (Pelletier, Frongillo, and Habicht 1993). This subsection considers the potential for disease control and prevention efforts to reduce undernutrition in young children.

Malaria is responsible for a large portion of childhood mortality in Sub-Saharan Africa. The effect of undernutrition on susceptibility to malaria has been discussed at length elsewhere (Caulfield, Richard, and Black 2004), but the nutritional deficiencies resulting from malaria have been insufficiently explored. Insecticide-treated bednets have been shown to prevent clinical episodes of malaria and decrease the prevalence of anemia in children (Lengeler 2003). Improvements in growth have also been documented.

Water, sanitation, and hygiene interventions decrease childhood malnutrition primarily by preventing diarrheal disease (Checkley and others 2004). Hand-washing interventions can reduce the risk of diarrheal diseases by about 45 percent. Hand-washing interventions can be included in water and sanitation programs or can exist as a single intervention, and they are both effective and cost-effective (Borghi and others 2002).

Vitamin A Deficiency

Even though the consequences of VAD had been defined by 1920, it was 1986 when vitamin A interventions were rigorously studied in a large, controlled community trial (Sommer and West 1996). A number of other community trials soon also demonstrated a significant decrease in child mortality with vitamin A supplementation (Beaton and others 1993). Supplementation can alleviate acute VAD quickly, whereas long-term strategies incorporate fortification and dietary diversification.

Supplementation can be either a curative or a preventive measure. If an individual presents with ocular symptoms of VAD, supplementation is part of the usual standard of care. Beyond the use of supplementation for symptoms that result directly from deficiency, its use as part of the treatment regimen for measles or severe malnutrition can improve health outcomes. In deficient areas, high-dose oral supplementation is recommended every four to six months for children under five and is highly efficacious in reducing ocular effects as well as

Box 28.1

Guiding Principles for Complementary Feeding of the Breastfed Child

1. Practice exclusive breastfeeding from birth to six months of age and introduce complementary foods at six months of age (180 days) while continuing to breastfeed.

2. Continue frequent, on-demand breastfeeding until two years of age or beyond.

3. Practice responsive feeding, applying the principles of psychosocial care. Specifically, do the following:
   - Feed infants directly and assist older children when they feed themselves, being sensitive to their hunger and satiety cues.
   - Feed slowly and patiently; encourage children to eat, but do not force them.
   - Experiment with different food combinations, tastes, textures, and methods of encouragement if children refuse many foods.
   - Minimize distractions during meals if the child loses interest easily.
   - Remember that feeding times are periods of learning and love, and talk to children during feeding, including making eye contact.

4. Practice good hygiene and proper food handling:
   - Wash hands before food preparation and eating (both caregivers and children).
   - Store foods safely and serve foods immediately after preparation.
   - Use clean utensils to prepare and serve food.
   - Use clean cups and bowls when feeding children.
   - Avoid the use of feeding bottles, which are difficult to keep clean.

5. Start at six months of age with small amounts of food and increase the quantity as the child gets older, while maintaining frequent breastfeeding. According to average breast milk intakes in developing countries, infants' needs from complementary foods are approximately 200 kilocalories per day at 6 to 8 months, 300 kilocalories per day at 9 to 11 months, and 550 kilocalories per day at 12 to 23 months.

6. Increase food consistency and variety gradually as the infant gets older, adapting to the infant's requirements and abilities. Infants can eat pureed, mashed, and semisolid foods beginning at six months. By eight months most infants can also eat finger foods—that is, snacks that they can eat unaided. By 12 months, most children can eat the same types of foods that the rest of the family consumes, keeping in mind the need for nutrient-dense foods. Avoid foods that cause choking.

7. Increase the frequency with which the child is fed complementary foods as he or she gets older. The appropriate number of feedings depends on the energy density of local foods and the usual amounts consumed at each feeding. For the average healthy, breastfed infant, meals should be provided two or three times a day at 6 to 8 months of age and three or four times a day at 9 to 23 months of age, with additional snacks.

8. Feed a variety of foods to ensure that nutrient needs are met. The child should eat meat, poultry, fish, or eggs daily, or as often as possible. Vegetarian diets cannot meet nutrient needs at this age unless nutrient supplements or fortified products are used.

9. Use fortified complementary foods or vitamin and mineral supplements for the infant, as needed. In some populations, breastfeeding mothers may also need vitamin and mineral supplements or fortified products for their own health and to ensure normal concentrations of certain nutrients in their breast milk.

10. Increase fluid intake during illness, including more frequent breastfeeding, and encourage the child to eat soft, varied, appetizing, favorite foods. After illness, give food more often than usual, and encourage the child to eat more.

Source: PAHO and WHO 2003.

---

mortality (Sommer and West 1996). A meta-analysis of controlled trials in children demonstrated a 23 percent reduction in mortality (Beaton and others 1993). High-dose vitamin A supplements are considered safe for infants younger than six months. Several studies suggest that giving vitamin A within 48 hours of birth reduces mortality in the first three months by 21 to 74 percent (D. Ross 2002).

A variety of foodstuffs have been fortified with vitamin A, including oil, monosodium glutamate, butter, wheat flour, sugar, and rice. Fortified white sugar has been successful in reducing VAD prevalence in Central America. In El Salvador and Guatemala, where fortified sugar is the primary source of vitamin A, it accounts for approximately 30 percent of the recommended dietary intake (RDI). Fortification of monosodium glutamate with vitamin A has been demonstrated to be biologically efficacious. Even though program implementation was flawed by unacceptable cost, discoloration of the monosodium glutamate, and packaging problems, indicators of VAD declined significantly during periods of fortification in both Indonesia and the Philippines (Dary and Mora 2002).

Vitamin A intakes can also be improved through dietary diversification, either by educating communities about important sources of vitamin A and beta-carotene that are available in the local diet or by increasing economic prosperity so that individuals have additional funds to spend on a wider variety of food. Education alone has not been demonstrated to affect the degree of VAD in a community, but it can be a powerful tool when incorporated in a broader strategy that also includes supplementation and fortification (Sommer and West 1996).

Iron Deficiency

Despite the public health community's enduring interest in preventing and treating iron deficiency anemia, little evidence suggests that the problem has been reduced. Indeed, in some regions the opposite may be true. From the 1970s to the 1980s, the iron density of people's diets decreased in every region except the Near East and North Africa as iron-poor cereals displaced legumes. During much of this period, iron deficiency anemia increased in South Asia and Sub-Saharan Africa, where the problem is most severe (Stoltzfus, Mullany, and Black 2004). Goals for reducing iron deficiency anemia were articulated for the 1990s at the 1990 World Summit for Children, and many countries adopted policies for providing supplementation for young children; however, few large programs have been developed to eliminate the problem.

The explanations for this failure to act include doubts among both scientific program planners and policy makers about the causes and consequences of iron deficiency and anemia; lack of political commitment; inadequate program planning, including mobilization and training of health staff members; insufficient community involvement; and, in particular, inherent difficulties with prolonged adherence to daily supplementation (Stoltzfus, Mullany, and Black 2004). Despite this bleak picture, guidelines for supplementation have been formulated for children ages 6 to 24 months and for low birthweight infants beginning at 2 months (Stoltzfus and Dreyfuss 1998). Also, various scientific documents synthesize and communicate current knowledge about the consequences of iron deficiency anemia and programming efforts.

Ample evidence indicates that iron deficiency is the principal cause of anemia in children; that iron supplements are efficacious in preventing and treating iron deficiency anemia, increasing hemoglobin concentrations by about 1 gram per deciliter on average in controlled trials; and that supplements reduce severe anemia even in malarious areas. The contribution of parasitic infections such as malaria and hookworm to anemia does not negate the usefulness of iron supplements; rather it underscores the need for multiple inputs to prevent severe anemia, given the risks of transfusion. Although current recommendations indicate daily supplements, less frequent delivery, such as intermittently or weekly, is commanding interest. Beaton and McCabe's (1999) meta-analysis concludes that both daily and weekly supplementation are efficacious if adherence is good.

In many countries, iron fortification of foods is the principal strategy for reducing iron deficiency and anemia. Fortified foodstuffs include wheat and maize flours, noodles, sugar, condiments, and complementary foods and milk for infants and children. Efficacy studies indicate the potential of fortification to increase iron intakes and reduce anemia, and effectiveness trials in Chile (dry milk for infants), Ghana (complementary food for young children), Guatemala (sugar), India (salt), Mexico (fortified weaning food and dry milk), and República Bolivariana de Venezuela (maize and wheat) have found improvements in hemoglobin concentration or reductions in anemia prevalence (Allen and Gillespie 2001; Rivera and others 2004). Nevertheless, few national iron fortification programs have evaluation results that are without controversy. Yip and Ramakrishnan (2002) argue that the strongest examples of the potential for fortification are found in the Chilean program of fortified dry milk for infants and in the U.S. program of iron-fortified infant cereals. A randomized trial in Mexico of a poverty alleviation program that distributes a complementary food fortified with multiple micronutrients, including iron, found positive effects on anemia rates (Rivera and others 2004). Evaluations of newly implemented iron fortification programs should gauge their contribution to anemia prevention.

Newer strategies, such as sprinkles (powders), spreads, or foodlets (a hybrid of a food and a tablet), appear promising, particularly for regions where the infrastructure will not support more traditional forms of fortification (Zlotkin and others 2003). Processed complementary foods and beverages offer additional vehicles for reducing iron and other micronutrient deficiencies and promoting well-being (Solon and others 2003). Implementing such strategies and documenting their cost-effectiveness are important activities for the next few years.

In many settings, promoting iron-rich organ meats and animal products and undertaking other food-based strategies may increase iron intakes and contribute to anemia reduction. Such approaches have been promoted for many years, but research is still needed to document their efficacy and effectiveness (Ruel and Levin 2000).

Iodine Deficiency Disorders

Interventions to diminish iodine deficiency using either supplementation or fortification are both efficacious and inexpensive, and WHO, the United Nations Children's Fund, and the International Council for the Control of Iodine Deficiency Disorders have pledged to eliminate iodine deficiency and the spectrum of IDD.

For regions with severe endemic iodine deficiency, high-dose iodine supplementation is indicated while longer-term solutions are put into place. Iodized oil and iodide tablets are the most common means of direct administration. Injections of iodized oil have been used with much success to decrease the prevalence of IDD and have been shown to be effective for three to four years, depending on the dosage (Hetzel 1989). Although injected oil is effective, it is also expensive, requires trained personnel to administer, and carries the risk of infectious disease transmission from contaminated needles. Because of those drawbacks, researchers began exploring oral administration as an alternative. Oral administration of iodized oil in liquid and tablet form has been successful in the long-term correction of clinical deficiency, and in Indonesia, oral administration was associated with a reduction in infant mortality (Cobra and others 1997).

Iodized or iodated salt is the primary strategy for correcting iodine deficiency because of the nearly universal consumption of salt regardless of socioeconomic status; the lack of an effect on consistency, color, or taste from the addition of iodine; and the limited number of producers in many countries. Large-scale salt fortification has been highly successful in many countries, and of the 130 countries with iodine deficiency, 75 percent have laws mandating salt iodization. The goal of universal salt iodization for consumption by both humans and livestock in all countries with endemic iodine deficiency was set at the 1990 World Summit for Children (WHO, UNICEF, and ICCIDD 2001). Some populations do not easily embrace salt iodization because of cultural preferences or because they have an ample supply of unprocessed salt, so other means of fortification are needed. One promising option is to add potassium iodate to irrigation water.

Zinc Deficiency

Although zinc deficiency is likely widespread and even mild deficiency probably has significant health consequences, few interventions have been developed to combat it in developing countries. Possible interventions include supplementation, fortification, and dietary diversification or modification. The strong evidence that the use of zinc supplements given during and for a short time after diarrhea improves the outcome of that episode and prevents future episodes has led to the recommendation that zinc, along with increased fluids and continued feeding, be used to treat all episodes of acute diarrhea (WHO and UNICEF 2004). Substantial efforts are under way to initiate programs in developing countries. Prophylactic zinc supplementation also improves growth and reduces diarrhea incidence (International Zinc Nutrition Consultative Group 2004).

Fortification interventions include the traditional method of adding zinc to a commercial food, consumer fortification using sprinkles, and plant-breeding techniques. For example, Mexico has introduced several large-scale programs, including the fortification of maize and wheat flours and the distribution of fortified complementary food and fortified milk to low-income children (Rivera and Sepulveda 2003). Researchers are investigating the possibility of home fortification of food using sprinkles containing iron and zinc (Zlotkin and others 2003), but further research is needed to determine whether sprinkles are a viable option. Through plant breeding and genetic engineering, staple crops may be made to contain more zinc or less phytate, resulting in increased zinc bioavailability (Ruel and Bouis 1998). Other dietary strategies target food preparation techniques, such as fermentation of unrefined flour to increase zinc bioavailability.

INTERVENTION COSTS AND COST-EFFECTIVENESS

Multiple strategies exist for preventing malnutrition in young children in the short and long term. This section considers the costs and cost-effectiveness of these interventions for preventing malnutrition or deaths attributable to each nutritional problem. Table 28.4 presents a compendium of cost information, including, where possible, the costs of preventing a child death or saving a DALY.

Horton and others (1996) use data from Brazil, Honduras, and Mexico to estimate the costs and cost-effectiveness of hospital-based programs to promote breastfeeding. Using standard costing methods, they examine the costs of breastfeeding promotion activities in each program and the additional inputs, as well as the savings. Savings accrued from the removal of infant formula where it was currently used. Using data on infant feeding practices and morbidity and mortality from Brazil, they estimated the costs of the programs per birth, per diarrhea case averted, and per death averted. As table 28.4 shows, the costs of such programs range from US$0.30 to US$0.40 per child, and from US$100 to US$200 per death averted, making them comparable in cost-effectiveness to measles and rotavirus vaccination. Assuming that deaths would otherwise have occurred around age one, and using average Latin American life expectancy at that age, yields a cost per DALY gained of only US$3 to US$7.

In many community-based strategies, multiple organizations work through a variety of communication channels to promote exclusive breastfeeding. Two studies in Ghana and Madagascar provide costs estimates for such programs (Chee, Makinen, and Sakagawa 2002; Chee and others 2003). The programs cost US$4 to US$16 per child, and given the effect on mothers' practices, the cost ranged from US$5 to

Table 28.4 Costs and Cost-Effectiveness of Nutrition Interventions

Type of deficiency and intervention	Source	Year	Country	Costs (US$)		
				Per child or per outcome	Per death averted	Per DALY gained
Underweight						
Breastfeeding support	Horton and others 1996	1996	Brazil, Honduras, Mexico	0.30–0.40 per birth; 0.65–1.10 per diarrhea case averted	100–200	3–7
Breastfeeding promotion	Ross, Loening, and Mbele 1987	1987	Mali	2–3 per child	282	11
Breastfeeding promotion	Chee, Makinen, and Sakagawa 2002	2002	Ghana	16 per child; 5–58 per adopter of exclusive breastfeeding	203[a]	7.80
	Chee and others 2003	2003	Madagascar	4.41 per child; 10–17 per adopter of exclusive breastfeeding	—	—
Child survival program with nutrition component	J. Ross 1997; WHO 2002	1997	Across programs	76–101 per undernourished child averted	1,200	41–43
Nutrition programs Less intensive More intensive				2–5 per child 5–10 per child		
Growth monitoring and counseling	Fiedler 2003	2003	Honduras	4 per child; 20 per undernourished child averted	240–320[b]	8–11
Vitamin A deficiency						
Capsule distribution	Rassas, Hottor, and others 2004	2004	Ghana	0.90 per child	277	11
	Rassas, Nakamba, and others 2004	2004	Zambia	1.23 per child	162	6–7
	Fiedler 2000	2000	Nepal	1.25 per child	327	11–12
	Fiedler and others 2000	1994				
Fortification Sugar Other	Institute of Medicine 1998; World Bank 1994		Guatemala	0.17 per child 0.05–0.15 per child	1,000	33–35
Iron deficiency						
Supplements	Institute of Medicine 1998; World Bank 1994	1994		3.17–5.30 per child	—	—
Fortification Salt	World Bank 1994	1994	India	0.12 per child	—	—
Sugar	World Bank 1994	1994	Guatemala	0.20–1.00 per child	—	—
Cereal	World Bank 1994			0.09 per child	2,000	66–70
Iodine deficiency	Institute of Medicine 1998; World Bank 1994					
Oil injection		1994	Peru	2.75 per child	—	—
			Zaire	0.80 per child	—	—
				1.25 per child	—	—
Fortification Water			Indonesia	0.05 per child		
Salt			Italy	0.02–0.05 per child	1,000	34–36
Salt			India	0.05 per child	—	—
Zinc deficiency						
Supplements with oral rehydration salts	Robberstad and others 2004	2004	n.a.	0.47 per child	2,100	73

— = Source did not include data from which to estimate deaths averted (and DALYs gained).

Note: Deaths prevented by promoting or supporting breastfeeding are assumed to occur around age one. Deaths prevented by other programs to reduce underweight and all programs to reduce micronutrient deficiency are assumed to occur between ages one and five. Authors' estimates of costs per DALY (in parentheses) using region-specific life expectancies at ages one and five, reflect this range.

a. Assumes that all the DALY gains come from preventing deaths.

b. Assumes that an undernourished child has a chance of 1 in 16 to 1 in 12 (6 to 8 percent) of dying before age five, the same as estimated for child survival programs.

US$58 per adopter of exclusive breastfeeding. In Ghana, an estimated 883 deaths were averted, yielding a program cost of US$7.80 per DALY gained or US$203 per death prevented. The range of costs within each program depended on the baseline prevalence of the behavior, the population density, and the characteristics of the implementing organizations themselves. Programs will be more cost-effective when the baseline prevalence is lower; the population density is higher; and the organizations involved are focused, highly motivated, and well organized.

Less information is available on the costs of community-based nutrition programs to prevent growth faltering, to control morbidity, and to improve survival. The costs of a program in Mali (Ross, Loening, and Mbele 1987), which included promotion of breastfeeding, counseling, and education on optimal child feeding; prevention of diarrheal disease; and growth monitoring, were estimated to be US$282 per death averted and US$11 per DALY gained. This estimate is consistent with others that nutrition programs cost US$2 to US$10 per child, depending on the intensity of nutrition counseling, including Fiedler's (2003) study of the Integrated Community Child Care Program in Honduras, which had an estimated cost of US$4 per child. (For a fuller analysis of such programs, including contextual and programmatic characteristics that affect outcomes, see chapter 56.)

In the past five years, investigators have undertaken several cost analyses of national programs to distribute vitamin A capsules. Two reports from Ghana and Zambia are particularly informative (Rassas, Hottor, and others 2004; Rassas, Nakamba, and others 2004). As table 28.4 shows, such programs cost US$0.90 to US$1.23 per child, with the costs per death averted ranging from US$162 to US$277. (Deaths from micronutrient deficiencies are assumed to occur between ages one and five, and estimates of cost per DALY ranging from US$6 to US$11 reflect this range, as well as region-specific life expectancies at those ages.) These costs are comparable with estimates of a vitamin A program in Nepal that cost US$1.25 per child and US$327 per death averted (Fiedler 2000). Ching and others (2000) examine the costs of incorporating vitamin A capsule distribution into immunization campaigns in 50 countries in 1998 and 1999. Their analysis finds that the total costs per death averted ranged from about US$150 to US$600, with the incremental costs for vitamin A distribution amounting to only about US$30 to US$150 per death averted. The costs per death averted depended on the country setting, the program's coverage, the delivery of vitamin A (one or two doses), and the underlying level of mortality. The incremental cost per DALY gained could be as low as US$1 or as high as US$6.

Fewer examples of vitamin A fortification programs are available, with the only clear example being sugar fortification in Central America. In 1994, estimates indicated that a program in Guatemala cost US$0.17 per child, and US$1,000 per death averted. Counting only the losses from mortality, the cost of saving a DALY was US$33 to US$35. However, for each death prevented, there were probably several cases of eye damage prevented and of improved general health; thus, taking full account of nonfatal effects would reduce the cost per DALY somewhat.

Iron supplementation is more costly than distribution of vitamin A capsules, as it involves a daily supplement over an extended period. Estimates indicate that such programs cost US$3.17 to US$5.30 per child. Numerous cost estimates are available for iron fortification programs, because these programs have been the principal strategy to prevent and control iron deficiency anemia. Such programs have traditionally cost US$0.09 to US$1.00 per child, depending on the country and the vehicle for fortification. These estimates are based on elemental iron as the fortifier. Even though this is the cheapest form available, critics have questioned the bioavailability of elemental iron, and many researchers now advocate using other forms of iron.

Iodine fortification programs cost little, about US$0.02 to US$0.05 per child. Iodized oil injections are more costly at US$0.80 to US$2.75 per beneficiary, but these programs may be recommended for settings where people consume little commercialized and easily fortified food.

Currently, no examples of zinc intervention programs are available from which to estimate cost-effectiveness. However, Robberstad and others' (2004) simulation analysis examines the potential costs and cost-effectiveness of providing zinc as an adjunct to oral hydration salts in treating diarrhea in young children. Providing zinc as part of case management carries an estimated incremental cost of US$0.47 per treatment, ranging from US$0.33 to US$0.62. Given the relationship between zinc provision and mortality risk, this addition to current management programs would cost, on average, US$2,100 per death adverted and US$73 per DALY gained.

Despite the enormity of the nutritional problems, the associated loss of DALYS, and the existence of programs to combat malnutrition, surprisingly little data on the costs or cost-effectiveness of nutritional programs are available. This problem represents a serious gap in information for health planning, implementation, and advocacy. Nonetheless, considerable evidence indicates that when programs to promote breastfeeding or child growth or to correct micronutrient deficiencies are delivered to populations with a relatively high prevalence of malnutrition, the cost per participating child is usually so low that deaths can be averted at a cost per DALY that is less than US$100, and often less than US$10, even in regions with low life expectancy. Few health interventions are comparably cost-effective.

ECONOMIC BENEFITS OF INTERVENTION

The previous sections outlined the costs to society in terms of deaths and disabilities resulting from growth faltering and micronutrient malnutrition, as well as the costs and cost-effectiveness of options for their alleviation and prevention; however, DALYs do not capture the full range of potential benefits to society from effective nutrition programs. For example, even though the effect of iron deficiency on mental retardation in children contributes to the attributable DALYs (Stoltzfus, Mullany, and Black 2004), the negative effects of iron deficiency on cognition that do not constitute retardation are not considered. Other effects of malnutrition on cognitive and physical functioning that ultimately affect labor productivity are also not considered, nor are other long-term health consequences of child undernutrition. Finally, because undernutrition increases the frequency and severity of disease, undernutrition is associated with considerable health care costs, which are also not captured in burden estimates.

Malnutrition and Human Capital Formation

Researchers have studied cognitive function using global measures of development and intelligence, such as IQ, along with school performance and more narrowly defined intellectual, psychomotor, and behavioral skills. A large body of research has examined whether undernutrition causes lasting cognitive deficits in later life and whether potential deficits are amenable to subsequent nutritional interventions. Acute malnutrition is associated with negative neuroanatomical, emotional, and behavioral effects on children's development. After recovery, results of behavioral and developmental tests generally improve, but the long-term developmental implications remain unclear. Many studies find IQ scores 8 to 18 points lower in children who suffered from severe malnutrition (Fishman and others 2004). Studies of chronic undernutrition also report deficits in IQ and school performance with stunting during early childhood. Evidence from nutritional interventions among high-risk or undernourished children suggests that early supplementary feeding (but no sooner than two years of age) improves developmental scores during the intervention, with some evidence of long-term benefits. For example, follow-up of Guatemalan children exposed to prenatal and early postnatal supplementation demonstrated long-term cognitive benefits even after adjusting for socioeconomic factors and educational experience (Pollitt and others 1995). These results argue strongly for preventing acute severe malnutrition and generalized growth faltering that leads to stunting in children.

Nutritional interventions may preserve or improve cognitive function through mechanisms other than preventing growth faltering or acute malnutrition. For example, breast-feeding confers some cognitive benefits. Anderson, Johnstone,

and Remley's (1999) meta-analysis estimates gains of 3.5 IQ points, adjusting for important covariates.

Iron deficiency has long been associated with developmental delays, and iron supplementation studies have demonstrated improvements in cognitive function. Whether the negative effects of iron deficiency and anemia on development are reversible remains controversial, which implies the need for strong preventive measures. More research is needed to learn about the effects of iron deficiency on development and to develop measures for evaluating programs that provide iron.

Multiple lines of evidence indicate that zinc influences development (Black 1998). Despite a clear biological role, epidemiological studies provide insufficient evidence to draw conclusions on the gain in human capital if zinc deficiency were reduced through public health interventions. Research to address this gap is under way.

The public health community has long recognized that iodine deficiency is the most common cause of preventable mental retardation. Even though the problem of maternal iodine deficiency and cretinism in the offspring is well recognized, evidence also suggests that deficiency in children is negatively associated with cognitive abilities. Bleichrodt and Born's (1994) meta-analysis finds losses of 13.5 IQ points in those with iodine deficiency. Some of these effects occur in the absence of goiter, the hallmark of IDD. More research is needed to fully understand the human consequences of milder forms of iodine deficiency that are probably still prevalent in developing countries.

Malnutrition and Loss of Productivity

Abundant evidence demonstrates that both anemia and iron deficiency decrease fitness and capacity for aerobic work by decreasing oxygen transport and respiratory efficiency in muscles. The consequences of iron deficiency are thus measurable in terms of loss of economic productivity. Aguayo, Scott, and Ross's (2003) case study in Sierra Leone estimates that anemia among women is associated with agricultural productivity losses of US$19 million per year. For children, the economic costs are not as clear, but those costs may be substantial depending on the children's ages and the types of work they perform.

Growth faltering that leads to stunting in early childhood translates into shortened adult stature. Adult height is related not only to total food consumption but also to protein intake (Jamison, Leslie, and Musgrove 2003), which reinforces the importance of dietary quality. Multiple levels of evidence link adult stature and worker productivity (Martorell 1996). Haddad and Bouis (1991) estimate that a 1 percent decrease in adult stature is associated with a 1.4 percent decrease in productivity. Others find that a 1 percent increase in adult stature is associated with a 2.0 to 2.4 percent increase in wages or earnings. Other things being equal, current programs to prevent stunting in early childhood can deliver about a third to a half of that 1 percent increase in adult stature. Thus, a lifetime of economic loss results from a failure to prevent stunting in early childhood and accompanying deficits in adult stature, and strategies to reduce this tremendous loss are available.

In addition, the impacts of malnutrition on cognitive development translate indirectly into deficits in productivity in adulthood. Children who are malnourished are more likely to start school late, to perform less well, and to stay in school for a shorter time (Behrman, Alderman, and Hoddinott 2004). Studies suggest that improvements in nutrition within the current range of benefits of programs for young children can lead to substantial increases in rates of school initiation and to more years of schooling (Alderman, Hoddinott, and Kinsey 2003; Alderman and others 2001; Behrman and others 2003). Both years of schooling and school performance affect wages and economic productivity. Alderman, Hoddinott, and Kinsey (2003) calculate that the effects of malnutrition during early childhood, with the accompanying effects on schooling, lead to a 12 percent reduction in lifetime earnings in Zimbabwe. Current programming could restore a significant proportion of those lost wages.

Resource Allocation

Malnutrition increases the likelihood that a child will be sick and, when sick, will become seriously ill. Thus, resources must be allocated to health care services to deal with the increased frequency and severity of illness caused by undernutrition and micronutrient deficiencies. To our knowledge, this increase in likelihood and severity of illness has never been quantified, but it is likely to be high, considering not only the costs of health care infrastructure, but also the time costs and costs of lost wages or schooling borne by the family for each episode of illness. Furthermore, to the extent that undernutrition or micronutrient deficiencies lead to deficits in cognitive development, resources need to be allocated to special education, rehabilitation, and vocational services. The costs associated with not providing such services are ultimately paid in mortality and economic statistics.

Adult Disease and Disability

In the past 10 years, a growing literature has identified associations between small size at birth; early patterns of postnatal growth; and adult conditions as diverse as diabetes, cardiovascular disease, and schizophrenia. More research is needed to provide evidence of causality for such associations and to create the evidence base for attributing those effects to malnutrition in burden-of-disease calculations. Given current knowledge, health care budgets in developing countries will likely be strained to deal with the burden of chronic diseases of adulthood caused by the failure to prevent maternal and child undernutrition.

PROGRAM IMPLEMENTATION: LESSONS OF EXPERIENCE

For decades, countries have implemented programs to alleviate growth faltering and micronutrient deficiencies in children; therefore, it is timely to consider what has been accomplished and what can be learned from successes and failures. The task is difficult, because nutrition programs are diverse, ranging from the simple fortification of salt with iodine to multifaceted programs to improve dietary intakes and prevent growth faltering. Nonetheless, some general statements about the state of programming in this area are possible.

Success in conceptualizing and implementing programs to reduce growth faltering by combining disease control strategies with the promotion of breastfeeding and optimal complementary feeding has been demonstrable. The focus has shifted away from growth monitoring and promotion (counseling) strategies to population-based assessment with more generalized dissemination of key messages for behavior change. Available data suggest high cost-effectiveness for such programs. Key challenges involve scaling up and sustainability, as well as strengthening of monitoring and evaluation systems. A gap in this knowledge concerns optimal feeding in the presence of HIV infection, and testing options and designing programs in such settings are of the highest priority.

Iodine fortification has been a clear success over decades, which underscores the need for continued and consistent funding and advocacy for such programs. Even when universal access to iodine becomes a reality, policy and programmatic supports will be necessary to maintain it.

The success of iodine fortification contrasts with other examples of fortification that have made slow and uneven progress. Fortification of foodstuffs with vitamin A is limited geographically, and even though many countries have embarked on iron fortification, these programs lag because of controversies about the effectiveness of existing programs, the evaluation methods used, and the lack of infrastructure for fortification in some settings. Concerted efforts to address the controversies and to provide evidence of the effectiveness of fortification in controlling iron deficiency are under way. In addition, recognition that fortification should address multiple micronutrient deficiencies, chiefly the B vitamins and zinc, has grown.

Programs to distribute vitamin A capsules twice a year are a reality in many areas characterized by VAD. Jones and others (2003) estimate that current coverage of supplementation for children living in areas with VAD is 55 percent. In the past few years, studies have provided solid data on the costs and cost-effectiveness of such programs in diverse settings.

In contrast, despite concerns about the health and developmental consequences of iron deficiency and anemia, few examples are available of even small-scale iron supplementation programs for young children. Supply and adherence continue to constrain progress, with adherence depending on program workers' and families' perceptions of benefits and their reluctance to continue the long-term use in children of what are often considered to be medicines. Similar constraints apply to programs to provide iron supplements to pregnant women, but operational research has overcome many obstacles, and the hope is that the lessons learned can inform the design and implementation of iron supplementation programs for young children.

Food-based strategies, particularly dietary diversification and the promotion of specific food groups for preventing micronutrient malnutrition, are less advanced than other programs. In part, this lack of advancement reflects the diverse nature of the behaviors to be changed and of the available options. Given this diversity and the fact that such strategies are more setting specific than, for example, capsule distribution, the lack of summary estimates of effectiveness is not surprising. Consensus is growing that improving dietary intakes through agricultural innovations and dietary diversification represents long-term answers to micronutrient malnutrition, but progress is slow because of the urgency of alleviating deficiencies in the short term. More research is needed to define the policies that will promote these strategies.

Research over the past decade has articulated a strong case for interventions to prevent zinc deficiency, with supplementation and fortification identified as important approaches. Experiences with zinc supplementation or fortification programs are needed to provide estimates of costs and cost-effectiveness. If the costs of providing zinc supplements to young children are in line with those reported earlier, then such programs would be highly cost-effective, considering the prevalence and burden of disease associated with zinc deficiency.

Child malnutrition results from multiple factors, and even though each context has its own unique features, the etiology has many more commonalities. Thus, for program planners and policy makers intent on alleviating malnutrition to begin designing and implementing programs in their particular settings from scratch is strikingly inefficient. In the past decade, this point has been recognized, and documents that articulate processes for program implementation and evaluation have mushroomed. These "road maps" permit policy makers and program planners to capitalize rapidly on interest in addressing nutrition problems. The road maps also communicate a sense of feasibility by streamlining the complex processes of program design and evaluation. Thus, their use can reduce the likelihood that programs will be diffuse (too many inputs), will be culturally inappropriate, will have unrealistic expectations, and will have no possibility of sustainability and no plans for process or impact evaluation.

Demonstrating that nutrition programs are effective is key to translating scientific findings into policies and programs as well as to ensuring the continuity and expansion of funding.

Despite decades of nutrition programs, with identifiable successes, uncertainty about their effectiveness persists. The value of publishing solid process and outcome evaluations in the scientific literature in addition to project reports has only recently been recognized and cannot be overstated. Whereas outcome evaluations provide data on program effects, process evaluations provide key information to maintain quality assurance and to support the plausibility of key outcomes. Consensus is growing on the need to evaluate a package of services rather than use complex strategies to tease apart the effects of specific program elements. Well-designed programs with process evaluation efficiently provide this information.

Although following standard scientific approaches to establish program effectiveness has enabled progress in many interventions, alternative designs can and should be used for this purpose. Scientists traditionally argue that randomized controlled trials are needed to establish causal evidence of effectiveness and that multiple trials are needed in diverse settings, perhaps followed by pooled or meta-analyses to provide summary estimates. Others argue that designs that provide plausible evidence of program effects or adequate information to support continued funding should be recognized as valid by funders and publishers in refereed journals and should be implemented more broadly (Victora, Habicht, and Bryce 2004).

RESEARCH AND DEVELOPMENT AGENDA

Despite progress, much work remains unfinished. Other chapters focus on research and development needs in relation to packaging services, scaling up, and ensuring sustainability. Here the focus is on research for strengthening the database for policy making.

Gaps in knowledge remain with respect to recognized strategies for intervention programs. Often information on intervention efficacy exists, yet little scientific literature on program effectiveness is available. Key gaps include the following:

- evaluation of the effectiveness of national iron fortification programs to reduce iron deficiency anemia
- implementation and evaluation of the effectiveness of iron supplementation programs for young children
- evaluation of the effect on child mortality of multifaceted programs to reduce child undernutrition
- evaluation of the effectiveness of programs based on the new guiding principles for reducing undernutrition and micronutrient malnutrition in young children
- implementation and evaluation of the effectiveness of food-based strategies to reduce micronutrient malnutrition
- implementation and evaluation of the effectiveness of early postnatal vitamin A supplementation to reduce infant mortality.

Costing studies should accompany the evaluations to allow estimates of cost-effectiveness for decision making.

Because of the logistical difficulties in developing fortification approaches in settings with little industry infrastructure, alternative fortification approaches are needed, such as micronutrient sprinkles or foodlets. In addition, operational research is needed to develop, implement, and evaluate programs to improve zinc status. Never has so much evidence been amassed on the consequences of a deficiency disorder without programmatic application. The challenge now is to develop and implement programs for preventing and treating zinc deficiency and to evaluate their effectiveness for child growth, health, and survival. The International Zinc Nutrition Consultative Group (2004) has laid out a research agenda with these aims in mind.

CONCLUSIONS

Undernutrition is a major cause of death and disability in young children. When ranked among other causes, growth faltering and micronutrient deficiencies figure prominently, both because they are prevalent and because their consequences are devastating. Not included in the numbers, however, are the losses of lifetime productivity associated with early malnutrition and the resources that must be allocated to confront the developmental and morbidity consequences of child malnutrition, which last a lifetime.

Success has been achieved in preventing and controlling iodine deficiency, and palpable progress has been made in the past 20 years in correcting vitamin A deficiency and promoting breastfeeding; however, for iron, articulated goals have not been translated into programs, and the problem has remained the same or worsened. Zinc deficiency is now recognized as an important new challenge.

As shown here, solid evidence shows that nutrition programs can be effective at addressing nutritional problems in young children. Increasingly available cost data, when combined with outcome evaluations, demonstrate that nutritional interventions rank favorably in terms of cost-effectiveness when compared with competing interventions. The case that further investment in nutrition interventions is warranted is thus compelling.

REFERENCES

Aguayo, V. M., S. Scott, and J. Ross. 2003. "Sierra Leone: Investing in Nutrition to Reduce Poverty—A Call for Action." *Public Health Nutrition* 6 (7): 653–57.

Alderman, H., J. Behrman, D. Ross, and R. Sabot. 2001. "Child Health and School Enrollment: A Longitudinal Analysis." *Journal of Human Resources* 36 (1): 185–205.

Alderman, H., J. Hoddinott, and B. Kinsey. 2003. *Long Term Consequences of Early Childhood Malnutrition.* Washington, DC: World Bank.

Allen, L., and S. Gillespie. 2001. *What Works? A Review of the Efficacy and Effectiveness of Nutrition Interventions.* Geneva: United Nations, Administrative Committee on Coordination and Subcommittee on Nutrition in collaboration with the Asian Development Bank.

Anderson, J. W., B. M. Johnstone, and D. T. Remley. 1999. "Breast-Feeding and Cognitive Development: A Meta-Analysis." *American Journal of Clinical Nutrition* 70 (4): 525–35.

Beard, J. L. 2001. "Iron Biology in Immune Function, Muscle Metabolism, and Neuronal Functioning." *Journal of Nutrition* 131 (2 Suppl. 2): S568–79.

Beaton, G. H., R. Martorell, K. J. Aronson, B. Edmonston, G. McCabe, A. C. Ross, and others. 1993. "Effectiveness of Vitamin A Supplementation in the Control of Young Child Morbidity and Mortality in Developing Countries." Geneva: United Nations, Administrative Committee on Coordination and Subcommittee on Nutrition.

Beaton, G. H., and G. McCabe. 1999. "Efficacy of Intermittent Iron Supplementation in the Control of Iron Deficiency Anaemia in Developing Countries: An Analysis of Experience—Final Report to the Micronutrient Initiative." Montreal: Micronutrient Initiative.

Becker S., R. E. Black, and K. H. Brown. 1991. "Relative Effects of Diarrhea, Fever, and Dietary Energy Intake on Weight Gain in Rural Bangladeshi Children." *American Journal of Clinical Nutrition* 53 (6): 1499–503.

Behrman, J., H. Alderman, and J. Hoddinott. 2004. *Hunger and Malnutrition.* Copenhagen: Copenhagen Consensus.

Behrman, J., J. Hoddinott, J. A. Maluccio, A. Quisumbing, R. Martorell, and A. D. Stein. 2003. *The Impact of Experimental Nutritional Interventions on Education into Adulthood in Rural Guatemala: Preliminary Longitudinal Analysis.* Philadelphia: University of Pennsylvania; Atlanta: Emory University; Washington, DC: International Food Policy Research Institute.

Black, M. M. 1998. "Zinc Deficiency and Child Development." *American Journal of Clinical Nutrition* 68 (Suppl. 2): S464–69.

Bleichrodt, N., and M. Born. 1994. "A Meta-Analysis of Research into Iodine and Its Relationship to Cognitive Development." In *The Damaged Brain of Iodine Deficiency*, ed. J. B. Stanbury, 195–200. New York: Communication Corporation.

Borghi, J., L. Guinness, J. Ouedraogo, and V. Curtis. 2002. "Is Hygiene Promotion Cost-Effective? A Case Study in Burkina Faso." *Tropical Medicine and International Health* 7 (11): 960–69.

Brown, K. H., K. G. Dewey, and L. H. Allen. 1998. *Complementary Feeding of Young Children in Developing Countries: A Review of Current Scientific Knowledge.* WHO/NUT/98.1. Geneva: World Health Organization.

Brown, K. H., J. M. Peerson, J. Rivera, and L. H. Allen. 2002. "Effect of Supplemental Zinc on the Growth and Serum Zinc Concentrations of Prepubertal Children: A Meta-Analysis of Randomized Controlled Trials." *American Journal of Clinical Nutrition* 75 (6): 1062–71.

Caballero, B. 2001. "Early Nutrition and Risk of Disease in the Adult." *Public Health Nutrition* 4 (6A): 1335–36.

Caulfield, L. E., and R. E. Black. 2004. "Zinc Deficiency." In *Comparative Quantification of Health Risks: Global and Regional Burden of Disease Attributable to Selected Major Risk Factors*, ed. M. Ezzati, A. D. Lopez, A. Rodgers, and C. J. L. Murray, vol. 1, 257–9. Geneva: World Health Organization.

Caulfield, L. E., S. L. Huffman, and E. G. Piwoz. 1999. "Interventions to Improve the Complementary Food Intakes of 6–12 Month Old Infants in Developing Countries: Impact on Growth, Prevalence of Malnutrition, and Potential Contribution to Child Survival." *Food and Nutrition Bulletin* 20 (2): 183–200.

Caulfield, L. E., S. A. Richard, and R. E. Black. 2004. "Undernutrition as an Underlying Cause of Malaria Morbidity and Mortality in Children." *American Journal of Tropical Medicine Hygiene* 71 (Suppl. 2): S55–63.

Checkley, W., P. R. Gilman, P. R. Black, L. D. Epstein, L. Cabrera, P. C. Sterling, and L. H. Moulton. 2004. "Effect of Water and Sanitation on Childhood Health in a Poor Peruvian Peri-Urban Community." *Lancet* 363 (9403): 112–18.

Chee, G., M. Makinen, and B. Sakagawa. 2002. *Cost and Effectiveness Analysis of LINKAGES' Breastfeeding Interventions in Ghana*. Bethesda, MD: Abt Associates.

Chee, G., K. Smith, M. Makinen, and Z. Rambeloson. 2003. *Cost and Effectiveness Analysis of LINKAGES' Infant and Young Child Feeding Program in Madagascar*. Bethesda, MD: Abt Associates.

Ching, P., M. Birmingham, T. Goodman, R. Sutter, and B. Loevinsohn. 2000. "Childhood Mortality Impact and Costs of Integrating Vitamin A Supplementation into Immunization Campaigns." *American Journal of Public Health* 90 (10): 1526–29.

Cobra, C., Muhilal, K. Rusmil, D. Rustama, Djatnika, S. S. Suwardi, and others. 1997. "Infant Survival Is Improved by Oral Iodine Supplementation." *Journal of Nutrition* 127 (4): 574–78.

Dary, O., and J. O. Mora. 2002. "Food Fortification to Reduce Vitamin A Deficiency: International Vitamin A Consultative Group Recommendations." *Journal of Nutrition* 132 (Suppl. 9): S2927–33.

Dewey, K. G. 2002. "Successful Intervention Programs to Promote Complementary Feeding." In *Public Health Issues in Infant and Child Nutrition*, Nestle Nutrition Workshop Series Pediatric Program, ed. R. E. Black and K. F. Michaelsen, vol. 48, 199–216. Philadelphia: Lippincott, Williams, and Wilkins.

Dewey, K. G., and K. H. Brown. 2003. "Update on Technical Issues Concerning Complementary Feeding of Young Children in Developing Countries and Implications for Intervention Programs." *Food and Nutrition Bulletin* 24 (1): 5–28.

Ezzati, M., A. D. Lopez, A. Rodgers, S. Vander Hoorn, C. J. Murray, and Comparative Risk Assessment Collaborating Group. 2002. "Selected Major Risk Factors and Global and Regional Burden of Disease." *Lancet* 360 (9343): 1342–43.

Fiedler, J. L. 2000. "The Nepal National Vitamin A Program: Prototype to Emulate or Donor Enclave?" *Health Policy Planning* 15 (2): 145–56.

———. 2003. *A Cost Analysis of the Honduras Community-Based Integrated Child Care Program*. Washington, DC: World Bank.

Fiedler, J. L., D. R. Dado, H. Maglalang, N. Juban, M. Capistrano, and M. V. Magpantay. 2000. "Cost Analysis as a Vitamin A Program Design and Evaluation Tool: A Case Study of the Philippines." *Social Science and Medicine* 51 (2): 223–42.

Fishman, S., L. Caulfield, M. de Onis, M. Blossner, A. Hyder, L. Mullany, and R. Black. 2004. "Childhood and Maternal Underweight." In *Comparative Quantification of Health Risks: Global and Regional Burden of Disease Attributable to Selected Major Risk Factors*, ed. M. Ezzati, A. D. Lopez, A. Rodgers, and C. J. L. Murray, . vol. 1, 39–162. Geneva: World Health Organization.

Gluckman, P. D., and M. A. Hanson. 2004. "Living with the Past: Evolution, Development, and Patterns of Disease." *Science* 305 (5691): 1733–36.

Grantham-McGregor, S. M., and C. C. Ani. 1999. "The Role of Micronutrients in Psychomotor and Cognitive Development." *British Medical Bulletin* 55 (3): 511–27.

Haddad, L. J., and H. E. Bouis. 1991. "The Impact of Nutritional Status on Agricultural Productivity: Wage Evidence from the Philippines." *Oxford Bulletin of Economics and Statistics*. 53: 45–68.

Hetzel, B. S. 1983. "Iodine Deficiency Disorders (IDD) and Their Eradication." *Lancet* 2 (8359): 1126–29.

———. 1989. "The Prevention and Control of Iodine Deficiency Disorders." Nutrition Policy Discussion Paper 3, United Nations, New York.

Hill, Z., B. Kirkwood, and K. Edmond. 2004. *Family and Community Practices That Promote Child Survival, Growth, and Development: A Review of the Evidence*. Geneva: World Health Organization.

Horton, S., T. Sanghvi, M. Phillips, J. Fiedler, R. Perez-Escamilla, C. Lutter, and others. 1996. "Breastfeeding Promotion and Priority Setting in Health." *Health Policy and Planning* 11 (2): 56–68.

Institute of Medicine. 1998. *Prevention of Micronutrient Deficiencies: Tools for Policy Makers and Public Health Workers*. Washington, DC: National Academy Press.

International Zinc Nutrition Consultative Group. 2004. "Developing Zinc Intervention Programs." *Food and Nutrition Bulletin* 24 (1): 163–86.

Jamison, D. T., J. Leslie, and P. Musgrove. 2003. "Malnutrition and Dietary Protein: Evidence from China and from International Comparisons." *Food and Nutrition Bulletin* 24 (2): 145–54.

Jones, G., R. W. Steketee, R. E. Black, Z. A. Bhutta, and S. S. Morris. 2003. "How Many Child Deaths Can We Prevent This Year?" *Lancet* 362 (9377): 65–71.

Kapil, U. 2002. "Integrated Child Development Services (ICDS) Scheme: A Program for Holistic Development of Children in India." *Indian Journal of Pediatrics* 69 (7): 597–601.

Lengeler, C. 2004. "Insecticide-Treated Bednets and Curtains for Preventing Malaria." *Cochrane Library* (2) CD000363.

Martorell, R. 1996. "The Role of Nutrition in Economic Development." *Nutrition Reviews* 54 (4 Part 2): S66–71.

PAHO and WHO (Pan American Health Organization and World Health Organization). 2003. *Guiding Principles for Complementary Feeding of the Breastfed Child*. Washington, DC: PAHO and WHO.

Pelletier, D. L., E. A. Frongillo Jr., and J. P. Habicht. 1993. "Epidemiologic Evidence for a Potentiating Effect of Malnutrition on Child Mortality." *American Journal of Public Health*. 83 (8): 1130–33.

Pollitt, E., K. S. Gorman, P. L. Engle, J. A. Rivera, and R. Martorell. 1995. "Nutrition in Early Life and the Fulfillment of Intellectual Potential." *Journal of Nutrition* 125 (Suppl. 4): S1111–18.

Ramakrishnan, U., N. Aburto, G. McCabe, and R. Martorell. 2004. "Multimicronutrient Interventions but Not Vitamin A or Iron Interventions Alone Improve Child Growth: Results from Three Meta-Analyses." *Journal of Nutrition* 134 (10): 2592–602.

Rassas, R., J. K. Hottor, O. A. Anerkai, M. M. Kwame, M. M. Agble, A. Nyaku, and T. Taylor. 2004. *Cost Analysis of the National Vitamin A Program in Ghana*. Arlington, VA: International Science and Technology Institute.

Rassas, R., P. M. Nakamba, C. M. Mwela, R. Mutemwa, B. Mulenga, W. Siamusantu, and T. Taylor. 2004. *Cost Analysis of the National Vitamin A Program in Zambia*. Arlington, VA: International Science and Technology Institute.

Rice, A. L., K. P. West Jr., and R. E. Black. 2004. "Vitamin A Deficiency." In *Comparative Quantification of Health Risks: Global and Regional Burden of Disease Attributable to Selected Major Risk Factors*, ed. M. Ezzati, A. D. Lopez, A. Rodgers, and C. J. L. Murray, vol. 1, 211–56. Geneva: World Health Organization.

Rivera, J. A., and A. J. Sepulveda. 2003. "Conclusions from the Mexican National Nutrition Survey 1999: Translating Results into Nutrition Policy." *Salud Publica Mexico*. 45 (Suppl. 4): S565–75.

Rivera, J. A., D. Sotres-Alvarez, J. P. Habicht, T. Shamah, and S. Villalpando. 2004. "Impact of the Mexican Program for Education, Health, and Nutrition (Progresa) on Rates of Growth and Anemia in Infants and Young Children: A Randomized Effectiveness Study." *Journal of the American Medical Association* 291 (21): 2563–70.

Robberstad, B., T. Strand, R. E. Black, and H. Sommerfelt. 2004. "Cost-Effectiveness of Zinc as Adjunct Therapy for Acute Childhood Diarrhea in Developing Countries." *Bulletin of the World Health Organization* 82 (7): 523–31.

Ross, D. A. 2002. "Recommendations for Vitamin A Supplementation." *Journal of Nutrition* 132 (Suppl. 9): S2902–6.

Ross, J. S. 1997. *Cost-Effectiveness of the Nutrition Communication Project in Mali*. Washington, DC: Academy for Educational Development.

Ross, S. M., W. E. Loening, and B. E. Mbele. 1987. "Breast-Feeding Support." *South African Medical Journal* 72 (5): 357–58.

Ruel, M. T., and H. E. Bouis. 1998. "Plant Breeding: A Long-Term Strategy for the Control of Zinc Deficiency in Vulnerable Populations." *American Journal of Clinical Nutrition* 68 (Suppl. 2): S488–94.

Ruel, M. T., and C. Levin. 2000. *Assessing the Potential for Food-Based Strategies to Alleviate Vitamin A and Iron Deficiencies: A Review of Recent Evidence.* Discussion paper 92, International Food Policy Research Institute, Washington, DC.

Shankar, A. H., and A. S. Prasad. 1998. "Zinc and Immune Function: The Biological Basis of Altered Resistance to Infection." *American Journal of Clinical Nutrition* 68 (Suppl. 2): S447–63.

Sikorski, J., M. J. Renfrew, S. Pindoria, and A. Wade. 2002. "Support for Breastfeeding Mothers." Cochrane Database System Reviews (1): CD001141.

Solon, F. S., J. N. Sarol, A. B. I. Bernardo, J. A. A. Solon, H. Mehansho, L. E. Sanchez-Fermin, and others. 2003. "Effect of a Multiple-Micronutrient Fortified Fruit Powder Beverage on the Nutrition Status, Physical Fitness, and Cognitive Performance of Schoolchildren in the Philippines." *Food and Nutrition Bulletin* 24 (Suppl. 4): S129–40.

Sommer, A., and K. P. West. 1996. *Vitamin A Deficiency Health, Survival, and Vision.* New York: Oxford University Press.

Stoltzfus, R. J., and M. L. Dreyfuss. 1998. *Guidelines for the Use of Iron Supplements to Prevent and Treat Iron Deficiency Anemia.* Washington, DC: ILSI Press.

Stoltzfus, R. J., L. Mullany, and R. E. Black. 2004. "Iron Deficiency Anemia." In *Comparative Quantification of Health Risks: Global and Regional Burden of Disease Attributable to Selected Major Risk Factors,* ed. M. Ezzati, A. D. Lopez, A. Rodgers, and C. J. L. Murray, vol. 1, 163–209. Geneva: World Health Organization.

Swindale, A., M. Deitchler, B. Cogill, and T. Marchione. 2004. "The Impact of Title II Maternal and Child Health and Nutrition Programs on the Nutritional Status of Children." Occasional Paper 4, Academy for Educational Development, Washington, DC.

Victora, C. G., J. P. Habicht, and J. Bryce. 2004. "Evidence-Based Public Health: Moving Beyond Randomized Trials." *American Journal of Public Health* 94 (3): 400–5.

WHO (World Health Organization). 1999. *Progress Towards Elimination of Iodine Deficiency Disorders.* WHO/NHD/99.4. Geneva: WHO.

———. 2002. *World Health Report 2002: Reducing Risks, Promoting Healthy Life.* Geneva: WHO.

WHO and UNICEF (United Nations Children's Fund). 2004. *WHO/UNICEF Joint Statement on the Clinical Management of Acute Diarrhea.* WHO/FCH/CAH/04.7. Geneva: WHO and UNICEF.

WHO, UNICEF, and ICCIDD (International Council for the Control of Iodine Deficiency Disorders). 2001. *Assessment of the Iodine Deficiency Disorders and Monitoring Their Elimination.* WHO/NHD/01.1. Geneva: WHO.

World Bank. 1994. *Enriching Lives: Overcoming Vitamin and Mineral Malnutrition in Developing Countries.* Washington, DC: World Bank.

Yip, R., and U. Ramakrishnan. 2002. "Experiences and Challenges in Developing Countries." *Journal of Nutrition* 132 (Suppl. 4): S827–30.

Zinc Investigators' Collaborative Group, Z. A. Bhutta, S. M. Bird, R. E. Black, K. H. Brown, J. M. Gardner, and others. 2000. "Therapeutic Effects of Oral Zinc in Acute and Persistent Diarrhea in Children in Developing Countries: Pooled Analysis of Randomized Controlled Trials." *American Journal of Clinical Nutrition* 72 (6): 1516–22.

Zinc Investigators' Collaborative Group, Z. A. Bhutta, R. E. Black, K. H. Brown, J. M. Gardner, S. Gore, and others. 1999. "Prevention of Diarrhea and Pneumonia by Zinc Supplementation in Children in Developing Countries: Pooled Analysis of Randomized Controlled Trials." *Journal of Pediatrics* 135 (6): 689–97.

Zlotkin, S., P. Arthur, C. Schauer, K. Y. Antwi, G. Yeung, and A. Piekarz. 2003. "Home-Fortification with Iron and Zinc Sprinkles or Iron Sprinkles Alone Successfully Treats Anemia in Infants and Young Children." *Journal of Nutrition* 133 (4): 1075–80.

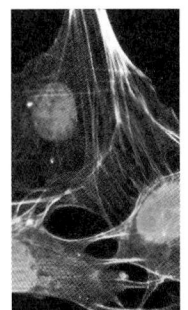

Chapter **29**

Health Service Interventions for Cancer Control in Developing Countries

Martin L. Brown, Sue J. Goldie, Gerrit Draisma, Joe Harford, and Joseph Lipscomb

INTRODUCTION

Cancer imposes a major disease burden worldwide, with considerable geographic variations in incidence; mortality; survival; overall disease burden; causative environmental factors; and mix of prevention, detection, treatment, and palliative programs that make up a country's cancer control strategy. Unless cancer prevention and screening interventions effectively reduce the incidence of cancer, the number of new cancer cases will increase from an estimated 10 million cases in 2000 to 15 million in 2020, 9 million of which would be in developing countries. By 2050, the cancer burden could reach 24 million cases per year worldwide, with 17 million cases occurring in developing countries (Parkin, Bray, and Devesa 2001).

Researchers have made numerous efforts to quantify the global burden of cancer and to estimate site-specific cancer mortality and morbidity (see, for example, Ferlay and others 2004; Parkin, Bray, and Devesa 2001). A recent report from the International Agency for Research on Cancer provides estimates of cancer incidence for Africa by site and country (Parkin and others 2003). In general, however, data on cancer incidence, prevalence, and mortality are less complete and less accurate in developing countries than in developed countries, because the latter have more resources to invest in population-based cancer registries and the infrastructure to maintain such registries.

Despite the limitations of current data for developing countries, the epidemiology of cancer in developing countries clearly differs from that in developed countries in some important respects. Developed countries often have relatively high rates of lung, colorectal, breast, and prostate cancer because of the earlier onset of the tobacco epidemic, the earlier exposure to occupational carcinogens, and the Western diet and lifestyle in such countries. In contrast, up to one-fourth of cancers in developing countries are associated with chronic infections. Liver cancer is often causally associated with infection by the hepatitis B virus (HBV), cervical cancer is associated with infection by certain types of human papillomavirus (HPV), and stomach cancer is associated with *Helicobacter pylori* infection.

This chapter focuses on interventions for controlling seven cancers that impose a particularly heavy burden of disease on developing countries: cervical cancer, liver cancer, stomach cancer, esophageal cancer, lung cancer, colorectal cancer, and breast cancer. In 2000, these seven types of cancer accounted for approximately 60 percent of all newly diagnosed cancer cases and cancer deaths in developing countries (Ferlay and others 2001). Four of the seven cancers—cervical, liver, stomach, and esophageal—have elevated incidence and mortality rates in developing countries. The other three—lung, colorectal, and breast—have lower incidence and mortality rates than the other four cancers, but they nonetheless impose a heavy disease burden and are increasing because of demographic and industrial transitions. Pediatric cancers and HIV-related cancers, two topics that are of great importance and concern, are beyond the scope of this chapter.

BURDEN OF CANCER IN DEVELOPING COUNTRIES

Data from Ferlay and others (2004) clearly illustrate the differing patterns of cancer incidence in developing and developed

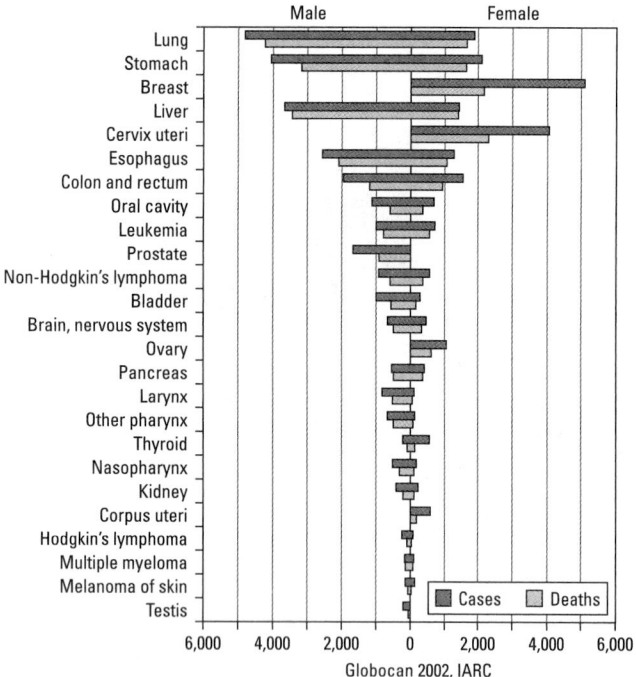

Source: Ferlay and others 2004.

Figure 29.1 Estimated Number of Cancer Cases of All Ages, Developing Regions, 2002
(hundreds)

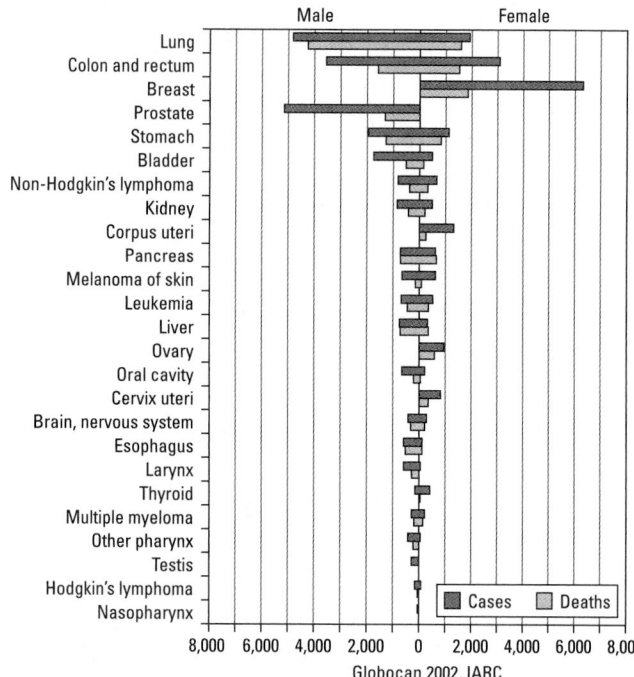

Source: Ferlay and others 2004.

Figure 29.2 Number of Cancer Cases of All Ages, Developed Regions, 2002
(hundreds)

countries (figures 29.1 and 29.2). In developing countries, the top five female cancers in rank order of incidence are breast, cervical, stomach, lung, and colorectal cancer; however, cervical cancer still accounts for more deaths than breast cancer in developing countries. The top five male cancers are lung, stomach, liver, esophageal, and colorectal cancer (figure 29.1). The incidence of cancers of the lung and breast is relatively high in both developed and developing countries. Colorectal cancer accounts for a smaller share of the burden in developing countries than in developed countries, but cancer of the stomach accounts for a higher share. Some cancers that are more common in developing than in developed countries, including stomach, liver, and cervical cancer, are related to the absence of a well-developed public health infrastructure for the control of cancer-causing infectious agents and contaminants, the lack of basic preventive health care and screening services for much of the population, and the poor-quality diets available to the most economically disadvantaged members of society in many developing countries. Cancer of the esophagus, also relatively common in developing countries, may reflect, in part, the consumption of traditional beverages at extremely high temperatures. Some cancers that are increasingly common in developing countries, including lung, breast, and colorectal cancer, may reflect the increasing Westernization of lifestyles, longer life expectancy, and globalization of markets for tobacco products.

For some cancers, including esophageal, liver, lung, and pancreatic cancer, survival rates vary little between developing and developed countries (Sankaranarayanan, Black, and Parkin 1998). Currently available methods of early detection and treatment have not been demonstrated to be effective for these cancers, so primary prevention remains the most practical intervention for control. For a second group of cancers, including large bowel, breast, ovarian, and cervical cancer, proven methods of early detection, diagnosis, and treatment are available that can, in principle, be delivered through district health care facilities. For these cancers, survival rates vary both between developing and developed countries as a whole and between specific countries within each of these groups. For a third group of cancers, including testicular cancer, leukemia, and lymphoma, the variability in survival between developing and developed countries is tremendous. Even though relatively effective treatments are available for these cancers, they are multimodal treatments that require a relatively high level of medical resources, a good health care infrastructure, and a level of sophisticated knowledge, which low- and middle-income developing countries may not have.

Table 29.1 shows estimated cancer deaths and the estimated disease burden in terms of disability-adjusted life years (DALYs) lost as a result of various types of cancers in developing and developed countries and by region in 2001. As the table

Table 29.1 Number of Cancer Deaths and DALYs Lost to Cancer, by World Bank Region and Country Income Level, 2001

Cancer site	East Asia and the Pacific		Europe and Central Asia		Latin America and the Caribbean		Middle East and North Africa		South Asia		Sub-Saharan Africa		Low- and middle-income countries		High-income countries	
	Deaths	DALYs lost	Deaths	DALYs lost	Deaths	DALYs lost	Deaths	DALYs lost	Deaths	DALYs lost	Deaths	DALYs lost	Deaths	DALYs lost	Deaths	DALYs lost
Trachea, bronchus, and lung cancers	387,000	5,333,000	165,000	2,323,000	55,000	728,000	20,000	283,000	129,000	1,807,000	15,000	225,000	771,000	10,701,000	456,000	5,397,000
Stomach cancer	442,000	6,134,000	101,000	1,376,000	57,000	735,000	18,000	252,000	45,000	629,000	33,000	487,000	696,000	9,616,000	146,000	1,628,000
Liver cancer	373,000	5,923,000	28,000	379,000	21,000	277,000	9,000	138,000	27,000	464,000	46,000	762,000	505,000	7,945,000	102,000	1,223,000
Esophageal cancer	232,000	3,217,000	21,000	288,000	16,000	215,000	5,000	72,000	80,000	1,116,000	24,000	343,000	380,000	5,252,000	58,000	702,000
Colorectal cancer	159,000	2,334,000	96,000	1,290,000	37,000	485,000	10,000	164,000	35,000	499,000	20,000	291,000	357,000	5,060,000	257,000	3,175,000
Breast cancer	93,000	1,730,000	63,000	1,058,000	37,000	642,000	14,000	273,000	76,000	1,246,000	34,000	574,000	317,000	5,527,000	155,000	2,509,000
Mouth and oropharyngeal cancers	66,000	1,064,000	27,000	426,000	14,000	204,000	5,000	78,000	140,000	2,020,000	19,000	284,000	271,000	4,078,000	41,000	576,000
Cervix uteri cancer	47,000	805,000	19,000	356,000	26,000	494,000	5,000	93,000	83,000	1,423,000	38,000	627,000	218,000	3,799,000	17,000	319,000
Lymphomas and multiple myeloma	42,000	753,000	23,000	375,000	24,000	383,000	12,000	232,000	82,000	1,401,000	34,000	622,000	216,000	3,770,000	115,000	1,362,000
Leukemia	76,000	1,652,000	27,000	462,000	22,000	444,000	14,000	307,000	38,000	851,000	14,000	245,000	190,000	3,965,000	73,000	919,000
Prostate cancer	16,000	164,000	25,000	283,000	37,000	340,000	6,000	64,000	21,000	210,000	40,000	416,000	145,000	1,479,000	119,000	1,212,000
Pancreatic cancer	37,000	544,000	35,000	481,000	20,000	248,000	4,000	55,000	13,000	176,000	8,000	117,000	117,000	1,621,000	110,000	1,232,000
Bladder cancer	30,000	348,000	24,000	300,000	9,000	100,000	15,000	214,000	30,000	408,000	10,000	133,000	117,000	1,504,000	59,000	670,000
Ovarian cancer	25,000	464,000	21,000	350,000	9,000	152,000	2,000	42,000	21,000	327,000	9,000	152,000	86,000	1,488,000	46,000	651,000
Corpus uteri cancer	8,000	175,000	17,000	349,000	12,000	254,000	1,000	22,000	4,000	66,000	3,000	41,000	44,000	908,000	27,000	586,000
Melanoma and other skin cancers	5,000	66,000	11,000	160,000	7,000	97,000	1,000	19,000	3,000	41,000	8,000	118,000	35,000	501,000	30,000	409,000
Other malignant neoplasms	104,000	1,640,000	123,000	1,901,000	82,000	1,263,000	26,000	440,000	26,000	1,444,000	55,000	844,000	490,000	7,538,000	257,000	3,316,000
Total (all malignant neoplasms)	2,142,000	32,346,000	826,000	12,157,000	485,000	7,061,000	167,000	2,748,000	853,000	14,128,000	410,000	6,281,000	4,955,000	74,752,000	2,068,000	25,886,000

Source: Mathers and others 2006.
Note: For an explanation of how DALYs are computed, see chapter 15 of this volume.

shows, the seven types of cancer that are the focus of this chapter account for seven of the first eight cancer sites ranked by number of deaths in developing countries. Considerable heterogeneity in the pattern of cancer burden across the six regions is apparent, and additional heterogeneity is apparent within these regions. Deaths from liver cancer are relatively high in East Asia and the Pacific and in Sub-Saharan Africa, probably because of the high prevalence of chronic HBV infection and the lack of adequate resources for food storage and preservation in those regions (Parkin and others 2003). The number of deaths from colorectal and breast cancer, as a proportion of all cancer deaths, is relatively high in Europe and Central Asia and in Latin America and the Caribbean, probably because those regions have increasingly adopted more Western lifestyle patterns of reproductive behavior, diet, and physical activity. The number of deaths from oral cancer is particularly high in South Asia, where the use of betel quid is common.

TYPES OF INTERVENTIONS FOR CANCER CONTROL

The World Health Organization (WHO) emphasizes that, when developing national strategies for controlling cancer, countries should consider the following four broad approaches (WHO 2002):

- *Primary prevention.* The goal of primary prevention is to reduce or eliminate exposure to cancer-causing factors, which include environmental carcinogens and lifestyle factors related to nutrition and physical activity. For the seven cancers considered here, approaches to primary prevention include immunization against, or treatment of, infectious agents that cause certain cancers; use of tobacco control programs; reduction of excessive alcohol consumption; dietary intervention; and pharmacological intervention.
- *Early detection and secondary prevention.* The main objective of early detection or secondary prevention through population-based screening programs is detection at a stage at which curative treatment is possible. Interventions for the early detection of cancer can help reduce mortality from cancer only if they are part of a wider cancer control strategy that includes effective diagnostic follow-up procedures and treatment (Anderson and others 2003). For cervical, colorectal, and breast cancer, effective methods of early detection and treatment are available, but their implementation has been uneven (Sankaranarayanan, Black, and Parkin 1998).
- *Diagnosis and treatment.* The primary modalities of cancer treatment are surgery, chemotherapy, and radiotherapy, and these modalities may be used alone or in combination.

There is increasing emphasis worldwide on the development of specialized cancer centers that apply evidence-based multimodal therapies, including rehabilitation and palliative care.

- *Palliative care.* The scope of palliative care has been expanded in recent years to encompass the alleviation of symptoms and treatment during all phases of disease—from diagnosis to death—and to address matters related to the psychological and quality-of-life aspects of disease, as well as the physiological aspects. Furthermore, palliative care has been expanded to include consideration for the well-being of the patient's family members as well as for the patient (Singer and Bowman 2002).

The discussion in this chapter focuses primarily on health service interventions for controlling the seven cancers that are the subject of this chapter. Other chapters deal with broad public health interventions involving the control of occupational and environmental exposures; health education; policy interventions such as regulation, labeling, and taxation related to tobacco consumption; diet; and physical activity.

COST-EFFECTIVENESS OF CANCER CONTROL INTERVENTIONS

There is a growing literature on the cost-effectiveness of interventions within each of the four categories above. In this section, we review published studies of the cost-effectiveness of health services–based cancer control interventions, and we present new analyses of the cost-effectiveness of screening interventions for cervical and breast cancer.

Primary Prevention

This subsection reviews studies of the effectiveness and cost-effectiveness of several interventions for the primary prevention of cancer.

Immunization against—or Treatment of—Infectious Agents That Cause Certain Cancers. Infectious agents are causally associated with three of the seven cancers that are the focus of this chapter—liver cancer (HBV), cervical cancer (HPV infection), and stomach cancer (*H. pylori* infection)—so eliminating these agents through immunization or other means offers hope for preventing such cancers.

The HBV vaccine was designed to prevent liver cancer and is currently the only such vaccine in widespread use. Long-term protection against acute and chronic infection has been demonstrated with the HBV vaccine in a wide range of settings (Coursaget and others 1994; Viviani and others 1999), and recent data support a reduction in hepatocellular carcinoma (Lee, Hsieh, and Ko 2003).

Infection with specific high-risk types of HPV plays a key role in causing cervical cancer. A double-blind placebo-controlled trial of an HPV 16 vaccine reported encouraging efficacy results in young female volunteers who had been fully vaccinated (three doses of vaccine or placebo) over a 1.7-year follow-up period (Koutsky and others 2002). In a more recent study, a bivalent HPV 16/18 vaccine prevented approximately 95 percent of persistent infections with HPV 16 and 18 (Harper and others 2004).

Several modeling studies have explored the potential benefits of HPV vaccination at the population level (Goldie and others 2003; Hughes, Garnett, and Koutsky 2002; Kulasingam and Myers 2003) and have elucidated several priorities for future research, including a better understanding of the heterogeneity of vaccine response and the effects of type-specific vaccination on other HPV types.

Hughes, Garnett, and Koutsky (2002) evaluate the potential effectiveness of HPV vaccination using a dynamic transmission model and find that, when both men and women were vaccinated—assuming 90 percent coverage, 75 percent effectiveness, and 10-year immunity—type-specific HPV prevalence was reduced by 44 percent. When only women were vaccinated, the reduction was 30 percent. The authors show that, if the vaccine targeted only certain types of high-risk HPV, cervical cancer incidence was not reduced proportionally because other high-risk types of HPV progressed to invasive cancer.

Goldie and others (2003) assess the impact of a type-specific HPV 16/18 vaccine calibrated to population-based data for Costa Rica. They find that a vaccine that prevented 98 percent of persistent HPV 16/18 was associated with an approximate equivalent reduction in HPV 16/18–associated cancer and a 51 percent reduction in total cervical cancer. The effect on total cancer was attenuated because of the competing risks associated with oncogenic types of HPV other than HPV 16/18.

Three studies have evaluated the potential cost-effectiveness of HPV vaccination in countries with cervical cancer screening programs (Goldie, Kohli, and others 2004; Kulasingam and Myers 2003; Sanders and Taira 2003). In general, these studies indicate that a program of HPV vaccination that permits a later age of screening initiation and a less frequent screening interval is likely to be a cost-effective use of health care resources in developed countries.

In Fujian province, China, a region of high mortality attributable to stomach cancer, a recently completed randomized controlled trial of *H. pylori* eradication with antibiotics provides some evidence that this approach may be effective in preventing stomach cancer in the subgroup of *H. pylori* carriers without precancerous lesions at the time of treatment (Wong and others 2004). A recent randomized trial of *H. pylori* eradication in Chiapas, Mexico, which used preneoplastic conditions as surrogate markers for the development of gastric cancer, found some evidence for the effectiveness of this treatment (Ley and others 2004).

Several studies, most of them in developed countries, have assessed the potential cost-effectiveness of screening individuals for infection with *H. pylori* and then eradicating *H. pylori* with antibiotic therapy as a means of preventing the later occurrence of stomach cancer. Roderick and others (2003) examine the cost-effectiveness of an *H. pylori* screening program conducted in the United Kingdom. Discounting costs and benefits at 6 percent, they find that the cost-effectiveness ratio for screening for *H. pylori*, initiated at age 40, is approximately US$28,000 per year of life saved (YLS). Optimal cost-effectiveness was not achieved until the *H. pylori* screening program had run for at least 40 years. Harris and others (1999) estimate the cost-effectiveness ratio associated with one-time screening for *H. pylori* at age 50 to be approximately US$50,000 per YLS (in 1995 dollars, 3 percent discount rate) when treatment for *H. pylori* infection results in a 15 percent reduction in stomach cancer risk. Assuming a 30 percent reduction, the figure was US$25,000 per YLS for the United States, but only a few hundred dollars per YLS in Colombia, which has a much higher rate of stomach cancer and lower health care costs.

Tobacco and Alcohol Control Programs. Tobacco consumption is the most important cause of lung and other cancers of the respiratory system, as well as of esophageal cancer, and may be a contributing factor for several other cancers. The most effective national tobacco control programs combine health promotion, education, and health service interventions with policies. Policy instruments include regulating tobacco advertising and promotion; enacting smoking bans in workplaces, restaurants, and public buildings and on public transportation; and increasing excise taxes on tobacco products (Fiore, Hatsukami, and Baker 2002; WHO 2002). Decreased rates of smoking uptake by children and adolescents would result in the greatest potential gain in life years. The WHO Framework Convention on Tobacco Control (WHO 2003b) summarizes tobacco control policies and programs related to regulation, taxation, and education. Da Costa e Silva (2003) shows prioritized treatment approaches for tobacco cessation, based on countries' levels of resources.

Excessive alcohol use accounts for 20 to 30 percent of liver and esophageal cancer (WHO 2001b). Interventions to reduce excessive consumption of alcohol have many principles in common with tobacco control, including the effectiveness of regulatory and taxation measures along with health promotion and addiction treatment programs.

Dietary and Related Interventions. The dietary ingestion of substances produced by the mold *Aspergillus flavus*, specifically aflatoxin B1, is causally associated with hepatocellular carcinoma. Exposure to aflatoxins may be synergistic with HBV infection in the development of this cancer. Effective means are available for preventing the contamination of grains and other types of food with aflatoxin during the growth, harvest, storage, and processing of such products (Kensler and others 2003; Turner and others 2002). Furthermore, chlorophyllin supplements have been found to reduce the carcinogenic properties of aflatoxin. That finding provides additional evidence for current dietary guidelines that meals should contain foods rich in chlorophylls—for example, spinach and other green, leafy vegetables (Kensler and others 2003).

Among those infected with *H. pylori,* diet is thought to play a critical role in the progression of superficial gastritis to chronic atrophic gastritis. Prolonged consumption of foods rich in salted, pickled, and smoked products increases the risk of stomach cancer, and increased consumption of fresh fruit and vegetables likely decreases the risk. Obesity is also a well-established risk factor for several cancers (Vainio and Bianchini 2002b). For that reason, WHO recommends that governments seeking to ensure compliance with nutritional objectives conduct appropriate school and public education campaigns on diet and work with the food and agriculture sectors (WHO 2002).

Pharmacological Interventions. *Chemoprevention* is defined as the reduction of the risk of cancer development through the use of micronutrients or pharmaceuticals. Clinical trials among high-risk individuals to establish the efficacy of chemoprevention via micronutrients (for instance, carotenoids and retinoids) and dietary fiber have been mainly negative (Alberts and others 2000; ATBC 1994; Omenn and others 1996; Schatzkin and others 2000). However, several ongoing clinical studies are examining the potential cancer preventive effects of calcium, vitamin D, folic acid, selenium, and vitamin E (Christensen 2004).

Both case-control and cohort studies show a reduced risk for colorectal cancer after prolonged use of aspirin (Vainio and Morgan 1999). Additional evidence indicates that aspirin has a preventive effect on several other types of cancer, including hormone receptor–positive breast cancer (Terry and others 2004), but questions remain about the balance between the clinical benefits and adverse side effects of long-term aspirin therapy, including gastrointestinal bleeding and hemorrhagic stroke (Imperiale 2003).

Some evidence suggests that the antiestrogen drug tamoxifen may reduce the risk of breast cancer (Gail and others 1999), but there is also conflicting evidence (Powles and others 1998; Veronesi and others 1998). The potential for primary prevention using other selective estrogen receptor modulators is a topic of current clinical research (Lippman, Lee, and Sabichi 1998). Preliminary analyses indicate that the use of tamoxifen to prevent breast cancer could be cost-effective in the United States (T. Smith and Hillner 2000).

Early Detection and Secondary Prevention

This subsection looks at studies of the effectiveness and cost-effectiveness of several interventions for the early detection and secondary prevention of cancer.

Screening for Liver Cancer. Screening methods for early detection of liver cancer include serum assays for alpha-fetoprotein and, potentially, ultrasound. A recently completed randomized controlled trial of liver cancer screening in China evaluated the use of two or six alpha-fetoprotein assays over a period of four years among men age 30 to 69 with chronic HBV (Chen and others 2003). Screening resulted in earlier diagnosis of liver cancer, but because treatment for established liver cancer is largely ineffective, screening did not reduce overall mortality.

Randomized trials that include ultrasound screening for liver cancer and that incorporate recent advances in antiviral preventive treatment have yet to be conducted. Sarasin, Giostra, and Hadengue's (1996) model-based cost-effectiveness analysis explores whether biannual screening of patients with Child-Pugh class A cirrhosis, under a set of assumptions systematically favorable to screening, would be cost-effective. The authors conclude that, even under best-case conditions, screening for liver cancer is not likely to be cost-effective.

Screening for Stomach Cancer. Mass screening programs for the early detection of invasive stomach cancer using radiological or endoscopic techniques have been widely implemented in Japan, where incidence rates of stomach cancer are high.

Babazono and Hillman (1995) compare the cost-effectiveness of three methods for the early detection of stomach cancer in the context of mass screening programs in Japan: indirect radiology (barium meal plus photofluoroscopy), direct radiology, and endoscopy. When screening for stomach cancer was started late in life, indirect radiology was the most cost-effective screening method. This analysis supports an increase in the recommended age for initiating screening for stomach cancer from age 40 to 50.

Screening for Lung Cancer. Investigators have carried out several cost-effectiveness analyses of the screening of high-risk individuals, such as current and former smokers, for lung cancer using helical computed tomography (Chirikos and others 2002; Mahadevia and others 2003; Marshall and others 2001). The results of these studies vary widely from quite favorable (US$19,000 per YLS) to extremely unfavorable (more than US$100,000 per YLS). The main reason for the wide variation in these studies is different assumptions about the clinical nature of early lung lesions detected by helical computed tomography—specifically, whether a large proportion of these

Table 29.2 Estimates of the Cost-Effectiveness of Colorectal Cancer Screening Interventions, United States
(cost-effectiveness ratios expressed as 2000 US$/YLS)

Colorectal screening test	Wagner and others 1996	Frazier and others 2000	Khandker and others 2000	Sonnenberg, Delco, and Inadomi 2000	Vijan and others 2001
Annual fecal occult blood test	11,725	17,805	13,656	10,463	5,691
Flexible sigmoidoscopy every 5 years	12,477	15,630	12,804	39,359	19,058
Flexible sigmoidoscopy every 5 years and annual fecal occult blood test	13,792	22,518	18,693	n.a.	17,942
Double-contrast barium enema every 5 years	11,168	21,712	25,624	n.a.	n.a.
Colonoscopy every 10 years	10,933	21,889	22,012	11,840	9,038

Source: Pignone and others 2002.
n.a. = not applicable.
Note: All costs and life years are discounted at 3 percent, except in the study by Wagner and others (1996), who use a discount rate of 5 percent.

small lung nodules represents "pseudo-disease" that will never progress to clinical lung cancer (Marcus and others 2000). The National Lung Cancer Screening Trial, currently under way (van Meerbeeck and Tournoy 2004), hopes to answer this question. Until results from the trial are available, no definitive statement can be made about the effectiveness or cost-effectiveness of lung cancer screening.

Screening for Colorectal Cancer. Screening methods for early detection of colorectal cancer include fecal occult blood testing, sigmoidoscopy, barium enema, and colonoscopy. Several studies of the cost-effectiveness of colorectal cancer screening in developed countries have been published (Pignone and others 2002). Table 29.2 presents estimates of the cost-effectiveness of colorectal cancer screening in the United States. Cost-effectiveness ratios for various modalities of colorectal cancer screening range from almost US$6,000 to about US$40,000 per YLS. Using models closely linked to European trials of biennial fecal occult blood testing to screen for colorectal cancer, Whynes and Nottingham Faecal Occult Blood Screening Trial (2004) report favorable cost-effectiveness ratios ranging from US$2,500 to US$4,000 per YLS. Studies of the cost-effectiveness of colorectal cancer screening in developed countries consistently conclude that such screening is cost-effective, but they do not totally agree on the relative rankings of different colorectal screening strategies (Pignone and others 2002).

Screening for Cervical Cancer. Cytology-based screening using the Papanicolaou smear has been the main screening method used for the secondary prevention of cervical cancer worldwide. In many low-income countries, however, cytology screening has proved difficult to sustain because of its reliance on highly trained cytotechnologists; good-quality laboratories; and infrastructure to support up to three visits for screening, evaluation of cytologic abnormalities with colposcopy, and treatment (Sankaranarayanan, Budukh, and Rajkumar 2001). Two alternative screening approaches replace the Pap smear

with simple visual screening methods, such as visual inspection after application of an acetic acid solution (VIA), or with HPV DNA testing (Denny and others 2000; Sankaranarayanan and others 1999; Schiffman and others 2000; Wright 2003; Wright and others 2000; Zimbabwe Project 1999). These newer options also eliminate colposcopy, potentially allowing screening and treatment to be performed during the same visit. In middle-income countries where cytology screening is available but cervical cancer mortality has not been reduced, key questions center around improving the quality of cytology-based programs; such improvement includes having adequate colposcopy and biopsy facilities and accessible treatment (Lazcano-Ponce and others 1999); making use of HPV DNA testing technology in a cost-effective manner; and targeting the appropriate age group for cervical cancer screening more accurately. The vast majority of published cost-effectiveness analyses of population-based cervical cancer screening performed during 1980–2003 focused on high-income countries. (A list of the 39 studies reviewed is available from the authors.) The detailed results of each study are somewhat difficult to compare. The types of costs included in each study varied substantially (patient time costs and programmatic costs often were omitted), studies frequently did not discount costs and benefits or did not note the discount rate used, and sensitivity analyses were not conducted consistently on all relevant variables. Despite those limitations, several themes emerge. The incremental cost-effectiveness of screening in the general population becomes increasingly less favorable as programs are intensified by shortening the screening interval. For example, Mandelblatt and others (2002) reported that for conventional cytology and HPV testing, compared with cytology alone, the incremental cost was more than US$300,000 when conducted annually compared to US$15,400 per YLS when conducted every 10 years. Maxwell and others (2002) reported that liquid-based cytology and HPV testing for equivocal results cost US$231,300 per YLS if conducted annually incremental to 14,300 per YLS if conducted every three years. Kim, Wright, and Goldie (2002) reported similar results for this same strategy (US$20,300 per YLS conducted every five years, US$59,600 per YLS every three years, and US$174,200 every two years). The analyses, which included strategies that employed both frequent screening and screening tests with higher sensitivity, often found the cost-effectiveness of frequent screening to be even less attractive. For example, Goldie, Kim, and Wright (2004) reported annual screening with combined cytology and HPV DNA testing in women over age 30 exceeded US$1 million per YLS compared to every two years. Although many analyses find that extending the age range to the very young, the very old, or both can be less cost-effective, for certain women in high-risk groups, including older, uninsured women who have never been screened, screening for cervical cancer at older ages can be cost-effective.

The analyses conducted in low-income countries focused on assessing the cost-effectiveness of an expanded set of strategies that included alternatives to conventional cytology. In addition, these analyses—unlike those in developed regions—often raised issues of feasibility, affordability, cultural context, accessibility, and equity.

In one of the earliest stochastic modeling evaluations of cervical cancer screening programs in developing regions, Sherlaw-Johnson, Gallivan, and Jenkins (1997) explored the effectiveness of cytology and HPV testing in the context of infrequent screening. They reported that the most efficient use of resources would be to concentrate cervical cancer screening efforts on women age 30 to 59 at least once per lifetime, because such blanket screening would reduce the incidence of invasive cervical cancer by up to 30 percent.

In an analysis focused on cervical cancer control in Vietnam, Suba and others (2001) reported that, because of the low direct medical costs associated with Vietnam's cervical cytology program, such a program appeared to be attractive for that country. They found that total costs to establish a nationwide Pap screening program based on five-year intervals averaged less than US$148,000 annually during the 10 years the authors assumed would be necessary to develop the program. Assuming 70 percent participation in the program, the authors found the cost-effectiveness ratio for cervical cytology screening, compared with no screening, to be US$725 per discounted YLS.

Goldie and others (2001) assessed the cost-effectiveness of several cervical cancer screening strategies in previously unscreened 30-year-old South African women. Screening tests included VIA, cytology, and HPV DNA testing. Strategies differed by the number of clinic visits required, frequency of screening and individual's age at the time of screening, and response to a positive test result. The authors found that when all strategies were considered to be equally available and were compared incrementally, HPV DNA testing was always more effective and less costly than cytology and generally more effec-

tive but more costly than VIA. They found that, in comparison with no screening, a single lifetime VIA screen at age 35, coupled with immediate treatment of women with positive results, resulted in a cost saving of US$39 per YLS as compared with a two-visit HPV, although programmatic costs were not considered. Using sensitivity analysis, the authors find the choice between using HPV DNA testing or VIA depended on the relative costs and sensitivity of the two tests and on the percentage of women lost to follow-up between the first and second visit.

Mandelblatt, Lawrence, Gaffikin, and others (2002) used a simulation model to compare seven cervical cancer screening techniques in Thailand. Comparing each strategy to the next less expensive alternative, the authors found that VIA performed at five-year intervals in women age 35 to 55, followed by immediate treatment of abnormalities, was the least expensive option and saved the greatest number of lives.

The Alliance for Cervical Cancer Prevention used primary data from studies conducted in India, Kenya, Peru, South Africa, and Thailand to develop a series of standardized, country-specific cost-effectiveness analyses. The costs and benefits associated with alternative strategies to reduce cervical cancer mortality were estimated for these five countries with different epidemiological profiles by integrating country-specific data from each site and using a standardized set of assumptions agreed on by an expert panel with experience in each country (Goldie, Gaffikin, and others 2004). In all five countries, lifetime cancer risk was reduced by approximately 25 to 35 percent with a single lifetime screen using either one-visit VIA or two-visit HPV DNA testing targeted at women age 35 to 40. Risk was reduced by more than 50 percent if screening was performed two or three times per lifetime. Although the cost of screening differed considerably between the countries, strategies were identified that, when performed two or three times per lifetime, would be considered extremely cost-effective depending on the individual country's per capita gross domestic product.

We conducted an exploratory analysis to evaluate the potential cost-effectiveness of cervical cancer screening strategies in Brazil, Madagascar, and Zimbabwe using computer-based simulation models calibrated to age-specific cervical cancer incidence and mortality in each country, along with published data. We evaluated once-in-a-lifetime screening between age 35 and 40 with (a) one-visit VIA, with screening and treatment conducted during the same visit; (b) two-visit HPV DNA screening, with HPV DNA testing during the first visit followed by treatment of screen-positive women during the second visit; and (c) three-visit cervical cytology screening, with a cytology sample obtained during the first visit, colposcopy for screen-positive women conducted during the second visit, and treatment provided during the third visit. We assumed that for the one- and two-visit strategies, women who screened positive and were eligible for cryotherapy were treated immediately, but

Table 29.3 Economic Outcomes of Once-in-a-Lifetime Cervical Cancer Screening Programs, Brazil, Madagascar, and Zimbabwe

Category	No screening	One-visit VIA	Two-visit HPV DNA testing	Three-visit cytology
Brazil				
Lifetime cost (international $)	68.41	75.08	77.43	121.12
Cost-effectiveness ratio (international $/YLS)*	n.a.	113	155	1430
Cost-effectiveness ratio (US$/YLS)	n.a.	54	118	572
Life expectancy gain per 1 million screened	n.a.	59,100	58,200	36,900
Number of deaths averted per 1 million screened	n.a.	10,399	10,235	6,411
Number of DALYs averted per 1 million screened	n.a.	56,646	55,751	35,174
Madagascar				
Lifetime cost (international $)	25.22	32.98	40.41	51.91
Cost-effectiveness ratio (international $/YLS)*	n.a.	167	332	921
Cost-effectiveness ratio (US$/YLS)	n.a.	52	162	368
Life expectancy gain per 1 million women screened	n.a.	46,500	45,800	29,000
Number of deaths averted per 1 million women screened	n.a.	8,815	8,676	5,438
Number of DALYs averted per 1 million women screened	n.a.	42,424	41,754	26,352
Zimbabwe				
Lifetime cost (international $)	31.10	39.69	44.81	61.93
Cost-effectiveness ratio (international $/YLS)*	n.a.	140	227	803
Cost-effectiveness ratio (US$/YLS)	n.a.	42	114	321
Life expectancy gain per 1 million screened	n.a.	61,300	60,400	38,400
Number of deaths averted per 1 million screened	n.a.	10,412	10,248	6,419
Number of DALYs averted per 1 million screened	n.a.	53,770	52,921	33,472

Source: Authors' calculations.
n.a. = not applicable.
*Converted from national currency, using purchasing power parity (PPP) exchange rates.

those ineligible for cryotherapy were referred for colposcopy and diagnostic workup.

We estimated direct medical costs using data from the literature and unit costs provided by the volume editors and WHO. All costs for the analysis are presented in 2000 dollars. We estimated patients' time costs and direct nonmedical costs using our own previous work and wage estimates based on World Bank data on per capita gross national income (WHO n.d.) and wage estimate regressions developed by the U.S. Department of Commerce. Table 29.3 presents the results of our analysis.

Lifetime costs per individual screened are given in international dollars. Cost-effectiveness ratios are provided in U.S. dollars as well as international dollars to facilitate comparison to other studies. The available data show that cervical cancer screening conducted once, twice, or three times in a lifetime can have a significant effect on the lifetime risk of cervical cancer compared with no screening. For countries with limited resources, screening efforts should target women age 35 or older; strategies should focus on screening all women at least once in their lifetime before increasing the frequency of screening; and countries should consider alternative approaches to the conventional three-visit cervical cytology screening techniques—for example, single-visit

VIA, followed by immediate treatment, or HPV DNA testing or cervical cytology followed by treatment at a second visit. Note that all screening tests may not be equally available in low-resource settings and that certain screening tests may be selected because of cultural preferences or for programmatic reasons. Implementing cervical cancer screening programs on the basis of VIA, HPV DNA testing, or cytology requires different types of resources, and the relative availability of these resources in different settings will affect the choice of strategy.

Screening for Breast Cancer. Methods for early detection of breast cancer include screening by mammography, clinical breast examination (CBE), and breast self-examination. Screening by mammography, CBE, or both may decrease breast cancer mortality, but uncertainty about the magnitude of the benefit remains because the quality of the evidence varies and results are inconsistent (Humphrey and others 2002). Recent controlled studies of organized breast self-examination programs indicate that this approach is not effective (Semiglazov and others 1999; Thomas and others 2002).

A randomized controlled trial of CBE screening for breast cancer began in Manila in 1995, but the intervention was discontinued after the first round because compliance with referral among women who were found to have a breast lump was extremely low (21 percent) and attempts to improve compliance failed. Analysis of the incidence of cancer cases in 1999 shows that the screening intervention succeeded in detecting more localized breast tumors, but the low compliance with referral and low yield of early cancers meant that the early detection program could not succeed in preventing deaths from breast cancer (International Agency for Research on Cancer n.d.).

Numerous cost-effectiveness studies of breast cancer screening programs have been conducted in developed countries (Vainio and Bianchini 2002a). Most cost-effectiveness studies of mammography screening in Europe yield cost-effectiveness ratios in the range of US$3,000 to US$10,000 per YLS, whereas those in the United States yield far less favorable cost-effectiveness ratios, ranging from US$20,000 to US$100,000 per YLS (table 29.4).

To investigate the potential cost-effectiveness of CBE and mammography for India, we used a microsimulation model of breast cancer screening (van Oortmarssen and others 1990). The model simulates individual life histories of disease states, and consequences of screening are calculated by comparing the histories with and without screening intervention for each individual. For our purposes, we assumed a population of 1 million Indian women with the age distribution of the country

Table 29.4 Estimates of the Cost-Effectiveness of Breast Cancer Screening Every Two Years for Women in Selected Developed Countries

Country	Age of women being screened (years)	Cost-effectiveness ratio (US$/YLS)[a]
Australia (de Koning 2000)	50–69	7,680
France (de Koning 2000)	50–69	4,580
Germany (de Koning 2000)	50–69	8,880
Netherlands (de Koning 2000)	50–69	3,140
Norway (Norum 1999)	50–69	14,790
Spain (de Koning 2000)	50–69	6,590
Spain, Catalonia (de Koning 2000)	50–69	4,400
Spain, Navarra (de Koning 2000)	45–65	2,450
United Kingdom (de Koning 2000)	50–69	2,680
United Kingdom (northwest) (de Koning 2000)	50–64	3,650
United States (M. Brown and Fintor 1993)	50–69	34,600
United States (Simpson and Snyder 1991)	50–64	20,611

Source: M. Brown and Fintor 1993; de Koning 2000; Norum 1999; Simpson and Snyder 1991.
Note: The discount rate used was 5 percent.
a. Converted from euros to U.S. dollars, using the exchange rate €1 = US$0.925.

in 2000 (United Nations Population Division 2003). We assumed that the screening program would last for 25 years and would have an attendance rate of 100 percent. We expressed the effects of screening as the reduction in the number of deaths caused by breast cancer and the number of life years gained because of the screening program. Costs and effects were discounted at a rate of 3 percent.

We estimated the model's parameters using data from Dutch screening projects (Collette and others 1992; Vervoort and others 2004). We used trial results to estimate the effectiveness of mammography in reducing breast cancer mortality (de Koning and others 1995). We based sensitivity estimates of CBE on data from Rijnsburger and others (2004) and based alternative (lower) estimates on data from Bobo, Lee, and Thames (2000) and Rijnsburger and others (forthcoming). We calibrated the model so that it would correctly predict the age-specific incidence and mortality of breast cancer in India (Ferlay and others 2001) and its stage distribution at clinical diagnosis (Sankaranarayanan, Black, and Parkin 1998). Details of these methods are available elsewhere (Lamberts and others 2004).

We calculated total costs by comparing the differential costs of breast cancer screening, diagnosis, initial therapy, adjuvant therapy, follow-up, and advanced disease in the case of screening versus no screening. We calculated component costs by multiplying the estimated resource use by the estimated costs per unit for each health care input. Reliable cost data for India were limited, so we extrapolated estimates from Dutch unit costs (Mulligan and others 2003). For the analysis discussed above, we calculated costs based on a market-basket approach.

The overall incidence of breast cancer is lower in India than in Western countries. The relationship between the incidence of breast cancer and age also differs: in Western countries, the incidence of breast cancer increases with age, whereas in India, it decreases with age, beginning at age 50. Investigators have generally attributed this finding to a cohort effect: breast cancer is more common among younger cohorts than older cohorts. The stage at which breast cancer is diagnosed is much less favorable in India than in Western countries.

Table 29.5 presents the results of our exploratory cost-effectiveness analysis of various breast cancer screening programs involving CBE or mammography for a population of 1 million women in India. As the table shows, biennial CBE from age 40 to 60 costs US$2.6 million, averts 358 breast cancer deaths, prevents the loss of 4,896 life years, and has a cost-effectiveness ratio of US$522 per YLS in comparison with no screening. Biennial CBE from age 50 to 70 is less favorable in terms of cost-effectiveness: US$582 per YLS.

The cost-effectiveness ratios for biennial mammography screening are not as favorable as those for biennial CBE screening. Annual CBE screening results in almost the same number of life years saved as biennial mammography screening at 36 percent of the cost.

Table 29.5 Cost-Effectiveness Analysis of Various Breast Cancer Screening Programs Involving Either CBE or Mammography for a Population of 1 Million Women, Compared with No Screening, India

Category	Base model: biennial CBE, ages 40–60	Annual CBE, ages 40–60	Biennial CBE, ages 50–70	CBE once every 5 years, ages 40–60	Biennial mammography, ages 40–60	Biennial mammography, ages 50–70	One lifetime mammogram, age 50
Effectiveness							
Number of screening tests performed	2,319,839	4,426,854	1,620,568	1,056,544	2,318,641	1,619,051	212,008
Number of cancers detected by screening	1,689	2,330	1,683	938	2,561	2,649	465
Number of deaths averted	358	528	313	184	599	557	105
Number of life years saved	4,896	7,242	3,464	2,462	7,955	6,180	1,422
Percentage reduction in mortality	7.8	11.4	6.8	4.0	13.0	12.1	2.3
Number of screening tests per death averted	6,473	8,385	5,170	5,730	3,868	2,909	2,028
Number of screening tests per life year saved	474	611	468	429	291	262	149
Number of screening tests per cancer detected	1,373	1,900	963	1,127	906	611	456
Cost-effectiveness							
Differential costs (2001 US$)	2,553,425	5,230,303	2,017,186	1,108,883	14,681,387	10,559,356	1,282,024
Cost per death prevented (2001 US$)	7,125	9,907	6,435	6,014	24,493	18,970	12,262
Cost per life year saved (2001 US$)	522	722	582	450	1,846	1,709	902

Source: Authors' calculations.
Note: The discount rate used was 3 percent.

Table 29.6 shows the results of our sensitivity analysis for the exploratory cost-effectiveness analysis of breast cancer screening in India. Cost-effectiveness ratios are lower when the incidence of cancer is higher, as in Bombay. Cost-effectiveness ratios are 32 and 16 percent higher, respectively, with a lower sensitivity of CBE and when the averted costs of palliative treatment are not included. Using alternative approaches to estimate screening program costs has a major effect, resulting in cost-effectiveness estimates 6 to 11 times higher than the base case analysis. This result underlines the need for economic studies that can obtain reliable data from primary sources on the true resource costs of cancer control interventions in developing countries. With data from such studies, researchers would not have to continue to rely on extrapolating cost estimates from data in developed countries.

These results depend critically on assumptions about the efficacy of CBE, for which the evidence is limited, highlighting the need for controlled studies of CBE in developing countries. Our estimates indicate that the cost-effectiveness of screening mammography in India compares favorably, in absolute terms, with breast cancer screening in developed countries. Nevertheless, screening mammography for breast cancer is likely to be less cost-effective in a country such as India than is screening for cervical cancer.

Cancer Treatment and Palliative Care

Barnum and Greenberg (1993) used an indirect approach to estimate the cost-effectiveness of initial cancer treatment in developing countries. They assumed that they could estimate the effectiveness of initial cancer treatment by comparing cancer survival in the United States for the period 1975–80 with the period 1940–45. The logic of such a comparison is that major advances in cancer diagnosis, surgery, radiation, and chemotherapy occurred during the intervening period, and thus survival in the 1940–45 period could be equated to outcomes expected to result from no treatment or ineffective treatment. Barnum and Greenberg's results indicated a cost-effectiveness ratio of the following:

- US$1,300 to US$6,200 per YLS for initial treatment of the more treatable cancers, that is, cervical, breast, oral cavity, and colorectal cancer
- US$53,000 to US$163,000 per YLS for initial treatment of the less treatable cancers, that is, liver, lung, stomach, and esophageal cancer.

The following subsections review cost-effectiveness studies performed on selected adjuvant or palliative cancer treatments that have been studied extensively in controlled clinical trials.

Table 29.6 Sensitivity Analysis for Changes in Breast Cancer Incidence and Attendance Rate, CBE Sensitivity, No Palliative Treatment, and Alternative Cost Estimates for a Population of 1 Million Women, Compared with No Screening, India

Category	Base model: biennial CBE, ages 40–60	Incidence of breast cancer, Bombay	Attendance rate, 70%	CBE sensitivity[a]	No palliative treatment	Alternative cost estimation Method 1[b]	Method 2[c]
Effectiveness							
Number of screening tests performed	2,319,839	2,319,991	1,624,401	2,320,051	2,319,839	2,319,839	2,319,839
Number of cancers detected by screening	1,689	1,921	1,229	1,370	1,689	1,689	1,689
Number of deaths averted	358	405	255	286	358	358	358
Number of life years saved	4,896	5,400	3,483	3,893	4,896	4,896	4,896
Percentage reduction in mortality	7.8	6.9	5.5	6.2	7.8	7.8	7.8
Number of screening tests per death averted	6,473	5,727	6,358	8,119	6,473	6,473	6,473
Number of screening tests per life year saved	474	430	466	596	474	474	474
Number of screening tests per cancer detected	1,373	1,208	1,322	1,693	1,373	1,373	1,373
Cost-effectiveness							
Differential costs (2001 US$)	2,553,425	2,505,274	1,798,662	2,684,628	2,983,754	28,814,056	16,532,879
Cost per death prevented (2001 US$)	7,125	6,184	7,040	9,395	8,325	80,396	46,130
Cost per life year saved (2001 US$)	522	464	516	690	609	5,885	3,377

Source: Authors' calculations.

Note: The discount rate used was 3 percent.

a. From Rijnsburger and others forthcoming.

b. Costs using 2001 prices in the Netherlands.

c. Costs using 2001 prices in the Netherlands multiplied by the ratio of gross domestic product shares spent on health care in India and the Netherlands, respectively.

Table 29.7 Cost-Effectiveness of Selected Breast Cancer Treatments for a Hypothetical Cohort of 45-Year-Old Premenopausal Women with Early-Stage Breast Cancer, United States
(cost in 2000 US$/quality-adjusted life year)

Treatment	Node-negative, estrogen receptor–positive	Node-negative, estrogen receptor–negative	Node-positive, estrogen receptor–positive	Node-positive, estrogen receptor–negative
Tamoxifen	17,400	326,800	6,600	88,300
Chemotherapy	17,400	7,600	14,000	7,500
Tamoxifen and chemotherapy	50,400	131,600	22,600	123,200

Source: T. Smith and Hillner 1993.

Breast Cancer Treatment Interventions. The following paragraphs review studies of the cost-effectiveness of adjuvant systemic therapy for early-stage breast cancer and of radiation therapy following mastectomy and chemotherapy to treat node-positive breast cancer in premenopausal women.

T. Smith and Hillner (2000), relying on results from the Early Breast Cancer Trialists' Collaborative Group (EBCTCG 1998), modeled the natural history of breast cancer in premenopausal 45-year-old women in the United States who were diagnosed with early-stage breast cancer and treated with tamoxifen, chemotherapy, or both. Table 29.7 summarizes the cost-effectiveness of various breast cancer treatments. Smith and Hillner's cost-effectiveness estimates for single-modality systemic adjuvant therapy for breast cancer are about the same order of magnitude as Barnum and Greenberg's (1993) estimates of cost-effectiveness for initial therapy of breast cancer (about US$7,300 per YLS in 2000 dollars). Other studies (Malin and others 2002; Norum 2000) have yielded cost-effectiveness estimates for chemotherapy and hormonal therapy two to three times more favorable than Smith and Hillner's estimates. The more favorable estimates are probably the result of the investigators' use of a discount rate of 3 percent instead of 5 percent and their assumption that the benefits of treatment continue over a longer period of time.

Two U.S. studies (Lee and others 2002; Marks and others 1999) have estimated the cost-effectiveness ratio for radiation therapy following mastectomy and chemotherapy for node-positive breast cancer in premenopausal women to be in the range of US$22,600 to US$43,000 per quality-adjusted life year (adjusted to 2000 U.S. dollars, with a discount rate of 3 percent). Results were sensitive to treatment costs, survival benefit, and patient time costs.

The clinical trials of postmastectomy radiation on which the two U.S. studies are based compared radiation following surgery plus chemotherapy with surgery plus chemotherapy alone. Love and others (2003), however, offer observational evidence that radiation treatment may also extend survival for Chinese and Vietnamese women when administered to patients with one to three positive nodes following mastectomy alone or mastectomy combined with oophorectomy and tamoxifen. If these benefits were confirmed, postmastectomy radiation might be cost-effective in developing countries, where the cost of radiation treatment is lower than in most developed countries.

Colorectal Cancer Treatment Interventions. As concerns colorectal cancer, investigators have carried out cost-effectiveness studies on surgical techniques, adjuvant treatment, follow-up monitoring for recurrence, and treatment of advanced disease (van den Hout and others 2002). Brown, Nayfield, and Shibley (1994) estimate that the cost-effectiveness of adjuvant chemotherapy for stage three colon cancer ranges from US$3,000 to US$7,000 per YLS (adjusted to 2000 U.S. dollars, with a discount rate of 6 percent). R. Smith and others' (1993) study conducted in the Australian health care setting obtains similar results in terms of cost per YLS but yields substantially higher costs per quality-adjusted life year.

Dahlberg and others' (2002) cost-effectiveness study, which relies on cost and clinical outcome data from the Swedish Rectal Cancer Trial (1997), demonstrates that rectal cancer patients receiving preoperative radiation therapy had improved cancer-specific and overall survival rates, as well as reduced local rectal cancer recurrence rates. They estimate the overall cost-effectiveness of preoperative radiation therapy for rectal cancer patients to be US$3,654 per YLS (in 2001 U.S. dollars, using a discount rate of 3 percent). In a sensitivity analysis, which varied the rates of local rectal cancer recurrence and the survival advantage with and without radiation treatment, cost-effectiveness ratios for preoperative radiation therapy for patients with rectal cancer ranged from US$908 to US$15,228 per YLS.

Cervical Cancer Treatment Interventions. Five recent phase 3 trials indicate that a new alternative therapy—cisplatin-based chemoradiation—is more effective than standard therapy using radiation alone in the treatment of advanced cervical cancer (Rose and Lappas 2000). Using an economic model, Rose and Lappas apply unit costs to resource allocation data derived from the cisplatin-based chemoradiation arms of the five randomized trials and examine the benefits in terms of increased median survival time. Costs per YLS for cisplatin-based chemoradiation regimens varied from US$2,384 to US$28,770 on the basis of published survival and from US$308 to US$3,712 on the basis of estimated survival. Although chemoradiation for advanced cervical cancer would probably be considered cost-effective in most developed countries, analyses that take local treatment settings into account are needed to determine if this result also holds for developing countries.

Palliative Care Interventions. The most basic approach to palliative care for terminally ill cancer patients, especially in low-resource settings, involves using inexpensive oral analgesics, ranging from aspirin to opiates, depending on individual patients' needs. Unfortunately, sufficient supplies of opioid drugs for use in palliative care are often not available in developing countries because of regulatory or pricing obstacles, ignorance, or false beliefs (for more information see http://www.medsch.wisc.edu/painpolicy/index.htm and chapter 52).

Appropriate palliative care for cancer patients may involve a variety of other treatment modalities, including antiemetic drugs to relieve the side effects of chemotherapy, radiation to effect temporary tumor regression, and physical therapy to alleviate disability related to lymphedema following breast cancer surgery. Berthelot and others' (2000) study combines information from several clinical trials and Canadian treatment cost information to perform cost-effectiveness analyses of different ambulatory chemotherapy regimens used for patients with metastatic non-small-cell lung cancer to palliate symptoms and modestly improve survival. They report that vinblastine plus cisplatin resulted in both better survival and lower health care expenditures than best supportive care because it resulted in fewer episodes of rehospitalization.

Van den Hout and others' (2003) study examines the cost-effectiveness of single-fraction versus multiple-fraction radiotherapy for palliative treatment of cancer patients with painful bone metastases. They find that overall medical and social costs for single-fraction radiotherapy for palliative therapy—US$1,144 per patient in medical costs and US$1,753 per patient in total social costs—were lower than comparable costs for multiple-fraction radiotherapy, despite the higher rate of retreatment associated with single-fraction radiotherapy. Whether those results are directly applicable to radiation treatment in developing countries, where single-fraction radiation treatment may be relatively less effective, is unknown. Nonetheless, the results strongly suggest that single-fraction radiotherapy may be an acceptable, if not preferred, choice of palliative treatment in settings where resources for radiation treatment are relatively scarce and the need for palliative treatment is relatively high.

APPLICABILITY OF COST-EFFECTIVENESS STUDIES FROM DEVELOPED TO DEVELOPING COUNTRIES

Many of the cost-effectiveness studies of cancer control interventions (prevention, screening, and treatment) have been performed in the context of high-income, developed countries; thus, the question arises whether such studies are applicable to health care delivery settings in developing countries. No simple rule is available to indicate how the results of cost-effectiveness studies in developed countries might translate to health care delivery settings in developing countries, but disease incidence and time horizon are major pertinent considerations in relation to cancer prevention and screening interventions. In relation to cancer treatment, other considerations have to be taken into account.

Factors Affecting the Applicability of Cost-Effectiveness Studies of Prevention and Screening

Cost-effectiveness analyses of cancer prevention and screening interventions are complex. Several parameters have a large influence on the results of these studies, including the following:

- age-specific cancer incidence
- all-cause life expectancy and temporal trends of major epidemics
- population age structure
- availability, effectiveness, and costs of cancer treatment
- health system costs of the prevention or screening intervention.

As illustrated by the several examples described in this chapter, those parameters are likely to vary widely between developed and developing countries.

For example, age-specific cancer incidence in the absence of a preventive or screening intervention can have a major influence on the potential cost-effectiveness of a cancer prevention or screening intervention. Generally, the higher the background incidence of the cancer, the more cost-effective the cancer prevention or screening intervention will be. For that reason, the relative cancer incidence patterns in developed and developing countries for the cancer screening interventions described earlier need to be considered.

Figure 29.3 shows age-specific cancer incidence patterns for cervical and breast cancer for developed and developing

countries. As the figure shows, the incidence of cervical cancer in developing countries is relatively high in comparison with the incidence of these cancers in developed countries, whereas the incidence of breast cancer is relatively low in developing countries compared with that in developed countries. Given the relatively high incidence of cervical cancer in developing countries, interventions for cervical cancer prevention and screening are likely to be more cost-effective in developing countries rather than developed countries, compared with interventions for breast cancer, all else being equal.

Factors Affecting the Applicability of Cost-Effectiveness Studies of Treatment

Many of the treatments for breast, colorectal, and lung cancer that have been shown to be efficacious in controlled clinical trials have been estimated to have cost-effectiveness ratios in the range of a few thousand U.S. dollars to a few tens of thousands

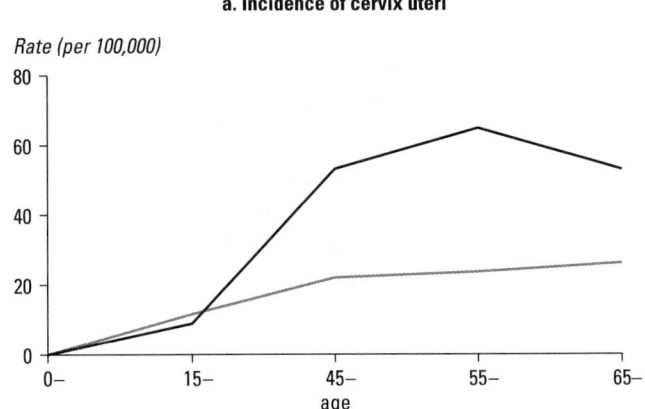

a. Incidence of cervix uteri

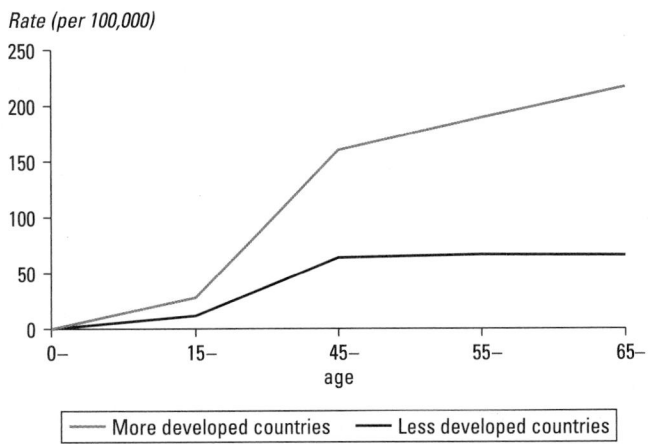

b. Incidence of breast cancer

Source: Ferlay and others 2001.

Figure 29.3 Age-Specific Incidence of Cervical and Breast Cancer, Developed and Developing Countries, 2000

of U.S. dollars per YLS. This range is considered quite favorable in developed countries but might be viewed as less favorable in low- and middle-income countries that face stringent constraints on health care resources. Disease incidence and time horizon do not loom as major considerations in the case of the cost-effectiveness of cancer treatment, because the cost of treatment applies only to those individuals already diagnosed with cancer and considered eligible for a specific treatment, not to a broader population considered to be at risk for developing cancer.

Thus, in low-income, low-cost countries with high mortality rates, because of the lack of primary treatment, the provision of basic cancer treatment may be a cost-effective first step toward cancer control, especially for highly treatable cancers with relatively low incidence in developing countries. For example, using a generalized cost-effectiveness approach, Ginsberg and others (2004) conclude that the provision of basic treatment for colorectal cancer in low-income African countries is likely to be a cost-effective first step toward cancer control.

Nevertheless, issues of economies of scale and scope may be associated with fixed investments in specialized medical equipment and skilled human capital. The centralization and regionalization of cancer treatment may be associated with a higher technical quality of care and might also be associated with the need to use these resources at economically efficient levels. Some cost elements, such as local labor and the availability of generic drugs since initial clinical trials were conducted, will clearly be lower in the contemporary setting of developing countries than in many of the cost-effectiveness studies reviewed earlier.

Finally, developments in cancer treatment, especially in relation to chemotherapy, are extremely dynamic. For example, the 1999 WHO list of essential drugs for cancer therapy (Sikora and others 1999; WHO 2003a), includes 5-fluorouracil as a priority one (essential) drug and irinotecan as a priority three (palliative benefit only) drug for the treatment of colorectal cancer. Just five years later, in many developed countries the following drugs, in addition to irinotecan, have been added to the basic regimen of 5-fluorouracil plus leucovorin for the treatment of colorectal cancer: oxaliplatin, bevacizumab, and cetuximab. Whereas 5-fluorouracil-based treatment of metastatic colorectal cancer increased median survival from 8 to 12 months, the newer drugs increase median survival to 21 months or more, at a significantly increased economic cost. In the United States, the drug cost of 5-fluorouracil-based therapy ranges from US$63 to US$263 for the initial eight weeks of therapy. Adding irinotecan or oxaliplatin increases the drug cost to about US$10,000, and adding bevacizumab or cetuximab adds another US$20,000 to US$30,000 to the cost of initial treatment. If the latter drugs are used over the longer term as envisioned, the average cost of supplying the drugs to a single patient could approach US$300,000. Those estimates do not consider the additional costs of chemotherapy preparation, administration, and supervision and supportive care (Schrag 2004). The situation is similar for other common cancers. Clearly, low- and middle-income countries cannot afford to make the newest cancer drugs widely available to cancer patients; however, this example illustrates the need for periodic updating of available chemotherapy options along with evaluations of the incremental costs and benefits associated with them.

RESEARCH AGENDA

Knowledge about the feasibility, effectiveness, and cost-effectiveness of cancer control interventions by health services in developing countries is extremely limited, partly because of the relative paucity of active research in this area. Work in the area of descriptive epidemiology, especially work based on cancer registry data, dominates the research literature on cancer in developing countries. A second body of literature consists of comparative epidemiology and case-control studies designed to assess the importance of various risk factors for cancer.

Although information from such studies is an essential first step for characterizing the nature and extent of the cancer burden and for monitoring the ultimate effect of cancer control interventions, it does not provide a sufficient knowledge base for designing and implementing cancer control programs. For progress to be made for developing countries, much more work is needed in the following areas:

- *Clinical evaluation studies of cancer control interventions in developing countries.* Clinical evaluation studies of preventive, screening, and treatment interventions that are specifically tailored to the needs and conditions of developing countries would be useful, including controlled clinical trials where possible.
- *Health services research in developing countries.* Health services research designed to characterize the amount, distribution, and organizational structure of health sector resources in developing countries would be helpful, along with research to fill the gaps between current resource endowments and the amount of funding that would be needed to implement the minimally acceptable level of effective cancer control. In developing countries, shortages of the equipment and personnel needed to administer radiotherapy for cancer, for example, have been well documented (Levin, Meghzifene, and Tatsuzaki 2001). However, no systematic analyses are available outside developed countries (Owen, Coia, and Hanks 1997) that project radiotherapy resource needs in terms of clinically effective applications of

radiotherapy, both by cancer site and by the known effectiveness of radiotherapy for primary treatment, adjuvant therapy, and palliative care. Similarly, even though researchers have carried out patterns of care studies that characterize the dissemination of radiation, chemotherapy, and hormonal therapy in many developed countries, comparable information for developing countries is generally unavailable. Health services research studies could also contribute important information about the current structure and organization of primary, secondary, and tertiary care in specific developing countries, with the ultimate aim of modeling and implementing cancer control delivery systems that either are integrated with or supplement existing care delivery systems. Studies of this type are needed to ensure that there is a balance, for example, between resources devoted to screening and those devoted to diagnostic follow-up and treatment. The disappointing performance of cervical cancer screening programs in many developing countries has been due in part to the lack of effective diagnostic follow-up and treatment following screening.

• *Country-specific economic evaluation studies.* Country-specific studies need to be done that assess resource requirements, economic costs, effectiveness, and ultimately cost-effectiveness of cancer control interventions adapted or tailored to the needs and requirements of low- and middle-income settings. Heuristic extrapolation is a first analytical step in this direction, but such studies can indicate only whether more direct and realistic studies are needed.

• *Studies of innovative health care information and communications technology.* More research is needed to determine if technological advances, such as computerized image reading or long-distance consultation by oncology specialists, facilitated by telemedicine communications technology, might alter the cost-effectiveness equation by raising quality, by lowering costs, or both. For remote localities or small, low-income developing countries, training and employing local expertise or advanced equipment for every aspect of cancer control may not be necessary if advanced communication and information technology could be used to facilitate virtual collaboration.

CONCLUSIONS

Our ability to draw any conclusions about the cost-effectiveness of cancer control interventions for low- and middle-income developing countries is limited, because most cost-effectiveness studies in this area have been conducted in high-income, developed countries. Cancer control interventions that appear to be cost-effective in high-income countries may not be cost-effective in low-income countries, even when the lower cost of providing health services is taken into account.

A useful way to draw inferences about the relative cross-country affordability of interventions is to translate cost-effectiveness ratios into percentage of per capita gross national product (GNP) per YLS (WHO 2001a). Our preliminary analysis of breast cancer screening in India, for example, suggesting an absolute cost-effectiveness level for screening mammography of about US$2,000 per YLS, compared with about US$3,000 per YLS in the Netherlands. At about 10 percent per capita GNP per YLS, screening mammography might be considered to be extremely cost-effective for the Netherlands. In India, however, we found a CE estimate equal to 400 percent per capita GNP per YLS suggesting that national policy makers would be much less likely to consider screening mammography as a viable intervention given India's health care budget constraints. However, they might well consider a CBE breast cancer screening program, at about 200 percent per capita GNP per YLS in India, to be moderately affordable if the program were definitively established to be effective.

For middle-income developing countries that have cancer incidence rates similar to those in high-income developed countries, the results of cost-effectiveness analyses from the developed countries may be more relevant, although further analysis clearly is needed. The case study of cervical cancer control that was cited earlier suggests that for low-income countries tailored cancer control interventions may need to be developed that would be both cost-effective and affordable. However, that suggestion does not imply that low-tech approaches should be uncritically embraced and assumed to be cost-effective. Until recently, education campaigns to promote breast self-examination were widely advocated as the low-tech alternative to screening mammography for breast cancer control in low-income countries; however, the best current evidence now indicates that such campaigns have no effect on breast cancer mortality (Semiglazov and others 1999; Thomas and others 2002).

In cancer treatment interventions, the cost-effectiveness of initial surgical treatment for treatable cancers, such as breast, cervical, and colorectal cancer, may be in the relatively favorable range of a few to several thousand dollars per YLS, which indicates that such interventions are likely to be cost-effective for middle-income countries and are possibly cost-effective for low-income countries. Although cost-effectiveness ratios for some of the approaches to adjuvant therapy that use conventional radiation and drugs also fall within this relatively favorable range, others are in the range of tens of thousands of dollars for each YLS. Thus, these forms of treatment would likely be considered potentially cost-effective and affordable in middle-income countries but not in low-income countries; however, more detailed examinations of specific cost conditions and available resource endowments for the delivery of cancer treatment services are needed to confirm these preliminary impressions. As with the case of cervical cancer control, treatment interventions that are tailored to the conditions of low-income countries might be shown to be efficacious and more economically attractive than treatment approaches that are transported directly from developed countries; however, research in this area is lacking.

Time Horizon and a Balanced Approach to Cancer Control Programs

The time horizon for cancer prevention and screening interventions is highly relevant to policy makers and health system planners, yet reports on the cost-effectiveness of such interventions often omit information about time horizons. For example, interventions that involve cancer control agents that prevent cancer cases that would have otherwise occurred many years after the preventive action, such as HPV vaccination, have a long time horizon. Similarly, the favorable cost-effectiveness of preventive screening for stomach cancer is not apparent until four decades following the initiation of the intervention. In the case of the 25-year program of CBE in India analyzed earlier, only about 10 percent of the benefits in terms of breast cancer deaths prevented would have been realized after 10 years of program operation. Decision makers must understand and take these time horizons into account when interpreting and acting on cost-effectiveness ratios; however, the long time horizon for cancer prevention and screening interventions is, in itself, not an argument against the application of such interventions. In some cases, countries that are more recent entrants into the field of cancer control may be able to benefit from the experience of developed countries and from the dynamic technical progress in this area to go directly to new innovations. For example, they might be able to implement HPV testing right away as the basis for cervical cancer screening, bypassing cervical cytology. Achieving the optimal temporal balance in comprehensive cancer control represents a daunting challenge to planning, evaluation, and implementation.

Start Small, Scale Up Smart

Because the current understanding of the effectiveness, optimal resource mix, and cost of many cancer control interventions is incomplete and uncertain, especially in relation to low- and middle-income countries, developing countries should start small. By starting small, they can gain knowledge from pilot programs that are well documented with regard to organizational and process factors; that are conducted in controlled settings, if possible; and that are monitored for efficiency, performance, and effectiveness. Thus, for example, new screening or treatment programs can be initiated in focused geographical areas or specific facilities with known and well-characterized target populations, and their performance and outcomes can be compared with matched control areas or facilities.

Developing countries should consider scaling up their regional or national programs only after the pilot programs have been shown to perform well.

Starting small also might entail applying an initial pilot program to a limited age range that is estimated to yield the most benefits per resource use or to a limited group of high-risk individuals defined by various risk characteristics, such as first-degree relatives of people with cancer. Indeed, various versions of this approach have characterized the dissemination of many cancer control interventions in developed countries. Organized breast cancer screening programs in some European countries, for example, were first implemented as pilot programs in specific regions and evaluated against control communities (Fracheboud and others 2001; Olsson and others 2000; van der Maas 2001), and regional and national programs were initially limited to the age groups, screening procedures, and screening frequencies estimated to be the most cost-effective. The programs were later extended, in terms of more intensive procedures, more frequent screening intervals, and wider age groups, after monitoring and analysis of initial program performance indicated that the incremental cost-effectiveness of these extensions would be favorable (Boer and others 1995; Shapiro and others 1998). The United Kingdom has taken a similar approach to colorectal cancer screening (Steele and others 2001).

ACKNOWLEDGMENTS

The authors would like to thank Rachel Ballard-Barbash, M.D.; Ted Trimble, M.D.; and Stephen Taplin, M.D., of the National Cancer Institute, and Deborah Schrag, M.D., of Memorial Sloan Kettering Cancer Institute for reading and commenting on early versions of this chapter. We thank Kerry Kemp and Penny Randall-Levy for editorial assistance. The exploratory analysis of breast cancer screening is the joint work of Quirine J. Lamberts, M.D., M.Sc.; Arno J. Der Kinderen, M.Sc.; Gerrit Draisma, Ph.D.; and Harry J. de Koning, M.D., of the Department of Public Health, Erasmus University Medical Center, Rotterdam. Steven Sweet, Jane Kim, and Jeremy Goldhaber-Fiebert of the Harvard Initiative for Global Health made invaluable contributions to the section on cervical cancer.

REFERENCES

Alberts, D. S., M. E. Martinez, D. J. Roe, J. M. Guillen-Rodriguez, J. R. Marshall, J. B. van Leeuwen, and others. 2000. "Lack of Effect of a High-Fiber Cereal Supplement on the Recurrence of Colorectal Adenomas: Phoenix Colon Cancer Prevention Physicians' Network." *New England Journal of Medicine* 342 (16): 1156–62.

Anderson, B. O., S. Braun, S. Lim, R. A. Smith, S. Taplin, and D. B. Thomas (Global Summit Early Detection Panel). 2003. "Early Detection of Breast Cancer in Countries with Limited Resources." *Breast Journal* 9 (Suppl. 2): S51–59.

ATBC (Alpha-Tocopherol, Beta Carotene Cancer Prevention Study Group). 1994. "The Effect of Vitamin E and Beta Carotene on the Incidence of Lung Cancer and Other Cancers in Male Smokers." *New England Journal of Medicine* 330 (15): 1029–35.

Babazono, A., and A. L. Hillman. 1995. "Declining Cost-Effectiveness of Screening for Disease: The Case of Gastric Cancer in Japan." *International Journal of Technology Assessment in Health Care* 11 (2): 354–64.

Barnum, H., and E. R. Greenberg. 1993. "Cancers." In *Disease Control Priorities in Developing Countries*, ed. D. T. Jamison, W. H. Mosley, A. R. Measham, and J. L. Bobadilla, 529–59. New York: Oxford University Press.

Berthelot, J. M., B. P. Will, W. K. Evans, D. Coyle, C. C. Earle, and L. Bordeleau. 2000. "Decision Framework for Chemotherapeutic Interventions for Metastatic Non-Small-Cell Lung Cancer." *Journal of the National Cancer Institute* 92 (16): 1321–29.

Bobo, J. K., N. C. Lee, and S. F. Thames. 2000. "Findings from 752,081 Clinical Breast Examinations Reported to a National Screening Program from 1995 through 1998." *Journal of the National Cancer Institute* 92 (12): 971–76.

Boer, R., H. J. de Koning, G. J. van Oortmarssen, and P. J. van der Maas. 1995. "In Search of the Best Upper Age Limit for Breast Cancer Screening." *European Journal of Cancer* 31A (12): 2040–43.

Brown, M. L., and L. Fintor. 1993. "Cost Effectiveness of Breast Cancer Screening: Preliminary Results of a Systematic Review of the Literature." *Breast Cancer Research and Treatment* 25 (2): 113–18.

Brown, M. L., S. G. Nayfield, and L. M. Shibley. 1994. "Adjuvant Therapy for Stage III Colon Cancer: Economic Returns to Research and Cost-Effectiveness of Treatment." *Journal of the National Cancer Institute* 86 (6): 424–30.

Chen, J. G., D. M. Parkin, Q. G. Chen, J. H. Lu, Q. J. Shen, B. C. Zhang, and Y. R. Zhu. 2003. "Screening for Liver Cancer: Results of a Randomised Controlled Trial in Qidong, China." *Journal of Medical Screening* 10 (4): 204–9.

Chirikos, T. N., T. Hazelton, M. Tockman, and R. Clark. 2002. "Screening for Lung Cancer with CT: A Preliminary Cost-Effectiveness Analysis." *Chest* 121 (5): 1507–14.

Christensen, D. 2004. "Dietary Prevention of Cancer: A Smorgasbord of Options for Moving Ahead." *Journal of the National Cancer Institute* 96 (11): 822–24.

Collette, C., H. J. Collette, J. Fracheboud, B. J. Slotboom, and F. de Waard. 1992. "Evaluation of a Breast Cancer Screening Programme—The DOM Project." *European Journal of Cancer* 28A (12): 1985–88.

Coursaget, P., D. Leboulleux, M. Soumare, P. le Cann, B. Yvonnet, J. P. Chiron, and others. 1994. "Twelve-Year Follow-up Study of Hepatitis B Immunization of Senegalese Infants." *Journal of Hepatology* 21 (2): 250–54.

da Costa e Silva, V. 2003. *Policy Recommendations for Smoking Cessation and Treatment of Tobacco Dependence: Tools for Public Health*. Geneva: World Health Organization.

Dahlberg, M., A. Stenborg, L. Pahlman, and B. Glimelius. 2002. "Cost-Effectiveness of Preoperative Radiotherapy in Rectal Cancer: Results from the Swedish Rectal Cancer Trial." *International Journal of Radiation Oncology, Biology, Physics* 54 (3): 654–60.

de Koning, H. J. 2000. "Breast Cancer Screening: Cost-Effective in Practice?" *European Journal of Radiology* 33 (1): 32–37.

de Koning, H. J., R. Boer, P. G. Warmerdam, P. M. Beemsterboer, and P. J. van der Maas. 1995. "Quantitative Interpretation of Age-Specific Mortality Reductions from the Swedish Breast Cancer Screening Trials." *Journal of the National Cancer Institute* 87 (16): 1217–23.

Denny, L., L. Kuhn, A. Pollack, H. Wainwright, and T. C. Wright Jr. 2000. "Evaluation of Alternative Methods of Cervical Cancer Screening for Resource-Poor Settings." *Cancer* 89 (4): 826–33.

EBCTCG (Early Breast Cancer Trialists' Collaborative Group). 1998. "Polychemotherapy for Early Breast Cancer: An Overview of the Randomised Trials." *Lancet* 352 (9132): 930–42.

Ferlay, J., F. Bray, P. Pisani, and D. M. Parkin. 2001. *GLOBOCAN 2000: Cancer Incidence, Mortality, and Prevalence Worldwide*, Version 1.0, IARC CancerBase No. 5. Lyon, France: International Agency for Research on Cancer and World Health Organization, IARC Press.

———. 2004. *GLOBOCAN 2002: Cancer Incidence, Mortality, and Prevalence Worldwide*, Version 2.0, IARC CancerBase No. 5. Lyon, France: International Agency for Research on Cancer and World Health Organization, IARC Press.

Fiore, M. C., D. K. Hatsukami, and T. B. Baker. 2002. "Effective Tobacco Dependence Treatment." *Journal of the American Medical Association* 288 (14): 1768–71.

Fracheboud, J., H. J. de Koning, R. Boer, J. H. Groenewoud, A. L. Verbeek, M. J. Broeders, and others (National Evaluation Team for Breast Cancer Screening in the Netherlands). 2001. "Nationwide Breast Cancer Screening Programme Fully Implemented in the Netherlands." *Breast* 10 (1): 6–11.

Frazier, A. L., G. A. Colditz, C. S. Fuchs, and K. M. Kuntz. 2000. "Cost-Effectiveness of Screening for Colorectal Cancer in the General Population." *Journal of the American Medical Association* 284 (15): 1954–61.

Gail, M. H., J. P. Costantino, J. Bryant, R. Croyle, L. Freedman, K. Helzlsouer, and V. Vogel. 1999. "Weighing the Risks and Benefits of Tamoxifen Treatment for Preventing Breast Cancer." *Journal of the National Cancer Institute* 91 (21): 1829–46.

Ginsberg, G. M., S. Lim, J. Lauer, C. Sepulveda, and T. Tantorres-Edeger. 2004. *Prevention, Screening, and Treatment of Colorectal Cancer: A Global and Regional Generalized Cost Effectiveness Analysis*. Geneva: World Health Organization.

Goldie, S., L. Gaffikin, A. Gordillo-Tobar, C. Levin, C. Mahé, J. Goldhaber-Fiebert, and T. Wright. 2004. "A Comprehensive Policy Analysis of Cervical Cancer Screening in Peru, India, Kenya, Thailand, and South Africa." Paper presented for the Alliance for Cervical Cancer Prevention at the 21st International Papillomavirus Conference, Mexico City, February 20–26.

Goldie, S. J., D. Grima, M. Kohli, T. C. Wright, M. Weinstein, and E. Franco. 2003. "A Comprehensive Natural History Model of HPV Infection and Cervical Cancer to Estimate the Clinical Impact of a Prophylactic HPV-16/18 Vaccine." *International Journal of Cancer* 106 (6): 896–904.

Goldie, S. J., J. J. Kim, and T. C. Wright. 2004. "Cost-Effectiveness of Human Papillomavirus DNA Testing for Cervical Cancer Screening in Women Aged 30 Years or More." *Obstetrics and Gynecology* 103 (4): 619–31.

Goldie, S. J., M. Kohli, D. Grima, M. C. Weinstein, T. C. Wright, X. C. Bosch, and E. Franco. 2004. "Projected Clinical Benefits and Cost-Effectiveness of a Human Papillomavirus 16/18 Vaccine." *Journal of the National Cancer Institute* 96 (8): 604–15.

Goldie, S. J., L. Kuhn, L. Denny, A. Pollack, and T. C. Wright. 2001. "Policy Analysis of Cervical Cancer Screening Strategies in Low-Resource Settings: Clinical Benefits and Cost-Effectiveness." *Journal of the American Medical Association* 285 (24): 3107–15.

Harper, D. M., E. L. Franco, C. Wheeler, D. G. Ferris, D. Jenkins, A. Schuind, and others. 2004. "Efficacy of a Bivalent L1 Virus-Like Particle Vaccine in Prevention of Infection with Human Papillomavirus Types 16 and 18 in Young Women: A Randomised Controlled Trial." *Lancet* 364 (9447): 1757–65.

Harris, R. A., D. K. Owens, H. Witherell, and J. Parsonnet. 1999. "*Helicobactor pylori* and Gastric Cancer: What Are the Benefits of Screening Only for the CagA Phenotype of *H. pylori*?" *Helicobactor* 4 (2): 69–76.

Hughes, J. P., G. P. Garnett, and L. Koutsky. 2002. "The Theoretical Population-Level Impact of a Prophylactic Human Papilloma Virus Vaccine." *Epidemiology* 13 (6): 631–39.

Humphrey, L. L., M. Helfand, B. K. Chan, and S. H. Woolf. 2002. "Breast Cancer Screening: A Summary of the Evidence for the U.S. Preventive Services Task Force." *Annals of Internal Medicine* 137 (5, Part 1): 347–60.

Imperiale, T. F. 2003. "Aspirin and the Prevention of Colorectal Cancer." *New England Journal of Medicine* 348 (10): 879–80.

International Agency for Research on Cancer. No date. "Cancer Mondial: DEP Scientific Programmes." http://www-dep.iarc.fr/thisunit/depproge.htm.

Kensler, T. W., G. S. Qian, J. G. Chen, and J. D. Groopman. 2003. "Translational Strategies for Cancer Prevention in Liver." *Nature Reviews: Cancer* 3 (5): 321–29.

Khandker, R. K., J. D. Dulski, J. B. Kilpatrick, R. P. Ellis, J. B. Mitchell, and W. B. Baine. 2000. "A Decision Model and Cost-Effectiveness Analysis of Colorectal Cancer Screening and Surveillance Guidelines for Average-Risk Adults." *International Journal of Technology Assessment in Health Care* 16 (3): 799–810.

Kim, J. J., T. Wright, and S. Goldie. 2002. "Cost Effectiveness of Alternative Triage Strategies for Atypical Squamous Cells of Undetermined Significance." *Journal of the American Medical Association* 287 (18): 2382–90.

Koutsky, L. A., K. A. Ault, C. M. Wheeler, D. R. Brown, E. Barr, F. B. Alvarez, and others (Proof of Principle Study Investigators). 2002. "A Controlled Trial of a Human Papillomavirus Type 16 Vaccine." *New England Journal of Medicine* 347 (21): 1645–51.

Kulasingam, S. L., and E. R. Myers. 2003. "Potential Health and Economic Impact of Adding a Human Papillomavirus Vaccine to Screening Programs." *Journal of the American Medical Association* 290 (6): 781–89.

Lamberts, Q. J., A. J. der Kinderen, G. Draisma, and H. J. de Koning. 2004. "Breast Cancer Screening in Developing Countries: A Cost-Effectiveness Analysis for India." Working Paper, Erasmus University Medical Center, Department of Public Health, Rotterdam, the Netherlands.

Lazcano-Ponce, E. C., S. Moss, P. Alonso de Ruiz, J. Salmeron Castro, and M. Hernandez Avila. 1999. "Cervical Cancer Screening in Developing Countries: Why Is It Ineffective? The Case of Mexico." *Archives of Medical Research* 30 (3): 240–50.

Lee, C. L., K. S. Hsieh, and Y. C. Ko. 2003. "Trends in the Incidence of Hepatocellular Carcinoma in Boys and Girls in Taiwan after Large-Scale Hepatitis B Vaccination." *Cancer Epidemiology, Biomarkers, and Prevention* 12 (1): 57–9.

Lee, J. H., H. A. Glick, J. A. Hayman, and L. J. Solin. 2002. "Decision-Analytic Model and Cost-Effectiveness Evaluation of Postmastectomy Radiation Therapy in High-Risk Premenopausal Breast Cancer Patients." *Journal of Clinical Oncology* 20 (11): 2713–25.

Levin, V., A. Meghzifene, and H. Tatsuzaki. 2001. "Improving Cancer Care: Increased Need for Radiotherapy in Developing Countries." *IAEA (International Atomic Energy Agency) Bulletin* 43: 25–32.

Ley, C., A. Mohar, J. Guarner, R. Herrera-Goepfert, L. S. Figueroa, D. Halperin, and others. 2004. "*Helicobacter pylori* Eradication and Gastric Preneoplastic Conditions: A Randomized, Double-Blind, Placebo-Controlled Trial." *Cancer Epidemiology, Biomarkers, and Prevention* 13 (1): 4–10.

Lippman, S. M., J. J. Lee, and A. L. Sabichi. 1998. "Cancer Chemoprevention: Progress and Promise." *Journal of the National Cancer Institute* 90 (20): 1514–28.

Lopez, Alan D., Colin D. Mathers, Majid Ezzati, Dean T. Jamison, and Christopher J. L. Murray, eds. 2006. *Global Burden of Disease and Risk Factors.* New York: Oxford University Press.

Love, R. R., N. Ba Duc, N. Cong Binh, P. A. Mahler, B. R. Thomadsen, N. Hong Long, and others. 2003. "Postmastectomy Radiotherapy in Premenopausal Vietnamese and Chinese Women with Breast Cancer Treated in an Adjuvant Hormonal Therapy Study." *International Journal of Radiation Oncology, Biology, Physics* 56 (3): 697–703.

Mahadevia, P. J., L. A. Fleisher, K. D. Frick, J. Eng, S. N. Goodman, and N. R. Powe. 2003. "Lung Cancer Screening with Helical Computed Tomography in Older Adult Smokers: A Decision and Cost-Effectiveness Analysis." *Journal of the American Medical Association* 289 (3): 313–22.

Malin, J. L., E. Keeler, C. Wang, and R. Brook. 2002. "Using Cost-Effectiveness Analysis to Define a Breast Cancer Benefits Package for the Uninsured." *Breast Cancer Research and Treatment* 74 (2): 143–53.

Mandelblatt, J. S., W. F. Lawrence, L. Gaffikin, K. K. Limpahayom, P. Lumbiganon, S. Warakamin, and others. 2002. "Costs and Benefits of Different Strategies to Screen for Cervical Cancer in Less-Developed Countries." *Journal of the National Cancer Institute* 94 (19): 1469–83.

Marcus, P. M., E. J. Bergstralh, R. M. Fagerstrom, D. E. Williams, R. Fontana, W. F. Taylor, and P. C. Prorok. 2000. "Lung Cancer Mortality in the Mayo Lung Project: Impact of Extended Follow-Up." *Journal of the National Cancer Institute* 92 (16): 1308–16.

Marks, L. B., P. H. Hardenbergh, E. T. Winer, and L. R. Prosnitz. 1999. "Assessing the Cost-Effectiveness of Postmastectomy Radiation Therapy." *International Journal of Radiation Oncology, Biology, Physics* 44 (1): 91–98.

Marshall, D., K. N. Simpson, C. C. Earle, and C. W. Chu. 2001. "Economic Decision Analysis Model of Screening for Lung Cancer." *European Journal of Cancer* 37 (14): 1759–67.

Mathers, C. D., A. D. Lopez, and C. J. L. Murray. "The Burden of Disease and Mortality by Condition: Data, Methods, and Results for 2001." In *Global Burden of Disease and Risk Factors,* eds. A. D. Lopez, C. D. Mathers, M. Ezzati, D. T. Jamison, and C. J. L. Murray. New York: Oxford University Press.

Maxwell, G. L., J. W. Carlson, M. Ochoa, T. Krivak, G. S. Rose, and E. R. Myers. 2002. "Costs and Effectiveness of Alternative Strategies for Cervical Cancer Screening in Military Beneficiaries." *Obstetrics and Gynecology* 100 (4): 740–48.

Mulligan, J., J. A. Fox-Rushby, T. Adam, B. Johns, and A. Mills. 2003. "Unit Costs of Delivering Health Interventions in Low- and Middle-Income Countries: Tertiary Unit Costs of Delivering Health Interventions in Low- and Middle-Income Countries." Working Paper 9, Disease Control Priorities Project, Bethesda, MD.

Norum, J. 1999. "Breast Cancer Screening by Mammography in Norway. Is It Cost-Effective?" *Annals of Oncology* 10 (2): 197–203.

———. 2000. "Adjuvant Cyclophosphamide, Methotrexate, Fluorouracil (CMF) in Breast Cancer: Is It Cost-Effective?" *Acta Oncologica* 39 (1): 33–39.

Olsson, S., I. Andersson, I. Karlberg, N. Bjurstam, E. Frodis, and S. Hakansson. 2000. "Implementation of Service Screening with Mammography in Sweden: From Pilot Study to Nationwide Programme." *Journal of Medical Screening* 7 (1): 14–18.

Omenn, G. S., G. E. Goodman, M. D. Thornquist, J. Balmes, M. R. Cullen, A. Glass, and others. 1996. "Effects of a Combination of Beta Carotene and Vitamin A on Lung Cancer and Cardiovascular Disease." *New England Journal of Medicine* 334 (18): 1150–55.

Owen, J. B., L. R. Coia, and G. E. Hanks. 1997. "The Structure of Radiation Oncology in the United States in 1994." *International Journal of Radiation Oncology, Biology, Physics* 39 (1): 179–85.

Parkin, D. M., F. I. Bray, and S. S. Devesa. 2001. "Cancer Burden in the Year 2000: The Global Picture." *European Journal of Cancer* 37 (Suppl. 8): S4–66.

Parkin, D. M., J. Ferlay, M. Hamdi-Cherif, F. Sitas, J. O. Thomas, H. Wabinga, and S. L. Whelan. 2003. *Cancer in Africa: Epidemiology and Prevention*. Lyon, France: International Agency for Research on Cancer and World Health Organization.

Pignone, M., S. Saha, T. Hoerger, and J. Mandelblatt. 2002. "Cost-Effectiveness Analyses of Colorectal Cancer Screening: A Systematic Review for the U.S. Preventive Services Task Force." *Annals of Internal Medicine* 137 (2): 96–104.

Powles, T., R. Eeles, S. Ashley, D. Easton, J. Chang, M. Dowsett, and others. 1998. "Interim Analysis of the Incidence of Breast Cancer in the Royal Marsden Hospital Tamoxifen Randomised Chemoprevention Trial." *Lancet* 352 (9122): 98–101.

Rijnsburger, A. J., G. J. van Oortmarssen, R. Boer, C. Baines, A. B. Miller, and H. J. de Koning. Forthcoming. "Clinical Breast Exams as a Screening Tool: Cost-Effectiveness."

Rijnsburger, A. J., G. J. van Oortmarssen, R. Boer, G. Draisma, T. To, A. B. Miller, and H. J. de Koning. 2004. "Mammography Benefit in the Canadian National Breast Screening Study-2: A Model Evaluation." *International Journal of Cancer* 110 (5): 756–62.

Roderick, P., R. Davies, J. Raftery, D. Crabbe, R. Pearce, P. Patel, and P. Bhandari. 2003. "Cost-Effectiveness of Population Screening for *Helicobactor pylori* in Preventing Gastric Cancer and Peptic Ulcer Disease, Using Simulation." *Journal of Medical Screening* 10 (3): 148–56.

Rose, P. G., and P. T. Lappas. 2000. "Analysis of the Cost-Effectiveness of Concurrent Cisplatin-Based Chemoradiation in Cervical Cancer: Implications from Five Randomized Trials." *Gynecologic Oncology* 78 (1): 3–6.

Sanders, G. D., and A. V. Taira. 2003. "Cost-Effectiveness of a Potential Vaccine for Human Papillomavirus." *Emerging Infectious Diseases* 9 (1): 37–48.

Sankaranarayanan, R., R. J. Black, and D. M. Parkin, eds. 1998. *Cancer Survival in Developing Countries*, IARC Scientific Publication 145. Lyon, France: International Agency for Research on Cancer Press and World Health Organization.

Sankaranarayanan, R., A. M. Budukh, and R. Rajkumar. 2001. "Effective Screening Programmes for Cervical Cancer in Low- and Middle-Income Developing Countries." *Bulletin of the World Health Organization* 79 (10): 954–62.

Sankaranarayanan, R., B. Shyamalakumary, R. Wesley, N. Sreedevi Amma, D. M. Parkin, and M. K. Nair. 1999. "Visual Inspection with Acetic Acid in the Early Detection of Cervical Cancer and Precursors." *International Journal of Cancer* 80 (1): 161–63.

Sarasin, F. P., E. Giostra, and A. Hadengue. 1996. "Cost-Effectiveness of Screening for Detection of Small Hepatocellular Carcinoma in Western Patients with Child-Pugh Class A Cirrhosis." *American Journal of Medicine* 101 (4): 422–34.

Schatzkin, A., E. Lanza, D. Corle, P. Lance, F. Iber, B. Caan, and others. 2000. "Lack of Effect of a Low-Fat, High-Fiber Diet on the Recurrence of Colorectal Adenomas." *New England Journal of Medicine* 342 (16): 1149–55.

Schiffman, M., R. Herrero, A. Hildesheim, M. E. Sherman, M. Bratti, S. Wacholder, and others. 2000. "HPV DNA Testing in Cervical Cancer Screening: Results from Women in a High-Risk Province of Costa Rica." *Journal of the American Medical Association* 283 (1): 87–93.

Schrag, D. 2004. "The Price Tag on Progress: Chemotherapy for Colorectal Cancer." *New England Journal of Medicine* 351 (4): 317–19.

Semiglazov, V. F., V. M. Moiseenko, A. G. Manikhas, S. A. Protsenko, R. S. Kharikova, R. T. Popova, and others. 1999. "Interim Results of a Prospective Randomized Study of Self-Examination for Early Detection of Breast Cancer." *Voprosy Onkologii* 45 (3): 265–71.

Shapiro, S., E. A. Coleman, M. Broeders, M. Codd, H. de Koning, J. Fracheboud, and others. 1998. "Breast Cancer Screening Programmes in 22 Countries: Current Policies, Administration, and Guidelines." *International Journal of Epidemiology* 27 (5): 735–42.

Sherlaw-Johnson, C., S. Gallivan, and D. Jenkins. 1997. "Evaluating Cervical Cancer Screening Programmes for Developing Countries." *International Journal of Cancer* 72 (2): 210–16.

Sikora, K., S. Advani, V. Koroltchouk, I. Magrath, L. Levy, H. Pinedo, and others. 1999. "Essential Drugs for Cancer Therapy: A World Health Organization Consultation." *Annals of Oncology* 10 (4): 385–90.

Simpson, K. N., and L. B. Snyder. 1991. "Informing the Mammography Coverage Debate. Results of Meta-Analysis, Computer Modeling, and Issue Analysis." *International Journal of Technology Assessment in Health Care* 7 (4): 616–31.

Singer, P. A., and K. W. Bowman. 2002. "Quality End-of-Life Care: A Global Perspective." *BMC Palliative Care* 1 (1): 4–13.

Smith, R. D., J. Hall, H. Gurney, and P. R. Harnett. 1993. "A Cost-Utility Approach to the Use of 5-Fluorouracil and Levamisole as Adjuvant Chemotherapy for Dukes' C Colonic Carcinoma." *Medical Journal of Australia* 158 (5): 319–22.

Smith, T. J., and B. E. Hillner. 1993. "The Efficacy and Cost-Effectiveness of Adjuvant Therapy of Early Breast Cancer in Premenopausal Women." *Journal of Clinical Oncology* 11 (4): 771–76.

———. 2000. "Tamoxifen Should Be Cost-Effective in Reducing Breast Cancer Risk in High-Risk Women." *Journal of Clinical Oncology* 18 (2): 284–86.

Sonnenberg, A., F. Delco, and J. M. Inadomi. 2000. "Cost-Effectiveness of Colonoscopy in Screening for Colorectal Cancer." *Annals of Internal Medicine* 133 (8): 573–84.

Steele, R. J., R. Parker, J. Patnick, J. Warner, C. Fraser, N. A. Mowat, and others (United Kingdom Colorectal Screening Pilot Group). 2001. "A Demonstration Pilot Trial for Colorectal Cancer Screening in the United Kingdom: A New Concept in the Introduction of Healthcare Strategies." *Journal of Medical Screening* 8 (4): 197–202.

Suba, E. J., C. H. Nguyen, B. D. Nguyen, and S. S. Raab (Viet/American Cervical Cancer Prevention Project). 2001. "De Novo Establishment and Cost-Effectiveness of Papanicolaou Cytology Screening Services in the Socialist Republic of Vietnam." *Cancer* 91 (5): 928–39.

Swedish Rectal Cancer Trial. 1997. "Improved Survival with Preoperative Radiotherapy in Resectable Rectal Cancer." *New England Journal of Medicine* 336 (14): 980–87.

Terry, M. B., M. D. Gammon, F. F. Zhang, H. Tawfik, S. L. Teitelbaum, J. A. Britton, and others. 2004. "Association of Frequency and Duration of Aspirin Use and Hormone Receptor Status with Breast Cancer Risk." *Journal of the American Medical Association* 291 (20): 2433–40.

Thomas, D. B., D. L. Gao, R. M. Ray, W. W. Wang, C. J. Allison, F. L. Chen, and others. 2002. "Randomized Trial of Breast Self-Examination in Shanghai: Final Results." *Journal of the National Cancer Institute* 94 (19): 1445–57.

Turner, P. C., A. Sylla, M. S. Diallo, J. J. Castegnaro, A. J. Hall, and C. P. Wild. 2002. "The Role of Aflatoxins and Hepatitis Viruses in the Etiopathogenesis of Hepatocellular Carcinoma: A Basis for Primary Prevention in Guinea-Conakry, West Africa." *Journal of Gastroenterology and Hepatology* 17 (Suppl.): S441–48.

United Nations Population Division. 2003. "India, Population by Five-Year Age Group and Sex (Thousands), Medium Variant, 2000–2004." In *World Population Prospects: The 2002 Revision Population Database, Tertiary World Population Prospects*. United Nations. http://esa.un.org/unpp.

Vainio, H., and F. Bianchini. 2002a. *Breast Cancer Screening*. IARC Handbooks of Cancer Prevention, Vol. 7. Lyon, France: International Agency for Research on Cancer Press and World Health Organization.

———. 2002b. *Weight Control and Physical Activity*. IARC Handbooks of Cancer Prevention, Vol. 6. Lyon, France: International Agency for Research on Cancer Press and World Health Organization.

Vainio, H., and G. Morgan. 1999. "Mechanisms of Aspirin Chemoprevention of Colorectal Cancer." *European Journal of Drug Metabolism and Pharmacokinetics* 24 (4): 289–92.

van den Hout, W. B., M. van den Brink, A. M. Stiggelbout, C. J. van de Velde, and J. Kievet. 2002. "Cost-Effectiveness Analysis of Colorectal Cancer Treatments." *European Journal of Cancer* 38 (7): 953–63.

van den Hout, W. B., Y. M. van der Linden, E. Steenland, R. G. Wiggenraad, J. Kievit, H. de Haes, and J. W. Leer. 2003. "Single- Versus Multiple-Fraction Radiotherapy in Patients with Painful Bone Metastases: Cost-Utility Analysis Based on a Randomized Trial." *Journal of the National Cancer Institute* 95 (3): 222–29.

van der Maas, P. J. 2001. "Breast Cancer Screening Programme in the Netherlands: An Interim Review." *Breast* 10 (1): 12–14.

van Meerbeeck, J. P., and K. G. Tournoy. 2004. "Screening and Diagnosis of NSCLC." *Annals of Oncology* 15 (Suppl. 4): iv 65–70.

van Oortmarssen, G. J., J. D. Habbema, P. J. van der Maas, H. J. de Koning, H. J. Collette, A. L. Verbeek, and others. 1990. "A Model for Breast Cancer Screening." *Cancer* 66 (7): 1601–12.

Veronesi, U., P. Maisonneuve, A. Costa, V. Sacchini, C. Maltoni, C. Robertson, and others. 1998. "Prevention of Breast Cancer with Tamoxifen: Preliminary Findings from the Italian Randomised Trial among Hysterectomised Women—Italian Tamoxifen Prevention Study." *Lancet* 352 (9122): 93–97.

Vervoort, M. M., G. Draisma, J. Fracheboud, L. V. van de Poll-Franse, and H. J. de Koning. 2004. "Trends in the Usage of Adjuvant Systemic Therapy for Breast Cancer in the Netherlands and Its Effect on Mortality." *British Journal of Cancer* 91 (2): 242–47.

Vijan, S., E. W. Hwang, T. P. Hofer, and R. A. Hayward. 2001. "Which Colon Cancer Screening Test? A Comparison of Costs, Effectiveness, and Compliance." *American Journal of Medicine* 111 (8): 593–601.

Viviani, S., A. Jack, A. J. Hall, N. Maine, M. Mendy, R. Montesano, and H. C. Whittle. 1999. "Hepatitis B Vaccination in Infancy in The Gambia: Protection against Carriage at 9 Years of Age." *Vaccine* 17 (23–24): 2946–50.

Wagner, J., S. Tunis, M. Brown, A. Ching, and R. Almeida. 1996. "Cost-Effectiveness of Colorectal Cancer Screening in Average-Risk Adults." In *Prevention and Early Detection of Colorectal Cancer,* ed. G. Young, P. Rozen, and B. Levin, 321–56. London: Saunders.

WHO (World Health Organization). 2001a. *Macroeconomics and Health: Investing in Health for Economic Development: Report of the Commission on Macroeconomics and Health.* Geneva: WHO.

———. 2001b. *World Health Report 2002: Reducing Risks, Promoting Healthy Life.* Geneva: WHO. http://www.who.int/whr/en/.

———. 2002. *National Cancer Control Programmes, Policies, and Managerial Guidelines,* 2nd ed. Geneva: WHO.

———. 2003a. "Essential Drugs and Medicines Policy: 13th Expert Committee on the Selection and Use of Essential Medicines, 31 March to 3 April 2003." Geneva: WHO. http://www.who.int/medicines/organization/par/edl/expertcomm.shtml.

———. 2003b. "WHO Framework Convention on Tobacco Control." Geneva: WHO. http://www.who.int/tobacco/fctc/en/fctc_booklet_english.pdf.

———. No date. "WHO Statistical Information System." Geneva: WHO. http://www3.who.int/whosis.

Whynes, D. K., and Nottingham Faecal Occult Blood Screening Trial. 2004. "Cost-Effectiveness of Screening for Colorectal Cancer: Evidence from the Nottingham Faecal Occult Blood Trial." *Journal of Medical Screening* 11 (1): 11–15.

Wong, B. C., S. K. Lam, W. M. Wong, J. S. Chen, T. T. Zheng, R. E. Feng, and others (China Gastric Cancer Study Group). 2004. "*Helicobacter pylori* Eradication to Prevent Gastric Cancer in High-Risk Region of China: A Randomized Controlled Trial." *Journal of the American Medical Association* 291 (2): 187–94.

Wright, T. C. Jr. 2003. "Chapter 10: Cervical Cancer Screening Using Visualization Techniques." *Journal of the National Cancer Institute Monographs* (31): 66–71.

Wright, T. C. Jr., L. Denny, L. Kuhn, A. Pollack, and A. Lorincz. 2000. "HPV DNA Testing of Self-Collected Vaginal Samples Compared with Cytologic Screening to Detect Cervical Cancer." *Journal of the American Medical Association* 283 (1): 81–86.

Zimbabwe Project. 1999. "Visual Inspection with Acetic Acid for Cervical-Cancer Screening: Test Qualities in a Primary-Care Setting: University of Zimbabwe/JHPIEGO Cervical Cancer Project." *Lancet* 353 (9156): 869–73.

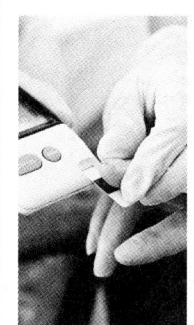

Chapter **30**

Diabetes: The Pandemic and Potential Solutions

K. M. Venkat Narayan, Ping Zhang, Alka M. Kanaya, Desmond E. Williams, Michael M. Engelgau, Giuseppina Imperatore, and Ambady Ramachandran

NATURE AND DISTRIBUTION OF DIABETES

Diabetes is a metabolic disease characterized by hyperglycemia resulting from defects in insulin secretion, insulin action, or both (American Diabetes Association 2004).

Classification of Diabetes

Diabetes takes three major forms. Type 1 diabetes results from destruction of the beta cells in the pancreas, leading to absolute insulin deficiency. It usually occurs in children and young adults and requires insulin treatment. Type 2 diabetes, which accounts for approximately 85 to 95 percent of all diagnosed cases, is usually characterized by insulin resistance in which target tissues do not use insulin properly. A third type of diabetes, gestational diabetes, is first recognized during pregnancy. Other rare types of diabetes include those caused by genetic conditions (for example, maturity-onset diabetes of youths), surgery, drug use, malnutrition, infections, and other illnesses.

The Burden of Diabetes

Diabetes affects persons of all ages and races. The disease reduces both a person's quality of life and life expectancy and imposes a large economic burden on the health care system and on families.

Secular Trend and Projections. In 2003, the worldwide prevalence of diabetes was estimated at 5.1 percent among people age 20 to 79 (table 30.1). The prevalence of diabetes was higher in developed countries than in developing countries. In the developing world, the prevalence was highest in Europe and Central Asia and lowest in Sub-Saharan Africa. Some of these variations may reflect differences in the age structures and level of urbanization of the various populations. By 2025, the worldwide prevalence is projected to be 6.3 percent, a 24 percent increase compared with 2003. The largest increase in prevalence by 2025 is expected to be in East Asia and the Pacific, and the smallest in Sub-Saharan Africa. In terms of those affected, the biggest increase in the developing countries is projected to take place among adults of working age.

In 2003, 194 million people worldwide ages 20 to 79 had diabetes, and by 2025, this number is projected to increase to 333 million, a 72 percent increase (table 30.1). The developing world accounted for 141 million people with diabetes (72.5 percent of the world total) in 2003. During the same period, the number of people with diabetes is projected to double in three of the six developing regions: the Middle East and North Africa, South Asia, and Sub-Saharan Africa.

Diabetes-Related Mortality and Disability. The death rate of men with diabetes is 1.9 times the rate for men without diabetes, and the rate for women with diabetes is 2.6 times that for women without diabetes (W. L. Lee and others 2000). Premature mortality caused by diabetes results in an estimated 12 to 14 years of life lost (Manuel and Schultz 2004; Narayan and others 2003). Cardiovascular disease

Table 30.1 Estimated Numbers of People Age 20 to 79 with Diabetes, Mortality, DALYs, and Direct Medical Costs Attributable to Diabetes, by Regions

Region	Number of people (thousands)		Prevalence (percent)		Direct medical costs, 2003 (US$ million)		Deaths, 2001 (thousands)	Disability-adjusted life years, 2001 (thousands)
	2003	2025	2003	2025	Low estimate	High estimate		
Developing countries	140,849	264,405	4.5	5.9	12,304	23,127	757	15,804
East Asia and the Pacific	31,363	60,762	2.6	3.9	1,368	2,656	234	4,930
Europe and Central Asia	25,764	33,141	7.6	9.0	2,884	5,336	51	1,375
Latin America and the Caribbean	19,026	36,064	6.0	7.8	4,592	8,676	163	2,775
Middle East and North Africa	10,792	23,391	6.4	7.9	2,347	4,340	31	843
South Asia	46,309	94,848	5.9	7.7	840	1,589	196	4,433
Sub-Saharan Africa	7,595	16,199	2.4	2.8	273	530	82	1,448
Developed countries	53,337	68,345	7.8	9.2	116,365	217,760	202	4,192
World	194,186	332,750	5.1	6.3	128,669	240,887	959	19,996

Source: Number of persons with diabetes, prevalence of diabetes, and direct medical costs of diabetes, International Diabetes Federation 2003b; all other information, WHO 2004.

(CVD) causes up to 65 percent of all deaths in developed countries of people with diabetes (Geiss, Herman, and Smith 1995).

The World Health Organization (WHO) estimates that, in 2001, 959,000 deaths worldwide were caused by diabetes, accounting for 1.6 percent of all deaths, and approximately 3 percent of all deaths caused by noncommunicable diseases. More recent estimates by WHO suggest that the actual number may be triple this estimate and that about two-thirds of these deaths occur in developing countries (WHO 2004). Within the developing regions, most deaths caused by diabetes occurred in East Asia and the Pacific and the fewest in Sub-Saharan Africa (table 30.1).

Diabetes-related complications include microvascular diseases (for example, retinopathy, blindness, nephropathy, and kidney failure) and macrovascular diseases (coronary heart disease, stroke, peripheral vascular disease, and lower-extremity amputation). Those complications result in disability. In the United States, a much higher proportion of people with diabetes than of people without diabetes have physical limitations: 66 percent compared with 29 percent (Ryerson and others 2003). Disabilities are even more pronounced among older people (Gregg and others 2000).

The World Health Organization estimated that, in 2001, diabetes resulted in 19,996,000 disability-adjusted life years (DALYs) worldwide. More than 80 percent of the DALYs resulting from diabetes were in developing countries (table 30.1). East Asia and the Pacific had the largest burden, and the Middle East and North Africa had the smallest burden. DALYs resulting from diabetes increased by 250 percent worldwide from 1990 to 2001 and by 266 percent for low- and middle-income countries (Mathers and others 2000).

Economic Burden of Diabetes

Diabetes imposes large economic burdens on national health care systems and affects both national economies and individuals and their families. Direct medical costs include resources used to treat the disease. Indirect costs include lost productivity caused by morbidity, disability, and premature mortality. Intangible costs refer to the reduced quality of life for people with diabetes brought about by stress, pain, and anxiety.

Direct Medical Costs. Good data on the direct medical costs of diabetes are not available for most developing countries. Extrapolation from developed countries suggests that, in 2003, the direct costs of diabetes worldwide for people age 20 to 79 totaled at least US$129 billion and may have been as high as US$241 billion (table 30.1). In the developing world, the costs were highest in Latin America and the Caribbean and lowest in Sub-Saharan Africa. The direct health care costs of diabetes range from 2.5 to 15.0 percent of annual health care budgets, depending on local prevalence and sophistication of the treatments available (International Diabetes Federation 2003b).

Indirect and Intangible Costs. In developing countries, the indirect costs of diabetes are at least as high, or even higher, than the direct medical costs (Barcelo and others 2003). Because the largest predicted rise in the number of people with diabetes in the next three decades will be among those in the economically productive ages of 20 to 64 (King, Aubert, and Herman 1998), the future indirect costs of diabetes will be even larger than they are now.

Diabetes lowers people's quality of life in many ways, including their physical and social functioning and their perceived physical and mental well-being. With a value of

1 representing the health-related quality of life without illness and 0 representing death, people with type 2 diabetes had a value of 0.77 in the population of the United Kingdom prospective diabetes study (Clarke, Gray, and Holman 2002).

Risk Factors for Diabetes

Risk factors for diabetes vary by disease type.

Type 1 Diabetes. Type 1 diabetes is most likely a polygenic disease, and a number of potential environmental risk factors have been implicated—including dietary factors; breastfeeding; initiation of bovine milk; infectious agents (for example, enterovirus, rotavirus, and rubella); chemicals; and toxins—but the results have been inconclusive (Akerblom and Knip 1998).

Type 2 Diabetes. The risk for type 2 diabetes is higher in monozygotic twins and people with a family history of diabetes (Rich 1990). This finding strongly suggests that genetic determinants play a role, but so far few genes have been associated with type 2 diabetes.

Environmental factors include prenatal factors, obesity, physical inactivity, and dietary and socioeconomic factors (Qiao and others 2004). Exposure to diabetes in utero increases the risk of developing type 2 diabetes in early adulthood (Dabelea and others 2000). Disproportionate growth and low birthweight increase the risk of developing diabetes and insulin resistance. In the postnatal environment, breastfeeding protects against the development of obesity, insulin resistance, and diabetes (Pettitt and others 1997; Young and others 2002).

The strongest and most consistent risk factors for diabetes and insulin resistance among different populations are obesity and weight gain (Haffner 1998): for each unit increase in body mass index, the risk of diabetes increases by 12 percent (Ford, Williamson, and Liu 1997). The distribution of fat around the trunk region, or central obesity, is also a strong risk factor for diabetes (Yajnik 2001). Diabetes risk may be reduced by increasing physical activity. Conversely, a sedentary lifestyle and physical inactivity are associated with increased risks of developing diabetes (Hu and others 2003). Some studies report a positive relationship between dietary fat and diabetes, but specific types of fats and carbohydrates may be more important than total fat or carbohydrate intake. Polyunsaturated fats and long-chain omega-3 fatty acids found in fish oils (Adler and others 1994) may reduce the risk of diabetes, and saturated fats and trans fatty acids may increase the risk of diabetes (Hu, van Dam, and Liu 2001). Sugar-sweetened beverages are associated with an increased risk of diabetes (Schulze and others 2004). High intakes of dietary fiber and of vegetables may reduce the risk of diabetes (Fung and others 2002; Stevens and others 2002).

Increased affluence and Westernization have been associated with an increase in the prevalence of diabetes in many indigenous populations and in developing economies (Rowley and others 1997; Williams and others 2001). Conversely, in developed countries, those in lower socioeconomic groups have a higher risk of obesity and consequently of type 2 diabetes (Everson and others 2002). Surrogates for socioeconomic status, such as level of education attained and income (Paeratakul and others 2002; Robbins and others 2001) are inversely associated with diabetes in high-income countries.

INTERVENTIONS AND DELIVERY MODES

Interventions against diabetes include those for preventing the disease, those for detecting the disease in its asymptomatic stage, and those for managing the disease to reduce its complications.

Preventing Type 1 Diabetes

Not enough scientific evidence is available to indicate that type 1 diabetes can be prevented, although various interventions have been explored. Examples of tested interventions include eliminating or delaying exposure to bovine protein and using insulin or nicotinamide for people at high risk of developing the disease.

Preventing Type 2 Diabetes

Four major trials—in China, Finland, Sweden, and the United States—have demonstrated that intensive lifestyle interventions involving a combination of diet and physical activity can delay or prevent diabetes among people at high risk (Eriksson and Lindgarde 1991; Knowler and others 2002; Pan and others 1997; Tuomilehto and others 2001). In the largest randomized, controlled trial to date, the Diabetes Prevention Program (Knowler and others 2002), the goals of the intensive lifestyle intervention were weight loss of 7 percent of baseline bodyweight through a low-calorie diet and moderate physical activity for at least 150 minutes per week. After 2.8 years of follow-up, the average weight loss was 4.5 kilograms for those in the lifestyle intervention group and less than 0.3 kilograms for those in the placebo group. The lifestyle intervention reduced the incidence of diabetes by 58 percent.

Pharmacological studies of diabetes prevention have been reviewed in detail elsewhere (Kanaya and Narayan 2003). In summary, a variety of specific medications have been tested (for example, metformin, acarbose, orlistat, troglitazone, angiotensin-converting enzyme [ACE] inhibitors, statins, estrogens, and progestins) and have been found to lower diabetes incidence, but the expense, side effects, and cumulative years of drug intervention are practical concerns. Except for the Diabetes Prevention Program (Knowler and others 2002), no trial of medication intervention has directly compared the effectiveness of a drug to that of lifestyle modification.

Screening for People with Diabetes or Prediabetes

The benefits of early detection of type 2 diabetes through screening are not clearly documented, nor is the choice of the appropriate screening test established. Questionnaires used alone tend to work poorly; biochemical tests alone or in combination with assessment of risk factors are a better alternative (Engelgau, Narayan, and Herman 2000).

Managing Diabetes

High-quality evidence exists for the efficacy of several current treatments in reducing morbidity and mortality in people with diabetes. These interventions are summarized in table 30.2.

In addition, a review of previous studies (Norris, Engelgau, and Narayan 2001) found positive effects for short follow-up (less than six months) of self-management training

Table 30.2 Effectiveness and Cost-Effectiveness of Interventions for Preventing and Treating Diabetes in Developed Countries

Strategy	Benefit	Quality of evidence[a]	Cost-effectiveness ratio (US$/QALY)[b]
Preventing diabetes			
• Lifestyle interventions for preventing type 2 diabetes	Reduction of 35–58 percent in incidence among people at high risk	I	1,100 (Diabetes Prevention Program Research Group forthcoming)
• Metformin for preventing type 2 diabetes	Reduction of 25–31 percent in incidence among people at high risk	I	31,200 (Diabetes Prevention Program Research Group forthcoming)
Screening for diabetes			
• Screening for type 2 diabetes in general population	Reduction of 25 percent in microvascular disease	III	73,500 (CDC Diabetes Cost-Effectiveness Study Group 1998)
Treating diabetes and its complications			
• Glycemic control in people with HbA1c greater than 9 percent	Reduction of 30 percent in microvascular disease per 1 percent drop in HbA1c	I	Cost saving (CDC Diabetes Cost-Effectiveness Study Group 1998)
• Glycemic control in people with HbA1c greater than 8 percent	Reduction of 30 percent in microvascular disease per 1 percent drop in HbA1c	I	34,400 (CDC Diabetes Cost-Effectiveness Study Group 1998; Klonoff and Schwartz 2000)
• Blood pressure control in people whose pressure is higher than 160/95 mmHg	Reduction of 35 percent in macrovascular and microvascular disease per 10 mmHg drop in blood pressure	I	Cost saving (CDC Diabetes Cost-Effectiveness Study Group 1998)
• Cholesterol control in people with total cholesterol greater than 200 milligrams/deciliter	Reduction of 25–55 percent in coronary heart diseases events; 43 percent fall in death rate	II-1	63,200 (CDC Diabetes Cost-Effectiveness Study Group 1998)
• Smoking cessation with recommended guidelines	16 percent quitting rate	I	12,500 (CDC Diabetes Cost-Effectiveness Study Group 1998)
• Annual screening for microalbuminuria	Reduction of 50 percent in nephropathy using ACE inhibitors for identified cases	III	47,400 (Klonoff and Schwartz 2000)
• Annual eye examinations	Reduction of 60 to 70 percent in serious vision loss	I	6,000 (Klonoff and Schwartz 2000; Vijan, Hofer, and Hayward 2000)
• Foot care in people with high risk of ulcers	Reduction of 50 to 60 percent in serious foot disease	I	Cost saving (Ragnarson and Apelqvist 2001)
• Aspirin use	Reduction of 28 percent in myocardial infarctions, reduction of 18 percent in cardiovascular disease	I	Not available
• ACE inhibitor use in all people with diabetes	Reduction of 42 percent in nephropathy; 22 percent drop in cardiovascular disease	I	8,800 (Golan, Birkmeyer, and Welch 1999)
• Influenza vaccinations among the elderly for type 2 diabetes	Reduction of 32 percent in hospitalizations; 64 percent drop in respiratory conditions and death	II-2	3,100 (Sorensen and others 2004)
• Preconception care for women of reproductive age	Reduction of 30 percent in hospital charges and 25 percent in hospital days	II-2	Cost saving (Klonoff and Schwartz 2000)

Source: Authors.

Note: mmHg = millimeters of mercury; QALY = quality-adjusted life year.

a. I indicates evidence from at least one randomized, controlled trial; II-1 indicates evidence from a well-designed, controlled trial without randomization; II-2 indicates evidence from cohort or case-control studies; and III indicates opinions of respected authorities (U.S. Preventive Services Task Force 1996).

b. We adjusted cost-effectiveness ratios to 2002 U.S. dollars using the consumer price index for medical care. In cases in which multiple studies evaluated the cost-effectiveness of an intervention, we report the median cost-effectiveness ratio.

on knowledge, frequency, and accuracy of self-monitoring of blood glucose; self-reported dietary habits; and glycemic control. Effects on lipids, physical activity, weight, and blood pressure varied.

COST-EFFECTIVENESS OF INTERVENTIONS AND PRIORITIES

Most of the interventions to prevent and treat diabetes and its complications significantly affect the use of health services. The limitations of clinical trials include their failure in most cases to capture the entire intervention effect over a lifetime and to include all segments of a population to whom the intervention may apply. Evaluating the cost-effectiveness of interventions often requires the use of computer simulation models, but data availability, technical complexity, and resource needs present a significant barrier to constructing such models for developing countries. Furthermore, data on interventions are often available only from developed countries, and these data are often extrapolated to developing countries.

Estimating the Cost-Effectiveness of Interventions in Developing Countries

To assess the cost-effectiveness of interventions in developing countries, we updated the results from Klonoff and Schwartz's (2000) comprehensive review by including studies that were published up to 2003. Table 30.2 summarizes the cost-effectiveness of interventions for the developed countries, mainly in the United States. The results show that the cost-effectiveness of interventions varies greatly—from cost saving (an intervention is both more effective and less expensive than the comparator) to US$73,500 per quality-adjusted life year (QALY) gained.

We estimated the cost-effectiveness ratio of diabetes interventions for the six developing regions shown in table 30.3. We assumed that the effectiveness of these interventions, as measured in QALYs, was the same as in developed countries but that the cost of interventions and other diabetes care differed between developed and developing countries and also among the six developing regions. Using this assumption, we estimated the cost-effectiveness ratio for a developing region as the cost-effectiveness ratio in the developed country, mainly represented by the United States, multiplied by the ratio of costs in the developing region to the cost in the developed countries, which we calculated as follows. These cost-effectiveness ratios are based on costs and benefits over a lifetime, except for preconception care for women of reproductive age.

We estimated that the cost of intervention and other diabetes care in the United States was 8.6 times the cost in Latin America and the Caribbean. This cost ratio was an average of four cost ratios—each weighted by its share (Barcelo and others 2003)—for outpatient care, inpatient care, drugs and laboratory tests, and treatment for diabetic complications. The cost ratio for each cost component was calculated as the cost of medical services or drugs in the United States divided by the cost of the same services or drugs in Latin America and the Caribbean. U.S. data for medical services and drugs for routine diabetes care, plus treatment cost for diabetes complications, were obtained from a 1998 cost-effectiveness Markov model of the U.S. Centers for Disease Control and Prevention (CDC). Data for laboratory service were obtained from the 2001 Clinical Diagnostic Laboratory Fee Schedule from the U.S. Centers for Medicare Services (available from http://www.cms.gov). Data for Latin America and the Caribbean were obtained from three countries—Argentina (Gagliardino and others 1993), Brazil (Health Policy Division of the Brazilian Ministry of Health), and Mexico (Villarreal-Rios and others 2000).

We applied Mulligan and others' framework (2003) to estimate the costs of intervention and diabetes care in each developing region. Assuming that cost estimates are available for one of the regions, this framework allows the development of a relative cost index for health care services that can then be used to obtain cost estimates for the other five regions. Using costs estimated by Mulligan and others (2003), we first estimated three health service indexes, including hospital bed days, outpatient and inpatient services, and laboratory tests and procedures. We then combined the three indexes into one overall index for diabetes care in accordance with the share of each component in developing countries (Barcelo and others 2003). Finally, we estimated the costs of intervention and diabetes care in the other five developing regions by multiplying the cost of care in the Latin America region by the overall regional relative cost index.

Ranking Implementation Priorities

We assessed the implementation priority and feasibility of interventions, as explained in table 30.3.

Level 1 Interventions. All three interventions in this category are cost saving and are also feasible in terms of all four aspects considered. The barrier to implementing these interventions may be a short-term hike in intervention costs.

Glycemic control in a population with poor control (hemoglobin A1c greater than 9 percent or another measure of glucose control in situations where HbA1c tests may be unaffordable) is cost saving because the reduction in medical care costs associated with both short-term and long-term complications is greater than is the cost of intervention. Glycemic control for people with type 1 diabetes involves insulin use and, for people with type 2 diabetes, depending on the stage and severity of the disease, consists of diet and physical activity, oral

Table 30.3 Cost-Effectiveness of Interventions for Preventing and Treating Diabetes and Its Complications in Developing Regions

Intervention	Cost/QALY (2001 US$)						Feasibility[a]	Implementing priority[b]
	East Asia and the Pacific	Europe and Central Asia	Latin America and the Caribbean	Middle East and North Africa	South Asia	Sub-Saharan Africa		
Level 1								
Glycemic control in people with HbA1c higher than 9 percent	Cost saving	Cost saving	Cost saving	Cost saving	Cost saving	Cost saving	++++	1
Blood pressure control in people with pressure higher than 160/95 mmHg	Cost saving	Cost saving	Cost saving	Cost saving	Cost saving	Cost saving	++++	1
Foot care in people with a high risk of ulcers	Cost saving	Cost saving	Cost saving	Cost saving	Cost saving	Cost saving	++++	1
Level 2								
Preconception care for women of reproductive age	Cost saving	Cost saving	Cost saving	Cost saving	Cost saving	Cost saving	++	2
Lifestyle interventions for preventing type 2 diabetes	80	100	130	110	60	60	++	2
Influenza vaccinations among the elderly for type 2 diabetes	220	290	360	310	180	160	++++	2
Annual eye examination	420	560	700	590	350	320	++	2
Smoking cessation	870	1,170	1,450	1,230	730	660	++	2
ACE inhibitor use for people with diabetes	620	830	1,020	870	510	460	+++	2
Level 3								
Metformin intervention for preventing type 2 diabetes	2,180	2,930	3,630	3,080	1,820	1,640	++	3
Cholesterol control for people with total cholesterol higher than 200 milligrams/deciliter	4,420	5,940	7,350	6,240	3,680	3,330	+++	3
Intensive glycemic control for people with HbA1c higher than 8 percent	2,410	3,230	4,000	3,400	2,000	1,810	++	3
Screening for undiagnosed diabetes	5,140	6,910	8,550	7,260	4,280	3,870	++	3
Annual screening for microalbuminuria	3,310	4,450	5,510	4,680	2,760	2,500	++	3

Source: Authors.

a. Feasibility was assessed based on difficulty of reaching the intervention population (the capacity of the health care system to deliver an intervention to the targeted population), technical complexity (the level of medical technologies or expertise needed for implementing an intervention), capital intensity (the amount of capital required for an intervention), and cultural acceptability (appropriateness of an intervention in terms of social norms and/or religious beliefs). ++++ indicates feasible for all four aspects, +++ indicates feasible for three of the four, ++ indicates feasible for two of the four, and + indicates feasible for one of the four.

b. Implementing priority was assessed by combining the cost-effectiveness of an intervention and its implementation feasibility; 1 represents the highest priority and 3 represents the lowest priority.

glucose-lowering agents, and insulin. Patient education is an essential component of these interventions to encourage patients to comply with medication regimes and to change to and maintain healthy lifestyles.

Glucose is generally poorly controlled in people with both type 1 and type 2 diabetes, mostly because of lack of access to insulin and other diabetes supplies in developing countries.

For example, the mean HbA1c level for people with diabetes in India was 8.9 percent in 1998 (Raheja and others 2001). A survey conducted by the International Diabetes Federation in 1997 (2003b) showed that no country in Africa had 100 percent accessibility to insulin. Ensuring adequate access to insulin should be an important priority for developing countries.

Blood pressure control for people with diabetes and hypertension reduces the incidence of both microvascular and macrovascular diseases. Major medication interventions include an ACE inhibitor, thiazide diuretics, or a beta blocker. Blood pressure control is cost saving mainly because of its large health benefits and relatively low intervention costs. Even in the United States, moderate blood pressure control costs less than US$250 per patient per year. Because many blood pressure medications are generic drugs, the costs are much lower in developing countries. In addition, the prevalence of people with poor control of blood pressure may be high in developing countries. For example, in Latin America and the Caribbean, 60 percent of people with type 2 diabetes in 2000 had blood pressure higher than 140/90 mmHg (Gagliardino, de la Hera and Siri 2001).

Complications related to foot problems are common among diabetics in developing countries. For example, in India, 43 percent of diabetes patients had foot-related complications (Raheja and others 2001). Interventions for foot care are low tech and require little capital. Interventions for foot care in developing countries should include educational programs for patients and professionals (for example, on foot hygiene, treatment of calluses, awareness of functional infections, and care for skin injuries); access to appropriate footwear; and multidisciplinary clinics. All three interventions could be cost saving, mainly because the cost of the interventions is low and the interventions can reduce the risk of foot ulceration and amputation, which are costly. Applying these interventions for high-risk patients, such as those with at least one previous foot ulcer or amputation, would yield even larger savings (Klonoff and Schwartz 2000).

Level 2 Interventions. The six interventions in this category are either cost saving and not feasible in one or more aspects or cost less than US$1,500 per QALY and are at least moderately feasible. Thus, interventions in this category represent good value for money but may present some difficulties in terms of feasibility.

Preconception care among women of reproductive age includes patient education and intensive glucose management. This intervention reduces short-term hospital costs for both mothers and infants and improves birth outcomes. However, the intervention may not be feasible in some developing countries because of the resources needed for the intervention and the difficulty of reaching the target population.

The lifestyle intervention for preventing type 2 diabetes costs US$60 to US$130 per QALY over a lifetime, depending on the region. The potential population eligible for a lifestyle intervention (those with impaired glucose tolerance or impaired fasting glucose) is large in developing countries. The International Diabetes Federation (2003b) estimates that the prevalence of impaired glucose tolerance was at least as high as the prevalence of diabetes in all regions. The expertise required for the intervention, such as dietitians and exercise physiologists, and the capacity of health care systems to handle the large populations eligible for the intervention may present a barrier to implementing the intervention in many developing countries.

People with diabetes are at higher risk of complications from influenza and pneumococcal infections than those without diabetes. Influenza vaccinations are a relatively cost-effective intervention, mainly because of the low intervention cost. However, the level of adoption for the intervention would depend on a country's ability to deliver the intervention to the targeted population.

The detection of proliferative diabetic retinopathy and macular edema by dilated eye examination followed by appropriate laser photocoagulation therapy prevents blindness. Annual screening and treatment programs for diabetic retinopathy cost US$700 or less per QALY gained in developing countries. The intervention is more cost-effective among older people, those who require insulin (Klonoff and Schwartz 2000), or those with poor glucose control (Vijan, Hofer, and Hayward 2000). In addition, screening less frequently, such as every two years, may be more cost-effective than screening every year (Vijan, Hofer, and Hayward 2000). Eye complications among people with diabetes are common in developing countries; for example, 39 percent of people with diabetes in India had eye-related complications (Rajala and others 1998). Although laser treatment is an effective intervention, such treatment may not be available in many developing countries or may be extremely costly.

ACE inhibitors can lower the blood pressure of those with hypertension and delay the onset or prevent further progression of renal disease for those with diabetes. Compared with screening for microalbuminuria and treating only those who have the condition, offering ACE inhibitors to all people with diabetes was more cost-effective at less than US$1,020 per QALY gained. This intervention was more cost-effective among younger people and was sensitive to the cost of drug. Thus, lowering the cost of the medication is a key factor for the success of this intervention in developing countries.

Smoking cessation includes both counseling and using medication such as a nicotine patch. Smoking cessation appears to be the least cost-effective among the level 2 interventions. However, the benefits of smoking cessation may be underestimated because our calculations only took the reduced risk of CVD into account (Earnshaw and others 2002). Adding the health benefits derived from preventing cancer and pulmonary diseases would improve the cost-effectiveness of smoking cessation. Considering the high prevalence of smoking in developing countries, smoking cessation should be a high-priority intervention, but the availability of the nicotine patch may be a barrier to implementing this intervention in developing countries.

Level 3 Interventions. The five interventions included in this category cost at least US$1,640 per QALY but could cost as much as US$8,550 per QALY. Compared with the level 1 and 2 interventions, those in this category are also less feasible. In general, depending on cost-effectiveness and feasibility, these interventions may not always be justifiable for all people in developing countries, given the limited health care resources. However, these interventions may be reasonable for selected subpopulation groups, such as those who can afford them.

Metformin therapy for preventing type 2 diabetes among people at high risk, such as those with prediabetes, is feasible because the drug is affordable in many developing countries; however, the intervention may not be good value for money. Cholesterol control intervention for people with diabetes falls into the same category. The cost-effectiveness of both these interventions would improve if the costs of the drug could be lowered.

The aim of intensive glucose control is to lower the glucose level of a person with diabetes to a level close to that of a person without diabetes. Implementing this intervention is a lower priority, mainly because of its relatively low cost-effectiveness in the context of the limited health care resources in developing countries. Although the U.K. Prospective Diabetes Study clearly demonstrates that lowering glucose levels can prevent or delay long-term diabetes complications (UKPDS Group 1998), the marginal return on very intensive glucose control in developing countries was relatively small.

Screening for undiagnosed diabetes is a low-priority intervention mainly because of its relatively high cost per QALY. However, screening for undiagnosed diabetes can be a worthwhile intervention for subpopulation groups, such as those that have a high prevalence of undiagnosed diabetes. In the United States, for example, screening for undiagnosed diabetes among African Americans was estimated to be 10 times more cost-effective than screening among other population groups (CDC Diabetes Cost-Effectiveness Study Group 1998). In addition, screening for undiagnosed diabetes may be a worthwhile intervention for patients with risk factors for other chronic diseases, such as hypertension, high lipid profiles, and prediabetes.

Annual screening for microalbuminuria was a low-priority intervention because screening added costs with no significant benefits. Treating all persons with diabetes with ACE inhibitors was a better treatment option than screening for microalbuminuria and treating only those who have the condition.

Cost-Effectiveness of a Polypill to Prevent CVD

A meta-analysis estimated that a hypothetical polypill could reduce the risk of CVD by 80 percent among all people over 55 or people with diabetes of any age (Wald and Law 2003). This hypothetical pill is a combination of three half-dose antihypertensive medications—aspirin, statin, and folic acid (see also chapter 33). Currently, neither is it available for use, nor have estimates of its benefits and adverse effects been confirmed in a formal, randomized, controlled trial. The idea is thus still theoretical. The cost-effectiveness of this hypothetical pill was, however, simulated using a computer model of people with newly diagnosed diabetes in the United States (Sorensen and others 2004), and the assessment found that a polypill intervention would cost US$11,000 per QALY gained. The intervention would be cost saving if such a pill cost US$1.28 or less per day. We estimated that the cost-effectiveness ratio of the polypill ranged from US$560 to US$1,280 per QALY gained for the six developing regions. This result was sensitive to changes in the cost of the intervention, but the intervention remained cost-effective within the most likely ranges of its cost (Sorensen and others 2004). A barrier to this intervention, in addition to the feasibility of producing such pill, is that its benefits and side effects would still have to be established in a randomized clinical trial.

Cost-Effectiveness of Diabetes Education

People with diabetes play a central role in managing their disease. Thus, diabetes education is an integral part of diabetes care. The goal of diabetes education is to support the efforts of people with diabetes to understand the nature of their illness and its treatment; to identify emergency health problems at early, reversible stages; to adhere to self-care practices; and to make necessary changes to their health habits (International Diabetes Federation 2003b). Health providers can deliver diabetes education programs in various settings. Evaluating the effectiveness of health education is challenging because of the difficulty of separating out its effect from that of other interventions. Nevertheless, a review of literature published in the United States suggests that self-management diabetes education may be cost-effective (Klonoff and Schwartz 2000).

Training in diabetes self-management reduces medical costs for diabetes care in developing countries in the short term. A multicenter intervention study in 10 Latin American countries demonstrated that an education program could reduce the cost of drugs by 62 percent (International Diabetes Federation 2003b), and another program in Argentina found a reduction in diabetes-related costs of 38 percent (Gagliardino and Etchegoyen 2001). Because the costs of education programs are generally low, the intervention may be cost-effective. Training patients to better manage their diabetes is also feasible because of its low technical complexity, low capital requirements, and cultural acceptability. Thus, diabetes education should be a high-priority intervention for all developing regions.

LESSONS AND EXPERIENCE

A number of lessons can be learned from the experiences in countries where the interventions described have been implemented.

Prevention

Data are sparse on community- or population-based strategies for preventing diabetes along with other chronic diseases such as CVD. Available studies on preventing type 2 diabetes have used clinic-based approaches targeted at high-risk groups, and researchers generally agree that type 2 diabetes can be prevented or its onset delayed. Putting these results into practice, however, is fraught with difficulties and unanswered questions, such as the following:

- Who would benefit from diabetes prevention?
- How can those who may benefit be identified?
- What are the costs and cost-effectiveness of diabetes prevention at a population level?
- How should results be extrapolated from developed countries to developing countries, whose priorities and approaches may be different?

Treatment

The quality of diabetes care generally remains suboptimal worldwide, regardless of a particular country's level of development, health care system, or population (Engelgau and others 2003; Garfield and others 2003). The Costs of Diabetes in Europe—Type 2 study, conducted in eight European countries, found suboptimal diabetes care in each country (Liebl, Mata, and Eschwege 2002). In the United States, population-based surveys in the 1990s among adults age 18 to 75 with diabetes found that only 63 percent of them had had a dilated eye examination and only 55 percent had had a foot examination within the past year, 18 percent had poor glycemic control, 42 percent had good cholesterol control, and 66 percent had a blood pressure within the normal range (Saaddine and others 2002).

The Diabcare-Asia project was conducted in the late 1990s. Results from India, Singapore, and Taiwan (China) found that in 1998, 32 to 50 percent of the diabetic population had poor glycemic control (equivalent to HbA1c > 8 percent), 43 to 67 percent had high cholesterol (greater than 5.2 millimoles per deciliter), and 47 to 54 percent had an abnormal level of triglyceride (greater than 1.7 millimoles per deciliter) (W. R. Lee and others 2001; Raheja and others 2001). Data from Latin America and the Caribbean showed that 41 percent of people with type 1 diabetes and 57 percent of those with type 2 diabetes had poor glucose control. Of those with type 2 diabetes, 56 percent

had hypertension, 53 percent had high cholesterol, and 45 percent had abnormal triglycerides (Gagliardino, de la Hera, and Siri 2001).

Quality of Diabetes Care

Small, single-site studies indicate that several interventions to improve quality of care at the patient, provider, or system levels are promising (Narayan and others 2004). A systematic review (Renders and others 2001) found that multifaceted professional interventions may enhance providers' performance in managing diabetes care; that organizational interventions involving regularly contacting and tracking patients by means of computerized tracking systems or through nurses can also improve diabetes management; that patient-oriented interventions can improve patients' outcomes; and that nurses can play an important role in patient-oriented interventions by educating patients and facilitating patients' adherence to treatment regimes. (See also chapter 70.)

Interventions that could modify providers' behavior include education as part of more complex interventions that also focus on systems and on the organization of practices—for example, feedback on performance, reminder systems, consensus development, and clinical practice guidelines. Potential systemic interventions include the use of continuous quality improvement techniques; feedback on performance; physician incentives for quality; nurses to provide diabetes care (which is typically provided by physicians); computerized reminder systems for providers, alone or in combination with a performance feedback program; patient-tracking or other reminder systems to improve regular follow-up; dedicated blocks of time set aside for diabetes patients in primary care practices; team care; electronic medical record systems; and other methods, such as telephone and mailing reminders, chart stickers, and flow sheets to prompt both providers and patients.

Interventions that empower patients can be successful components of diabetes programs. A systems-oriented approach using manual or computerized systems that remind patients to make follow-up appointments and that prompt staff members to generate reminder cards for patients can improve compliance with follow-up and enhance efficiency of office practices. In addition, comprehensive implementation of multiple risk-factor interventions in real-life settings has been shown to reduce vascular events by more than 50 percent among people with diabetes (Gaede and others 2003).

The Institute of Medicine Committee on Quality of Health Care in America (2001) argues strongly that newer systems of care and newer ways of thinking are needed to tackle complex diseases such as diabetes. Furthermore, the model of the process of change in a simple mechanical system is woefully inadequate for dealing with the complex, interactive, and interconnected adaptive systems in which diabetes is prevented and treated. Applied research, designed to encompass the system as a whole and not simply its component parts, can enhance our understanding of complex health care dynamics for chronic diseases (Fraser and Greenhalgh 2001; Plsek and Greenhalgh 2001).

RESEARCH AND DEVELOPMENT AGENDA

The following subsections discuss the major issues for research and development.

Prevention

Well-designed community-based studies of primary prevention for type 2 diabetes are needed, especially as part of multifactorial interventions, in developing countries. Research is also needed into safer and cheaper drugs to prevent diabetes when lifestyle intervention either is not feasible or has failed. In addition, we need to know the long-term effects of diabetes prevention on CVD and other outcomes. More effective and cheaper ways to prevent the major complications of diabetes are also needed. Other areas also deserving of research include noninvasive methods for monitoring blood glucose and more effective and efficient ways of screening for prediabetes, diabetes, and early diabetes complications. Evidence of the benefits of diabetes education on outcomes is lacking, and organized research to assess effective components of diabetes education and their impact on control of risk factors and long-term outcomes should be a priority.

Epidemiological and Economics Research

Scant data are available on the future burden of diabetes and its complications in developing countries. Data on trends in and the effects of risk factors for diabetes in developing countries—obesity; birthweight; physical inactivity; television viewing; dietary factors; fast foods; socioeconomic factors; and effects of urbanization, industrialization, globalization, and stress—are also sparse. Low-cost ways to obtain such data in a standardized manner may be worth considering. More data are also needed on the costs of diabetes, the impact of the disease on quality of life, and the cost-effectiveness of various interventions in the context of developing countries (International Diabetes Federation 2003a).

Health Systems and Operational Research

Greater emphasis on translation research is needed. Well-designed and standardized studies of quality of care and outcomes will help (TRIAD Study Group 2002). Research aimed at understanding system-level complexity and finding ways to deliver chronic disease care that takes such complexity into account is also likely to yield profitable results (Institute of Medicine Committee on Quality of Health Care in America 2001). Computer models suitable for assessing cost-effectiveness and for forecasting the burden in developing countries are needed. Operational research aimed at understanding the tradeoffs and the best mix of resource allocation for diabetes and chronic disease care in developing countries is also needed.

Basic Research

Further strategic unraveling of the genetic basis of type 2 diabetes and gene-environment interactions may help explain the diabetes epidemic and provide better understanding of the pathophysiology of the disease. It may also may lead to better prevention and treatment strategies. Understanding the role of prenatal influences, especially in developing countries, may offer productive opportunities for interventions. Because of the increasing occurrence of type 2 diabetes in children, as well as the role of obesity in accelerating the onset of type 1 diabetes, further research into the typology and classification of diabetes is vital. The rapid industrialization and economic development being experienced by several developing countries may make research into the role of socioeconomic factors, urban stress, and lifestyle factors on the causation of diabetes productive.

CONCLUSIONS

A growing diabetes pandemic is unfolding with rapid increases in the prevalence of type 2 diabetes. The direct health care costs of diabetes worldwide amount to 2003 US$129 billion per year. Estimates indicate that developing countries spend between 2.5 and 15.0 percent of their annual direct health budgets on diabetes care, and families with diabetic members spend 15 to 25 percent of their incomes on diabetes care.

A whole array of effective interventions to prevent diabetes and its complications is available, and we have attempted to assess their potential cost-effectiveness in developing regions. Using these estimations and a qualitative assessment of the feasibility of implementation, we have prioritized available interventions into the following three categories:

- level 1—cost saving and highly feasible
- level 2—cost saving or cost less than US$1,500 per QALY but pose some feasibility challenges
- level 3—cost between US$1,640 and US$8,550 per QALY and pose significant feasibility challenges.

Table 30.4 presents a summary of all major diabetes interventions, major health effects of the interventions, and level of implementation priority.

In addition, we propose diabetes education as an essential intervention. However, more organized research into the precise components of diabetes education and its effect on

Table 30.4 Key Cost-Effective Interventions for Preventing and Treating Diabetes and Its Complications

Intervention	Description	Applicable population	Major effect
Level 1[a]			
• Glycemic control in people with poor control	Insulin, oral glucose-lowering agents, diet and exercise	People with diabetes, all ages, HbA1c greater than 9 percent	Reduction in microvascular disease
• Blood pressure control	Blood pressure control medications	People with diabetes, hypertensive, all ages	Reduction in macrovascular disease, microvascular disease, and mortality
• Foot care	Patient and provider education, foot examination, foot hygiene, and appropriate footwear	People with diabetes, middle-aged or older	Reduction in serious foot diseases and amputations
Level 2[b]			
• Preconception care for women of reproductive age	Patient self-management	Women with diabetes who plan to become pregnant	Reduction in HbA1c level and hospital expenses of the mother and baby
• Lifestyle intervention to prevent diabetes	Behavioral change, including diet and physical activity, to reduce bodyweight	People who are at high risk (for example, prediabetes for type 2 diabetes)	Reduction in type 2 diabetes incidence by 58 percent
• Influenza vaccination	Vaccination	Elderly people with diabetes	Reduction in hospitalizations, respiratory conditions, and mortality
• Detection and treatment of eye diseases	Eye examination to screen for and treat eye diseases	People with diabetes, middle-aged or older	Reduction in serious vision loss
• ACE inhibitors	Angiotensin-converting enzyme medication	People with diabetes	Reduction in nephropathy, cardiovascular disease, and death
• Smoking cessation	Physician counseling and nicotine replacement therapy	People with diabetes, all ages, smokers	Increase in quitting rate and reduction in cardiovascular disease
Level 3[c]			
• Metformin therapy for preventing diabetes	Metformin medication	People who are at high risk (for example, prediabetes for type 2 diabetes)	Reduction in type 2 diabetes incidence by 33 percent
• Intensive glucose control	Insulin, oral glucose-lowering agents, or both	Diabetes, all ages, with HbA1c less than 9 percent	Reduction in microvascular disease
• Lipid control	Cholesterol-lowering medication	Diabetes, all ages, with high cholesterol	Reduction in cardiovascular disease events and mortality
• Screening for microalbuminuria	Screening for microalbuminuria and treating those who test positive	Diabetes, all ages	Reduction in kidney diseases
• Screening for undiagnosed diabetes	Screening for undiagnosed diabetes and treating those who test positive	People who are at high risk for type 2 diabetes	Reduction in microvascular disease
Essential background intervention[d]			
Diabetes education	Patient self-management	Diabetes, all ages	Reduction in HbA1c level and better compliance with lifestyle changes
Other promising intervention[e]			
Polypill	Hypothetical pill combining low doses of antihypertensive medication, aspirin, statin, and folate	Diabetes, all ages	Reduction in cardiovascular disease

Source: Authors.

a. Level 1 interventions are cost saving and highly feasible.

b. Level 2 interventions are cost saving or cost less than US$1,500 per quality-adjusted life year but pose feasibility challenges.

c. Level 3 interventions cost between US$1,640 and US$8,550 per quality-adjusted life year and pose significant feasibility challenges.

d. Diabetes education is the backbone on which many diabetes interventions depend, but empirical data on the effectiveness of diabetes education on outcomes and on the precise components of diabetes education are still lacking.

e. An intervention that appears promising but needs further research to document its effectiveness and/or safety. The polypill is only a theoretical concept at this time and is not available for implementation.

long-term outcomes is needed. We also propose that further research be launched in relation to the novel and potentially promising polypill.

Finally, this chapter suggests a number of interventions at the level of the patient, provider, and system that could help address the overall suboptimal quality of diabetes care; notes the possible benefits of making important drugs available at cheaper costs in developing countries; and suggests some research priorities for developing regions.

REFERENCES

Adler, A. I., E. J. Boyko, C. D. Schraer, and N. J. Murphy. 1994. "Lower Prevalence of Impaired Glucose Tolerance and Diabetes Associated with Daily Seal Oil or Salmon Consumption among Alaska Natives." *Diabetes Care* 17 (12): 1498–1501.

Akerblom, H. K., and M. Knip. 1998. "Putative Environmental Factors in Type 1 Diabetes." *Diabetes/Metabolism Review* 14 (1): 31–67.

American Diabetes Association. 2004. "Diagnosis and Classification of Diabetes Mellitus." *Diabetes Care* 27 (Suppl. 1): S5–10.

Barcelo, A., C. Aedo, S. Rajpathak, and S. Robles. 2003. "The Cost of Diabetes in Latin America and the Caribbean." *Bulletin of the World Health Organization* 81 (1): 19–27.

CDC (U.S. Centers for Disease Control and Prevention) Diabetes Cost-Effectiveness Study Group. 1998. "The Cost-Effectiveness of Screening for Type 2 Diabetes." *Journal of the American Medical Association* 280 (20): 1757–63.

Clarke, P., A. Gray, and R. Holman. 2002. "Estimating Utility Values for Health States of Type 2 Diabetic Patients Using the EQ-5D (UKPDS 62)." *Medical Decision Making* 22 (4): 340–49.

Dabelea, D., R. L. Hanson, R. S. Lindsay, D. J. Pettitt, G. Imperatore, M. M. Gabir, and others. 2000. "Intrauterine Exposure to Diabetes Conveys Risks for Type 2 Diabetes and Obesity: A Study of Discordant Sibships." *Diabetes* 49 (12): 2208–11.

Diabetes Prevention Program Research Group. Forthcoming. "The Cost-Effectiveness of Diet and Physical Activity or Metformin in the Prevention of Type 2 Diabetes among Adults with Impaired Glucose Tolerance." *Annals of Internal Medicine.*

Earnshaw, S. R., A. Richter, S. W. Sorensen, T. J. Hoerger, K. A. Hicks, M. Engelgau, and others. 2002. "Optimal Allocation of Resources across Four Interventions for Type 2 Diabetes." *Medical Decision Making* 22 (Suppl. 5): S80–91.

Engelgau, M. M., K. M. Narayan, and W. H. Herman. 2000. "Screening for Type 2 Diabetes." *Diabetes Care* 23 (10): 1563–80.

Engelgau, M. M., K. M. Narayan, J. B. Saaddine, and F. Vinicor. 2003. "Addressing the Burden of Diabetes in the 21st Century: Better Care and Primary Prevention." *Journal of the American Society of Nephrology* 14 (7 Suppl. 2): S88–91.

Eriksson, K. F., and F. Lindgarde. 1991. "Prevention of Type 2 (Non-Insulin-Dependent) Diabetes Mellitus by Diet and Physical Exercise. The 6-Year Malmo Feasibility Study." *Diabetologia* 34 (12): 891–98.

Everson, S. A., S. C. Maty, J. W. Lynch, and G. A. Kaplan. 2002. "Epidemiologic Evidence for the Relation between Socioeconomic Status and Depression, Obesity, and Diabetes." *Journal of Psychosomatic Research* 53 (4): 891–95.

Ford, E. S., D. F. Williamson, and S. Liu. 1997. "Weight Change and Diabetes Incidence: Findings from a National Cohort of US Adults." *American Journal of Epidemiology* 146 (3): 214–22.

Fraser, S. W., and T. Greenhalgh. 2001. "Coping with Complexity: Educating for Capability." *British Medical Journal* 323 (7316): 799–803.

Fung, T. T., F. B. Hu, M. A. Pereira, S. Liu, M. J. Stampfer, G. A. Colditz, and others. 2002. "Whole-Grain Intake and the Risk of Type 2 Diabetes: A Prospective Study in Men." *American Journal of Clinical Nutrition* 76 (3): 535–40.

Gaede, P., P. Vedel, N. Larsen, G. V. Jensen, H. H. Parving, and O. Pedersen. 2003. "Multifactorial Intervention and Cardiovascular Disease in Patients with Type 2 Diabetes." *New England Journal of Medicine* 348 (5): 383–93.

Gagliardino, J. J., H. M. de la Hera, and F. Siri. 2001. "Evaluation of the Quality of Care for Diabetic Patients in Latin America" (in Spanish). *Revista Panamericana de Salud Pública* 10 (5): 309–17.

Gagliardino, J. J., and G. Etchegoyen. 2001. "A Model Educational Program for People with Type 2 Diabetes: A Cooperative Latin American Implementation Study (PEDNID-LA)." *Diabetes Care* 24 (6): 1001–7.

Gagliardino, J. J., E. M. Olivera, H. Barragan, and R. A. Puppo. 1993. "A Simple Economic Evaluation Model for Selecting Diabetes Health Care Strategies." *Diabetic Medicine* 10 (4): 351–54.

Garfield, S. A., S. Malozowski, M. H. Chin, K. M. Venkat Narayan, R. E. Glasgow, L. W. Green, and others. 2003. "Considerations for Diabetes Translational Research in Real-World Settings." *Diabetes Care* 26 (9): 2670–74.

Geiss, L. S., W. H. Herman, and P. J. Smith. 1995. "Mortality among Persons with Non-Insulin Dependent Diabetes." In *Diabetes in America*, 2nd ed., ed. National Diabetes Data Group, 233–58. Bethesda, MD: National Institutes of Health.

Golan, L., J. D. Birkmeyer, and H. G. Welch. 1999. "The Cost-Effectiveness of Treating All Patients with Type 2 Diabetes with Angiotensin-Converting Enzyme Inhibitors." *Annals of Internal Medicine* 131 (9): 660–67.

Gregg, E. W., G. L. Beckles, D. F. Williamson, S. G. Leveille, J. A. Langlois, M. M. Engelgau, and others. 2000. "Diabetes and Physical Disability among Older U.S. Adults." *Diabetes Care* 23 (9): 1272–77.

Haffner, S. M. 1998. "Epidemiology of Type 2 Diabetes: Risk Factors." *Diabetes Care* 21 (Suppl. 3): C3–6.

Hu, F. B., T. Y. Li, G. A. Colditz, W. C. Willett, and J. E. Manson. 2003. "Television Watching and Other Sedentary Behaviors in Relation to Risk of Obesity and Type 2 Diabetes Mellitus in Women." *Journal of the American Medical Association* 289 (14): 1785–91.

Hu, F. B., R. M. van Dam, and S. Liu. 2001. "Diet and Risk of Type II Diabetes: The Role of Types of Fat and Carbohydrate." *Diabetologia* 44 (7): 805–17.

Institute of Medicine Committee on Quality of Health Care in America. 2001. *Crossing the Quality Chasm: A New Health System for the 21st Century*. Washington, DC: National Academy Press.

International Diabetes Federation. 2003a. *Cost-Effective Approaches to Diabetes Care and Prevention*. Brussels: International Diabetes Federation.

———. 2003b. *Diabetes Atlas*. 2nd ed. Brussels: International Diabetes Federation.

Kanaya, A. M., and K. M. Narayan. 2003. "Prevention of Type 2 Diabetes: Data from Recent Trials." *Primary Care* 30 (3): 511–26.

King, H., R. E. Aubert, and W. H. Herman. 1998. "Global Burden of Diabetes, 1995–2025: Prevalence, Numerical Estimates, and Projections." *Diabetes Care* 21 (9): 1414–31.

Klonoff, D. C., and D. M. Schwartz. 2000. "An Economic Analysis of Interventions for Diabetes." *Diabetes Care* 23 (3): 390–404.

Knowler, W. C., E. Barrett-Connor, S. E. Fowler, R. F. Hamman, J. M. Lachin, E. A. Walker, and others. 2002. "Reduction in the Incidence of Type 2 Diabetes with Lifestyle Intervention or Metformin." *New England Journal of Medicine* 346 (6): 393–403.

Lee, W. L., A. M. Cheung, D. Cape, and B. Zinman. 2000. "Impact of Diabetes on Coronary Artery Disease in Women and Men: A Meta-analysis of Prospective Studies." *Diabetes Care* 23 (7): 962–68.

Lee, W. R., H. S. Lim, A. C. Thai, W. L. Chew, S. Emmanuel, L. G. Goh, and others. 2001. "A Window on the Current Status of Diabetes Mellitus in Singapore—The Diabcare-Singapore 1998 Study." *Singapore Medical Journal* 42 (11): 501–507.

Liebl, A., M. Mata, and E. Eschwege. 2002. "Evaluation of Risk Factors for Development of Complications in Type II Diabetes in Europe." *Diabetologia* 45 (7): S23–28.

Manuel, D. G., and S. E. Schultz. 2004. "Health-Related Quality of Life and Health-Adjusted Life Expectancy of People with Diabetes in Ontario, Canada, 1996–1997." *Diabetes Care* 27 (2): 407–14.

Mathers, C. D., C. Stein, D. Ma Fat, C. Rao, M. Inoue, N. Tomijima, and others. 2000. *Global Burden of Disease 2000: Version 2 Methods and Results.* Global Programme on Evidence for Health Policy Discussion Paper Series. Geneva: World Health Organization.

Mulligan, J., J. A. Fox-Rushby, T. Adam, B. Johns, and A. Mills. 2003. "Unit Costs of Health Care Inputs in Low and Middle Income Regions." Disease Control Priorities Project Working Paper 9, Fogarty International Center, National Institutes of Health, Bethesda, MD.

Narayan, K. M., E. Benjamin, E. W. Gregg, S. L. Norris, and M. M. Engelgau. 2004. "Diabetes Translation Research: Where Are We and Where Do We Want to Be?" *Annals of Internal Medicine* 140 (11): 958–63.

Narayan, K. M., J. P. Boyle, T. J. Thompson, S. W. Sorensen, and D. F. Williamson. 2003. "Lifetime Risk for Diabetes Mellitus in the United States." *Journal of the American Medical Association* 290 (14): 1884–90.

Norris, S. L., M. M. Engelgau, and K. M. Narayan. 2001. "Effectiveness of Self-Management Training in Type 2 Diabetes: A Systematic Review of Randomized Controlled Trials." *Diabetes Care* 24 (3): 561–87.

Paeratakul, S., J. C. Lovejoy, D. H. Ryan, and G. A. Bray. 2002. "The Relation of Gender, Race, and Socioeconomic Status to Obesity and Obesity Comorbidities in a Sample of U.S. Adults." *International Journal of Obesity and Related Metabolic Disorders* 26 (9): 1205–10.

Pan, X. R., G. W. Li, Y. H. Hu, J. X. Wang, W. Y. Yang, Z. X. An, and others. 1997. "Effects of Diet and Exercise in Preventing NIDDM in People with Impaired Glucose Tolerance: The Da Qing IGT and Diabetes Study." *Diabetes Care* 20 (4): 537–44.

Pettitt, D. J., M. R. Forman, R. L. Hanson, W. C. Knowler, and P. H. Bennett. 1997. "Breastfeeding and Incidence of Non-Insulin-Dependent Diabetes Mellitus in Pima Indians." *Lancet* 350 (9072): 166–68.

Plsek, P. E., and T. Greenhalgh. 2001. "Complexity Science: The Challenge of Complexity in Health Care." *British Medical Journal* 323 (7313): 625–28.

Qiao, Q., D. E. Williams, G. Imperatore, K. M. Venkat Narayan, and J. Tuomilehto. 2004. "Epidemiology and Geography of Type 2 Diabetes Mellitus." In *International Textbook of Diabetes Mellitus*, 3rd ed., ed. R. A. DeFronzo and others, 33–56. Chichester, U.K.: John Wiley & Sons.

Ragnarson, T. G., and J. Apelqvist. 2001. "Prevention of Diabetes-Related Foot Ulcers and Amputations: A Cost-Utility Analysis Based on Markov Model Simulations." *Diabetologia* 44 (11): 2077–87.

Raheja, B. S., A. Kapur, A. Bhoraskar, S. R. Sathe, L. N. Jorgensen, S. R. Moorthi, and others. 2001. "DiabCare Asia—India Study: Diabetes Care in India—Current Status." *Journal of the Association of Physicians of India* 49: 717–22.

Rajala, U., M. Laakso, Q. Qiao, and S. Keinanen-Kiukaanniemi. 1998. "Prevalence of Retinopathy in People with Diabetes, Impaired Glucose Tolerance, and Normal Glucose Tolerance." *Diabetes Care* 21 (10): 1664–69.

Renders, C. M., G. D. Valk, S. J. Griffin, E. H. Wagner, V. J. Eijk, and W. J. Assendelft. 2001. "Interventions to Improve the Management of Diabetes in Primary Care, Outpatient, and Community Settings: A Systematic Review." *Diabetes Care* 24 (10): 1821–33.

Rich, S. S. 1990. "Mapping Genes in Diabetes. Genetic Epidemiological Perspective." *Diabetes* 39 (11): 1315–19.

Robbins, J. M., V. Vaccarino, H. Zhang, and S. V. Kasl. 2001. "Socioeconomic Status and Type 2 Diabetes in African American and Non-Hispanic White Women and Men: Evidence from the Third National Health and Nutrition Examination Survey." *American Journal of Public Health* 91 (1): 76–83.

Rowley, K. G., J. D. Best, R. McDermott, E. A. Green, L. S. Piers, and K. O'Dea. 1997. "Insulin Resistance Syndrome in Australian Aboriginal People." *Clinical and Experimental Pharmacology and Physiology* 24 (9–10): 776–81.

Ryerson, B., E. F. Tierney, T. J. Thompson, M. M. Engelgau, J. Wang, E. W. Gregg, and others. 2003. "Excess Physical Limitations among Adults with Diabetes in the U.S. population, 1997–1999." *Diabetes Care* 26 (1): 206–10.

Saaddine, J. B., M. M. Engelgau, G. L. Beckles, E. W. Gregg, T. J. Thompson, and K. M. Narayan. 2002. "A Diabetes Report Card for the United States: Quality of Care in the 1990s." *Annals of Internal Medicine* 136 (8): 565–74.

Schulze, M. B., J. E. Manson, D. S. Ludwig, G. A. Colditz, M. J. Stampfer, W. C. Willett, and others. 2004. "Sugar-Sweetened Beverages, Weight Gain, and Incidence of Type 2 Diabetes in Young and Middle-Aged Women." *Journal of the American Medical Association* 292 (8): 927–34.

Sorensen, S., M. Engelgau, T. Hoerger, K. Hicks, K. Narayan, D. Williamson, and others. 2004. "Assessment of the Benefits from a Polypill to Reduce Cardiovascular Disease among Persons with Type 2 Diabetes Mellitus." Poster presented at the 64th Annual Scientific Sessions of the American Diabetes Association, Orlando, Florida, June 4–8, 2004.

Stevens, J., K. Ahn, Juhaeri, D. Houston, L. Steffan, and D. Couper. 2002. "Dietary Fiber Intake and Glycemic Index and Incidence of Diabetes in African-American and White Adults: The ARIC Study." *Diabetes Care* 25 (10): 1715–21.

TRIAD Study Group. 2002. "The Translating Research into Action for Diabetes (TRIAD) Study: A Multicenter Study of Diabetes in Managed Care." *Diabetes Care* 25 (2): 386–89.

Tuomilehto, J., J. Lindstrom, J. G. Eriksson, T. T. Valle, H. Hamalainen, P. Ilanne-Parikka, and others. 2001. "Prevention of Type 2 Diabetes Mellitus by Changes in Lifestyle among Subjects with Impaired Glucose Tolerance." *New England Journal of Medicine* 344 (18): 1343–50.

UKPDS (U.K. Prospective Diabetes Study) Group. 1998. "Intensive Blood-Glucose Control with Sulphonylureas or Insulin Compared with Conventional Treatment and Risk of Complications in Patients with Type 2 Diabetes (UKPDS 33)." *Lancet* 352 (9131): 837–53.

U.S. Preventive Services Task Force. 1996. *Guide to Clinical Preventive Services: Report of the U.S. Preventive Services Task Force*, 2nd ed. Washington, DC: Office of Disease Prevention and Health Promotion, U.S. Government Printing Office.

Vijan, S., T. P. Hofer, and R. A. Hayward. 2000. "Cost-Utility Analysis of Screening Intervals for Diabetic Retinopathy in Patients with Type 2 Diabetes Mellitus." *Journal of the American Medical Association* 283 (7): 889–96.

Villarreal-Rios, E., A. M. Salinas-Martinez, A. Medina-Jauregui, M. E. Garza-Elizondo, G. Nunez-Rocha, and E. R. Chuy-Diaz. 2000. "The Cost of Diabetes Mellitus and Its Impact on Health Spending in Mexico." *Archives of Medical Research* 31 (5): 511–14.

Wald, N. J., and M. R. Law. 2003. "A Strategy to Reduce Cardiovascular Disease by More Than 80%." *British Medical Journal* 326 (7404): 1419.

Williams, D. E., W. C. Knowler, C. J. Smith, R. L. Hanson, J. Roumain, A. Saremi, and others. 2001. "The Effect of Indian or Anglo Dietary Preference on the Incidence of Diabetes in Pima Indians." *Diabetes Care* 24 (5): 811–16.

WHO (World Health Organization). 2004. "Global Burden of Disease for the Year 2001 by World Bank Region, for Use in Disease Control Priorities in Developing Countries." 2nd ed. http://www.fic.nih.gov/dcpp/gbd.html.

Yajnik, C. S. 2001. "The Insulin Resistance Epidemic in India: Fetal Origins, Later Lifestyle, or Both?" *Nutrition Reviews* 59 (1, part 1): 1–9.

Young, T. K., P. J. Martens, S. P. Taback, E. A. Sellers, H. J. Dean, M. Cheang, and others. 2002. "Type 2 Diabetes Mellitus in Children: Prenatal and Early Infancy Risk Factors among Native Canadians." *Archives of Pediatrics and Adolescent Medicine* 156 (7): 651–55.

Chapter **31**

Mental Disorders

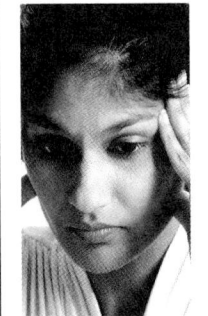

Steven Hyman, Dan Chisholm, Ronald Kessler, Vikram Patel,
and Harvey Whiteford

Mental disorders are diseases that affect cognition, emotion, and behavioral control and substantially interfere both with the ability of children to learn and with the ability of adults to function in their families, at work, and in the broader society. Mental disorders tend to begin early in life and often run a chronic recurrent course. They are common in all countries where their prevalence has been examined. Because of the combination of high prevalence, early onset, persistence, and impairment, mental disorders make a major contribution to total disease burden. Although most of the burden attributable to mental disorders is disability related, premature mortality, especially from suicide, is not insignificant. Table 31.1 summarizes discounted disability-adjusted life years (DALYs) for selected psychiatric conditions in 2001.

Mental disorders have complex etiologies that involve interactions among multiple genetic and nongenetic risk factors. Gender is related to risk in many cases: males have higher rates of attention deficit hyperactivity disorder, autism, and substance use disorders; females have higher rates of major depressive disorder, most anxiety disorders, and eating disorders. Biochemical and morphological abnormalities of the brain associated with schizophrenia, autism, mood, and anxiety disorders are being identified using approaches such as postmortem analysis and noninvasive neuroimaging. Major worldwide efforts under way to identify risk-conferring genes for mental disorders are proving challenging, but initial results are promising. Identifying the gene or genes causing or creating vulnerability for a disorder should help us understand what goes wrong in the brain to produce mental illness and should have a clinical effect by contributing to improved diagnostics and therapeutics (Hyman 2000).

Twin studies make it clear that environmental risk factors also play an important role in mental disorders; concordance for disease among identical twins, although substantially higher than among nonidentical twins, is still well below 100 percent (Kendler and others 2003). However, as is the case for genetic factors, investigation of environmental risk factors has proved difficult. For schizophrenia, where nongenetic components of risk may include obstetrical complications and season of birth (Mortensen and others 1999), perhaps as a proxy for infections early in life, research has been hampered by the modest proven effect of the nongenetic risk factors identified to date. For depression, anxiety, and substance use disorders, where environmental risk factors are more robust, adverse circumstances associated with risk, such as early childhood abuse, violence, poverty, and stress (Patel and Kleinman 2003) correlate with multiple disorders and could be affected by selection bias as well as by bias associated with self-reporting. Generalizable, prospective cross-cultural studies are needed to delineate nongenetic risk factors more clearly. Posttraumatic stress disorder (PTSD) is the mental disorder for which clear environmental triggers are best documented. Even here, though, enormous interindividual variability occurs in the threshold of stress severity associated with PTSD as well as in the evidence from twin studies of genetic influences on stress reactivity in triggering PTSD.

The last half of the 20th century saw enormous progress in the development of treatments for mental disorders. Beginning in the early 1950s, effective psychotropic drugs were discovered that treated the symptoms of schizophrenia, bipolar disorder, major depression, anxiety disorders, obsessive-compulsive disorder, attention deficit hyperactivity disorder, and others. The safety and efficacy of antipsychotic, mood-stabilizing,

Table 31.1 Disease Burden of Selected Major Psychiatric Disorders, by World Bank Region

	World Bank region							
	Sub-Saharan Africa	Latin America and the Caribbean	Middle East and North Africa	Europe and Central Asia	South Asia	East Asia and the Pacific	High-income countries	World
Total population (millions)	668	526	310	477	1,388	1,851	929	6,159
Total disease burden (thousands of DALYs)	344,754	104,287	65,570	116,502	408,655	346,941	149,161	1,535,870
Total neuropsychiatric disease burden (thousands of DALYs)	15,151	18,781	8,310	14,106	37,734	42,992	31,230	168,304
Total burden (thousands of discounted DALYs per year)								
Schizophrenia	1,146	1,078	696	778	2,896	3,934	1,115	11,643
Bipolar disorder	1,204	883	567	668	2,237	3,118	1,056	9,733
Depression	3,275	5,219	2,027	4,268	14,582	14,054	8,408	51,833
Panic disorder	519	409	264	340	1,081	1,401	536	4,550
Total burden (DALYs per year per 1 million population)								
Schizophrenia	1,716	2,049	2,247	1,630	2,087	2,126	1,201	1,894
Bipolar disorder	1,803	1,678	1,830	1,400	1,612	1,685	1,137	1,583
Depression	4,905	9,919	6,544	8,944	10,507	7,594	9,054	8,431
Panic disorder	777	777	852	713	779	757	577	740
Percentage of total disease burden								
Schizophrenia	0.33	1.03	1.06	0.67	0.71	1.13	0.75	0.76
Bipolar disorder	0.35	0.85	0.86	0.57	0.55	0.90	0.71	0.63
Depression	0.95	5.00	3.09	3.66	3.57	4.05	5.64	3.37
Panic disorder	0.15	0.39	0.40	0.29	0.26	0.40	0.36	0.30
Percentage of neuropsychiatric disease burden								
Schizophrenia	7.56	5.74	8.38	5.52	7.67	9.15	3.57	6.92
Bipolar disorder	7.95	4.70	6.82	4.74	5.93	7.25	3.38	5.78
Depression	21.62	27.79	24.39	30.26	38.64	32.69	26.92	30.80
Panic disorder	3.43	2.18	3.18	2.41	2.86	3.26	1.72	2.70

Source: WHO Global Burden of Disease 2001 estimates recalculated by World Bank region (http://www.fic.nih.gov/dcpp/gbd.html).

antidepressant, anxiolytic, and stimulant drugs have been established through a large number of randomized clinical trials. Psychosocial treatments have been developed and tested using modern methodologies. Brief, symptom-focused psychotherapies such as cognitive-behavioral therapies have been shown to be efficacious for panic disorder, phobias, obsessive-compulsive disorder, and major depression.

There is, however, an important caveat about the current knowledge base for treatment. As is the case for almost all of medicine, randomized clinical trials have been performed largely with highly selected populations in specialized research settings in industrial countries. A need exists to subject existing treatments to effectiveness trials in more representative populations and diverse settings, especially in developing countries. That limitation notwithstanding, a substantial body of knowl-

edge exists to guide treatment. It is particularly unfortunate, therefore, that timely diagnoses and the application of research-based treatments significantly lag behind the state of knowledge in industrial and developing countries alike. As a result, substantial opportunities exist to decrease the enormous burden attributable to mental disorders worldwide by closing the gap between *what we know* and *what we do.*

Mental disorders are stigmatized in many countries and cultures (Weiss and others 2001). Stigma has been facilitated by the slow emergence of convincing scientific explanations for the etiologies of mental disorders and by the mistaken belief that symptoms are caused by a lack of will power or reflect some moral taint. Recent scientific findings combined with educational efforts in some countries have begun to reduce the stigma (Rahman and others 1998), but shame and fear associated with mental illness remain substantial obstacles to help seeking, to diagnosis, and to treatment worldwide. The stigmatization of mental illness has resulted in disparities, compared with other illnesses, in the availability of care, in research, and in abuses of the human rights of people with these disorders.

This chapter focuses on the attributable and avoidable burden of four leading contributors to mental ill health globally: schizophrenia and related nonaffective psychoses, bipolar affective disorder (manic-depressive illness), major depressive disorder, and panic disorder. The choice of these disorders is determined not only by their contribution to disease burden, but also by the availability of data for the cost-effectiveness analyses. Even where such data are available, they are often from industrial countries and extrapolation has been necessary. The exclusion of other mental disorders, such as childhood disorders, from analysis is not because the authors consider these disorders unimportant but because of the paucity of data. Also, this chapter does not specifically deal with the important issue of suicide. A background paper on suicide in developing countries has been developed as part of the Disease Control Priorities Project (DCPP) and is available (Vijayakumar, Nagaraj, and John 2004). The economic analysis presented in this chapter uses the cost-effectiveness analysis methodology specifically developed for the DCPP. The authors recognize that mental disorders impose costs and burdens on families as well as individuals that are not captured by the DALY. Treatment will alleviate some of this burden in addition to alleviating symptoms and disability.

A description of the major clinical features, natural course, epidemiology, burden, and treatment effectiveness for each group of disorders is given in the next section. For diagnostic criteria, readers are referred to *The ICD-10 Classification of Mental and Behavioral Disorders* (ICD-10) (WHO 1992) or *Diagnostic and Statistical Manual of Mental Disorders* (DSM-IVTR) (American Psychiatric Association 2000). A discussion follows of population-level costs and cost-effectiveness of interventions capable of reducing the current burden associated with four disorders in different developing regions of the world (tables 31.2–31.6), before moving to a discussion of key issues and implications for mental health policy and improvement of services in developing regions of the world.

SCHIZOPHRENIA AND NONAFFECTIVE PSYCHOSES

Schizophrenia is a chronic disorder punctuated by episodes of florid psychotic symptoms, such as hallucinations and delusions. Hallucinations are sensory perceptions that occur in the absence of appropriate stimuli. Hallucinations may occur in any sensory modality but in schizophrenia are most commonly auditory—for example, hearing voices or noises. Delusions are fixed false beliefs that are not explained by the person's culture and that the patient holds despite all reasonable evidence to the contrary.

Patients also exhibit *negative symptoms*—that is, deficits in normal capacities, such as marked social deficits, impoverishment of thought and speech, blunting of emotional responses, and lack of motivation. Additionally, patients typically have cognitive symptoms, such as disorganized or illogical thinking and an inability to hold goal information in mind to make decisions or plan actions.

Natural History and Course

Schizophrenia, as defined in current diagnostic manuals, is almost certainly heterogeneous, but still does not comprise all nonaffective psychoses (NAPs). In addition to schizophrenia, NAPs include schizophreniform disorder, characterized by schizophrenia-like symptoms of inadequate duration to qualify as schizophrenia. Because they cannot be readily disentangled in community epidemiological surveys, schizophrenia and other NAPs are considered together. Because of the data available, however, the cost-effectiveness analyses reported below are restricted to schizophrenia. Despite likely etiological heterogeneity, schizophrenia exhibits consistency in its symptom pattern across those countries and cultures studied (Jablensky and others 1992).

Incidence studies show that onset of schizophrenia and other NAPs is typically in middle to late adolescence for males and late adolescence to early adulthood for females, although later onsets are observed. Childhood-onset cases are quite rare but particularly severe (Nicolson and Rapoport 1999). Often, schizophrenia is first diagnosed with the occurrence of an acute episode of florid psychotic symptoms. The first psychotic episode is often preceded by prodromal symptoms such as social withdrawal, irritability or dysphoria, increasing academic or work-related difficulties, and increasing eccentricity. However, such symptoms are not specific; studies of whether early diagnosis and intervention can improve outcomes are under way (McGorry and others 2002).

The course of schizophrenia is typically one of acute exacerbations of severe psychotic symptoms, followed by full or partial remission. Psychotic episodes may be followed by a full remission after the first and occasionally other early episodes, but over time, residual symptoms and disability typically continue between relapses (Robinson and others 1999). The time between relapses is markedly extended by maintenance treatment with antipsychotic drugs, generally at lower doses than are needed to treat acute episodes. Cognitive and occupational functioning tends to decline over the first years of the illness and then to plateau at a level that is generally well below what would have been expected for the individual. Residual impairment, though, has substantial cross-cultural variation for reasons that are not well understood. Schizophrenia has consistently been found in epidemiological surveys to be highly comorbid, usually with anxiety disorders, mood disorders, and substance use disorders (Kendler and others 1996).

Epidemiology and Burden

A great many studies of NAP incidence have been carried out in clinical samples. In a review of these studies, Jablensky (2000) found incidence estimates to be in the range of 0.002 to 0.011 percent per year for schizophrenia and 0.016 to 0.042 percent per year for overall NAP. Those annual estimates can be multiplied by the number of birth cohorts at risk to yield an estimate of lifetime risk in any one cohort. Assuming conservatively that the main age range of risk is between ages 15 and 55, researchers estimate lifetime risk is in the range of 0.08 to 0.44 percent for schizophrenia and in the range of 0.64 to 1.68 percent for NAPs. Lifetime prevalence estimates from community epidemiological surveys of NAPs are quite consistent with those from clinical studies, in the range of 0.3 to 1.6 percent (see, for example, Hwu, Yeh, and Cheng 1989; Kendler and others 1996).

Although schizophrenia is a relatively uncommon disorder, aggregate estimates of disease burden are high—around 2,000 DALYs lost per 1 million total population (table 31.1)—because the condition is associated with early onset, long duration, and severe disability.

Interventions

A substantial body of evidence exists on the efficacy of various treatments for schizophrenia and NAP and on the effectiveness of various models of health care delivery for persons with these disorders. This evidence comes primarily from industrial countries. The efficacy data show conclusively that antipsychotic drugs reduce severity of the episodes, hasten resolution of florid symptoms, and reduce duration of hospitalization. Maintenance treatment with antipsychotic drugs prolongs the period between relapses (Joy, Adams, and Lawrie 2001).

A second generation of antipsychotic medications (also called *atypical*) is replacing older *neuroleptic* antipsychotic drugs throughout the industrial world. In some clinical trials, second-generation drugs show small advantages in efficacy over first-generation drugs, but their widespread adoption results from marked improvement in tolerability. Their relative lack of side effects compared with first-generation drugs has led to improved quality of life and improved treatment adherence. Second-generation drugs are not without side effects, however; for example, some are associated with substantial weight gain and increased risk of diabetes. One drug, clozapine, has greater efficacy than other antipsychotic drugs, but because of a 1 percent risk of agranulocytosis, its use requires weekly blood counts and is cumbersome and expensive.

Psychosocial interventions also play an important role in managing schizophrenia (Bustillo and others 2001). Cognitive-behavioral approaches to managing specific symptoms and improving medication adherence, group therapy, and family interventions all have demonstrated efficacy in improving clinical outcomes. Community-based models of mental health care delivery with case management and assertive outreach programs have been shown in health systems of industrial countries to be effective ways of managing schizophrenia in the community, for example, by reducing the need for hospital admissions. However, the applicability of these models to developing countries, as is discussed later, is hard to estimate because of differences in health system characteristics. Long-term remission rates for schizophrenia in developing countries appear to be significantly higher than those reported in industrial countries (Harrison and others 2001), likely resulting from such factors as strong family social support.

Despite their clear usefulness, current treatments do not prevent schizophrenia, and no clear evidence demonstrates that they induce full recovery or prevent premature mortality. Instead, treatment reduces time in episode of florid psychosis and increases time between episodes; thus treatment effects can be understood in terms of improvements in disability. Reported treatment effect sizes from meta-analyses in the literature, converted into improvements in the average level of disability (Andrews and others 2003; Sanderson and others 2004), show improvements (compared with no treatment) of 18 to 19 percent (antipsychotic drugs alone) and 30 to 31 percent (antipsychotic drugs with adjunctive psychosocial treatment). Placed on a disability scale of 0 to 1, where 0 equals no disability, an "average" case of schizophrenia moves from a disability level of 0.63 (untreated weight from the Global Burden of Disease study, Murray and Lopez 1996) to 0.43 to 0.54 (treated).

MOOD DISORDERS

The cardinal features of mood disorders are pervasive abnormalities in the predominant emotional state of the person, such as depressed, elated, or irritable. In mood disorders, these core emotional symptoms are accompanied by abnormalities in physiology, such as changes in patterns of sleep, appetite, and energy, and by changes in cognition and behavior. In developing countries, concurrent somatic symptoms are also commonly reported and may be the chief complaint. A generally accepted subclassification of mood disorders distinguishes unipolar depressive disorders from bipolar disorder (defined by the occurrence of mania). This distinction is based on symptoms, course of illness, patterns of familial transmission, and treatment response.

Bipolar Disorder

Bipolar disorder is characterized by episodes of mania and depression, often followed by relative periods of healthy mood (euthymia). Mixed states with symptoms of both mania and depression also occur. Mania is typically characterized by euphoria or irritability, a marked increase in energy, and a decreased need for sleep. Individuals with mania often exhibit intrusive, impulsive, and disinhibited behaviors. They may be excessively involved in goal-directed behaviors characterized by poor judgment; for example, a person might spend all funds to which he or she has access and more. Self-esteem is typically inflated, frequently reaching delusional proportions. Speech is often rapid and difficult to interrupt. Individuals with mania also may exhibit cognitive symptoms; patients cannot stick to a topic and may jump rapidly from idea to idea, making comprehension of their train of thought difficult. Psychotic symptoms are common during manic episodes. The depressive episodes of people with bipolar disorder are symptomatically indistinguishable from those who have unipolar depressions alone. Unlike anxiety and unipolar mood disorders, which are more common in women, bipolar disorder has an equal gender ratio of lifetime prevalence, although the ratio of depressive-to-manic episodes is higher among bipolar women than men.

Natural History and Course. Retrospective reports from community epidemiological surveys consistently show that bipolar disorder has an early age of onset (in the late teens through mid-20s). Onset in childhood is increasingly recognized, although it remains controversial. Late onset is less common. The vast majority of patients with bipolar disorder have recurrent episodes of illness, both mania and depression. Classic descriptions of bipolar disorder suggest recovery to baseline functioning between episodes, but many patients have residual symptoms that may cause significant impairment (Angst and Sellaro 2000). These states of mania, depression, and lesser (or absent) symptoms are used in the intervention analysis below.

The rate of cycling between mania and depression varies widely among individuals. One common pattern of illness is for episodes initially to be separated by a relatively long period, perhaps a year, and then to become more frequent with age. A minority of patients with four or more cycles per year, termed *rapid cyclers,* tend to be more disabled and less responsive to existing treatments. Once cycles are established, most acute episodes start without an identifiable precipitant; the best documented exception is that manic episodes may be initiated by sleep deprivation, making a regular daily sleep schedule and avoidance of shift work important in management (Frank, Swartz, and Kupfer 2000).

Bipolar disorder has consistently been found in epidemiological surveys to be highly comorbid with other psychiatric disorders, especially anxiety and substance use disorders (ten Have and others 2002). The extent of comorbidity is much greater than for unipolar depressive disorders or anxiety disorders. Some individuals with classic symptoms of bipolar disorder also exhibit chronic psychotic symptoms superimposed on their mood syndrome. These individuals are said to have schizoaffective disorder. Their prognosis tends to be less favorable than for the usual bipolar patient, although somewhat better than for individuals with schizophrenia. Schizoaffective disorder may also be diagnosed when chronic psychotic symptoms are superimposed on unipolar depression. Individuals with this combination of symptoms have outcomes similar to patients with schizophrenia (Tsuang and Coryell 1993).

Epidemiology and Burden. Lifetime and 12-month prevalence estimates of bipolar disorder have been reported from a number of community psychiatric epidemiological surveys. Lifetime prevalence estimates are in the range 0.1 to 2.0 percent (Vega and others 1998; Vicente and others 2002), with a weighted mean across surveys of 0.7 percent. Prevalence estimates for past-year episodes have a similarly wide range (0.1 to 1.3 percent) (Vega and others 1998) and a weighted mean of 0.5 percent. It is important to note that good evidence exists suggesting that bipolar disorder has a wide subthreshold spectrum that includes people who are often seriously impaired even though they do not meet full DSM or ICD criteria for the disorder (Perugi and Akiskal 2002). This spectrum might include as much as 5 percent of the general population. The ratio of recent-to-lifetime prevalence of bipolar disorder in community surveys is quite high (0.71), indicating that bipolar disorder is persistent.

Epidemiological data show that bipolar disorder is associated with substantial impairments in both productive and social roles (Das Gupta and Guest 2002). Epidemiological evidence documents consistent delays in patients initially seeking professional treatment (Olfson and others 1998), especially among early-onset cases, as well as substantial undertreatment of current cases. Each of these characteristics—chronic, recurrent course; significant impairments to functioning; modest treatment rates—contributes to estimates of aggregate disease burden that approach those for schizophrenia (1,200 to 1,800 DALYs lost per 1 million population, making up more than 5 percent of the burden attributable to neuropsychiatric disorders as a whole—see table 31.1).

Interventions. Analyses of the primary treatment approaches for bipolar disorder are based on the three health states that characterize the disorder—mania, depression, and euthymia. Robust evidence from controlled trials shows that antipsychotic drugs and some benzodiazepines produce a relatively rapid reduction in symptoms of a manic phase. Mood-stabilizing drugs act more slowly, but they reduce the severity and duration of acute manic episodes. Maintenance treatment with two mood-stabilizing drugs—lithium and valproic acid (administered as sodium valproate)—has been shown to have significant, albeit partial, efficacy in reducing rates of both manic and depressive relapses. The drawback of lithium is that toxic levels are not much greater than therapeutic levels; thus, serum-level monitoring is required.

For the cost-effectiveness analyses, lithium and valproic acid, which have empirical data supporting their efficacy in treating and preventing manic and depressive episodes, were considered. Because evidence suggests that psychosocial approaches enhance compliance with medication (Huxley, Parikh, and Baldessarini 2000), adjuvant strategies also were assessed. The primary treatment effect was a change in the population-level disability associated with bipolar disorder (a weighted average of time spent in a manic, depressed, or euthymic phase of illness). Both an acute treatment effect—calculated as the product of initial response and reduced episode duration—and a prophylactic treatment effect were ascribed to lithium and valproic acid, resulting in an estimated improvement of close to 50 percent over the untreated composite disability weight of 0.445 (Chisholm and others forthcoming). This estimate then was adjusted for expected nonadherence to treatment in real-world clinical settings—slightly lower for lithium than for valproic acid (Bowden and others 2000). A secondary effect of treatment—reduction of the case fatality rate by two-thirds—was also ascribed to lithium, though, because of an absence of current evidence, not to valproic acid (Goodwin and others 2003). This reduction was derived through a change in the standardized mortality ratio from 2.5 to 1.5, estimated on the basis of natural history studies reported for the prelithium era (for example, Astrup, Fossum, and Holmboe 1959; Helgason 1964) to the postlithium era (for example, Goodwin and others 2003).

Major Depressive Disorder

The core symptom of major depression is a disturbance of mood; sadness is most typical, but anger, irritability, and loss of interest in usual pursuits may predominate. Often the affected person is unable to experience pleasure (anhedonia) and may feel hopeless. In many countries of the developing world, patients will not complain of such emotional symptoms, but rather of physical symptoms, such as fatigue or multiple aches and pains.

Typical physiological symptoms that occur across cultures include sleep disturbance (most often insomnia with early morning awakening, but occasionally excessive sleeping); appetite disturbance (usually loss of appetite and weight loss, but occasionally excessive eating); and decreased energy. Behaviorally, some individuals with depression exhibit slowed motor movements (psychomotor retardation), whereas others may be agitated. Cognitive symptoms may include thoughts of worthlessness and guilt, suicidal thoughts, difficulty concentrating, slow thinking, and poor memory. Psychotic symptoms occur in a minority of cases.

Natural History and Course. Major depression is an episodic disorder that generally begins early in life (median age of onset in the mid to late 20s in community epidemiological surveys), although new onsets can be observed across the lifespan. Childhood onset is being increasingly recognized, although not all childhood precursors of adult depression take the form of a clear depressive disorder. Most individuals suffering from a depressive episode will have a recurrence (Mueller and others 1999), with recurrence risk greater among those with early-onset disease. Many individuals do not recover completely from their acute episodes and have chronic milder depression punctuated by acute exacerbations (Judd and others 1998). The current term for chronic, milder depression lasting more than two years is *dysthymia*. Although the symptoms of minor depression are, by definition, less severe than those of a major depressive episode, chronicity ultimately makes even this lesser form of the illness very disabling in many cases (Judd, Schettler, and Akiskal 2002). Depression has consistently been found in epidemiological surveys to be highly comorbid with other mental disorders, with roughly half the people who have a history of depression also having a lifetime anxiety disorder. Comorbidities of depression and anxiety disorders are generally strongest with generalized anxiety disorder and panic disorder (Kessler and others 1996).

Epidemiology and Burden. Prevalence of nonbipolar depression has been estimated in a number of large-scale community epidemiological surveys. Lifetime prevalence estimates of having either major depressive disorder or dysthymia in these surveys are in the range 4.2 to 17.0 percent (Andrade and others 2003; Bijl and others 1998), with a weighted mean of 12.1 percent. Six- to 12-month prevalence estimates have a similarly wide range (1.9 to 10.9 percent) (Andrade and others 2003; Robins and Regier 1991), with a weighted mean of 5.8 percent. These wide differences in prevalence likely represent the difficulties inherent in self-reporting of conditions that are invariably stigmatized across cultures. Prevalence estimates are consistently highest in North America and lowest in Asia (with prevalence estimates of major depressive disorders generally a good deal higher than those of dysthymia).

Epidemiological data document consistent delays in patients initially seeking professional treatment for depression, especially among early-onset cases (Olfson and others 1998), as well as substantial undertreatment. For example, World Mental Health surveys in six Western European countries found that only 36.6 percent of people with active nonbipolar depression in the 12 months before the survey received any professional treatment for this disorder during the subsequent year

(ESEMeD/MHEDEA 2000 Investigators 2004). The situation is even worse in developing countries, where the vast majority of people with depression who seek help do so in general health care settings and complain of nonspecific physical symptoms. Such individuals receive a correct diagnosis in less than one-quarter of cases and typically are treated with medicines of doubtful efficacy (Linden and others 1999).

Depression is consistently found in community surveys to be associated with substantial impairments in both productive and social roles (Wang, Simon, and Kessler 2003). As with bipolar depression, but exacerbated by its high incidence, the recurrent nature and disabling consequences of (unipolar) depression mean that overall disease burden estimates are high in all regions of the world (5,000 to 10,000 DALYs per 1 million population, as much as 5 percent of the total burden of disease from all causes; table 31.1). Depression is, in fact, ranked as the fourth leading cause of disease burden globally and represents the single largest contributor to nonfatal burden (Ustun and others 2004).

Interventions. Efficacy has been demonstrated for several classes of antidepressant drugs and for two psychosocial treatments for depression (Paykel and Priest 1992). The older tricyclic antidepressants (TCAs) and newer drugs, including the selective serotonin reuptake inhibitors (SSRIs), have similar efficacy. The newer drugs have milder side-effect profiles and are consequently more likely to be tolerated at therapeutic doses (Pereira and Patel 1999). SSRIs have not been widely used in developing countries because of their higher cost, although as the patent protection expires, this situation is likely to change (Patel 1996). Of the psychosocial treatments with demonstrated efficacy, the most widely accepted are cognitive-behavioral approaches. Alone or in combination, drug and psychosocial treatments speed recovery from acute episodes. Maintenance treatment with drugs decreases relapse risk (Geddes and others 2003). Some evidence suggests that a course of psychotherapy may also delay relapses. Although most of the clinical trials have been carried out in industrial countries, at least three high-quality trials have demonstrated the efficacy of antidepressants, group therapy, or both in developing countries (Araya and others 2003; Bolton and others 2003; Patel and others 2003).

For the cost-effectiveness analyses, depression was modeled as an episodic disorder with a high rate of remission and subsequent recurrence, and with excess mortality from suicide (Chisholm and others 2004). None of the selected depression interventions was accorded a reduction in case fatality, however, owing to the lack of robust clinical evidence that antidepressants or psychotherapy in themselves alter the relative risk of death by suicide (Storosum and others 2001). The main modeled impact of intervention targeted toward episodic treatment of a new depressive episode was a reduction in the duration of time depressed, equivalent to an increase in the remission rate (25 to 40 percent improvement over no treatment; Malt and others 1999; Solomon and others 1997). In addition, all interventions were attributed a modest improvement in the level of disability for an unremitted depressive episode (10 to 15 percent), resulting from increased proportions of cases moving from more to less severe health states. For the estimated 56 percent of prevalent cases eligible for maintenance treatment (at least two lifetime episodes), an additional effect of efficacious maintenance treatment was incorporated into the analysis by reducing the incidence of recurrent episodes by 50 percent (Geddes and others 2003). Estimates of intervention effectiveness include the positive change that would occur naturally and also incorporate any placebo effect, which, in the treatment of depression, is not inconsiderable (Andrews 2001).

ANXIETY DISORDERS

Anxiety disorders are a group of disorders that have as their central feature the inability to regulate fear or worry. Although anxiety in itself is likely to feature in the clinical presentation of most patients, somatic complaints such as chest pain, palpitations, respiratory difficulty, headaches, and the like are also common, and these symptoms may be more common in developing countries. A number of different types of anxiety disorder exist, some of which are now briefly described.

The central feature of *panic disorder* is an unexpected panic attack, which is a discrete period of intense fear accompanied by physiologic symptoms such as a racing heart, shortness of breath, sweating, or dizziness. The person may have an intense fear of losing control or of dying. Panic disorder is diagnosed when panic attacks are recurrent and give rise to anticipatory anxiety about additional attacks. People with panic disorder may progressively restrict their lives to avoid situations in which panic attacks occur or situations from which it might be difficult to escape should a panic attack occur. They commonly avoid crowds, traveling, bridges, and elevators, and ultimately some individuals may stop leaving home altogether. Pervasive phobic avoidance is described as agoraphobia.

Generalized anxiety disorder is characterized by chronic unrealistic and excessive worry. These symptoms are accompanied by specific anxiety-related symptoms such as sympathetic nervous system arousal, excessive vigilance, and motor tension. *Posttraumatic stress disorder* follows serious trauma. It is characterized by emotional numbness, punctuated by intrusive reliving of the traumatic episode, generally initiated by environmental cues that act as reminders of the trauma; by disturbed sleep; and by hyperarousal, such as exaggerated startle responses.

Social anxiety disorder (*social phobia*) is characterized by a persistent fear of social situations or performance situations that expose a person to potential scrutiny by others. The affected person has intense fear that he or she will act in a way that will be humiliating. Separating social anxiety disorder from extremes of normal temperament, such as shyness, is difficult. Nonetheless, social anxiety disorder can be quite disabling. *Simple phobias* are extreme fear in the presence of discrete stimuli or cues, such as fear of heights.

The core features of *obsessive-compulsive disorder* are obsessions (intrusive, unwanted thoughts) and compulsions (performance of highly ritualized behaviors intended to neutralize the negative thoughts and emotions resulting from the obsessions). One symptom pattern might be repetitive hand washing beyond the point of skin damage to neutralize fears of contamination.

Natural History and Course

The anxiety disorders differ in their age of onset, course of illness, and symptom triggers. One of these disorders, PTSD, is dependent for its etiology on one or more powerfully negative life events. Although the anxiety disorders are discussed as a group, panic disorder is chosen because of the available data for the purposes of the cost-effectiveness analysis.

Prevalence estimates of anxiety disorders based on community epidemiological surveys vary widely, from a low of 2.2 percent (Andrade and others 2003) to a high of 28.5 percent (Kessler and others 1994), with a weighted mean across surveys of 15.6 percent. Prevalence estimates for anxiety disorders in the past 6 to 12 months have a similarly wide range (1.2 to 19.3 percent) (Andrade and others 2003; Kessler and others 1994), with a weighted mean of 9.4 percent. Despite wide variation in overall prevalence, several clear relative prevalence patterns can be seen across surveys. Specific phobia is generally the most prevalent lifetime anxiety disorder, with social phobia generally the second most prevalent lifetime anxiety disorder. Panic disorder and obsessive-compulsive disorder are generally the least prevalent.

These surveys also provide evidence about the persistence of anxiety disorders, indirectly defined as the ratio of 6-month or 12-month to lifetime prevalence. This ratio averages approximately 60 percent for overall anxiety disorders, indicating a high rate of persistence across the life course. The highest persistence is generally found for social phobia, and the lowest for agoraphobia. These estimates of high persistence are consistent with results obtained from longitudinal studies of patients (Yonkers and others 2003).

Anxiety disorders have consistently been found in epidemiological surveys to be highly comorbid both among themselves and with mood disorders (for example, de Graaf and others 2003). The vast majority of people with a history of one anxiety disorder typically also have a second anxiety disorder, while more than half the people with a history of either anxiety or mood disorder typically have both types of disorder. Retrospective reports from community surveys consistently show that anxiety disorders have early average ages of onset. An impressive cross-national consistency can be seen in these patterns, with an estimated median age of onset of anxiety at approximately 15.

Epidemiological surveys have also looked at the treatment of anxiety disorders. As with depression, consistent evidence in these surveys suggests that delays in initially seeking professional treatment for an anxiety disorder are widespread after first onset (Olfson and others 1998). This finding is especially true among early-onset cases. Epidemiological data also show that only a minority of current cases receive any formal treatment in Western countries, whereas treatment of anxiety disorders is virtually nonexistent in many developing countries. The most recently published surveys, the World Mental Health surveys in six Western European countries, found that only 26.3 percent of people with an active anxiety disorder in the 12 months before the survey received any professional treatment (ESEMeD/MHEDEA 2000 Investigators 2004).

Anxiety disorders have consistently been found to be associated with substantial impairments in both productive roles (for example, work absenteeism, work performance, unemployment, and underemployment) and social roles (social isolation, interpersonal tensions, and marital disruption, among others) (see, for example, Kessler and Frank 1997). As noted earlier, for the purposes of this chapter, one of the anxiety disorders—panic disorder—has been chosen to describe interventions and undertake cost-effectiveness analysis. Panic disorder is as disabling as obsessive-compulsive disorder and PTSD, accounts for about one-third of all seriously impairing anxiety disorders, is one of the most common anxiety disorders presenting for treatment, and imposes an estimated burden of 600 to 800 DALYs per 1 million population.

Good evidence exists that both drug and psychosocial treatments are effective for managing anxiety disorders. Antidepressant drugs (both older TCAs and SSRIs) have been shown to be effective for the treatment of several anxiety disorders, including panic disorder, reducing the duration and intensity of the disorder. Although high-potency benzodiazepines are efficacious for panic disorder, these drugs carry a risk of dependence and are not considered the first line of treatment. Psychosocial treatments, especially cognitive-behavioral therapy, are also effective in diminishing both panic attacks and phobic avoidance.

Interventions for Panic Disorder

Although evidence-based interventions for panic disorder have yet to be evaluated or made widely available in developing countries, the potential population-level impact of a number of interventions—including older and newer antidepressants, anxiolytic drugs (benzodiazepines), and psychosocial treatments—was examined. Interventions reduce the severity of panic attacks and improve the probability of making a full recovery. Effect sizes for symptom improvement were drawn from a meta-analysis of the long-term effects of intervention of panic disorder (Bakker and others 1998) and converted into an equivalent change in disability weight (Sanderson and others 2004). Concerning remission, a number of controlled and naturalistic studies (for example, Faravelli, Paterniti, and Scarpato 1995; Yonkers and others 2003) reveal a consistent remission rate of 12 to 13 percent for pharmacological and combination strategies—except for benzodiazepine use, for which the evidence is that longer-term recovery is actually worse than placebo (Katschnig and others 1995)—which represents a 62 percent improvement in efficacy over the untreated remission rate (7.4 percent).

COST-EFFECTIVENESS METHODS AND RESULTS

This section estimates the burden attributed to schizophrenia, bipolar disorder, depression, and panic disorder that could be averted (through scaling up) by proven, efficacious treatments. It is followed by calculations of the expected cost and cost-effectiveness of such treatments. Analysis is conducted at the level of six low- and middle-income geographical World Bank regions.

Estimation of Population-Level Effectiveness of Treatments

In modeling the impact of mental health interventions, we used a state-transition model (Lauer and others 2003) that traces the development of a population, taking into account births, deaths, and the disease in question. In addition to population size and structure, the model makes use of a number of epidemiological parameters (incidence and prevalence, remission, and cause-specific and residual rates of mortality) and assigns age- and gender-specific disability weights to both the disease in question and the general population. The output of the model is an estimate of the total healthy life years experienced by the population over a lifetime period (100 years). The model was run for a number of possible scenarios, including no treatment at all (natural history), current treatment coverage, and scaled-up coverage of current as well as potential new interventions. For the treatment scenarios, an implementation period of 10 years was used (thereafter, epidemiological rates and health state valuations return to natural history levels). The model derived the number of additional healthy years gained (equivalent to DALYs averted) each year in the population compared with the outcome for no treatment at all. DALYs averted in future years were discounted at a rate of 3 percent

(reflecting a societal preference for health benefits to be realized sooner), but no age-weighting was used.

Estimation of the baseline epidemiological situation that would prevail without treatment used incidence and prevalence estimates from the Global Burden of Disease 2000 study of the World Health Organization (WHO) (see online Global Burden of Disease documentation for the four disorders at http://www.who.int/evidence/bod). Current pharmacological or psychosocial treatments do not exert a primary preventive effect on the onset of the four conditions (although some evidence exists that treating depression in parents may reduce risk for offspring), indicating that currently observed incidence rates coincide with those that would pertain under no treatment. Prevention of recurrences of acute episodes (secondary prevention) has been demonstrated for maintenance treatments for major depression and bipolar disorder. Maintenance treatment with antipsychotic drugs decreases the risk of recurrent acute episodes of schizophrenia. For each condition, a range of treatment strategies was considered and assessed, including older (and widely available) psychotherapeutic drugs, newer pharmacotherapies, psychosocial treatments, and combination treatments (see table 31.2 for a list of interventions included).

Estimation of Population-Level Treatment Costs

Cost estimation followed the principles and procedures described in chapter 7 for carrying out economic analyses of disease control priorities in developing countries. For depression and panic disorder, treatment was assumed to occur in a primary care setting, whereas for schizophrenia and bipolar disorder, which often produce highly disruptive behaviors, both hospital- and community-based outpatient service models were derived and compared. Both program- and patient-level costs were identified and estimated. Program-level costs included the infrastructure and administrative support for implementing mental health treatments, as well as training inputs (for example, two to three days per trainee were estimated for training primary care doctors and case managers in psychotropic medication management). Patient-level resource inputs included medication regimens (for example, fluoxetine, 20 milligrams daily), laboratory tests (for example, lithium blood levels), primary care visits (including any contacts with a case manager), and hospital outpatient and inpatient care. Estimated patient-level resource inputs for each of the four disorders were informed by empirical economic evaluative studies (for example, Patel and others 2003; Srinivasa Murthy and others 2005) as well as a multinational Delphi consensus study of resource use for psychiatric disorders in seven developing countries (Ferri and others 2004). Region-specific unit costs or prices were applied to all resource inputs (see Mulligan and others 2003) to give an annual cost for each case as well as for all cases at the specified level of treatment

Table 31.2 Interventions for Reducing the Burden of Major Psychiatric Disorders in Developing Countries

Disorder	Intervention	Example
Schizophrenia	Older (neuroleptic) antipsychotic drug	Haloperidol
Treatment setting: hospital outpatient	Newer (atypical) antipsychotic drug	Risperidone
Treatment coverage (target): 80 percent	**Older antipsychotic drug and psychosocial treatment**	Haloperidol plus family psychoeducation
	Newer antipsychotic drug and psychosocial treatment	Risperidone plus family psychoeducation
Bipolar affective disorder	Older mood-stabilizing drug	Lithium carbonate
Treatment setting: hospital outpatient	Newer mood-stabilizing drug	Sodium valproate
Treatment coverage (target): 50 percent	**Older mood-stabilizing drug and psychosocial treatment**	Lithium plus family psychoeducation
	Newer mood-stabilizing drug and psychosocial treatment	Valproate plus family psychoeducation
Depression	Episodic treatment	
Treatment setting: primary health care	**Older TCA**	Imipramine or amitriptyline
Treatment coverage (target): 50 percent	**Newer antidepressant drug (SSRI; generic)**	Fluoxetine
	Psychosocial treatment	Group psychotherapy
	Older antidepressant drug and psychosocial treatment	Amitriptyline plus group psychotherapy
	Newer antidepressant drug and psychosocial treatment	Fluoxetine plus group psychotherapy
	Maintenance treatment	
	Older antidepressant drug and psychosocial treatment	Imipramine plus group psychotherapy
	Newer antidepressant drug and psychosocial treatment	Fluoxetine plus group psychotherapy
Panic disorder	Benzodiazepines	Alprazolam
Treatment setting: primary health care	**Older TCA**	Amitriptyline
Treatment coverage (target): 50 percent	**Newer antidepressant drug (SSRI; generic)**	Fluoxetine
	Psychosocial treatment	Cognitive therapy
	Older antidepressant drug and psychosocial treatment	Amitriptyline plus cognitive therapy
	Newer antidepressant drug and psychosocial treatment	Fluoxetine plus cognitive therapy

Source: Authors' own estimates and recommendations.
Note: Interventions in **bold** are the most cost-effective treatments of choice.

coverage. Costs incurred over the 10-year implementation period were discounted at 3 percent and expressed in U.S. dollars (rather than international dollars, which attempt to adjust for differences in purchasing power between countries).

Coverage

In each World Bank region, treatment costs and effects were ascribed to the population in need, both at current levels of intervention coverage and at a scaled-up, target level of coverage (80 percent for schizophrenia, 50 percent for the other conditions). Target coverage levels were predicated on the basis of what could feasibly be achieved given existing rates of treatment (Ferri and others 2004; Kohn and others 2004), as well as on prerequisites for increased coverage, such as recognition of common mental disorders in primary care. Estimation of current regional levels of effective coverage is hampered by lack of data; nevertheless, an attempt was made to approximate the expected proportion of the diseased population receiving

evidence-based pharmacological and psychosocial treatments (Ferri and others 2004; Kohn and others 2004), plus those in contact with traditional healers (the effectiveness of which was conservatively approximated by ascribing a placebo effect size for each disorder).

Results

Tables 31.3 through 31.6 provide estimates of the population-level effects (measured in DALYs averted), costs, and cost-effectiveness of each intervention by world region for the four types of psychiatric disorder considered in this chapter. A number of key findings emerge from this analysis.

Treatment Effectiveness. Results for schizophrenia and bipolar disorder are similar (albeit at differing coverage levels), ranging from less than 100 DALYs averted per 1 million population under the current situation in Sub-Saharan Africa and South Asia to 350 to 400 DALYs averted per 1 million population for

Table 31.3 Cost-Effectiveness Results: Schizophrenia

Model definition: Treatment setting: (a) hospital-based; (b) community-based Treatment coverage: 80 percent	World Bank region					
	Sub-Saharan Africa	Latin America and the Caribbean	Middle East and North Africa	Europe and Central Asia	South Asia	East Asia and the Pacific
Total effect (DALYs averted per year per 1 million population)						
Current situation	74	136	115	258	87	148
Older (neuroleptic) antipsychotic drug	149	219	214	254	177	231
Newer (atypical) antipsychotic drug	160	235	230	273	190	248
Older antipsychotic drug plus psychosocial treatment	254	373	364	353	300	392
Newer antipsychotic drug plus psychosocial treatment	261	383	373	364	308	403
Total cost (US$ million per year per 1 million population)						
Current situation	0.42	2.07	1.31	3.13	0.51	1.11
Hospital-based service model						
Older (neuroleptic) antipsychotic drug	0.60	3.09	2.40	2.24	0.74	1.18
Newer (atypical) antipsychotic drug	2.80	6.33	5.41	6.16	3.36	4.63
Older antipsychotic drug plus psychosocial treatment	0.67	3.27	2.56	2.36	0.81	1.26
Newer antipsychotic drug plus psychosocial treatment	2.87	6.56	5.61	6.31	3.44	4.73
Community-based service model						
Older (neuroleptic) antipsychotic drug	0.40	1.58	1.42	1.17	0.44	0.66
Newer (atypical) antipsychotic drug	2.59	4.85	4.45	5.11	3.07	4.12
Older antipsychotic drug plus psychosocial treatment	0.47	1.81	1.61	1.32	0.52	0.75
Newer antipsychotic drug plus psychosocial treatment	2.67	5.09	4.66	5.28	3.16	4.22
Cost-effectiveness (US$ per DALY averted)						
Current situation	5,695	15,192	11,400	12,134	5,900	7,533
Hospital-based service model						
Older (neuroleptic) antipsychotic drug	4,047	14,123	11,205	8,793	4,164	5,120
Newer (atypical) antipsychotic drug	17,433	26,893	23,543	22,530	17,702	18,700
Older antipsychotic drug plus psychosocial treatment	2,623	8,781	7,040	6,685	2,693	3,212
Newer antipsychotic drug plus psychosocial treatment	10,996	17,146	15,027	17,329	11,164	11,746
Community-based service model						
Older (neuroleptic) antipsychotic drug	2,668	7,230	6,618	4,595	2,499	2,855
Newer (atypical) antipsychotic drug	16,174	20,583	19,352	18,685	16,178	16,622
Older antipsychotic drug plus psychosocial treatment	**1,839**	**4,847**	**4,431**	**3,745**	**1,743**	**1,917**
Newer antipsychotic drug plus psychosocial treatment	10,232	13,313	12,485	14,481	10,239	10,484

Source: Authors' own estimates.
Note: Intervention data in **bold** are the most cost-effective treatments of choice.

Table 31.4 Cost-Effectiveness Results: Bipolar Disorder

Model definition: Treatment setting: (a) hospital-based; (b) community-based Treatment coverage: 50 percent	World Bank region					
	Sub-Saharan Africa	Latin America and the Caribbean	Middle East and North Africa	Europe and Central Asia	South Asia	East Asia and the Pacific
Total effect (DALYs averted per year per 1 million population)						
Current situation	79	128	97	199	93	153
Older mood-stabilizing drug (lithium)	292	336	296	381	319	389
Newer mood-stabilizing drug (valproate)	211	300	273	331	278	351
Older mood-stabilizing drug plus psychosocial treatment	312	365	322	413	346	422
Newer mood-stabilizing drug plus psychosocial treatment	232	330	300	365	306	386
Total cost (US$ million per year per 1 million population)						
Current situation	0.31	1.22	0.74	1.27	0.42	0.67
Hospital-based service model						
Older mood-stabilizing drug (lithium)	0.61	2.77	1.92	2.03	0.82	1.30
Newer mood-stabilizing drug (valproate)	0.79	2.87	2.04	2.20	1.03	1.53
Older mood-stabilizing drug plus psychosocial treatment	0.63	2.79	1.95	2.05	0.84	1.32
Newer mood-stabilizing drug plus psychosocial treatment	0.81	2.90	2.08	2.22	1.06	1.55
Community-based service model						
Older mood-stabilizing drug (lithium)	0.46	1.78	1.20	1.37	0.59	0.93
Newer mood-stabilizing drug (valproate)	0.64	1.91	1.36	1.57	0.82	1.17
Older mood-stabilizing drug plus psychosocial treatment	0.48	1.80	1.23	1.39	0.62	0.95
Newer mood-stabilizing drug plus psychosocial treatment	0.67	1.95	1.39	1.59	0.85	1.19
Cost-effectiveness (US$ per DALY averted)						
Current situation	3,967	9,518	7,668	6,398	4,463	4,373
Hospital-based service model						
Older mood-stabilizing drug (lithium)	2,091	8,246	6,478	5,341	2,553	3,348
Newer mood-stabilizing drug (valproate)	3,727	9,579	7,501	6,648	3,709	4,358
Older mood-stabilizing drug plus psychosocial treatment	2,016	7,644	6,036	4,957	2,424	3,119
Newer mood-stabilizing drug plus psychosocial treatment	3,480	8,800	6,937	6,100	3,459	4,016
Community-based service model						
Older mood-stabilizing drug (lithium)	1,587	5,295	4,068	3,608	1,862	2,394
Newer mood-stabilizing drug (valproate)	3,057	6,386	4,971	4,727	2,943	3,338
Older mood-stabilizing drug plus psychosocial treatment	**1,545**	**4,928**	**3,823**	**3,359**	**1,787**	**2,241**
Newer mood-stabilizing drug plus psychosocial treatment	2,874	5,908	4,645	4,359	2,765	3,092

Source: Authors' own estimates.

Note: Intervention data in **bold** are the most cost-effective treatments of choice.

Table 31.5 Cost-Effectiveness Results: Depression

Model definition: Treatment setting: primary health care Treatment coverage: 50 percent	World Bank region					
	Sub-Saharan Africa	Latin America and the Caribbean	Middle East and North Africa	Europe and Central Asia	South Asia	East Asia and the Pacific
Total effect (DALYs averted per year per 1 million population)						
Current situation	133	264	218	308	218	243
Episodic treatment: older antidepressant drug (TCA)	599	995	920	874	987	891
Episodic treatment: newer antidepressant drug (SSRI)	632	1,049	971	925	1,042	941
Episodic psychosocial treatment	624	1,036	958	936	1,028	927
Episodic psychosocial treatment plus older antidepressant	745	1,237	1,144	1,100	1,228	1,107
Episodic psychosocial treatment plus newer antidepressant	745	1,237	1,144	1,100	1,228	1,107
Maintenance psychosocial treatment plus older antidepressant	1,174	1,953	1,806	1,789	1,937	1,747
Maintenance psychosocial treatment plus newer antidepressant	1,174	1,953	1,806	1,789	1,937	1,747
Total cost (US$ million per year per 1 million population)						
Current situation	0.36	0.90	0.63	0.74	0.56	0.67
Episodic treatment: older antidepressant drug (TCA)	0.30	1.28	0.96	0.81	0.47	0.47
Episodic treatment: newer antidepressant drug (SSRI)	0.66	1.86	1.47	1.39	1.04	0.99
Episodic psychosocial treatment	0.37	1.67	1.27	0.97	0.55	0.53
Episodic psychosocial treatment plus older antidepressant	0.50	1.96	1.53	1.21	0.77	0.72
Episodic psychosocial treatment plus newer antidepressant	0.90	2.60	2.10	1.85	1.40	1.29
Maintenance psychosocial treatment plus older antidepressant	0.96	3.44	2.77	2.19	1.45	1.38
Maintenance psychosocial treatment plus newer antidepressant	1.80	4.80	3.99	3.56	2.81	2.59
Cost-effectiveness (US$ per DALY averted)						
Current situation	2,692	3,414	2,905	2,391	2,546	2,777
Episodic treatment: older antidepressant drug (TCA)	**505**	**1,288**	**1,039**	**929**	**478**	**533**
Episodic treatment: newer antidepressant drug (SSRI)	1,042	1,771	1,516	1,501	1,003	1,048
Episodic psychosocial treatment	592	1,611	1,330	1,035	537	570
Episodic psychosocial treatment plus older antidepressant	674	1,586	1,335	1,104	627	653
Episodic psychosocial treatment plus newer antidepressant	1,203	2,101	1,834	1,682	1,140	1,161
Maintenance psychosocial treatment plus older antidepressant	**817**	**1,760**	**1,533**	**1,226**	**749**	**788**
Maintenance psychosocial treatment plus newer antidepressant	1,535	2,459	2,211	1,990	1,449	1,481

Source: Authors' own estimates.
Note: Intervention data in **bold** are the most cost-effective treatments of choice.

Table 31.6 Cost-Effectiveness Results: Panic Disorder

Model definition: Treatment setting: primary health care Treatment coverage: 50 percent	World Bank region					
	Sub-Saharan Africa	Latin America and the Caribbean	Middle East and North Africa	Europe and Central Asia	South Asia	East Asia and the Pacific
Total effect (DALYs averted per year per 1 million population)						
Current situation	49	94	64	88	57	90
Anxiolytic drug (benzodiazepine)	144	182	170	183	168	195
Older antidepressant drug (TCA)	232	290	272	290	269	312
Newer antidepressant drug (SSRI; generic)	245	307	287	307	284	330
Psychosocial treatment (cognitive-behavioral therapy)	233	292	273	292	270	313
Older antidepressant plus psychosocial treatment	262	329	308	329	304	353
Newer antidepressant plus psychosocial treatment	276	346	324	346	320	372
Total cost (US$ million per year per 1 million population)						
Current situation	0.06	0.13	0.08	0.07	0.05	0.10
Anxiolytic drug (benzodiazepine)	0.10	0.20	0.15	0.15	0.10	0.12
Older antidepressant drug (TCA)	0.09	0.18	0.14	0.14	0.08	0.11
Newer antidepressant drug (SSRI; generic)	0.15	0.27	0.21	0.23	0.16	0.20
Psychosocial treatment (cognitive-behavioral therapy)	0.11	0.27	0.21	0.17	0.09	0.11
Older antidepressant plus psychosocial treatment	0.15	0.32	0.26	0.23	0.13	0.17
Newer antidepressant plus psychosocial treatment	0.22	0.41	0.34	0.32	0.22	0.26
Cost-effectiveness (US$ per DALY averted)						
Current situation	1,192	1,378	1,208	824	948	1,109
Anxiolytic drug (benzodiazepine)	681	1,075	892	842	572	629
Older antidepressant drug (TCA)	**369**	**619**	**508**	**474**	**305**	**339**
Newer antidepressant drug (SSRI; generic)	**630**	**865**	**747**	**741**	**567**	**606**
Psychosocial treatment (cognitive-behavioral therapy)	468	927	786	594	338	365
Older antidepressant plus psychosocial treatment	556	977	844	685	443	474
Newer antidepressant plus psychosocial treatment	788	1,188	1,050	918	671	709

Source: Authors' own estimates.
CBT = cognitive behavioral therapy
Note: Intervention data in **bold** are the most cost-effective treatments of choice.

combination drug and psychosocial interventions in Europe and Central Asia and East Asia and the Pacific. Second-generation (atypical) antipsychotic drugs were considered slightly more effective than first-generation drugs (on the basis of a modest intrinsic efficacy difference and differences in tolerability and adherence); lithium was considered modestly more effective as a mood-stabilizing drug than valproate (on the basis of its additional positive effect on suicide rates). Adjuvant psychosocial treatment in combination with pharmacotherapy significantly added to expected population-level health gain.

With the exception of Europe and Central Asia, less than 10 percent of the disease burden currently is being averted, whereas the implementation of combined interventions at a scaled-up level of coverage is expected to avert 14 to 22 percent of the burden of schizophrenia (coverage level, 80 percent) and 17 to 29 percent of the burden of bipolar disorder (coverage level, 50 percent).

For primary care treatment of common mental disorders, including depression and panic disorder, current levels of effective coverage avert only 3 to 8 percent of the existing disease burden, whereas scaling up of the most effective interventions to a coverage level of 50 percent could be expected to avert more than 20 percent of the burden of depression and up to one-third of the burden of panic disorder. Considered at a population level, episodic treatments for depressive episodes did not differ substantially within regions (averting 10 to15 percent of current burden); more substantial health gain is expected by providing maintenance treatment to individuals with recurrent depression (approximately 1,200 to 1,900 DALYs averted per 1 million population; 18 to 23 percent of burden). Such an approach has been found to reduce the risk of relapse by half. Although the evidence to date from developing regions is meager, our results suggest that SSRIs such as fluoxetine, alone or in combination with psychosocial treatment, are the most effective treatments for panic disorder, with health gains considerably better than those estimated for benzodiazepine anxiolytic drugs such as alprazolam.

Treatment Costs. Community-based service models for schizophrenia and bipolar disorder were found to be appreciably less costly than hospital-based service models (for example, interventions for bipolar disorder were 25 to 40 percent less costly). The total cost per capita of community-based outpatient treatment with first-generation antipsychotic or mood-stabilizing drugs, including all patient-level resource needs as well as infrastructural support, ranged from US$0.40 to US$0.50 in Sub-Saharan Africa and South Asia to US$1.20 to US$1.90 in Latin America and the Caribbean and in Europe and Central Asia (equivalent patient costs per year, US$170 to US$300 and US$300 to US$800, respectively). The cost per capita for interventions using second-generation (atypical) antipsychotic drugs still under patent is much higher (US$2.50 to US$5.00). By contrast, some of the newer antidepressant drugs (SSRIs) are now off patent, and their use in treating depression and panic disorder was accordingly costed at their generic, nonbranded price. The patient-level cost of treating a 6-month episode of depression ranged from as little as US$30 (older antidepressants in Sub-Saharan Africa or South Asia) to US$150 (newer antidepressants in combination with brief psychotherapy in Latin America and the Caribbean). Total annual costs for all incidents of depressive episodes receiving treatment, including training and other program-level costs, were as much as US$2 to US$5 per capita for a maintenance treatment program using newer antidepressants, three times more costly than episodic treatment with newer antidepressant drugs only. Patient-level resource inputs for panic disorder interventions cost US$50 to US$200 per case per year, and overall costs including program costs of training and administration amounted to US$0.10 to US$0.30 per capita.

Cost-Effectiveness. Compared with both the current situation and the epidemiological situation of no treatment (natural history), the most cost-effective strategy for averting the burden of psychosis and severe affective disorders in developing countries is expected to be a combined intervention of first-generation antipsychotic or mood-stabilizing drugs with adjuvant psychosocial treatment delivered through a community-based outpatient service model, with a cost-effectiveness ratio of below US$2,000 in Sub-Saharan Africa and South Asia, rising to US$5,000 in Latin America and the Caribbean (equivalent to more than 500 DALYs averted per US$1 million expenditure in Sub-Saharan Africa and South Asia and 200 DALYs averted in Latin America and the Caribbean). Currently, the high acquisition price of second-generation antipsychotic drugs makes their use in developing regions questionable on efficiency grounds, although this situation can be expected to change as these drugs come off patent. By contrast, evidence indicates that the relatively modest additional cost of adjuvant psychosocial treatment reaps significant health gains, thereby making such a combined strategy for schizophrenia and bipolar disorder treatment more cost-effective than pharmacotherapy alone.

For more common mental disorders treated in primary care settings (depressive and anxiety disorders), the single most cost-effective strategy is the scaled-up use of older antidepressants (because of their lower cost but similar efficacy compared with newer antidepressants). However, as the price margin between older and generic newer antidepressants continues to diminish, generic SSRIs—which have milder side effects and are more likely to be taken at a therapeutic dose (Pereira and Patel 1999)—can be expected to be at least as cost-effective and, therefore, the pharmacological treatment of choice in the future. Because depression is often a recurring condition, proactive care management, including long-term maintenance treatment with antidepressant drugs, represents a cost-effective way of significantly reducing the enormous burden of depression that exists in developing regions now (400 to 1,300 DALYs averted per US$1 million expenditure).

POLICY AND SERVICE IMPLICATIONS

Many attempts have been made during the past 50 years to have mental health care placed higher on national and international agendas. In 1974, a WHO Expert Committee on the

Organization of Mental Health Services in Developing Countries (WHO 1975) made the following recommendations:

- Develop a national mental health policy and create a unit within the Health Ministry to implement it.
- Budget for workforce development, essential drug procurement, infrastructure development, data collection, and research.
- Decentralize service provision and integrate mental health into primary health care.
- Train and supervise primary health care providers in mental health using specialist mental health staff.

Thirty years later, international agencies, nongovernmental organizations, and professional bodies continue to make those exact recommendations. One reason for the lack of action in mental health has been the paucity of information on the cost-effectiveness of mental health interventions. Advocacy without the necessary science can readily be ignored in countries with massive health problems and meager resources. This chapter aims to address this deficiency.

Symptoms of mental disorders are often attributed to other illnesses, and mental disorders are often not considered health problems (Jacob 2001). Many nonscientific explanations for mental illness exist, and stigma exists to varying degrees everywhere (Weiss and others 2001) with widespread delays or failure to seek appropriate care (James and others 2002).

When care is sought, a hierarchy of interventions comes into play, ranging from self-help, informal community support, traditional healers, primary health care, specialist community mental health care, and psychiatric units in general hospitals to specialist long-stay mental hospitals. The mix of interventions depends on the availability of resources within a country or region (Saxena and Maulik 2003). The more resource-constrained the country or region is, the greater is the reliance on self-help, informal community support (especially family-based), and primary health care.

Traditional healers are often the first source individuals with mental illness and their families turn to for professional assistance (see, for example, Abiodun 1995). A recent review of common mental disorders among primary health clinics and traditional healers in urban Tanzania showed that the prevalence of common mental disorders among those attending traditional healers was double that of patients at primary health care centers (Ngoma, Prince, and Mann 2003). Traditional healers are a heterogeneous group and include faith healers, spiritual healers, religious healers, and practitioners of indigenous or alternative systems of medicine. In some countries, they are part of the informal health sector, but in other countries, traditional healers charge for their services and should be considered part of the private health care sector. Often, traditional healers have high acceptability and are accessible; at times, traditional healers

work closely (and apparently effectively) with conventional mental health services (Thara, Padmavati, and Srinivasan 2004). Alternatively, animosity and competition can exist, and recent examples of human rights violations by traditional healers demonstrate the heterogeneity of this group of providers.

The formal diagnosis and treatment of mental disorders occur in both primary and specialist health services. Examples in nearly a dozen countries now show it is feasible and practicable to treat common mental disorders in primary health care settings (for example, Chisholm and others 2000; De Jong 1996; Mohit and others 1999). The challenge is to enhance systems of care by taking effective local models and disseminating them throughout a country.

Concern has been expressed that the more sophisticated psychotherapies used in mental health care are beyond the human resources of developing countries. However, basic psychological therapies can be effective, though there is some evidence, at least for depression, that the newer drug therapies are more cost-effective than psychological therapies (Patel and others 2003). Psychoeducational family intervention has been shown to be suitable for rehabilitation in schizophrenia in rural China (Ran and others 2003) and to be cost-effective compared with other standard treatment (Xiong and others 1994). Evidence also shows that nurses can replace physicians as primary health care providers in certain circumstances without loss of effectiveness (Climent and others 1978). Primary care practitioners need support to develop skills and experience in diagnosing and treating mental disorders: they need a sustainable supply of medicines, access to supervision, and incentives to see patients with mental illness (Abas and others 2003). Community approaches using low-cost, locally available resources may improve treatment adherence and clinical outcomes even in rural and underresourced settings (Chatterjee and others 2003; Srinivasa Murthy and others 2005).

In most countries, acute inpatient beds are being moved from mental hospitals into general or district hospitals. Although this policy potentially improves accessibility and increases the links with, and support provided to, primary mental health care, concerns can be raised as to whether general hospitals can adapt to provide adequate services to people with severe mental disorders. However, such services have been effectively established in a number of countries (see, for example, Alem and others 1999; Kilonzo and Simmons 1998), showing this form of service delivery to be feasible when it is clinically indicated.

Nongovernmental organizations are important providers of mental health care. An estimated 93 percent of African and 80 percent of Southeast Asian countries have nongovernmental organizations in the mental health sector. They provide diverse services—including advocacy, informal support, housing, suicide prevention, substance misuse counseling, dementia support, rehabilitation, research, and other programs—that complement, or in some cases substitute for, public and private clinical services (Levkoff, Macarthur, and Bucknall 1995; Patel and Thara 2003).

Services for children and adolescents, the majority of the population in many developing countries, are even more deficient than those for adults. Priority needs to be given to these services (Rahman and others 2000). At the other end of the life spectrum, many developing countries are facing aging populations with grossly underdeveloped aged care services (Levkoff, Macarthur, and Bucknall 1995). The high level of civil conflict and natural disasters requires attention to postconflict and posttrauma mental health conditions. The prevalence of these disorders is demonstrated by a recent study (Livanou, Basoglu, and Kalendar 2002) showing that, of 1,000 survivors of the August 1999 earthquake in Turkey, the incidence of PTSD was 63 percent and of depression was 42 percent.

Specialist mental health providers, especially mental hospitals, tend to focus the services they provide on the lower-prevalence, higher-disability disorders, such as schizophrenia and bipolar disorder. Modern treatments, if available and used, allow most patients to be treated effectively out of hospital. Specifically, the use of antipsychotic and mood-stabilizing drugs and the development of strategies for community-based treatment have led to the closing of large numbers of psychiatric inpatient beds in many countries and their replacement with community services and general hospital psychiatric units (for example, Larrobla and Botega 2001).

However, in some countries, the majority of psychotic patients remain in long-term inpatient facilities that engage in custodial care, which is often of poor quality; moreover, basic rights are often violated at such facilities (van Voren and Whiteford 2000). Even if the quality of care is reasonable, accessibility is a problem: these hospitals are often situated in urban areas, but populations are largely rural and have limited transportation (Saraceno and others 1995). Furthermore, the concentration of resources in these facilities can leave little for other service components (Gallegos and Montero 1999). For example, in Indonesia, 97 percent of the mental health budget is spent on public mental hospitals (Trisnantoro 2002). For many developing countries, the debate about the role of, or problems with, mental hospitals is subsumed within a gross deficiency of psychiatric beds of any kind.

The priority for virtually all countries is generating sufficient resources for primary mental health care and deciding how to expand and best use scarce specialist resources. The quality of care is often very poor, and huge variations exist in resource availability between countries (Saxena and Maulik 2003; WHO 2001). Very few countries have what could be considered an optimal mix of these services, and there are no universally accepted planning parameters. However, conceptual models for developing national mental health policy and guidelines for service planning exist that can be useful in developing countries (Tansella and Thornicroft 1998; Townsend and others 2004; WHO 2003).

CONCLUSION: PUBLIC SUPPORT FOR A COST-EFFECTIVE INTERVENTION PACKAGE

In developing countries, much of the mental health care spending is reported to be out of pocket. Individuals purchase modern and traditional treatments if they can afford to do so. Although a large private health sector exists in low-income countries (Mills and others 2002), the quality and cost vary. Although unregulated markets fail in health, they fail even more in mental health. It is unlikely that a country will be able to rely on an unregulated private sector to deliver services that will reduce the burden of mental disorders.

In addition to being a large and growing component of disease burden, mental disorders meet virtually all the criteria by which we determine the need for government involvement in health care (Beeharry and others 2002). They affect the poor, cause externalities, and inflict catastrophic costs; moreover, private demand is inadequate. Indeed, the authors recognize that the main measure of outcome used in this and other chapters—the disability-adjusted life year—is limited to capturing change in service user–level symptoms, disability, recovery, and case-fatality. The DALY does *not* capture the positive change that treatment may have on a number of other significant consequences of mental disorders, including family burden (in particular, productive time and household resources given up in the care of the sick family member) and lost productivity, at the level of both the individual and the household (treatment accelerates return to paid work or usual household activities) and, by implication, at the level of society in general. The evidence base for these productivity increases, although modest in volume, constitutes an important additional argument alongside "cost per DALY" considerations for investing in mental health.

The total budgetary requirements and health consequences of a cost-effective package of mental health care can begin to be mapped out by selecting one intervention for each of the four disorders considered in this chapter. Although the data available for this exercise have limitations and will need to be refined with further research, table 31.7 summarizes the estimated costs and effects of a package consisting of (a) outpatient-based treatment of schizophrenia and bipolar disorder with first-generation antipsychotic or mood-stabilizing drugs and adjuvant psychosocial treatment, (b) proactive care of depression in primary care with generic SSRIs (including maintenance treatment of recurrent episodes), and (c) treatment of panic disorder in primary care with generic SSRIs. The estimated benefit of such a package would be an annual reduction of 2,000 to 3,000 DALYs per 1 million population, at a cost of US$3 million to US$9 million (that is, US$3 to US$4 per capita in Sub-Saharan

Table 31.7 Costs and Effects of a Specified Mental Health Care Package

	World Bank region					
	Sub-Saharan Africa	Latin America and the Caribbean	Middle East and North Africa	Europe and Central Asia	South Asia	East Asia and the Pacific
Total effect (DALYs averted per year per 1 million population)						
Schizophrenia: older antipsychotic drug plus psychosocial treatment	254	373	364	353	300	392
Bipolar disorder: older mood-stabilizing drug plus psychosocial treatment	312	365	322	413	346	422
Depression: proactive care with newer antidepressant drug (SSRI; generic)	1,174	1,953	1,806	1,789	1,937	1,747
Panic disorder: newer antidepressant drug (SSRI; generic)	245	307	287	307	284	330
Total effect of interventions	1,985	2,998	2,779	2,862	2,867	2,891
Total cost (US$ million per year per 1 million population)						
Schizophrenia: older antipsychotic drug plus psychosocial treatment	0.47	1.81	1.61	1.32	0.52	0.75
Bipolar disorder: older mood-stabilizing drug plus psychosocial treatment	0.48	1.80	1.23	1.39	0.62	0.95
Depression: proactive care with newer antidepressant drug (SSRI; generic)	1.80	4.80	3.99	3.56	2.81	2.59
Panic disorder: newer antidepressant drug (SSRI; generic)	0.15	0.27	0.21	0.23	0.16	0.20
Total cost of interventions	2.9	8.7	7.0	6.5	4.1	4.5
Cost-effectiveness (DALYs averted per US$1 million expenditure)						
Schizophrenia: older antipsychotic drug plus psychosocial treatment	544	206	226	267	574	522
Bipolar disorder: older mood-stabilizing drug plus psychosocial treatment	647	203	262	298	560	446
Depression: proactive care with newer antidepressant drug (SSRI; generic)	652	407	452	502	690	675
Panic disorder: newer antidepressant drug (SSRI; generic)	1,588	1,155	1,339	1,350	1,765	1,649

Source: Authors' own estimates.

Africa and South Asia, and US$7 to US$9 per capita in Latin America and the Caribbean). Accordingly, for every US$1 million invested in such a mental health care package, 350 to 700 healthy years of life would be gained over what would occur without intervention.

At a country level, data such as those presented in this chapter can be used to estimate the proportion of burden currently averted, the proportion that can be averted with current knowledge and optimal coverage, and the burden not able to be averted with current knowledge. Such modeling has been done for some countries (for example, Andrews and others 2004).

Although much remains to be learned about the etiology and treatment of mental disorders, the potential clearly exists for a considerable reduction in the burden caused by them. For these gains to be made, the challenge is to overcome the cultural, financial, and structural barriers that prevent people from seeking and receiving treatment. We need to close the gap between what we know and what we do in treating mental disorders. We can alleviate the substantial burden of these disorders and reverse or limit many of the devastating social and economic impacts.

REFERENCES

Abas, M., L. Mbengeranwa, I. Chagwedera, P. Maramba, and J. Broadhead. 2003. "Primary Care Services for Depression in Harare, Zimbabwe." *Harvard Review of Psychiatry* 11 (3): 157–65.

Abiodun, O. 1995. "Pathways to Mental Health Care in Nigeria." *Psychiatric Services* 46 (8): 823–26.

Alem, A., L. Jacobsson, M. Araya, D. Kebede, and G. Kullgren. 1999. "How Are Mental Disorders Seen, and Where Is Help Sought in a Rural

Ethiopian Community?" *Acta Psychiatrica Scandinavica* 100 (Suppl. 397): 40–47.

American Psychiatric Association. 2000. *Diagnostic and Statistical Manual of Mental Disorders*. 4th ed., text revision. Washington, DC: American Psychiatric Association.

Andrade, L., J. J. Caraveo-Anduaga, P. Berglund, R. V. Bijl, E. Dragomirecka, R. Kohn, and others. 2003. "The Epidemiology of Major Depressive Episodes: Results from the International Consortium of Psychiatric Epidemiology (ICPE) Surveys." *International Journal of Methods in Psychiatric Research* 12 (1): 3–21.

Andrews, G. 2001. "Placebo Response in Depression: Bane of Research, Boon to Therapy." *British Journal of Psychiatry* 178 (3): 192–94.

Andrews, G., C. Issakidis, K. Sanderson, J. Corry, and H. Lapsley. 2004. "Utilizing Survey Data to Inform Public Policy: Comparison of the Cost-Effectiveness of Treatment of Ten Mental Disorders" *British Journal of Psychiatry* 184 (6): 526–33.

Andrews, G., K. Sanderson, J. Corry, C. Issakidis, and H. Lapsley. 2003. "Cost-Effectiveness of Current and Optimal Treatment for Schizophrenia." *British Journal of Psychiatry* 183 (5): 427–35.

Angst, J., and R. Sellaro. 2000. "Historical Perspectives and Natural History of Bipolar Disorder." *Biological Psychiatry* 48 (6): 445–57.

Araya, R., G. Rojas, R. Fritsch, J. Gaete, M. Rojas, and T. J. Peters. 2003. "Treating Depression in Primary Care in Low-Income Women in Santiago, Chile: A Randomised Controlled Trial." *Lancet* 361 (9362): 995–1000.

Astrup, C., A. Fossum, and R. Holmboe. 1959. "A Follow-up Study of 270 Patients with Acute Affective Psychoses." *Acta Psychiatrica Scandinavica* 34 (Suppl. 135): 1–65.

Bakker, A., A. J. L. M. van Balkom, P. Spinhoven, B. M. Blaauw, and R. van Dyck. 1998. "Follow-up on the Treatment of Panic Disorder with or without Agoraphobia: A Quantitative Review." *Journal of Nervous and Mental Disease* 186 (7): 414–19.

Beeharry, G., H. Whiteford, D. Chambers, and F. Baingana. 2002. "Outlining the Scope for Public Sector Involvement in Mental Health." Health Nutrition and Population Discussion Paper, World Bank, Washington, DC.

Bijl, R. V., G. van Zessen, A. Ravelli, C. de Rijk, and Y. Langendoen. 1998. "The Netherlands Mental Health Survey and Incidence Study (NEMESIS): Objectives and Design." *Social Psychiatry and Psychiatric Epidemiology* 33 (12): 581–86.

Bolton, P., J. Bass, R. Neugebauer, H. Verdeli, K. Clougherty, P. Wickramaratne, and others. 2003. "Group Interpersonal Psychotherapy for Depression in Rural Uganda." *Journal of the American Medical Association* 289 (23): 3117–24.

Bowden, C. L., J. R. Calabrese, S. L. McElroy, L. Gyulai, A. Wassef, F. Petty, and others. 2000. "A Randomized, Placebo-Controlled 12-Month Trial of Divalproex and Lithium in Treatment of Outpatients with Bipolar I Disorder: Divalproex Maintenance Study Group." *Archives of General Psychiatry* 57 (5): 481–89.

Bustillo, J. R., J. Lauriello, W. P. Horan, and S. J. Keith. 2001. "The Psychosocial Treatment of Schizophrenia: An Update." *American Journal of Psychiatry* 158 (2): 163–75.

Chatterjee, S., V. Patel, A. Chatterjee, and H. Weiss. 2003. "Evaluation of a Community-Based Rehabilitation Model for Chronic Schizophrenia in Rural India." *British Journal of Psychiatry* 182 (1): 57–62.

Chisholm, D., K. Sanderson, J. L. Ayuso-Mateos, and S. Saxena. 2004. "Reducing the Burden of Depression: A Population-Level Analysis of Intervention Cost-Effectiveness in 14 Epidemiologically Defined Sub-Regions (WHO-CHOICE)." *British Journal of Psychiatry* 184 (5): 393–403.

Chisholm, D., K. Sekar, K. K. Kumar, K. Saeed, S. James, M. Mubbashar, and R. S. Murthy. 2000. "Integration of Mental Health Care into Primary Care: Demonstration Cost-Outcome Study in India and Pakistan." *British Journal of Psychiatry* 176 (6): 581–88.

Chisholm, D., M. Van Ommeren, J. L. Ayuso-Mateos, and S. Saxena. Forthcoming. "Cost-Effectiveness of Clinical Interventions for Reducing the Global Burden of Bipolar Disorder: A Global Analysis (WHO-CHOICE)." *British Journal of Psychiatry*.

Climent, C. E., M. V. De Arango, R. Plutchick, and C. A. Leon. 1978. "Development of an Alternative, Efficient Low Cost Mental Health Delivery System in Cali, Colombia, 1: The Auxiliary Nurse." *Social Psychiatry* 13 (1): 29–35.

Das Gupta, R., and J. F. Guest. 2002. "Annual Cost of Bipolar Disorder to U.K. Society." *British Journal of Psychiatry* 180 (3): 227–33.

de Graaf, R., R. V. Bijl, J. Spijker, A. T. Beekman, and W. A. Vollebergh. 2003. "Temporal Sequencing of Lifetime Mood Disorders in Relation to Comorbid Anxiety and Substance Use Disorders—Findings from the Netherlands Mental Health Survey and Incidence Study." *Social Psychiatry and Psychiatric Epidemiology* 38 (1): 1–11.

De Jong, J. 1996. "A Comprehensive Public Mental Health Programme in Guinea-Bissau: A Useful Model for African, Asian, and Latin-American Countries." *Psychological Medicine* 26 (1): 97–108.

ESEMeD/MHEDEA 2000 Investigators. 2004. "Use of Mental Health Services in Europe: Results from the European Study of Epidemiology of Mental Disorders, ESEMeD Project." *Acta Psychiatrica Scandinavica* 109 (Suppl. 420): 47–54.

Faravelli, C., S. Paterniti, and A. Scarpato. 1995. "5-Year Prospective, Naturalistic Follow-up Study of Panic Disorder." *Comprehensive Psychiatry* 36 (4): 271–77.

Ferri, C., D. Chisholm, M. Van Ommeren, and M. Prince. 2004. "Resource Utilisation for Neuropsychiatric Disorders in Developing Countries: A Multinational Delphi Consensus Study." *Social Psychiatry and Psychiatric Epidemiology* 39 (3): 218–27.

Frank, E., H. A. Swartz, and D. J. Kupfer. 2000. "Interpersonal and Social Rhythm Therapy: Managing the Chaos of Bipolar Disorder." *Biological Psychiatry* 48 (6): 593–604.

Gallegos, A., and F. Montero. 1999. "Issues in Community Based Rehabilitation for Persons with Mental Illness in Costa Rica." *International Journal of Mental Health* 28: 25–30.

Geddes, J., S. M. Carney, T. A. Furukawa, D. J. Kupfer, and G. M. Goodwin. 2003. "Relapse Prevention with Antidepressant Drug Treatment in Depressive Disorders: A Systematic Review." *Lancet* 361 (9358): 653–61.

Goodwin, F. K., B. Fireman, G. E. Simon, E. Hunkeler, J. Lee, and D. Revicki. 2003. "Suicide Risk in Bipolar Disorder during Treatment with Lithium and Divalproex." *Journal of the American Medical Association* 290 (11): 1467–73.

Harrison, G., K. Hopper, T. Craig, E. Laska, C. Diegel, J. Wanderling, and others. 2001. "Recovery from Psychotic Illness: A 15- and 25-Year International Follow-up Study." *British Journal of Psychiatry* 178 (6): 506–17.

Helgason, T. 1964. "Epidemiology of Mental Disorders in Iceland: A Psychiatric and Demographic Investigation of 5,395 Icelanders." *Acta Psychiatrica Scandinavica* 40 (Suppl. 173): 1–180.

Huxley, N. A., S. V. Parikh, and R. J. Baldessarini. 2000. "Effectiveness of Psychosocial Treatments in Bipolar Disorder: State of the Evidence." *Harvard Review of Psychiatry* 8 (3): 126–40.

Hwu, H. G., E. K. Yeh, and L. Y. Cheng. 1989. "Prevalence of Psychiatric Disorders in Taiwan Defined by the Chinese Diagnostic Interview Schedule." *Acta Psychiatrica Scandinavica* 79 (2): 136–47.

Hyman, S. E. 2000. "The Genetics of Mental Illness: Implications for Practice." *Bulletin of the World Health Organization* 78 (4): 455–63.

Jablensky, A. N. 2000. "Epidemiology of Schizophrenia: The Global Burden of Disease and Disability." *European Archives of Psychiatry and Clinical Neuroscience* 250 (6): 274–85.

Jablensky, A. N., G. Sartorius, M. Ernberg, A. Anker, J. E. Korten, R. Cooper, and others. 1992. "Schizophrenia: Manifestations, Incidence, and Course in Different Cultures: A World Health Organization Ten-Country Study." *Psychological Medicine* (Suppl 20): 1–97.

Jacob, K. 2001. "Community Care for People with Mental Disorders in Developing Countries." *British Journal of Psychiatry* 178 (4): 296–98.

James, S., D. Chisholm, R. S. Murthy, K. Sekar, K. Saeed, and M. Mubbashar. 2002. "Demand for, Access to, and Use of Community Mental Health Care: Lessons from a Demonstration Project in India and Pakistan." *International Journal of Social Psychiatry* 48 (3): 163–76.

Joy, C. B., C. E. Adams, and S. M. Lawrie. 2001. "Haloperidol versus Placebo for Schizophrenia." Cochrane Database of Systematic Reviews (2) D003082. http://www.mediscope.ch/cochrane-abstracts/ab003082.htm.

Judd, L. L., H. S. Akiskal, J. D. Maser, P. J. Zeller, J. Endicott, W. Coryell, and others. 1998. "A Prospective 12-Year Study of Subsyndromal and Syndromal Depressive Symptoms in Unipolar Major Depressive Disorders." *Archives of General Psychiatry* 55 (8): 694–700.

Judd, L. L., P. J. Schettler, and H. S. Akiskal. 2002. "The Prevalence, Clinical Relevance, and Public Health Significance of Subthreshold Depressions." *Psychiatric Clinics of North America* 25 (4): 685–98.

Katschnig, H., M. Amering, J. M. Stolk, G. L. Klerman, J. C. Ballenger, A. Briggs, and others. 1995. "Long-Term Follow-up after a Drug Trial for Panic Disorder." *British Journal of Psychiatry* 167 (4): 487–94.

Kendler, K. S., T. J. Gallagher, J. M. Abelson, and R. C. Kessler. 1996. "Lifetime Prevalence, Demographic Risk Factors, and Diagnostic Validity of Nonaffective Psychosis as Assessed in a U.S. Community Sample: The National Comorbidity Survey." *Archives of General Psychiatry* 53 (11): 1022–31.

Kendler, K. S., C. A. Prescot, J. Myers, and M. C. Neale. 2003. "The Structure of Genetic and Environmental Risk Factors for Common Psychiatric and Substance Use Disorders in Men and Women." *Archives of General Psychiatry* 60 (9): 929–37.

Kessler, R. C., and R. G. Frank. 1997. "The Impact of Psychiatric Disorders on Work Loss Days." *Psychological Medicine* 27 (4): 861–73.

Kessler, R. C., K. A. McGonagle, S. Zhao, C. B. Nelson, M. Hughes, S. Eshleman, and others. 1994. "Lifetime and 12-Month Prevalence of DSM-III-R Psychiatric Disorders in the United States: Results from the National Comorbidity Survey." *Archives of General Psychiatry* 51 (1): 8–19.

Kessler, R. C., C. B. Nelson, K. A. McGonagle, J. Liu, M. Swartz, and D. G. Blazer. 1996. "Comorbidity of DSM-III-R Major Depressive Disorder in the General Population: Results from the U.S. National Comorbidity Survey." *British Journal of Psychiatry* 168 (Suppl. 30): 17–30.

Kilonzo, G., and N. Simmons. 1998. "Development of Mental Health Services in Tanzania: A Reappraisal for the Future." *Social Science and Medicine* 47 (4): 419–28.

Kohn, R., S. Saxena, I. Levav, and B. Saraceno. 2004. "The Treatment Gap in Mental Health Care." *Bulletin of the World Health Organization* 82 (11): 858–66.

Larrobla, C., and N. Botega. 2001. "Restructuring Mental Health: A South American Survey." *Social Psychiatry and Psychiatric Epidemiology* 36 (5): 256–59.

Lauer, J. A., C. J. L. Murray, K. Roehrich, and H. Wirth. 2003. "PopMod: A Longitudinal Population Model with Two Interacting Disease States." *Cost Effectiveness and Resource Allocation* 1: 6.

Levkoff, S., I. Macarthur, and J. Bucknall. 1995. "Elderly Mental Health in the Developing World." *Journal of Social Science and Medicine* 41 (7): 983–1003.

Linden, M., Y. Lecrubier, C. Bellantuono, O. Benkert, S. Kisely, and G. Simon. 1999. "The Prescribing of Psychotropic Drugs by Primary Care Physicians: An International Collaborative Study." *Journal of Clinical Psychopharmacology* 19 (2): 132–40.

Livanou, M., M. Basoglu, and D. Kalendar. 2002. "Traumatic Stress Responses in Treatment-Seeking Earthquake Survivors in Turkey." *Journal of Nervous and Mental Disorders* 190 (12): 816–23.

Malt, U. F., O. H. Robak, H-P. Madsbu, and M. Loeb. 1999. "The Norwegian Naturalistic Treatment Study of Depression in Primary Practice (NORDEP)—I: Randomised Double Blind Study." *British Medical Journal* 318 (7192): 1180–84.

McGorry, P. D., A. R. Yung, L. J. Phillips, H. P. Yuen, S. Francey, E. M. Cosgrave, and others. 2002. "Randomized Controlled Trial of Interventions Designed to Reduce the Risk of Progression to First-Episode Psychosis in a Clinical Sample with Subthreshold Symptoms." *Archives of General Psychiatry* 59 (10): 921–28.

Mills, A., R. Brugha, K. Hanson, and B. McPake. 2002. "What Can Be Done about the Private Health Sector in Low-Income Countries." *Bulletin of the World Health Organization* 80 (4): 325–30.

Mohit, A., K. Saeed, D. Shahmohamadi, and J. Bolhari. 1999. "Mental Health Manpower Development in Afghanistan: Report of a Training Course for Primary Health Care Physicians." *Eastern Mediterranean Health Journal* 5 (2): 215–19.

Mortensen, P. B., C. B. Pedersen, T. Westergaard, J. Wohlfahrt, H. Ewald, O. Mors, and others. 1999. "Effects of Family History and Place and Season of Birth on the Risk of Schizophrenia." *New England Journal of Medicine* 340 (8): 603–8.

Mueller, T. I., A. C. Leon, M. B. Keller, D. A. Solomon, J. Endicott, W. Coryell, and others. 1999. "Recurrence after Recovery from Major Depressive Disorder during 15 Years of Observational Follow-up." *American Journal of Psychiatry* 156 (7): 1000–6.

Mulligan, J-A., J. A. Fox-Rushby, T. Adam, B. Johns, and A. Mills. 2003. "Unit Costs of Health Care Inputs in Low and Middle Income Regions." Working Paper 9, Disease Control Priorities Project, Fogerty International Center, National Institutes of Health, Bethesda, MD. http://www.fic.nih.gov/dcpp/wps.html.

Murray, C. J. L., and A. D. Lopez. 1996. *The Global Burden of Diseases: A Comprehensive Assessment of Mortality and Disability from Diseases, Injuries, and Risk Factors in 1990 and Projected to 2020.* Boston: Harvard School of Public Health; Geneva: World Health Organization; Washington, DC: World Bank.

Ngoma, M., M. Prince, and A. Mann. 2003. "Common Mental Disorders among Those Attending Primary Health Clinics and Traditional Healers in Urban Tanzania." *British Journal of Psychiatry* 183 (4): 349–55.

Nicolson, R., and J. L. Rapoport. 1999. "Childhood-Onset Schizophrenia: Rare but Worth Studying." *Biological Psychiatry* 46 (10): 1418–28.

Olfson, M., R. C. Kessler, P. A. Berglund, and E. Lin. 1998. "Psychiatric Disorder Onset and First Treatment Contact in the United States and Ontario." *American Journal of Psychiatry* 155 (10): 1415–22.

Patel, V. 1996. "Influences on Cost-Effectiveness." *British Journal of Psychiatry* 169 (3): 381.

Patel, V., D. Chisholm, S. Rabe-Hesketh, F. Dias-Saxena, G. Andrew, and A. Mann. 2003. "Efficacy and Cost-Effectiveness of Drug and Psychological Treatments for Common Mental Disorders in General Health Care in Goa, India: A Randomised Controlled Trial." *Lancet* 361 (9351): 33–39.

Patel, V., and A. Kleinman. 2003. "Poverty and Common Mental Disorders in Developing Countries." *International Journal of Public Health* 81 (8): 609–15.

Patel, V., and R. Thara, eds. 2003. *Meeting Mental Health Needs of Developing Countries: NGO Innovations in India.* New Delhi: Sage.

Paykel, E. S., and R. Priest. 1992. "Recognition and Management of Depression in General Practice: Consensus Statement." *British Medical Journal* 305 (6863): 1198–202.

Pereira, J., and V. Patel. 1999. "Which Antidepressants Are Best Tolerated in Primary Care? A Pilot Randomized Trial in Goa." *Indian Journal of Psychiatry* 41 (4): 358–63.

Perugi, G., and H. S. Akiskal. 2002. "The Soft Bipolar Spectrum Redefined: Focus on the Cyclothymic, Anxious-Sensitive, Impulse-Dyscontrol, and Binge-Eating Connection in Bipolar II and Related Conditions." *Psychiatric Clinics of North America* 25 (4): 713–37.

Rahman, A., M. Mubbashar, R. Gater, and D. Goldberg. 1998. "Randomised Trial of Impact of School Mental Health Programme in Rural Rawalpindi, Pakistan." *Lancet* 352 (9133): 1022–25.

Rahman, A., M. Mubbashar, R. Harrington, and R. Gater. 2000. "Annotation: Developing Child Mental Health Services in Developing Countries." *Journal of Child Psychology and Psychiatry* 41 (5): 539–46.

Ran, M. S., M. Z. Xiang, C. L. W. Chan, J. Leff, P. Simpson, M. S. Huang, and others. 2003. "Effectiveness of Psychoeducational Intervention for Rural Chinese Families Experiencing Schizophrenia." *Social Psychiatry and Psychiatric Epidemiology* 38 (2): 69–75.

Robins, L. N., and D. A. Regier. 1991. *Psychiatric Disorders in America: The Epidemiologic Catchment Area Study.* New York: Free Press.

Robinson, D., M. G. Woerner, J. M. Alvir, R. Bilder, R. Goldman, S. Geisler, and others. 1999. "Predictors of Relapse Following Response from a First Episode of Schizophrenia or Schizoaffective Disorder." *Archives of General Psychiatry* 56 (3): 241–47.

Sanderson, K., G. Andrews, J. Corry, and H. Lapsley. 2004. "Modeling Change in Preference Values from Descriptive Health Status Using the Effect Size." *Quality of Life Research* 13 (7): 1255–64.

Saraceno, B., E. Terzian, F. Barquero, and G. Tognoni. 1995. "Mental Health Care in the Primary Health Care Setting: A Collaborative Study in Six Countries of Central America." *Health Policy and Planning* 10 (2): 133–43.

Saxena, S., and P. K. Maulik. 2003. "Mental Health Services in Low- and Middle-Income Countries: An Overview." *Current Opinion in Psychiatry* 16 (4): 437–42.

Solomon, D. A., M. B. Keller, A. C. Leon, T. I. Mueller, M. T. Shea, M. Warshaw, and others. 1997. "Recovery from Depression: A 10-Year Prospective Follow-up across Multiple Episodes." *Archives of General Psychiatry* 54 (11): 1001–6.

Srinivasa Murthy, R., K. Kishore Kumar, D. Chisholm, S. Kumar, T. Thomas, K. Sekar, and C. Chandrashekar. 2005. "Community Outreach for Untreated Schizophrenia in Rural India: A Follow-up Study of Symptoms, Disability, Family Burden, and Costs." *Psychological Medicine* 35: 341–51.

Storosum, J. G., B. J. van Zweiten, W. van den Brink, B. Gersons, and M. D. Broekmans. 2001. "Suicide Risk in Placebo-Controlled Studies of Major Depression." *American Journal of Psychiatry* 158 (8): 1271–75.

Tansella, M., and G. Thornicroft. 1998. "A Conceptual Framework for Mental Health Services: The Matrix Model." *Psychological Medicine* 28 (3): 503–8.

ten Have, M., W. Vollebergh, R. Bijl, and W. A. Nolen. 2002. "Bipolar Disorder in the General Population in the Netherlands (Prevalence, Consequences, and Care Utilisation): Results from the Netherlands Mental Health Survey and Incidence Study (NEMESIS)." *Journal of Affective Disorders* 68 (2–3): 203–13.

Thara, R., R. Padmavati, and T. Srinivasan. 2004. "Focus on Psychiatry in India." *British Journal of Psychiatry* 184 (4): 366–73.

Townsend, C., H. Whiteford, F. Baingana, W. Gulbinat, R. Jenkins, A. Baba, and others. 2004. "A Mental Health Policy Template: Domains and Elements for Mental Health Policy Formulation." *International Review of Psychiatry* 16 (1–2): 18–23. http://www.qcmhr.uq.edu.au/template/.

Trisnantoro, L. 2002. "Decentralization Policy on Public Mental Hospitals in Indonesia: A Financial Perspective." Paper presented at the Seminar on Mental Health and Health Policy in Developing Countries, May 15, Harvard University.

Tsuang, D., and W. Coryell. 1993. "An 8-Year Follow-up of Patients with DSM-III-R Psychotic Depression, Schizoaffective Disorder, and Schizophrenia." *American Journal of Psychiatry* 150 (8): 1182–88.

Ustun, T. B., J. L. Ayuso-Mateos, S. Chatterji, C. Mathers, and C. J. L. Murray. 2004. "Global Burden of Depressive Disorders: Methods and Data Sources." *British Journal of Psychiatry* 184 (5): 386–92.

van Voren, R., and H. Whiteford. 2000. "Reform of Mental Health in Eastern Europe." *Eurohealth* Special Issue 6 (2): 63–65.

Vega, W. A., B. Kolody, S. Aguilar-Gaxiola, E. Alderete, R. Catalana, and J. J. Caraveo-Anduaga. 1998. "Lifetime Prevalence of DSM-III-R Psychiatric Disorders among Urban and Rural Mexican Americans in California." *Archives of General Psychiatry* 55 (9): 771–78.

Vicente, B., P. Rioseco, S. Saldivia, R. Kohn, and S. Torres. 2002. "Chilean Study on the Prevalence of Psychiatric Disorders (DSM-III-R/CIDI) (ECPP)." *Revista Medica de Chile* 130 (5): 527–36.

Vijayakumar, L., K. Nagaraj, and S. John. 2004. "Suicide and Suicide Prevention in Developing Countries." Working Paper 27, Disease Control Priorities Project, Fogerty International Center, National Institutes of Health, Bethesda, MD. http://www.fic.nih.gov/dcpp/wps.html.

Wang, P. S., G. E. Simon, and R. C. Kessler. 2003. "The Economic Burden of Depression and the Cost-Effectiveness of Treatment." *International Journal of Methods in Psychiatric Research* 12 (1): 22–33.

Weiss, M. G., S. Jadhav, R. Raguram, P. Vounatsou, and R. Littlewood. 2001. "Psychiatric Stigma across Cultures: Local Validation in Bangalore and London." *Anthropology and Medicine* 8 (1): 71–87.

WHO (World Health Organization). 1975. *Organization of Mental Health Services in Developing Countries: Sixteenth Report of the WHO Expert Committee on Mental Health.* Technical Report Series 564, WHO, Geneva.

———. 1992. *The ICD-10 Classification of Mental and Behavioral Disorders.* Geneva: WHO.

———. 2001. "Mental Health Resources: Project Atlas." WHO, Geneva. http://www.who.int/mip/2003/other_documents/en/EAARMentalHealthATLAS.pdf.

———. 2003. "Mental Health Policy and Services Development Project." WHO, Geneva. http://www.who.int/mental_health/policy/en/.

Xiong, W., M. R. Phillips, X. Hu, R. Wang, Q. Dai, J. Kleinman, and A. Kleinman. 1994. "Family-Based Intervention for Schizophrenic Patients in China: A Randomised Controlled Trial." *British Journal of Psychiatry* 165 (2): 239–47.

Yonkers, K. A., S. E. Bruce, I. R. Dyck, and M. B. Keller. 2003. "Chronicity, Relapse, and Illness-Course of Panic Disorder, Social Phobia, and Generalized Anxiety Disorder: Findings in Men and Women from 8 Years of Follow-up." *Depression and Anxiety* 17 (3): 173–79.

Chapter **32**

Neurological Disorders

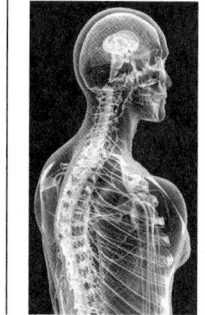

Vijay Chandra, Rajesh Pandav, Ramanan Laxminarayan,
Caroline Tanner, Bala Manyam, Sadanand Rajkumar,
Donald Silberberg, Carol Brayne, Jeffrey Chow, Susan Herman,
Fleur Hourihan, Scott Kasner, Luis Morillo, Adesola Ogunniyi,
William Theodore, and Zhen-Xin Zhang

Historically, policy makers and researchers have used mortality statistics as the principal measure of the seriousness of diseases, based on which countries and organizations have launched disease control programs. Mortality statistics alone, however, underestimate the suffering caused by diseases that may be non-fatal but cause substantial disability. Many neurological and psychiatric conditions belong in this category. The absence of some neurological disorders from lists of leading causes of death has contributed to their long-term neglect. When the relative seriousness of diseases is assessed by time lived with disability rather than by mortality, several neurological disorders appear as leading causes of suffering worldwide.

World Health Organization data suggest that neurological and psychiatric disorders are an important and growing cause of morbidity. The magnitude and burden of mental, neurological, and behavioral disorders is huge, affecting more than 450 million people globally. According to the Global Burden of Disease Report, 33 percent of years lived with disability and 13 percent of disability-adjusted life years (DALYs) are due to neurological and psychiatric disorders, which account for four out of the six leading causes of years lived with disability (Mathers and others 2003).

Unfortunately, the burden of these disorders in developing countries remains largely unrecognized. Moreover, the burden imposed by such chronic neurological conditions in general can be expected to be particularly devastating in poor populations. Primary manifestations of the impact on the poor—including the loss of gainful employment, with the attendant loss of family income; the requirement for caregiving, with further potential loss of wages; the cost of medications; and the need for other medical services—can be expected to be particularly devastating among those with limited resources. In addition to health costs, those suffering from these conditions are also frequently victims of human rights violations, stigmatization, and discrimination. Stigmatization and discrimination further limit patients' access to treatment. These disorders, therefore, require special attention in developing countries.

This chapter addresses Alzheimer's disease (AD) and other dementias, epilepsy, Parkinson's disease (PD), and acute ischemic stroke. These conditions are current or emerging public health problems in developing countries, as assessed by high prevalence, large numbers of people who are untreated, and availability of inexpensive but effective interventions that could be applied on a large scale through primary care. Unfortunately, reliable population-based data from developing countries on the epidemiology of these and other neurological disorders are extremely limited. Some other important neurological conditions that cause high morbidity, such as headache, are not covered because of difficulties in recommending evidence-based interventions in developing countries.

ALZHEIMER'S DISEASE AND OTHER DEMENTIAS

Dementia is a deterioration of intellectual function and other cognitive skills that is of sufficient severity to interfere with social or occupational functioning. Of the many diseases that lead to dementia, AD is the most common cause worldwide among people age 65 and older, followed by vascular dementia, mixed dementia consisting of AD plus vascular dementia, and dementia caused by general medical conditions. Although distinguishing AD from other causes of dementia is important, particularly for treatment with acetylcholinesterase inhibitors, the burden from all causes of dementia is similar. Although the discussion in this chapter deals mostly with AD, the role of treatable dementias in developing countries is important as it can reduce the burden of caring in families.

Prevalence and Incidence Rate

More than 100 prevalence studies of AD and other dementias have been reported throughout the world. The prevalence of dementia has generally been found to double with every five-year increase in age, from 3 percent at age 70 to 20 to 30 percent at age 85 (Henderson and Jorm 2000). Studies in developing countries have shown a prevalence of dementia ranging from 0.84 to 3.50 percent (Chandra and others 1998; Hendrie and others 1995; Rajkumar, Kumar, and Thara 1997). Several studies have reported the incidence rate of AD and other dementias in Europe and the United States (Jorm and Jolley 1998). Compared with incidence rates in developed countries, very low age-specific incidence rates of AD and other dementias have been reported from developing countries (Chandra and others 2001; Hendrie and others 2001).

A comparison of data from developed and developing countries raises several important questions. The reported differences in the prevalence of AD and other dementias across countries could be due partly to methodological differences or could be due to genuine differences caused by variations in diet, education, life expectancy, sociocultural factors, and other risk factors. The low incidence reported from Ballabgarh, India, and Ibadan, Nigeria, raises the possibility of environmental factors or gene-environment interactions in the causation of AD. At the same time, multi-infarct dementia is more common than primary degenerative dementia in China (Li and others 1991), which also suggests variation in risk factors across countries.

Risk and Protective Factors and Survivorship

Three separate genes (APP, PS1, and PS2) are linked to early-onset, familial AD. Another gene (APO E4) is a risk factor for late-onset, nonfamilial cases (Henderson and Jorm 2000). Other genes have been implicated but not confirmed in large studies. Other risk factors reported in the literature include increasing age, positive family history of dementia, female gender (but this factor is controversial), lower level of education, several medical conditions, and exposure to such environmental factors as organic solvents and aluminum (Henderson and Jorm 2000).

Protective factors reported in the literature include a higher level of education, a specific gene (APO E2), the intake of antioxidants, and the use of some anti-inflammatory medications (Henderson and Jorm 2000). The use of estrogen supplements for women was believed to be a protective factor for AD (Henderson 1997), but a recent study of women taking a combination of estrogen and progesterone showed that these women had twice the risk of developing dementia than women taking a placebo (Shumaker and others 2003).

Studies from developed countries have reported median survival after the onset of dementia symptoms ranging from 5.0 years to 9.3 years (Walsh, Welch, and Larson 1990). In developing countries, the reported median survival was 3.3 years for all demented subjects and 2.7 years for those with AD (Chandra and others 1998).

Burden of Disease

Burden of disease estimates of AD and other dementias include vascular dementia, unspecified dementias, and other unclassified degenerative diseases of the nervous system. Mathers and others (2003) estimate DALYs for all dementias as 17,108,000, with the burden being almost twice as much for females (11,016,000) as for males (6,092,000). Because dementia is a disease of older ages, the burden from dementia is generally greater in high-income countries, where life expectancy is higher, diagnosis is better, and better treatment leads to increased longevity. Note, however, the relatively high burden in East Asia and the Pacific and South Asia relative to their level of economic development (table 32.1).

The bulk of care for those with dementia in developing countries is provided by the family at home, where the main caregivers are spouses (36 percent) and children (42 percent) (Prince 2000). Women in both developed and developing countries are usually the main caregivers (Prince 2000). Studies in developed countries indicate that caregivers' psychological well-being is a key factor in patients' admission to nursing or residential care (Levin, Moriarty, and Gorbach 1994).

In estimating the overall costs of care for dementia, one must emphasize the value of reducing the burden on caregivers. Caregiving can result in social isolation, psychological stress, and high rates of depression (Buck and others 1997). However, the methodology for estimating the costs of informal care needs to be standardized.

Interventions

As of now, there is no cure for AD, but some measures can provide symptomatic relief to patients and caregivers.

Population-Based Interventions. No firm evidence indicates that any form of population-based intervention can prevent AD or that the progression of cognitive decline in old age can

Table 32.1 Disability-Adjusted Life Years by Cause and Region, 2001
(thousands)

Condition	Global total			East Asia and the Pacific	Europe and Central Asia	Latin America and the Caribbean	Middle East and North Africa	South Asia	Sub-Saharan Africa	High-income countries
	Both sexes	Males	Females							
AD and other dementias	17,108	6,092	11,016	4,110	1,612	1,215	292	1,955	450	7,468
Epilepsy	6,223	3,301	2,922	1,303	354	737	248	1,741	1,373	464
PD	2,325	1,124	1,202	435	228	90	81	303	100	1,086
Cerebrovascular disease	72,024	35,482	36,542	25,832	12,616	3,936	1,948	13,184	5,125	9,354

Source: Mathers and others 2006.

be halted or reduced. However, growing inferential evidence suggests that reducing the risk of brain trauma in earlier life, for example, by mandating seat belt and crash helmet use, may help prevent dementia in later life (Gentleman, Graham and Roberts 1993).

Personal Interventions. There is a reduction in brain levels of the neurotransmitter acetylcholine in patients suffering from AD. Drugs that inhibit acetylcholinesterase, the enzyme responsible for metabolizing acetylcholine, cause an increase in brain acetylcholine. Evidence from randomized trials has confirmed that, for patients with mild to moderate AD, cognitive performance benefits, at least in the short term, from the use of acetylcholinesterase inhibitors (Foster and others 1996). Despite this benefit to patients, the practical benefits of treatment with acetylcholinesterase inhibitors are mainly attributable to the lowered caregiver burden. The benefits of using acetylcholinesterase inhibitors for other dementias have yet to be proven.

The behavioral and psychological symptoms of dementia are a major source of stress to family members providing care to patients. Training family caregivers in behavioral management techniques, including problem solving, memory training, and reality orientation, has been shown to reduce the level of agitation and anxiety in people with dementia (Brodaty and Gresham 1989; Haupt, Karger, and Janner 2000). Use of low doses of antipsychotic medications, which calm the patient and reduce symptoms such as aggression and wandering, have been shown to reduce caregiver stress, but these improvements have not been quantified (Melzer and others 2004).

Interventions that have specifically targeted stress and depression among caregivers and have shown positive results include caregiver training, counseling and support for caregivers, and cognitive and behavioral family interventions (Marriott and others 2000). Limitations to the implementation of such strategies include the need for training by specialists, which makes these strategies less suitable for developing countries. The challenge for developing countries is to develop culturally appropriate interventions that can be delivered within existing resources, such as supporting families in their role as caregivers.

Treating underlying disease and risk factors for cardiovascular disease can help prevent future cerebrovascular disease that could lead to multi-infarct dementia. Other conditions, such as hypothyroidism or vitamin B_{12} deficiency, which could lead to or aggravate dementia, are easily treatable, and the costs of treatment are much lower than the costs of dementia care.

In Western countries, the model of care for patients with moderate to severe dementia is based on skilled, long-term care in institutions. However, such long-term care institutions do not exist in developing countries, and if they were set up, they would be extremely expensive and beyond the reach of most patients and their families. Thus, the model of care in developing countries should be based on home care, along with providing training and support for family caregivers.

Interventions that should not be pursued include the use of multiple medications, which can be detrimental in older age groups, particularly unproven medications such as cerebral activators and neurotropic agents. In addition, in many developing countries, dementia is still equated with "madness," and patients are sometimes taken to traditional healers. Community education has a role to play in eliminating such practices.

EPILEPSY

Epilepsy is a common brain disorder characterized by two or more unprovoked seizures. Seizures are discrete events caused by transient, hypersynchronous, abnormal neuronal activity. Seizures may occur in close temporal association with a variety of acute medical and neurological diseases, such as acute stroke, sepsis, or alcohol withdrawal. However, the vast majority of seizures have no immediate identifiable cause.

Epilepsy can be broadly divided into three categories: idiopathic epilepsy (for example primary generalized childhood-onset absence epilepsy), which is thought to have a genetic basis; secondary or symptomatic epilepsy, which is caused by a known central nervous system injury or disorder, such as infection, stroke, traumatic brain injury, or cerebral dysgenesis; and cryptogenic epilepsy, for which there is no clear evidence of an etiological factor. Idiopathic and cryptogenic cases represent approximately 70 percent of epilepsy cases; the remaining 30 percent are symptomatic (secondary).

Prevalence, Incidence Rate, Remission, and Mortality

The generally accepted estimate of the prevalence of active epilepsy globally is in the range of 5 to 8 per 1,000 population, but investigators from African and Latin American countries report at least double the prevalence reported elsewhere (Leonardi and Ustun 2002).

The incidence rate of epilepsy in developed countries is approximately 43 per 100,000 (Kotsopoulos and others 2002). In developing countries, the incidence rate of epilepsy is higher, with a median of 69 per 100,000 (Kotsopoulos and others 2002).

Based on follow-up of patients under treatment by general practitioners in the United Kingdom, Cockerell and others (1997) report that after nine years 86 percent of epilepsy patients had achieved a remission of three years, and 68 percent had achieved a remission of five years. Thus, data from developed countries suggest a good outcome of seizure control in most patients with treatment. In developing countries, although many people with new onset seizures do not receive treatment, some proportion of patients go into spontaneous remission even without treatment (Mani and others 1993). However, the actual remission rate in developing countries is yet to be documented in population-based studies.

The risk of premature death in people with epilepsy is two to three times higher than for the general population. In addition to sudden unexplained death, which occurs in up to 1 in 100 patients with severe refractory epilepsy, additional mortality results from accidents and suicide. However, the exact cause of the increased risk is not known in most cases.

Risk Factors

A reported risk factor for idiopathic (presumed genetic) epilepsy is family history of epilepsy. Reported risk factors for symptomatic epilepsy include prenatal or perinatal causes (obstetric complications, prematurity, low birthweight, neonatal asphyxia). Recent data suggest that the effect of obstetric complications or neonatal asphyxia may have been overemphasized. Prematurity, low birthweight, and neonatal seizures may be independent risk factors as well as markers of underlying disease. Other causes include traumatic brain injuries, central nervous system infections, cerebrovascular disease, brain tumors, and neurodegenerative diseases. Developmental

disabilities are not a risk factor for epilepsy in themselves, but they may be associated with seizure disorder (Casetta and others 2002; Leone and others 2002).

Treatment Gap

Epilepsy affects about 50 million people worldwide, of whom approximately 80 percent live in developing countries (WHO 2000). The difference between the number of people with active epilepsy and the number who are being appropriately treated in a given population at a given point in time is known as the *treatment gap*. Meinardi and others (2001) estimate that 90 percent of people with epilepsy in developing countries are inadequately treated. Possible reasons for the high treatment gap include fear of stigmatization, cultural beliefs, lack of knowledge about the medical nature of epilepsy, illiteracy, economic issues, distance to health facilities, inadequate supply of antiepileptic drugs (AEDs), and lack of prioritization by health authorities (Wang and others 2003). Even in the developed world, patients who live in isolated rural regions or inner-city slums and those who are isolated from the majority because of cultural factors may suffer a treatment gap.

Faith Healers

Many people with epilepsy seek treatment from faith healers, to whom they pay large sums in cash or in kind for treatment with no beneficial medical effects. Karaagac and others (1999) find that in Silivri, Turkey, 65 percent of 49 people with epilepsy had visited religious figures at the onset or during the course of the disease. A study from rural India revealed that 44 percent of children with epilepsy had sought help from traditional practitioners, whereas approximately 33 percent had received help from both qualified and traditional practitioners (Pal and others 2002). Native Americans still seek traditional healing ceremonies for epilepsy instead of—or in addition to—Western medicine.

Patient Compliance

In a study in rural Thailand, only 57 percent of people with epilepsy were 100 percent compliant with treatment, possibly because of misunderstanding of the instructions (48 percent), forgetfulness (16 percent), and economic limitations (13 percent) (Asawavichienjinda, Sitthi-Amorn, and Tanyanont 2003). To improve compliance in a rural African community, medical personnel visited the community every 6 months and provided a long-term supply of medications; this effort led to a substantial increase in compliance at 20 months (Kaiser and others 1998). In India, Desai and others (1998) demonstrate the dependency of compliance on access to free treatment. Inadequate communication between doctors and patients influences compliance negatively (Gopinath and others 2000).

Burden of Disease

The burden of disease (BOD) estimates for epilepsy include epilepsy and status epilepticus. Mathers and others (2003) estimate the DALYs for epilepsy as 6,223,000, with slightly higher rates for males (3,301,000) than for females (2,922,000). Many risk factors for epilepsy are linked with a lower level of economic development; thus, the burden is highest in South Asia followed by Sub-Saharan Africa (table 32.1). A notable observation is the reportedly low burden in the Middle East and North Africa, despite parts of that region being relatively underdeveloped. Epilepsy imposes a large economic burden on patients and their families. It also imposes a hidden burden associated with stigmatization and discrimination against patients and even their families in the community, workplace, school, and home. Social isolation, emotional distress, dependence on family, poor employment opportunities, and personal injury add to the suffering of people with epilepsy.

Interventions

Currently, there are no preventive measures for idiopathic or cryptogenic epilepsy; however, much can be done to prevent secondary seizures.

Population-Based Interventions. Public health policies, such as better perinatal care by well-trained birth attendants (particularly in rural areas) and strategies to control severe head injuries (for example, by means of laws requiring motorcyclists to wear helmets and prohibiting drunk driving), can modify risk factors for epilepsy and thereby reduce the incidence and prevalence of epilepsy. Policies to control neurocysticercosis (for instance, building latrines in rural areas) can serve to prevent such infections. Mass deworming for neurocysticercosis has not been shown to be effective in the long term (Pal, Carpio, and Sander 2000) but was effective in a campaign in Ecuador (M. Cruz, personal communication, 2004).

Estimates indicate that 70 to 80 percent of people in developing countries live in rural and remote areas and have no easy access to skilled medical care. Strategies that involve training community-based health care providers who practice in these communities to identify and manage patients with epilepsy should be considered.

Policies are needed to ensure the continuous availability of cheap and efficacious medications, such as phenobarbital, to all epilepsy patients. Campaigns to educate communities about the medical nature of epilepsy and to dispel myths and misconceptions about epilepsy could reduce stigma against epilepsy and thereby encourage patients to seek medical treatment.

Personal Interventions. Researchers, primarily in high-income countries, have tested (a) the efficacy of both older AEDs (such as phenobarbital, phenytoin, carbamazepine, and valproic acid) and newer AEDs (such as lamotrigine, oxcarbazepine, and topiramate) in controlling seizure frequency and (b) the safety of these AEDs when prescribed alone or in combination. Some, but not all, of the new AEDs may be better tolerated in monotherapy and have fewer long-term adverse effects than older AEDs. However, no study has shown any difference in efficacy between the older and newer medications (Aldenkamp, De Krom, and Reijs 2003). Newer medications are more expensive and, for people in most developing countries, are practically impossible to access. In some low-income countries, however, even older AEDs are not available, and when they are, their supply is irregular.

Newer AEDs are generally recommended as add-on or adjunctive drugs for better seizure control in patients with refractory epilepsy already on AEDs. The first AED will render approximately 50 percent of patients seizure free. Approximately 20 to 40 percent of patients who do not respond to the first AED will respond to the introduction of a second AED, with a greater than 50 percent decrease in seizure frequency (Schapel and others 1993).

The Global Campaign against Epilepsy, which is jointly sponsored by the World Health Organization, International League against Epilepsy, and International Bureau for Epilepsy, advocates using phenobarbital to close the high treatment gap in low-income countries. As a first step, all patients with epilepsy should be given phenobarbital, so that the majority of patients responsive to phenobarbital will be appropriately treated. In resource-poor countries, phenobarbital can be provided for as little as US$5 to US$10 per year. Phenobarbital has extremely low abuse potential. Its side effects—predominantly sedation, possible mild cognitive impairment, and depression—have limited its use in industrial countries. In developing countries, however, side effects are less important than uncontrolled seizures, and they can be diminished by using the lowest possible effective doses. Thus, phenobarbital is the drug of choice for large-scale, community-based programs, particularly in rural and remote areas of developing countries.

In recent years, some centers in both developed and developing countries have been performing surgery on cases of *refractory epilepsy,* that is, on patients who do not respond to any AEDs. Before centers can undertake such surgery, however, they must have the requisite expertise, facilities, and equipment, including a skilled neurosurgeon. Proper selection of patients—for example, those with mesial temporal pathology on MRI—is extremely important. A meta-analysis of studies of people who underwent epilepsy surgery in developed countries shows that 58 percent are seizure free and 10 to 15 percent have reduced seizure frequency (Engel and others 2003). After surgery, even if patients are seizure free, medication should be continued for one to two years (Engel and others 2003).

PARKINSON'S DISEASE

PD is characterized by bradykinesia, resting tremor, cogwheel rigidity, postural reflex impairment, progressive course, and good response to dopaminergic therapy. Other distinct forms of parkinsonism include relatively rare genetic forms and the less common neurodegenerations with multiple system involvement or significant striatal lesions (for example, progressive supranuclear palsy or multiple system atrophy). Parkinsonism secondary to external causes, such as manganese poisoning or carbon monoxide poisoning, although now rare, is referred to as secondary parkinsonism. Because the burden of these diseases to the patient is similar to or greater than that for PD and there is no evidence for addressing these disorders separately, they will not be distinguished here.

Prevalence, Incidence Rate, and Mortality

Prevalence estimates vary widely across populations (Tanner and Goldman 1996; Zhang and Roman 1993). Recent reports, contrary to previous reports, suggest that the prevalence in developing and developed countries may be similar (Marras and Tanner 2002). Few incidence studies have been performed, and none in developing countries. Van Den Eeden and others (2003) report the incidence rate of PD in the United States as approximately 13 per 100,000 person-years. Men are affected more commonly than women (Tanner and Goldman 1996). Lower PD incidence in African Americans—and by extension Africans—has been suggested but is controversial (Van Den Eeden and others 2003). Most mortality estimates available for developed countries show about a twofold overall increased mortality, independent of age, in those with PD (Berger and others 2000).

Causes and Risk Factors

The cause of PD is unknown. A specific environmental risk factor has not been identified. Pure genetic forms account for 10 to 15 percent of cases or fewer. Increasing age and male gender are risk factors worldwide (Marras and Tanner 2002). Exposure to toxins, head trauma, frequent infections, diets high in animal fat, and midlife adiposity have been reported to increase PD risk, but none do so consistently (Tanner and Goldman 1996). The most consistent association is an inverse association with cigarette smoking and caffeine consumption, suggesting a protective effect (Ascherio and others 2001).

Burden of Disease

The BOD estimates for PD include Parkinson's disease and secondary parkinsonism. Mathers and others (2003) estimate the DALYs for PD as 2,325,000, with the burden being slightly higher in females (1,202,000) than males (1,124,000). Though male gender is a risk factor for PD, the higher burden in females may reflect their longer life span. As PD is a disease of older ages, the burden from PD is generally higher in high-income countries, where life expectancy is higher, diagnosis is better, and better treatment leads to increased longevity. However, the burden is high in East Asia and the Pacific and South Asia relative to that in other regions (table 32.1).

The economic burden of PD includes direct costs, such as for medication, physicians, hospitals, and chronic care facilities. Estimated indirect costs resulting from the loss of labor of both patients and caregivers typically exceed direct costs. The quality of life of both patients and caregivers is adversely affected.

Interventions

Treatment of PD is based on symptomatic relief, except for preventing secondary parkinsonism caused by neurotoxins.

Population-Based Interventions. No determinants of PD amenable to population-based interventions have been identified.

Personal Interventions. Specific curative or neuroprotective treatments for PD have not been established. Interventions are primarily directed at palliation of symptoms and include pharmaceuticals, surgery, physical therapy, and—in some countries—traditional medicines.

Levo-dopa (l-dopa), l-dopa/decarboxylase inhibitor is the most widely used therapy for PD. It provides partial relief of all PD symptoms. Despite its benefits, chronic side effects after long-term use can cause significant morbidity.

Researchers in developing countries have studied the use of traditional medicines for PD. Clinical trials have shown that the seeds of *Mucuna pruriens,* which contain l-dopa, are a safe and effective treatment for PD (Parkinson's Disease Group 1995), and in animal studies, they are two to three times more effective than synthetic l-dopa dose per dose (Hussain and Manyam 1997). This substance is available in ayurvedic formulations in India at a much lower cost than that of synthetic antiparkinsonian drugs. Another traditional medicine is derived from *Banisteriopsis caapi,* which tribal societies of the Amazonian jungle use to make a potent hallucinogenic brew. It reportedly showed dramatic positive effects on rigidity and akinesia in 15 patients with postencephalitic parkinsonism (Lewin and Schuster 1929). A third traditional option is tai chi, a basic exercise in traditional Chinese medicine that may help with some of the motor deficits of PD.

Surgical treatment for PD by deep brain stimulation is generally recommended to address the loss of efficacy of dopaminergic drugs. For most patients, it is not effective independent of drugs. Although a few will have dramatic improvement and may be able to reduce or stop drugs, this effect is generally temporary. Criteria for selection of patients for deep brain stimulation include those with advanced disease who are responsive to l-dopa, not demented, and in good general health. Additional considerations are the high cost of the equipment, the need for trained personnel to program the device, and—in most cases—the need for several visits to a medical center to program the stimulator correctly, with periodic returns to adjust the settings.

STROKE

Stroke, also known as *cerebrovascular accident* or *brain attack,* is a syndrome caused by an interruption in the flow of blood to part of the brain caused either by occlusion of a blood vessel (*ischemic stroke*) or rupture of a blood vessel (*hemorrhagic stroke*). The interruption in blood flow deprives the brain of nutrients and oxygen, resulting in injury to cells in the affected vascular territory of the brain. The occlusion of a blood vessel can sometimes be temporary and present as a reversible neurological deficit, which is termed a *transient ischemic attack.* Even though stroke is a clinical diagnosis, brain imaging is required to distinguish ischemic stroke from hemorrhagic stroke. When imaging is unavailable, clinical scores can be useful to identify patients with intracerebral hemorrhage (Allen 1983; Poungvarin, Viriyavejakul, and Komontri 1991).

Frequency of Types of Strokes, Prevalence, Incidence Rate, Mortality, and Disability after Stroke

In most parts of the world, about 70 percent of strokes are due to ischemia, 27 percent are due to hemorrhage, and 3 percent are of unknown cause (Gunatilake, Jayasekera, and Premawardene 2001). Approximately 25 percent of all ischemic strokes are due to cardioembolic causes, with the proportion being higher among younger individuals. In some parts of the world—for instance, China and Japan—hemorrhagic strokes account for a greater proportion of all strokes, ranging from 17.1 to 39.4 percent in China (Zhang and others 2003) to 38.7 percent in Japan (Fukiyama and others 2000).

Comparable data do not exist for all parts of the world. Most morbidity data from Southeast Asian countries, for example, are hospital based and are, thus, likely to be underestimates, because many stroke patients die before they are brought to the hospital. Mortality data are also likely to be underestimates, because verifying the cause of death is usually difficult.

In India, the prevalence of stroke has been estimated at 203 per 100,000 population older than 20 (Anand and others 2001). The male-to-female ratio was one to seven. In Taiwan, China, the crude point prevalence was 592 per 100,000 (Huang, Chiang, and Lee 1997).

He and others (1995) report the age-adjusted stroke incidence of 117 per 100,000 population in China. The annual incidence of stroke in China is reported to have increased in both men and women, with an average annual percentage change of 4.5 and 4.2 percent, respectively (Wang, Zhao, and Wu 2001). In Japan, the age-adjusted annual incidence of stroke was 105 per 100,000 (Fukiyama and others 2000). Wide variation within these countries and a high risk of death after the first stroke in the first year in Japan have been reported. Investigators believe that those observations are due to variations in the prevalence of hypertension and the consequent larger proportion of hemorrhagic stroke (Kiyohara and others 2003).

Walker and others (2000) report the yearly age-adjusted mortality rate per 100,000 for age group 15 to 64 ranged from 35 to 65 in men and 27 to 88 in women in Tanzania. When compared with the rates in England and Wales—11 for men and 9 for women—these rates are extremely high. The authors postulate that the high rates in Tanzania are due to untreated hypertension. Many developed countries have experienced a steep decline in stroke mortality in recent decades, but the rate of decline has fallen substantially in recent years (Liu, Ikeda, and Yamori 2001; Sarti and others 2000). Mortality from stroke has increased in some Eastern European countries (Sarti and others 2000).

Approximately 15 percent of patients die shortly after a stroke. Of the remaining 85 percent, approximately 10 percent recover almost completely, and 25 percent recover with minor impairments (National Stroke Association 2002). Thus, approximately 40 percent experience moderate to severe impairments that require special rehabilitative care. About 10 percent will require care in a nursing home or other long-term facility.

Risk Factors

Risk factors for stroke in general are similar to those for cardiovascular disease. Moreover, risk factors for first stroke and recurrence of stroke are also similar if they remain uncontrolled after the first attack (see chapter 33).

Increasing age, particularly after 55, is one of the most important risk factors for stroke (Thorvaldsen and others 1995). Although stroke is more prevalent among men, stroke-related fatality rates are higher among women (Goldstein and others 2001). Hypertension is the most important modifiable determinant of both first and recurrent stroke (Eastern Stroke and Coronary Heart Disease Collaborative Research Group 1998). The association between blood pressure and stroke in East Asian populations seems stronger than in Western populations (Eastern Stroke and Coronary Heart Disease Collaborative Research Group 1998). Other risk factors include smoking, environmental exposure to tobacco smoke, dyslipidemia, atrial fibrillation, diabetes and impaired glucose tolerance, generalized and abdominal obesity, physical inactivity, excess alcohol consumption, increased homocysteine levels, drug abuse, hemostatic factors, and existing cerebrovascular disease (Goldstein and others 2001).

In developing countries, rheumatic heart disease leading to embolic stroke is also a major cause. This risk factor is declining in importance with the control of rheumatic fever. Dehydration in postpartum women can lead to a stroke, particularly in remote areas where deliveries are conducted at home.

Burden of Disease

The BOD estimates for stroke include subarachnoid hemorrhage, intracerebral hemorrhage, cerebral infarction, and sequelae of cerebrovascular disease. Mathers and others (2003) estimate the DALYs for cerebrovascular disease as 72,024,000, with the burden being almost similar for females (36,542,000) and males (35,482,000). The burden is highest in East Asia and the Pacific, followed by South Asia and by Europe and Central Asia (table 32.1). The burden in Sub-Saharan Africa is higher than in the Middle East and North Africa, which may suggest an etiology for stroke other than atherosclerotic disease.

Health experts anticipate that the number of stroke cases will increase, particularly in developing countries, because of aging populations and increased exposure to major risk factors. Corresponding to this increase in the number of stroke cases will be an increase in the number of people with disabilities surviving after stroke.

Interventions

Several intervention strategies are available for stroke, but only a few can be applied in developing countries.

Population-Based Interventions. Public health policies to address risk factors for stroke include tobacco and alcohol control, laws to provide labels showing the fat content of foods, and public education about the harm caused by high-fat foods. Public health programs to control rheumatic fever will reduce rheumatic heart disease and the subsequent risk of embolic strokes. Better training of birth attendants will reduce the risk of peripartum hemorrhage, which leads to puerperal strokes.

Personal Interventions. Modification of adverse lifestyle and major risk factors such as hypertension, diabetes, high lipid levels, smoking, and alcohol abuse is beneficial both for primary prevention and recurrence of stroke. Some evidence indicates that the decline in the incidence of stroke observed in many countries is due to better management of hypertension (MacWalter and Shirley 2002). Special consideration should be given to the profile of risk factors in developing countries,

which include not only recognized risk factors in developed countries but also locally relevant risk factors, such as rheumatic heart disease and puerperal stroke.

Treatment strategies for acute ischemic stroke include the following:

- *General management.* Overall medical care of patients with an acute stroke is important. Attention to complications such as bronchoaspiration, fluid and electrolyte imbalance, and control of blood sugar, as well as prevention of deep vein thrombosis, is crucial. Experience in developed countries suggests that specialized stroke units provide the best care for acute stroke patients (Smaha 2004), but in developing countries, particularly in rural areas, where hospital beds are scarce and most patients are attended by general physicians, such units are impractical.
- *Platelet antiaggregants.* Aspirin can prevent early stroke recurrence if given during the acute phase of stroke (within 48 hours) (Chinese Acute Stroke Trial Collaborative Group 1997; International Stroke Trial Collaborative Group 1997). The adverse effects of aspirin (cerebral hemorrhage and gastrointestinal complications) appear to be dose related, and most agree that using a low dose of aspirin is prudent (Antithrombotic Trialists' Collaboration 2002). Since aspirin can aggravate a hemorrhagic stroke, simple guidelines for the use of platelet antiaggregants should be developed and could be based on scales such as the Siriraj score to rule out hemorrhage (Poungvarin, Viriyavejakul, and Komontri 1991).
- *Thrombolytic therapy.* Tissue plasminogen activator and recombinant tissue plasminogen activator (rt-PA) can be used to halt a stroke by dissolving the blood clot that is blocking blood flow to the brain (National Institute of Neurological Disorders and Stroke rt-PA Stroke Study Group 1995). Thrombolytic therapy can increase bleeding and must be used only after careful patient screening, with a CT scan of the brain within three hours of stroke symptom onset, to exclude an intracranial bleed. It also requires appropriately trained physicians to administer the medication. These prerequisites for the administration of thrombolytic agents restrict its use to selected centers in developing countries.

Strategies for prevention of recurrence of stroke apply equally to individuals who have experienced a transient ischemic attack and to those who have experienced a complete stroke. These strategies include the following:

- *Platelet antiaggregants.* Aspirin therapy is effective in preventing recurrence of stroke, with low daily doses being at least as effective as higher daily doses (Antithrombotic Trialists' Collaboration 2002). When compared with aspirin, clopidogrel has a slight benefit among those who have had a previous stroke, myocardial infarction, or symptomatic peripheral arterial disease. Clopidogrel is an effective and safe alternative for patients who do not tolerate aspirin. Although clopidogrel may be slightly more effective than aspirin, it is also more expensive. Antiplatelet combination therapy using agents with different mechanisms of action, such as the combination of extended release dipyridamole and aspirin, has been shown to reduce the risk of stroke over aspirin alone (Sacco, Sivenius, and Diener 2005). In contrast, combination therapy with aspirin and clopidogrel offers no advantage over aspirin alone and also increases the risk of hemorrhage (Diener and others 2004).

- *Anticoagulant therapy.* Anticoagulation with warfarin should be considered in stroke patients with atrial fibrillation, because of its clear efficacy in preventing embolic strokes, provided that patients are appropriately monitored (European Atrial Fibrillation Trial Study Group 1993; Mohr and others 2001). Anticoagulant therapy also reduces the risk of embolic stroke in patients with rheumatic heart disease. However, anticoagulation can be hazardous in developing countries because of the lack of monitoring facilities.

- *Surgical treatment.* In patients with symptomatic carotid disease with stenosis of 70 percent and in asymptomatic patients with high-grade stenosis, carotid endarterectomy has been shown to be more beneficial than medical care alone (Asymptomatic Carotid Atherosclerosis Study 1995; Asymptomatic Carotid Surgery Trial Collaborative Group 2004; North American Symptomatic Carotid Endarterectomy Trial Collaborators 1991). However, inappropriate selection of patients or high intraoperative complications could obviate such benefits. Carotid angioplasty has been suggested as an alternative to carotid endarterectomy in management of severe internal carotid artery disease, but its advantages and disadvantages have yet to be clearly established (Naylor, London, and Bell 1997). Carotid endarterectomy for stroke prevention is available at only a few centers in developing countries, which makes its widespread use impractical.

The goal of rehabilitation after a stroke is to enable individuals who have experienced a stroke to reach the highest feasible level of independence as soon as possible. Successful rehabilitation depends on the extent of brain damage, skill of the rehabilitation team, length of time before rehabilitation is started, and support provided by caregivers. Because each stroke patient has specific rehabilitation needs, customizing the rehabilitation program is important. Rehabilitation therapies include several complementary approaches:

- physical therapy, which helps stroke patients relearn simple motor activities, such as walking

- occupational therapy, which helps patients relearn everyday activities, such as eating and drinking
- speech therapy, which helps patients relearn language and speaking skills
- counseling, which can help alleviate some of the mental and emotional problems that result from stroke.

Comprehensive rehabilitation in a multidisciplinary stroke unit reduces deaths, disability, and the need for long-term institutional care (Smaha 2004), but such facilities are extremely limited in developing countries. Home-based rehabilitation services can prevent long-term deterioration in activities of daily living, although the absolute impact is relatively modest (Outpatient Service Trialists 2002). However, in developing countries, the vast majority of patients will be treated either at home by a general physician or in a small community hospital where no skilled rehabilitation therapist is available.

COST-EFFECTIVENESS OF INTERVENTIONS IN DEVELOPING COUNTRIES

We determined incremental cost-effectiveness ratios (ICERs) for selected interventions for each condition by calculating total DALYs lost by a population because of the condition with and without treatment and then dividing the difference by the treatment cost. The disability weights used are presented in table 32.2. All analyses in this section followed the volume editors' standardized guidelines for economic analysis, region-specific age structures, and underlying mortality rates. We converted nontradable inputs into U.S. dollars at the market exchange rate. We assumed that the costs of tradable inputs were internationally consistent, as were costs associated with surgical treatments. Table 32.3 presents the costs of drugs and medical services. No fixed costs were assumed; therefore, our results are not linked with the extent of treatment coverage.

Table 32.2 Disability Weights Used in ICER Analysis

Weight	AD and other dementias	Epilepsy	PD	Acute stroke	Recurrent stroke
Untreated	0.627	0.15	0.392[a]	0.278[b]	0.556
Treated	0.627[c]	0	0.316	0.235[b]	n.a.[d]

Source: Mathers and others 2006.
n.a. = not applicable.
a. Treatment for PD is assumed to be effective for a maximum of 10 years. We also assume that a patient reverts to the untreated disability weight after 10 years.
b. Disability is assumed to last a maximum of 10 years; then we assume the patient recovers fully.
c. The patient is assumed to experience no benefit from treatment. Benefits are in the form of reduced caregiver hours.
d. Treatment does not change the disability weight following a recurrent stroke; only the likelihood of experiencing a second stroke is reduced.

Table 32.3 Input Requirements for Interventions by Condition

Condition	Visits to primary health care doctor in outpatient department		Primary health care worker visits to patient in home or patient visits to see the worker in outpatient department		Specialist care in outpatient department		Inpatient care		Annual drug costs (US$)
	Patients using the service[a] (percent)	Visits per year	Patients using the service (percent)	Visits per year	Patients using the service (percent)	Visits per year	Patients using the service (percent)	Length of stay	
AD and other dementias									
Acetylcholinesterase inhibitors	100	4	100	12	100	2	5	7	638
Antipsychotics	100	12	100	12	25	6	5	7	10
Epilepsy									
Phenobarbital	100	2	100	6	10	2	1	3	1
Lamotrigine[b]	100	2	100	6	10	2	1	3	144
Surgery	n.a.	n.a.	n.a.	n.a.	n.a.	n.a.	n.a.	n.a.	2,600[c]
PD									
Levodopa/carbidopa	100	3	100	6	100	2	1	5	71
Ayurvedic preparations	100	3	100	6	100	2	1	5	19
Deep brain stimulation	n.a.	n.a.	n.a.	n.a.	n.a.	n.a.	n.a.	n.a.	37,000
Stroke (acute attack)									
Aspirin	n.a.	n.a.	100	1	100	1	100	14	3
Heparin	n.a.	n.a.	100	1	100	1	100	14	691
rt-PA	n.a.	n.a.	100	1	100	1	1	7	1,777[d]
Stroke (prevention of recurrence)									
Aspirin	100	4	100	6	100	1	n.a.	n.a.	3
Dipyridamole and aspirin	100	4	100	6	100	1	n.a.	n.a.	64
Carotid endarterectomy	n.a.	n.a.	n.a.	n.a.	n.a.	n.a.	n.a.	n.a.	6,216

Source: Authors.

n.a. = not applicable.

a. Percentage of patients receiving the specified treatment.

b. Nondrug treatment costs for lamotrigine are not included in the cost-effectiveness analyses because they are accounted for in the phenobarbital treatment costs. Lamotrigine is taken in addition to phenobarbital.

c. Epilepsy surgery also requires screening at a cost of US$600 per screened patient. Because only half of screened patients are eligible for surgery, the cost amounts to US$1,200 per treated patient.

d. This treatment requires testing for eligible patients. The costs of screening ineligible patients include all the same hospital and doctor costs as treatment, as well as 80 percent of the drug cost to account for the diagnostic CT.

AD and Other Dementias

We analyzed the use of acetylcholinesterase inhibitors in the treatment of AD on the basis of the following assumptions: first, only patients who were older than 60 at the time of onset were considered; second, the treatment has no long-term benefits—that is, it does not reduce patient disability and has no effect on mortality.

We computed the benefits of reduced caregiver hours on the basis of reports that the improvement in cognitive function in AD patients associated with treatment using acetylcholinesterase inhibitors was a 1.2 point change in the global assessment scale for cognitive function, as measured by the Mini Mental State Examination. A 1 point improvement in the score was associated with a 0.56 hour per day reduction in caregiver hours, or roughly 205 hours per year (Marin and others 2003).

The cost of using acetylcholinesterase inhibitors per hour of caregiver time saved averaged US$13 across low- and middle-income countries (LMICs) and was at least US$11 in specific regions (the regions are the same as those in table 32.1). This amount is substantially more than the wage rate in these regions, which would generally not exceed US$1 to US$1.50 per hour, even for hired caregivers specifically trained to care for AD patients. We, therefore, conclude that the use of acetylcholinesterase inhibitors in developing countries is not efficient from an economic perspective. Calculating the cost per DALY averted for acetylcholinesterase inhibitors would not be meaningful, because we assume no benefit to the patient. Finally, the use of acetylcholinesterase inhibitors is uncommon in developing countries; therefore, reducing its use is not an important concern.

Epilepsy

We analyzed the cost-effectiveness of phenobarbital in the treatment of epilepsy, and the results are shown in table 32.4. We assumed that phenobarbital was provided to all patients. The cost of using phenobarbital per DALY gained in LMICs was US$89. Table 32.4 shows that the benefits of phenobarbital are large relative to its cost.

We did not look at other AEDs, such as phenytoin or carbamazepine, because the costs of those medications are much greater than that of phenobarbital, but their effectiveness is essentially the same (Aldenkamp, De Krom, and Reijs 2003). Although their use may be justified for specific medical reasons, phenobarbital is much more cost-effective.

We analyzed treatment options for patients who are refractory to treatment with phenobarbital. We assumed that such cases were treated either with a combination of phenobarbital and lamotrigine or with a combination of phenobarbital and surgery. We used the cost for epilepsy surgery of US$2,600, in accordance with a study from Colombia, and applied it to all regions (Malmgren and others 1996; Tureczek, Fandino-

Franky, and Wieser 2000). We assumed that roughly half of surgery recipients experience no more seizures and that the remaining half continue to take phenobarbital despite undergoing surgery. Our evaluation of the surgical option included the costs of diagnostic services and the costs associated with screening patients who ultimately may not be eligible for surgery. For patients in LMICs who are refractory to phenobarbital, the ICER of the add-on drug lamotrigine was US$3,000, and the ICER of the surgical option plus phenobarbital was US$3,100. The difference between phenobarbital and the other two options was significant in all regions.

Among refractory epilepsy patients eligible for surgery and according to postoperative outcome studies conducted in developed countries, surgery may be of comparable cost-effectiveness to treatment with a combination of phenobarbital and lamotrigine. Because effectiveness data for developing countries are not available, this calculation is based on cost estimates from a study in Colombia and estimates of the effectiveness of surgery from developed countries. If the surgical outcome in developing countries were worse than in developed countries, the cost-effectiveness of surgery would be lower. Furthermore, we note a number of limitations to the use of surgery in refractory epilepsy, particularly in developing countries, along with the lack of long-term follow-up data on the outcome of surgery. We stress that the primary treatment of epilepsy is with phenobarbital, and effective treatment of epilepsy lies in more efficient use of this highly cost-effective medication to close the treatment gap.

Parkinson's Disease

We evaluated three interventions for PD: a combination of l-dopa and carbidopa, traditional medicines such as the ayurvedic treatment used in India, and deep brain stimulation. We assumed that treatment for all three modalities was effective for 10 years from the onset of treatment. The ICERs in LMICs for these three modalities were US$1500, US$750 and US$31,000, respectively (table 32.4). On the basis of the cost of medication and evidence from clinical trials of effectiveness (Parkinson's Disease Group 1995) and from animal studies (Hussain and Manyam 1997), we found that ayurvedic treatment was the most cost-effective option. The relatively favorable ICER for ayurvedic treatment is due to the extremely low medication cost of this intervention. The relatively high ICER for deep brain stimulation was largely attributable to the extremely high cost of surgery. Table 32.4 shows DALYs gained for US$1 million of health expenditure.

Stroke

We evaluated two sets of interventions for stroke: treatment of acute stroke and prevention of secondary stroke. We assumed

Table 32.4 Results from Cost-Effectiveness Analysis of Interventions for Alzheimer's Disease, Epilepsy, Parkinson's Disease, and Stroke, by World Bank Region

Condition	Low- and middle-income countries	East Asia and the Pacific	Europe and Central Asia	Latin America and the Caribbean	Middle East and North Africa	South Asia	Sub-Saharan Africa
AD							
Cost per care hour reduced using acetylcholinesterase inhibitors (US$)	11	11	12	13	12	11	11
Epilepsy							
Incremental costs of DALYs gained per year of treatment compared with no treatment (US$)							
Phenobarbital	89	78	122	261	165	54	25
Phenobarbital and lamotrigine	2,994	3,306	2,945	4,301	3,344	2,872	1,490
Phenobarbital and surgery	3,060	3,411	3,049	3,477	2,904	3,097	1,788
Number of DALYs gained per US$1 million per year							
Phenobarbital	11,262	12,799	8,185	3,828	6,072	18,581	39,632
Phenobarbital and lamotragine	334	302	340	232	299	348	671
Phenobarbital and surgery	327	293	328	288	344	323	559
PD							
Incremental costs of DALYs gained per year of treatment compared with no treatment (US$)							
Levodopa/carbidopa	1,512	1,398	1,760	2,254	1,944	1,311	1,281
Ayurvedic preparation	751	638	1,000	1,494	1,184	551	520
Levodopa/carbidopa and deep brain stimulation	31,114	26,941	29,310	29,444	30,770	31,347	34,069
Number of DALYs gained per US$1 million per year							
Levodopa/carbidopa	662	715	568	444	514	763	781
Ayurvedic preparation	1,331	1,568	1,000	669	845	1,815	1,922
Levodopa/carbidopa and deep brain stimulation	32	37	34	34	32	32	29

Stroke (treatment of acute attack)

Incremental costs of DALYs gained per year
of treatment compared with no treatment (US$)

Aspirin	149	109	104	574	534	118	112
Heparin	2,675	2,185	1,318	4,952	5,443	2,967	2,940
rt-PA	1,278	1,169	648	2,158	2,516	1,630	1,623

Number of DALYs gained per US$1 million per year

Aspirin	6,691	9,209	9,633	1,742	1,873	8,463	8,942
Heparin	374	458	759	202	184	337	340
rt-PA	783	856	1,543	463	398	613	616

Stroke (prevention of recurrence)

Incremental costs of percent recurrence risk
averted after 2 years of treatment (US$)

Aspirin	4	3	6	9	7	2	2
Dipyridamole and aspirin	5	5	6	8	7	4	4
Carotid endarterectomy	87	87	87	87	87	87	87

Incremental costs of DALYs gained per 2 years
of treatment compared with no treatment (US$)

Aspirin	70	60	59	233	196	52	34
Dipyridamole and aspirin	93	95	63	194	186	96	69
Carotid endarterectomy	1,458	1,614	836	2,001	2,234	1,759	1,284

Number of DALYs gained per US$1 million
per 2 years of treatment

Aspirin	14,313	16,569	16,866	4,285	5,093	19,348	29,373
Dipyridamole and aspirin	10,752	10,555	15,969	5,150	5,384	10,369	14,572
Carotid endarterectomy	686	620	1,197	500	448	568	779

Source: Authors.

that stroke sufferers have fully recovered 10 years after their last stroke.

We evaluated aspirin, heparin, and rt-PA for the treatment of acute stroke. The International Stroke Trial Collaborative Group (1997) reports that, within 14 days of the onset of stroke, mortality with heparin treatment is less than with a placebo; however, after six months, mortality is actually greater for patients treated with heparin than with a placebo—that is, there is a negative cost per DALY gained if this effect is incorporated. The estimates presented here are based on the change in the short-term mortality risk. For LMICs, the cost per DALY averted using aspirin was US$150 (table 32.4). The equivalent costs of interventions using rt-PA and heparin were US$1,300 and US$2,700, respectively. The costs of heparin are higher than the costs of rt-PA, despite the expensive equipment required for rt-PA, because of the lower effectiveness of heparin.

Table 32.4 presents DALYs averted for US$1 million of health expenditure for the three treatments. The cost per DALY gained using aspirin is a conservative estimate, because the use of aspirin has additional benefits in terms of preventing a recurrence of stroke.

Table 32.4 shows the costs of preventing a second stroke within two years of the first stroke. For LMICs, aspirin was the least expensive option at US$3.80 per single percentage point decrease in the risk of a second stroke within two years of the first. This rate translates to roughly US$70 per DALY gained (table 32.4). Combining dipyridamole with aspirin, because of higher cost, was slightly more expensive at roughly US$5.20 per single percentage point decrease in recurrent stroke risk for a single individual, or about US$93 per DALY. In contrast, carotid endarterectomy was US$87 for an equivalent decrease in individual recurrence risk or almost US$1,500 per DALY. The aspirin monotherapy option for preventing a recurrence of stroke was the most cost-effective approach only in South Asia and Sub-Saharan Africa, largely because of the relatively low costs of nontradable inputs, such as hospital and doctors' fees, in those regions. Low input costs of nontradables increase the relative importance of drug costs in determining the most cost-effective intervention; therefore, the cheaper drug, aspirin, was most cost-effective. Table 32.4 shows that, though US$1 million would be most effectively spent on aspirin alone in South Asia and Sub-Saharan Africa, investment in aspirin and dipyridamole treatment would result in a greater DALY gain in the other regions.

RECOMMENDATIONS

The use of acetylcholinesterase inhibitors for treating patients with AD, as assessed by the number of caregiver hours saved, suggests that this intervention is not cost-effective. This finding, combined with the limited efficacy of acetylcholinesterase

inhibitors, suggests that they should not be widely used in developing countries. Instead, giving low doses of antipsychotic medication to patients with any form of dementia who also have behavioral problems may be a better option for reducing caregiver stress, although this possibility has not been systematically evaluated.

Phenobarbital is by far the most cost-effective intervention for managing epilepsy and should be recommended for widespread use in public health campaigns against epilepsy in LMICs. For those patients who do not respond to phenobarbital, the addition of lamotrigine is advisable rather than surgery, because of the resource-intensive evaluation and infrastructure required for epilepsy surgery.

Indigenous systems of medicine, such as the ayurvedic medicines used in India, are much more cost-effective than Western medications or surgical procedures for managing patients with PD. Other countries may wish to test and standardize such medications for their own use.

Aspirin is by far the most cost-effective intervention both for treating acute stroke and for preventing a recurrence of stroke. It is easily available in developing countries, even in rural areas.

RESEARCH AND DEVELOPMENT AGENDA

The populations of most developing countries are aging rapidly. Many neurological disorders frequently occur in the elderly, posing an emerging public health problem. As a result, developing countries should begin or expand their research and development agendas to address issues related to the prevention, identification, and management of neurological disorders. In the short term, they should focus on early identification, optimum treatment, and amelioration of distress and handicaps and on reduction of the social and economic burden on patients and their families. In the long term, they should develop and implement strategies for primary prevention of neurological disorders. Specific areas for research and development include the following:

- *Conducting population-based epidemiological studies in developing countries.* Population-based data from developing countries are insufficient, which limits evidence-based planning. In addition, such data may also suggest important hypotheses for research if they identify genuine differences across regions (for example, the reported difference in the incidence of AD in developed and developing countries). In addition, the identification of risk or protective factors would be useful in the primary prevention of such diseases.
- *Enhancing existing health care delivery systems.* In most developing countries, approximately 70 to 80 percent of patients live in rural areas, where medical care is frequently provided by nonphysician health care providers or, at best,

by a general physician. Limitations in the availability of health care have resulted in a huge treatment gap for many neurological disorders. For such situations, a simple model for the management of neurological disorders by existing community-based health care providers, trained to provide such services, would be helpful. Research is needed on optimum referral systems for more difficult cases that local communities will accept and can afford. Strategies for home-based care of patients need to be systematically evaluated.

- *Developing cheaper and more efficacious medicines.* Many currently available medications have significant side effects and are too expensive for many patients in developing countries. Newer medications need to be developed with lower costs, fewer side effects, better efficacy, and less frequent dose schedules.
- *Promoting the use of indigenous systems of medicine.* Many people in developing countries use local indigenous medicines. More research needs to be done on the pharmacological properties of those medications (see chapter 69).
- *Launching stigma removal campaigns.* The stigmatization of patients with neurological disorders and of their families is still prevalent, particularly in rural and remote areas, and it often prevents patients from seeking and obtaining appropriate medical care. Effective strategies to address this issue need to be developed and implemented on a large scale.

MISSED OPPORTUNITIES

Many research studies have reported that the incidence of AD is lower in developing countries than in Western countries. Migration studies, such as those looking at the migration of Africans to the United States, have shown a change in the risk for AD within one or two generations. This finding suggests that developing countries may have some protective factors that rapidly change on migration to developed countries. Despite this information being available for more than 25 years, no systematic efforts have been made to identify these protective factors. Given the rapid adaptation of Western lifestyles in developing countries, identifying these factors is important before the opportunity is permanently lost.

The successful use of phenobarbital for treating epilepsy was first described in 1912. Not only is it effective for many types of epilepsy, but it is also inexpensive. Nevertheless, despite its availability for more than 90 years and its modest cost, the treatment gap for epilepsy still exceeds 90 percent in many developing countries.

Indigenous systems of medicine, such as for the treatment of PD, have been used for centuries in developing countries. However, their utility has not been fully exploited.

Despite evidence of the benefit of control of hypertension in the primary prevention of stroke, most efforts in developing countries are directed at treatment of stroke. This approach not only is more expensive but also is less beneficial to the patient.

ACKNOWLEDGMENTS

The lead author would like to acknowledge with gratitude the support provided by the regional director and director of program management of the South-East Asia Regional Office of the World Health Organization. Special mention must be made of Dr. Daniel Chisholm, who provided input into the cost-effectiveness analysis, particularly that dealing with epilepsy, and of Dr. Donald Silberberg, who served as the senior adviser to the chapter. The authors wish to thank the many reviewers for their valuable suggestions, which have been incorporated into the chapter.

REFERENCES

Aldenkamp, A. P., M. De Krom, and R. Reijs. 2003. "Newer Antiepileptic Drugs and Cognitive Issues." *Epilepsia* 44 (Suppl. 4): 21–29.

Allen, C. M. C. 1983. "Clinical Diagnosis of Acute Stroke Syndrome." *Quarterly Journal of Medicine* 42: 515–23.

Anand, K., D. Chowdhury, K. B. Singh, C. S. Pandav, and S. K. Kapoor. 2001. "Estimation of Mortality and Morbidity Due to Strokes in India." *Neuroepidemiology* 20 (3): 208–11.

Antithrombotic Trialists' Collaboration. 2002. "Collaborative Meta-Analysis of Randomised Trials of Antiplatelet Therapy for Prevention of Death, Myocardial Infarction, and Stroke in High Risk Patients." *British Medical Journal* 324 (7329): 71–86.

Asawavichienjinda, T., C. Sitthi-Amorn, and W. Tanyanont. 2003. "Compliance with Treatment of Adult Epileptics in a Rural District of Thailand." *Journal of Medical Association Thailand* 86 (1): 46–51.

Ascherio, A., S. M. Zhang, M. A. Hernan, I. Kawachi, G. A. Colditz, F. E. Speizer, and others. 2001. "Prospective Study of Caffeine Consumption and Risk of Parkinson's Disease in Men and Women." *Annals of Neurology* 50 (1): 56–63.

Asymptomatic Carotid Atherosclerosis Study. 1995. "Endarterectomy for Asymptomatic Carotid Artery Stenosis." *Journal of the American Medical Association* 273 (18): 1421–28.

Asymptomatic Carotid Surgery Trial Collaborative Group. 2004. "Prevention of Disabling and Fatal Strokes by Successful Carotid Endarterectomy in Patients without Recent Neurological Symptoms: Randomised Controlled Trial." *Lancet* 363: 1491–502.

Berger, K., M. M. Breteler, C. Helmer, D. Inzitari, L. Fratiglioni, C. Trenkwalder, and others. 2000. "Prognosis with Parkinson's Disease in Europe: A Collaborative Study of Population-Based Cohorts: Neurologic Diseases in the Elderly Research Group." *Neurology* 54 (11 Suppl. 5): S24–27.

Brodaty, H., and M. Gresham. 1989. "Effect of a Training Programme to Reduce Stress in Carers of Patients with Dementia." *British Medical Journal* 299 (6712): 1375–79.

Buck, D., B. A. Gregson, C. H. Bamford, P. McNamee, G. N. Farrow, J. Bond, and others. 1997. "Psychological Distress among Informal Supporters of Frail Older People at Home and in Institutions." *International Journal of Geriatric Psychiatry* 12 (7): 737–44.

Casetta, I., V. C. Monetti, S. Malagu, E. Paolino, V. Govoni, E. Fainardi, and others. 2002. "Risk Factors for Cryptogenic and Idiopathic Partial Epilepsy: A Community-Based Case-Control Study in Copparo, Italy." *Neuroepidemiology* 21 (5): 251–54.

Chandra, V., M. Ganguli, R. Pandav, J. Johnston, S. Belle, and S. T. DeKosky. 1998. "Prevalence of Alzheimer's Disease and Other Dementias in Rural India: The Indo-U.S. Study." *Neurology* 51 (4): 1000–8.

Chandra, V., R. Pandav, H. H. Dodge, J. M. Johnston, S. H. Belle, S. T. DeKosky, and others. 2001. "Incidence of Alzheimer's Disease in a Rural Community in India: The Indo-U.S. Study." *Neurology* 57 (6): 985–89.

Chinese Acute Stroke Trial Collaborative Group. 1997. "CAST: Randomised Placebo-Controlled Trial of Early Aspirin Use in 20,000 Patients with Acute Ischaemic Stroke: CAST (Chinese Acute Stroke Trial) Collaborative Group." *Lancet* 349 (9066): 1641–49.

Cockerell, O. C., A. L. Johnson, J. W. Sander, and S. D. Shorvon. 1997. "Prognosis of Epilepsy: A Review and Further Analysis of the First Nine Years of the British National General Practice Study of Epilepsy: A Prospective Population-Based Study." *Epilepsia* 38 (1): 31–46.

Desai, P., M. V. Padma, S. Jain, and M. C. Maheshwari. 1998. "Knowledge, Attitudes, and Practice of Epilepsy: Experience at a Comprehensive Rural Health Services Project." *Seizure* 7 (2): 133–38.

Diener, H. C., J. Bogousslavsky, L. M. Brass, C. Cimminiello, L. Csiba, M. Kaste, and others. 2004. "Aspirin and Clopidogrel Compared with Clopidogrel Alone after Recent Ischaemic Stroke or Transient Ischaemic Attack in High-Risk Patients (MATCH): Randomised, Double-Blind, Placebo-Controlled Trial." *Lancet* 364 (9431): 301–7.

Eastern Stroke and Coronary Heart Disease Collaborative Research Group. 1998. "Blood Pressure, Cholesterol, and Stroke in Eastern Asia: Eastern Stroke and Coronary Heart Disease Collaborative Research Group." *Lancet* 352 (9143): 1801–7.

Engel, J. Jr., S. Wiebe, J. French , M. Sperling, P. Williamson, D. Spencer, and others. 2003. "Practice Parameter: Temporal Lobe and Localized Neocortical Resections for Epilepsy." *Epilepsia* 44 (6): 741–51.

European Atrial Fibrillation Trial Study Group. 1993. "Secondary Prevention in Non-Rheumatic Atrial Fibrillation after Transient Ischaemic Attack or Minor Stroke." *Lancet* 342 (8882): 1255–62.

Foster, N. L., R. C. Petersen, S. I. Gracon, and K. Lewis. 1996. "An Enriched-Population, Double-Blind, Placebo-Controlled, Crossover Study of Tacrine and Lecithin in Alzheimer's Disease: The Tacrine 970-6 Study Group." *Dementia* 7 (5): 260–66.

Fukiyama, K., Y. Kimura, K. Wakugami, and H. Muratani. 2000. "Incidence and Long-Term Prognosis of Initial Stroke and Acute Myocardial Infarction in Okinawa, Japan." *Hypertension Research* 23 (2): 127–35.

Gentleman, S. M., D. I. Graham, and G. W. Roberts. 1993. "Molecular Pathology of Head Trauma: Altered Beta APP Metabolism and the Aetiology of Alzheimer's Disease." *Progress in Brain Research* 96: 237–46.

Goldstein, L. B., R. Adams, K. Becker, C. D. Furberg, P. B. Gorelick, G. Hademenos, and others. 2001. "Primary Prevention of Ischemic Stroke: A Statement for Healthcare Professionals from the Stroke Council of the American Heart Association." *Stroke* 32 (1): 280–99.

Gopinath, B., K. Radhakrishnan, P. S. Sarma, D. Jayachandran, and A. Alexander. 2000. "A Questionnaire Survey about Doctor-Patient Communication, Compliance, and Locus of Control among South Indian People with Epilepsy." *Epilepsy Research* 39 (1): 73–82.

Gunatilake, S. B., B. A. Jayasekera, and A. P. Premawardene. 2001. "Stroke Subtypes in Sri Lanka: A Hospital-Based Study." *Ceylon Medical Journal* 46 (1): 19–20.

Haupt, M., A. Karger, and M. Janner. 2000. "Improvement of Agitation and Anxiety in Demented Patients after Psychoeducative Group Intervention with Their Caregivers." *International Journal of Geriatric Psychiatry* 15 (12): 1125–29.

He, J., M. J. Klag, Z. Wu, and P. K. Whelton. 1995. "Stroke in the People's Republic of China: II. Meta-Analysis of Hypertension and Risk of Stroke." *Stroke* 26 (12): 2228–32.

Henderson, A. S., and A. F. Jorm. 2000. "Definition of Epidemiology of Dementia: A Review." In *Dementia*, ed. M. Mario and N. Sartorius, 1–34. West Sussex, U.K.: John Wiley.

Henderson, V. W. 1997. "The Epidemiology of Estrogen Replacement Therapy and Alzheimer's Disease." *Neurology* 48 (5 Suppl. 7): S27–35.

Hendrie, H. C., A. Ogunniyi, K. S. Hall, O. Baiyewu, F. W. Unverzagt, O. Gureje, and others. 2001. "Incidence of Dementia and Alzheimer Disease in 2 Communities: Yoruba Residing in Ibadan, Nigeria, and African Americans Residing in Indianapolis, Indiana." *Journal of the American Medical Association* 285 (6): 739–47.

Hendrie, H. C., B. O. Osuntokun, K. S. Hall, A. O. Ogunniyi, S. L. Hui, F. W. Unverzagt, and others. 1995. "Prevalence of Alzheimer's Disease and Dementia in Two Communities: Nigerian Africans and African Americans." *American Journal of Psychiatry* 152 (10): 1485–92.

Huang, Z. S., T. L. Chiang, and T. K. Lee. 1997. "Stroke Prevalence in Taiwan: Findings from the 1994 National Health Interview Survey." *Stroke* 28 (8): 1579–84.

Hussain, G., and B. V. Manyam. 1997. "Mucuna Pruriens Proves More Effective than L-DOPA in Parkinson's Disease Animal Model." *Phytotherapy Research* 11: 419–23.

International Stroke Trial Collaborative Group. 1997. "The International Stroke Trial (IST): A Randomised Trial of Aspirin, Subcutaneous Heparin, Both, or Neither among 19,435 Patients with Acute Ischaemic Stroke: International Stroke Trial Collaborative Group." *Lancet* 349 (9065): 1569–81.

Jorm, A. F., and D. Jolley. 1998. "The Incidence of Dementia: A Meta-Analysis." *Neurology* 51 (3): 728–33.

Kaiser, C., G. Asaba, C. Mugisa, W. Kipp, S. Kasoro, T. Rubaale, and others. 1998. "Antiepileptic Drug Treatment in Rural Africa: Involving the Community." *Tropical Doctor* 28 (2): 73–77.

Karaagac, N., S. N. Yeni, M. Senocak, M. Bozluolcay, F. K. Savrun, H. Ozdemir, and others. 1999. "Prevalence of Epilepsy in Silivri, a Rural Area of Turkey." *Epilepsia* 40 (5): 637–42.

Kiyohara, Y., M. Kubo, I. Kato, Y. Tanizaki, K. Tanaka, K. Okubo, and others. 2003. "Ten-Year Prognosis of Stroke and Risk Factors for Death in a Japanese Community: The Hisayama Study." *Stroke* 34 (10): 2343–47.

Kotsopoulos, I. A., T. van Merode, F. G. Kessels, M. C. de Krom , and J. A. Knottnerus. 2002. "Systematic Review and Meta-Analysis of Incidence Studies of Epilepsy and Unprovoked Seizures." *Epilepsia* 43 (11): 1402–9.

Leonardi, M., and T. B. Ustun. 2002. "The Global Burden of Epilepsy." *Epilepsia* 43 (Suppl. 6): 21–25.

Leone, M., E. Bottacchi, E. Beghi, E. Morgando, R. Mutani, R. Cremo, and others. 2002. "Risk Factors for a First Generalized Tonic-Clonic Seizure in Adult Life." *Neurological Sciences* 23 (3): 99–106.

Levin, E., J. Moriarty, and P. Gorbach. 1994. "Better for the Break." London: Her Majesty's Stationery Office, National Institute of Social Work Research Unit.

Lewin, L., and P. Schuster. 1929. "Ergebnisse von Banisterinversuchen an Kranken." *Deutsche Medizinische Wochenschrift* 55: 419.

Li, G., Y. C. Shen, C. H. Chen, Y. W. Zhau, S. R. Li, and M. Lu. 1991. "A Three-Year Follow-up Study of Age-Related Dementia in an Urban Area of Beijing." *Acta Psychiatrica Scandanavica* 83 (2): 99–104.

Liu, L., K. Ikeda, and Y. Yamori. 2001. "Changes in Stroke Mortality Rates for 1950 to 1997: A Great Slowdown of Decline Trend in Japan." *Stroke* 32 (8): 1745–49.

MacWalter, R. S., and C. P. Shirley. 2002. "A Benefit-Risk Assessment of Agents Used in the Secondary Prevention of Stroke." *Drug Safety* 25 (13): 943–63.

Malmgren, K., A. Hedstrom, R. Granqvist, H. Malmgren, and E. Ben-Menachem. 1996. "Cost Analysis of Epilepsy Surgery and of Vigabatrin Treatment in Patients with Refractory Partial Epilepsy." *Epilepsy Research* 25 (3): 199–207.

Mani, K., G. Rangan, H. V. Srinivas, and S. Narendran. 1993. "Natural History of Untreated Epilepsy: A Community-Based Study in Rural South India." *Epilepsia* 34 (Suppl. 2): 166.

Marin, D., K. Amaya, R. Casciano, K. L. Puder, J. Casciano, S. Chang, and others. 2003. "Impact of Rivastigmine on Costs and on Time Spent in Caregiving for Families of Patients with Alzheimer's Disease." *International Psychogeriatics* 15 (4): 385–98.

Marras, C., and C. Tanner. 2002. "The Epidemiology of Parkinson's Disease." In *Movement Disorders Neurologic Principles and Practice*, ed. R. L. Watts and W. C. Koller, 177–96. New York: McGraw-Hill.

Marriott, A., C. Donaldson, N. Tarrier, and A. Burns. 2000. "Effectiveness of Cognitive-Behavioural Family Intervention in Reducing the Burden of Care in Carers of Patients with Alzheimer's Disease." *British Journal of Psychiatry* 176 (1): 557–62.

Mathers, C. D., A. D. Lopez, and C. J. L. Murray. "The Burden of Disease and Mortality by Condition: Data, Methods, and Results for 2001." In *Global Burden of Disease and Risk Factors*, eds. A. D. Lopez, C. D. Mathers, M. Ezzati, D. T. Jamison, and C. J. L. Murray. New York: Oxford University Press.

Meinardi, H., R. A. Scott, R. Reis, J. W. Sander, and ILAE Commission on the Developing World. 2001. "The Treatment Gap in Epilepsy: The Current Situation and Ways Forward." *Epilepsia* 42 (1): 136–49.

Melzer, D., K. Pearce, B. Cooper, and C. Brayne. 2004. "Alzheimer's Disease and Other Dementias." Department of Public Health and Epidemiology, University of Birmingham, U.K. http://hcna.radcliffe-oxford.com/dementiaframe.htm.

Mohr, J. P., J. L. P. Thompson, R. M. Lazar, B. Levin, R. L. Sacco, K. L. Furie, and others. 2001. "A Comparison of Warfarin and Aspirin for the Prevention of Recurrent Ischemic Stroke." *New England Journal of Medicine* 345 (20): 1444–51.

National Institute of Neurological Disorders and Stroke rt-PA Stroke Study Group. 1995. "Tissue Plasminogen Activator for Acute Ischemic Stroke: The National Institute of Neurological Disorders and Stroke rt-PA Stroke Study Group." *New England Journal of Medicine* 333 (24): 1581–87.

National Stroke Association. 2002. "Recovery and Rehabilitation." National Stroke Association, Englewood, CO. http://www.stroke.org/HomePage.aspx?P=435435784753465.

Naylor, A. R., N. J. M. London, and P. R. Bell. 1997. "Carotid Endarterectomy versus Carotid Angioplasty." *Lancet* 349 (9046): 203–24.

North American Symptomatic Carotid Endarterectomy Trial Collaborators. 1991. "Beneficial Effect of Carotid Endarterectomy in Symptomatic Patients with High-Grade Carotid Stenosis: North American Symptomatic Carotid Endarterectomy Trial Collaborators." *New England Journal of Medicine* 325 (7): 445–53.

Outpatient Service Trialists. 2002. "Therapy-Based Rehabilitation Services for Stroke Patients at Home." *Cochrane Database of Systematic Reviews* (2) CD002925.

Pal, D. K., A. Carpio, and J. W. Sander. 2000. "Neurocysticercosis and Epilepsy in Developing Countries." *Journal of Neurology Neurosurgery Psychiatry* 68 (2): 137–43.

Pal, D. K., T. Das, S. Sengupta, and G. Chaudhury. 2002. Help-Seeking Patterns for Children with Epilepsy in Rural India: Implications for Service Delivery. *Epilepsia* 43 (8): 904–11.

Parkinson's Disease Group. 1995. "An Alternative Medicine Treatment for Parkinson's Disease: Results of a Multicenter Clinical Trial: HP-200 in Parkinson's Disease Study Group." *Journal of Alternative Complementary Medicine* 1 (3): 249–55.

Poungvarin, N., A. Viriyavejakul, and C. Komontri. 1991. "Siriraj Stroke Score and Validation Study to Distinguish Supratentorial Intracerebral Haemorrhage from Infarction." *British Medical Journal* 302: 1565–67.

Prince, M. 2000. "Dementia in Developing Countries: A Consensus Statement from the 10/66 Dementia Research Group." *International Journal of Geriatric Psychiatry* 15 (1): 14–20.

Rajkumar, S., S. Kumar, and R. Thara. 1997. "Prevalence of Dementia in a Rural Setting: A Report from India." *International Journal of Geriatric Psychiatry* 12 (7): 702–27.

Sacco, R., J. Sivenius, and H. C. Diener. 2005. "Efficacy of Aspirin Plus Extended-Release Dipyridamole in Preventing Recurrent Stroke in High-Risk Populations." *Archives of Neurology* 62: 403–8.

Sarti, C., D. Rastenyte, Z. Cepaitis, and J. Tuomilehto. 2000. "International Trends in Mortality from Stroke, 1968 to 1994." *Stroke* 31 (7): 1588–601.

Schapel, G. J., R .G. Beran, F. J. Vajda, S. F. Berkovic, M. L. Mashford, F. M. Dunagan, and others. 1993. "Double-Blind, Placebo Controlled, Crossover study of Lamotrigine in Treatment Resistant Partial Seizures." *Journal of Neurology Neurosurgery Psychiatry* 56 (5): 448–53.

Shumaker, S. A., C. Legault, S. R. Rapp, L. Thal, R. B. Wallace, J. K. Ockene, and others. 2003. "Estrogen Plus Progestin and the Incidence of Dementia and Mild Cognitive Impairment in Postmenopausal Women: The Women's Health Initiative Memory Study—A Randomized Controlled Trial." *Journal of the American Medical Association* 289 (20): 2651–62.

Smaha, L. A. 2004. "The American Heart Association Get with the Guidelines Program." *American Heart Journal* 148 (Suppl. 5): S46–48.

Tanner, C., and S. Goldman. 1996. "Epidemiology of Parkinson's Disease." *Neurology Clinics* 14: 317–35.

Thorvaldsen, P., K. Asplund, K. Kuulasmaa, A. M. Rajakangas, and M. Schroll. 1995. "Stroke Incidence, Case Fatality, and Mortality in the WHO MONICA Project: World Health Organization Monitoring Trends and Determinants in Cardiovascular Disease." *Stroke* 26 (3): 361–67.

Tureczek, I. E., J. Fandino-Franky, and H. G. Wieser. 2000. "Comparison of the Epilepsy Surgery Programs in Cartagena, Colombia, and Zurich, Switzerland." *Epilepsia.* 41 (Suppl. 4): S35–40.

Van Den Eeden, S. K., C. M. Tanner, A. L. Bernstein, R. D. Fross, A. Leimpeter, D. A. Bloch, and others. 2003. "Incidence of Parkinson's Disease: Variation by Age, Gender, and Race/Ethnicity." *American Journal of Epidemiology* 157 (11): 1015–22.

Walker, R. W., D. G. McLarty, H. M. Kitange, D. Whiting, G. Masuki, D. M. Mtasiwa, and others. 2000. "Stroke Mortality in Urban and Rural Tanzania: Adult Morbidity and Mortality Project." *Lancet* 355 (9216): 1684–87.

Walsh, J. S., H. G. Welch, and E. B. Larson. 1990. "Survival of Outpatients with Alzheimer-Type Dementia." *Annals of Internal Medicine* 113 (6): 429–34.

Wang, W. Z., J. Z. Wu, D. S. Wang, X. Y. Dai, B. Yang, T. P. Wang, and others. 2003. "The Prevalence and Treatment Gap in Epilepsy in China: An ILAE/IBE/WHO Study." *Neurology* 60 (9): 1544–45.

Wang, W., D. Zhao, and G. Wu. 2001. "The Trend of Incidence Rate of Acute Stroke Event in Urban Areas, Beijing from 1984 to 1999" (in Chinese). *Zhonghua Liu Xing Bing Xue Za Zhi* 22 (4): 269–72.

WHO (World Health Organization). 2000. *The Global Campaign against Epilepsy* (information pack). Geneva: WHO.

Zhang, L. F., J. Yang, Z. Hong, G. G. Yuan, B. F. Zhou, L. C. Zhao, and others. 2003. "Proportion of Different Subtypes of Strokes in China." *Stroke* 34 (9): 2091–96.

Zhang, Z. X., and G. C. Roman. 1993. "Worldwide Occurrence of Parkinson's Disease: An Updated Review." *Neuroepidemiology* 12 (4): 195–208.

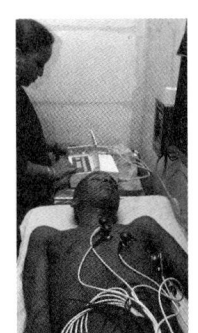

Chapter **33**

Cardiovascular Disease

Thomas A. Gaziano, K. Srinath Reddy, Fred Paccaud, Sue Horton, and Vivek Chaturvedi

Cardiovascular disease (CVD) is the number one cause of death worldwide (Mathers and others 2006; Murray and Lopez 1996; WHO 2002b). CVD covers a wide array of disorders, including diseases of the cardiac muscle and of the vascular system supplying the heart, brain, and other vital organs. This chapter reviews the epidemiological transition that has made CVD the world's leading cause of death, assesses the status of the transition by region, and indicates regional differences in the burden of CVD. It also reviews the cost-effectiveness of various interventions directed at the most relevant causes of CVD morbidity and mortality.

EPIDEMIOLOGY OF CVD

At the beginning of the 20th century, CVD was responsible for less than 10 percent of all deaths worldwide, but by 2001 that figure was 30 percent. About 80 percent of the global burden of CVD death occurs in low- and middle-income countries. Murray and Lopez (1996) predicted that CVD will be the leading cause of death and disability worldwide by 2020 mainly because it will increase in low- and middle-income countries. By 2001, CVD had become the leading cause of death in the developing world, as it has been in the developed world since the mid 1900s (Mathers and others 2006; WHO 2002a). Nearly 50 percent of all deaths in high-income countries and about 28 percent of deaths in low- and middle-income countries are the result of CVD (Mathers and others 2006). Other causes of death, such as injuries, respiratory infections, nutritional deficiencies, and HIV/AIDS, collectively still play a predominant role in certain regions, but even in those areas CVD is now a significant cause of mortality.

Predominant Cardiovascular Diseases

This chapter focuses on the most common causes of CVD morbidity and mortality:

- ischemic heart disease (IHD)
- stroke
- congestive heart failure (CHF).

These diseases account for at least 80 percent of the burden of CVD in all income regions, which share many of the same common risk factors; accordingly, similar interventions are appropriate. A fourth manifestation, rheumatic heart disease (RHD), which accounts for 3 percent of all disability-adjusted life years (DALYs) lost as a result of CVD, does not contribute significantly to the overall global burden of CVD. The burden of RHD will likely continue to diminish, but it is still an important inflammatory cause of heart disease in developing countries and accordingly is addressed in this chapter. We do not address many other forms of CVD because of the scope of this volume; the regional rather than global nature of some inflammatory diseases, such as Chagas disease; or the congenital abnormalities or genetically based cardiomyopathies for which prevention and treatment options remain limited.

Ischemic Heart Disease. IHD is the single largest cause of death in the developed countries and is one of the main contributors to the disease burden in developing countries. The two leading manifestations of IHD are angina and acute myocardial infarction. In 2001, IHD was responsible for 7.3 million deaths and 58 million DALYs lost worldwide (WHO 2002b). Seventy-five percent of global deaths and 82 percent of the total DALYs resulting from IHD occurred in the low- and middle-income countries.

Glossary

ACE inhibitors (angiotensin-converting enzyme inhibitors): a group of antihypertensive drugs that exert their influence through the renin-angiotensin-aldosterone system.

Antiplatelets: drugs that interfere with the blood's ability to clot.

Atheroschlerosis: a chronic disease characterized by thickening and hardening of the arterial walls.

Atrial fibrillation: an abnormal rhythm of the heart that can result in an increased risk of stroke because of the formation of emboli (blood clots) in the heart.

Beta-blockers: a group of drugs that decrease the heart rate and force of contractions and lower blood pressure.

Cardiogenic shock: poor tissue perfusion resulting from failure of the heart to pump an adequate amount of blood.

Cardiomyopathy: a disorder of the muscle limiting the heart's function.

Chagas disease: a tropical American disease caused by a parasitic infection. Chronic symptoms include cardiac problems, such as an enlarged heart, altered heart rate or rhythm, heart failure, or cardiac arrest.

Dyslipidemia: a condition marked by abnormal concentrations of lipids or lipoproteins in the blood.

Embolus: a blood clot that moves through the bloodstream until it lodges in a narrowed vessel and blocks circulation.

Endocarditis: inflammation of the lining of the heart and its valves.

Hypertension: abnormally high arterial blood pressure.

Reperfusion: restoration of the flow of blood to a previously ischemic tissue or organ.

Statins: a group of drugs that inhibit the synthesis of cholesterol and promote the production of low-density lipoprotein (LDL)–binding receptors in the liver, resulting in a decrease in the level of LDL and a smaller increase in the level of high-density lipoprotein (HDL).

Thrombolysis: the breaking up of a blood clot.

Thrombus: a blood clot that forms inside a blood vessel or cavity of the heart.

Transient ischemic attack: transient reduced blood flow to the brain that produces strokelike symptoms but no lasting damage.

Angina is the characteristic pain of IHD. It is caused by atherosclerosis leading to stenosis (partial occlusion) of one or more coronary arteries. Patients with chronic stable angina have an average annual mortality of 2 percent or less. Acute myocardial infarction (AMI) is the total occlusion of a major coronary artery with a complete lack of oxygen and nutrients leading to cardiac muscle necrosis. AMI is usually diagnosed by changes in the electrocardiogram; by elevated serum enzymes, such as creatine phosphokinase and troponin T or I; and by pain similar to that of angina. Thirty-day mortality after an AMI is high: even with best medical therapy it remains at about 33 percent, with half the deaths occurring before the individual reaches the hospital. Even in a hospital with a coronary care unit where advanced care options are available, mortality is still 7 percent. In a hospital without such facilities or therapies, the mortality rate is closer to 30 percent. Even though mortality among patients who have recovered from an AMI has declined in recent decades, approximately 4 percent of patients who survive initial hospitalization die in the first year following the event (Antman and others 2004).

Stroke. Stroke is caused by a disruption in the flow of blood to part of the brain either because of the occlusion of a blood vessel (ischemic stroke) or the rupture of a blood vessel (hemorrhagic stroke). Many of the same risk factors for IHD apply to stroke; in addition, atrial fibrillation is an important risk factor for stroke. The annual risk of stroke in patients with non-valvular atrial fibrillation is 3 to 5 percent, with 50 percent of thromboembolic stroke being attributable to atrial fibrillation (Wolf, Abbott, and Kannel 1991). Chapter 32 discusses the diagnosis and management of the clinical syndromes in greater detail.

Congestive Heart Failure. CHF is the end stage of many heart diseases. It is characterized by abnormalities in myocardial function and neurohormonal regulation resulting in fatigue, fluid retention, and reduced longevity. CHF is caused by pathological processes that affect the heart; IHD and hypertension-related heart disease are the most common etiologies. The risk of developing CHF is two times more in hypertensive men and three times more in hypertensive women compared with those who are normotensive. CHF is five times more common in those who have had an AMI than in those who have not. The prognosis for those with established CHF is generally poor and worse than for those with most malignancies (McMurray and Stewart 2000) or AIDS, with a one-year mortality rate as high as 40 percent and a five-year mortality between 26 and 75 percent.

The worldwide burden of CHF is substantial and continues to rise. Throughout the developed world the prevalence is about 2 to 3 percent, with an annual incidence rate of 0.1 to 0.2 percent (McMurray and Stewart 2000). However, the incidence and prevalence of CHF rise dramatically with age. Prevalence is 27 per 1,000 population for those older than 65, compared with 0.7 per 1,000 for those younger than 50 (McKelvie 2003). CHF occurs more frequently in men, and incidence and mortality differ substantially according to gender and socioeconomic status. CHF causes 53,000 deaths in the United States each year and contributes to another 213,000, and the death rate attributed to CHF rose by 155 percent from 1979 to 2001 in the United States (American Heart Association 2002). CHF is the first-listed diagnosis in 1 million hospitalizations.

Rheumatic Heart Disease. RHD is the consequence of an acute rheumatic fever (ARF)—that is, a poorly adapted autoimmune response to group A β-hemolytic streptococci. It affects the connective tissue, mainly the joints and the heart valves. The most serious complications are valvular stenosis, regurgitation following the valvulitis, or both (Ephrem, Abegaz, and Muhe 1990). RHD is also a predisposing factor for infective endocarditis, a disease of younger adults, predominantly males (Koegelenberg and others 2003).

According to 2001 estimates, RHD accounts for 338,000 deaths per year worldwide, two-thirds of them in Southeast Asia and the Western Pacific (WHO 2002b). About 12 million people in developing countries, most of them children, suffer from RHD (WHO 1995). Steer and others' (2002) review of developing countries suggests that RHD prevalence in children is between 0.7 and 14 per 1,000, with the highest rates in Asia. RHD and ARF are the most common causes of cardiac disease among children in developing countries (Ephrem, Abegaz, and Muhe 1990; Schneider and Bezabih 2001; Steer and others 2002) and account for almost 10 percent of sudden cardiac deaths (Kaplan 1985).

Until the 1950s, ARF accounted for a substantial portion of cardiovascular problems among schoolchildren in developed countries, and even though it is now far less common, outbreaks still occur (Carapetis, Currie, and Kaplan 1999), suggesting that neither antibiotics nor other public health measures have been totally effective in controlling ARF.

The Epidemiological Transition

Over the past two centuries, the industrial and technological revolutions have resulted in a dramatic shift in the causes of illness and death. Before 1900, infectious diseases and malnutrition were the most common causes of death; however, primarily because of improved nutrition and public health measures, they have gradually been supplanted in most high-income countries by CVD and cancer. As improvements continue to spread to developing countries, CVD mortality rates are increasing.

Known as the epidemiological transition, this shift is highly correlated with changes in personal and collective wealth (the economic transition), social structure (the social transition), and demographics (the demographic transition). Omran (1971) provides an excellent model of the epidemiological transition that divides it into three basic ages: pestilence and famine, receding pandemics, and degenerative and human-created diseases (table 33.1). Olshansky and Ault (1986) add a fourth stage: delayed degenerative diseases.

The consistent pattern for most high-income countries going through the epidemiological transition has been initially high rates of stroke, mostly hemorrhagic. Only in the third phase, with the presence of increased resources, but coupled with increased diabetes and smoking rates and adverse lipid profiles, do rates of IHD climb. This phase is also accompanied by better control of severe hypertension, reducing the rates of hemorrhagic stroke, which is then replaced by ischemic stroke. Most regions appear to be following this pattern and have a predominance of IHD. The two exceptions are East Asia and the Pacific and Sub-Saharan Africa. The pattern in East Asia and the Pacific is dominated by China and appears to be a result of China's stage in the transition but may also be following a pattern similar to Japan's—that is, dominated by more strokes and fewer IHD deaths—whereas Sub-Saharan Africa is in an earlier phase of the epidemiological transition.

Even though countries tend to enter these stages at different times, the progression from one stage to the next tends to proceed in a predictable manner. The six World Bank regions are at various phases of the epidemiological transition (table 33.1), and where development has occurred, it has often been at a more compressed rate than in the high-income countries. Although rates of IHD and stroke fell 2 to 3 percent per year in the high-income countries during the 1970s and 1980s, the rate of decline has since slowed. Overweight and obesity are escalating at an alarming pace, while rates of type 2 diabetes, hypertension, and lipid abnormalities associated with obesity are on the rise. This trend is not unique to the developed countries, however. According to the World Health Organization, worldwide more than 1 billion adults are overweight and 300 million are clinically obese. Even more disturbing are increases in childhood obesity that have led to large increases in diabetes and hypertension. If these trends continue, age-adjusted CVD mortality rates could increase in the high-income countries in the coming years. These trends are discussed in greater detail in chapter 45.

Table 33.1 Stages of the Epidemiological Transition and Its Global Status, by Region

Stage	Description	Life expectancy (years)	Dominant form of CVD	Percentage of deaths attributable to CVD	Percentage of the world's population in this stage	Regions affected
Pestilence and famine	Predominance of malnutrition and infectious diseases	35	RHD, cardiomyopathy caused by infection and malnutrition	5–10	11	Sub-Saharan Africa, parts of all regions excluding high-income regions
Receding pandemics	Improved nutrition and public health leads to increase in chronic diseases, hypertension	50	Rheumatic valvular disease, IHD, hemorrhagic stroke	15–35	38	South Asia, southern East Asia and the Pacific, parts of Latin America and the Caribbean
Degenerative and human-created diseases	Increased fat and caloric intake, widespread tobacco use, chronic disease deaths exceed mortality from infections and malnutrition	60	IHD, stroke (ischemic and hemorrhagic)	>50	35	Europe and Central Asia, northern East Asia and the Pacific, Latin America and the Caribbean, Middle East and North Africa, and urban parts of most low-income regions (especially India)
Delayed degenerative diseases	CVD and cancer are leading causes of morbidity and mortality, prevention and treatment avoids death and delays onset; age-adjusted CVD declines	>70	IHD, stroke (ischemic and hemorrhagic), CHF	<50	15	High-income countries, parts of Latin America and the Caribbean

Source: Adapted from Olshanksy and Ault 1986; Omran 1971; WHO 2003b.

Risk Factors

The risk of developing CVD depends to a large extent on the presence of several risk factors. The major risk factors for CVD include tobacco use, high blood pressure, high blood glucose, lipid abnormalities, obesity, and physical inactivity. The global variations in CVD rates are related to temporal and regional variations in these known risk factors. Discussions of the strength of the associations of the various factors with CVD are found elsewhere (chapters 30, 44, and 45). Although some risk factors, such as age, ethnicity, and gender, obviously cannot be modified, most of the risk is attributable to lifestyle and behavioral patterns, which can be changed.

BURDEN OF DISEASE

CVD is the leading cause of death in all World Bank regions with the exception of Sub-Saharan Africa (figure 33.1), where HIV/AIDS has emerged as the leading cause of mortality (Mathers and others 2006). Between 1990 and 2020, IHD is anticipated to increase by 120 percent for women and 137 percent for men in developing countries, compared with age-related increases of 30 to 60 percent in developed countries (Leeder and others 2004). Even though 80 percent of CVD deaths occur in low- and middle-income countries, the death rates for most regions are still below the rate for high-income countries, which is 320 per 100,000 population annually. The marked exception is Europe and Central Asia, which has a rate of 690 CVD deaths per 100,000 population.

Regional Burdens

The majority of the burden occurs in East Asia and the Pacific, Europe and Central Asia, and South Asia because a large pro-

portion of the world's population lives in East Asia and the Pacific and South Asia and the incidence of IHD is high in Europe and Central Asia.

East Asia and the Pacific. The status and character of the epidemiological transition across the region reflects the diversity of economic circumstances in East Asia and the Pacific. Since the 1950s, life expectancy in China has nearly doubled from 37 years to 71 years (WHO 2003b). Approximately 60 percent of the population still lives outside urban centers, and as is the case in most developing countries, rates of IHD, stroke, and hypertension are higher in urban centers. China appears to be straddling the second and third stages of a Japanese-style epidemiological transition, with CVD rates higher than 35 percent, though dominated by stroke, not IHD. However, in urban China, the death rate from IHD rose by 53 percent from 1988 to 1996.

Europe and Central Asia. The emerging market economies, which consist of the former socialist states of Europe, are largely in the third phase of the epidemiological transition. As a group, they have the highest rates of CVD mortality in the world, similar to those seen in the United States in the 1960s when CVD was at its peak. Belarus, Croatia, Kazakhstan, Romania, and Ukraine have seen significant increases in IHD death rates (figure 33.2). In the Russian Federation, life expectancy for men has dropped precipitously since 1986 from 71.6 years to about 59 years in 2004, in large part because of CVD. In the Czech Republic, Hungary, Poland, and Slovenia, age-adjusted CVD rates have been declining. Nevertheless, CVD rates generally remain higher than in Western Europe.

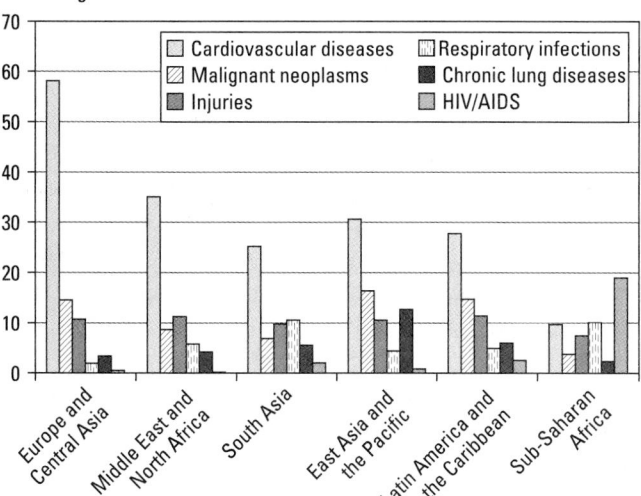

Percentage of total deaths

Source: Mathers and others 2006.

Figure 33.1 Major Causes of Death in Persons of All Ages in Low- and Middle-Income Regions

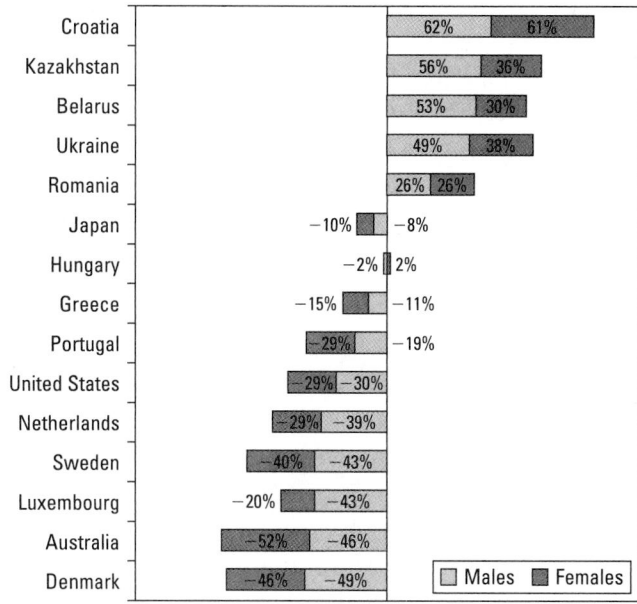

Source: Mackay and Mensah 2004.

Figure 33.2 Percentage Change in Ischemic Heart Disease Death Rates in People Age 35 to 74, 1988–98, Selected Countries

Latin America and the Caribbean. In 2001, CVD accounted for about 31 percent of all deaths in Latin America and the Caribbean, but that figure is expected to rise to 38 percent by 2020 (Murray and Lopez 1996). In recent decades, average life expectancy in Latin America and the Caribbean has risen from 51 to 71 years, and the quality of nutrition has improved steadily. At the same time, the region has seen a switch from vegetables as a source of protein to animal protein and an increase in fat intake as a percentage of energy. As a whole, the region seems to be in the third phase, but in South America, some areas are still in the first phase of the transition.

Middle East and North Africa. Increasing economic wealth in the Middle East and North Africa has been characteristically accompanied by urbanization. The rate of CVD has been increasing rapidly and is now the leading cause of death, accounting for 25 to 45 percent of total deaths. Over the past few decades, daily per capita fat consumption has increased in most countries in the region, ranging from a 13.6 percent increase in Sudan to a 143.3 percent increase in Saudi Arabia (Musaiger 2002). IHD is the predominant cause of CVD, with about three IHD deaths for every stroke death. RHD remains a major cause of morbidity and mortality, but the number of hospitalizations for RHD is declining rapidly.

South Asia. Some regions of India appear to be in the first phase of the transition, whereas others are in the second or even the third phase. Nonetheless, India is experiencing an alarming increase in heart disease, which seems to be linked to changes in lifestyle and diet, rapid urbanization, and possibly an underlying genetic component. Diabetes is also a major health issue. India has 31.6 million diabetics, and the number is expected to reach 57.2 million by 2025 (Ghaffar, Reddy, and Singhi 2004). The World Health Organization estimates that, by 2010, 60 percent of the world's cardiac patients will be in India. About 50 percent of CVD-related deaths occur among people younger than 70, compared with about 22 percent in the West. Between 2000 and 2030, about 35 percent of all CVD deaths in India will occur among those age 35 to 64, compared with only 12 percent in the United States and 22 percent in China (Leeder and others 2004).

Sub-Saharan Africa. In Sub-Saharan Africa, deaths attributable to CVD are projected to more than double in between the years 1990 and 2020. Although HIV/AIDS is the leading overall cause of death in this region, CVD is the second-leading killer and is the first among those over the age of 30. Stroke is the dominant form, in keeping with patterns characteristic of earlier phases of the epidemiological transition. With increasing urbanization, levels of average daily physical activity are falling and smoking rates are increasing. Hypertension has emerged as a major public health concern, and hypertensive

disease accounts for the dominance of stroke (Bertrand 1999). RHD and cardiomyopathies, the latter caused mostly by malnutrition, various viral illnesses, and parasitic organisms, are also important causes of CVD mortality and morbidity.

Social and Economic Impact

Leeder and others' (2004) report highlights the economic impact of cardiovascular diseases in developing economies, which arises largely because working-age adults account for a high proportion of the CVD burden. Conservative estimates in Brazil, China, India, Mexico, and South Africa indicate that each year at least 21 million years of future productive life are lost because of CVD. In South Africa, for example, costs for the direct treatment of CVD were equivalent to 2 to 3 percent of gross domestic product, or roughly 25 percent of all health care expenditures (Pestana and others 1996).

Current expenditures in developed countries are indicators of possible future expenditure in developing countries. For example, Hodgson and others (2001) estimated that in 2003 the direct and indirect costs of CVD in the United States would amount to US$350 billion. They also estimated that in 1998 Americans spent US$109 billion on hypertension, equivalent to about 13 percent of the health care budget. Studies are limited but suggest that obesity-related diseases are responsible for 2 to 8 percent of all health care expenditures in developed countries.

COST-EFFECTIVENESS OF INTERVENTIONS

CVD remains one of the most studied and written about subjects in medicine. As a result, many interventions exist with strong evidence for significant reductions in morbidity and mortality associated with CVD.

Intervention Effectiveness by Disease

This chapter addresses those interventions believed to have the largest effect because they result in large reductions in CVD events, are inexpensive, or the prevalence or incidence of the diseases to which they are directed is significant. The omission of an intervention does not imply that it is not cost-effective but rather that either it had an effect on a smaller percentage of people or the chapter was unable to encompass all such interventions.

Acute Myocardial Infarction. Treatment of AMI involves medical therapies that reduce myocardial oxygen demand and fatal arrhythmias (beta-blockers), that restore blood flow by inhibiting platelet aggregation (aspirin), or that dissolve the thrombus occluding the arterial lumen (thrombolytics) or an invasive intervention with cardiac catheterization and angioplasty.

Beta-blockers are used both during and after an AMI. Benefits persist for at least 6 years and up to 15 years after the first AMI. The second Thrombolysis in Myocardial Infarction trial showed significant benefits when beta-blockers were used within two hours of symptoms (Roberts and others 1991).

Aspirin, an antiplatelet agent, and thrombolytic agents, the standard treatments for reopening the artery in AMI, have demonstrated an additive effect in reducing mortality (GISSI 1986), with a benefit irrespective of age, sex, blood pressure, heart rate, or previous history of AMI or diabetes (Fibrinolytic Therapy Trialists' Collaborative Group 1994). The benefits are greater the closer the thrombolytics are given to the time of onset, and the risk of bleeding is greater the later they are given. The risk of adverse events following administration of thrombolytics is low during the first 24 hours; trials with thrombolytics show that the benefits are greatest when they are administered less than 12 hours after an AMI and preferably less than 6 hours (Antman and others 2004).

The invasive alternative to immediate medical reperfusion of an occluded coronary artery is angioplasty or percutaneous coronary intervention. Its superiority over thrombolysis in developed countries remains a matter of debate. Issues that remain important in relation to the choice of strategy are overall severity or location of the AMI and the time from symptom onset to initiation of treatment. In patients presenting late or with a high risk of mortality, such as those in cardiogenic shock, percutaneous coronary intervention may be beneficial (Hochman and others 1999). However, as with thrombolytic agents, the benefits of percutaneous coronary intervention diminish significantly with time between the onset of symptoms and the opening of the artery (De Luca and others 2004; D. O. Williams 2004).

The invasive strategy requires a facility and individual physicians who conduct enough of the procedures annually to remain proficient. In the absence of these conditions, the American Heart Association recommends that treatment focus on thrombolytics (Antman and others 2004). Given either a lack of facilities and operators for percutaneous interventions or long distances to such facilities in many developing countries, we did not evaluate this procedure.

Long-Term Management of Existing Vascular Disease. The management of individuals with chronic vascular disease consists of invasive techniques, pharmacotherapy, lifestyle and behavioral changes, and rehabilitative measures. It also involves addressing such issues as adherence to treatment, regular follow-ups to determine compliance and assess risk, and treatment of comorbidities that are likely to have an impact on the progression of vascular disease (for instance, renal disease).

Invasive Interventions The three most common procedures are coronary artery bypass graft (CABG), percutaneous trans-luminal coronary angioplasty (PTCA), and PTCA with stents. CABG is the placement of grafts, usually from the saphenous vein or internal mammary artery, to bypass stenosed coronary arteries while maintaining cerebral and peripheral circulation by cardiopulmonary bypass. CABG is a major operative procedure requiring appropriate surgical and anesthetic environments and has a perioperative mortality of 1 to 3 percent, with later complication rates of 15 to 20 percent.

Almost 1 million CABGs per year are performed worldwide, with about 519,000 interventions in the United States alone in 2000 (American Heart Association 2002). The main indication for CABG is for those with left main coronary artery stenosis or those with involvement of multiple coronary arteries with reduced left ventricular function, particularly among diabetics. The prevalence estimates of those with left main coronary artery stenosis or involvement of three coronary arteries has varied over time, but current estimates range from 7 to 20 percent of survivors of myocardial infarction (Kuntz and others 1996; Rogers and others 1991; Topol, Holmes, and Rogers 1991) For these cases, investigators have shown that CABG is more beneficial than medical treatment, both in terms of symptoms and of mortality (Eagle and others 1999).

Both developed and developing countries are increasingly using PTCA (Denbow and others 1997). The main indications for its use are low-risk patients with single- or double-vessel disease and poor response to medical treatment. The success rate of PTCA is more than 95 percent; however, because it has no mortality benefit when compared with medical therapy or CABG, we did not evaluate new analyses of the cost-effectiveness of this intervention, but instead provided information from experience in developed countries. The addition of stents to PTCA has lead to a decrease in restenosis rates and readmissions to hospitals but shows no change in mortality compared with medical therapy.

Pharmacological Interventions The pharmacological interventions either prevent thrombosis, as does aspirin, or target the individual risk factors, as do the antihypertensives (diuretics, beta-blockers, and ACE inhibitors) or statins targeting cholesterol. Furthermore, these agents may possibly have additional properties of reducing the risk of fatal arrhythmias, improving repair after AMI (remodeling), or stabilizing the atherosclerotic plaque.

Overall, the long-term administration of antiplatelet agents in those with vascular disease leads to a 25 percent reduction in the risk of major vascular events: 33 percent for nonfatal AMI, 25 percent for nonfatal stroke, and 16 percent for any vascular death. The use of aspirin has produced similar benefits in individuals with IHD or prior stroke. Antiplatelet treatment in individuals with a previous AMI has been shown to prevent 18 nonfatal myocardial infarctions, 5 nonfatal strokes, and 14 vascular deaths for every 1,000 patients treated for two years (Antithrombotic Trialists' Collaboration 2002).

The benefits of antiplatelet agents for those with vascular disease far outweigh the risks. The risk of intracranial bleeding increases by nearly 25 percent with the use of antiplatelet agents, but in absolute terms this risk comes to only one or two intracranial bleeds per 1,000 patients treated per year. The risk of major extracranial bleeding, mostly gastrointestinal, also increases by 60 percent, or one or two excess events per 1,000 patients per year.

The most established and commonly used agent is aspirin, although other agents (for example, clopidogrel or ticlopidine) with similar efficacy but much greater cost are available. Low doses of aspirin—75 to 100 milligrams (mg) per day—are as beneficial as higher doses.

Lowering LDL and elevating HDL cholesterol levels is one of the cornerstones of treatment of cardiovascular disease, and investigators have suggested that suboptimal levels of cholesterol contribute to almost two-thirds of the global cardiovascular risk (WHO 2002b). Although the usual target of lipid-lowering therapy has been lowering total or LDL cholesterol, medical experts are increasingly recognizing the importance of increasing HDL cholesterol and lowering triglyceride levels, especially in high-risk individuals, such as those with diabetes or metabolic syndrome, as well as in ethnic populations like Southeast Asians.

Recent evidence has demonstrated that the relationship between cholesterol levels and vascular events is continuous and occurs at much lower cholesterol thresholds than previously believed. The clinical trials have consistently demonstrated a 25 to 30 percent reduction in the risk of cardiovascular morbidity and mortality. Furthermore, the evidence suggests that more aggressive reductions in cholesterol have higher benefits than mild or moderate reductions (Cannon and others 2004; Knatterud and others 2000). No increased risk of cancers appears to exist, as was previously believed, although a small increase exists in the risk of inflammation of noncardiac muscle (myopathy) (Pfeffer and others 2002).

As with cholesterol, the relationship between blood pressure and vascular events is continuous and is discussed further in chapter 45. Even patients with presumed "normal" blood pressure and prior vascular disease benefit from lowering blood pressure (Nissen and others 2004), confirming earlier evidence that individuals with a history of AMI who have lower blood pressure are less likely to have future vascular events. Furthermore, investigators have established mortality and morbidity benefits for several specific classes of drugs to reduce blood pressure in patients with vascular disease, namely, beta-blockers, calcium-channel blockers, and ACE inhibitors (Fox 2003).

In patients with a prior history of stroke or transient ischemic attack (transient occlusion of artery supplying the brain), the long-term benefits of lowering blood pressure have been clearly established. Lowering blood pressure reduces the overall risk of future stroke by 28 percent and of other vascular events and CHF by 26 percent in patients with a history of stroke disease, irrespective of their hypertension status. The benefits are even more pronounced for individuals with a history of hemorrhagic stroke. Larger reductions in blood pressure confer greater benefits, and benefits are present across different age groups, genders, and ethnicities and with varying comorbid status.

Beta-blockers are one of the cornerstones of long-term treatment of individuals with IHD, especially those with a history of AMI. Long-term use of beta-blockers has been associated with 23 percent relative risk reduction in mortality (Freemantle and others 1999), 25 percent relative risk reduction in nonfatal myocardial infarction, and 30 percent relative risk reduction in sudden cardiac death (Yusuf and others 1985). The benefits are larger for those at highest risk of sustaining a vascular event in the future and are present across all age groups and sexes. Furthermore, beta-blockers provide clear benefits in patients with chronic stable angina, where they provide symptom relief as well as reductions in vascular events (Heidenreich and others 1999).

ACE inhibitors have proved invaluable in preventing cardiovascular events and CHF in those with IHD. The extent to which the benefits conferred by their use are caused by their ability to lower blood pressure or by their other properties, such as cardiac remodeling and neurohormonal modulation, is not clear. Long-term use of ACE inhibitors in those with a history of myocardial infarction and in other individuals at high risk of vascular disease reduces vascular mortality by 25 percent and other nonfatal events, such as recurrent myocardial infarction, revascularization, hospitalization, progression or new onset of CHF, and stroke (Teo and others 2002). In those with asymptomatic or symptomatic left ventricular dysfunction after myocardial infarction, ACE inhibitors reduce the risk of a variety of vascular endpoints by 20 to 26 percent. Similarly, the use of ACE inhibitors even in those with no evident left ventricular dysfunction confers a 21 percent reduction in risk for major coronary events (Dagenais and others 2001), 32 percent for stroke (Bosch and others 2002), and 20 to 22 percent for composite vascular outcomes (Fox 2003).

Nonpharmacological Interventions Cessation of smoking and dietary modifications are important goals of secondary prevention of CVD. Cardiac rehabilitation, including exercise, is useful for a wide range of patients with IHD and reduces future vascular events by about 15 percent. Exercise alone reduces vascular mortality by 24 percent and vascular endpoints by 15 percent (Jolliffe and others 2000). Results of trials for psychological interventions targeted at stress, depression, low social support, and so on have been conflicting.

Congestive Heart Failure. Diuretics are standard therapy for CHF, with the loop and thiazide diuretics most commonly used. Diuretics provide relief of symptoms more rapidly than any other CHF medication because they are the only drugs that can adequately control the fluid retention associated with CHF. Using spironolactone, a neurohormonal antagonist, together with a diuretic decreased the risk of mortality by 30 percent and of hospitalization by 35 percent, compared with a placebo in patients with severely advanced heart failure (Pitt and others 1999); however, this combination requires intensive monitoring of electrolytes and testing to follow patients and thus was not included in our cost-effectiveness analyses.

Investigators have shown that ACE inhibitors reduce risks related to a variety of endpoints, including mortality, hospitalization, major coronary events, deterioration of symptoms, and progression from asymptomatic to symptomatic left ventricular dysfunction, by 25 to 33 percent. The benefit is conferred irrespective of the etiology of systolic failure; begins soon after the start of treatment; persists over the long term; and is independent of age, sex, and baseline use of other medications. Furthermore, the use of ACE inhibitors has proved to be highly cost-effective in developed countries.

Beta-blockers improve symptoms, decrease hospitalization and deterioration of heart function, and improve mortality. They should be used even when the patient becomes asymptomatic. Beta-blockers are beneficial at all stages of CHF, reducing the morbidity and mortality associated with CHF by 25 to 33 percent. Because most patients with CHF die of sudden cardiac death, the protective effects of beta-blockers are probably related to their antiarrhythmic properties.

Digitalis decreases hospitalization rates in individuals with CHF but has no effect on vascular or total mortality (Digitalis Investigation Group 1997). Given that it also has a narrow therapeutic-toxic window and requires careful monitoring, its role in standard treatment for CHF has diminished and has not been included in our cost-effectiveness analyses.

Rheumatic Heart Disease. The management of patients with ARF includes providing antistreptococcal treatment, managing clinical manifestations, and screening children. In the acute stage, all patients with ARF should be treated as if they have a group A streptococcal infection—that is, with a 10-day course of penicillin. Anti-inflammatory agents provide symptomatic relief during ARF but do not prevent RHD. Secondary prophylaxis prevents colonization of the upper respiratory tract and consists of penicillin or sulfadiazine for the first five years (and for life for patients with valvular heart disease). Noncompliance is frequent, reaching rates as high as one-third of patients (Bassili and others 2000). Tertiary treatment entails surgery for valve replacement or valvuloplasty.

Linking Costs and Effectiveness in Developing Countries

Few intervention trials have been carried out solely in developing countries, but investigators have extrapolated estimates of cost-effectiveness ratios for the developing world in general based on changes in key input prices (Goldman and others 1991); however, this process is limited by the fact that both the underlying epidemiology and the costs can differ significantly across and within countries and regions. Thus, our results reflect models that used prices and epidemiological data for World Bank regions where applicable. Intervention effects were, however, based on systematic reviews of randomized trials or meta-analyses in developed countries. Until intervention trials are conducted in developing countries, this option remains the best for evaluating the cost-effectiveness of various interventions in the developing regions. In cases in which models for diseases in selected regions were not developed, we present results of cost-effectiveness analyses from high-income countries.

We used estimates of life expectancy for the model from data supplied by the volume editors. The model includes only the costs related to the intervention itself and to CVD events and their sequelae. Costs include personnel salaries, health care visits, diagnostic tests, and hospital stays as provided by the volume editors. Our analysis does not include indirect costs, such as those arising from lost work time or family assistance. Drug costs are from McFayden (2003). All are in U.S. dollars unless otherwise specified. Disability weights were taken from Mathers and others (2006).

Ischemic Heart Disease.

Acute Myocardial Infarction We evaluated four incremental strategies for the treatment of AMI and compared them with a strategy of no treatment as a base case. The four treatment strategies were aspirin (162.5 mg per day for 30 days); aspirin and atenolol (100 mg per day for 30 days); aspirin, atenolol, and streptokinase (1.5 million units); and aspirin, atenolol, and tissue plasminogen activator (100 mg accelerated regimen). Doses for the aspirin and streptokinase were those used by the Second International Study of Infarct Survival Collaborative Group (ISIS-2 Collaborative Group 1988), the atenolol regimen was that of the First International Study of Infarct Survival (ISIS-1 Collaborative Group 1986), and the tissue plasminogen activator dosing was that used in the Global Use of Strategies to Open Occluded Coronary Arteries (GUSTO)–I trial (GUSTO Investigators 1993). The relative risk of dying from AMI was reduced for all patients receiving the medications. Patients receiving the thrombolytics faced increased risks of major bleeds and hemorrhagic strokes. Because the effectiveness of streptokinase diminishes over time, we carried out two further sensitivity analyses to compare its use for patients over and under the age of 75 and for patients who receive the intervention sooner or later than six hours after the onset of symptoms.

Table 33.2 presents incremental cost-effectiveness ratios (ICERs) for each therapy by region. The incremental cost per DALY averted was less than US$25 for all six regions for the aspirin and aspirin plus atenolol interventions; US$634 to US$734 for aspirin, atenolol, and streptokinase; and slightly less than US$16,000 for aspirin, atenolol, and tissue plasminogen activator. Minor variations occurred between regions because of small differences in follow-up care costs. The results for an analysis that evaluated ICERs as cost per life year saved showed no significant differences.

Table 33.3 displays the results of the secondary analysis for streptokinase and tissue plasminogen activator. Giving the streptokinase sooner than six hours following onset reduces the incremental cost per DALY to less than US$440 compared with more than US$1,300 if given after six hours. Similar effects are seen when streptokinase is given to those under 75 compared with those 75 years or older.

According to meta-analyses, nitroglycerin has a modest effect on mortality in AMI: a 3 percent reduction. However, given that it can have profound effects on blood pressure that could limit the use of beta-blockers that confer more significant benefits, its use should be limited to patients with ongoing ischemic pain and systolic blood pressures greater than 90 millimeters of mercury who do not have ongoing right ventricular infarction. When modeled, it had a reasonable cost-effectiveness ratio of US$70 per life year saved, but we did not include the analysis in the incremental analysis because of the blood pressure effects of the multiple agents.

Secondary Prevention Four medical therapies—aspirin, beta-blockers, statins, and ACE inhibitors—have been the mainstay of treatment for those with IHD in the developed world. To evaluate the best medical intervention, we used incremental cost-effectiveness analysis to examine the 15 different possible combinations of the four standard medical therapies. The four therapies were 75 to 100 mg per day of aspirin, 100 mg per day of atenolol, 10 mg per day of enalapril, and 40 mg per day of lovastatin. In addition, CABG surgery provides an invasive option that gives added mortality benefit when compared with conventional medical therapy in patients with certain anatomical obstructions in coronary circulation. Thus, we evaluated CABG in addition to all four medications for those with left main coronary artery disease or with three-vessel coronary artery disease and reduced left ventricular function. Because these therapies also have significant effects on the incidence of stroke, we included the effect on DALYs and costs for stroke in the analyses.

In addition to the mortality benefits demonstrated by trials of the individual medications or surgery, they also resulted in significant reductions in hospitalizations in developed countries. The cost savings from these reduced hospitalizations make the cost-effectiveness of such interventions quite favor-

able in developed countries; however, given that hospital facilities may not be available to most patients in many developing regions, we undertook two separate analyses, one with hospital costs and one without.

In a setting where hospitals are available, a combination of aspirin and atenolol dominated no therapy and was cost saving in all regions (table 33.2). The ICERs for the addition of enalapril ranged from US$660 per DALY in Sub-Saharan Africa to US$866 per DALY in Europe and Central Asia. The combination of all four medications ranged from US$1,720 per DALY to US$2,026 per DALY. For CABG the costs per DALY ranged from about US$24,000 to more than US$72,000. Despite having similar benefits as aspirin and atenolol in relation to mortality, enalapril and lovastatin demonstrated higher per DALY costs because of the added costs of monitoring renal and liver function, respectively, as is required for these two medications.

When we assumed that hospitals were not readily available (table 33.2), no therapy combination was cost saving compared with no therapy. The combination of aspirin and atenolol was the next best strategy, with ICERs ranging from US$386 per DALY in South Asia to US$545 per DALY in Latin America and the Caribbean. The addition of enalapril increased the range of ICERs to US$783 per DALY to US$1,111 per DALY, and the addition of lovastatin increased them still further. CABG was not evaluated because of the underlying assumption that hospitals were not available.

Table 33.4 shows the number of events prevented with the four-drug combination medical therapy compared with no therapy and the additional number of events averted with CABG compared with the four-drug combination. The medical regimen alone would prevent some 2,000 CVD deaths, about 4,000 myocardial infarctions, and approximately 200 strokes per million persons treated in each region. The use of CABG in addition to the medical regimen would prevent an additional 65–70 deaths, nearly 300 myocardial infarctions, and up to 30 strokes per million population.

Congestive Heart Failure. The interventions examined for CHF were the addition of the ACE inhibitor enalapril, the beta-blocker metoprolol, or both to a baseline of diuretic treatment. As for the IHD interventions, we performed separate analyses for each assumption of whether or not hospital facilities would be available. For the model of treatment for CHF assuming hospitalization (table 33.2), the addition of enalapril is cost saving and the ICER for the addition of metoprolol ranges from US$124 to US$219 per DALY depending on the region. When the availability of hospitals is limited (table 33.2), the enalapril plus diuretics strategy is no longer cost saving, but it costs only US$31 per DALY or less, and the ICER for enalapril, metoprolol, and diuretics increases only to about US$275 per DALY. These figures are probably underestimates of the cost per

Table 33.2 ICERs for Treatment Compared with No Treatment, by Region
US$/DALY

Region	Medical therapy for AMI compared with baseline of no treatment				Medical therapy and CABG for IHD compared with baseline of no treatment, hospital access				Medical therapy and CABG for IHD compared with baseline of no treatment, limited hospital access			ACE inhibitors and beta-blockers for CHF compared with baseline of diuretics, hospital access		ACE inhibitors and beta-blockers for CHF compared with baseline of diuretics, limited hospital access	
	ASA	ASA, BB	ASA BB, SK	ASA, BB, TPA	ASA, BB	ASA, BB, ACEI	ASA, BB, ACEI, Statin	CABG	ASA, BB	ASA, BB, ACEI	ASA, BB, Statin	ACEI	ACEI, MET	ACEI	ACEI, MET
East Asia and the Pacific	13	15	672	15,867	Cost saving	781	1,914	33,846	461	942	2,220	Cost saving	189	27	274
Europe and Central Asia	19	21	722	15,878	Cost saving	866	2,026	47,942	530	1,097	2,470	Cost saving	144	30	275
Latin America and the Caribbean	20	22	734	15,887	Cost saving	821	1,942	62,426	545	1,111	2,497	Cost saving	124	31	275
Middle East and North Africa	17	20	715	15,893	Cost saving	672	1,686	72,345	527	996	2,305	Cost saving	128	29	275
South Asia	9	11	638	15,860	Cost saving	715	1,819	24,040	386	828	2,034	Cost saving	219	25	273
Sub-Saharan Africa	9	11	634	15,862	Cost saving	660	1,720	26,813	389	783	1,955	Cost saving	218	25	273

Source: Authors' calculations.

ASA = aspirin, BB = atenolol, SK = streptokinase, TPA = tissue plasminogen activator, ACEI = enalapril, Statin = lovastatin, MET = metoprolol.

Note: The intervention in the first column of each set of strategies is compared with the baseline; each successive intervention for each set of strategies is compared with the intervention immediately to its left.

Table 33.3 Sensitivity Analyses: Effect of Time to Treatment and Age on Use of Thrombolytics in AMI (All Regions Combined)

	SK[a] (US$/DALY)	TPA[a] (US$/DALY)
Time to thrombolysis		
<6 hours	374–437	15,800
6–12 hours	1,300–1,440	15,700
Age at treatment		
<75	559–650	14,800
75 or older	1,260–1,350	21,000

Source: Authors' calculations.
SK = streptokinase; TPA = tissue plasminogen activator.
a. In addition to aspirin and atenolol.

DALY, given some loss in the mortality benefit for the hospitalization that the model does not capture.

Rheumatic Heart Disease. For RHD, except in epidemics, secondary prevention is more effective than primary prevention. Primary prevention by means of antibiotic treatment of streptococcus infections of the pharynx is not highly cost-effective in endemic situations, given that only 10 to 20 percent of such infections are from streptococcus, less than 3 percent of these will evolve into rheumatic fever, and only a proportion of these continue on to RHD (Strasser 1985). The development of a rapid antigen test for diagnosing group A streptococcal pharyngitis may make primary prevention more cost-effective (Majeed and others 1993). Similarly, in an epidemic in which the proportion of infections from streptococcus is higher or the rate of progression to rheumatic fever is higher, primary prevention

may be cost-effective. Secondary prevention using benzathine penicillin injections is cost-saving according to Strasser (1985) and should be considered for all developing countries with the infrastructure to perform the required follow-up.

Cost-Effectiveness Analyses in High-Income Countries

Table 33.5 summarizes the results of cost-effectiveness analyses for CVD interventions in high-income countries. These results include analyses that are similar to ours. The differences are that they reflect costs and treatment patterns in the high-income countries studied, mostly the United States. Costs in developing countries are roughly one-fifth of those in developed countries (but closer to one-third in Latin America and approaching one-half in South Africa). However, where patented drugs are involved and patent laws are enforced, the costs may be much closer to U.S. levels.

Because the cost-effectiveness studies have been undertaken largely in the United States, the results do not always readily transfer to developing countries. In some U.S. studies, the alternative procedure considered is medical management; such facilities simply may not exist in developing countries. Similarly, interventions that are cost saving in the United States may not be cost saving in developing countries but may well be cost-effective in terms of cost per DALY saved. Furthermore, the cost-effectiveness analyses reflect morbidity and mortality rates in developed countries.

Interventions that Kupersmith and others (1995) classify as highly cost-effective in the United States (less than US$20,000 per life year saved or quality-adjusted life year saved) may be cost-effective in many developing countries. Interventions that

Table 33.4 Number of Deaths and CVD Events Prevented by the Use of a Four-Component Medical Regimen and CABG per 100,000 Myocardial Infarction Survivors over 10 Years, by Region

Region	Number of events prevented with four-component medical regimen compared with no therapy[a]				Number of incremental events prevented with CABG compared with medical therapy			
	IHD deaths averted	Stroke deaths averted	Myocardial infarctions prevented	Strokes prevented	IHD deaths averted	Stroke deaths averted	Myocardial infarctions prevented	Strokes prevented
East Asia and the Pacific	1,900	104	4,077	209	79	11	248	22
Europe and Central Asia	1,990	89	3,964	179	83	1	294	7
Latin America and the Caribbean	1,913	83	4,040	118	62	4	258	18
Middle East and North Africa	1,908	95	4,294	118	62	1	296	22
South Asia	1,930	97	4,043	122	34	2	275	30
Sub-Saharan Africa	1,909	91	4,233	173	69	12	254	1

Source: Authors' calculations.
a. Aspirin, atenolol, enalapril, and lovastatin.

Table 33.5 Cost-Effectiveness Analyses for CVD Interventions in High-Income Countries

Intervention	Alternative	Cost-effectiveness	Source
IHD			
Lovastatin, 20 mg/day	Diet	Cost saving (males age 45–54); US$4,700/life year saved (females age 45–54)	Goldman and others 1991[a]
Defibrillators in emergency vehicles	No defibrillators	US$47 to US$551/life year saved; up to US$2,600 in rural areas	Jermyn 2000; Ornato and others 1988; Rowley, Garner, and Hampton 1990[b]
Propranolol for postmyocardial infarction (beta-blocker)	No beta-blockers	US$2,400 for high-risk patients; US$23,400 for low-risk patients	Goldman and others 1988[a]
CABG for left main disease	Medical management	US$2,700 to US$6,700/life year saved	Weinstein and Stason 1982;[b] A. Williams 1985[a]
PTCA (men age 55 with severe angina)	Medical management	US$6,400 to US$8,800/life year saved (US$28,000 to US$132,000 for mild angina)	Wong and others 1990[b]
Primary angioplasty	No intervention after AMI	US$12,000/quality-adjusted life year	Parmley 1999
Three-vessel CABG	Medical management	US$14,000/life year saved	Weinstein and Stason 1982
Streptokinase (reperfusion), with PTCA available	No intervention after AMI	US$15,000/quality-adjusted life year	Parmley 1999
Tissue plasminogen activator (AMI)	Steptokinase	US$33,500/life year saved	Lorenzoni and others 1998
Primary stenting, one-vessel, men over age 55	PTCA	US$32,000/life year saved	Cohen and others 1993
Three-vessel CABG for severe angina	PTCA	US$41,000/life year saved	Wong and others 1990[b]
Two-vessel CABG	Medical management	US$33,000 to US$90,000/life year saved	Weinstein and Stason 1982; A. Williams 1985
Angiography for coronary artery disease	CABG	US$45,000/quality-adjusted life year	Doubilet, McNeil, and Weinstein 1985[a]
Stroke			
Anticoagulants (warfarin) for chronic nonvascular atrial fibrillation	Aspirin	Warfarin dominates for high-risk patients; US$10,000/quality-adjusted life year for medium-risk patients; US$462,000/quality-adjusted life year for low-risk patients	Gage, Cardinalli, and Owens 1998[c]
Anticoagulants for mitral stenosis and atrial fibrillation	No anticoagulants	US$5,500/quality-adjusted life year	Eckman, Levine, and Pauker 1992[c]
Carotid endarterectomy (symptomatic patients)	Aspirin	US$5,100 to US$51,000/life year saved	Kuntz and Kent 1996; Matchar, Pauk, and Lipscomb 1996[c]
Cardiac transplant	No transplant	US$54,000/life year saved	Evans 1986[a]
Arrhythmias			
Implantable cardioverter-defibrillator for cardiac arrest (long term)	Medical management	US$28,000/life year saved	King, Aubert, and Herman 1998; Kuppermann and others 1990
RHD			
Benzathine penicillin injections	No injections	Cost saving	Strasser 1985

Source: Authors.
Note: All costs have been converted to 2001 U.S. dollars.
a. Surveyed in Kupersmith and others 1995.
b. Surveyed in Tengs and others 1995.
c. Surveyed in Holloway and others 1999.

Kupersmith and others (1995) classify as cost-effective in the United States (US$20,000 to US$40,000 per life year saved or quality-adjusted life year saved) are probably borderline cost-effective for developing countries. Interventions that Kupersmith and others (1995) classify as borderline, expensive, or very expensive in the United States are unlikely to merit public funding in developing countries.

Thus, medical interventions that are likely to be cost-effective in developing countries include benzathine penicillin injections as secondary prevention for those who have had rheumatic fever (usually for five years); ACE inhibitors for CHF; and various drugs (beta-blockers, off-patent statins) for long-term care following a myocardial infarction, confirming our earlier analyses. Other therapies that are probably cost-effective but that we did not analyze include antithrombotic agents (aspirin, heparin) to prevent venous thromboembolism; anticoagulants for medium- and high-risk nonvalvular atrial fibrillation (stroke); and anticoagulants for mitral stenosis and atrial fibrillation (stroke).

Selected invasive interventions that might possibly be cost-effective for CVD in certain developing countries include pacemaker implants for atrioventricular heart block, primary angioplasty for acute myocardial infarction, and reperfusion with streptokinase. Of course, the ability to undertake these interventions assumes a cost-effective infrastructure for diagnosis and referral and an adequate volume of cases. For example, the American Heart Association recommends acute angioplasty in centers where the physician conducts at least 75 such procedures each year and the hospital conducts at least 200 per year. For stroke, carotid endarterectomy is potentially cost-effective for symptomatic patients compared with aspirin alone, again in an environment with an adequate volume of cases. Cost-effectiveness is much lower for asymptomatic cases.

Interventions that rank as cost-effective for heart disease in the U.S. context and that are borderline cost-effective in developing countries include implantable cardioverter-defibrillator for cardiac arrest, primary stenting for single-vessel disease (the study was for men over age 55), CABG for two-vessel disease, and angiography for patients with a high probability of coronary artery disease.

RESEARCH AND DEVELOPMENT

Even though most of the interventions currently available appear to be expensive and complex for developing countries, the demand for effective care for cardiovascular diseases will exert major pressure on health systems in coming decades. Increased use of these procedures is already documented in China and India (Murray and Lopez 1994, 1997; Unger 1999). In this context, cardiovascular research should be concentrated in the fields of primary prevention, health services, clinical guidelines, clinical research, and epidemiology.

Primary Prevention

Because the control of many cardiovascular risk factors is strongly related to the legislative environment—for example, that pertaining to tobacco use or nutrition—the design and implementation of appropriate laws and regulations is likely to increase in developing countries. However, any such initiatives need to be monitored and systematically evaluated, especially to estimate the magnitude of the reduction achieved.

Another area of research is the assessment of chemoprophylaxis in primary prevention. Multidrug combinations such as the hypothetical "polypill" are likely to be the first practical initiative of a long list of important innovations. Both the efficacy and the effectiveness of new interventions in primary prevention should be evaluated as a matter of urgency, because no results of large-scale clinical trials in developing countries are as yet available.

Health Services

Capacity building—more specifically, education and training—of health care workers in developing countries, is a major issue for the future, along with critical evaluations of the performance of health workers. Such evaluations should compare various capacity-building strategies; for instance, they could compare the delivery of simplified regimens of care by community health workers versus delivery of care by trained health professionals.

The dissemination of innovations deserves special attention in a context of scarce resources (Berwick 2003). The transfer of technologies to developing countries should be made on cost-effectiveness criteria, which implies analysis conducted in the specific situation of developing countries—for example, cost-effectiveness for thrombolytics in a developing country might be much worse than in the United States if getting to a hospital on time is a problem. Sensitivity analysis of the cost-effectiveness of surgical and medical interventions in developing countries is also needed.

Furthermore, the appropriate incentives for technological changes in health care should be investigated (McClellan and Kessler 1999). This line of research includes analyses of the pricing of technologies (including drugs) or of new designs for services, such as point-of-care devices for use by community health workers.

The long period of incubation of CVD opens up opportunities for extensive screening based on preclinical signs and biomarkers. However, strong lines of research are needed to secure effective and safe screening programs and should include opportunistic screening for places where visits to health centers are limited.

Finally, all assessments made in relation to health services research should take into account the costs related to scaling up any procedure evaluated.

Clinical Guidelines

The diffusion of health technologies usually leads to a widening of the clinical indication beyond the evidence-based scope of the intervention (PTCA is a classic example) (Dravik 1998), corresponding to a decrease not only in the procedure's efficacy, but also in its effectiveness (Anderson and Lomas 1988; Blustein 1993). Several studies suggest that overuse and underuse tend to coexist in the same community and that even severe scarcity of resources does not protect against overuse of cardiological interventions, at least among certain segments of the population (Joorabchi 1979; Soumerai and others 1997).

The consequences of such trends are more dramatic in developing than developed countries. Therefore, the introduction of costly care should be accompanied by a corresponding effort in relation to the provision of formal education to providers and prescribers, complemented by the development of clinical guidelines aimed at avoiding both the overuse and the underuse of procedures.

Clinical guidelines are already numerous, but all have been established in affluent countries. A new, specific effort should be made in developing countries to address local issues, such as problems related to the availability of procedures or drugs or to accessibility of services, and the development and maintenance of these guidelines should follow best available standards.

Clinical Research

In most situations, health care innovations should be introduced as experimental interventions to permit proper monitoring and evaluation. These experiments do not have to address the efficacy of the procedure (many innovations will already have been tested), but rather issues pertaining to their effectiveness and efficiency in the specific context of developing countries.

Another reason for the experimental approach is the rapidity with which the field of CVD is evolving. It is not reasonable, at the local level, to wait until the publication of trial results and meta-analyses, which often takes place years after changes have occurred in everyday practice. For this reason, a new culture of clinical research should be developed in which every innovation should be taken as an opportunity for systematic experimental evaluation.

Among various topics in clinical research, adherence deserves special mention. On average, 50 percent of patients in developed countries do not take their prescribed medicines after one year, despite having full access to medicines. In developing countries, this poor adherence is made worse by poor access to health services and drugs, to lack of education, and to other factors (Bovet and others 2002; WHO 2003a). Options for improving adherence should be designed and experimented with.

Epidemiological Research

A basic task of epidemiological research is to assess geographic and secular trends in the distribution of risk factors. Of special relevance is the movement from regional to country levels and the trend within a country. The impact of poor health status in early life should be assessed from the impact of poor fetal health to the consequence of multiple childhood infections on the risk for CVD. Because of the scarce availability of resources, the development and maintenance of health care should be supported by a comprehensive information system. Simple, affordable health information systems are preferable along the lines of the framework developed by the World Health Organization.

CONCLUSIONS: PITFALLS AND PROMISES

A global CVD epidemic is rapidly evolving, and the burden of disease is shifting. Twice as many deaths from CVD now occur in developing as in developed countries. The vast majority of CVD can be attributed to conventional risk factors. Even in Sub-Saharan Africa, high blood pressure, high cholesterol, extensive tobacco and alcohol use, and low vegetable and fruit consumption are already among the top risk factors for disease. Because of the time lag associated with CVD risk factors, especially in children, the full effect of exposure to these factors will be seen only in the future. Information from more than 100 countries shows that more 13- to 15-year-olds smoke than ever before, and studies show that obesity levels in children are increasing markedly in countries as diverse as Brazil, China, India, and almost all island states (Leeder and others 2004). Populationwide efforts now to reduce risk factors through multiple economic and educational policies and programs will reap savings later in medical and other direct costs as well as indirectly in terms of improved quality of life and economic productivity.

REFERENCES

American Heart Association. 2002. *Heart Disease and Stroke Statistics—2003 Update.* http://www.americanheart.org/downloadable/heart/10461207852142003HDSStatsBook.pdf.

Anderson, G. M., and J. Lomas. 1988. "Monitoring the Diffusion of a Technology: Coronary Artery Bypass Surgery in Ontario." *American Journal of Public Health* 78 (3): 251–54.

Antithrombotic Trialists' Collaboration. 2002. "Collaborative Meta-analysis of Randomised Trials of Antiplatelet Therapy for Prevention of Death, Myocardial Infarction, and Stroke in High Risk Patients." *British Medical Journal* 324 (7329): 71–86.

Antman, E. M., D. T. Anbe, P. W. Armstrong, E. R. Bates, L. A. Green, M. Hand, and others. 2004. "ACC/AHA Guidelines for the Management of Patients with ST-Elevation Myocardial Infarction—Executive Summary: A Report of the American College of Cardiology/American Heart Association Task Force on Practice Guidelines (Writing Committee to Revise the 1999 Guidelines for the Management of Patients with Acute Myocardial Infarction)." *Circulation* 110 (5): 588–636.

Bassili, A., S. R. Zaher, A. Zaki, M. Abdel-Fattah, and G. Tognoni. 2000. "Profile of Secondary Prophylaxis among Children with Rheumatic Heart Disease in Alexandria, Egypt." *Eastern Mediterranean Health Journal* 6 (2–3): 437–46.

Bertrand, E. 1999. "Cardiovascular Disease in Developing Countries." In *Cardiology*, ed. S. Dalla Volta. New York: McGraw-Hill.

Berwick, D. M. 2003. "Disseminating Innovations in Health Care." *Journal of the American Medical Association* 289 (15): 1969–75.

Blustein, J. 1993. "High-Technology Cardiac Procedures. The Impact of Service Availability on Service Use in New York State." *Journal of the American Medical Association* 270 (3): 344–49.

Bosch, J., S. Yusuf, J. Pogue, P. Sleight, E. Lonn, B. Rangoonwala, and others. 2002. "Use of Ramipril in Preventing Stroke: Double Blind Randomised Trial." *British Medical Journal* 324 (7339): 699–702.

Bovet, P., M. Burnier, G. Madeleine, B. Waeber, and F. Paccaud. 2002. "Monitoring One-Year Compliance to Antihypertension Medication in the Seychelles." *Bulletin of the World Health Organization* 80 (1): 33–39.

Cannon, C. P., E. Braunwald, C. H. McCabe, D. J. Rader, J. L. Rouleau, R. Belder, and others. 2004. "Intensive versus Moderate Lipid Lowering with Statins after Acute Coronary Syndromes." *New England Journal of Medicine* 350 (15): 1495–504.

Carapetis, J. R., B. J. Currie, and E. L. Kaplan. 1999. "Epidemiology and Prevention of Group A Streptococcal Infections: Acute Respiratory Tract Infections, Skin Infections, and Their Sequelae at the Close of the Twentieth Century." *Clinical Infectious Diseases* 28 (2): 205–10.

Cohen, D. J., J. A. Breall, K. K. Ho, R. M. Weintraub, R. E. Kuntz, M. C. Weinstein, and others. 1993. "Economics of Elective Coronary Revascularization. Comparison of Costs and Charges for Conventional Angioplasty, Directional Atherectomy, Stenting, and Bypass Surgery." *Journal of the American College of Cardiology* 22 (4): 1052–59.

Dagenais, G. R., S. Yusuf, M. G. Bourassa, Q. Yi, J. Bosch, E. M. Lonn, and others. 2001. "Effects of Ramipril on Coronary Events in High-Risk Persons: Results of the Heart Outcomes Prevention Evaluation Study." *Circulation* 104 (5): 522–26.

De Luca, G., H. Suryapranata, J. P. Ottervanger, and E. M. Antman. 2004. "Time Delay to Treatment and Mortality in Primary Angioplasty for Acute Myocardial Infarction: Every Minute of Delay Counts." *Circulation* 109 (10): 1223–25.

Denbow, C. E., E. E. Chung, W. Foster, H. Gist, and R. E. Vlietstra. 1997. "Percutaneous Transluminal Coronary Angioplasty (PTCA) in Jamaica. Preliminary Results." *West Indian Medical Journal* 46 (4): 115–19.

Digitalis Investigation Group. 1997. "The Effect of Digoxin on Mortality and Morbidity in Patients with Heart Failure." *New England Journal of Medicine* 336 (8): 525–33.

Doubilet, P., B. J. McNeil, and M. C. Weinstein. 1985. "The Decision Concerning Coronary Angiography in Patients with Chest Pain: A Cost-Effectiveness Analysis." *Medical Decision Making* 5 (3): 293–309.

Dravik, V. 1998. "PTCA Increase." *Canadian Journal of Cardiology* 14 (Suppl. A): 27A–31A.

Eagle, K. A., R. A. Guyton, R. Davidoff, G. A. Ewy, J. Fonger, T. J. Gardner, and others. 1999. "ACC/AHA Guidelines for Coronary Artery Bypass Graft Surgery: Executive Summary and Recommendations—A Report of the American College of Cardiology/American Heart Association Task Force on Practice Guidelines (Committee to Revise the 1991 Guidelines for Coronary Artery Bypass Graft Surgery)." *Circulation* 100 (13): 1464–80.

Eckman, M. H., H. J. Levine, and S. G. Pauker. 1992. "Decision Analytic and Cost-Effectiveness Issues Concerning Anticoagulant Prophylaxis in Heart Disease." *Chest* 102 (4 Suppl.): 538S–549S.

Ephrem, D., B. Abegaz, and L. Muhe. 1990. "Profile of Cardiac Diseases in Ethiopian Children." *East African Medical Journal* 67 (2): 113–17.

Evans, R. W. 1986. "Cost-Effectiveness Analysis of Transplantation." *Surgical Clinics of North America* 66 (3): 603–16.

Fibrinolytic Therapy Trialists' Collaborative Group. 1994. "Indications for Fibrinolytic Therapy in Suspected Acute Myocardial Infarction: Collaborative Overview of Early Mortality and Major Morbidity Results from All Randomised Trials of More Than 1,000 Patients. Fibrinolytic Therapy Trialists' (FTT) Collaborative Group." *Lancet* 343 (8893): 311–22.

Fox, K. M. 2003. "Efficacy of Perindopril in Reduction of Cardiovascular Events among Patients with Stable Coronary Artery Disease: Randomised, Double-Blind, Placebo-Controlled, Multicentre Trial (the EUROPA Study)." *Lancet* 362 (9386): 782–88.

Freemantle, N., J. Cleland, P. Young, J. Mason, and J. Harrison. 1999. "Beta Blockade after Myocardial Infarction: Systematic Review and Meta Regression Analysis." *British Medical Journal* 318 (7200): 1730–37.

Gage, B. F., A. B. Cardinalli, and D. K. Owens. 1998. "Cost-Effectiveness of Preference-Based Antithrombotic Therapy for Patients with Nonvalvular Atrial Fibrillation." *Stroke* 29 (6): 1083–91.

Ghaffar, A., K. S. Reddy, and M. Singhi. 2004. "Burden of Non-communicable Diseases in South Asia." *British Medical Journal* 328 (7443): 807–10.

GISSI (Gruppo Italiano per lo Studio della Streptochinasi nell'Infarto Miocardico). 1986. "Effectiveness of Intravenous Thrombolytic Treatment in Acute Myocardial Infarction. Gruppo Italiano per lo Studio della Streptochinasi nell'Infarto Miocardico (GISSI)." *Lancet* 1 (8478): 397–402.

Goldman, L., S. T. Sia, E. F. Cook, J. D. Rutherford, and M. C. Weinstein. 1988. "Costs and Effectiveness of Routine Therapy with Long-Term Beta-Adrenergic Antagonists after Acute Myocardial Infarction." *New England Journal of Medicine* 319 (3): 152–57.

Goldman, L., M. C. Weinstein, P. A. Goldman, and L. W. Williams. 1991. "Cost-Effectiveness of HMG-CoA Reductase Inhibition for Primary and Secondary Prevention of Coronary Heart Disease." *Journal of the American Medical Association* 265 (9): 1145–51.

GUSTO (Global Use of Strategies to Open Occluded Coronary Arteries) Investigators. 1993. "An International Randomized Trial Comparing Four Thrombolytic Strategies for Acute Myocardial Infarction." *New England Journal of Medicine* 329 (10): 673–82.

Heidenreich, P. A., K. M. McDonald, T. Hastie, B. Fadel, V. Hagan, B. K. Lee, and others. 1999. "Meta-analysis of Trials Comparing Beta-Blockers, Calcium Antagonists, and Nitrates for Stable Angina." *Journal of the American Medical Association* 281 (20): 1927–36.

Hochman, J. S., L. A. Sleeper, J. G. Webb, T. A. Sanborn, H. D. White, J. D. Talley, and others. 1999. "Early Revascularization in Acute Myocardial Infarction Complicated by Cardiogenic Shock." *New England Journal of Medicine* 341 (9): 625–34.

Hodgson, T. A., and L. Cai. 2001. "Medical Care Expenditures for Hypertension, its Complications, and its Comorbidities." *Medical Care* 39 (6): 599–615.

Holloway, R. G., C. G. Benesch, C. R. Rahilly, and C. E. Courtright. 1999. "A Systematic Review of Cost-Effectiveness Research of Stroke Evaluation and Treatment." *Stroke* 30 (7): 1340–49.

ISIS-1 (First International Study of Infarct Survival) Collaborative Group. 1986. "Randomised Trial of Intravenous Atenolol among 16,027 Cases of Suspected Acute Myocardial Infarction: ISIS-1 (First International Study of Infarct Survival Collaborative Group)." *Lancet* 2 (8498): 57–66.

ISIS-2 (Second International Study of Infarct Survival) Collaborative Group. 1988. "Randomised Trial of Intravenous Streptokinase, Oral Aspirin, Both, or Neither among 17,187 Cases of Suspected Acute Myocardial Infarction: ISIS-2. ISIS-2 (Second International Study of Infarct Survival) Collaborative Group." *Lancet* 2 (8607): 349–60.

Jermyn, B. D. 2000. "Cost-Effectiveness Analysis of a Rural/Urban First-Responder Defibrillation Program." *Prehospital Emergency Care* 4 (1): 43–47.

Jolliffe, J. A., K. Rees, R. S. Taylor, D. Thompson, N. Oldridge, and S. Ebrahim. 2000. "Exercise-Based Rehabilitation for Coronary

Heart Disease." *Cochrane Database of Systematic Reviews* (4) CD001800.

Joorabchi, B. 1979. "The Emergence of Cardiac Nondisease among Children in Iran." *Israel Journal of Medical Sciences* 15 (3): 202–6.

Kaplan, E. L. 1985. "Epidemiological Approaches to Understanding the Pathogenesis of Rheumatic Fever." *International Journal of Epidemiology* 14 (4): 499–501.

King, H., R. E. Aubert, and W. H. Herman. 1998. "Global Burden of Diabetes, 1995–2025: Prevalence, Numerical Estimates, and Projections." *Diabetes Care* 21 (9): 1414–31.

Knatterud, G. L., Y. Rosenberg, L. Campeau, N. L. Geller, D. B. Hunninghake, S. A. Forman, and others. 2000. "Long-Term Effects on Clinical Outcomes of `Aggressive Lowering of Low-Density Lipoprotein Cholesterol Levels and Low-Dose Anticoagulation in the Post Coronary Artery Bypass Graft Trial: Post CABG Investigators." *Circulation* 102 (2): 157–65.

Koegelenberg, C. F., A. F. Doubell, H. Orth, and H. Reuter. 2003. "Infective Endocarditis in the Western Cape Province of South Africa: A Three-Year Prospective Study." *QJM* 96 (3): 217–25.

Kuntz, K. M., and K. C. Kent. 1996. "Is Carotid Endarterectomy Cost-Effective? An Analysis of Symptomatic and Asymptomatic Patients." *Circulation* 94 (9 Suppl.): II194–98.

Kuntz, K. M., J. Tsevat, L. Goldman, and M. C. Weinstein. 1996. "Cost-Effectiveness of Routine Coronary Angiography after Acute Myocardial Infarction." *Circulation* 94 (5): 957–65.

Kupersmith, J., M. Holmes-Rovner, A. Hogan, D. Rovner, and J. Gardiner. 1995. "Cost-Effectiveness Analysis in Heart Disease, Part III: Ischemia, Congestive Heart Failure, and Arrhythmias." *Progress in Cardiovascular Diseases* 37 (5): 30–46.

Kuppermann, M., B. R. Luce, B. McGovern, P. J. Podrid, J. T. Bigger Jr., and J. N. Ruskin. 1990. "An Analysis of the Cost Effectiveness of the Implantable Defibrillator." *Circulation* 81 (1): 91–100.

Leeder, S., S. Raymond, H. Greenberg, H. Liu, and K. Esson. 2004. *A Race against Time: The Challenge of Cardiovascular Disease in Developing Countries.* New York: Trustees of Columbia University.

Lorenzoni, R., D. Pagano, G. Mazzotta, S. D. Rosen, G. Fattore, R. De Caterina, and others. 1998. "Pitfalls in the Economic Evaluation of Thrombolysis in Myocardial Infarction: The Impact of National Differences in the Cost of Thrombolytics and of Differences in the Efficacy across Patient Subgroups." *European Heart Journal* 19 (10): 1518–24.

Mackay, J., and G. A. Manesh. 2004. *The Atlas of Heart Disease and Stroke.* Geneva: WHO.

Majeed, H. A., L. al-Doussary, M. M. Moussa, A. R. Yusuf, and A. H. Suliman. 1993. "Office Diagnosis and Management of Group A Streptococcal Pharyngitis Employing the Rapid Antigen Detecting Test: A 1-Year Prospective Study of Reliability and Cost in Primary Care Centres." *Annals of Tropical Paediatrics* 13 (1): 65–72.

Matchar, D., J. Pauk, and J. Lipscomb. 1996. "A Health Policy Perspective on Carotid Endarterectomy: Cost, Effectiveness, and Cost-Effectiveness." In *Surgery for Cerebrovascular Disease,* 2nd ed., ed. W. Moore. Philadelphia: W. B. Saunders.

Mathers, C. D., A. D. Lopez, and C. J. L. Murray. "The Burden of Disease and Mortality by Condition: Data, Methods, and Results for 2001." In *Global Burden of Disease and Risk Factors,* eds. A. D. Lopez, C. D. Mathers, M. Ezzati, D. T. Jamison, and C. J. L. Murray. New York: Oxford University Press.

McClellan, M., and D. Kessler. 1999. "A Global Analysis of Technological Change in Health Care: The Case of Heart Attacks—The TECH Investigators." *Health Affairs* 18 (3): 250–55.

McFayden, J. E., ed. 2003. *International Drug Price Indicator Reference Guide.* Boston: Management Sciences for Health.

McKelvie, R. 2003. "Heart Failure." *Clinical Evidence* 9: 95–118.

McMurray, J. J., and S. Stewart. 2000. "Heart Failure: Epidemiology, Aetiology, and Prognosis of Heart Failure." *Heart* 83 (5): 596–602.

Murray, C. J., and A. D. Lopez. 1994. *Global Comparative Assessments in the Health Sector: Disease Burden, Expenditures, and Intervention Packages.* Geneva: World Health Organization.

———. 1996. *Global Burden of Disease and Injury Series, Vols. I and II, Global Health Statistics.* Boston: Harvard School of Public Health.

———. 1997. "Mortality by Cause for Eight Regions of the World: Global Burden of Disease Study." *Lancet* 349 (9061): 1269–76.

Musaiger, A. O. 2002. "Diet and Prevention of Coronary Heart Disease in the Arab Middle East Countries." *Medical Principles and Practice* 11 (Suppl. 2): 9–16.

Nissen, S. E., E. M. Tuzcu, P. Libby, P. D. Thompson, M. Ghali, D. Garza, and others. 2004. "Effect of Antihypertensive Agents on Cardiovascular Events in Patients with Coronary Disease and Normal Blood Pressure: The CAMELOT Study: A Randomized Controlled Trial." *Journal of the American Medical Association* 292 (18): 2217–25.

Olshansky, S. J., and A. B. Ault. 1986. "The Fourth Stage of the Epidemiologic Transition: The Age of Delayed Degenerative Diseases." *Milbank Memorial Fund Quarterly* 64: 355–91.

Omran, A. R. 1971. "The Epidemiologic Transition: A Theory of the Epidemiology of Population Change." *Milbank Memorial Fund Quarterly* 49: 509.

Ornato, J. P., E. J. Craren, E. R. Gonzalez, A. R. Garnett, B. K. McClung, and M. M. Newman. 1988. "Cost-Effectiveness of Defibrillation by Emergency Medical Technicians." *American Journal of Emergency Medicine* 6 (2): 108–12.

Parmley, W. W. 1999. "Cost-Effectiveness of Reperfusion Strategies." *American Heart Journal* 138 (2, part 2): S142–52.

Pestana, J. A., K. Steyn, A. Leiman, and G. M. Hartzenberg. 1996. "The Direct and Indirect Costs of Cardiovascular Disease in South Africa in 1991." *South African Medical Journal* 86 (6): 679–84.

Pfeffer, M. A., A. Keech, F. M. Sacks, S. M. Cobbe, A. Tonkin, R. P. Byington, and others. 2002. "Safety and Tolerability of Pravastatin in Long-Term Clinical Trials: Prospective Pravastatin Pooling (PPP) Project." *Circulation* 105 (20): 2341–46.

Pitt, B., F. Zannad, W. J. Remme, R. Cody, A. Castaigne, A. Perez, and others. 1999. "The Effect of Spironolactone on Morbidity and Mortality in Patients with Severe Heart Failure." *New England Journal of Medicine* 341 (10): 709–17.

Roberts, R., W. J. Rogers, H. S. Mueller, C. T. Lambrew, D. J. Diver, H. C. Smith, and others. 1991. "Immediate versus Deferred Beta-Blockade Following Thrombolytic Therapy in Patients with Acute Myocardial Infarction: Results of the Thrombolysis in Myocardial Infarction (TIMI) II-B Study." *Circulation* 83 (2): 422–37.

Rogers, W. J., J. D. Babb, D. S. Baim, J. H. Chesebro, J. M. Gore, R. Roberts, and others. 1991. "Selective versus Routine Predischarge Coronary Arteriography after Therapy with Recombinant Tissue-Type Plasminogen Activator, Heparin, and Aspirin for Acute Myocardial Infarction: TIMI II Investigators." *Journal of the American College of Cardiology* 17 (5): 1007–16.

Rowley, J. M., C. Garner, and J. R. Hampton. 1990. "The Limited Potential of Special Ambulance Services in the Management of Cardiac Arrest." *British Heart Journal* 64 (5): 309–12.

Schneider, J., and K. Bezabih. 2001. "Causes of Sudden Death in Addis Ababa, Ethiopia." *Ethiopian Medical Journal* 39 (4): 323–40.

Soumerai, S. B., T. J. McLaughlin, D. Spiegelman, E. Hertzmark, G. Thibault, and L. Goldman. 1997. "Adverse Outcomes of Underuse of Beta-Blockers in Elderly Survivors of Acute Myocardial Infarction." *Journal of the American Medical Association* 277 (2): 115–21.

Steer, A. C., J. R. Carapetis, T. M. Nolan, and F. Shann. 2002. "Systematic Review of Rheumatic Heart Disease Prevalence in Children in Developing Countries: The Role of Environmental Factors." *Journal of Paediatrics and Child Health* 38 (3): 229–34.

Strasser, T. 1985. "Cost-Effective Control of Rheumatic Fever in the Community." *Health Policy* 5 (2): 159–64.

Tengs, T. O., M. E. Adams, J. S. Pliskin, D. G. Safran, J. E. Siegel, M. C. Weinstein, and others. 1995. "Five-Hundred Life-Saving Interventions and Their Cost-Effectiveness." *Risk Analysis* 15 (3): 369–90.

Teo, K. K., S. Yusuf, M. Pfeffer, C. Torp-Pedersen, L. Kober, A. Hall, and others. 2002. "Effects of Long-Term Treatment with Angiotensin-Converting-Enzyme Inhibitors in the Presence or Absence of Aspirin: A Systematic Review." *Lancet* 360 (9339): 1037–43.

Topol, E. J., D. R. Holmes, and W. J. Rogers. 1991. "Coronary Angiography after Thrombolytic Therapy for Acute Myocardial Infarction." *Annals of Internal Medicine* 114 (10): 877–85.

Unger, F. 1999. "Cardiac Interventions in Europe 1997: Coronary Revascularization Procedures and Open Heart Surgery." *Cor Europaeum* 7: 177–89.

Weinstein, M. C., and W. B. Stason. 1982. "Cost-Effectiveness of Coronary Artery Bypass Surgery." *Circulation* 66 (5, part 2): III56–66.

WHO (World Health Organization). 1995. "Strategy for Controlling Rheumatic Fever/Rheumatic Heart Disease, with Emphasis on Primary Prevention." *Bulletin of the World Health Organization* 73 (5): 583–87.

———. 2002a. *Integrated Management of Cardiovascular Risk.* Geneva: WHO CVD Program.

———. 2002b. *The World Health Report 2002: Reducing Risks, Promoting Healthy Life.* Geneva: WHO.

———. 2003a. "Adherence to Long-Term Therapies: Evidence for Action." WHO, Geneva. http://www.who.int/chronic_conditions/adherence_report.pdf.

———. 2003b. *World Health Report 2003: Shaping the Future.* Geneva: WHO.

Williams, A. 1985. "Economics of Coronary Artery Bypass Grafting." *British Medical Journal* 291 (6491): 326–29.

Williams, D. O. 2004. "Treatment Delayed Is Treatment Denied." *Circulation* 109 (15): 1806–8.

Wolf, P. A., R. D. Abbott, and W. B. Kannel. 1991. "Atrial Fibrillation as an Independent Risk Factor for Stroke: The Framingham Study." *Stroke* 22 (8): 983–88.

Wong, J. B., F. A. Sonnenberg, D. N. Salem, and S. G. Pauker. 1990. "Myocardial Revascularization for Chronic Stable Angina. Analysis of the Role of Percutaneous Transluminal Coronary Angioplasty Based on Data Available in 1989." *Annals of Internal Medicine* 113 (11): 852–71.

Yusuf, S., R. Peto, J. Lewis, R. Collins, and P. Sleight. 1985. "Beta Blockade during and after Myocardial Infarction: An Overview of the Randomized Trials." *Progress in Cardiovascular Diseases* 27 (5): 335–71.

Chapter 34

Inherited Disorders of Hemoglobin

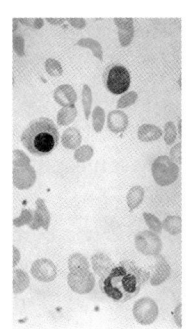

David Weatherall, Olu Akinyanju, Suthat Fucharoen, Nancy Olivieri, and Philip Musgrove

As a result of carrier protection against malaria, the inherited hemoglobin disorders are the commonest diseases attributable to single defective genes. Approximately 7 percent of the world's population is a carrier, and 300,000 to 500,000 babies with severe forms of such disorders are born each year (WHO 1989). Although these disorders are most frequent in tropical regions, they are now encountered in most countries because of migrations of populations.

INTRODUCTION

If untreated, many of the inherited hemoglobin disorders result in death during the first few years of life. Their effect on the burden of disease has only recently been recognized, following an epidemiological transition caused by improvements in hygiene, nutrition, and control of infection that has reduced childhood mortality. Babies with severe hemoglobin disorders are now able to survive long enough to present for diagnosis and treatment. The impact of these diseases is being felt throughout the Indian subcontinent and much of Asia. Although the situation will worsen in Sub-Saharan Africa as it undergoes a similar transition, such diseases are already responsible for a major health burden. International health agencies and the governments of affected countries need to understand the future extent of the problem and to develop programs to control and manage these diseases.

Normal Hemoglobin

Hemoglobin (Hb), the pigment in the red blood cells that transfers oxygen to the tissues, changes structure during human development. In adults two components exist: a major hemoglobin, Hb A, and a minor hemoglobin, Hb A_2. The bulk of the hemoglobin during later fetal life is Hb F. These hemoglobins each consist of two pairs of unlike globin chains. The adult hemoglobins and fetal hemoglobin have α chains combined with β (Hb A, $\alpha_2\beta_2$), δ (Hb A_2, $\alpha_2\delta_2$), or γ chains (Hb F, $\alpha_2\gamma_2$). Each of the different globin chains is controlled by distinct genes; two genes exist for the α and γ chains and one for each of the other chains. Their structure and the regions of the genes that control the production of the different globin chains have been determined (Steinberg and others 2001; Weatherall and Clegg 2001b).

Spectrum of Inherited Hemoglobin Disorders

Inherited hemoglobin disorders fall into two main groups: the structural hemoglobin variants and the thalassemias, which are caused by defective globin production. They all follow a recessive form of inheritance. Those with a single defective globin gene—carriers or heterozygotes—are symptomless. If two carriers marry, a one in four chance exists that each child they produce will receive defective genes from each parent—that is, they are homozygous for the particular disorder.

The structural variants result mostly from single amino acid substitutions in the α or β chains. Often these are innocuous, but in some cases they may alter the stability or functional properties of the hemoglobin and lead to a clinical disorder. They are designated by letters of the alphabet or by the place names where the condition was first discovered. Even though researchers have identified more than 700 structural hemoglobin variants, only three (Hb S, Hb C, and Hb E) are widespread.

The homozygous state for the sickle cell gene results in sickle cell anemia, whereas the compound heterozygous state for the sickle cell and Hb C genes results in Hb SC disease. Hb SC disease, although milder, also has important public health implications. Hb E, the commonest variant globally, is innocuous in its heterozygous and homozygous states, but because it is synthesized less effectively than Hb A, it interacts with β thalassemia to produce an extremely common condition called Hb E β thalassemia, which is becoming an increasingly important health burden in many parts of Asia.

The thalassemias are classified according to the ineffectively synthesized globin chains. From a public health viewpoint, only the α and β thalassemias are sufficiently common to be important.

Clinical Features

The inherited hemoglobin disorders are characterized by an extremely diverse series of clinical syndromes of varying severity.

Sickle Cell Anemia and Related Disorders. The clinical features of sickle cell disorders reflect the red blood cells' propensity to assume a sickle shape in deoxygenated blood, leading to shortened red cell survival and a tendency to block small blood vessels (Bunn 1997; Serjeant 1992). Even though patients may adapt to their anemia, their illness is interspersed with acute episodes, including: attacks of bone pain; sequestration of blood into the lungs, liver, or spleen; or thrombosis of cerebral vessels, which may cause a stroke. They are extremely prone to infection, particularly during early childhood, and to a wide range of chronic complications. For reasons not yet understood, the severity of the disease varies extensively. Even in populations in eastern Saudi Arabia and parts of India, which have a high frequency of α thalassemia and an unusual ability to produce Hb F in adult life, both of which, when inherited with sickle cell disease, result in a milder form of the illness, morbidity is still high.

Although little is known about mortality from "sickling" disorders in developing countries, in Sub-Saharan Africa many children die early because of these conditions (Akinyanju 2001; Fleming and others 1979). Fleming and others, working in rural Nigeria, found that even though more than 2 percent of all newborns had sickle cell anemia, it was absent in the adolescent and adult populations. At the same time, they found that urban centers in Nigeria, where medical care was available, had an increasing number of affected adults, and by the late 1970s, a significant improvement in survival had clearly followed the introduction of antimalarial measures (Molineaux and others 1979). Both in Jamaica and in the United States, death appears to peak between one and three years of age, usually from infection. Recent U.S. data suggest that the median age of adult death is 42 for men and 48 for women (Dover and

Platt 1998). Even though Hb SC disease is milder than sickle cell anemia, it is associated with many complications, including a higher frequency of proliferative retinopathy.

Thalassemias. The homozygous or compound heterozygous states for β thalassemia also run a variable course, although without transfusion, death usually occurs in the first few years (Weatherall and Clegg 2001b). With adequate transfusions and the administration of drugs to remove iron, children may develop well and survive to adulthood. However, these drugs are expensive, and even when they are available in poorer countries, many children receive inadequate dosages and die in childhood or adolescence from iron overload. The situation is further complicated because the common β thalassemias of intermediate severity—notably Hb E β thalassemia—exhibit a clinical spectrum ranging from transfusion-dependent disease to a condition compatible with normal survival and growth into adult life without treatment.

The α thalassemias are equally heterogeneous. The extremely common milder forms (termed α+ thalassemias because some α chains are produced) produce only a mild hypochromic anemia in homozygotes. In contrast, the α° thalassemias, so called because of the absence of α chain synthesis, result in stillbirth in their homozygous states following pregnancies with toxemic and postpartum complications. The compound heterozygous states for α+ and α° thalassemias result in Hb H disease, which varies in severity and may be transfusion dependent.

The thalassemias are extremely heterogeneous at the molecular level: more than 200 different mutations of the β globin genes have been found, and the α thalassemias are almost as varied. Every severely affected population in the world has a few common mutations unique to a particular region, together with varying numbers of rare ones.

Population Genetics and Dynamics

The high gene frequencies for the hemoglobin disorders are attributable to the effects of natural selection. Although severely affected homozygotes would, in the absence of medical interventions, have died early in life, asymptomatic heterozygotes for Hb S, Hb C, and probably β thalassemia and Hb E, as well as those with mild forms of α thalassemia, are more resistant to severe malarial infection than normal persons. Hence, in environments in which malaria was common, carriers were protected and survived to have more children, and the gene frequencies rose until they were balanced by loss of severely affected homozygotes from the population. Although some decline in frequency among immigrant populations may occur because of lack of exposure to malaria and outbreeding, this decline will occur over many generations, and even if malaria were completely eradicated, an equally long time would pass before any significant fall occurred in the global frequency.

Changes resulting from variation in selection or in population dynamics will, however, be small compared with the effect of the demographic and epidemiological transitions that many countries have recently undergone. For example, thalassemia was not identified in Cyprus until 1944, when major improvements in public health revealed that the disease was common. By the early 1970s, estimates indicated that, in the absence of steps to control the disease, in about 40 years approximately 78,000 units of blood would be required each year to treat all the severely affected children, 40 percent of the population would be carriers, and the cost to the health system would equal or exceed the island's health budget (Weatherall and Clegg 2001b).

Global Distribution and Frequency of the Hemoglobinopathies

Figures 34.1a and 34.1b show the global distributions of the hemoglobinopathies. Table 34.1 shows approximate carrier frequencies by region.

The gene for Hb S is distributed throughout Sub-Saharan Africa, the Indian subcontinent, and the Middle East, where carrier frequencies range from 5 to 40 percent or more. Hb E is found in the eastern half of the Indian subcontinent and throughout Southeast Asia, where carrier rates may exceed 60 percent. Thalassemia is frequent in a broad band from the Mediterranean basin and parts of Africa, throughout the Middle East, the Indian subcontinent, Southeast Asia, and Melanesia and into the Pacific islands. The α^+ thalassemias occur right across the tropical zone, reaching extremely high frequencies in some populations, whereas the α^0 thalassemias are restricted to parts of Southeast Asia and the Mediterranean basin (table 34.1).

Several World Health Organization (WHO) workshops have attempted to estimate the global burden of the thalassemias and important structural hemoglobin variants (Angastiniotis and Modell 1998; Weatherall and Clegg 2001b; WHO 1989, 1994). There are perhaps 270 million carriers and 300,000 to 500,000 annual births of infants with sickle cell

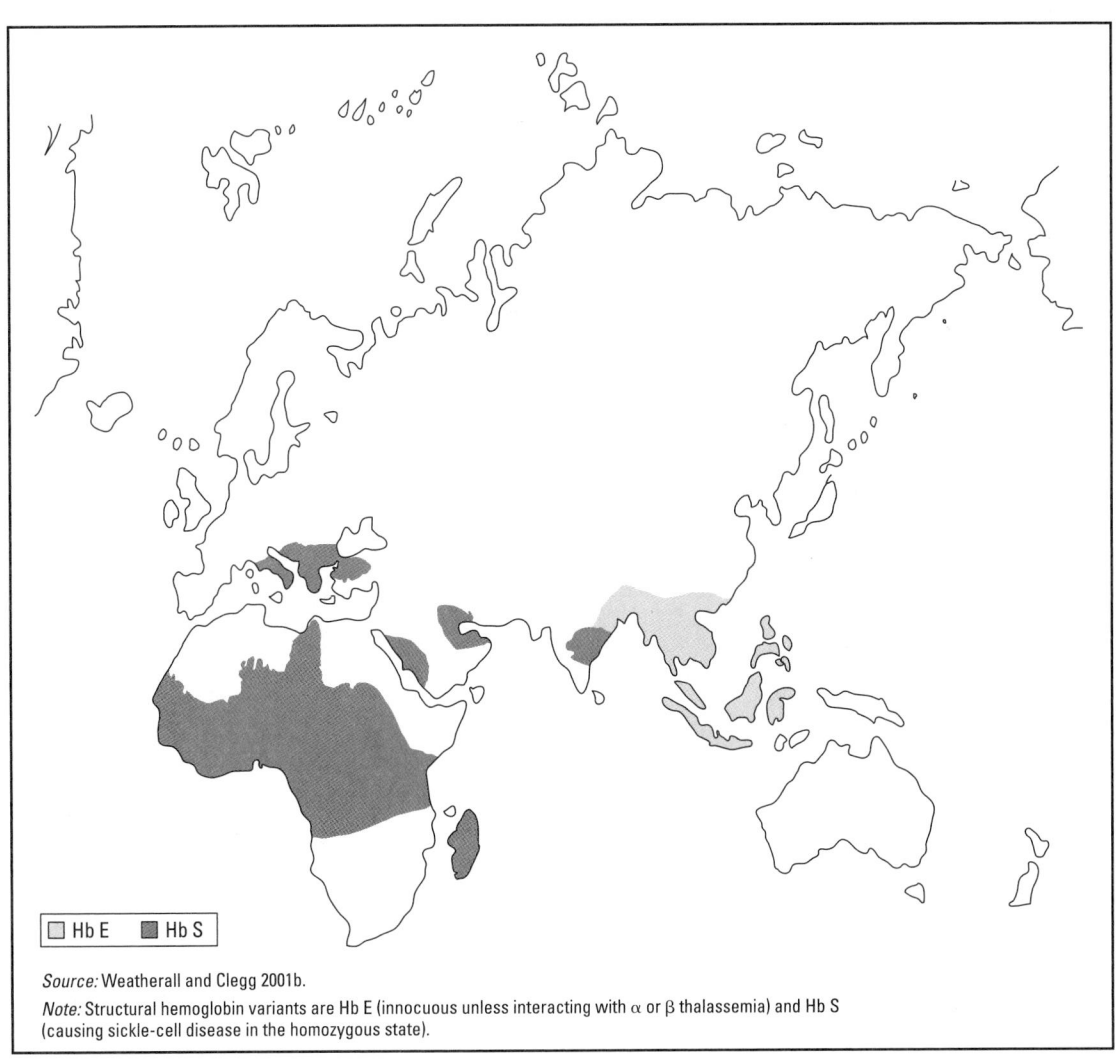

Source: Weatherall and Clegg 2001b.

Note: Structural hemoglobin variants are Hb E (innocuous unless interacting with α or β thalassemia) and Hb S (causing sickle-cell disease in the homozygous state).

Figure 34.1a Global Distribution of Hemoglobinopathies Hb E and Hb S

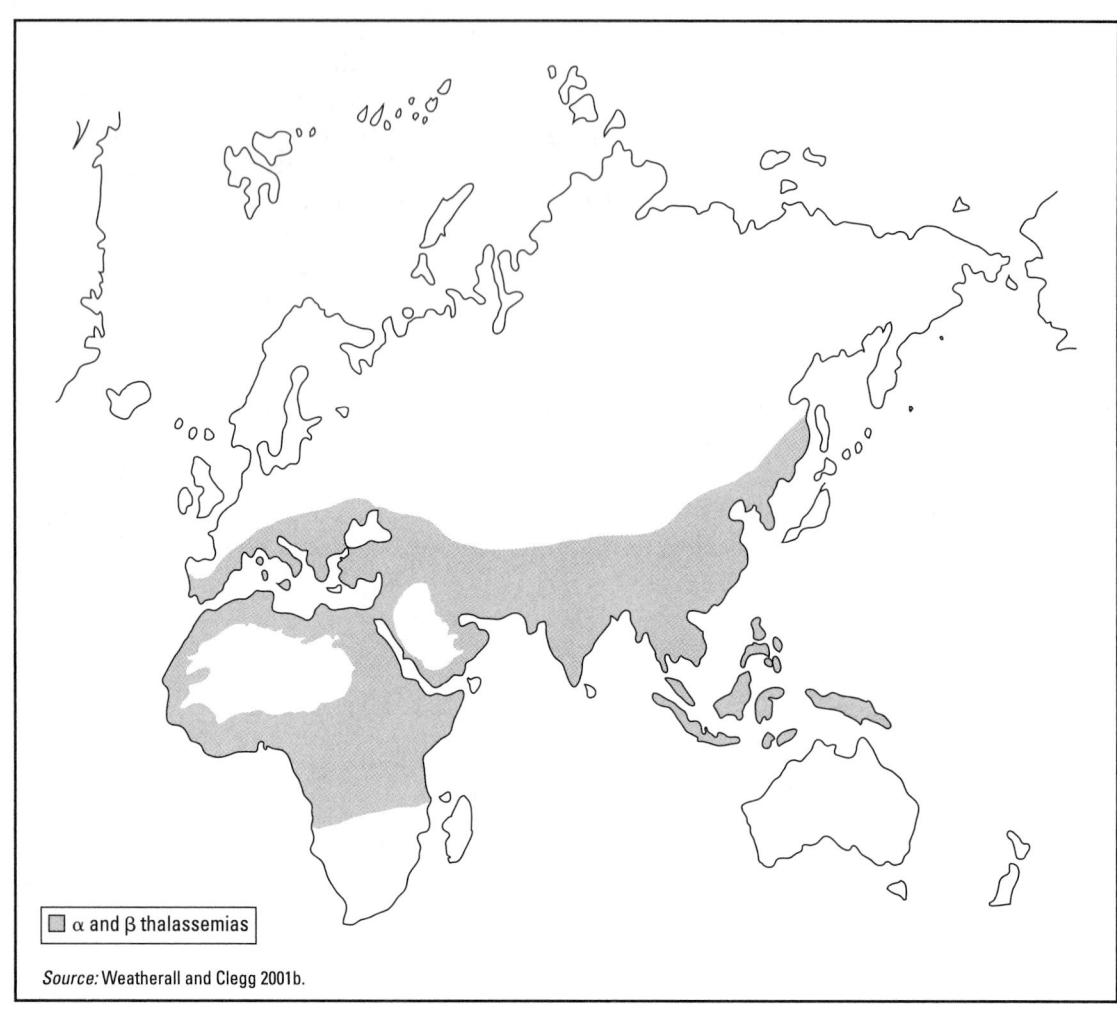

Figure 34.1b Global Distribution of Hemoglobinopathies α and β Thalassemias

Source: Weatherall and Clegg 2001b.

Table 34.1 Carrier Frequencies for Common Hemoglobin Disorders, by World Health Organization Region, 2001 *(percent)*

Region	Hb S	Hb C	Hb E	β thalassemia	α° thalassemia	α⁺ thalassemia
Americas	1–20	0–10	0–20	0–3	0–5	0–40
Eastern Mediterranean	0–60	0–3	0–2	2–18	0–2	1–60
Europe	0–30	0–5	0–20	0–19	1–2	0–12
Southeast Asia	0–40	0	0–70	0–11	1–30	3–40
Sub-Saharan Africa	1–38	0–21	0	0–12	0	10–50
Western Pacific	0	0	0	0–13	0	2–60

Sources: Livingstone 1985; Weatherall and Clegg 2001a, 2001b.
Note: Many of these data are derived from small population samples.

anemia or serious forms of thalassemia. Southeast Asia, where the thalassemias and Hb E predominate, is most severely affected. Sub-Saharan Africa has the second-highest burden, reflecting the high incidence of Hb S. Weatherall and Clegg (2001b)

summarize information about the different thalassemia mutations in those regions.

These data only approximate the problems for health care services that the hemoglobin disorders will pose in the future.

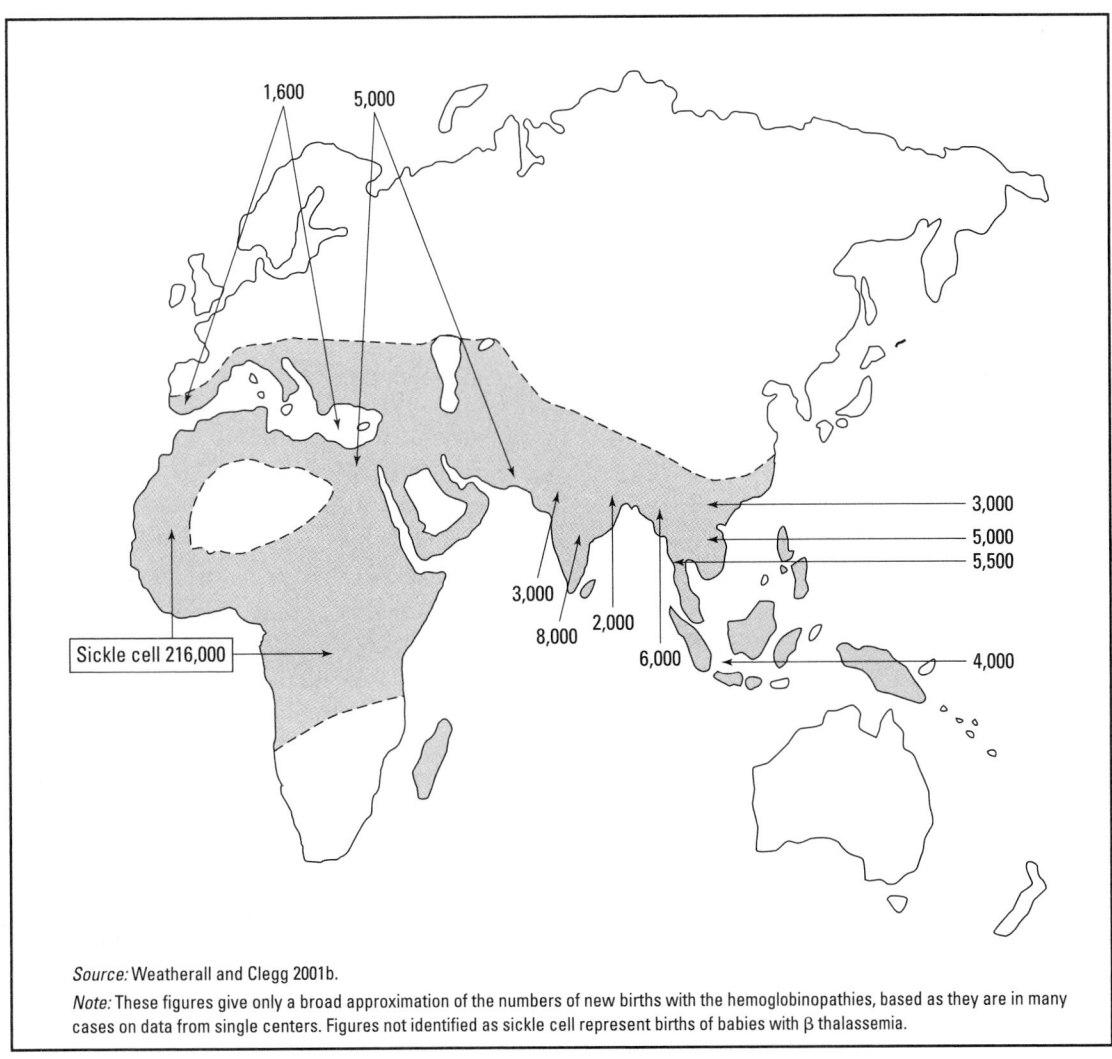

Figure 34.2 Approximate Annual Births of Babies with Sickle Cell Anemia and β Thalassemia

Source: Weatherall and Clegg 2001b.

Note: These figures give only a broad approximation of the numbers of new births with the hemoglobinopathies, based as they are in many cases on data from single centers. Figures not identified as sickle cell represent births of babies with β thalassemia.

Unfortunately, few of the data are based on micromapping of incidence in different populations. Weatherall and Clegg's (2001b) review of studies in Indonesia, Sri Lanka, and Thailand reveals the extent of variability of incidence within relatively short geographic distances, suggesting that the number of annual births of babies with β thalassemia major or Hb E β thalassemia may be underestimated. Similarly, published data for the annual births of babies with sickle cell anemia in India and the Middle East are almost certainly too low, because estimates based on gene frequency suggest that the figure may be close to 100,000. The data in table 34.1 and figure 34.2, therefore, represent a minimal estimate of the future likely health burden resulting from inherited hemoglobin disorders. Furthermore, in many cases, the data are not based on projected increases in birth rates.

Because of these uncertainties, including how long countries will take to pass through the epidemiological transition,

assessing the burden that the disorders will impose on health services is difficult. As more babies survive and present for treatment, the population on long-term therapy will steadily expand; the more effective the treatment, the greater the burden will be on health services. For example, from 2005 to 2025, an estimated 100,000 cases of Hb E β thalassemia will be added to the Thai population, and 20,000 β thalassemia homozygotes will be born each year in southern China (Weatherall and Clegg 2001b). If these children all survive to adulthood, they will account for a large proportion of health service expenditure.

BURDEN OF DISEASE

WHO disease burden estimates do not include the incidence or prevalence of the hemoglobin disorders, nor the deaths or disability-adjusted life year (DALY) losses from sickle cell disease or thalassemia. Neither do they treat these disorders as risk factors for anemia, infection, stroke, and other conditions or estimate the prevalence (frequency) of the underlying genetic factors. Thus, the estimates provided here are necessarily incomplete and speculative.

For severe β thalassemia, figure 34.2 suggests 43,100 births per year, nearly all in low- and middle-income countries, where affected babies are likely to die before reaching two years of age. At least 41,500 deaths probably occur each year, or 0.3 percent of all deaths of children under five. This estimate may be too low, because it does not include the estimated 20,000 births per year in China. Thus, the severe β thalassemias probably account for 50,000 to 100,000 deaths per year, or 0.5 to 0.9 percent of all deaths of children under five in low- and middle-income countries. Each death accounts for 29.2 DALYs if it occurs before the child reaches the age of one. Taken together, all the deaths contribute 1.46 million to 2.92 million DALYs to the world burden.

Treated β thalassemia victims who survive to age 40 or older contribute much less to the disease burden because they are fewer and their residual disability weight is only 0.02 to 0.10 (chapter 15 provides an explanation of disability weights). Living with poorly treated thalassemia has a weight equal to or greater than 0.1. No global estimates of the number of treated survivors are available, but estimates indicate that 500,000 may exist in Thailand alone, of which perhaps 55,000 are transfusion dependent with severe disabilities. Their total DALY loss, including disability for those with milder Hb H disease, would be only some 15,000 per year, trivial relative to the DALYs resulting from premature mortality. Deaths by age 10 from homozygous β thalassemia or by age 30 from Hb E β thalassemia would add 53,600 DALYs in Thailand.

α° thalassemia contributes to the burden of disease primarily through stillbirths or deaths shortly following birth and secondarily through mothers' disability during pregnancy. WHO does not count stillbirths, and no data on affected births are available except for an estimate of 1,250 per year in Thailand, which adds 37,242 DALYs. Assuming that mothers suffer a disability weight of 0.3 during the last trimester would add only 100 DALYs. Every 1,000 homozygous α° thalassemia pregnancies contribute about 30,000 DALYs, but insufficient information is available on incidence elsewhere to use the Thai estimate to project global or regional levels.

For sickle cell disease, the burden is harder to estimate because of the higher survival rate and the disability during crises. Figure 34.2 shows an estimated 216,000 births per year in Africa alone, but reliable data on survival are not available. Early studies suggested a mortality rate greater than 80 percent by age five, but more recent estimates indicate that the figure is probably greater than 50 percent, with the improvement resulting from treatment and from control of the infections that cause most early sickle cell deaths. Mortality of 50 to 80 percent at ages one to five implies at least 21,600 to 34,500 deaths

per year and possibly as many as 173,000. These translate into 0.5 million to 4.5 million DALYs, accounting for less than 1 percent, but perhaps as much as 2 percent, of the burden for children under five. Life expectancies and the extent of disabilities among survivors in Africa are unknown, so the low DALY number is no doubt underestimated.

Outside Africa, Weatherall and Clegg (2001b) estimate 60,000 sickle cell births per year concentrated in India and the Middle East and among descendants of Africans in the Americas. The actual figure may be as high as 100,000. Without treatment, deaths peak in the first 2 years of life, and half of all deaths occur in the first 20 years. If 25 percent of sufferers die at age 1 and 25 percent at age 10, those deaths would contribute almost 14,000 DALYs for every 1,000 births in a low- or middle-income country. Including deaths after age 20 and disability might double the estimate.

Survival elsewhere is greater than in Africa, because of lower risks of infection and greater access to treatment. The United Kingdom has about 10,000 survivors (Davies and others 2000), and the United States has some 50,000 (Ashley-Koch, Yang, and Olney 2000). No good estimates are available of the numbers or age distribution of survivors in most of the rest of the world, but Hambleton's (2004b) cohort study in Jamaica shows how treatment increased survival: 70 percent of those enrolled starting in 1973 survived to age 20, as did 80 percent of those enrolled three to six years later.

Of 1,000 babies born with sickle cell disease, Jamaican clinic records and follow-up show how many would die at each age in each year, allowing an estimate of the burden from premature mortality (Hambleton 2004a). Table 34.2 presents those results: 560 deaths per year represent almost 14,000 DALYs. Deaths after age 50 contribute less because they are fewer, and life expectancy and DALYs per death decline with age. Thus, 18,000 to 22,000 DALYs per year for deaths at all ages is a reasonable estimate of the mortality burden from 1,000 sickle cell births per year at Jamaican levels of treatment coverage and effectiveness. Applied to the estimated 60,000 to 100,000 births per year outside Africa, this figure implies at least 1.08 to 2.20 million DALYs, or 0.1 percent of the total burden in low- and middle-income countries.

Three sources of disability also contribute to the burden: anemia without painful crises or other complications; disability from mild or severely painful crises; and other clinical events, both acute and chronic (for example, leg ulcers and retinopathy).

For the first source, the disability weight is assumed to average 0.04. This source adds a constant 0.04 DALYs for every year a sickle cell patient survives. The loss per year per 1,000 births in Jamaica is multiplied by 2.5 for deaths during each five-year interval (because deaths are assumed to occur at the midpoint of the interval) and by 5.0 for survivors, who suffer disability for the entire five years. This loss adds about 10 percent to the loss from premature mortality.

Table 34.2 Burden of Sickle Cell Disease by Age Group, Assuming 1,000 Births per Year and Survival to Various Ages, Jamaica, Starting in 1973

Category	0–4	5–9	10–14	15–19	20–24	25–29	30–34	35–39	40–44	45–49	Total or average
Number of survivors	876	834	807	777	727	680	627	564	491	440	682.3
Number of deaths	124	42	27	30	50	47	53	63	73	51	560
Death rate (percent/year)	2.61	0.98	0.66	0.75	1.32	1.33	1.61	2.10	2.73	2.17	1.63
Number of DALYs lost/death	28.90	28.59	27.77	26.84	25.82	24.69	23.43	22.00	20.39	18.58	24.70
Total DALY losses from deaths	3,584	1,201	750	805	1,291	1,161	1,242	1,386	1,488	948	13,856
Number of DALYs lost from background (chronic) anemia	188	171	164	158	150	141	130	119	106	93	1,420
Total DALYs lost from deaths and chronic anemia	3,772	1,372	914	963	1,441	1,302	1,372	1,505	1,594	1,041	15,276
Number of pain crises/year	242.7	381.0	383.8	584.4	866.7	600.5	523.6	473.4	309.6	182.2	4,548
Number of other acute clinical events	77.5	22.2		182.2							281.9
Number of other chronic clinical events	49.8	14.8	12.8	10.9							88.3

Source: Authors' calculations based on Hambleton 2004a, 2004b.

Note: The number of DALYs lost per death is calculated assuming all deaths occur at the midpoint of the age interval. Life expectancies by age are those for all low- and middle-income countries together. The number of pain crises is the total during one year for all the individuals in an age group. Those who die during the interval are assumed to die in equal numbers at the midpoint of each of the five years and, therefore, to suffer half as much disability from chronic anemia and half as many pain crises in that year as those of the same age who survive the year. Blanks in the table indicate that clinical events are rare in the corresponding age groups and their numbers are not well recorded. The totals of acute and chronic clinical events are therefore probably slight under-estimates.

For the second source of disability, even mild crises should be weighted considerably worse than background anemia, and severe crises requiring hospitalization should be weighted worse still: values of 0.2 and 0.5, respectively, are assumed. The number of crises and the share that are severe vary with age, with peak severity at ages 21 to 45 for a mean disability weight of 0.35. Because each crisis lasts only 7 to 10 days, or about 0.023 year, the loss per 1,000 births in each five-year age group never exceeds 10 DALYs and makes no difference to the total burden.

The third source of disability may carry disability weights of 0.135 for a leg ulcer, 0.276 for stroke survivors, 0.279 for acute chest syndrome, and 0.567 for retinopathy, but disability weights for a number of other conditions are unknown. Even if acute conditions last one month with an average disability weight of 0.5, they add less than 10 DALYs in any five-year interval. These conditions occur much less frequently than painful crises, but chronic ones may last much longer, contributing more or less to the burden than pain crises but adding little to mortality losses. Table 34.2 therefore includes only the estimated losses from background anemia and the frequencies, but not the DALY losses, of painful crises and other events that add negligibly to the burden.

CONTROL AND TREATMENT

With the exception of the few patients who can obtain a bone marrow transplant, no cure exists for the inherited disorders of hemoglobin. Even though research directed at their correction by means of somatic cell gene therapy is ongoing, this technology will probably not be generally applicable for some time, and when it is developed, it may be extremely expensive. Thus, for the moment, the major approaches to the control and management of these diseases are population screening, genetic counseling and prenatal diagnosis, and management of symptoms.

Prevention

Programs to reduce the number of seriously affected individuals follow two approaches. First, population screening and counseling programs can be established to educate populations about the risks of having children with similarly affected partners. Data about the effectiveness of this approach are extremely limited. In an early study in Greece, people's knowledge of their genetic makeup had no effect on marriage patterns (Stamatoyannopoulos 1973); however, a recent study in the Islamic Republic of Iran found that about 50 percent of affected couples decided to separate, and births with severe β thalassemia fell to about 30 percent of those expected (Samavat and Modell 2004). The reasons for this remarkable discrepancy require further investigation.

The second preventive approach also involves population screening or screening in prenatal clinics. If women are found to be carriers, their partners are screened, and following counseling they are offered a prenatal diagnosis and termination of affected fetuses. This method has been used widely in the Mediterranean region and elsewhere, resulting in a major reduction in newborns with serious forms of thalassemia (Cao, Galanello, and Rosatelli 1998; Weatherall and Clegg 2001b). Prenatal diagnosis programs are available in China, India, the Islamic Republic of Iran, Lebanon, Pakistan, Singapore, Thailand, the United Arab Emirates, the United States, and many European countries; several other countries are establishing similar programs.

Because severe thalassemia is incompatible with survival without regular blood transfusions, prenatal diagnosis is a logical approach where acceptable until more definitive treatments become available. The situation with sickle cell anemia is different. First, it is not uniformly fatal in early life, and morbidity and mortality during this period can be controlled. Second, the clinical course of the condition is unpredictable: some patients' symptoms are relatively mild, whereas others develop life-threatening complications. Hence, even though some countries are practicing prenatal diagnosis, in others neither communities nor doctors consider that it should be applied widely. This complex issue would be clarified if the reasons for the phenotypic variability of the sickling disorders were better defined.

Whether or not screening programs are backed up with an offer of prenatal diagnosis, they require an intense period of education of the population about the nature of inherited hemoglobin disorders. This education requires input from many sectors of society, including the media, public health workers, local volunteer societies, and the medical community. Programs of this type require careful planning as well as availability of facilities for screening and counseling when the program is initiated. Their development also requires prior discussion between the government, health care workers, and members of the community—including religious leaders.

Treatment

The treatment of the hemoglobinopathies varies widely depending on the disease. The severe forms of β thalassemia require lifelong blood transfusions. The family of β thalassemia intermediate diseases ranges from transfusion-dependent forms to symptomless carrier traits. Hb E β thalassemia, the commonest hemoglobinopathy in Asia, varies in severity from forms that require regular or intermittent transfusions to milder anemia that does not require lifelong transfusions unless complications arise, particularly hypersplenism. Weatherall and Clegg's (2001b) review of studies in Asia indicates that the medical community does not always appreciate these subtleties and that many patients who receive regular transfusions might well have survived without transfusions had their early management been more effective.

Thus, those managing patients with severe forms of β thalassemia must make absolutely sure in infancy that regular transfusions are required. If so, babies and children require transfusion at monthly intervals using washed red cells rather than whole blood. In addition, blood must be screened for hepatitis B and C, for HIV, and—in some countries—for malaria. Because patients accumulate iron from transfusions, they also require lifelong treatment with a chelating agent, the most effective being desferrioxamine delivered subcutaneously overnight using a pump. Oral chelating agents, which would undoubtedly improve compliance, are available, but their efficacy and safety have yet to be verified. Some children with the major form of β thalassemia—and many with the intermediate varieties—will at some point require splenectomy, to be preceded by appropriate vaccinations and followed by prophylactic penicillin. They also require regular assessments of their iron status by measurements of serum ferritin or, better, by hepatic iron concentrations. Various complications occur, particularly for those not adequately transfused, including endocrine deficiencies, bone disease, and infection. Bloodborne infections, particularly hepatitis C and HIV/AIDS, are an increasing hazard. Most children with β thalassemia also require regular folate supplementation and vitamin C with their chelation therapy.

The serious forms of α thalassemia, $α^o$ thalassemia, cause stillbirth late in pregnancy and several maternal complications. Although some infants have been given exchange transfusion or transfusion in the immediate neonatal period and survived, they have gone on to a transfusion-dependent life. Because of the increased risk of congenital malformations as a result of the disease—and particularly because of maternal complications—this course of action is not recommended, and this disease is an important indication for prenatal diagnosis. Those who inherit $α^o$ thalassemia from one parent and $α^+$ thalassemia from the other have a moderately severe form called Hb H disease that is usually compatible with a life independent of transfusions except for periods of stress, such as infection. The $α^+$ thalassemias cause no clinical problems, either in their homozygous or heterozygous states.

Patients with sickle cell anemia are at high risk from infection early in life; therefore, diagnosis as early as possible is vital. Excellent evidence, at least in developed countries, indicates that prophylactic penicillin significantly reduces early morbidity and mortality.

Even though many children adapt well to their anemia, many eventually develop sickle cell crises (Ballas 1998). The most common form, the so-called painful crisis, is characterized by severe bone pain that often requires hospital admission and treatment with analgesics, oxygen, and infection control. More life-threatening crises, including stroke, marrow aplasia associated with viral illness, and pulmonary crises with severe hypoxia, require urgent hospital treatment. Regular Doppler testing of the cerebral blood flow can anticipate neurological complications that can be prevented by regular transfusions (Adams and others 1998), which can be continued indefinitely.

Because most aplastic crises result from human parvovirus infection, the development of a vaccine would be a great advantage. The other acute complication, splenic sequestration causing rapid enlargement of the spleen, is associated with profound anemia. It necessitates urgent hospital admission and blood transfusion, plus sometimes splenectomy. A variety of other complications require hospital treatment, including priapism, aseptic necrosis of the femoral or humoral heads, renal failure, and recurrent hematuria. At every age patients with sickling disorders seem to be more prone to infection that often requires hospital admission. In most sickling disorders, crises are more frequent and anemia worsens during pregnancy. A review of extensive clinical trials in the United States shows that the long-term administration of hydroxyurea reduces the frequency of crises and prolongs life in adult sufferers (Weatherall 2003).

Although milder, Hb SC disease is clinically important, particularly because of the relatively high incidence of ocular complications.

Requirements

Screening and diagnosis for the hemoglobin disorders requires relatively simple laboratory techniques combined with a well-organized program for their application in the community.

Screening and Carrier Detection. Unlike many genetic diseases, carrier screening for the main hemoglobin disorders is well established, accurate, and inexpensive. The initial screening for thalassemia usually measures the mean cell volume and the mean cell hemoglobin. Thresholds below which the likelihood of some form of thalassemia is great are well established. The diagnosis of β thalassemia is confirmed by finding a raised level of Hb A_2 using high-performance liquid chromatography (HPLC) or cheaper forms of chromatography or quantitative hemoglobin electrophoresis. Ideally, the initial blood count should use an electronic cell counter, and the Hb A_2 should be measured using HPLC. However, the equipment for HPLC analysis is expensive, and the cost per sample is approximately US$2. For this reason, several more economical approaches have been developed (Fucharoen and others 2004). The initial screening can be done using a single-tube osmotic fragility test, which, even though it may result in a relatively high number of false positive results, usually gives fewer false negatives. Commercial kits for osmotic fragility testing have recently been produced, and at least one variety has been validated in Thailand. Further validation of this approach is required before it can be recommended. Various cheaper methods for measuring the Hb A_2 level are available.

When the red cell indices suggest thalassemia or an osmotic fragility test is positive but the Hb A_2 level is normal, it is vital to distinguish between iron deficiency and α thalassemia.

Several simple, cheap tests are available for diagnosing iron deficiency, but α thalassemia presents more of a problem. Screening tests will identify those heterozygous for α^o thalassemia or homozygous for α^+ thalassemia but will miss most cases of heterozygosity for α^+ thalassemia. However, given the restricted distribution of α^o thalassemia, these distinctions are clinically important only in areas where α^o thalassemia is common. Further diagnosis of the α thalassemias requires DNA analysis.

Several simple and cheap screening tests are available for sickling disorders, but all of them require confirmation of the genotype by hemoglobin electrophoresis. Neonatal screening requires electrophoresis because the solubility test, which is used widely for adult screening, is unreliable in the first months of life.

Throughout Asia, screening for Hb E is also necessary, either with a one-tube dye test or by hemoglobin electrophoresis. The Hb E trait is missed by measuring cell size or osmotic fragility.

Initial Diagnosis of More Severe Hemoglobinopathies. The initial diagnosis of β thalassemia is usually clinical. It can be confirmed by finding typical thalassemic changes of the peripheral blood, together with an elevated level of Hb F. A variety of cheap tests for measuring Hb F levels are available, or HPLC analysis can be used. Hemoglobin electrophoresis or HPLC is used to diagnose α^o thalassemia homozygotes and children with Hb H disease.

Sickle cell anemia, Hb SC disease, or combinations of the sickle cell gene with forms of β thalassemia can all be identified by hemoglobin electrophoresis and can be confirmed by a family study.

Further Analysis. More detailed confirmatory analysis, including identification of the underlying mutation, is required for the β thalassemias as a prerequisite for prenatal diagnosis. A variety of approaches to mutation analysis based on the polymerase chain reaction, which amplifies particular regions of DNA, are available, but because every population has a number of less common mutations, a central reference laboratory in each country must be able to sequence the β globin genes. Rapid DNA-based techniques for identifying the different deletion and nondeletion forms of α thalassemia are also available (Weatherall and Clegg 2001b).

Facilities and Organization. To provide an adequate laboratory service, each country with a high incidence of β thalassemia or sickle cell anemia (a carrier rate equal to or greater than 1 to 2 percent) requires at least one central reference laboratory to carry out accurate hemoglobin and DNA analyses. Peripheral hospital laboratories with expertise in screening tests and their quality control are also required.

General pediatricians, pediatricians with a special interest in blood diseases, or pediatricians or other clinicians who devote their entire time to the management of such diseases may care for children with severe hemoglobin disorders. A problem arises for older patients, who must often change their doctors during adolescence. There is a serious dearth of physicians trained to care for older patients. Ideally, every country with a high incidence of inherited hemoglobin disorders should have centers specially designated for treating patients of all ages. Such centers require outpatient transfusion facilities, space for parents to wait while their children are being transfused, inpatient facilities, and access to basic laboratory diagnostic services. Centers involved in prenatal diagnosis require access to appropriate obstetric services. The advantage of specialist centers is continuity of care. Patients with chronic disease must have confidence in their medical advisers. Such confidence can be achieved only if they see the same staff over the entire course of their illness.

As concerns personnel, a WHO working group has recommended one doctor, three nurses, one laboratory technician, one counselor, and one administrative assistant for every 50 to 100 patients (WHO 1994). Overall, the workload is higher in centers for thalassemia than for sickle cell anemia, largely because of the lesser need for regular blood transfusions for those with the latter condition. However, sickle cell anemia is associated with more acute inpatient episodes per year.

The other major role of centers of this type is education, including training other clinicians, medical students, counselors, nurses, and others needed to provide information to local communities.

A number of publications describe treatment protocols to use in managing patients (Weatherall and Clegg 2001b; WHO 1985, 1987, 1989, 1994). Treatments include the following:

- *Blood transfusion.* Although regular transfusion is required most frequently for managing the thalassemias, it is increasingly being applied for the prophylaxis of serious complications of sickle cell anemia. Treatment centers need to cooperate closely with national blood transfusion programs. Washed or otherwise leukocyte-depleted blood should always be used. Blood has to be screened for hepatitis B, hepatitis C, HIV, and—in some populations—malarial parasites. Blood requirements for patients with thalassemia range from 500 to 1,500 liters per 100 patients per year, depending on their age distribution.
- *Iron chelation.* Transfusion-dependent thalassemic patients and patients with sickle cell anemia maintained on transfusion for prophylactic purposes require 30 to 50 milligrams per kilogram per day of desferrioxamine infused subcutaneously by pump. One pump is required per patient. Regular assessment of body iron and assessment for complications are essential.
- *Immunization and other prophylactic measures.* Every child with sickle cell anemia should receive oral prophylactic penicillin from the time of diagnosis. Some centers now

routinely immunize patients with polyvalent pneumococcal, meningococcal, and *Haemophilus influenzae* vaccines. However, the effectiveness of regimens of this type has not been clearly established even for splenectomized patients.

- *Splenectomy.* Each year, 2 to 3 percent of patients with severe β thalassemia require splenectomy. When patients who have received suboptimal treatment first receive standard treatment, the proportion needing splenectomy can be much higher—up to 30 percent in the first one or two years (WHO 1994). Because of the spleen's natural tendency to atrophy, splenectomy is required only in patients with sickle cell anemia who are having repeated splenic sequestration episodes or who develop hypersplenism.
- *Bone marrow transplantation.* Given the continuing improvement in results, bone marrow transplantation is now a realistic option for patients with severe forms of β thalassemia and sickle cell anemia who have histocompatible related donors and, in particular, are relatively free of complications, particularly chronic hepatitis and severe iron loading (Giardini 1997). Marrow transplantation requires specialized facilities and a trained staff, and the initial capital expenditure is high, but it should be considered wherever the serious hemoglobinopathies are a major problem if the alternative is lifetime treatment.
- *Prenatal diagnosis programs.* If prenatal diagnosis programs are part of an existing genetic and diagnosis service, fetal sampling will involve only marginal costs. If they must be set up from scratch, they require at least two obstetricians trained in fetal medicine, access to ultrasound, and a specialist nurse. Disposable or reusable sampling equipment is also required, together with suitable sterile facilities for amniocentesis, facilities for termination of pregnancy in the first or second trimesters, and access to experienced bereavement counselors. Access to a laboratory able to carry out mutation analysis is also required.
- *Other treatments.* Patients with hemoglobinopathies require folate supplements. Those infected with hepatitis C require treatment with antiviral agents. Those with endocrine damage caused by iron loading may require hormone replacement therapy.

In addition, centers for hemoglobin disorders require a trained counselor or clinical psychologist to handle both genetic and social issues. They should interact with local public health organizations to disseminate information about inherited hemoglobin diseases to schools and to the community at large. Many countries have parent support groups. The Thalassemia International Federation, an international body run largely by parents and lay members, provides advice and support for national parent associations and hemoglobinopathy programs.

COSTS AND EFFECTIVENESS OF DIAGNOSIS AND MANAGEMENT

Defining the full costs of treating patients with inherited disorders of hemoglobin is difficult, and comparing them between countries is even harder. The variables that confound such estimates include different health care systems, varying methods of obtaining donated blood, widely varying practices in screening blood for pathogens, and differing costs of drugs and equipment. WHO working parties and others have produced approximate data (Alwan and Modell 1997; WHO 1985, 1987, 1989, 1994).

Thalassemias

Information about the economic aspects of the thalassemias is sparse, including the costs and effectiveness of different interventions, three of which are discussed here: screening and counseling, treatment using transfusions and chelation, and cure by means of bone marrow transplant.

Screening and Counseling. Screening and counseling are cost-effective to the extent that they avert an affected birth or ensure early and adequate treatment of an affected child. Several studies, beginning with community screening programs in Montreal (Scriver and others 1984), have provided strong evidence that screening and prenatal diagnosis are highly effective in relation to control of the thalassemias. Alwan and Modell (1997), Davies and others (2000), and Modell and Kuliev (1991, 1993) provide detailed discussions of the issues involved, together with estimates of the costs of screening and counseling programs compared with the treatment of established disease, and even though the estimates are based mainly on studies in developed countries, the findings are probably more generally applicable.

The effectiveness of prenatal diagnosis programs can be quite high if more than 2 percent of the population is a carrier and the public education programs that precede their establishment are well designed. In Europe, 80 to 90 percent of counseled at-risk couples now request prenatal diagnosis, and a rapid reduction in affected births has been observed. The thalassemia birth rate fell almost 100 percent between the late 1970s and the late 1980s in Cyprus and Sardinia and about 80 percent in mainland Greece and Italy (Modell and Kuliev 1991). Between 1974 and 1986, such births fell by 40 percent in the United Kingdom (Modell and Kuliev 1991).

In terms of cost-effectiveness, terminating a pregnancy cannot be compared with improving the health of a child carried to term, but it is clearly cost saving compared with treatment. Modell and Kuliev (1991) estimate the cost of replacement (when a couple terminates an affected pregnancy and subsequently has a normal child) at only 30 percent of the annual cost of treatment, or 2 percent of the discounted lifetime cost. Similarly, Scriver and others (1984) estimate the costs of preventing an affected birth in Canada as less than annual treatment costs and about 4 percent of lifetime costs.

Treatment. Investigators have made several estimates of the costs of treating the β thalassemias. Approximate annual costs of care in Thailand in 2003 were as follows (authors' estimates updated from unpublished Thai sources):

- homozygous β thalassemia: US$19.84 million for patients in their first year of treatment and US$17.7 million per year for patients in subsequent years of treatment
- Hb E β thalassemia: US$100.3 million for patients in the first year of treatment and US$92.4 million for patients in subsequent years of treatment
- homozygous α^0 thalassemia: US$727,000
- Hb H disease: US$7.49 million.

The life expectancy of a child in Thailand homozygous for β thalassemia is only 10 years, reflecting an inability to provide the bulk of patients with expensive chelating drugs. These costs are therefore not fully comparable to those from more developed countries, where better care means that children live longer. Han, Han, and Myint (1992) provide data for Myanmar that are comparable to those for Thailand.

Table 34.3 shows the annual costs for a program in Toronto that offers a high level of symptomatic care, and table 34.4 presents treatment costs for the eastern Mediterranean, taking into account the increasing expenditure required as children grow and require higher doses of maintenance drugs and more units of blood each year. Despite the difficulties of making comparisons, tables 34.3 and 34.4 indicate that the costs for managing β thalassemia in the eastern Mediterranean are roughly similar to those in Toronto, exclusive of transfusion, and are therefore probably reasonable estimates of the costs of managing thalassemias in developed countries.

Transfusion is required to keep a child with severe thalassemia alive beyond age one or two, but by itself prolongs life only to age 10 to 15. The gain is the added 9 to 14 years lived with disability weights of 0.1 to 0.5, implying 0.50 DALY gained for the last years and 0.75 to 0.90 per year earlier. Table 34.4 shows the costs of transfusion at ages 7 to 11, and figures in parentheses in the table show the costs at age 2 and for adults. Costs and health gains run parallel, so it makes little difference whether they are discounted when summed over an interval. Table 34.5 shows discounted total costs and DALYs gained for death at age 10 or 15 and using disability values of 0.1 and 0.25. For both ages, the cost per DALY is about US$2,000 for low disability and about US$3,000 for high disability for transfusion only.

Table 34.3 Annual Costs of Hemoglobinopathy per Outpatient, Excluding Transfusion, Toronto
(2001 US$)

Category	Thalassemia Chelated	Thalassemia Nonchelated	Sickle cell disease Chelated	Sickle cell disease Nonchelated
Clinic staff salaries	1,011.95	183.68	1,011.95	252.99
Clinic supplies	930.19	25.15	930.19	34.65
Medical and surgical outpatient unit	2,069.57	n.a.	2,069.57	n.a.
Consultations	92.58	88.39	92.58	11.94
Diagnostic tests	742.58	281.44	905.89	210.99
Laboratory costs	413.96	31.04	414.01	42.74
Laboratory costs (medical dayunit visits)	665.81	n.a.	665.81	n.a.
Total	5,926.64	609.70	6,090.00	553.31

Source: Estimated costs provided by Nancy Oliveri of the University of Toronto.
Note: n.a. = not applicable.

Table 34.4 Costs of Treatment of Thalassemia for One Patient Age 7 to 11, Eastern Mediterranean
(2001 US$)

Category	Minimum treatment		Full treatment	
Costs other than iron chelation				
Day transfusion: hotel and nursing	375		375	
12 transfusions/year	1,088	(600–1,575)	2,250	(1,390–3,150)
Investigations	135	(135–435)	278	(278–870)
Occasional costs (such as operations)	150		645	
Staff salaries	300		620	
Total if no desferrioxamine therapy	2,048	(1,560–2,835)	n.a.	n.a.
Desferrioxamine therapy (iron chelation)	3,080	(1,440–4,725)	6,165	(2,880–9,450)
Total with desferrioxamine therapy	5,128	(3,000–7,560)	10,333	(6,190–15,110)

Source: Alwan and Modell 1997.
Note: n.a. = not applicable. The figures in parentheses show the range of costs for a two-year-old and an adult; where no range is shown, the cost is independent of age. Both minimum and full treatment include transfusion and chelation. *Full treatment* means more frequent transfusion and consultations, more laboratory work, and more surgery.

A thalassemic patient can be kept alive beyond adolescence, possibly for a normal life span, if also chelated. This treatment means added annual costs of about US$3,000, or about US$6,000 (table 34.4) for full treatment, plus higher costs of transfusion and other components. Besides prolonging life, full treatment is assumed to reduce disability from 0.10 to 0.02 and from 0.25 to 0.10. Table 34.5 also shows discounted incremental costs, DALY gains, and cost per DALY of full treatment compared with those of minimal treatment. The incremental cost per DALY is high up to age 15 because of the modest gain compared with prolonging life with greater disability. From age 15, the cost drops because the child would otherwise die. If a life expectancy of 80 years is assumed, lifetime costs are some US$9,000 to US$11,000 per DALY at a disability weight of 0.1 and roughly US$10,000 to US$12,000 at a disability weight of 0.25.

Comparing full treatment to none, annual costs rise with age from US$6,190 to US$15,110 (table 34.4). As table 34.5 shows, up to age 15, 10.8 to 11.8 discounted DALYs are gained at a total cost of US$121,284 and a cost per DALY of approximately US$10,300 to US $11,200, comparable to lifetime incremental costs. Beyond age 15, the cost per DALY is some US$16,000 to US$17,000, and over the lifetime it is between US$13,000 and US$15,000. Because costs and gains run parallel—and also because of discounting—the lifetime cost per DALY is not sensitive to age at death of 45 or older, so differences in regional life expectancies do not matter.

These cost estimates come from the eastern Mediterranean. In Thailand, the first-year costs are much higher than the costs shown in table 34.5 and include the costs of delivering the child and protecting it from infection. Thereafter, the cost per year of treating the 6,250 survivors of each birth cohort

Table 34.5 Cost-Effectiveness of Treatment for Homozygous β and Transfusion-Dependent Hb E β Thalassemia

Category	Cost/patient (US$)	DALYs gained/patient		Cost/DALY (US$)	
		Disability weight = 0.1	Disability weight = 0.25	Disability weight = 0.1	Disability weight = 0.25
Minimal treatment, transfusion only					
Until death at age 10	17,368	6.96–7.60	6.00–6.39	2,285–2,495	2,718–2,896
Until death at age 15	23,840	10.25–10.81	7.52–7.87	2,206–2,325	3,029–3,170
Full treatment with chelation: incremental compared with minimal treatment					
Until age 15	60,467	1.03–3.80	0.55–2.03	15,912–58,706	29,787–109,940
Beyond age 15 to maximum age 80	132,901	17.25	16.35	7,704	8,129
Total lifetime	193,368	18.28–21.05	16.90–18.38	9,186–10,578	10,520–11,442
Full treatment with chelation: total compared with no treatment					
Until age 15	121,284	11.81	10.84	10,273	11,186
Beyond age 15 to maximum age 80	274,662	17.25	16.35	15,922	16,799
Total lifetime	395,946	29.06	27.19	13,625	14,578

Source: Authors' calculations. All costs and DALYs gained are discounted at 3 percent annually, starting at birth.

Note: Differences in DALYs gained for a given age range and disability weight depend on how rapidly health is assumed to deteriorate in the years immediately preceding death.

with transfusion alone (assuming they live only 10 years) drops, implying a cost per DALY of US$3,146 to US$3,776. Half the 97,500 people with Hb E β thalassemia are assumed to require treatment, leading to a cost per DALY of US$2,100 to US$2,500, consistent with costs in the eastern Mediterranean. For chelated patients in Toronto, the estimate of US$5,927 per year (table 34.3) implies a cost per DALY of US$6,600 to US$8,000, considerably less than in the eastern Mediterranean, but the costs do not include transfusion. Thus, data from three different regions on the cost-effectiveness of full therapy for victims of the common treatable forms of thalassemia are roughly comparable.

De Silva and others' (2000) study provides approximate costs for treating thalassemia in Sri Lanka. If we assume that a prevention program will probably not be developed in the near future, the data suggest that management of the disease will consume approximately 5 to 8 percent of the country's health budget based on 1999 figures. Those estimates have not been used to derive cost-effectiveness results.

Bone Marrow Transplantation. Angelucci and Lucarelli (2001) discuss the economic aspects of bone marrow transplantation. The 1991 cost was US$73,250, excluding follow-up but including the expense of setting up a program. This amount is almost certainly cost saving compared with lifelong transfusion and chelation, and it is also more cost-effective, given the reduction in disability from curing the disease.

Sickle Cell Disease

Extensive data on the costs of sickle cell anemia come from Davis, Moore, and Gergen's (1997) analysis in the United States. An estimated 75,000 hospitalizations of both children and adults occurred each year from 1989 through 1993. The average cost of hospitalization in 1996 was estimated at US$6,300, resulting in a total direct cost of US$575 million per year. In this and subsequent studies, the bulk of hospitalizations was confined to a subset of about 10 percent of the total patient population.

In the United States, specialized treatment centers provide a cost-saving approach to the care of sickle cell anemia. Patients enrolled in these centers used emergency rooms and inpatient units significantly less frequently than those cared for in the general hospital community, resulting in significantly lower health care costs (Nietert, Silverstein, and Abboud 2002; Yang and others 1995). Currently, only a small proportion of patients are treated in centers of this kind, even in developed countries. A pilot study in Benin found that the development of a comprehensive clinical care program reduced the frequency and severity of acute complications related to sickle cell anemia (Rahimy and others 2003). The annual cost per family using the program was US$40, and the annual cost for each hospitalization was US$100.

Neonatal Screening and Prophylaxis. Extensive controlled trials in several developed countries have demonstrated the

Table 34.6 Cost-Effectiveness of Penicillin Prophylaxis for Sickle Cell Disease Detected by Newborn Screening, Jamaica

Category	Monthly injection	Daily oral dose	Total/1,000 children
Monthly cost of penicillin (J$)	22	250	26,560
Nurse's time, 10 minutes/month (J$)	90	n.a.	88,200
Clinician's time, 20 minutes 4–6 times/year (J$)	152.67–229.00	152.67–229.00	152,670–229,000
Total year 1, 8 treatments (J$)	2,117–2,728	3,221–3,832	2,140,000–2,750,000
Total, each of years 2–4, 12 treatments (J$)	3,176–4,092	4,832–5,748	3,210,000–4,130,000
Discounted total (discount rate of 3 percent), first 4 years	11,101–14,303	16,889–20,091	11,220,000–14,420,000
Equivalent in U.S. dollars[a]			
US$1 = J$49.8	223–287	339–407	220,000–290,000
US$1 = J$59.8	186–239	282–336	190,000–240,000
Number of deaths averted by prophylaxis	0.024/child	0.024/child	24 deaths
Costs per death averted (US$)	7,750–11,958	11,750–16,958	7,830–12,058
Costs per DALY gained (US$)	267–412	405–585	270–416

Source: Authors' calculations based on data from Hambleton 2004a, 2004b.

Note: n.a. = not applicable. The results are based on a cohort study of 315 cases.

a. Two exchange rates are shown because the exchange rate changed during the course of the study.

life-saving effect of giving prophylactic penicillin from birth. A randomized trial suggested that this approach would save significantly more lives than starting prophylactic penicillin when an infant presents with symptoms of the disease. Without treatment, pneumococcal infection is the leading cause of death before age five. Penicillin by monthly injection or daily oral dose from about age four months to four years reduces bacteremia by 83 to 86 percent (D. Bonds, personal communication, September 28, 2004; Gill and others 1989, 1995; Panepinto and others 2000). Prophylaxis also reduces the case-fatality rate from infection from 27 to 18 percent.

Data from the United States show that neonatal screening for sickle cell disease followed by the use of appropriate prophylactic treatment prevents deaths (Tsevat and others 1991). With 16 percent of the U.S. population being African American, without screening and treatment 13 deaths would occur per million infants. Six of these deaths could be prevented by targeting only African Americans, and two more could be prevented by universal screening. Ignoring disability and discounting at 3 percent, we find that targeted screening costs US$6,709 per life year saved, or somewhat more per DALY. At more than US$30,000 per life year saved, universal screening would not be cost-effective compared with targeted testing (Panepinto and others 2000).

Data from a Jamaican cohort of 315 children with sickle cell disease allow for a similar cost-effectiveness analysis in a middle-income country (Hambleton 2004a, 2004b). They suggest that treatment averts seven to eight deaths, or that a newly diagnosed child's chances of dying before age four are reduced by 2.4 percentage points. Because bacteremia becomes less frequent with age, few cases occur—and little is known about the mortality risk—after childhood.

In the Jamaican cohort, up to 2 percent of children take prophylactic penicillin orally; the rest receive monthly injections requiring 10 minutes of a nurse's time. A clinician sees each child for 20 minutes four to six times a year. Table 34.6 shows the costs of personnel and penicillin. Other recurrent costs, such as those for syringes, will be low in comparison. No allowance is made for capital costs. The marginal cost of detecting sickle cell disease in newborns who have already been screened for other conditions such as phenylketonuria is only about US$3.30 (D. Bonds, personal communication, September 28, 2004). The cost of screening children who do not have sickle cell disease depends on prevalence and is not included in the estimates. It becomes unimportant as more of the population is at risk.

On average, preventing a death costs about US$8,000 to US$12,000 by means of injection and about US$5,000 more when oral penicillin is used. Because death would typically occur between one and two years of age, each death averted saves 29 DALYs and costs about US$270 to US$400 per DALY. Penicillin prophylaxis is probably more cost-effective than any other intervention. It is standard practice in Jamaica and the United States and can be recommended for middle-income countries where the prevalence is high enough—in the general population or in those of African origin—to justify screening.

Application to Other Countries. The limited data available indicate that specialized treatment centers and neonatal screening programs are effective approaches toward the control of sickle cell anemia. Although these conclusions should be valid for developing countries, many uncertainties remain. In particular, data on the causes of infection in infants with sickle cell disease in Africa are sparse. Because the spectrum of infection may be different, the value of penicillin prophylaxis in Africa is unknown.

Laboratory diagnosis is well defined, is cheap, and does not differ depending on the level of available technology. The major uncertainty is whether the increasing indications for prophylactic transfusion in developed countries will be mirrored in other populations.

Other Treatments. As indicated in the discussion of the burden of disease, sickle cell patients suffer various clinical events for which treatment may be life saving, such as transfusion for aplastic crises. For painful crises, intervention (analgesics and possibly hospitalization) is only palliative. Because of the lack of information on costs and of consensus on the associated disabilities with and without treatment, we have not assessed the cost-effectiveness of any of these treatments.

OPTIONS FOR CONTROL AND MANAGEMENT OF INHERITED HEMOGLOBIN DISORDERS

Even though much more work is needed on both the scientific and the economic aspects of the hemoglobinopathies, certain issues are now clear. Until more definitive ways of treating them are available, reliable knowledge exists on how they can best be managed symptomatically. Furthermore, compelling evidence suggests that population screening programs combined with prenatal diagnosis can reduce the financial burden these increasingly common diseases impose on health services. Defining several options for their control and management is therefore possible. These are based, with some modifications, on Alwan and Modell (1997).

Severe β Thalassemias

This list provides most of the possible options for the control and management of β thalassemia in developing countries.

- *Option one:* best possible patient care, together with retrospective genetic counseling after the first affected child is diagnosed
- *Option two:* best possible patient care, together with retrospective genetic counseling and the option of prenatal diagnosis for subsequent pregnancies
- *Option three:* best possible patient care, together with retrospective genetic counseling and prospective (premarital) carrier screening and counseling, but no prenatal diagnosis
- *Option four:* best possible patient care with premarital, family-based, and population-based prospective carrier screening and genetic counseling, but no prenatal diagnosis
- *Option five:* best possible patient care, premarital and prenatal prospective carrier screening and genetic counseling, and the option of prenatal diagnosis

- *Option six:* based on option four or five but includes the availability of a bone marrow transplant program.

Options one and two, though still commonly practiced in many countries, offer little prospect of reducing the frequency of serious forms of thalassemia. Overall, that reduction is best achieved by option five, which combines maximum possibilities for reducing the frequency of severe disease with the best possible care for affected children. Although thalassemia births have fallen sharply in some developed countries, the effect of prenatal screening is likely to be lower for the large mainland populations of Asia if this policy is implemented, which is why this option includes best-practice treatment. Limited studies also suggest that families that undergo prenatal diagnosis tend to settle at the population norm for the number of children that they subsequently have and that their views on their ability to have unaffected children are extremely positive. For those countries or groups in which termination of pregnancy is unacceptable for religious or cultural reasons, option four is recommended. Option six, which is possible only in countries where bone marrow transplantation is available, should be exploited by any country with a high frequency of the disease, because it offers a potentially cost-effective approach to managing some proportion of affected children.

For the extremely heterogeneous intermediate forms of β thalassemia, notably Hb E β thalassemia, options three and four would probably be best, at least until a better understanding has been gained of the clinical heterogeneity of these thalassemias.

α Thalassemias

Few options are available for the α° thalassemias. Homozygous babies with this condition are stillborn. However, because of the serious maternal complications of carrying these babies, this condition should be screened for prenatally, and affected babies should be identified by prenatal diagnosis with a view to terminating the pregnancy.

Hb H disease, the compound heterozygous state between α$^+$ and α° thalassemia, is generally a relatively mild disorder that simply requires careful follow-up and treatment of complications. Although some have suggested that screening and prenatal diagnosis may be relevant for the more severe forms, more data are required to reach a conclusion.

Sickle Cell Disorders

These options for the management of the sickle cell disorders are directed particularly at the populations of developing countries, although, overall, they are relevant to most countries:

- *Option one:* best possible patient care with the use of prophylactic penicillin following diagnosis, together with retrospective genetic counseling

- *Option two:* best possible patient care, together with a neonatal screening program and the use of penicillin for all homozygous babies, together with retrospective screening and counseling
- *Option three:* best possible patient care, together with neonatal screening and the use of prophylactic penicillin from birth for homozygotes, together with population screening and prospective genetic counseling
- *Option four:* as for option three, plus the availability of prenatal diagnosis, bone marrow transplantation, or both.

Option three would be required to combine best management with the possibility of reducing the frequency of the disease, although whether this option would have any effect by altering the pattern of marriage is not clear. Whether prenatal screening of mothers would be valuable is also not clear: it would reduce the number of neonates who require screening, but because the cost of screening for sickle cell trait is so small, the issue is probably not important. Prenatal diagnosis can be developed (option four), but this option does not seem to be a high priority for sickling disorders in many developed countries, at least until more is known about the reasons for their phenotypic heterogeneity. By contrast, demand is greater in developing countries with limited facilities for the care of these patients. Some developed countries are beginning to immunize children with sickling disorders against infections with pneumococcus, *H. influenzae,* and meningococcus, but in developing countries, this treatment would add enormously to the burden of management programs. Clinical trials to test the efficacy of prophylactic penicillin with or without these vaccine regimens are urgently needed. Similarly, more information about the pathogens that cause early deaths in developing countries is required before the widespread use of prophylactic penicillin can be recommended.

Bone Marrow Transplantation

Experience in developed countries indicates that bone marrow transplantation may offer a cost-effective approach to managing a subset of patients with inherited disorders of hemoglobin (Borgna-Pignatti 1985). In developing countries, if this service is available at all, it is usually confined to the private sector or to those who can pay the fees teaching hospitals require. Given this context, defining the role of bone marrow transplantation in the global control of these diseases is difficult.

International and National Support Groups

Largely through the efforts of parents with affected children and clinicians who have taken an interest in the hemoglobin disorders, many countries have developed national thalassemia or sickle cell anemia societies that provide support for parents, workshops for doctors, and a variety of other important inputs.

In the case of thalassemia, the Thalassemia International Federation acts as an international coordinating body that helps countries develop workshops for training in diagnosis and treatment and organizes international meetings at which experts from different countries share their research and clinical experiences. In 1996, a group of doctors formed the Fédération des Associations de Lutte contre la Drépanocytose en Afrique (Federation of Associations to Control Sickle Cell Anemia in Africa). The membership has grown to 13 Sub-Saharan countries. The federation represents a major initiative in relation to regional training in both the diagnosis and the treatment of sickle cell disease in Sub-Saharan Africa. Unfortunately, it has been unable to raise sufficient funds to equip and run even a modest secretariat. Considering the success of the Thalassemia International Federation, particularly in countries with limited facilities for managing the hemoglobin disorders, the lack of support for this initiative in Africa is a clear indication of the importance of educating nongovernmental organizations and similar bodies about the increasing public health problems resulting from the inherited hemoglobin disorders.

Ethical and Social Issues

The various options for controlling and managing the hemoglobin disorders raise many ethical and social issues (see Weatherall and Clegg 2001b for more details). These issues arise most often in developing countries, where the level of education is often low and understanding of genetic diseases is limited. Serious genetic diseases such as thalassemia are associated with social problems such as patient stigmatization and broken marriages because one partner blames the other for the birth of an affected child. In countries where arranged marriages are still common, screening programs for heterozygotes may make it difficult for female carriers to find husbands. In addition, cultural and religious objections about interfering with nature arise when pregnancies are terminated because children have serious genetic diseases. At the same time, if governments perceive prenatal diagnosis and termination of pregnancy to be a highly cost-effective way of controlling these diseases, which they are, the danger arises that governments will pressure women to undergo these procedures. Therefore, before any programs are established, extensive discussions between governments, the medical profession, and the community about how to control these diseases are vital.

FURTHER RESEARCH

Despite the progress made toward understanding the molecular pathology, pathophysiology, and management of the inherited hemoglobin disorders, many gaps persist:

- First, much better data are required about their frequency and distribution in many developing countries.

- Second, more information is required about the reasons, both genetic and environmental, for the remarkable clinical heterogeneity of these conditions.
- Third, much better criteria are required for the management of the intermediate forms of thalassemia and of sickle cell anemia.
- Fourth, much more work is required on the role of the environment, a topic that has been badly neglected compared with research on the genetics of these conditions.
- Finally, further studies are required on better methods for their symptomatic management or a definitive cure.

One important approach toward progress in controlling these diseases is further development of North-South partnerships (WHO 2002). Arrangements of this kind have been extremely successful for thalassemia but have not evolved for sickle cell anemia research. In both cases such partnerships should evolve and lead to local South-South networks allowing individual countries to share their expertise about these increasingly important conditions.

Finally, a great deal more work needs to be carried out, particularly in developing countries, to investigate the economic aspects of these diseases, in terms of both their overall health burden and their control and management.

CONCLUSIONS

The inherited hemoglobin disorders are posing an increasing global health problem, killing thousands of children because of the inadequacy or unavailability of treatment. With appropriate therapy, many children can survive and have an excellent quality of life, despite requiring lifelong treatment. Even though the full economic burden of managing these disorders is currently unknown, in the case of thalassemia, screening and prenatal diagnosis are cost-effective means of prevention. Penicillin prophylaxis provides cost-effective protection from infection for babies with sickle cell disease and should be standard practice wherever it is affordable.

ACKNOWLEDGMENTS

The authors thank Bernadette Modell for reprints and preprints of her work in this field and Liz Rose for preparing the manuscript.

REFERENCES

Adams, R. J., V. C. McKie, L. Hsu, B. Files, E. Vichinsky, C. Pegelow, and others. 1998. "Prevention of a First Stroke by Transfusions in Children with Sickle Cell Anemia and Abnormal Results on Transcranial Doppler Ultrasonography." *New England Journal of Medicine* 339 (1): 5–11.

Akinyanju, O. 2001. "Issues in the Management and Control of Sickle Cell Disorder." *Archives of Ibadan Medicine* 2 (2): 37–41.

Alwan, A., and B. Modell. 1997. *Community Control of Genetic and Congenital Disorders.* Eastern Mediterranean Region Office Technical Publication Series 24. Alexandria, VA: World Health Organization.

Angastiniotis, M., and B. Modell. 1998. "Global Epidemiology of Hemoglobin Disorders." *Annals of the New York Academy of Sciences* 850: 251–69.

Angelucci, E., and G. Lucarelli. 2001. "Bone Marrow Transplantation in Thalassemia." In *Disorders of Hemoglobin,* ed. M. H. Steinberg, B. G. Forget, D. R. Higgs, and R. L. Nagel, 1052–72. New York: Cambridge University Press.

Ashley-Koch, A., Q. Yang, and R. S. Olney. 2000. "Sickle Hemoglobin (HbS) Allele and Sickle Cell Disease: A HuGE Review." *American Journal of Epidemiology* 151 (9): 839–45.

Ballas, S. K. 1998. "Sickle Cell Disease: Clinical Management." *Clinical Haematology* 11 (1): 185–214.

Borgna-Pignatti, C. 1985. "Marrow Transplantation for Thalassemia." *Annual Review of Medicine* 36: 329–36.

Bunn, H. F. 1997. "Pathogenesis and Treatment of Sickle Cell Disease." *New England Journal of Medicine* 337 (11): 762–69.

Cao, A., R. Galanello, and M. C. Rosatelli. 1998. "Prenatal Diagnosis and Screening of the Haemoglobinopathies." *Clinical Haematology* 11 (1): 215–38.

Davies, S. C., E. Cronin, M. Gill, P. Greengross, M. Hickman, and C. Normand. 2000. "Screening for Sickle Cell Disease and Thalassaemia: A Systematic Review with Supplementary Research." *Health Technology Assessment* 4 (3): i–99.

Davis, H., R. M. Moore Jr., and P. J. Gergen. 1997. "Cost of Hospitalizations Associated with Sickle Cell Disease in the United States." *Public Health Report* 112 (1): 40–43.

De Silva, S., C. A. Fisher, A. Premawardhena, S. P. Lamabadusuriya, T. E. A. Peto, G. Perera, and others (Sri Lanka Thalassaemia Study Group). 2000. "Thalassaemia in Sri Lanka: Implications for the Future Health Burden of Asian Populations." *Lancet* 355 (9206): 786–91.

Dover, G. J., and O. S. Platt. 1998. "Sickle Cell Disease." In *Hematology in Infancy and Childhood,* ed. D. G. Nathan and S. H. Orkin, 762–801. Philadelphia: W. B. Saunders.

Fleming, A. F., J. Storey, L. Molineaux, E. A. Iroko, and E. D. Attai. 1979. "Abnormal Haemoglobins in the Sudan Savanna of Nigeria: I. Prevalence of Haemoglobins and Relationships between Sickle Cell Trait, Malaria, and Survival." *Annals of Tropical Medicine and Parasitology* 73 (2): 161–72.

Fucharoen, G., K. Sanchaisuriya, N. Sae-Ung, S. Dangwibul, and S. Fucharoen. 2004. "A Simplified Screening Strategy for Thalassaemia and Haemoglobin E in Rural Communities in South-East Asia." *Bulletin of the World Health Organization* 82 (5): 364–72.

Giardini, C. 1997. "Treatment of B-Thalassemia." *Current Opinion in Hematology* 4: 79–87.

Gill, F., A. Brown, D. Gallagher, S. Diamond, E. Goins, R. Grover, and others. 1989. "Newborn Experience in the Cooperative Study of Sickle Cell Disease." *Pediatrics* 83 (5, pt. 2): 827–29.

Gill, F., L. Sleeper, S. Weiner, A. Brown, R. Bellevue, R. Grover, and others. 1995. "Clinical Events in the First Decade in a Cohort of Infants with Sickle Cell Disease." *Blood* 86 (11): 776–83.

Hambleton, I. 2004a. "Lifetime Survival Estimates for People with SS Disease in Jamaica." Note prepared for the Disease Control Priorities Project, University of the West Indies, Mona, Jamaica.

———. 2004b. "Mortality among People with Homozygous Sickle Cell Disease in Jamaica." Note prepared for the Disease Control Priorities Project, University of the West Indies, Mona, Jamaica.

Han, A. M., K. E. Han, and T. T. Myint. 1992. "Thalassemia in the Outpatient Department of the Yangon Children's Hospital in Myanmar: Cost Analysis of the Day-Care-Room Services for Thalassemia." *Southeast Asian Journal of Tropical Medicine and Public Health* 23 (2): 273–77.

Livingstone, F. B. 1985. *Frequencies of Hemoglobin Variants: Thalassemia, the Glucose-6-Phosphate Dehydrogenase Variants, and Ovalocytosis in Human Populations.* Oxford, U.K.: Oxford University Press.

Modell, B., and A. M. Kuliev. 1991. "Services for Thalassaemia as a Model for Cost-Benefit Analysis of Genetics Services." *Journal of Inherited Metabolic Disorders* 14 (4): 640–51.

———. 1993. "A Scientific Basis for Cost-Benefit Analysis of Genetics Services." *Trends in Genetics* 9 (2): 46–52.

Molineaux, L., A. F. Fleming, R. Cornille-Brogger, I. Kagan, and J. Storey. 1979. "Abnormal Haemoglobins in the Sudan Savanna of Nigeria: III. Malaria, Immunoglobulins, and Antimalarial Antibodies in Sickle Cell Disease." *Annals of Tropical Medicine and Parasitology* 73 (4): 301–10.

Nietert, P. J., M. D. Silverstein, and M. R. Abboud. 2002. "Sickle Cell Anaemia: Epidemiology and Cost of Illness." *Pharmacoeconomics* 20 (12): 357–66.

Panepinto, J. A., D. Magid, M. J. Rewers, and P. A. Lane. 2000. "Universal versus Targeted Screening of Infants for Sickle Cell Disease: A Cost-Effectiveness Analysis." *Journal of Pediatrics* 136 (2): 201–8.

Rahimy, M. C., A. Gangbo, G. Ahouignan, R. Adjou, C. Deguenon, S. Goussanou, and E. Alihonou. 2003 "Effect of a Comprehensive Clinical Care Program on Disease Course in Severely Ill Children with Sickle Cell Anemia in a Sub-Saharan African Setting." *Blood* 102 (3): 834–38.

Samavat, A., and B. Modell. 2004. "Iranian National Thalassaemia Screening Programme." *British Medical Journal* 329 (7475): 1134–37.

Scriver, C. R., M. Bardanis, L. Cartier, C. L. Clow, G. A. Lancaster, and J. T. Ostrowsky. 1984. "Beta-Thalassemia Disease Prevention: Genetic Medicine Applied." *American Journal of Human Genetics* 36 (5): 1024–38.

Serjeant, G. R. 1992. *Sickle Cell Disease.* Oxford, U.K.: Oxford University Press.

Stamatoyannopoulos, G. 1973. "Problems of Screening and Counseling in the Hemoglobinopathies." In *Fourth International Congress on Birth Defects,* ed. A. G. Motulsky and W. Lenz, 268–76. Amsterdam: Excerpta Medica.

Steinberg, M. H., B. G. Forget, D. R. Higgs, and R. L. Nagel, eds. 2001. *Disorders of Hemoglobin.* New York: Cambridge University Press.

Tsevat, J., J. B. Wong, S. G. Pauker, and M. H. Steinberg. 1991. "Neonatal Screening for Sickle Cell Disease: A Cost-Effectiveness Analysis." *Journal of Pediatrics* 118 (4, pt. 1): 546–54.

Weatherall, D. J. 2003. "Pharmacological Treatment of Monogenic Disease." *Pharmacogenomics Journal* 3 (5): 264–66.

Weatherall, D. J., and J. B. Clegg. 2001a. "Inherited Haemoglobin Disorders: An Increasing Global Health Problem." *Bulletin of the World Health Organization* 79 (8): 704–12.

———. 2001b. *The Thalassaemia Syndromes.* 4th ed. Oxford, U.K.: Blackwell Science.

WHO (World Health Organization). 1985. *Report of the Third and Fourth Annual Meeting of the WHO Working Group for the Community Control of Hereditary Anaemias.* HMG/WG/85.8. Geneva: WHO.

———. 1987. *Report of the Fifth WHO Working Group on the Feasibility Study on Hereditary Disease Community Control Programmes, Heraklion, Crete, 24–25 October 1987.* WHO/HDP/WG/HA/89.2. Geneva: WHO.

———. 1989. *Report of the Fifth WHO Working Group on the Feasibility Study on Hereditary Disease Community Control Programmes (Hereditary Anaemias) Cagliari, Sardinia.* WHO/HDP/WG/HA/89.2. Geneva: WHO.

———. 1994. *Guidelines for the Control of Haemoglobin Disorders. Report of the Sixth Annual Meeting of the WHO Working Group on Haemoglobinopathies, Cagliari, Sardinia, 8–9 April 1989.* Geneva: WHO.

———. 2002. *Genomics and World Health.* Geneva: Advisory Committee on Health Research, WHO.

Yang, Y. M., A. K. Shah, M. Watson, and V. N. Mankad. 1995. "Comparison of Costs to the Health Sector of Comprehensive and Episodic Health Care for Sickle Cell Disease Patients." *Public Health Report* 110 (1): 80–86.

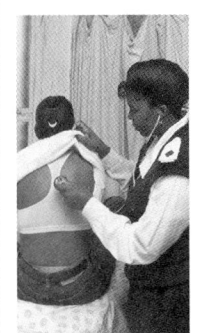

Chapter **35**

Respiratory Diseases of Adults

Frank E. Speizer, Susan Horton, Jane Batt, and Arthur S. Slutsky

Adult respiratory diseases in the developing world are a major burden in terms of morbidity and mortality and, particularly as related to chronic respiratory disease, are of increasing concern (Murray and Lopez 1996). For many years, the leading cause of adult respiratory disease mortality has been tuberculosis, which still kills far more people than it should, given the increased efficacy of treatment and preventive regimens (see chapter 16). However, the burden of other acute and chronic adult respiratory diseases, which is the focus of this chapter, has been rising throughout the world. These diseases fall into four categories: acute diseases, such as pneumonia and influenza; chronic diseases, such as chronic obstructive pulmonary disease (COPD) and asthma; occupational lung diseases, such as byssinosis, asbestosis, and coal worker's pneumoconiosis; and other parenchymal lung diseases, such as immune-related lung diseases. Lung cancer, tuberculosis, and AIDS-related lung diseases are dealt with in chapters 29, 16, and 18, respectively.

ACUTE DISEASES: PNEUMONIA AND INFLUENZA

Obtaining figures on the incidence and burden of pneumonia and influenza in adults throughout the developing world has been surprisingly difficult. Much of the research and surveillance has been directed toward the pediatric age group (see chapter 25). In 2000, fatal lower respiratory infections, as a class that represents serious pneumonia and influenza, were reported as the cause of 120 deaths per million men and 76 deaths per million women worldwide for the 15 to 59 age group (WHO 2000). For both sexes in this age group, this statistic represents approximately one-third of the deaths caused by tuberculosis. However, for the age groups over 60, rates of death from lower respiratory disease more than double

for each decade of life, whereas rates of death from tuberculosis remain relatively constant. Notably, acute respiratory diseases—in addition to tuberculosis—remain major concerns among adults with AIDS.

The diagnosis of pneumonia varies according to the patient's access to medical care. Often the diagnosis is made simply on the basis of cough and fever. For patients with access to a hospital, the likelihood of obtaining a chest x-ray increases; generally the infection is bacteriologically confirmed only in the most sophisticated medical centers. The natural history of pneumonia without antibiotic treatment varies with the etiologic agent and the patient's underlying comorbid conditions and age. Mortality resulting from these lower respiratory diseases is approximately 10-fold higher in people age 60 to 69 than in people age 15 to 59 (WHO 2000). Comorbid conditions, malnutrition, low socioeconomic status, and cigarette smoking each play a role in increasing the incidence of disease and worsening the prognosis, both with and without treatment.

From studies conducted in the developed world, it would be reasonable to conclude that common antibiotics for pneumonias that occur outside a hospital setting would effectively reduce days lost from work and, in the absence of other morbid conditions, mortality. The few studies in which sputum specimens have been cultured suggest that *Streptococcus pneumoniae* is found in between 40 and 50 percent of the cases. Gram-negative organisms or mixed infections are often isolated, and thus, the use of broad-spectrum antibiotics is warranted (Hooi, Looi, and Ng 2001; Hui and others 1993; Lieberman and others 1996). As would be expected, increased use of antibiotics has resulted in increased resistance to common antibiotics. In addition, 10 to 15 percent of these cases may be tuberculosis (Dolin, Raviglione, and Kochi 1994).

Scott and others (2000) suggested that, despite the similarity of the mortality rates for hospital-treated pneumonia in developing and developed countries, there are important differences in the age distributions. The median age at death among Kenyan adults was 33 years, in contrast to more than 65 years in more developed countries. Many patients in developing countries present late in the course of the disease. Often they die before an appropriate diagnostic workup can be completed, thus leading to an underestimate of case-fatality rates.

Signs and symptoms of influenza can vary from trivial to explosive. Although the disease is usually self-limiting, it can result in both severe incapacity and, when not properly treated, potentially fatal secondary pneumonia. Clearly, patients with comorbid conditions, the very young, pregnant women, and the elderly are at greater risk of suffering from complications from influenza. Those criteria, along with the adequacy of supply, form the basis for choosing who should be considered for vaccination each year. Because the symptoms of influenza can be quite similar to those of bacterial pneumonia, influenza may often be misdiagnosed as pneumonia. Generally, influenza is more self-limiting than pneumonia, although the infectivity and transmission of influenza from person to person can be substantial. The current threat of H5N1 influenza has resulted in increased human and avian surveillance and preparations for a possible pandemic (box 35.1).

The recent 2003 outbreak of severe acute respiratory syndrome (SARS; see chapter 53) emphasizes the importance of accurate and open surveillance and a coordinated response in

---

Box 35.1

H5N1 Influenza

Clearly, of even greater concern is the potential for a new influenza A pandemic, as occurred in 1918 and more recently in 1958 and 1968, from a newly altered strain of avian influenza. With each additional bird-to-human case, modest genetic mutation or re-assortment increases the chance for the avian virus to be altered to become established and virulent in mammalian species. This may result in the establishment of sustained transmission among humans. While the pandemics of 1958 and 1968 were together responsible for approximately 3 million deaths, mostly in the very young, the elderly, and in those with comorbid conditions, the 1918 episode is believed to have caused over 40 million deaths, mostly in the age group 15 to 35 years. This potential for greatly increased mortality among such a robust population has fueled recent concern (WHO 2005a).

This concern has become more immediate with the identification of a sub-strain of influenza A, H5N1, first identified in 1997 in Hong Kong when it jumped from poultry to humans and killed six of 18 infected people. Virtually all of the original cases were believed to have been bird-to-human transmission. Since that time there have been a few hundred serologically confirmed cases in Cambodia, Indonesia, Thailand, and Vietnam, with high case fatality but no sustained evidence of ongoing human-to-human transmission (WHO 2005b).

The H5N1 strain is highly pathogenic among poultry. During 2003–2004 it resulted in outbreaks in 8 countries in Asia, with over 100 million birds dying from disease or being culled. More recently, though an additional 150 million birds have been culled, because much of the developing world's poultry economy depends on rural backyard sources, it is not clear how effective these control measures have been. Although these efforts were thought to help control the spread of the virus, permanent ecological reservoirs appear to have become established in wild fowl and domestic chickens over a relatively broad region of Southeast Asia. WHO authorities have expressed concern about the finding that migratory birds that are infected with H5N1 but are relatively asymptomatic have spread viable viruses over large regions with subsequent infection in domestic poultry. Furthermore, more recently there has been evidence of disease in wild and zoo mammals as well as isolated cases of infection in domestic cats. Recent reports from Vietnam include two cases in humans infected through the consumption of uncooked duck blood. Further investigation of possible person-to-person transmission is underway. Recently, WHO (2005b) stated, "The possible spread of H5N1 avian influenza to poultry in additional countries cannot be ruled out. WHO recommends heightened surveillance for outbreaks in poultry and die-offs in migratory birds, and rapid introduction of *containment measures*, as recommended by FAO and OIE. Heightened vigilance for cases of respiratory disease in persons with a history of exposure to infected poultry is also recommended in countries with known poultry outbreaks. The provision of clinical specimens and viruses, from humans and animals, to WHO and OIE/FAO reference laboratories allows studies that contribute to the assessment of pandemic risk and helps ensure that work towards vaccine development stays on course."

Humans have little natural immunity to the H5N1 viruses. Thus, in contrast to the usual influenza epidemics, which affect the very young, elderly, and those with

---

comorbid conditions, virtually the entire population in an exposed community is at risk. In human cases of avian influenza, following the initial respiratory infection, mortality results from two distinct processes. One process begins with relatively rapid onset of respiratory distress from hypoxia associated with ARDS.[a] The alternative process results from secondary bacterial infection with a variety of organisms. In the documented H5N1 influenza infections in humans, respiratory symptoms are most prominent. However, in one case of encephalitis in a child from Vietnam, H5N1 influenza virus was identified in cerebrospinal fluid and fecal matter, and in throat and serum samples. Isolates from several cases were resistant to two commonly used antiviral medications (amantadine and rimantadine), while two other antiviral medications (oseltamivir and zanamivir) still appear to be effective.

There is no way to predict the outcome of these ongoing events. What seems evident is that if human-to-human transmission becomes established, a pandemic will follow.

Given the lack of natural immunity, there is considerable concern that even if adequate vaccines were available, distribution on a worldwide basis would be limited by economic considerations as well as distribution problems in the developing world. Efforts are underway to identify the genetic make-up of the strains of H5N1 that will yield the most effective vaccines and to produce such vaccines in a cost-effective manner. Testing H5N1 vaccines based on recently identified viruses in normal healthy volunteers suggests the immunologic response may be adequate, but several months of production would be necessary to produce adequate supplies for one region, let alone for worldwide distribution. Stockpiles of effective antiviral medications are being generated in some countries. In the interim, WHO has encouraged the rapid reporting of cases and the establishment of procedures for better public health intervention strategies before and during a pandemic (WHO 2005c). Many countries have developed pandemic influenza preparedness plans in anticipation of such an event.

Source: Authors.
a. ARDS is defined as Acute Respiratory Distress Syndrome resulting from multiple causes, the most likely in this situation being an immunological reaction to the virus.

Table 35.1 Public Health Measures in the SARS Episode, 2003

Procedure	Comment
1. Isolation of patients	Isolate rapidly after onset of symptoms.
2. Quarantine of contacts	Usually at home, but separate from patients. When in contact with unexposed subjects, wear masks and avoid public transportation and visits to crowded places.
3. Education	Reduce delay between onset of symptoms and isolation. In endemic areas, get subject to monitor temperature daily. Use fever hotlines, fever evaluation clinics.
4. Thermal screening	Monitor temperature of travelers from endemic areas (not proven effective).
5. Increased social distance	Cancel mass gatherings. Close schools, theaters, public facilities. Require use of masks in public settings.
6. Disinfection	Practice frequent hand washing. Use aerosol disinfectant agents.
7. Travel advisories	Postpone unessential travel. Screen travelers at entry and exit (not proven effective). Distribute health notices to travelers.

Source: Data compiled and summarized from Bell 2004.

controlling the spread of newly active influenza strains. The potential for global spread and the occurrence of worldwide epidemics of influenza (presumed to be transmitted to humans from domesticated or wild animals and then through close proximity to humans with symptomatic disease—generally to caregivers) points out the importance of continued surveillance for such episodes (Low and McGeer 2004). The lessons learned from the SARS epidemic reinforce the importance of proven traditional public health measures, such as finding and isolating cases, quarantining close contacts, and improving infection control practices (Bell 2004). Those methods, along with several other, less traditional efforts, were presumed to be

part of the reason the epidemic was contained as promptly as it was (see table 35.1). However, because of the high case-fatality rate, the disease caused significant disruption throughout the world.

Economic Impact of Influenza and Cost-Effectiveness of Interventions in the Developed World

Influenza is common in developed countries. Annually, it affects 10 to 20 percent of the U.S. population (Lee and others 2002); those affected experience on average a loss of 2.8 workdays per episode. Those over 65 years of age are more susceptible to complications, increased costs of hospitalization, and even death. The cost of outbreaks can be large. The costs of the 1996–97 epidemic in Germany were estimated at US$1,045 million, and the annual costs of outbreaks at US$11 million to US$18 million (WHO 2002a).

For those over age 65, many countries encourage preventive vaccinations annually, on the basis of studies suggesting that vaccination (either opportunistic or in a campaign) is cost-effective in elderly populations (for example, see the model of Scuffham and West 2002). Given a good antigenic match, inactivated influenza vaccines prevent laboratory-confirmed illness in 70 to 90 percent of healthy adult vaccine recipients (WHO 2002a). Vaccination is less costly than chemoprophylaxis (with ion-channel inhibitors such as amantadine and rimantadine, or with neuraminidase inhibitors such as zanamivir and oseltamivir) or early treatment with the same drugs. In both the institutionalized and the healthy elderly, vaccination substantially reduces overall mortality from influenza (by 40 to 68 percent).

The cost-effectiveness of vaccination for healthy working-age adults, taking into account workdays lost, is a matter of debate. Demicheli and others (2000) concluded that the most cost-effective option for healthy adults age 14 to 60 was to take no action. However, these authors include only medical costs in their calculations. Postma and others (2002) reviewed 11 studies. Only one shows cost savings on the basis of medical costs alone, but nine of them implied cost savings from vaccination if the value of lost work is included. Because of differences in costs and health care usage patterns, data on cost savings in developed countries cannot be helpfully extrapolated to developing countries.

Economic Impact of Influenza in the Developing World

In Hong Kong, China (where there is a milder year-round pattern of infection, little influenza-related mortality, and low reported work losses), a model suggested that vaccination was not cost saving, even if targeted to the elderly (Fitzner and others 2001). The only case for vaccination was if it controlled the emergence of highly virulent strains and prevented transmission to the rest of the world. According to the World Health Organization (WHO), much less is known about the impact of influenza in the developing world. However, in the tropics, where viral transmission normally continues year-round, influenza outbreaks tend to have high attack and case-fatality rates. For example, during an influenza outbreak in Madagascar in 2002, more than 27,000 cases were reported within three months and 800 deaths occurred despite rapid intervention. An investigation of this outbreak, coordinated by WHO, found that health consequences were severe in poorly nourished populations with limited access to adequate health care (WHO 2002b). It is not possible to extrapolate the exact annual burden of influenza in the tropics from data on such occasional and severe outbreaks. Because many areas (for example, Sub-Saharan Africa) do not have surveillance centers, not enough is known at this point to make policy recommendations. There are also no readily available estimates of the cost-effectiveness of influenza vaccination in those environments. (For further discussion of the role of vaccination, see chapter 20.)

CHRONIC RESPIRATORY DISEASES: NATURE, CAUSES, AND BURDEN

COPD and asthma have very different diagnoses and causes; hence, they are discussed in separate sections. However, the treatments for these different chronic respiratory diseases share similarities, and that discussion is therefore combined. One of the difficulties in defining COPD on a worldwide basis is that three distinct levels are used, depending on the sophistication of the health care system in the country where the patient is being evaluated:

- *Chronic bronchitis* with and without obstruction, which may be part of the COPD diagnosis, is defined by the presence of chronic cough and phlegm for three months per year for two or more years and is generally assessed by standardized questionnaires.
- *Obstructive airways disease* is often assessed by reduced pulmonary function as measured by simple spirometry and the presence of a reduced ratio of the forced expiratory volume in one second (FEV_1) divided by the vital capacity (VC).
- For *emphysema*, which is also part of the syndrome of COPD, pulmonary function (changes in lung volume and reduced diffusion capacity), x-ray evidence of bullae formation, hyperinflation of the chest, and (with the use of high-resolution CT scanning) the presence of characteristic changes in lung architecture all may contribute to the diagnosis.

What is apparent is that not all these diagnostic procedures are applied equally, particularly in the developing world; thus, COPD may be seriously underreported. The 1998 Workshop Report by the WHO and the National Institutes of Health (NIH) on "Global Strategy for the Diagnosis, Management, and Prevention of COPD," developed as part of the Global Initiative for Chronic Obstructive Lung Disease (GOLD 2001), uses an international standard for defining the level of obstruction from COPD. This strategy should improve worldwide estimates. This standard definition will still require the use of equipment that measures pulmonary function (Buist 2002). Over the next several years, as the price and distribution of this equipment becomes more favorable and as more groups

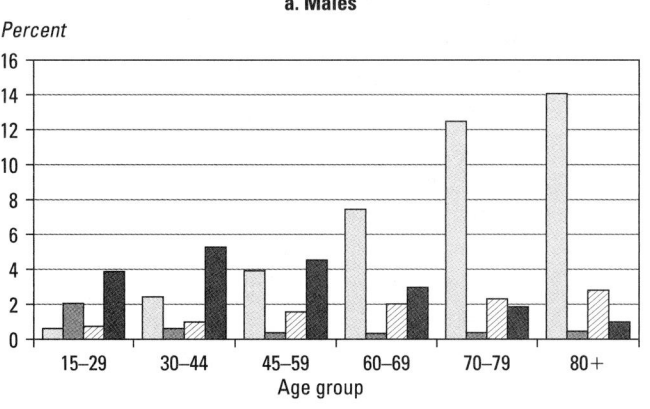

a. Males

Percent

b. Females

Percent

COPD ▨ Asthma ▢ Other respiratory diseases ■ Tuberculosis

Source: WHO 2000.

Figure 35.1 Chronic Respiratory Diseases DALYs as a Percentage of World Totals

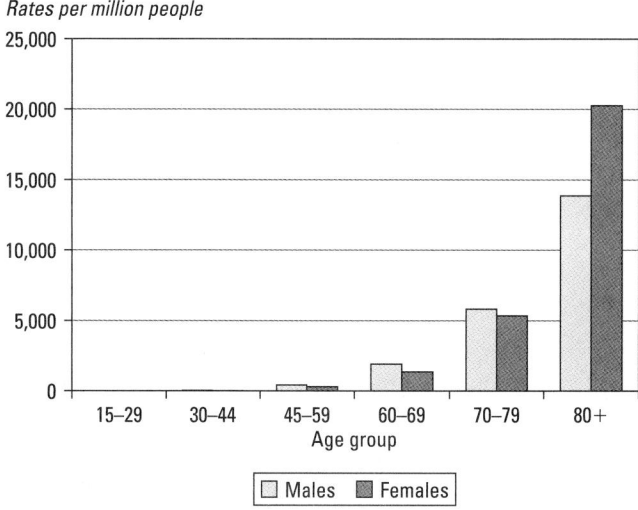

Rates per million people

□ Males ■ Females

Source: WHO 2000.

Figure 35.2 COPD by Age and Sex, Worldwide

undertake the training in its use and in the interpretation of results from the tests, diagnostic uniformity will improve. Unfortunately, as pointed out by Aït-Khaled, Enarson, and Bousquet (2001), the applicability of these guidelines has not been effectively tested in developing countries.

In adults, COPD dominates all other chronic respiratory diseases in accounting for 2 percent to more than 10 percent of lost disability-adjusted life years (DALYs) on a worldwide basis. Its incidence increases dramatically with age (figures 35.1a and 35.1b). Of note, mortality from COPD is low before age 45. Over age 45, death rates increase from 50 to 200 per 10,000 individuals and are consistent across age groups in men and women, with the exception of death rates in women over age 80, which exceed those in men in that age group (figure 35.2).

Much of COPD in the developed world is related to cigarette smoking, and there is no question that progression of the disease is related to the number of cigarettes smoked and the years of smoking. Smoking cessation has been associated with

reduced mortality from COPD, presumably through a mechanism that results in a modest improvement in pulmonary function that appears to be related primarily to the extent of chronic bronchitis and mucus hypersecretion (Scanlon and others 2000; Speizer and others 1989). Within a few years of stopping smoking, smokers' rate of decline of pulmonary function (that is, FEV_1) returns to the rate found in nonsmokers, although little of the lost pulmonary function is regained (Fletcher and others 1976). Similar effects are seen in the developing world. However, because smoking is far less prevalent in developing countries, especially among women, other exposures are related to the development of disease (see also chapter 46). One of the most important exposures, particularly for women, is to unvented coal-fired cooking stoves, starting during childhood and continuing into adult life (see chapter 42).

Because the interventions and treatments for COPD overlap with those for asthma, they will be treated together.

The diagnosis of asthma has been debated for centuries. Health care providers can generally agree on the diagnosis in the individual patient who is wheezing and in whom other etiologic factors are ruled out. They would also agree on the definition of the disease as an inflammatory response in the airways that results in variable and generally reversible airflow obstruction with or without treatment. However, depending on the training of health care providers, the nature of surveillance, the characteristics of a given community, and the particular environment of the community, the accuracy of the estimate of the prevalence of asthma in a community may vary much more. The reported prevalence of the disease may be based on no more than an answer to this question: "Has a provider ever told you that you (or your child) has had asthma?" The response to this question has been validated in a number of studies. In contrast, the diagnosis may depend on examination of the patient's chest, physiological testing, responsiveness to provocative stimuli to the airways, and specific response to therapy. Thus, estimates of community burden from asthma may depend on the threshold used in making the diagnosis.

Despite variations in diagnostic criteria, worldwide estimates of the asthma burden among adults have generally come from surveys within selected communities. In contrast to other adult respiratory diseases, the prevalence of asthma is relatively low (figures 35.1a and 35.1b). In adults, the DALYs for asthma are at a peak of about 2 percent of the total worldwide in people age 15 to 29, and they decline in each older age group. This pattern is also reflected in mortality rates, with the highest rates occurring in young people and equal rates in men and women about age 60. After age 60, reported rates of death caused by asthma in men begin to exceed those in women, and both become substantial. That shift reflects primarily either increasingly questionable diagnostic accuracy or misclassification of other obstructive respiratory diseases such as COPD.

Economic Impact of Asthma and COPD in the Developed World

In the United Kingdom (where asthma rates are particularly high), respiratory disease accounts for 6.5 percent of hospital admissions. Fifteen percent of the working population report work-limiting health problems caused by respiratory disease, and 18.3 million workdays were lost to asthma problems in 1995–96 (Chung and others 2002).

In the Netherlands, annual costs associated with asthma and COPD (direct and indirect) were estimated to exceed US$500 million for a population of about 14 million (data for the 1980s). Asthma or COPD was responsible for 3 percent of absenteeism caused by illness, and asthma was also the main reason for absence from school among children age 4 to 12 (Rutten–van Mölken and others 1992).

In the United States in the early 1990s, health care costs attributable to respiratory disease were US$11 billion (about 2 percent of total health care costs), and an estimated 3 million workdays and 10 million schooldays were lost to respiratory disease (Stoloff, Poinsett-Holmes, and Dorinsky 2002).

Another survey (Weiss and Sullivan 2001) estimated the costs of asthma in 1991 US dollars for four developed countries (Australia, Sweden, the United Kingdom, and the United States) and one state (New South Wales in Australia). Per patient costs of asthma ranged from US$326 (Australia) to US$1,315 (Sweden) annually, with direct costs accounting, in most cases, for more than half of total costs.

Economic Impact of Asthma in the Developing World

Data for developing countries are much scarcer. For Estonia, Kiivet and others (2001, cited in Lee and Weiss 2002) estimated the direct annual costs of asthma to be US$104 per year per asthma patient, equivalent to 1.4 percent of direct health care costs. In Singapore, medical costs for asthma constitute 1.3 percent of total health care costs (Chew, Goh, and Lee 1999, cited in WHO 2001).

One study (Aït-Khaled, Enarson, and Bousquet 2001, cited in Weiss and Sullivan 2001) found that asthma drugs cost between 3.8 and 25 percent of the patient's monthly income in 24 developing countries in Asia and Africa. K. R. Smith (2000) estimates the burden of respiratory disease in India that is attributable to indoor air pollution (only a fraction of all respiratory disease) as 1.6 billion to 2 billion sick days per year. Of that total, asthma is responsible for about one-third, acute respiratory infection is responsible for about one-third, and the remainder is attributable to COPD, tuberculosis, and ischemic heart disease. Asthma and COPD combined account for 44 percent of the burden.

Cost Effectiveness of Interventions for COPD and Asthma in Developed Countries

Five recent overviews of the economics of chronic respiratory disease, COPD, and asthma (Friedmann and Hilleman 2001; Lee and Weiss 2002; Ruchlin and Dasbach 2001; Sullivan and Weiss 2001; Weiss and Sullivan 2001), in addition to many individual studies, focus on developed countries.[1] Only a limited number of studies use cost- or quality-adjusted life years (QALYs) saved as the outcome (others use life years saved). (Studies focusing on intermediate health outcomes and on cost minimization are not discussed here.) In general, costs in developing countries would be about 20 percent of those reported here, according to detailed unit cost data by region from WHO-CHOICE (Choosing Interventions That Are Cost-Effective) and on comparisons of respiratory drug prices from online pharmacies in the United States and from the International Drug Price Indicator Guide (http://erc.msh.org). The exceptions are interventions involving nondiscounted drugs that are still under strictly enforced patents, for which the costs in developing countries would be closer to those in the United States. Table 35.2 summarizes the results.

Inhaled salbutamol (short-acting beta-2 agonist) is the first line of treatment for both intermittent asthma (daytime symptoms less than once per week, nocturnal symptoms less than twice per month, and normal spirometry between episodes) and COPD (mild to severe) in both developed and developing countries. This treatment became standard practice beginning in the 1970s, so there are no cost-effectiveness studies of salbutamol compared with placebo. This medical intervention is likely the most cost-effective one, but it is still likely to cost

Table 35.2 Cost-Effectiveness of Interventions for Asthma and COPD in 2001

Reference	Intervention	Alternative	Cost-effectiveness
Pharmacological			
Authors' estimates	Inhaled ipratropium bromide	Placebo	US$6,700–US$8,900/QALY for moderate COPD
Paltiel and others 2001	Quick relievers[a] and inhaled corticosteroids	Quick relievers only	US$13,900/QALY in adults with mild to moderate asthma: US$10,600 for moderate only
Van den Boom and others 2001	Inhaled corticosteroid (fluticasone propionate)	Placebo	US$13,400/QALY COPD treatment
Akins and O'Malley 2000	A-1 antitrypsin augmentation therapy	Standard care[b]	US$14,400/QALY, severely deficient individuals
Hay and Robin 1991, in Ruchlin and Dasbach 2001	A-1 antitrypsin augmentation therapy	Standard care[b]	US$45,000–US$215,000/life year, depends on age, efficacy, and so forth
Education			
Toevs, Kaplan, and Atkins 1984, in Ruchlin and Dasbach 2001	Education and exercise program	Exercise program only	US$71,500/QALY
Long-term oxygen			
Authors' estimate	Home oxygen therapy for COPD	No oxygen	US$19,000/life year (US$26,700–US$38,000/QALY)
Mechanical ventilation			
Schmidt and others 1983, in Rutten–van Mölken	Mechanical ventilation	Standard hospital care[c] (excluding ventilation)	US$6,400–US$23,600/life year (COPD, asthma, cardiac patients) excluding physician costs
Anon and others 1999 in Ruchlin and Dasbach 2001	Mechanical ventilation in intensive care unit, asthma, and COPD patients	Standard hospital care[c] (excluding ventilation)	US$35,000–US$60,700/QALY
Surgery			
Al and others 1998, in Ruchlin and Dasbach 2001	Lung transplant in end-stage disease	No transplant	US$464,000/QALY
Ramsey and others 1995, in Ruchlin and Dasbach 2001	Lung transplant in those eligible	No transplant	US$238,200/QALY

a. *Quick relievers* refer to rapid-acting bronchodilators (for example, salbutamol) that act to relieve bronchoconstriction and accompanying acute symptoms of wheeze, chest tightness, and cough.
b. Standard care includes medical management (ipratropium bromide, beta-2 agonist, steroid) and home oxygen as needed.
c. Standard care includes medical management and oxygen.

some thousands of dollars per life year saved in the United States.

The next line of treatment currently recommended for developing countries is inhaled corticosteroids (for example, beclomethasone) for mild to severe persistent asthma (disease ranging from daytime symptoms greater than once per week, nocturnal symptoms more than twice a month, and normal spirometry between episodes to daily frequent symptoms associated with severe obstruction) and inhaled ipratropium bromide for COPD. Both first-generation corticosteroids and ipratropium bromide are off patent. However, as pointed out by Chan-Yeung and others (2004), the use of corticosteroids either intermittently or chronically is commonly recommended in developed countries, where the background level of tuberculosis among patients is considerably lower. In developing countries with higher tuberculosis rates, corticosteroids must be used with greater caution.

Inhaled steroids cost about US$13,900 per QALY for mild to moderate asthma or when used in early treatment of

COPD. The cost per QALY is likely to be lower for severe asthma, but ethical considerations render random controlled trials unfeasible.

No cost-effectiveness study could be found for ipratropium bromide compared with placebo. We estimate that the cost per QALY saved would be between one-half and two-thirds of that for a new-generation inhaled steroid such as fluticasone propionate. This estimate, which is based on the relative cost of the two drugs in the United States and assumes similar effectiveness of the two drugs, would put the cost of ipratropium bromide between US$6,700 and US$8,900 per QALY.

Most of the other interventions summarized in table 35.2 have a higher cost per QALY. For individuals who develop COPD related to a severe deficiency in alpha-1 antitrypsin, alpha-1 antitrypsin therapy is sometimes considered, at a cost of between US$45,000 and US$215,000 per life year.[2] The use of long-acting beta-2 agonists and leukotriene modifiers is now an accepted and integrated component of the treatment of moderate to severe asthma in the developed world. However, the cost savings for the developing world are difficult to demonstrate because the endpoints of studies using those drugs are often changes in spirometric testing, improved quality-of-life measures, steroid-sparing effects, or altered hospital admission rates.

Likewise, oral or intravenous steroids play a crucial role in the treatment of acute exacerbations in both asthma and COPD, but endpoint assessments in studies typically address decreases in the duration of hospital stays and increases in the use of emergency department facilities, which result in decreases in health costs in the developed world. Oral steroids are inexpensive, even by standards in developing countries, and in the short term might appear to be cost-effective, but they are associated with major medium- to long-term consequences and are not recommended as standard therapy.

Educational programs tend to be cost saving in developed countries, where uncontrolled exacerbations are extremely costly in terms of hospital care (six such programs are surveyed in Van Mölken and others 1992 and one in Ruchlin and Dasbach 2001). Similarly, exercise rehabilitation programs (six surveyed in Ruchlin and Dasbach 2001) can also be cost saving. WHO (2001) has commented on cost savings achieved by education programs for asthma from four different U.S. studies. Only one of these studies addressed cost per well year, which was estimated at US$71,500 in 2001 (Toevs, Kaplan, and Atkins 1984, cited in Ruchlin and Dasbach 2001). However, there are likely to be monetary savings from fewer workdays lost, which are not factored into this analysis.

WHO (2001) surveyed one self-management training program for chronic asthma in India (Ghosh and others 1998), which resulted in improvements in health status, reduced use of emergency departments and hospitals, and savings on health costs. Sudre and others (1999) pointed out that studies of education programs tend not to provide a good description of the actual program content and that a more systematic description of these interventions needs to be promoted to replicate best practice.

Long-term oxygen therapy is a life-prolonging intervention in advanced stages of COPD. Recent studies do not quantify the cost per QALY but instead compare different methods of oxygen delivery (cylinder or concentrator). These authors' crude estimate for long-term oxygen use is US$19,000 per life year saved.[3] If the quality-of-life scores of patients on long-term oxygen were 0.8 or 0.6, the cost per QALY would be US$22,750 or US$31,700, respectively. (K. J. Smith and Pesce 1994, cited in the Harvard Catalogue of Preference Scores, assign a median score of 0.4 to quality of life for patients with severe COPD with high supportive care needs and poor functional status.)

In hospitals, mechanical ventilation in the intensive care unit has been estimated to cost US$35,000 to US$60,700 per QALY in 2001 (Anon and others 1999, cited in Ruchlin and Dasbach 2001). Studies suggest that noninvasive positive pressure ventilation, where it is feasible, is less costly than invasive mechanical ventilation for specific indications. Finally, costs of lung transplants are at a level scarcely affordable even in developed countries; Al and others (1998, cited in Ruchlin and Dasbach 2001) estimated costs at US$464,000 per QALY, and Ramsey and others (1995, cited in Ruchlin and Dasbach 2001) estimated costs at US$238,000 per QALY (in 2000 U.S. dollars).

All those interventions compare unfavorably with the cost-effectiveness of smoking prevention for preventing COPD (discussed in chapter 46). Smoking prevention is one of the most cost-effective health interventions that exists, and there is a strong case for moving resources from expensive curative interventions to that intervention. Likewise, prevention of COPD by switching the cooking source from unventilated stoves that burn biomass to either improved stoves or kerosene stoves is more cost-effective than treatment (see chapter 42).

Cost-Effectiveness of Interventions for COPD and Asthma in Developing Countries

It is difficult to transfer the costs per QALY saved in developed countries to developing countries. The cost of patented drugs in developing countries should be the same as that in developed countries, whereas the costs of education and of the time of medical personnel should be substantially lower (on the order of 20 percent of U.S. levels). In practice, the costs of off-patent drugs also vary considerably. Beclomethasone dipropionate (one of the older, off-patent inhaled steroids) is available for about US$15 per 200-dose inhaler in Canada in online pharmacies but is quoted at US$1 to US$3 by agencies and suppliers on the International Drug Price Indicator Guide (http://erc.msh.org). A similar price difference exists for salbutamol inhalers. Hence, the most cost-effective therapies in developed countries (inhaled salbutamol and first-generation corticosteroids for asthma and ipratropium bromide for COPD) are also likely to be cost-effective in the wealthier developing countries—or more broadly if inexpensive drug supplies are available. Those drugs are likely to be particularly cost-effective for those with severe and moderately severe asthma or COPD but less cost-effective for those with mild disease. Recent practice suggests that a combination of long-acting beta agonists and inhaled corticosteroids can control moderate to severe disease more rapidly. However, to make this form of therapy cost-effective, the patient needs to be reevaluated to determine whether one or the other drug can be removed. Because of cost considerations, that may not be feasible in the developing world.

Once control has been obtained, education alone appears to be ineffective when only respiratory outcomes are considered (although education on the benefits of exercise has other health benefits: see chapter 44 on lifestyles). However, education addressing the appropriate use of medication is extremely important, particularly in developing countries, where timely emergency care for severe exacerbations may not be readily available. Although the cost of educational efforts would be expected to be considerably lower in developing countries, this area requires more systematic research.

Long-term oxygen is also an option for high-income households in middle-income developing countries. The costs are likely to be lower than in developed countries. In Brazil the monthly cost for supplemental home oxygen therapy is close to US$150 (Sant'Anna and others 2003), compared with US$400 per month paid by Medicare, which would bring the cost-effectiveness to US$7,000 per life year by these authors' crude estimates, or between US$8,750 and US$11,700 per QALY. Publicly funded systems are unlikely to be able to pay this rate, although private insurers and wealthy households might pay because such therapy prolongs life.

The other interventions in table 35.2 are likely to be too expensive for most developing countries to use at present.

OCCUPATIONAL LUNG DISEASE AND OTHER RESPIRATORY DISEASES

Although occupational lung diseases are often considered diseases of the industrial world, they are occurring with increased frequency in the developing world, where guidelines for worker safety are generally more lax or nonexistent. In addition, because of increased migration from rural areas to more urbanized centers and the transfer of major manufacturing activities from the developed market economy countries to the less developed countries, the number of employees with potentially harmful occupational exposures has increased exponentially in the past 30 years. The general discussion of occupation-related diseases is reviewed in chapter 60. We focus here on specific occupation-related lung diseases.

Occupational lung diseases are, for the most part, characterized as related to particular occupational exposures and generally fall into two broad pathophysiological types. One type may result in pulmonary fibrosis, which is manifested by restricted lung volume and decreased diffusion capacity on pulmonary function testing and increased interstitial pulmonary markings on chest x-ray. Certain occupational lung diseases, such as silicosis, are complicated by a substantially increased risk of tuberculosis, which contributes to the overall burden of respiratory disease in the developing world. The second pattern of occupational lung disease is that of obstructive airways disease, which may be reversible (occupational asthma) or irreversible (chronic bronchitis with or without obstruction or emphysema or COPD), in which the chest x-ray often is negative and the diagnosis is dependent largely on reported histories of exposures, symptoms, and pulmonary function testing.

There are few reliable estimates of the global burden of occupation-related respiratory diseases. Because of the lack of systematic surveillance in most developing countries, the few published estimates of occupation-related respiratory diseases have relied on selected studies involving particular industries that investigators have had unique opportunities to explore. For example, Trapido and others (1996) conducted a survey in a relatively small group of former mineworkers and found that approximately 55 percent had pneumoconiosis with or without tuberculosis. They estimated that about 25 percent of migrant and former mineworkers in South African gold mines with 15 to 25 years of exposure had occupational lung diseases. Loewenson (1999) pointed out the difficulties in making assessments of occupational risk throughout the African countries and suggested a series of methodological issues that need to be considered.

Leigh and others (1999) estimated the global burden of diseases related to occupational factors at 4.2 million to 10.0 million cases per year. If one subtracts the rates for established market economy countries, the total burden for the rest of the world is approximately 3.4 million to 9.1 million cases per year. Using limited data and applying rates from individual nations and regional groups of countries, the authors made an indirect calculation for the expected number of cases of occupation-related diseases globally. Figure 35.3 summarizes their estimates for pneumoconiosis and other chronic respiratory diseases by age and gender. Notably, these two categories of disease account for approximately 30 percent of all occupational diseases. The prevalence of these diseases increases with age and is higher among men.

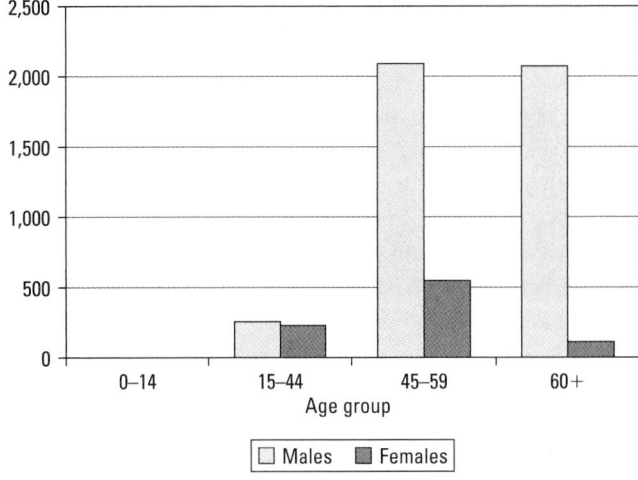

Rates per million people

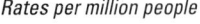

Source: Leigh and others 1999.

Figure 35.3 Estimated Combined Pneumoconiosis and Other Occupation-Related Chronic Respiratory Diseases

Asbestosis and asbestos-related cancers present a particular problem in developing countries. Asbestosis can manifest both as other interstitial lung disease, as described above, and as obstructive airways disease. In addition, occupational exposure is associated with the occurrence of lung cancer, and according to studies in developed countries, the rate of occurrence is synergistically associated with smoking. Because the cost of health care compensation in the developed world exceeds the potential profit from mining and manufacturing of asbestos products, much of the industry has moved to the developing world.

LaDou (2004) has recently summarized the status of the potential for reducing occupational exposure on a worldwide basis and suggests that upward of 10 million lives will be lost if the current lack of controls and continued increases in mining and manufacturing are not changed. In 2000, more than 2 million tons of asbestos products were produced, whereas 25 years earlier the total production was 350,000 tons each year. Except for the Russian Federation and Canada, virtually all the larger producers are in the developing world, where the recognition and reporting of health effects are less well established. The likelihood of reversing this trend and developing an international ban on asbestos use is small, particularly because it is the nations that produce more asbestos products that are, in fact, increasing consumption.

The economic burden of occupational lung diseases is surprisingly difficult to document. Most developed countries and some developing countries (for example, South Africa) have legislation protecting workers from exposure and compensating those who have contracted chronic conditions. In the United States, compensation payments from the Social Security Administration and the Department of Labor for black lung disease totaled US$1.6 billion in 1996 (NIOSH 1999). Data exist on compensation for claims for various occupational lung diseases for the United States and the European Union countries. However, claims data represent only a small fraction of the true economic cost (for example, not all workers make claims; compensation payments lag considerably). For the United States, the annual costs of complying with the revised respirator standards for 1993 were US$111 million for about 5 million workers needing to use a respirator (presumably these costs of prevention were far lower than the economic cost of unprotected work) (OSHA 1998). The primary treatment for affected workers is to remove them from the inciting exposures. (See chapter 60 for discussion of preventive strategies that need to be considered to reduce the risk of occupational disease.)

Some of the other major classes of adult respiratory diseases are discussed in other chapters: tuberculosis, in chapter 16; AIDS-related lung disease, in chapter 18; and lung cancer, in chapter 29. Other diseases that have been studied, particularly in the developed world, include the hypersensitivity or immunologically related pulmonary diseases most often associated with environmental exposures to specific inhaled antigens or interstitial inflammation and fibrosis, often of unknown origin. In the developing world, little systematic work has been done on these diseases to assess incidence or prevalence. These conditions probably occur considerably less frequently than asthma and COPD. However, they are likely to have a higher prevalence in developing countries than is reported in the developed world simply because of the presumed associations with exposures to organic dusts and the increased prevalence of malnutrition (see chapter 56), both of which are likely to occur in more rural and less developed areas of the world.

See chapters 16, 18, and 29 for interventions for tuberculosis, AIDS-related lung disease, and lung cancer, respectively. Managing immunologic and fibrotic respiratory diseases with medication is extremely difficult and expensive. Therapeutic trials often fail, presumably because the treatments are not aimed at a particular antigen. The most effective way of managing these respiratory diseases is to reduce exposure to the inciting agents, an approach that hinges on two strong premises, which are not always applicable in the developed world. First, the disease must be recognized as related to a common environmental contaminant encountered in an occupational or avocational exposure—for example, exposure to thermophilic actinomycetes in moldy hay or sugarcane results in farmer's lung, and exposure to bird feathers or droppings results in bird fancier's disease. Second, community resources must be directed toward educating the public about the importance of limiting exposure to these agents.

GENERAL APPROACH TO LOWERING RISK OF ADULT RESPIRATORY DISEASE

Although interventions of various sorts are indicated for each of the disease categories discussed, these interventions are often costly and sometimes ineffective in lowering or preventing premature mortality. Thus, from an operational perspective, it is important to consider preventive and therapeutic strategies that will have greater societal effect than will the management of the manifestations of diseases as they arise in individuals. This approach applies to acute diseases (vaccination schemes to reduce the burden of influenza, in contrast to individual management of community-acquired pneumonia) and chronic diseases (smoking prevention and reduction programs, compared with availability of routine asthma medication). Primary prevention strategies should include efforts by multiple agencies of government and the community coming together to establish appropriate priorities for action. Four sources of exposure stand out: tobacco smoke, indoor smoke, outdoor air pollutants, and occupational exposure (see chapters 46, 42, 43, and 60, respectively). Of these, the most pressing and cost-effective is a cohesive policy to control tobacco smoking.

In conjunction with the International Union against Tuberculosis and Lung Disease (IUATLD) and selected universities and health institutions in various countries, WHO is developing the Practical Approach to Lung Health (PAL, previously known as the Adult Lung Health Initiative). The program is focused on improving primary care services, as well as appropriate referral to secondary health care facilities, for individuals with tuberculosis, acute respiratory infections (especially pneumonia), asthma, and COPD. Four countries (Chile, Morocco, Nepal, and South Africa) are serving as the pilot implementation sites (WHO 2003).

In Chile, where respiratory symptoms account for one-third of primary health care visits, a respiratory disease program was initiated in 2001 as part of ongoing efforts to strengthen primary health care. The pilot program was implemented in 15 centers. Standard formats are used to devise scores to determine follow-up for asthma and COPD. Sentinel centers are used to provide epidemiologic information. Influenza immunization coverage of the elderly and at-risk population has reached 85 percent (WHO 2003).

In Morocco, survey work done before establishing a PAL strategy showed that 31 percent of patients who consult primary health care centers present with respiratory symptoms. Of those patients, 85 percent have acute respiratory infections, 14 percent have chronic conditions, and 1 percent have tuberculosis. In Mexico, an IUATLD study implementing asthma control measures was shown to be cost-effective. Control of asthma improved, and the majority of patients experienced a decrease in the severity of asthma. The cost of asthma management decreased because of lower costs for emergency services and hospitalizations (WHO 2003).

FUTURE RESEARCH NEEDS

One of the difficulties in quantifying the burden of respiratory diseases in adults is the inability to apply uniform methods of diagnosis across economies in which sophisticated diagnostic procedures are possible, let alone across less developed economies. The problems relate in part to differences in the language describing the same symptoms, levels of registration of census and disease reporting, availability of diagnostic procedures, and reluctance to make accurate estimates because of the cost of intervention strategies. Furthermore, unless controls on cigarette smoking are initiated, little progress in stemming the increasing burden of chronic respiratory diseases can be expected.

There are still a number of unanswered questions related to COPD, which remains the dominant respiratory disease in adults. The developing world provides some unique opportunities for research that go beyond the primary prevention that would result from better smoking control policies. Because not all smokers are at increased risk, the interaction of smoking with nutritional status (including micronutrient status), with genetic factors that determine susceptibility, and with respiratory infections may act as a precursor of susceptibility to environmental (ambient or occupational) pollution and personal (smoking) pollution. Similarly, the role of immunologic stimulation or immunocompetence needs further exploration as it relates to the development of asthma. Synergies between the conditions discussed in this chapter and other infections (particularly tuberculosis, but possibly others) may be especially important in the developing world. Finally, specific environmental conditions—such as altitude, heat and cold stress, and increased ambient pollution from rapid urbanization—and their effects on asthma and COPD should be explored.

Acute respiratory infections, specifically bacterial pneumonia, have not been addressed nearly as well for adults as they have been for children. For example, simple data on the prevalence of infecting organisms, typical susceptibilities, the ability to train ancillary workers in clinical diagnosis, and the correlation of clinical assessment with verified disease would be helpful in establishing the feasibility of assessment and treatment at home versus at a clinic or hospital, specifically in the developing world. Common etiologic agents in North America are common elsewhere; therefore, treatment of disease would be relatively inexpensive. Most community-acquired acute disease responds relatively well. Certainly, penicillin should be recommended as a first-line drug for community-acquired pneumonia. Educating local healers on the importance of initiating treatment earlier in the course of disease would translate into savings with respect to decreased days of work lost and reduced case-fatality rates. Follow-up monitoring and the development of hospital-based bacteriologic testing should be expanded to identify and control for the emergence of resistant bacterial strains.

Studies of asthma in the developed world have been extensive and of extremely high quality but are directed specifically toward the health care structures in which they are tested. Specific cost-effectiveness studies in the developing world should be done to see, for example, whether a focus on disease education and modification of risk factors in addition to medications outweighs simple administration of medications (with instructions on use). In the developed world, there is no question that an approach that is multitiered and involves multiple health care providers is the best, but we still do not have concrete evidence of where monies are best spent in the developing world. Another possible fruitful area of research is on education programs. Most of the literature relates to education programs for specific entities (for example, "asthma triggers") and their costs in developed countries. Education programs in developing countries that are multidimensional (smoking cessation, indoor air quality, vaccination) are likely to be relatively inexpensive and cost-effective. Better methods of educating local healers through the use of demonstration projects should be tested, as should more efficient distribution systems to make relatively inexpensive medication available. General increased awareness of the impact of symptoms on adults and of the potential for earlier intervention in a disease should also be explored and tested for their effects on reducing respiratory disease burdens.

NOTES

1. The survey of the cost-effectiveness of interventions below is based on a review of the University of York database (http://www.york.ac.uk/inst/crd), combined with a Medline search (focusing mainly on data after 1996).

2. According to Hay and Robin (1991), cited in Ruchlin and Dasbach (2001). Akins and O'Malley (2000) have a much lower estimate, which probably does not include all the costs of screening and the like.

3. This estimate was calculated as follows: the MRC (1981) trials suggest that over five years the mortality in a randomized trial for patients with severe hypoxemia is 667 per 100,000 for those not treated with long-term oxygen, compared with 548 per 100,000 for those treated with long-term oxygen (reviewed in Crockett and others 2001). The cost per month of home oxygen is taken as US$400 (based on U.S. Medicare reimbursements in the early 1990s).

REFERENCES

Aït-Khaled, N., D. Enarson, and J. Bousquet. 2001. "Chronic Respiratory Diseases in Developing Countries: The Burden and Strategies for Prevention and Management." *Bulletin of the World Health Organization* 79 (10): 971–79.

Akins, S. A., and P. O'Malley. 2000. "Should Health-Care Systems Pay for Replacement Therapy in Patients with Alpha(1)-Antitrypsin Deficiency? A Critical Review and Cost-Effectiveness Analysis." *Chest* 117 (3): 875–80.

Al, M. J., M. A. Koopmanschap, P. J. van Enckevort, A. Geertsma, W. van der Bij, W. J. de Boer, E. M. TenVergert. 1998. "Cost-Effectiveness of Lung Transplantation in the Netherlands." *Chest* 113: 124–40.

Anon, J. M., A. Garcia de Lorenzo, A. Zarazaga, V. Gomez-Tello, and G. Garrido. 1999. "Mechanical Ventilation of Patients on Long-Term Oxygen Therapy with Acute Exacerbations of Chronic Obstructive Pulmonary Disease: Prognosis and Cost-Utility Analysis." *Intensive Care Medicine* 25 (5): 452–57.

Bell, D. M. 2004. "World Health Organization Working Group on Prevention of International and Community Transmission of SARS. Public Health Interventions and SARS Spread, 2003." *Emerging Infectious Diseases* 10 (11). http://www.cdc.gov/ncidod/EID/vol10no11/04-0729.htm.

Buist, A. S. 2002. "Guidelines for the Management of Chronic Obstructive Pulmonary Disease." *Respiratory Medicine* 96 (Suppl. C): S11–16.

Chan-Yeung, M., N. Aït-Khaled, N. White, K. W. Tsang, and W. C. Tan. 2004. "Management of Chronic Pulmonary Disease in Asia and Africa." *International Journal of Tuberculosis and Lung Disease* 8 (2): 159–70.

Chew, F. T., D. Y. Goh, and B. W. Lee. 1999. "The Economic Cost of Asthma in Singapore." *Australian and New Zealand Journal of Medicine* 29 (2): 228–33.

Chung, F., N. Barnes, M. Allen, R. Angus, P. Corris, A. Knox, and others. 2002. "Assessing the Burden of Respiratory Disease in the U.K." *Respiratory Medicine* 96: 963–75.

Crockett, A. J., J. M. Cranston, J. R. Moss, and J. H. Alpers. 2001. "A Review of Long-Term Oxygen Therapy for Chronic Obstructive Pulmonary Disease." *Respiratory Medicine* 95: 437–43.

Demicheli, V., T. Jefferson, D. Rivetti, and J. Deeks. 2000. "Prevention and Early Treatment of Influenza in Healthy Adults." *Vaccine* 18: 957–1030.

Dolin, P. J., M. C. Raviglione, and A. Kochi. 1994. "Global Tuberculosis Incidence and Mortality during 1990–2000." *Bulletin of the World Health Organization* 72: 212–20.

Fitzner, K. A., K. F. Shortridge, S. M. McGhee, and A. J. Hedley. 2001. "Cost-Effectiveness Study on Influenza Prevention in Hong Kong." *Health Policy* 56: 215–34.

Fletcher, C. M., R. Peto, C. M. Tinker, and F. E. Speizer. 1976. *The Natural History of Chronic Bronchitis: An Eight Year Follow-up Study of Working Men in London.* New York: Oxford University Press.

Friedmann, M., and D. E. Hilleman. 2001. "Economic Burden of Chronic Obstructive Pulmonary Disease: Impact of New Treatment Options." *Pharmacoeconomics* 19 (3): 245–54.

Ghosh, C. S., P. Ravindran, M. Joshi, and S. C. Stearns. 1998. "Reductions in Hospital Use from Self Management Training for Chronic Asthmatics." *Social Science and Medicine* 46 (8): 1087–93.

GOLD (Global Initiative for Chronic Obstructive Lung Disease). 2001. "Global Strategy for the Diagnosis, Management and Prevention of GOLD." National Heart, Lung, and Blood Institute–WHO Workshop Report, NHLBI Publication 2701, National Institutes of Health, Bethesda, MD.

Hay, J. W., and E. C. Robin. 1991. "Cost-Effectiveness of Alpha-1 Antitrypsin Replacement Therapy in Treatment of Congenital Chronic Obstructive Pulmonary Disease." *American Journal of Public Health* 81: 427–33.

Hooi, L. N., I. Looi, and A. J. Ng. 2001. "A Study on Community Acquired Pneumonia in Adults Requiring Hospital Admission in Penang." *Medical Journal of Malaysia* 56: 275–84.

Hui, K. P., N. K. Chin, K. Chow, A. Brownlee, T. C. Yeo, G. Kumarasinghe, and others. 1993. "Prospective Study of the Etiology of Adult Community Acquired Bacterial Pneumonia Needing Hospitalisation in Singapore." *Singapore Medical Journal* 34: 329–34.

Kiivet, R. A., I. Kaur, A. Lang, A. Aaviksoo, and L. Nirk. 2001. "Costs of Asthma Treatment in Estonia." *European Journal of Public Health* 11: 89–92.

LaDou, J. 2004. "The Asbestos Cancer Epidemic." *Environmental Health Perspectives* 112: 285–90.

Lee, P. Y., D. V. Matchar, D. A. Clements, J. Huber, J. D. Hamilton, and E. D. Peterson. 2002. "Economic Analysis of Influenza Vaccination and Antiviral Treatment for Healthy Working Adults." *Annals of Internal Medicine* 137: 225–31.

Lee, T. A., and K. B. Weiss. 2002. "An Update on the Health Economics of Asthma and Allergy." *Current Opinion in Allergy and Clinical Immunology* 2: 195–200.

Leigh, J., P. Macaskill, E. Kuosma, and J. Mandryk. 1999. "Global Burden of Disease and Injury Due to Occupational Factors." *Epidemiology* 10: 626–31.

Lieberman, D., F. Schlaeffer, I. Boldur, D. Lieberman, S. Horowitz, M. G. Friedman, and others. 1996. "Multiple Pathogens in Adult Patients Admitted with Community-Acquired Pneumonia: A One Year Prospective Study of 346 Consecutive Patients." *Thorax* 51: 179–84.

Loewenson, R. 1999. "Assessment of the Health Impact of Occupational Risk in Africa: Current Situation and Methodological Issues." *Epidemiology* 10: 632–9.

Low, D. E., and A. McGeer. 2004. "SARS—One Year Later." *New England Journal of Medicine* 349: 2381–2.

MRC (Medical Research Council Working Group). 1981. "Long-Term Domiciliary Oxygen Therapy in Chronic Hypoxic Cor Pulmonale Complicating Chronic Bronchitis and Emphysema." *Lancet* 1 (8222): 681–86.

Murray, C. J. L., and A. D. Lopez, eds. 1996. *The Global Burden of Disease: A Comprehensive Assessment of Mortality and Disability from Diseases, Injuries and Risk Factors in 1990 and Projected to 2020.* Cambridge, MA: Harvard University Press.

NIOSH (National Institute of Occupational Safety and Health). 1999. *Work-Related Lung Disease Surveillance Report 1999.* NIOSH Publication 2000-105. http://www.cdc.gov/niosh/docs/2000-105/2000-105.html.

OSHA (Occupational Safety and Health Administration). 1998. *Respiratory Protection Regulations. Section 6: Summary of the Final Economic Analysis.* http://www.osha.gov/pls/oshaweb/owadisp.show_document?p_id=1052&p_table=PREAMBLES.

Paltiel, A. D., A. L. Fuhlbrigge, B. T. Kitch, B. Liljas, S. T. Weiss, P. J. Neumann, and K. M. Kuntz. 2001. "Cost-Effectiveness of Inhaled Corticosteroids in Adults with Mild-to-Moderate Asthma: Results from the Asthma Policy Model." *Journal of Allergy and Clinical Immunology* 108 (1): 39–49.

Postma, M. J., P. Jansema, M. L. L. van Genugten, M.-L. A. Heijnen, J. C. Jager, and L. T. W. de Jong-van den Berg. 2002. "Pharmacoeconomics of Influenza Vaccination for Healthy Working Adults." *Drugs* 62 (7): 1013–24.

Ramsey, S. D., D. L. Patrick, R. K. Albert, E. B. Larson, D. E. Wood, and G. Raghu. 1995. "The Cost-Effectiveness of Lung Transplantation: A Pilot Study." *Chest* 108: 1594–601.

Ruchlin, H. S., and E. J. Dasbach. 2001. "An Economic Overview of Chronic Obstructive Pulmonary Disease." *Pharmacoeconomics* 19 (6): 623–42.

Rutten–van Mölken, M. P., E. K. Van Doorslaer, and F. F. Rutten. 1992. "Economic Appraisal of Asthma and COPD Care: A Literature Review 1980–1991." *Social Science and Medicine* 35 (2): 161–75.

Sant'Anna, C. A., R. Stelmach, M. I. Zanetti Feltrin, W. J. Filho, T. Chiba, and A. Cukier. 2003. "Evaluation of Health-Related Quality of Life in Low-Income Patients with COPD Receiving Long-Term Oxygen Therapy." *Chest* 123 (1): 136–41.

Scanlon, P. D., J. E. Connett, L. A. Waller, M. D. Altose, W. C. Bailey, A. S. Buist, and D. P. Tashkin. 2000. "Smoking Cessation and Lung Function in Mild-to-Moderate Chronic Obstructive Pulmonary Disease: The Lung Health Study." *American Journal of Respiratory and Critical Care Medicine* 161: 381–90.

Schmidt, C. D., C. G. Elliott, D. Carmelli, R. L. Jensen, M. Gengiz, J. C. Schmit, and others. 1983. "Prolonged Mechanical Ventilation for Respiratory Failure: A Cost-Benefit Analysis." *Critical Care Medicine* 11: 407.

Scott, J. A. G., A. J. Hall, C. Muyodi, B. Lowe, M. Ross, B. Chohan, and others. 2000. "Aetiology, Outcome, and Risk Factors for Mortality among Adults with Acute Pneumonia in Kenya." *Lancet* 355: 1225–30.

Scuffham, P. A., and P. A. West. 2002. "Economic Evaluation of Strategies for the Control and Management of Influenza in Europe." *Vaccine* 20: 2562–78.

Smith, K. J., and R. R. Pesce. 1994. "Pulmonary Artery Catheterization in Exacerbations of COPD Requiring Mechanical Ventilation: A Cost-Effectiveness Analysis." *Respiratory Care* 39: 961–7.

Smith, K. R. 2000. "National Burden of Disease in India from Indoor Air Pollution." *Proceedings of the National Academy of Sciences of the United States of America* 97 (24): 13286–93.

Speizer, F. E., M. E. Fay, D. W. Dockery, and B. G. Ferris Jr. 1989. "Chronic Obstructive Pulmonary Disease Mortality in Six U.S. Cities." *American Review of Respiratory Disease* 140: S49–55.

Stoloff, S., K. Poinsett-Holmes, and P. M. Dorinsky. 2002. "Combination Therapy with Inhaled Long-Acting β2-Agonists and Inhaled Corticosteroids: A Paradigm Shift in Asthma Management." *Pharmacotherapy* 22 (2): 212–26.

Sudre, P., S. Jacquemet, C. Uldry, and T. V. Perneger. 1999. "Objectives, Methods, and Content of Patient Education Programmes for Adults with Asthma: Systematic Review of Studies Published between 1979 and 1998." *Thorax* 54: 681–7.

Sullivan, S. D., and K. B. Weiss. 2001. Health Economics of Asthma and Rhinitis: II. Assessing the Value of Interventions. *Journal of Allergy and Clinical Immunology* 107: 203–10.

Toevs, C. D., R. M. Kaplan, and C. J. Atkins. 1984. "The Costs and Effects of Behavioral Programs in Chronic Obstructive Pulmonary Disease." *Medical Care* 22: 1088–100.

Trapido, A. S., N. P. Mqoqi, C. M. Macheke, B. G. Williams, J. C. Davies, and C. Panter. 1996. "Occupational Lung Disease in Ex-Mineworkers—Sound a Further Alarm!" *South African Medical Journal* 86 (5): 559.

Van den Boom, G., M. P. Rutten–van Mölken, J. Molema, P. R. Tirimanna, C. van Weel, and C. P. van Schayck. 2001. "The Cost Effectiveness of Early Treatment with Fluticasone Propionate 250 Microg Twice a Day in Subjects with Obstructive Airway Disease. Results of the DIMCA Program." *American Journal of Respiratory and Critical Care Medicine* 164 (11): 2057–66.

Weiss, K. B., and S. D. Sullivan. 2001. "The Health Economics of Asthma and Rhinitis: I. Assessing the Economic Impact." *Journal of Allergy and Clinical Immunology* 107: 3–8.

WHO (World Health Organization). 2000. "Global Burden of Disease 2000: Deaths by Age, Sex and Cause for the Year 2000." WHO, Geneva.

———. 2001. "Innovative Care for Chronic Conditions: Building Blocks for Action." WHO/MNC/CCH/02.01. WHO, Geneva.

———. 2002a. "Influenza." *Weekly Epidemiological Record* 77.28 (July 12): 229–40.

———. 2002b. "Outbreak of Influenza, Madagascar, July–August 2002." *Weekly Epidemiological Record* 77.46 (November 15): 381–88.

———. 2003. "Report of the First International Review Meeting, Practical Approach to Lung Health (PAL) Strategy." http://whqlibdoc.who.int/hq/2003/WHO_CDS_TB_2003.324.pdf.

———. 2005a. "Strengthening Pandemic Influenza Preparedness and Response." Report by the Secretariat. 58th World Health Assembly, A58/13, April 7.

———. 2005b. "Communicable Disease Surveillance & Response." Confirmed Human Cases of Avian Influenza A (H5N1). http://www.who.int/csr/don/en/. (This site provides weekly updates "Disease Outbreak News" of reported cases to WHO by specific countries and latest assistance with regard to potential pandemic status and preparedness. (*Last accessed August 19, 2005, Updated 28*[2]).

———. 2005c. "WHO Global Influenza Preparedness Plan." The Role of WHO and Recommendations for National Measures before and during Pandemics. WHO/CDS/CSR/GIP/2005.5, pp. 1–49.

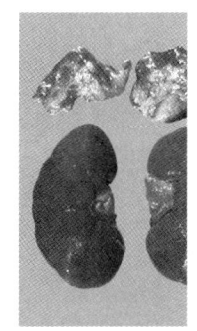

Chapter **36**

Diseases of the Kidney and the Urinary System

John Dirks, Giuseppe Remuzzi, Susan Horton, Arrigo Schieppati, and S. Adibul Hasan Rizvi

CAUSES AND CHARACTERISTICS OF THE BURDEN OF DISEASES

Estimates of the global burden of disease indicate that diseases of the kidney and urinary tract account for approximately 830,000 deaths and 18,467,000 disability-adjusted life years annually, ranking them 12th among causes of death (1.4 percent of all deaths) and 17th among causes of disability (1.0 percent of all disability-adjusted life years). This ranking is similar across World Bank regions (table 36.1).

Recent research suggests that the data shown in table 36.1 underestimate the global prevalence of kidney disease. Chronic kidney disease (CKD) patients often suffer from cardiovascular or cerebrovascular disease, and their deaths may be attributed to either complication (Hostetter 2004). Altered kidney function is often found in patients with hypertensive and ischemic heart disease, both of which are associated with increased cardiovascular morbidity and mortality. Approximately 30 percent of patients with diabetes have diabetic nephropathy, with higher rates found in some ethnic groups (King, Aubert, and Herman 1998). Table 36.2 shows that both genders are similarly affected by kidney disease (Coresh and others 2003).

Generally, renal diseases progress to a final stage as end-stage renal disease (ESRD) and function is substituted by renal replacement therapy (RRT), hemodialysis, peritoneal dialysis, or transplantation. National and international registries of patients on RRT are useful for providing information on the prevalence of renal diseases in a given country. Data combined from different sources show that more than 1.5 million people

worldwide are on RRT, 80 percent of whom live in Japan, Europe, and North America (Weening 2004).

The percentage of patients on regular dialysis varies across countries as a consequence of the capacity of health care systems to provide treatment. Europe is an example. Whereas in the 15 countries of the European Union (before 2004) the prevalence rate of RRT was approximately 650 patients per 1 million people, in Central and Eastern Europe it was only 160 patients per 1 million people, reflecting differences in gross national product.

Much less is known about the prevalence of earlier stages of CKD, when symptoms may be mild, ignored, or undiagnosed. A lack of standardization of the stages of CKD has hampered assessments of the burden of CKD. In an attempt to carry out such an assessment, the National Center for Health Statistics of the Centers for Disease Control and Prevention in the United States conducted a survey from 1988 to 1994. The center analyzed a sample of 15,625 noninstitutionalized individuals age 20 and older and defined five stages of renal dysfunction according to estimates of renal function and urine albumin level. Coresh and others (2003) found that the estimated prevalence of CKD in the United States is 11 percent of the adult population, or 19.8 million people. Nationally representative data on U.S. adults older than 20 show that 6.3 percent, or 11 million people, have stage 1 CKD, or kidney damage (proteinuria) with normal kidney function (Glomerular Function Rate (GFR) at least 90 milliliters per minute in 1.73 per meter squared) or stage 2 CKD, that is, mildly reduced kidney function (60 to 89 ml/min/1.73 m^2). Furthermore, 4.3 percent, or 7.6 million people, exhibit stage 3 CKD, or moderately

Table 36.1 Contribution of Diseases of the Kidney and Urinary System to the Global Burden of Disease by Gender and Region *(thousands)*

Gender and region	Population	Deaths	Disability-adjusted life years	Years lived with disability	Years of life lost
Females	3,056,384	397	8,008	2,546	5,450
Males	3,093,849	433	10,459	4,493	5,960
World	6,150,233	830	18,647	7,039	11,415
East Asia and the Pacific	1,850,775	233	5,400	1,858	3,530
Europe and Central Asia	447,180	53	1,417	623	793
Latin America and the Caribbean	526,138	70	1,667	779	888
Middle East and North Africa	309,762	57	1,283	460	823
South Asia	1,387,873	156	3,991	1,373	2,619
Sub-Saharan Africa	667,663	107	2,623	1,046	1,576

Source: Mathers and others 2006.

Table 36.2 Global Deaths Caused by Diseases of the Genitourinary System by Gender and Age

Gender	Age (years)							
	Birth–4	5–14	15–29	30–44	45–59	60–69	70–79	80+
Male deaths								
Number (thousands)	11	7	24	43	80	86	110	88
Percent	3	2	5	10	18	19	24	20
Female deaths								
Number (thousands)	10	6	21	29	61	66	85	98
Percent	3	2	5	8	16	18	23	24

Source: WHO 2002.

reduced kidney function (30 to 59 ml/min/1.73 m^2), and 0.2 percent, or 400,000, have stage 4 CKD, or severely reduced kidney function (15 to 29 ml/min/1.73 m^2) (Coresh and others 2003; Coresh, Astor, and Sarnak 2004; National Kidney Foundation 2002). A sizable proportion (360,000) of these patients eventually progress toward ESRD (stage 5, or less than 15 ml/min/1.73 m^2) and require RRT. Early detection of CKD is, therefore, important to retard or arrest the loss of renal function. Late detection of CKD is a lost opportunity for making lifestyle changes and initiating therapeutic measures.

CAUSES OF DISEASES OF THE KIDNEY AND URINARY SYSTEM

Kidney disease leading to ESRD has many causes. The prevalence varies by country, region, ethnicity, gender, and age.

Genetic Diseases

Knowledge of inherited kidney disease has changed radically with advances in molecular biology and gene-sequencing technology. The characterization of inherited kidney diseases has improved, and novel mutations leading to selective renal defects have been described. Inherited kidney diseases are rare, with the exception of autosomal dominant polycystic kidney disease, the fourth most common cause of ESRD in developed countries. This disease has a prevalence of 1 in 1,000 people and affects approximately 10 million people worldwide (Grantham 1997). Autosomal recessive polycystic kidney disease is less frequent, with an incidence of 1 in 40,000, but is an important hereditary disease of childhood (Guay-Woodford, Jafri, and Bernstein 2000). Many other inherited diseases can lead to ESRD, but together they account for only a small percentage of all people with ESRD.

Glomerulonephritis

Glomerulonephritides are a group of kidney diseases that affect the glomeruli. They fall into two major categories: *glomerulonephritis* refers to an inflammation of the glomeruli and can be primary or secondary, and *glomerulosclerosis* refers to scarring of the glomeruli. Even though glomerulonephritis and glomerulosclerosis have different causes, both can lead to ESRD. Glomerulonephritis ranks second after diabetes as the foremost cause of ESRD in Europe. (Stengel and others 2003) and is the second leading cause of ESRD in the United States, according to the United States Renal Data System (http://www.ifrr.net/). Approximately 20 to 35 percent of patients requiring RRT have a glomerular disease.

Glomerular diseases are more prevalent and severe in tropical regions and low-income countries (Seedat 2003). A common mode of presentation is the nephrotic syndrome, with the age of onset at five to eight years. Estimates indicate that 2 to 3 percent of medical admissions in tropical countries are caused by renal-related complaints, most resulting from glomerulonephritis.

A number of kidney diseases that result from infectious diseases, such as malaria, schistosomiasis, leprosy, filariasis, and hepatitis B virus, are exclusive to the tropics. HIV/AIDS can be complicated by several forms of kidney disease; however, patient data are sparse (Seedat 2003).

Acute poststreptococcal nephritis following a throat or skin infection caused by Group A streptococcus has almost disappeared in high-income countries because of improved hygiene and treatment but remains an important glomerular disease in India and Africa, where epidemics have been reported (Seedat 2003).

The eradication of endemic infections, along with improvements in socioeconomic status, education, sanitation, and access to treatment, is a crucial step toward decreasing the incidence of glomerular diseases in developing countries.

Infections, Stones, and Obstructive Uropathy

Infections of the urinary tract are a common health problem worldwide and can be categorized as either uncomplicated or complicated. Uncomplicated infections include bladder infections such as cystitis, seen almost exclusively in young women (Hooton 2000). Among sexually active women, the incidence of cystitis is 0.5 episodes per person annually, and recurrence develops in 27 to 44 percent of cases. Acute, uncomplicated pyelonephritis, involving the kidney, is less frequent in women than is cystitis. Males are less susceptible to acute, uncomplicated infections of the bladder or the kidney, with an incidence of five to eight episodes per 10,000 men annually. Even though uncomplicated urinary tract infections are considered benign, they have significant medical and financial implications estimated at approximately US$1.6 billion per year (Foxman 2003).

As for complicated urinary tract infections, hospitalization results in almost 1 million such infections per year in the United States. Bladder catheterization is the most important cause.

Developing countries exhibit a different pattern of urinary tract infection. Obstructive or reflux nephropathy is often attributed to urinary schistosomiasis (Barsoum 2003). Worldwide, 200 million people are affected and an estimated 300 million are at risk. The disease causes lesions in the bladder and predisposes those with the condition to secondary infections, bladder cancers, and chronic pyelonephritis.

Some 15 to 20 million people have tuberculosis (TB) worldwide, of whom 8 million to 10 million are infectious. Genitourinary TB is a common form of extrapulmonary TB and is always secondary to the primary lesion, which usually occurs in the lung (Pasternak and Rubin 1997). Lesions referred to as *ulcero-cavernous* or *miliary* affect the kidneys. If left untreated, such lesions may progress to kidney destruction. Early recognition of and effective therapy for TB substantially decrease the consequences in relation to kidney function.

In the industrial countries, kidney stones are a common problem (Morton, Iliescu, and Wilson 2002), affecting 1 person in 1,000 annually, and the incidence is increasing in tropical developing countries (Robertson 2003). Factors such as age, sex, and ethnic and geographic distribution determine prevalence. The peak age of onset is in the third decade, and prevalence increases with age until 70.

Although largely idiopathic, the following risk factors are associated with stone disease: low urine volume, hyperuricosuria, hyperoxaluria, hypomagnesuria, and hypocitraturia. Diarrhea, malabsorption, low protein, low calcium, increased consumption of oxalate-rich foods, and low fluid intake may play a role in the genesis of stone disease. In developing countries, 30 percent of all pediatric urolithiasis cases occur as bladder stones in children. The formation of bladder stones in children is caused by a poor diet high in cereal content and low in animal protein, calcium, and phosphates.

Kidney stones can have different clinical presentations, ranging from asymptomatic to large obstructing calculi in the upper urinary tract that can severely impair renal function and lead to ESRD. Although specific causes of kidney stones should be treated appropriately, general treatment includes increased fluid intake, limited daily salt intake, moderate animal protein intake, and medical treatment with alkali and thiazides.

The Afro-Asian stone-forming belt stretches from Sudan, the Arab Republic of Egypt, Saudi Arabia, the United Arab Emirates, the Islamic Republic of Iran, Pakistan, India, Myanmar, Thailand, and Indonesia to the Philippines. The disease affects all age groups from less than 1 year old to more than 70, with a male to female ratio of 2 to 1. The prevalence of calculi ranges from 4 to 20 percent (Hussain and others 1996). Urolithiasis accounts for some 50 percent of the urological workload and the bulk of urological emergencies. Patients may present with major complications leading to eventual ESRD and resulting in significant morbidity and mortality. In developed countries, only about 1 percent of patients are on dialysis because of obstructive uropathy, whereas in developing countries such as Indonesia and Thailand, obstructive uropathy is often the leading cause of ESRD, accounting for 20 percent or more of patients on dialysis. The availability of appropriately trained medical and surgical personnel and of equipment essential for treating stone disease promptly would reduce the incidence of obstructive uropathy and ESRD. Cost analyses indicate that the medical prevention of stones saves more than US$2,000 per person annually (Parks and Coe 1996).

Benign Prostatic Hypertrophy

Benign prostatic hypertrophy is a major cause of lower urinary tract symptoms and leads to obstructive renal failure and ESRD. By age 80, 80 percent of men have benign prostatic hypertrophy. The World Health Organization quotes a mortality rate of 0.5 to 1.5 per 100,000 (La Vecchia, Levi, and Lucchini 1995). The actual incidence of benign prostatic hypertrophy is difficult to assess because of the lack of epidemiological data. In the developed world, the incidence varies between 0.24 and 10.90 per 1,000 annually from age 50 to 80, and the probability of prostate surgery for benign prostatic hypertrophy ranges from 1.4 to 6.0 percent (Oishi and others 1998).

Acute Renal Failure

Acute renal failure refers to a sudden and usually temporary loss of kidney function that may be so severe that RRT is needed until kidney function recovers. Even though acute renal failure can be a reversible condition, it carries a high mortality rate. Acute renal failure is a prominent feature of major earthquakes, where many suffer from crush syndrome accompanied by severe dehydration and rapid release of muscle cell contents, including potassium. Kidney function shuts down unless body fluid and blood pressure are rapidly corrected and frequent hemodialysis is available. Recent earthquake rescues in the Islamic Republic of Iran and Turkey have demonstrated the benefits of rapid hydration and dialysis (Sever and others 2001).

Diabetes

Diabetes is one of the most common noncommunicable diseases (see chapter 30). With the serious complication of nephropathy, diabetes has become the single most important cause of ESRD in the United States and Europe, according to Stengel and others (2003) and the United States Renal Data System (http://www.ifrr.net/). Diabetes may account for one-third of all ESRD cases.

Family-based studies and segregation analyses suggest that inherited factors play a major role in people's susceptibility to diabetic renal complications (Seaquist and others 1989). In the United States, the burden of ESRD is threefold to fivefold greater among African Americans, Mexican Americans, and Native Americans than other Americans, and Imperatore and others (2000) find a 200 percent greater possibility of the occurrence of inherited diabetic nephropathy. A family history of

hypertension has also been associated with an increased risk of diabetic nephropathy. When specific markers of risk are found, high-risk individuals can be identified early and monitored for the development of proteinuria and kidney dysfunction.

The earliest sign of diabetic nephropathy is the appearance of small amounts of protein in the urine (*proteinuria*). As proteinuria increases and blood pressure rises, kidney function declines. The complete loss of kidney function occurs at different rates among type 2 diabetes patients, but it eventually occurs in 30 percent of proteinuria cases. The latter have a 10-fold increased risk of dying from associated coronary artery disease, which may obviate the progression of diabetic nephropathy to ESRD. As therapies and interventions for coronary artery disease improve, patients with type 2 diabetes may survive long enough to develop kidney failure.

Hypertension

Hypertension and kidney disease are closely related. Most primary renal diseases eventually produce hypertension. Arterial hypertension accelerates many forms of renal disease and hastens the progression to ESRD (Luke 1999). Recent studies have firmly established the importance of continuous blood pressure reduction to slow the progression of many forms of renal injury, particularly glomerular disease (Agodoa and others 2001; Peterson and others 1995). Over the long term, damage to the heart and cardiovascular system resulting from hypertension represents the major cause of morbidity and mortality among ESRD patients (Martinez-Maldonado 1998).

Before the development of effective antihypertensive agents, 40 percent of hypertensive patients developed kidney damage and 18 percent developed renal insufficiency over time (Johnson and Feehally 2000). Elevated serum creatinine develops in 10 to 20 percent of hypertensive patients, with African Americans and Africans at particularly high risk. In 2 to 5 percent of hypertensive patients, progression toward ESRD will occur in 10 to 15 years. Despite the relatively low rate of progression, hypertension remains the most common cause of ESRD after diabetes in the United States, is the foremost cause of death in all developed countries, and is a likely primary cause in developing countries given its high global prevalence rate. Native Americans and Hispanic Americans are disproportionately affected relative to Caucasian Americans.

GLOBAL PERSPECTIVES IN RELATION TO RRT

Despite the lack of uniform data worldwide, the medical community is aware that the total number of patients requiring RRT is growing in all high- and middle-income countries. In the United States, for example, 360,000 people with ESRD were on RRT in 2003, compared with 150,000 in 1994, and according to a recent forecast, by 2014 the figure will have increased to 650,000 (Xue and others 2001). This increase represents a linear growth in new cases combined with longer survival by existing patients.

Levels in middle-income countries are lower, but rising. In Eastern Europe between 1990 and 1996, following economic changes, the number of hemodialysis and peritoneal dialysis centers increased by 56 and 296 percent, respectively (Rutkowski 2002), and the number of patients rose by 78 and 306 percent, respectively.

Overall, the incidence of ESRD is increasing worldwide at an annual growth rate of 8.0 percent, far in excess of the annual population growth rate of 1.3 percent. Nearly 1.6 million people, or only 15 percent of those affected, are receiving RRT, 80 percent of them in developed countries. The remaining 20 percent are treated in more than 100 developing countries, whose populations account for more than 50 percent of the world's population. A large proportion of people living in the poorest countries die of uremia because of a complete lack of RRT.

Risk Factors for Kidney Disease

The identification of risk factors can prevent or limit disease through lifestyle modifications or specific therapeutic interventions (Appel 2003; McClellan and Flanders 2003). For example, familial predisposition for a disease, which is not amenable to modification, can be used to identify high-risk populations for future monitoring.

Low socioeconomic status and limited access to health care are strong risk factors for kidney failure but account for only part of the excess of ESRD among African Americans (Perneger, Whelton, and Klag 1995), whereas racial and social factors account for most ESRD incidence (Pugh and others 1988; Rostand 1992). Factors associated with the progression of CKD include the following:

- unmodifiable variables
  - old age
  - gender
  - genetics
  - ethnicity
- risk factors susceptible to social and educational interventions
  - low birthweight
  - smoking
  - alcohol abuse
  - illicit drug abuse
  - analgesic abuse and exposure to toxic substance such as lead
  - sedentary lifestyle
- risk factors susceptible to pharmacological interventions
  - hypertension

- dyslipidemia
- poor glycemic control in diabetic patients
- proteinuria
- biological markers
  - hemoglobin
  - insulin-resistant syndrome
  - proteinuria
  - serum creatinine.

Growing evidence suggests that fetal exposure to an abnormal intrauterine environment leads to an increased risk of chronic disease later in life. For example, children of diabetic mothers are prone to obesity and diabetes at a young age, and intrauterine growth retardation can lead to ischemic heart disease, diabetes, hypertension, and kidney disease. Disadvantaged racial minorities in developed countries and the impoverished in developing countries are at risk of intrauterine growth retardation caused by malnutrition (Nelson 2001; Nelson, Morgenstern, and Bennett 1998). Attention to maternal nutrition and other factors that would reduce low birthweight and impaired nephron development may have long-term implications for the development of CKD.

In low-income countries, poverty is associated with increased exposure to infectious diseases that increase susceptibility to CKD, including glomerulonephritis and parasitic diseases. Obesity caused by a diet rich in saturated fats and high in salt are risk factors for diabetic nephropathy and hypertensive kidney disease. Change in dietary habits and physical activity can reduce the overall incidence of diabetes (see chapter 44). Smoking and excessive alcohol consumption increase the risk of ESRD (McClellan and Flanders 2003), and analgesic abuse and exposure to toxic substances such as lead may affect progressive renal insufficiency (Lin and others 2001).

Interventions to Delay CKD

During the past 20 years, human and animal research has developed our understanding of CKD and led to preventive measures. The notion of renoprotection has resulted in a dual approach to renal diseases based on effective and sustained pharmacological control of blood pressure and reduction of proteinuria. Lowering blood lipids, stopping smoking, and maintaining tight glucose control for diabetes form part of the multimodal protocol for managing renal patients monitored by specific biological markers (Ruggenenti, Schieppati, and Remuzzi 2001).

Abnormal urinary excretion of protein is strongly associated with the progression of CKD in both diabetic and nondiabetic renal diseases. Clinical studies have established that a reduction in proteinuria is associated with a decreased rate of kidney function loss. A specific category of drugs that lower blood pressure, the angiotensin-converting enzyme (ACE) inhibitors or angiotensin receptor blockers, appear to be more effective than other antihypertensive drugs in slowing the progression of both diabetic and nondiabetic CKDs (Brenner and Zagrobelny 2003). The administration of an ACE inhibitor (or of an angiotensin receptor blocker) is an important treatment for controlling blood pressure and slowing the rate of progression of chronic kidney failure. Other drugs to lower blood pressure are added as necessary to achieve current targets of 120/80 to 130/80 millimeters of mercury. Concurrent diuretic therapy is often necessary in patients with renal insufficiency, because fluid overload is an important determinant of hypertension in such cases.

Dyslipidemia accelerates atherosclerosis and may promote the progression of renal disease. Careful control of the blood glucose level in diabetic patients can be beneficial and may limit other complications. Obesity has not been directly linked to the progression of CKD but is an important risk factor for diabetes and cardiovascular morbidity and mortality. Many patients and health care professionals do not appreciate the benefits of smoking cessation, an important measure in protecting the kidneys from progressive disease resulting from cardiovascular disease (CVD). Additional elements of secondary prevention measures include the treatment of anemia and of abnormal calcium and phosphorus metabolism.

The International Society of Nephrology is developing a program that can be implemented according to the specific needs of a given developing country. The program has two objectives: (a) to identify the prevalence of renal disease among seemingly healthy subjects using a communitywide screening program, especially among populations at risk, and (b) to initiate interventions to prevent the progression of renal disease and affect both renal and CVD outcomes in subjects with or at risk of developing renal disease based on the screening program (Weening 2004). The Kidney Help Trust of Chennai, India, has undertaken a screening program for a population of 25,000. All those who tested positive for high blood pressure, diabetes, or both (about 15 percent) were further studied and then treated with inexpensive antihypertensive and antidiabetic drugs. The cost of the one-year program was Rs 300,000 (US$7,500) or a per capita cost of US$0.27, well within the limits of the Indian government's per capita annual health expenditure of US$7.67 (Mani 2003). A similar program in Bolivia examined a population of 14,000 and also found that 15 percent were hypertensive, diabetic, or both.

An extremely successful program of detection and treatment of renal and cardiovascular diseases among Australian Aborigines was conducted from 1995 to 2000. The ESRD rate among Aborigines is 3 to 10 times that in developed countries. Treatment consisted of long-acting ACE inhibitors to lower blood pressure. After an average of 3.4 years of follow-up, the incidence of ESRD was reduced by 63 percent and nonrenal deaths were reduced by 50 percent. Hoy and others (2003) estimate that this two-year program may have saved US$500,000 to US$2.7 million in avoided or delayed dialysis costs.

Trained staff members can carry out screening programs inexpensively. Economic analysis, however, suggests that large-scale programs should be restricted to screening and treating only specific high-risk populations. Screening programs can be implemented using simple, cheap, and reliable tests consisting of measurements of bodyweight, blood pressure, blood glucose, and creatinine. Screening includes testing urine for hemoglobin, glucose, leukocytes, and protein (repeat tests may be necessary on a spot urine sample); calculating albumin to creatinine ratios; testing positive results for increased serum creatinine and fasting glucose (or glycosylated hemoglobin A1c test); and reassessing the urine protein excretion rate, a cornerstone of kidney assessment. Resulting albumin to creatinine ratio categories would indicate a scale of severity of glomerular disease, with a cardiovascular risk score based on body mass index, hypertension, fasting glucose level, microalbuminuria or gross albuminuria, and serum creatinine. Patients with positive markers for kidney disease would receive the best treatment available at the screening center. Incorporating screening for kidney disease within screening programs developed for CVD and diabetes is important because proteinuria and renal dysfunction are early sensitive markers of vascular dysfunction and CVD patients are at significantly higher risk of kidney disease than the general population.

Resultant medical treatment would focus on the use of ACE inhibitors or angiotensin receptor blockers with a target blood pressure of 120/80 to 130/80 millimeters of mercury. The greater the level of proteinuria, the more treatment is required; thus, the ACE inhibitor dose would be titrated up as proteinuria levels increased. Diuretics and other antihypertensives would be added to meet blood pressure targets. Efforts should be made to obtain low-cost (off-patent) ACE inhibitors or other low-cost antihypertensives. Such treatment should delay or stop the progression of kidney disease and reduce the risk of CVD. Other preventive measures include serum glucose and lipid control and low-dose aspirin if a risk of CVD exists (see chapter 44).

ECONOMIC BENEFITS OF INTERVENTION

An abundance of literature is available on the economics of ESRD. In the industrial world, treatment is usually readily available and is covered by government or private health insurance. Previous restrictions—for example, treatment being limited to certain age groups—have been removed (Chugh and Jha 1995). Dialysis treatment accounts for 0.7 to 1.8 percent of health care budgets in European countries, even though dialysis patients account for only 0.02 to 0.05 percent of the population (Schiepatti, Perico, and Remuzzi 2003).

The most cost-effective option is prevention. Population screening is not particularly cost-effective, given the low incidence of ESRD—namely, 100 to 200 per million population worldwide (Kher 2002)—and given that testing is not highly accurate. According to Kiberd and Jindal (1998), screening costs around US$20 per test, but the positive predictive value for a single test is only 0.3. Even repeat testing does not improve predictive value dramatically. Screening strategies have, therefore, focused on specific populations at higher risk of ESRD than the general population. Whereas only 2 to 5 percent of more than 1 billion hypertensive patients will ultimately develop nephropathy, approximately 30 percent of type 1 and type 2 diabetic patients will develop overt nephropathy (Satko and Freedman 2001). The conclusion is that treating all diabetics in developed countries with ACE inhibitors is a cost-saving strategy. The modest outlay for ACE inhibitors, which amounts to US$320 per year in the United States and is likely to come down as more ACE inhibitor treatments come off patent, offsets the much larger future costs of dialysis and transplant (Golan, Birkmeyer, and Welch 1999; Kiberd and Jindal 1998).

We undertook a crude cost-effectiveness calculation for treating diabetics in developing countries with ACE inhibitors in those cases in which no treatment of ESRD is undertaken. If we use Clark and others' (2000) assumptions, 82 percent of diabetic patients not using ACE inhibitors would survive for 11 years from the onset of macroproteinuria to ESRD, whereas 72 percent of those using ACE inhibitors would survive for 18 years from the onset of macroproteinuria to ESRD (the annualized death rate for both groups is 1.8 percent). If we make the gross assumption that all patients with ESRD in poor developing countries die, this assumption suggests that, at a discount rate of 3 percent and an annual cost for ACE inhibitors of US$320, the cost per quality-adjusted life year (QALY) saved would be about US$1,100 for treating diabetic patients with macroproteinuria. Because of the lack of data, these calculations apply survival rates in developed countries to developing countries; thus, the rates are likely too high. Using survival rates in developing countries would probably increase the cost per QALY saved, but treatment with ACE inhibitors is nevertheless likely to be an attractive investment (table 36.3).

Satko and Freedman (2001) suggest that screening first- and second-degree relatives of ESRD patients may be cost-effective. They cite one study that found 38 percent of first-degree relatives of African-American patients with hypertensive ESRD had some form of renal disease (Bergman and others 1996). Satko and Freedman also cite a study by Freedman, Soucie and McClellan (1997) revealing that in 4,365 incident ESRD patients in the southeastern United States, 14 percent of white patients and 23 percent of black patients had first- or second-degree relatives with ESRD (the rates would probably have been higher if subclinical nephropathy had been included). Satko and Freedman (2001) recommend annual screening for blood pressure, urinalysis, measurement of serum creatinine and blood urea nitrogen concentration, and testing for diabetes mellitus, when appropriate, for first- and second-degree

Table 36.3 Cost-Effectiveness of Selected Interventions for Kidney Disease

Intervention	Alternative	Outcome (2000 US$)
Center hemodialysis[a]	No RRT	55,000–80,000/life year 79,000–114,000/QALY
Home hemodialysis[a]	No RRT	33,000–50,000/life year 47,000–71,000/QALY
Kidney transplant[a]	No RRT	10,000/life year 11,000/QALY
ACE inhibitors for all type 1 diabetics with macroproteinuria[b]	No RRT	1,100/QALY
Screening diabetic relatives of nephropathy patients[c]	No screening	Screening potentially cost saving
Treat all type 2 diabetics with ACE inhibitors[d]	Screening for microalbuminuria and treating those who test positive	Incremental cost-effectiveness ratio is 7,500/QALY for treating all type 2 diabetics
Treat all insulin-dependent diabetics with ACE inhibitors[e]	Screening for microalbuminuria or macroproteinuria and treating those who test positive	Treating all insulin-dependent diabetics dominates under a plausible range of parameters

Sources: [a]Winkelmayer and others 2002 (review); [b]authors' rough estimates; [c]Satko and Freedman 2001; [d]Golan, Birkmeyer, and Welch 1999; [e]Kiberd and Jindal 1998.

relatives of ESRD patients. They did not calculate any formal cost-effectiveness results (table 36.3).

Kidney transplants are the most cost-effective intervention for ESRD. Transplant costs in developed countries have declined steadily from about US$60,000 in 1970 to about US$10,000 currently (Winkelmayer and others 2002). In addition to facing transplant costs, patients face ongoing costs for immunosuppressive drugs, which start at about US$3,000 per year initially but can decline thereafter to US$300 per year (Kher 2002). Kidney transplants are cheaper in India than in the United States, ranging from US$1,500 in government hospitals to as much as US$7,000 in private hospitals. Such costs, combined with a higher quality of life than obtained with dialysis, make renal transplantation the most cost-effective option (table 36.3). However, the availability of kidneys is a major limiting factor. Developed countries tend to have well-organized organ retrieval programs, and cadaveric donor transplants are more common than they are in developing countries. Japan, with its extremely low transplant rates, is an exception, perhaps because of difficulties in obtaining permission for organ donation.

Developing countries have limited access to cadaveric donor programs but better living donor programs. Unrelated living donors are more common than in developed countries because poverty increases the willingness of donors to offer kidneys in exchange for payment. The Philippines recently restricted donations to "emotionally related" donors, but that limitation does not prevent abuses, such as men marrying women of the appropriate blood type in the hope of obtaining a kidney. Developing countries face particular transplantation problems, such as patients' inability to continue paying for immunosuppressive drugs and the transmission of hepatitis B and C, malaria, and TB through organ transplant (Kher 2002).

Long-term hemodialysis was introduced in 1960 and is the most costly treatment option at approximately US$60,000 per year at a center and US$40,000 at home in developed countries. It is most cost-effective if used as an interim measure before kidney transplant. Peritoneal dialysis—for example, continuous ambulatory peritoneal dialysis—was developed in the late 1970s and is less expensive—approximately US$20,000 per year (Winkelmayer and others 2002). Most economies continue to rely on hemodialysis for dialysis patients, except for those mandating that continuous ambulatory peritoneal dialysis be the first choice—that is, Hong Kong (China), Mexico, New Zealand, and the United Kingdom. Switching to continuous ambulatory peritoneal dialysis has the potential of reducing costs for developing countries, especially if they manufacture the consumables domestically rather than importing them. Nevertheless, dialysis remains costly and is not a viable long-term solution in places where health budgets are limited.

More than 120 countries have dialysis programs (Moeller, Gioberge, and Brown 2002). The following data from India highlight the stark economics of dialysis (Kher 2002). Government hospitals will provide hemodialysis only for acute renal failure or pretransplant stabilization (Li and Chow 2001), and with an incidence of 100 per million population, approximately 100,000 patients develop ESRD each year. Of the 10,000 who consult a nephrologist, RRT is initiated for 9,000. Of the 8,500 who begin hemodialysis, about 60 percent are lost to follow-up within three months, probably because of the costs involved. Few remain on dialysis after 24 months. Between 17 and 23 percent of those on dialysis for two to three months receive transplants.

IMPLEMENTATION OF CONTROL STRATEGIES: LESSONS OF EXPERIENCE

Measures for primary and secondary prevention of CKD are now well documented and will eventually reduce the number of patients requiring dialysis. Until recently, the focus has been on RRT to save lives, and considerable efforts are being made to improve the quality of dialysis. In the United States, guidelines derived from the Kidney Disease Outcomes Quality Initiative have added greatly to the quality of dialysis in terms of access (graft or fistula), adequacy, treatment of anemia, treatment of secondary hyperparathyroidism, and—more recently—greater

emphasis on CVD, all of which contribute to quality-of-life outcomes, but at an increased cost (National Kidney Foundation 2002).

The high mortality rate of dialysis approximates 10 percent per year and has changed little over the past decade; however, new approaches are emerging for dealing with CVD in RRT facilities. More patients with kidney disease die before they get to the point at which they need treatment for renal failure, because early kidney disease is a major marker for CVD and reinfarction, congestive heart failure, and stroke.

In middle-income countries such as Thailand and Turkey and in middle-income countries in Latin America (Zatz, Romão, and Noronha 2003), extensive dialysis facilities are available, as they are in some low-income countries. For example, in 2003, Pakistan had 110 centers with 2,400 patients on hemodialysis; India had 100 centers with 6,000 patients mostly on hemodialysis; and China had 75,000 patients on dialysis. Those figures show that needs and markets for dialysis are expanding. However, in poorer countries, such as Nicaragua and Tanzania, options for RRT are limited because of the lack of equipment, trained staff, and costly consumables. In addition, many low-income countries lack health insurance to defray treatment expenditures, keeping dialysis out of reach. In such countries—for example, Nigeria—dialysis directed at preparation for renal transplantation is the best policy. Recent findings concerning primary prevention through lifestyle changes and secondary prevention by means of pharmaceutical treatment should eventually reduce, but not eliminate, the burden of ESRD.

The acknowledgment by the World Bank and the World Health Organization that chronic conditions, particularly those resulting from diabetes and hypertension, will increase to become a leading cause of death by 2028 has intensified the need for prevention and RRT programs. The need to increase awareness, launch targeted screening and intervention studies, provide training for staff, maintain education for physicians in kidney and urological disease, and assist centers for RRT is urgent.

Developed nations have well-established nephrology and urology centers attached to academic medical institutions and regional public and private secondary and tertiary referral hospitals. They have training programs to meet national requirements for health professionals—including renal physicians, primary care physicians, and nurses—specializing in kidney and urological disorders. Their centers incorporate the results of up-to-date research developments pertaining to kidney disease and clinical applications of the latest advances in care and technology. Numerous publications arise from academic endeavors, and a close association exists between health care delivery and pharmaceutical industries. Each country and region has societies of nephrology and urology for adults and children.

Middle-income countries may have both public academic centers and private hospitals that offer specialized equipment, such as lithotripters and imaging technology, and dialysis and transplant programs. Although facilities and trained staff for RRT are more limited than in developed countries, some developing countries, such as Turkey, have excellent facilities.

In lower-income countries, facilities and staff are in short supply, and assistance is needed. Large countries, such as China, India, and Pakistan, have kidney centers available but have considerable unevenness in development of kidney centers and health care in general. Some lower-income countries possess remarkable institutions; for instance, the Sindh Institute of Urology and Transplantation in Karachi, Pakistan, which is supported mainly by charitable donations, provides every patient who presents with ESRD an opportunity for accessing RRT. Overall, however, centers of excellence are urgently needed in developing countries. All the "players," from governments and international organizations to societies and foundations, need to be congregated in conjunction with national institutions to focus on the continued advantages—through treatment—that can be delivered to those developing cardiovascular, diabetic, and kidney disease.

RESEARCH AND DEVELOPMENT AGENDA

Significant progress in knowledge about the geographic burden of kidney and urological diseases has taken place during the past three or four decades as a result of more accurate registries. An international kidney disease data center, in partnership with the World Bank and the World Health Organization, is now required to progressively increase the amount and quality of data collected worldwide.

Basic Knowledge of Kidney Disease

Recent research findings have advanced the understanding and treatment of kidney disease. A continuing emphasis on understanding the basic mechanisms of glomerulonephritic, vasculitic, and autoimmune disease and the detailed mechanisms of the progression of kidney disease to kidney failure is required, as well as research into improved therapies. Well-developed research centers are best equipped to deal with these requirements, aided by national governments, charitable organizations and foundations, international organizations, and centers in the developing world.

Prevention of Kidney Failure

Prevention of acute and chronic kidney disease should be a global priority. During the past decade, an array of clinical trials has been directed at assessing the benefits of interventional therapy, particularly the success of ACE inhibitors. Such trials can play an important role in increasing knowledge and improving the implementation of prevention of kidney disease

in developing countries. Training epidemiologists and physicians to execute screening strategies and clinical trials in their own settings is urgently needed. The cooperation of global funding agencies and training centers; the consistent availability of effective, inexpensive pharmaceuticals; and the assessment of the efficacy and side effects of multiple drug therapy must be coordinated. The priority is to make low-cost drugs available, using as a model the recent process that allowed universal access to inexpensive antiretrovirals for HIV infection.

Renal Replacement Therapy

Successful RRT outcomes depend on reducing morbidity and mortality among dialysis patients. RRT costs escalate in concert with the rising costs of pharmaceuticals—for example, erythropoietin compounds to treat anemia and vitamin D metabolites and calcimimetics to treat secondary hyperparathyroidism and bone disease. Strategies that will result in less expensive dialysis systems and pharmaceuticals are needed (Schieppati, Perico, and Remuzzi 2003). Costs relating to renal transplantation have reached a steady state, but the lack of availability of donor kidneys is a serious—and perhaps irresolvable—limitation.

Establishment of Teaching and Research Centers

Most high-quality training and research centers for kidney and urinary diseases are in the developed world, where training is expensive. Important centers of clinical care have emerged in countries such as Argentina, China, Mexico, South Africa, Thailand, and Turkey. The ability to obtain high-quality training at the local level would be advantageous to developing countries. For example, the International Society of Nephrology has identified and supported a major clinical training center in South Africa that plays a leading role in training nephrologists and urologists for South Africa and other Sub-Saharan African countries to world standards at lower costs than in developed countries and with increased retention of local physicians. Such local centers should be a national priority in developing countries and should be closely linked to international centers for cardiovascular and diabetic disease, meeting approved international standards for training while recognizing national differences in the pattern of kidney disease. Financial assistance is required to enhance the education and training of health professionals, improve baseline infrastructure, and initiate research studies directed at critical clinical questions and at current and new knowledge relating to the prevention of kidney disease. The centers should have excellent data collection methods and a computer infrastructure that would connect them to current knowledge and allow them to communicate freely on a global scale. Major priority should be given to developing leading centers in selected regions.

Cost-Effectiveness of Treatment

More work is needed in the area of screening and treatment in both developed and developing countries. Work on the cost-effectiveness of screening and treating particular subpopulations would be useful, as would the development of better predictive tests for microalbuminuria. In addition, cohort studies of hypertensive and diabetic populations might help develop better indicators that predict susceptibility to progression toward nephropathy.

CONCLUSIONS: PROMISES AND PITFALLS

Kidney disease and kidney failure, especially as a complication of type 2 diabetes mellitus and hypertension, are rising globally and are rising faster in developing countries. Kidney failure patients account for a small fraction of the disease burden but a disproportionately high cost. CKD, along with all chronic diseases, is placing long-term demands on health care. On a global scale, RRT is rising sharply in terms of costs and is usually unavailable in developing countries. Hemodialysis and peritoneal dialysis are life saving, but in the long term they require coupling with newer, proven, interventional pharmacological treatments that frequently delay or stop continuing progression to ESRD. Advances in the past decade have proven that primary and secondary prevention measures can now reduce the burden of ESRD, and if they are not widely disseminated, the need for RRT will increase along with the certainty that the requirements of kidney disease patients cannot be met.

The following guidelines for diseases of the kidney and urinary system are recommended:

- Expand surveillance of the prevalence of various kidney and urological diseases in developing countries. Provide support for further epidemiological studies in selected countries for assessing the prevalence of kidney disease and interventions to address it and for establishing an international kidney disease data center.
- Promote public awareness in developing countries about the nature and early signs of kidney disease along with knowledge of prevention measures and therapies.
- Focus more attention on the increasing prevalence of diabetes and hypertension, and develop kidney disease programs in that context. Measures of kidney function and protein excretion should be taken. The implementation of primary and secondary prevention to reduce the prevalence of ESRD should be expanded.
- Increase coordination and resources for efficient and timely distribution of supplies and equipment, assessment of patients, and frequent dialysis for acute renal failure patients caused by crush injuries during such major disasters as earthquakes. Countries in earthquake-prone regions should

develop emergency policies and practices and be linked with the appropriate international agencies.

- Have the World Bank and the World Health Organization establish a policy advisory group with relevant international groups, such as the International Society of Nephrology, to address and advise national and regional health ministries on kidney and urological strategies as requested.
- Make major health and medical education programs available on an annual basis through existing societies and agencies to train and update physicians, nurses, technicians, and other relevant health professionals.
- Develop selected centers of excellence for education, training, clinical care, and prevention of kidney and urological disease and clinical care of renal failure. At least 10 such centers should be developed in the next decade and located in the countries of the former Soviet Union, Africa, Asia, Eastern Europe, and Latin America. Funds should be provided by international and national agencies and national government organizations and be sustained for up to 10 years.

REFERENCES

Agodoa, L. Y., L. Appel, G. L. Bakris, G. Beck, J. Bourgoignie, J. P. Briggs, and others (African American Study of Kidney Disease and Hypertension Study Group). 2001. "Effect of Ramipril vs. Amlodipine on Renal Outcomes in Hypertensive Nephrosclerosis: A Randomized Controlled Trial." *Journal of the American Medical Association* 285: 2719–28.

Appel, L. J. 2003. "Lifestyle Modification as a Means to Prevent and Treat High Blood Pressure." *Journal of the American Society of Nephrology* 14: S99–102.

Barsoum, R. S. 2003. "End-Stage Renal Disease in North Africa." *Kidney International* 63 (Suppl. 83): S111–14.

Bergman, S., B. O. Key, K. Kirk, D. G. Warnock, and S. G. Rostand. 1996. "Kidney Disease in the First-Degree Relatives of African-Americans with Hypertensive End-Stage Renal Disease." *American Journal of Kidney Diseases* 27: 341–46.

Brenner, B. M., and J. Zagrobelny. 2003. "Clinical Renoprotection Trials Involving Angiotensin II–Receptor Antagonists and Angiotensin-Converting-Enzyme Inhibitors." *Kidney International* 63 (Suppl. 83): S77–85.

Chugh, K. S., and V. Jha. 1995. "Differences in the Care of ESRD Patients Worldwide: Required Resources and Future Outlook." *Kidney International* 48: S7–13.

Clark, W. F., D. N. Churchill, L. Forwell, G. Macdonald, and S. Foster. 2000. *Canadian Medical Association Journal* 162 (2): 195–98.

Coresh, J., B. C. Astor, A. T. Greene, G. Eknoyan, and A. S. Levey. 2003. "Prevalence of Chronic Kidney Disease and Decreased Kidney Function in the Adult U.S. Population: Third National Health and Nutrition Examination Survey." *American Journal of Kidney Diseases* 41: 1–12.

Coresh, J., B. Astor, and M. Sarnak. 2004. "Evidence for Increased Cardiovascular Disease Risk in Patients with Chronic Kidney Disease." *Current Opinion in Nephrology and Hypertension* 13 (1): 73–81.

Foxman, B. 2003. "Epidemiology of Urinary Tract Infections: Incidence, Morbidity, and Economic Costs." *Disease-a-Month* 49: 53–70.

Freedman, B. I., J. M. Soucie, and W. M. McClellan. 1997. "Family History of End-Stage Renal Disease among Incident Dialysis Patients." *Journal of the American Society of Nephrology* 8: 1942–45.

Golan, L., J. D. Birkmeyer, and H. G. Welch. 1999. "The Cost-Effectiveness of Treating All Patients with Type 2 Diabetes with Angiotensin-Converting Enzyme Inhibitors." *Annals of Internal Medicine* 131 (9): 660–67.

Grantham, J. 1997. "Pathogenesis of Autosomal Dominant Polycystic Kidney Disease: Recent Developments." In *Hereditary Kidney Diseases,* ed. A. Sessa, F. Conte, M. Meroni, and G. Battini, vol. 122, 1–9, *Contributions to Nephrology.* Basel, Switzerland: Karger.

Guay-Woodford, L. M., Z. H. Jafri, and J. Bernstein. 2000. "Other Cystic Kidney Diseases." In *Comprehensive Clinical Nephrology,* ed. R. J. Johnson and J. Feehally, 50.1–12. London: Mosby.

Hooton, T. 2000. "Urinary Tract Infections in Adults." In *Comprehensive Clinical Nephrology,* ed. R. J. Johnson and J. Feehally, 56.1–12. London: Mosby.

Hostetter, T. H. 2004. "Chronic Kidney Disease Predicts Cardiovascular Disease." *New England Journal of Medicine* 351 (13): 1344–46.

Hoy, W. E., Z. Wang, P. R. A. Baker, and A. M. Kelly. 2003. "Secondary Prevention of Renal and Cardiovascular Disease: Results of a Renal and Cardiovascular Treatment Program in an Australian Aboriginal Community." *Journal of the American Society of Nephrology* 14: S178–85.

Hussain, M., M. Lai, B. Ali, S. Ahmed, N. Zafar, A. Naqvi, and A. Rizvi. 1996. "Management of Urinary Calculi Associated with Renal Failure." *Journal of the Pakistan Medical Association* 45 (8): 205–8.

Imperatore, G., W. C. Knowler, D. J. Pettitt, S. Kobes, P. H. Bennett, and R. L. Hanson. 2000. "Segregation Analysis of Diabetic Nephropathy in Pima Indians." *Diabetes* 49: 1049–56.

Johnson, R., and J. Feehally. 2000. "Introduction to Glomerular Disease: Clinical Presentation." In *Comprehensive Clinical Nephrology,* ed. R. J. Johnson and J. Feehally, 20.1–14. London: Mosby.

Kher, V. 2002. "End-Stage Renal Disease in Developing Countries." *Kidney International* 62: 350–62.

Kiberd, B. A., and K. K. Jindal. 1998. "Routine Treatment of Insulin-Dependent Diabetic patients with ACE Inhibitors to Prevent Renal Failure: An Economic Evaluation." *American Journal of Kidney Diseases* 31 (1): 49–54.

King, H., R. E. Aubert, and W. H. Herman. 1998. "Global Burden of Diabetes, 1995–2025: Prevalence, Numerical Estimates, and Projection." *Diabetes Care* 21: 1414–31.

La Vecchia, C., F. Levi, and F. Lucchini. 1995. "Mortality from Benign Prostatic Hyperplasia: Worldwide Trends 1950–92." *Journal of Epidemiology and Community Health* 49: 379.

Li, P. K. T., and K. M. Chow. 2001. "The Cost Barrier to Peritoneal Dialysis in the Developing World: An Asian Perspective." *Peritoneal Dialysis International* 21: S307–13.

Lin, J. L., D. T. Tan, K. H. Hsu, and C. C. Yu. 2001. "Environmental Lead Exposure and Progressive Renal Insufficiency." *Archives of Internal Medicine* 161: 264–71.

Luke, R. G. 1999. "Hypertensive Nephrosclerosis: Pathogenesis and Prevalence. Essential Hypertension Is an Important Cause of End-Stage Renal Disease." *Nephrology Dialysis Transplantation* 14: 2271–78.

Mani, M. K. 2003. "Prevention of Chronic Renal Failure at the Community Level." *Kidney International* 63 (Suppl. 83): S86–89.

Martinez-Maldonado, M. 1998. "Hypertension in End-Stage Renal Disease." *Kidney International* 54 (68): 67–72.

Mathers, C. D., A. D. Lopez, and C. J. L. Murray. "The Burden of Disease and Mortality by Condition: Data, Methods, and Results for 2001." In *Global Burden of Disease and Risk Factors,* eds. A. D. Lopez, C. D.

Mathers, M. Ezzati, D. T. Jamison, and C. J. L. Murray. New York: Oxford University Press.

McClellan, W. M., and W. D. Flanders. 2003. "Risk Factors for Progressive Chronic Kidney Disease." *Journal of the American Society of Nephrology* 14: S65–70.

Moeller, S., S. Gioberge, and G. Brown. 2002. "ESRD Patients in 2001: Global Overview of Patients, Treatment Modalities, and Development Trends." *Nephrology Dialysis Transplantation* 17: 2071–76.

Morton, A. R., E. A. Iliescu, and J. W. Wilson. 2002. "Nephrology: 1. Investigation and Treatment of Recurrent Kidney Stones." *Canadian Medical Association Journal* 166: 213–18.

National Kidney Foundation. 2002. "K/DOQI Clinical Practice Guidelines for Chronic Kidney Disease: Evaluation, Classification, and Stratification." *American Journal of Kidney Diseases* 39 (Suppl. 1): S1–266.

Nelson, R. G. 2001. "Diabetic Renal Disease in Transitional and Disadvantaged Populations." *Nephrology* 6: 9–17.

Nelson, R. G., H. Morgenstern, and P. H. Bennett. 1998. "Birth Weight and Renal Disease in Pima Indians with Type 2 Diabetes Mellitus." *American Journal of Epidemiology* 148: 650–56.

Oishi, K., P. Boyle, M. J. Barry, R. Farah, F. L. Gu, S. Jacobson, and others. 1998. "Epidemiology and Natural History of Benign Prostatic Hyperplasia." In *Fourth International Consultation on BPH, Proceedings,* ed. L. Denis, K. Griffiths, S. Khoury, A. T. K. Cockett, J. McConnell, C. Chatelain, G. Murphy, O. Yoshida (Health Publication Ltd.), 23–59. Plymouth, U.K.: Plymbridge Distributors Ltd.

Parks, J., and F. L. Coe. 1996. "The Financial Effects of Kidney Stone Prevention." *Kidney International* 50 (5): 1706–12.

Pasternak, M. S., and R. H. Rubin. 1997. "Urinary Tract Tuberculosis." In *Diseases of the Kidney,* 6th ed., ed. R. W. Schrier and C. W. Gottschalk, 989–1009. Boston: Little, Brown.

Perneger, T. V., P. K. Whelton, and M. J. Klag. 1995. "Race and End-Stage Renal Disease. Socioeconomic Status and Access to Health Care as Mediating Factors." *Archives of Internal Medicine* 155: 1201–8.

Peterson, J. C., S. Adler, J. M. Burkart, T. Greene, L. A. Hebert, L. G. Hunsicker, and others. 1995. "Blood Pressure Control, Proteinuria, and the Progression of Renal Disease: The Modification of Diet in Renal Disease Study." *Annals of Internal Medicine* 123: 754–62.

Pugh, J. A., M. P. Stern, S. M. Haffner, C. W. Eifler, and M. Zapata. 1988. "Excess Incidence of Treatment of End-Stage Renal Disease in Mexican Americans." *American Journal of Epidemiology* 127: 135–44.

Robertson, W. G. 2003. "Renal Stones in the Tropics." *Seminars in Nephrology* 23: 77–87.

Rostand, S. G. 1992. "U. S. Minority Groups and End-Stage Renal Disease: A Disproportionate Share." *American Journal of Kidney Diseases* 19: 411–13.

Ruggenenti, P., A. Schieppati, and G. Remuzzi. 2001. "Progression, Remission, Regression of Chronic Renal Diseases." *Lancet* 357: 1601–8.

Rutkowski, B. 2002. "Changing Pattern of End-Stage Renal Disease in Central and Eastern Europe." *Nephrology Dialysis Transplantation* 15: 156–60.

Satko, S. G., and B. I. Freedman. 2001. "Screening for Subclinical Nephropathy in Relatives of Dialysis Patients." *Seminars in Dialysis* 14 (5): 311–12.

Schieppati, A., N. Perico, and G. Remuzzi. 2003. "The Potential Impact of Screening and Intervention for Renal Diseases in Developing Countries." *Nephrology Dialysis Transplantation* 18: 858–59.

Seaquist, E. R., F. C. Goets, S. Rich, and J. Barbosa. 1989. "Familial Clustering of Diabetic Kidney Disease: Evidence for Genetic Susceptibility to Diabetic Nephropathy." *New England Journal of Medicine* 320: 1161–65.

Seedat, Y. K. 2003. "Glomerular Disease in the Tropics." *Seminars in Nephrology* 23: 12–20.

Sever, M. S., E. Erek, R. Vanholder, E. Akoglu, M. Yavuz, H. Ergin, and others (Marmara Earthquake Study Group). 2001. "The Marmara Earthquake: Epidemiological Analysis of the Victims with Nephrological Problems." *Kidney International* 60: 1114–23.

Stengel, B., S. Billon, P. van Dijk, K. Jager, F. Dekker, K. Simpson, and others. 2003. "Trends in the Incidence of Renal Replacement Therapy for End-Stage Renal Disease in Europe, 1990–1999." *Nephrology Dialysis Transplantation* 18: 1824–33.

Weening, J. 2004. "Advancing Nephrology around the Globe: An Invitation to Contribute." *Journal of the American Society of Nephrology* 15: 2761–62.

WHO (World Health Organization). 2002. "Reducing Risks, Promoting Healthy Life." In *The World Health Report 2002*, ed. WHO. Geneva: WHO. http://www.who.int/whr/en/.

Winkelmayer, W. C., M. C. Weinstein, M. A. Mittleman, R. J. Glynn, and J. S. Pliskin. 2002. "Health Economic Evaluations: The Special Case of End-Stage Renal Disease Treatment." *Medical Decision Making* 22: 417–30.

Xue, J. L., J. Z. Ma, T. A. Louis, and A. J. Collins. 2001. "Forecast of the Number of Patients with End-Stage Renal Disease in the United States to the Year 2010." *Journal of the American Society of Nephrology* 12: 2753–58.

Zatz, R., J. E. Romão Jr., and I. L. Noronha. 2003. "Nephrology in Latin America, with Special Emphasis on Brazil." *Kidney International* 63 (Suppl. 83): S131–34.

Chapter 37

Skin Diseases

Roderick Hay, Sandra E. Bendeck, Suephy Chen, Roberto Estrada, Anne Haddix, Tonya McLeod, and Antoine Mahé

In assigning health priorities, skin diseases are sometimes thought of, in planning terms, as small-time players in the global league of illness compared with diseases that cause significant mortality, such as HIV/AIDS, community-acquired pneumonias, and tuberculosis. However, skin problems are generally among the most common diseases seen in primary care settings in tropical areas, and in some regions where transmissible diseases such as tinea imbricata or onchocerciasis are endemic, they become the dominant presentation. For instance, the World Health Organization's 2001 report (Mathers 2006) on the global burden of disease indicated that skin diseases were associated with mortality rates of 20,000 in Sub-Saharan Africa in 2001. This burden was comparable to mortality rates attributed to meningitis, hepatitis B, obstructed labor, and rheumatic heart disease in the same region. Using a comparative assessment of disability-adjusted life years (DALYs) from the same report, the World Health Organization recorded an estimated total of 896,000 DALYs for the region in the same year, similar to that attributed to gout, endocrine disease, panic disorders, and war-related injuries. As noted later, those figures require confirmation by more detailed studies, and their practical application to health interventions needs to be tested.

Assessing the impact of skin disease on the quality of life in comparison with that of chronic nondermatological diseases is difficult; however, the study by Mallon and others (1999), which was not carried out in a developing country, compares the common skin disease acne with chronic disorders such as asthma, diabetes, and arthritis and finds comparable deficits in objective measurements of life quality. Skin disease related to HIV, which may constitute an important component of the skin disease burden in developing countries, particularly in Sub-Saharan Africa, leads to a similar impact on life quality compared with non-HIV-related skin problems, although the use of antiretroviral therapy significantly improves quality of life (Mirmirani and others 2002). Those findings indicate that skin diseases have a significant impact on quality of life.

Although mortality rates are generally lower than for other conditions, people's needs for effective remedies for skin conditions should be met for a number of important reasons.

- First, skin diseases are so common and patients present in such large numbers in primary care settings that ignoring them is not a viable option. Children, in particular, tend to be affected, adding to the burden of disease among an already vulnerable group.
- Second, morbidity is significant through disfigurement, disability, or symptoms such as intractable itch, as is the reduction in quality of life. For instance, the morbidity from secondary cellulitis in lymphatic filariasis, which may lead to progressive limb enlargement, is severe, and subsequent immobility contributes to social isolation.
- Third, the relative economic cost to families of treating even trivial skin complaints limits the uptake of therapies. Generally, families must meet such costs from an overstretched household budget, and such expenses in turn reduce the capacity to purchase such items as essential foods (Hay and others 1994).
- Fourth, screening the skin for signs of disease is an important strategy for a wide range of illnesses, such as leprosy, yet a basic knowledge of the simple features of disease whose presenting signs occur in the skin is often lacking at the primary care level.

A shortage of elementary skills in the management of skin diseases is a further confounding problem. A number of studies assessing success in the management of skin diseases in primary care settings in the developing world find that treatment failure rates of more than 80 percent are common (Figueroa and others 1998; Hiletework 1998). An additional point, often overlooked, is that skin diseases in the developing world are often transmissible and contagious but are readily treatable (Mahé, Thiam N'Diaye, and Bobin 1997).

A number of common diseases account for the vast majority of the skin disease burden; therefore implementing effective treatments targeted at those conditions results in significant gains for both personal and public health. Even where eradication is impossible, control measures may be important in reducing the burden of illness; yet few systematic attempts have been made to validate control programs for skin diseases as public health interventions.

PREVALENCE OF SKIN DISEASES

Few studies aimed at estimating the prevalence of skin diseases have been carried out in Western societies. However, Rea, Newhouse, and Halil's (1976) study in Lambeth, south London, which used a questionnaire-based, population-centered approach backed by random examination, reveals an overall 52 percent prevalence of skin disease, of which the investigators judged that just over half the cases required treatment. Studies from developing countries have generally adopted a more inclusive approach that uses systematic, community-based surveys backed by examination. Published figures for the prevalence of skin diseases in developing countries range from 20 to 80 percent.

In a study in western Ethiopia, between 47 and 53 percent of the members of two rural communities claimed to have a skin disease (Figueroa and others 1998), but when they were examined, 67 percent of those who denied having skin problems were found to have treatable skin conditions, most of which were infections. However, prevalence alone does not equate with disease burden. For instance, most communities recognize scabies as a problem because of its intractable itching and secondary infection, whereas they may ignore tinea capitis, which is equally common among the same populations, because they are aware that it follows a benign and asymptomatic course in many patients.

Researchers agree about the main risk factors associated with skin disease in developing countries, the most important of which appears to be household overcrowding. In primary schools in western Ethiopia, more than 80 percent of randomly examined schoolchildren had at least one skin disease, which was usually caused by one of four conditions: scabies,

pediculosis capitis, tinea capitis, or pyoderma (Figueroa and others 1996). Those figures mirror work carried out elsewhere. For instance, in Tanzania, in a survey of two village communities, Gibbs (1996) found that 27 percent of patients had a treatable skin disease, and once again, infections were the most common diseases. Overcrowding was a major risk factor in that survey. A similar community-based survey in Sumatra, Indonesia, showed a 28 percent prevalence of skin disease (Saw and others 2001). What seems to influence the overall prevalence and pattern of skin conditions in certain areas is the existence of a number of common contagious diseases, notably, scabies and tinea capitis. Hot and humid climatic conditions may also predispose populations to pyoderma, thereby affecting the distribution of disease.

PATTERNS OF SKIN DISEASES AT THE COMMUNITY LEVEL

A recent (unpublished) survey by the International Foundation of Dermatology designed to provide information about community patterns of skin disease in nine different countries across the world—Australia (Northwest Territory), Ethiopia, Indonesia, Mali, Mexico, Mozambique, Senegal, Tanzania, and Thailand)—and poor regions in other tropical environments from Mexico to Madagascar indicates that the following were the main skin conditions at community level:

- *Scabies.* Although scabies was often the commonest skin disease, it was completely absent in some regions.
- *Superficial mycoses.* This group of infections was usually reported as one of the three commonest diseases.
- *Pyoderma.* This disease was often, but not invariably, associated with scabies.
- *Pediculosis.* This disease was the subject of much variation but is often overlooked in surveys. Firm, community-level data on the prevalence of pediculosis are deficient; thus, this disease is not discussed further in this chapter.
- *Eczema or dermatitis.* Although this disease was usually unclassified, irritant dermatitis and chronic lichen simplex were often cited.
- *HIV-related skin disease.* This disease was reported mainly in Africa. The pruritic papular dermatitis of AIDS is a specific problem.
- *Pigmentary anomalies.* Three different problems were cited: hypopigmentation, often diagnosed as pityriasis alba, a form of eczema; melasma; and dermatitis caused by cosmetic bleaching agents (Mahé and others 2003).
- *Acne.* This disease was reported as an emerging and common problem.

These diseases are the same as those recorded in the literature described previously. Other skin conditions cited by different members of the group surveyed follow:

- *Tropical ulcer.* The incidence was highly variable, but tropical ulcer can account for a huge workload in primary care centers in endemic areas.
- *Nonfilarial lymphoedema.* This condition was mainly confined to Ethiopia.
- *Onchodermatitis, filarial lymphoedema, endemic treponematoses, Buruli ulcers, and leprosy.* These conditions are discussed in detail elsewhere in this book, but note that they often present with skin changes and symptoms.

According to World Bank (2002) figures for low-income populations in 2000, the estimated numbers of individuals infected with pyoderma and scabies, based on the highest prevalence figures from community surveys in the developing world, are 400 million and 600 million, respectively. Based on the lowest prevalence figures, these estimated numbers are 40 million and 50 million, respectively. For tinea capitis, the estimated number of cases based on the highest estimates of prevalence for Sub-Saharan Africa alone is 78 million.

Overall, these data suggest that significant changes could be made in reducing the burden of skin diseases by focusing on the small group of conditions, particularly infections, that account for the bulk of the community case load. This chapter concentrates on those conditions for which such a strategy could be implemented—namely, scabies, pyoderma, fungal infections, tropical ulcers, HIV/AIDS-related dermatoses, and pigmentary disorders.

EFFECTIVE THERAPIES

In considering the evidence for effective treatment, a subgroup of the team (Bendeck, Chen, and McLeod) undertook a data search to establish the evidence base for treatment of the common conditions. They carried out comprehensive searches of the MEDLINE (1966–April 2003) and EMBASE (1980–April 2003) databases to identify therapeutic studies on scabies, pyodermas, and superficial mycoses (but note that many of the studies were performed in industrial countries). They used foreign-language articles if an English abstract was provided. Table 37.1 shows search terms for each of the skin diseases common in the developing world and for treatment.

The team members reviewed study titles and abstracts to select relevant articles and scrutinized the bibliographies of selected articles to identify pertinent studies not captured in the initial literature search. They defined admissible evidence as primary therapeutic studies, based on clinical evaluation, of the treatment of each disease.

Table 37.1 Search Strategy for Therapies

Disease	Search term for disease	Search term for treatment
Scabies	["scabies"]	["treatment of" or "ivermectin" or "permethrin" or "Lindane" or "malathion" or "benzoyl benzoate" or "crotamiton" or "sulfur"]
Pyoderma or bacterial skin infections	["skin diseases, bacterial" or "ecthyma" or "staphylococcal skin infections" or "impetigo" or "pyoderma" or "folliculitis"]	["drug therapy" or "prevention & control" or "therapy"]
Tinea capitis:	["tinea capitis"]	["drug therapy" or "therapy" or "prevention & control"]
Tinea imbricata:	["tinea imbricata.mp"]	
Tropical ulcer	["tropical ulcer$.ti"] or ["skin ulcer(explode)" and "tropic$.mp"]	

Source: Authors.
Note: Terms in brackets are medical subject heading terms. If no standard medical subject heading terms were available, databases were searched either using the title option (denoted as ".ti") or the keyword option (denoted as ".mp").

SKIN DISEASES

Scabies

Scabies is a common ectoparasitic infestation caused by *Sarcoptes scabei,* a human-specific mite that is highly prevalent in some areas of the developing world. Scabies is transmitted by direct contact. In industrial societies, it is usually seen in sexually active adults, although it may also appear in the form of clusters of cases among the elderly in residential homes. Peaks of infection in communities may be cyclical. The ease of transmission appears to depend, in part, on the parasitic load, and some patients, including the elderly, may have large numbers of parasites present. By contrast, in healthy adults, the total parasite load may be low, but they, nonetheless, may suffer from highly itchy lesions. The organisms can also reach high densities in patients suffering from a severe depression of immunological responses, as in HIV infection. In this crusted or Norwegian form of scabies, lesions may present with atypical crusted lesions that itch little.

In developing countries, transmission commonly occurs in young children and infants and their mothers and is related to close contact, overcrowding, and shared sleeping areas. Sexual contact is less important as a means of transmission. Scabies is also a scourge of prisons in developing countries, where it is associated with overcrowding (Leppard and Naburi 2000). No evidence exists that transfer is related to inadequate hygiene.

The most important complication of scabies is secondary bacterial infection, usually caused by Group A streptococci. Evidence from studies among the indigenous population of northern Australia indicates that this infection is not always benign and that persistent proteinuria is associated with past scabies infestation, suggesting that nephritis related to secondary infection of scabies may cause long-lasting renal damage (White, Hoy, and McCredie 2001).

The disease presents with itchy papules and sinuous linear tracks in the skin that can be highly pruritic and particularly troublesome at night. Often more than one member of a household has the disease.

Treatment. The treatments used for scabies are mainly applied topically. Treatment is not based on treating just affected individuals, both because of the ease with which scabies spreads and because symptoms may develop days or weeks after infection. The advice given to patients always includes a recommendation to treat the entire household with a similar medication, a difficult problem when many people live in the same dwelling. The treatments commonly available include the following:

- *Sulfur ointments.* There are no controlled clinical studies of the use of this cheap medication, which is usually made up in an ointment base. Soap containing sulfur is available in some areas. Anecdotally, sulfur ointment needs to be applied for at least one week to the entire body. Irritation is a common side effect, and lower concentrations, such as 2.5 percent, are applied to infants.
- *Benzyl benzoate.* A 10 to 25 percent benzyl benzoate emulsion is applied over the entire body and left on the skin for up to 24 hours before washing off. Current recommendations suggest that one to three applications may be sufficient, but consensus on the optimal treatment regimen would be useful. Benzyl benzoate emulsion is an irritant and can lead to secondary eczema in some patients.
- *Gamma benzene hexachloride (Lindane).* This product is widely available and is used as a single application washed off after 12 to 24 hours. Concerns have arisen about the increasing risk of drug resistance and the absorption of the drug through the skin. It is also not used in children because of reports of neurotoxicity and fits. This product is not available in many countries.
- *Malathion (0.5 percent) in an aqueous base.* The highly purified commercial forms are effective after a single application, although a second is advised. No data are available on the use of this preparation in developing countries.
- *Crotamiton cream or monosulfiram 25 percent.* These alternative therapies have highly variable efficacy rates.

- *Permethrin 5 percent cream.* This effective, nonirritant treatment is usually administered as a cream applied all over the body. A single application washed off after 8 to 12 hours is used. The tubes are small, and adequate quantities should be prescribed. This treatment is also the most costly of the topical therapies.

Treatment failures in developing countries may be related to the lack of a suitable place in many communities where patients can apply treatment effectively over the entire body from the neck down in privacy.

Oral ivermectin, which is an important drug in the treatment of onchocerciasis, has also been used in patients with scabies, particularly those with the crusted form or in places such as prisons, where large numbers of infected individuals live in close proximity. It has also been applied as a community-based treatment and is reported to be effective as such (Hegazy and others 1999). It is not licensed for the treatment of scabies, and the lack of safety data on the use of ivermectin in infants limits its use. In addition, insufficient evaluations of its efficacy and cost-effectiveness in developing countries have been carried out.

Evidence for Effective Therapies. The team identified 56 articles on therapies for scabies and found the following to be the viable ones: oral and topical ivermectin, permethrin, gamma benzene hexachloride, benzyl benzoate, crotamiton, malathion, and topical sulfur. Table 37.2 summarizes the evidence for ivermectin versus a placebo or permethrin and for topical ivermectin, as well as for the less expensive topical sulfur.

Community-Based Treatments for Scabies. Few studies have addressed the problem of community-administered treatments for scabies, despite the argument that without a community approach to therapy in many developing countries, the successful management of scabies in areas where it affects more than 5 to 6 percent of the population is doomed to failure. Taplin and others' (1991) study of the use of 5 percent permethrin cream in the San Blas Islands, Panama, confirms this view. A three-year program of treatments backed by surveillance reduced the prevalence of scabies from 33 percent to less than 1 percent; however, a three-week break in regular treatment was followed by a rapid increase in prevalence to 3 percent. The results of treatments involving the application of similar protocols, but using other topical agents, are not available. Oral ivermectin lends itself to a community-based treatment approach and has been used in this way (Hegazy and others 1999; Usha and Gopalakrishnan Nair 2000), but insufficient follow-up data are currently available to comment further on this approach.

Bacterial Skin Infections or Pyoderma

Bacterial skin infections or pyoderma are common in most developing countries (Mahé, Thiam N'Diaye, and Bobin 1997).

Table 37.2 Evidence of the Efficacy of Treatments for Scabies

Treatment and average wholesale price	Strongest evidence	Number of people in study	Results	Comments
Ivermectin oral US$5.20 (3 mg), given at 200 μg/kg, one or two doses	Randomized clinical trial (versus placebo) (Hegazy and others 1999)	55	79.3 percent cure with single dose of ivermectin 200 μg/kg versus 16.0 percent cure with placebo ($p < 0.001$)	• Will treat concomitant strongyloidiasis and onchocerciasis • Not approved for scabies by the U.S. Food and Drug Administration • Safety not established for children under five and pregnant women
	Randomized clinical trial (versus permethrin) (Taplin and others 1991)	85	Single dose: 70.0 percent cure with ivermectin 200 μg/kg versus 97.8 percent cure with permethrin 5 percent Second dose (two-week interval): 95.0 percent cure with ivermectin 200 μg/kg (statistically equivalent cure rates with ivermectin and permethrin used as single dose/application)	• A single application of permethrin is superior to a single dose of ivermectin, which suggests that ivermectin may not be effective at all stages in the life cycle of the parasite
Ivermectin (topical)	Open-label, prospective, single group (Macotela-Ruiz and Ramos 1996)	32	100 percent cure rate with two doses of ivermectin 1 percent solution at six weeks (no statistics reported)	• Subjects treated with 1 percent ivermectin in a solution of propylene glycol at 400 μg/kg repeated once after one week • Well tolerated
Sulfur compounds (topical) Ointment (480 grams) US$2.32	Open-label, nonrandomized, prospective cohort (Usha and Gopalakrishnan Nair 2000)	102	71 percent cure at four weeks using sulfur, 5 percent in children younger than 12 months, and 10 percent in children older than 12 months	• Typically used as 5 percent to 10 percent in petrolatum • Messy and smelly • Must be applied repetitively for three nights • Mild local irritation may occur

Source: Authors.
μg = microgram; kg = kilogram; mg = milligram; p = probability.

Generally these infections arise as primary infections of the skin known as impetigo or as secondary infections of other lesions such as scabies or insect bites. The usual bacterial causes are Group A streptococci or *Staphylococcus aureus*. Bacterial infections are common in communities. In many cases, no bacteriological confirmation is available from cultures, but surveys show that Group A streptococci account for a substantial number of cases (Carapetis, Currie, and Kaplan 1999; Taplin and others 1973), which is not often the case in similar infections in temperate climates, where *S. aureus* dominates. This finding carries implications for the selection of treatment options. The reasons for this finding are not clear, although humidity and heat are associated with increased risk of bacterial skin infection. In addition to these superficial infections, *S. aureus* also causes folliculitis, or hair follicle infections and abscesses. Rarer causes of skin infection in developing countries include cutaneous diphtheria and anthrax, as well as necrotizing infection caused by *Vibrio vulnificus*.

Bacterial infection causes irritation and some discomfort. In some cases, the infection penetrates deep down through the epidermis, causing a necrotic ulcer—a condition known as ecthyma. However, some evidence suggests that streptococcal infection may cause additional long-term damage through the development of prolonged proteinuria, as described earlier in relation to scabies.

Treatment. Treatment with topical antibacterials, such as fusidic acid or mupirocin, is expensive; thus, the use of cheaper agents, such as antiseptics, is an important option but one that has been evaluated in only a few instances. Chlorhexidine and povidone iodine have both been used, but potassium permanganate is also said to be clinically effective. Gentian violet at concentrations of 0.5 to 1.0 percent is a cheap agent that is widely used, with proven in vitro efficacy against agents commonly involved in pyoderma. Most of those compounds have been used to prevent rather than to treat infections. The most extensively evaluated topical preparations are fusidic acid ointment and mupirocin, which are given daily for up to 10 days. Those drugs are effective in eradicating bacterial infections but, as noted, are not cheap options. Group A streptococci are still sensitive to penicillin, which can be used for treatment, with alternatives for staphylococcal infections being cloxacillin, flucloxacillin, and erythromycin. Industrial countries largely view methicillin resistance among staphylococci as a nosocomial problem, yet it has now spread to the community, and skin infections provide an ideal medium for the spread of resistance, even in developing countries. *S. aureus* strains isolated from skin sites, even in remote tropical areas, are now resistant to beta-lactam penicillins and tetracyclines through the spread of resistance genes. Tetracycline ointment is still available in many rural pharmacies and is widely used to treat superficial skin lesions, even though some bacterial infections will be unresponsive. Topical neomycin and bacitracin are widely available, are associated with identifiable levels of treatment failure, and also carry a risk of sensitization or adverse effects.

Evidence for Effective Treatment. The team reviewed 727 studies of therapies for pyoderma or bacterial skin infections. These studies could be grouped into either prophylactic regimens or therapeutic trials. For the prevention of pyoderma, the studies surveyed included the following effective therapies: chlorhexidine solution, hexachlorophene scrubbing, and neomycin/polymyxin B-bacitracin (Neosporin) cream. For

the treatment of pyodermas, a number of studies reported effective topical therapies, namely: povidone-iodine solution, hydrogen peroxide cream, electrolyzed strong acid aqueous solution, tea ointment, Soframycin ointment, honey, fusidic acid cream, trimethoprim-polymyxin B sulfate cream, rifaximin cream, sulconazole cream, miconazole cream, neomycin/polymyxin B-bacitracin (Neosporin) cream, terbinafine cream, and mupirocin. Systemic agents cited were cephalexin, erythromycin, penicillin, Augmentin, amoxicillin, sultamicillin, (di)cloxacillin, azithromycin, cefadroxil, cefpodoxime, cefaclor, ceftizoxime, clindamycin, clarithromycin, tetracycline, fluoroquinolones, and fusidic acid.

Table 37.3 presents the evidence for commonly used antiseptics and some of the specific antibacterial agents. In practice, topical treatments such as chlorhexidine, povidone, and in some cases neomycin or mupirocin will provide the most cost-effective control measures. For extensive infection, cloxacillin or erythromycin provides alternatives. However, current evaluations are subject to some weaknesses, such as a lack of large, comparative studies, particularly of the topical therapies, including antiseptics, used in developing countries.

Community-applied measures for managing skin infections have not been evaluated, but measures such as early treatment of scabies or basic wound care of sores might provide

Table 37.3 Evidence of the Efficacy of Topical Treatments for Pyoderma

Treatment, level of evidence, cost (manufacturer, formulation, average wholesale price)	Evidence	Number of people in study	Results	Comments[a]
Chlorhexidine gluconate (4 percent) detergent solution Level of evidence: VI Cost: • Clay-Park • Liquid, topical, 4 percent • 120 ml, US$7.01	Open-label, prospective cohort (versus nothing) (Taplin and others 1973)	3,602	6.3 percent clinical pyoderma on postdischarge in the chlorhexidine group; 24 percent in the nonchlorhexidine group (no statistics reported)	• Neonatal cord pyoderma • Prophylaxis study
	Open-label, prospective cohort (versus 70 percent ethanol and versus nothing) (Taplin and others 1973)	5,220	Hospital A: 15.2 percent of group without and 2.1 percent with chlorhexidine prevented cord pyoderma; hospital B: 21.0 percent with ethanol and 1.0 percent with chlorhexidine prevented pyoderma (no statistics reported)	• Neonatal cord pyoderma • Prophylaxis study • Performed and reported at two different hospitals
Povidone-iodine solution (Betadine) Level of evidence: II Cost: • Alpharma U.S. Pharmaceutical Directory • Solution, topical product, 10 percent, • 400 ml, US$5.46	Double-blind RCT (fusidic acid cream plus povidone iodine versus placebo cream plus povidone iodine) (Seeberg and others 1984)	160	92 percent improvement with fusidic acid and 88 percent with placebo	• Impetigo • 14 percent of placebo group versus 4 percent in fusidic acid group may have received antibiotics in weeks 2 and 4, potentially explaining the lack of difference in efficacy
	Open-label, prospective cohort (versus salicylic acid) (Linder 1978)	25	12/12 Betadine responded; 0/13 salicylic acid responded	• Disinfection of chronic wounds of lymphedematous patients • Outcome measure and statistics not clear

Table 37.3 Continued

Treatment, level of evidence, cost (manufacturer, formulation, average wholesale price)	Evidence	Number of people in study	Results	Comments[a]
Potassium permanganate Level of evidence: none Cost: • A-A Spectrum • Crystal, NA • 500 gm, US$16.10				
Mupirocin Level of evidence: I Summary: Efficacy supported by two RCTs and several comparison studies; some concern about resistance Cost: • GlaxoSmithKline (GSK) Pharmaceuticals • Ointment, TP, 2 percent • 22 gm, US$41.36	Double-blind RCT (versus placebo vehicle) (Koning and others 2002)	52	100 percent of mupirocin patients versus 85 percent of placebo (difference not significant)	• Impetigo/ecthyma • Outcome: cure or improvement • 38 in final evaluation; no ITT
	Double-blind, RCT (versus vehicle) (Daroczy 2002)	106	85 percent of mupirocin versus 53 percent vehicle-treated patients ($p = 0.007$)	• Secondarily infected dermatoses with *S. aureus* or *S. pyogenes* • Outcome: marked or moderate improvement • 92 in final evaluation; no ITT
	Open-label RCT (versus oral erythromycin) (Eells and others 1986)	97	90 percent of erythromycin and 96 percent for mupirocin (no statistics given); long-term follow-up: 9 erythromycin versus 3 mupirocin patients developed new lesions ($p = 0.05$)	• Impetigo contagiosa • Outcome: cure or clinical improvement • Also looked at long-term (up to one month) follow-up
	Open-label RCT (versus oral erythromycin) (Barton, Friedman, and Portilla 1988; Breneman 1990)	60	No significant difference in various evaluations of clinical efficacy except investigator's global evaluation (efficiency/safety performance) ($p = 0.01$)	• Impetigo • Both articles present the same research • More adverse effects with erythromycin
	Investigator-blinded, RCT (versus oral erythromycin) (McLinn 1988)	75	93 percent mupirocin versus 96 percent erythromycin (no statistical difference) Recurrence with erythromycin: 10 percent of patients with *S. aureus* and 6 percent of patients with *S. pyogenes*; recurrence with mupirocin: none.	• Impetigo • Also looked at bacterial recurrences • 53 patients clinically and bacteriologically assessable; no ITT

Source: Authors.
gm = gram; ITT = intent to treat; ml = milliliter; *p* = probability; RCT = randomized clinical trial; TP = topical product.
a. Comments include type of skin infection; indication of prophylaxis, otherwise therapeutic trial; ITT analysis; and other comments.

significant benefits. In this area, carefully designed pilot control programs would provide extremely valuable data.

Fungal Infections

Fungal infections that affect the skin and adjacent structures are common in all environments. They include infections such as ringworm or dermatophytosis; superficial candidosis and infections caused by lipophilic yeasts and *Malassezia* species;

and some other common causes of foot infection, such as *Scytalidium*. The clinical and social impact of fungal infections on individuals varies with local conditions. For instance, tinea pedis is a treatable condition that causes cracking and inflammation with itching between the toes. It is generally viewed as a nuisance that only marginally affects the quality of life; however, under certain conditions its significance is far greater. For example, fungal infections of the web spaces and toenails in diabetics provide a portal of entry for *S. aureus*, an event closely related to the development of serious foot complications in patients with peripheral vascular disease and neuropathy. Similarly, foot infections originally caused by dermatophytes can develop into more serious disabling infections through secondary Gram-negative bacterial infection among certain occupational groups in the tropics, such as workers in heavy industry, the police, or the armed forces. Wearing heavy footwear is a risk factor for the emergence of this problem.

Other infections, such as oropharyngeal candidosis, are important complications of HIV. This commonest infectious complication of AIDS is a potential early marker. Whereas in many patients it may simply have nuisance value, in others it has a more serious impact and leads to dysphagia and loss of appetite. *Malassezia* infections such as pityriasis versicolor are also common in the developing world and often occur in more than 50 percent of the population; however, they are generally asymptomatic but cause patches of depigmentation, and patients seldom seek treatment.

Some fungal infections are extremely widely distributed or common in defined endemic areas. They include tinea capitis and tinea imbricata.

Tinea Capitis. Tinea capitis is a common, contagious disease of childhood that can spread extensively in schools. It is caused by dermatophyte fungi of the genera *Trichophyton* and *Microsporum* (Elewski 2000). Infections can spread from child to child (*anthropophilic infections*) or from animals to children (*zoophilic infections*). Anthropophilic infections tend to be endemic or epidemic, whereas the zoophilic forms occur sporadically. The commonest sources and causes of zoophilic infections are cats and dogs (*Microsporum canis*), cattle and camels (*Trichophyton verrucosum*), and rodents (*T. mentagrophytes*). The causes of the anthropophilic form of this infection vary in different areas of the world. Although in areas of the developing world this condition is endemic at high levels, in many parts of Africa it is a common condition affecting more than 30 percent of children in primary schools. The main African species are *M. audouinii, T. soudanense*, and *T. violaceum*. The last is also found in the Middle East and India. *T. tonsurans*, the form of tinea capitis endemic in the United States (Wilmington, Aly, and Frieden 1996) and in parts of Europe, such as France and the United Kingdom (Hay and others 1996), is extremely resistant to treatment. No evidence indicates that this form has spread to Africa yet, although this possibility exists.

Families of children with tinea capitis seldom present for treatment. However, in a small proportion of individuals, tinea capitis produces a highly inflammatory lesion with suppuration on the scalp along with permanent scarring and local hair loss. The numbers of infected individuals showing this highly symptomatic change are not known with any accuracy, but it is believed to occur in about 5 percent of cases, more

with *T. tonsurans*. This factor poses a dilemma in management, because where the disease is common and endemic, a regular source will always exist for new, severe, inflammatory infections in children. Therefore, addressing this issue by tackling individual cases without addressing the reservoir, albeit illogical, may ultimately be the most practical approach.

The diagnosis of tinea capitis is difficult to make clinically in mild cases because the main presenting signs are localized patches of hair loss with fine scaling. In some children, the hair loss is more diffuse. With the inflammatory forms, circumscribed patches of hair loss with erythema and pustulation also occur, and the whole area is raised into a boggy mass. The only way to confirm the diagnosis accurately is to take hair samples for culture and microscopy, which is not possible in many areas because they lack laboratory diagnostic facilities. One specific form of tinea capitis, favus, is clinically recognizable and distinct, because the scalp is covered with white plaques called *scutula*. The infection is chronic and can develop into permanent, scarring alopecia. Inhabitants of endemic areas often recognize favus as a distinct condition that causes chronic illness, and as a result, the uptake of consultation for treatment is higher.

Highly effective, topically applied treatments for tinea capitis are unavailable, and even though simple remedies such as benzoic acid compound (Whitfield's ointment) may lead to clinical improvements, relapse is almost universal. Nevertheless, the use of topical therapies may limit the spread of tinea capitis. Treatment depends on the use of oral therapies. The most widely available of these is griseofulvin, which is given to children in doses of 10 to 20 milligrams per kilogram daily for a minimum of six weeks. Noncontrolled studies show that a single dose of 1 gram of griseofulvin given under supervision can eradicate infection in more than 70 percent of individuals, but such regimens have not been adequately assessed under trial conditions to determine their effect on community levels of infection, nor are follow-up data available.

Recent years have seen the development of a number of effective, new, oral antifungals, including terbinafine, itraconazole, and fluconazole. Terbinafine is a highly active agent that is effective in the treatment of dermatophyte infections. It is given in doses of 62.5 milligrams for those under 10 kilograms, 125 milligrams for those weighing 10 to 40 kilograms, and 250 milligrams for those over 40 kilograms. Evidence indicates that it is effective after one week of therapy in *T. violaceum* and *T. tonsurans* infections, but the best responses are seen when it is used for four weeks. Unfortunately, at these doses it is less effective for *Microsporum* infections, although some data suggest that responses are significant if the doses are doubled. This drug is, therefore, difficult to administer in standardized protocols when the cause of infection is uncertain. Itraconazole is also effective, but no suitable pediatric formulation is available because it is marketed in a capsule form that is difficult to administer to young children. Fluconazole is also effective, although comparative studies of its use are not available. All three drugs are costly, and a community-based program that uses them would be difficult to fund and implement.

The team found a total of 432 articles for the treatment of tinea capitis. Table 37.4 presents key references for the oral therapies, the mainstay of therapy. The effective treatments included topical therapies (benzoic acid, bifonazole, selenium sulfide, ketaconazole shampoo, and miconazole shampoo) as well as systemic agents (griseofulvin, terbinafine, itraconazole, fluconazole, and ketoconazole). The results of topical treatments appear inferior to those of oral therapy, although they have not been directly compared, and some of the topical agents were applied to prevent transmission rather than to treat infection.

Attempts at community control of tinea capitis have been devised but have not been monitored adequately. The methods have been based on surveillance through culture and treatment of all infected children. Culture-based diagnosis is difficult to implement regularly in developing countries. The treatment used for community therapy has been griseofulvin in conventional daily or large single doses, but those approaches have not been compared. In addition, control protocols usually advise treating carriers with topically applied agents such as selenium sulfide (which is relatively cheap) or a miconazole shampoo (which is moderately priced). In practice, some "carriers" are really patients with extremely localized and hard-to-detect infections, and such patients will not respond to topical treatment in the long term. A second problem is the absolute reliance on laboratory confirmation of cultures to direct treatment of carriers. Therefore, other strategies need to be evaluated, such as reducing the community load, perhaps by topical therapy or single-dose griseofulvin, to reduce the risk of spread. An alternative would be to continue with the existing practice of treating individual cases while recognizing that this process ignores the community reservoir.

Tinea Imbricata (Tokelau Ringworm). In many parts of the developing world, tinea imbricata is an exotic and unusual infection, with isolated foci occurring in remote areas of Brazil, India, Indonesia, Malaysia, Mexico, and the western Pacific. However, in some specific locations, it is common and endemic, reaching prevalence rates of more than 30 percent in some communities in the western Pacific. For example, extrapolating from a school survey in Goodenough Island, Papua New Guinea, Hay and others (1984) estimate that more than 7,000 people out of a population of about 20,000 were infected.

The disease presents in the form of widespread scaling, often arranged in concentric rings or with large sheets of desquamation. The infection may develop early in life and persist into old age without the development of effective immunity. Tinea imbricata often affects wide areas of the body, sparing only body folds and scalp skin. In those areas where it is endemic, it can be a significant problem occupying much of the time of health aid post staff.

Individual treatments have depended on the antifungals described earlier, including griseofulvin. Terbinafine and itraconazole are highly effective, but their cost has constrained their use. As table 37.5 shows, the relapse rates after itraconazole are also higher than after terbinafine (Budimulja and others 1994). Topical agents such as benzoic acid compound (Whitfield's ointment) are helpful, but are seldom curative and are difficult to apply over such large areas. Some patients may be treated with locally derived treatments, such as the sipoma paint used in Papua New Guinea, which contains salicylic acid, brilliant green, and kerosene. Traditional treatments have also been used, but never evaluated. The leaves of *Cassia alata,* for instance, are widely used in the western Pacific.

The team found studies of the use of griseofulvin, terbinafine, and itraconazole for tinea imbricata. Some studies did mention sipoma paint and *Cassia alata,* but no studies evaluating their efficacy have been performed. The team also found case reports supporting the use of griseofulvin.

Different treatments for use on a community basis need to be evaluated because the impact of this condition on local health services in areas of high prevalence is heavy in terms of both time and staff workload.

Tropical Ulcer

Tropical ulcer is a common condition found mainly in children and teenagers in well-defined tropical regions. It usually affects the lower limbs (Bulto, Maskel, and Fisseha 1993), causing the sudden appearance of regular and deep ulceration. It is mainly seen in Africa, India, and the western Pacific and in parts of Indonesia and the Philippines. The disease is caused by a combined infection of a number of different bacteria together with a fusiform bacterium, *Fusobacterium ulcerans,* and an as yet unidentified spirochete. The disease is associated with poor living conditions and exposure to water, particularly flood or stagnant water and mud. In endemic areas, it is a constant drain on resources. Morris and others' (1989) study of aid posts in East Sepik province, Papua New Guinea, shows that management of tropical ulcer was occupying a third of the posts' time and almost half their health care budgets.

The lesion usually starts with mild discomfort and overlying hyperpigmentation on the skin that progresses rapidly over a few days until the skin breaks down and sloughs, revealing an underlying ulcer. The lesion is often clean on first presentation and round with smooth edges. It generally starts on the lower leg or ankle, and in about 10 percent of cases, it progresses to become an irregular, enlarged, and chronic ulcer.

The condition heals well in most patients with simple cleansing and treatment with penicillin; however, early grafting

Table 37.4 Evidence of the Efficacy of Different Regimens for Tinea Capitis

Treatment, level of evidence, cost (manufacturer, formulation, average wholesale price)	Evidence	Number of people in study	Results	Comments
Benzoic acid compound (Whitfield's ointment) Level of evidence: III Cost: not found	Investigator-blinded RCT (versus miconazole cream) (Wilmington, Aly, and Frieden 1996)	41	Mycological cure: 12/20 using benzoic acid compound and 10/19 using miconazole cream	• Neither treatment is fully efficacious
	Observational study (Hay and others 1996)		Prevalence dropped from 7.8 percent to 5.8 percent ($p < 0.05$)	• Prevalence study of dermatophytomycoses in rural schools • After institution of treatment by 12 trained community health workers, only prevalence of tinea capitis dropped significantly
Griseofulvin Level of evidence: III Cost: • Pedinol, tablets, 125 mg, US$63.00 for 100 tablets • Martec, tablets, 125 mg, US$34.10 for 100 tablets	Multicenter, single-blinded, RCT (versus terbinafine, itraconazole, and fluconazole) (Wright and Robertson 1986)	200	Effective treatment: 46/50 (92 percent) griseofulvin, 47/50 (94 percent) terbinafine, 43/50 (86 percent) itraconazole, 42/50 (84 percent) fluconazole ($p = 0.33$)	• ITT analysis performed • Griseofulvin for six weeks similar in efficacy to terbinafine, itraconazole, and fluconazole for two to three weeks
	Single-cohort retrospective analysis (Schmeller, Baumgartner, and Dzikus 1997)	474	60.7 percent responded well; 39.3 percent returned less than eight months later; 10.7 percent had a recurrence later	• Observation over a two-year period • Conclusions: griseofulvin may be ineffective in one-third or more patients
	Multicenter, open-label, RCT (four weeks terbinafine versus eight weeks griseofulvin) (Gupta and others 2001)	210	No statistically significant differences (cure = 67 percent in both groups); however, graphical presentation of data demonstrates a slightly higher proportion of patients in terbinafine group achieved "cure" earlier	• 147 patients were evaluable; no ITT • Four weeks of treatment with oral terbinafine had a similar efficacy to eight weeks of treatment with griseofulvin
	Parallel-group, multi-center, double-blind RCT (versus terbinafine) (Abdel-Rahman, Nahata, and Powell 1997)	134	Terbinafine for six weeks had a similar efficacy to griseofulvin	• Four oral terbinafine groups (6, 8, 10, or 12 weeks) compared with 12 weeks of griseofulvin • ITT analysis performed • Six weeks of terbinafine could represent an alternative to griseofulvin
	Double-blind RCT (versus terbinafine) (Fuller and others 2001)	50	Week 8: 76 percent griseofulvin and 72 percent terbinafine (not statistically significant); week 12: 44 percent griseofulvin and 76 percent terbinafine ($p < 0.05$)	• Outcome: cure rates at weeks 8 and 12 • Terbinafine is a good alternative for less-frequent recurrences
	Double-blind RCT (versus itraconazole) (Lipozencic and others 2002)	35	88 percent itraconazole versus 88 percent griseofulvin	• Tinea corporis and tinea capitis evaluated together • Outcome measure: cure • 34 patients evaluable for efficacy; no ITT • Two griseofulvin patients discontinued therapy because of vomiting • Itraconazole has the same efficacy as griseofulvin and fewer side effects

Source: Authors.

ITT = intention to treat; p = probability; RCT = randomized clinical trial.

Table 37.5 Evidence of the Efficacy of Terbinafine for Tinea Imbricata

Treatment, level of evidence, cost (manufacturer, brand name, formulation, average wholesale price)	Evidence	Number of people in study	Results	Comments
Terbinafine Level of evidence: II Cost: • Novartis • Lamisil • Tablets, 250 mg, US$260.51 for 30 tablets (AWP) • Tablets, 250 mg, US$868.16 for 100 tablets (AWP) • Cream, TP, 1 percent, 15 gm, US$32.61 (AWP) • Cream, TP, 1 percent, 30 gm, US$58.40 (AWP)	Double-blind randomized clinical trial (terbinafine versus itraconazole) (Lopez-Gomez and others 1994)	83	Clinical and mycological cure rate: • 37/37 for terbinafine, 31/35 for itraconazole ($p = 0.05$) At week 17 follow-up, reinfection or relapse: • 6/37 (16 percent) evaluable terbinafine patients • 24/31 (75 percent) evaluable itraconazole patients ($p < 0.001$)	• Terbinafine has a slightly higher cure rate and a lower reinfection and relapse rate than itraconazole • 72 patients eligible for follow-up

Source: Authors.
AWP = average wholesale price; gm = gram; mg = milligram; p = probability.

may be necessary if healing is delayed. Treatment, therefore, consists of early treatment with penicillin, a strategy that may also fit with a syndromic approach to ulceration, because it will also be effective for yaws. The alternative is oral metronidazole, but no evidence of the comparative efficacy of these two approaches is available.

In searching the literature for effective remedies for tropical ulcer, the team found little evidence. The team did find studies evaluating metronidazole and topical dressings, and several articles mentioned the efficacy of penicillin and split skin grafting, but no randomized controlled trials have been performed. A single case report supports the use of co-trimoxazole. The management strategy thereafter depends on keeping the wound clean to allow appropriate healing using local antisepsis and cleansing, such as potassium permanganate solution, chlorhexidine, or even saline, and protecting the area from further abrasion or secondary infection with sterile dressings. Clinical experience suggests that if this regimen is not followed, the risk of developing chronic leg ulceration is substantial.

No community strategies for preventing tropical ulcer are known, although the process of infection suggests that simple, hygienic measures to disinfect and clean the affected limb, perhaps modified from those used in lymphatic filariasis, might be effective as a simple preventive regimen. The possible use of vaccines has been substantially researched for the animal counterpart, sheep foot rot, which is caused by a similar combination of organisms.

HIV-Related Skin Diseases

A wide range of skin conditions may develop as a consequence of HIV infection, but most are beyond the scope of this chapter. They include conditions that are a significant drain on scarce resources. These include Kaposi's sarcoma and toxic epidermal necrolysis, a potentially life-threatening form of skin failure that is often drug induced and requires the level of care and attention that would be deployed for patients with severe burns.

The commonest skin-related complication of HIV, particularly in Africa, is the itchy papular eruption or papular pruritic eruption of HIV. It presents with fiercely itchy multiple papules on the face and upper trunk. It is of unknown etiology and responds only to symptomatic treatment—for instance, antipruritic preparations such as antihistamines—although simple topical preparations, such as calamine or menthol creams, may alleviate the itching. Recognizing this condition is important, because it is seen only in HIV/AIDS cases and is often mistakenly treated as acne. It does not respond to treatments for acne.

Pigmentary Disorders

The development of pigmentary change is an important source of concern in many communities (Taylor 1999). Disorders associated with pigmentary changes are common and range from hereditary defects such as albinism (Lookingbill,

Lookingbill, and Leppard 1995) to increased pigmentation, or *hyperpigmentation*, associated with inflammatory skin lesions such as acne. Albinism is a significant cause of life-threatening skin cancer in the developing world.

For many of these conditions, no effective remedies are available. For instance, hyperpigmentation secondary to inflammation cannot be removed effectively, although it may fade with time. Similarly, no effective cure exists for vitiligo, a common disease involving loss of pigment, although experimental treatments such as melanocyte grafting do produce localized repigmentation. Therefore, advising patients of the current comparative ineffectiveness of treatments for these conditions is important. Preventing the use of therapies that do not lead to effective outcomes should be an important part of the strategy for treating skin diseases.

Some forms of increased pigmentation, such as melasma, which is hyperpigmentation of the cheek and forehead areas and is seen mainly in women, respond to the application of hydroquinone derivatives. However, because such treatments are often misused, they would not be used at the community level and would be used only with advice from a trained practitioner. Depigmenting creams, lotions, and emulsions are widely available as cosmetic preparations in many local markets and shops, and in a study in Dakar, Senegal, more than 50 percent of women questioned stated that they were regularly using bleaching creams ranging from hydroquinones to corticosteroids (Mahé and others 2003). Hydroquinones are potentially damaging to the skin and with continuous use cause patchy increased pigmentation and scarring of the facial skin. Similarly, misuse of corticosteroids is associated with a range of secondary effects from skin thinning to increased infection rates. Warning people about the potential risks of depigmenting creams would be a useful health promotion strategy in many communities.

Skin depigmentation is also a feature of leprosy. Thus, teaching health care workers responsible for leprosy surveillance to recognize skin patterns is a practical strategy of great potential value in continuing progress toward eliminating this disease.

ECONOMIC ASSESSMENTS AND SKIN DISEASES IN DEVELOPING COUNTRIES

Apart from the studies mentioned here in relation to families' costs for treating community-acquired skin diseases in Mexico (Hay and others 1994) and costs to health posts of managing tropical ulcer in Papua New Guinea (Morris and others 1989), no published studies are available of the economic burden of skin disease. An extensive literature search did reveal some studies related to diseases that affect the skin but discussed elsewhere in this work (Buruli ulcer and onchocercal skin disease), as well as a paper on the direct costs of treating scabies in Italy. These studies are shown in table 37.6.

Examples of drug costs (tables 37.2 to 37.4) for tinea capitis, scabies, and pyoderma can be estimated as follows:

- Treatment of a single case of scalp ringworm using griseofulvin purchased from two differently priced U.S. sources to achieve the published efficacy rates (table 37.4) with a conventional therapeutic course of six weeks, assuming a daily dose of 250 milligrams, would provide between 61 and 92 percent efficacy at a drug cost per individual of US$29 or US$53, depending on the drug source. Alternatively, a single supervised dose of 1 gram would cost US$1.40 or US$2.50. With supervision of treatment, the total cost per cure using daily treatment ranges from US$35 to US$88 per patient.
- Treatment of 100 people with scabies using sulfur ointment, assuming 500 grams per individual, would cost US$58 or US$0.58 per person. This regimen would provide a 71 percent cure rate at three months and a cost per cure of $1.30 per patient.
- Treatment with povidone of an individual with pyoderma would cost US$0.68, assuming that 400 milliliters would treat eight people. This regimen would provide a cure rate of 88 percent at three months and a cost per cure of US$1.10 per patient.

These calculations have taken into account ideal community treatment conditions, where the recurrence rate is negligible. However, if such a community-based scheme is not effectively developed, more than 50 percent of those with scabies are likely to be reinfected. The figures are lower for tinea capitis (15 percent) and pyoderma (10 percent). Table 37.7 shows the costs of treating large populations.

Although little information is currently available, in particular about the effect of local pricing of medications on overall effective treatment costs, the studies cited in this chapter indicate that the financial burden of skin diseases within families may well be significant and that producing a series of robust analyses of the cost implications of both treatment and failure to provide adequate management strategies for these common conditions is critical.

The 1990 global burden of disease study estimated that the disability weighting associated with skin disease was at least 0.02. However, the disability weighting for severe scabies (25 percent of cases) and patients with ecthyma (10 percent of pyoderma cases) is 0.10. If we take skin cases with the lower disability estimates—for example, mild to moderate scabies and pyoderma—the cost per DALY gained would be about US$1.00 to US$1.50 (table 37.7). For tinea capitis, the cost per DALY gained using daily treatment would be considerably higher, US$175 at the lower drug cost.

Table 37.6 Literature Review on the Economic Impact of Skin Diseases

Disease	Author	Year of research	Country	Study type and population	Cost categories and indicators	Results
Buruli ulcer	Asiedu	1998	Ghana	Retrospective study of 102 cases at a district hospital in the Ashanti region	• Health care costs (inpatient services including medicines, surgery, laboratory) • Indirect costs (loss of productivity, food, miscellaneous)	• Total costs: US$783.27 per patient • Health care costs: US$233.78 per patient • Indirect costs: US$549.49 per patient • Percentage of total health care cost relative to district budget: 40 percent
Onchocerciasis (OSD)	Workneh	1993	Ethiopia	Males age 18 to 54 working at a coffee plantation with OSD and without OSD	• Days of leave • Income	• Those with OSD had significantly more days of leave and less income than controls
Onchocerciasis (OSD)	Oladepo	1997	Nigeria	Matched pairs of male farmers with OSD and without OSD	• Current cultivated farm size • Personal wealth	• Those with OSD had significantly smaller farm sizes and less personal wealth
Onchocerciasis (OSD)	Benton	1998	Ethiopia, Nigeria, and Sudan	Communities	• Educational impact • Direct costs • Indirect functional capacity costs, for example, from disability	• Children of OSD heads of household had double the risk of dropping out of school • People with severe OSD spend US$20 more per year on health (15 percent of their incomes) • People with severe OSD spend longer time seeking care
Scabies	Papini	1999	Italy	Outbreaks in two nursing homes	• Health care costs (medical consults, treatment, disinfestation procedures, laundry, extra staffing, disposable materials)	• US$151.17 per resident

Source: Asiedu 1998; Workneh 1993; Oladepo 1997; Benton 1998; and Papini 1999.
OSD = onchocercal skin disease.

Table 37.7 Cost of Cure and Impact on DALYs for the Three Most Common Skin Diseases, Using the Cheapest Effective Treatments

Disease	Cost of cure (US$/million population)	Number of people cured for US$1 million	Cost per DALY gained (US$)	Comment
Tinea capitis	5,250,000	285,000	175 (assuming cost per drug of US$29 for course of treatment)	Estimated on the basis of a high-prevalence (15 percent) region such as Ethiopia
Scabies	58,000	1,700,000	1.00–1.50	Estimated on the basis of a high-prevalence (10 percent) region
Pyoderma	55,000	900,000	1.00–1.50	Estimated on the basis of a high-prevalence (5 percent) region.

Source: Authors.

The benefits of devising control measures for treatable skin disease are also affected by the high prevalence figures for skin diseases in low-income countries with total populations of between 40 million and 600 million affected, depending on variations in disease prevalence.

CURRENT STATUS OF COMMUNITY CONTROL MEASURES IN DERMATOLOGY

Despite the logic of developing community-focused services for dermatology, such services have seldom been achieved (Hay, Andersson, and Estrada 1991). Perhaps the best current example of a concerted, community-based approach is the Regional Training Center for Dermatology in Moshi, Tanzania, which focuses on developing a primary care skills base in African countries for the care of patients with skin and sexually transmitted diseases (Kopf 1993). The program has now trained more than 100 medical assistants and nurses, who were placed in 15 different countries at the primary care level and who, in many cases, play key roles in developing local health programs. A key issue is that action proportional to the severity of the problem is needed. For instance, one option would be to help nonspecialized health workers significantly improve their skills in managing common skin diseases. That option would present a new challenge for the teaching of dermatology. Along those lines, a recent initiative to effect change through a control and education program in Mali targeted at pyoderma, scabies, and tinea capitis is currently being evaluated. Early assessments indicate that the teaching methods have been effective in instilling recognition skills among primary care health workers. The effect on community levels of skin diseases is not yet known.

Skin diseases remain a low priority for many health authorities, despite the large demand for services. Addressing the potential for controlling skin problems by means of simple and effective public health measures should be a realistic target for alleviating a common and solvable source of ill health. An effective plan, team, and basic dermatological formulary can do much to improve matters (Estrada and others 2000). This chapter outlines some of the challenges for such programs and some of the deficiencies of current provision.

REFERENCES

Abdel-Rahman, S. M., M. C. Nahata, and D. A. Powell. 1997. "Response to Initial Griseofulvin Therapy in Pediatric Patients with Tinea Capitis." *Annals of Pharmacotherapy* 31: 406–10.

Asiedu, K., and S. Etuaful. 1998. "Socioeconomic Implications of Buruli Ulcer in Ghana: A Three-year Review." *American Journal of Tropical Medicine & Hygiene* 59: 1015–22.

Barton, L. L., A. D. Friedman, and M. G. Portilla. 1988. "Impetigo Contagiosa: A Comparison of Erythromycin and Dicloxacillin Therapy." *Pediatric Dermatology* 5: 88–91.

Benton, B. 1998. "Economic Impact of Onchocerciasis Control through the African Programme for Onchocerciasis Control: An Overview." *Annals of Tropical Medicine & Parasitology* 92 Suppl 1: S33–39.

Breneman, D. L. 1990. "Use of Mupirocin Ointment in the Treatment of Secondarily Infected Dermatoses." *Journal of the American Academy of Dermatology* 22: 886–92.

Budimulja, U., K. Kuswadji, S. Bramono, J. Basuki, L. S. Jadanarso, S. Untung, and others. 1994. "A Double-Blind, Randomized, Stratified Controlled Study of the Treatment of Tinea Imbricata with Oral Terbinafine or Itraconazole." *British Journal of Dermatology* 130: 29–31.

Bulto, T., F. H. Maskel, and G. Fisseha. 1993. "Skin Lesions in Resettled and Indigenous Populations in Gambela, with Special Emphasis on the Epidemiology of Tropical Ulcer." *Ethiopian Medical Journal* 31: 75–82.

Carapetis, J. R., B. J. Currie, and E. L. Kaplan. 1999. "Epidemiology and Prevention of Group A Streptococcal Infections: Acute Respiratory Tract Infections, Skin Infections, and Their Sequelae at the Close of the 20th Century." *Clinical Infectious Diseases* 28: 205–10.

Daroczy, J. 2002. "Antiseptic Efficacy of Local Disinfecting Povidone-Iodine (Betadine) Therapy in Chronic Wounds of Lymphedematous Patients." *Dermatology* 204: 75–78.

Eells, L. D., P. M. Mertz, Y. Piovanetti, G. M. Pekoe, and W. H. Eaglestein. 1986. "Topical Antibiotic Treatment of Impetigo with Mupirocin." *Archives of Dermatology* 122: 1273–76.

Elewski, B. 2000. "Tinea Capitis: A Current Perspective." *Journal of the American Academy of Dermatology* 42: 1–20.

Estrada, R., M. Romero, G. Chavez, and G. Estrada. 2000. "Dermatologia communitaria: diez años de experiencia. Estudio epidemiológico comparativo entre población urbana y rural del estado de Guerrero." *Dermatologia Revista Mexicana* 44: 268–73.

Figueroa, J. I., L. C. Fuller, A. Abraha, and R. J. Hay. 1996. "The Prevalence of Skin Disease among Schoolchildren in Rural Ethiopia: A Preliminary Assessment of Dermatologic Needs." *Pediatric Dermatology* 13: 378–81.

———. 1998. "Dermatology in Southwestern Ethiopia: Rationale for a Community Approach." *International Journal of Dermatology* 37: 752–58.

Fuller, L. C., C. H. Smith, R. Cerio, R. A. Marsden, G. Midgley, A. L. Beard, and others. 2001. "A Randomized Comparison of Four Weeks of Terbinafine versus Eight Weeks of Griseofulvin for the Treatment of Tinea Capitis." *British Journal of Dermatology* 144: 321–27.

Gibbs, S. 1996. "Skin Disease and Socioeconomic Conditions in Rural Africa: Tanzania." *International Journal of Dermatology* 35: 633–39.

Gupta, A. K., P. Adam, N. Dlova, C. W. Lynde, S. Hofstader, N. Morar, and others. 2001. "Therapeutic Options for the Treatment of Tinea Capitis Caused by Trichophyton Species: Griseofulvin versus the New Oral Antifungal Agents, Terbinafine, Itraconazole, and Fluconazole." *Pediatric Dermatology* 18: 433–38.

Hay, R. J., N. Andersson, and R. Estrada. 1991. "Mexico: Community Dermatology in Guerrero." *Lancet* 337: 906–7.

Hay, R. J., Y. M. Clayton, N. De Silva, G. Midgley, and E. Rossor. 1996. "Tinea Capitis in Southeast London: A New Pattern of Infection with Public Health Implications." *British Journal of Dermatology* 135: 955–58.

Hay, R. J., R. Estrada, H. Alarcon, G. Chavez, L. F. Lopez, S. Paredes, and N. Andersson. 1994. "Wastage of Family Income on Skin Disease in Mexico." *British Medical Journal* 309: 848.

Hay, R. J., S. Reid, E. Talwat, and K. MacNamara. 1984. "Endemic Tinea Imbricata: A Study on Goodenough Island, PNG." *Transactions of the Royal Society of Tropical Medicine and Hygiene* 78: 246–51.

Hegazy, A. A., N. M. Darwish, I. A. Abdel-Hamid, and S. M. Hammad. 1999. "Epidemiology and Control of Scabies in an Egyptian Village." *International Journal of Dermatology* 38: 291–95.

Hiletework, M. 1998. "Skin Diseases Seen in Kazanchis Health Center." *Ethiopian Medical Journal* 36: 245–54.

Koning S., L. W. van Suijlekom-Smit, J. L. Nouwen, C. M. Verduin, R. M. Bernsen, A. P. Oranje, and others. 2002. "Fusidic Acid Cream in the Treatment of Impetigo in General Practice: Double-Blind Randomised Placebo Controlled Trial." *British Medical Journal* 324: 203–6.

Kopf, A. W. 1993. "International Foundation for Dermatology: A Challenge to Meet the Dermatologic Needs of Developing Countries." *Dermatologic Clinics* 11: 311–14.

Leppard, B., and A. E. Naburi. 2000. "The Use of Ivermectin in Controlling an Outbreak of Scabies in a Prison." *British Journal of Dermatology* 143: 520–23.

Linder, C. W. 1978. "Treatment of Impetigo and Ecthyma." *Journal of Family Practice* 7: 697–700.

Lipozencic, J., M. Skerlev, R. Orofino-Costa, V. C. Zaitz, A. Horvath, E. Chouela, and others. 2002. "A Randomized, Double-Blind, Parallel-Group, Duration-Finding Study of Oral Terbinafine and Open-Label, High-Dose Griseofulvin in Children with Tinea Capitis Due to Microsporum Species." *British Journal of Dermatology* 146 (5): 816–23.

Lookingbill, D. P., G. L. Lookingbill, and B. Leppard. 1995. "Actinic Damage and Skin Cancer in Albinos in Northern Tanzania: Findings in 164 Patients Enrolled in an Outreach Skin Care Program." *Journal of the American Academy of Dermatology* 32: 653–58.

Lopez-Gomez, S., A. Del Palacio, J. Van Cutsem, M. Soledad Cuetara, L. Iglesias, and A. Rodriguez-Noriega. 1994. "Itraconazole versus Griseofulvin in the Treatment of Tinea Capitis: A Double-Blind Randomized Study in Children." *International Journal of Dermatology* 33: 743–47.

Macotela-Ruiz, E. I. C., and Q. F. B. E. N. Ramos. 1996. "Tratamiento de escabiasis con Ivermectina por via oral en una comunidad rural cerrada: Implicaciones epidemiológicas." *Dermatologia Revista Mexicana* 40: 179–84.

Mahé, A., F. Ly, G. Aymard, and J. M. Dangou. 2003. "Skin Diseases Associated with the Cosmetic Use of Bleaching Products in Women from Dakar, Senegal." *British Journal of Dermatology* 148: 493–500.

Mahé, A., H. Thiam N'Diaye, and P. Bobin. 1997. "The Proportion of Medical Consultations Motivated by Skin Diseases in the Health Centers of Bamako (Republic of Mali)." *International Journal of Dermatology* 36: 185–86.

Mallon, E., J. N. Newton, A. Klassen, S. L. Stewart-Brown, T. J. Ryan, and A. Y. Finlay. 1999. "The Quality of Life in Acne: A Comparison with General Medical Conditions Using Generic Questionnaires." *British Journal of Dermatology* 140: 672–76.

Mathers, C. D., A. D. Lopez, and C. J. L. Murray. "The Burden of Disease and Mortality by Condition: Data, Methods, and Results for 2001." In *Global Burden of Disease and Risk Factors*, eds. A. D. Lopez, C. D. Mathers, M. Ezzati, D. T. Jamison, and C. J. L. Murray. New York: Oxford University Press.

McLinn, S. 1988. "Topical Mupirocin versus Systemic Erythromycin Treatment for Pyoderma." *Pediatric Infectious Disease Journal* 7: 785–90.

Mirmirani, P., T. A. Maurer, T. G. Berger, L. P. Sands, and M. M. Chren. 2002. "Skin-Related Quality of Life in HIV-Infected Patients on Highly Active Antiretroviral Therapy." *Journal of Cutaneous Medicine and Surgery* 6: 10–15.

Morris, G. E., R. J. Hay, A. Srinavasa, and A. Bunat. 1989. "The Diagnosis and Management of Tropical Ulcer in East Sepik Province of Papua New Guinea." *Journal of Tropical Medicine and Hygiene* 92: 215–20.

Oladepo, O., W. R. Brieger, S. Otusanya, O. O. Kale, S. Offiong, and M. Titiloye. 1997. Farm Land Size and Onchocerciasis Status of Peasant Farmers in South-western Nigeria. *Tropical Medicine & International Health* 2: 334–340.

Papini, M., R. Maccheroni, and P. L. Bruni. 1999. "O Tempora o Mores: The Cost of Managing Institutional Outbreaks of Scabies." *International Journal of Dermatology* 38: 638–39.

Rea, J. N., M. L. Newhouse, and T. Halil. 1976. "Skin Disease in Lambeth: A Community Study of Prevalence and Use of Medical Care." *British Journal of Preventive and Social Medicine* 30: 107–14.

Saw, S. M., D. Koh, M. R. Adjani, M. L. Wong, C. Y. Hong, J. Lee, and others. 2001. "A Population-Based Prevalence Survey of Skin Diseases in Adolescents and Adults in Rural Sumatra, Indonesia, 1999." *Transactions of the Royal Society of Tropical Medicine and Hygiene* 95: 384–88.

Schmeller, W., S. Baumgartner, and A. Dzikus. 1997. "Dermatophytomycoses in Children in Rural Kenya: The Impact of Primary Health Care." *Mycoses* 40: 55–63.

Seeberg, S., B. Brinkhoff, E. John, and I Mer. 1984. "Prevention and Control of Neonatal Pyoderma with Chlorhexidine." *Acta Paediatrica Scandinavica* 73: 498–504.

Taplin D., L. Lansdell, A. A. Allen, R. Rodriguez, and A. Corets. 1973. "Prevalence of Streptococcal Pyoderma in Relation to Climate and Hygiene." *Lancet* 1: 501–3.

Taplin, D., S. L. Porcelain, T. L. Meinking, R. L. Athey, J. A. Chen, P. M. Castillero, and R. Sanchez. 1991. "Community Control of Scabies: A Model Based on Use of Permethrin Cream." *Lancet* 337: 1016–18.

Taylor, S. C. 1999. "Cosmetic Problems in Skin of Color." *Skin Pharmacology and Applied Skin Physiology* 12: 139–43.

Usha, V., and T. V. Gopalakrishnan Nair. 2000. "A Comparative Study of Oral Ivermectin and Topical Permethrin Cream in the Treatment of Scabies." *Journal of the American Academy of Dermatology* 42: 236–40.

White, A. V., W. E. Hoy, and D. A. McCredie. 2001. "Childhood Post-Streptococcal Glomerulonephritis as a Risk Factor for Chronic Renal Disease in Later Life." *Medical Journal of Australia* 174: 492–96.

Wilmington, M., R. Aly, and I. J. Frieden. 1996. "Trichophyton Tonsurans Tinea Capitis in the San Francisco Bay Area: Increased Infection Demonstrated in a 20-Year Survey of Fungal Infections from 1974 to 1994." *Journal of Medical and Veterinary Mycology* 34: 285–87.

Workneh, W., M. Fletcher, and G. Olwit. 1993. "Onchocerciasis in Field Workers at Baya Farm, Teppi Coffee Plantation Project, Southwestern Ethiopia: Prevalence and Impact on Productivity." *Acta Tropica* 54: 89–97.

World Bank. 2002. *World Development Indicators*. Washington, DC: World Bank.

Wright, S., and V. J. Robertson. 1986. "An Institutional Survey of Tinea Capitis in Harare, Zimbabwe, and a Trial of Miconazole Cream versus Whitfield's Ointment in Its Treatment." *Clinical and Experimental Dermatology* 11: 371–77.

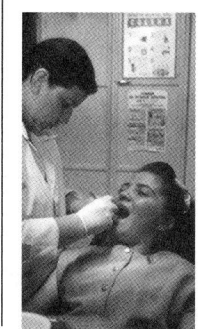

Chapter **38**

Oral and Craniofacial Diseases and Disorders

Douglas Bratthall, Poul Erik Petersen, Jayanthi Ramanathan Stjernswärd, and L. Jackson Brown

The oral cavity is an essential part of the body and contributes to total health and well-being. Recent research indicates that poor oral health affects general health and that some systemic diseases can affect oral health. A variety of diseases involve the oral cavity; the two main oral diseases present worldwide and lead to tooth destruction or tooth loss:

- dental caries, the disease that leads to cavities in the teeth
- periodontal disease, which leads to loosening of teeth.

Both diseases are preventable, and strong efforts have been made to control them. Other diseases and conditions are much less prevalent, yet serious, and sometimes even life threatening: oral precancer and cancer, oral manifestations of HIV and AIDS, noma, developmental disorders, and fluorosis of teeth.

DENTAL CARIES

Dental caries develops by the localized dissolution of the tooth hard tissues, caused by acids that are produced by bacteria in the biofilms (dental plaque) on the teeth and eventually lead to "cavities." The biofilm consists of microorganisms, including the highly cariogenic mutans streptococci, and a matrix made up mainly of extracellular polysaccharides. The destructive acids are produced when fermentable carbohydrates (sugars) reach these biofilms, each episode resulting in tooth damage (attack). If this process does not occur frequently, then the natural capacity of the body (through saliva) to remineralize will

prevent formation of a cavity. Thus, the main risk factors include presence of cariogenic biofilms and frequent consumption of fermentable carbohydrates. Exposure to fluorides in optimum concentrations reduces the risk, and normal saliva flow and saliva protective systems are also important to counteract the cariogenic factors.

Untreated caries can give rise to infection of the tooth pulp, which can spread to the supporting tissues and the jaws, culminating in advanced disease conditions that are often painful. For example, in Thailand, recent surveys of a sample of 12-year-old children revealed that 53 percent had suffered from pain or discomfort from teeth over the past year (Petersen and others 2001). The corresponding figures in China were 34 percent for 12-year-olds (Peng, Petersen, Fan, and others 1997) and 74 percent for adults (Petersen, Peng, and Tai 1997).

Tooth decay is a public health problem worldwide. According to the U.S. Surgeon General's report (U.S. Public Health Service 2000), dental caries is the single most common chronic childhood disease in the United States. Epidemiological data for almost 200 countries are available in the World Health Organization (WHO) Country/Area Profile Programme (CAPP) oral health database (http://www.whocollab.od.mah.se/index.html) (see table 38.1 for examples). Caries prevalence of permanent teeth is expressed by the decayed, missing, and filled teeth (DMFT) index (calculated by counting the number of DMFT of individuals and taking the mean for the group examined). One indicator age group used for international comparisons is 12-year-old children. The WHO oral health goal was to achieve three DMFT or fewer among 12-year-olds

723

Table 38.1 Mean DMFT and SiC Index of 12-Year-Olds for Some Countries, by Ascending Order of DMFT

Country	Mean DMFT	SiC Index	Year	Sample size	Reference
Australia	0.8	2.4	1999	29,130	Armfield, Roberts-Thomson, and Spencer 2003
Nepal	0.8	2.5	2000	623	Data from WHO, courtesy P. E. Petersen
Sweden	0.9	2.6	2001	71,896	Sundberg 2002
Jamaica	1.0	2.8	1995	362	Data from PAHO, courtesy E. D. Beltran and S. Estupinan-Day
China	1.0	3.0	1996	23,452	Data from WHO, courtesy P. E. Petersen
Senegal	1.2	2.8	1994	300	Sembene, Kane, and Bourgeois 1999
Sri Lanka	1.4	3.6	1994–95	2,003	Abayaratna and Krishnarasa 1997
England, U.K. (Northwest)	1.4	3.2	2000–1	12,029	Pitts and others 2002
United States	1.4	3.6	1988–91	176	Data from PAHO, courtesy E. D. Beltran and S. Estupinan-Day
Portugal	1.5	3.6	1999	800	Data from WHO, courtesy P. E. Petersen
Germany	1.7	4.1	1997	1,043	Micheelis and Reich 1999
Israel	1.7	4.1	2002	1,327	Courtesy S. P. Zusman, Division of Dental Health, Israel
South Africa	1.7	4.3	1988–89	1,571	van Wyk 1994
Greece (Northeastern province) (11-year-olds)	1.8	4.2	2001	2,217	Demertzi and Topitsoglou 2002
Scotland (U.K.)	1.8	4.3	1996–97	6,165	Data from K. Woods from the study Pitts, Evans, and Nugent 1998
France	2.0	4.7	1998	6,000	Hescot and Roland 2000
Thailand	2.4	4.9	2001	1,116	Data from WHO, courtesy P. E. Petersen
Mexico (state of Mexico)	2.5	5.0	1997	1,138	Irigoyen and Sanchez-Hinojosa 2000
Uruguay	2.5	5.3	1999	596	Sector Público 1999
Comoros	2.6	6.1	2000	142	Data from WHO, courtesy P. E. Petersen
Belarus	2.7	5.4	1999	2,537	Data from WHO, courtesy P. E. Petersen
Romania	2.7	5.8	2001	785	Data from WHO, courtesy P. E. Petersen
Nicaragua	2.8	5.7	1997	365	Data from PAHO, courtesy E. D. Beltran and S. Estupinan-Day
Greenland	3.5	7.0	2002	236	Data from WHO, courtesy P. E. Petersen
Latvia	3.8	7.1	1998	416	Data from WHO, courtesy P. E. Petersen
Poland	3.9	7.2	1997	1,732	Data from WHO, courtesy P. E. Petersen
Honduras	4.0	7.5	1997	307	Data from PAHO, courtesy E. D. Beltran and S. Estupinan-Day
Bolivia	4.7	8.8	1995	389	Data from PAHO, courtesy E. D. Beltran and S. Estupinan-Day
Slovak Republic	5.9	14.3	1998	1,589	Data from WHO, courtesy P. E. Petersen
Costa Rica	8.5	13.7	1988	1,349	Data from PAHO, courtesy E. D. Beltran and S. Estupinan-Day

Source: Authors.
PAHO = Pan American Health Organization; SiC = Significant caries.

by 2000. According to the CAPP database, 70 percent of the countries had achieved three DMFT or fewer by 2001, representing 85 percent of the world population. Several developing economies, however, have reported a trend toward higher levels of dental caries.

A detailed analysis of caries data for many countries, both industrial and developing, shows skewed distributions of the disease—that is, a proportion of a population of children showing a high or very high number of caries and the rest showing a low number of caries or none. Expressing caries prevalence as mean DMFT may, therefore, not accurately describe the disease

level in populations with skewed distribution. The Significant Caries (SiC) Index was proposed to bring attention to those hidden high caries groups (Bratthall 2000). The SiC Index is calculated by simply taking the mean DMFT of the one-third of the group having the highest DMFT in a population (figure 38.1). Table 38.1 shows several countries having fewer than three mean DMFT but high SiC Index values, thus illustrating the hidden caries burden for children (Nishi and others 2002).

Dental caries is found not only in children and young adults but also in all age groups. The elderly, in particular those with exposed tooth root surfaces, constitute a special risk

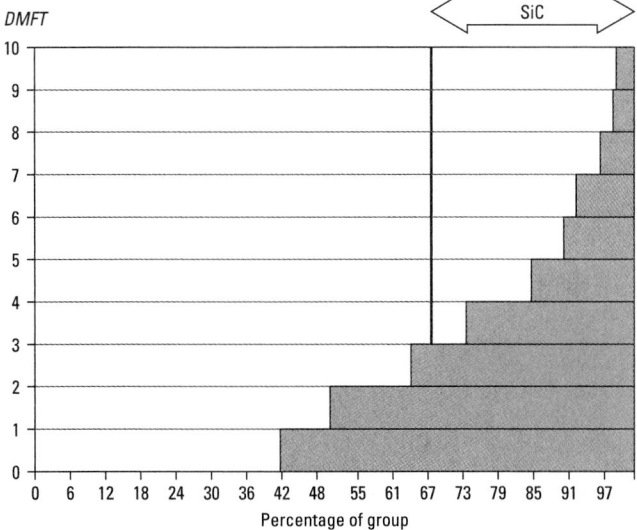

DMFT

SiC

Percentage of group

Source: Adyatmaka and others 1998.

Note: The mean DMFT is 2.3. The Significant Caries Index is 5.4. Arrow indicates the proportion of individuals who are included in the calculation of the index. West Kalimantan is one of the most caries-affected provinces in Indonesia.

Figure 38.1 DMFT for 331 12-Year-Olds, West Kalimantan, Indonesia

population (Barmes 2000). A Swedish study reported DMFT values of 21.4 and 24.4 for 50- and 70-year-olds, respectively, indicating that nearly all teeth were affected in these age groups (Hugoson and others 1995). Thomson (2004), reviewing longitudinal studies of older adults (age 50+), found an incidence of root surface caries varying from 29 to 59 percent and concluded that older people are a caries-active group, experiencing new caries at a rate comparable to that of adolescents. With increasing numbers of people becoming 50 years of age or older in some developing countries, root surface caries may become a significant problem.

When we consider the global epidemiology of dental caries, the main patterns seem to be the following:

- Countries with low mean sugar consumption (less than 10 to 15 kilograms of sugar per person per year) generally have low mean caries prevalence.
- Countries with high mean sugar consumption (more than 20 to 25 kilograms of sugar per person per year) and without effective preventive programs generally have high mean caries prevalence.
- Countries with high mean sugar consumption (more than 20 to 25 kilograms of sugar per person per year) using effective preventive programs have been able to reduce the caries prevalence.

If we consider the prevalence of caries *within* a population, the main patterns seem to be as follows:

- Disadvantaged or poor population groups have higher dental caries experience than advantaged groups.

- Individuals with poor oral hygiene and frequent sugar intake are at increased risk.
- Individuals not exposed to fluorides—for example, from fluoridated water or toothpastes—are at increased risk of caries.
- Persons with individual risk factors, such as reduced saliva flow or exposed tooth root surfaces, or with certain general diseases are also at increased risk of caries.

Caries Intervention Programs

Since the discovery of the caries-preventive effect of fluorides in the 1930s, different forms of fluoride administration programs have been implemented, often with remarkable caries-reducing effects. Fluoride has been added to different vehicles, such as water, salt, toothpaste, and milk. Fluoride tablets and fluoride mouth rinsing have been used among young children and in schools, and more recently even among adults at high caries risk (Petersen 1989, 1990). For individual use, fluoride in high concentrations has been added to various forms of gels and varnishes to be applied on the teeth. Furthermore, fluoride in chewing gum is available in some countries. When a group of international experts on cariology were asked in a study to identify the main causes of the caries decline seen in several Western countries during recent decades, practically all the experts pointed to fluoride dentifrice as the most significant factor (Bratthall, Hänsel-Petersson, and Sundberg 1996).

According to WHO (1994), community water fluoridation is safe and cost-effective in preventing dental caries in every age group, benefiting all residents served by the community water regardless of their social or economic status (Burt 2002; Petersen and Lennon 2004; White, Antczak-Bouckoms, and Weinstein 1989). Examples of countries with fluoridated water supplies for significant parts of the populations are Argentina, Brazil, Brunei Darussalam, Canada, Chile, Ireland, New Zealand, the United Kingdom, and the United States. In many developing countries, lack of community water supplies makes water fluoridation impossible.

Effective fluoride toothpastes have been available for about 40 years (WHO 1994). They have been tested in numerous studies, in particular in school-based programs. The most commonly used concentrations are 1,000 or 1,500 parts per million (ppm). Because most studies have been conducted in developed countries, WHO launched a program testing a so-called "affordable fluoridated toothpaste" in developing countries. In the West Kalimantan Province of Indonesia, a supervised school-based toothbrushing program was implemented over a period of three years, resulting in a reduction of 12 to 40 percent of caries incidence in the study groups when compared to control groups (Adyatmaka and others 1998).

Domestic salt fluoridation is another method of automatic fluoridation. In the early 1950s, Switzerland and Austria introduced this approach by offering their populations fluoridated salt for the table and for cooking. The fluoride concentration in the salt originally was 90 ppm and was later increased to 250 ppm. Fluoridated salt is now available in several countries in Europe and in South and Central America. A comparison of caries data for Jamaica in 1984 (before salt fluoridation) and 1995 (after salt fluoridation) showed a reduction of caries experience of 69 percent, 84 percent, and 87 percent among 15-, 12-, and 6-year-olds, respectively (Estupinan-Day and others 2001).

Milk fluoridation projects are being conducted in several countries, including Bulgaria, China, the Russian Federation, Thailand, and the United Kingdom. In Bulgaria, a milk fluoridation project resulted in a 79 percent lower DMFT in those children who had participated in the full five years of the program than in the control children (Pakhomov and others 1995).

Fluoride tablets and fluoride mouth-rinsing programs under supervision in schools have been implemented in several countries, including the Scandinavian countries, the United Kingdom, and the United States. The requirement that teachers and students be motivated has limited such approaches. In recent years, many national fluoride programs have been adjusted as the additional caries-reducing effects of topical applications with daily use of fluoridated toothpaste have been questioned (Petersen and Torres 1999).

Oral Health Education and Promotion Programs

The WHO Global Oral Health Programme has developed a manual for integration of oral health with school health programs (WHO 2003). In many industrial countries, school health education programs have included oral health, and researchers have shown that children's self-care capacity improved in regard to regular toothbrushing with the use of fluoridated toothpaste (Flanders 1987; Honkala, Kannas, and Rise 1990; Petersen and Torres 1999; Sogaard and Holst 1988; Wang and others 1998). Examples also exist from school oral health education in developing countries. Some programs have been organized within the context of the WHO Health Promoting Schools Initiative. In Madagascar, the evaluation of program outcomes has shown remarkably good results in reducing dental caries risk, improving self-care capacity of children and mothers, and introducing higher levels of dental knowledge and attitudes (Razanamihaja and Petersen 1999). Other successful examples are available from Tanzania (Petersen and others 2002; van Palenstein Helderman and others 1997), Zimbabwe (Frencken and others 2001), and Namibia (Priwe 1998).

In China, principles from the WHO Health Promoting Schools Initiative have been applied in certain provinces; positive effects of programs were obtained regarding health-related knowledge and behavior, but the clinical outcome measures were less evident (Petersen and others 2004; Tai and others

2001). The Chinese health authorities have emphasized preventive oral care and oral health education since the late 1980s. The nationwide mass campaign "Love Teeth Day" has been conducted annually since 1989, and the effective transmission of oral health messages to the public has shown improved oral health knowledge and behavior in children as well as in adults (Peng, Petersen, Tai, and others 1997).

In addition, various dental organizations (Cohen 1990) and private companies have developed and carried out successful oral health programs worldwide. For example, toothpaste manufacturers have donated toothpastes, toothbrushes, and educational material promoting oral health in several countries.

Effectiveness of the Oral Health Programs

In countries with systematic national oral disease prevention programs, the total cumulative effect of these programs is reflected in the epidemiological figures demonstrating caries decline (table 38.2) and in the growing proportions of caries-free individuals. However, singling out the effects of specific activities or methods of programs is difficult because several program components often operate simultaneously. For example, in industrial countries, practically all individuals use fluoridated toothpaste, and removing this preventive measure from a group of individuals just to evaluate the effect of another fluoride program would be unethical. In addition, other factors affect caries reduction, such as changing lifestyles, changing patterns of sugar consumption, and improving living conditions.

The current trend in clinical health care and public health is to base recommendations on evidence derived from systematic reviews of the literature and critical assessment of the quality of results (U.S. Public Health Service 2000). The office of the U.S. Surgeon General (U.S. Public Health Service 2000) and the Swedish Council on Technology Assessment in Health Care (SBU 2002) are examples of entities that have attempted to determine the effectiveness in public health of evidence-based approaches and technologies.

Oral Health in America, the U.S. Surgeon General's report (U.S. Public Health Service 2000), reviewed experiences from the administration of fluorides. Primarily based on U.S. studies, the report had these conclusions:

- Strong evidence exists supporting the effectiveness of water fluoridation in preventing crown and root caries in children and adults.
- Strong evidence exists of the effectiveness of the school-based fluoride supplement (tablets) program. The program, with motivated supervising personnel, such as teachers, is recommended for children at high risk for caries.
- Evidence supports the effectiveness of school-based fluoride (0.2 percent sodium fluoride) mouth-rinsing programs conducted before 1985 (before the introduction of fluoride

Table 38.2 Declining Caries Experience in Some Countries

Country	Year	DMFT in 12-year-olds	Reference
African region			
Côte d'Ivoire	1996	1.8	Guinan and others 1999
	1993	2.6	Data from Oral Health Programme, WHO
Niger	1997	1.3	Petersen and Kaka 1999
	1992	1.5	Data from Oral Health Programme, WHO
	1988	1.7	Woodward and Walker 1994
American region			
Colombia	1998	2.3	Data from PAHO
	1984	4.8	Woodward and Walker 1994
Costa Rica	1999	2.3	Data from PAHO
	1996	4.8	Data from Ministry of Health
	1993	4.9	Data from PAHO
Guyana	1995	1.3	Beltran-Aguilar, Estupinan-Day, and Baez 1999
	1983	2.7	Woodward and Walker 1994
Haiti	2000	1.0	Data from PAHO
	1994	2.2	Data from PAHO
Honduras	*1997*	*3.7*	Beltran-Aguilar, Estupinan-Day, and Baez 1999
	1987	*5.7*	Beltran-Aguilar, Estupinan-Day, and Baez 1999
Jamaica	1995	1.1	Beltran-Aguilar, Estupinan-Day, and Baez 1999
	1984	6.7	Beltran-Aguilar, Estupinan-Day, and Baez 1999
Nicaragua	1997	2.8	Beltran-Aguilar, Estupinan-Day, and Baez 1999
	1983	6.9	Beltran-Aguilar, Estupinan-Day, and Baez 1999
Panama	*1997*	*3.6*	Beltran-Aguilar, Estupinan-Day, and Baez 1999
	1989	*4.2*	Beltran-Aguilar, Estupinan-Day, and Baez 1999
United States	1992–94	1.28	NHANES III, Courtesy D. Bruce
	1988–91	1.4	Beltran-Aguilar, Estupinan-Day, and Baez 1999
	1986–87	1.8	Beltran-Aguilar, Estupinan-Day, and Baez 1999
Venezuela, R. B. de	1997	2.1	Beltran-Aguilar, Estupinan-Day, and Baez 1999
	1986	3.6	Data from PAHO
Middle Eastern region			
Saudi Arabia	1995	1.7	Data from Oral Health Programme, WHO
	1991	2.1	Data from Oral Health Programme, WHO
United Arab Emirates	1995	1.6	Nithila and others 1998
	1993	2.0	Data from Oral Health Programme, WHO
European region			
Belarus	2000	2.7	Leous and Petersen 2002
	1994	3.8	Leous and Petersen 2002
Denmark	2002	0.9	Data from National Board of Health, Denmark
	1995	1.2	Data from National Board of Health, Denmark
	1980	5.0	Data from National Board of Health, Denmark

(Continues on the following page.)

Table 38.2 Continued

Country	Year	DMFT in 12-year-olds	Reference
France	1998	1.9	Hescot and Roland 2000
	1993	2.1	Hescot and Roland 2000
	1990	3.0	Hescot and Roland 2000
Hungary	*1996*	*3.8*	Szoke and Petersen 2000
	1991	*4.3*	Szoke and Petersen 2000
	1985	*5.0*	Szoke and Petersen 2000
Israel	2002	1.66	Data from Dr S. P. Zusman, Division of Dental Health, Israel
	1989	3.0	Zadik, Zusman, and Kelman 1992
Latvia	*2000*	*3.9*	Latvia, State Dentistry Centre 2000
	1998	*4.2*	Latvia, State Dentistry Centre 2000
Norway	2000	1.5	Data from Norwegian Board of Health
	1992	2.2	von der Fehr 1994
	1986	3.1	Haugejorden 1994
Poland	*2000*	*3.8*	Wierzbicka and others 2002
	1991	*5.1*	Wierzbicka and others 2002
Portugal	1999	1.5	de Almeida and others 2003
	1990	3.2	de Almeida and others 2003
	1984	3.7	de Almeida and others 2003
Romania	2000	2.7	Petersen and Rusu 2002
	1990	3.9	Petersen and others 1994
Sweden	2001	0.9	Sundberg 2002
	1995	1.4	Sundberg 2002
	1985	3.1	Sundberg 2002
United Kingdom	1996–97	1.1	Pitts, Evans, and Nugent 1998
	1983	3.1	Downer 1994
Asian region			
Bangladesh	2000	1.0	Ullah 2001
	1981	1.5	Data from Oral Health Programme, WHO
Sri Lanka	1994–95	1.4	Abayaratna and Krishnarasa 1997
	1983–84	1.9	Sri Lanka, Ministry of Health 1985
Western Pacific region			
Australia	1999	0.8	Armfield, Roberts-Thomson, and Spencer 2003
	1990	1.4	Armfield, Roberts-Thomson, and Spencer 2003
	1980	3.6	Carr 1988
Hong Kong (China)	2001	0.8	Hong Kong, Department of Health 2003
	1986	1.5	Lo, Evans, and Lind 1990
Japan	1999	2.4	Data from Ministry of Health and Welfare
	1993	3.6	Miyazaki and Morimoto 1996
	1987	4.9	Miyazaki and Morimoto 1996
Malaysia	1997	1.6	Malaysia, Dental Services Division 1997
	1988	2.4	Malaysia, Dental Services Division 1997

Source: Authors.

PAHO = Pan American Health Organization; NHANES III = Third U.S. National Health and Nutritional Examination Survey.

Note: Numbers in italics indicate that the country did not achieve the WHO global goal of fewer than three DMFT by 2000 but shows caries decline.

toothpastes) in preventing caries in children. The cost-effectiveness of this intervention is reduced with the current decline in prevalence of caries. It is recommended for use in high-risk children consistently over a period of time.

- Strong evidence supports the effectiveness of sealants in preventing pits and fissure caries. The report recommends that the programs be limited to high-risk children and high-risk teeth.
- Fluoride varnishes were not approved for use in the United States until 1994; hence, investigations are ongoing of the effectiveness of this intervention.

The Swedish Council on Technology Assessment in Health Care (SBU 2002) applied strict criteria of evidence of effectiveness; that is, the study had to be randomized and have a sample representing the total population. For permanent teeth, a three-year follow-up was necessary. The number of studies meeting all the criteria was not very high. Here are some conclusions of this review:

- Daily use of fluoridated toothpaste is an effective method to reduce caries in permanent teeth among children and adolescents. Daily, weekly, or biweekly fluoride mouth rinsing can reduce caries, but together with daily fluoride toothpaste use, the additional effects are not strong.
- Daily fluoride mouth rinsing can reduce root surface caries in the elderly, and professional application of fluoride varnish twice a year has a caries-reducing effect in permanent teeth among youth, as does the use of fluoridated toothpaste.
- Fissure sealants have a caries-reducing effect.

According to the SBU report, it was difficult to interpret the effect of programs aimed at reducing the intake of sugars or the effect of so-called sugar substitutes. Systematic evaluation of community preventive programs should be carried out in the future, particularly to help identify appropriate alternatives for developing countries.

ASPECTS OF TREATMENT OF CAVITIES AND OF CARIES DISEASE

One has to differentiate between treatment of cavities and treatment of the disease process resulting in cavities. The normal treatment of a tooth with a cavity is a filling or, if the cavity is large, a crown. Large cavities may involve "root-fillings" or even extraction of the tooth. A variety of materials are used globally: composites, amalgam, gold, porcelain, and others. Options for replacing extracted teeth include removable prostheses, fixed bridges, or implants. The more complex treatments are costly, and no country has been able to afford to introduce systems in which all dental costs are covered by public funds. Moreover, a filling does not affect the disease process causing the cavities. Treatment must be directed against the causative factors (described earlier). For the individual case, several options are available in addition to the various fluoride programs mentioned: dietary counseling, sugar substitutes, antimicrobial agents to reduce plaque and specific bacteria, and the use of saliva-stimulating products.

In many developing countries, the lack of dental manpower means that carious teeth remain untreated. The ratio of dentists to population is particularly unfavorable in the African region compared with Western European countries. For instance, according to CAPP, the ratio is 1 to 1.2 million in Ethiopia, 1 to 225,000 in Mali, and 1 to 166,000 in Zambia, against about 1 to 1,000 in Scandinavian countries and 1 to 2,100 in the United Kingdom (see http://www.whocollab.od.mah.se/index.html). In India, the ratio is 1 to 27,000 in the urban areas but 1 to 300,000 in the rural areas (Shah 2001). Such ratios mean that neither dental caries disease nor the cavities will receive proper attention.

After taking into consideration the high costs for dental treatment and the lack of dentists, atraumatic restorative treatment (ART) was introduced. This approach requires only hand instruments rather than sophisticated electric dental drills, and trained dental auxiliaries can deliver ART. The public dental health services in South Africa adopted the approach as an appropriate and economic means of providing basic restorative care in certain communities. A randomized clinical trial conducted in Tanzania showed no statistically significant differences between the retention of occlusal amalgam (74 percent) and ART occlusal restorations (67 percent) after a six-year follow-up (1992–98) (Mandari, Frencken, and Van't Hof 2003). A potentially affordable treatment procedure that could prevent untreated carious teeth from being extracted, ART may have relevance to some middle-income countries, although the method is not realistic for most low-income countries, where sustainability of such programs would be low.

PERIODONTAL DISEASES: CHRONIC GINGIVITIS AND CHRONIC PERIODONTITIS

Gingivitis, the inflammation of gum tissue caused by bacteria accumulating in the plaque along the gingival margin, precedes chronic periodontitis. The more destructive form of periodontal disease, which breaks down the supporting tissues of the teeth, progressively leading to loosening of teeth and tooth loss, affects 10 to 15 percent of most adult populations (Papapanou 1999). Cigarette smoking and diabetes mellitus (with poorly controlled diabetes) are two major risk factors associated with periodontal disease and appear markedly to affect the initiation and progression of the disease (Genco 1996; Papapanou 1999).

In recent years there has been a growing awareness of the association between some systemic diseases and oral disease, especially periodontal diseases. For example, a national study in the United States found that the prevalence of diabetes mellitus in patients with periodontitis was significantly greater (twofold) than in nonperiodontal patients (Soskolne and Klinger 2001). Periodontal disease may be considered one of the complications of diabetes. Effective control of periodontal infection in diabetics appears to reduce the levels of advanced glycogen end-products in the serum.

Proper oral hygiene practices can prevent both gingivitis and advanced periodontal disease. All intervention programs leading to improved oral hygiene are instrumental in the control of periodontal disease and will reduce risk of future tooth loss. The school-based oral health educational programs previously discussed are effective in preventing gingivitis, but no community-based intervention program addresses periodontal disease, especially among adults. Tobacco cessation programs are also important in the prevention of periodontal diseases. Treatment of periodontal diseases consists of plaque removal, scaling, and sometimes surgery, plus motivation and instruction in oral hygiene. Dental hygienists can perform parts of the treatment program.

ORAL PRECANCER AND CANCER

The most frequent form of oral precancerous lesion, leukoplakia, appears as a white patch that cannot be rubbed off, typically in the buccal mucosa, lateral borders of the tongue, and floor of the mouth. The prevalence of leukoplakia among those 15 years old and above ranged from 1.1 percent in Cambodia, to 1.7 percent in Myanmar, to 3.6 percent in Sweden (Axell 1976; Ikeda and others 1995). Malignant transformation varies in different populations; nearly 5 percent of lesions are found to be malignant at first biopsy, and 5 percent develop into malignancy at a later stage. Erythroplakias appear as red patches and are less common but have a higher tendency (90 percent or more) than leukoplakias to transform into malignancies (Sudbo and Reith 2003).

Oral cancers affect about 300,000 people worldwide annually (Ferlay and others 2001) and often develop from oral precancerous lesions (Sudbo and Reith 2003). Early detection of oral precancerous lesions, notably oral leukoplakia and erythroplakia, could easily prevent the development of the disfiguring disease oral cancer and premature death.

Tobacco use in any form (smoking or chewing) and excessive alcohol consumption remain the primary risk factors in the development of these precancerous lesions ("Early Diagnosis and Prevention of Oral Cancer and Precancer" 1995; Reichart 2001). Factors such as local irritation, *Candida albicans* infection, and nutritional deficiencies are also associated with the presence of leukoplakia.

Screening populations and routine examination in dental and medical clinics for oral precancer and early cancer lesions would reduce the mortality, morbidity, and cost of treatment associated with oral cancers. Not all oral premalignancies show malignant transformation, and detection of these oral lesions by biopsies are straightforward, not requiring sophisticated equipment. Tobacco cessation programs aimed at younger and older age groups and control of excessive alcohol intake are definitely beneficial in the prevention of oral cancer.

ORAL MANIFESTATIONS OF HIV/AIDS

The scarce epidemiological data available on oral manifestations of HIV in developing countries are difficult to interpret because these studies are not standardized (Holmes and Stephan 2002). In the study groups, the prevalence of oral lesions in Africa ranged from 15 percent to more than 90 percent of infected individuals; in India the prevalence was 72 percent; and in Thailand it was 82 percent. Reviews are available on the different studies performed on oral manifestations of HIV and AIDS (Naidoo and Chikte 1999; Patton and others 2002).

Candida infections, oral hairy leukoplakia, oral ulcers, and Kaposi's sarcoma are some of the common oral manifestations of HIV and AIDS. Notably, Kaposi's sarcomas were never detected in the Asian populations studied in India, Singapore, and Thailand but were seen in South African, Zambian, and Zimbabwean studies (Arendorf and others 1998; Hodgson 1997; Holmes and Stephan 2002; Lim and others 2001; Nittayananta and Chungpanich 1997; Ranganathan and others 2000). The presence of oral candidiasis and hairy leukoplakia alone or at the same time in an apparently healthy individual could be an early indicator of the undetected HIV infection progressing to AIDS. Those signs may be used as indicators during clinical examinations in developing countries where technology for laboratory tests is not available or is too expensive (Greenspan and Greenspan 2002; Holmes and Stephan 2002).

NOMA (CANCRUM ORIS)

Noma usually begins as a small ulcer of the gingiva and develops into a rapidly spreading gangrenous condition of the oral and facial tissues. Seen mainly in debilitated and malnourished children, it is disfiguring and deadly. The condition is reported in developing countries in several regions of the world, particularly in Sub-Saharan Africa (Enwonwu, Falkler, and Idigbe 2000; Naidoo and Chikte 2000; Petersen 2003). Noma disappeared from the industrial world in the 20th century except during World War II. In contrast, risk factors such as poverty, poor hygiene, and malnutrition, eventually in combination with infectious diseases such as HIV and AIDS, may have recently increased the prevalence of this disease in Sub-Saharan Africa (Enwonwu 1995; Naidoo and Chikte 2000). Most important, 90 percent of infected children die without having received any care.

Although the specific etiologic factors for noma are not known, poverty has been identified as the single most important risk indicator. Accordingly, improving the overall socio-economic conditions can prevent noma. Public health approaches such as providing a high-protein diet, clean water, and sanitation and preventing communicable diseases such as diphtheria, dysentery, and tuberculosis would be needed for effective prevention of noma in Africa. Prognosis of noma is considerably better with timely administration of antibiotics.

DEVELOPMENTAL DISORDERS

Developmental disorders involve teeth and the craniofacial structures. A few of these disorders are congenital diseases of the enamel or dentin; problems related to the number, size, or shape of teeth; and craniofacial birth defects, such as cleft lip and palate (CL/P). Among the most common congenital malformations seen in humans, cardiovascular malformation is ranked as the first and CL/P as the second. Unilateral CL/P occurs six times more frequently than the bilateral form. Females are more prone to get cleft palates, whereas cleft lip or CL/P is most common in males (U.S. Public Health Service 2000).

The incidence of CL/P differs from 0.18 to 3.74 per 1,000 live births, the highest incidence being seen in Native Americans at 3.74 per 1,000, closely followed by the Japanese at 3.36 per 1,000 live births. A fairly uniform incidence of 1 per 600 to 700 live births is reported among Europeans. Overall, the incidence rates appear high among Asians (0.82 to 3.36 per 1,000 live births), intermediate in Caucasians (0.9 to 2.69 per 1,000 live births), and often very low in black Africans (0.18 to 1.67 per 1,000 live births) (Hewson and McNamara 2000; Vanderas 1987; Wantia and Rettinger 2002).

The causes of CL/P are complex, involving multiple genetic and environmental risk factors. Not all cases of CL/P are inherited. A number of risk factors, such as folic acid deficiencies, maternal smoking, and maternal age, have been implicated in the formation of clefts (Wantia and Rettinger 2002).

Advanced surgery, specific prosthetic appliances, and orthodontic treatment can improve the quality of life for those born with clefts. However, such treatment is not accessible to children of several developing countries. Tobacco cessation programs aimed at pregnant mothers are essential in the prevention of CL/P.

FLUOROSIS OF TEETH

Fluorosis of teeth develops during formation of teeth when children are young. Drinking water having more than 1.5 ppm of fluoride can give rise to enamel defects and discoloration of teeth, leading to endemic fluorosis in the population. These effects may vary from mild to severe. For example, in the Great Rift Valley area of East Africa, the ground water has high levels of fluoride, leading to high rates of dental fluorosis—nearly 90 percent in some parts of Kenya (Chibole 1987). Some individuals in developed countries can acquire fluorosis of teeth as a result of the widespread use of different forms of fluorides in the prevention of caries, though the degree of fluorosis often is mild compared with endemic fluorosis.

Defluoridation of the central water supplies is possible when naturally occurring fluoride is excessive in the drinking water. However, most developing countries do not have central water distribution systems, and the cost of defluoridation equipment and its maintenance can be high. WHO encourages effective and inexpensive methods that are useful for individual households or community defluoridation of drinking water (WHO 1994). Such methods exist, but a number of operational problems have been identified, requiring further initiatives in this field (Kloos and Haimanot 1999).

COMMON-RISK-FACTOR INTERVENTION PROGRAMS

New research is pointing to associations between chronic oral infections—particularly periodontitis—and heart and lung diseases, stroke, osteoporosis, low birthweight, and premature births in addition to diabetes. Such findings strengthen WHO health promotion strategies that are based on the common-risk-factor approach, which controls essential risk factors that contribute to a large number of chronic diseases (Petersen 2003). Risk behaviors such as smoking; alcohol; diets rich in fats and sugars and low in fiber, fruit, and vegetables; stress; poor hygiene; and sedentary lifestyle are factors leading to such major chronic diseases as cardiovascular diseases, cancers, diabetes, obesity, osteoporosis, dental caries, and periodontal disease. These principal risk factors for major chronic diseases are often seen to cluster in the same individuals.

The WHO Global Oral Health Programme recommends the common-risk-factors approach (Petersen 2003), which implies development of integral activities in health promotion and disease prevention, involving health education, community empowerment, and legislative policy development. For example, such programs could aim at reducing the caries levels among preschool children and simultaneously improving general health. Promoting the reduction of sugar consumption would improve not only oral health but also general health

Table 38.3 Prevention Strategies for Oral Health

Disease or condition	Causes	Actions needed and methods
Dental caries	High or frequent sugar consumption, plaque present, highly cariogenic microorganisms, nonuse of fluorides, reduced saliva flow, systemic diseases, and other individual risk factors	Targeted actions against causative factors on community and individual levels Health education toward self-care capacity, fluoride programs, sugar restriction, actions based on risk assessment of individuals and groups
Periodontal diseases	Plaque present, pathogenic bacteria, influence of systemic diseases, tobacco use	Improved oral hygiene, professional cleaning, antibiotics, identification and treatment of systemic diseases Elimination of pockets if present and removal of local dental irritants, such as rough fillings Tobacco cessation
Oral precancer and cancer	Tobacco and alcohol use; see chapter 29	Tobacco cessation; see chapter 29
Oral manifestations of HIV/AIDS	See chapter 18	See chapter 18. Special oral care
Noma (cancrum oris)	Probably bacterial in connection with severe malnourishment	Antibiotics together with nutritional support; surgery sometimes necessary
Developmental disorders	Various genetic or environmental causes such as tobacco use	Tobacco cessation programs aimed at pregnant mothers
Fluorosis of teeth	Too high concentration of fluoride in drinking waters or from other sources	Identification of water sources and reduction of fluoride or recommendation of other water sources

Source: Authors; partly based on Bratthall and Barmes 1993.
Note: This table is by no means complete. Many other oral diseases or conditions are important and need attention. The listed ones are of special relevance for developing countries.

through better quality of children's diet. Some prevention strategies for oral health, suitable for developing countries are outlined in table 38.3.

RESEARCH AND FUTURE ACTIONS

Several promising actions against factors causing the two major oral diseases, caries and periodontal disease, are ongoing: attempts to control the formation of the biofilm with its microflora are of high priority. One research line is to identify pathogenic bacteria and try to replace them with genetically modified, less pathogenic bacteria or to eradicate them by antibiotics or antiseptics. Preventing dental caries by a vaccine is not a new idea, and efforts continue. Among other ideas is the use of plantibodies (plant-derived therapeutic antibodies) or genetically modified bacteria, releasing components targeting pathogens. Functional foods, which include various elements in food, may be another future option to control oral diseases. Although pilot or small-scale studies seem promising, it will be several years before such methods can possibly be of use in populations because large clinical trials have not even started.

Saliva is believed to be usable as a diagnostic tool, providing noninvasive assessment of a number of oral and systemic diseases. Devices are being designed to identify in saliva various bacteria and their virulence factors, drugs, metabolic products,

hormones, biomarkers for oral cancer, inflammatory mediators, and more. Future developments may result in other affordable and effective devices.

Continuous attempts are being made to assess the sociobehavioral factors in oral health and the information on risk factors. Caries risk assessment models are tested also for the individual cases. Through present knowledge, individuals in need of targeted actions can be identified. Another strong trend is to use evidence-based reviews. This type of research is, of course, not restricted to oral health. Several reviews have already been done, and a frequent conclusion is that the number of randomized clinical trials is limited, in particular for common clinical procedures. This trend will change as the quality of future oral health research improves, but not all research problems can be solved by such studies. Community-based participatory research is another approach that may be used to improve oral health studies (O'Fallon and Dearry 2002).

Within the management of dental diseases—in particular, caries—is the "minimally invasive dentistry" approach, which promotes the concept that large restorations (crowns, bridges) are not as necessary as believed. Risk assessment, preventive measures, and improved dental materials with good adhesion capacity are some of the several components in this approach.

Research in transfer of knowledge using the Internet or other electronic media is another strongly expanding area, from which developing countries should be able to benefit.

COST-EFFECTIVENESS OF ORAL HEALTH CARE

Using the evidence available, the U.S. Surgeon General's report (U.S. Public Health Service 2000) and the report of the Swedish Council on Technology Assessment in Health Care (SBU 2002; see also Kallestal and others 2003) have attempted to determine the cost-effectiveness of oral health intervention programs from developed countries.

Among the findings in the U.S. report were the following:

- Water fluoridation costs about a dollar per person per year for water serving most individuals in the United States. Community water fluoridation is believed to be an effective and cost-effective caries preventive method.
- Economic analyses of community dental sealant programs suggest that they are cost-effective and may even provide cost savings when used in high-risk populations.

The Swedish report (SBU 2002), reviewing original studies on economic evaluation of caries prevention (a total of 17 selected from 1966 to 2003 MEDLINE and manual Internet searches), commented that no conclusion could be drawn owing to the low evidence values and contradictory results. This comment prompted the group to present its own calculation for cost-effectiveness based on Swedish caries prevalence and charges used in Swedish dental care. The group found that the cost-effectiveness for fluoridated toothpaste is extremely good (cost per prevented DMFT very low), which, of course, is not surprising, given the significant caries-reducing results in combination with low cost for society.

No clear correlation appears to exist between caries experience and health care investment for individual countries. Some countries with the lowest health care expenditures have values for caries experience (DMFT) that are similar to or even lower than those countries having the highest expenditures on health (figure 38.2). Those low-income countries often have low per capita sugar consumption and, therefore, do not need to install expensive measures for treatment or prevention.

It may seem surprising that so few studies are available regarding the cost-effectiveness of caries prevention, or of any other oral disease. In a critical review article, Schwarz (1998) analyzed the issue. He wrote, "Several decades after considerable improvements in the oral disease situation were documented in Scandinavia, doubts are still expressed about whether preventive measures are cost-effective." In addition, he recommended that four elements be considered when a preventive effect was evaluated: the definition of prevention, the practical perception of effective prevention, the appropriateness of traditional cost-effectiveness analysis, and the time factor. He pointed out that "caries prevention is not uniformly defined by the profession, that dental research is casting doubt

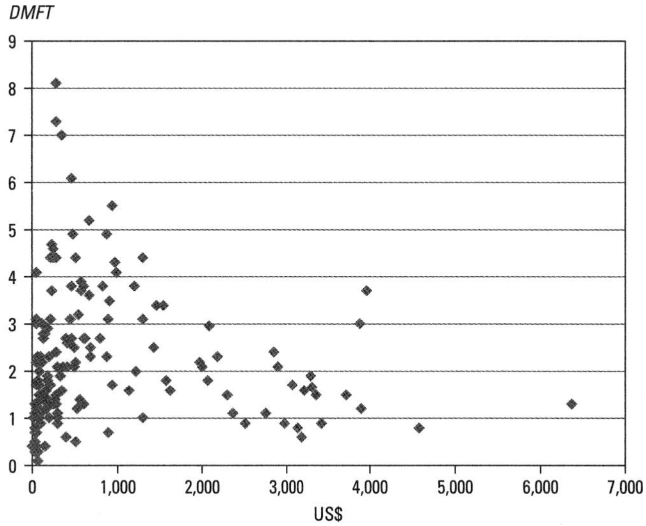

Source: For health expenditure: http://www.who.int/en/; for DMFT: http://www.whocollab.od.mah.se/index.html, both for June 2003.

Note: Original data for health expenditures were in international dollars and were converted to U.S. dollars using the exchange rate of US$1 = 0.70681 (period average June 2003). Because the exchange rate varies over time, the data should be taken as approximate values.

Figure 38.2 DMFT as Related to Health Care Expenditure per Capita for 12-Year-Olds in 149 Countries

on the effectiveness of traditionally accepted preventive measures, that political pressures on health care are motivated by economic pressures." Finally, he stated that traditional cost-benefit and cost-effectiveness analyses have not been able to help the decision makers choose wisely and that the time perspective for the real effects of prevention lies beyond the interests of decision makers.

However, without proper prevention, the alternative strategy is restorative dentistry—that is, to make fillings, crowns, and dentures. Is this a feasible alternative for developing countries? Yee and Sheiham (2003) give some examples: In Nepal, a simple amalgam filling would cost about US$4, which does not include the many additional expenses for impoverished rural families, who may have to travel by bus or walk for a day or two to get to the clinic. The total expenses incurred, including dental fees, meals, and lodging but not including lost wages, would amount to US$12, an enormous sum considering the average Nepalese's earning of US$0.75 per day, and it is enough to buy food for a month. Yee and Sheiham conclude that treating caries with the traditional method of restorative dentistry is beyond the financial capabilities of most low-income nations because three-quarters of these countries do not even have sufficient resources to finance an essential package of health care services for their children. Yee and Sheiham (2003) estimate that treating dental caries by the traditional amalgam restorative dentistry in the permanent dentition of the child population would cost about US$2,000 for 1,000 children of mixed ages from 6 to 18 years, which would require financial resources beyond the capabilities of low-income nations. Hence, they propose a public health and health promotion approach to reduce caries burden instead of the restorative approach.

Although several studies evaluating the effectiveness of intervention and oral health promotion programs in developing countries are becoming available (Estupinan-Day and others 2001; Pakhomov and others 1995; Petersen and others 2004), a definite need exists for further cost-effectiveness analysis on such programs, which should be addressed in the future. It would also be useful if studies were commenced on intervention programs using the common-risk approach suggested by WHO (Petersen 2003).

CONCLUSIONS

Dental caries and periodontal diseases are the most known oral diseases, but other conditions can strongly and negatively influence the quality of life. Effective programs to reduce the burden of oral diseases—in particular, caries—are available in principle, but to run these programs in developing countries, new approaches are needed. The WHO strategy of identifying common risk factors seems promising for health promotion. In broad terms, the most important challenges for oral health in the 21st century relate to the transfer of knowledge and experiences in preventive oral care to the poor and disadvantaged population groups in both developing and developed countries.

ACKNOWLEDGMENTS

We acknowledge with great appreciation comments and suggestions from Dr. Lois Cohen, Dr. Kevin Hardwick, Dr. Jeanne C. Sinkford, and Thomas Wall. Sir George Alleyne, our editor, is to be congratulated for his constructive ideas and patience.

REFERENCES

Abayaratna, S., and K. Krishnarasa. 1997. *National Oral Health Survey 1994–95.* Colombo: Ministry of Health.

Adyatmaka, A., U. Sutopo, P. Carlsson, D. Bratthall, and G. Pakhomov. 1998. *School-Based Primary Preventive Programme for Children: Affordable Toothpaste as a Component in Primary Oral Health Care—Experiences from a Field Trial in Kalimantan Barat, Indonesia.* Geneva: World Health Organization.

Arendorf, T. M., B. Bredekamp, C. A. Cloete, and G. Sauer. 1998. "Oral Manifestations of HIV Infection in 600 South African Patients." *Journal of Oral Pathology and Medicine* 27: 176–79.

Armfield, J. M., K. F. Roberts-Thomson, and A. J. Spencer. 2003. *The Child Dental Health Survey, Australia 1999: Trends across the 1990s.* Adelaide: Australian Institute of Health and Welfare. http://www.cecdo.org/pages/database%20intro.html.

Axell, T. 1976. "A Prevalence Study of Oral Mucosal Lesions in an Adult Swedish Population." *Odontologisk Revy* 27 (Suppl. 36): 1–103.

Barmes, D. E. 2000. "Public Policy on Oral Health and Old Age: A Global View." *Journal of Public Health Dentistry* 60: 335–37.

Beltran-Aguilar, E. D., S. Estupinan-Day, and R. Baez. 1999. "Analysis of Prevalence and Trends of Dental Caries in the Americas between the 1970s and 1990s." *International Dental Journal* 49: 322–29.

Bratthall, D. 2000. "Introducing the Significant Caries Index Together with a Proposal for a New Global Oral Health Goal for 12-Year-Olds." *International Dental Journal* 50: 378–84.

Bratthall, D., and D. E. Barmes. 1993. "Oral Health." In *Disease Control Priorities in Developing Countries,* ed. D. T. Jamison, W. H. Mosley, A. R. Measham, and J. L. Bobadilla, 647–59. Washington, DC: World Bank.

Bratthall, D., G. Hänsel-Petersson, and H. Sundberg. 1996. "Reasons for the Caries Decline: What Do the Experts Believe?" *European Journal of Oral Sciences* 104: 416–22.

Burt, B. A. 2002. "Fluoridation and Social Equity." *Journal of Public Health Dentistry* 62: 195–200.

Carr, L. M. 1988. "Dental Health of Children in Australia, 1977–1985." *Australian Dental Journal* 33: 205–11.

Chibole, O. 1987. "Epidemiology of Dental Fluorosis in Kenya." *Journal of the Royal Society of Health* 107: 242–43.

Cohen, L. K. 1990. "Promoting Oral Health: Guidelines for Dental Associations." *International Dental Journal* 40: 79–102.

de Almeida, C. M., P. E. Petersen, S. J. Andre, and A. Toscano. 2003. "Changing Oral Health Status of 6- and 12-Year-Old Schoolchildren in Portugal." *Community Dental Health* 20: 211–16.

Demertzi, A., and V. Topitsoglou. 2002. "Caries Prevalence of 11-Year-Olds between 1989–2001." Abstract. *Community Dental Health* 19: 203.

Downer, M. C. 1994. "The 1993 National Survey of Children's Dental Health: A Commentary on the Preliminary Report." *British Dental Journal* 176: 209–14.

"Early Diagnosis and Prevention of Oral Cancer and Precancer: Report of Symposium III." 1995. *Advanced Dental Research* 9: 134–37.

Enwonwu, C. O. 1995. "Noma: A Neglected Scourge of Children in Sub-Saharan Africa." *Bulletin of the World Health Organization* 73: 541–45.

Enwonwu, C. O., W. A. Falkler, and E. O. Idigbe. 2000. "Oro-Facial Gangrene (Noma/Cancrum Oris): Pathogenetic Mechanisms." *Critical Reviews in Oral Biology and Medicine* 11: 159–71.

Estupinan-Day, S. R., H. Baez, R. Horowitz, R. Warpeha, B. Sutherland, and M. Thamer. 2001. "Salt Fluoridation and Dental Caries in Jamaica." *Community Dentistry and Oral Epidemiology* 29: 247–52.

Ferlay, J., F. Bray, P. Pisani, and D. M. Parkin. 2001. *GLOBOCAN 2000: Cancer Incidence, Mortality and Prevalence Worldwide.* Version 1.0. IARC CancerBase, International Agency for Research on Cancer, Lyon. http://wwwdep.iarc.fr/globocan/globocan.htm.

Flanders, R. A. 1987. "Effectiveness of Dental Health Educational Programs in Schools." *Journal of the American Dental Association* 114: 239–42.

Frencken, J. E., K. Borsum-Andersson, F. Makoni, F. Moyana, S. Mwashaenyi, and J. Mulder. 2001. "Effectiveness of an Oral Health Education Programme in Primary Schools in Zimbabwe after 3.5 Years." *Community Dentistry and Oral Epidemiology* 29: 253–59.

Genco, R. J. 1996. "Current View of Risk Factors for Periodontal Diseases." *Journal of Periodontology* 67: 1041–49.

Greenspan, J. S., and D. Greenspan. 2002. "The Epidemiology of the Oral Lesions of HIV Infection in the Developed World." *Oral Diseases* 8 (Suppl. 2): 34–39.

Guinan, J. C., R. Bakayoko-Ly, M. Samba, A. L. Kattie, and A. E. Oka. 1999. "Caries Assessment of School Children 12 Years of Age in 1996 in Ivory Coast." *Tropical Dental Journal* 22: 48–54.

Haugejorden, O. 1994. "Changing Time Trend in Caries Prevalence in Norwegian Children and Adolescents." *Community Dentistry and Oral Epidemiology* 22: 220–25.

Hescot, P., and E. Roland. 2000. *La santé dentaire en France, 1998.* L'Union Française pour la Santé Bucco-Dentaire, Paris.

Hewson, A. R., and C. M. McNamara. 2000. "Cleft Lip and/or Palate in the West of Ireland, 1980–1996." *Special Care in Dentistry* 20: 143–46.

Hodgson, T. A. 1997. "HIV-Associated Oral Lesions: Prevalence in Zambia." *Oral Diseases* 3 (Suppl. 1): 46–50.

Holmes, H. K., and L. X. G. Stephan. 2002. "Oral Lesions of HIV Infection in Developing Countries." *Oral Diseases* 8 (Suppl. 2): 40–43.

Hong Kong, Department of Health. 2003. *Oral Health Survey 2001.* http://www.info.gov.hk/tooth_club/survey_eng.htm.

Honkala, E., L. Kannas, and J. Rise. 1990. "Oral Health Habits in 11 European Countries." *International Dental Journal* 40: 211–17.

Hugoson, A., G. Koch, T. Bergendal, A. L. Hallonsten, C. Slotte, B. Thorstensson, and H. Thorstensson. 1995. "Oral Health of Individuals Aged 3–80 Years in Jönköping, Sweden, in 1973, 1983 and 1993." *Swedish Dental Journal* 19: 243–60.

Ikeda, N., Y. Handa, S. P. Khim, C. Durward, T. Axell, T. Mizuno, and others. 1995. "Prevalence Study of Oral Mucosal Lesions in a Selected Cambodian Population." *Community Dentistry and Oral Epidemiology* 23: 49–54.

Irigoyen, M. E., and G. Sanchez-Hinojosa. 2000. "Changes in Dental Caries Prevalence in 12-Year-Old Students in the State of Mexico after 9 Years of Salt Fluoridation." *Caries Research* 34: 303–7.

Kallestal, C., A. Norlund, B. Soder, G. Nordenram, H. Dahlgren, L. G. Petersson, and others. 2003. "Economic Evaluation of Dental Caries Prevention: A Systematic Review." *Acta odontologica Scandinavica* 61: 341–46.

Kloos, H., and R. T. Haimanot. 1999. "Distribution of Fluoride and Fluorosis in Ethiopia and Prospects for Control." *Tropical Medicine and International Health* 4: 355–64.

Latvia, State Dentistry Centre. 2000. *Annual Report of Dental Health Care in Latvia.* Riga: State Dentistry Centre.

Leous, P., and P. E. Petersen. 2002. *Oral Health Status of Schoolchildren in Belarus, 2000.* Copenhagen: WHO Regional Office for Europe.

Lim, A. A., Y. S. Leo, C. C. Lee, and A. N. Robinson. 2001. "Oral Manifestations of Human Immunodeficiency Virus (HIV)–Infected Patients in Singapore." *Annals of the Academy of Medicine, Singapore* 30: 600–6.

Lo, E. C., R. W. Evans, and O. P. Lind. 1990. "Dental Caries Status and Treatment Needs of the Permanent Dentition of 6–12-Year-Olds in Hong Kong." *Community Dentistry and Oral Epidemiology* 18: 9–11.

Malaysia, Dental Services Division. 1997. *Dental Services.* Kuala Lumpur: Ministry of Health.

Mandari, G. J., J. E. Frencken, and M. A. Van't Hof. 2003. "Six-Year Success Rates of Occlusal Amalgam and Glass-Ionomer Restorations Placed Using Three Minimal Intervention Approaches." *Caries Research* 37: 246–53.

Micheelis, W., and E. Reich. 1999. *The Third German Oral Health Study (DMS III).* Cologne, Germany: Deutscher Aerzte-Verlag.

Miyazaki, H., and M. Morimoto. 1996. "Changes in Caries Prevalence in Japan." *European Journal of Oral Sciences* 104: 452–58.

Naidoo, S., and U. M. Chikte. 1999. "HIV/AIDS—The Evolving Pandemic and Its Impact on Oral Health in Sub-Saharan Africa." *South African Dental Journal* 54: 616–30.

———. 2000. "Noma (Cancrum Oris): Case Report in a 4-Year-Old HIV-Positive South African Child." *South African Dental Journal* 55: 683–86.

Nishi, M., J. Stjernsward, P. Carlsson, and D. Bratthall. 2002. "Caries Experience of Some Countries and Areas Expressed by the Significant Caries Index." *Community Dentistry and Oral Epidemiology* 30: 296–301.

Nithila, A., D. Bourgeois, D. E. Barmes, and H. Murtomaa. 1998. "WHO Global Oral Data Bank, 1986–96: An Overview of Oral Health Surveys at 12 Years of Age." *Bulletin of the World Health Organization* 76: 237–44.

Nittayananta, W., and S. Chungpanich. 1997. "Oral Lesions in a Group of Thai People with AIDS." *Oral Diseases* 3 (Suppl. 1): S41–45.

O'Fallon, L. R., and A. Dearry. 2002. "Community-Based Participatory Research as a Tool to Advance Environmental Health Sciences." *Environmental Health Perspectives* 110 (Suppl. 2): 155–59.

Pakhomov, G. N., K. Ivanova, I. J. Moller, and M. Vrabcheva. 1995. "Dental Caries-Reducing Effects of a Milk Fluoridation Project in Bulgaria." *Journal of Public Health Dentistry* 55: 234–37.

Papapanou, P. N. 1999. "Epidemiology of Periodontal Diseases: An Update." *Journal of the International Academy of Periodontology* 1: 110–16.

Patton, L. L., J. A. Phelan, F. J. Ramos-Gomez, W. Nittayananta, C. H. Shiboski, and T. L. Mbuguye. 2002. "Prevalence and Classification of HIV-Associated Oral Lesions." *Oral Diseases* 8 (Suppl. 2): 98–109.

Peng, B., P. E. Petersen, M. W. Fan, and B. J. Tai. 1997. "Oral Health Status and Oral Health Behaviour of 12-Year-Old Urban Schoolchildren in the People's Republic of China." *Community Dental Health* 14: 238–44.

Peng, B., P. E. Petersen, B. J. Tai, B. Y. Yuan, and M. W. Fan. 1997. "Changes in Oral Health Knowledge and Behaviour 1987–95 among Inhabitants of Wuhan City, PR China." *International Dental Journal* 47: 142–47.

Petersen, P. E. 1989. "Evaluation of a Dental Preventive Program for Danish Chocolate Workers." *Community Dentistry and Oral Epidemiology* 17: 53–59.

———. 1990. "Self-Administered Use of Fluoride among Danish Chocolate Workers." *Scandinavian Journal of Dental Research* 98: 189–91.

———. 2003. "The World Oral Health Report 2003: Continuous Improvement of Oral Health in the 21st Century—The Approach of the WHO Global Oral Health Programme." *Community Dentistry and Oral Epidemiology* 31 (Suppl. 1): 1–21.

Petersen, P. E., I. Danila, A. Delean, O. Grivu, G. Ionita, M. Pop, and A. Samolia. 1994. "Oral Health Status among Schoolchildren in Romania, 1992." *Community Dentistry and Oral Epidemiology* 22: 90–3.

Petersen, P. E., N. Hoerup, N. Poomviset, J. Prommajan, and A. Watanapa. 2001. "Oral Health Status and Oral Health Behaviour of Urban and Rural Schoolchildren in Southern Thailand." *International Dental Journal* 51: 95–102.

Petersen, P. E., and M. Kaka. 1999. "Oral Health Status of Children and Adults in the Republic of Niger, Africa." *International Dental Journal* 49: 159–64.

Petersen, P. E., and M. A. Lennon. 2004. "Effective Use of Fluorides for the Prevention of Dental Caries in the 21st Century: The WHO Approach." *Community Dentistry and Oral Epidemiology* 32: 319–21.

Petersen, P. E., U. Nyandindi, E. N. Kikiwilu, L. Mabelya, B. S. Lembariti, and V. J. Poulsen. 2002. *Oral Health Status and Oral Health Behaviour of Schoolchildren, Teachers, and Adults in Tanzania.* Geneva: World Health Organization.

Petersen, P. E., B. Peng, and B. J. Tai. 1997. "Oral Health Status and Oral Health Behaviour of Middle-Aged and Elderly People in PR China." *International Dental Journal* 47: 305–12.

Petersen, P. E., B. Peng, B. Tai, Z. Bian, and M. Fan. 2004. "Effect of a School-Based Oral Health Education Programme in Wuhan City, People's Republic of China." *International Dental Journal* 54: 33–41.

Petersen, P. E., and M. Rusu. 2002. *Oral Health Status of Romanian Schoolchildren—National Survey 2000.* Copenhagen: WHO Regional Office for Europe.

Petersen, P. E., and A. M. Torres. 1999. "Preventive Oral Health Care and Health Promotion Provided for Children and Adolescents by the Municipal Dental Health Service in Denmark." *International Journal of Paediatric Dentistry* 9: 81–91.

Pitts, N. B., D. J. Evans, and Z. J. Nugent. 1998. "The Dental Caries Experience of 12-Year-Old Children in the United Kingdom: Surveys Coordinated by the British Association for the Study of Community Dentistry in 1996/97." *Community Dental Health* 15: 49–54.

Pitts, N. B., D. J. Evans, Z. J. Nugent, and C. M. Pine. 2002. "The Dental Caries Experience of 12-Year-Old Children in England and Wales: Surveys Coordinated by the British Association for the Study of Community Dentistry in 2000/2001." *Community Dental Health* 19: 46–53.

Priwe, C. 1998. *The Smiling School Project: A School Based Oral Health Promotion Programme: Mid-Term Progress Report.* Windhoek: Ministry of Health and Social Services.

Ranganathan, K., B. V. Reddy, N. Kumarasamy, S. Solomon, R. Viswanathan, and N. W. Johnson. 2000. "Oral Lesions and Conditions Associated with Human Immunodeficiency Virus Infection in 300 South Indian Patients." *Oral Diseases* 6: 152–57.

Razanamihaja, N., and P. E. Petersen. 1999. "School Based Oral Health Promotion Programmes in Madagascar." In *Health Care Systems in Africa—Patterns and Perspectives*, ed. L. Blegvad, 123–29. Copenhagen: University of Copenhagen Press.

Reichart, P. A. 2001. "Identification of Risk Groups for Oral Precancer and Cancer and Preventive Measures." *Clinical Oral Investigations* 5: 207–13.

SBU (Swedish Council on Technology Assessment in Health Care). 2002. *Att förebygga karies: En systematisk litteraturöversikt.* Gothenburg: Swedish Council on Technology Assessment in Health Care.

Schwarz, E. 1998. "Is Caries Prevention Cost-Effective? Does Anybody Care?" *Acta odontologica Scandinavica* 56: 187–92.

Sector Público. 1999. *Encuesta de salud bucal, En escolares de 11 a 14 años.* Montevideo: Ministry of Public Health.

Sembene, M., A. W. Kane, and D. Bourgeois. 1999. "Caries Prevalence in 12-Year-Old Schoolchildren in Senegal in 1989 and 1994." *International Dental Journal* 49: 73–75.

Shah, N. 2001. "Geriatric Oral Health Issues in India." *International Dental Journal* 51: 212–18.

Sogaard, A. J., and D. Holst. 1988. "The Effect of Different School Based Dental Health Education Programmes in Norway." *Community Dental Health* 5: 169–84.

Soskolne, W. A., and A. Klinger. 2001. "The Relationship between Periodontal Diseases and Diabetes: An Overview." *Annals of Periodontology* 6: 91–98.

Sri Lanka, Ministry of Health. 1985. *National Oral Health Survey, 1983–84.* Colombo: Ministry of Health.

Sudbo, J., and A. Reith. 2003. "Which Putatively Pre-Malignant Oral Lesions Become Oral Cancers? Clinical Relevance of Early Targeting of High-Risk Individuals." *Journal of Oral Pathology and Medicine* 32: 63–70.

Sundberg, H. 2002. *Tandhälsan hos barn och ungdomar 1985–2001.* Newsletter. Swedish National Board of Health and Welfare, Stockholm.

Szoke, J., and P. E. Petersen. 2000. "Evidence for Dental Caries Decline among Children in an East European Country (Hungary)." *Community Dentistry and Oral Epidemiology* 28: 155–60.

Tai, B., M. Du, B. Peng, M. Fan, and Z. Bian. 2001. "Experiences from a School-Based Oral Health Promotion Programme in Wuhan City, PR China." *International Journal of Paediatric Dentistry* 11: 280–91.

Thomson, W. M. 2004. "Dental Caries Experience in Older People over Time: What Can the Large Cohort Studies Tell Us?" *British Dental Journal* 196: 89–92.

Ullah, M. S. 2001. *An Epidemiological Oral Health Study on 12-Year-Old Bangladeshi Schoolchildren.* Thesis, Faculty of Dentistry, Oslo.

U.S. Public Health Service. 2000. *Oral Health in America: A Report of the Surgeon General.* Washington, DC: U.S. Public Health Service. http://www.nidr.nih.gov/sgr/sgrohweb/TOC.htm.

Vanderas, A. P. 1987. "Incidence of Cleft Lip, Cleft Palate, and Cleft Lip and Palate among Races: A Review." *Cleft Palate Journal* 24: 216–25.

van Palenstein Helderman, W. H., L. Munck, S. Mushendwa, M. A. van't Hof, and F. G. Mrema. 1997. "Effect Evaluation of an Oral Health Education Programme in Primary Schools in Tanzania." *Community Dentistry and Oral Epidemiology* 25: 296–300.

van Wyk, P. J. 1994. *National Oral Health Survey, South Africa, 1988/89.* Pretoria: Department of Health.

von der Fehr, F. R. 1994. "Caries Prevalence in the Nordic Countries." *International Dental Journal* 44 (Suppl. 1): 371–78.

Wang, N. J., C. Kalletstal, P. E. Petersen, and I. B. Arnadottir. 1998. "Caries Preventive Services for Children and Adolescents in Denmark, Iceland, Norway and Sweden: Strategies and Resource Allocation." *Community Dentistry and Oral Epidemiology* 26: 263–71.

Wantia, N., and G. Rettinger. 2002. "The Current Understanding of Cleft Lip Malformations." *Facial Plastic Surgery* 18: 147–53.

White, B. A., A. A. Antczak-Bouckoms, and M. C. Weinstein. 1989. "Issues in the Economic Evaluation of Community Water Fluoridation." *Journal of Dental Education* 53: 646–57.

WHO (World Health Organization). 1994. *Fluorides and Oral Health.* Technical Report Series No. 846. Geneva: WHO.

———. 2003. *School Oral Health Promotion.* WHO School Health Information Series 11. Geneva: WHO.

Wierzbicka, M., P. E. Petersen, F. Szatko, E. Dybizbanska, and I. Kalo. 2002. "Changing Oral Health Status and Oral Health Behaviour of Schoolchildren in Poland." *Community Dental Health* 19: 243–50.

Woodward, M., and A. R. Walker. 1994. "Sugar Consumption and Dental Caries: Evidence from 90 Countries." *British Dental Journal* 176: 297–302.

Yee, R., and A. Sheiham. 2003. "Is Treating Caries in Children in Developing Countries by the Restorative Approach a Rational Objective?" *Developing Dentistry* 3: 10–17.

Zadik, D., S. P. Zusman, and A. M. Kelman. 1992. "Caries Prevalence in 5- and 12-Year-Old Children in Israel." *Community Dentistry and Oral Epidemiology* 20: 54–55

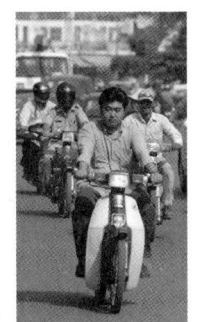

Chapter 39

Unintentional Injuries

Robyn Norton, Adnan A. Hyder, David Bishai, and Margie Peden

This chapter examines the issue of unintentional injuries and focuses on a selected number of cause-specific unintentional injuries. Injuries have traditionally been defined as damage to a person caused by an acute transfer of energy (mechanical, thermal, electrical, chemical, or radiation) or by the sudden absence of heat or oxygen. Unintentional injuries consist of that subset of injuries for which there is no evidence of predetermined intent. The cause-specific unintentional injuries examined here include those that the World Health Organization (WHO) routinely analyzes and publishes data on and that individually account for the greatest unintentional injury burden in terms of mortality and disability-adjusted life years (DALYs). These include road traffic injuries (RTIs), poisonings, falls, burns, and drowning (figure 39.1).

BURDEN AND CAUSES OF UNINTENTIONAL INJURIES

This section provides a brief outline of the burden of unintentional injuries and then reviews the available evidence about known and potential causes of such injuries.

Burden of Unintentional Injuries

Worldwide, unintentional injuries accounted for more than 3.5 million deaths in 2001, or about 6 percent of all deaths and 66 percent of all injury deaths. Unintentional injuries were also responsible for more than 113 million DALYs in 2001, or about 8 percent of all DALYs and some 70 percent of all injury DALYs. More than 90 percent of unintentional injury deaths occurred in low- and middle-income countries (LMICs),

accounting for around 7 percent of all deaths in those countries. Similarly, more than 90 percent of DALYs that were attributed to unintentional injuries occurred in LMICs, accounting for about 8 percent of all DALYs in those countries. Injury death rates per 100,000 population were higher in LMICs (62 per 100,000) than globally (57 per 100,000).

Males accounted for almost two-thirds of the deaths attributed to unintentional injuries in LMICs in 2001, with rates of both injury death and DALY losses higher among males than females (table 39.1). Compared with other age groups, young people age 15 to 29 accounted for the largest proportion of deaths from unintentional injuries in LMICs (figure 39.2).

RTIs accounted for the greatest burden of deaths from unintentional injuries in LMICs in 2001, or about 34 percent of the total burden, and the greatest burden of DALYs from unintentional injuries in LMICs in 2001, accounting for 28 percent of the burden (figure 39.1). Whereas young people age 15 to 29 years accounted for the highest proportion of all unintentional injuries, those age 45 to 59 accounted for the highest proportion of injuries from poisonings, while those age 70 to 79 accounted for the highest proportion of injuries from falls (figure 39.2).

Economic Burden of Unintentional Injuries. Estimates of the burden of unintentional injuries as measured in terms of economic costs are almost nonexistent. The best estimates available are for RTIs. Using road crash costs from 21 developed and developing countries, the Transport Research Laboratory Ltd. finds that the average annual cost of road crashes was equivalent to about 1.0 percent of gross national product in developing countries, 1.5 percent in transition countries, and 2.0 percent in highly motorized countries. The annual burden

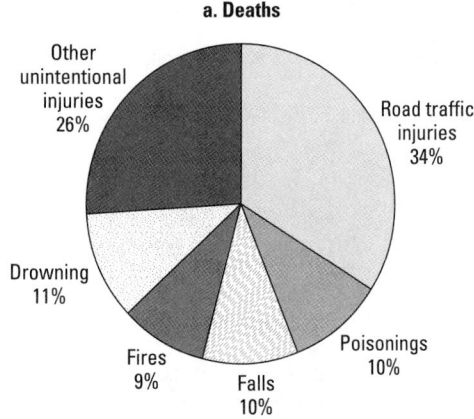

a. Deaths

Other unintentional injuries 26%

Road traffic injuries 34%

Drowning 11%

Fires 9%

Falls 10%

Poisonings 10%

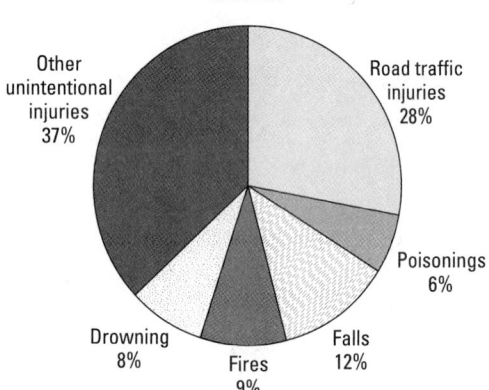

b. DALYs

Other unintentional injuries 37%

Road traffic injuries 28%

Drowning 8%

Fires 9%

Falls 12%

Poisonings 6%

Source: Authors.

Figure 39.1 Distribution of Unintentional Injuries, Low- and Middle-Income Countries, 2001

Table 39.1 Cause-Specific Death Rates and DALYs Lost because of Unintentional Injuries, by Gender, Worldwide and in LMICs, 2001

Category	Global			LMICs		
	Total	Males	Females	Total	Males	Females
Deaths (per 100,000 population)						
All unintentional injuries	57	75	41	61	80	44
RTIs	19	28	11	20	30	11
Poisonings	6	7	4	6	8	5
Falls	6	8	5	6	8	5
Fires	5	4	6	6	4	7
Drowning	6	9	4	7	10	5
Other unintentional injuries	15	19	11	16	20	11
DALY losses (per 1,000 population)						
All unintentional injuries	20	25	14	22	28	16
RTIs	6	8	3	6	9	4
Poisonings	1	2	1	1	2	1
Falls	2	3	2	3	3	2
Fires	2	1	2	2	2	2
Drowning	2	2	1	2	2	1
Other unintentional injuries	7	9	5	8	10	6

Source: Authors.
Note: All figures are rounded to the nearest 1,000.

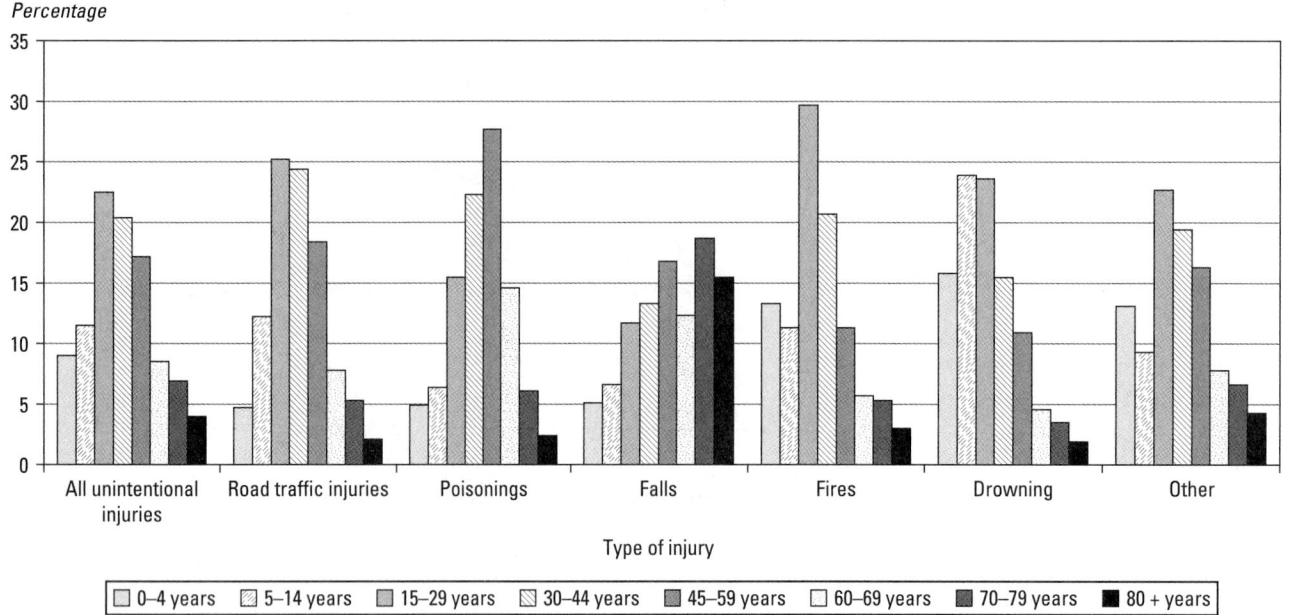

Percentage

All unintentional injuries | Road traffic injuries | Poisonings | Falls | Fires | Drowning | Other

Type of injury

☐ 0–4 years   ▨ 5–14 years   ▨ 15–29 years   ▨ 30–44 years   ■ 45–59 years   ☐ 60–69 years   ▨ 70–79 years   ■ 80 + years

Source: Authors.

Figure 39.2 Distribution of Unintentional Injuries by Type of Injury and Age Group, LMICs, 2001

of road crash costs is about US$518 billion globally and about US$65 billion in LMICs, exceeding the total annual amount these countries receive in development assistance (Jacobs, Aeron-Thomas, and Astrop 2000).

Causes of Unintentional Injuries in LMICs

As in the case of most diseases, unintentional injuries are caused by multiple factors. The traditional epidemiological paradigm of host, vector, and environmental factors that in combination contribute to the incidence of disease has been adapted and applied in determining the causes of unintentional injury. However, this paradigm has been extended to consider each factor in relation to the time of the injury—that is, factors operating before, during, and after the injury that might be associated with both its incidence and its severity (Haddon 1968). Although the matrix, called the *Haddon matrix,* was initially developed to address the problem of RTIs only, it provides a comprehensive framework in which researchers can consider the multitude of factors that may play a role in the causal injury pathway, as outlined in table 39.2.

In the past two decades, the evidence base for the identification of risk factors for unintentional injuries in high-income countries (HICs) has increased dramatically as the number of injury researchers and research institutions has increased. However, because of the paucity of injury researchers and research institutions in LMICs, the evidence base for the identification of risk factors for unintentional injuries in these countries is growing more slowly.

Although knowledge about risk factors for injuries in HICs may also be relevant for LMICs, the material presented in the following section focuses on information that has been obtained from studies in LMICs. However, the section also considers the extent to which information obtained from studies conducted in HICs may be relevant.

Risk Factors for Road Traffic Injuries. The increasing volume of traffic is one of the main factors contributing to the increase in RTIs in LMICs. Motorization rates rise with income (Kopits and Cropper 2005), and a number of LMICs experiencing growth have seen a corresponding increase in the number of motor vehicles (Ghaffar and others 1999). In some LMICs, this growth has been led by an increase in motorized two-wheeled vehicles, one of the least safe forms of travel, which has resulted in concurrent increases in related injuries (Zhang and others 2004).

The rapid growth in motor vehicles in many LMICs has not been accompanied by improvements in facilities for these road users or by facilities that respond to the continued predominance of nonmotorized traffic (Khayesi 2003). Many of the technical aspects of planning, highway design, traffic engineering, and traffic management that are the hallmarks of transportation systems in many HICs are absent in LMICs, which need to plan for a level of heterogeneity in traffic that HICs do not encounter (Tiwari 2000).

Studies undertaken primarily in HICs show a strong relationship between the increase in vehicle speeds and increased risk of crash and injury, both for motor vehicle occupants and for vulnerable road users, particularly pedestrians (European Road Safety Action Program 2003). This relationship is likely to be true for LMICs, and indeed, data obtained from routinely collected police reports in a number of LMICs show that speed is listed as the leading cause of road traffic crashes, accounting for up to 50 percent of all crashes (Afukaar 2003; Odero, Khayesi, and Heda 2003; Wang and others 2003).

Several case-control studies in HICs have confirmed the role of alcohol in the increasing risk of road crashes (Peden and

Table 39.2 The Haddon Matrix as Applied to Road Traffic Injuries

| Phase | Nature of intervention | Factors | | |
		Human	Vehicles and equipment	Environment
Precrash	Crash prevention	Information Attitudes Impairment Police enforcement	Roadworthiness Lighting Braking Handling Speed management	Road design Road layout Speed limits Pedestrian facilities
Crash	Injury prevention during crash	Use of restraints Impairment	Occupant restraints Other safety devices Crash-protective design	Forgiving roadside (for example, crash barriers)
Postcrash	Life sustaining	First-aid skill Access to medical personnel	Ease of access Fire risk	Rescue facilities Congestion

Source: Authors.

others 2004). Studies conducted in LMICs showed that drivers had consumed alcohol in 33 to 69 percent of crashes in which drivers were fatally injured and in 8 to 29 percent of crashes in which drivers were not fatally injured (Odero and Zwi 1995). Alcohol consumption by pedestrians also increases their risk of injuries in HICs; moreover, in at least some LMICs, more than 50 percent of fatally injured pedestrians had consumed alcohol (Peden and others 1996).

Other factors that increase the risks of road crashes in HICs include fatigue, use of hand-held mobile telephones, and inadequate visibility of vulnerable road users (Peden and others 2004), all of which are equally likely to increase risks in LMICs. Indeed, a recent case-control study from China shows that the risks of a crash doubled with chronic sleepiness on the part of the driver (G. F. Liu and others 2003), and surveys of commercial and public road transport in a number of African countries have shown that drivers often work long hours and go to work exhausted (Mock, Amegashi, and Darteh 1999; Nafukho and Khayesi 2002). Studies in Malaysia clearly show that motorcyclists who use daytime running lights have a crash risk about 10 to 29 percent lower than those who do not because of their greater visibility (Radin Umar, Mackay, and Hills 1996).

Road- and vehicle-related factors may also increase the risk of crash involvement. Specific factors related to road planning include traffic passing through residential areas, conflicts between pedestrians and vehicles, schools located on busy roads, lack of median barriers to prevent dangerous passing on two-lane roads, and lack of barriers to prevent pedestrian access onto high-speed roads, although few studies have specifically examined the risks associated with those factors (Ross and others 1991).

Although the severity of crash injuries is related to in-vehicle crash protection, evidence indicates that many engineering advances found in vehicles in HICs are not present in vehicles in LMICs (Odero, Garner, and Zwi 1997). Perhaps one of the most important factors contributing to injury severity relates to crash protection for vulnerable road users. However, few HICs, let alone LMICs, require the fronts of cars or buses to be designed in a way that would protect vulnerable road users (Mohan 2002).

A significant risk factor for increased severity of injuries of users of motorized two-wheeled vehicles is riders' failure to use motorcycle helmets (B. Liu and others 2004). Studies in a number of Asian countries have shown that failure to use helmets, use of nonstandard helmets, and use of improperly secured helmets are not uncommon, even in countries with mandatory helmet laws (Conrad and others 1996; Kulanthayan and others 2000). Failure to wear helmets is also a risk factor for increased injury severity among bicyclists (Attewell, Glase, and McFadden 2001). Although the failure to use seat belts is a significant risk factor associated with injury severity among vehicle occupants, many LMICs have no requirements for seat belts to be fitted or used (Peden and others 2004).

Studies in HICs suggest that roadside hazards, such as trees, poles, and road signs, may contribute to between 18 and 42 percent of road crashes and increase injury severity (Kloeden and others 1998), although the extent to which this is also true in LMICs has not been determined.

Risk Factors for Poisonings. The literature on poisonings in LMICs includes comprehensive information about intentional poisonings; significant information about occupation-related poisonings, especially pesticide poisonings; and a growing body of information about lead poisoning. Each of these types of poisoning is covered elsewhere in this book. This chapter focuses on risk factors for other types of poisoning in LMICs, and, in particular, focuses on risk factors for poisonings in young children.

The literature's focus on risk factors for childhood poisoning probably reflects the fact that child poisoning victims are seen more often than adults in most hospital settings (Ellis and others 1994; Nhachi and Kasilo 1992). This fact is in stark contrast to the data presented earlier, which clearly show that middle-aged individuals sustain the vast majority of deaths and DALYs from poisonings in LMICs. Those numbers no doubt reflect the importance of work-related poisonings.

Young males consistently appear to be at higher risk of poisonings than females (Ellis and others 1994; Fernando and Fernando 1997; Soori 2001). The most common agents involved in childhood poisonings are paraffin (or kerosene) and other household chemicals; pesticides; and various plants or animals, including snakes (Fernando and Fernando 1997).

Several case-control studies in LMICs indicate the importance of a number of sociodemographic risk factors, including young parents, residential mobility, and limited adult supervision of children (Azizi, Zulkifli, and Kasim 1993; Soori 2001). The studies also suggest that previous poisoning may be a risk factor (Soori 2001). Another important factor seems to be storage, including the number of storage containers used in the residence; the use of nonstandard containers for storage (for example, beverage bottles for storing kerosene); and the storage of poisons at ground level (Azizi, Zulkifli, and Kasim 1993; Chatsantiprapa, Chokkanapitak, and Pinpradit 2001; Soori 2001).

Risk Factors for Fall-Related Injuries. Risk factors for fall-related injuries in older people are generally considered in terms of risk factors for falling, risk factors associated with the severity of the impact following the fall, and risks factors associated with low levels of bone mineral density—insofar as almost all fall-related injuries in older people involve broken bones. The risk factors associated with the latter two categories are generally related to aspects of the aging process and, as a consequence, are considered in more detail in chapter 51.

Analytical studies conducted in a variety of LMICs have tended to show that risk factors for fall-related injuries, especially hip fractures, are consistent with the risk factors identified in HICs. Those risk factors include low bone density; poor nutritional status and low body mass index; low calcium intake; comorbid conditions, such as hypertension and diabetes; poor performance in activities of daily living; low levels of engagement in physical activity; poor cognitive function; poor perceived health status; poor vision; environmental factors affecting balance or gait; family history of hip fracture; and alcohol consumption (Boonyaratavej and others 2001; Clark and others 1998; Jitapunkul, Yuktananandana, and Parkpian 2001).

Some studies have identified other factors that may be more relevant in the context of LMICs. For example, studies in Thailand suggest that factors associated with poor socioeconomic status may increase risk—for example, not having electricity in the house and living in Thai-style houses or huts (Jitapunkul, Yuktananandana, and Parkpian 2001).

The literature specifically identifying risk factors for falls in younger people in LMICs is sparse, but the information there is indicates that such falls usually occur in and around the home, with a significant proportion being associated with falls from heights, including rooftops and trees (Adesunkanmi, Oseni, and Badru 1999; Bangdiwala and Anzola-Perez 1990; Kozik and others 1999; Raja, Vohra, and Ahmed 2001). However, falls other than from heights predominate and are frequently related to engagement in vigorous levels of physical activity.

Risk Factors for Burn-Related Injuries. Despite the focus of WHO's data on burn-related injuries sustained as a result of fires, a number of country-specific surveys conducted in medical facilities suggest that scalds from hot water may be equally important or more important causes of burn-related injuries (Chan and others 2002; Delgado and others 2002; Forjuoh, Guyer, and Smith 1995; Rossi and others 1998). However, in some countries, including China and particularly India, fire-related injuries clearly outweigh scald-related injuries (Ahuja and Bhattacharya 2002; Jie and Ren 1992).

Overall, women are at greater risk of fire-related burn injuries than are men; however, data from population-based and medical center surveys suggest that in some settings (excluding India), males may be at greater risk of burns than are females (Chan and others 2002; Zhu, Yang, and Meng 1988). In many studies, burn-related injuries account for a much higher proportion of injuries in young children compared with other age groups (Jie and Ren 1992; E. H. Liu and others 1998).

Rural location appears to be a consistent risk factor for burn-related injuries (Courtright, Haile, and Kohls 1993; Zhu, Yang and Meng 1988), as is the home (Delgado and others 2002; Forjuoh, Guyer, and Smith 1995; E. H. Liu and others 1998).

Investigators have undertaken case-control studies aimed at identifying risk and protective factors for burn-related injuries in Africa, Asia, and South America, and all focus on identifying risk factors for children. Environmental risk factors that have been identified include lack of a water supply, storage of a flammable substance in the home, cooking equipment in the kitchen within reach of children, and housing that is located in slums and congested areas. Persons with personal and socioeconomic risk factors included children who were not the first born, who had a pregnant mother, whose mother recently was dismissed from a job, who had recently moved, who had a pre-existing impairment, whose sibling died from a burn or had a history of burn, whose parents lacked alertness to burns, whose clothing was made of synthetic fabrics, whose parents were illiterate, and whose parents were of low economic status. Protective factors included the presence of a living room, better maternal education, and a history of previous injury among males who lived in good environmental conditions (Daisy and others 2001; Delgado and others 2002; Forjuoh and others 1995; Werneck and Reichenheim 1997).

Risk Factors for Drowning. Most drowning incidents in LMICs are not associated with recreation or leisure, as is commonly the case in HICs, but instead are associated with everyday activities near bodies of water, including rivers, wells, and buckets (Celis 1997; Hyder and others 2003; Kobusingye, Guwatudde, and Lett 2001).

As noted earlier, men account for a higher proportion of drowning incidents than women, and children age one to four and young people appear to be at greatest risk, with drowning accounting for a high proportion of injury-related deaths in those age groups (Celis 1997; Kibel and others 1990; Kozik and others 1999; Tan, Li, and Bu 1998). Some surveys also suggest that older people may be at particularly high risk (Tan, Li, and Bu 1998).

Descriptive surveys indicate that those living in rural areas are at greater risk than those living in urban areas (Kobusingye, Guwatudde, and Lett 2001), probably indicating greater exposure to unprotected water surfaces. A number of studies find that most adult drowning incidents appear to be associated with positive blood alcohol tests (Carlini-Cotrim and da Matta Chasin 2000; Celis 1997).

Case-control studies of drowning in young children have identified both sociodemographic risk factors and risk factors associated with proximity to bodies of water. Ahmed, Rahman, and van Ginneken's (1999) study in Bangladesh shows that the risk of drowning increased with the age of the mother and increased much more sharply the larger the number of children in the family. Celis's (1997) case-control study in Mexico finds that the risk of drowning associated with having a well at home was almost seven times that for children in homes without a well.

INTERVENTIONS

Interventions to prevent unintentional injuries have traditionally been considered in terms of the three E's—education, enforcement, and engineering—and within the framework of the Haddon matrix. That is, interventions are considered in terms of preventing the occurrence of the injury, minimizing the severity of injury at the time of the injury, and minimizing the severity of injury following the injury event.

Although randomized controlled trials are the gold standard for assessing the effectiveness of injury interventions, such trials are still relatively rare in relation to injuries, and in many cases such trials may be impractical to implement. Studies comparing the incidence of injury before and after the implementation of an intervention, sometimes with reference to a control population in which the intervention has not been introduced, more commonly provide the only evidence of effectiveness. In some areas, findings from observational studies, such as case-control studies, provide the best available evidence. However, randomized controlled trials are clearly not needed for some interventions because their benefits are obvious. Other interventions, particularly those that may have modest but important benefits, may require rigorous evaluation methods.

Evidence of the effectiveness of interventions in LMICs, as opposed to HICs, is also relatively uncommon. Although the proven efficacy of some interventions in HICs does not require replication in LMICs—for example, the use of motorcycle helmets—strategies that may be effective in increasing the rates of helmet wearing in HICs may not necessarily be appropriate in LMICs. Thus, WHO and others increasingly endorse tailoring interventions found to be effective in HICs to LMICs, followed by rigorous evaluation (Peden and others 2004). Table 39.3 provides a summary of promising and recommended interventions, as well as interventions that have specifically been shown to be effective in LMICs.

Road Traffic Injuries

Many working to reduce RTIs use the "safer roads, safer vehicles, safer people, and safer systems" motto. A recent augmentation of this motto derives from the recognition of the important

Table 39.3 Promising and Effective Interventions for Injuries in LMICs

Injury	Promising interventions	Interventions shown to be effective in LMICs (references)
RTIs	Reducing motor vehicle traffic: efficient fuel taxes, changes in land-use policy, safety impact assessment of transportation and land-use plans, provision of shorter and safer routes, trip reduction measures	Increasing the legal age of motorcyclists from 16 to 18 years (Norghani and others 1998)
	Making greater use of safer modes of transport	
	Minimizing exposure to high-risk scenarios: restricting access to different parts of the road network, giving priority to higher occupancy vehicles or to vulnerable road users, restricting the speed and engine performance of motorized two-wheelers, increasing the legal age for operating a motorcycle, using graduated driver's licensing systems	
	Safer roads	
	Safety awareness in planning road networks, safety features in road design, and remedial action in high-risk crash sites: making provisions for slow-moving traffic and vulnerable road users; providing passing lanes, median barriers, and street lighting	
	Traffic calming measures, such as speed bumps	Speed bumps in reducing pedestrian injuries (Afukaar, Antwi, and Ofosu-Amaah 2003)
	Speed cameras	
	Safer vehicles	
	Improving the visibility of vehicles, including requiring automatic daytime running lights	Daytime running lights on motorcycles (Radin Umar, Mackay, and Hills 1996; Yuan 2000)
	Incorporating crash protective design into vehicles, including installing seat belts	
	Mandating vehicle licensing and inspection	
	Safer people	
	Legislating strategies and increasing enforcement of, for example, speed limits, alcohol-related limits, hours of driving for commercial drivers, seat belt use, bicycle and motorcycle helmet use	Increases in fines and suspension of driver's licenses (Poli de Figueiredo and others 2001)
		Legislation and enforcement of motorcycle helmets (Ichikawa, Chadbunchachai, and Marui 2003; Supramaniam, Belle, and Sung 1984).

Table 39.3 Continued

Injury	Promising interventions	Interventions shown to be effective in LMICs (references)
Poisonings	Better storage, including positioning and nature of storage vessels	Free distribution of child-resistant containers (Krug and others 1994)
	Use of child-resistant containers	
	Warning labels	
	First-aid education	
	Poison control centers	
Fall-related injuries	*Older people*	
	Muscle strengthening and balance retraining, individually prescribed	
	Tai chi group exercise	
	Home hazard assessment and modification for high-risk individuals	
	Multidisciplinary, multifactorial screening for health and environmental risk factors	
	Younger people	
	Multifaceted community programs of the Children Can't Fly type	
Burn-related injuries	*Fire-related injuries*	
	Introducing programs to install smoke alarms	
	Separating cooking areas from living areas	
	Locating cooking surfaces at heights	
	Reducing the storage of flammable substances in households	
	Supervising children more effectively	
	Introducing, monitoring, and enforcing standards and codes for fire-resistant garments	
	Scald-related injuries	
	Separating cooking areas from play areas	
	Improving the design of cooking vessels	
	Fire- and scald-related injuries	
	Increasing awareness of burns prevention	
	Providing first-aid education	
Drowning	Limiting exposure to bodies of water close to dwellings, such as by fencing	
	Providing learn-to-swim programs	
	Providing education about risks for drowning	
	Increasing supervision and providing lifeguards at recreational facilities	
	Equipping boats with flotation devices and ensuring their use	
	Legislating and enforcing rules about the numbers of individuals carried on boats	
	Having trained and responsive coast guard services	

Source: Authors.

role of appropriate transport and land-use policies in managing exposure to the risk of an RTI (Peden and others 2004).

Managing exposure to risk involves strategies aimed at reducing motor vehicle traffic, encouraging the use of safer modes of travel, and minimizing exposure to high-risk scenarios, as outlined in greater detail in table 39.3. Evidence from Malaysia shows that increasing the legal age of motorcyclists from 16 to 18 has been beneficial (Norghani and others 1998), but evidence of the effectiveness of many of the other strategies is not yet available for LMICs.

Safer Roads. Intervention strategies focusing on safer roads should incorporate safety awareness in planning road networks, safety features in road design, and remedial action for high-risk crash sites. HICs have adopted many of these strategies, and though they have not been examined in rigorously controlled studies, such strategies form the basis of best-practice guidelines and manuals now being used in LMICs (Ross and others 1991).

Traffic calming measures are among the strategies recommended for incorporating safety features into road design.

Although evidence from randomized controlled trials is not yet available (Bunn and others 2003), a before-and-after study conducted in Ghana suggested that speed bumps were effective in reducing traffic injuries, especially pedestrian injuries (Afukaar, Antwi, and Ofosu-Amaah 2003). A recent summary of research findings also suggests that automated speed enforcement virtually eliminates speeding (ICF Consulting Ltd. and Imperial College Centre for Transport Studies 2003).

Safer Vehicles. Strategies focusing on safer vehicles include improving the visibility of vehicles, incorporating crash protective design into vehicles, and promoting further development of "intelligent" vehicles. However, in LMICs, strategies that simply ensure regular maintenance of older vehicles or removal of vehicles in poor condition from the roads, as well as vehicle licensing and inspection, have the potential to be cost-effective (Peden and others 2004).

Meta-analyses of the effects of automatic daytime running lights on cars consistently show that they reduce road crashes (Elvik and Vaa 2004). Studies in both Malaysia and Singapore show similar positive effects for daytime running lights on motorcycles (Radin Umar, Mackay, and Hills 1996; Yuan 2000).

Although the fitting of seat belts—probably the most well-known and effective safer vehicle strategy—is covered by technical standards worldwide and is mandatory in most countries, anecdotal evidence suggests that vehicles in many LMICs lack functioning seat belts (Forjuoh 2003).

Safer People. Intervention strategies aimed at improving road user behavior are increasingly focusing on the introduction and enforcement of relevant legislation rather than on educational efforts. For example, Poli de Figueiredo and others' (2001) research in Brazil indicates that increasing fines and suspending drivers' licenses immediately reduced RTIs and deaths.

A large body of research, although little of it conducted in LMICs, shows that setting and enforcing speed limits reduces RTIs by up to 34 percent. It also shows that RTIs are reduced in varying magnitudes by setting and enforcing legal blood alcohol limits and minimum drinking-age laws, using alcohol checkpoints, and running mass media campaigns aimed at reducing drinking and driving (Peden and others 2004).

The introduction and enforcement of mandatory seat belt and child restraint laws reduces occupant deaths and injuries by up to 25 percent; however, such laws have not been introduced in all LMICs (Peden and others 2004).

Both bicycle and motorcycle helmets reduce head injuries among riders by up to 85 percent. Though education may be effective in increasing helmet use, the effect is greater when combined with legislation and enforcement, as demonstrated in Malaysia and Thailand (Ichikawa, Chadbunchachai, and Marui 2003; Supramaniam, Belle, and Sung 1984).

Poisonings

The prevention of unintentional poisonings includes consideration of both occupational and nonoccupational poisonings; however, chapter 60 provides a fuller discussion of effective interventions in relation to work-related poisonings, so these are not discussed here.

Suggested interventions to reduce exposure to nonoccupational poisonings include better storage of poisons in terms of both the location and the nature of the storage vessels used. Specific interventions include storing poisons outside the home and above children's head height and reducing the use of secondhand household containers—for example soda bottles—along with introducing and enforcing legislation to prohibit the sale of poisons in such containers (Nhachi and Kasilo 1994).

The efficacy of child-resistant containers in preventing access to poisons has been demonstrated, and data from a controlled before-and-after study in South Africa suggest that free distribution of child-resistant containers is a highly effective means of preventing poisoning in children (Krug and others 1994).

Fall-Related Injuries

Interventions proven effective for preventing falls by older people in HICs include muscle strengthening and balance retraining that is individually prescribed at home by a trained health professional; tai chi group exercise; home hazard assessment and modification that is professionally prescribed for older people with a history of falling; and multidisciplinary, multifactorial health and environmental risk factor screening and intervention programs, both for community-dwelling older people in general and for older people with known risk factors (Chang and others 2004).

In relation to fall-related injuries among young children, other than general recommendations about increased supervision of children and the importance of height reductions and appropriate ground surfacing to prevent playground injuries, only one intervention provides evidence of effectiveness that may be relevant for LMICs. The Children Can't Fly Program has four major components, which include surveillance and follow-up, media campaigns, community education, and the provision of free, easily installed window guards to families with young children living in high-risk areas (Spiegel and Lindaman 1977). The program has been shown to be effective in reducing falls in low-income areas.

Burn-Related Injuries

Evidence of the effectiveness of interventions to prevent fire-related injuries is limited. A randomized controlled trial of a smoke detector giveaway program in inner London was unable to show evidence of the program's effectiveness on the incidence of fires and fire-related injuries (DiGuiseppi and others 2002). However, a more recent study suggests that installation programs may be more effective in increasing the use of these alarms than giveaway programs alone (Harvey and others 2004).

Interventions that have been proposed but whose effectiveness has not yet been proven include separating cooking areas from living areas (including efforts to reduce the use of indoor fires for cooking), ensuring that cooking surfaces are at heights, reducing the storage of flammable substances in households, and supervising young children more effectively (Forjuoh 2004). The introduction, monitoring, and enforcement of standards and codes for and the wearing of fire-retardant garments have also been proposed (Bawa Bhalla, Kale, and Mohan 2000).

Evidence of the effectiveness of interventions to prevent scald injuries is minimal but promising, although such interventions primarily focus on education, legislation, and enforcement of efforts to regulate the temperature of water flowing from household taps (Macarthur 2003).

Finally, interventions directed at increasing awareness of burn prevention have been proposed, largely because of the success of safe community interventions involving a multitude of strategies (Ytterstad and Sogaard 1995).

Drowning

Evidence for the effectiveness of interventions to prevent drowning is almost nonexistent. The only available data come from case-control studies undertaken in HICs that suggest that fencing domestic swimming pools reduces the risks of drowning (Thompson and Rivara 2000). Extrapolation of those findings to a low-income setting suggests that covering wells with grills, fencing nearby lakes or riverbanks, and building flood control embankments might be effective in reducing drowning.

COSTS, COST-EFFECTIVENESS, AND ECONOMIC BENEFITS OF INTERVENTION

Data on effective interventions for preventing unintentional injuries in LMICs and on the economic costs of these injuries are limited. As a result, published data on the costs, cost-effectiveness, and economic benefits of interventions to prevent unintentional injuries in LMICs are virtually nonexistent. The economic evaluation of interventions and the measurement of the economic costs of injuries therefore remain a high research priority.

Some data are available from HICs on the costs and, in particular, the net economic benefits of interventions for RTIs. Also, a body of evidence suggests that many of the interventions designed to provide safer roads and vehicles, and to improve driver behavior, have clear net economic benefits

(Peden and others 2004). Some data are also starting to emerge from HICs with respect to the cost-effectiveness of fall-related injury prevention programs for older people. However, data on either the costs or the cost-effectiveness of interventions to prevent poisonings, burns, or drownings are limited.

Cost-effectiveness studies done in HICs can only be suggestive for LMICs, because the costs of property losses, disability, and medical care are so vastly different. Furthermore, basic efficacy is not always guaranteed when a control strategy that worked in a modern city is exported to a poor LMIC village. Consequently, the ability to extrapolate from high-income to low-income countries is severely limited. Yet as middle-income countries progress, they will begin to consider interventions that have already been proven.

Despite the methodological challenges, we modeled the cost-effectiveness of five potential interventions to prevent unintentional injuries using information presented earlier on known effective interventions in LMICs. In each case, the evidence for effectiveness in an LMIC setting was strong. However, because so few interventions have been evaluated in LMICs, we had to make certain assumptions to extrapolate findings about costs and effectiveness in one LMIC setting to other settings (for an outline of the assumptions associated with this modeling, see Bishai and Hyder 2004). Our economic analyses are highly generalized and indicative of what might be achieved with the interventions considered.

For the analyses, we present all cost estimates in local currency converted to U.S. dollars (2001 exchange rates). We adopt a societal perspective for each intervention, but if appropriate, we comment on cost-effectiveness from a government perspective. The time horizon for each intervention is one year of sustaining the intervention. Costs are annualized so that a typical year of operating the intervention is known. As with any intervention, annual operating costs may fall as those involved learn ways to carry out their tasks more efficiently. Each year of program operation prevents an estimated number of deaths and injuries. In each case, we present estimates of the raw numbers of deaths and the undiscounted numbers of life years they represent. However, from an economic perspective, the life years and DALYs of those who sustain nonfatal injuries count less than the deaths. For comparability with other economic estimates, and in accordance with the economic analysis guidelines provided to authors, we discount estimates of DALYs using both a 3 percent and a 6 percent discount rate. The 3 percent discount rate is standard for economic evaluations in HICs; however, a higher discount rate may be appropriate in LMICs.

Increased Penalties for Speeding and Other Effective Road Safety Regulations

Poli de Figueiredo and others (2001) provide evidence from Brazil on the effectiveness of an intervention to publicize and enforce traffic speed and other road safety regulations. This intervention required three components—legislation to impose stiffer penalties, media coverage of the new regime, and better enforcement—and achieved a 25 percent reduction in traffic fatalities between 1997 and 1998.

On the basis of a model of the costs of media coverage and of better police enforcement, we estimate that implementing such an intervention in a population of 1 million people might range from as low US$8,100 in South Asia to US$196,000 in LMICs in Europe and Central Asia (table 39.4). Those intervention costs are incremental costs that assume that the population already has 50 percent of the necessary police strength. We define adequacy as one officer for every 5,000 vehicles and use regional data on vehicles per 1 million people to estimate the number of police officers and amount of equipment needed to enforce traffic laws. The assumption is that after the intervention the population will have enough officers to issue citations to one-third of their beat's 5,000 vehicles each year. This effort would require them to write about 7 to 10 citations per workday. Using the estimates of traffic injury burdens in the regions listed in the table and the potential to lower traffic deaths by 25 percent, as reported in the Brazilian study, we estimate potential DALY reductions and cost per DALY averted (table 39.4; for details of the calculations see Bishai and Hyder 2004).

The cost estimates shown in table 39.4 do not include potential cost offsets from savings derived by preventing expenditures on medical care or vehicle repair. Including those potential savings would lower the societal cost and enhance the estimated cost-effectiveness. Those cost offsets will vary widely by region. To demonstrate the importance of cost offsets, we use data from Bangladesh, for which the Transport Research Laboratory Ltd. (2003) has estimated the medical and property costs of traffic crashes. On the basis of these estimates, we calculate 1 fatality, 8 serious injuries, and 28 slight injuries occur for every fatal crash in Bangladesh. Each serious injury is associated with US$2,016 in costs for property, administration, lost output, medical care, and pain and suffering, and each slight

injury incurs US$929 in similar costs (Bishai and Hyder 2004). Thus, if we associate 1 prevented traffic fatality with preventing 8 serious injuries worth US$16,128 (8 × US$2,016) and 28 slight injuries worth US$26,012 (28 × US$929), then total additional cost savings would amount to US$42,140.

If intervention costs in Bangladesh were close to the US$8,105 shown in table 39.4 for South Asia, then the intervention would save society more than it cost if it prevented only one death and the expected proportion of nonfatal injuries. If an enforcement intervention in Bangladesh were as effective as the one documented in Brazil, it could lower fatalities by 25 percent. With 83 traffic fatalities per 1 million population, the intervention could prevent 21 deaths and lead to net savings of US$876,835—or (21 × US$42,140) − US$8,105— for every million population receiving this intervention.

Speed Bumps

A study in Ghana (Afukaar, Antwi and Ofosu-Amah 2003) showed that road traffic fatalities fell by more than 50 percent following the introduction of speed bumps. Because speed bumps are usually most effective when installed at the most hazardous junctions or near pedestrian crossings, planners need to know which junctions are the most hazardous. We assumed that half of a city's crashes occur at junctions and that cities have different numbers of treatable junctions. A few junctions would have multiple fatalities per year, but most would have one or zero fatalities per year. We assumed that the number of fatalities per junction would be distributed as a negative exponential to calculate how many junctions might lack effective speed control modifications and could thereby be targeted as those responsible for 10 percent or 25 percent of a city's preventable fatalities. Assuming a 10-year useful life for a speed bump and using regionalized estimates of speed bump construction costs, we modeled the annualized cost of constructing speed bumps at junctions responsible for 10 percent or 25 percent of fatalities. As before, we lacked an evidence

Table 39.4 Costs, DALYs, and Costs per DALY of an Intervention to Improve and Publicize Traffic Enforcement by Region (2001 US$)

Region	Cost to intervene in a population of 1,000,000 for 1 year[a]	Present value of annual DALYs averted		Cost per DALY averted	
		Discounted at 3 percent per year	Discounted at 6 percent per year	Discounted at 3 percent per year	Discounted at 6 percent per year
East Asia and the Pacific	11,817	1,517	956	8	12
Europe and Central Asia	195,971	1,433	903	137	217
Latin American and the Caribbean	225,513	1,333	840	169	268
Middle East and North Africa	114,915	2,166	1,365	53	84
South Asia	8,105	1,528	963	5	8
Sub-Saharan Africa	24,518	2,003	1,370	12	18

Source: Authors' calculations.

a. Costs do not include cost offsets from prevented medical care and prevented vehicle repair.

Table 39.5 Annualized Costs and DALYs of an Intervention to Build Speed Bumps for the Top 10 Percent of the Most Lethal Junctions in a City of 1 Million, by Region

Region	Cost to intervene in population of 1,000,000 for 1 year[a]	Present value of annual DALYs averted (2001 US$)		Cost per DALY averted (2001 US$)	
		Discounted at 3 percent per year	Discounted at 6 percent per year	Discounted at 3 percent per year	Discounted at 6 percent per year
East Asia and the Pacific	725	167	105	4.34	6.89
Europe and Central Asia	708	158	99	4.48	7.11
Latin American and the Caribbean	299	147	92	2.04	3.23
Middle East and North Africa	1,070	238	150	4.49	7.12
South Asia	324	168	106	1.93	3.06
Sub-Saharan Africa	498	220	151	2.26	3.30

Source: Authors' calculations.

a. Annual costs in local currency converted to US$ around 2001. Costs do not include cost offsets from prevented medical care and prevented vehicle repair.

base from which to estimate cost offsets from prevented medical care or vehicle repair and could not include those potential savings.

Table 39.5 presents the costs of DALYs saved and costs per DALY saved by building speed bumps at the top 10 percent of the most lethal junctions in a city of 1 million people. We assumed the speed bumps could lower injuries by 50 percent, as observed in the Ghana study. Given the low costs per DALY averted and the typical high expenditures for medical care for crash victims, we are confident that the medical savings to society would more than offset the intervention's costs, but we lack the data to prepare complete estimates.

Bicycle Helmet Legislation and Enforcement

Thompson, Rivara, and Thompson's (1989) case-control study indicates that the effectiveness of a bicycle helmet for a single rider is 85 percent. The effect on lives saved and DALYs averted depends on how many people in a population ride bicycles and the roadway environment for riders. Although the degree of energy transferred to the brain in a crash and the clinical efficacy of helmets may be the same worldwide, few data are available on exposure and the bicycle crash burden in LMICs. Thus, in modeling the effects of bicycle helmet legislation, we were limited to assessing the case of the one country with adequate data on bicycle injury epidemiology: China. In China, bicycle-related deaths kill 22 people per 1 million population per year (Li and Baker 1997). Given estimates of the annualized cost of helmet acquisition for all the bicyclists in a Chinese population of 1 million and of the enforcement costs of penalizing unhelmeted riders, we estimate that protecting bicyclists with helmets would cost US$265,000. Assuming that China could convert from zero to 100 percent adherence to helmet use, it could achieve an 85 percent reduction in head injuries from this intervention and would avert

2,478 DALYs at a 3 percent discount rate and 1,562 DALYs at a 6 percent discount rate. Thus, the cost-effectiveness of going from zero to 100 percent helmet use in China would be US$107 (US$265,000/2,478) per DALY at a 3 percent discount rate or US$170 (US$265,000/1,562) per DALY at a 6 percent discount rate.

Motorcycle Helmet Legislation and Enforcement

As with bicycles, we have epidemiological data for China, where motorcycle-related deaths kill 16 people per 1 million population per year (Zhang and others 2004). We assume that a population of 1 million in China has 125,000 regular motorcyclists, which will require the equivalent of half the time of a police officer to cite 1 percent of them for helmet violations. At Chinese salary levels, this effort would cost the equivalent of US$7,500 per year. The helmets for this population would cost US$250,000 at US$2 per year of helmet use. Thus, the total cost of the intervention would be US$257,500. Assuming a mean age of injury of 20 years and a disability weight of 0.4 for head injury, we estimate the DALYs averted by motorcycle helmet legislation as 589 at a 3 percent discount rate and 357 at a 6 percent discount rate. This intervention therefore costs US$437 (US$257,500/589) per DALY based on a 3 percent discount rate or US$721 (US$257,500/357) per DALY based on a 6 percent discount rate.

Childproof Paraffin Containers

The use of childproof paraffin containers is relevant primarily in Sub-Saharan Africa, where households use paraffin as a cooking fuel and frequently store it in bottles previously used to store beverages. Studies from South Africa have significantly enhanced our understanding of the cost-effectiveness of distributing child-resistant containers. According to Krug and others'

(1994) findings, a population of 1 million who used paraffin regularly in South Africa experienced 1,040 poisonings a year. After child-resistant containers were distributed, the incidence dropped to 540, indicating that 500 poisonings per year had been prevented. We therefore assume that (a) in a population of 1 million, child-resistant containers would need to be distributed to 200,000 households; (b) each child-resistant container costs R 0.85 (US$0.33), including the costs of distribution; and (c) total direct costs would be US$66,000 (200,000 × US$0.33).

The average cost of treating a poisoned child in a South African hospital was R 256.13 (US$100). Thus, indirect cost savings would be US$50,000 (500 × US$100), which would partially offset the US$66,000 in direct costs, leading to a net cost of US$16,000 to intervene. The mean age of children who suffered poisoning in South Africa was 12 to 24 months. Although no deaths were reported among children in the South African study, the most common figure in the literature is a 2 percent case fatality rate (Krug and others 1994), suggesting that the prevention of 500 poisonings averted 10 deaths among children around two years old. Life tables provided to the authors for Sub-Saharan Africa show life expectancy at age 2 is 49 years; thus, the US$16,000 intervention could save 490 life years. Therefore, a rough estimate of the cost-effectiveness of child-resistant containers as a way of preventing paraffin poisoning in South Africa would be US$1,600 (US$16,000/10) per death averted.

Most survivors of paraffin poisoning do not suffer permanent disability, and because we lack any objective means for assigning disability weights to those who are disabled, we neglect years lived with a disability in calculating DALYs. The investment of US$16,000 thus results in 10 children surviving for 49 more years. Undiscounted, this is 490 (10 × 49) life years. The impact is 263 DALYs averted at a 3 percent discount rate or 166 DALYs averted at a 6 percent discount rate. The cost-effectiveness is US$61 (US$16,000/263) per DALY at a 3 percent discount rate or US$96 (US$16,000/166) per DALY at a 6 percent discount rate.

Summary

Estimated costs per DALY from the interventions considered here range from negative (that is, savings) to a few hundred U.S. dollars per DALY. The order of magnitude of the costs per DALY averted using these injury countermeasures suggests that they could be categorized as highly cost-effective (Murray and others 2000). Our estimates of intervention costs neglect the potential savings from prevented medical spending but still appear quite promising. Although our estimates provide some indicative information about the economic properties of counterinjury interventions, these findings point primarily to the lack of information about the global economic burden of injury that could enable more comprehensive estimates.

IMPLEMENTATION OF PREVENTION AND CONTROL STRATEGIES

Investments in the health sector to address specific problems are a critical indicator of political commitment, sectoral efforts, and priorities at the national and international levels. In some cases, investments are so low that they provide a useful reference point for assessing the returns on additional investments in the future. Such a situation has been described as a null point in health systems, and current expenditures on injury prevention and control in LMICs approximate this concept (Murray and others 2000).

This concept can be illustrated by considering investments in preventing RTIs, which are responsible for the majority of the burden of unintentional injuries and about which much is known regarding effective interventions, even though such interventions have not been examined in the context of rigorously controlled studies in LMICs (see box 39.1).

Peden and others (2004) recognize that, despite the global burden of RTIs, the levels of investment are pitifully small, largely because of a lack of awareness of the scale of the problem and a lack of awareness that interventions can prevent and reduce the levels of harm. As a consequence, the report directs a number of recommendations at governments and communities in the hope that these recommendations will enable countries, particularly LMICs, to begin a sustainable process that will eventually lead to the adaptation and implementation of effective preventive strategies. The recommendations include the following:

- Identify a lead government agency to guide the national road safety effort.
- Assess the problems, policies, and institutional settings relating to RTIs and the capacity for preventing RTIs in each country.
- Prepare a national road safety strategy and plan of action.
- Allocate financial and human resources to address the problem.
- Implement specific actions to prevent crashes, minimize injuries and their consequences, and evaluate the effect of those actions.
- Support the development of national capacity and international cooperation.

Although few data are available to show the levels of investment in other areas of unintentional injury prevention, those levels are no doubt considerably lower than for RTIs. With increases in the proportions and numbers of older people in many LMICs, the burden of fall-related injuries is likely to increase significantly in the coming years. Recognition of the changing demographics in countries such as China, Mexico, and Thailand plus a growing body of evidence on effective

Implementation: Case Study of RTIs

Bishai and others (2003) quantify the magnitude of government investment in road safety and the extent of RTIs in Pakistan and Uganda. They estimate that Pakistan spent $0.07 per capita, or 0.015 percent of gross domestic product (GDP) per capita, on road safety in 1998 and that Uganda spent $0.09 per capita, or 0.02 percent of GDP per capita. This type of evidence stands in stark contrast with the high burden of RTIs in these countries.

These findings occur in the context of public expenditure on health of 1.8 percent of GDP by Pakistan and 1.6 percent by Uganda (UNDP 1998). Per capita health spending by households in Uganda was $7.70 in 1995/96, and public spending on health at the district level was $4.84 per capita in 1997/98 (Hutchinson 1999). Public spending on road safety amounts to about 1 percent of public spending on health in each country. It is equivalent to 0.2 percent of military spending in Pakistan and 1.1 percent of Uganda's military budget.

A review of road safety initiatives in Benin, Côte d'Ivoire, Kenya, Tanzania, and Zimbabwe found similar underinvestment in road safety and attributes this insuffi-cient investment to conflicts between government ministries, inefficient civil services, and corruption rather than to a lack of knowledge about possible road crash countermeasures (Assum 1998).

RTIs have an inverted U-shaped relationship to economic development—injuries rise early during development, then plateau with investments in road safety, and then fall as appropriate interventions succeed (van Beeck, Borsboom, and Mackenbach 2000). This biphasic pattern is known as a Kuznets curve. Attempts to estimate a Kuznets curve for road fatalities suggest that the inflection point at which fatalities begin to decline occurs at GDP per capita in the range of $5,000 to $10,000 (Bishai and others, forthcoming; Kopits and Cropper 2005). This relationship, although based on historical records from HICs, has an important lesson for LMICs: they do not need to experience massive death and disability from RTIs provided that they undertake safety investments now. Waiting for overall economic development before implementing specific interventions will result in the needless loss of millions of lives.

Note: All dollars in box 39.1 are 1998 international dollars.

---

interventions to prevent falls suggest that investments in this area could lead to significant benefits. Similarly, increasing recognition of the significance of the burden of drowning in children is leading to growing awareness of the need to invest in that area. However, the absence of any effective evidence-based interventions may be a barrier to further investment, suggesting that research into the burden of drowning must be a priority.

Investment in prevention and control activities in other areas of unintentional injuries is minimal in most LMICs, in large part because the burden of those injuries is unrecognized and because evidence of effective interventions is lacking. Therefore, there is clearly a need to consider the development, implementation, and evaluation of prevention strategies in combination, so that effective interventions can be identified and promulgated and so that ineffective interventions can be identified and discarded.

RESEARCH AND DEVELOPMENT AGENDA

The Global Forum for Health Research (2002) estimates that of the US$73.5 billion spent on health research globally in 1998,

less than 10 percent was spent on addressing problems related to 90 percent of the world's population. Analyses revealed that RTIs were a highly neglected area for investment compared with the burden of disease RTIs represented as measured in U.S. dollars per DALY. As a result, increasing the level of investment for research and development (R&D) on RTIs and other injuries should be a focus of global advocacy efforts, and investment is critical for promoting an R&D agenda on injuries in LMICs.

Developing and prioritizing a global R&D agenda for unintentional injuries, though, is challenging, and such an exercise may be more useful at national or large subnational levels. However, a number of issues requiring R&D are likely to be common across a range of LMICs.

Epidemiological research to describe the existing burden, causes, and distribution of unintentional injuries in LMICs is still needed. Often the data are most limited for areas with the greatest potential burden of injuries. Assessing the loss of health and life from unintentional injuries—whom they affect, how, and under what specific circumstances—is thus a continuing research agenda for LMICs. Problems of underreporting and other biases in available data also need to be addressed.

The lack of intervention research in LMICs is a huge gap in global health research. For the most part, no scientific trials of injury interventions have been conducted in LMICs, and existing and new interventions need to be modified, adapted, and tested in those specific settings. Three broad domains should be the foci of intervention research:

- R&D to enhance the efficiency of currently available efficacious interventions. For example, increasing the use of helmets would prevent motorcycle injuries in East Asia.
- R&D to enhance the cost-effectiveness of interventions that are currently not being implemented or that could be used more widely. For example, seat belts and child restraints are known effective interventions, and reducing the cost of such interventions might enhance their wide-scale implementation in LMICs.
- R&D to develop new interventions for unintentional injuries and to respond to that proportion of the burden that is not currently being addressed. For example, childhood falls from rooftops in South Asia have been recognized as an issue, but a locally derived intervention is currently unavailable.

Although some might argue that intervention research should be the priority in most LMICs, unless the basic underpinning research on the burden and determinants of unintentional injuries has been undertaken, the political and financial support for such research will not be forthcoming.

The dearth of economic and policy analysis of unintentional injuries in LMICs is an embarrassment for the global health research community. A recent review of economic analysis of road traffic interventions found a complete absence of any detailed studies from the developing world (Waters, Hyder and Phillips 2004). This gap in health systems research would need to be addressed to develop and implement successful injury prevention programs.

Defining a research agenda is necessary but is not by itself sufficient to conduct research or to implement the results. Two key conditions are required for moving forward: a critical mass of people to conduct research and appropriate funds to support R&D. Developing human resources for all aspects of injury prevention and control in the developing world should be a high priority. Individuals need to be trained and institutions supported and empowered to conduct quality scientific research in their own countries and on issues relevant to their locations, which would then be used within their countries. This approach involves paying attention to the issue of strengthening the capacity for research, a major cross-cutting theme for the health sector in the developing world.

Funding is and always will be a limiting factor for research; however, the mismatch between the burden of injuries and R&D investments can be corrected. Unintentional injuries are a major health problem. They cause preventable loss of life and health, and they have major economic implications. As a result, R&D investments are a health and economic imperative for developing countries and donor organizations.

CONCLUSIONS: PROMISES AND PITFALLS

Unintentional injuries are an important contributor to global death and disability burdens, especially in LMICs. However, the significance of the burden is not matched by substantive knowledge about risk factors or effective interventions in LMICs. Nevertheless, the models outlined in this chapter indicate that several interventions for preventing unintentional injuries are highly cost-effective and in some cases could result in significant cost savings.

Recent evidence shows that public efforts in injury control, such as traffic safety, are poorly funded in developing countries (Bishai and others 2003). The low expenditure compares unfavorably with expenditure on other health conditions and with expenditures in more developed nations, where government efforts in relation to such issues as traffic safety are well funded. Even adjusting for the 20-fold to 30-fold difference in gross domestic product per capita between HICs and LMICs, the investment disparities suggest that LMICs attach a low priority to injury prevention.

Given the current low level of investment, initial investments in safety, if chosen with care, could turn out to be extremely beneficial to public health and welfare. If, in the first instance, investments were to be made only in the interventions modeled here, then injury reductions would likely be significant. The next step would be to modify other interventions that have proven effective in HICs and to combine the introduction of such interventions with evaluations of their effects. Policy makers will be concerned that many of the cost-effective interventions are not low-cost interventions. They save many lives but require an extensive upfront investment. Using cost-effectiveness analyses of these interventions to document high returns would encourage financing of these interventions and widespread replication efforts.

Policy makers would be unwise to wait for advanced stages of economic development to attend to the problem of road safety or other unintentional injuries. Indeed, given the limited but growing knowledge that low-cost, effective interventions exist, for governments not to intervene would be unethical. Even though institutional obstacles are formidable in developing countries, governments routinely overcome them to address other perceived threats to public well-being—such as crime, terrorism, and war—that disrupt fewer lives than unintentional injuries. The real enigma is that such a profound loss of life can take place each year in LMICs without an outcry that would trigger sustained and effective political commitment by governments and civil society.

ACKNOWLEDGMENTS

We would like to acknowledge the assistance of Kristina McDaid and Kylie Monro of the George Institute for International Health in preparing this chapter. We would also like to acknowledge useful comments on the initial draft of the chapter provided by David Sleet of the Centers for Disease Control and Prevention, National Center for Injury Prevention and Control, and by Tony Bliss of the World Bank.

REFERENCES

Adesunkanmi, A. R., S. A. Oseni, and O. S. Badru. 1999. "Severity and Outcome of Falls in Children." *West African Journal of Medicine* 18 (4): 281–85.

Afukaar, F. K. 2003. "Speed Control in LMICs: Issues, Challenges, and Opportunities in Reducing Road Traffic Injuries." *Injury Control and Safety Promotion* 10 (1–2): 77–81.

Afukaar, F. K., P. Antwi, and S. Ofosu-Amaah. 2003. "Pattern of Road Traffic Injuries in Ghana: Implications for Control." *Injury Control and Safety Promotion* 10 (1–2): 69–76.

Ahmed, M. K., M. Rahman, and J. van Ginneken. 1999. "Epidemiology of Child Deaths Due to Drowning in Matlab, Bangladesh." *International Journal of Epidemiology* 28 (2): 306–11.

Ahuja, R. B., and S. Bhattacharya. 2002. "An Analysis of 11,196 Burn Admissions and Evaluations of Conservative Management Techniques." *Burns* 28 (6): 555–61.

Assum, T. 1998. "Road Safety in Africa: Appraisal of Road Safety Initiatives in Five African Countries." Sub-Saharan Africa Transport Policy Program. Working Paper 33, World Bank, Washington, DC.

Attewell, R. G., K. Glase, and M. McFadden. 2001. "Bicycle Helmet Efficacy: A Meta-Analysis." *Accident Analysis and Prevention* 33 (3): 345–52.

Azizi, B. H., H. I. Zulkifli, and M. S. Kasim. 1993. "Risk Factors for Accidental Poisoning in Urban Malaysian Children." *Annals of Tropical Paediatrics* 13 (2): 183–88.

Bangdiwala, S. I., and E. Anzola-Perez. 1990. "The Incidence of Injuries in Young People: II. Log-Linear Multivariable Models for Risk Factors in a Collaborative Study in Brazil, Chile, Cuba, and Venezuela." *International Journal of Epidemiology* 19 (1): 125–32.

Bawa Bhalla, S., S. R. Kale, and D. Mohan. 2000. "Burn Properties of Fabrics and Garments Worn in India." *Accident Analysis and Prevention* 32 (3): 407–20.

Bishai, D., and A. Hyder. 2004. "Modeling the Cost Effectiveness of Injury Interventions in Lower and Middle Income Countries." Disease Control Priorities Working Paper 29, Johns Hopkins Bloomberg School of Public Health, Baltimore.

Bishai, D., A. A. Hyder, A. Ghaffar, R. H. Morrow, and O. Kobusingye. 2003. "Rates of Public Investment for Road Safety in Developing Countries: Case Studies of Uganda and Pakistan." *Health Policy and Planning* 18 (2): 232–35.

Bishai, D., A. Qureshi, P. James, and A. Ghaffar. Forthcoming. "National Road Fatalities and Economic Development." *Health Economics.*

Boonyaratavej, N., P. Suriyawongpaisal, A. Takkinsatien, S. Wanvarie, R. Rajatanavin, and P. Apiyasawat. 2001. "Physical Activity and Risk Factors for Hip Fractures in Thai Women." *Osteoporosis International* 12 (3): 244–48.

Bunn, F., T. Collier, C. Frost, K. Ker, I. Roberts, and R. Wentz. 2003. "Area-Wide Traffic Calming for Preventing Traffic-Related Injuries." *Cochrane Database of Systematic Reviews* (1) CD003110.

Carlini-Cotrim, B., and A. A. da Matta Chasin. 2000. "Blood Alcohol Content and Death from Fatal Injury: A Study in Metropolitan Area of São Paulo, Brazil." *Journal of Psychoactive Drugs* 32 (3): 269–75.

Celis, A. 1997. "Home Drowning among Preschool Age Mexican Children." *Injury Prevention* 3 (4): 252–56.

Chan, K. Y., O. Hairol, H. Imtiaz, M. Zailani, S. Kunar, S. Somasundaram, and others. 2002. "A Review of Burns Patients Admitted to the Burns Unit of Hospital Universiti Kebangsaan Malaysia." *Medical Journal of Malaysia* 57 (4): 418–25.

Chang, J. T., S. C. Morton, L. Z. Rubinstein, W. A. Mojica, M. Maglione, M. J. Suttorp, and others. 2004. "Interventions for the Prevention of Falls in Older Adults: Systematic Review and Meta-Analysis of Randomised Clinical Trials." *British Medical Journal* 328 (7441): 653–54.

Chatsantiprapa, K, J. Chokkanapitak, and N. Pinpradit. 2001. "Host and Environment Factors for Exposure to Poisons: A Case Control Study of Preschool Children in Thailand." *Injury Prevention* 7 (3): 214–17.

Clark P., F. de la Pena, F. Gomez Garcia, J. A. Orozco, and P. Tugwell. 1998. "Risk Factors for Osteoporotic Hip Fractures in Mexicans." *Archives of Medical Research* 29 (3): 253–57.

Conrad, P., Y. S. Bradshaw, R. Lamsudin, N. Kasniyah, and C. Costello. 1996. "Helmets, Injuries, and Cultural Definitions: Motorcycle Injury in Urban Indonesia." *Accident Analysis and Prevention* 28: 193–200.

Courtright, P., D. Haile, and E. Kohls. 1993. "The Epidemiology of Burns in Rural Ethiopia." *Journal of Epidemiology and Community Health* 47 (1): 19–22.

Daisy, S., A. K. Mostaque, T. S. Bari, R. R. Kahn, and Q. Quamruzzaman. 2001. "Socioeconomic and Cultural Influence in the Causation of Burns in the Urban Children of Bangladesh." *Journal of Burn Care and Rehabilitation* 22 (4): 269–73.

Delgado J., M. E. Ramirez-Cardich, R. H. Gilman, R. Lavarello, N. Dahodwala, A. Bazan, and others. 2002. "Risk Factors for Burns in Children: Crowding, Poverty, and Poor Maternal Education." *Injury Prevention* 8 (1): 38–41.

DiGuiseppi, C., I. Roberts, A. Wade, M. Sculpher, P. Edwards, C. Godward, and others. 2002. "Incidence of Fires and Related Injuries after Giving Out Free Smoke Alarms: Cluster Randomized Controlled Trial." *British Medical Journal* 325 (7371): 995.

Ellis, J. B., A. Krug, J. Robertson, I. T. Hay, and U. MacIntyre. 1994. "Paraffin Ingestion—The Problem." *South African Medical Journal* 84 (11): 727–30.

Elvik, R., and T. Vaa. 2004. *Handbook of Road Safety Measures.* Amsterdam: Elsevier.

European Road Safety Action Program. 2003. *Halving the Number of Road Accident Victims in the European Union by 2010: A Shared Responsibility.* Brussels: European Commission.

Fernando, R., and D. N. Fernando. 1997. "Childhood Poisoning in Sri Lanka." *Indian Journal of Pediatrics* 64 (4): 457–60.

Forjuoh, S. N. 2003. "Traffic-Related Injury Prevention Interventions for Low Income Countries." *Injury Control and Safety Promotion* 10 (1–2): 109–18.

———. 2004. "Preventing Burns in Low and Middle-Income Countries." Disease Control Priorities Working Paper.

Forjuoh S. N., B. Guyer, and G. S. Smith. 1995. "Childhood Burns in Ghana: Epidemiological Characteristics and Home-Based Treatment." *Burns* 21 (1): 24–28.

Forjuoh S. N., B. Guyer, D. M. Strobino, P. M. Keyl, M. Diener-West, and G. S. Smith. 1995. "Risk Factors for Childhood Burns: A Case-Control Study of Ghanaian Children." *Journal of Epidemiology and Community Health* 49 (2): 189–93.

Ghaffar, A., A. A. Hyder, M. I. Mastoor, and I. Shaikh. 1999. "Injuries in Pakistan: Directions for Future Health Policy." *Health Policy and Planning* 14 (1): 11–17.

Global Forum for Health Research. 2002. *The 10/90 Report on Health Research 2001–2002.* Geneva: Global Forum for Health Research.

Haddon, W. Jr. 1968. "The Changing Approach to the Epidemiology, Prevention, and Amelioration of Trauma: The Transition to Approaches Etiologically Rather Than Descriptively Based." *American Journal of Public Health and the Nation's Health* 58 (8): 1431–38.

Harvey, P. A, M. Aitken, G. W. Ryan, L. A. Demeter, J. Givens, R. Sundararaman, and others 2004. "Strategies to Increase Smoke Alarm Use in High-Risk Households." *Journal of Community Health* 29 (5): 375–85.

Hutchinson, P. 1999. "Health Care in Uganda." Discussion Paper 404, World Bank, Washington, DC.

Hyder, A. A., S. Arifeen, N. Begum, S. Fishman, S. Wali, and A. H. Baqui. 2003. "Death from Drowning: Defining a New Challenge for Child Survival in Bangladesh." *Injury Control and Safety Promotion* 10 (4): 205–10.

ICF Consulting Ltd. and Imperial College Centre for Transport Studies. 2003. "Cost-Benefit Analysis of Road Safety Improvements." Final report. London: ICF Consulting Ltd. and Imperial College Centre for Transport Studies.

Ichikawa, M., W. Chadbunchachai, and E. Marui. 2003. "Effect of the Helmet Act for Motorcyclists in Thailand." *Accident Analysis and Prevention* 35 (2): 83–89.

Jacobs, G., A. Aeron-Thomas, and A. Astrop. 2000. "Estimating Global Road Fatalities." TRL Report 445, Transport Research Laboratory, Crowthorne, U.K.

Jie, X., and C. B. Ren. 1992. "Burn Injuries in the Dong Bei Area of China: A Study of 12,606 Cases." *Burns* 18 (3): 228–32.

Jitapunkul, S., P. Yuktananandana, and V. Parkpian. 2001. "Risk Factors of Hip Fracture among Thai Female Patients." *Journal of the Medical Association of Thailand* 84 (11): 1576–81.

Khayesi, M. 2003. "Liveable Streets for Pedestrians in Nairobi: The Challenge of Road Traffic Accidents." In *The Earthscan Reader on World Transport Policy and Practice*, ed. J. Whitelegg and G. Haq, 35–41. London: Earthscan.

Kibel, S. M., F. O. Nagel, J. Myers, and S. Cywes. 1990. "Childhood Near-Drowning—A 12-Year Retrospective Review." *South African Medical Journal* 78 (7): 418–21.

Kloeden, C. N., A. J. McLean, M. R. J. Baldock, and A. J. T. Cockington. 1998. "Severe and Fatal Car Crashes Due to Roadside Hazards: A Report to the Motor Accident Commission." Adelaide, Australia: National Health and Medical Research Council Road Accident Research Unit, University of Adelaide.

Kobusingye, O., D. Guwatudde, and R. Lett. 2001. "Injury Patterns in Rural and Urban Uganda." *Injury Prevention* 7 (1): 46–50.

Kopits, E., and M. Cropper. 2005. "Traffic Fatalities and Economic Growth." *Accident Analysis and Prevention* 37 (1): 169–78.

Kozik, C. A., S. Suntayakorn, D. W. Vaughn, C. Suntayakorn, R. Snitbhan, and B. L. Innis. 1999. "Causes of Death and Unintentional Injury among Schoolchildren in Thailand." *Southeast Asian Journal of Tropical Medicine and Public Health* 30 (1): 129–35.

Krug, A., J. B. Ellis, I. T. Hay, N. F. Mokgabudi, and J. Robertson. 1994. "The Impact of Child-Resistant Containers on the Incidence of Paraffin (Kerosene) Ingestion in Children." *South African Medical Journal* 84 (11): 730–34.

Kulanthayan, S., R. S. Umar, H. A. Hariza, M. T. Nasir, and S. Harwant. 2000. "Compliance of Proper Safety Helmet Usage in Motorcyclists." *Medical Journal of Malaysia* 55 (1): 40–44.

Li, G., and S. P. Baker. 1997. "Injuries to Bicyclists in Wuhan, People's Republic of China." *American Journal of Public Health* 87 (6): 1049–52.

Liu, B., R. Ivers, R. Norton, S. Blows, and S. K. Lo. 2004. "Helmets for Preventing Injury in Motorcycle Riders." Cochrane Database of Systematic Reviews (4) CD004333.

Liu, E. H., B. Khatri, Y. M. Shakya, and B. M. Richard. 1998. "A 3 Year Prospective Audit of Burns Patients Treated at the Western Regional Hospital of Nepal." *Burns* 24 (2): 129–33.

Liu, G. F., S. Han, D. H. Liang, F. Z. Wang, X. Z. Shi, J. Yu, and others. 2003. "Driver Sleepiness and Risk of Car Crashes in Shenyang, a Chinese Northeastern City: Population-Based Case-Control Study." *Biomedical and Environmental Sciences* 16 (3): 219–26.

Macarthur, C. 2003. "Evaluation of Safe Kids Week 2001: Prevention of Scald and Burn Injuries in Young Children." *Injury Prevention* 9 (2): 112–16.

Mock, C., J. Amegashi, and K. Darteh. 1999. "Role of Commercial Drivers in Motor Vehicle Related Injuries in Ghana." *Injury Prevention* 5 (4): 268–71.

Mohan, D. 2002. "Road Safety in Less-Motorized Environments: Future Concerns." *International Journal of Epidemiology* 31 (3): 527–32.

Murray, C. J. L., D. B. Evans, A. Acharya, and B. Baltussen. 2000. "Development of WHO Guidelines on Generalized Cost-Effectiveness Analysis." *Health Economics* 9 (3): 235–51.

Nafukho, F. M., and M. Khayesi. 2002. "Livelihood, Conditions of Work, Regulation, and Road Safety in the Small-Scale Public Transport Sector: A Case of the Matatu Mode of Transport in Kenya." In *Urban Mobility for All: Proceedings of the Tenth International CODATU Conference, Lomé, Togo, 12–15 November 2002*, ed. X. Godard and I. Fatonzoun, 241–45. Lisse, the Netherlands: AA Balkema.

Nhachi, C. F., and O. M. Kasilo. 1992. "The Pattern of Poisoning in Urban Zimbabwe." *Journal of Applied Toxicology* 12 (6): 435–38.

Nhachi, C. F., and O. M. Kasilo. 1994. "Household Chemicals Poisoning Admissions in Zimbabwe's Main Urban Centres." *Human and Experimental Toxicology* 13 (2): 69–72.

Norghani, M., A. Zainuddin, R. S. Radin Umar, and H. Hussain. 1998. *Use of Exposure Control Methods to Tackle Motorcycle Accidents in Malaysia.* Research Report 3/98. Serdang, Malaysia: Road Safety Research Center, University Putra Malaysia.

Odero, W., P. Garner, and A. B. Zwi. 1997. "Road Traffic Injuries in Developing Countries: A Comprehensive Review of Epidemiological Studies." *Tropical Medicine and International Health* 2 (5): 445–60.

Odero W., M. Khayesi, and P. M. Heda. 2003. "Road Traffic Injuries in Kenya: Magnitude, Causes, and Status of Intervention." *Injury Control and Safety Promotion* 10 (1–2): 53–61.

Odero, W. O., and A. B. Zwi. 1995. "Alcohol-Related Traffic Injuries and Fatalities in LMICs: A Critical Review of Literature." In *Proceedings of the 13th International Conference on Alcohol, Drugs, and Traffic Safety, Adelaide, 13–18 August 1995*, ed. C. N. Kloeden and A. J. McLean, 713–20. Adelaide, Australia: Road Accident Research Unit.

Peden, M., D. Knottenbelt, J. Van der Spuy, R. Oodit, M. J. Scholtz, and J. M. Stokol. 1996. "Injured Pedestrians in Cape Town: The Role of Alcohol." *South African Medical Journal* 86 (9): 1103–5.

Peden, M., R. Scurfield, D. Sleet, D. Mohan, A. A. Hyder, E. Jarawan, and others, eds. 2004. *World Report on Road Traffic Injury Prevention.* Geneva: World Health Organization.

Poli de Figueiredo, L. F., S. Rasslan, V. Bruscagin, R. Cruz, and M. Rocha e Silva. 2001. "Increases in Fines and Driver Licence Withdrawal Have Effectively Reduced Immediate Deaths from Trauma on Brazilian Roads: First-Year Report on the New Traffic Code." *Injury* 32 (2): 91–94.

Radin Umar, R. S., G. M. Mackay, and B. L. Hills. 1996. "Modelling of Conspicuity-Related Motorcycle Accidents in Seremban and Shah Alam, Malaysia." *Accident Analysis and Prevention* 28 (3): 325–32.

Raja, I. A., A. H. Vohra, and M. Ahmed. 2001. "Neurotrauma in Pakistan." *World Journal of Surgery* 25 (9): 1230–37.

Ross, A., C. Baguley, V. Hills, M. McDonald, and D. Silcock. 1991. *Towards Safer Roads in Developing Countries: A Guide for Planners and Engineers*. Crowthorne, U.K.: Transport Research Laboratory.

Rossi, L. A., E. C. Braga, R. C. Barruffini, and E. C. Carvalho. 1998. "Childhood Burn Injuries: Circumstances of Occurrences and Their Prevention in Ribeirão Preto, Brazil." *Burns* 24 (5): 416–19.

Soori, H. 2001. "Developmental Risk Factors for Unintentional Childhood Poisoning." *Saudi Medical Journal* 22 (3): 227–30.

Spiegel, C. N., and F. C. Lindaman. 1977 "Children Can't Fly: A Program to Prevent Childhood Morbidity and Mortality from Window Falls." *American Journal of Public Health* 67 (12): 1143–47.

Supramaniam, V., V. Belle, and J. Sung. 1984. "Fatal Motorcycle Accidents and Helmet Laws in Peninsular Malaysia." *Accident Analysis and Prevention* 16 (3): 157–62.

Tan, Z., X. Li, and Q. Bu. 1998. "Epidemiological Study on Drowning in Wujin, Jiangsu, 1997." *Zhonghua Liu Xing Bing Xue Za Zhi* 19 (4): 208–10.

Thompson, D. C., and F. P. Rivara. 2000. "Pool Fencing for Preventing Drowning in Children." Cochrane Database of Systematic Reviews (2) CD001047.

Thompson, R. S., F. P. Rivara, and D. C. Thompson. 1989. "A Case-Control Study of the Effectiveness of Bicycle Safety Helmets." *New England Journal of Medicine* 320 (21): 1361–67.

Tiwari, G. 2000. "Traffic Flow and Safety: Need for New Models for Heterogeneous Traffic." In *Injury Prevention and Control*, ed. D. Mohan and G. Tiwari, 71–88. London: Taylor and Francis.

Transport Research Laboratory Ltd. 2003. *Guidelines for Estimating the Cost of Road Crashes in Developing Countries*. Department for International Development, Project R7780. London: Babtie, Ross, Silcock.

UNDP (United Nations Development Programme). 1998. *Human Development Report 1998*. New York: Oxford University Press.

van Beeck, E. F., G. J. Borsboom, and J. P. Mackenbach. 2000. "Economic Development and Traffic Accident Mortality in the Industrialized World, 1962–1990." *International Journal of Epidemiology* 29 (3): 503–9.

Wang, S., G. B. Chi, C. X. Jing, X. M. Dong, C. P. Wu, and L. P. Li. 2003. "Trends in Road Traffic Crashes and Associated Injury and Fatality in the People's Republic of China, 1951–1999." *Injury Control and Safety Promotion* 10 (1–2): 83–87.

Waters, H. R., A. A. Hyder, and T. L. Phillips. 2004. "Economic Evaluation of Interventions for Reducing Road Traffic Injuries—A Review of Literature with Applications to Low and Middle-Income Countries." *Asia Pacific Journal of Public Health* 16 (1): 23–31.

Werneck, G. L., and M. E. Reichenheim. 1997. "Paediatric Burns and Associated Risk Factors in Rio de Janeiro, Brazil." *Burns* 23 (6): 478–83.

Ytterstad, B., and A. J. Sogaard: 1995. "The Harstad Injury Prevention Study: Prevention of Burns in Small Children by a Community-Based Intervention." *Burns* 21 (4): 259–66.

Yuan, W. 2000. "The Effectiveness of the 'Ride Bright' Legislation for Motorcycles in Singapore." *Accident Analysis and Prevention* 32 (4): 559–63.

Zhang, J., R. Norton, K. C. Tang, S. K. Lo, J. Zhuo, and W. Geng. 2004. "Motorcycle Ownership and Injury in China." *Injury Control and Safety Promotion* 11 (3): 159–63.

Zhu, Z. X., H. Yang, and F. Z. Meng. 1988. "The Epidemiology of Childhood Burns in Jiamusi, China." *Burns, Including Thermal Injury* 14 (5): 394–96.

Chapter **40**

Interpersonal Violence

Mark L. Rosenberg, Alexander Butchart, James Mercy, Vasant Narasimhan, Hugh Waters, and Maureen S. Marshall

Violence kills more than 1.6 million people each year. The impact of nonfatal violence cannot be quantified, but it is even more pernicious given resultant disabilities and long-term physical, psychological, economic, and social consequences.

The direct and indirect costs of violence are enormous. Violence directly affects health care expenditures worldwide. Indirectly, violence has a negative effect on national and local economies—stunting economic development, increasing economic inequality, eroding human and social capital, and increasing law enforcement expenditures (Waters and others 2004).

The U.S.-based Centers for Disease Control and Prevention identified violence as a leading public health problem in the mid 1980s and early 1990s (Rosenberg 1985; Rosenberg and Fenley 1991), as did the World Health Assembly in 1996 (Resolution WHA49.25). Contributing to the World Health Organization (WHO) report on global violence and health, Dahlberg and Krug (2002) divided violence into the following categories:

- self-directed violence, or violence in which the perpetrator is the victim (for example, suicide)
- interpersonal violence, or violence inflicted by another individual or a small group of individuals
- collective violence, or violence committed by larger groups, such as states, organized political groups, militia groups, and terrorist organizations.

This chapter focuses on interpersonal violence, which disproportionately affects low- and middle-income countries (LMICs).[1] The WHO report on violence and health estimates that more than 90 percent of all violence-related deaths occur in LMIC countries (Dahlberg and Krug 2002). The estimated rate of violent death in LMICs was 32.1 per 100,000 people in 2000, compared with 14.4 per 100,000 in high-income countries.

This chapter is based on a public health approach to preventing interpersonal violence. A public health approach has three overriding characteristics: it applies scientific methodology, emphasizes prevention, and encourages collaboration.

Applying a scientific methodology to a public health approach involves collecting and analyzing data to define the magnitude, scope, and characteristics of the problem, examining the factors that increase or decrease the risk for violence, and identifying the factors that can be modified through interventions. Interventions are designed, tested, and evaluated. Efficacious and promising interventions are implemented, and their effects and cost-effectiveness are evaluated. Ongoing monitoring of intervention effects on risk factors and target problems builds the database to allow quantitative assessment of successes and clear identification of remaining needs.

Fundamentally, public health is focused on prevention of harm caused by disease or violence. Although criminal justice systems have traditionally focused on capturing perpetrators of violence and punishing them for their actions (typically through incarceration), the public health system attempts to prevent violence from occurring and concentrates on identifying ways to keep people from committing acts of violence. Interventions may eliminate or reduce the underlying risk factors and shore up protective factors. Prevention strategies are conceived and implemented with reference to the interaction of risk factors among people at different stages of the life cycle (Mercy and Hammond 1999; additional sources online).

A public health approach must be collaborative, drawing on contributions from different sectors and disciplines. Public health analyses of violence aim to encourage integrated actions by diverse sectors such as health, education, social services, and justice. Each sector has a role to play, and collectively their actions have the potential to reduce violence.

THE NATURE, BURDEN, AND CAUSES OF INTERPERSONAL VIOLENCE

WHO (WHO Global Consultation on Violence and Health 1996, 2–3) defines *violence* as follows: "The intentional use of physical force or power, threatened or actual, against oneself, another person, or against a group or community that either results in or has a high likelihood of resulting in injury, death, psychological harm, mal-development, or deprivation." This definition emphasizes that, for the act to be classified as violence, a person or group must intend to use force or power against another person. Thus, violence is distinguished from unintended incidents that result in injury or harm.

The nature or mode of violence may be physical, sexual, or psychological, or it may involve deprivation and neglect. Given the difficulties of measuring deprivation and neglect, this chapter concentrates on the physical, sexual, and psychological modes.

Acts of interpersonal violence are classified as family violence or community violence. Family violence is further categorized by victim: child, intimate partner, or elder. *Child abuse,* as defined by WHO (1999, 15), is "physical and/or emotional ill-treatment, sexual abuse, neglect or negligent treatment or commercial or other exploitation, resulting in actual or potential harm to the child's health, survival, development, or dignity in the context of a relationship of responsibility, trust, or power." Behavior within an intimate relationship that causes physical, psychological, or sexual harm is typically labeled *intimate partner violence* or *domestic violence. Elder abuse* is mistreatment of older people, generally those older than age 60 or 65, in the home or in an institutional setting.

Community violence is categorized by two types of perpetrators: acquaintances and strangers. It includes sexual assault by strangers and violence in institutional environments, such as residential care facilities, jails, workplaces, and schools. Youth violence, with perpetrators and victims typically 10 to 29 years of age, is also a form of community violence.

Outcomes of Interpersonal Violence

Identifying the outcomes of interpersonal violence helps to determine the magnitude of the problem.

Data. As noted earlier, a fundamental aspect of the public health approach is the collection of accurate information, such as demographic characteristics of victims and perpetrators, weapon involvement, settings in which violence occurs, situational determinants, and nature and severity of resultant injuries and other harm. Data sources include death certificates, vital statistics records, medical examiners' reports, hospital and other medical records, police and judiciary records, and self-reported information from victim surveys and special studies. Multiple data sources, with their inherent strengths and limitations, are essential.

The most widely encountered sources of information are from the health and criminal justice sectors. Reliable data on violent deaths are not routinely collected in most countries. Where data collection systems are in place, coroner and mortuary reports, death certificates, and vital statistics records usually provide additional data about the victim. The health sector typically documents characteristics of the decedent and the cause, location, circumstances, and time of death. The criminal justice sector documents deaths or arrests resulting from interpersonal violence, including sometimes recording information about the relationship between the victim and the offender, the circumstances surrounding the violence, and the demographics of the perpetrator.

Theoretically, health and criminal justice sector data include information about nonfatal violence at all levels of severity, including threats of violence and instances of psychological violence, deprivation, and neglect. In practice, however, only data about violence-related injuries presenting at hospital emergency departments are collected. Studies from a variety of countries show that for every victim reporting violence to the police, at least two more present only at health agencies (Houry and others 1999; Kruger and others 1998; Sutherland, Sivarajasingam, and Shepherd 2002; additional sources online). Victims of nonfatal violence treated by the health sector may provide information about the perpetrator-victim relationship, about the circumstances surrounding the attack, and about contextual and developmental risk factors. However, the health sector is frequently restricted in recording information about perpetrators.

In LMICs, population-based surveys are a more useful source of information about violence-related injuries at all severity levels (Sethi, Habibula, and others 2004). Such surveys have been conducted in Bangladesh (Rahman, Andersson, and Svanstrom 1998); Colombia (Duque, Klevens, and Ramirez 2003); Iraq (Roberts and others 2004); Pakistan (Ghaffar 2001); South Africa (Butchart, Kruger, and Lekoba 2000; additional sources online); and Uganda (Kobusingye, Guwatudde, and Lett 2001). Demographic and health surveys with questions about violent victimization also collect information about the relationship between violence and other health conditions, but they can provide only limited insight into the perpetrators.

Hospital emergency departments have been used in some postconflict settings to monitor weapons-related injuries and evaluate the relative contributions of collective and interpersonal violence to the caseload (Meddings and

O'Connor 1999; Michael and others 1999). Some developing countries, such as Bangladesh, Kenya, and Uganda, also use violence and injury surveillance systems based in health facilities to monitor hospitalizations resulting from violence and other causes of injury (Kobusingye and Lett 2000; Odero and Kibosia 1995; Rahman and others 2001). Where emergency and forensic medical services are reasonably well developed and where access to such services is equitable, violence and injury surveillance tools have been integrated into hospital emergency departments (Hasbrouck and others 2002; additional sources online), prenatal clinics (Dunkle and others 2004), forensic service centers for rape victims (Swart and others 2000), and mortuaries (Butchart and others 2001). Those efforts have proven effective in obtaining victim-based, descriptive epidemiological information and insights into the relationships between victims and perpetrators.

Deaths Resulting from Interpersonal Violence. Global burden of disease estimates indicate that, in 2001, approximately 1.6 million people died as a result of violence. Of those deaths, 34 percent were due to interpersonal violence (table 40.1).

Rates and patterns of violent death vary by country and region (figure 40.1). Homicide rates were highest in developing countries in Sub-Saharan Africa and Latin America and the Caribbean and lowest in East Asia, the western Pacific, and some countries in northern Africa. Studies show a strong, inverse relationship between homicide rates and both economic development and economic equality (Butchart and Engstrom 2002; Fajnzylber, Lederman, and Loayza 2000). Poorer countries, especially those with large gaps between the rich and the poor, tend to have higher rates of homicide than wealthier countries.

Table 40.1 Estimated Violence-Related Deaths, by Type and Region, 2001

Category	Number[a]	Rate per 100,000 population[b]	Proportion of total (percent)
Suicide	875,000	15.2	53.3
Homicide	557,000	9.3	34.0
War-related fatality	208,000	3.5	12.7
Total	1,640,000	28.0	100.0
LMICs	1,489,000	31.0	90.8
High-income countries	150,000	14.3	9.2

Source: Mathers and others 2006.
a. Rounded to the nearest thousand.
b. Age standardized.

Homicide rates differ markedly by age and sex (table 40.2). Gender differences were least marked for children. For the 15 to 29 age group, male rates were nearly six times those for female rates; for the remaining age groups, male rates were from two to four times those for females. Female homicide rates doubled after age 14 and gradually but steadily increased with age, and male rates increased more than 14 times after age 14, peaked in the 15 to 29 age group, and then gradually decreased with age. Overall, homicides resulted in the deaths of 3.4 males per female.

Violence-Related Burden of Disease. The sum of years of potential life lost because of premature mortality and years of productive life lost because of disability is not a particularly useful measure of the burden of violence. Disability-adjusted life years rely, in part, on estimates of nonfatal events. In the case of violence, those estimates are restricted to injuries and

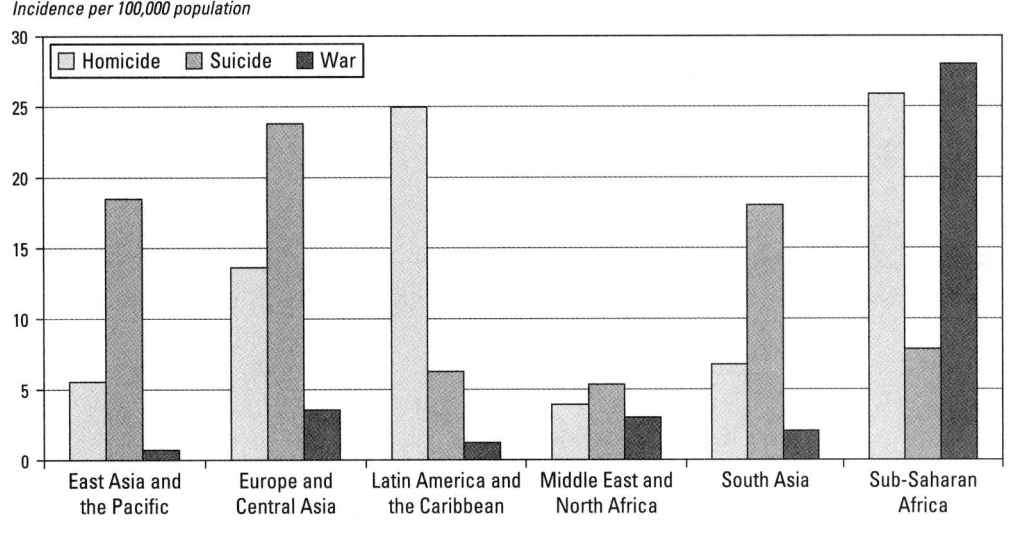

Incidence per 100,000 population

Source: Mathers and others 2006.

Figure 40.1 Homicide, Suicide, and War-Related Fatality Rates, by Region, 2001

Table 40.2 Estimated Global Homicide and Suicide Rates,
by Age Group, 2001
(number per 100,000 population)

Age	Homicides		Suicides	
	Males	Females	Males	Females
0–4 years	2.1	2.0	0.0	0.0
5–14 years	1.6	1.5	1.4	1.1
15–29 years	23.1	3.9	18.9	13.2
30–44 years	20.9	4.7	22.9	13.0
45–59 years	16.5	5.0	29.0	15.8
60+ years	12.6	5.4	41.7	20.8
Total	14.3	3.7	17.7	10.7

Source: Mathers and others 2006.

physical disabilities, both markedly underreported. In addition, given that psychological and other noninjury health consequences of violence are substantial, failure to include them in the measurement of disability-adjusted life years means that estimates of the nonfatal burden of violence may be grossly underestimated.

Violence-related morbidity can be analyzed as four distinct, but often co-occurring, outcome clusters: injuries and disabilities, mental health and behavioral consequences, reproductive health consequences, and other health consequences.

Studies in a number of countries show that, for every homicide among young people age 10 to 24, 20 to 40 other young people receive hospital treatment for a violent injury (Mercy and others 2002). Injuries range from minor, which can be self-treated, to severe. Severe injuries are those that may require resource-intensive emergency medical treatment and inpatient care and may result in lifelong disabilities, such as amputations, brain damage, or paraplegia. Few countries have information systems for monitoring nonfatal violent injuries, and existing systems typically record only data on violent injuries presenting at hospital emergency departments. Data from those sites cannot be directly compared, given the marked differences between and within countries in the availability and accessibility of emergency medical services.

The mental health consequences of violence are far reaching. Child abuse has well-documented sequelae of psychiatric disorders and suicidal behaviors (Runyan and others 2002). Both short- and long-term sequelae have been demonstrated (Mercy and others 2002, Heise and Garcia-Moreno 2002), including depression, anxiety disorders, substance abuse disorders, aggression, cognitive problems, sleep disorders, and posttraumatic stress disorder. The severity and duration of those consequences vary with the child's age and the length of time the child suffers the abuse, as well as the duration and intensity of the abuse, the child's relationship to the abuser, and the treatment received (Runyan and others 2002).

Intimate partner violence results in an increased incidence of suicide and suicide attempts, as well as in depression, anxiety, and phobias (Heise and Garcia-Moreno 2002). Additional consequences include substance abuse, eating and sleep disorders, poor self-esteem, posttraumatic stress disorder, psychosomatic disorders, and risky sexual behaviors. Sexual assault results in consequences that can be long lasting and severe, including posttraumatic stress disorder, depression, and conduct disorders, as well as sleep and eating disorders (Jewkes, Sen, and Garcia-Moreno 2002).

According to Jewkes, Sen, and Garcia-Moreno (2002), among adolescents and women age 12 to 45, the frequency of pregnancy as a result of rape varies from 5 to 18 percent. In addition, younger rape victims often have an increased rate of later, unintended pregnancies. Rape frequently results in gynecological problems, problems of sexual functioning, and sexually transmitted diseases, including HIV infection. HIV infection and the stigma it carries put both female and male victims of sexual assault at increased risk of further violence. A similar range of reproductive health consequences may also follow intimate partner violence.

A strong, graded relationship exists between the breadth of exposure to abuse or household dysfunction during childhood and the presence of adult diseases, including ischemic heart disease, cancer, chronic lung disease, skeletal fractures, and liver disease (Felitti and others 1998). In developed countries, abuse and other violent events of childhood have been associated with a 4- to 12-fold increased risk for alcoholism, drug abuse, depression, and suicide attempt; a 2- to 4-fold increased risk for smoking, poor self-rated health, 50 or more sexual intercourse partners, and sexually transmitted disease; and a 1.4- to 1.6-fold increased risk for physical inactivity and severe obesity (Anda and others 1999; Dietz and others 1999; Dube and others 2001, 2002; Hillis and others 2000, 2001; Williamson and others 2002). Similar exposures to violence in developing countries may have different, yet equally wide-ranging, impacts beyond direct physical and psychological injuries.

Data on Violence in Developing Countries

Studies documenting the human and economic toll of violence in LMICs are strikingly scarce. In addition to disparate levels of economic development, other differences between countries strongly influence levels and patterns of interpersonal violence and the toll that such violence takes on society. Countries with weak governments and institutions are at considerably higher risk for interpersonal violence than countries with developed institutions, and countries at war are likewise at higher risk than countries at peace. The same factors that lead to high levels of interpersonal violence—lack of economic development; weak social, political, and judicial institutions; social disturbances; and warfare—also adversely affect nations' ability to collect data and to address the causes or consequences of this violence.

Table 40.3 Risk Factors for Becoming a Victim or Perpetrator of Violence

Level of the ecological model	Risk factors
Individual (biological and personal history factors that influence how individuals behave)	Early developmental experience
	Demographic characteristics (for example, age, education, family, or personal income)
	Victim of child abuse and neglect
	Psychological and personality disorders
	Physical health and disabilities
	Alcohol or substance abuse problems
	History of violent behavior
	Youth
	Male
	Gun ownership
Relationship (with family members, friends, intimate partners, peers)	Marital conflicts around gender roles and resources
	Association with friends who engage in violent or delinquent behavior
	Poor parenting practices
	Parental conflict involving use of violence
	Low socioeconomic status of household
Community (neighborhoods, schools, workplaces)	High residential mobility
	High unemployment
	High population density
	Social isolation
	Proximity to drug trade
	Inadequate victim care services
	Poverty
	Weak policies and programs in, for example, workplaces, schools, residential care facilities
Societal (broad factors that reduce inhibitions against violence)	Rapid social change
	Economic inequality
	Gender inequality
	Policies that create and sustain or increase economic and social inequalities
	Norms that give priority to parents' rights over child welfare
	Norms that entrench male dominance over women
	Poverty
	Weak economic safety nets
	Poor rule of law
	Poor criminal justice system that supports the use of excessive violence by police officers against citizens and leaves perpetrators immune from prosecution
	Social or cultural norms that support violence
	Availability of means (for example, firearms)
	Conflict or postconflict situation

Source: Krug and others 2002a.

Risk Factors for Understanding Violence

Risk factors for violence are conditions that increase the possibility of becoming a victim or perpetrator of violence. No single factor explains why a person or group is at a high or low risk of violence. Rather, violence is an outcome of a complex interaction among many factors. This relationship is captured in an ecological model that classifies risk factors for violence by four levels: individual, relationship, community, and societal (Dahlberg and Krug 2002). Although some risk factors may be unique to a particular type of violence, the various types of violence more commonly share a number of risk factors (table 40.3).

ECONOMIC IMPACT OF VIOLENCE

Violence exacts an extraordinary economic toll.

Costs of Violence

Estimates of the costs of violence vary broadly, with many of the differences resulting from the inclusion or exclusion of different categories. Cost categories can be broadly grouped into direct costs, which result directly from acts of violence or attempts to prevent them, and indirect costs, which include the opportunity cost of time, lost productivity, and impaired quality of life.

Those and other methodological issues lead to differing estimates of the costs of violence.[2] Researchers have calculated the value of a human life using lost wages, estimates of the quality of life, wage premiums for risky jobs, willingness to pay for safety measures, and individual behavior related to safety measures. The value of human life used in U.S. studies ranges from US$3.1 million to US$6.8 million (Fisher, Chestnut, and Violette 1989; Viscusi 1993; additional sources online). The rate used to discount future costs and benefits also varies, generally from 2 to 10 percent.[3]

Fromm (2001) reviews a variety of sources and calculates an aggregate total of US$94 billion in annual costs to the U.S. economy resulting from child abuse, which is equal to 1 percent of gross domestic product (GDP). The estimate includes direct medical costs and related costs of legal services, policing, and incarceration, as well as the value of indirect productivity losses, psychological costs, and future criminality. Using secondary sources, Courtney (1999) calculates direct costs of US$14 billion, including counseling and child welfare services, resulting from child abuse in the United States.

The Centers for Disease Control and Prevention (CDC 2003) cite an estimated 5.3 million victimizations involving intimate partner violence each year in the United States among women 18 and older, resulting in nearly 2 million injuries. More than 550,000 of those injuries require medical attention. The costs of intimate partner violence, including medical care, mental health care, and lost productivity, exceed US$5.8 billion annually.

As a percentage of GDP, estimates of the costs of intimate partner violence are considerably higher in LMICs than in high-income countries. Morrison and Orlando (1999) calculate the costs of domestic violence against women on the basis of stratified random samples of women. Using only the lost productive capacity of the women, they extrapolate total costs of US$1.73 billion in Chile and US$32.7 million in Nicaragua. In a subsequent publication, Buvinic and Morrison (1999) calculate that the direct medical costs plus lost productivity are equivalent to 2.0 percent of GDP in Chile and 1.6 percent of GDP in Nicaragua.

Several studies have used the U.S. National Crime Victimization Survey, an annual survey based on 100,000 inter-views with crime victims, to estimate the incidence and calculate the direct costs of sexual assault. For example, Miller, Cohen, and Rossman (1993) calculate average psychological costs of US$66,600 for each rape and total costs of US$85,000 for sexual assault resulting in physical injury. Psychological costs, also referred to as "pain and suffering," are considered indirect costs. Because many studies do not include those types of costs, cost estimates vary widely.

Violence at the workplace also extracts an economic toll, but studies of its magnitude are not well developed and are hampered by measurement difficulties and nonstandardized methodologies. Biddle and Hartley (2002) study homicides in the workplace in the United States and calculate an annual cost of approximately US$970 million. An international report commissioned by the International Labour Organization on the costs of violence and stress in work environments estimates that losses from stress and violence at work are equivalent to 1.0 to 3.5 percent of GDP over a range of countries (Hoel, Sparks, and Cooper 2001). All those studies use a broad definition of *workplace violence,* including psychological violence such as sexual harassment and bullying.

Violence committed by juveniles is particularly costly to society. Miller's (2001) analysis of violent crimes committed in Pennsylvania in 1993 finds that juvenile violence accounted for 24.7 percent of all violent crimes and 46.6 percent of total victim costs from violent crime. Cohen (1988) calculates that the total cost to society of a youth engaging in a life of crime ranges from US$1.9 million to US$2.6 million.

Proximate Risk Factors

Alcohol, drugs, and guns contribute to the costs of interpersonal violence. According to estimates by the Children's Safety Network Economics and Insurance Resource Center (1997), the cost of violent crime committed under the influence of alcohol equaled US$33.3 million in 1995, or 8.3 percent of the cost of all violent crime in the United States. The National Crime Prevention Council (1999) estimates that the cost of all drug-related crime, including productivity costs, amounts to US$60 billion to US$100 billion annually in the United States, with violent crime accounting for approximately 10 percent of this figure.

Cook and Ludwig (2000) estimate that the annual costs of gun violence in the United States are on the order of US$100 billion. Miller and Cohen (1997) calculate a significantly higher estimate for the toll of gun-related violence in the United States: US$155 billion (including psychological costs and the value of quality of life). They also calculate that, on a per capita basis, the cost of gun violence in Canada equals one-third of the U.S. cost. Peden and van der Spuy's (1998) study at the Groote Schurr Hospital in Cape Town, South Africa, finds that direct medical costs averaged R 30,628 (US$10,308) per gunshot victim.

Effects on Public Finances

The public sector (and thus society in general) bears many of the costs of interpersonal violence. Several studies (Klein and others 1999; Payne and others 1993; additional sources online) find that 56 to 80 percent of U.S. health care costs for stabbing and gun injuries are either directly paid by public financing or are not paid at all. In the latter case, government and society absorb the costs in the form of uncompensated care financing and overall higher payment rates. In LMICs, society likely also absorbs the costs of violence through direct public expenditures and negative effects on investment and economic growth.

INTERVENTIONS

The evidence base of ways to prevent violence is expanding rapidly, but huge gaps remain in relation to effective strategies for reducing the health burden associated with interpersonal violence. The greatest strides have come in the areas of youth violence and child abuse, and almost all the prevention knowledge has been developed in high-income countries. Despite those limitations, an understanding of the epidemiology and etiology of violence and prevention provides important insights into the spectrum of policies and interventions that can be drawn on to prevent violence in LMICs.

Violence Prevention Strategies

The many commonalities among the various forms of violence in relation to their epidemiology and etiology suggest that common pathways to prevention may be available (Reza, Mercy, and Krug 2001). A typology of prevention strategies is useful in sorting through the complexities and commonalities of this problem to identify the range of strategies that might be incorporated into effective violence prevention plans. We propose a typology of prevention based on two key dimensions: the stages of human development and the ecological model mentioned earlier.

The epidemiology of violence, including its onset, desistance, and continuity, is closely related to the stages of human development (Williams, Guerra, and Elliott 1997). Increasing evidence points to the existence of discrete developmental pathways to violent behavior (Loeber and others 1993; Tolan and Gorman-Smith 1998; U.S. Department of Health and Human Services 2001; additional sources online). Thus, intervening at early developmental stages may reduce the likelihood that violence is expressed during later developmental stages.

The ecological model is also an important dimension of the typology, because violence is the product of multiple and overlapping levels of influence on behavior. The ecological model assumes that violent behavior is influenced by social contexts and the individual attributes brought to these contexts. Intervention may therefore attempt to influence aspects or risk factors at any or all of the model's four levels (Dahlberg and Krug 2002; Mercy and Hammond 1999).

Table 40.4 presents our typology of prevention strategies. The examples presented are not exhaustive, nor have all the strategies proven effective. Rather, they illustrate the breadth of potential solutions and emphasize the need to consider addressing the problem simultaneously at different stages of human development and through different social contexts. In many cases, an intervention might have an effect on multiple forms of violence. At this time, data to prove or disprove the effectiveness of most of these interventions are insufficient, and in those cases in which sufficient data are available, they are almost always from high-income countries.

Strategic Focuses for Prevention

A simple understanding of the approaches illustrated in table 40.4 is insufficient for developing a comprehensive violence prevention strategy. A public health approach to violence prevention concentrates on identifying ways to keep people from committing violent acts. Interventions may eliminate or reduce the underlying risk factors and shore up protective factors. Interventions are typically classified in terms of three levels of prevention: primary, secondary, and tertiary (Dahlberg and Krug 2002).

Primary Prevention. Primary prevention interventions focus on preventing violence before it occurs. The literature has given rise to several strategic focuses for the primary prevention of violence that are important considerations in violence prevention planning. Some have been successfully implemented at the community level in LMICs.

The cultural context plays an important role in violent behavior. Cultural traditions are sometimes used to justify such social practices as female genital mutilation and severe physical punishment of children (Mercy and others 2003). Conversely, cultural norms can be a source of protection against violence, such as traditions that promote the equality of women or respect for the elderly. Although evidence-based approaches for changing cultural traditions as a violence prevention strategy are not yet available, some countries have adopted this strategy. In South Africa, the Soul City health promotion campaign makes residents aware of the extent and consequences of violence and encourages better parenting through role models and improved communication among family members. Evaluations have found shifts in attitudes and social norms concerning intimate partner violence and domestic relations. Willingness to change behavior and take action to stop violence has increased in urban and rural areas among both men and women (Krug and others 2002b,

Table 40.4 Prevention Strategies, by Developmental Stage and Ecological Context

Level of the ecological model	Developmental stage			
	Infant and toddler years (age birth–3)	**Childhood (age 4–11)**	**Adolescence (age 12–19)**	**Adulthood (age 20+)**
Individual	• Reduction in unintended pregnancies • Access to prenatal and postnatal services • Treatment programs for child witnesses of violence and victims of maltreatment to reduce consequences	• Social development training[a] • Preschool enrichment programs[a] • Drug-resistance education[b] • School-based programs to prevent child maltreatment • Community-based prevention of child sexual abuse • Gun safety training	• Social development training[a] • Drug-resistance education[b] • Educational incentives for at-risk, disadvantaged students[a] • Individual counseling[b] • Supervised exposure to prison and morgue (shock or scare high-risk youth[b]) • Residential programs in psychiatric or correctional institutions[b] • Academic enrichment programs • Gun safety training • Boot camps[b] • Waivers to try in adult court[b] • School-based violence prevention programs[a]	• Incentives for postsecondary education or vocational training • Services for adults abused as children • Treatment for child and intimate partner abuse offenders • Waiting periods for firearm purchases • Owner liability for damage by guns
Relationship	• Home visitation services[a] • Parenting training[a] • Therapeutic foster care	• Parenting training[a] • Mentoring • Partnership programs between homes and schools to promote parental involvement	• Mentoring[a] • Peer mediation and counseling[b] • Temporary foster care programs for serious and chronic delinquents • Family therapy[a]	• Programs to strengthen ties to family • Programs to strengthen ties to jobs • Couples therapy • Relationship education
Community	• Lead monitoring and toxin removal • Screening by health care providers for maltreatment	• Safe havens for children on high-risk routes to and from school • After school programs to extend adult supervision • Recreational programs	• Recreational programs • Multicomponent gang prevention programs[b] • Health care professionals trained in identification and referral of high-risk youth and victims of sexual violence • Community policing • Improvements in emergency response, trauma care, and access to health services • Programs to buy back guns[b] • Metal detectors in schools	• Adult recreation programs • Shelters and crisis centers for battered women and victims of elder abuse • Criminal justice reforms to criminalize child maltreatment, intimate partner violence, and elder abuse • Mandatory arrest policies for intimate partner violence • Public shaming of intimate partner violence offenders • Services for identifying and treating elder abuses • Health care professional training in identification and referral of victims of elder abuse and sexual violence

Table 40.4 Continued

Level of the ecological model	Developmental stage			
	Infant and toddler years (age birth–3)	Childhood (age 4–11)	Adolescence (age 12–19)	Adulthood (age 20+)
	• Community policing • Emergency response and trauma care improvements • Health care providers trained in the detection and reporting of child maltreatment • Programs to buy back guns[b] • Promotion of safe storage of firearms and other lethal means of inflicting violence • Prevention and education campaigns to increase awareness of child maltreatment • Child protection service programs		• Community policing • Emergency response and trauma care improvements • Programs to buy back guns[b] • Disruption of illegal gun markets • Prohibition of firearm sales to high-risk purchasers • Mandatory sentences for gun use in crimes • Coordinated community interventions for violence prevention • Prevention and education campaigns to increase awareness of youth violence, intimate partner violence, sexual violence, and elder abuse	
Societal	• Promote cultural norms to value and protect life • Promote strength-based cognitive and socio-emotional skills from birth	• Reduce violent content of movies, television, video games, and Internet sites available to children • Launch public information campaigns to promote pro-social norms	• Reduce violent content of movies, television, video games, and Internet sites available to children • Enforce laws prohibiting illegal transfers of guns to youths	• Establish job creation programs for the chronically unemployed
		• Strengthen police and judicial systems • Deconcentrate poverty • Reduce income inequality	• Strengthen police and judicial systems • Promote safe storage of firearms • Deconcentrate poverty • Reduce income inequality • Change cultural norms that support violence and abuse of children and adults	

Source: Authors.

a. These programs have been demonstrated to be effective in reducing violence or risk factors for violence.

b. These programs have been found to be ineffective in reducing violence.

box 9.1). In the Kapchorwa district of Uganda, a community health program has enlisted the support of elders in adopting alternative practices to female genital mutilation that are consistent with their cultural traditions (United Nations Population Fund 1998).

The lethality of interpersonal violence is affected by the means people use to carry out this violence. Reducing access to lethal means, such as firearms, may help minimize the health consequences of violence. A wide variety of strategies have been used to restrict access to firearms, such as mandating waiting periods before purchase, promoting safe storage of firearms, and limiting where firearms can and cannot be carried. In the mid 1990s, Colombian officials in Bogotá and Cali, noting that homicide rates increased during weekends following paydays, on national holidays, and near elections, implemented a ban on carrying handguns during those times, which resulted in a 13 to 14 percent reduction in homicide rates (Villaveces and others 2000). In the Australian state of Victoria, firearm-related suicides, assaults, and unintentional deaths decreased following the 1988 implementation of legislation that required the registration of all firearms and strengthened licensing regulations; a mandatory waiting period was added in 1996 (Ozanne-Smith and others 2004). However, the evidence to determine whether such strategies are effective in reducing firearm-related homicides is currently insufficient (Hahn and others 2003), although several policies hold promise (Hemenway 2004; Ludwig and Cook 2003).

Inadequate parental involvement in children's and adolescents' activities and lack of supervision are well-established risk factors for youth violence (U.S. Department of Health and Human Services 2001). Evidence indicates that a supportive relationship with parents or other adults is protective against antisocial behavior. Although not widely evaluated, some mentoring programs that match high-risk youths with a positive adult role model appear to be effective in reducing youth violence (Grossman and Garry 1997; Thornton and others 2002); however, negative findings have also been reported for mentoring, particularly when mentors receive little training and when the relationships between adults and youths break down. The design of mentoring programs varies considerably, and participation by both mentors and youths can be uneven.

Programs that target those who influence children are more effective than interventions that target all adults. For example, preschool enrichment, home visitation, and parenting programs have been found to have both short- and long-term effects on preventing violence (Farrington 2003; Mercy and others 2002; Utting 2003; additional sources online). Early intervention can help shape attitudes, knowledge, and behavior of children at a time when they are more open to positive influences and can affect their behavior over their lifetime (Mercy and others 1993).

Income inequality is a risk factor universally associated with interpersonal and collective violence (Butchart and Engstrom 2002; Zwi, Garfield, and Loretti 2002; additional sources online). Poverty itself does not appear to be consistently associated with violence, but the juxtaposition of extreme poverty with extreme wealth appears to be a key ingredient in recipes for violence. Economic programs or policies that reduce or minimize the effects of income inequality may be strategic in violence prevention, although the evidence base for such interventions has not been established.

Secondary and Tertiary Prevention. Although an emphasis on primary prevention is essential for reducing the health burden associated with violence, secondary prevention programs and services are necessary for addressing the immediate consequences of violent actions and behaviors, and tertiary programs focus on long-term care. Efforts targeted at victims of violence are extremely important for mitigating the physical and psychological consequences of the various forms of violence and abuse and for reducing victims' risks for future violence (National Center for Injury Prevention and Control 2002).

Physicians and other health professionals are gatekeepers in efforts to monitor, identify, treat, and intervene in cases of interpersonal violence. As previously noted, more cases of interpersonal violence come to the attention of health care providers than of police. The role of health care providers in prevention efforts is neither widely understood nor embraced, and many institutional and educational barriers limit their effectiveness (Cohen, De Vos, and Newberger 1997). Programs to educate health care providers are under way worldwide. Many hospital emergency departments, doctors' offices, and clinic settings use screening programs to identify victims of intimate partner violence, child abuse, or elder abuse, although the effectiveness of those interventions in reducing subsequent violence is not well understood (Heise and Garcia-Moreno 2002; Runyan and others 2002; Wolf, Daichman, and Bennett 2002).

Therapeutic approaches have been implemented in many parts of the world to reduce child abuse. Though some research suggests that these interventions can improve the mental health of victims, less information is available on other benefits (Runyan and others 2002; additional sources online). One approach to preventing child sexual abuse in the United States challenges social norms by offering help to those at risk of offending and by encouraging adults to watch for and act on warnings of child sexual abuse before an offense is committed (CDC 2001). Under such programs, individuals voluntarily turn themselves in for treatment and thereby prevent potential future violence.

The outcome of injury from interpersonal violence depends not only on its severity, but also on the speed and appropriateness of treatment (Committee on Trauma Research 1985). Establishment of trauma systems designed to treat and manage injured victims efficiently and effectively is an important factor in reducing the health burden of violence. Research suggests that reductions in criminal assaults resulting in death in the United States are partly explained by the increased survival of victims. Developments in medical technology and trauma services may be reducing the number of interpersonal violence fatalities (Harris and others 2002). Hospital emergency departments may also provide an opportunity to intervene with victims who might otherwise seek revenge against their attackers or victims who are at greater risk for revictimization (Muelleman and others 1996).

COST-EFFECTIVENESS OF INTERVENTIONS

Studies show that implementing preventive interventions costs less than dealing with the outcomes of violence, in some cases by several orders of magnitude.

Examples of Cost-Saving Interventions

To date, most evaluations of preventive interventions measure cost and effects in high-income countries. Although cost savings may not be comparable in LMICs, effects may be greater.

Legislation and Shelter for Abused Women. The 1994 Violence against Women Act in the United States has resulted in an estimated net benefit of US$16.4 billion, including US$14.8 billion in averted victims' costs (Clark, Biddle, and Martin 2002). This wide-ranging legislation introduced programs aimed at deterring crimes against women and providing assistance to female victims of crimes. Interventions include penalties for repeat offenders, use of sexual history in criminal and civil cases, programs for victims of child abuse, safe homes for women, confidentiality of the abused person's address, and pretrial detention in sex offense cases. Chanley, Chanley, and Campbell's (2001) analysis shows that providing shelters for victims of domestic violence results in an estimated cost-benefit ratio of 18.4 to 6.8.

Parent Training and Home Visitation. Caldwell (1992) estimates that the costs of child abuse and neglect in Michigan are US$1 billion a year, including the costs of crimes committed by the victims of child abuse later in life and the costs of their incarceration. The study estimates that prevention costs, including a home visitor program for every family and a comprehensive parent education program, are just one-nineteenth of the cost of child abuse. Armstrong's (1983) cost-benefit analysis of a child abuse prevention program in Yeardon, Pennsylvania, finds net savings of US$647,000 per year and a cost-benefit ratio of 1.86.

Registering Firearms. Chapdelaine and Maurice (1996) quantify the costs and benefits of a Canadian law that required gun owners to register their firearms by January 1, 2001. Implementing a universal licensing and registration system cost approximately US$70 million (2001 U.S. dollars), including a significant one-time expense, compared with annual direct health care costs of gun-related violence of US$50 million. When the indirect costs of gun violence are included, the economic benefits of the law are much clearer. Miller (1995) estimates the total costs of firearm-related injuries in Canada at US$5.6 billion, including lost productivity and psychological costs, equivalent to 1 percent of Canada's GDP.

Youth Intervention. Greenwood and others (1996) compare interventions to reduce youth crime in the United States and find that providing high school students with incentives to graduate, which costs US$14,100 per program participant, is the most cost-effective intervention, resulting in an estimated 258 serious crimes prevented per US$1 million spent. Parent training prevents an estimated 157 serious crimes per US$1 million, compared with 72 for delinquent supervision programs and 11 for home visits and day care. All those interventions (excluding home visits) are more cost-effective than California's "three strikes" law, which incarcerates for life those individuals convicted of three serious crimes.

Need for LMIC Cost-Benefit Data

Though violence disproportionately affects LMICs, studies of the economic effects of violence in those countries are scarce. Comparisons with high-income countries are complicated by the tendency to undervalue economic losses related to productivity in lower-income countries, because such losses are typically based on forgone wages and income. Thus, when the costs of violent homicides are calculated, the estimates range from US$15,319 per homicide in South Africa, to US$829,000 in New Zealand, to more than US$2 million in the United States. Given the existing methodological differences and widespread gaps in the literature, systematic research into the costs of

violence and the costs versus benefits of prevention efforts is urgently needed.

IMPLEMENTATION OF PREVENTION STRATEGIES

Promoting violence prevention involves encouraging and supporting the development, implementation, and evaluation of programs explicitly designed to stop the perpetration of violence at local, regional, and national levels.

The 2003 World Health Assembly Resolution (WHA56.24) on implementing the recommendations of the *World Report on Violence and Health* (Krug and others 2002b; see also Butchart and others 2004) advocates a five-point strategy.

Increasing Capacity for Collecting and Managing Data

Increased capacity for collecting health, criminal justice, and social service sector data on violence and its consequences is fundamental to building a sustained, high-level policy and intervention programming response in LMICs. Population-level data are needed to design and evaluate community-level intervention trials. Health sector data can cover a larger and often different subset of violence-related injuries than police statistics and, with criminal justice and social service data, can strengthen abilities to define the problem, identify causes and risk factors, design appropriate interventions, and monitor the interventions' effectiveness.

Information systems play a large role in recent efforts to address infectious diseases such as tuberculosis and HIV, allowing better identification of high-risk populations and appropriate interventions. A similar role is imminent for violence prevention. As previously stated, information systems must integrate data from the criminal justice, labor, education, social services, and health sectors and must be linked with systems housed at multilateral agencies or regional joint initiatives. Sharing information regionally allows countries to identify opportunities for collaboration and to share best practices.

Support for Research

Supporting research on the causes, consequences, and prevention of violence has proven effective in mobilizing prevention responses in developing countries. In South Africa, the 1997 Essential National Health Research Conference identified research for improved violence prevention and control as a top priority, and in 2001, the Medical Research Council established a program to give violence prevention research the same priority as research into HIV/AIDS, tuberculosis, and malaria (Jeenah and others 1997; Medical Research Council of South Africa 2004). South Africa also has applied research data in various prevention contexts, including establishment of a national violence and injury mortality surveillance system, passage of firearms legislation, assessment of national and municipal-level burden-of-disease estimates, and design of prevention programs (Butchart and others 2001; Groenewald and others 2003).

The currently limited evidence base and understanding of the causes of all types of violence must be expanded through planned, documented, evaluated, and shared research. Some developing countries have opportunities to develop and document prevention programs in special settings, such as for refugees, orphans, nomadic, displaced, and homeless populations.

Promoting Primary Prevention

An important first step in promoting primary prevention is systematic documentation of existing prevention programs. Records can include information on the types of violence and risk factors addressed, target populations served, interventions used, and any monitoring and measurement of the effects. Such information can help make the programs more visible to policy makers and development partners and can be used to promote increased investment in programs that apply proven and promising interventions.

WHO has outlined a methodology for systematic documentation (Sethi, Marais, and others 2004, 22–33) and has initiated a project to evaluate the feasibility and utility of such documentation in selected cities and provinces in Brazil, India, Jamaica, Jordan, the former Yugoslav Republic of Macedonia, Mozambique, the Russian Federation, and South Africa.

Strengthening Support Services for Victims

A situational analysis of the accessibility and organization of emergency, acute, long-term, and rehabilitative services can identify needs and help strengthen care and support services for victims of violence. The establishment and adequate funding of first responder systems, such as police and ambulance teams, may lower the costs of violence and contribute to prevention. Maps showing hospitals and clinics with specialized systems for treating victims of violence can help these first responders. Ready access to legal resources empowers victims. Mock and others (2004) offer guidelines for strengthening victim care and support services.

Claramunt and Cortes's (2003) assessment in Belize, Costa Rica, El Salvador, Guatemala, Honduras, and Nicaragua established baseline information that could be used to advocate for strengthened medical and legal services for victims of sexual violence. Their findings included a lack of adequate medical and legal information systems, the insufficient training of medical staff, and a lack of clear protocols for moving patients through the system. Services in associated sectors—medical, forensic, social, and legal—should be examined, because integrated efforts can improve access to and value of services that previously existed in isolation. Training of medical and legal service providers in activities aimed at preventing violence may also affect the success of long-term prevention; however, this training strategy has not been extensively evaluated.

Developing Action Plans

A national plan of action for preventing interpersonal violence and improving victim support and care is the blueprint that provides a set of common goals, a shared time frame, a strategy for coordinating activities, and a framework for evaluating the different sectors involved. Such a plan is therefore central to organizing national and community-level interventions that involve more than one objective and that depend on input from many different sectors. Strong political support from the highest levels of government is important in aligning the various players and ensuring that the plan is implemented and that associated programs are maintained. Nongovernmental organizations may provide support and continuity in countries where programs may be interrupted because of unstable, changing governments.

Collaboration among national governments and health-related nongovernmental and multilateral organizations can establish the importance of formally addressing violence through public health approaches. Though legal and criminal justice approaches provide a deterrent, experience in high-income countries suggests that a proactive public health approach can reduce the negative health, social, and economic consequences of interpersonal violence.

CONCLUSIONS: PROMISES AND PITFALLS

Violence prevention may be seen as a luxury rather than a public health priority in LMICs; however, the magnitude of the problem and the associated health burden negate this view. Resolutions on violence prevention passed by the World Health Assembly and codified in the *World Report on Violence and Health* and reports from the United Nations Crime Prevention Council present frameworks for approaching violence prevention. The first World Health Assembly resolution was cosponsored by a developing country, South Africa, and a developed country, the United States. Both recognized the importance of making violence prevention a global public health priority even before evidence of effectiveness could be collected. Seven years after the resolution, both developing and developed countries applauded and adopted the *World Report on Violence and Health*, signaling the beginning of an exciting new agenda for public health.

The public health model for violence prevention focuses on primary prevention and intervention for victims and emphasizes the value of integrating efforts across sectors. However, the model is weakened by a paucity of sustained interventions and measured outcomes in LMICs.

Currently, the best approach may be to take small, incremental steps, focusing on relatively discrete and easily implemented interventions that address a prevalent problem. LMICs should build on programs for which some evidence of effectiveness exists in high-income countries and adopt a "learn as you go" approach.

Many LMICs face the daunting challenges of the spreading HIV/AIDS epidemic and ongoing intergroup conflict or war. Those problems can destroy the infrastructure of civil society, increase stress and economic hardship, and lead to increases in suicide and interpersonal violence of all kinds—in both sexes and at all ages. In prioritizing violence prevention efforts, policy makers and health care professionals may mitigate some of the secondary repercussions of these deadly factors.

A great deal of progress has been made in violence prevention. There is strong reason to believe that the interventions under way and the capacity to implement violence prevention will make a difference. The lessons learned to date during the public health community's short experience with violence prevention are consistent with the lessons from the community's much longer experience with the prevention of infectious and chronic diseases. Violence can be prevented in LMICs if their governments, their citizens, and the global community start now, act wisely, and work together.

ACKNOWLEDGMENTS

The editors thank Linda I. Dahlberg for her thoughtful contributions and Angela Browne for her review.

NOTES

1. The World Bank (2004) classifies countries by annual gross national income (2001 U.S. dollars) per capita as follows: low-income, US$735 or less; lower-middle-income, US$736 to US$2,935; upper-middle-income, US$2,936 to US$9,075; and high-income, US$9,076 or more.

2. Cost estimates have been converted to 2001 U.S. dollars to facilitate comparisons.

3. Whenever possible, we have cited results calculated using a 3 percent discount rate, as recommended by the U.S. Panel on Cost-Effectiveness in Medicine (Gold, Siegel, and Weinstein 2001).

REFERENCES

Anda, R. F., J. B. Croft, V. J. Felitti, D. Nordenberg, W. H. Giles, D. F. Williamson, and others. 1999. "Adverse Childhood Experiences and Smoking during Adolescence and Adulthood." *Journal of the American Medical Association* 282 (17): 1652–58.

Armstrong, K. A. 1983. "Economic Analysis of a Child Abuse Program." *Child Welfare* 62 (1): 3–13.

Biddle, E., and D. Hartley. 2002. "The Cost of Workplace Homicides in the USA, 1980–1997." Abstract submitted for the World Health Organization's Sixth World Conference on Injury Prevention and Control, Montreal, May 12–15.

Butchart, A., and K. Engstrom. 2002. "Sex- and Age-Specific Effects of Economic Development and Inequality on Homicide Rates in 0 to 24 Year Olds: A Cross-Sectional Analysis." *Bulletin of the World Health Organization* 80: 797–805.

Butchart, A., J. Kruger, and R. Lekoba. 2000. "Perceptions of Injury Causes and Solutions in a Johannesburg Township: Implications for Prevention." *Social Science and Medicine* 50: 331–44.

Butchart, A., M. Peden, R. Matzopoulos, S. Burrows, R. Phillips, N. Bhagwandin, and others. 2001. "The South African National Non-natural Mortality Surveillance System: Rationale, Pilot Results, and Evaluation." *South African Medical Journal* 91 (5): 408–17.

Butchart, A., A. Phinney, P. Check, and A. Villaveces. 2004. *Preventing Violence: A Guide to Implementing the Recommendations of the* World Report on Violence and Health. Geneva: Department of Injuries and Violence Prevention, World Health Organization.

Buvinic M., and A. Morrison. 1999. *Violence as an Obstacle to Development.* 1–8. Washington, DC: Inter-American Development Bank.

Caldwell, R. A. 1992. *The Costs of Child Abuse vs. Child Abuse Prevention: Michigan's Experience.* East Lansing: Michigan Children's Trust Fund.

CDC (Centers for Disease Control and Prevention). 2001. "Evaluation of a Child Sexual Abuse Prevention Program: Vermont, 1995–1997." *Morbidity and Mortality Weekly Report* 50 (5): 77–78, 87.

———. 2003. *Costs of Intimate Partner Violence against Women in the United States.* Atlanta: National Center for Injury Prevention and Control.

Chanley, S. A., J. J. Chanley, and H. E. Campbell. 2001. "Providing Refuge: The Value of Domestic Violence Shelter Services." *American Review of Public Administration* 31: 393–413.

Chapdelaine, A., and P. Maurice. 1996. "Firearms Injury Prevention and Gun Control in Canada." *Canadian Medical Association Journal* 155 (9): 1285–89.

Children's Safety Network Economics and Insurance Resource Center. 1997. *Cost of Violent Crime and of Alcohol-Involved and Drug-Involved Violent Crime in the USA, 1995.* Landover, MD: National Public Services Research Institute.

Claramunt, M. C., and M. V. Cortes. 2003. *Situación de los servicios medico-legales y de salud para víctimas de violencia sexual en Centroamérica.* Serie genero y salud publica 14. San José, Costa Rica: Pan-American Health Organization.

Clark, K. A., A. K. Biddle, and S. L. Martin. 2002. "A Cost-Benefit Analysis of the Violence against Women Act of 1994." *Violence against Women* 8 (4): 417–28.

Cohen, M. A. 1988. "The Monetary Value of Saving a High-Risk Youth." *Journal of Quantitative Criminology* 14 (1): 5–33.

Cohen, S., E. De Vos, and E. Newberger. 1997. "Barriers to Physician Identification and Treatment of Family Violence: Lessons from Five Communities." *Academic Medicine* 72 (Suppl. 1): S19–25.

Committee on Trauma Research, National Research Council, Institute of Medicine. 1985. *Injury in America: A Continuing Public Health Problem.* Washington, DC: National Academy Press.

Cook, P. J., and J. Ludwig. 2000. *Gun Violence: The Real Costs.* New York: Oxford University Press.

Courtney, M. E. 1999. "National Call to Action: Working toward the Elimination of Child Maltreatment. The Economics." *Child Abuse and Neglect* 23 (10): 975–86.

Dahlberg, L. L., and E. G. Krug. 2002. "Violence: A Global Public Health Problem." In *World Report on Violence and Health,* ed. E. G. Krug, L. L. Dahlberg, J. A. Mercy, A. B. Zwi, and R. Lozano, 1–21. Geneva: World Health Organization.

Dietz, P. M., A. M. Spitz, R. F. Anda, D. F. Williamson, P. M. McMahon, J. S. Santelli, and others. 1999. "Unintended Pregnancy among Adult Women Exposed to Abuse or Household Dysfunction during Their Childhood." *Journal of the American Medical Association* 282: 1359–64.

Dube, S. R., R. F. Anda, V. J. Felitti, D. P. Chapman, D. F. Williamson, and W. H. Giles. 2001. "Childhood Abuse, Household Dysfunction, and the Risk of Attempted Suicide throughout the Life Span: Findings from the Adverse Childhood Experiences Study." *Journal of the American Medical Association* 286: 3089–96.

Dube, S. R., R. F. Anda, V. J. Felitti, V. J. Edwards, and J. B. Croft. 2002. "Adverse Childhood Experiences and Personal Alcohol Abuse as an Adult." *Addictive Behaviors* 27: 713–25.

Dunkle, K. L., R. K. Jewkes, H. C. Brown, G. E. Gray, J. A. McIntryre, and S. D. Harlow. 2004. "Gender-Based Violence, Relationship Power, and Risk of HIV Infection in Women Attending Antenatal Clinics in South Africa." *Lancet* 363 (9419): 1415–21.

Duque, L. F., J. Klevens, and C. Ramirez. 2003. "Cross Sectional Survey of Perpetrators, Victims, and Witnesses of Violence in Bogotá, Colombia." *Journal of Epidemiology and Community Health* 57 (5): 355–60.

Ezzati, M., S. Vander Hoorn, A. D. Lopez, G. Danaei, A. Rodgers, C. Mathers, and C. J. L. Murray. 2006. "Comparative Quantification of Mortality and the Burden of Disease Attributable to Selected Major Risk Factors for 2001." In A. D. Lopez, C. D. Mathers, M. Ezzati, D. T. Jamison, and C. J. L. Murray, eds. *Global Burden of Disease and Risk Factors.* New York: Oxford University Press.

Fajnzylber, P., D. Lederman, and N. Loayza. 2000. "Crime and Violence: An Economic Perspective." *Economia* 1: 219–78.

Farrington, D. P. 2003. "Advancing Knowledge about the Early Prevention of Adult Antisocial Behaviour." In *Early Prevention of Adult Antisocial Behaviour,* ed. D. P. Farrington and J. W. Coid, 1–31. Cambridge, U.K.: Cambridge University Press.

Felitti, V. J., R. F. Anda, D. Nordenberg, D. F. Williamson, A. M. Spitz, V. Edwards, and others. 1998. "Relationship of Childhood Abuse and Household Dysfunction to Many of the Leading Causes of Death in Adults: The Adverse Childhood Experiences (ACE) Study." *American Journal of Preventive Medicine* 14: 245–58.

Fisher, A., L. Chestnut, and D. Violette. 1989. "The Value of Reducing Risks to Death: A Note on New Evidence." *Journal of Policy Analysis and Management* 8 (1): 88–100.

Fromm, S. 2001. "Total Estimated Cost of Child Abuse and Neglect in the United States: Statistical Evidence." Prevent Child Abuse America. http://www.preventchildabuse.org/learn_more/research_docs/cost_analysis.pdf.

Ghaffar, A. 2001. *National Injury Survey of Pakistan, 1997–1999.* Islamabad: National Injury Research Centre.

Gold, M. R., J. E. Siegel, and M. C. Weinstein. 2001. *Cost-Effectiveness in Health and Medicine.* New York: Oxford University Press.

Greenwood, P. W., K. E. Model, C. P. Rydell, and J. Chiesa. 1996. *Diverting Children from a Life of Crime: Measuring Costs and Benefits.* Santa Monica, CA: Rand.

Groenewald, P., D. Bradshaw, B. Nojilana, D. Bourne, J. Nixon, H. Mahomed, and J. Daniels. 2003. *Cape Town Mortality, 2001, Part I, Cause of Death and Premature Mortality.* Cape Town, South Africa: City of Cape Town, South African Medical Research Council, and University of Cape Town.

Grossman, J. B., and E. M. Garry. 1997. "Mentoring: A Proven Delinquency Prevention Strategy." *Juvenile Justice Bulletin* NCJ 164386. Washington, DC: United States Department of Justice, Office of Justice Programs.

Hahn, R. A., O. O. Bilukha, A. Crosby, M. T. Fullilove, A. Liberman, E. K. Moscicki, and others. 2003. "First Reports Evaluating the Effectiveness of Strategies for Preventing Violence: Firearms Laws." *Morbidity and Mortality Weekly Report* 52 (RR14): 11–20.

Harris, A. R., S. H. Thomas, G. A. Fisher, and D. J. Hirsch. 2002. "Murder and Medicine: The Lethality of Criminal Assault 1960–1999." *Homicide Studies* 6 (2): 128–66.

Hasbrouck, L. M., T. Durant, E. Ward, and G. Gordon. 2002. "Surveillance of Interpersonal Violence in Kingston, Jamaica: An Evaluation." *Injury Control and Safety Promotion* 9 (4): 249–53.

Heise, L., and C. Garcia-Moreno. 2002. "Violence by Intimate Partners." In *World Report on Violence and Health,* ed. E. G. Krug, L. L. Dahlberg, J. A. Mercy, A. B. Zwi, and R. Lozano, 87–121. Geneva: World Health Organization.

Hemenway, D. 2004. *Private Guns, Public Health.* Ann Arbor: University of Michigan Press.

Hillis, S. D., R. F. Anda, V. J. Felitti, and P. A. Marchbanks. 2001. "Adverse Childhood Experiences and Sexual Risk Behaviors in Women: A Retrospective Cohort Study." *Family Planning Perspectives* 33 (5): 206–11.

Hillis, S. D., R. F. Anda, V. J. Felitti, D. Nordenberg, and P. A. Marchbanks. 2000. "Adverse Childhood Experiences and Sexually Transmitted Diseases in Men and Women: A Retrospective Study." *Pediatrics* 106: E11.

Hoel, H., K. Sparks, and C. L. Cooper. 2001. "Estimating the Costs." In *The Cost of Violence/Stress at Work and the Benefits of a Violence/Stress-Free Working Environment,* 38–51. Geneva: International Labour Organization. http://www.ilo.org/public/english/protection/safework/whpwb/econo/costs.pdf.

Houry, D., K. M. Feldhaus, S. R. Nyquist, J. Abbot, and P. T. Pons. 1999. "Emergency Department Documentation in Cases of Intentional Assault." *Annals of Emergency Medicine* 34: 715–19.

Jeenah, M. S., Y. Dada, C. Househam, and D. Harrison. 1997. *Essential National Health Research in South Africa.* Document 97.1. Geneva: Council for Health Research and Development.

Jewkes, R., P. Sen, and C. Garcia-Moreno. 2002. "Sexual Violence." In *World Report on Violence and Health,* ed. E. G. Krug, L. L. Dahlberg, J. A. Mercy, A. B. Zwi, and R. Lozano, 147–81. Geneva: World Health Organization.

Klein, S. R., I. J. Kanno, D. A. Gilmore, and S. E. Wilson. 1999. "The Socioeconomic Impact of Assault Injuries on an Urban Trauma Center." *American Surgeon* 57 (12): 793–97.

Kobusingye, O. C., D. Guwatudde, and R. R. Lett. 2001. "Injury Patterns in Rural and Urban Uganda." *Injury Prevention* 7 (1): 46–50.

Kobusingye, O. C., and R. R. Lett. 2000. "Hospital-Based Trauma Registries in Uganda." *Journal of Trauma* 48 (3): 498–502.

Krug, E. G., L. L. Dahlberg, J. A. Mercy, A. B. Zwi, and R. Lozano. 2002a. *World Report on Violence and Health.* Geneva: World Health Organization.

Krug, E. G., L. I. Dahlberg, J. A. Mercy, A. B. Zwi, and A. Wilson. 2002b. "The Way Forward: Recommendations for Action." In *World Report on Violence and Health,* ed. E. G. Krug, L. L. Dahlberg, J. A. Mercy, A. B. Zwi, and R. Lozano, 243–60. Geneva: World Health Organization.

Kruger, J., A. Butchart, M. Seedat, and A. Gilchrist. 1998. "A Public Health Approach to Violence Prevention in South Africa." In *The Dynamics of Aggression and Violence in South Africa,* ed. R. van Eeden and M. Wentzel, 399–424. Pretoria: Human Sciences Research Council.

Loeber, R., P. Wung, K. Keenan, B. Biroux, M. Stouthamer-Loeber, W. B. Van Kammen, and others. 1993. "Developmental Pathways in Disruptive Child Behavior." *Development and Psychopathology* 5: 103–33.

Ludwig, J., and P. J. Cook, eds. 2003. *Evaluating Gun Policy.* Washington, DC: Brookings Institution.

Mathers, C. D., A. D. Lopez, and C. J. L. Murray. 2006. "The Burden of Disease and Mortality by Condition: Data, Methods, and Results for 2001." In A. D. Lopez, C. D. Mathers, M. Ezzati, D. T. Jamison, and C. J. L. Murray, eds. *Global Burden of Disease and Risk Factors.* New York: Oxford University Press.

Meddings, D. R., and S. M. O'Connor. 1999. "Circumstances around Weapon Injury in Cambodia after Departure of a Peacekeeping Force: Prospective Cohort Study." *British Medical Journal* 319 (7207): 412–15.

Medical Research Council of South Africa. 2004. "Crime, Violence, and Injury Lead Programme." http://www.mrc.ac.za/crime/about.htm.

Mercy, J. A., A. Butchart, D. Farrington, and M. Cerda. 2002. "Youth Violence." In *World Report on Violence and Health*, ed. E. G. Krug, L. L. Dahlberg, J. A. Mercy, A. B. Zwi, and R. Lozano, 25–56. Geneva: World Health Organization.

Mercy, J. A., and W. R. Hammond. 1999. "Preventing Homicide: A Public Health Perspective." In *Studying and Preventing Homicide: Issues and Challenges*, ed. M. D. Smith and M. Zahn, 274–94. Thousand Oaks, CA: Sage.

Mercy, J. A., E. G. Krug, L. L. Dahlberg, and A. B. Zwi. 2003. "Violence and Health: The United States in a Global Perspective." *American Journal of Public Health* 93 (2): 256–61.

Mercy, J. A., M. L. Rosenberg, K. E. Powell, C. V. Broome, and W. L. Roper. 1993. "Public Health Policy for Preventing Violence." *Health Affairs* 12 (4): 7–29.

Michael, M., D. R. Meddings, S. Ramez, and J. L. Gutierrez-Fisac. 1999. "Incidence of Weapon Injuries Not Related to Interfactional Combat in Afghanistan in 1996: Prospective Cohort Study." *British Medical Journal* 319 (7207): 415–17.

Miller, T. R. 1995. "Costs Associated with Gunshot Wounds in Canada in 1991." *Canadian Medical Association Journal* 153 (9): 1261–68.

———. 2001. "Costs of Juvenile Violence: Policy Implications." *Pediatrics* 107 (1): 1–7.

Miller, T. R., and M. A. Cohen. 1997. "Costs of Gunshot and Cut/Stab Wounds in the United States, with Some Canadian Comparisons." *Accident Analysis and Prevention* 29 (3): 329–41.

Miller, T. R., M. A. Cohen, and S. B. Rossman. 1993. "Victim Costs of Violent Crime and Resulting Injuries." *Health Affairs* 12 (4): 186–97.

Mock, C., J. D. Lormand, J. Goosen, M. Joshipura, and M. Peden. 2004. *Guidelines for Essential Trauma Care.* Geneva: World Health Organization.

Morrison, A. R., and M. B. Orlando. 1999. "Social and Economic Costs of Domestic Violence: Chile and Nicaragua." In *Too Close to Home: Domestic Violence in the Americas*, ed. A. R. Morrison and M. L. Biehl, 51–80. New York: Inter-American Development Bank.

Muelleman, R. L., J. Reuwer, T. G. Sanson, L. Gerson, R. H. Woolard, A. H. Yancy, and others. 1996. "An Emergency Medicine Approach to Violence throughout the Life Cycle." *Academic Emergency Medicine* 3 (7): 708–15.

National Center for Injury Prevention and Control. 2002. *CDC Injury Research Agenda.* Atlanta: Centers for Disease Control and Prevention.

National Crime Prevention Council. 1999. *Saving Money while Stopping Crime.* Washington, DC: National Crime Prevention Council.

Odero, W. O., and J. C. Kibosia. 1995. "Incidence and Characteristics of Injuries in Eldoret, Kenya." *East African Medical Journal* 72 (11): 706–10.

Ozanne-Smith, J., K. Ashby, S. Newstead, V. Z. Stathakis, and A. Clapperton. 2004. "Firearm Related Deaths: The Impact of Regulatory Reform." *Injury Prevention* 10: 280–86.

Payne, J. E., T. V. Berne, R. L. Kaufman, and R. Dubrowskij. 1993. "Outcome of Treatment of 686 Gunshot Wounds of the Trunk at Los Angeles County–USC Medical Center." *Journal of Trauma* 34 (2): 276–81.

Peden, M., and J. van der Spuy. 1998. "The Cost of Treating Firearm Victims." *Trauma Review* 6 (2): 4–5.

Rahman, F., Y. Ali, R. Andersson, and L. Svanstrom. 2001. "Epidemiology of Injury: Results from Injury Registration at District Level Hospital in Bangladesh: Implications for Injury Surveillance in Low-Income Countries." *Injury Control and Safety Promotion* 8 (1): 29–36.

Rahman, F., R. Andersson, and L. Svanstrom. 1998. "Medical Help Seeking Behaviour of Injury Patients in a Community in Bangladesh." *Public Health* 112 (1): 31–35.

Reza, A., J. A. Mercy, and E. G. Krug. 2001. "The Epidemiology of Violent Deaths in the World." *Injury Prevention* 7 (2): 104–11.

Roberts, L., R. Lafta, R. Garfield, J. Khudhairi, and G. Burnham. 2004. "Mortality before and after the 2003 Invasion of Iraq: Cluster Sample Survey." *Lancet* 364 (9448): 1857–64.

Rosenberg, M. L., ed. 1985. *Violence as a Public Health Problem: Background Papers for the Surgeon General's Workshop on Violence and Public Health.* Leesburg, VA. October.

Rosenberg, M. L., and M. A. Fenley, eds. 1991. *Violence in America: A Public Health Approach.* New York: Oxford University Press.

Runyan, D., C. Wattam, R. Ikeda, F. Hassan, and L. Ramiro. 2002. "Child Abuse and Neglect by Parents and Other Caregivers." In *World Report on Violence and Health*, ed. E. G. Krug, L. L. Dahlberg, J. A. Mercy, A. B. Zwi, and R. Lozano, 57–86. Geneva: World Health Organization.

Sethi, D., S. Habibula, K. McGee, M. Peden, S. Bennett, A. A. Hyder, and others. 2004. *Guidelines for Conducting Community Surveys on Injuries and Violence.* Geneva: World Health Organization.

Sethi, D., S. Marais, M. Seedat, J. Nurse, and A. Butchart. 2004. *Handbook for the Documentation of Interpersonal Violence Prevention Programmes.* Geneva: World Health Organization, Department of Injuries and Violence Prevention.

Sutherland, I., V. Sivarajasingam, and J. P. Shepherd. 2002. "Recording of Community Violence by Medical and Police Services." *Injury Prevention* 8: 246–47.

Swart, L., A. Gilchrist, A. Butchart, M. Seedat, and L. Martin. 2000. "Rape Surveillance through District Surgeon Offices in Johannesburg, 1996–1998: Findings, Evaluation, and Prevention Implications." *South African Journal of Psychology* 30 (2): 1–10.

Thornton, T. A., C. A. Craft, L. L. Dahlberg, B. S. Lynch, and K. Baer. 2002. *Best Practices of Youth Violence Prevention: A Sourcebook for Community Action.* Rev. ed. Atlanta: Centers for Disease Control and Prevention, National Center for Injury Prevention and Control.

Tolan, P. H., and D. Gorman-Smith. 1998. "Development of Serious and Violent Offending Careers." In *Serious and Violent Juvenile Offenders: Risk Factors and Successful Interventions*, ed. R. Loeber and D. P. Farrington, 13–29. Thousand Oaks, CA: Sage.

United Nations Population Fund. 1998. "Reproductive Health Effects of Gender-Based Violence." *UNFPA Annual Report 1998*, 20–21. http://www.unfpa.org/about/report/report98/ppgenderbased.htm.

U.S. Department of Health and Human Services. 2001. *Youth Violence: A Report of the Surgeon General.* Rockville, MD: U.S. Department of Health and Human Services. http://www.mentalhealth.org/youthviolence/surgeongeneral/SG_Site/home.asp.

Utting, D. 2003. "Prevention through Family and Parenting Programs." In *Early Prevention of Adult Antisocial Behaviour*, ed. D. P. Farrington and J. W. Coid, 243–64. Cambridge, U.K.: Cambridge University Press.

Villaveces, A., P. Cummings, V. E. Espitia, T. D. Koepsell, B. McKnight, and A. L. Kellermann. 2000. "Effect of a Ban on Carrying Firearms on Homicide Rates in 2 Colombian Cities." *Journal of the American Medical Association* 283 (9): 1205–9.

Viscusi, W. K. 1993. "The Value of Risks to Life and Health." *Journal of Economic Literature* 31 (4): 1912–46.

Waters, H., A. Hyder, Y. Rajkotia, S. Basu, and A. Butchart. 2004. *The Economic Dimensions of Interpersonal Violence*. Geneva: World Health Organization, Department of Injuries and Violence Prevention.

WHO (World Health Organization). 1999. *Report of the Consultation on Child Abuse Prevention*. WHO/HSC/PVI/99.1. Geneva: WHO.

WHO Global Consultation on Violence and Health. 1996. *Violence: A Public Health Priority*. WHO/EHA/SPI.POA.2. Geneva: WHO.

Williams, K. R., N. G. Guerra, and D. S. Elliott. 1997. *Human Development and Violence Prevention: A Focus on Youth*. Boulder: University of Colorado, Center for the Study and Prevention of Violence, Institute of Behavioral Science.

Williamson, D. F., T. J. Thompson, R. F. Anda, W. H. Dietz, and V. J. Felitti. 2002. "Body Weight and Obesity in Adults and Self-Reported Abuse in Childhood." *International Journal of Obesity and Related Metabolic Disorders* 26: 1075–82.

Wolf, R., L. Daichman, and G. Bennett. 2002. "Abuse of the Elderly." In *World Report on Violence and Health*, ed. E. G. Krug, L. L. Dahlberg, J. A. Mercy, A. B. Zwi, and R. Lozano, 125–45. Geneva: World Health Organization.

World Bank. 2004. "List of World Economies." Washington, DC: World Bank. http://www.worldbank.org.

Zwi, A. B., R. Garfield, and A. Loretti. 2002. "Collective Violence." In *World Report on Violence and Health*, ed. E. G. Krug, L. L. Dahlberg, J. A. Mercy, A. B. Zwi, and R. Lozano, 213–39. Geneva: World Health Organization.

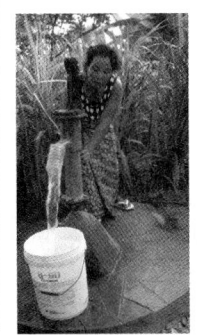

Chapter **41**

Water Supply, Sanitation, and Hygiene Promotion

Sandy Cairncross and Vivian Valdmanis

Water supply in the context of this chapter includes the supply of water for domestic purposes, excluding provision for irrigation or livestock. *Sanitation* is used here in the narrow sense of excreta disposal, excluding other environmental health interventions such as solid waste management and surface water drainage.

The effect of these other measures on disease burden is largely confined to urban areas and is considerably less than that of water supply, sanitation, and hygiene promotion (Cairncross and others 2003). More fundamentally, expenditure on solid waste disposal and drainage is rarely seen as forming part of a portfolio of investments in public health or competing with public health investments. Rather, it is generally perceived by decision makers as comparable with other investments in municipal infrastructure and services, such as roads or public transportation, which are not considered to be public health interventions.

This chapter focuses on water supply, excreta disposal, and hygiene promotion and considers the costs and benefits of each in turn. Water supply and sanitation can be provided at various levels of service, and those levels have implications for benefits. Water supply and sanitation offer many benefits in addition to improved health, and those benefits are considered in detail because they have important implications for the share of the cost that is attributable to the health sector. From the point of view of their effect on burden of disease, the main health benefit of water supply, sanitation, and hygiene is a reduction in diarrheal disease, although the effects on other diseases are substantial. In the concluding sections, the percentage reductions arrived at in the discussion throughout the chapter are used

together with data on existing levels of coverage to derive estimates of the potential effects of water supply and excreta disposal on the burden of disease, globally and by region, and with cost data to derive cost-effectiveness estimates.

WATER SUPPLY

What constitutes a perfectly satisfactory water supply to some consumers leaves others, even in developing countries, considering themselves unserved. In much of rural Africa, a hand pump 500 meters from the household is a luxury, but most residents in urban Latin America would not consider themselves served by a water supply unless they had a house connection. In Asia, urban planners would consider a community served if there were sufficient standposts on the street corner; however, if the water only flows for a few hours per week, producing lengthy nighttime queues, the residents may regard this situation as a lack of service and opt to buy water expensively from itinerant vendors. As these examples illustrate, water supply is not a single, well-defined intervention, such as immunization, but can be provided at various levels of service with varying benefits and differing costs.

Levels of Service and Their Costs

Many public health workers unfamiliar with the water sector assume that the most important characteristic of a water supply is its improved *quality*. However, most of the benefit is attributable to improved convenience of access to water in *quantity.* Moreover, global statistics are not available on the coverage and costs of provision of water in terms of its quality. The *Global Water Supply and Sanitation Assessment 2000 Report* (WHO and UNICEF 2000), the most recent compilation of global statistics on water supply, changed the way that such data are compiled, from the previous unreliable estimates by provider agencies to consumers' responses in population-based surveys. The change required a departure from the old definition of *reasonable access to safe water,* because most consumers cannot tell whether their water supply is safe. They can, however, state the type of technology involved, and that fact was used to define a new indicator of *improved* water supply. In the main, improved water supplies could be expected to provide water of better quality and with greater convenience than traditional *not improved* sources. The report treated the following technologies as improved: household connection, public standpipe, borehole, protected (lined) dug well, protected spring, and rainwater collection. Unprotected wells and springs, vendors, and tanker-trucks were considered unimproved. Bottled water was also considered unimproved because of concerns about the quantity of water supplied, not because of concerns over the water quality.

Reasonable access was defined as the availability of at least 20 liters per capita per day from a source within 1 kilometer of the user's dwelling. Within the broad category of those with reasonable access to an improved water supply, two significantly different levels of service can be distinguished:

- house connections
- public or community sources.

In most settings, these subcategories correspond to very different levels of water consumption, different amounts of time spent collecting water, and as discussed in later sections, different health benefits.

The *Global Water Supply and Sanitation Assessment 2000 Report* also gives median construction costs per person served for the various technologies in the three main regions of the developing world. These costs are shown in figure 41.1. However, local conditions, such as the size of the community to be served and the presence of suitable aquifers, can cause tremendous variations in the unit cost of water supply.

For a community of given size, there are no significant returns to scale in the number of house connections made. Most of the investment in major works must be made before house connections can be offered, so that the marginal cost of each connection is only a fraction of the total. For those and other reasons, water supply is a natural monopoly requiring "lumpy" investments, which makes the unit costs difficult to calculate.

The cost of house connections may be representative in Latin America and the Caribbean, where they are often provided in rural areas. In Asia and Africa, however, the reported

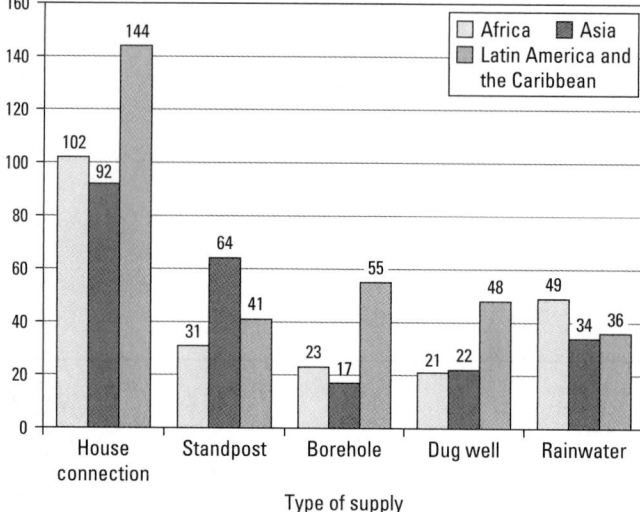

Cost per capita (US$)

Source: WHO/UNICEF 2000.

Figure 41.1 Median Construction Cost of Water Supply Facilities for Africa, Asia, and Latin America and the Caribbean

costs of house connections relate almost exclusively to urban areas because such connections are only rarely provided in smaller communities. The smaller size of rural communities means that piped systems in general—and house connections in particular—will tend to be more expensive per capita there than in urban areas. An overall unit cost figure of US$150, just above the highest of the three continental medians, is therefore taken for house connections in the cost-effectiveness calculations.

For public water points corresponding to improved water supply, hydrogeological and other constraints mean that the cheapest technology is not feasible in every community. A cost figure of US$40 per capita is about the middle of the range offered by different technologies (standpost, borehole, and dug well) providing this level of service for each continent (figure 41.1) and, therefore, seems reasonable for this level of service, although it can be expected to vary between US$15 and US$65 or more, depending on local conditions. The range of costs reported by individual countries for the *Global Water Supply and Sanitation Assessment 2000 Report* varied by more than an order of magnitude.

In calculating the cost-effectiveness of investment in water supplies, one must amortize these capital costs over an appropriate lifetime. Most major components of an urban water supply system have a potential lifetime of 50 years or more, but a prudent utility would aim to amortize them within about 20 years. A reasonable basis for calculation, for both urban and rural supplies, is to allow an amount of 5 percent of the capital cost as an annual straight-line amortization of the construction cost of the water supply.

Construction costs do not represent the full cost of water supplies. The *Global Water Supply and Sanitation Assessment 2000 Report* also gives median reported production costs per cubic meter for urban (house connection) water supplies as US$0.20 for Asia and US$0.30 for Africa and Latin America and the Caribbean. If we assume a mean daily water consumption of 100 liters per capita by those with household connections, those figures give annual per capita operation and maintenance costs of US$7.30 and US$10.95, respectively, or 8 to 10 percent of the capital cost of construction. In this chapter, a generic figure of US$10 is used for the annual per capita operation and maintenance cost.

Reliable figures for the annual maintenance costs for rural water supplies are harder to find, particularly because much of the maintenance is carried out by the volunteer labor of villagers. Arlosoroff and others (1987), after reviewing a wide range of rural water supply projects in various countries, concluded that with a centralized maintenance system, the annual per capita cost of maintenance of a hand pump–based supply can range from US$0.50 to US$2.00, while well-planned, community-level maintenance can bring that figure down as low as US$0.05 per capita per year. A nominal annual figure of US$1.00 per capita is therefore used in this chapter. A similar figure can be applied to urban public standposts, for which volunteer labor is less forthcoming but transport costs are lower. This maintenance cost represents 2.5 percent of the construction cost arrived at above.

The Time-Saving Benefit

Benefits to health are not normally foremost in the minds of those provided with new water supplies. An exhaustive study of the economics of rural water supply by the World Bank concluded that "the most obvious benefit is that water is made available closer to where rural households need it. . . . It is not clear that rural populations think much about the relationship between water and health" (Churchill and others 1987, 21–22).

The Value of Time. The saving in time and drudgery of carrying water home from the source is substantial, and several reasons exist to attribute a money value to it. The most powerful argument for the money value of poor women's time is that households often pay others to deliver their water, or pay to collect from nearby rather than from more distant sources that are free of charge. Thompson and others (2001) found that, of urban East African households lacking a piped supply, the proportion paying for water had increased from 53 percent to 80 percent over 30 years. In a survey of 12 sites in 10 countries, Zaroff and Okun (1984) found that households were spending a median of over 20 percent of their income on the purchase of water from vendors. The prices charged by vendors are typically more than 10 times—and can be up to 50 times—the normal tariff charged by the formal water supply utility.

Cairncross and Kinnear (1992) found that vendor prices increased with the time required to collect the water, showing that households pay more as the alternative of collecting water themselves becomes more burdensome. If the amount paid to the vendor for bringing the water is divided by the time saved from collecting it, the implicit value that people ascribe to their time can be calculated. Whittington, Mu, and Roche (1990), working in rural Kenya, showed in this way that the implicit value of the time saved was roughly US$0.38 per hour, very close to the average imputed wage rate for such households of US$0.35 per hour.

Because the poorest urban households typically spend more than 90 percent of their household budget on food, the money they spend on water is sacrificed from their food budget (Cairncross and Kinnear 1992). The provision of water more cheaply thus offers a substantial nutritional benefit to the poorest.

Assessing the Time Saved. The cost of water collection in rural areas is usually in time and effort rather than in money paid to vendors. The saving in time and drudgery underlies many social benefits. Given the relevance of the time-saving benefit to water supply policy and the fact that the benefit is usually uppermost in the mind of the consumer, it is remarkable how few data have been collected on the amounts of time spent collecting water.

Working in 334 study sites in Kenya, Tanzania, and Uganda, Thompson and others (2001) found a mean distance from rural unpiped households to their water sources of 622 meters. In urban areas, the distance was only 204 meters, but queuing at the tap meant that a water collection journey took almost as long.

Feachem and others (1978) found in 10 villages of the densely populated lowlands of Lesotho that the installation of a water supply had saved the average adult woman 30 minutes per day. In one-third of the villages, the saving per woman was more than an hour a day. Lesotho has many springs, so that time saving is likely to be on the low side compared with Africa as a whole.

These time-saving benefits are confirmed by the Multi-Indicator Cluster Surveys of the United Nations Children's Fund (UNICEF). A recent analysis of the responses in 23 African countries has produced a more representative account of water collection journey times in that continent (G. Keast, UNICEF, personal communication 2003). Nearly half the households interviewed (44 percent) required a journey of more than 30 minutes to collect water, implying that the women in such households spent an hour or more each day in water collection. At almost any reasonable level of service, most of that time would be saved by an improved water supply.

In Asia, an Indian national survey for UNICEF found that women spent an average of 2.2 hours per day collecting water from rural wells (Mukherjee 1990). A study in Sri Lanka, which is generally considered to be well provided with water sources, found that 10 percent of women had to travel more than 1 kilometer to their nearest source (Mertens and others 1990).

Valuation of the Time-Saving Benefit. Putting a precise figure on the money value of the time of poor people is a tricky task, even for the most self-confident economist. In 1987, Churchill and others took US$0.125 per hour as an illustrative but not unrealistic figure. To take the same figure today could hardly be described as extravagant. Assuming this valuation of an hour of time—and that a water supply bestows a mean saving of only 15 minutes per person per day—yields a conservative estimate of the value of the time-saving benefit of US$11.40 per year. The data presented earlier indicate that, at least in Africa, the true figure is nearer to double that amount, enough to justify the full construction cost of a dug well or borehole supply in a single year. In Latin America and the Caribbean, costs are higher, and time savings may be less, but rural incomes are also higher—and so, therefore, is the value of people's time. Little doubt exists that, in all three regions of the developing world, the value of time saved is sufficient on its own to justify both the investment costs (at any reasonable rate of amortization) and the operation and maintenance costs of water supplies.

Even in settings where water vending is not common, contingent valuation surveys have widely demonstrated a willingness to pay for water supplies, particularly at the level of service of house connections (World Bank Water Demand Research Team 1993). In general, such measured willingness to pay has exceeded the cost of providing the supplies, and payment to vendors often exceeds it by many times.

Policy Implications. Whether the consumers actually pay for the full value of the time-saving benefit, it is what makes water supplies popular and largely it is what motivates politicians to invest in them. More than half the total annual investment in water supply in the developing countries of Africa, Asia, and Latin America and the Caribbean is from domestic sources (WHO and UNICEF 2000). Most of the investment is from the public sector. In general, investments in water supply—whether by the governments of developing countries or by external support agencies—do not come from health sector budgets and are not compared with other health interventions when investment decisions are made, even though health benefits do arise from water supply improvements.

Water supply is thus a health-related intervention that comes without cost to the budgets of the health sector. Although it undoubtedly offers health benefits, it has a sufficient economic and political rationale in other social benefits associated with time saving. The health benefits are a positive externality to this rationale. However, this fact does not mean that the authorities responsible for public health should ignore the water sector. The function of the health sector is one of regulation, advocacy, and provision of supplementary inputs, as appropriate, to ensure that potential health benefits of water supply are realized to the optimal extent.

For example, the regulatory role of the health sector in quality surveillance of drinking water is well known and widely accepted. Substantial and largely unexploited additional potential is present in this role if quality is interpreted in the wider sense of *quality of service* rendered by the water supply utility, in terms not only of water quality but also of quantity, continuity, coverage, control of sanitary hazards, and cost. Those other aspects, as will be argued in the following sections, are no less important for health.

Where a regulatory role is not available to the health sector or agencies concerned with public health, advocacy can be no less cost-effective. For example, connection charges are a major barrier to house connections for low-income groups. In many cities of the developing world, the individual connection charge is about a month's basic wage. Advocacy of lower connection charges, with the amount recovered from the monthly water tariffs, can therefore help achieve an increase in the number of people who have house connections and who can benefit from the corresponding health gain at no cost to the public purse. Finally, the health sector can provide important complementary services, such as hygiene promotion and promotion of low-cost sanitation to increase coverage; because of the nature of such services, the water sector, with its focus on technology, is ill-equipped to offer them.

The unit costs of such regulation and advocacy are minimal. One example is the case of UNICEF's participation over the past 30 years in India's rural water supply program. UNICEF's investment has represented no more than 1 percent of the total, but its influence has played a central part in the evolution of the technical and institutional model of the program that supplies water to 1 in 10 members of the human race.

An example of the effectiveness of such measures is provided by the interventions of the Mexican Ministry of Health in June 1991. Fostered by fear of the devastating effects of cholera, these measures included the chlorination of water supplied for human consumption and the prohibition of sewage irrigation of fruit and vegetables. As a result, the incidence of diarrhea in children under five years of age fell from 4.5 to 2.2 episodes per child-year, and the corresponding mortality rate fell from 101.6 to 62.9 per 100,000 children (Gutiérrez and others 1996).

The current rate of annual investment per capita in water supply and sanitation, including both national investment and external aid funds, is reportedly US$2.25 in Asia, US$7.53 in Africa, and US$8.87 in Latin America and the Caribbean (WHO and UNICEF 2000). One percent of the water sector's investment would, therefore, be US$0.02 to US$0.10 per capita. If each ministry of health in the developing world were to invest such a sum in public health advocacy and regulation related to water supply, the sector's performance, at least where low-income groups are concerned, could be transformed. It is hard to put a figure on the health effects of such investment, but the Mexican example suggests that they would be substantial. For the sake of cost-effectiveness estimation, such spending is arbitrarily assumed to have the effect of ensuring improved water supplies for an additional 10 percent of the population to which it refers.

Direct Health Effects

The full list of water-related infections is large and varied, but most are only marginally affected by water supply improvements. The first effort to simplify the relationship between water supplies and health in developing countries was made by David Bradley (White, Bradley, and White 1972), who developed a classification of disease transmission routes in terms of whether they were

- *waterborne,* in the strict sense in which the pathogen is ingested in drinking water
- *water-washed*—that is, favored by inadequate hygiene conditions and practices and susceptible to control by improvements in hygiene
- *water-based,* referring to transmission by means of an aquatic invertebrate host
- *water-related insect vector* routes, involving an insect vector that breeds in or near to water.

Whereas the prevention of waterborne disease transmission requires improvements in water quality, water-washed transmission is interrupted by improvements in the availability—and hence the quantity—of water used for hygiene and the purposes to which it is put. Water supply may affect water-based transmission (for example, if it reduces the need for people to enter schistosomiasis-infected water bodies) or water-related insect vectors of disease (for example, if a more reliable supply averts the need for the water-storage vessels in which dengue vectors breed), though that will depend on the precise life cycle of the parasite involved and the preferred breeding sites and behavior of the vector.

Classification and Burden of Water-Related Diseases. Before Bradley's classification can be applied to diseases (rather than transmission routes), it requires a small adjustment (Cairncross and Feachem 1993) to allow for the fact that practically all potentially waterborne infections that are transmitted by the feco-oral route can potentially be transmitted by other means (contamination of fingers, food, fomites, field crops, other fluids, flies, and so on) all of which are water-washed routes. In addition to the feco-oral infections, a number of infections of the skin and eyes can be considered water washed but not waterborne. The final classification is shown in table 41.1.

The classification can now be used to assess how the disease burden prevented by water supply is distributed among disease groups. Bradley himself did this, a time long before the disability-adjusted life year (DALY) had been invented as a unit of benefit measurement (White, Bradley, and White 1972, 191). He used official statistics on the number of cases of each disease diagnosed and treated by health services in East Africa and combined them with notional percentages by which morbidity and mortality caused by each condition could be expected to fall if water supply were "excellent."

Those notional reductions were based on subjective assessments of the literature available at the time and were described by their author as "little more than guesses," but it is hard to prove many of them seriously at fault, even today. A selection is presented in table 41.2.

The result of these calculations was that the feco-oral disease group accounted for 91 percent of the deaths preventable by water supply, 50 percent of inpatient bed nights, and 33 percent

Table 41.1 The Bradley Classification of Water-Related Infections

Transmission route	Description	Disease group	Examples
Waterborne	The pathogen is in water that is ingested	Feco-oral	Diarrheas, dysenteries, typhoid fever
Water-washed (or water-scarce)	Person-to-person transmission because of a lack of water for hygiene	Skin and eye infections	Scabies, trachoma
Water-based	Transmission via an aquatic intermediate host (for example, a snail)	Water-based	Schistosomiasis, guinea worm
Water-related insect vector	Transmission by insects that breed in water or bite near water	Water-related insect vector	Dengue, malaria, trypanosomiasis

Source: Cairncross and Feachem 1993.

Table 41.2 Percentage Reductions in Disease Rates Assumed by Bradley

Diagnosis	Percentage reduction expected from excellent water supply
Most diarrhea and dysentery	50
Typhoid fever	80
Paratyphoid, other *Salmonella*	40
Trachoma	60
Scabies	80
Skin and subcutaneous infections	50
Urinary schistosomiasis	80
Intestinal schistosomiasis	40
Malaria	0

Source: White, Bradley, and White 1972.

of outpatient consultations. Rosen and Vincent (2001) have made a similar calculation for the whole of Africa in 1990 and found that the feco-oral group accounted for 85 percent of the preventable DALYs. When measured in terms of deaths or DALYs, feco-oral infections account for the vast majority of the impact, because of the high mortality caused by diarrheal diseases among young children. Most deaths from diarrheal diseases are of children younger than age five, and most of those are among children younger than two. A child death averted is worth 30 DALYs. Varley, Tarvid, and Chao (1998) have calculated that for diarrhea morbidity reduction to have the same effect in DALYs as averting one such death, it would have to prevent 115,000 child-days of diarrhea. After the diarrheal diseases, the next most important category in terms of DALYs (12 percent of the total) is the water-based group, primarily schistosomiasis. The purely water-washed diseases, mainly skin infections, represent a more conspicuous portion only when compared in terms of the burden placed on health services by inpatients or outpatients.

How representative is this African breakdown of the developing world as a whole? Diarrheal disease among poor communities is cosmopolitan. A global review of studies of the incidence of diarrhea morbidity could find no clear geographic or climatic trend (Bern and others 1992), so the burden of disease is no doubt similar around the developing world. The second most important disease group is represented by schistosomiasis, which is absent from much of Asia and Latin America. The relative importance of feco-oral disease is, therefore, likely to be still greater in the poor communities of Asia and the Western Hemisphere than it is in Africa.

Epidemiological Questions and Problems. The predominant contribution of feco-oral diseases to the burden of disease attributable to water supply raises an important question,

because this group can be transmitted by both waterborne and water-washed routes. It is important for the water engineer to know whether scarce funding should be spent on improved water treatment and measures to protect water quality or instead on providing a limitless supply of water at a high level of access and convenience and encouraging its use for improved hygiene practices. We need to know, that is, whether the feco-oral infections endemic in poor communities are mainly waterborne or mainly water washed.

Moreover, the fact that some diarrheal diseases are still prevalent in communities with a high level of water supply service indicates that water supply alone cannot completely prevent these diseases. A further question then, is this: by how much do water supply improvements reduce diarrheal diseases?

Numerous studies have sought to answer these questions, but they are hard to answer rigorously, for several reasons. First, it is almost impossible, ethically and politically, to randomize the intervention. Where the intervention is an improvement in the level of access to water, it cannot be blinded; no placebo exists for a standpost. Where quasi-experimental studies have been used—opportunistically exploiting an intervention allocated by political or technical means—significant confounding has frequently been found (Briscoe, Feachem, and Rahaman 1985).

Confounding has been especially intractable in studies in which the allocation of facilities has been on a household basis, so that the exposure groups are self-selected—for instance, studies in which individual households that have chosen to install a private tap are compared with others that have chosen not to do so. The former households are likely to be wealthier, better educated, and more conscious of hygiene than their neighbors, so it would not be surprising if they were also more likely do many other things that protect their families from feco-oral disease. The more sophisticated studies have used multivariate models to control for confounding, but where relative risks are low and the exposure groups are self-selected, even those models do not guarantee that confounding is eliminated (Cairncross 1990).

A further difficulty arises from the fact that cases of feco-oral disease in a given community cannot be considered independent events, because such diseases are infectious. The sample size, it can be argued, is the number of such villages rather than the number of individuals enrolled in the study. Yet a number of important studies in the literature compare a single intervention area with only one control area.

Other epidemiological weaknesses exist in the data. Blum and Feachem (1983) reviewed 50 studies of the health effect of water supply and sanitation projects and noted that every one contained one or more of these basic errors of methodology. A further weakness in the evidence for the effect of water supply on diarrheal disease burden is that most of it relates to diarrheal disease morbidity, and significant assumptions are

Table 41.3 Median Reductions in Diarrhea Morbidity Reported from Different Water Supply and Sanitation Interventions

Intervention (object of improvement)	Number of rigorous studies from which morbidity reductions could be calculated	Median reduction in diarrheal morbidity (percent)
Water quality only	4	15
Water quantity only	5	20
Water quantity and quality	2	17
Sanitation only	5	36
Water and sanitation	2	30
Hygiene promotion only	6	33

Source: Esrey and others 1991.

needed to extrapolate such evidence to an effect on diarrheal mortality.

Effect on Diarrheal Disease. Esrey and Habicht (1985) and Esrey and others (1991) reviewed the same literature from a different perspective. Though conscious of the methodological shortcomings of most studies, they sought to assess the overall reductions in diarrheal disease that water supply could be expected to cause. They applied a number of criteria of epidemiological rigor and took the median reduction in morbidity reported from each type of intervention. Their conclusions are summarized in table 41.3.

For more than a decade, this review has remained the most authoritative on the subject. However, the small reductions in disease that it reports for water supply conceal an important heterogeneity. Though these overall results are frequently quoted, the following remark by Esrey and others (1991, 613) has usually been overlooked:

> In the studies reporting a health benefit, the water supply was piped into or near the home, whereas in those studies reporting no benefit, the improved water supplies were protected wells, tubewells, and standpipes.

In the studies in the two reviews by Esrey and Habicht (1985) and Esrey and others (1991) in which the water supply was provided in the home, the median reduction in diarrheal disease is 49 percent (from 12 studies), and the reduction from the two better studies is 63 percent. Those reductions are several times greater than the overall median impacts in table 41.3. The 63 percent figure will be used in the burden of disease calculations that follow. In the two better studies, the members of the comparison group were using not an unimproved water supply, but a protected water source away from the home. The reductions they found are, therefore, in addition to those resulting from a public standpost level of service.

Some subsequent studies have confirmed this pattern. For example, Bukenya and Nwokolo (1991) showed in Papua New Guinea that use of a household tap was associated with 56 percent less diarrhea than use of public standposts providing water of good quality.

Conditions for Health Effect. Providing a public water point appears to have little effect on health, even where the water provided is of good quality and replaces a traditional source that was heavily contaminated with fecal material. By contrast, moving the same tap from the street corner to the yard produces a substantial reduction in diarrheal morbidity. How is this pattern to be understood?

The first step to an explanation is an understanding that most endemic diarrheal disease is transmitted by water-washed routes and is not waterborne. Although waterborne epidemics of diarrheal diseases such as cholera and typhoid have been notorious in the history of public health, the endemic pattern of transmission seems to be different, particularly in poor communities. Five types of evidence support this view:

- *Negative health impact studies.* As mentioned earlier, Esrey and Habicht (1985) and Esrey and others (1991) cite a number of studies of the health impact of water supplies in which water quality improvements have failed to have a significant effect on diarrheal disease incidence.
- *Food microbiology.* Studies of the microbiology of foods in developing countries—particularly the weaning foods fed to children in the age group most susceptible to diarrheal disease—have shown such food to be far more heavily contaminated with fecal bacteria than is drinking water (Lanata 2003), even when the water has been stored in open pots.
- *Seasonality of diarrhea.* In countries with a seasonal variation in temperature, bacterial diarrheas peak in the warmer season, whereas viral diarrheas peak in the winter. This pattern suggests that the bacterial pathogens show environmental regrowth at some stage in their transmission route, which means that they must have a nutritional substrate. Water is, thus, a less likely vehicle than food.

- *Fly-control studies.* Trials in rural Asia and Africa have shown that fly control can reduce diarrheal disease incidence by 23 percent (Chavasse and others 1999).
- *Hand-washing studies.* A recent systematic review of the effect of hand washing with soap has shown that this simple measure is associated with a reduction of 43 percent in diarrheal disease and 48 percent in diarrheas with the more life-threatening etiologies (Curtis and Cairncross 2003).

Those five types of evidence suggest that domestic hygiene—particularly food and hand hygiene—is the principal determinant of endemic diarrheal disease rates and not drinking water quality.

The second step is an understanding of how the level of service and convenience of a water supply influence such hygiene practices in the home. Taking the amount of water used per capita as an indicator of hygiene changes, other things being equal, one finds that providing a source of water closer to the home—and therefore more convenient to use—has very little effect on water consumption unless the old source was more than 1 kilometer (30 minutes' roundtrip journey) away from the user's dwelling (Feachem and others 1978).

However, water consumption doubles or triples when house connections are provided (White, Bradley, and White 1972), and reason exists to believe that much of the additional consumption is used for hygiene purposes. For example, Curtis and others (1995) found that provision of a yard tap nearly doubled the odds of a mother washing her hands after cleaning her child's anus and more than doubled the odds that she would wash any fecally soiled linen immediately.

In conclusion, water supplies are likely to have an effect on diarrheal disease when they lead to hygiene behavior change—that is, when the old source of water was more than 30 minutes' roundtrip away or when house connections are provided.

By a happy coincidence, then, the health benefits of water supply are most likely to be realized in exactly those cases in which the time-saving benefit is greatest—when the old source of water is farthest away, and when the new one is on the plot of the individual household. Though water supplies offering house connections are more expensive, the additional time savings offered by this level of service mean that people are willing to pay more for them. Moreover, collecting revenue from households with private connections is far simpler than collecting it from public taps because the sanction of disconnection can be used against households that default on payment of the tariff.

Calculating the burden of disease associated with inadequate water supply requires a figure for the reduction associated with the levels of service for which coverage statistics are available. The following burden of disease calculations are based on a reduction of 17 percent from an improved public water supply (table 41.3) and of a further 63 percent from house connections.

The effect of water supply improvements (and of hygiene practices such as hand washing) on diarrhea mortality can be expected to be at least as great as—and probably greater than—their effect on morbidity for several reasons. A theoretical argument for this improvement pattern is given by Esrey, Feachem, and Hughes (1985) in terms of infectious doses. Esrey and others (1991) also reported a median reduction of 65 percent in diarrhea mortality attributable to water supply, sanitation, or both in three studies, compared with 22 percent from 49 studies of morbidity. The effect of hand washing on life-threatening diarrheas—shigellosis, typhoid, cholera, and hospitalized cases—is greater than that on diarrhea morbidity as a whole (Curtis and Cairncross 2003). Finally, the two known direct studies in the literature of the effect of house connections on diarrhea mortality ("Serviço Especial da Saúde Pública," an unpublished study in Palmares, Pernambuco, Brazil, cited by Wagner and Lanoix 1959; Victora and others 1988) found reductions of 65 percent (relative to a public standpost) and 80 percent (relative to various communal sources, some polluted), respectively.

Effect on Other Disease Categories. Water supplies have a beneficial effect on a number of disease groups other than diarrhea, although the corresponding burden of disease is far less. The median reductions in morbidity from other water-related conditions, reported by Esrey and others (1990), are shown in table 41.4.

Table 41.4 Median Reductions in Morbidity Associated with Improved Water Supply and Sanitation: Conditions Other Than Diarrhea, Related Most Closely to Water Supply

Disease	All studies		Better studies		
	Number of studies	Median reduction (percent)	Number of studies	Median reduction (percent)	Range (percent)
Dracunculiasis	7	76	2	78	75–81
Schistosomiasis	4	73	3	77	59–87
Trachoma	13	50	7	27	0–79

Source: Esrey and others 1990.

To be effective in controlling schistosomiasis, the water supply must be so convenient as to discourage water contact for laundry and bathing. It is unlikely that this level of convenience can be achieved without house connections.

Evidence suggests that water availability and hygiene can produce substantial reductions in trachoma (Emerson and others 2000). Because the reductions come from hygiene improvements such as hand and face washing, they are also likely to be greatest with house connections. Dracunculiasis is affected by water quality, but the simplest improved water supply is adequate to prevent transmission.

Conflicting evidence exists about whether water supply or improved water-washed hygiene affects the transmission of intestinal helminths. On one hand, Henry (1981) found in an intervention study in St. Lucia that piped water supplies were associated with a 30 percent reduction in ascariasis among children under age three over a two-year period. On the other hand, Han and others (1988) showed in Burma that an intervention to promote hand washing with soap had no effect on prevalence or intensity of infection with *Ascaris* spp. However, the potential contribution of water supply to reducing the burden of disease through its effect on these other infections is relatively minor when compared with its effect on diarrheal disease.

EXCRETA DISPOSAL

In much the same way as with water supply, care is needed to ensure that different people who talk about sanitation are referring to the same thing. When the WHO-UNICEF Joint Monitoring Program was compiling the *Global Water Supply and Sanitation Assessment 2000 Report* (WHO and UNICEF 2000), a major effort was needed to persuade some of the Latin American partners that a pit latrine, considered a status symbol in much of rural Africa, was an acceptable form of excreta disposal. In some countries, even engineered sewerage systems are considered unacceptable if not connected to a functioning wastewater treatment plant.

Levels of Service, Technologies, and Their Costs

A wide range of technologies is used, particularly for settings in which low-cost solutions are required, and this variation has led some to inquire whether the different types of latrine might confer differing health benefits. In the early 1980s, the World Bank established a Technology Advisory Group for low-cost sanitation, and this question was among those it was asked to investigate. Using field studies and a thorough literature review, the group concluded that all types of systems can be operated hygienically, and that

> The greatest determinants of the efficacy of alternative facilities are, first, whether they are used by everyone all the

time, and second, whether they are adequately maintained. . . . Pit latrines would, from the viewpoint of health rather than convenience, approximate the same rating as a waterborne sewerage system. (Feachem and others 1983, 49–50)

The group therefore judged it most appropriate not to distinguish between sanitation technologies and to consider all of them as providing adequate access to sanitation as long as they were private or shared (but not public) and hygienically separated human excreta from human contact. This definition was followed in the *Global Water Supply and Sanitation Assessment 2000 Report,* which accepted only sewerage, septic tanks with soakaways, pour-flush latrines, and pit latrines as improved technologies. Service or bucket latrines and latrines with an open pit were not accepted. The effect of technology type on health benefit is discussed further in the sections that follow.

Public latrines, however, do not provide an adequate solution to the excreta disposal needs of a community. Quite apart from the notorious and widespread inadequacies in their maintenance, they are not usually accessible at night or by the elderly, by those with disabilities, or—if there is an entry charge—by young children. Thus, some promiscuous defecation continues to be practiced, particularly by children, in communities where public latrines are the only level of service available.

Figure 41.2 shows the regional median construction costs per capita of the various sanitation technologies found by the *Global Water Supply and Sanitation Assessment 2000 Report.* Although the simple, on-site systems tend to be cheaper than systems such as sewerage and septic tanks, the difference is less than might be expected. For example, a World Bank survey in several developing countries found the mean cost of conventional sewerage to be 10 times that for on-site systems such as improved pit latrines and pour-flush toilets (Kalbermatten, Julius, and Gunnerson 1982). It is likely that the off-site costs of sewered systems and the cost of the additional water needed for them to function have not been fully included in national reports to the *Global Water Supply and Sanitation Assessment 2000 Report.* For the purposes of calculating cost-effectiveness, a construction cost of US$60 per capita seems adequate for basic sanitation facilities (a household pit latrine, ventilation-improved latrine, or a pour-flush toilet) in any region of the developing world. Taking a relatively short lifetime of five years for a latrine and straight-line amortization gives an annual cost of US$12 per capita per year. In such a short lifetime, very little maintenance is normally required, other than occasional cleaning; the cost of maintenance is, therefore, considered to be included in the amortized annual cost.

That said, it should be borne in mind that substantially cheaper solutions are often feasible, such as the "15 taka latrine"

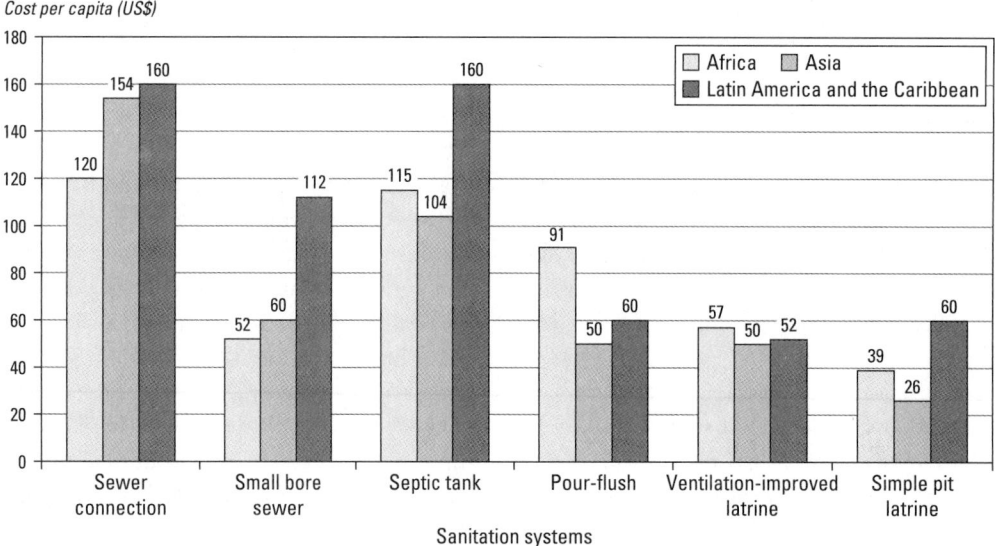

Cost per capita (US$)

Figure 41.2 Median Construction Cost of Sanitation Technologies in Africa, Asia, and Latin America and the Caribbean

Source: WHO/UNICEF 2000.

(costing only US$0.27 per household) developed in Bangladesh, which includes a pour-flush pan made of tin sheet and an odor- and insect-proof seal made of flexible plastic pipe.

Social Benefits

Like water supply, sanitation offers a number of social benefits in addition to direct health gains, which tend to feature more prominently in the minds of the users. This outcome is illustrated by the responses given by a sample of householders in rural Benin when asked to rate the importance they ascribed to the various benefits of latrines on a scale of 1 to 4 (table 41.5). Health-related benefits (shown bold in table 41.5) were rarely mentioned spontaneously and generally rated among the less important benefits.

With sanitation as with water supply, strong gender differences exist in the perception of the social benefits of sanitation. For male heads of household in Benin as in other countries around the world, enhanced social status figures highly among the benefits of latrine ownership, whereas for women, security, convenience, and aesthetic factors count for more. Women who lack sanitation often risk sexual harassment on the way to and from their defecation site. In some cultural settings, women are constrained to go out for defecation and urination only during the hours of darkness, effectively becoming prisoners of daylight. Though no systematic study has been made of the health implications of such practices, they are likely to include an increased prevalence of urinary tract infections. The emancipation that a latrine bestows on such women cannot lightly be dismissed.

Table 41.5 Benefits of Latrine Ownership as Perceived by 320 Households in Rural Benin

Benefit	(Average importance rating, scale 1–4)
Avoid discomforts of the bush	3.98
Gain prestige from visitors	3.96
Avoid dangers at night	3.86
Avoid snakes	3.85
Reduce flies in compound	3.81
Avoid risk of smelling or seeing feces in bush	3.78
Protect my feces from enemies	3.71
Have more privacy to defecate	3.67
Keep my house or property clean	3.59
Feel safer	3.56
Save time	3.53
Make my house more comfortable	3.50
Reduce my family's health care expenses	**3.32**
Leave a legacy for my children	3.16
Have more privacy for household affairs	3.00
Make my life more modern	2.97
Feel royal	2.75
Make it easier to defecate because of age or sickness	2.62
Be able to increase my tenants' rent	1.17
For health (spontaneous mention)	**1.27**

Source: Jenkins 1999.

Willingness to Pay. The governments of developing countries cannot afford to provide heavily subsidized sanitation to all—or even to the majority—of their populations. The 2.6 billion people in Africa, Asia, and Latin America who do have adequate sanitation—53 percent of the population of those regions—have paid most of the cost themselves. Even those of the urban poor who do not have sanitation have expressed a willingness to pay for its full cost—or at least the local cost (excluding major interceptor sewers and treatment works, if required)—in a number of surveys, as long as credit is available on reasonable terms to smooth the cash flow (Altaf 1994). With regard to the rural poor, the success of well-conceived sanitation promotion programs in achieving coverage close to 100 percent, without a substantial subsidy, in some of the poorest rural communities in the world (Allan 2003) shows that people are willing to pay for sanitation if a suitable product is offered to them on suitable terms.

Why then do 2.4 billion people still lack sanitation? Several factors constrain the expression of the existing demand.

The constraint most frequently mentioned by unserved householders is cost, but this factor is usually more a perceived constraint than an objective one, for several reasons. First, many households are unaware of the true cost of latrines in their area, or the lower-cost models are not offered because local suppliers and artisans do not know about them or are attracted by the greater margins to be made on the more expensive technologies. Second, the high cost of capital to the poor rules out their borrowing the cost of a latrine, which to them would be a substantial investment. Third, they may be wary of investing in a property that belongs to their landlord, lest it be used as an excuse for a rent increase or even eviction. They may also feel, with some reason, that it is for the landlord to make the investment, rather than themselves, and they may be waiting for the landlord to do so. This belief has a similar effect to the common misapprehension of citizens, often encouraged by politicians, that the local government is responsible for sanitation and will eventually come to their aid; in either case, the outcome is inaction.

Other constraints include lack of ready access to necessary techniques and skills or to specific building materials and components. Where the skills exist locally, residents may lack confidence in the quality of work and value for money offered by the local artisans, or they may not know how to contact the right artisans. In many urban areas, local building regulations make low-cost sanitation technologies illegal.

Those constraints are compounded by the fragmentation of governmental responsibility for sanitation. Often it is devolved to local governments with little capacity to implement sanitation improvements. At the national level, one ministry may be responsible for sewerage and another for low-cost technologies; one may be responsible for construction, another for promotion, and a third for enforcing building codes and planning regulations.

Policy Implications. There are important externalities to households' investment in sanitation. Households are protected from their own feces by their sanitation facilities, but so, too, are their neighbors, and this factor is probably more important in epidemiological terms. If households are not fully aware of the health benefit—or if much of it accrues to others—a case exists for public intervention to increase coverage because these externalities exist.

This public intervention need not be in the form of subsidy. Strong arguments can be marshaled against a subsidy for low-cost sanitation (Cairncross 2003a). Subsidy limits the number of facilities that are built to the size of the subsidy budget; it encourages the design and marketing of unaffordable sanitation systems; it frequently leads to capture by the better-off, who install expensive toilets while the poor go without; and it distorts the market, diverting the efforts of latrine builders who would otherwise be seeking to meet the needs of low-income groups.

The intervention can be by regulation. National and local governments have substantial regulatory powers that can be used to increase sanitation coverage without significantly increasing costs or public expenditure. For example, more than 90 percent of households in the town of Bobo Dioulasso, Burkina Faso, have their own latrine (Traoré and others 1994) as a direct result of the local administration's practice in the past of withdrawing rights of land tenure from owners who did not build a latrine on their plot within a specified time. Another regulatory intervention is to enforce the obligation of landlords to provide sanitation for their tenants.

An alternative strategy is to provide support to the marketing of sanitation. This strategy can be undertaken in a number of ways that are not feasible for the existing producers, mainly artisan builders and small component manufacturing workshops. Those interventions would aim principally at overcoming the constraints to the expression of effective demand for sanitation and could include the following:

- advertising and other forms of promotion
- facilitation of building regulation approval
- brokerage to put potential purchasers in touch with providers
- quality assurance and guarantee schemes
- training in low-cost construction techniques and in marketing
- centralized production of essential components
- provision of pit emptying and desludging services.

Promotion of improved hygiene practices, including appropriate use and maintenance of the sanitation facilities, is another possible intervention by the public sector. All of those measures will help increase sanitation coverage and health benefits and are appropriate interventions for the health sector. The costs of several of them are recoverable (after an initial launch period) as fees, so that public intervention need not require public expenditure.

Costs of Promotion. The costs of promotion and administration found in two government-run rural sanitation programs documented by the World Bank were US$16.80 (Zimbabwe) and $20.00 (the Philippines) per latrine, respectively (Cairncross 1992). Because these costs are largely fixed, the cost per unit falls as the number of units built increases. Unit costs will therefore be high in relatively unsuccessful programs. Successful programs, on the other hand, often engender the construction of more latrines than they can account for, which also gives an upward bias to the promotional costs per unit built. For example, for every latrine built by Lesotho's rural sanitation program in the late 1980s, four others were built independently but as a result of its promotional activities.

More recently, successful sanitation programs managed by nongovernmental organizations (NGOs) have documented slightly lower unit costs for promotion. For example, the Zimbabwean NGO AHEAD (Applied Health Education and Development), working through district-level health staff and a network of community health clubs, achieved the construction of 3,400 latrines in Makoni district within two years at a total promotional cost of US$45,660, or US$13.43 per unit, equivalent to US$2.24 per household member served (Waterkeyn 2003). In Bangladesh, WaterAid and its partner, a local NGO named VERC (Village Education Resource Centre), have developed an approach that has successfully achieved 100 percent sanitation coverage and the elimination of open defecation in more than 100 villages in six districts at a cost of US$8 per household, or US$1.50 per capita (Allan 2003). Both pro-grams also promoted domestic hygiene practices in addition to the construction and use of latrines. In Bangladesh, all (and in Zimbabwe, most) of the costs of latrine construction were paid by the population themselves.

The programs in Bangladesh and Zimbabwe were particularly successful and well managed. The promotion cost is taken as US$2.50 per capita for cost-effectiveness calculations, which is slightly above the higher of the two, to allow for the imperfections of sanitation programs in the real world.

Direct Health Benefits

Evidence supports the claim that improved excreta disposal helps prevent a number of diseases, including diarrhea, intestinal worm parasites, and trachoma. Of these, the effect that accounts for the largest burden of DALYs is that on diarrheal disease.

Diarrheal Disease. The effect of sanitation on diarrhea morbidity has already been mentioned. Table 41.3 shows the results of Esrey and others' (1991) review, attributing a median reduction in incidence of 36 percent to sanitation. Although this figure is the median of the five "better" studies, it must be interpreted with great care because almost all the known studies on the health effects of sanitation are observational studies that use self-selected exposure groups. Confounding by a sense of hygiene is likely to be a significant problem in any such study. From Brazil to Bangladesh, the owners of latrines have been observed to behave more hygienically than their neighbors in practices such as hand washing that are not affected by the presence of a latrine (Hoque and others 1995—see table 41.6;

Table 41.6 Factors Associated with Hand-Washing Behavior by 90 Women in Bangladesh

Associated factor	Hand-washing behavior observed after defecation		Ratio of prevalences of good practice (95 percent confidence interval)
	Good	Poor	
Uses own sanitary latrine			
Yes	22	11	1.73
No	22	35	(1.15–2.59)
Uses tubewell water exclusively			
Yes	18	10	1.53
No	26	36	(1.03–2.29)
Owns agricultural land			
Yes	36	24	2.25
No	8	22	(1.20–4.22)
Believes that washing hands prevents diseases			
Yes	26	27	1.01
No	21	18	(0.66–1.55)

Source: Hoque and others 1995.

Strina and others 2003). It is thus impossible to prove, except by an intervention study, that any health benefit associated with latrine ownership is due to the latrine and not to the hygiene habits of latrine owners.

The overall reduction in diarrhea from sanitation quoted by Esrey and others (1991) likely disguises considerable heterogeneity in terms of the context rather than the type of sanitation technology. For example, sanitation is likely to have a greater effect on diarrheal disease in high-density urban areas, where open defecation leads to gross fecal pollution of the neighborhood, and less effect in rural communities, where all but the youngest children use communal defecation sites some distance away from their homes.

For example, Moraes and others (2003), working in urban *favelas* in northeast Brazil, found that diarrhea incidence among children in households with a toilet was half that in households that did not have one. This comparison is likely to be affected by confounding because the households with toilets were a self-selected group. Comparison between communities is less likely to be affected by confounding, but Moraes and others found a greater reduction. The mean incidence of diarrhea in young children in communities with sewers was only one-third of that in the communities that, for administrative and technical reasons, did not have sanitary drainage.

Thus, although the quality of the studies reviewed by Esrey and others (1991) was in general poor and the range of reductions wide, little doubt exists that excreta disposal can be associated with significant reductions in diarrhea morbidity. Studies showing that proximity to open or overflowing sewers (Moraes and others 2003), failure to dispose hygienically of children's stools (Traoré and others 1994), or the presence of excreta on the ground in the household compound (Bukenya and Nwokolo 1991) is a risk factor for fecal-oral infections provide supporting evidence for the likely effect of sanitation infrastructure, particularly in urban settings, on diarrheal disease transmission.

In conclusion, there are some reasons, such as the likelihood of confounding, to believe that Esrey and others' (1991) median reduction is an overestimate, but reasons exist also to believe that the reductions measured were not as great as they might have been had the provision of sanitation been accompanied by hygiene promotion to ensure that the facilities were fully and appropriately used (especially by young children) and maintained. A systematic review of the effect of sanitation on diarrheal disease is urgently required. Meanwhile, and on balance, Esrey and others' median reduction of 36 percent in diarrhea incidence is the most authoritative estimate available.

Interaction with Water Supply. The results of Esrey and others' (1991) review suggest that the effect of water supply and sanitation combined is no greater than that of either on its own. However, that conclusion is based on only two studies, and the percentage reductions found in the individual studies of each type of intervention exhibit a wide range. Reflection on how in practice each of the two interventions interrupts the transmission of fecal-oral pathogens would suggest that their effects would be largely independent: whereas water supply helps prevent contamination of drinking water, hands, and food, excreta disposal helps prevent contamination of the household yard and surroundings, including children's play areas. Esrey and others (1990) reported three other studies in which sanitation and water supply had a greater effect together than individually, but the reductions in diarrhea incidence in those studies could not be calculated.

For the purpose of burden of disease calculations, therefore, the effects of water supply and sanitation improvements on diarrhea are considered here to be independent and additive, which has the advantage of simplicity.

Effect on Other Disease Categories. The first evidence for the health benefits of excreta disposal related not to its effect on diarrheal disease but on intestinal helminths.

A prolonged series of in-depth studies from 1920 to 1930 by researchers of the Rockefeller Foundation established beyond doubt that promiscuous defecation, especially in the household surroundings and particularly by children, played a major role in the transmission of *Ascaris* spp., *Trichuris* spp., and hookworms in a range of settings from Panama to China and the southeastern United States. By implication, the use of sanitary toilets should interrupt transmission by that route.

However, more recent attempts to measure the reductions in parasite prevalence or intensity attributable to improved sanitation have often suffered from the same shortcomings as the studies of their impact on diarrheal disease; many have been cross-sectional studies and, therefore, subject to confounding.

Esrey and others (1991), in reviewing this literature, found that water supply and sanitation reduced the prevalence of ascariasis by a median of 28 percent (range 0 to 83 percent) and of hookworm infection by 4 percent (0 to 100 percent). Those reductions are likely caused by the sanitation rather than by the water-supply improvements. Indeed, three of the nine positive studies of ascariasis and three of the five positive studies of hookworm involved sanitation alone. It is also likely that the effect of excreta disposal on *Trichuris* infection is similar to that on ascariasis (Henry 1981).

Much emphasis has been placed in recent years on chemotherapy as a control intervention for intestinal helminths, particularly the chemotherapy of schoolchildren. However, that option is not always sustainable because the children are quickly reinfected by the eggs and larvae that remain in the environment. Sanitation, particularly school sanitation, has been adopted by the major international donor agencies as an integral component of the FRESH (Focusing Resources on Effective School Health) framework to ensure its sustainability.

A study in Bangladesh (Mascie-Taylor and others 1999) suggested that chemotherapy was more cost-effective (though less effective) as a helminth control intervention than a health education program that included the promotion of sanitation. However, the health education program was excessively labor intensive and, therefore, expensive; it involved the constant deployment of six health educators and a supervisor in each study area of only 550 households, resulting in a cost of Tk 1600 (US$30) per household, compared with Tk 330 (US$6) per year for chemotherapy. That cost compares with the total cost of US$8 per family for WaterAid's successful "100 percent sanitation" approach in rural Bangladesh (Allan 2003). Whereas the promotion of sanitation is a one-time cost, the cost of chemotherapy is a recurrent annual expenditure. Allowing for such a sanitation promotion initiative once every five years—and using the chemotherapy costing of Mascie-Taylor and others (1999)—sanitation promotion is more cost-effective against helminths in Bangladesh than is chemotherapy. If the cost were apportioned between the effect on diarrheal disease and the effect on helminths, sanitation would be far more cost-effective than chemotherapy.

Sanitation can also help prevent trachoma. More than 70 percent of the incidence of this infection has been shown to be caused by flies, mainly of the species *Musca sorbens*, which breeds preferentially in scattered human feces. Pit latrines have been shown to reduce the population of these flies by depriving them of their breeding sites (Emerson and others 2004).

HYGIENE PROMOTION

To a greater degree than with water supply and sanitation, lamentably little reliable evidence exists on the cost or the effectiveness of interventions to change hygiene behavior and still less on the relative cost-effectiveness of different approaches to the design of such interventions.

The Shortage of Evidence

With regard to effectiveness, Loevinsohn (1990) reviewed health education interventions in developing countries and applied four relatively modest criteria of scientific rigor to the 67 published studies he found:

- a description of the intervention in sufficient detail to allow its replication
- an objective outcome measure, based either on health status or on behavior change
- a control group and a sample size greater than two clusters or 60 individuals

- a description of the target population (in terms of their level of education and other factors) adequate to permit a judgment of the relevance of the study to other contexts.

Only three studies were found to meet all four criteria. One (Stanton and Clemens 1987) dealt with environmental hygiene promotion and raises some doubts—although the hygiene behavior of the intervention group was better than the control, both were significantly worse than they had been before the intervention.

A subsequent review of 31 studies (Cave and Curtis 1999) found 5 more studies that could be considered methodologically sound, but none showed a clear effect on behavior. Of a further 11 studies of "reasonable" rigor, only two showed a major effect on behavior.

Shortcomings also exist in the cost data. Many costings are based on budget forecasts and not on real expenditures. Even when actual expenditures are used, major difficulties exist in apportioning the overhead costs that make up a significant proportion of the total. Health educators and the resources they use (such as vehicles) are rarely dedicated exclusively to health education. A further problem in the derivation of unit costs is agreeing on the denominator, which can be the number of people attending health education sessions, the number of members in their households, or the number of people in the target catchment area. For those reasons, different analysts are likely to derive different unit costs from the same data; indeed, the same authors have on occasion arrived at widely differing unit cost figures from the same data.

Time adds a further dimension to this discussion. Do interventions to promote hygiene behavior change have to be implemented continuously, or at least annually, if their effect is to be sustained, or are such changes self-sustaining?

Sustainability

We will take the last question first. Wilson and Chandler (1993) returned after two years to a population in which a four-month intervention to promote hand washing with soap had included provision of free soap. They found that 79 percent of mothers, the original target group, had continued the practice despite the fact that they now had to buy the soap.

Further evidence of the sustainability of new hygiene behaviors was found by Cairncross and Shordt (2003) in a collaborative study with partner organizations in six developing countries in Africa and South Asia. Target populations of previous hygiene promotion projects were visited at 12-month intervals, and various indicators of hygiene behavior were assessed and compared. In four of the six countries, indicators for populations in which the intervention had ended relatively recently were also compared with those in areas where the last intervention had ended several years previously. Those two types of comparison, with the various indicators assessed in each country, allowed a total of 46 comparisons to be made. Only in three such comparisons was there any indication of a falling-off of hygiene with time since the intervention ended; in one case, the falling-off was attributable to the deteriorating condition of the latrines from wear and tear rather than to a decline in compliance.

In some cases, new hygiene practices have become stronger or more prevalent after the ending of external intervention to promote them, as they become self-propagating and consolidated in the community's material culture (Allan 2003).

It is likely that hygiene promotion activities need to be repeated from time to time—say, every five years—but are not required on a continuous basis. It follows from this observation that calculations of cost-effectiveness should take into account the morbidity and mortality averted not only during the implementation of the intervention, but also for a number of years—perhaps five—thereafter.

Costs

Cases in which the costs as well as the effectiveness of hygiene promotion programs have been documented objectively are few indeed. In the absence of suitable data, Varley, Tarvid, and Chao (1998) calculated a costing for a typical program from first principles, arriving at a cost of US$3 (range US$2 to US$3) per household per year, or US$0.60 per capita.

One of the few cases in which data exist is a program in urban Burkina Faso described by Borghi and others (2002). Their data show that the total cost to the provider of the three-year intervention was US$0.65 per capita, or US$4.54 per seven-person household, after deducting the cost of the international research component. Of this total, 63 percent is composed of administration and undifferentiated start-up costs of the project. Most of the remaining costs were accounted for in roughly equal measure by house-to-house visits, discussions in health centers, hygiene lessons in schools, and street theater presentations.

Additional costs were incurred by the 18.5 percent of households that complied, practicing improved hygiene as a result of the program, amounting to US$8 per household per year. More than 90 percent of that sum was the cost of soap for hand washing.

However, on the basis of the observed increase in prevalence of hand washing with soap, the intervention was estimated to have averted sufficient diarrhea morbidity and mortality to save US$2.80 per household per year (US$15 per compliant household per year) in direct costs of medical care and indirect costs attributable to lost productivity. Of this total, 93 percent represented the lost future productivity associated with the deaths of young children.

Waterkeyn (2003) provides an example from rural Zimbabwe. In the two districts in which the Community Health Clubs approach was examined, it was successful in increasing the prevalence of hand washing with soap among the club members by 6 percent and 37 percent, respectively, and it was successful in reducing the prevalence of open defecation by 29 percent and 98 percent, respectively. The marginal cost of the intervention, which used existing health staff, was US$4.00 per club member, or an average of US$0.67 per member of an affected household. Including the salaries of staff members would roughly double the figure to about US$1.40 per capita.

Those figures can be compared with an estimate of US$5.00 per mother (in 1982 dollars) by Phillips and others (1987) based on a review of several programs. Assuming that roughly 1 in 10 members of the population are mothers of young children, this cost is equivalent to about US$0.50 per capita. For cost-effectiveness analysis, a nominal cost of US$1.00 per capita is, therefore, taken because it is roughly the midpoint of the range of recent estimates.

Effect on Diarrhea

Esrey and others (1991) found only six studies of the effect of hygiene promotion interventions on diarrhea morbidity, with a median reduction of 33 percent. A subsequent review by Huttly, Morriss, and Pisani (1997) arrived at a similar result—a median reduction of 35 percent.

The interventions promoting the single hygiene practice of washing one's hands with soap tended to achieve greater reductions in disease than those that promoted several different behaviors. That finding was confirmed by a systematic review of the literature on hand washing (Curtis and Cairncross 2003), which concluded that hand washing with soap—and interventions to promote it—could reduce diarrhea morbidity by 43 percent and life-threatening diarrhea by 48 percent. Because the effect of diarrhea prevention in DALYs is mainly attributable to the prevention of diarrhea deaths, the higher of these two figures is more appropriate for calculating the effect of hygiene promotion on the burden of disease.

It is not surprising that interventions advocating more behavior changes should have less effect, because numerous messages dilute one another in the minds of the target audience. Because some of the interventions in the systematic review were planned without an adequate prior program of formative research, it is possible that they could have had a still greater effect if they were better conceived.

Effect on Respiratory Infections

Reasons exist to believe that hand washing with soap could be a cost-effective intervention not only against diarrheal diseases, but also for the prevention of acute respiratory infections (ARIs). The intervention is plausible, given what is known about the transmission routes of ARIs, and there is also epidemiological evidence, in that all six published studies of the effect of hand washing on ARIs show a significant reduction (Cairncross 2003b).

These two disease groups are the most important causes of child mortality worldwide, and respiratory infections also cause significant adult mortality, for which no alternative preventive intervention is yet available, field-tested, and ready for implementation. A randomized, controlled trial of the efficacy of hand-washing promotion on an ARI outcome is an urgent priority for future research.

Interactions with Water Supply and Sanitation

It can be argued that there is little point in encouraging people to wash their hands if they do not have access to water or to use a latrine if they do not have one.

The argument has only limited validity where sanitation is concerned; an important role for any hygiene promotion is to promote sanitation itself. With regard to water, in the studies reviewed by Curtis and Cairncross (2003), the reductions in disease achieved by hand washing in settings with indoor piped water supply were not significantly different from those achieved elsewhere. Given that the rationale is ambivalent and the evidence inconclusive, the simplest plausible assumption is that the effects of water supply, sanitation, and hygiene promotion on diarrhea are independent and additive to one another.

EFFECT ON BURDEN OF DISEASE

The effect of water supply, sanitation, and hygiene on the global burden of disease can now be estimated, in two stages. First, the evidence presented in this chapter is used to arrive at the reductions in diarrhea that are expected to result from the various combinations and levels of service and that are assumed for the calculation. Then, these figures are applied to the coverage levels for individual countries and the burden of diarrheal disease prevailing in the different regions of the world. Because such a calculation has been done before by Prüss and others (2002) from rather different premises, it was desirable to examine the comparability of the results.

Assumptions: Reductions in Diarrheal Disease

In summary of the discussion of health effects in this chapter, water supply, sanitation, and hygiene promotion are considered to be associated, under typical conditions, with the reductions in diarrheal disease morbidity shown in table 41.7. These reductions are considered to be independent of one another, so that the relative risks for several interventions can be multiplied.

Table 41.7 Assumed Reductions in Diarrhea Attributable to Water Supply, Sanitation, and Hygiene Promotion

Intervention	Reduction in diarrhea (percent)	Corresponding relative risk
Water supply		
Public source	17	1.20
Additional, for house connection	63	2.70
Excreta disposal	36	1.56
Hygiene promotion	48	1.92

Source: Authors.

These assumptions can be compared as follows with the assumptions underlying a previous calculation of the global burden of disease from water, sanitation, and hygiene (Prüss and others 2002; WHO 2002). For that calculation, the following seven scenarios were considered:

VI. No improved water supply or basic sanitation
Va. Basic sanitation only
Vb. Improved water supply only
IV. Improved water supply and basic sanitation
III. Improved water supply and basic sanitation plus house connection water supply, or improved hygiene or water disinfected at point of use
II. "Regulated" water supply (presumably house connection) and full sanitation
I. Ideal situation, corresponding to absence of disease transmission through water, sanitation, and hygiene.

Scenario II is essentially the position prevailing in industrial countries. Leaving out scenarios I and III, which apply to only a small proportion of the population, the following scenarios are broadly equivalent to the categories considered earlier in this chapter:

VI. No improved water or sanitation
Va. Sanitation only
Vb. Improved water supply (public source)
IV. Both improved water supply and sanitation
II. House connection water supply, and sanitation.

In the Prüss model, the relative risks associated with transition from scenarios Va and Vb to VI are taken as 1.26 and 1.60, respectively, comparable with the figures of 1.20 and 1.56 in table 41.7. However, Prüss and others (2002) assume equal risks in scenarios IV and Va, whereas a relative risk of 1.20 follows from the assumption in this chapter that the effects of water supply and sanitation are independent. The Prüss model assumes a relative risk of 1.54 between scenarios III and IV, corresponding to the diarrhea reduction of 35 percent from hygiene promotion found by Huttly, Morriss, and Pisani (1997). Scenario III is essentially a theoretical construct, and between it and scenario II a further relative risk of 1.8 is assumed (in what Prüss and others term their *realistic approach*), on the basis of some recent trials of home disinfection of water, giving a total of 2.76 between scenarios IV and II. The latter figure is close to the corresponding value of 2.70 implied by the assumptions made here, for different reasons. Scenario I, like scenario III, is included not because it is prevalent in reality, but to illustrate a point. Its equivalent would be the generalized and effective implementation of a well-conceived hygiene promotion intervention. Because such hygiene promotion has hardly ever been provided to whole populations, it is similarly hypothetical. From that perspective, the corresponding relative risks of 2.5 (Prüss and others 2002) and 1.92 (table 41.7) are of a similar order of magnitude.

The similarity of the two sets of assumptions, based on rather different premises, is illustrated in figure 41.3.

To allow for the uncertainty in their assumptions, Prüss and others (2002) calculated the burden of disease attributable to water supply, sanitation, and hygiene using two approaches. The *realistic approach* used the assumptions described above and shown in figure 41.3. The *minimal approach* assumed no difference in risk between scenarios II and III. Given the ideal and hypothetical nature of scenario I and the low probability of intensive hygiene promotion being funded for a population that already benefits from high levels of water supply and sanitation provision, we consider the model on the right of figure 41.3 as *optimistic* and prefer to take for our more *realistic* approach the less ambitious baseline of house connections and full sanitation, which approximates the current position in most of Western Europe and North America. This approach responds to recent calls for "baselines and counterfactuals which should include alternative, operationalizable policy/program options (including the status quo)" (Ezzati 2003, 458). It also has the advantage of providing an estimate of burden of

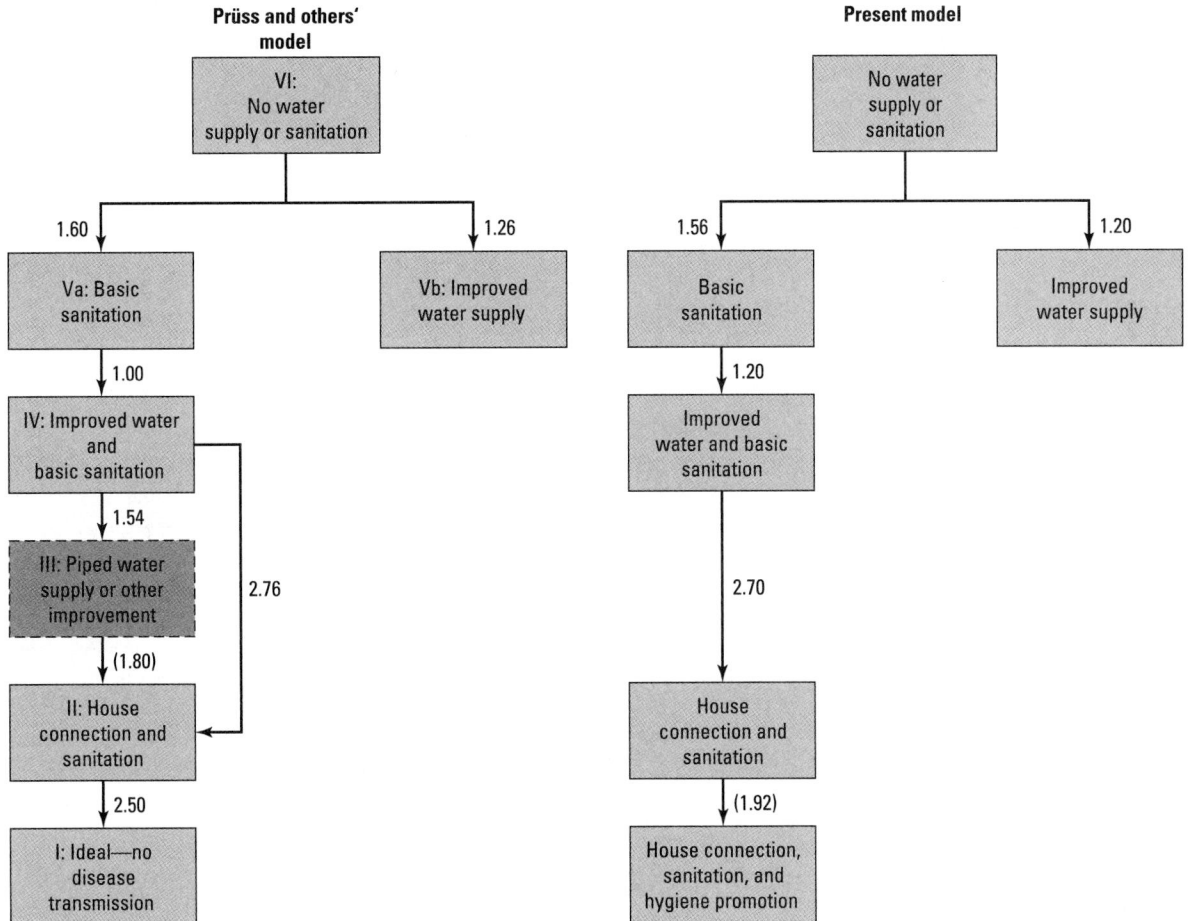

Source: Authors and Prüss and others 2002.

Note: The numbers show relative risk of diarrhea in upper relative to lower boxes. Relative risks in parentheses are set to 1.0 for the minimal version of the Prüss model and for the realistic version of the present model.

Figure 41.3 Comparison of Assumptions Made by Prüss and others (2002) and in this chapter.

disease to which the industrial countries contribute only a negligible amount.

Calculation of Burden of Disease

Prüss and others (2002) worked with water and sanitation coverage data for individual countries (WHO and UNICEF 2000) to derive distributions of the population in each region between five of the seven scenarios, as shown in table 41.8. They then combined these figures with the relative risks in figure 41.3 and diarrhea incidence and case fatality rates from Murray and Lopez (1996) to derive estimates of the number of DALYs attributable to water supply, sanitation, and hygiene in each region and mortality subregion. The results are shown, for their realistic and minimal models, in the first two columns of table 41.9. The realistic estimates are those presented in the *World Health Report 2002* (WHO 2002, 225).

Using the same spreadsheets but the relative risks on the right of figure 41.3, we derive the results in the third and fourth columns of table 41.9 for the optimistic and realistic versions of

the present model. The figures for the burden of disease attributable to deficient water supply, sanitation, and hygiene in the industrial countries of Europe, North America, and the Pacific are very different, but the global totals are remarkably similar.

It should be no surprise to find that the attributable burden in the industrial (that is, low-mortality) countries of Europe, North America, and the Pacific is zero or very close to zero. The realistic model was deliberately designed to take as its baseline the conditions prevailing in those countries. This finding does not mean that no diarrheal disease in those countries can be attributed to deficient water supply, sanitation, or hygiene; rather, it means that the baseline there is the current condition, because no realistic policy option is available to reduce the burden of such disease in the immediate future.

Table 41.10 shows the two realistic assessments of DALYs attributable to water supply, sanitation, and hygiene in terms of percentages of the total DALYs in each region and subregion. Again, the two estimates are close. The proportion of the total disease burden attributable to water, sanitation, and hygiene is greatest in the high-mortality countries of the Eastern

Table 41.8 Distribution of the Population between Scenarios of Water Supply and Sanitation Provision *(percent)*

Region (mortality in children and adults)	Scenario				
	II	IV	Va	Vb	VI
African					
Child high, adult high	0	54	5	6	35
Child high, adult very high	0	42	10	9	38
American (Western Hemisphere)					
Child very low, adult very low	99.8	0	0	0	0.2
Child low, adult low	0	76	1	9	14
Child high, adult high	0	68	0	7	25
Eastern Mediterranean					
Child low, adult low	0	83	5	8	4
Child high, adult high	0	66	0	16	18
European					
Child very low, adult very low	100	0	0	0	0
Child low, adult low	0	79	8	1	12
Child low, adult high	0	94	5	0	1
Southeast Asian					
Child low, adult low	0	70	3	7	19
Child high, adult high	0	35	0	53	12
Western Pacific					
Child very low, adult very low	100	0	0	0	0
Child low, adult low	0	42	1	33	24

Source: Prüss and others 2002.

Table 41.9 Distribution of DALYs Attributable to Diarrhea Caused by Poor Water Supply, Sanitation, and Hygiene by Subregion, According to Various Assumptions
(thousands)

Region (mortality in children and adults)	WHO 2002 (realistic)	Prüss 2002 (minimal)	Present model (optimistic)	Present model (realistic)
African				
Child high, adult high	6,916	6,198	6,747	5,727
Child high, adult very high	11,720	10,473	11,402	9,678
American				
Child very low, adult very low	61	61	49	1
Child low, adult low	1,290	1,143	1,232	1,009
Child high, adult high	756	673	725	613
Eastern Mediterranean				
Child low, adult low	629	548	599	482
Child high, adult high	8,303	7,318	7,983	6,653
European				
Child very low, adult very low	66	66	52	0
Child low, adult low	550	483	528	426
Child low, adult high	121	105	115	91
Southeast Asian				
Child low, adult low	1,241	1,096	1,195	982
Child high, adult high	18,487	16,595	17,856	15,545
Western Pacific				
Child very low, adult very low	27	27	21	0
Child low, adult low	3,991	3,574	3,619	3,303
Total, industrial countries	825	742	765	518
Total, developing countries	53,333	47,618	51,358	43,992
Global total	54,158	48,360	52,123	44,510

Source: See Acknowledgments.

Mediterranean region, reaching 6 to 7 percent of the total. They are followed by the high-mortality countries of Southeast Asia and Africa, where the water and sanitation complex accounts for 4 to 5 percent of the total. Globally, improvements in water supply, sanitation, and hygiene could eliminate 3 to 4 percent of the global burden of disease.

Cost-Effectiveness

The assumptions regarding effect on diarrheal disease are summarized in table 41.7. Because the effect on diarrheal disease accounts for the vast majority of the effect, no effort is made to apportion the costs between their effectiveness in preventing the other diseases affected by water supply, sanitation, and hygiene. The costs derived in this chapter are summarized in table 41.11.

The annual costs used for water supply included both the amortized construction cost and operation and maintenance costs. Given that investments in water supply and sanitation are made largely by other sectors (and for other motives) than health, an alternative cost-effectiveness estimate is made that is based only on the costs of regulation, advocacy, and promotion.

The other assumptions used to calculate the cost-effectiveness of improved water supply—of house connections, of sanitation, and of hygiene promotion—other than those set out above, are as described by Varley, Tarvid, and Chao (1998). The key parameters are as follows:

- proportion of population under age five: 17 percent
- diarrhea incidence: five cases per child under age five per year

Table 41.10 DALYs Due to Diarrhea Attributable to Poor Water Supply, Sanitation, and Hygiene by Subregion, as a Percentage of Total DALYs

Region (mortality in children and adults)	WHO 2002 (realistic)	Present model (realistic)
African		
Child high, adult high	4.7	3.9
Child high, adult very high	5.6	4.6
American (Western Hemisphere)		
Child very low, adult very low	0.1	0.0
Child low, adult low	1.6	1.2
Child high, adult high	4.3	3.5
Eastern Mediterranean		
Child low, adult low	2.7	2.1
Child high, adult high	7.3	5.9
European		
Child very low, adult very low	0.1	0.0
Child low, adult low	1.4	1.1
Child low, adult high	0.2	0.2
Southeast Asian		
Child low, adult low	2.0	1.6
Child high, adult high	5.2	4.3
Western Pacific		
Child very low, adult very low	0.2	0.0
Child low, adult low	1.7	1.4
Total, industrial countries	0.4	0.2
Total, developing countries	4.3	3.5
Global total	3.7	3.0

Source: See Acknowledgments.

- median age at onset of disease: 1 year
- average duration: 8 days
- case fatality rate: 0.5 percent
- coverage by oral rehydration therapy: 30 percent
- oral rehydration therapy reduction in case fatality rate: 50 percent

On this basis, we arrived at the cost-effectiveness values in table 41.12.

All of these figures underestimate the cost-effectiveness of investments in water and sanitation, for several reasons:

- The effects of these interventions on diseases other than diarrhea have not been taken into account; they seem to be relatively minor for water supply but may be substantial if hand washing proves to affect ARI.
- Effects on diarrhea mortality, which account for 98 percent of the DALYs, are likely to be greater than the reductions in morbidity shown in table 41.7.
- The cost figures have generally been taken so as to be sufficient for all contexts, whereas water supply and sanitation can be implemented more cheaply in favorable settings—such as where a convenient aquifer or reliable rainfall exists.
- Potential economies exist in combining the interventions; for example, sanitation promotion can be combined with hygiene promotion and water pipes laid with sewers.
- The current global initiative to promote hand washing, involving commercial marketing expertise, may identify more cost-effective approaches to hygiene promotion.
- If a sustainable low-cost sanitation industry can be developed, it will have an interest in promoting its own product.

As they stand, the cost-effectiveness values above, except for house connections and construction of latrines, are well below the US$150/DALY cutoff value proposed by the World Bank

Table 41.11 Costs Assumed for Cost-Effectiveness Calculations (US$ per capita)

Intervention	Construction cost (US$ per capita)	Amortization lifetime (years)	Amortized annual cost (US$ per capita)	Operation and maintenance cost (US$ per capita)
Water supply				
House connections	150.00	20	7.50	10.00
Hand pump or standpost	40.00	20	1.00	1.00
Water regulation and advocacy		US$0.02 to US$0.10 per capita per year		
Sanitation	≤60.00	5	≤12.00	n.a.
Sanitation promotion	2.50	5	0.50	n.a.
Hygiene promotion	1.00	5	0.20	n.a.

Source: Authors.
n.a. = not applicable.

Table 41.12 Cost-Effectiveness of Water Supply, Sanitation, and Hygiene Promotion (US$/DALY)

Intervention	Cost-effectiveness
Water supply	
Hand pump or standpost	94.00
House connection	223.00
Water sector regulation and advocacy	47.00
Basic sanitation	
Construction and promotion	≤270.00
Promotion only	11.15
Hygiene promotion	3.35

Source: Authors.

(1993) as a criterion of cost-effectiveness. Allowing only for the cost component that should fall to the health sector puts them all well within this ceiling. For comparison, the cost-effectiveness of promoting oral rehydration therapy, the principal other measure available to prevent diarrhea mortality, has been estimated at US$23/DALY. The cost-effectiveness of promoting sanitation and hygiene as derived above (US$11.15 and US$3.35, respectively, per DALY) compares favorably with that figure.

ACKNOWLEDGMENTS

The calculations of the burden of disease were made by Dr. D. Campbell-Lendrum, using spreadsheets derived by Annette Prüss-Üstün. Their collaboration is gratefully acknowledged.

REFERENCES

Allan, S. 2003. "The WaterAid Bangladesh/VERC 100% Sanitation Approach; Cost, Motivation and Subsidy." M.Sc. dissertation, London School of Hygiene and Tropical Medicine.

Altaf, M. A. 1994. "Household Demand for Improved Water and Sanitation in a Large Secondary City: Findings from a Study in Gujranwala, Pakistan." *Habitat International* 18 (1): 45–55.

Arlosoroff S., G. Tchannerl, D. Gray, W. Journey, A. Karp, O. Langenegger, and R. Roche. 1987. *Community Water Supply: The Handpump Option.* Washington, DC: World Bank.

Bern, C., J. Martines, I. de Zoysa, and R. I. Glass. 1992. "The Magnitude of the Global Problem of Diarrheal Disease: A Ten-Year Update." *Bulletin of the World Health Organization* 70 (6): 705–14.

Blum, D., and R. G. Feachem. 1983. "Measuring the Impact of Water Supply and Sanitation Investments on Diarrheal Diseases: Problems of Methodology." *International Journal of Epidemiology* 12 (3): 357–65.

Borghi, J., L. Guinness, J. Ouedraogo, and V. Curtis. 2002. "Is Hygiene Promotion Cost-Effective? A Case Study in Burkina Faso." *Tropical Medicine and International Health* 7 (11): 960–69.

Briscoe, J., R. G. Feachem, and M. M. Rahaman. 1985. "Measuring the Impact of Water Supply and Sanitation Facilities on Diarrhea Morbidity: Prospects for Case-Control Methods." Offset publication WHO/CWS/85.3, World Health Organization, Geneva.

Bukenya, G. B., and N. Nwokolo. 1991. "Compound Hygiene, Presence of Standpipe, and Risk of Childhood Diarrhea in an Urban Settlement in Papua New Guinea." *International Journal of Epidemiology* 20 (2): 534–39.

Cairncross, S. 1990. "Health Impacts in Developing Countries: New Evidence and New Prospects." *Journal of the Institution of Water and Environmental Management* 4 (6): 571–77.

———. 1992. "Sanitation and Water Supply: Practical Lessons from the Decade." Water and Sanitation Discussion Paper 9, World Bank, Washington, DC.

———. 2003a. "Sanitation in the Developing World: Current Status and Future Solutions." *International Journal of Environmental Health Research* 13 (Suppl. 1): S123–31.

———. 2003b. "Handwashing with Soap: A New Way to Prevent ARIs?" *Tropical Medicine and International Health* 8 (8): 677–79.

Cairncross, S., and R. Feachem. 1993. *Environmental Health Engineering in the Tropics.* 2nd ed. Chichester, U.K.: John Wiley & Sons.

Cairncross, S., and J. Kinnear. 1992. "Elasticity of Demand for Water in Khartoum, Sudan." *Social Science and Medicine* 34 (2): 183–89.

Cairncross, S., D. O'Neil, A. McCoy, and D. Sethi. 2003. *Health, Environment, and the Burden of Disease: A Guidance Note.* London: Department for International Development.

Cairncross, S., and K. Shordt. 2003. "It Does Last! Some Findings from a Multi-Country Study of Hygiene Sustainability." *Waterlines* 22 (3): 4–7.

Cave, B., and V. Curtis. 1999. "Effectiveness of Promotional Techniques in Environmental Health." WELL Study 165, London School of Hygiene and Tropical Medicine for Department for International Development.

Chavasse, D. C., R. P. Shier, O. A. Murphy, S. R. Huttly, S. N. Cousens, and T. Akhtar. 1999. "Impact of Fly Control on Childhood Diarrhea in Pakistan: Community-Randomised Trial." *Lancet* 353 (9146): 22–25.

Churchill, A. A., D. de Ferranti, R. Roche, C. Tager, A. A. Walters, and A. Yazer. 1987. "Rural Water Supply and Sanitation: Time for a Change." World Bank Discussion Paper 18, Washington, DC, World Bank.

Curtis, V., and S. Cairncross. 2003. "Effect of Washing Hands with Soap on Diarrhea Risk in the Community: A Systematic Review." *Lancet Infectious Diseases* 3 (5): 275–81.

Curtis, V., B. Kanki, T. Mertens, E. Traore, I. Diallo, F. Tall, and S. Cousens. 1995. "Potties, Pits and Pipes: Explaining Hygiene Behaviour in Burkina Faso." *Social Science and Medicine* 41 (3): 383–93.

Emerson, P. M., S. Cairncross, R. L. Bailey, and D. C. Mabey. 2000. "Review of the Evidence Base for the 'F' and 'E' Components of the SAFE Strategy for Trachoma Control." *Tropical Medicine and International Health* 5 (8): 515–27.

Emerson, P. M., S. W. Lindsay, N. Alexander, M. Bah, S.-M. Dibba, H. B. Faal, and others. 2004. "Role of Flies and Provision of Latrines in Trachoma Control: Cluster-Randomised Controlled Trial." *Lancet* 363: 1093–98.

Esrey, S. A., R. G. Feachem, and J. M. Hughes. 1985. "Interventions for the Control of Diarrheal Diseases among Young Children: Improving Water Supplies and Excreta Disposal Facilities." *Bulletin of the World Health Organization* 63 (4): 757–72.

Esrey, S. A., and J-P. Habicht. 1985. *The Impact of Improved Water Supplies and Excreta Disposal Facilities on Diarrheal Morbidity, Growth, and Mortality among Children.* Cornell International Nutrition Monograph Series 15. Ithaca, NY: Division of Nutritional Sciences, Cornell University.

Esrey, S. A., J. B. Potash, L. Roberts, and C. Shiff. 1990. "Health Benefits from Improvements in Water Supply and Sanitation: Survey and Analysis of the Literature on Selected Diseases." WASH Technical Report 66, Environmental Health Project, Rosslyn, VA, for USAID.

————. 1991. "Effects of Improved Water Supply and Sanitation on Ascariasis, Diarrhea, Dracunculiasis, Hookworm Infection, Schistosomiasis, and Trachoma." *Bulletin of the World Health Organization* 69 (5): 609–21.

Ezzati, M. 2003. "Complexity and Rigour in Assessing the Health Dimensions of Sectoral Policies and Programmes." *Bulletin of the World Health Organization* 81 (6): 458–59.

Feachem, R. G., D. J. Bradley, H. Garelick, and D. D. Mara. 1983. *Sanitation and Disease: Health Aspects of Excreta and Wastewater Management.* Chichester, U.K.: John Wiley & Sons.

Feachem, R. G., E. Burns, S. Cairncross, A. Cronin, P. Cross, D. Curtis, and others. 1978. *Water, Health, and Development: An Interdisciplinary Evaluation.* London: Tri-Med Books.

Gutiérrez, G., R. Tapie-Conyer, H. Guiscafré, H. Reyes, H. Martínez, and J. Kumate. 1996. "Impact of Oral Rehydration and Selected Public Health Interventions on Reduction of Mortality from Childhood Diarrheal Diseases in Mexico." *Bulletin of the World Health Organization* 74 (2): 189–97.

Han, A. M., T. Hlaing, M. L. Kyin, and T. Saw. 1988. "Hand Washing Intervention to Reduce Ascariasis in Children." *Transactions of the Royal Society of Tropical Medicine and Hygiene* 82 (1): 153.

Henry, F. J. 1981. "Environmental Sanitation Infection and Nutritional Status of Infants in Rural St. Lucia, West Indies." *Transactions of the Royal Society of Tropical Medicine and Hygiene* 75 (4): 507–13.

Hoque, B. A., D. Mahalanabis, M. J. Alam, and M. S. Islam. 1995. "Post-Defecation Handwashing in Bangladesh: Practice and Efficiency Perspectives." *Public Health* 109 (1): 15–24.

Huttly, S. R. A., S. S. Morriss, and V. Pisani. 1997. "Prevention of Diarrhea in Young Children in Developing Countries." *Bulletin of the World Health Organization* 75 (2): 165–74.

Jenkins, M. W. 1999. "Sanitation Promotion in Developing Countries: Why the Latrines of Benin Are Few and Far Between." Ph.D. thesis, University of California–Davis, Department of Civil and Environmental Engineering.

Kalbermatten, J. D., D. S. Julius, and C. G. Gunnerson. 1982. *Appropriate Sanitation Alternatives: A Technical and Economic Appraisal.* Baltimore: Johns Hopkins University Press.

Lanata, C. F. 2003. "Studies of Food Hygiene and Diarrheal Disease." *International Journal of Environmental Health Research* 13 (Suppl. 1): S175–83.

Loevinsohn, B. P. 1990. "Health Education Interventions in Developing Countries: A Methodological Review of Published Articles." *International Journal of Epidemiology* 19 (4): 788–94.

Mascie-Taylor, C. G. N., M. Alam, R. M. Montanari, R. Karim, T. Ahmed, E. Karim, and S. Akhtar. 1999. "A Study of the Cost-Effectiveness of Selective Health Interventions for the Control of Intestinal Parasites in Rural Bangladesh." *Journal of Parasitology* 85 (1): 6–11.

Mertens, T. E., M. A. Fernando, T. F. Marshall, B. R. Kirkwood, S. Cairncross, and A. Radalowicz. 1990. "Determinants of Water Quality, Availability, and Use in Kurunegala, Sri Lanka." *Tropical Medicine and Parasitology* 41 (1): 89–97.

Moraes, L. R. S., J. A. Cancio, S. Cairncross, and S. Huttly. 2003. "Impact of Drainage and Sewerage on Diarrhea in Poor Urban Areas in Salvador, Brazil." *Transactions of the Royal Society of Tropical Medicine and Hygiene* 97 (2): 153–58.

Mukherjee, N. 1990. *People, Water, and Sanitation: What They Know, Believe, and Do in Rural India.* New Delhi: National Drinking Water Mission, Government of India.

Murray, C. J. L., and A. D. Lopez. 1996. *Global Health Statistics.* Cambridge, MA: Harvard School of Public Health for WHO and World Bank.

Phillips, M. A., R. G. A. Feachem, and A. Mills. 1987. *Options for Diarrhoel Disease Control: The Cost and Cost-Effectiveness of Selected Interventions for the Prevention of Diarrhea.* London: Evaluation and Planning Centre for Health Care.

Prüss, A., D. Kay, L. Fewtrell, and J. Bartram. 2002. "Estimating the Burden of Disease from Water, Sanitation, and Hygiene at a Global Level." *Environmental Health Perspectives* 110 (5): 537–42.

Rosen, S., and J. R. Vincent. 2001. "Household Water Resources and Rural Productivity in Sub-Saharan Africa: A Review of the Evidence." African Economic Policy Discussion Paper 69, John F. Kennedy School of Government, Harvard University, Cambridge, MA.

Stanton, B. F., and J. D. Clemens. 1987. "An Educational Intervention for Altering Water-Sanitation Behaviors to Reduce Childhood Diarrhea in Urban Bangladesh: II. A Randomized Trial to Assess the Impact of the Intervention on Hygienic Behaviors and Rates of Diarrhea." *American Journal of Epidemiology* 125 (2): 292–301.

Strina, A., S. Cairncross, M. L. Barreto, C. Larrea, and M. S. Prado. 2003. "Childhood Diarrhea and Observed Hygiene Behavior in Salvador, Brazil." *American Journal of Epidemiology* 157 (11): 1032–38.

Thompson, J., I. T. Porras, J. K. Tumwine, M. R. Mujwahuzi, M. Katui-Katua, N. Johnstone, and L. Wood. 2001. *Drawers of Water II: 30 Years of Change in Domestic Water Use and Environmental Health in East Africa.* London: International Institute for Environment and Development.

Traoré, E., S. Cousens, V. Curtis, T. Mertens, F. Tall, A. Traoré, and others. 1994. "Child Defecation Behaviour, Stool Disposal Practices, and Childhood Diarrhea in Burkina Faso: Results from a Case-Control Study." *Journal of Epidemiology and Community Health* 48 (3): 270–75.

Varley, R. C. G., J. Tarvid, and D. N. W. Chao. 1998. "A Reassessment of the Cost-Effectiveness of Water and Sanitation Interventions in Programmes for Controlling Childhood Diarrhea." *Bulletin of the World Health Organization* 76 (6): 617–31.

Victora, C. G., P. G. Smith, J. P. Vaughan, L. C. Nobre, C. Lombardi, A. M. Teixeira, and others. 1988. "Water Supply, Sanitation, and Housing in Relation to the Risk of Infant Mortality from Diarrhea." *International Journal of Epidemiology* 17 (3): 651–54.

Wagner, E. G., and J. N. Lanoix. 1959. *Water Supply for Rural Areas and Small Communities.* WHO Monograph Series 42. Geneva: World Health Organization.

Waterkeyn, J. 2003. "Cost-Effective Health Promotion: Community Health Clubs." In *Proceedings of the 29th WEDC Conference, Abuja, Nigeria.* Loughborough, U.K.: Water Engineering and Development Centre.

White, G. F., D. J. Bradley, and A. U. White. 1972. *Drawers of Water: Domestic Water Use in East Africa.* Chicago: University of Chicago Press.

Whittington, D., X. Mu, and R. Roche. 1990. "Calculating the Value of Time Spent on Collecting Water: Some Estimates for Ukunda, Kenya." *World Development* 18 (2): 269–80.

WHO (World Health Organization). 2002. *Reducing Risks, Promoting Healthy Life: World Health Report 2002.* Geneva: WHO.

WHO and UNICEF (World Health Organization and United Nations Children's Fund). 2000. *Global Water Supply and Sanitation Assessment 2000 Report.* Geneva: WHO with UNICEF.

Wilson, J. M., and G. N. Chandler. 1993. "Sustained Improvements in Hygiene Behaviour amongst Village Women in Lombok, Indonesia." *Transactions of the Royal Society of Tropical Medicine and Hygiene* 87 (6): 615–16.

World Bank. 1993. *World Development Report 1993: Investing in Health.* New York: Oxford University Press.

World Bank Water Demand Research Team. 1993. "The Demand for Water in Rural Areas: Determinants and Policy Implication." *World Bank Research Observer* 8 (1): 47–70.

Zaroff, B., and D. A. Okun. 1984. "Water Vending in Developing Countries." *Aqua* 5: 284–95.

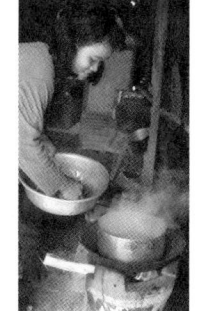

Chapter **42**

Indoor Air Pollution

Nigel Bruce, Eva Rehfuess, Sumi Mehta, Guy Hutton, and Kirk Smith

Access to modern energy sources has been described as a "necessary, although not sufficient, requirement for economic and social development" (IEA 2002). It is, therefore, of great concern that almost half the world's population still relies for its everyday household energy needs on inefficient and highly polluting solid fuels, mostly biomass (wood, animal dung, and crop wastes) and coal.

The majority of households using solid fuels burn them in open fires or simple stoves that release most of the smoke into the home. The resulting indoor air pollution (IAP) is a major threat to health, particularly for women and young children, who may spend many hours close to the fire. Furthermore, the reliance on solid fuels and inefficient stoves has other, far-reaching consequences for health, the environment, and economic development.

NATURE, CAUSES, AND BURDEN OF CONDITION

About 3 billion people still rely on solid fuels, 2.4 billion on biomass, and the rest on coal, mostly in China (IEA 2002; Smith, Mehta, and Feuz 2004). There is marked regional variation in solid fuel use, from less than 20 percent in Europe and Central Asia to 80 percent and more in Sub-Saharan Africa and South Asia.

This issue is inextricably linked to poverty. It is the poor who have to make do with solid fuels and inefficient stoves, and many are trapped in this situation: the health and economic consequences contribute to keeping them in poverty, and their poverty stands as a barrier to change. Where socioeconomic circumstances improve, households generally move up the energy ladder, carrying out more activities with fuels and appliances that are increasingly efficient, clean, convenient, and more expensive. The pace of progress, however, is extremely slow, and for the poorest people in Sub-Saharan Africa and South Asia, there is little prospect of change.

Illustrated in figures 42.1 and 42.2 are findings for Malawi and Peru, respectively, from Demographic and Health Surveys (ORC Macro 2004). The examples are selected from available national studies with data on main cooking fuel use to represent the situation in poor African and South American countries. The main rural and urban cooking fuels are illustrated in figures 42.1a and 42.2a; the findings are then broken down nationally by level of education of the principal respondent (woman of childbearing age) in figures 42.1b and 42.2b, and in urban areas by her level of education in figures 42.1c and 42.2c.

Biomass is predominantly, though not exclusively, a rural fuel: indeed, in many poor African countries, biomass is the main fuel for close to 100 percent of rural homes. Marked socioeconomic differences (indicated by women's education) exist in both urban and rural areas. During the 1990s, use of traditional fuels (biomass) in Sub-Saharan Africa increased as a percentage of total energy use, although in most other parts of the world the trend has generally been the reverse (World Bank 2002).

In many poorer countries, the increase in total energy use accompanying economic development has occurred mainly through increased consumption of modern fuels by better-off minorities. In Sub-Saharan Africa, however, the relative increase in biomass use probably reflects population growth in rural and poor urban areas against a background of weak (or negative) national economic growth. Reliable data on trends in

a. Primary household fuel use in urban and rural areas

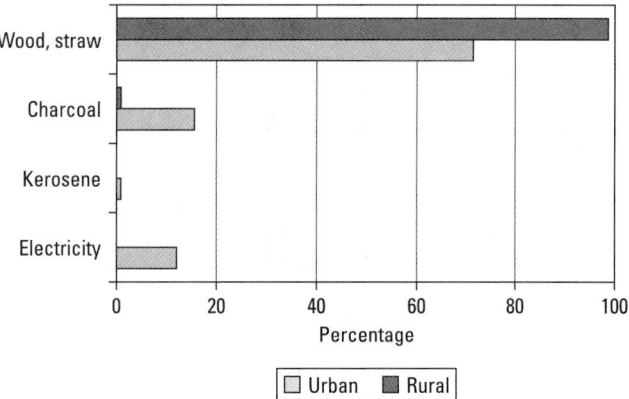

a. Primary household fuel use in urban and rural areas

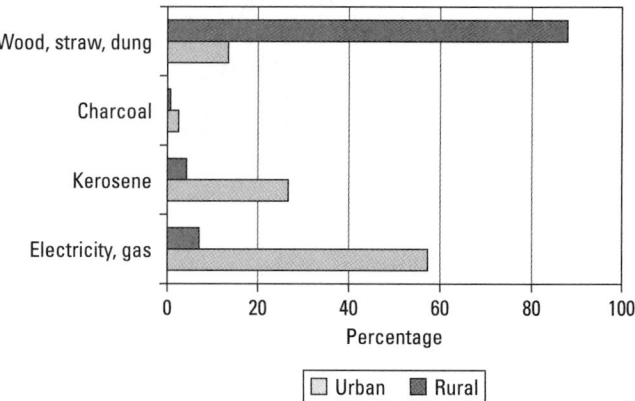

b. Primary household fuel use, by level of education of respondent

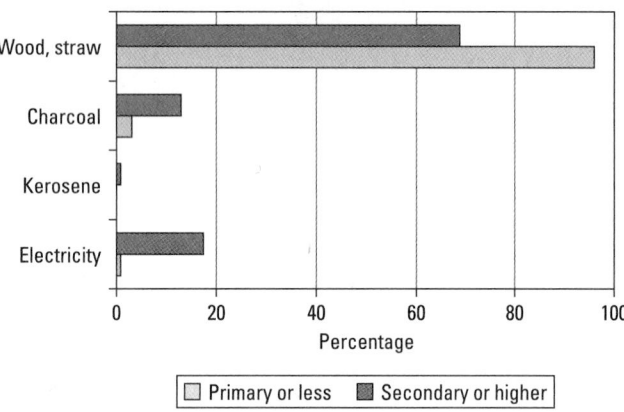

b. Primary household fuel use, by level of education of respondent

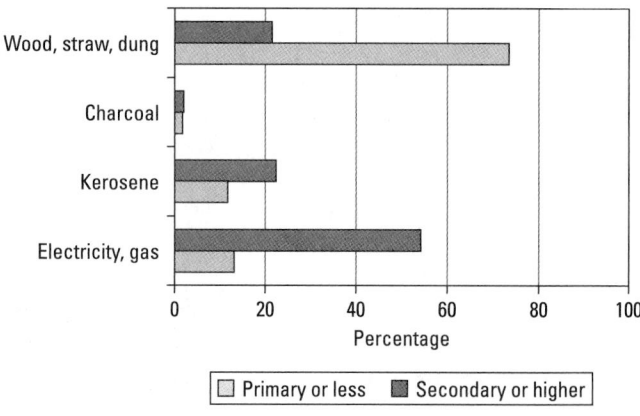

c. Primary household fuel use in urban areas, by level of education of respondent

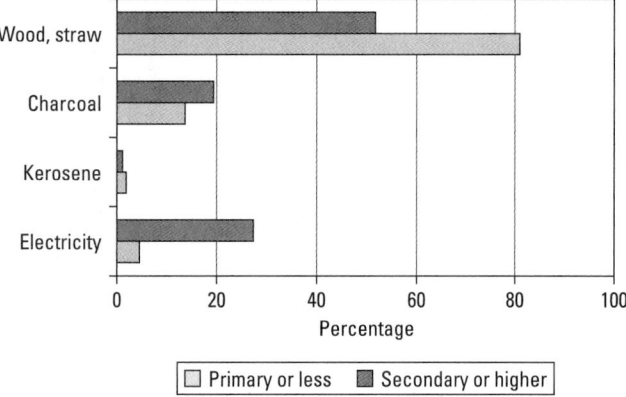

c. Primary household fuel use in urban areas, by level of education of respondent

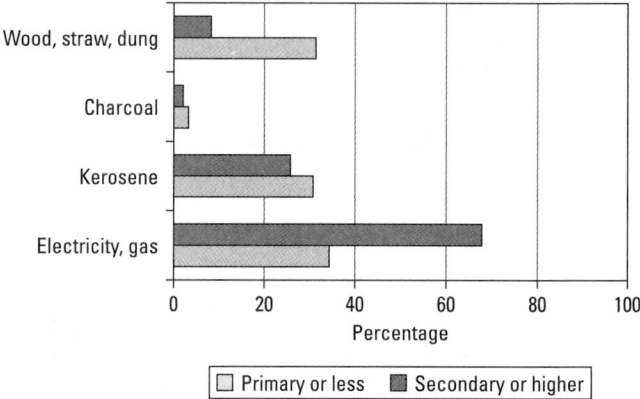

Source: Unpublished data derived from Demographic and Health Survey.

Figure 42.1 Patterns of Household Fuel Use in Malawi, 2000

Source: Unpublished data derived from Demographic and Health Survey.

Figure 42.2 Patterns of Household Fuel Use in Peru, 2000

household energy use are not available for most countries. Information is available from India, where the percentage of rural homes using firewood fell from 80 percent in 1993–94 to 75 percent in 1999–2000 (D'Sa and Narasimha Murthy 2004). Nationally, liquid petroleum gas (LPG) use increased from 9 to 16 percent over the same period, with a change from 2 percent to 5 percent in rural areas, and it is expected to reach 36 percent nationally and 12 percent for rural homes by 2016. International Energy Agency projections to 2030 show that, although a reduction in residential biomass use is expected in most developing countries, in Africa and South Asia the decline will be small, and the population relying on biomass will increase from 2.4 billion to 2.6 billion, with more than 50 percent of residential energy consumption still derived from this source(OECD and IEA 2004). The number of people without access to electricity is expected to fall from 1.6 billion to 1.4 billion. Because electricity is used by poor households for lighting and not as a cleaner substitute for cooking, electrification will not, at least in the short to medium term, bring about substantial reductions in IAP.

Levels of Pollution and Exposure

Biomass and coal smoke emit many health-damaging pollutants, including particulate matter (PM),[1] carbon monoxide (CO), sulfur oxides, nitrogen oxides, aldehydes, benzene, and polyaromatic compounds (Smith 1987). These pollutants mainly affect the lungs by causing inflammation, reduced ciliary clearance, and impaired immune response (Bruce, Perez-Padilla, and Albalak 2000). Systemic effects also result, for example, in reduced oxygen-carrying capacity of the blood because of carbon monoxide, which may be a cause of intrauterine growth retardation (Boy, Bruce, and Delgado 2002). Evidence is emerging, thus far only from developed countries, of the effects of particulates on cardiovascular disease (Pope and others 2002, 2004).

Saksena, Thompson, and Smith (2004) have recently compiled data on several of the main pollutants associated with various household fuels from studies of homes in a wide range of developing countries. Concentrations of PM_{10}, averaged over 24-hour periods, were in the range 300 to 3,000 (or more) micrograms per cubic meter ($\mu g/m^3$). Annual averages have not been measured, but because these levels are experienced almost every day of the year, the 24-hour concentrations can be taken as a reasonable estimate. By comparison, the U.S. Environmental Protection Agency's annual air pollution standard for PM_{10} is 50 $\mu g/m^3$, one to two orders of magnitude lower than levels seen in many homes in developing countries. During cooking, when women and very young children spend most time in the kitchen and near the fire, much higher levels of PM_{10} have been recorded—up to 30,000 $\mu g/m^3$ or more. With use of biomass, CO levels are generally not as high in comparison, typically with 24-hour averages of up to 10 parts per million (ppm), somewhat below the World Health Organization (WHO) guideline level of 10 ppm for an eight-hour period of exposure. Much higher levels of CO have been recorded, however. For example, a 24-hour average of around 50 ppm was found in Kenyan Masai homes (Bruce and others 2002), and one Indian study reported carboxyhemoglobin levels similar to those for active cigarette smokers (Behera, Dash, and Malik 1988). The health effects of chronic exposure of young children and pregnant women to levels of CO just below current WHO guidelines have yet to be studied. For additional information on levels of other pollutants in biomass and coal smoke, see Saksena, Thompson, and Smith (2004).

Fewer studies of personal exposure have been done than of area pollution, mainly because measurement of personal PM typically requires wearing a pump, a cumbersome procedure. CO can be measured more easily and has been used as a proxy: time-weighted (for example, 24-hour average) CO correlates well with PM if a single main biomass stove is used (Naeher and others 2001). Time-activity and area pollution information can also be combined to estimate personal exposure (Ezzati and Kammen 2001). These various methods indicate that personal 24-hour PM_{10} exposures for cooks range from several hundred $\mu g/m^3$ to more than 1,000 $\mu g/m^3$ (Ezzati and Kammen 2001), with even higher exposures during cooking (Smith 1989). Few studies have measured personal PM exposures of very young children: one study in Guatemala found levels a little lower than those of their mothers (Naeher, Leaderer, and Smith 2000).

Health Impacts of IAP

A systematic review of the evidence for the impact of IAP on a wide range of health outcomes has recently been carried out (Smith, Mehta, and Feuz 2004; see table 42.1). This review identified three main outcomes with sufficient evidence to include in the burden-of-disease calculations and a range of other outcomes with as yet insufficient evidence.

Studies for the key outcomes used in the burden-of-disease calculations—acute lower respiratory infection (ALRI), chronic obstructive pulmonary disease (COPD), and lung cancer—had to be primary studies (not reviews or reanalyses), written or abstracted in English (and for lung cancer, Chinese), that reported an odds ratio and variance (or sufficient data to estimate them) and provided some proxy for exposure to indoor smoke from the use of solid fuels for cooking and heating purposes.

A limitation of almost all studies has been the lack of measurement of pollution or exposure: instead, proxy measures have been used, including the type of fuel or stove used, time spent near the fire, and whether the child is carried on the mother's back during cooking. The studies do not, therefore, provide data on the exposure-response relationship, although a recent study from Kenya has gone some way to addressing this omission (Ezzati and Kammen 2001).

In some countries, household fuels carry locally specific risks. It has been estimated that more than 2 million people in China suffer from skeletal fluorosis, in part resulting from use of fluoride-rich coal (Ando and others 1998). Arsenic, another contaminant of coal, is associated with an increased risk of lung cancer in China (Finkelman, Belkin, and Zheng 1999). There has been concern, however, that reducing smoke could increase risk of vectorborne disease, including malaria. Some

Table 42.1 Status of Evidence Linking Biomass Fuels and Coal with Child and Adult Health Outcomes

Health outcome	Age	Status of evidence
Sufficient evidence for burden-of-disease calculation		
Acute lower respiratory infections	Children < 5 years	*Strong.* Some 15–20 observational studies for each condition, from developing countries. Evidence is consistent (significantly elevated risk in most though not all studies); the effects are sizable, plausible, and supported by evidence from outdoor air pollution and smoking.
Chronic obstructive pulmonary disease	Adult women	
Lung cancer (coal exposure)	Adult women	
Chronic obstructive pulmonary disease	Adult men	*Moderate-I.* Smaller number of studies, but consistent and plausible.
Lung cancer (coal exposure)	Adult men	
Not yet sufficient evidence for burden-of-disease calculation		
Lung cancer (biomass exposure)	Adult women	*Moderate-II.* Small number of studies, not all consistent (especially for asthma, which may reflect variations in definitions and condition by age), but supported by studies of outdoor air pollution, smoking, and laboratory animals.
Tuberculosis	Adult	
Asthma	Child and adult	
Cataracts	Adult	
Adverse pregnancy outcomes	Perinatal	*Tentative.* Adverse pregnancy outcomes include low birthweight and increased perinatal mortality. One or a few studies at most for each of these conditions, not all consistent, but some support from outdoor air pollution and passive-smoking studies.
Cancer of upper aerodigestive tract	Adult	
Interstitial lung disease	Adult	
Ischemic heart disease	Adult	Several studies from developed countries have shown increased risk for exposure to outdoor air pollution at much lower levels than IAP levels seen in developing countries. As yet, no studies from developing countries.

Source: Smith, Mehta, and Feuz 2004.

studies have shown that biomass smoke can repel mosquitoes and reduce biting rates (Palsson and Jaenson 1999; Paru and others 1995; Vernede, van Meer, and Alpers 1994). Few studies have examined the impact of smoke on malaria transmission: one from southern Mexico found no protective effect of smoke (adjusted odds ratio 1.06 [0.72–1.58]; Danis-Lozano and others 1999), and another from The Gambia found that wood smoke did not protect children in areas of moderate transmission (Snow and others 1987).

Method Used for Determining Attributable Disease Burden

Smith, Mehta, and Feuz (2004) have provided a full explanation of the calculation of the disease burden associated with IAP. Summarized here are the methods they used to estimate the two most critical components of these calculations: the number of people exposed and the relative risks.

Exposure. The absence of pollution or exposure measurement in health studies required use of a binary classification: the use or nonuse of solid fuels. The authors obtained estimates of solid fuel use for 52 countries from a range of sources, mostly household surveys, and statistical modeling was used for countries with no data (the majority) (Smith, Mehta, and Feuz 2004). They assumed, conservatively, that all

countries with a 1999 per capita gross national product (GNP) greater than US$5,000 had made a complete transition either to electricity or cleaner liquid and gaseous fuels or to fully ventilated solid fuel devices. To account for differences in exposure caused by variation in the quality of stoves, they applied a *ventilation factor* (VF), set from 1 for no ventilation to 0 for complete ventilation. In China, a VF of 0.25 was used for child health outcomes and 0.5 for adult outcomes, reflecting a period of higher exposure (to open fires) before the widespread introduction of chimney stoves. Countries with a 1999 GNP per capita greater than US$5,000 were assigned a VF of 0, and all other countries a value of 1, reflecting the very low rates of use of clean fuels or effective ventilation technologies. The authors obtained the final point estimate for exposure by multiplying the percentage of solid fuel use by the VF. They arbitrarily assigned an uncertainty range of ±5 percent to the estimates.

Risk. Smith, Mehta, and Feuz (2004) carried out meta-analyses for the three health outcomes with sufficient evidence (table 42.2). They used fixed-effects models and sensitivity analysis that took account of potential sources of heterogeneity, including the way in which exposure was defined and whether adjustment had been made for confounders (Smith, Mehta, and Feuz 2004).

Table 42.2 Summary of Relative Risk Estimates for Health Outcomes Used in Burden-of-Disease Estimates

Health outcome	Age and sex group	Number of studies	Relative risk	95 percent confidence interval
ALRI	Children < 5 years	8	2.3	1.9–2.7
COPD	Women > 30 years	8	3.2	2.3–4.8
	Men > 30 years[a]	2	1.8	1.0–3.2
Lung cancer (coal)	Women > 30 years	9	1.9	1.1–3.5
	Men > 30 years	3	1.5	1.0–2.5

Sources: Smith, Mehta, and Feuz 2004.

a. Because of the limited quantity and quality of available evidence, the male COPD relative risk and range have been fixed to include 1.0 (no effect) as the lower estimate.

The Burden of Disease from Solid Fuel Use

Information on the proportions exposed and risk of key disease outcomes was combined with total burden-of-disease data to obtain the population attributable fractions associated with IAP (WHO 2002b). Globally, solid fuels were estimated to account for 1.6 million excess deaths annually and 2.7 percent of disability-adjusted life years (DALYs) lost, making them the second most important environmental cause of disease, after contaminated water, lack of sanitation, and poor hygiene (table 42.3). Approximately 32 percent of this burden (DALYs) occurs in Sub-Saharan Africa, 37 percent in South Asia, and 18 percent in East Asia and the Pacific. In developing countries with high child and adult mortality, solid fuel use is the fourth most important risk factor behind malnutrition, unsafe sex, and lack of water and sanitation, and it is estimated to account for 3.7 percent of DALYs lost (WHO 2002b).

Overall, there are more female deaths but similar numbers of male and female DALYs (table 42.3b). The reason can be found by looking further at the health outcomes. Deaths and DALYs from ALRI in children under five years of age are slightly greater for males (table 42.3c). Women experience twice the DALYs and three times the deaths from COPD (male smoking-attributable COPD deaths excluded). Far fewer cases of lung cancer are attributable to IAP, but women experience about three times the burden of men.

Table 42.3 also shows how the poorest regions of the world carry by far the greatest burden, particularly for ALRI. More than half of all the deaths and 83 percent of DALYs lost attributable to solid fuel use occur as a result of ALRI in children under five years of age. In high-mortality areas, such as Sub-Saharan Africa, these estimates indicate that approximately 30 percent of mortality and 40 percent of morbidity caused by ALRI can be attributed to solid fuel use, as can well over half of the deaths from COPD among women. Because they derive from WHO risk assessments, these estimates include age weights, such that years of life lost at very young or advanced

ages count less than years lost in the prime of adult life. Age weighting makes little difference to the DALYs lost per death up to age five; how much it affects the DALY cost of adult deaths depends on the age distribution of deaths from COPD. Because these are likely to occur at age 45 or beyond, the DALY losses are underestimated compared with estimates without age weighting that follow the usual practice in this volume.

Other Effects of Household Energy Use in Developing Countries

A number of other health impacts—for example, burns from open fires—were not assessed because the burden-of-disease assessment process allowed inclusion of only those health effects resulting directly from pollution. Children are at risk of burns and scalds, resulting from falling into open fires and knocking over pots of hot liquid (Courtright, Haile, and Kohls 1993; Onuba and Udoidiok 1987). Modern fuels are not always safe either, because children are also at risk of drinking kerosene, which is often stored in soft drink bottles (Gupta and others 1998; Reed and Conradie 1997; Yach 1994).

Families—mainly the women and children—can spend many hours each week collecting biomass fuels, particularly where environmental damage and overpopulation have made them scarce. This time could be spent more productively on child care and household or income-generating tasks. There are also risks to health from carrying heavy loads and dangers from mines, snake bites, and violence (Wickramasinghe 2001). Inefficient stoves waste fuel, draining disposable income if fuel is bought. Although women carry out most of the household activities requiring fuels, they often have limited control over how resources can be spent to change the situation (Clancy, Skutsch, and Batchelor 2003). These conditions can combine to restrict income generation from home-based activities that require fuel energy (for example, processing and preparing food for sale).

Homes that are heavily polluted and dark can hinder productivity of householders, including children doing homework and others engaged in home-based income-generating activities such as handicrafts. In many poor homes, lighting is obtained from the open fire and simple kerosene wick lamps, which provide poor light and add to pollution.

Solid fuel use has important environmental consequences. Domestic use of solid fuels in high-density rural and urban environments contributes to outdoor air pollution. Many low-income urban populations rely on charcoal, the production of which can place severe stress on forests. The use of wood as fuel can contribute to deforestation, particularly where it is combined with population pressure, poor forest management, and clearance of land for agriculture and building timber. Damage to forest cover can increase the distance traveled to obtain wood and can result in the use of freshly cut (green) wood, dung, and

Table 42.3 Deaths and DALYs Lost Because of Solid Fuel Use

a. Overall

World Bank region	Deaths (thousands)	DALYs (thousands)	Total burden (percent)
East Asia and the Pacific	540	7,087	18.4
Europe and Central Asia	21	544	1.4
Latin America and the Caribbean	26	774	2.0
Middle East and North Africa	118	3,572	9.3
South Asia	522	14,237	36.9
Sub-Saharan Africa	392	12,318	32.0
World	1,619	38,532	100.0

b. All causes, by sex

World Bank region	Deaths (thousands)			DALYs (thousands)		
	Male	Female	All	Male	Female	All
East Asia and the Pacific	152	388	540	3,028	4,060	7,087
Europe and Central Asia	9	13	21	251	293	544
Latin America and the Caribbean	12	14	26	368	405	774
Middle East and North Africa	57	61	118	1,849	1,724	3,572
South Asia	218	304	522	6,641	7,596	14,237
Sub-Saharan Africa	211	181	392	6,901	5,417	12,318
World	658	961	1,619	19,037	19,495	38,532

c. From ALRI (children under age five)

World Bank region	Deaths (thousands)			DALYs (thousands)		
	Male	Female	All	Male	Female	All
East Asia and the Pacific	40	41	81	1,502	1,535	3,036
Europe and Central Asia	7	6	13	235	204	439
Latin America and the Caribbean	8	7	15	324	281	605
Middle East and North Africa	51	44	95	1,794	1,571	3,365
South Asia	177	178	355	6,228	6,278	12,506
Sub-Saharan Africa	198	153	351	6,777	5,191	11,967
World	481	429	910	16,860	15,058	31,918

d. From COPD (men and women 30 years and over)

World Bank region	Deaths (thousands)			DALYs (thousands)		
	Male	Female	All	Male	Female	All
East Asia and the Pacific	105	338	443	1,461	2,430	3,891
Europe and Central Asia	2	7	9	16	89	104
Latin America and the Caribbean	4	7	11	44	125	168
Middle East and North Africa	6	17	23	55	153	208
South Asia	41	126	167	410	1,314	1,724
Sub-Saharan Africa	13	28	41	124	227	351
World	171	522	693	2,110	4,336	6,446

Source: Modified by authors to World Bank regions, from Smith, Mehta, and Feuz 2004.

twigs, which are more polluting and less efficient. In some urban communities, poverty and supply problems are resulting in the use of plastic and other wastes for household fuel (IEA 2002).

Stoves with inefficient combustion produce relatively more products of incomplete combustion, such as methane, which have a markedly higher global-warming potential than carbon dioxide (Smith, Uma, and others 2000). It has, therefore, been argued that, although the energy use and greenhouse gas emissions from homes in developing countries are small relative to the emissions generated in industrial countries, cleaner and more efficient energy systems could provide the double benefit of reduced greenhouse gas emissions (with opportunities for carbon trading) and improved health through reduced IAP (Wang and Smith 1999).

The evidence available for assessing these effects, which together could have a substantial influence on health and economic development, is patchy at best. This area is important for research (Larson and Rosen 2002).

INTERVENTIONS AND POLICY

The uses of energy in the home—for example, for cooking and keeping warm and as a focus of social activities—have important attributes that are specific to the locality, culture, and individual households and are often associated with established traditions and deeply held beliefs. Encouraging the use of cleaner and more efficient energy technologies by populations that are among the poorest in the world has not been easy, but recent years have seen progress being made with respect to suitable technology that meets the needs of households and with respect to the development of supportive policy.

Poverty Reduction and the Millennium Development Goals

Given the close relationship between socioeconomic conditions and solid fuel use, poverty reduction must be a key element of policy to alleviate IAP. The United Nations Millennium Development Goals set targets for poverty eradication, improvements in health and education, and environmental protection; they represent the accepted framework for the world community to achieve measurable progress (United Nations Statistics Division 2003). Although reducing IAP can contribute to achieving a number of these goals, it is particularly relevant to reducing child mortality (Goal 4) from ALRI.

Goal 7, Target 9, aims at integrating sustainable development into country policies and programs. The proportion of population using solid fuels has been adopted as an indicator for Target 9. Alleviating drudgery resulting from collecting fuel and using inefficient stoves, together with the involvement of women in implementing changes, can promote gender equality and empower women (Goal 3). Household energy interventions can also contribute to eradicating extreme poverty (Goal 1) through health improvements, time saving, and better environments for education and facilitating income generation (WHO 2004a).

Interventions

Although the main focus of this chapter is IAP, the many other ways in which household energy can affect health and development emphasize why interventions should aim to achieve a range of benefits, including the following:

- reduced levels of IAP and human exposure
- increased fuel efficiency
- reduced time spent collecting fuel and using inefficient stoves
- reduced stress on the local environment
- increased opportunities for income generation
- contribution to an overall improvement in the quality of the home environment—in particular, the working environment and conditions for women.

Interventions for reducing IAP can be grouped under three headings: those acting on the *source of pollution*, those improving the *living environment* (aspects of the home), and changes to *user behaviors* (table 42.4).

It should not be assumed that an intervention that reduces IAP will necessarily achieve other aims listed previously. For example, in colder areas, an enclosed stove with a flue that reduces IAP may reduce radiant heat and light, forcing households to use other fuels for those purposes. If not addressed with households, such problems may well result in disappointing reductions in IAP exposure, poor acceptance of interventions, and lack of motivation to maintain them.

Policy Instruments

Although a range of interventions is available, poor households face many barriers to their adoption, and enabling policy is needed (table 42.5). This area of practice is complex and evolving, often requiring solutions that are highly setting specific.

INTERVENTION COSTS AND EFFECTIVENESS

The cost-effectiveness analysis discussed in this chapter is based on recent work by Mehta and Shahpar (2004). The key components of this analysis are described here, with particular emphasis on the underlying assumptions.

Table 42.4 Interventions for Reducing Exposure to IAP

Source of pollution	Living environment	User behaviors
Improved cooking devices	*Improved ventilation*	*Reduced exposure through operation of source*
• Improved biomass stoves without flues • Improved stoves with flues attached	• Hoods, fireplaces, and chimneys built into the structure of the house • Windows and ventilation holes (such as in roof), which may have cowls to assist extraction	• Fuel drying • Using pot lids to conserve heat • Properly maintaining stoves and chimneys and other appliances
Alternative fuel-cooker combinations • Briquettes and pellets • Charcoal • Kerosene • Liquid petroleum gas • Biogas, producer gas • Solar cookers (thermal) • Other low-smoke fuels • Electricity	*Kitchen design and placement of the stove* • Kitchen separate from house to reduce exposure of family (less so for cook) • Stove at waist height to reduce direct exposure of cook leaning over fire	*Reductions by avoiding smoke* • Keeping children away from smoke—for example, in another room (if available and safe to do so)
Reduced need for the fire • Insulated fireless cooker (haybox) • Efficient housing design and construction • Solar water heating		

Source: Modified from Ballard-Tremeer and Mathee 2000.

Table 42.5 Policy Instruments for Promoting Implementation of Effective Household Energy Interventions

Policy instruments	Examples	Applications
Information, education, and communication	Schools	Learning about household energy, health, and development should be integrated in school curricula, particularly in countries where these topics are a priority for health and economic development. This goal can be achieved through programs such as the WHO Global School Health Initiative, which promotes environmental health education, including education about IAP.
	Media	Local and national radio, television, and newspapers can be used to raise awareness and disseminate information on technologies and opportunities to support implementation, such as promotions and microcredit. These media can be directed at a range of audiences, including decision makers, professionals, and the public where radio is widely used.
	Community education	Opportunities such as adult literacy programs can be used to raise awareness and share experience of interventions, and innovative methods can be used (for example theater).
Taxes and subsidies	Tax on fuels and appliances	Reduced tax on fuels and appliances may promote development of distribution networks and uptake, and it may be seen as efficient if there is evidence of health, education, and economic benefits.
	Subsidy on fuels and appliances	General (for example, national) subsidies on fuels such as kerosene have been applied to promote use by poor households. Subsidies have been found to be inefficient instruments, however, often benefiting the better off rather than the poor. Time-limited subsidy on specific products (for example, clean fuel appliances, connection to grid) may be a useful method for promoting initial uptake, generating demand, and thereby providing market conditions for lower prices and more consistent quality.
Regulation and legislation	Air quality standards	Although some developing countries have air quality standards for urban air, none have them for indoor air in settings where solid fuels are widely used. Routine monitoring and enforcement is not practical, but it may be useful to set standards and targets linked to specific assessments. For more routine use, information from censuses and surveys, such as fuel type, stove type, and venting for smoke, offers a practical alternative for setting air quality standards for IAP in developing countries.
	Design standards for appliances	Design standards can be applied to safety (prevention of burns, gas leaks, and explosions); venting of emissions; and efficiency. Although such standards may be difficult to enforce in an informal economy, they could become valuable with wider-scale production.
Direct expenditures	Public program provision of appliances	Large-scale public provision of appliances, such as improved stoves or clean-fuel appliances, has generally been found unsuitable. Some form of targeted provision or partial subsidy where households have made informed choices and commit to cost sharing may be useful to stimulate demand and act in favor of equity.

Table 42.5 Continued

Policy instruments	Examples	Applications
	Funding of finance schemes	Experience has shown that credit is most likely to be made available and adopted for energy applications that contribute directly to productive, income-generating activities (such as food processing for sale). Meeting everyday cooking and space-heating needs is seen as a lower priority. Good opportunities may exist where biomass fuel is purchased and where cost saving combines with other valued benefits, such as increased prestige and cleaner kitchens. Support for such schemes, mainly in the form of raising awareness, skills training in managing funds, and seed funding (the main source of funds being from users) may be cost-effective.
Research and development	Surveys	Surveys of fuel and appliance use, knowledge of risks to health, willingness to pay for interventions, knowledge of and confidence in credit schemes, and the like are important for planning interventions.
	Development and evaluation of interventions	Evaluation of interventions should be conducted in a range of settings, using harmonized methods, if possible, that allow local flexibility but permit comparison with other types of interventions and other locations.
	Studies of health effects	Stronger and better-quantified evidence of the effects on health of reducing IAP, which includes exposure measurement, is required not only for key outcomes such as ALRI, but also for other health outcomes for which evidence is currently tentative.
	Research capacity development	Capacity for carrying out a wide range of research—from national and local surveys, to monitoring and evaluation of interventions, to more complex health studies—requires strengthening in those countries where the problems associated with household energy and IAP are most pressing.

Source: Authors.

Costs

Intervention costs have a number of components, the relative importance of which will vary with the type of fuel and device (box 42.1).

The level of costs incurred by consumers and others, including government, depends not only on the type of intervention but also on how it is delivered, supplied, and adopted.

Experience indicates that successful interventions are sustainable in local markets, implying that the consumer pays the majority of initial and recurrent costs. The contributions of the government, utilities, nongovernmental organizations (NGOs), and the commercial sector will depend on many factors, including the type of intervention and fuel, location (urban or rural), existing level of supply and distribution

---

Box 42.1

Cost Components for Household Energy Interventions

- *Fuels,* which vary from zero (in direct cash terms, though not in opportunity cost) for collected biomass to a U.S. dollar or so per week for kerosene and several U.S. dollars per week for electricity (where used for cooking).
- *Stove appliances,* which vary from zero for a simple three-stone fire (stones arranged on the floor to support cooking pots, with the fire lit between the stones), to US$50 (and in some cases more than US$100) for a good-quality woodstove with a chimney and up to several hundred U.S. dollars for a biogas installation.

- *Additional appliances*—for example, an LPG storage bottle has a moderately high initial cost but should last for many years.
- *Maintenance costs,* which vary from zero for a three-stone fire up to modest, but not negligible, costs of repairing (and periodically replacing) woodstoves and chimneys. Appliances for using kerosene, LPG, and electricity also require maintenance and periodic replacement.
- *Program costs,* which apply to various aspects of provision of energy services, particularly LPG and electricity, but may also include costs of, for example, establishing more sustainable biomass reserves and administrative costs.

Source: Authors.

Cost Issues in Switching to Cleaner Fuels for a "Typical" Poor Kenyan Family

Ruth[1] and her family live 3 kilometers from a small town on the main road about one hour by bus from Kisumu. They are subsistence farmers, with a small income from selling vegetables, from irregular laboring work obtained by her husband, and from making and selling handicrafts. Ruth, a mother of five, cooks over a three-stone fire using mostly wood, which she collects every other day from plots up to two hours walking distance from home. She spends 8 to 12 hours each week collecting wood. Ruth and her family use about 2 liters of kerosene each week for wick lamps and for cooking. They use dry cell batteries for the radio; grid electricity runs nearby, but connection is far too expensive. In all, the family spends an equivalent of US$1 to US$2 per week on fuel and batteries.

Through her women's group, Ruth hears that a few families are using LPG, now available at a nearby petrol station. The women say it is very quick and easy to use, and it keeps pots, clothes, and walls clean. The women and children seem to feel better, with less cough, runny eyes, and headaches. But those families run small shops and

have been able to find the money to buy the gas bottle and cooker.

She talks with her husband about LPG, and although quite supportive, her husband thinks they cannot afford it. They could spend a little more on fuel, but income is irregular. Why abandon free fuel when they are so poor? Ruth thinks she could earn more money from her handicrafts in the time she saves collecting wood. On balance, they reckon they could probably afford the cost of the gas if they could be sure of more regular income, but they do not know where they could find the money to pay for the cooker and bottle.

Ruth then learns about a revolving fund set up by her women's group with the help of an NGO. If she can make small regular payments, she and her husband could get a loan to buy the stove and gas bottle next year. But they have never saved before, and what if they need money for medicines or for the children at school? Will they be able to keep saving each week to make sure they have enough to refill the gas bottle when needed?

1. Not her real name.
Source: Authors.

---

networks, and support for credit (for example, seed funds and fund capital) and targeted subsidies.

Some degree of market support may be required to stimulate demand and to encourage adoption by poor households, particularly those using three-stone fires (and other simple stoves) and collected biomass, because those methods do not incur direct monetary costs. Some countries have applied subsidies on fuels such as kerosene to assist poor families, but general subsidies are now considered to be an inefficient instrument for this purpose (von Schirnding and others 2002). Targeted subsidy and small-scale credit may be more appropriate ways of helping poor families acquire new household energy technologies and can have low default rates. Experience shows, however, that households are more likely to access credit for directly productive (with regard to income) uses of energy, rather than for everyday cooking and space-heating needs. Because the latter are the most important sources of IAP, more promotion of other benefits is needed, such as improved family health; fuel cost savings; time saved by faster cooking and reduced need for biomass; greater prestige; and cleaner homes, clothes, and utensils. A number of these benefits may result in reduced expenditure or increased income generation.

Box 42.2 illustrates how these various issues can influence the decisions of a "typical" poor rural African household considering transition from gathered biomass to predominant use of a commercial fuel (LPG).

Effectiveness

Most evidence available for assessing intervention effectiveness deals with the effect on IAP levels and in some cases personal exposure. No experimentally derived evidence is available, however, on the effect of reducing IAP exposure on incidence of ALRI or the course of COPD in adults. A randomized trial of an improved chimney stove is currently under way in Guatemala, focusing on ALRI in children up to 18 months of age (Dooley 2003). A cohort study in Kenya by Ezzati and Kammen (2001) describes significant exposure-response relationships for all acute respiratory infections—and for ALRI specifically—associated with the use of traditional and improved woodstoves and charcoal. However, those effect estimates require confirmation because the study has small numbers of children (93 children under age five, living in 55 homes). For the other major health outcome, lung cancer, Lan and others (2002) reported adjusted hazard ratios of 0.59 (95 percent confidence interval: 0.49 to 0.71) for men and 0.54 (0.44 to 0.65) for women using improved coal stoves compared with traditional open coal fires in a 16-year retrospective cohort study in rural China.

Measuring evidence on reductions in pollution and exposure is nonetheless an important step in assessing effectiveness. Summarized here are the main findings of studies that have measured pollution levels in homes using traditional open fires, various improved stoves, kerosene, and LPG (see also Saksena, Thompson, and Smith 2004) and one that examined the effect of rural electrification in South Africa (Rollin and others 2004).

Effect of Improved Stoves. In East Africa, cheap improved stoves without flues, burning either wood or charcoal, are popular. These wood-burning stoves can reduce kitchen pollution by up to 50 percent, but levels still remain high (Ezzati, Mbinda, and Kammen 2000). Charcoal emits much less PM (but with a higher CO-to-PM ratio than wood), and stoves such as the Kenyan *jiko* yield particulate levels in the region of 10 percent of those from wood fires.

In a number of Asian and Latin American countries, improved stoves with flues have been promoted quite extensively, although many such stoves are found to be in poor condition after a few years. Some studies from India have shown minimal or small reductions in PM (Ramakrishna 1988; Smith, Aggarwal, and Dave 1983). Other studies, from Nepal, have shown reductions of about two-thirds, although the very high baseline levels mean that homes with stoves still recorded total suspended particulate values of 1,000 to 3,000 $\mu g/m^3$ during cooking (Pandey and others 1990; Reid, Smith, and Sherchand 1986). Results from Latin American countries are similar, although the IAP levels are generally lower. Studies have shown that *plancha*-type stoves (made of cement blocks, with a metal plate and flue) reduce PM by 60 to 70 percent and by as much as 90 percent when they are in good condition. Typical 24-hour PM levels (PM_{10}, $PM_{3.5}$ [respirable], and $PM_{2.5}$ have variously been reported) with open fires of 1,000 to 2,000 $\mu g/m^3$ have been reduced to 300 to 500 $\mu g/m^3$, and in some cases to less than 100 $\mu g/m^3$ (Albalak and others 2001; Brauer and others 1996; Naeher, Leaderer, and Smith 2000). One study from Mexico found little difference between homes with open fires and with improved stoves (Riojas-Rodriguez and others 2001), but the 16-hour levels of PM_{10} at about 300 $\mu g/m^3$ with open fires were relatively low.

Improved stoves with flues have so far had little success in Sub-Saharan Africa, although recent work developing hoods with flues for highly polluted Kenyan Masai homes reported reductions in 24-hour mean respirable PM of 75 percent from more than 4,300 $\mu g/m^3$ to about 1,000 $\mu g/m^3$ (Bruce and others 2002).

Personal exposures were usually found to have been reduced proportionately less than area pollution levels. For example, in Kenya, where hoods with flues achieved a 75 percent reduction in 24-hour mean kitchen $PM_{3.5}$ and CO, the woman's mean 24-hour CO exposure was reduced by only 35 percent (Bruce and others 2002). Similar results were found for child exposures in a study of improved wood stoves in Guatemala (Bruce and others 2004). We are aware of only one study that has used direct measurement of personal particulate exposure in very young children (Naeher, Leaderer, and Smith 2000). This study, also in Guatemala, reported mean 10- to 12-hour (daytime) $PM_{2.5}$ levels for children under 15 months of age of 279 $\mu g/m^3$ (+SD of 19.5) for the open fire and 170 $\mu g/m^3$ (+154) for the *plancha* stoves, a 40 percent reduction.

Impact of Cleaner Fuels. Good evidence shows that kerosene and LPG can deliver much lower levels of pollution, although it is important to determine the extent to which the cleaner fuel is substituting for biomass. For example, a study in rural Guatemala comparing LPG with open fires and *plancha* chimney stoves found that LPG-using households typically also used an open fire for space heating and cooking with large pots. As a result, the *plancha* stoves achieved the lowest pollution levels in that setting (Albalak and others 2001). Still, a number of studies, mainly from India, show that introducing kerosene and LPG dramatically reduces kitchen pollution, which perhaps reflects different cooking requirements and less need for space heating. In rural Tamil Nadu, two-hour (mealtime) kitchen respirable PM levels of 76 $\mu g/m^3$ using kerosene and of 101 $\mu g/m^3$ using gas contrasted with levels of 1,500 to 2,000 $\mu g/m^3$ using wood and animal dung (Parikh and others 2001). Personal (cook) 24-hour exposure to respirable PM was 132 $\mu g/m^3$ with the use of kerosene as opposed to 1,300 and 1,500 $\mu g/m^3$, respectively, with the use of wood and dung (Balakrishnan and others 2002). Other studies confirm those findings, for example, with the use of gas in Mexico (Saatkamp, Masera, and Kammen 2000).

Delivering electricity to rural homes requires extensive infrastructure, and most poor people with access to electricity can afford to use it only for lighting and running low-demand electrical appliances. Without marked improvements in socioeconomic conditions, electrification has little potential to bring about substantial reductions in IAP. South Africa is one of the few countries with a large rural population traditionally dependent on biomass that has the resources for rural electrification. An investigation of three rural villages with similar socioeconomic characteristics, two not electrified and one electrified, in the North West province found that 3.6 years (average) after connection to the grid, 44 percent of the electrified homes had never used an electric cooker (Rollin and others 2004). Only 27 percent of electrified homes cooked primarily with electricity; the remainder used a mix of electricity, kerosene, and solid fuels. Despite the mixed fuel use, households cooking with electricity had the lowest pollution levels. Overall, homes in the electrified village had significantly lower 24-hour mean respirable PM and CO levels and significantly lower mean 24-hour CO exposure for children under 18 months of age than homes in the nonelectrified villages.

Effect of Other Interventions. Little systematic evaluation has been made of other interventions listed in table 42.4. Investigation of the potential of improving ventilation has, overall, shown that although enlarging eaves can be quite effective (Bruce and others 2002), removing smoke generally requires a well-functioning flue or chimney. Behavioral changes are currently the subject of an intervention study in South Africa (Barnes and others 2004a, 2004b).

Cost-Effectiveness Analysis

Although clean fuels can be expected to have a greater health effect than improved stoves (even those with flues), clean fuels may be too expensive and inaccessible for many poor communities over the short to medium term. Furthermore, even though clean fuels may be the best longer-term goal, an intermediate stage of improved biomass stoves may promote change by raising awareness of benefits and thus creating demand by improving health, saving time, and mitigating poverty. For those reasons, this cost-effectiveness analysis (CEA) examines both improved biomass stove and clean fuel options in the following scenarios:

- access to improved stoves (stoves with flues that vent smoke to the exterior), with coverage of 95 percent
- access to cleaner fuels (LPG or kerosene), with coverage of 95 percent
- part of the population with access to cleaner fuels (50 percent) and part with improved stoves (45 percent).

In each case, the intervention is compared with the current level of coverage of the respective technology or fuel.

Cost Assumptions. The assumptions for costs include program costs, fixed costs (including stoves), and recurrent fuel costs. Household costs for each region were drawn from the most comprehensive estimates available in the literature (von Schirnding and others 2002; Westoff and Germann 1995). For LPG, costs include the initial price of a cooker and cylinder and the recurrent refill costs. Assumed household annual costs, discounted at 3 percent, range from US\$1 to US\$10 for improved stoves and from US\$3 to US\$4 for kerosene or up to US\$30 for LPG. Recurrent costs of fuel were found to be the most significant cost for the cleaner fuel interventions. Wood fuel costs are estimated at US\$0.25 per week and assumed to be the same for traditional and improved stoves.

Costs were estimated separately for cleaner fuel and improved stove programs, using an "ingredients" approach (Johns, Baltussen, and Hutubessy 2003) and a costing template developed by WHO (2003). In summary, all the ingredients—including administrative, training, and operational costs—necessary to set up and maintain a given program must be added up. For regional estimates, costs of all traded goods were in U.S. dollars, whereas nontraded (local) costs were estimated in local currency and converted to U.S. dollars using relevant exchange rates. All costs were annualized using a 3 percent discount rate. Costs for tradable goods are scaled, using region-specific standardized price multipliers to reflect the increasing costs of expanding coverage caused by higher transportation costs to more remote areas (Johns, Baltussen, and Hutubessy 2003). Price multipliers were not applied to improved stoves because they tend to be manufactured locally with mainly local materials. Program costs were found to make up a small proportion of the overall intervention costs. Savings from averted health care costs are not included; because many of these cases currently go untreated, it can be argued that including treatment costs could result in inflated cost-effectiveness ratios (CERs).

Effectiveness and Health Outcome Assumptions. For this analysis, cleaner fuels are assumed to remove exposure completely, whereas improved stoves are assumed to reduce exposure by 75 percent (ventilation factor of 0.25). The effect on health of the exposure reduction will vary from region to region, because it depends on current levels of exposure as well as region-specific rates of morbidity and mortality. A number of assumptions have been made about households in carrying out analyses at the regional level. First, regional estimates of household composition (numbers of people, by age group and sex) and, hence, the effect of interventions on exposure and health apply at the level of individual households. Second, the age distribution of household members is similar in exposed and nonexposed groups; for example, the number of children per household is the same irrespective of household fuel use and ventilation characteristics. That assumption is likely to be conservative, since poorer, more polluted homes will typically have higher fertility and more children under five; all other factors being equal, such households would therefore experience a higher burden of disease from IAP exposure.

The health outcomes included are ALRI and COPD, because they were responsible for nearly all of the 1.6 million deaths attributable to IAP. The risk estimates used are those derived from the meta-analyses, as summarized in table 42.2. Smoking is an important confounding variable for COPD, particularly with men, because they generally smoke more than women do in developing countries. At present, information is sparse on the independent effect of solid fuel use on COPD in the presence of smoking. To avoid possible overestimation of the impact of IAP on COPD, attributable fractions for COPD from solid fuel use were applied to disease burdens remaining after removal of smoking-attributable burdens (Ezzati and Lopez 2004). Current estimates of exposure are used in combination with estimates of disease burden to obtain region-specific disease burdens for exposed and unexposed populations. Regional patterns of disease for 2000 have been used, including incidence, mortality, remission, duration, and case-fatality rate, obtained from WHO (2004b). In contrast to the estimates of burden in table 42.3, no age weighting has been used in the cost-effectiveness analysis. Health impacts are discounted at 3 percent.

Implementation Period. The implementation period is 10 years, although effects have been evaluated over 100 years in order to approximate the benefits for an entire population cohort. Thus, health effects are calculated for a cohort with a typical age structure for the population concerned that experiences the intervention for 10 years. It is assumed that after 100 years, all of the cohort (including children born during the 10-year implementation period) will have died.

The implementation period has critical implications, particularly in situations in which it takes several years to establish an intervention (for example, developing local markets for cleaner fuel), in which there are high start-up costs, and in which disease prevention is experienced in the distant future. This is especially true for chronic health effects (for example, COPD) that result from exposure over many years. If the intervention is implemented and exposure reduced for only 10 years, the disease burden is effectively deferred by 10 years, whereas longer-term implementation would result in many more cases being averted. For this analysis, using the 10-year intervention scenario specified for the Disease Control Priorities Project-2, incident cases are deferred by 10 years. For COPD, it is assumed that reduced exposure results in a milder form of COPD, accounted for by using a lower severity weighting.

Findings for Cost-Effectiveness Analysis. Findings from the CEA are expressed, for the four intervention scenarios with differing coverage (50 percent, 80 percent, 95 percent), by region, as (a) total healthy years gained in each region, (b) CERs in U.S. dollars per healthy year gained, and (c) healthy years gained per US$1 million (table 42.6). For all regions, the cleaner fuels yield the greatest gain in healthy years, but improved stoves also have a significant effect. The largest total population gains in healthy years are in Sub-Saharan Africa and South Asia for all types of interventions and in East Asia and the Pacific (mainly China) for cleaner fuels.

In the two regions with the largest burden of disease attributable to solid fuel use (Sub-Saharan Africa and South Asia), CERs are lowest (most favorable) for improved stoves, although in both regions kerosene has CERs just over twice those of improved stoves. In East Asia and the Pacific, kerosene is most cost-effective, followed by improved stove and clean fuel combinations and then by LPG (for coverage over

50 percent). In Latin America and the Caribbean, kerosene has the most favorable CER, followed by kerosene in combination with improved stoves. When the 50 percent and 80 percent coverage scenarios are compared, large differences in the ratio are seen in regions where coverage for that intervention is already substantial, and there is much less health gain at lower levels of coverage. Where no result is given, the specified coverage of the intervention has already been reached.

Multivariate sensitivity analysis was conducted to assess the effect of uncertainty in cost and effectiveness estimates. Costs were assumed to vary with a standard deviation of 5 percent, and effectiveness by the range of the confidence interval around the relative risk for each health endpoint. Results for Southeast Asia are shown in figure 42.3: the "clouds," or uncertainty regions, illustrate the range of possible point estimates emerging from the sensitivity analysis. This example is representative because other regions show essentially similar results. Despite the uncertainty, the ranking of the interventions remains the same (Mehta and Shahpar 2004).

Discussion. Results of this cost-effectiveness analysis indicate that an improved biomass stove is the most cost-effective intervention for South Asia and Sub-Saharan Africa, the two regions with the highest solid fuel–related disease burden. This finding is important given International Energy Agency projections to 2030, which indicate that biomass will remain the principal household fuel for the poor in South Asia and Sub-Saharan Africa and that actual numbers of users will increase over that period (IEA 2002). Cleaner fuels (particularly kerosene) are the most cost-effective options for East Asia and the Pacific, the other region with a high burden of solid fuel–related disease. Cleaner fuels, in particular LPG, appear relatively costly for South Asia and Sub-Saharan Africa, but circumstances in individual countries may vary considerably and in ways that make this fuel much more cost-effective. Sudan, for example, has abundant cheap supplies of LPG and favorable excise arrangements for imported appliances, which would result in a lower CER for LPG than in other countries in the region. Furthermore, as will be discussed later, costs and benefits from the user's perspective will differ markedly, depending on whether the starting point is free fuel collection or purchased biomass fuel.

In interpreting the results, one should bear in mind the assumptions underlying the CEA. Much of the evidence indicates that, although improved biomass stoves may reduce kitchen pollution by up to 75 percent, the reduction in exposure of women and children is typically no more than 30 to 40 percent (equivalent to VF of 0.6 to 0.7). Achievement of the 75 percent reduction in exposure (VF = 0.25) assumed for this analysis is consistent only with well-designed and -maintained chimney stoves that meet most of the cooking and heating energy needs of the household and high population coverage (to avoid exposure from neighbors and others). Those conditions may be

Table 42.6 Intervention Scenarios for World Bank Regions

a. Healthy years gained

Intervention	Coverage (percent)	Sub-Saharan Africa	Latin America and the Caribbean	Middle East and North Africa	Europe and Central Asia	South Asia	East Asia and the Pacific
LPG	50	22,160,000	160,000	n.a.	n.a.	44,810,000	2,560,000
	80	60,370,000	4,670,000	15,570,000	1,330,000	149,300,000	228,710,000
	95	75,630,000	11,260,000	22,510,000	4,810,000	184,940,000	568,640,000
Kerosene	50	22,160,000	160,000	n.a.	n.a.	44,810,000	2,560,000
	80	60,370,000	4,670,000	15,570,000	1,330,000	149,300,000	228,710,000
	95	75,630,000	11,260,000	22,520,000	4,810,000	184,940,000	568,640,000
Improved stove	50	18,010,000	n.a.	n.a.	n.a.	48,880,000	1,120,000
	80	40,270,000	1,380,000	6,630,000	n.a.	101,670,000	6,980,000
	95	51,540,000	2,600,000	11,640,000	n.a.	128,380,000	32,760,000
Combined (with stove)	LPG	69,250,000	8,650,000	19,540,000	3,230,000	170,340,000	427,350,000
	Kerosene	69,250,000	8,650,000	19,540,000	3,230,000	170,340,000	427,350,000

b. Cost-effectiveness ratios (US$ per healthy year gained)

Intervention	Coverage (percent)	Sub-Saharan Africa	Latin America and the Caribbean	Middle East and North Africa	Europe and Central Asia	South Asia	East Asia and the Pacific
LPG	50	715	1,405	n.a.	n.a.	542	1,695
	80	518	783	756	1,221	312	115
	95	518	814	762	1,321	314	100
Kerosene	50	84	631	n.a.	n.a.	63	225
	80	60	115	95	183	36	14
	95	60	106	95	167	36	12
Improved stove	50	25	n.a.	n.a.	n.a.	15	297
	80	21	947	457	n.a.	13	587
	95	20	1,101	368	n.a.	13	327
Combined (with stove)	LPG	295	761	606	1,375	177	83
	Kerosene	45	296	220	507	26	25

c. Healthy years gained per US$1 million

Intervention	Coverage (percent)	Sub-Saharan Africa	Latin America and the Caribbean	Middle East and North Africa	Europe and Central Asia	South Asia	East Asia and the Pacific
LPG	50	1,400	710	n.a.	n.a.	1,840	590
	80	1,930	1,280	1,320	820	3,210	8,680
	95	1,930	1,230	1,310	760	3,190	10,040
Kerosene	50	11,970	1,580	n.a.	n.a.	16,000	4,440
	80	16,600	8,690	10,500	5,470	27,850	72,840
	95	16,620	9,470	10,560	6,000	27,680	85,840
Improved stove	50	39,640	n.a.	n.a.	n.a.	67,330	3,360
	80	47,940	1,060	2,190	n.a.	74,750	1,700
	95	49,510	910	2,720	n.a.	76,300	3,060
Combined (with stove)	LPG	3,390	1,310	1,650	5,660	5,660	12,020
	Kerosene	22,250	3,380	4,550	38,590	35,590	40,730

Source: Authors.

n.a. = not applicable because the specified coverage of the intervention has already been reached.

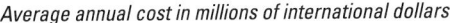

Average annual cost in millions of international dollars

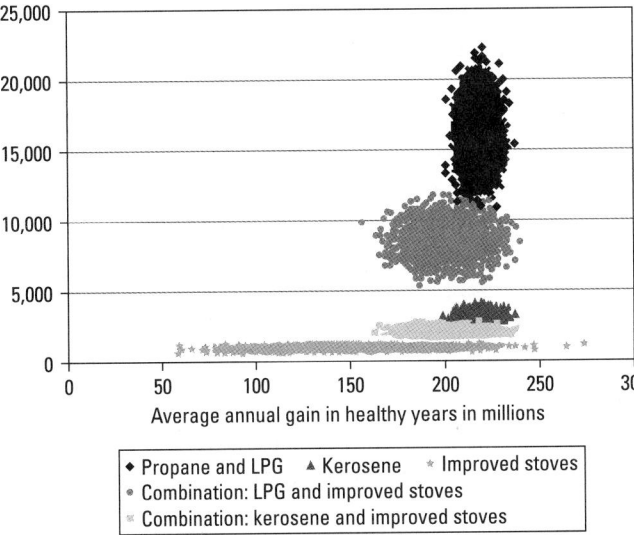

Average annual gain in healthy years in millions

◆ Propane and LPG ▲ Kerosene ＊ Improved stoves
● Combination: LPG and improved stoves
× Combination: kerosene and improved stoves

Source: Mehta and Shahpar 2004.

Figure 42.3 Multivariate Sensitivity Analysis for Three Types of Interventions and Combined Intervention Scenarios, Southeast Asia Region

achievable and should be the goal, but they are not currently widespread. The relative cost-effectiveness advantage for improved stoves over cleaner fuel reported here should therefore be viewed as relating more to what might be achievable with good biomass stoves rather than to what is currently being achieved. The assumption that kerosene and LPG are equally clean and achieve zero exposure (VF = 0) presumes, at the very least, the use of high-quality kerosene fuel and pressurized burners. In many places, kerosene is of low quality, and the types of kerosene stoves and lamps used result in poor combustion.

Cost comparisons for the various fuels also need careful consideration. For example, the cost of solid fuel has been assumed to be constant for traditional open fires and improved stoves. As a general assumption this is reasonable, because the efficiency of "improved" stoves varies, and some may even be less fuel efficient than are open fires. However, new stove technology is markedly improving efficiency, and some designs reduce daily fuel consumption by 40 percent or more, resulting in savings of time (where fuel is collected) and money (where fuel is bought) (Boy and others 2000).

Transition from biomass (collected free) or charcoal (typically paid for daily in small amounts) to LPG would almost certainly require changes in saving and budgeting habits for a poor household (see also box 42.2). Those changes may entail arranging a loan to purchase the gas bottle and stove and saving money for the relatively large, periodic outlay to refill the cylinder. Such changes are very likely to have other consequences for the family that should not be overlooked. However, those consequences are complex and difficult to allow for within the current CEA framework. Empirical data are required on how

household budgets change with various interventions and approaches to implementation.

The calculations have been undertaken for whole regions and provide no indication of how CERs differ among countries and specific communities. As local data on exposure, risk factors, health outcomes, and intervention effectiveness become available, similar analyses should be conducted at national and subnational levels.

Averted treatment costs have not been included on the grounds that most users of solid fuel are poor and have limited access to health services; many do not seek medical care for ALRI and even fewer do so for COPD. Inclusion of averted costs would increase cost-effectiveness. However, efforts to raise awareness about health risks and the importance of seeking care for ALRI (and COPD), which should accompany an intervention program, may increase care seeking and costs to the consumer. As more complete information becomes available, future CEAs should include treatment costs, with the option of allowing for an increase in care seeking associated with the intervention.

Interpretation of the results of this CEA, particularly with respect to comparisons with other types of intervention, needs to acknowledge that, although public organizations and other agencies will (or may) have some involvement in funding intervention programs, most of the cost of market-based interventions will be borne by households and those involved in production and marketing. Furthermore, it is hoped that, in addition to reducing IAP, interventions (and the means of accessing them) will have other positive effects, including on household budgets, in creating opportunities for income generation and empowering women in decisions about how energy is used. The promotion of market-based solutions implies new opportunities for artisans and entrepreneurs, but also the loss of traditional employment. The balance sheet for interventions is therefore complex, is specific to the setting, and will evolve as markets and enterprise develop.

Cost-Benefit Analysis

The CER gives cost per unit of health gained (healthy year) based on reduced risk of specified disease outcomes (ALRI, COPD). As discussed earlier, however, household energy interventions can affect a wide range of social, economic, and environmental issues, with important implications for health and development. In an economic analysis of water and sanitation interventions, Hutton and Haller (2004) found that time saved was the most important benefit. Those other effects cannot easily be expressed in units of health gain. Cost-benefit analysis (CBA) offers an alternative approach that may be better suited to environmental health interventions, given that health arguments alone will not motivate the multiple sectors involved in financing and implementing household energy interventions.

All main benefits in CBA are expressed in a common unit of monetary value and compared with costs in the cost-benefit ratio (CBR). The assessment of costs in CBA would have many assumptions and methods in common with CEA. The key differences lie in the selection of effects for inclusion as benefits and the methods for valuing them. In principle, there is no reason all the full range of effects discussed earlier could not be included (table 42.7), although in practice some, such as global climate effects, may be too uncertain. Where disadvantages of interventions are identified, they should also be included.

Benefit valuation presents particular challenges: effects are highly setting specific; evidence for some is limited, and their effects poorly quantified; and valuation in monetary units of benefits, such as lost working time averted for women, is difficult because women frequently are unpaid or work in informal markets. As a result, methods of valuation based on human capital may not be suitable, and alternative approaches such as contingent valuation, in which communities are involved in agreeing on market values for nontradable commodities, may be preferable. A related issue is valuing benefits that relate to

sustainability and health, which would be experienced after many years and by subsequent generations. Larson and Rosen (2002) used a mix of valuation of statistical life and contingent valuation methods to examine the CBRs for improved stoves with respect to mortality (Guatemala, East Africa) and morbidity (Pakistan), concluding that ratios appeared favorable. Although they discuss other benefits, those benefits were not included in their valuations. Their observation that the favorable CBRs are not reflected in the generally low adoption of improved stoves led them to conclude that the information required for assessing household demand correctly is not currently available.

IMPLEMENTATION OF CONTROL STRATEGIES: LESSONS FROM EXPERIENCE

The past 30 to 40 years have seen many diverse programs on household energy, from small-scale NGO- and community-led

Table 42.7 Possible Data Requirements for Quantifying Benefits

Impact category	Variables or elements to identify
Direct benefits related to specific health outcomes	
Expenditure and time for health care–seeking	Health service use of those with diseases caused by IAP (number of cases, visits or days per case)
	Health service use of those having accidents or injuries due to reasons related to fuel use:
	Direct: burns, poisoning
	Indirect: injuries in collecting fuel
	Access features to get to health services (distance, mode of transport, time; average visits per case)
	Other consumption related to health care–seeking
	Time loss of seeking health care, both of the patient and of those accompanying patient
Other direct benefits in and around the home	
Time gained owing to less illness and death	Activities of those with diseases caused by IAP
	Impact of disease on activities (time input, productivity)
	Value of time of various occupations
Time saving of changed technology	Reduced time spent collecting fuel
	Reduced time spent cooking and on other tasks requiring fire or stove
	Value of time of various occupations
	Income-generating activities achieved through increased time
	Impact on household cleanliness and hygiene and need for cleaning
Change in household environment and production	Effect of improved lighting on evening activities (education, production)
	Effect of availability of electricity and other fuels on household production activities
	Impact on ergonomics related to cooking
Consequences of process of acquiring new technology and related changes	Increased confidence in capacity of the household to save for immediate or future needs
	More involvement of women in decision making with respect to changes in household energy use and related issues
Indirect benefits related to the environment	
Local environment	Impact of fuel scarcity on local environment, average fuel collection time
	Increased risk of environmental effects (such as soil fertility) or disasters (such as flooding, landslides)
Global environment	Contribution of local area to greenhouse gases

Source: Authors.

initiatives to ambitious national programs, the largest of which has been the installation of some 200 million improved stoves in rural China. Although few have been subjected to rigorous evaluation, an assessment has been made of the Indian national stove program (box 42.3; ESMAP and World Bank 2001); the Chinese national stove program (box 42.4; Sinton and others 2004; Smith and others 1993); and LPG promotion (box 42.5; UNDP and ESMAP 2002). Experience with a number of smaller initiatives has also been reported—for example, the ceramic and metal stoves in East Africa, which have proved popular and provided local employment (Njenga 2001), and improved stove interventions in Guatemala (UNDP and ESMAP 2003).

Implementation of the Chinese national program differed substantially from that in India. Although the Chinese rural populations concerned are poor, they do have greater effective purchasing power than the poor in many developing countries, allowing development of a program with the majority of con-sumers purchasing stoves at close to full cost (Smith and others 1993). Among the key features of the Chinese program reported to have contributed to its success are decentralization of administration; a commercialization strategy that provided subsidies to rural energy enterprise development and quality control through the central production of critical components, such as parts of the combustion chamber; and engagement of local technical institutions in modifying national stove designs to local needs. National-level stove competitions were held among counties for contracts, ensuring local interest and allowing the best-placed counties to proceed first; financial payments were provided to counties only after completion of an independent review of their achievements. No large flows of funds came from the central government (in contrast, for example, to India); local governments provided the major financial contributions. As a result, delays and other problems associated with transferring large amounts of money have been

---

Box 42.3

Key Features and Lessons from India's National Stove Program

The Indian National Programme of Improved Cookstoves was established in 1983 with goals common to many such initiatives:

- conserving fuel
- reducing smoke emissions in the cooking area and improving health conditions
- reducing deforestation
- limiting the drudgery of women and children and reducing cooking time
- improving employment opportunities for the rural poor.

Although the Ministry of Non-Conventional Energy Sources was responsible for planning, setting targets, and approving stove designs, state-level agencies relayed this information to local government agencies or NGOs. A technical backup unit in each state trained rural women or unemployed youths to become self-employed workers to construct and install the stoves.

Between 1983 and 2000, the program distributed more than 33 million improved stoves. Despite extensive gov-ernment promotion efforts, improved stoves now account for less than 7 percent of all stoves. Among those that have been adopted, poor quality and lack of maintenance have resulted in a life span of two years at most and typically much less. Evaluation of the program identified four main problems:

- Most states placed inadequate emphasis on commer-cialization, now seen as crucial for effective and sustainable uptake.
- Overall, there was insufficient interaction with users, self-employed workers, and NGOs, so the designs did not meet needs of households, and there was very poor acceptance of user training.
- Quality control for installation and maintenance of the stove and its appropriate use was lacking.
- High levels of subsidy (about 50 percent of the stove cost) were found to reduce household motivation to use and maintain the stove.

Some more successfully managed areas of the program focused resources on technical assistance, research and development, marketing, and information dissemination. Recently, the government of India decentralized the pro-gram and transferred all implementation responsibility to state level. Since 2000, the program promotes only durable cement stoves with chimneys that have a minimum life span of five years. The introduction of these stoves will make adhesion to technical specifications and quality con-trol much easier.

Source: Authors, based on ESMAP and World Bank 2001.

Box 42.4

Household Effects of China's National Improved Stove Program

In 2002, an independent multidisciplinary evaluation was undertaken by a team of U.S. and Chinese researchers to evaluate (a) implementation methods used to promote improved stoves; (b) commercial stove production and marketing organizations that were created; and (c) effects of the program on households, including health, stove performance, socioeconomic factors, and monitoring of indoor air quality. The first two objectives were assessed through a facility survey of 108 institutions at all levels. The third objective was assessed through a household survey of nearly 4,000 households in three provinces: Zhejiang, Hubei, and Shaanxi. Key findings were as follows:

- The household survey revealed highly diverse fuel usage patterns: 28 and 34 different fuel combinations were used in kitchens in winter and summer, respectively. Most households owned at least one or more coal and one or more biomass stoves. Of the biomass stoves 77 percent, but only 38 percent of the coal stoves, were classified as improved. On average, improved stoves had a mean efficiency of 14 percent, which is well below the program target of between 20 and 30 percent, but above the mean efficiency of 9 percent for traditional stoves.
- With respect to air quality (measured with PM_4, the "thoracic fraction" of particulate matter, and CO), coal stoves showed significantly higher concentrations than biomass stoves during the summer, but not during the winter. Among households using biomass fuels (but

not among households using combinations of fuels that included coal or LPG), improved stoves showed significantly lower PM_4 and CO concentrations than traditional stoves.
- In both children and adults, coal use was associated with higher levels of exposure (as measured by CO in exhaled breath) and improved biomass stoves with lower levels. Reported childhood asthma and adult respiratory disease were negatively associated with use of improved stoves and good stove maintenance. These results should, however, be treated as indicative because of limited sample size.

Overall, several important conclusions emerge with relevance to future improved stove programs:

- A wide range of combinations of different fuel and stove types may limit the effect of an improved stove program.
- Given the importance of space heating, making available an improved biomass stove for cooking may not be a sufficient strategy to reduce IAP. Improved coal stoves need to be promoted among rural Chinese households.
- Even among households using improved stoves, PM_4 and CO levels were higher than Chinese national indoor air standards, implying that a large fraction of China's rural population is still chronically exposed to pollution levels substantially above those determined by the Chinese government to harm human health.

Source: Authors, based on Sinton and others 2004.

---

avoided. The Chinese program succeeded in shifting norms: most biomass stoves now available on the market have flues and other technical features that classify them as improved.

Experience in the promotion of LPG has also been reported, for example, from the Indian Deepam Scheme (ESMAP and World Bank 2004; UNDP and ESMAP 2002) and from the LPG Rural Energy Challenge (UNDP 2005). The latter initiative, developed by UNDP and the World LPG Association in 2002, is promoting the development of new, viable markets for LPG in developing countries. Key elements include developing partnerships in countries; enabling regulatory environments that facilitate LPG business development and product delivery; reducing barriers, for example, by introducing smaller (more affordable) gas bottles; and raising government and consumer

awareness of costs and benefits. McDade (2004) has recently identified a number of key lessons emerging from experience with the promotion of LPG markets (box 42.5).

Electrification has an important role in development (IEA 2002). Evidence from South Africa suggests that communities with grid access experience lower IAP exposure (Rollin and others 2004). Electricity is not expected to bring about large reductions in IAP exposure in most low-income countries, however, because most poor households can afford it only for uses such as lighting and running entertainment appliances and not for cooking and space heating. The International Energy Agency has recently carried out a detailed review of electrification, including the issues involved in supply and cost recovery among poor (and especially rural) communities (IEA 2002).

Box 42.5

Key Lessons Learned in the Promotion of New Markets for LPG in Developing Countries

- LPG can be affordable outside of urban areas, where wood fuel is currently purchased. On the other hand, for many consumers who do not participate in the monetized economy, it will be premature to promote LPG markets.
- One-time subsidies on appliances could be a good use of government (or other) resources.
- Microcredit initiatives should emphasize the cost-saving and productive potential and should seek to package both the gas (and appliances) and the financing.
- Concerns about safe handling, cylinder refilling, and transportation can be serious barriers to market

expansion. These issues need to be addressed by raising awareness among consumers and strengthening regulatory environments.

- Appliances for a range of end uses required by consumers must be available.
- Government leadership is essential, backed up by policy that sets the basic parameters for successful market expansion and avoids conflict between, for example, subsidies on competing fuels that undermine efforts to promote LPG markets.
- Specific initiatives, such as integrated energy centers (as in Morocco and South Africa) offer an effective means of developing markets in rural areas.

Source: Authors, based on McDade 2004.

The key lessons from experience with interventions to date may be summarized as follows:

- Too often, intervention technologies have been developed without adequate reference to users' needs and, as a result, have been poorly used and maintained or abandoned. Consequently, it is important to involve users—particularly women—in assessing needs and developing suitable interventions.
- Sustainable adoption should also be promoted through greater availability of a choice of appropriately priced interventions through local commercial outlets (artisans, shops, markets). This situation will come about only if demand is sufficient and if producers and distributors recognize this demand.
- All too commonly, communities most at risk exhibit low awareness, low demand, and poverty (often extreme poverty). A combination of user involvement and market approaches is needed, supported by the promotion and availability of targeted subsidies or microcredit facilities or both. The nature and extent of such financial support should depend on the purchasing power of the community.
- Local initiatives such as those outlined above must be led by national (and subnational) policy that acknowledges the contributions of a range of actors (government, business, NGOs, and so on) and sectors (energy, health, environment, finance, and so on) and that results in coordinated action. The instruments listed in table 42.5 should be considered when developing national policy.

In a recent review of the situation in Guatemala, the United Nations Development Programme and Energy Sector

Management Assistance Programme (UNDP and ESMAP 2003) found that, despite the almost total reliance of the rural population on biomass, a marked lack of national policy, leadership, and coordinated action existed in relation to household energy. Countries need to develop mechanisms for action and coordination in light of local needs, available institutional capacity, and leadership potential.

THE RESEARCH AND DEVELOPMENT AGENDA

WHO has, through a process involving multistakeholder meetings and reviews, developed some consensus on research and development priorities for household energy, IAP, and health (see for example WHO 2002a). Effective coordination is a prerequisite because of the need for input from, and collaboration between, many different organizations and "actors" that have generally not previously worked in partnership on this issue. One recent response to this need has been the establishment of the Partnership for Clean Indoor Air, following the Johannesburg World Summit on Sustainable Development in 2002 (EPA 2004; http://www.pciaonline.org/).

The evidence base on health effects requires further strengthening, particularly to quantify the effect of a measured reduction in IAP exposure on the risk of key outcomes (for example, ALRI). A randomized controlled trial is currently under way in Guatemala, focusing primarily on ALRI in children up to 18 months of age (Dooley 2003); however, at least one other such trial on another continent would be desirable. Also required are observational studies for outcomes for which few studies currently exist, including tuberculosis, low birthweight and perinatal mortality, cataracts, asthma, and cardiovascular disease. A small number of such studies are in progress, but further effort is required, with perinatal outcomes being a particular priority.

Despite limitations in the evidence on health effects, what is known about the health, social, and economic consequences of current patterns of household energy use in poor countries is of sufficient concern to press ahead with an active program of research and development regarding interventions. This activity should address both the technology (and associated knowledge and behavior) and the approaches taken for implementation. Although some development and innovation in technology and fuels (for example, clean fuels derived from biomass) are likely to be valuable, the single greatest challenge is to promote wider access to—and adoption of—existing knowledge and interventions. Projects and programs currently in progress or being developed should be carefully evaluated using quantitative and qualitative methods to assess a range of effects. Work is currently under way to develop suitable methods and tools for this purpose (WHO 2005). Experience and lessons learned need to be disseminated widely to ensure that they reach governments, donors, researchers, NGOs, and communities. As part of this effort, WHO is developing a resource for countries that offers information on the effectiveness of interventions as well as the enabling factors that facilitate long-term, sustained adoption and use of suitable improved technologies in different settings (WHO 2004c).

Economic assessment, including cost-effectiveness analysis, has a valuable part to play. Critical issues resulting from limited evidence have been identified about estimations and assumptions for costs, exposure reductions, health effects, and averted treatment costs, as well as the current inability to assess national and subnational cost-effectiveness. CBA may be more suitable for interventions in this and similar areas but will require better description of environmental, social, and economic effects and further development of valuation methods. New health studies and broadly based evaluations of interventions should help fill some of these gaps.

Determination of the macroeconomic costs to countries of current household energy use and the potential gains resulting from change to more efficient and cleaner options could substantially add to the case for action.

Monitoring progress requires the development and testing of standard indicators for use in such policy documents as the *World Development Report* and for routine application at national and subnational levels. The Millennium Development Goal Indicator on the proportion of the population using solid fuels is a key starting point, and WHO, the reporting agency, is working to broaden the monitoring of this indicator through international surveys, such as demographic and health surveys (ORC Macro 2004), the Multiple Indicator Cluster Survey (UNICEF 2004), and the World Health Survey (WHO 2004d),

as well as through work on regional and national indicators conducted under the Global Initiative on Children's Environmental Health Indicators (WHO 2004e). Future reporting will need to be further refined by taking into account differences in cooking practices (for example, type of stove and cooking location), as well as in fuel use for lighting and heating.

Advocacy for stronger action, internationally and in countries, is required. Products and guidance for a range of audiences should be prepared, with clear messages on the extent of the problem, the population groups most affected, what works, and what should be avoided. Tools such as the recently published guidelines on estimating the national burden of disease from solid fuels will help provide local evidence to argue for greater attention and action (Desai, Mehta, and Smith 2004).

CONCLUSIONS

IAP from solid fuel use is responsible for a large burden of disease among the world's poorest and most vulnerable populations. Inefficient and polluting household energy systems hold back development through resulting ill health, constraints on women's time and income generation, environmental impacts, and other factors. Although there is a trend toward cleaner and more efficient energy with increasing prosperity, little improvement is in prospect for more than 2 billion of the world's poorest people, particularly in South Asia and Sub-Saharan Africa. The number of people relying on traditional biomass is actually expected to increase until 2030.

Although the development of new energy technologies has a part to play in addressing this problem, many effective interventions are already available. The single greatest challenge is to dramatically increase the access of poor households to cleaner and more efficient household energy systems. Much valuable experience has been gained from successful—and unsuccessful—programs in household energy over the past three to four decades. Despite this experience, coherent, evidence-based policy is lacking in most of the countries concerned, where the lessons from experience now need to be implemented. Implementation will require greater awareness of the problem at international and national levels, provision of support for national collaborative action, and a focus on supporting appropriate, mainly market-based interventions.

Better information is crucial to this effort, including stronger evidence of the health effects of IAP exposure; assessment of the social, economic, and environmental benefits of interventions; and indicators to monitor progress. Economic analysis can help bring the case for action into policy, but it needs to be applied at country level and to include a wider range of benefits. Results from analysis at the regional level show that interventions can be cost-effective, particularly improved stoves, as long as these interventions can deliver substantial exposure reductions in practice. This conclusion, as well as its qualification, is important given the expectation that biomass will remain the principal household fuel in many developing countries for more than 20 years. The balance of effort and resources put into promoting cleaner biomass interventions rather than cleaner fuels, or vice-versa, will be an important policy issue for many countries and for the international community (Smith 2002).

With a range of innovative projects and programs under way in a number of countries and regions of the world, now is an important time to focus attention and effort on achieving the health, social, and economic gains that should result from improvements in household energy systems in developing countries.

NOTE

1. Particles are typically described according to the aerodynamic diameter, and although the devices used to separate particles of a given size do not yield a very sharp cutoff, this classification is functionally useful because smaller particles are able to penetrate farther into the lungs. Total suspended particles (TSP) include suspended particles of all sizes. Commonly defined smaller particles include PM_{10} (up to 10 microns diameter); respirable PM (includes all very small particles, about 50 percent of those 4 microns in diameter, and none above 10 microns in diameter); and $PM_{2.5}$ (up to 2.5 microns in diameter).

REFERENCES

Albalak, R., N. G. Bruce, J. P. McCracken, and K. R. Smith. 2001. "Indoor Respirable Particulate Matter Concentrations from an Open Fire, Improved Cookstove, and LPG/Open Fire Combination in a Rural Guatemalan Community." *Environmental Science and Technology* 35 (13): 2650–55.

Ando, M., M. Tadano, S. Asanuma, K. Tamura, S. Matsushima, T. Watanabe, and others. 1998. "Health Effects of Indoor Fluoride Pollution from Coal Burning in China." *Environmental Health Perspectives* 106 (5): 239–44.

Balakrishnan, K., J. Parikh, S. Sankar, R. Padmavathi, K. Srividya, V. Venugopal, and others. 2002. "Daily Average Exposures to Respirable Particulate Matter from Combustion of Biomass Fuels in Rural Households of Southern India." *Environmental Health Perspectives* 110 (11): 1069–75.

Ballard-Tremeer, G., and A. Mathee. 2000. "Review of Interventions to Reduce the Exposure of Women and Young Children to Indoor Air Pollution in Developing Countries." Paper prepared for USAID/WHO International Consultation on Household Energy, Indoor Air Pollution and Health, Washington, DC, May 4–6.

Barnes, B., A. Mathee, L. Shafritz, L. Krieger, L. Sherburne, and M. Favin. 2004a. "Testing Selected Behaviours to Reduce Indoor Air Pollution Exposure in Young Children." *Health Education Research* 19 (5): 543–50.

Barnes, B., A. Mathee, L. Shafritz, L. Krieger, and S. A. Zimicki. 2004b. "A Behavioural Intervention to Reduce Child Exposure to Indoor Air Pollution: Identifying Possible Target Behaviours." *Health Education and Behaviour* 13 (3): 306–17.

Behera, D., S. Dash, and S. Malik. 1988. "Blood Carboxyhaemoglobin Levels Following Acute Exposure to Smoke of Biomass Fuel." *Indian Journal of Medical Research* 88 (December): 522–24.

Boy, E., N. G. Bruce, and H. Delgado. 2002. "Birthweight and Exposure to Kitchen Wood Smoke during Pregnancy." *Environmental Health Perspectives* 110 (1): 109–14.

Boy, E., N. G. Bruce, K. R. Smith, and R. Hernandez. 2000. "Fuel Efficiency of an Improved Wood Burning Stove in Rural Guatemala: Implications for Health, Environment, and Development." *Energy for Sustainable Development* 4 (2): 21–29.

Brauer, B., K. Bartlett, J. Regaldo-Pineda, R. Perez-Padilla. 1996. "Assessment of Particulate Concentrations from Domestic Biomass Combustion in Rural Mexico." *Environmental Science and Technology* 30: 104–9.

Bruce, N. G., E. Bates, R. Nguti, S. Gitonga, J. Kithinji, and A. Doig. 2002. "Reducing Indoor Air Pollution through Participatory Development in Rural Kenya." In *Proceedings of 9th International Conference on Indoor Air Quality and Climate, Monterey, CA*, 590–95.

Bruce, N. G., J. P. McCracken, R. Albalak, M. Schei, K. R. Smith, V. Lopez, and C. West. 2004. "The Impact of Improved Stoves, House Construction, and Child Location on Levels of Indoor Air Pollution and Exposure in Young Guatemalan Children." *Journal of Exposure Analysis and Environmental Epidemiology* 14 (Suppl. 1): S110–17.

Bruce, N. G., R. Perez-Padilla, and R. Albalak. 2000. "Indoor Air Pollution in Developing Countries: A Major Environmental and Public Health Challenge." *Bulletin of the World Health Organization* 78 (9): 1078–92.

Clancy, J. S., M. Skutsch, and S. Batchelor. 2003. *The Gender-Energy-Poverty Nexus: Finding the Energy to Address Gender Concerns in Development*. Project report CNTR998521. London: Department for International Development.

Courtright, P., D. Haile, and E. Kohls. 1993. "The Epidemiology of Burns in Rural Ethiopia." *Journal of Epidemiology and Community Health* 47 (1): 19–22.

Danis-Lozano, R., M. H. Rodriguez, L. Gonzalez-Ceron, and M. Hernandez-Avila. 1999. "Risk Factors for Plasmodium Vivax Infection in the Lacandon Forest, Southern Mexico." *Epidemiology of Infection* 122 (3): 461–69.

Desai, M. A., S. Mehta, and K. R. Smith. 2004. *Indoor Smoke from Solid Fuels: Assessing the Environmental Burden of Disease at National and Local Levels*. Environmental Burden of Disease Series 4. Geneva: World Health Organization.

Dooley, E. E. 2003. "New Stoves for Better Children's Health?" *Environmental Health Perspectives* 111 (1): A33.

D'Sa, A., and K. V. Narasimha Murthy. 2004. "LPG as a Cooking Fuel Option for India." *Energy for Sustainable Development* 8 (3): 91–106.

EPA (U.S. Environmental Protection Agency). 2004. *Partnership for Clean Indoor Air*. Washington, DC: EPA. http://www.epa.gov/iaq/pcia.html.

ESMAP (Energy Sector Management Assistance Programme) and World Bank. 2001. *Indoor Air Pollution: Energy and Health for the Poor*, Issue 5 (September). Delhi: World Bank.

———. 2004. *Clean Household Energy for India: Reducing the Risks to Health*. Delhi: World Bank.

Ezzati, M., and D. M. Kammen. 2001. "Quantifying the Effects of Exposure to Indoor Air Pollution from Biomass Combustion on Acute Respiratory Infections in Developing Countries." *Environmental Health Perspectives* 109 (5): 481–88.

Ezzati, M., and A. Lopez. 2004. "Mortality and Morbidity Due to Smoking and Oral Tobacco Use: Global and Regional Estimates for 2000." In *Comparative Quantification of Health Risks: The Global Burden of Disease Due to Selected Risk Factors*, ed. M. Ezzati, A. D. Lopez, A. Rodgers, and C. J. L. Murray. Geneva: World Health Organization.

Ezzati, M., M. B. Mbinda, and D. M. Kammen. 2000. "Comparison of Emissions and Residential Exposure from Traditional and Improved Cookstoves in Kenya." *Environmental Science and Technology* 34 (4): 578–83.

Finkelman, R. B., H. E. Belkin, and B. Zheng. 1999. "Health Impacts of Domestic Coal Use in China." *Proceedings of the National Academy of Science* 96 (7): 3427–31.

Gupta, S., Y. C. Govil, P. K. Misra, R. Nath, and K. L. Srivastava. 1998. "Trends in Poisoning in Children: Experience at a Large Referral Teaching Hospital." *National Medical Journal of India* 11 (4): 166–68.

Hutton, G., and L. Haller. 2004. *Evaluation of the Costs and Benefits of Water and Sanitation Improvements at the Global Level.* Geneva: World Health Organization.

IEA (International Energy Agency). 2002. "Energy and Poverty." In *World Energy Outlook 2002.* Paris: International Energy Agency.

Johns, B., R. Baltussen, and R. Hutubessy. 2003. "Programme Costs in the Economic Evaluation of Health Interventions. *Cost Effectiveness and Resource Allocation* 1 (1). http://www.resource-allocation.com/content/1/1/1.

Lan, Q., R. S. Chapman, D. M. Schreinemachers, L. Tian, and X. He. 2002. "Household Stove Improvement and Risk of Lung Cancer in Xuanwei, China." *Journal of the National Cancer Institute* 94 (11): 826–35.

Larson, B. A., and S. Rosen. 2002. "Understanding Household Demand for Indoor Air Pollution Control in Developing Countries." *Social Science and Medicine* 55 (4): 571–84.

McDade, S. 2004. "Fueling Development: The Role of LPG in Poverty Reduction and Growth." *Energy for Sustainable Development* 8 (3): 74–81.

Mehta, S., and C. Shahpar. 2004. "The Health Benefits of Interventions to Reduce Indoor Air Pollution from Solid Fuel Use: A Cost-Effectiveness Analysis." *Energy for Sustainable Development* 8 (3): 53–59.

Naeher, L., B. Leaderer, and K. R. Smith. 2000. "Particulate Matter and Carbon Monoxide in Highland Guatemala: Indoor and Outdoor Levels from Traditional and Improved Wood Stoves and Gas Stoves." *Indoor Air* 10 (3): 200–205.

Naeher, L., K. R. Smith, B. Leaderer, L. Neufeld, and D. Mage. 2001. "Carbon Monoxide as a Tracer for Assessing Exposures to Particulate Matter in Wood and Gas Cookstove Households in Highland Guatemala." *Environmental Science and Technology* 35 (3): 575–81.

Njenga, B. K. 2001. "Upesi Rural Stoves Project." In *Generating Opportunities: Case Studies on Energy and Women,* ed. G. V. Karlsson and S. Misana, 45–51. Washington, DC: United Nations Development Programme.

OECD and IEA (Organisation for Economic Co-operation and Development and International Energy Agency). 2004. "Energy and Development." In *World Energy Outlook 2004.* Paris: OECD and IEA.

Onuba, O., and E. Udoidiok. 1987. "The Problems of Burns and Prevention of Burns in Developing Countries." *Burns* 13 (5): 382–85.

ORC Macro. 2004. "Demographic and Health Survey." ORC Macro. http://www.measuredhs.com/.

Palsson, K., and T. G. Jaenson. 1999. "Plant Products Used as Mosquito Repellants in Guinea Bissau, West Africa." *Acta Tropica* 72 (1): 39–52.

Pandey, M., R. Neupane, A. Gautam, and I. Shrestha. 1990. "The Effectiveness of Smokeless Stoves in Reducing Indoor Air Pollution in a Rural Hill Region of Nepal." *Mountain Research and Development* 10 (4): 313–20.

Parikh, J., K. Balakrishnan, V. Laxmi, and B. Haimanti. 2001. "Exposures from Cooking with Biofuels: Pollution Monitoring and Analysis for Rural Tamil Nadu, India." *Energy* 26: 949–62.

Paru, R., J. Hii, D. Lewis, and M. P. Alpers. 1995. "Relative Repellancy of Woodsmoke and Topical Applications of Plant Products against Mosquitoes." *Papua New Guinea Medical Journal* 38 (3): 215–21.

Pope, C. A. III, R. T. Burnett, M. J. Thun, E. E. Calle, D. Krewski, K. Ito, and G. D. Thurston. 2002. "Lung Cancer, Cardiopulmonary Mortality, and Long-Term Exposure to Fine Particulate Air Pollution." *Journal of the American Medical Association* 287 (9): 1132–41.

Pope, C. A. III, M. L. Hansen, R. W. Long, K. R. Nielsen, N. L. Eatough, W. E. Wilson, and D. J. Eatough. 2004. "Ambient Particulate Air Pollution, Heart Rate Variability, and Blood Markers of Inflammation in a Panel of Elderly Subjects." *Environmental Health Perspectives* 112 (3): 339–45.

Ramakrishna, J. 1988. "Patterns of Domestic Air Pollution in Rural India." Ph.D. dissertation. University of Hawaii, Honolulu.

Reed, R. P., and F. M. Conradie. 1997. "The Epidemiology and Clinical Features of Paraffin (Kerosene) Poisoning in Rural African Children." *Annals of Tropical Paediatrics* 17 (1): 49–55.

Reid, H., K. R. Smith, and B. Sherchand. 1986. "Indoor Smoke Exposures from Traditional and Improved Cookstoves: Comparisons among Rural Nepali Women." *Mountain Research and Development* 6 (4): 293–304.

Riojas-Rodriguez, H., P. Romano-Riquer, C. Santos-Burgoa, and K. R. Smith. 2001. "Household Firewood Use and the Health of Children and Women of Indian Communities in Chiapas, Mexico." *International Journal of Occupational and Environmental Health* 7 (1): 44–53.

Rollin, H., A. Mathee, N. G. Bruce, J. Levin, and Y. E. R. von Schirnding. 2004. "Comparison of Indoor Air Quality in Electrified and Un-Electrified Dwellings in Rural South African Villages." *Indoor Air* 14 (3): 208–16.

Saatkamp, B. D., O. R. Masera, and D. M. Kammen. 2000. "Energy and Health Transitions in Development: Fuel Use, Stove Technology, and Morbidity in Jarácuaro, Mexico." *Energy for Sustainable Development* 4 (2): 5–14.

Saksena, S., L. Thompson, and K. R. Smith. 2004. "Indoor Air Pollution and Exposure Database: Household Measurements in Developing Countries." http://ehs.sph.berkeley.edu/hem/page.asp?id=33.

Sinton, J. E., K. R. Smith, J. Peabody, L. Yaping, Z. Ziliang, R. Edwards, and G. Quan. 2004. "An Assessment of Programs to Promote Improved Household Stoves in China." *Energy for Sustainable Development* 8 (3): 33–52.

Smith, K. R. 1987. *Biofuels, Air Pollution, and Health: A Global Review.* New York: Plenum Press.

———. 1989. "Dialectics of Improved Stoves." *Economic and Political Weekly* 24 (10): 517–22.

———. 2002. "In Praise of Petroleum?" *Science* 298: 1847.

Smith, K. R., A. L. Aggarwal, and R. M. Dave. 1983. "Air Pollution and Rural Biomass Fuels in Developing Countries: A Pilot Village Study in India and Implications for Research and Policy." *Atmospheric Environment* 17 (11): 2343–62.

Smith, K. R., S. Mehta, and M. Feuz. 2004. "Chapter 18: Indoor Smoke from Household Use of Solid Fuels." In *Comparative Quantification of Health Risks: The Global Burden of Disease Due to Selected Risk Factors,* ed. M. Ezzati, A. D. Lopez, A. Rodgers, and C. J. L. Murray, vol 2, 1435–93. Geneva: World Health Organization.

Smith, K. R., G. Shuhua, H. Kun, and Q. Daxiong. 1993. "One Hundred Million Improved Cookstoves in China: How Was It Done?" *World Development* 21 (6): 941–61.

Smith, K. R., R. Uma, V. V. N. Kishore, J. Zhang, V. Joshi, and M. A. K. Khalil. 2000. "Greenhouse Implications of Household Stoves: An Analysis for India." *Annual Review Energy Environment* 25: 741–63.

Snow, R. W., A. K. Bradley, R. Hayes, P. Byass, and B. M. Greenwood. 1987. "Does Woodsmoke Protect against Malaria?" *Annals of Tropical Medical Parasitology* 81 (4): 449–51.

UNDP (United Nations Development Programme). 2005. "LP Gas Rural Challenge." http://www.undp.org/energy/lpg.htm.

UNDP and ESMAP (United Nations Development Programme and Energy Sector Management Assistance Programme). 2002. *India: Household Energy, Indoor Air Pollution, and Health.* Delhi: UNDP and World Bank.

———. 2003. *Health Impacts of Traditional Fuel Use in Guatemala.* Washington, DC: UNDP and World Bank.

UNICEF (United Nations Children's Fund). 2004. "Monitoring the Situation of Women and Children: The Multiple Indicator Cluster Survey." http://www.childinfo.org.

United Nations Statistics Division. 2003. "Millennium Development Goals." http://millenniumindicators.un.org/unsd/mi/mi_goals.asp.

Vernede, R., M. M. van Meer, and M. P. Alpers. 1994. "Smoke as a Form of Personal Protection against Mosquitoes: A Field Study in Papua New Guinea." *Southeast Asian Journal of Tropical Medicine and Public Health* 25 (4): 771–75.

von Schirnding, Y. E. R., N. G. Bruce, K. R. Smith, G. Ballard-Tremeer, M. Ezzati, and K. Lvovsky. 2002. "Addressing the Impact of Household Energy and Indoor Air Pollution on the Health of the Poor: Implications for Policy Action and Intervention Measures." Paper prepared for the Commission on Macroeconomics and Health, WHO/HDE/HID/02.9. World Health Organization, Geneva.

Wang, X., and K. R. Smith. 1999. "Secondary Benefits of Greenhouse Gas Control: Health Impacts in China." *Environmental Science and Technology* 33 (18): 3056–61.

Westoff, B., and D. Germann. 1995. *Stove Images: A Documentation of Improved and Traditional Stoves in Africa, Asia and Latin America.* Brussels: Commission of the European Communities, Directorate-General for Development.

WHO (World Health Organization). 2002a. "Addressing the Links between Indoor Air Pollution, Household Energy, and Human Health: Based on the WHO-USAID Global Consultation on the Health Impact of Indoor Air Pollution and Household Energy in Developing Countries." Meeting Report WHO/HDE/HID/02.10. WHO, Geneva.

———. 2002b. *Reducing Risks, Promoting Healthy Life: World Health Report 2002.* Geneva: WHO.

———. 2003. *Making Choices in Health: WHO Guide to Cost-Effectiveness Analysis.* Geneva: WHO.

———. 2004a. "Indoor Air Thematic Briefing 1: Indoor Air Pollution, Household Energy and the Millennium Development Goals." Geneva: WHO. http://www.who.int/indoorair/info/en/iabriefing1rev.pdf.

———. 2004b. "Burden of Disease Statistics. Burden of Disease Unit." Geneva: WHO. http://www.who.int/research/en/.

———. 2004c. "Evidence for Policy Makers: Indoor Air Pollution." Geneva: WHO. http://www.who.int/indoorair/policy/en/.

———. 2004d. "The World Health Survey." Geneva: WHO. http://www3.who.int/whs/.

———. 2004e. "From Theory to Action: Implementing the WSSD Global Initiative on Children's Environmental Health Indicators." Geneva: WHO. http://www.who.int/ceh/publications/924159188_9/en/.

———. 2005. "Development of a Catalogue of Methods: Indoor Air Pollution." Geneva: WHO. http://www.who.int/indoorair/interventions/methodology/en/.

Wickramasinghe, A. 2001. "Gendered Sights and Health Issues in the Paradigm of Biofuel in Sri Lanka." *Energia News* 4 (4): 14–16.

World Bank. 2002. "Energy Efficiency and Emissions." In *World Development Indicators.* Washington, DC: World Bank.

Yach, D. 1994. "Paraffin Poisoning: Partnership Is the Key to Prevention." *South African Medical Journal* 84 (11): 717.

Chapter **43**

Air and Water Pollution: Burden and Strategies for Control

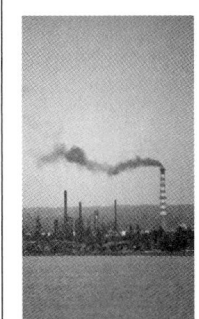

Tord Kjellstrom, Madhumita Lodh, Tony McMichael, Geetha Ranmuthugala, Rupendra Shrestha, and Sally Kingsland

Environmental pollution has many facets, and the resultant health risks include diseases in almost all organ systems. Thus, a chapter on air and water pollution control links with chapters on, for instance, diarrheal diseases (chapter 19), respiratory diseases in children and adults (chapters 25 and 35), cancers (chapter 29), neurological disorders (chapter 32), and cardiovascular disease (chapter 33), as well as with a number of chapters dealing with health care issues.

NATURE, CAUSES, AND BURDEN OF AIR AND WATER POLLUTION

Each pollutant has its own health risk profile, which makes summarizing all relevant information into a short chapter difficult. Nevertheless, public health practitioners and decision makers in developing countries need to be aware of the potential health risks caused by air and water pollution and to know where to find the more detailed information required to handle a specific situation. This chapter will not repeat the discussion about indoor air pollution caused by biomass burning (chapter 42) and water pollution caused by poor sanitation at the household level (chapter 41), but it will focus on the problems caused by air and water pollution at the community, country, and global levels.

Estimates indicate that the proportion of the global burden of disease associated with environmental pollution hazards ranges from 23 percent (WHO 1997) to 30 percent (Smith, Corvalan, and Kjellstrom 1999). These estimates include infectious diseases related to drinking water, sanitation, and food hygiene; respiratory diseases related to severe indoor air pollution from biomass burning; and vectorborne diseases with a major environmental component, such as malaria. These three types of diseases each contribute approximately 6 percent to the updated estimate of the global burden of disease (WHO 2002).

As the World Health Organization (WHO) points out, outdoor air pollution contributes as much as 0.6 to 1.4 percent of the burden of disease in developing regions, and other pollution, such as lead in water, air, and soil, may contribute 0.9 percent (WHO 2002). These numbers may look small, but the contribution from most risk factors other than the "top 10" is within the 0.5 to 1.0 percent range (WHO 2002).

Because of space limitations, this chapter can give only selected examples of air and water pollution health concerns. Other information sources on environmental health include Yassi and others (2001) and the Web sites of or major reference works by WHO, the United Nations Environment Programme (UNEP), Division of Technology, Industry, and Economics (http://www.uneptie.org/); the International Labour Organization (ILO), the United Nations Industrial Development Organization (UNIDO; http://www.unido.org/), and other relevant agencies.

Table 43.1 indicates some of the industrial sectors that can pose significant environmental and occupational health risks to populations in developing countries. Clearly, disease control measures for people working in or living around a smelter may be quite different from those for people living near a tannery or a brewery. For detailed information about industry-specific

Table 43.1 Selected Industrial Sectors and Their Contribution to Air and Water Pollution and to Workplace Hazards

Industrial sector	Air	Water	Workplace[a]
Base metal and iron ore mining	PM	Toxic metal sludge	Silica
Cement manufacturing	PM	Sludge	Silica
Coalmining and production	PM, coal dust	Sludge	Coal dust, silica
Copper smelting	Arsenic	Arsenic	Arsenic, cadmium
Electricity generation	PM, SO_2	Hot water	SO_2
Foundries	PM	Solvents	Silica, solvents
Iron and steel smelting	PM	Sludge	Carbon monoxide, nickel
Lead and zinc smelting	PM, SO_2, lead, cadmium, arsenic	Lead, cadmium, arsenic	PM, SO_2, lead, cadmium, arsenic
Meat processing and rendering	Odor	High biological oxygen demand	Infections
Oil and gas development	SO_2, carcinogens	Oil	Hydrocarbons
Pesticide manufacturing	Pesticides and toxic intermediates	Pesticides and toxic intermediates	Pesticides and toxic intermediates
Petrochemicals manufacturing	SO_2	Oil	Hydrocarbons
Petroleum refining	SO_2	Sludge, hydrocarbons	Hydrocarbons
Phosphate fertilizer plants	PM	Nutrients	
Pulp and paper mills	Odor	High biological oxygen demand, mercury	Chlorine
Tanning and leather finishing	Odor	Chromium, acids	Chromium, acids
Textile manufacturing		Toxic dyes	

Source: World Bank 1999.

a. In all the cases, the workplaces are subject to risk of injury, noise, dust, and excessively hot or cold temperatures.

pollution control methods, see the Web sites of industry sector organizations, relevant international trade union organizations, and the organizations listed above.

Air Pollution

Air pollutants are usually classified into suspended particulate matter (PM) (dusts, fumes, mists, and smokes); gaseous pollutants (gases and vapors); and odors.

Suspended PM can be categorized according to total suspended particles: the finer fraction, PM_{10}, which can reach the alveoli, and the most hazardous, $PM_{2.5}$ (median aerodynamic diameters of less than 10.0 microns and 2.5 microns, respectively). Much of the $PM_{2.5}$ consists of secondary pollutants created by the condensation of gaseous pollutants—for example, sulfur dioxide (SO_2) and nitrogen dioxide (NO_2). Types of suspended PM include diesel exhaust particles; coal fly ash; wood smoke; mineral dusts, such as coal, asbestos, limestone, and cement; metal dusts and fumes; acid mists (for example, sulfuric acid); and pesticide mists.

Gaseous pollutants include sulfur compounds such as SO_2 and sulfur trioxide; carbon monoxide; nitrogen compounds such as nitric oxide, NO_2, and ammonia; organic compounds such as hydrocarbons; volatile organic compounds; polycyclic aromatic hydrocarbons and halogen derivatives such as aldehydes; and odorous substances. Volatile organic compounds are released from burning fuel (gasoline, oil, coal, wood,

charcoal, natural gas, and so on); solvents; paints; glues; and other products commonly used at work or at home. Volatile organic compounds include such chemicals as benzene, toluene, methylene chloride, and methyl chloroform. Emissions of nitrogen oxides and hydrocarbons react with sunlight to eventually form another secondary pollutant, ozone, at ground level. Ozone at this level creates health concerns, unlike ozone in the upper atmosphere, which occurs naturally and protects life by filtering out ultraviolet radiation from the sun.

Sources of Outdoor Air Pollution. Outdoor air pollution is caused mainly by the combustion of petroleum products or coal by motor vehicles, industry, and power stations. In some countries, the combustion of wood or agricultural waste is another major source. Pollution can also originate from industrial processes that involve dust formation (for example, from cement factories and metal smelters) or gas releases (for instance, from chemicals production). Indoor sources also contribute to outdoor air pollution, and in heavily populated areas, the contribution from indoor sources can create extremely high levels of outdoor air pollution.

Motor vehicles emit PM, nitric oxide and NO_2 (together referred to as NO_x), carbon monoxide, organic compounds, and lead. Lead is a gasoline additive that has been phased out in industrial countries, but some developing countries still use leaded gasoline. Mandating the use of lead-free gasoline is an important intervention in relation to health. It eliminates

Box 43.1

The Bhopal Catastrophe

The Bhopal plant, owned by the Union Carbide Corporation, produced methyl isocyanate, an intermediate in the production of the insecticide carbaryl. On December 2, 1984, a 150,000-gallon storage tank containing methyl isocyanate apparently became contaminated with water, initiating a violent reaction and the release of a cloud of toxic gas to which 200,000 people living near the plant were exposed. Low wind speed and the high vapor pressure of methyl isocyanate exacerbated the severity of toxic exposure, resulting in the immediate death of at least 6,000 people.

The dominating nonlethal effects of this emission were severe irritation of the eyes, lungs, and skin. Effects on the nervous system and reproductive organs were also reported. The reaction of methyl isocyanate with water had a corrosive effect on the respiratory tract, which resulted in extensive necrosis, bleeding, and edema. Treatment was impeded by the unknown and disputed composition of the gas cloud and a lack of knowledge about its health effects and about antidotes.

Source: Dhara and Dhara 2002.

---

vehicle-related lead pollution and permits the use of catalytic converters, which reduce emissions of other pollutants.

Catastrophic emissions of organic chemicals, as occurred in Bhopal, India, in 1984 (box 43.1), can also have major health consequences (McGranahan and Murray 2003; WHO 1999).

Another type of air pollution that can have disastrous consequences is radioactive pollution from a malfunctioning nuclear power station, as occurred in Chernobyl in 1986 (WHO 1996). Radioactive isotopes emitted from the burning reactor spread over large areas of what are now the countries of Belarus, the Russian Federation, and Ukraine, causing thousands of cases of thyroid cancer in children and threatening to cause many cancer cases in later decades.

Exposure to Air Pollutants. The extent of the health effects of air pollution depends on actual exposure. Total daily exposure is determined by people's time and activity patterns, and it combines indoor and outdoor exposures. Young children and elderly people may travel less during the day than working adults, and their exposure may therefore be closely correlated with air pollution levels in their homes. Children are particularly vulnerable to environmental toxicants because of their possibly greater relative exposure and the effects on their growth and physiological development.

Meteorological factors, such as wind speed and direction, are usually the strongest determinants of variations in air pollution, along with topography and temperature inversions. Therefore, weather reports can be a guide to likely air pollution levels on a specific day.

Workplace air is another important source of air pollution exposure (chapter 60). Resource extraction and processing industries, which are common in developing countries, emit dust or hazardous fumes at the worksite (table 43.1). Such industries include coalmining, mineral mining, quarrying, and cement production. Developed countries have shifted much of their hazardous production to developing countries (LaDou 1992). This shift creates jobs in the developing countries, but at the price of exposure to air pollution resulting from outdated technology. In addition, specific hazardous compounds, such as asbestos, have been banned in developed countries (Kazan-Allen 2004), but their use may still be common in developing countries.

Impacts on Health. Epidemiological analysis is needed to quantify the health impact in an exposed population. The major pollutants emitted by combustion have all been associated with increased respiratory and cardiovascular morbidity and mortality (Brunekreef and Holgate 2002). The most famous disease outbreak of this type occurred in London in 1952 (U.K. Ministry of Health 1954), when 4,000 people died prematurely in a single week because of severe air pollution, followed by another 8,000 deaths during the next few months (Bell and Davis 2001).

In the 1970s and 1980s, new statistical methods and improved computer technology allowed investigators to study mortality increases at much lower concentrations of pollutants. A key question is the extent to which life has been shortened. Early loss of life in elderly people, who would have died soon regardless of the air pollution, has been labeled *mortality displacement,* because it contributes little to the overall burden of disease (McMichael and others 1998).

Long-term studies have documented the increased cardiovascular and respiratory mortality associated with exposure to PM (Dockery and others 1993; Pope and others 1995).

A 16-year follow-up of a cohort of 500,000 Americans living in different cities found that the associations were strongest with $PM_{2.5}$ and also established an association with lung cancer mortality (Pope and others 2002). Another approach is ecological studies of small areas based on census data, air pollution information, and health events data (Scoggins and others 2004), with adjustments for potential confounding factors, including socioeconomic status. Such studies indicate that the mortality increase for every 10 micrograms per cubic meter (μg per m^3) of $PM_{2.5}$ ranges from 4 to 8 percent for cities in developed countries where average annual $PM_{2.5}$ levels are 10 to 30 μg/m^3. Many urban areas of developing countries have similar or greater levels of air pollution.

The major urban air pollutants can also give rise to significant respiratory morbidity (WHO 2000). For instance, Romieu and others (1996) report an exacerbation of asthma among children in Mexico City, and Xu and Wang (1993) note an increased risk of respiratory symptoms in middle-aged non-smokers in Beijing.

In relation to the very young, Wang and others (1997) find that PM exposure, SO_2 exposure, or both increased the risk of low birthweight in Beijing, and Pereira and others (1998) find that air pollution increased intrauterine mortality in São Paulo.

Other effects of ambient air pollution are postneonatal mortality and mortality caused by acute respiratory infections, as well as effects on children's lung function, cardiovascular and respiratory hospital admissions in the elderly, and markers for functional damage of the heart muscle (WHO 2000). Asthma is another disease that researchers have linked to urban air pollution (McConnell and others 2002; Rios and others 2004). Ozone exposure as a trigger of asthma attacks is of particular concern. The mechanism behind an air pollution and asthma link is not fully known, but early childhood NO_2 exposure may be important (see, for example, Ponsonby and others 2000).

Leaded gasoline creates high lead exposure conditions in urban areas, with a risk for lead poisoning, primarily in young children. The main concern is effects on the brain from low-level exposure leading to behavioral aberrations and reduced or delayed development of intellectual or motoric ability (WHO 1995). Lead exposure has been implicated in hypertension in adults, and this effect may be the most important for the lead burden of disease at a population level (WHO 2002). Other pollutants of concern are the carcinogenic volatile organic compounds, which may be related to an increase in lung cancer, as reported by two recent epidemiological studies (Nyberg and others 2000; Pope and others 2002).

Urban air pollution and lead exposure are two of the environmental hazards that WHO (2002) assessed as part of its burden-of-disease calculations for the *World Health Report 2002*. The report estimates that pollution by urban PM causes as much as 5 percent of the global cases of lung cancer, 2 percent of deaths from cardiovascular and respiratory conditions,

and 1 percent of respiratory infections, adding up to 7.9 million disability-adjusted life years based on mortality only. This burden of disease occurs primarily in developing countries, with China and India contributing the most to the global burden. Eastern Europe also has major air pollution problems, and in some countries, air pollution accounts for 0.6 to 1.4 percent of the total disability-adjusted life years from mortality.

The global burden of disease caused by lead exposure includes subtle changes in learning ability and behavior and other signs of central nervous system damage (Fewthrell, Kaufmann, and Preuss 2003). WHO (2002) concludes that 0.4 percent of deaths and 0.9 percent (12.9 million) of all disability-adjusted life years may be due to lead exposure.

Water Pollution

Chemical pollution of surface water can create health risks, because such waterways are often used directly as drinking water sources or connected with shallow wells used for drinking water. In addition, waterways have important roles for washing and cleaning, for fishing and fish farming, and for recreation.

Another major source of drinking water is groundwater, which often has low concentrations of pathogens because the water is filtered during its transit through underground layers of sand, clay, or rocks. However, toxic chemicals such as arsenic and fluoride can be dissolved from the soil or rock layers into groundwater. Direct contamination can also occur from badly designed hazardous waste sites or from industrial sites. In the United States in the 1980s, the government set in motion the Superfund Program, a major investigation and cleanup program to deal with such sites (U.S. Environmental Protection Agency 2000).

Coastal pollution of seawater may give rise to health hazards because of local contamination of fish or shellfish—for instance, the mercury contamination of fish in the infamous Minamata disease outbreak in Japan in 1956 (WHO 1976). Seawater pollution with persistent chemicals, such as polychlorinated biphenyls (PCBs) and dioxins, can also be a significant health hazard even at extremely low concentrations (Yassi and others 2001).

Sources of Chemical Water Pollution. Chemicals can enter waterways from a point source or a nonpoint source. Point-source pollution is due to discharges from a single source, such as an industrial site. Nonpoint-source pollution involves many small sources that combine to cause significant pollution. For instance, the movement of rain or irrigation water over land picks up pollutants such as fertilizers, herbicides, and insecticides and carries them into rivers, lakes, reservoirs, coastal waters, or groundwater. Another nonpoint source is storm-water that collects on roads and eventually reaches rivers or lakes. Table 43.1 shows examples of point-source industrial chemical pollution.

Paper and pulp mills consume large volumes of water and discharge liquid and solid waste products into the environment. The liquid waste is usually high in biological oxygen demand, suspended solids, and chlorinated organic compounds such as dioxins (World Bank 1999). The storage and transport of the resulting solid waste (wastewater treatment sludge, lime sludge, and ash) may also contaminate surface waters. Sugar mills are associated with effluent characterized by biological oxygen demand and suspended solids, and the effluent is high in ammonium content. In addition, the sugarcane rinse liquid may contain pesticide residues. Leather tanneries produce a significant amount of solid waste, including hide, hair, and sludge. The wastewater contains chromium, acids, sulfides, and chlorides. Textile and dye industries emit a liquid effluent that contains toxic residues from the cleaning of equipment. Waste from petrochemical manufacturing plants contains suspended solids, oils and grease, phenols, and benzene. Solid waste generated by petrochemical processes contains spent caustic and other hazardous chemicals implicated in cancer.

Another major source of industrial water pollution is mining. The grinding of ores and the subsequent processing with water lead to discharges of fine silt with toxic metals into waterways unless proper precautions are taken, such as the use of sedimentation ponds. Lead and zinc ores usually contain the much more toxic cadmium as a minor component. If the cadmium is not retrieved, major water pollution can occur. Mining was the source of most of the widespread cadmium poisoning (Itai-Itai disease) in Japan in 1940–50 (Kjellstrom 1986).

Other metals, such as copper, nickel, and chromium, are essential micronutrients, but in high levels these metals can be harmful to health. Wastewater from mines or stainless steel production can be a source of exposure to these metals. The presence of copper in water can also be due to corrosion of drinking water pipes. Soft water or low pH makes corrosion more likely. High levels of copper may make water appear bluish green and give it a metallic taste. Flushing the first water out of the tap can minimize exposure to copper. The use of lead pipes and plumbing fixtures may result in high levels of lead in piped water.

Mercury can enter waterways from mining and industrial premises. Incineration of medical waste containing broken medical equipment is a source of environmental contamination with mercury. Metallic mercury is also easily transported through the atmosphere because of its highly volatile nature. Sulfate-reducing bacteria and certain other micro-organisms in lake, river, or coastal underwater sediments can methylate mercury, increasing its toxicity. Methylmercury accumulates and concentrates in the food chain and can lead to serious neurological disease or more subtle functional damage to the nervous system (Murata and others 2004).

Runoff from farmland, in addition to carrying soil and sediments that contribute to increased turbidity, also carries nutrients such as nitrogen and phosphates, which are often added in the form of animal manure or fertilizers. These chemicals cause eutrophication (excessive nutrient levels in water), which increases the growth of algae and plants in waterways, leading to an increase in cyanobacteria (blue-green algae). The toxics released during their decay are harmful to humans.

The use of nitrogen fertilizers can be a problem in areas where agriculture is becoming increasingly intensified. These fertilizers increase the concentration of nitrates in groundwater, leading to high nitrate levels in underground drinking water sources, which can cause methemoglobinemia, the life-threatening "blue baby" syndrome, in very young children, which is a significant problem in parts of rural Eastern Europe (Yassi and others 2001).

Some pesticides are applied directly on soil to kill pests in the soil or on the ground. This practice can create seepage to groundwater or runoff to surface waters. Some pesticides are applied to plants by spraying from a distance—even from airplanes. This practice can create spray drift when the wind carries the materials to nearby waterways. Efforts to reduce the use of the most toxic and long-lasting pesticides in industrial countries have largely been successful, but the rules for their use in developing countries may be more permissive, and the rules of application may not be known or enforced. Hence, health risks from pesticide water pollution are higher in such countries (WHO 1990).

Naturally occurring toxic chemicals can also contaminate groundwater, such as the high metal concentrations in underground water sources in mining areas. The most extensive problem of this type is the arsenic contamination of groundwater in Argentina, Bangladesh (box 43.2), Chile, China, India, Mexico, Nepal, Taiwan (China), and parts of Eastern Europe and the United States (WHO 2001). Fluoride is another substance that may occur naturally at high concentrations in parts of China, India, Sri Lanka, Africa, and the eastern Mediterranean. Although fluoride helps prevent dental decay, exposure to levels greater than 1.5 milligrams per liter in drinking water can cause pitting of tooth enamel and deposits in bones. Exposure to levels greater than 10 milligrams per liter can cause crippling skeletal fluorosis (Smith 2003).

Water disinfection using chemicals is another source of chemical contamination of water. Chlorination is currently the most widely practiced and most cost-effective method of disinfecting large community water supplies. This success in disinfecting water supplies has contributed significantly to public health by reducing the transmission of waterborne disease. However, chlorine reacts with naturally occurring organic matter in water to form potentially toxic chemical compounds,

Arsenic in Bangladesh

The presence of arsenic in tube wells in Bangladesh because of natural contamination from underground geological layers was first confirmed in 1993. Ironically, the United Nations Children's Fund had introduced the wells in the 1960s and 1970s as a safe alternative to water contaminated with microbes, which contributed to a heavy diarrheal disease burden. Estimates indicate that 28 million to 35 million people of Bangladesh's population of 130 million are exposed to arsenic levels exceeding 50 micrograms per liter, the prescribed limit for drinking water in Bangladesh (Kinniburgh and Smedley 2001).

This number increases to 46 million to 57 million if the WHO guideline level of 10 micrograms per liter is used. The most common sign of arsenic poisoning in Bangladesh is skin lesions characterized by hyperkeratosis and melanosis. Other effects reported, but not epidemiologically confirmed, include cancer (particularly of the skin, lungs, and bladder); liver damage; diabetes; hypertension; and reproductive effects (spontaneous abortions and stillbirths). Cancer and vascular effects are the dominating effects in other arsenic-polluted areas (WHO 2001).

Source: Authors.

known collectively as disinfection by-products (International Agency for Research on Cancer 2004).

Exposure to Chemical Water Pollution. Drinking contaminated water is the most direct route of exposure to pollutants in water. The actual exposure via drinking water depends on the amount of water consumed, usually 2 to 3 liters per day for an adult, with higher amounts for people living in hot areas or people engaged in heavy physical work. Use of contaminated water in food preparation can result in contaminated food, because high cooking temperatures do not affect the toxicity of most chemical contaminants.

Inhalation exposure to volatile compounds during hot showers and skin exposure while bathing or using water for recreation are also potential routes of exposure to water pollutants. Toxic chemicals in water can affect unborn or young children by crossing the placenta or being ingested through breast milk.

Estimating actual exposure via water involves analyzing the level of the contaminant in the water consumed and assessing daily water intake (WHO 2003). Biological monitoring using blood or urine samples can be a precise tool for measuring total exposure from water, food, and air (Yassi and others 2001).

Health Effects. No published estimates are available of the global burden of disease resulting from the overall effects of chemical pollutants in water. The burden in specific local areas may be large, as in the example cited in box 43.2 of arsenic in drinking water in Bangladesh. Other examples of a high local burden of disease are the nervous system diseases of methylmercury poisoning (Minamata disease), the kidney and

bone diseases of chronic cadmium poisoning (Itai-Itai disease), and the circulatory system diseases of nitrate exposure (methemoglobinemia) and lead exposure (anemia and hypertension).

Acute exposure to contaminants in drinking water can cause irritation or inflammation of the eyes and nose, skin, and gastrointestinal system; however, the most important health effects are due to chronic exposure (for example, liver toxicity) to copper, arsenic, or chromium in drinking water. Excretion of chemicals through the kidney targets the kidney for toxic effects, as seen with chemicals such as cadmium, copper, mercury, and chlorobenzene (WHO 2003).

Pesticides and other chemical contaminants that enter waterways through agricultural runoff, stormwater drains, and industrial discharges may persist in the environment for long periods and be transported by water or air over long distances. They may disrupt the function of the endocrine system, resulting in reproductive, developmental, and behavioral problems. The endocrine disruptors can reduce fertility and increase the occurrence of stillbirths, birth defects, and hormonally dependent cancers such as breast, testicular, and prostate cancers. The effects on the developing nervous system can include impaired mental and psychomotor development, as well as cognitive impairment and behavior abnormalities (WHO and International Programme on Chemical Safety 2002). Examples of endocrine disruptors include organochlorines, PCBs, alkylphenols, phytoestrogens (natural estrogens in plants), and pharmaceuticals such as antibiotics and synthetic sex hormones from contraceptives. Chemicals in drinking water can also be carcinogenic. Disinfection by-products and arsenic have been a particular concern (International Agency for Research on Cancer 2004).

INTERVENTIONS

The variety of hazardous pollutants that can occur in air or water also leads to many different interventions. Interventions pertaining to environmental hazards are often more sustainable if they address the driving forces behind the pollution at the community level rather than attempt to deal with specific exposures at the individual level. In addition, effective methods to prevent exposure to chemical hazards in the air or water may not exist at the individual level, and the only feasible individual-level intervention may be treating cases of illness.

Figure 43.1 shows five levels at which actions can be taken to prevent the health effects of environmental hazards. Some would label interventions at the driving force level as policy instruments. These include legal restrictions on the use of a toxic substance, such as banning the use of lead in gasoline, or community-level policies, such as boosting public transportation and reducing individual use of motor vehicles.

Interventions to reduce pressures on environmental quality include those that limit hazardous waste disposal by recycling hazardous substances at their site of use or replacing them with

less hazardous materials. Interventions at the level of the state of the environment would include air quality monitoring linked to local actions to reduce pollution during especially polluted periods (for example, banning vehicle use when pollution levels reach predetermined thresholds). Interventions at the exposure level include using household water filters to reduce arsenic in drinking water as done in Bangladesh. Finally, interventions at the effect level would include actions by health services to protect or restore the health of people already showing signs of an adverse effect.

Interventions to Reduce Air Pollution

Reducing air pollution exposure is largely a technical issue. Technologies to reduce pollution at its source are plentiful, as are technologies that reduce pollution by filtering it away from the emission source (end-of-pipe solutions; see, for example, Gwilliam, Kojima, and Johnson 2004). Getting these technologies applied in practice requires government or corporate policies that guide technical decision making in the right direction. Such policies could involve outright bans (such as requiring lead-free gasoline or asbestos-free vehicle brake linings or building materials); guidance on desirable technologies (for example, providing best-practice manuals); or economic instruments that make using more polluting technologies more expensive than using less polluting technologies (an example of the polluter pays principle).

Examples of technologies to reduce air pollution include the use of lead-free gasoline, which allows the use of catalytic converters on vehicles' exhaust systems. Such technologies significantly reduce the emissions of several air pollutants from vehicles (box 43.3). For trucks, buses, and an increasing number of smaller vehicles that use diesel fuel, improving the quality of the diesel itself by lowering its sulfur content is another way to reduce air pollution at the source. More fuel-efficient vehicles, such as hybrid gas-electric vehicles, are another way forward. These vehicles can reduce gasoline consumption by about 50 percent during city driving. Policies that reduce "unnecessary" driving, or traffic demand management, can also reduce air pollution in urban areas. A system of congestion fees, in which drivers have to pay before entering central urban areas, was introduced in Singapore, Oslo, and London and has been effective in this respect.

Power plants and industrial plants that burn fossil fuels use a variety of filtering methods to reduce particles and scrubbing methods to reduce gases, although no effective method is currently available for the greenhouse gas carbon dioxide. High chimneys dilute pollutants, but the combined input of pollutants from a number of smokestacks can still lead to an overload of pollutants. An important example is acid rain, which is caused by SO_2 and NO_x emissions that make water vapor in the

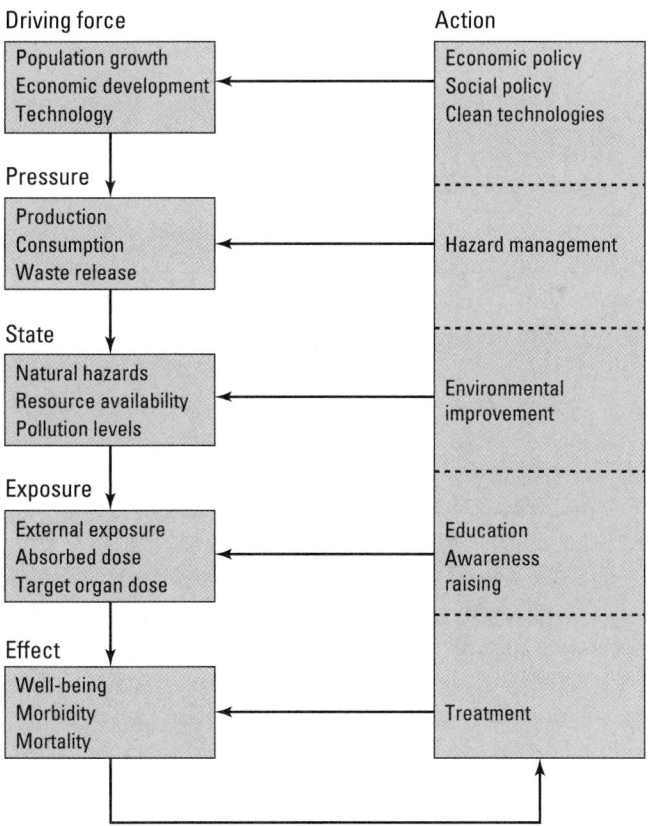

Driving force

Action

Source: Kjellstrom and Corvalan 1995.

Figure 43.1 Framework for Environmental Health Interventions

Box 43.3

Air Pollution Reduction in Mexico City

Mexico City is one of the world's largest megacities, with nearly 20 million inhabitants. Local authorities have acknowledged its air quality problems since the 1970s. The emissions from several million motor vehicles and thousands of industries created major concerns about health effects. Annual average particulate matter (PM_{10}) levels of 50 to 100 $\mu g/m^3$ have been measured in the worst-polluted central area and can be associated with annual mortality excess of 15 to 30 percent. Even if only 20 percent of the population were exposed to such high levels, that exposure would account for 6,000 to 12,000 additional deaths per year. To tackle the problem, Mexico City started air quality monitoring and health studies in the 1980s. High-risk groups were the 2.2 million children, 250,000 street vendors, and 250,000 commercial drivers. After 20 years of policies and actions, interventions for better health have borne fruit.

The first intervention was lead-free gasoline in 1990, which enabled the government to require catalytic converters on new cars, thus dramatically reducing carbon monoxide, NO_x, and hydrocarbon emissions. In 1997, leaded gasoline was completely phased out. The annual average concentration of lead in the air in the worst-polluted area was reduced from 1.2 $\mu g/m^3$ in 1990 to less than 0.1 $\mu g/m^3$ in 2000. Surveys of blood lead levels in children showed reductions from 200 to 100 $\mu g/liter$ during the same period, implying that the intervention had protected thousands of children from lead poisoning. Another key concern was SO_2 emissions from industry and diesel vehicles. Heavy fuel oil was phased out in the mid 1990s, and the sulfur content of diesel was reduced. In addition, power plants and some industry shifted to natural gas in the early 1990s. The result was a 90 percent reduction of SO_2 in ambient air in five years.

Air quality standards, emission standards for vehicles, and other technical actions to reduce air emissions were tightened during the 1990s, contributing to downward trends of carbon monoxide, NO_x, and ozone levels. Levels of emissions were reduced by half at some sites, resulting in an estimated reduction of 3,000 to 6,000 excess deaths.

Sources: Fernandez 2002; McMichael, Kjellstrom, and Smith 2001; WHO 2000.

---

atmosphere acidic (WHO 2000). Large combined emissions from industry and power stations in the eastern United States drift north with the winds and cause damage to Canadian ecosystems. In Europe, emissions from the industrial belt across Belgium, Germany, and Poland drift north to Sweden and have damaged many lakes there. The convergence of air pollutants from many sources and the associated health effects have also been documented in relation to the multiple fires in Indonesia's rain forest in 1997 (Brauer and Hisham-Hashim 1998); the brown cloud over large areas of Asia, which is mainly related to coal burning; and a similar brown cloud over central Europe in the summer, which is caused primarily by vehicle emissions.

Managing air pollution interventions involves monitoring air quality, which may focus on exceedances of air quality guidelines in specific hotspots or on attempts to establish a specific population's average exposure to pollution. Sophisticated modeling in combination with monitoring has made it possible to start producing detailed estimates and maps of air pollution levels in key urban areas (World Bank 2004), thus providing a powerful tool for assessing current health impacts and estimated changes in the health impacts brought about by defined air pollution interventions.

Interventions to Reduce Water Pollution

Water pollution control requires action at all levels of the hierarchical framework shown in figure 43.1. The ideal method to abate diffuse chemical pollution of waterways is to minimize or avoid the use of chemicals for industrial, agricultural, and domestic purposes. Adapting practices such as organic farming and integrated pest management could help protect waterways (Scheierling 1995). Chemical contamination of waterways from industrial emissions could be reduced by cleaner production processes (UNEP 2002). Box 43.4 describes one project aimed at effectively reducing pollution.

Other interventions include proper treatment of hazardous waste and recycling of chemical containers and discarded products containing chemicals to reduce solid waste buildup and leaching of toxic chemicals into waterways. A variety of technical solutions are available to filter out chemical waste from industrial processes or otherwise render them harmless. Changing the pH of wastewater or adding chemicals that flocculate the toxic chemicals so that they settle in sedimentation ponds are common methods. The same principle can be used at the individual household level. One example is the use of iron chips to filter out arsenic from contaminated well water in Bangladeshi households (Kinniburgh and Smedley 2001).

Water Pollution Control in India

In 1993, the Demonstration in Small Industries for Reducing Wastes Project was started in India with support from the United Nations Industrial Development Organization. International and local experts initiated waste reduction audits in four pulp and paper plants, four textile dyeing and finishing factories, and four pesticide production units. The experts identified priority areas, estimated the likely reduction in the pollutant load, and came up with more than 500 pollution prevention options. The 12 companies spent a total of US$300,000 to implement pollution prevention options and saved US$3 million in raw materials and wastewater treatment costs.

The most impressive savings were in the pulp and paper sector. For instance, the Ashoka Pulp and Paper Company participated in the project with the dual objectives of reducing production costs and complying with environmental regulations in a cost-effective manner. Pressure from the public to improve environmental performance and the need to conserve water, especially during the summer, added urgency to the project. The company implemented 24 waste minimization options, with 13 additional options under consideration, resulting in net annual savings of about US$160,000. The payback period for the implemented options was less than seven months, and the annual savings will continue.

The project demonstrated that waste minimization can cut pollution and business costs at the same time, especially when the environmental protection effort is directed toward the production process itself rather than to end-of-pipe treatment. The key to success lies in the sustained involvement of local experts and committed factory managers.

Source: United Nations 1997.

INTERVENTION COSTS AND COST-EFFECTIVENESS

This chapter cannot follow the detailed format for the economic analysis of different preventive interventions devised for the disease-specific chapters, because the exposures, health effects, and interventions are too varied and because of the lack of overarching examples of economic assessments. Nevertheless, it does present a few examples of the types of analyses available.

Comparison of Interventions

A review of more than 1,000 reports on cost per life year saved in the United States for 587 interventions in the environment and other fields (table 43.2) evaluated costs from a societal perspective. The net costs included only direct costs and savings. Indirect costs, such as forgone earnings, were excluded. Future costs and life years saved were discounted at 5 percent per year. Interventions with a cost per life year saved of less than or equal to zero cost less to implement than the value of the lives saved. Each of three categories of interventions (toxin control, fatal injury reduction, and medicine) presented in table 43.2 includes several extremely cost-effective interventions.

The cost-effective interventions in the air pollution area could be of value in developing countries as their industrial and transportation pollution situations become similar to the United States in the 1960s. The review by Tengs and

others (1995) does not report the extent to which the various interventions were implemented in existing pollution control or public health programs, and many of the most cost-effective interventions are probably already in wide use. The review did create a good deal of controversy in the United States, because professionals and nongovernmental organizations active in the environmental field accused the authors of overestimating the costs and underestimating the benefits of controls over chemicals (see, for example, U.S. Congress 1999).

Costs and Savings in Relation to Pollution Control

A number of publications review and discuss the evidence on the costs and benefits of different pollution control interventions in industrial countries (see, for example, U.S. Environmental Protection Agency 1999). For developing countries, specific data on this topic are found primarily in the so-called gray literature: government reports, consultant reports, or reports by the international banks.

Air Pollution. Examples of cost-effectiveness analysis for assessing air quality policy include studies carried out in Jakarta, Kathmandu, Manila, and Mumbai under the World Bank's Urban Air Quality Management Strategy in Asia (Grønskei and others 1996a, 1996b; Larssen and others 1996a, 1996b; Shah, Nagpal, and Brandon 1997). In each city, an emissions inventory was established, and rudimentary dispersion modeling was carried out. Various mitigation measures for

Table 43.2 Median Cost Per Life Year Saved, Selected Relatively Low-Cost Interventions
(1993 U.S. dollars)

Intervention	Cost per life year saved
Toxin control	
Control coal-fired power plant emissions through high chimneys and other means	≤ 0
Reduce lead in gasoline from 1.1 to 0.1 grams per gallon	≤ 0
Ban amitraz pesticide on apples	≤ 0
Introduce a chloroform emission standard at selected pulp mills	≤ 0
Control SO_2 by desulfuring residual fuel oil	≤ 0
Initiate sedimentation, filtration, and chlorination of drinking water	4,200
Introduce radon remediation in homes with levels greater than 21.6 picocuries per liter	6,100
Ban asbestos in brake linings	29,000
Set arsenic emission standards at selected copper smelters	36,000
Fatal injury reduction	
Make motorcycle helmet laws mandatory	≤ 0
Install automatic seat belts in cars	≤ 0
Require bad drivers to attend driving improvement schools	≤ 0
Pass a law requiring smoke detectors in homes	≤ 0
Improve standards for concrete construction	≤ 0
Ban residential growth in tsunami-prone areas	≤ 0
Make seat belt use in cars mandatory	69
Install smoke detectors in airplane lavatories	30,000
Medicine	
Require all common types of early childhood vaccinations	≤ 0
Implement annual stool colon cancer screening for people age 55 and older	≤ 0
Introduce detoxification or methadone maintenance for heroin addicts	≤ 0
Screen newborns for phenylketonuria	≤ 0
Recommend cervical cancer screening every three years for women age 65 and older	≤ 0
Introduce universal prenatal care for expectant mothers	≤ 0
Vaccinate all citizens against influenza	140
Screen men age 45–54 for hypertension	5,200
Institute annual mammography and breast examinations for women age 40–64	17,000
Perform three-vessel coronary artery bypass surgery for severe angina	23,000

Source: Based on Tengs and others 1995.
Note: The fatal injury reduction and medicine categories are included for comparison purposes.

reducing PM_{10} and health impacts were examined in terms of reductions in tons of PM_{10} emitted, cost of implementation, time frame for implementation, and health benefits and their associated cost savings. Some of the abatement measures that have been implemented include introducing unleaded gasoline, tightening standards, introducing low-smoke lubricants for two-stroke engine vehicles, implementing inspections of vehicle exhaust emissions to address gross polluters, and reducing garbage burning.

Transportation policies and industrial development do not usually have air quality considerations as their primary objec-

tive, but the World Bank has developed a method to take these considerations into account. The costs of different air quality improvement policies are explored in relation to a baseline investment and the estimated health effects of air pollution. A comparison will indicate the cost-effectiveness of each policy. The World Bank has worked out this "overlay" approach in some detail for the energy and forestry sectors in the analogous case of greenhouse gas reduction strategies (World Bank 2004).

Water Pollution. The costs and benefits associated with interventions to remove chemical contaminants from water need to be assessed on a local or national basis to determine specific needs, available resources, environmental conditions (including climate), and sustainability. A developing country for which substantial economic analysis of interventions has been carried out is China (Dasgupta, Wang, and Wheeler 1997; Zhang and others 1996).

Another country with major concerns about chemicals (arsenic) in water is Bangladesh. The arsenic mitigation programs have applied various arsenic removal technologies, but the costs and benefits are not well established. Bangladesh has adopted a drinking water standard of 50 µg/L (micrograms per liter) for arsenic in drinking water. The cost of achieving the lower WHO guideline value of 10 µg/L would be significant. An evaluation of the cost of lowering arsenic levels in drinking water in the United States predicts that a reduction from 50 to 10 µg/L would prevent a limited number of deaths from bladder and lung cancer at a cost of several million dollars per death prevented (Frost and others 2002).

Alternative water supplies need to be considered when the costs of improving existing water sources outweigh the benefits. Harvesting rainwater may provide communities with safe drinking water, free of chemicals and micro-organisms, but contamination from roofs and storage tanks needs to be considered. Rainwater collection is relatively inexpensive.

ECONOMIC BENEFITS OF INTERVENTIONS

One of the early examples of cost-benefit analysis for chemical pollution control is the Japan Environment Agency's (1991) study of three Japanese classical pollution diseases: Yokkaichi asthma, Minamata disease, and Itai-Itai disease (table 43.3). This analysis was intended to highlight the economic aspects of pollution control and to encourage governments in developing countries to consider both the costs and the benefits of industrial development. The calculations take into account the 20 or 30 years that have elapsed since the disease outbreaks occurred and annualize the costs and benefits over a 30-year period. The

pollution damage costs are the actual payments for victims' compensation and the cost of environmental remediation. The compensation costs are based on court cases or government decisions and can be seen as a valid representation of the economic value of the health damage in each case. As table 43.3 shows, controlling the relevant pollutants would have cost far less than paying for damage caused by the pollution.

A few studies have analyzed cost-benefit aspects of air pollution control in specific cities. Those analyses are based mainly on modeling health impacts from exposure and relationships between doses and responses. Voorhees and others (2001) find that most studies that analyzed the situation in specific urban areas used health impact assessment to estimate impacts avoided by interventions. Investigators have used different methods for valuing the economic benefits of health improvements, including market valuation, stated preference methods, and revealed preference methods. The choice of assumptions and inputs substantially affected the resulting cost and benefit valuations.

One of the few detailed studies of the costs and benefits of air pollution control in a specific urban area (Voorhees and others 2000) used changing nitric oxide and NO_2 emissions in Tokyo during 1973–94 as a basis for the calculations. The study did not use actual health improvement data but calculated likely health improvements from estimated reductions in NO_2 levels and published dose-response curves. The health effects included respiratory morbidity (as determined by hospital admissions and medical expenses), and working days lost for sick adults, and maternal working days lost in the case of a child's illness. The results indicated an average cost-benefit ratio of 1 to 6, with a large range from a lower limit of 3 to 1 to an upper limit of 1 to 44. The estimated economic benefits of reductions in nitric oxide and NO_2 emissions between 1973 and 1994 were considerable: US$6.78 billion for avoided medical costs, US$6.33 billion for avoided lost wages of sick adults, and US$0.83 billion for avoided lost wages of mothers with sick children.

Blackman and others' (2000) cost-benefit analysis of four practical strategies for reducing PM_{10} emissions from

Table 43.3 Comparison of Actual Pollution Damage Costs and the Pollution Control Costs That Would Have Prevented the Damage, for Three Pollution-Related Disease Outbreaks, Japan
(¥ millions, 1989 equivalents)

| Pollution disease | Main pollutant | Pollution control costs | Pollution damage costs | | | |
			Health damage	Livelihood damage	Environmental remediation	Total
Yokkaichi asthma	SO_2, air pollution	14,800	21,000 (1,300)[a]	Not estimated	Not estimated	21,000
Minamata disease	Mercury, water pollution	125	7,670	4,270	690	12,630
Itai-Itai disease	Cadmium, water and soil pollution	600	740	880	890	2,510

Source: Japan Environment Agency 1991.
Note: US$1 = ¥150.
a. Based on actual compensation payments to a fraction of the population. The larger figure is what it would have cost to compensate all those who were affected.

traditional brick kilns in Ciudad Juárez in Mexico suggests that, given a wide range of modeling assumptions, the benefits of three control strategies would be considerably higher than the costs. Reduced mortality was by far the largest component of benefits, accounting for more than 80 percent of the total.

Pandey and Nathwani (2003) applied cost-benefit analysis to a pollution control program in Canada. Their study proposed using the life quality index as a tool for quantifying the level of public expenditure beyond which the use of resources is not justified. The study estimated total pollution control costs at US$2.5 billion per year against a monetary benefit of US$7.5 billion per year, using 1996 as the base year for all cost and benefit estimates. The benefit estimated in terms of avoided mortality was about 1,800 deaths per year.

El-Fadel and Massoud's (2000) study of urban areas in Lebanon shows that the health benefits and economic benefits of reducing PM concentration in the air can range from US$4.53 million to US$172.50 million per year using a willingness-to-pay approach. In that study, the major monetized benefits resulted from reduced mortality costs.

Aunan and others (1998) assessed the costs and benefits of implementing an energy saving and air pollution control program in Hungary. They based their monetary evaluation of benefits on local monitoring and population data and took exposure-response functions and valuation estimates from Canadian, U.S., and European studies. The authors valued the average total benefits of the interventions at US$1.56 billion per year (with 1994 as the base year), with high and low bounds at US$7.6, billion and US$0.4 billion, respectively. They estimated the cost-benefit ratio at 1 to 3.4, given a total cost of interventions of US$0.46 billion per year. Many of the benefits resulted from reduced mortality in the elderly population and from reduced asthma morbidity costs.

Misra (2002) examined the costs and benefits of water pollution abatement for a cluster of 250 small-scale industries in Gujarat, India. Misra's assessment looked at command-and-control, market-based solutions and at effluent treatment as alternatives. In a cost-benefit analysis, Misra estimated the net present social benefits from water pollution abatement at the Nandesari Industrial Estate at Rs 0.550 billion at 1995–96 market prices using a 12 percent social discount rate. After making corrections for the prices of foreign exchange, unskilled labor, and investment, the figure rose to Rs 0.62 billion. It rose still further to about Rs 3.1 billion when distributional effects were taken into account.

IMPLEMENTATION OF CONTROL STRATEGIES: LESSONS OF EXPERIENCE

The foregoing examples demonstrate that interventions to protect health that use chemical pollution control can have an attractive cost-benefit ratio. The Japan Environment Agency (1991) estimates the national economic impact of pollution control legislation and associated interventions. During the 1960s and early 1970s, when the government made many of the major decisions about intensified pollution control interventions, Japan's gross domestic product (GDP) per capita was growing at an annual rate of about 10 percent, similar to that of the rapidly industrializing countries in the early 21st century. At that time, Japan's economic policies aimed at eliminating bottlenecks to high economic growth, and in the mid 1960s, industry was spending less than ¥50 billion per year on pollution control equipment. By 1976, this spending had increased to almost ¥1 trillion per year. The ¥5 trillion invested in pollution control between 1965 and 1975 accounted for about 0.9 percent of the increase in GDP per capita during this period. The Japan Environment Agency concluded that the stricter environmental protection legislation and associated major investment in pollution control had little effect on the overall economy, but that the resulting health benefits are likely cumulative.

Air

The broadest analysis of the implementation of control strategies for air pollution was conducted by the U.S. Environmental Protection Agency in the late 1990s (Krupnick and Morgenstern 2002). The analysis developed a hypothetical scenario for 1970 to 1990, assuming that the real costs for pollution control during this period could be compared with the benefits of reduced mortality and morbidity and avoided damage to agricultural crops brought about by the reduction of major air pollutant levels across the country during this period. The study estimated reduced mortality from dose-response relationships for the major air pollutants, assigning the cost of each death at the value of statistical life and the cost of morbidity in relation to estimated health service utilization. The study used a variety of costing methods to reach the range of likely present values presented in table 43.4. It assumed that the reduction of air pollution resulted from the implementation of the federal Clean Air Act of 1970 and associated state-level regulations and air pollution limits.

The analysis showed a dramatically high cost-benefit ratio and inspired debate about the methodologies used and the results. One major criticism was of the use of the value of statistical life for each death potentially avoided by the reduced air pollution. A recalculation using the life-years-lost method reduced the benefits for deaths caused by PM from US$16,632 billion to US$9,100 billion (Krupnick and Morgenstern 2002). The recalculated figure is still well above the fifth percentile estimate of benefits and does not undermine the positive cost-benefit ratio reported. Thus, if a developing country were to implement an appropriate control strategy for urban air pollution, it might derive significant

Table 43.4 Present Value of Monetary Benefits and Costs Associated with Implementation of the U.S. Clean Air Act, 1970–90 *(1990 US$ billions)*

Category	Pollutant	Present value, 5th percentile	Present value, mean	Present value, 95th percentile
Mortality	PM	2,369	16,632	40,957
Mortality	Lead	121	1,339	3,910
Chronic bronchitis	PM	409	3,313	10,401
IQ reduction	Lead	271	399	551
Other morbidity	Several	227	337	501
Soil damage	PM	6	74	192
Visibility reduction	PM	38	54	71
Agricultural damage	Ozone	11	23	35
Total benefits	All	3,452	22,171	56,618
Total costs	All	Not estimated	523	Not estimated
Net benefits (total benefits − total costs)	All	Not estimated	21,648	Not estimated

Source: Krupnick and Morgenstern 2002.

economic benefits over the subsequent decades. The country's level of economic development, local costs, and local benefit valuations will be important for any cost-benefit assessment. WHO's (2000) air quality guidelines are among the documents that provide advice on analytical approaches.

Water

We were unable to find an analysis for water similar to the broad analysis presented for air, but the examples of water pollution with mercury, cadmium, and arsenic described earlier indicate the economic benefits that can be reaped from effective interventions against chemical water pollution. Since the pollution disease outbreaks of mercury and cadmium poisoning in Japan, serious mercury pollution situations have been identified in Brazil, China, and the Philippines, and serious cadmium pollution has occurred in Cambodia, China, the Lao People's Democratic Republic, and Thailand. Arsenic in groundwater is an ongoing, serious problem in Bangladesh, India, and Nepal and a less serious problem in a number of other countries.

WHO has analyzed control strategies for biological water pollution and water and sanitation improvements in relation to the Millennium Development Goals (Hutton and Haller 2004). The analysis demonstrated the considerable benefits of water and sanitation improvements: for every US$1 invested, the economic return was in the range of US$5 to US$28 for a number of intervention options. Careful analysis of the same type is required for populations particularly vulnerable to chemical water pollution to assess whether control of chemical pollution can also yield significant benefits.

RESEARCH AND DEVELOPMENT AGENDA

Even though a good deal of information is available about the health risks of common air and water pollutants, further research is needed to guide regulations and interventions. The pollutants that were most common in developed countries in the past are still major problems in developing countries; however, direct application of the experiences of developed countries may not be appropriate, because exposed populations in developing countries may have a different burden of preexisting diseases, malnutrition, and other factors related to poverty. Research on specific vulnerabilities and on relevant dose-response relationships for different levels of economic development and for various geographic conditions would therefore be valuable for assessing risks and targeting interventions. In addition, global chemical exposure concerns, such as endocrine disruptors in air, water, and food, require urgent research to establish the need for interventions in both industrial and developing countries.

An important research topic is to clearly describe and quantify the long-term health effects of exposure to air pollution. The existing literature indicates that long-term exposure may have more adverse health effects than short-term exposure and, hence, have higher cost implications. Another topic is to assess the health issue pertaining to greenhouse gases and climate change, which are related to the same sources as urban air pollution (Intergovernmental Panel on Climate Change 2001). Research and policy analysis on how best to develop interventions to reduce health risks related to climate change need to be considered together with the analysis of other air pollutants.

In addition, to improve analysis of the economic costs of health impacts, better estimates are needed of the burden of disease related to chemical air and water pollution at local, national, and global levels. Cost-effectiveness analysis of air and water pollution control measures in developing countries needs to be supported by further research, as cost levels and benefit valuations will vary from country to country, and solutions that are valid in industrial countries may not work as well in developing countries. Strategies for effective air and water resource management should include research on the potential side effects of an intervention, such as in Bangladesh, where tube wells drilled to supply water turned out to be contaminated with arsenic (see box 43.2). Research is also needed that would link methodologies for assessing adverse health effects with exposure and epidemiological studies in different settings to permit the development of more precise forecasting of the health and economic benefits of interventions.

The variety of health effects of urban air pollution and the variety of sources create opportunities for ancillary effects that need to be taken into account in economic cost-effectiveness and cost-benefit analysis. These are the beneficial effects of reducing air pollution on other health risks associated with the sources of air pollution. For example, if the air pollution from transportation emissions is reduced by actions that reduce the use of private motor vehicles by, say, providing public transportation, not only are carbon dioxide levels reduced; traffic crash injuries, noise, and physical inactivity related to the widespread use of motor vehicles also decline (Kjellstrom and others 2003).

One of the key challenges for policies and actions is to find ways to avoid a rapid buildup of urban air pollution in countries that do not yet have a major problem. The health sector needs to be involved in assessing urban planning, the location of industries, and the development of transportation systems and needs to encourage those designing public transportation and housing to ensure that new sources of air pollution are not being built into cities.

Decades of economic and industrial growth have resulted in lifestyles that increase the demands on water resources simultaneous with increases in water pollution levels. Conflicts between household, industrial, and agricultural water use are a common public health problem (UNESCO 2003). The developing countries need to avoid the experiences of water pollution and associated disease outbreaks in industrial countries. Strategies to ensure sufficient pollution control must be identified at the same time as strategies to reduce water consumption. High water use depletes supplies and increases salinity in groundwater aquifers, particularly in coastal regions. The impact of climate change must also be taken into consideration (Vorosmarty and others 2000).

CONCLUSION: PROMISES AND PITFALLS

Evidence shows that a number of chemicals that may be released into the air or water can cause adverse health effects. The associated burden of disease can be substantial, and investment in research on health effects and interventions in specific populations and exposure situations is important for the development of control strategies. Pollution control is therefore an important component of disease control, and health professionals and authorities need to develop partnerships with other sectors to identify and implement priority interventions.

Developing countries face major water quantity and quality challenges, compounded by the effects of rapid industrialization. Concerted actions are needed to safely manage the use of toxic chemicals and to develop monitoring and regulatory guidelines. Recycling and the use of biodegradable products must be encouraged. Technologies to reduce air pollution at the source are well established and should be used in all new industrial development. Retrofitting of existing industries and power plants is also worthwhile. The growing number of private motor vehicles in developing countries brings certain benefits, but alternative means of transportation, particularly in rapidly growing urban areas, need to be considered at an early stage, as the negative health and economic impacts of high concentrations of motor vehicles are well established. The principles and practices of sustainable development, coupled with local research, will help contain or eliminate health risks resulting from chemical pollution. International collaboration involving both governmental and nongovernmental organizations can guide this highly interdisciplinary and intersectoral area of disease control.

REFERENCES

Aunan, K., G. Patzay, H. A. Aaheim, and H. M. Seip. 1998. "Health and Environmental Benefits from Air Pollution Reductions in Hungary." *Science of the Total Environment* 212: 245–68.

Bell, M. L., and D. I. Davis. 2001. "Reassessment of the Lethal London Fog of 1952: Novel Indicators of Acute and Chronic Consequences of Acute Exposure to Air Pollution." *Environmental Health Perspectives* 109 (Suppl. 3): 389–94.

Blackman, A., S. Newbold, J. S. Shih, and J. Cook. 2000. "The Benefits and Costs of Informal Sector Pollution Control: Mexican Brick Kilns." Discussion Paper 00–46, Resources for the Future, Washington, DC.

Brauer M., and J. Hisham-Hashim. 1998. "Indonesian Fires: Crisis and Reaction." *Environmental Science and Technology* 32: 404A–7A.

Brunekreef, B., and S. T. Holgate. 2002. "Air Pollution and Health." *Lancet* 360: 1233–42.

Constantinides, G. 2000. *Cost-Benefit Analysis Case Studies in Eastern Africa for the GPA Strategic Action Plan on Sewage.* Nairobi: United Nations Environmental Programme. http://www.gpa.unep.org/documents/other/casestudies/east_africa_case_studies_final_draft.pdf.

Dasgupta, S., H. Wang, and D. Wheeler. 1997. "Surviving Success: Policy Reform and the Future of Industrial Pollution in China." Working Paper 1856, World Bank, Washington, DC.

Dhara, V. R., and R. Dhara. 2002. "The Union Carbide Disaster in Bhopal: A Review of Health Effects." *Archives of Environmental Health* 57 (5): 391–404.

Dockery, D. W., C. A. Pope, X. Xu, J. D. Spengler, J. H. Ware, M. E. Fay, and others. 1993. "An Association between Air Pollution and Mortality in Six U.S. Cities." *New England Journal of Medicine* 329 (24): 1753–59.

El-Fadel, M., and M. Massoud. 2000. "Particulate Matter in Urban Areas: Health-Based Economic Assessment." *Science of the Total Environment* 257: 133–46.

Fernandez, A. 2002. *Mexico City: Air Pollution Case Study*. Environment course. Cambridge, MA: Harvard University. http://courses.dce.harvard.edu/environment/week10em1_new.html.

Fewthrell, L., R. B. Kaufmann, and A. Preuss. 2003. *Assessing the Environmental Burden of Disease at the National and Local Level: Lead*. Environmental Burden of Disease Series 2. Geneva: World Health Organization.

Frost, F. J., K. Tollestrup, G. F. Craun, R. Raucher, J. Chwirka, and J. Stomp. 2002. "Evaluation of Costs and Benefits of a Lower Arsenic MCL." *Journal AWWA (American Water Works Association)* 94 (3): 71–82.

Grønskei, K. E., F. Gram, L. O. Hagen, S. Larssen, H. Jansen, X. Olsthoorn, and others. 1996a. *URBAIR Urban Air Quality Management Strategy in Asia: Jakarta Report*. Washington, DC: World Bank.

———. 1996b. *URBAIR Urban Air Quality Management Strategy in Asia: Kathmandu Valley Report*. Washington, DC: World Bank.

Gwilliam, K., M. Kojima, and T. Johnson. 2004. *Reducing Air Pollution from Transport*. Washington, DC: World Bank.

Hutton, G., and L. Haller. 2004. *Evaluation of the Costs and Benefits of Water and Sanitation Improvements at the Global Level*. WHO/SDE/WSH/04.04. Geneva: World Health Organization. http://www.who.int/water_sanitation_health/wsh0404/en/.

Intergovernmental Panel on Climate Change. 2001. *Climate Change 2001*. Geneva: World Meteorological Organization, Intergovernmental Panel on Climate Change. http://www.ipcc.ch.

International Agency for Research on Cancer. 2004. *Some Drinking Water Disinfectants and Contaminants, Including Arsenic*. Monograph 84. Lyon, France: International Agency for Research on Cancer.

Japan Environment Agency. 1991. *Pollution in Japan—Our Tragic Experience* (in Japanese, with English translation available). Tokyo: Japan Environment Agency, Study Group for Global Environment and Economics, Office of Planning and Research.

Kazan-Allen, L. 2004. "The Asbestos War." *International Journal of Occupational and Environmental Health* 9: 173–93.

Kinniburgh, D. G., and P. A. Smedley, eds. 2001. *Arsenic Contamination of Groundwater in Bangladesh*. BGS Technical Report WC/00/19. Keyworth, U.K.: British Geological Survey; Dhaka: Department of Public Health Engineering.

Kjellstrom, T. 1986. "Itai-Itai Disease." In *Cadmium and Health*, ed. L. Friberg, G. F. Nordberg, T. Kjellstrom, and C. G. Elinder, vol. 2, 257–90. Boca Raton, FL: CRC Press.

Kjellstrom, T., and C. Corvalan. 1995. "Framework for the Development of Environmental Health Indicators." *World Health Statistics Quarterly* 48: 144–54.

Kjellstrom, T., L. van Kerkhoff, G. Bammer, and T. McMichael. 2003. "Comparative Assessment of Transport Risks: How It Can Contribute to Health Impact Assessment of Transport Policies." *Bulletin of the World Health Organization* 81: 451–57.

Krupnick, A., and R. Morgenstern. 2002. "The Future of Benefit-Cost Analysis of the Clean Air Act." *Annual Review of Public Health* 23: 427–48.

LaDou, J. 1992. "The Export of Hazards to Developing Countries." In *Occupational Health in Developing Countries*, ed. J. Jeyaratnam, 340–60. Oxford, U.K.: Oxford University Press.

Larssen, S., F. Gram, L. O. Hagen, H. Jansen, X. Olsthoorn, R. V. Aundhe, and U. Joglekar. 1996a. *URBAIR Urban Air Quality Management Strategy in Asia: Greater Mumbai Report*. Washington, DC: World Bank.

Larssen, S., F. Gram, L. O. Hagen, H. Jansen, X. Olsthoorn, R. Lesaca, and others. 1996b. *URBAIR Urban Air Quality Management Strategy in Asia: Metro Manila Report*. Washington, DC: World Bank.

McConnell, R., K. Berhane, F. Gilliland, S. J. London, T. Islam, W. J. Gauderman, and others. 2002. "Asthma in Exercising Children Exposed to Ozone: A Cohort Study." *Lancet* 359 (9304): 386–91.

McGranahan, G., and F. Murray. 2003. "Air Pollution and Health in Rapidly Developing Countries." London: Earthscan.

McMichael, A. J., H. R. Anderson, B. Brunekreef, and A. Cohen. 1998. "Inappropriate Use of Daily Mortality Analyses to Estimate Longer-Term Mortality Effects of Air Pollution." *International Journal of Epidemiology* 27: 450–53.

McMichael, A. J., T. Kjellstrom, and K. Smith. 2001. "Environmental Health." In *International Public Health*, ed. M. H. Merson, R. E. Black, and A. J. Mills, 379–438. Gaithersburg, MD: Aspen.

Misra, S. 2002. "An Empirical Investigation of Collective Action Possibilities for Industrial Water Pollution Abatement: Case Study of a Cluster of Small-Scale Industries in India." *World Bank Economists' Forum* 2: 89–113.

Murata, K., P. Weihe, E. Budtz-Jorgensen, P. J. Jorgensen, and P. Grandjean. 2004. "Delayed Brainstem Auditory Evoked Potential Latencies in 14-Year-Old Children Exposed to Methylmercury." *Journal of Pediatrics* 144: 177–83.

Nyberg, F., P. Gustavsson, L. Jarup, T. Bellander, N. Berglind, R. Jacobsson, and others. 2000. "Urban Air Pollution and Lung Cancer in Stockholm." *Epidemiology* 11: 487–95.

Pandey, M. D., and J. S. Nathwani. 2003. "Canada Wide Standard for Particulate Matter and Ozone: Cost-Benefit Analysis Using a Life Quality Index." *Risk Analysis* 23 (1): 55–67.

Pereira, L. A., D. Loomis, G. M. Conceição, A. L. Braga, R. M. Arcas, K. S. Kishi, and others. 1998. "Association between Air Pollution and Intrauterine Mortality in São Paulo, Brazil." *Environmental Health Perspectives* 106: 325–29.

Ponsonby, A. L., D. Couper, T. Dwyer, A. Carmichael, A. Kemp, and J. Cochrane. 2000. "The Relation between Infant Indoor Environment and Subsequent Asthma." *Epidemiology* 11: 128–35.

Pope, C. III, R. Burnett, M. Thun, E. Calle, D. Krewski, K. Ito, and G. D. Thurston. 2002. "Lung Cancer, Cardiopulmonary Mortality, and Long-Term Exposure to Fine Particulate Air Pollution." *Journal of the American Medical Association* 287 (9): 1132–41.

Pope, C. III, M. J. Thun, M. M. Namboodiri, D. W. Dockery, J. S. Evans, F. E. Speizer, and others. 1995. "Particulate Air Pollution as a Predictor of Mortality in a Prospective Study of U.S. Adults." *American Journal of Respiratory Critical Care Medicine* 151 (3, part 1): 669–74.

Rios, J. L. M., J. L. Boechat, C. C. Sant'Anna, and A. T. Franca. 2004. "Atmospheric Pollution and the Prevalence of Asthma: Study among Schoolchildren in Two Areas of Rio de Janeiro, Brazil." *Annals of Allergy, Asthma, and Immunology* 92 (6): 629–34.

Romieu, I., F. Meneses, S. Ruiz, J. J. Sienra, J. Huerta, M. C. White, and R. A. Etzel. 1996. "Effects of Air Pollution on the Respiratory Health of Asthmatic Children Living in Mexico City." *American Journal of Respiratory Critical Care Medicine* 154: 300–7.

Scheierling, S. 1995. "Overcoming Agricultural Pollution of Water: The Challenge of Integrating Agricultural and Environmental Policies in the European Union." Technical Paper 269, World Bank, Washington, DC.

Scoggins, A., T. Kjellstrom, G. Fisher, J. Connor, and N. Gimson. 2004. "Spatial Analysis of Annual Air Pollution and Mortality." *Science of the Total Environment* 321: 71–85.

Shah, J., T. Nagpal, and C. Brandon, eds. 1997. *Urban Air Quality Management Strategy in Asia: Guidebook.* Washington, DC: World Bank.

Smith, K. R., C. Corvalan, and T. Kjellstrom. 1999. "How Much Global Ill Health Is Attributable to Environmental Factors?" *Epidemiology* 10: 573–84.

Smith, R. S. 2003. "Naturally Occurring Hazards." Article prepared for World Water Day, March 22, World Health Organization, Geneva. http://www.worldwaterday.org/2001/thematic/natural.html.

Tengs, T. O., M. E. Adams, J. S. Pliskin, D. G. Safran, J. E. Siegel, M. C. Weinstein, and J. D. Graham. 1995. "Five-Hundred Life-Saving Interventions and Their Cost-Effectiveness." *Risk Analysis* 15: 369–90.

U.K. Ministry of Health. 1954. *Mortality and Morbidity during the London Fog in December 1952.* London: U.K. Ministry of Health.

UNEP (United Nations Environment Programme). 2002. "Cleaner Production. Seventh International High-Level Seminar, Prague." *Industry and Environment* 25 (3–4): 1–109.

UNESCO (United Nations Educational, Scientific and Cultural Organization). 2003. *Water for People, Water for Life.* Paris: UNESCO.

United Nations. 1997. *Success Stories from India: Minimizing Waste by DESIRE.* Report for the special session of the General Assembly, Earth Summit+5, New York, June 23–27. http://www.un.org/esa/earthsummit/unido3.htm.

U.S. Congress. Senate. Governmental Affairs Committee. 1999. *Testimony of Professor Lisa Heinzerling Concerning the Nomination of John D. Graham to Be Administrator of the Office of Budget and Regulatory Affairs, Office of Management and Budget.* http://www.citizen.org/congress/regulations/graham/heinzerling_testimony.html.

U.S. Environmental Protection Agency. 1999. *The Benefits and Costs of the Clean Air Act 1990 to 2010.* Report to Congress. Washington, DC: U.S. Environmental Protection Agency. http://www.epa.gov/oar/sect812/.

———. 2000. *Superfund: 20 Years of Protecting Human Health and the Environment.* EPA 540-R-00-007. Washington, DC: U.S. Environmental Protection Agency. http://www.epa.gov/superfund.

Voorhees, A. S., S. Araki, R. Sakai, and H. Sato. 2000. "An Ex Post Cost-Benefit Analysis of the Nitrogen Dioxide Air Pollution Control Program in Tokyo." *Journal of the Air and Waste Management Association* 50: 391–410.

Voorhees, A. S., R. Sakai, S. Araki, H. Sato, and A. Otsu. 2001. "Cost-Benefit Analysis Methods for Assessing Air Pollution Control Programs in Urban Environments: A Review." *Environmental Health and Preventive Medicine* 6: 63–73.

Vorosmarty, C. J., P. Green, J. Salisbury, and R. B. Lammers. 2000. "Global Water Resources: Vulnerability from Climate Change and Population Growth." *Science* 289: 283–88.

Wang, X., H. Ding, L. Ryan, and X. Xu. 1997. "Association between Air Pollution and Low Birth Weight: A Community-Based Study." *Environmental Health Perspectives* 105: 514–20.

WHO (World Health Organization). 1976. *Mercury.* Environmental Health Criteria 1. Geneva: WHO.

———. 1990. *Public Health Impact of Pesticides Used in Agriculture.* Geneva: WHO.

———. 1995. *Lead, Inorganic.* Environmental Health Criteria 165. Geneva: WHO.

———. 1996. *Health Consequences of the Chernobyl Accident: Scientific Report.* Geneva: WHO.

———. 1997. *Health and Environment in Sustainable Development.* Document WHO/EHG/97.8. Geneva: WHO.

———. 1999. *Public Health and Chemical Incidents: Guidance for National and Regional Policy Makers.* Cardiff, U.K.: University of Wales Institute, WHO Collaborating Centre for Chemical Incidents. http://www.who.int/ipcs/publications/en/Public_Health_Management.pdf.

———. 2000. *Air Quality Guidelines for Europe.* 2nd ed. Copenhagen: WHO.

———. 2001. *Arsenic and Arsenic Compounds.* Environmental Health Criteria 224. Geneva: WHO.

———. 2002. *World Health Report 2002.* Geneva: WHO.

———. 2003. *Guidelines for Drinking Water Quality.* 3rd ed. Geneva: WHO. http://www.who.int/water_sanitation_health/dwq/guidelines3rd/en/.

WHO and International Programme on Chemical Safety. 2002. *Global Assessment of the State of Science of Endocrine Disruptors.* Document WHO/PCS/EDC/02.2. Geneva: WHO and the International Programme on Chemical Safety.

World Bank. 1999. *Pollution Prevention and Abatement Handbook 1998.* Washington, DC: World Bank. http://wbln0018.worldbank.org/essd/essd.nsf/GlobalView/PPAH.

———. 2004. *Air Pollution Calculation Toolkit.* Washington, DC: World Bank. http://lnweb18.worldbank.org/essd/essdext.nsf/46ByDocName/ToolkitsGlobalOverlay.

Xu, X., and L. Wang. 1993. "Association of Indoor and Outdoor Particulate Level with Chronic Respiratory Disease." *American Review of Respiratory Diseases* 148: 1516–22.

Yassi, A-L., T. Kjellstrom, T. deKok, and T. Guidotti. 2001. *Basic Environmental Health.* New York: Oxford University Press.

Zhang, C., M. Huq, S. Dasgupta, and D. Wheeler. 1996. "Water Pollution Abatement by Chinese Industry: Cost Estimates and Policy Implications." Working Paper 1630, World Bank, Washington, DC.

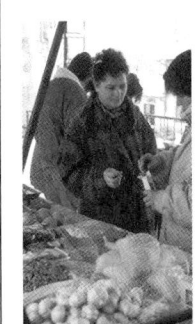

Chapter **44**

Prevention of Chronic Disease by Means of Diet and Lifestyle Changes

Walter C. Willett, Jeffrey P. Koplan, Rachel Nugent, Courtenay Dusenbury, Pekka Puska, and Thomas A. Gaziano

Coronary artery disease (CAD), ischemic stroke, diabetes, and some specific cancers, which until recently were common only in high-income countries, are now becoming the dominant sources of morbidity and mortality worldwide (WHO 2002). In addition, rates of cancers and cardiovascular disease (CVD) among migrants from low-risk to high-risk countries almost always increase dramatically. In traditional African societies, for example, CAD is virtually nonexistent, but rates among African Americans are similar to those among Caucasian Americans. These striking changes in rates within countries over time and among migrating populations indicate that the primary determinants of these diseases are not genetic but environmental factors, including diet and lifestyle. Thus, considerable research has been aimed at identifying modifiable determinants of chronic diseases.

Prospective epidemiological studies, some randomized prevention trials, and many short-term studies of intermediate endpoints such as blood pressure and lipids have revealed a good deal about the specific dietary and lifestyle determinants of major chronic diseases. Most of these studies have been conducted in Western countries, in part because of the historical importance of these diseases in the West, but also because they have the most developed research infrastructure. A general conclusion is that reducing identified, modifiable dietary and lifestyle risk factors could prevent most cases of CAD, stroke, diabetes, and many cancers among high-income populations (Willett 2002). These findings are profoundly important, because they indicate that these diseases are not inevitable consequences of a modern society. Furthermore, low rates of these diseases can be attained without drugs or expensive medical

facilities, an outcome that is not surprising, because their rates have historically been extremely low in developing countries with few medical facilities. However, preventing these diseases will require changes in behaviors related to smoking, physical activity, and diet; investments in education, food policies, and urban physical infrastructure are needed to support and encourage these changes (see box 44.1).

CHRONIC DISEASE PREVENTION

In this section, we briefly review dietary and lifestyle changes that reduce the incidence of chronic disease. The potential magnitude of benefit is also discussed.

Recommended Lifestyle Changes

Specific changes in diet and lifestyle and likely benefits are summarized in table 44.1. These relationships and supporting evidence are summarized here.

Avoid Tobacco Use. Avoidance of smoking by preventing initiation or by cessation for those who already smoke is the single most important way to prevent CVD and cancer (chapter 46). Avoiding the use of smokeless tobacco will also prevent a good deal of oral cancer.

Maintain a Healthy Weight. Obesity is increasing rapidly worldwide (chapter 45). Even though obesity—a body mass index (BMI) of 30 or greater—has received more attention

Table 44.1 Convincing and Probable Relationships between Dietary and Lifestyle Factors and Chronic Diseases

Dietary and lifestyle factors	CVD	Type 2 diabetes	Cancer	Dental disease	Fracture	Cataract	Birth defects	Obesity	Metabolic syndrome	Depression	Sexual dysfunction
Avoid smoking	↓	↓	↓	↓	↓	↓		↑			↓
Pursue physical activity	↓	↓	↓		↓			↓	↓	↓	↓
Avoid overweight	↓	↓	↓		↑	↓			↓		↓
Diet											
Consume healthy types of fats[a]	**↓**	**↓**							↓		
Eat plenty of fruits and vegetables	**↓**		↓		↓	↓	↓	↓			
Replace refined grains with whole grains	↓	↓						↓	↓		
Limit sugar intake[b]	↓	↓		↓				↓	↓		
Limit excessive calories								↓	↓		
Limit sodium intake	↓										

Source: Authors' summary of a review by the WHO and FAO 2003; Bacon and others 2003; Fox 1999; IARC 2002.
Note: **Bold** = convincing; Standard = probable relation; ↑ = increase in risk; ↓ = decrease in risk.
a. Replace trans and saturated fats with mono- and polyunsaturated fats, including a regular source of N-3 fatty acids.
b. Includes limiting sugar-based beverages.

than overweight, overweight (BMI of 25 to 30) is typically even more prevalent and also confers elevated risks of many diseases. For example, overweight people experience a two- to threefold elevation in the risks of CAD and hypertension and a more than tenfold increase in the risk of type 2 diabetes compared with lean individuals (BMI less than 23) (Willett, Dietz, and Colditz 1999). Both overweight and obese people also experience elevated mortality from cancers of the colon, breast (postmenopausal), kidney, endometrium, and other sites (Calle and others 2003).

Many people with a BMI of less than 25 have gained substantial weight since they were young adults and are also at increased risk of these diseases, even though they are not technically overweight (Willett, Dietz, and Colditz 1999). For example, in rural China, where the average BMI was less than 21 for both men and women, F. B. Hu and others (2000) found that the prevalence of hypertension was nearly five times greater for those with a BMI of approximately 25 than for the leanest people. Because many Asians are experiencing adverse consequences of excess body fat with a BMI of less than 25, the definition of overweight for Asia has recently been expanded to include a BMI of 23 to 25 (WHO 2000). For most people, unless obviously malnourished as an adolescent or young adult, bodyweight should ideally not increase by more than 2 or 3 kilograms after age 20 to maintain optimal health (Willett, Dietz, and Colditz 1999). Thus, a desirable weight for most people should be within the BMI range of 18.5 to 25.0, and preferably less than 23.

Additional valuable information can be obtained by measuring waist circumference, which reflects abdominal fat accumulation. In many studies, waist circumference is a strong predictor of CAD, stroke, and type 2 diabetes, even after controlling for BMI (Willett, Dietz, and Colditz 1999). A waist circumference of approximately 100 centimeters for men and 88 centimeters for women has been used as the criterion for the upper limit of the healthy range in the United States, but for many people this extent of abdominal fat would be far above optimal. Because abdominal circumference is easily assessed, even where scales may not be available, further work to develop locally appropriate criteria could be worthwhile. In the meantime, increases of more than 5 centimeters can be used as a basis for recommending changes in activity patterns and diet.

Views about the causes of obesity and ways to prevent or reduce it have been controversial. Diets low in fat and high in carbohydrates were believed to limit caloric intake spontaneously and thus to control adiposity, but such diets have not reduced bodyweight in trials that have lasted for a year or more (Willett and Leibel 2002). Some researchers have suggested that diets with a high energy density, referring to the amount of energy per volume, offer an alternative explanation for the observed increases in obesity (Swinburn and others 2004), but long-term studies have not examined this theory. Sugar-sweetened beverages contribute significantly to the overconsumption of calories, in part because calories in fluid form appear to be poorly regulated by the body (E. A. Bell, Roe, and Rolls 2003). In children, an increase in soda consumption of one serving per day was associated with an odds ratio of 1.6 for incidence of obesity (Ludwig, Peterson, and Gortmaker 2001), and in a randomized trial, replacement of a standard soda with a zero-calorie diet soda was associated with significant weight loss (Raben and others 2002). Reductions in dietary fiber and increases in the dietary glycemic load (large amounts of rapidly absorbed carbohydrates from refined starches and sugar) may also contribute to obesity (Ebbeling and others 2003; Swinburn and others 2004).

Aspects of the food supply unrelated to its macronutrient composition are also likely to be contributing to the global rise in obesity. Inexpensive food energy from refined grains, sugar, and vegetable oils has become extremely plentiful in most countries. Food manufacturers and suppliers use carefully researched methods to make products based on these cheap ingredients maximally convenient and attractive.

Maintain Daily Physical Activity and Limit Television Watching. Contemporary life in developed nations has markedly reduced people's opportunities to expend energy, whether in moving from place to place, in the work environment, or at home (Koplan and Dietz 1999). Dramatic reductions in physical activity are also occurring in developing countries because of urbanization, increased availability of motorized transportation to replace walking and bicycle riding, and mechanization of labor. However, regular physical activity is a key element in weight control and prevention of obesity (IARC 2002; Swinburn and others 2004). For example, among middle-aged West African women, more walking was associated with a three-unit lower BMI (Sobngwi, Gautier, and Mbanya 2003), and in China, car owners are 80 percent more likely to be obese (Hu 2002).

In addition to its key role in maintaining a healthy weight, regular physical activity reduces the risk of CAD, stroke, type 2 diabetes, colon and breast cancer, osteoporotic fractures, osteoarthritis, depression, and erectile dysfunction (table 44.1). Important health benefits have even been associated with walking for half an hour per day, but greater reductions in risk are seen with longer durations of physical activity and more intense activity.

The number of hours of television watched per day is associated with increased obesity rates among both children and adults (Hernandez and others 1999; Ruangdaraganon and others 2002) and with a higher risk of type 2 diabetes and gallstones (F. B. Hu and others 2001; Leitzmann and others 1999). This association is likely attributable both to reduced physical activity and to increased consumption of foods and beverages high in calories, which are typically those promoted on television. Decreases in television watching reduce weight (Robinson 1999), and the American Academy of Pediatrics recommends a maximum of two hours of television watching per day.

Eat a Healthy Diet. Medical experts have long recognized the effects of diet on the risk of CVD, but the relationship between diet and many other conditions, including specific cancers, diabetes, cataracts, macular degeneration, cholelithiasis, renal stones, dental disease, and birth defects, have been documented more recently. The following list discusses six aspects of diet for which strong evidence indicates important health implications (table 44.1). These goals are consistent with a detailed

2003 World Health Organization (WHO) report (WHO and FAO 2003).

- *Replace saturated and trans fats with unsaturated fats, including sources of omega-3 fatty acids.* Replacing saturated fats with unsaturated fats will reduce the risk of CAD (F. B. Hu and Willett 2002; Institute of Medicine 2002; WHO and FAO 2003) by reducing serum low-density lipoprotein (LDL) cholesterol. Also, polyunsaturated fats (including the long-chain omega-3 fish oils and probably alpha-linoleic acid, the primary plant omega-3 fatty acid) can prevent ventricular arrhythmias and thereby reduce fatal CAD. In a case-control study in Costa Rica, where fish intake was extremely low, the risk of myocardial infarction was 80 percent lower in those with the highest alpha-linoleic acid intake (Baylin and others 2003). Intakes of omega-3 fatty acids are suboptimal in many populations, particularly if fish intake is low and the primary oils consumed are low in omega-3 fatty acids (for example, partially hydrogenated soybean, corn, sunflower, or palm oil). These findings have major implications, because changes in the type of oil used for food preparation are often quite feasible and not expensive.

  Trans fatty acids produced by the partial hydrogenation of vegetable oils have uniquely adverse effects on blood lipids (F. B. Hu and Willett 2002; Institute of Medicine 2002) and increase risks of CAD (F. B. Hu and Willett 2002); on a gram-for-gram basis, both the effects on blood lipids and the relationship with CAD risk are considerably more adverse than for saturated fat. In many developing countries, trans fat consumption is high because partially hydrogenated soybean oil is among the cheapest fats available. In South Asia, vegetable ghee, which has largely replaced traditional ghee, contains approximately 50 percent trans fatty acids (Ascherio and others 1996). Independent of other risk factors, higher intakes of trans fat and lower intakes of polyunsaturated fat increase risk of type 2 diabetes (F. B. Hu, van Dam, and Liu 2001).

- *Ensure generous consumption of fruits and vegetables and adequate folic acid intake.* Strong evidence indicates that high intakes of fruits and vegetables will reduce the risk of CAD and stroke (Conlin 1999). Some of this benefit is mediated by higher intakes of potassium, but folic acid probably also plays a role (F. B. Hu and Willett 2002). Supplementation with folic acid reduces the risk of neural tube defect pregnancies. Substantial evidence also suggests that low folic acid intake is associated with greater risk of colon—and possibly breast—cancer and that use of multiple vitamins containing folic acid reduces the risk of these cancers (Giovannucci 2002). Findings relating folic acid intake to CVD and some cancers have major implications for many parts of the developing world. In many areas, consumption of fruits and vegetables is low. For example, in northern China, approximately half the adult population is deficient in folic acid (Hao and others 2003).

- *Consume cereal products in their whole-grain, high-fiber form.* Consuming grains in a whole-grain, high-fiber form has double benefits. First, consumption of fiber from cereal products has consistently been associated with lower risks of CAD and type 2 diabetes (F. B. Hu, van Dam, and Liu 2001; F. B. Hu and Willett 2002), which may be because of both the fiber itself and the vitamins and minerals naturally present in whole grains. High consumption of refined starches exacerbates the metabolic syndrome and is associated with higher risks of CAD (F. B. Hu and Willett 2002) and type 2 diabetes (F. B. Hu, van Dam, and Liu 2001). Second, higher consumption of dietary fiber also appears to facilitate weight control (Swinburn and others 2004) and helps prevent constipation.

- *Limit consumption of sugar and sugar-based beverages.* Sugar (free sugars refined from sugarcane or sugar beets and high-fructose corn sweeteners) has no nutritional value except for calories and, thus, has negative health implications for those at risk of overweight. Furthermore, sugar contributes to the dietary glycemic load, which exacerbates the metabolic syndrome and is related to the risk of diabetes and CAD (F. B. Hu, van Dam, and Liu 2001; F. B. Hu and Willett 2002; Schulze and others 2004). WHO has suggested an upper limit of 10 percent of energy from sugar, but lower intakes are usually desirable because of the adverse metabolic effects and empty calories.

- *Limit excessive caloric intake from any source.* Given the importance of obesity and overweight in the causation of many chronic diseases, avoiding excessive consumption of energy from any source is fundamentally important. Because calories consumed as beverages are less well-regulated than calories from solid food, limiting the consumption of sugar-sweetened beverages is particularly important.

- *Limit sodium intake.* The principle justification for limiting sodium is its effect on blood pressure, a major risk factor for stroke and coronary disease (chapter 33). WHO has suggested an upper limit of 1.7 grams of sodium per day (5 grams of salt per day) (WHO and FAO 2003).

Potential of Dietary and Lifestyle Factors to Prevent Chronic Diseases

Several lines of evidence indicate that realistic modifications of diet and lifestyle can prevent most CAD, stroke, diabetes, colon cancer, and smoking-related cancers. Less progress has been made in identifying practically modifiable causes of breast and prostate cancers.

Success in Finland

Finland provides one of the best-documented examples of a community intervention. In 1972, Finland had the world's highest CVD mortality rate. Planners examined the policy and environmental factors contributing to CVD and sought appropriate changes, such as increased availability of low-fat dairy products, antismoking legislation, and improved school meals. They used the media; schools; worksites; and spokespersons from sports, education, and agriculture to educate residents. After five years, signifi-

cant improvements were documented in smoking, cholesterol, and blood pressure. By 1992, CVD mortality rates for men age 35 to 64 had dropped by 57 percent. The program was so successful that it was expanded to include other lifestyle-related diseases. Twenty years later, major reductions in CVD risk-factor levels, morbidity, and mortality were attributed to the project. Recent data show a 75 percent decrease in CVD mortality (Puska and others 1998).

One line of evidence is based on declines in CAD in countries that have implemented preventive programs. Rates of CAD mortality have been cut in half in several high-income countries, including Australia, the United Kingdom, and the United States. The most dramatic example is that of Finland (box 44.2).

Other evidence derives from randomized intervention studies. These often have serious limitations for estimating the potential magnitude of benefits, because typically only one or a few factors are modified, durations are usually only a few years, and noncompliance with lifestyle change is often substantial. Nevertheless, some examples are illustrative of the potential benefit. In two randomized studies among adults at high risk of type 2 diabetes, those assigned to a program emphasizing dietary changes, weight loss, and physical activity experienced only half the risk of incident diabetes (Knowler and others 2002; Tuomilehto and others 2001). The Lyon Heart Study, conducted among those with existing heart disease, found a Mediterranean-type diet high in omega-3 fatty acids reduced recurrent infarction by 70 percent compared with an American Heart Association diet (de Lorgeril and others 1994).

A third approach is to estimate the percentage of disease that is potentially preventable by reducing multiple behavioral risk factors using prospective cohort studies. Among U.S. adults, more than 90 percent of type 2 diabetes, 80 percent of CAD, 70 percent of stroke, and 70 percent of colon cancer are potentially preventable by a combination of nonsmoking, avoidance of overweight, moderate physical activity, healthy diet, and moderate alcohol consumption (Willett 2002).

Collectively, these findings indicate that the low rates of these diseases suggested by international comparisons and time trends are attainable by realistic, moderate changes that are compatible with 21st-century lifestyles.

INTERVENTIONS

Interventions aimed at changing diet and lifestyle factors include educating individuals, changing the environment, modifying the food supply, undertaking community interventions, and implementing economic policies. In most cases, quantifying the effects of the intervention is difficult, because behavioral changes may take many years and synergies are potentially important but hard to estimate in formal studies. Substantial nihilism often exists regarding the ability to change populations' diets or behaviors, but major changes are possible over extended periods of time. For example, per capita egg consumption in the United States decreased from approximately 420 to 270 per year between 1940 and 1990 following recommendations for preventing CAD (though in reality, the evidence for benefits was meager). Similarly, the prevalence of smoking, despite its being a physically addictive behavior, halved among men in the United States between 1965 and 2000. Because changing behaviors related to diet and lifestyle require sustained efforts, long-term persistence is needed. However, opportunities exist that do not require individual behavior changes, and these can lead to more rapid benefits.

Educational Interventions

Efforts to change diets, physical activity patterns, and other aspects of lifestyle have traditionally attempted to educate individuals through schools, health care providers, worksites, and general media. These efforts will continue to play an important role, but they can be strongly reinforced by policy and environmental changes.

School-Based Programs. School-based programs include the roles of nutrition and physical activity in maintaining physical

The Planet Health Program

Planet Health, developed for middle school students, in the United States, has an immediate goal of reducing television viewing time with the long-range goal of preventing unhealthy weight gain (Gortmaker and others 1999). Teachers incorporate messages about reducing television watching, nutrition, and increasing fitness into mathematics, social studies, science, and language arts lessons. Fitness units and periodic "FitChecks" during physical education complement the classroom lessons. Teacher training, student self-assessment using graphs, and student reflection about enjoyable activities that could replace at least a portion of the time they spend watching television are key elements. This program has reduced television watching and weight in girls (Gortmaker and others 1999). Because the program is integrated into existing classes, its cost is minimal.

Live for Life®

Johnson & Johnson introduced Live for Life in 1979 with the goal of making its employees the healthiest in the world (Bly, Jones, and Richardson 1986). In 1993, the company integrated its health and wellness program with its disability management, employee assistance, and occupational medicine programs. Instead of using physicians and nurses to treat symptoms, the combined program sought to use a variety of health professionals to change individual behavior and improve health status. Employees were offered US$500 in benefit credits for participation. The program included routine health risk assessment, health promotion after recovery from a medical event, and support when returning to work after a major illness. Even though the intervention program had little effect on body-weight, physical fitness did increase. By the end of the third year, savings to the company were more than US$400 per year per employee.

and mental health (box 44.3). School food services should provide healthy meals, both because they directly affect health and because they provide a special opportunity to teach by example. In many countries, school-based physical education remains a significant source of physical activity for young people. In China, 72 percent of children age 6 to 18 engage in moderate to vigorous physical activity for a median of 90 to 100 minutes per week (Tudor-Locke and others 2003). Maintaining these programs should be a high priority because they have likely contributed to the historically low rates of obesity in such countries.

Worksite Interventions. Worksite interventions can efficiently include a wide variety of health promotion activities because workers spend a large portion of their waking hours and eat a large percentage of their food there. Interventions can include educating employees; screening them for behavioral risk factors; offering incentive programs to walk, ride a bicycle, or take public transportation to work; offering exercise programs during breaks or after work; improving the physical environment to promote activity; and providing healthier foods in cafeterias (box 44.4). Worksite health promotion can result in a positive return on investment through lower health costs and fewer sick days.

Interventions by Health Care Providers. Controlled intervention trials for smoking cessation and physical activity have shown that physician counseling, especially when accompanied by supporting written material, can be efficacious in modifying behavior. Studies of dietary counseling by physicians indicate that even brief messages about nutrition can influence behavior and that the magnitude of the effect is related to the intensity of the intervention (Pignone and others 2003). Identifying patients who are overweight or obese, or who are gaining weight but are not yet overweight, is an initial step in preventing and treating overweight. However, many physicians are not well trained to measure and calculate BMI and identify weight problems.

Reducing Automobile Use in Brazil

Curitiba, Brazil, provides an example of the benefits of a strategy that reduces automobile use and increases use of public transportation. In 1965, city planners adopted a master plan that promoted development along designated corridors along with a bus system so efficient that it has virtually eliminated the need for automobiles. Minibuses are used to quickly and efficiently transport individuals from residential neighborhoods to express bus lines. These bus lines run almost every 90 seconds and can carry up to 270 passengers each. Compared with other Brazilian cities of its size, Curitiba uses 30 percent less gasoline per capita, and its air pollution is among the lowest in the nation.

Transportation Policy and Environmental Design

Transportation policies and the design of urban environments are fundamental determinants of physical activity and therefore influence the risks of obesity and other chronic diseases. Countries can take a number of steps to make positive changes.

Limit the Role of Automobiles. In wealthy countries, the automobile has strongly influenced the trend toward low-density, automobile-based suburban developments, many built without sidewalks. These sprawling settlements tend to have few services within walking distance and are usually not linked to public transporationt. Dependence on automobiles affects physical activity, because those who use public transportation tend to walk more. In a prospective study in eight provinces in China, 14 percent of households acquired a car between 1889 and 1997, and the likelihood of men becoming obese during the same period was twice as great in households that acquired a car than in those that did not (A. C. Bell, Ge, and Popkin 2002).

National policies strongly influence automobile use and dependency. In the United States, low taxes on gasoline, free parking, and wide streets encourage car ownership: almost 92 percent of U.S. households own at least one car, and 59 percent own two or more cars (Pucher and Dijkstra 2003). In contrast, in most of Western Europe, narrow streets, limited parking, and high gasoline prices make the costs of automobile use almost double those in the United States (Pucher and Dijkstra 2003). As a result, Europeans walk or bike more and use their cars approximately 50 percent less than their American counterparts. Investment in roads rather than in public transportation creates a vicious cycle: poor public transportation systems lead to more dependency on the automobile.

As car use grows, injuries and deaths associated with automobile accidents also grow. In China, the number of four-wheeled vehicles increased from about 60,000 to more than 50 million between 1951 and 1999, and traffic fatalities increased from about 6,000 to more than 413,000 (S. Y. Wang and others 2003). Many innovative strategies have been developed to discourage private automobile use and to promote public transportation, walking, and bicycling (see box 44.5). Singapore has long been in the lead in relation to such efforts: a combination of limiting the number of licenses issued, implementing a vehicle quota system, and introducing a road pricing system has limited personal car ownership and congestion throughout the country. Other nations and regions are now enacting similar road pricing systems or congestion taxes. For example, London's congestion charging system levies a fee of approximately US$8 per day for cars entering central London. Since its inception in 2003, the charge has reduced congestion in the city and is expected to channel funds back into the city's transportation facilities.

Unfortunately some countries, particularly China, have taken a different approach to their future transportation needs. Government initiatives that encourage families to buy automobiles include lowering taxes, simplifying registration procedures, and allowing foreign financing. In Beijing alone, residents purchased 400,000 cars in 2003.

Promote Walking and Bicycle Riding. Walking or cycling for transportation and leisure are effective and practical means of engaging in physical activity and are still the most common ways to travel in many developing countries. In Bangkok and Manila, only 25 percent of travel is by car, motorcycle, or taxi, compared with 75 percent by public transportation or walking (Pendakur 2000). In Madras, India, only 8 percent of the population travels by private, motorized transportation; 22 percent of people walk; 20 percent bike; and the rest use public transportation (Pendakur 2000). In China, approximately 90 percent of the urban population walks or rides a bicycle to work, shopping, or school each day (G. Hu and others 2002). Walking or biking is more likely to be prevalent in smaller cities—that is, those with 1 million to 5 million people—than in larger ones.

Bicycle riding and walking are also important for children's health. Most American children do not walk or bike to school, even when distances are short (box 44.6). In contrast, almost

90 percent of Chinese children under 12 walk or ride a bicycle to school (Hu 2002).

In many areas, the shift toward private car use has not yet begun and can perhaps be forestalled by policies that benefit walkers and cyclists rather than drivers. Such policies include implementing road designs that promote a safe and well-lit environment for walking and cycling, including traffic-calming measures to reduce automobile speeds.

Many Western European countries have taken steps to increase safety for cyclists and walkers. In Germany and the Netherlands, bike paths serve as travel routes, not just weekend recreational destinations as they do in the United States. The former countries have invested heavily in bike paths and have also created extensive car-free areas in cities, with well-lit sidewalks, clearly marked crosswalks, and pedestrian islands that have improved safety. Both countries have increased the number of bicycle-friendly streets (on which cars are permitted but bicycles have the right of way) and have created systems to separate streams of traffic, including cars, pedestrians, and bicycles. A meta-analysis of selected traffic-calming studies in many countries reported reductions in traffic speed, accidents, injuries, and fatalities and an increase in bicycle use and walking (Bunn and others 2003).

Design Cities and Towns to Promote Health. Handy and others' (2002) comprehensive assessment of recent research on urban planning concludes that a combination of urban design, land-use patterns, and transportation systems that promotes walking and bicycling will help create active, healthier, and more livable communities. In densely developed cities that have been built around public transportation rather than away from it, individuals are much more likely to take public transit, walk, or bicycle than in other areas and to weigh less and be less likely to suffer from hypertension (Ewing, Schieber, and Zegeer 2003; Lopez 2004; Saelens, Sallis, and Frank 2003).

Those living in walker-friendly neighborhoods also appear to be more mentally healthy and are more likely to know their neighbors, to be socially active, and to participate in the political process (Leyden 2003). In contrast, urban sprawl has been linked to decreases in mental health and social capital (Frumkin 2002) as well as anger and frustration over long commutes (Surface Transportation Policy Project 1999). Sprawl adversely affects the elderly in particular because they are unable to walk to places of interest and many cannot drive. Such isolation does not promote good physical or mental health.

The so-called smart growth movement has resulted from concerns about urban sprawl and unsustainable development and is encouraging governments worldwide to rethink how they develop new areas and redevelop older suburbs and cities. Smart growth principles include mixing land uses, using compact building designs, including a range of transportation and housing choices, building walker-friendly neighborhoods in attractive communities with a distinctive sense of place, and implementing a philosophy of directing development toward existing communities and the preservation of open space (Office of the Administrator 2001) (box 44.7).

The involvement of public health practitioners in transportation planning and building design is becoming more common. In Edinburgh, a health impact assessment conducted on proposed options for transportation policy showed the effects of specific choices on both affluent members of the community and the poor. Its recommendations, now adopted, included new spending on pedestrian safety, a citywide bicycle network, more greenways and park-and-ride programs, and more rail transportation or bus services. Priorities are to benefit pedestrians first, cyclists second, public transportation users third, freight and delivery people fourth, and car users last. Establishing criteria for building design can also lead to increases in physical activity. For example, increasing signage promoting stair use, as well as the attractiveness of the facilities themselves, encourages people to use the stairs (Boutelle and others 2001) (box 44.8).

Improved Food Supply

People's diets can be enhanced by improving the food supply. The usual position of the food industry is that it simply

Enhancing Urban Life in the Republic of Korea

In Seoul, the government is managing growth by creating six satellite communities with high-rise residential buildings outside the city center. These communities are intended to become new job-creation centers and to shift the balance of employment away from one centralized location to provide a more regional balance. Major expressways are being removed to create parks, sidewalks, and bikeways (http://www.itdp.org/STe/ste6/#seoul).

Promoting Physical Activity in Brazil

One successful example of increasing activity is Agita São Paulo, a multilevel physical activity initiative designed for the 34 million citizens of Brazil's São Paulo state (Matsudo and others 2002). The program was launched in 1996 to increase the public's knowledge of the benefits of exercise and expand participation in physical fitness activities by encouraging people to do 30 minutes of moderate activity at least five times a week. As elsewhere, program designers perceived a lack of time as the major factor preventing daily exercise. They chose three settings as places to promote activity: home (gardening, chores, avoidance of television watching); transportation (walking, taking the stairs); and leisure time (dancing). Agitol, a prescription for exercise, was developed for physicians to dispense. Its message is displayed on electricity bills and stickers, and it is touted by radio stations and other media outlets.

After four years, 55.7 percent of those surveyed had heard about Agita, 37 percent knew its purpose, and those who knew of the program's purpose were more likely to be active. Agita appears to have played a role in increasing activity in the region (Matsudo and others 2002). It is closely linked to a national program to promote healthy diets and active lifestyles by nutritional content labeling, promotion of healthy diets in schools, communication of guidelines for healthy eating, and encouragement of innovative community-based initiatives (Coitinho, Monteiro, and Popkin 2002).

provides whatever consumers demand, but this argument is misleading, because the industry spends more than US$12 billion annually to influence consumer choices just within the United States and many times this amount globally. Much of this sum goes to promote foods with adverse health effects, and children are primary targets.

Improving Processing and Manufacturing. Altering the manufacturing process can rapidly and effectively improve diets because such action does not require the slow process of behavioral change. One example is eliminating the partial hydrogenation of vegetable oils, which destroys essential omega-3 fatty acids and creates trans fatty acids. European manufacturers have largely eliminated trans fatty acids from their food supply by altering production methods.

Regulations can facilitate changes in manufacturing directly or indirectly by providing an incentive for manufacturers to change their processes. For example, in 2003, the U.S. Food and Drug Administration announced that food manufacturers had to include trans fatty acid content on the standard food label. Following imposition of this requirement, several large food companies said that they would reduce or eliminate trans fats, and many more are planning to do so (U.S. Food and Drug Administration 2003). In Mauritius, the government required a change in the commonly used cooking oil from mostly palm oil to soybean oil, which changed people's fatty acid intake and reduced their serum cholesterol levels (Uusitalo and others 1996). Changes in types of fat can often be almost invisible and inexpensive. Omega-3 fatty acid intakes can be increased by incorporating oils from rapeseed, mustard, or soybean into manufactured foods, cooking oils sold for use at home, or both. Selective breeding and genetic engineering provide alternative ways to improve the healthfulness of oils by modifying their fatty acid composition.

When the consumption of processed food is high, a reduction in salt consumption will usually require changes at the manufacturing level, because processed food is a major salt source. If the salt content of foods is reduced gradually, the change is imperceptible to consumers. Coordination among manufacturers or government regulation is needed; otherwise producers whose foods are lower in salt may be placed at a disadvantage. Unfortunately, good examples are not available. Another example of improved processing would be to reduce the refining of grain products, which can be done in small, almost invisible decrements.

Fortifying Food. Food fortification has eliminated iodine deficiency, pellagra, and beriberi in much of the world. In regions where iodine deficiency remains a serious problem, fortification should be a high priority. Folic acid intake is suboptimal in many regions of both developing and developed countries. Fortifying foods with folic acid is extremely inexpensive and could substantially reduce the rates of several chronic diseases. Grain products—such as flour, rice, and pasta—are usually the best foods to fortify, and in many countries, they are already being fortified with other B vitamins. Since 1998, grain products in the United States have been fortified with folic acid, which has almost eliminated folate deficiency, and rates of neural tube defect pregnancies have declined by about 19 percent (Honein and others 2001). Where intakes of vitamins B12 and B6 are also low and contribute to elevations of homocysteine, as among vegetarian populations in India, simultaneous fortification of food with these vitamins should be considered. The effects of fortification on reducing CVD are not considered proven, but the potential benefits are huge; therefore, intervention trials to evaluate the effects of fortification should be a high priority.

Increasing the Availability and Reducing the Cost of Healthy Foods. Policies regarding the production, importation, distribution, and sale of specific foods can influence their cost and availability. Policies may be directed at the focus of agricultural research and the types of production promoted by extension services. Policies often promote grains, dairy products, sugar, and beef, whereas those that encourage the production and consumption of fruits, vegetables, nuts, legumes, whole grains, and healthy oils would tend to enhance rather than reduce health.

Promoting Healthy Food Choices and Limiting Aggressive Marketing to Children. Almost every national effort to improve nutrition incorporates the promotion of healthy food choices, such as fruits, vegetables, and legumes. Ideally, such efforts are coordinated among government groups, retailers, professional groups, and nonprofit organizations, and investment in such efforts should include the careful testing and refining of social-marketing strategies.

Another strategy is to protect consumers from aggressive marketing of unhealthy foods. Producers spend billions of dollars a year encouraging children to consume foods that are detrimental to their health. Manufacturers and fast-food chains personify food products with cartoon characters; display food brands on toys; and issue "educational" card games that subvert children's natural gift for play, story telling, and make believe. The willingness to limit advertising depends on a country's political culture, but the public clearly distinguishes between advertising aimed at adults and that targeted at children. For example, in the United States, 46 percent of adults surveyed supported restrictions on advertising to children (Blendon 2002). Restrictions can range from banning advertising to children to limiting the types of products that advertisers may promote to this audience.

Initiatives at the Community Level

Nations and regions can promote a variety of initiatives to encourage greater physical activity and better nutrition. These initiatives are likely to be most effective when they are multifaceted and coordinated and when they are developed with the active involvement of individuals and organizations within communities (Puska and others 1998).

Many countries are undertaking efforts to educate their populations about healthy lifestyles. In the Islamic Republic of Iran, the Isfahan Healthy Heart Program, a WHO collaborating center for research and training for CVD control, prevention, and rehabilitation for cardiac patients, has developed a comprehensive, integrated community intervention that involves schools, worksites, health care facilities, food services, urban planners, and the media. Physical activity is promoted by creating safe routes for walking and bicycle riding and by organizing recreational walking that involves entire families (http://ihhp.mui.ac.ir).

South Africa's Community Health Intervention Programme, a partnership between an insurance company and an academic institution, has created programs targeted to specific age groups, including children and older adults. The program's twice-weekly classes have reduced blood pressure and increased strength and balance (Lambert, Bohlmann, and Kolbe-Alexander 2001) (box 44.9).

Singapore's Fit and Trim Program uses a multidisciplinary approach to increase physical activity and healthy diets among schoolchildren. Between 1992 and 2000, the rate of obesity declined by 13.1 to 16.6 percent for children age 11 to 12 and 15 to 16 (Toh, Cutter, and Chew 2002) (box 44.10 outlines the national program for adults).

Economic Policies

Economic policies can have important effects on behavior and choices, and these policies have been particularly useful in

Box 44.9

A Comprehensive Intervention Approach in South Africa

The Coronary Risk Factor Study in South Africa (Rossouw and others 1993) tested community interventions at different levels of intensity in two communities with a third control community. The target population was Caucasian South Africans. Interventions included direct media campaigns, public health messages delivered in a variety of ways, and home mailings. Also included were community activities, such as fun walks, public meetings, involvement of community-based organizations, free screening for blood pressure, small-group personal interventions, and encouragement of food substitution in stores and restaurants. The results showed an improvement in the community risk factor profile for CAD in the intervention communities, especially in relation to blood pressure, smoking, and overall risk. The results indicate no additional benefit of the personal intervention for high-risk individuals beyond that already offered by the mass media program. Estimated per capita costs of the heavy intervention program were roughly four times as much as for the mild intervention program (US$22 per capita compared with US$5 per capita), and the low-intervention community received almost the same level of benefits as the high-intervention community.

Box 44.10

The Singapore National Healthy Lifestyle Program

Because CVD and cancer had become the major causes of death in Singapore, the government adopted the National Healthy Lifestyle Program in 1992 (Cutter, Tan, and Chew 2001). This coordinated, multisectoral approach involved government ministries, health professionals, employers, unions, and community organizations. The program aimed at improving the social and physical environment so as to promote healthy living. Healthy diets, regular physical exercise, and nonsmoking were emphasized. The program used the mass media; legislative measures to discourage smoking; and widespread school, workplace, and community health promotion packages.

In a follow-up survey after six years, cigarette smoking had decreased from 34 to 27 percent among men, the proportion of adults who exercised regularly had increased from 14 to 17 percent, and the prevalence of obesity was stable. However, hypertension and high LDL cholesterol levels had increased modestly. From 1991 to 1999, the age-standardized incidence of myocardial infarction declined from 98.2 to 83.0 per 100,000 residents (Mak and others 2003) and age-standardized mortality from CAD decreased from 60.8 to 47.2 per 100,000 residents.

reducing the prevalence of smoking (see chapter 46). Policies that could influence diet and physical activity deserve careful consideration because they are rarely neutral and often support unhealthy behaviors. Consider the following examples:

- Subsidies can favor the consumption of less healthy foods, such as sugar, refined grains, beef, and high-fat dairy products as opposed to fruits, vegetables, whole grains, nuts, legumes, and fish. Poland provides a striking example of how changes in subsidies can affect health (box 44.11). Governments often subsidize foods indirectly by sheltering them from sales taxes in the recognition that they are essential; however, this logic should not extend to foods with adverse health effects, such as sugar-sweetened beverages and those high in trans fats. Legislation can make this distinction, providing a modest economic incentive for healthier choices and at the same time conveying important nutritional messages (see chapter 11).

- Use of individual automobiles is often subsidized by building and maintaining highways, providing inexpensive parking, and imposing low taxes on petroleum products that do not fully reflect their societal and environmental costs. Increasing taxes on petroleum products and subsidizing public transportation could have an important effect on choice of transportation modality, which as noted earlier, has major effects on health.

- Walking, riding bicycles, and using public transportation can be promoted by economic policies that, in addition

Poland: A Dramatic Decline in Heart Disease

After Poland's transition to a democratic government in the early 1990s, the government removed large subsidies for butter and lard, and consumption of nonhydrogenated vegetable fat increased rapidly (Zatonski, McMichael, and Powles 1998). The ratio of dietary polyunsaturated to saturated fat increased from 0.33 in 1990 to 0.56 in 1999, and during this period mortality rates from CAD dropped by 28 percent (data provided by W. Zatonski). Changes in smoking and in the consumption of fruits and vegetables probably played a minor role in this decrease (see figure).

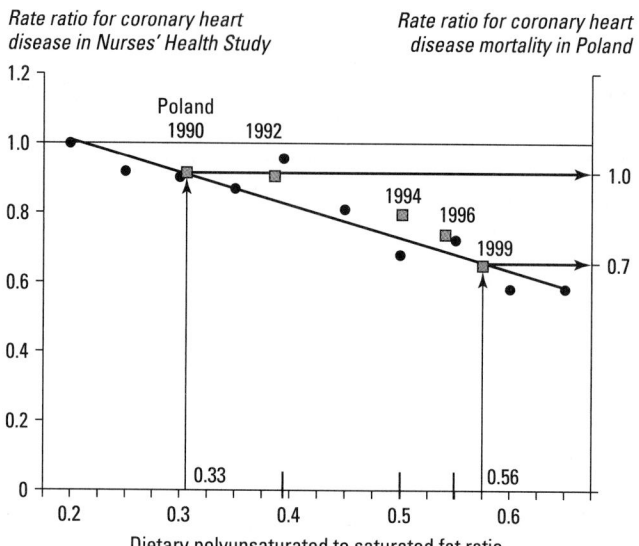

Risk of Coronary Heart Disease According to Polyunsaturated to Saturated Fat Ratio

Notes: Squares represent data for Poland from 1990 to 1999. Circles are for deciles of polyunsaturated fat to saturated fat and for risk of coronary heart disease in the Nurses' Health Study (Hu 1999), which closely predict the observed changes in Poland.

to providing better infrastructure, include discounts on transportation fares, provide secure bicycle parking, and reduce health insurance premiums.

COST-EFFECTIVENESS OF INTERVENTIONS

Only a few studies have described interventions for lifestyle diseases in developing countries.

Modeling Likely Interventions

Primary targets for reducing lifestyle diseases include changing the fat composition of the diet, limiting sodium intake, and engaging in regular physical activity.

Using available data, we calculated a range of estimates under given assumptions for the cost-effectiveness of replacing dietary saturated fat with monounsaturated fat, replacing trans fat with polyunsaturated fat, and reducing salt intake. An increase in moderate physical activity by three to five hours per week is considered likely to lower the risk of many diseases, but data to model the cost-effectiveness of this intervention are not currently available. For further details of methods and assumptions underlying the analyses presented here, see the Web site version of this book.

Reducing Saturated Fat Content. In the base case, assuming a 3 percent drop in cholesterol and a US$6 per person cost of the intervention, averting one disability-adjusted life year (DALY) would cost as little as US$1,865 in South Asia and as much as US$4,012 in the Middle East and North Africa. The intervention's effectiveness could be increased by replacing part of the saturated fat with polyunsaturated fat, which has additional beneficial effects mediated by mechanisms other than LDL cholesterol (see tables 44.2 and 44.3).

Replacing Dietary Trans Fat from Partial Hydrogenation with Polyunsaturated Fat. We could not use the model for saturated fat to estimate the effects of replacing trans fat with polyunsaturated fat because only a small part of the benefit is attributable to reducing LDL cholesterol (F. B. Hu and Willett 2002). Trans fats also adversely affect high-density lipoprotein (HDL) cholesterol, triglycerides, endothelial function, and inflammatory markers. In addition, increases in polyunsaturated fat (assuming a mix of N-6 and omega-3 fatty acids) will reduce LDL cholesterol, insulin resistance, and probably fatal cardiac arrhythmias.

In calculations that are based only on the adverse effects on LDL and HDL, replacing 2 percent of the energy from trans fat

Table 44.2 Incremental Cost-Effectiveness Ratios, Selected Interventions, by Region
(US$/DALY averted)

Region	Media campaign to reduce saturated fat content	Substituting 2 percent of energy from trans fat with polyunsaturated fat				Reducing salt content by means of legislation plus public education
		7 percent CAD reduction		**40 percent CAD reduction**		
		Intervention cost of US$0.50/adult[a]	Intervention cost of US$6.00/adult	Intervention cost of US$0.50/adult[a]	Intervention cost of US$6.00/adult	
East Asia and the Pacific	2,769	73	1,583	Cost saving	227	2,056
Europe and Central Asia	2,929	65	1,670	Cost saving	228	2,170
Latin America and the Caribbean	3,297	40	1,865	Cost saving	225	2,476
Middle East and North Africa	4,012	25	2,259	Cost saving	252	3,056
South Asia	1,865	38	1,014	Cost saving	138	1,325
Sub-Saharan Africa	2,356	53	1,344	Cost saving	184	1,766

Source: Authors' calculations.
a. Based on the U.S. Food and Drug Administration's analysis of the costs of the intervention in the United States.

Table 44.3 Two-Way Sensitivity Analysis of the Costs of the Intervention to Reduce Saturated Fat Content and of the Relative Risk Reduction in CAD Events, South Asia
(US$/DALY averted)

Relative risk reduction in CAD events (percent)	Cost per individual		
	US$0.25	US$3.00	US$6.00[a]
10	Cost saving	318	680
5	Cost saving	680	1,403
4[b]	Cost saving	911	1,865
1	258	3,572	7,188

Source: Authors' calculations.
a. Threshold analysis reveals that at the base assumption of US$6 for the intervention, no level in the range of assumed CAD reduction is cost saving.
b. Threshold analysis reveals that at a cost below US$0.36 per individual and a 4 percent reduction in CAD (base assumption), the intervention is cost saving.

with polyunsaturated fat was estimated to reduce CAD by 7 to 8 percent (Grundy 1992; Willett and Ascherio 1994). Epidemiological studies, which include the contributions of the additional causal pathways, suggest a much greater reduction, from about 25 to 40 percent (F. B. Hu and others 1997; Oomen and others 2001). Another likely benefit is a reduction in the incidence of type 2 diabetes: estimates indicate that the same 2 percent reduction would reduce incidence by 40 percent (Salmeron and others 2001).

Because voluntary action by industry (as has nearly been achieved in the Netherlands) or by regulation (as occurred in Denmark) can eliminate partially hydrogenated fat from the diet, this initiative does not require consumer education, and the costs can be extremely low. In an analysis required before implementing food labeling, the U.S. Food and Drug Administration (2003) estimated that trans fat labeling would be highly cost-effective. Even though the effect of labeling itself

was estimated to have only a modest effect on consumer behavior, as noted earlier, it is having a major effect on manufacturers' behavior.

The potential for reducing CVD rates by replacing trans fats with polyunsaturated fats will depend on the diets of specific populations. Whereas the intake of trans fat is low in China, it is likely to be high in parts of India, Pakistan, and other Asian countries because of the extraordinarily high content in commonly used cooking fats.

Table 44.2 presents the results of a cost-effectiveness analysis assuming the two different estimates for CAD reduction: 7 percent and 40 percent. We used costs of US$0.50 per adult per year, which was the maximal cost in the U.S. Food and Drug Administration analysis, and of US$6.00 per adult per year using traditional health education approaches. The lower estimate—or one even lower—is possible because trans fat can be eliminated at the source rather than depending entirely on changes in individual behavior. With the lower cost, the smaller effect estimate leads to a cost-effectiveness ratio of between US$25 and US$73 per DALY averted, depending on the region, and with the higher-effect estimate, the intervention can be cost saving.

Reducing the Salt Content of Manufactured Foods through Legislation and an Accompanying Education Campaign. Table 44.2 shows the base-case cost-effectiveness of a legislated reduction in salt content. The intervention appears to be relatively cost-effective, with a cost per DALY averted of US$1,325 in South Asia to US$3,056 in the Middle East and North Africa. Those regional variations are attributable to differing risk profiles across regions as well as to price differentials for the costs of treating disease sequelae.

The actual blood pressure reduction from lower salt consumption could vary from the base-case assumption, as could the costs of the education campaign. Table 44.4 shows the

Table 44.4 Two-Way Sensitivity Analysis of the Costs of the Intervention to Reduce Salt Content and Its Effectiveness, South Asia
(US$/DALY averted)

Blood pressure reduction (millimeters of mercury)	Cost per individual		
	US$1a	US$3	US$6
4	9	308	608
3	49	448	847
2b	129	727	1,326
1	368	1,565	2,761

Source: Authors' calculations.

a. Threshold analysis reveals that at a cost of US$1 per individual, a blood pressure reduction would have to be greater than 5 millimeters of mercury for the intervention to be cost saving. At the base-case assumption of a cost of US$6 for the intervention, there is no cost saving threshold level of reduction.

b. Threshold analysis reveals that at a cost of less than US$0.47 per individual the intervention is cost-saving.

results of lower costs of the education campaign and higher or lower effects of the intervention on blood pressure. These results may argue for initial efforts to focus on reductions in the use of salt during the manufacturing process with no public education campaign. The cost-effectiveness of such a change is high and could be augmented with a public education campaign only if needed to support the legislated change. At lower implementation costs, the intervention is highly cost-effective, even with half the assumed effect on blood pressure.

Adopting Physical Activity Interventions. Even though health experts believe that physical activity interventions are effective in reducing the risk of lifestyle diseases, no studies of their cost-effectiveness are available from developing countries. If people walk voluntarily (the model assumes no opportunity cost), a net economic benefit would accrue to all segments of the U.S. population. If we project the economic benefits to the entire U.S. population and assume 25 percent compliance by the sedentary population, the voluntary program would generate US$6.8 billion in savings (in 2001 U.S. dollars).

Aggregate Costs of Obesity and Unhealthy Lifestyles

A series of U.S. studies appears to confirm that the avoidable costs of chronic diseases are substantial, although many developing countries have not yet experienced the full demands on their health sectors resulting from these conditions. Colditz (1999) estimates that obesity is responsible for 7 percent of all U.S. direct health care costs and that inactivity is responsible for an additional 2.4 percent of all health care costs. Indirect costs associated with obesity and inactivity account for another 5 percent of health care costs. Pronk and others (1999) assess the difference in health care costs between adult patients with

and without risk factors for noncommunicable diseases (physical activity, BMI, and smoking status) and find that a healthier lifestyle of physical activity three times per week, a moderate BMI, and nonsmoking status reduce health care costs by 49 percent compared with an unhealthy lifestyle.

Cost-Effectiveness of Community-Based Interventions

Populationwide and community-based interventions appear to be cost-effective if they reach large populations, address high-mortality and high-morbidity diseases, and are multipronged and integrated efforts. The full costs of achieving changes in behavior and policy are often complex and difficult to estimate. Interventions may yield additional spinoff benefits. For instance, decisions to reduce children's television viewing could easily improve school outcomes as well as reduce childhood obesity. Similarly, increasing walking and bicycle riding for transportation could reduce air pollution.

RESEARCH AND DEVELOPMENT PRIORITIES

A number of research and development priorities have been identified:

- Conduct randomized trials of the use of folic acid and alpha-linoleic acid to prevent CAD in developing countries. These interventions cost little, and the potential benefits are large and rapid.
- Develop prospective cohort studies of dietary and lifestyle factors in developing and transition countries to refine the understanding of risk factors in those contexts. To date, almost all such studies have taken place in Europe and North America.
- Develop surveillance systems for chronic diseases and for major risk factors, such as obesity, in developing countries.
- Develop additional multifaceted, community-based demonstration programs in developing countries to document the feasibility of lifestyle changes and to learn more about effective strategies.
- Conduct detailed cost-effectiveness analyses of various prevention strategies to modify dietary and lifestyle factors.

RECOMMENDED PRIORITY INTERVENTIONS

An overall objective is to develop comprehensive national and local plans that take advantage of every opportunity to encourage and promote healthy eating and active living. These plans would involve health care providers; worksites; schools; media; urban planners; all levels of food production, processing, and preparation; and governments. The goal is cultural change in the direction of healthy living. An important element in cultural change is national leadership by individuals and by professional organizations. Specific interventions will depend on local physical and cultural conditions and should be based on careful analysis of existing dietary and activity patterns and their determinants; however, the following interventions can be considered (specific interventions for control of smoking are discussed elsewhere):

- Physical activity:
  - Develop transportation policies and a physical environment to promote walking and riding bicycles. This intervention includes constructing sidewalks and protected bicycle paths and lanes that are attractive, safe, well-lighted, and functional with regard to destinations.
  - Adopt policies that promote livable, walker-friendly communities that include parks and are centered around access to public transportation.
  - Encourage the use of public transportation and discourage overdependence on private automobiles.
  - Promote the use of stairs. Building codes can require the inclusion of accessible and attractive stairways.
- Healthy diets:
  - Develop comprehensive school programs that integrate nutrition into core curricula and healthy nutrition into school food services. Regional or national standards to promote healthy eating should be developed for school food services. Programs should also aim at limiting television watching, in part by promoting attractive alternatives.
  - Work with the agriculture sector and food industries to replace unhealthy fats with healthy fats, including adequate amounts of omega-3 fatty acids. This goal can be achieved through a combination of education, regulation, and incentives. Specific actions will depend on local sources of fat and on regional production and distribution. For example, in areas where palm oil is dominant, research could focus on developing strains that are lower in saturated fat and higher in unsaturated fat through selective breeding or genetic alteration. Labeling requirements or regulation can be used to discourage or eliminate the use of partially hydrogenated vegetable oils and to promote the use of nonhydrogenated unsaturated oils instead.
  - Require clear labeling of energy content for all packaged foods, including fast food.
  - Use tax policies to encourage the consumption of healthier foods. For example, high-sugar sodas could be fully taxed and not subsidized in the same way as healthier foods.
  - Emphasize the production and consumption of healthy food products in agriculture support and extension programs.

- Implement folic acid fortification if folic acid intake is low.
- Ensure that health providers regularly weigh both children and adult patients, track their weights over time, and provide counseling regarding diet and activity if they are already overweight or if unhealthy weight gain is occurring during adulthood. Those activities should be integrated with programs that address undernutrition. Health care providers should be encouraged to set a good example by not smoking, by exercising regularly, and by eating healthy diets.
- Promote healthy foods at worksite food services. Worksites can also promote physical activity by providing financial incentives for using public transportation or riding bicycles (and by not subsidizing automobiles by providing free parking). Providing areas for exercise during work breaks and showers may be useful.
- Set standards that restrict the promotion of foods high in sugar, refined starch, and saturated and trans fats to children on television and elsewhere.
- Set national standards for the amount of sodium in processed foods.
- National campaigns:
  - Invest in developing locally appropriate health messages related to diet, physical activity, and weight control. This effort is best done in cooperation with government agencies, nongovernmental organizations, and professional organizations so that consistent messages can be used on television and radio; at health care settings, schools, and worksites; and elsewhere. This effort should use the best social-marketing techniques available, with messages continuously evaluated for effectiveness.
  - Develop a sustainable surveillance system that monitors weight and height, physical activity, and key dietary variables.

Implementation of the recommended policies to promote health and well-being is often not straightforward because of opposition by powerful and well-funded political and economic forces, such as those involved in the tobacco, automobile, food, and oil industries (Nestle 2002). The solutions will depend on a country's specific political landscape. However, experiences in many countries indicate that alliances of public interest groups, professional organizations, and motivated individuals can overcome such powerful interests. Strategies should start with sound science and can use a mix of mass media, lobbying efforts, and lawsuits. Also, the food industry is far from monolithic, and elements can often be identified whose interests coincide with health promotion, which can create valuable partnerships. As an example, the willingness of some margarine manufacturers to invest in developing products free of trans fatty acids greatly helped the effort to reduce these fats, because these producers then became proponents for labeling the trans fat content of foods. Protection of children can be a powerful lever because of almost universal concern about their welfare and the recognition that they cannot be responsible for the long-term consequences of their diet and lifestyle choices.

CONCLUSIONS

Many of the ongoing diet and lifestyle interventions in low- and middle-income countries are relatively recent, and few have documented reductions in the rates of major chronic diseases. However, the successes of Finland, Singapore, and many other high-income countries in reducing rates of CAD, stroke, and smoking-related cancers strongly suggest that similar benefits will emerge in the developing countries.

ACKNOWLEDGMENTS

The authors appreciate Hilary Farmer's assistance in preparing this manuscript.

REFERENCES

Ascherio, A., E. Cho, K. Walsh, F. M. Sacks, W. C. Willett, and A. Faruqui. 1996. "Premature Coronary Deaths in Asians" (letter). *British Medical Journal* 312: 508.

Bacon, C. G., M. A. Mittleman, I. Kawachi, E. Giovannucci, D. B. Glasser, and E. B. Rimm. 2003. "Sexual Function in Men Older Than 50 Years of Age: Results from the Health Professionals Follow-up Study." *Annals of Internal Medicine* 139: 161–68.

Ball, D., S. Ellison, J. Adamy, and G. Fowler. 2004. "Recipes without Borders?" *Wall Street Journal*, August 18, 2004, p. 1.

Baylin, A., E. K. Kabagambe, A. Ascherio, D. Spiegelman, and H. Campos. 2003. "Adipose Tissue Alpha-Linolenic Acid and Nonfatal Acute Myocardial Infarction in Costa Rica." *Circulation* 107: 1586–91.

Bell, A. C., K. Ge, and B. M. Popkin. 2002. "The Road to Obesity or the Path to Prevention: Motorized Transportation and Obesity in China." *Obesity Research* 10: 277–83.

Bell, E. A., L. S. Roe, and B. J. Rolls. 2003. "Sensory-Specific Satiety Is Affected More by Volume Than by Energy Content of a Liquid Food." *Physiology and Behavior* 78: 593–600.

Blendon, R. J. 2002. *Welfare of Children in America*. Cambridge, MA: Cogent Research.

Bly, J. L., R. C. Jones, and J. E. Richardson. 1986. "Impact of Worksite Health Promotion on Health Care Costs and Utilization. Evaluation of Johnson & Johnson's Live for Life Program." *Journal of the American Medical Association* 256: 3235–40.

Boutelle, K, R. Jeffery, D. McMurray, and K. Schmitz. 2001. "Using Signs, Artwork, and Music to Promote Stair Use in a Public Building." *American Journal of Public Health* 91: 2004–6.

Bunn, F., T. Collier, C. Frost, K. Ker, I. Roberts, and R. Wentz. 2003. "Traffic Calming for the Prevention of Road Traffic Injuries: Systematic Review and Meta-Analysis." *Injury Prevention* 9: 200–4.

Buss, D. 2004. "Is the Food Industry the Problem or the Solution?" *New York Times*, August 29, 2004, p. 5.

Calle, E. E., C. Rodriguez, K. Walker-Thurmond, and M. J. Thun. 2003. "Overweight, Obesity, and Mortality from Cancer in a Prospectively Studied Cohort of U.S. Adults." *New England Journal of Medicine* 348: 1625–38.

Coitinho, D., C. A. Monteiro, and B. M. Popkin. 2002. "What Brazil Is Doing to Promote Healthy Diets and Active Lifestyles." *Public Health Nutrition* 5: 263–67.

Colditz, G. A. 1999. "Economic Costs of Obesity and Inactivity." *Medicine Science and Sports Exercise* 31: S663–67.

Conlin, P. R. 1999. "The Dietary Approaches to Stop Hypertension (Dash) Clinical Trial: Implications for Lifestyle Modifications in the Treatment of Hypertensive Patients." *Cardiology Review* 7: 284–88.

Cutter, J., B. Y. Tan, and S. K. Chew. 2001. "Levels of Cardiovascular Disease Risk Factors in Singapore Following a National Intervention Programme." *Bulletin of the World Health Organization* 79: 908–15.

de Lorgeril, M., S. Renaud, N. Mamelle, P. Salen, J. L. Martin, I. Monjaud, and others. 1994. "Mediterranean Alpha-Linolenic Acid–Rich Diet in Secondary Prevention of Coronary artery disease." *Lancet* 343: 1454–59. (Erratum in *Lancet* 1995, 345: 738.)

Dickinson, S., S. Colagiuri, E. Faramus, P. Petocz, and J. C. Brand-Miller. 2002. "Postprandial Hyperglycemia and Insulin Sensitivity Differ among Lean Young Adults of Different Ethnicities." *Journal of Nutrition* 132: 2574–79.

Ebbeling, C. B., M. M. Leidig, K. B. Sinclair, J. P. Hangen, and D. S. Ludwig. 2003. "A Reduced-Glycemic Load Diet in the Treatment of Adolescent Obesity." *Archives of Pediatric and Adolescent Medicine* 157: 773–79.

Ewing, R, R. Schieber, and C. Zegeer. 2003. "Urban Sprawl as a Risk Factor in Motor Vehicle Occupant and Pedestrian Facilities." *American Journal of Public Health* 93: 1541–45.

Fox, K. R. 1999. "The Influence of Physical Activity on Mental Well-Being." *Public Health Nutrition* 2: 411–18.

Frumkin, H. 2002. "Urban Sprawl and Public Health." *Public Health Reports* 117: 201–17.

Giovannucci, E. 2002. "Epidemiologic Studies of Folate and Colorectal Neoplasia: A Review." *Journal of Nutrition* 132: 2350–55S.

Gortmaker, S. L., K. Peterson, J. Wiecha, A. M. Sobol, S. Dixit, M. K. Fox, and N. Laird. 1999. "Reducing Obesity via a School-Based Interdisciplinary Intervention among Youth: Planet Health." *Archives of Pediatric and Adolescent Medicine* 153: 409–18.

Grundy, S. M. 1992. "How Much Does Diet Contribute to Premature Coronary Heart Disease?" In *Atherosclerosis IX: Proceedings of the Ninth International Symposium on Atherosclerosis*, ed. O. Stein, S. Eisenberg, and Y. Stein, 471–78. Tel Aviv: Creative Communications.

Handy, S. L., M. G. Boarnet, R. Ewing, and R. E. Killingsworth. 2002. "How the Built Environment Affects Physical Activity: Views from Urban Planning." *American Journal of Preventive Medicine* 23: 64–73.

Hao, L., J. Ma, M. J. Stampfer, A. Ren, Y. Tian, Y. Tang, and others. 2003. "Geographical, Seasonal, and Gender Differences in Folate Status among Chinese Adults." *Journal of Nutrition* 133: 3630–35.

Harris, M. I., K. M. Flegal, C. C. Cowie, M. S. Eberhardt, D. E. Goldstein, R. R. Little, and others. 1998. "Prevalence of Diabetes, Impaired Fasting Glucose, and Impaired Glucose Tolerance in U.S. Adults: The Third National Health and Nutrition Examination Survey, 1988–1994." *Diabetes Care* 21: 518–24.

Hernandez, B., S. L. Gortmaker, G. A. Colditz, K. E. Peterson, N. M. Laird, and S. Parra-Cabrera. 1999. "Association of Obesity with Physical Activity, Television Programs, and Other Forms of Video Viewing among Children in Mexico City." *International Journal of Obesity and Relational Metabolism Disorders* 23: 845–54.

Honein, M. A., L. J. Paulozzi, T. J. Mathews, J. D. Erickson, and L. Y. Wong. 2001. "Impact of Folic Acid Fortification of the U.S. Food Supply on the Occurrence of Neural Tube Defects." *Journal of the American Medical Association* 285: 2981–86.

Hu. 2002.

Hu, F. B., M. F. Leitzmann, M. J. Stampfer, G. A. Colditz, W. C. Willett, and E. B. Rimm. 2001. "Physical Activity and Television Watching in Relation to Risk for Type 2 Diabetes Mellitus in Men." *Archives of Internal Medicine* 161: 1542–48.

Hu, F. B., M. J. Stampfer, J. E. Manson, E. B. Rimm, A. Wolk, G. A. Colditz, and others. 1999. "Dietary Intake of Alpha-Linolenic Acid and Risk of Fatal Ischemic Heart Disease among Women." *American Journal of Clinical Nutrition* 69: 890–97.

Hu, F. B., M. J. Stampfer, J. E. Manson, E. Rimm, G. A. Colditz, B. A. Rosner, and others. 1997. "Dietary Fat Intake and the Risk of Coronary Heart Disease in Women." *New England Journal of Medicine* 337: 1491–99.

Hu, F. B., R. M. van Dam, and S. Liu. 2001. "Diet and Risk of Type 2 Diabetes: The Role of Types of Fat and Carbohydrate." *Diabetologia* 44: 805–17.

Hu, F. B., B. Wang, C. Chen, Y. Jin, J. Yang, M. J. Stampfer, and X. Xu. 2000. "Body Mass Index and Cardiovascular Risk Factors in a Rural Chinese Population." *American Journal of Epidemiology* 151: 88–97.

Hu, F. B., and W. C. Willett. 2002. "Optimal Diets for Prevention of Coronary Heart Disease." *Journal of the American Medical Association* 288: 2569–78.

Hu, G., H. Pekkarinen, O. Hanninen, Z. J. Yu, H. G. Tian, Z. Y. Guo, and A. Nissinen. 2002. "Physical Activity during Leisure and Commuting in Tianjin, China." *Bulletin of the World Health Organization* 80: 933–38.

IARC (International Agency for Research on Cancer). 2002. *Weight Control and Physical Activity.* Lyon, France: IARC Press.

Institute of Medicine. 2002. *Dietary Reference Intakes for Energy, Carbohydrate, Fiber, Fat, Fatty Acids, Cholesterol, Protein, and Amino Acids (Macronutrients): A Report of the Panel on Macronutrients, Subcommittees on Upper Reference Levels of Nutrients and Interpretation and Uses of Dietary Reference Intakes, and the Standing Committee on the Scientific Evaluation of Dietary Reference Intakes.* Washington, DC: National Academy of Sciences. http://www.nap.edu/catalog/10490.html.

Jones, T. F., and C. B. Eaton. 1994. "Cost-Benefit Analysis of Walking to Prevent Coronary Heart Disease." *Archives of Family Medicine* 3: 703–10.

Keeler, E. B., W. G. Manning, J. P. Newhouse, E. M. Sloss, and J. Wasserman. 1989. "The External Costs of a Sedentary Life-Style." *American Journal of Public Health* 79: 975–81.

Knowler, W. C., E. Barrett-Connor, S. E. Fowler, R. F. Hamman, J. M. Lachin, E. A. Walker, and D. M. Nathan. 2002. "Reduction in the Incidence of Type 2 Diabetes with Lifestyle Intervention or Metformin." *New England Journal of Medicine* 346 (6): 393–403.

Koplan, J. P., and W. H. Dietz. 1999. "Caloric Imbalance and Public Health Policy." *Journal of the American Medical Association* 282: 1579–81.

Lambert, E. V., I. Bohlmann, and T. Kolbe-Alexander. 2001. "'Be Active': Physical Activity for Health in South Africa." *South African Journal of Clinical Nutrition* 14: S12–16.

Law, M. R., C. D. Frost, and N. J. Wald. 1991. "By How Much Does Dietary Salt Reduction Lower Blood Pressure? III—Analysis of Data from Trials of Salt Reduction." *British Medical Journal* 302 (6780): 819–24.

Leitzmann, M. F., E. B. Rimm, W. C. Willett, D. Spiegelman, F. Grodstein, M. J. Stampfer, and others. 1999. "Recreational Physical Activity and the Risk of Cholecystectomy in Women." *New England Journal of Medicine* 341: 777–84.

Leyden, K. 2003. "Social Capital and the Built Environment: The Importance of Walkable Neighborhoods." *American Journal of Public Health* 93: 1546–51.

Lopez, R. 2004. "Urban Sprawl and Risk for Being Overweight or Obese." *American Journal of Public Health* 94: 1574–79.

Ludwig, D. S., K. E. Peterson, and S. L. Gortmaker. 2001. "Relation between Consumption of Sugar-Sweetened Drinks and Childhood Obesity: A Prospective, Observational Analysis." *Lancet* 357: 505–8.

Mak, K. H., K. S. Chia, J. D. Kark, T. Chua, C. Tan, B. H. Foong, and others. 2003. "Ethnic Differences in Acute Myocardial Infarction in Singapore." *European Heart Journal* 24: 151–60.

Matsudo, V., S. Matsudo, D. Andrade, T. Araujo, E. Andrade, L. Carlos de Oliveira, and G. Braggion. 2002. "Promotion of Physical Activity in a Developing Country: The Agita São Paulo Experience." *Public Health Nutrition* 5: 253–61.

Nestle, M. 2002. *Food Politics: How the Food Industry Influences Nutrition and Health.* Berkeley. CA: University of California Press.

Nissinen, A., X. Berrios, and P. Puska. 2001. "Community-Based Noncommunicable Disease Interventions: Lessons from Developed Countries for Developing Ones." *Bulletin of the World Health Organization* 79: 963–70.

Office of the Administrator. 2001. *What Is Smart Growth?* Washington, DC: Environmental Protection Agency. http://www.epa.gov/smartgrowth/pdf/whtissg4v2.pdf.

Oomen, C. M., M. C. Ocke, E. J. Feskens, M. A. van Erp-Baart, F. J. Kok, and D. Kromhout. 2001. "Association between Trans Fatty Acid Intake and 10-Year Risk of Coronary Heart Disease in the Zutphen Elderly Study: A Prospective Population-Based Study." *Lancet* 357: 746–51.

Pendakur, V. S. 2000. *World Bank Urban Transport Strategy Review.* Yokohama, Japan: Pacific Policy and Planning Associates.

Petrella, R., J. Koval, D. Cunningham, and D. Paterson. 2003. "Can Primary Care Doctors Prescribe Exercise to Improve Fitness: The Step Test Exercise Prescription (STEP) Project." *American Journal of Preventive Medicine* 24: 316–22.

Pignone, M. P., A. Ammerman, L. Fernandez, C. T. Orleans, N. Pender, S. Woolf, and others. 2003. "Counseling to Promote a Healthy Diet in Adults: A Summary of the Evidence for the U.S. Preventive Services Task Force." *American Journal of Preventive Medicine* 24: 75–92.

Pratt, M., C. A. Macera, and G. Wang. 2000. "Higher Direct Medical Costs Associated with Physical Inactivity." *Physician and Sports Medicine* 28:63–70. http://www.physsportsmed.com/issues/2000/10_00/pratt.htm.

Pronk, N. P., M. J. Goodman, P. J. O'Connor, and B. C. Martinson. 1999. "Relationship between Modifiable Health Risks and Short-Term Health Care Charges." *Journal of the American Medical Association* 282: 2235–39.

Pucher, J., and L. Dijkstra. 2003. "Promoting Safe Walking and Cycling to Improve Public Health: Lessons from the Netherlands and Germany." *American Journal of Public Health* 93: 1509–16.

Puska, P., E. Vartiainen, J. Tuomilehto, V. Salomaa, and A. Nissinen. 1998. "Changes in Premature Deaths in Finland: Successful Long-Term Prevention of Cardiovascular Diseases." *Bulletin of the World Health Organization* 76: 419–25.

Raben, A., T. H. Vasilaras, A. C. Moller, and A. Astrup. 2002. "Sucrose Compared with Artificial Sweeteners: Different Effects on Ad Libitum Food Intake and Body Weight after 10 Weeks of Supplementation in Overweight Subjects." *American Journal of Clinical Nutrition* 76: 721–29.

Robinson, T. N. 1999. "Reducing Children's Television Viewing to Prevent Obesity: A Randomized Controlled Trial." *Journal of the American Medical Association* 282: 1561–67.

Rossouw, J. E., P. L. Jooste, D. O. Chalton, E. R. Jordaan, M. L. Langenhoven, P. C. Jordaan, and others. 1993. "Community-Based Intervention: The Coronary Risk Factor Study (Coris)." *International Journal of Epidemiology* 22: 428–38.

Ruangdaraganon, N., N. Kotchabhakdi, U. Udomsubpayakul, C. Kunanusont, and P. Suriyawongpaisal. 2002. "The Association between Television Viewing and Childhood Obesity: A National Survey in

Thailand." *Journal of the Medical Association of Thailand* 85 (Suppl. 4): S1075–80.

Saelens, B. E., J. F. Sallis, and L. D. Frank. 2003. "Environmental Correlates of Walking and Cycling: Findings from the Transportation, Urban Design, and Planning Literatures." *Annals of Behavioral Medicine* 25: 80–91.

Salmeron, J., F. B. Hu, J. E. Manson, M. J. Stampfer, G. A. Colditz, E. B. Rimm, and W. C. Willett. 2001. "Dietary Fat Intake and Risk of Type 2 Diabetes in Women." *American Journal of Clinical Nutrition* 73: 1019–26.

Schulze, M. B., J. E. Manson, D. S. Ludwig, G. A. Colditz, M. J. Stampfer, W. C. Willett, and F. B. Hu. 2004. "Sugar-Sweetened Beverages, Weight Gain, and Incidence of Type 2 Diabetes in Young and Middle-Aged Women." *Journal of the American Medical Association* 292: 927–34.

Selmer, R., I. Kristiansen, A. Haglerod, S. Graff-Iverson, H. Larsen, H. Meyer, and others. 2000. "Cost and Health Consequences of Reducing the Population Intake of Salt." *Journal of Epidemiology and Community Health* 54: 697–702.

Sobngwi, E., J. F. Gautier, and J. C. Mbanya. 2003. "Exercise and the Prevention of Cardiovascular Events in Women" (author reply). *New England Journal of Medicine* 348: 77–79.

Staunton, C., D. Hubsmith, and W. Kallins. 2003. "Promoting Safe Walking and Biking to School: The Marin County Success Story." *American Journal of Public Health* 93: 1431–34.

Surface Transportation Policy Project. 1999. "Aggressive Driving: Where You Live Matters." Washington, DC. http://www.transact.org/report.asp?id=56.

Swinburn, B. A., I. Caterson, J. C. Seidell, and W. P. James. 2004. "Diet, Nutrition, and the Prevention of Excess Weight Gain and Obesity." *Public Health Nutrition* 7: 123–46.

Toh, C. M., J. Cutter, and S. K. Chew. 2002. "School-Based Intervention Has Reduced Obesity in Singapore." *British Medical Journal* 324: 427.

Tosteson, A., M. Weinstein, M. Hunink, M. A. Mittleman, L. Williams, P. Goldman, and L. Goldman. 1997. "Cost-Effectiveness of Population-Wide Educational Approaches to Reduce Serum Cholesterol Levels." *Circulation* 95: 24–30.

Tudor-Locke, C., B. E. Ainsworth, L. S. Adair, S. Du, and B. M. Popkin. 2003. "Physical Activity and Inactivity in Chinese School-Aged Youth: The China Health and Nutrition Survey." *International Journal of Obesity* 27: 1093–99.

Tuomilehto, J., J. Lindstrom, J. G. Eriksson, T. T. Valle, H. Hamalainen, P. Ilanne-Parikka, and others. 2001. "Prevention of Type 2 Diabetes Mellitus by Changes in Lifestyle among Subjects with Impaired Glucose Tolerance." *New England Journal of Medicine* 344: 1343–50.

Unwin, N., P. Setel, S. Rashid, F. Mugusi, J. C. Mbanya, H. Kitange, and others. 2001. "Noncommunicable Diseases in Sub-Saharan Africa: Where Do They Feature in the Health Research Agenda?" *Bulletin of the World Health Organization* 79: 947–53.

U.S. Food and Drug Administration, Center for Food and Safety and Applied Nutrition. 2003. "Food Labeling: Trans Fatty Acids in Nutrition." *Federal Register* 68, no. 133, 41433–506 (July 11, 2003). http://www.cfsan.fda.gov/~lrd/fr03711a.html (see also http://vm.cfsan.fda.gov/~lrd/fr991117.html).

Uusitalo, U., E. J. Feskens, J. Tuomilehto, G. Dowse, U. Haw, D. Fareed, and others. 1996. "Fall in Total Cholesterol Concentration over Five Years in Association with Changes in Fatty Acid Composition of Cooking Oil in Mauritius: Cross-Sectional Survey." *British Medical Journal* 313: 1044–46.

Wang, G., C. Macera, B. Scudder-Soucie, T. Schmid, M. Pratt, and D. Buchner. 2004. "Cost Effectiveness of a Bicycle/Pedestrian Trail Development in Health Promotion." *Preventive Medicine* 38: 237–42.

Wang, S. Y., G. B. Chi, C. X. Jing, X. M. Dong, C. P. Wu, and L. P. Li. 2003. "Trends in Road Traffic Crashes and Associated Injury and Fatality in the People's Republic of China, 1951–1999." *Injury Control and Safety Promotion* 10: 83–87.

WHO (World Health Organization). 2000. *Obesity: Preventing and Managing the Global Epidemic.* WHO Technical Report 894. Geneva: WHO.

———. 2002. *The World Health Organization Report 2002: Reducing Risks, Promoting Healthy Life.* Geneva: WHO.

WHO and FAO (World Health Organization and Food and Agriculture Organization of the United Nations). 2003. *Diet, Nutrition, and the Prevention of Chronic Diseases: Report of a Joint WHO/FAO Expert Consultation.* Report 916. Geneva: WHO.

Willett, W. C. 2002. "Balancing Lifestyle and Genomics Research for Disease Prevention." *Science* 296: 695–98.

Willett, W. C., and A. Ascherio. 1994. "Trans-Fatty Acids: Are the Effects Only Marginal?" *American Journal of Public Health* 84: 722–24.

Willett, W. C., W. H. Dietz, and G. A. Colditz. 1999. "Guidelines for Healthy Weight." *New England Journal of Medicine* 341: 427–34.

Willett, W. C., and R. L. Leibel. 2002. "Dietary Fat Is Not a Major Determinant of Body Fat." *American Journal of Medicine* 113 (Suppl. 9B): 47–59S.

World Bank. 2003. *Noncommunicable Diseases in Pacific Island Countries: Disease Burden, Economic Cost, and Policy Options.* Nouméa, New Caledonia: World Bank.

Zatonski, W. A., A. J. McMichael, and J. W. Powles. 1998. "Ecological Study of Reasons for Sharp Decline in Mortality from Ischaemic Heart Disease in Poland since 1991." *British Medical Journal* 316: 1047–51.

Chapter **45**

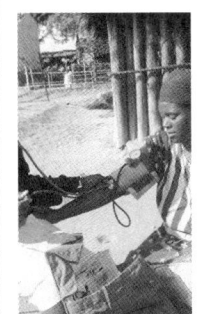

The Growing Burden of Risk from High Blood Pressure, Cholesterol, and Bodyweight

Anthony Rodgers, Carlene M. M. Lawes,
Thomas Gaziano, and Theo Vos

High blood pressure, cholesterol, and bodyweight are responsible for a large and increasing proportion of the global burden of disease. Although historically these risks have been regarded as "Western," their impact is now recognized as global: they are already leading causes of disease in middle-income countries and of emerging importance in low-income countries (Ezzati and others 2004; WHO 2002). This chapter presents an evidenced-based review of the impact of high blood pressure, cholesterol, and bodyweight; the cost-effectiveness of relevant interventions; and the economic benefits of interventions. The chapter focuses on personal interventions—that is, those that are mediated largely by interpersonal actions and take place at the individual level. As such, the chapter should be considered as complementary to chapter 44 on lifestyles, which addresses populationwide interventions.

Prevention strategies have been broadly classified as individual based (also known as high risk) or population based (Rose 1985). The former typically involve screening to detect individuals above a certain threshold level of an individual risk factor—for example, people with hypertension—followed by personal interventions for those individuals. In contrast, the population-based approach aims at lowering mean risk-factor levels and shifting the population distribution of exposure in a favorable direction (Rose 1985). One example would be by reducing salt content in manufactured foods, thereby lowering blood pressure levels on a populationwide basis. Such an approach has the potential to produce large and lasting changes in disease incidence but requires substantial sociopolitical

investments. Another approach is an evolution of the individual-based strategy in which treatments are targeted to those at high absolute risk of cardiovascular disease (CVD) rather than those with single risk-factor levels above traditional thresholds, such as hypertension or obesity (Jackson and others 1993). Such an approach appears to be highly cost-effective, with the potential to substantially reduce CVD rates when combined with populationwide interventions (Murray and others 2003).

EPIDEMIOLOGY

Elevated blood pressure, cholesterol, and bodyweight are all established risk factors for CVD and, in the case of bodyweight, for other diseases, such as diabetes, certain cancers, and osteoarthritis. The associations between blood pressure (Asia Pacific Cohort Studies Collaboration 1999, 2003a; Prospective Studies Collaboration 2002); cholesterol (Asia Pacific Cohort Studies Collaboration 2003b; Law, Wald, and Thompson 1994; Prospective Studies Collaboration 1995); and body mass index (BMI) (Asia Pacific Cohort Studies Collaboration 2004; Willett and others 1995) and CVD are direct and continuous from relatively low levels, indicating that optimal levels are about 115/75 millimeters of mercury (mmHg), 3.8 millimoles per liter (mmol/l), and 21 kilograms per square meter (kg/m^2), respectively (figure 45.1).

Although some studies suggest *J*- or *U*-shaped associations (Calle and others 1999; Cruickshank 1994; D'Agostino and

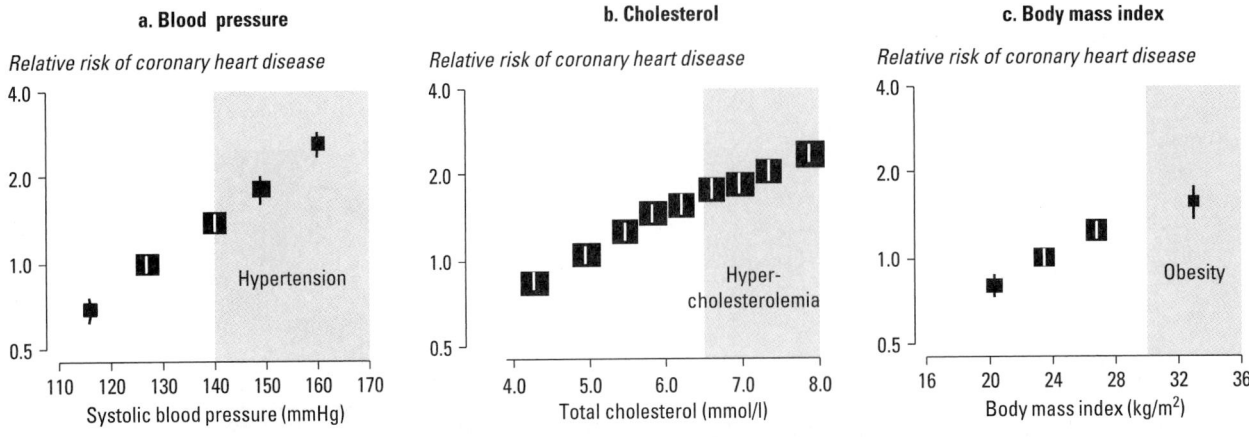

a. Blood pressure

Relative risk of coronary heart disease

Hypertension

Systolic blood pressure (mmHg)

b. Cholesterol

Relative risk of coronary heart disease

Hyper-
cholesterolemia

Total cholesterol (mmol/l)

c. Body mass index

Relative risk of coronary heart disease

Obesity

Body mass index (kg/m²)

Figure 45.1 Continuous Risks of Blood Pressure, Cholesterol, and Body Mass and Coronary Heart Disease Risk

others 1991; Farnett and others 1991; Field and others 2001; Iso and others 1989; Kannel, D'Agostino, and Silbershatz 1997; Stewart 1979; Troiano and others 1996), low levels of these risk factors are unlikely to cause CVD. Rather, such associations more likely reflect incipient disease, which itself produces both a fall in risk-factor levels and an increase in CVD risk (Alderman 1996; Flack and others 1995; MacMahon and others 1997; Manson, Willett, and Stampfer 1995; Neaton and Wentworth 1992; Sleight 1997a, 1997b; Stevens and others 1998). No trial evidence points to a J-curve association for blood pressure, despite including patients with below average blood pressure (Hansson and others 1999; McMurray and McInnes 1992; Pfeffer 1993; Staessen and others 1997).

The continuous associations between blood pressure, cholesterol, and bodyweight and CVD demonstrate the lack of a biological justification for current threshold levels, such as those that define hypertension. Indeed, most of the disease burden resulting from these three risk factors occurs in the large majority of the population with nonoptimal levels but without hypertension, hypercholesterolemia, or obesity. Hence, this chapter avoids those terms and instead uses high blood pressure, high cholesterol, and high bodyweight, defined as nonoptimal levels of these risk factors (that is, over 115/75 mmHg, 3.8 mmol/l, or 21 kg/m², respectively).

The strength of the proportional associations of these risk factors with CVD is similar for most population subgroups. Although they attenuate with age, they remain strong and positive in the oldest age groups. Overall, in middle-aged populations, a 10 mmHg lower systolic blood pressure (SBP) is associated with a roughly 30 to 40 percent lower stroke risk and 20 to 25 percent lower ischemic heart disease (IHD) risk, a 1 mmol/l lower cholesterol level is associated with about a 15 to 20 percent lower stroke risk and 20 to 25 percent lower IHD risk, and a 2 kg/m² lower BMI is associated with an 8 to

12 percent lower stroke and IHD risk and an approximately 20 to 30 percent lower diabetes risk.

BURDEN OF THE DISEASE, CONDITION, OR RISK FACTOR

Epidemiological data on blood pressure, cholesterol, and body-weight levels are predominantly available from developed countries; however, evidence indicates that these risk factors are important and increasing in many other countries. Surveys in developing countries suggest increases in these risks occur early in the path to industrialization (Bobak and others 1997; Evans and others 2001; Suh 2001; Wu and others 1996). Good evidence also documents risk-factor levels rising after people migrate to more urbanized settings (Poulter and Sever 1994) in Africa (Poulter 1999; Poulter, Khaw, and Sever 1988), China (He, Klag, and others 1991; He, Tell, and others 1991), and the Pacific islands (Joseph and others 1983; Salmond and others 1985; Salmond, Prior, and Wessen 1989). The World Health Organization's *Global Burden of Disease* study demonstrated that CVD was a leading cause of death in many regions and that most adults in developed and developing countries have nonoptimal blood pressure, cholesterol, and bodyweight levels (Ezzati and others 2004; WHO 2002). Indeed, even using traditional cutoff points, these risk factors are prevalent: of 140 subgroups defined by age, sex, and region, 45 percent had a mean SBP equal to or greater than 140 mmHg, 25 percent had mean cholesterol levels over 5.5mmol/l, and 45 percent had mean BMI levels of at least 25 kg/m².

Health Burden

The *Global Burden of Disease* study assessed the burden attributable to nonoptimal levels of these risks (table 45.1) (Ezzati

Table 45.1 Global Burden of Disease Attributable to Nonoptimal Blood Pressure, Cholesterol, and BMI by Region, 2000

Condition	High-mortality developing countries[a]	Low-mortality developing countries[b]	Developed countries[c]	World total
Attributable deaths (thousands)				
Blood pressure	1,969	2,205	2,966	7,140 (12.8%)
Cholesterol	1,405	849	2,161	4,415 (7.9%)
BMI	399	775	1,417	2,591 (4.6%)
Attributable DALYs (thousands)				
Blood pressure	20,630	20,277	23,363	64,270 (4.4%)
Cholesterol	15,602	8,609	16,227	40,438 (2.8%)
BMI	6,408	11,115	15,892	33,415 (2.3%)

Sources: Ezzati and others 2004; WHO 2002b.

Note: The burden of disease estimated to be attributable to nonoptimal blood pressure (mean SBP > 115 mmHg), cholesterol (mean > 3.8 mmol/l), and body mass index (mean > 21 kg/m²) in 2000.
A, B, C and D designations in specific notes below are as follows: A = very low child mortality and very low adult mortality; B = low child mortality and low adult mortality; C = low child mortality and high adult mortality; D = high child mortality and high adult mortality; E = high child mortality and very high adult mortality.
a. The high-mortality developing countries include those in Africa, America D, the Eastern Mediterranean D, and Southeast Asia D.
b. The low-mortality developing countries include those in America B, Eastern Mediterranean B, Southeast Asia B, and the Western Pacific B.
c. The developed countries include those in America A, Europe, and the Western Pacific A.

and others 2004; WHO 2002). The burden for blood pressure was related to deaths and disability-adjusted life years (DALYs) from IHD, stroke, hypertensive disease, and other CVD; endpoints for cholesterol included IHD and stroke; and endpoints for BMI were IHD, stroke, hypertensive disease, diabetes, certain cancers, and osteoarthritis. Globally, 7.1 million deaths were attributed to high blood pressure in 2000, 4.4 million to high cholesterol, and 2.6 million to high BMI. This burden was shared approximately equally among the sexes. A large fraction occurred in middle age, especially in developing countries, and this factor, together with the frequently debilitating nature of nonfatal CVD, accounted for a large number of DALYs.

More of the DALY burden was experienced in developing countries than in developed countries, reflecting the large populations in developing countries and their already high risk-factor levels. In all regions, most CVD is attributable to the combined effects of high blood pressure, cholesterol, and bodyweight levels (figure 45.2).

Table 45.2 shows the burden resulting from the overlapping or multicausal etiology of diseases. Analyses of the combined impact of these and other major cardiovascular risks indicate that the joint contribution of established risks is responsible for 83 to 89 percent of the IHD burden and 70 to 76 percent of the stroke burden worldwide (Ezzati and others 2003; Ezzati and others 2004).

Financial Burden

The economic impact of high blood pressure, cholesterol, and bodyweight levels can be estimated indirectly using the foregoing data—namely, that more than two-thirds of the CVD

burden can be attributed to those risks. In addition, more than three-quarters of type 2 diabetes is caused by high bodyweight (Ezzati and others 2004; WHO 2002). Hence the economic impact of nonoptimal levels of those risks will be at least two-thirds that due to CVD and diabetes. A recent report highlighted the economic impact of CVD in developing economies, noting that a high proportion of the CVD burden occurs among adults of working age (Leeder and others 2004). In Brazil, China, India, Mexico, and South Africa, conservative

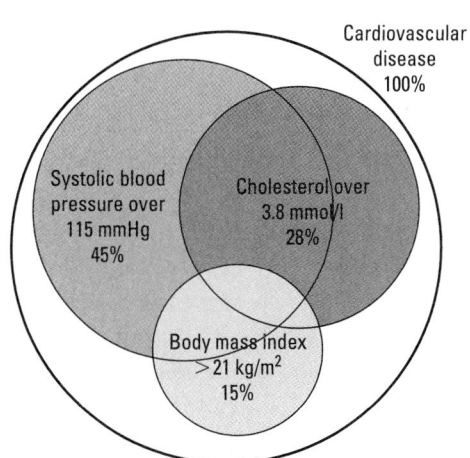

Source: Ezzati and others 2004; WHO 2002.

Note: Individual and joint contributions of high blood pressure, cholesterol, and body weight to global cardiovascular burden are shown, with the size of each circle proportional to the size of burden (as measured in DALYs) (WHO 2002). The percentages indicate the attributable burden for each risk factor, and the overlap shows disease caused by joint or mediated effects.

Figure 45.2 Global CVD Burden Caused by High Blood Pressure, Cholesterol, and Bodyweight

Table 45.2 Individual and Joint Contributions of Seven Selected Risk Factors to the Burden of CVD by Region

Disease	Percentage of the regional disease burden	Population attributable fractions for individual risk factors (percentages)	Overall population attributable fraction (percent)
High-mortality developing countries			
Stroke	1.6	High blood pressure (56), high cholesterol (18), high BMI (7), low fruit and vegetable intake (12), physical inactivity (6), tobacco (7), alcohol (2)	65–71
IHD	3.0	High blood pressure (44), high cholesterol (54), high BMI (11), low fruit and vegetable intake (33), physical inactivity (21), tobacco (8), alcohol (4)	80–87
Low-mortality developing countries			
Stroke	4.7	High blood pressure (58), high cholesterol (13), high BMI (11), low fruit and vegetable intake (10), physical inactivity (5), tobacco (8), alcohol (7)	67–74
IHD	3.2	High blood pressure (45), high cholesterol (48), high BMI (22), low fruit and vegetable intake (31), physical inactivity (22), tobacco (8), alcohol (3)	79–87
Developed countries			
Stroke	6.0	High blood pressure (72), high cholesterol (27), high BMI (23), low fruit and vegetable intake (12), physical inactivity (9), tobacco (22), alcohol (0)	81–86
IHD	9.4	High blood pressure (58), high cholesterol (63), high BMI (33), low fruit and vegetable intake (28), physical inactivity (22), tobacco (22), alcohol (−0.2)	89–93
World			
Stroke	3.1	High blood pressure (62), high cholesterol (18), high BMI (13), low fruit and vegetable intake (11), physical inactivity (7), tobacco (12), alcohol (4)	70–76
IHD	4.0	High blood pressure (49), high cholesterol (56), high BMI (21), low fruit and vegetable intake (31), physical inactivity (22), tobacco (12), alcohol (2)	83–89

Source: Ezzati and others 2003.
Note: See notes to table 45.1 for a breakdown of the regional groupings.

estimates indicated that at least 21 million years of future productive life are lost because of CVD each year. Although no detailed data exist on the direct economic burden of the individual risk factors, the costs of CVD treatment in developing countries are significant. In South Africa, for example, 2 to 3 percent of gross domestic product was devoted to the direct treatment of CVD, or roughly 25 percent of all health care expenditures (Pestana and others 1996). For many middle-income countries, high body mass is already an important cause of health inequities (Monteiro and others 2004).

Current expenditure in developed countries provides an indication of possible future expenditure in developing countries. For example, estimated direct and indirect costs of CVD in the United States were US$350 billion in 2003. In 1998, US$109 billion was spent on hypertension, or about 13 percent of the health care budget (Hodgson and Cai 2001). Studies are limited but suggest that obesity-related diseases are responsible for 2 to 8 percent of all health care expenditures in developed countries. For example, in 1991, 2.5 percent of health care costs in New Zealand were attributable to obesity (Swinburn and others 1997), and in 1996, US$22 billion was attributed to obesity-related CVD in the United States, equivalent to 17 percent of CVD-related health expenditures (G. Wang and others 2002).

INTERVENTIONS

Data on the choice of interventions for blood pressure, cholesterol, and bodyweight and their effectiveness are now presented.

Choice and Classification of Interventions

A variety of population-based and personal interventions could potentially be used to address the risks associated with high blood pressure, cholesterol, and bodyweight. Of the personal interventions discussed in this section—lifestyle and dietary, pharmacological, and surgical interventions—two main strategies exist for choosing whom to treat: those above certain threshold values of *single* risk-factor levels and those above certain values of absolute cardiovascular (or global) risk, which is determined by the levels of *multiple* factors.

Targeting treatments by levels of a single risk factor (such as hypertension) does not effectively focus on overall risk of developing CVD, which is mainly determined by the net effects of other risk factors. For example, the predicted 10-year CVD risk for someone with an SBP of 140/90 mmHg can vary from 5 to 50 percent depending on the number of concomitant risk factors. The number of people who would need to be treated to prevent an event can therefore vary by an order of magnitude, even if they have the same blood pressure levels. Thus, a treatment strategy based only on individual risk-factor levels is likely to result in high-risk patients being undertreated and many patients at relatively low risk being treated with little absolute benefit, which is unlikely to be the best allocation of scarce health care resources.

The absolute-risk strategy was developed in New Zealand (Jackson and others 1993) and has been adopted extensively elsewhere, for example, by the British Hypertension Society (Ramsay and others 1999) and the Joint Task Force of European and other Societies on Coronary Prevention (Wood and others 1998). The absolute CVD risk is estimated using risk assessments such as the Framingham risk function (Anderson and others 1991) or the Prospective Cardiovascular Munster Study score (Assmann, Cullen, and Schulte 2002) on the basis of the number and severity of CVD risk factors. Targeting treatments at those at high absolute risk rather than those above arbitrary thresholds ensures a favorable ratio of benefits to risks. It can be expected to reduce events in the large proportion of people who are, for example, nonhypertensive but who still have nonoptimal blood pressure (Rose 1981). Combinations of personal interventions targeted at those at high absolute risk also have the potential of being highly cost-effective.

The simplest indicator of high absolute risk is established CVD, principally myocardial infarction, angina, stroke, or transient ischemic attack. For example, without preventive treatment, people who have had a myocardial infarction face an annual risk of death from coronary heart disease of about 5 percent (Law, Watt, and Wald 2002). That risk persists indefinitely—probably for the rest of a person's life—and varies little with age or sex.

However, many individuals with no history of CVD are at similar elevated risk for future CVD as a result of constellations of elevated risks. Thus, the distinction between primary and secondary prevention is somewhat artificial and could lead to undertreatment of many high-risk individuals. While recognizing that the distinction is somewhat arbitrary, this chapter discusses the cost-effectiveness of efforts to manage those without previous CVD, and chapter 33 reviews the management of those with known vascular disease. A unifying system targeting treatments at those at highest risk, either with CVD or multiple risk factors, is likely to be highly cost-effective because more than 75 percent of events occur in the 5 to 10 percent of people with CVD or specific clusters of risk factors (Haq and others 1999; Tosteson and others 1997).

The limitations of the individual-risk-factor approach, together with increasing evidence that the thresholds do not have any biological justification, have motivated the adoption of strategies that take other risk factors into account. Although the most complete way of doing so is using the absolute-risk strategy outlined earlier, one intermediate strategy involves lowering the thresholds of blood pressure or lipid levels at which treatment is initiated if one or more additional CVD risk factors, such as diabetes, are present (Chobanian and others 2003).

Intervention Effectiveness

This section summarizes data on the effectiveness of population-based interventions and personal interventions (lifestyle and dietary interventions and pharmacological and surgical interventions). The studies concerned have mainly been conducted in developed countries.

Population-Based Interventions. Investigators have undertaken a variety of population-based community intervention studies, mostly in developed countries in the 1970s and 1980s (for further details see chapter 44). These studies have tended to be multifactorial projects testing whether comprehensive community programs could produce favorable changes in such risk factors as bodyweight, cholesterol, and blood pressure and in CVD morbidity and mortality (Schooler and others 1997). In general, they included a combination of populationwide and individual interventions, including messages disseminated through local associations, sports clubs, the media, and food associations; healthy food options at restaurants and worksite cafeterias; food labeling at supermarkets; face-to-face communication at meetings and distribution of educational materials; smoking restrictions; and competitions to develop healthy food. Except in Finland, the projects had mixed results, although many demonstrated significant effects with respect to individual components of the interventions. The limitations of many of the projects include inability to detect small but potentially important changes in risk factors, short duration of intervention and follow-up, and issues with outcome measures. Some have also suggested that those trials with less favorable results may have lacked adequate community support and public policy initiatives (Feinleib 1996; Mittelmark and others 1993; Schooler and others 1997; Susser 1995).

A number of population-based interventions have also taken place in developing countries, including the following:

- In China, the Tianjin Project showed a significant reduction in sodium intake in men after three years of intervention, and after five years, the prevalence rates of both hypertension and obesity decreased among 45- to 65-year-olds (Schooler and others 1997).
- In Chile, the Mirame Project was a three-year intervention program designed to provide and evaluate strategies to promote healthy lifestyles among schoolchildren and their families. Nissinen, Berrios, and Puska (2001) report a significant positive effect on some risk factors for the intervention schools.
- In Mauritius, government-led initiatives resulted in a change in the composition of cooking oil from mostly palm oil, which is high in saturated fatty acids, to wholly soybean oil, which is high in unsaturated fatty acids. From 1987 to 1992, total cholesterol concentrations fell significantly, and the estimated intake of saturated fatty acids decreased, with much of this finding reportedly resulting from the change in cooking oil (Uusitalo and others 1996).

An effective populationwide intervention draws together different kinds of feasible activities that combined produce a synergistic effect (Nissinen, Berrios, and Puska 2001; Puska 1999). Even though the projects and trials were undertaken in a range of different communities and used a variety of methods and interventions, several common themes emerge. Some of the important elements of a successful program that enables individuals to adopt healthier lifestyles include the following:

- clear responsibility for coordinating prevention efforts, with credible agencies with good communication methods carrying out long-term education programs
- intersectoral collaboration, with multiple messages sourced from different organizations, including health sector entities, nonhealth government agencies, schools, workplaces, religious organizations, and voluntary agencies
- collaboration with the food industry to ensure the availability of reasonably priced healthier food options, with food labeling that presents relevant information in a clear, reliable, and standardized format
- realistic multiyear time frames.

Lifestyle and Dietary Personal Interventions. Many guidelines have concluded that lifestyle modifications, such as weight loss, healthy diet (such as one rich in potassium and low in sodium), physical activity, and moderate alcohol consumption are effective in reducing blood pressure (see, for example, Chobanian and others 2003). Trials indicate that a reduction of

salt intake lowers blood pressure, with larger blood pressure reductions in the elderly and in those with higher initial blood pressure levels (Law, Frost, and Wald 1991; Whelton and others 1998). An increase in daily fruit and vegetable intake may also lower blood pressure, and when combined with an increase in low-fat dairy products and a reduction in saturated and total fat, may lower blood pressure even more (Appel and others 1997). Weight reduction lowers blood pressure in proportion to the amount of weight lost (Whelton and others 1998), and physical activity appears to lower blood pressure in a way that may be independent of weight loss. High levels of alcohol intake are associated with blood pressure elevation, which is reversible by reducing intake (Kaplan 1995).

Dietary approaches to lowering total cholesterol and low-density lipoprotein (LDL) cholesterol typically involve reduced intake of dietary fats, particularly saturated fats. Evidence suggests a dose-response relationship between saturated fatty acid intake and LDL cholesterol levels (NCEP Expert Panel 2002). Plant sterols and stanols have recently been incorporated into foods such as margarine and can reduce LDL cholesterol by about 10 percent; however, this approach is currently relatively expensive (Law 2000). Dietary advice may also suggest increasing the intake of viscous fiber—for instance, in the form of cereal grains, fruits, and vegetables—because these dietary sources may enhance the lowering of LDL cholesterol. Maintaining bodyweight in the desirable range and engaging in moderate physical activity complement these dietary strategies (NCEP Expert Panel 2002).

Increases in obesity have been related to declines in energy expenditure (for example, reductions in physical activity and adoption of a more sedentary lifestyle) and a higher intake of energy-dense but micronutrient-poor foods, such as most processed foods (WHO 2003b). A variety of trials have recorded beneficial health effects, with weight reduction achieved by a combination of interventions (NHLBI Obesity Education Initiative Expert Panel 1998). These interventions include dietary counseling and therapy that involves a decrease in daily caloric intake and a reduction in saturated fats and total fats. An increase in physical activity is an important component of weight-loss therapy. Behavioral strategies revolving around self-monitoring of eating habits, stress management, problem solving, and social support may also complement these approaches. Overall, however, the effects of lifestyle modifications to reduce weight and maintain the weight loss are relatively poor, with many reports finding that weight returns to baseline levels after several years.

Pharmacological and Surgical Personal Interventions. Randomized trials have shown that medications to lower blood pressure effectively reduce the risk of stroke, IHD, and heart failure. Results from meta-analyses of more than 40 different trials published in 2003 included about 210,000 participants and more than 8,000 stroke and 11,000 IHD events (Blood Pressure Lowering Treatment Trialists' Collaboration 2003; Fox and EUROPA Investigators 2003; Law, Wald, and Rudnicka 2003; Lawes and others 2004; Pepine and others 2003). The trials may be broadly classified into three groups: (a) drug versus placebo trials, (b) more intensive regimens to lower blood pressure versus less intensive regimens, and (c) drug versus drug trials.

The drug versus placebo trials achieved the greatest reductions in blood pressure, and a dose-response relationship was apparent between blood pressure reduction and reduced risk of stroke. Overall, the trials indicated that a 10 mmHg reduction in SBP would result in a 32 percent reduction in stroke risk and a 14 percent relative reduction in IHD risk. This finding is consistent with the size of associations observed in cohort studies.

Clear evidence indicates that all the major drug classes have similar effects on the risk of stroke and coronary heart disease per mmHg reduction in blood pressure (Blood Pressure Lowering Treatment Trialists' Collaboration 2003; Lawes and others 2004). The only clear evidence of clinically important, class-specific effects are with agents that block the renin-angiotensin system, which reduce diabetes incidence by about one-quarter, and with calcium channel blockers, which reduce heart failure less than other agents (although this result may be partly caused by misclassification, because a known side effect of calcium channel blockers is ankle edema, which is a diagnostic component of heart failure). Because all agents lower blood pressure by about the same modest amount and because their effects on blood pressure are additive (Law and others 2003), the key issue seems to be which combinations of two or more drugs should be provided and how long-term adherence can be maximized.

Over the past three decades, numerous trials have assessed the effect of different cholesterol-lowering interventions (Law, Wald, and Rudnicka 2003; Law, Wald, and Thompson 1994). The placebo-controlled trials can be broadly classified into those testing fibrates, statins, and other interventions (mostly dietary interventions, but also some other interventions such as resins and niacin). The statins are the most effective in lowering total and LDL cholesterol, with reductions of more than 1 mmol/l in most trials. A good correlation has been found between reduction in total cholesterol and relative risk reduction. This finding suggests, as for trials investigating blood pressure lowering, that even though some drugs are more effective in achieving greater reductions in risk factors, their effect on disease outcomes is similar per unit reduction of cholesterol. Overall, a 1 mmol/l reduction in total cholesterol is associated with a 21 percent relative risk reduction in IHD and a 17 percent reduction in risk of stroke. Again, this finding is consistent with the epidemiology, with the proviso that the vast majority of strokes in clinical trials were ischemic.

In clinical trials of statins, the relative risk reduction in cardiovascular events is similar at all levels of baseline cholesterol, extending to levels below 5 mmol/l total cholesterol, and is also consistent among patients who are and are not taking concurrent blood pressure lowering and other medications (Heart Protection Study Collaborative Group 2002). Similar findings are observed with treatments to lower blood pressure (Progress Collaborative Group 2001), indicating that these treatment effects are independent. This finding is plausible, because they act through different mechanisms and because observational studies do not suggest a large interaction (Neaton and Wentworth 1992).

The benefits of lowering blood pressure and cholesterol are achieved surprisingly rapidly: for most outcomes, risk appears to be fully reversed within 6 to 18 months of beginning treatment. For example, individuals with cholesterol lowered in the past two or more years are at approximately the same coronary heart disease risk as otherwise identical individuals whose cholesterol has been at that level for decades (Law, Wald, and Thompson 1994).

Pharmacological agents for weight loss that have been subject to randomized controlled trials include dexfenfluramine, sibutramine, orlistat, and phentermine/fenfluramine (although the last has been withdrawn because of a reported association between the drugs and valvular heart disease). Overall, trials suggest only modest weight-loss effects, with an average net weight loss of 1.5 kg after eight weeks and 2 to 3 kg after one year (NHLBI Obesity Education Initiative Expert Panel 1998). A systematic review of orlistat trials indicated a pooled net weight loss of 1.2 kg at 12 weeks, 2.9 to 3.4 kg at one year, and 2.5 to 2.4 kg at two years (O'Meara and others 2001). Results of a systematic review of trials assessing sibutramine were similar (O'Meara and others 2002), with fewer data available on long-term sustained weight loss.

Investigators have also undertaken several randomized controlled trials to assess the effects of different surgical interventions, generally in individuals with a BMI equal to or greater than 35 or 40 kg/m^2. Weight loss resulting from gastric bypass varied from 50 to 100 kg six months to a year following surgery (NHLBI Obesity Education Initiative Expert Panel 1998). Overall, several trials suggest that surgery resulted in about 23 to 37 kg more weight loss than conventional treatment and that this loss was maintained for eight years (Clegg and others 2002). Furthermore, gastric bypass surgery appears to be more beneficial than gastroplasty or jejunoileal bypass.

In relation to compliance and adherence with pharmacological therapy, population surveys have demonstrated that, even in industrial countries, high blood pressure is either untreated or inadequately controlled in about 70 to 75 percent of patients and that adherence to medications among patients suffering from chronic disease is only about 50 percent (WHO 2003a). The extent of poor adherence is likely to be even greater in developing countries given the relative lack of health services and inequities in access. Pharmacotherapy faces a variety of potential barriers, including the symptomless nature of the conditions, a lack of knowledge or denial of risk, the complicated nature of drug regimens, the risk of side effects (real and perceived), and the costs of treatment.

Health providers may use multiple strategies to increase compliance and adherence. Patient-centered interventions include involving individuals in the decision-making process; providing individualized patient education and disease counseling and adapting treatment to patients' lifestyles; simplifying dosing schedules; providing drug information leaflets, medication charts, and special reminder packaging for medications; holding group sessions for education and family-oriented disease management therapies; and implementing automated telephone assessment and self-care education calls with nurse follow-up (Haynes and others 2003).

Strategies may also aim to increase physician adherence, and interventions may include the use of guidelines, peer review and audit, and prompts to remind physicians to review risks and medications (Ebrahim 1998; NCEP Expert Panel 2002). These strategies obviously do not address issues pertaining to resources and access in poor countries.

Several trials and overviews have attempted to assess the value of different interventions to improve compliance and adherence; however, issues have arisen in connection with the generalizability of the interventions, the low statistical power in many trials, the lack of description of all parts of interventions, and the assessment of complex interventions without assessment of the separate effects of the intervention components. Haynes and others' (2003) systematic review concludes that, overall, no single approach to improving adherence can be recommended. Simpler treatment regimens can sometimes improve adherence and treatment outcomes for both short- and long-term treatments. Several complex strategies, including combinations of more thorough patient instructions and counseling, easier access to care, reminders, close follow-up, supervised self-monitoring, family therapy, and rewards for success can improve adherence and treatment outcomes in some patients. However, even the most effective interventions did not lead to large improvements in adherence or treatment outcomes and were relatively resource intensive. By contrast, Connor, Rafter, and Rodgers's (2004) systematic review indicates improved adherence and clinical outcomes with fixed-dose combination treatment or unit-of-use packaging.

Few good, evidence-based strategies to improve obesity management are currently available, although reminder systems, brief training interventions, shared care, inpatient care, and dietitian-led treatments may all be worth further investigation (Harvey and others 2003). Thus, a clear need for innovations still exists to help people follow medication prescriptions as well as dietary and lifestyle advice.

COST-EFFECTIVENESS OF INTERVENTIONS

Costs include expenditures required to identify and treat risk factors as well as expenditures for treating CVD when it is not prevented. Where possible, this chapter deals with the separate sources of costs for several reasons. First, the costs for identifying those requiring treatment vary significantly by level of economic development and by urban versus rural location. In many situations in developing countries, such costs will make most or all forms of screening beyond a determination of CVD history unaffordable. Second, in some countries, such as India, that are large producers of generic drugs, prices are reported to be lower than in most other drug-producing or -importing countries. Third, this approach allows researchers and policy makers to understand the constituent costs so that they can examine where cost reductions may be most beneficial. Fourth, it clarifies what expenditures may be required as a result of changes in decisions about the treatment of risk factors. Finally, many people in developing countries do not have access to hospitals for acute management of CVD events. Nonetheless, increased expenditure on treating risk factors may lead to significant reductions in the costs of treating subsequent CVD events for many countries. Ultimately, the net effect is reflected in cost-effectiveness analyses. Unless otherwise stated, costs are in 2001 U.S. dollars.

The costs of personal interventions include the costs of patient screening (identifying high-risk patients), drugs and their acquisition, clinic visits, health care workers' time, laboratory tests, and travel. Annual drug costs for medications to lower blood pressure and cholesterol vary widely by country and depend on whether generics are available and used. For example, according to the *International Drug Price Indicator Guide* (Management Sciences for Health 2004), annual costs in 2002 of generic 40 mg lovastatin ranged from US$14 in Barbados to US$217 in Costa Rica, and on-patent statins can cost almost a US$1,000 a year in the United States. Because drug costs vary by up to two orders of magnitude across countries, results of cost-effectiveness analyses are particularly sensitive to their input prices. Table 45.3 presents some sample prices. The costs of these medications have dropped considerably in recent years, and now the annual costs for hydrochlorothiazide (25 mg), atenolol (50 mg), and captopril (50 mg), are US$2, US$4, and US$9, respectively (Management Sciences for Health 2004). Statins will become increasingly affordable as simvastatin joins lovastatin in coming off patent (2006 in the United States and already off patent in Germany and the United Kingdom).

The estimated number of visits to manage high blood pressure and cholesterol, under traditional paradigms, ranges from two to six per year at costs ranging from US$3 to US$20 per visit across the six regions assessed, but note that generally many fewer tests and less follow-up is required with a strategy

Table 45.3 Annual Costs of Selected Cardiovascular Medications

Medication	United States (2002 US$)[a]	Average international price (2002 US$)	Projected polypill[b]
Beta-blocker	32–365	3–15	n.a.
Diuretic	6–37	1–3	n.a.
Statin	180–864	11–147	n.a.
Aspirin	2	1–6	n.a.
Angiotensin-converting enzyme inhibitor	65–365	1–19	n.a.
Total	285–1,633	17–190	20–40

Sources: U.S. prices: Murray 2004; international prices: Management Sciences for Health 2004.
n.a. = not applicable.
a. Based on average wholesale prices.
b. Based on a moderate increase from the sum of the lowest-cost generic components.

based on absolute risk. Diagnostic testing for cholesterol in the United States using a general laboratory is reimbursed at US$6 for total cholesterol, US$16 for a complete lipoprotein cholesterol fractionation analysis, and US$6 for triglycerides (Xact Medicare Services 2003). Point-of-care one-step enzymatic strips that require only a few drops of blood from a finger stick and that can process total cholesterol in minutes cost less than US$3 per test (Greenland and others 1987). A basic metabolic panel for those on diuretics or for measuring renal function is US$12. The costs attributed to patient time and travel for visits have not been estimated for many countries, but they were recently estimated at US$12 to US$26 per visit in the United States, depending on age and sex (Prosser and others 2000).

A review of studies to date highlights several issues regarding cost-effectiveness analyses, including the significant variations in terms of calculations of cost per life year saved. The two most important aspects of the cost-effectiveness of any primary intervention are the future risk for CVD of the population treated and the costs of the medications.

Population-Based Interventions

Given the strong association between CVD and high blood pressure, cholesterol, and body mass, most guidelines for those risk factors begin by recommending lifestyle modifications. Although these benefits can lead to changes in risk factors, their effect on CVD events is not well documented. However, on the basis of assumptions about cholesterol and blood pressure reduction from population-based lifestyle education programs and given the relatively low cost of the interventions—US$5 to US$17 per person per year (Tosteson and others 1997)—the cost-effectiveness of such programs may be reasonable. However, the cost-effectiveness ratios of these interventions were sensitive to the cost of the intervention as well as to the expected reduction in the risk factor. For example, a commu-

nity intervention that expects a 4 percent reduction in total serum cholesterol and costs US$5 per person annually targeted would save more than US$2 billion over 25 years of the program. When the North Karelia (Puska 1999) estimates were used in a cost-effectiveness analysis in the United States (Tosteson and others 1997), the cost-effectiveness ratios ranged from being cost saving to US$88,000 (in 1985 U.S. dollars) per life year saved, depending on the percentage reduction in cholesterol (1 to 4 percent).

Personal Interventions to Lower Blood Pressure or Cholesterol in Developed Countries

A common finding of cost-effectiveness analyses of primary prevention of CVD by means of lowering blood pressure and cholesterol is the wide variability in cost-effectiveness ratios, depending on underlying risk, age, and costs of medications. For personal interventions using drug treatment for lowering blood pressure and cholesterol levels, no single cost-effectiveness analysis adequately summarizes experience in the developed countries. Collectively, the studies evaluating hypertension treatment in Australia, New Zealand, the United States, and the Scandinavian countries suggest a range of cost-effectiveness ratios from US$4,600 to more than US$100,000 per life year gained when applied to the entire adult population without further risk stratification (Kupersmith and others 1995). Compared with the entire population, for those at high risk with diastolic blood pressures over 105 mmHg and older than 45, hypertension treatment can cost as little as a few hundred dollars per life year gained or can even be cost saving (Johannesson and others 1991).

Investigators have reported that primary prevention with cholesterol-reducing medications is less attractive overall than other interventions, such as hypertension treatment, from a cost-effectiveness perspective, although once again this finding is likely to differ considerably now that statins are off patent.

Reported cost-effectiveness ratios have ranged from US$10,000 to US$2 million per life year gained (Hay, Yu, and Ashraf 1999), whereas dietary interventions for cholesterol reduction are more favorable, with ratios of around US$2, 000 per quality-adjusted life year (QALY) (Prosser and others 2000). For cholesterol treatment, Prosser and others (2000) find cost-effectiveness ratios of US$50,000 per QALY for on-patent statins among those at highest risk (high cholesterol levels and multiple risk factors) and up to US$1.4 million per QALY among low-risk females when compared with dietary strategy alone. The cost per life year gained in the primary prevention trial of the West of Scotland Coronary Prevention Study among high-risk individuals treated with pravastatin was about US$30,000 (Caro and others 1997). Using the same criteria, Downs and others (1998) find that the cost per life year saved in the Air Force/Texas Coronary Atherosclerosis Prevention Study cohort with average cholesterol levels was more than US$100,000. In general, younger and older age groups tend to have the least favorable cost-effectiveness ratios. For younger groups, this finding probably reflects their overall lower risk and the many years of treatment required before realizing a benefit. For the elderly, high cost-effectiveness ratios may reflect other competing causes of death and the delay of up two years between treatment and benefit seen in most primary prevention trials.

Personal Interventions to Lower Blood Pressure or Cholesterol in Developing Countries

No trials of blood pressure, cholesterol, or body mass lowering have been conducted solely in developing countries. As a result, we have derived assessments of cost-effectiveness by extrapolating from results in developed countries presented earlier. Goldman and others (1991) report that a decline in the cost of lovastatin by 40 percent, once generic, would result in a roughly 30 percent reduction in the cost-effectiveness ratio. However, this finding does not take into account that both the underlying epidemiology and the costs can be quite different across and within countries and regions.

Murray and others (2003) compare 17 nonpersonal and personal health service interventions or combinations of interventions in the 14 epidemiological subregions defined by the World Health Organization (WHO) as part of its Choosing Interventions That Are Cost-Effective (WHO-CHOICE) initiative. The nonpersonal interventions included health education through the mass media and legislative efforts to reduce salt intake, improve blood pressure generally, and reduce cholesterol and obesity levels. The personal interventions included treatment with statins of those above two different cholesterol-level thresholds (greater than 6.2 mmol/l or greater than 5.7 mmol/l), treatment with beta-blockers and diuretics of those above two different hypertension thresholds (greater than 160 mmHg or greater than 140 mmHg), and treatment of individuals with

both hypertension and increased cholesterol with all three medications. Finally, the effects of combination treatment with a beta-blocker, diuretic, statin, and aspirin were modeled for four groups defined on the basis of absolute risk (10-year probability of a cardiovascular event of 5, 15, 25, or 35 percent).

Intervention effects were based on systematic reviews of randomized trials or meta-analyses. Population health effects caused by the interventions were based on stochastically simulating populations on the basis of age, sex, and risk factor distribution of smoking, hypertension, cholesterol, BMI, and smoking in the 14 subregions, both with and without the various treatments to determine the effect. The effects of the intervention were then translated into DALYs using a standard multistate modeling tool. Costs include both program-level costs (media, training, and administration) and patient-level costs (medicines, health care visits, diagnostic tests). All costs were based on a standard ingredients approach and on regional estimations. The costs of CVD events were not included.

The results are summarized in table 45.4. The incremental cost-effectiveness ratios for the strategy assessing absolute risk and using the triple combination of beta-blocker, statin, and aspirin with or without the addition of health education and salt legislation ranged from US$138 per DALY saved (absolute risk greater than 35 percent) in the Africa E region to US$4,319 per DALY saved (absolute risk greater than 5 percent) in the Latin America and the Caribbean B region. These estimates are in international or purchasing-power parity dollars (see chapter 15 for an explanation). Table 45.4 also shows the approximate equivalent costs in U.S. dollars and explains the conversion from the WHO-CHOICE estimates. The nonpersonal interventions, including efforts to reduce salt intake in processed foods, were less costly than the personal interventions. Personal interventions based on treatment guidelines were cost-effective; however, when the strategies for treating high cholesterol or hypertension were compared with the absolute-risk approach, they were not favorable and were dominated by the latter, meaning that the absolute-risk approach of treating those with a greater than 35 percent risk averted more DALYs and cost less than either the blood pressure or cholesterol strategies. For an example of a country-specific analysis, see box 45.1.

Several recent publications have suggested that combination treatments of medications to lower blood pressure, statin, aspirin, and perhaps other agents such as folate could more than halve cardiovascular risk (Wald and Law 2003; WHO 2002; Yusuf 2002). This suggestion is especially relevant for developing countries, given that suitable components are all now off patent. Good evidence indicates that single-pill combinations increase adherence to drug regimens (Connor, Rafter, and Rodgers 2004) and reduce supply and transport costs. We used a Markov model to evaluate the cost-effectiveness of such a hypothetical pill or combination packaging of the individual medications. We modeled the effect of a pill that included half

Table 45.4 Comparison of the Cost-Effectiveness of Absolute Risk with Treatment According to Either Blood Pressure or Lipid Targets Alone in Addition to Population-Based Strategies, Selected WHO Regions

Region	Strategy	Risk (percent)	Incremental cost-effectiveness ratio (cost/DALY saved)[a]	
			International $	US$
Africa E	Prevention (SL and/or HE)		Dominated[b]	
	Targeted risk factors[c]		Dominated[b]	
	Absolute risk[c] (TRI)	35	138	42
		25	778	295
		15	1,445	639
Latin America and the Caribbean B	Prevention (SL)		127	65
	Prevention (SL + HE)		145	74
	Targeted risk factors[c]		Dominated[b]	
	Absolute risk[d] (TRI + SL + HE)	35	286	178
		25	1,598	1,058
		15	2,391	1,664
		5	4,319	3,075
Southeast Asia B	Prevention (SL)		70	18
	Prevention (SL + HE)		127	32
	Targeted risk factors[c]		Dominated[b]	
	Absolute risk[d] (TRI + SL + HE)	35	301	133
		25	1,197	578
		15	2,094	1,120
		5	3,952	2,233
Western Pacific B	Prevention (SL)		97	18
	Targeted risk factors[c]		Dominated[b]	
	Absolute risk[d] (TRI + SL + HE)	35	1,124	423
		25	1,278	564
		15	2,092	1,042
		5	4,028	2,135

Source: Murray and others 2003.

B = low child mortality and low adult mortality; E = high child mortality and very high adult mortality; HE = health education through the mass media to reduce cholesterol; SL = legislation to decrease the salt content of processed foods, including appropriate labeling and enforcement; TRI = treatment with aspirin, beta-blockers, and a statin.

a. Costs of prevention and nondrug costs for treatment according to absolute risk are converted at an estimated regional average ratio of exchange rate to purchasing-power parity rate; drug costs are not converted, assuming drugs to be imported at world prices. The share of drug costs in total treatment cost, as a function of risk, is taken from the estimates for India in table 45.6 and assumed to be the same for all regions.

b. Dominated strategies were both less effective and more costly than comparator strategies.

c. Treating SBP greater than 140 mmHg or 160 mmHg or total cholesterol greater than 5.7 mmol/l or 6.2 mmol/l (220 or 240 mg/dlL).

d. Risk refers to 10-year risk of CVD greater than or equal to the number listed.

of the standard doses of hydrochlorothiazide, atenolol, lisinopril, lovastatin, and aspirin on overall morbidity and mortality in treating those without prior CVD. We did not include folate because no randomized trials had shown that it reduced CVD events at the time of the analysis. The assumptions of the relative risk reductions were based on those of Wald and Law (2003). The strategies compared were for treating various high-risk populations (absolute risk for CVD greater than 15, 25, and 35 percent over 10 years. We applied the model to a population of 1 million adults over the age of 35, with the costs and bene-

fits seen from a societal perspective and with the intervention run for 10 years. We calculated estimates for one representative country from each region where demographic and risk factor data existed. Unlike the WHO-CHOICE analysis, this analysis separated use of the intervention according to those with and without established CVD. Table 45.5 presents the results.

Table 45.6 shows the breakdown of events averted and costs for India. Even though the absolute numbers differ for other countries, the relative differences between the different groups receiving the "polypill" compared with the groups not receiving

Box 45.1

Example of Country-Specific Analysis: South Africa

In another analysis, researchers (Gaziano 2001) compared the approach based on absolute risk with blood pressure guidelines in South Africa. The analysis used country-specific epidemiology and, where available, applied local cost data. The study compared six strategies for initiating drug treatment—two different blood pressure levels (160/95 mmHg and 140/90 mmHg) and four different levels of absolute CVD risk over 10 years (40, 30, 20, and 15 percent)—to a strategy of no treatment. The methodology differed from the WHO-CHOICE study because of the availability of local data. Data on diabetes prevalence were included to further refine risk estimates. Also the actual mix of medications was used to assess costs with actual current drug-use patterns, which included the use of some nongeneric medications.

The table displays the results. The four absolute-risk strategies had the four lowest incremental cost-effectiveness ratios. The strategy of initiating antihypertensive therapy for those individuals with a predicted 10-year CVD risk greater than 40 percent had an incremental cost-effectiveness ratio of US$700 per QALY gained compared with no treatment. The absolute risk of CVD greater than 30, 20, and 15 percent had larger and increasing cost-effectiveness ratios. Treatments based on the 1995 South African guidelines and the Joint National Commission VI guidelines were both more costly and resulted in fewer QALY gains than the 15 percent absolute-risk strategy and were therefore dominated by the less costly absolute-risk treatment strategies.

Furthermore, the results showed that the cost-effectiveness ratios were quite sensitive to the costs of treatment for hypertension, especially medication costs. Further analysis revealed a threshold point for an annual treatment cost of US$53. Below this threshold, the 40 percent absolute-risk strategy cost less and increased the number of life years gained compared with the no primary prevention strategy and is therefore cost saving. In South Africa, annual treatment with diuretics and beta-blockers could be provided for less than US$40.

Incremental Cost-Effectiveness Ratios for Selected Hypertension Management Strategies over 10 Years, South Africa

Treatment	Incremental cost-effectiveness ratio[a]	
	US$/QALY	US$/life year saved[b]
No treatment	n.a.	n.a.
Absolute risk of CVD > 40 percent	700	900
Absolute risk of CVD > 30 percent	1,600	2,100
Absolute risk of CVD > 20 percent	4,900	6,700
Absolute risk of CVD > 15 percent	11,000	18,000
Target level 160/95 mmHg (1995 South African guidelines)[c]	Dominated[d]	Dominated[d]
Target level 140/90 mmHg (Joint National Commission VI guidelines)	Dominated[d]	Dominated[d]

Source: Gaziano and others 2005.
n.a. = not applicable.
a. Each strategy's costs and effects are compared with those of the preceding less costly strategy.
b. Total and incremental life years not shown.
c. Compared with an absolute risk of CVD greater than 15 percent because the 1995 South African guidelines are dominated by the former.
d. A dominated strategy is one that is both more expensive and less effective than the preceding strategy to which it is compared.

Table 45.5 Incremental Cost-Effectiveness Ratios of a Multidrug Regimen by World Bank Region Compared with a Baseline of No Drug Treatment *(2001 US$/DALY)*

Region	35 percent risk	25 percent risk	15 percent risk	5 percent risk
East Asia and the Pacific	830	1,440	2,320	3,820
Europe and Central Asia	940	1,450	1,960	3,620
Latin America and the Caribbean	920	1,470	2,420	3,740
Middle East and North Africa	720	1,290	2,190	4,030
South Asia	670	1,250	1,932	3,020
Sub-Saharan Africa	610	1,170	1,920	2,960

Source: Authors' calculations.
Note: The regimen includes aspirin, a beta-blocker, a thiazide diuretic, an angiotensin-converting enzyme inhibitor, and a statin. The risk refers to a 10-year risk of CVD.

Table 45.6 Polypill Cost-Effectiveness Estimates for a Population of 1 Million Adults at Varying Levels of Risk for CVD Treated for 10 Years in India

Costs and effects	Comparison with no polypill	Absolute risk of a CVD event over 10 years			
		> 35 percent	> 25 percent	> 15 percent	> 5 percent
Total cost (2001 US$ millions)	23.5	34.5	51.4	92.2	205.2
Profile of total costs					
Percentage attributable to inpatient stay	12.0	6.0	3.0	1.0	0.3
Percentage attributable to ambulatory care	0	29.0	40.0	49.0	54.0
Percentage attributable to labor	75.0	36.0	21.0	9.0	2.0
Percentage attributable to pharmaceuticals	0	23.0	31.0	38.0	42.0
Percentage attributable to laboratory expenses	12.0	6.0	3.0	1.0	0.0
Effects[a]					
Number of myocardial infarction cases averted	n.a.	10,200	14,400	21,300	31,800
Number of stroke cases averted	n.a.	5,200	7,000	12,400	19,600
Number of coronary heart disease deaths averted	n.a.	10,500	13,500	19,600	25,900
Number of stroke deaths averted	n.a.	5,900	7,500	10,500	14,200
Number of life years saved	n.a.	39,000	51,000	67,000	98,000
Number of DALYs gained	n.a.	41,000	57,000	86,000	134,000
Incremental cost-effectiveness (US$/DALY)	n.a.	300	990	1,500	2,430

Source: Authors' calculations.
n.a. = not applicable.
a. Each strategy compared with no polypill.

it are similar for all countries. Although the total costs for treating lower-risk patients increase, so do the benefits, and the overall incremental cost-effectiveness ratio remains relatively favorable. The proportion of costs shifts away from those attributable to hospital care when no primary prevention is initiated to costs attributable to ambulatory care and pharmaceuticals when more lower-risk patients are treated.

Interventions to Reduce Bodyweight

No large-scale randomized trials of weight reduction as an isolated intervention are available on which to base estimates of the benefits of weight loss in lowering the risk of coronary heart disease. Thus, costs per life year saved would have to be modeled to project benefits. In one such analysis, a school-based educational program to reduce obesity among middle school students reported a cost of US$4,300 per QALY (L. Wang and others 2003). However, this analysis assumed that the weight loss would be maintained throughout adulthood, but the high relapse rates found in weight reduction studies do not bear out this assumption (Serdula and others 1999). Further research is needed to evaluate the benefits of weight reduction in relation to reducing CVD events and the long-term sustainability of weight loss before reliable cost-effectiveness estimates can be made.

Distributional and Equity Consequences

Failing to translate available evidence from industrial countries about CVD prevention strategies into practicable solutions for developing countries would have clear equity implications, especially when CVD is a large and growing problem in developing countries and when safe and effective interventions that were once extremely expensive are now available for a few cents a day. Because access to cardiovascular health care in developing countries often depends on patients' ability to pay, the poor would stand to benefit the most from a low-cost intervention such as a polypill.

Some see CVD as exclusively a disease of the affluent in developing countries; however, in many developing countries, the transition of CVD to becoming a disease of the poor has already begun—a transition already seen in developed countries around the world. A recent analysis of the distribution of major cardiovascular risks by poverty levels has shown that many cardiovascular risks already affect the poor in the world's poorest countries (Ezzati and others 2004; WHO 2002). Combating the trend requires highly effective, low-cost solutions relevant for most or all of those at risk in developing countries, in contrast to the investments in high-tech treatment interventions that have commonly occurred to date.

ECONOMIC BENEFITS OF INTERVENTION

In the cost-effectiveness analyses, most of the gains are reported in cost savings either from particular interventions, such as decreased hospitalizations resulting from the improved combination therapy of the polypill, or from a more efficient means of screening those at highest risk through an absolute-risk approach. Those who do not die from the sequelae of poorly controlled risk factors for CVD suffer from serious chronic illness, such as stroke and congestive heart failure. Those chronic diseases can result in significant impairments, thereby preventing those affected from continuing to work and sometimes also requiring the services of other family members, who themselves end up having to leave the workforce. Further losses resulting from disability include the loss of wages for major wage earners and their families and the state's losses in terms of disability compensation. Leeder and others (2004) estimate that in 2000 the cost of CVD disability payments in South Africa equaled US$70 million.

However, many other indirect economic gains or losses are not included in the economic analysis, such as gains or losses in productivity. Leeder and others (2004) report that, at current CVD mortality rates, the potential productive years of life lost (defined as those years between the ages of 35 and 64) will nearly double by 2030. Those later adult working years are particularly important, given the many years of investment in skills through formal education and experience that would be lost. Preventing CVD would therefore improve the size and skills of the workforce and would therefore aid economic development. For those reasons, the Commission for Macroeconomics and Health has recommended that any intervention that costs less than triple a country's per capita gross domestic product be regarded as cost-effective (WHO 2001). Many of the combination cardiovascular preventive approaches outlined in this chapter comfortably satisfy that criterion.

RESEARCH AND DEVELOPMENT AGENDA

The cost-effectiveness data reviewed in this chapter indicate that the best use of resources for personal-level interventions for preventing CVD mediated by high blood pressure, cholesterol, and bodyweight would be combination medications targeted to those at high absolute risk. This strategy represents a considerable departure from existing paradigms, such as hypertension treatment. Research and development is therefore required in several areas to develop, implement, and evaluate this strategy. This research could include several themes as follows:

- Refine absolute risk-based treatment in developing country settings:
  - Evaluate optimal communications to the public and to health professionals that explain the rationale for this

new paradigm and its advantages over traditional paradigms, such as hypertension treatment. One barrier to adopting preventive therapy based on absolute risk has been its relative complexity compared with dichotomous diagnosis-based strategies, such as hypertension–no hypertension.
  - Develop simple methods for predicting absolute risk using straightforward, inexpensive, direct measures, such as physical examination, clinical history, and on-site tests. These methods would likely involve low-cost algorithms completed by a multipurpose health care worker involving, for example, the collection of data on age, sex, tobacco use, blood pressure, waist circumference, and urine dipstick results. The development of different levels of screening protocol may also be needed in certain settings.
  - Calibrate existing algorithms for different disease rates and cardiovascular profiles in developing countries.
  - Develop treatment algorithms that can easily be adopted in resource-poor settings by, for example, multipurpose health care workers.
  - Develop methods for predicting absolute risk on the basis of the probability of lost healthy life years as well as the probability of a clinical event. This strategy could mean developing an index of healthy life years at risk from a cardiovascular event in the next five years, which would require taking case fatalities into consideration and discounting. A major barrier to adopting a strategy based on absolute risk has been the absence of a time-based measure and, hence, the equal value placed on preventing an event at a young and at an old age.
- Develop and evaluate combination treatments:
  - Carry out new research on the ideal combinations for different patient groups and populations at different stages of the health transition. Local initiatives would be needed to determine the ideal combination of medications based principally on cost, tolerability, and ability to lower risk-factor levels. One default set of interventions could be an angiotensin-converting enzyme inhibitor (for example, enalapril or lisinopril); a diuretic (such as hydrochlorothiazide or chlothalidone); a statin (for instance, simvastatin or lovastatin); and low-dose aspirin.
  - Measure the potential costs and benefits of adding other active agents, such as vitamins or diabetic medications.
  - Quantify the extent of improved access, acceptability, and tolerability for people with symptomatic vascular disease who have established indications for those medications.
  - Evaluate the benefits and costs in developing countries with large-scale clinical trials and demonstration projects, both among patients who have established indications (compared with usual care) and among those

who do not have clear indications but are still at high risk (compared with a placebo).

- o Evaluate the advantages and disadvantages of a polypill versus unit-of-use packs and other novel delivery strategies.
- Investigate weight-loss initiatives:
  - o Develop strategies to improve the effectiveness of personal interventions to reduce bodyweight in developing countries.
  - o Evaluate the use of gastric surgery for weight loss in the extremely obese in selected settings.
- Assess technology:
  - o Screen which technologies should be transferred to developing countries on the basis of cost-effectiveness criteria.
  - o Design new technologies specifically for use by community health workers (for example, point-of-care devices).
- Review public and personal health services:
  - o Carry out a critical evaluation of community health workers versus trained health professionals in delivering simplified screening and treatment regimens.
  - o Provide guideline assistance for CVD prevention and management to regional and country-specific ministers of health and policy makers.
  - o Support demonstration projects to determine the limitations for managing chronic conditions in resource-poor settings.

CONCLUSIONS

The analyses presented in this chapter indicate that providing off-patent blood pressure and cholesterol-lowering medications targeted at those at high absolute risk seems to be a cost-effective strategy. Currently available personal interventions to prevent or reduce high BMI are likely to be much less cost-effective.

An approach based on absolute risk will still involve choosing some level below which people are not recommended for personal treatments, which will leave some people at risk of progression of vascular disease. This issue exists with current paradigms and underscores the need for parallel improvements in population-based prevention. The strategy based on absolute risk must be regarded as complementary to populationwide initiatives that address the root causes of CVD—in particular, the societal determinants that lead to high salt and saturated fat in the diet in relation to high blood pressure and cholesterol and high-energy diets coupled with decreasing physical activity in relation to high bodyweight. Preventing and reducing those risks in developing countries will reduce the need for medication-based prevention strategies in the coming decades.

REFERENCES

Alderman, M. H. 1996. "Blood Pressure J-Curve: Is It Cause or Effect?" *Current Opinion in Nephrology and Hypertension* 5 (3): 209–13.

Anderson, K. M., P. M. Odell, P. W. Wilson, and W. B. Kannel. 1991. "Cardiovascular Disease Risk Profiles." *American Heart Journal* 121 (1, part 2): 293–98.

Appel, L. J., T. J. Moore, E. Obarzanek, W. M. Vollmer, L. P. Svetkey, F. M. Sacks, and others. 1997. "A Clinical Trial of the Effects of Dietary Patterns on Blood Pressure: DASH Collaborative Research Group." *New England Journal of Medicine* 336 (16): 1117–24.

Asia Pacific Cohort Studies Collaboration. 1999. "Determinants of Cardiovascular Disease in the Asia Pacific Region: Protocol for a Collaborative Overview of Cohort Studies." *CVD Prevention* 2: 281–89.

———. 2003a. "Blood Pressure and Cardiovascular Disease in the Asia Pacific Region." *Journal of Hypertension* 21: 707–16.

———. 2003b. "Cholesterol, Coronary Heart Disease, and Stroke in the Asia Pacific Region." *International Journal of Epidemiology* 32: 563–72.

———. 2004. "Body Mass Index and Cardiovascular Disease in the Asia-Pacific Region: An Overview of 33 Cohorts Involving 305,000 Participants." *International Journal of Epidemiology* 33: 1–8.

Assmann, G., P. Cullen, and H. Schulte. 2002. "Simple Scoring Scheme for Calculating the Risk of Acute Coronary Events Based on the 10-Year Follow-up of the Prospective Cardiovascular Munster (PROCAM) Study." *Circulation* 105: 310–15.

Blood Pressure Lowering Treatment Trialists' Collaboration. 2003. "Effects of Different Blood-Pressure-Lowering Regimens on Major Cardiovascular Events: Results of Prospectively Designed Overviews of Randomised Trials: Blood Pressure Lowering Treatment Trialists' Collaboration." *Lancet* 362 (9395): 1527–35.

Bobak, M., Z. Skodova, Z. Pisa, R. Poledne, and M. Marmot. 1997. "Political Changes and Trends in Cardiovascular Risk Factors in the Czech Republic, 1985–92." *Journal of Epidemiology and Community Health* 51 (3): 272–77.

Calle, E. E., M. J. Thun, J. M. Pettrelli, C. Rodriguez, and C. Heath. 1999. "Body Mass Index and Mortality in a Prospective Cohort of U.S. Adults." *New England Journal of Medicine* 341 (15): 1097–1105.

Caro, J., W. Klittich, A. McGuire, I. Ford, J. Norrie, and D. Pettitt. 1997. "The West of Scotland Coronary Prevention Study: Economic Benefit Analysis of Primary Prevention with Pravastatin." *British Medical Journal* 315: 1577–82.

Chobanian, A. V., G. L. Bakris, H. R. Black, W. C. Cushman, L. A. Green, I. L. Izzo Jr., and others. 2003. "The Seventh Report of the Joint National Committee on Prevention, Detection, Evaluation, and Treatment of High Blood Pressure: The JNC 7 Report." *Journal of the American College of Cardiology* 289 (19): 2560–72.

Clegg, A. J., J. Colquitt, M. K. Sidhu, P. Royle, E. Loveman, and A. Walker. 2002. "The Clinical Effectiveness and Cost-Effectiveness of Surgery for People with Morbid Obesity: A Systematic Review and Economic Evaluation." *Health Technology Assessment* (Winchester, U.K.) 6 (12): 1–153.

Connor, J., N. Rafter, and A. Rodgers. 2004. "Do Fixed-Dose Combination Pills or Unit-of-Use Packaging Improve Adherence? A Systematic Review." *Bulletin of World Health Organization* 82: 935–39.

Cruickshank, J. M. 1994. "J-Curve in Antihypertensive Therapy: Does It Exist? A Personal Point of View." *Cardiovascular Drugs and Therapy* 8 (5): 757–60.

D'Agostino, R. B., A. J. Belanger, W. B. Kannel, and J. M. Cruickshank. 1991. "Relation of Low Diastolic Blood Pressure to Coronary Heart Disease Death in Presence of Myocardial Infarction: The Framingham Study." *British Medical Journal* 303 (6799): 385–89.

Downs, J. R., M. Clearfield, S. Weis, E. Whitney, D. R. Shapiro, P. A. Beere, and others. 1998. "Primary Prevention of Acute Coronary Events with Lovastatin in Men and Women with Average Cholesterol

Levels: Results of AFCAPS/TexCAPS—Air Force/Texas Coronary Atherosclerosis Prevention Study." *Journal of the American Medical Association* 279 (20): 1615–22.

Ebrahim, S. 1998. "Detection, Adherence, and Control of Hypertension for the Prevention of Stroke: A Systematic Review." *Health Technology Assessment* (Winchester, U.K.) 2 (11): i–iv, 1–78.

Evans, A., H. Tolonen, H. W. Hense, M. Ferrario, S. Sans, K. Kuulasmaa, and others. 2001. "Trends in Coronary Risk Factors in the WHO MONICA Project." *International Journal of Epidemiology* 30 (Suppl. 1): S35–40.

Ezzati, M., A. Lopez, A. Rodgers, S. Vander Hoorn, and C. J. L. Murray, eds. 2004. *Comparative Quantification of Health Risks: Global and Regional Burden of Disease Attributable to Selected Major Risk Factors.* Geneva: World Health Organization.

Ezzati, M., S. Vander Hoorn, A. Rodgers, A. D. Lopez, C. D. Mathers, C. J. L. Murray, and others. 2003. "Estimates of Global and Regional Potential Health Gains from Reducing Multiple Major Risk Factors." *Lancet* 362: 271–80.

Farnett, L., C. D. Mulrow, W. D. Linn, C. R. Lucey, and M. R. Tuley. 1991. "The J-Curve Phenomenon and the Treatment of Hypertension. Is There a Point Beyond Which Pressure Reduction Is Dangerous?" *Journal of the American Medical Association* 265 (4): 489–95.

Feinleib, M. 1996. "New Directions for Community Intervention Studies." *American Journal of Public Health* 86 (12): 696–98.

Field, A. E., E. H. Coakley, A. Must, J. L. Spadano, N. Laird, W. H. Dietz, and others. 2001. "Impact of Overweight on the Risk of Developing Common Chronic Diseases during a 10-Year Period." *Archives of Internal Medicine* 161: 1581–86.

Flack, J. M., J. Neaton, R. Grimm Jr., J. Shih, J. Cutler, K. Ensrud, and others. 1995. "Blood Pressure and Mortality among Men with Prior Myocardial Infarction: Multiple Risk Factor Intervention Trial Research Group." *Circulation* 92 (9): 2437–45.

Fox, K. M. and EUROPA (European Trial on Reduction of Cardiac Events with Perindopril in Stable Coronary Artery Disease) Investigators. 2003. "Efficacy of Perindopril in Reduction of Cardiovascular Events among Patients with Stable Coronary Artery Disease: Randomised, Double-Blind, Placebo-Controlled, Multicentre Trial (the EUROPA Study)." *Lancet* 362 (9386): 782–88.

Gaziano, T. A., K. Steyn, D. J. Cohen, M. C. Weinstein, and L. H. Opie. 2005. "Cost-Effectiveness Analysis of Hypertension Guidelines in South Africa: Absolute Risk versus Blood Pressure Level." *Circulation* 112 (23): 3569–76.

Goldman, L., M. C. Weinstein, P. A. Goldman, and L. W. Williams. 1991. "Cost-Effectiveness of HMG-CoA Reductase Inhibition for Primary and Secondary Prevention of Coronary Heart Disease." *Journal of the American Medical Association* 265: 1145–51.

Greenland, P., J. C. Levenkron, M. G. Radley, J. G. Baggs, R. A. Manchester, and N. L. Bowley. 1987. "Feasibility of Large-Scale Cholesterol Screening: Experience with a Portable Capillary-Blood Testing Device." *American Journal of Public Health* 77: 73–75.

Hansson, L., L. H. Lindholm, T. Ekbom, B. Dahlof, J. Lanke, B. Schersten, and others. 1999. "Randomised Trial of Old and New Antihypertensive Drugs in Elderly Patients: Cardiovascular Mortality and Morbidity—The Swedish Trial in Old Patients with Hypertension-2 Study." *Lancet* 354 (9192): 1751–56.

Haq, I. U., L. E. Ramsay, W. W. Yeo, P. R. Jackson, and E. J. Wallis. 1999. "Is the Framingham Risk Function Valid for Northern European Populations? A Comparison of Methods for Estimating Absolute Coronary Risk in High Risk Men." *Heart* 81 (1): 40–46.

Harvey, E. L., A. M. Glenny, S. F. L. Kirk, and C. D. Summerbell. 2003. "Improving Health Professionals' Management and the Organisation of Care for Overweight and Obese People." Cochrane Database of Systematic Reviews (1).

Hay, J. W., W. M. Yu, and T. Ashraf. 1999. "Pharmacoeconomics of Lipid-Lowering Agents for Primary and Secondary Prevention of Coronary Artery Disease." *Pharmacoeconomics* 15: 47–74.

Haynes, R. B., H. McDonald, A. X. Garg, and P. Montague. 2003. "Interventions for Helping Patients to Follow Prescriptions for Medications." Cochrane Database of Systematic Reviews (1).

He, J., M. J. Klag, P. K. Whelton, J. Y. Chen, J. P. Mo, M. C. Qian, and others. 1991. "Migration, Blood Pressure Pattern, and Hypertension: The Yi Migrant Study." *American Journal of Epidemiology* 134 (10): 1085–1101.

He, J., G. S. Tell, Y. C. Tang, P. S. Mo, and G. Q. He. 1991. "Effect of Migration on Blood Pressure: The Yi People Study." *Epidemiology* 2 (2): 88–97.

Heart Protection Study Collaborative Group. 2002. "MRC/BHF Heart Protection Study of Cholesterol Lowering with Simvastatin in 20,536 High-Risk Individuals: A Randomised Placebo-Controlled Trial." *Lancet* 360 (9326): 7–22.

Hodgson, T. A., and L. Cai. 2001. "Medical Care Expenditures for Hypertension, Its Complications, and Its Comorbidities." *Medical Care* 39: 599–615.

Iso, H., D. R. Jacobs Jr., D. Wentworth, J. D. Neaton, and J. D. Cohen. 1989. "Serum Cholesterol Levels and Six-Year Mortality from Stroke in 350,977 Men Screened for the Multiple Risk Factor Intervention Trial." *New England Journal of Medicine* 320 (14): 904–10.

Jackson, R., P. Barham, J. Bills, T. Birch, L. McLennan, S. MacMahon, and others. 1993. "Management of Raised Blood Pressure in New Zealand: A Discussion Document." *British Medical Journal* 307: 107–10.

Johannesson, M., L. Borgquist, B. Jonsson, and L. Rastam. 1991. "The Costs of Treating Hypertension: An Analysis of Different Cutoff Points." *Health Policy* 18 (2): 141–50.

Joseph, J. G., I. A. Prior, C. E. Salmond, and D. Stanley. 1983. "Elevation of Systolic and Diastolic Blood Pressure Associated with Migration: The Tokelau Island Migrant Study." *Journal of Chronic Diseases* 36 (7): 507–16.

Kannel, W. B., R. B. D'Agostino, and H. Silbershatz. 1997. "Blood Pressure and Cardiovascular Morbidity and Mortality Rates in the Elderly." *American Heart Journal* 134 (4): 758–63.

Kaplan, N. M. 1995. "Alcohol and Hypertension." *Lancet* 345 (8965): 1588–89.

Kupersmith, J., M. Holmes-Rovner, A. Hogan, D. Rovner, and J. Gardiner. 1995. "Cost-Effectiveness Analysis in Heart Disease, Part II: Preventive Therapies." *Progress in Cardiovascular Diseases* 37: 243–71.

Law, M. 2000. "Plant Sterol and Stanol Margarines and Health." *British Medical Journal* 320: 861–64.

Law, M., C. Frost, and N. Wald. 1991. "By How Much Does Dietary Salt Reduction Lower Blood Pressure? III: Analysis of Data from Trials of Salt Reduction." *British Medical Journal* 302: 819–24.

Law, M. R., N. J. Wald, J. K. Morris, and R. E. Jordan. 2003. "Value of Low Dose Combination Treatment with Blood Pressure Lowering Drugs: Analysis of 354 Randomised Trials." *British Medical Journal* 326 (7404): 1427.

Law, M. R., N. J. Wald, and A. R. Rudnicka. 2003. "Quantifying Effect of Statins on Low Density Lipoprotein Cholesterol, Ischaemic Heart Disease, and Stroke: Systematic Review and Meta-Analysis." *British Medical Journal* 326 (7404): 1423.

Law, M. R., N. J. Wald, and S. G. Thompson. 1994. "By How Much and How Quickly Does Reduction in Serum Cholesterol Concentration Lower Risk of Ischaemic Heart Disease?" *British Medical Journal* 308 (6925): 367–72.

Law, M. R., H. C. Watt, and N. J. Wald. 2002. "The Underlying Risk of Death after Myocardial Infarction in the Absence of Treatment." *Archives of Internal Medicine* 162 (21): 2405–10.

Lawes, C. M. M., D. A. Bennett, V. L. Feigin, and A. Rodgers. 2004. "Blood Pressure and Stroke: An Overview of Published Reviews." *Stroke* 35: 776–85.

Leeder, S., S. Raymond, H. Greenburg, H. Liu, and K. Esson. 2004. *A Race against Time: The Challenge of Cardiovascular Disease in Developing Economies.* New York: Columbia University.

MacMahon, S., A. Rodgers, B. Neal, and J. Chalmers. 1997. "Blood Pressure Lowering for the Secondary Prevention of Myocardial Infarction and Stroke." *Hypertension* 29: 537–38.

Management Sciences for Health. 2004. *International Drug Price Indicator Guide.* Washington, DC: Management Sciences for Health.

Manson, J. E., W. C. Willett, and M. J. Stampfer. 1995. "Body Weight and Mortality among Women." *New England Journal of Medicine* 333 (11): 677–85.

McMurray, J., and G. T. McInnes. 1992. "The J-Curve Hypothesis." *Lancet* 339 (8792): 561–62.

Mittelmark, M. B., M. K. Hunt, G. W. Heath, and T. L. Schmid. 1993. "Realistic Outcomes: Lessons from Community-Based Research and Demonstration Programs for the Prevention of Cardiovascular Diseases." *Journal of Public Health Policy* 14 (4): 437–62.

Monteiro, C. A., W. L. Conde, B. Lu, and B. M. Popkin. 2004. "Obesity and Inequities in Health in the Developing World." *International Journal of Obesity* 28: 1181–86.

Murray, C. J. L., J. A. Lauer, R. C. W. Hutubessy, L. Niessen, N. Tomijima, A. Rodgers, and others. 2003. "Reducing the Risk of Cardiovascular Disease: Effectiveness and Costs of Interventions to Reduce Systolic Blood Pressure and Cholesterol: A Global and Regional Analysis." *Lancet* 361: 717–25.

Murray, L., ed. 2004. *Red Book.* Montvale, NJ: Thomson Physicians Desk Reference.

NCEP (National Cholesterol Education Program) Expert Panel. 2002. Third Report of the Expert Panel on Detection, Evaluation, and Treatment of High Blood Cholesterol in Adults (Adult Treatment Panel III). Bethesda, MD: National Institutes of Health, National Heart, Lung, and Blood Institute.

Neaton, J. D., and D. Wentworth 1992. "Serum Cholesterol, Blood Pressure, Cigarette Smoking, and Death from Coronary Heart Disease: Overall Findings and Differences by Age for 316,099 White Men—Multiple Risk Factor Intervention Trial Research Group." *Archives of Internal Medicine* 152 (1): 56–64.

NHLBI (National Heart, Lung, and Blood Institute) Obesity Education Initiative Expert Panel 1998. *Clinical Guidelines on the Identification, Evaluation, and Treatment of Overweight and Obesity in Adults.* Bethesda, MD: National Institutes of Health, NHLBI.

Nissinen, A., X. Berrios, and P. Puska. 2001. "Community-Based Noncommunicable Disease Interventions: Lessons from Developed Countries for Developing Ones." *Bulletin of the World Health Organization* 79 (10): 963–70.

O'Meara, S., R. Riemsma, L. Shirran, L. Mather, and G. ter Riet. 2001. "A Rapid and Systematic Review of the Clinical Effectiveness and Cost-Effectiveness of Orlistat in the Management of Obesity." *Health Technology Assessment* (Winchester, U.K.) 5 (18): 1–81.

———. 2002. "The Clinical Effectiveness and Cost-Effectiveness of Sibutramine in the Management of Obesity: A Technology Assessment." *Health Technology Assessment* (Winchester, U.K.) 6 (6): 1–97.

Pepine, C. J., E. M. Handberg, R. M. Cooper-DeHoff, R. G. Marks, P. Kowey, F. H. Messerli, and others. 2003. "A Calcium Antagonist vs. a Non-Calcium Antagonist Hypertension Treatment Strategy for Patients with Coronary Artery Disease—The International Verapamil-Trandolapril Study (INVEST): A Randomized Controlled Trial." *Journal of the American Medical Association* 290 (21): 2805–16.

Pestana, J. A., K. Steyn, A. Leiman, and G. M. Hartzenberg. 1996. "The Direct and Indirect Costs of Cardiovascular Disease in South Africa in 1991." *South African Medical Journal* 86 (6): 679–84.

Pfeffer, M. A. 1993. "Angiotensin-Converting Enzyme Inhibition in Congestive Heart Failure: Benefit and Perspective." *American Heart Journal* 126 (3, part 2): 789–93.

Poulter, N. R. 1999. "Coronary Heart Disease Is a Multifactorial Disease." *American Journal of Hypertension* 12 (10, part 2): 92–95S.

Poulter, N. R., K. T. Khaw, and P. S. Sever. 1988. "Higher Blood Pressures of Urban Migrants from an African Low-Blood Pressure Population Are Not Due to Selective Migration." *American Journal of Hypertension* 1 (3 Pt. 3): 143S–45S.

Poulter, N. R., and P. Sever. 1994. "Blood Pressure in Other Populations: A. Low Blood Pressure Populations and the Impact of Rural-Urban Migration." In *Textbook of Hypertension,* ed. J. Swales, 22–36. Oxford, U.K.: Blackwell Scientific Publications.

Progress Collaborative Group. 2001. "Randomised Trial of a Perindopril-Based Blood-Pressure-Lowering Regimen among 6,105 Individuals with Previous Stroke or Transient Ischaemic Attack." *Lancet* 358 (9287): 1033–41.

Prospective Studies Collaboration. 1995. "Cholesterol, Diastolic Blood Pressure, and Stroke: 13,000 Strokes in 45,000 People in 45 Prospective Cohorts." *Lancet* 346: 1647–53.

———. 2002. "Age-Specific Relevance of Usual Blood Pressure to Vascular Mortality: A Meta-Analysis of Individual Data for One Million Adults in 61 Prospective Studies." *Lancet* 360: 1903–13.

Prosser, L. A., A. A. Stinnett, P. A. Goldman, L. W. Williams, M. G. Hunink, and L. Goldman. 2000. "Cost-Effectiveness of Cholesterol-Lowering Therapies According to Selected Patient Characteristics." *Annals of Internal Medicine* 132: 769–79.

Puska, P. 1999. "The North Karelia Project: From Community Intervention to National Activity in Lowering Cholesterol Levels and CHD Risk." *European Heart Journal* 1 (Suppl.): S9–13.

Ramsay, L. E., B. Williams, G. D. Johnston, G. A. MacGregor, L. Poston, J. F. Potter, and others. 1999. "British Hypertension Society Guidelines for Hypertension Management 1999: Summary." *British Medical Journal* 319 (7210): 630–35.

Rose, G. 1981. "Strategy of Prevention: Lessons from Cardiovascular Disease." *British Medical Journal* 282: 1847–51.

———. 1985. "Sick Individuals and Sick Populations." *International Journal of Epidemiology* 14: 32–38.

Salmond, C. E., J. G. Joseph, I. A. Prior, D. G. Stanley, and A. F. Wessen. 1985. "Longitudinal Analysis of the Relationship between Blood Pressure and Migration: The Tokelau Island Migrant Study." *American Journal of Epidemiology* 122 (2): 291–301.

Salmond, C. E., I. A. Prior, and A. F. Wessen. 1989. "Blood Pressure Patterns and Migration: A 14-Year Cohort Study of Adult Tokelauans." *American Journal of Epidemiology* 130 (1): 37–52.

Schooler, C., J. W. Farquhar, S. P. Fortmann, and J. A. Flora. 1997. "Synthesis of Findings and Issues from Community Prevention Trials." *Annals of Epidemiology* 7 (Suppl.): S54–68.

Serdula, M., A. Mokad, D. Williamson, D. Galuska, J. Mendlein, and G. Heath. 1999. "Prevalence of Attempting Weight Loss and Strategies for Controlling Weight." *Journal of the American Medical Association* 282 (14): 1353–58.

Sleight, P. 1997a. "Lowering of Blood Pressure and Artery Stiffness." *Lancet* 349 (9048): 362.

———. 1997b. "Lowering of Blood Pressure and Artery Stiffness." *Lancet* 349 (9056): 955–56.

Staessen, J., R. Fagard, L. Thijs, H. Celis, G. Arabidze, W. Birkenhager, and others. 1997. "Randomised Double-Blind Comparison of Placebo and Active Treatment for Older Patients with Isolated Systolic Hypertension." *Lancet* 350: 757–64.

Stevens, J., J. Cai, E. R. Pamuk, D. F. Williamson, M. J. Thun, and J. L. Wood. 1998. "The Effect of Age on the Association between Body-Mass Index and Mortality." *New England Journal of Medicine* 338 (1): 1–7.

Stewart, I. M. 1979. "Relation of Reduction in Pressure to First Myocardial Infarction in Patients Receiving Treatment for Severe Hypertension." *Lancet* 1 (8121): 861–65.

Suh, I. 2001. "Cardiovascular Mortality in Korea: A Country Experiencing Epidemiologic Transition." *Acta Cardiologica* 56 (2): 75–81.

Susser, M. 1995. "The Tribulations of Trials—Intervention in Communities." *American Journal of Public Health* 85 (2): 156–58.

Swinburn, B., T. Ashton, J. Gillespie, B. Cox, A. Menon, D. Simmons, and others. 1997. "Health Care Costs of Obesity in New Zealand." *International Journal of Obesity and Related Metabolic Disorders: Journal of the International Association for the Study of Obesity* 21: 891–96.

Tosteson, A. N. A., M. C. Weinstein, M. G. M. Hunink, M. A. Mittleman, L. W. Williams, P. A. Goldman, and others. 1997. "Cost-Effectiveness of Populationwide Educational Approaches to Reduce Serum Cholesterol Levels." *Circulation* 95: 24–30.

Troiano, R. P., E. A. Frongillo, J. Sobal, and D. A. Levitsky. 1996. "The Relationship between Body Weight and Mortality: A Quantitative Analysis of Combined Information from Existing Studies." *International Journal of Obesity and Related Metabolic Disorders* 20: 63–75.

Uusitalo, U., E. J. Feskens, J. Tuomilehto, G. Dowse, U. Haw, D. Fareed, and others. 1996. "Fall in Total Cholesterol Concentration over Five Years in Association with Changes in Fatty Acid Composition of Cooking Oil in Mauritius: Cross-Sectional Survey." *British Medical Journal* 313 (7064): 1044–46.

Wald, N. J., and M. R. Law 2003. "A Strategy to Reduce Cardiovascular Disease by More Than 80 Percent." *British Medical Journal* 326 (7404): 1419.

Wang, G., Z. J. Zheng, G. Heath, C. Macera, M. Pratt, and D. Buchner. 2002. "Economic Burden of Cardiovascular Disease Associated with Excess Body Weight in U.S. Adults." *American Journal of Preventive Medicine* 23: 1–6.

Wang, L. Y., Q. Yang, R. Lowry, and H. Wechsler. 2003. "Economic Analysis of a School-Based Obesity Prevention Program." *Obesity Research* 11: 1313–24.

Whelton, P. K., L. J. Appel, M. A. Espeland, W. B. Applegate, W. H. Ettinger Jr., J. B. Kostis, and others. 1998. "Sodium Reduction and Weight Loss in the Treatment of Hypertension in Older Persons: A Randomized Controlled Trial of Nonpharmacologic Interventions in the Elderly (TONE): TONE Collaborative Research Group." *Journal of the American Medical Association* 279 (11): 839–46.

WHO (World Health Organization). 2001. *Macroeconomics and Health: Investing in Health for Economic Development—Report of the Commission on Macroeconomics and Health.* Geneva: WHO. http://www.cmhealth.org/.

———. 2002. *World Health Report 2002: Reducing Risks, Promoting Healthy Life.* Geneva: WHO.

———. 2003a. *Adherence to Long-Term Therapies: Evidence for Action.* Geneva: WHO.

———. 2003b. *Diet, Nutrition, and the Prevention of Chronic Diseases.* Geneva: WHO.

Willett, W. C., J. E. Manson, M. J. Stampfer, G. A. Colditz, B. Rosner, F. E. Speizer, and others. 1995. "Weight, Weight Change, and Coronary Heart Disease in Women: Risk within the 'Normal' Weight Range." *Journal of the American Medical Association* 273 (6): 461–65.

Wood, D., G. De Backer, O. Faergeman, I. Graham, G. Mancia, K. Pyorala, and others. 1998. "Prevention of Coronary Heart Disease in Clinical Practice: Summary of Recommendations of the Second Joint Task Force of European and other Societies on Coronary Prevention." *Journal of Hypertension* 16: 1404–14.

Wu, X., Z. Huang, J. Stamler, Y. Wu, Y. Li, A. R. Folsom, and others. 1996. "Changes in Average Blood Pressure and Incidence of High Blood Pressure 1983–1984 to 1987–1988 in Four Population Cohorts in the People's Republic of China: The PRC-USA Cardiovascular and Cardiopulmonary Epidemiology Research Group." *Journal of Hypertension* 14 (11): 1267–74.

Xact Medicare Services. 2003. *Medicare Clinical Laboratory Fee Schedule.* Camp Hill, PA: Xact Medicare Services.

Yusuf, S. 2002. "Two Decades of Progress in Preventing Vascular Disease." *Lancet* 360 (9326): 2–3.

Chapter **46**

Tobacco Addiction

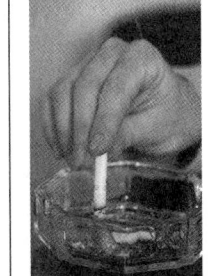

Prabhat Jha, Frank J. Chaloupka, James Moore, Vendhan
Gajalakshmi, Prakash C. Gupta, Richard Peck, Samira Asma,
and Witold Zatonski

Cigarette smoking and other forms of tobacco use impose a large and growing global public health burden. Worldwide, tobacco use is estimated to kill about 5 million people annually, accounting for 1 in every 5 male deaths and 1 in 20 female deaths of those over age 30. On current smoking patterns, annual tobacco deaths will rise to 10 million by 2030. The 21st century is likely to see 1 billion tobacco deaths, most of them in low-income countries. In contrast, the 20th century saw 100 million tobacco deaths, most of them in Western countries and the former socialist economies.

Hundreds of millions of premature tobacco deaths could be avoided if effective interventions were widely applied in low- and middle-income countries. Numerous studies from high-income countries and a growing number from low- and middle-income countries provide robust evidence that tobacco tax increases, timely dissemination of information about the health risks of smoking, restrictions on smoking in public and workplaces, comprehensive bans on advertising and promotion, and increased access to cessation therapies are effective in reducing tobacco use and its consequences. Cessation by the 1.1 billion current smokers is central to meaningful reductions in tobacco deaths over the next five decades. New analyses presented here find that higher tobacco taxes could prevent 3 million tobacco deaths by 2030 among smokers alive today. Reduced uptake of smoking by children would yield benefits chiefly after 2050. Price and non-price interventions are, for the most part, highly cost-effective.

This chapter begins with an overview of smoking trends and tobacco's health consequences, followed by a discussion of the economic rationale for government intervention, with a focus on the uniquely addictive properties of nicotine. A review of the effectiveness of tobacco-control policies in reducing tobacco initiation and in increasing cessation follows. A cost-effectiveness analysis of these interventions is provided. Finally, the constraints to implementing tobacco-control policies are discussed.

SMOKING TRENDS

Tobacco use, in both smoked and nonsmoked forms, is common worldwide. This chapter focuses on smoked tobacco, chiefly cigarettes and *bidis* (tobacco hand rolled in the leaf of another plant, *temburi*, which is popular in India and parts of Southeast Asia), because smoked tobacco is more common—accounting for about 65 to 85 percent of all tobacco produced worldwide (WHO 1997)—and causes more disease and more diverse types of disease than does oral tobacco use.

Prevalence

A systematic review of 139 studies on adult smoking prevalence (Jha and others 2002) found that more than 1.1 billion people worldwide smoke, with about 82 percent of smokers residing in low- and middle-income countries. Table 46.1 provides an update of these estimates for the population in 2000. Globally, male smoking far exceeds female smoking, with a smaller gender difference in high-income countries. Smoking prevalence is highest in Europe and Central Asia, where 35 percent of all adults are smokers.

While overall smoking prevalence continues to increase in many low- and middle-income countries, many high-income countries have witnessed decreases, most clearly in men. A

Table 46.1 Estimated Smoking Prevalence (by Gender) and Number of Smokers, 15 Years of Age and Older, 2000

World Bank region	Smoking prevalence (percent)			Total smokers	
	Males	Females	Overall	Millions	Percentage of all smokers
East Asia and the Pacific	63	5	34	429	38
Europe and Central Asia	56	17	35	122	11
Latin America and the Caribbean	40	24	32	98	9
Middle East and North Africa	36	5	21	37	3
South Asia	32	6	20	178	15
Sub-Saharan Africa	29	8	18	56	6
Low- and middle-income economies	49	8	29	920	82
High-income economies	37	21	29	202	18

Source: Authors.

study in 36 mostly Western countries, from early 1980 to the mid 1990s, suggested that the decrease in smoking prevalence observed among men was caused by the higher prevalence in younger age groups of those who have never smoked. Among women, there was little overall change in smoking prevalence because the increasing prevalence of smokers in younger cohorts counterbalanced increasing cessation in older age groups (Molarius and others 2001).

Cessation

Ex-smoking rates are a good measure of cessation at a population level. In *some* high-income countries, the prevalence rates of ex-smokers have increased over the past two to three decades. For example, in the United Kingdom, smoking prevalence among males over age 30 fell from 70 percent in the 1950s to 30 percent in 2000; female smoking prevalence fell from 40 to 20 percent over the same period. Much of the decrease arose from cessation. Today, two times as many ex-smokers as smokers exist among those age 50 or over. Currently, 30 percent of the U.K. male population is made up of former smokers (Peto and others 2000). Polish male cessation rates have also increased, partly because of control programs. One of every four adult Polish males described himself as an ex-smoker (Zatonski and Jha 2000). In contrast, the prevalence of male ex-smokers in most developing countries is low: 10 percent in Vietnam, 5 percent in India, and 2 percent in China (Jha and others 2002). Even those low figures may be falsely elevated because they include people who quit because either they were too ill to continue or they had early symptoms of tobacco-related illness (Martinson and others 2003).

HEALTH CONSEQUENCES OF SMOKING

The health consequences of smoking are often assumed to be widely understood. In fact, ignorance of the magnitude of tobacco hazards is widespread in terms of both individual health and population policy. Thus, the salient aspects of tobacco epidemiology are outlined in this section.

Key Messages for the Individual Smoker

More than 50 years of epidemiology on smoking-related diseases have led to three key messages for individual smokers worldwide (Doll and others 2004; Peto and others 2003).

- The eventual risk of death from smoking is high, with about one-half to two-thirds of long-term smokers eventually being killed by their addiction.
- These deaths involve a substantial number of life years forgone. About half of all tobacco deaths occur at ages 35 to 69, resulting in the loss of about 20 to 25 years of life, compared with the life expectancy of nonsmokers.
- Cessation works: those adults who quit before middle age avoid almost all the excess hazards of continued smoking.

Worldwide, about 80 percent of deaths among the 2.7 billion adults over age 30 involve vascular, respiratory, or neoplastic disease. Smoking is associated with an increase in the frequency of many of these diseases, although important differences exist between and across populations. The following discussion focuses on the consequences of smoking on adult mortality. Detailed epidemiological reviews of worldwide mortality from smoking are found elsewhere (C. Gajalakshmi and others 2000; V. Gajalakshmi and others 2003; Gupta and Mehta 2000; Liu and others 1998; Niu and others 1998; Peto and others 1994).

Current Mortality and Disability from Smoking

Recent updates of indirect estimates of global tobacco mortality (Ezzati and Lopez 2003; M. Ezzati, personal communication, November 2004) indicate that in 2000, 5.0 million premature deaths were caused by tobacco. About half (2.6 million) of those deaths were in low-income countries. Males accounted

Table 46.2 Tobacco Mortality and Total DALYs by Gender, 2000
(thousands)

World Bank region	Tobacco deaths		Total DALYs	
	Males	**Females**	**Males**	**Females**
East Asia and the Pacific	829	274	13,116	4,128
Europe and Central Asia	754	161	12,407	2,686
Latin America and the Caribbean	177	97	2,789	1,613
Middle East and North Africa	97	28	1,676	554
South Asia	768	187	12,397	3,285
Sub-Saharan Africa	105	66	1,659	1,091
Low- and middle-income economies	2,730	813	44,044	13,357
High-income economies	929	548	12,304	6,866
World	3,659	1,361	56,347	20,222

Source: Ezzati and Lopez 2003; Mathers and others 2006.

Note: The terms *high-income* and *former socialist economies* as used in the text correspond roughly to high-income and Europe and Central Asia regions using the World Bank classification. *Low-income countries* corresponds roughly to East Asia and the Pacific, Latin America and the Caribbean, Middle East and North Africa, South Asia, and Sub-Saharan Africa.

for 3.7 million deaths, or 72 percent of all tobacco deaths. About 60 percent of male and 40 percent of female tobacco deaths were of middle-aged persons (ages 35 to 69).

In high-income countries and former socialist economies, the 1 million middle-aged male tobacco deaths were largely composed of cardiovascular disease (0.45 million) and lung cancer (0.21 million). In contrast, in low-income countries, the leading causes of death among the 1.3 million male tobacco deaths were cardiovascular disease (0.4 million), chronic obstructive pulmonary disease (0.2 million), other respiratory disease (chiefly tuberculosis, 0.2 million), and lung cancer (0.18 million). The specific numbers of deaths from tobacco and of total disability-adjusted life years (DALYs) by gender and World Bank region are shown in table 46.2. Disability estimates are not discussed here; however, disability is highly correlated with mortality in most settings.

Past and Future Trends in Mortality

In high-income and former socialist economies with more complete and reliable mortality statistics, one can measure the effects of increased smoking prevalence and subsequent decreases that have been observed among large numbers of adults. These changes are best documented by examining lung cancer mortality rates among young adults because lung cancer is not often misclassified with other causes of death at young ages and it is almost entirely attributable to smoking.

Age-Standardized Lung Cancer Mortality Rates

Age-standardized male lung cancer rates at ages 35 to 44 per 100,000 men in the United Kingdom had fallen from 18 in 1950 to 4 by 2000. In contrast, comparable French male lung cancer rates show the reverse pattern (Peto and others 2003; figure 46.1). In France, the increase in smoking occurred some decades later than in the United Kingdom, and declines in smoking began only after

1990. Similarly, a large increase in female lung cancer at young ages was avoided in the United Kingdom, but female lung cancer at young ages continues to rise in France.

Future increases in tobacco deaths worldwide are expected to arise from increased smoking by males in developing countries and by women worldwide. Such increases are a product of population growth and increased age-specific tobacco mortality rates, the latter relating to both smoking duration and the amount of tobacco smoked. Peto and others (1994) have made the following calculation: if the proportion of young people taking up smoking continues to be about half of men and one-tenth of young women, there will be about 30 million new long-term smokers each year. As previously noted, epidemiological studies in developed and developing countries suggest that half of these smokers will eventually die from smoking. However, if we conservatively assume that "only" about one-third of smokers die as a result of smoking, then smoking will eventually kill about 10 million people a year. Thus, for the 25-year period from 2000 to 2025, there would be about 150 million tobacco deaths, or about 6 million deaths per year on average; from 2025 to 2050, there would be about 300 million tobacco deaths, or about 12 million deaths per year.

Further estimations are more uncertain, but current smoking trends and projected population growth indicate that from 2050 to 2100 there will be an additional 500 million tobacco deaths. These projections for the next three to four decades are comparable to retrospective and early prospective epidemiological studies in China (Liu and others 1998; Niu and others 1998), which suggest that annual tobacco deaths will rise to 1 million before 2010 and to 2 million by 2025, when the young adult smokers of today reach old age. Similarly, results from a large retrospective study in India suggest that 1 million annual deaths can be expected from male smokers by 2025 (V. Gajalakshmi and others 2003). With other populations in Asia, Eastern

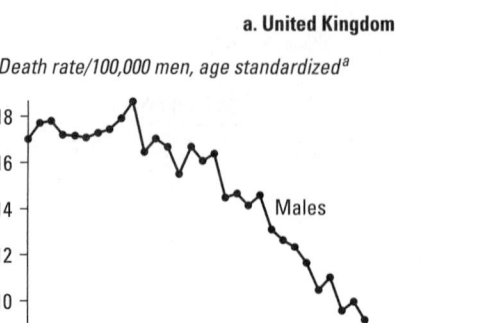

a. United Kingdom

Death rate/100,000 men, age standardized[a]

b. France

Death rate/100,000 men, age standardized[a]

Source: Peto and others 2003.

a. Mean of annual rates in component five-year age groups (35–39, 40–44).

Figure 46.1 Changes in Lung Cancer Mortality at Age 35 to 44 in the United Kingdom and France, 1950–99

Europe, Latin America, the Middle East, and (less certainly) Sub-Saharan Africa showing similar growth in population and age-specific tobacco death rates, the estimate of some 450 million tobacco deaths over the next five decades appears plausible. Almost all of these deaths will be among current smokers.

Benefits of Cessation

Current tobacco mortality statistics reflect past smoking behavior, given the long delay between the onset of smoking and the development of disease. The prevention of a substantial proportion of these tobacco deaths before 2050 requires adult cessation. For example, halving the per capita adult consumption of tobacco by 2020 (akin to the declines in adult smoking in the United Kingdom) would avert about 180 million tobacco deaths. Continuing to reduce the percentage of children who start to smoke will prevent many deaths, but its main effect will be on mortality rates in 2050 and beyond (figure 46.2; Jha and Chaloupka 2000a; Peto and Lopez 2001).

Substantial evidence indicates that smoking cessation reduces the risk of death from tobacco-related diseases. Among doctors in the United Kingdom, those who quit smoking before the onset of major disease avoided most of the excess hazards of smoking (Doll and others 2004). The benefits of quitting were largest in those who quit before middle age (between ages 25 and 34 years) but were still significant in those who quit later (between ages 45 and 54 years).

Cessation before middle age avoids more than 90 percent of the lung cancer risk attributable to tobacco, with quitters possessing a pattern of survival similar to that of persons who

Tobacco deaths (million)

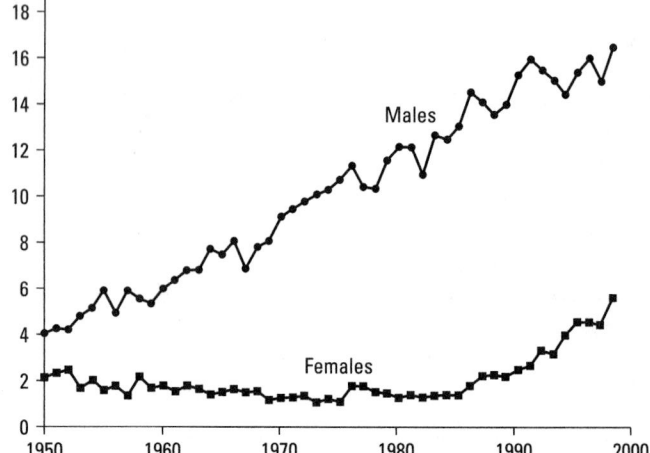

Source: Jha and Chaloupka 2000a; Peto and Lopez 2001.

Note: Peto and others (1994) estimate 60 million tobacco deaths between 1950 and 2000 in industrial countries. This figure estimates an additional 10 million tobacco deaths between 1990 and 2000 in developing countries. The figure also assumes no tobacco deaths before 1990 in developing countries and minimal tobacco deaths worldwide before 1950. Projections for deaths from 2000 to 2050 are based on Peto and Lopez (2001).

Figure 46.2 Tobacco Deaths in the Next 50 Years under Current Smoking Patterns

have never smoked. In the United Kingdom, among those who stopped smoking, the risk of lung cancer fell steeply with time since cessation. For men who stopped at ages 60, 50, 40, and 30, the cumulative risks of lung cancer by age 75 were

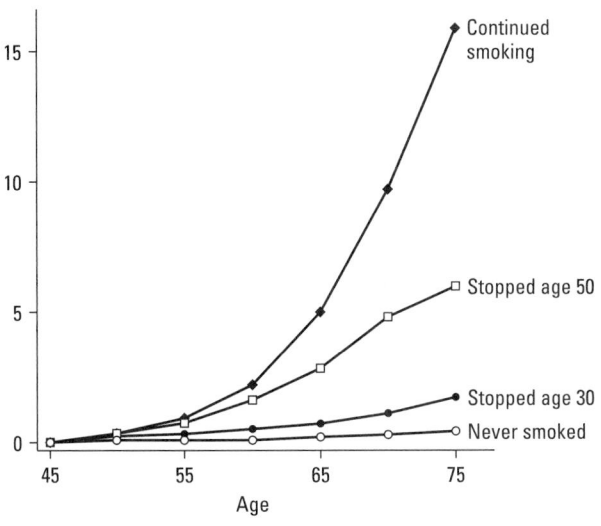

Lung cancer mortality (percent)

Source: Peto and others 2000.

Figure 46.3 Stopping Works: Cumulative Risk of Lung Cancer Mortality in U.K. Males, 1990 rates

10 percent, 6 percent, 3 percent, and 2 percent, respectively (Peto and others 2000; figure 46.3). These results have been supported by a recent multicenter study of men in four European countries; for men who quit smoking at age 40, the study found that the excess lung cancer risk avoided was 85 percent, 91 percent, and 80 percent in the United Kingdom, Germany, and Italy, respectively (Crispo and others 2004). Smoking cessation is uncommon in most developing countries, but some evidence exists that, among Chinese men, quitting also reduces the risks of total and vascular mortality (Lam and others 2002).

RATIONALE FOR GOVERNMENT INTERVENTION

In addition to the public health burden caused by tobacco, an economic rationale exists for government to intervene to reduce tobacco use:

- Consumers have inadequate information about the health consequences of tobacco use (Jha and others 2000; Warner and others 1995). Specifically, the decision to initiate smoking is made primarily by youths, whose ability to make fully informed, appropriately forward-looking decisions is questioned by society in many different contexts (minimum ages for drinking, driving, and voting, for instance). In industrial countries, about 80 percent of adult smokers begin smoking before age 20. Even if children and young adults have information on future risks, they tend to discount that future risk greatly.

- The addictive nature of tobacco is underappreciated and poorly understood. Although general awareness of risks is better in high-income countries, many people still underestimate tobacco's danger relative to other health risks, and many smokers fail to fully internalize these risks (Weinstein 1998).

- Smokers may impose costs on others from passive tobacco smoke or, more controversially, from higher health care costs (Lightwood and others 2000; Warner 2003).

The reader is referred to more detailed discussions on the welfare economics of tobacco (Barnum 1994; Jha and others 2000; Peck and others 2000; Warner and others 1995; and several background papers in the Disease Control Priorities Project Working Paper Series). We discuss nicotine addiction because this newer evidence has profound implications for explaining smoking behavior and for devising control policies.

Nicotine Addiction

Before the landmark 1988 U.S. Surgeon General's report, which suggested that cigarettes and other forms of tobacco are addictive and that nicotine is the major agent in tobacco responsible for addiction, the prevailing view was that tobacco use was largely a voluntary behavior or personal choice (Koop 2003). Since that time, clinicians, behavioral scientists, researchers, and public health experts have increasingly recognized manufactured tobacco products as some of the most addictive and deadly dependence-producing substances available. Although numerous factors have been identified that can contribute to the reinforcement of the smoking habit—for example, the synergistic and independent effects of other compounds in tobacco smoke (such as tar and acetaldehyde) or the sensory and environmental stimuli associated with smoking (such as tobacco advertising)—little debate exists that nicotine is a significant contributor to the development and maintenance of the smoking habit (Markou and Henningfield 2003). In most aspects of dependence, nicotine is on par with other powerfully addictive drugs, such as heroin and cocaine. Newer evidence has converged on the following key points.

Biological Aspects. Nicotine is a psychoactive drug that triggers a cascade of neurobiological events in the reward areas of the brain and throughout the body that can, in turn, act in concert to reinforce tobacco use (Markou and Henningfield 2003). Even a short-term exposure to nicotine has been shown to induce long-lasting changes of the excitatory input into the brain's reward system, which may be an important early step in the path to addiction (Laviolette and van der Kooy 2004). Notably, in some experimental models, if nicotine's neurobiological effects are blocked pharmacologically, or if nicotine is removed from cigarette smoke, smoking eventually ceases

(Jarvis 2004). The overwhelming property of nicotine that leads to its frequent use is the occurrence of nicotine withdrawal, for which cigarette smoke provides rapid relief. Though each individual differs greatly in his or her sensitivity to nicotine dependence, evidence suggests that most adults are susceptible to the biological effects of nicotine and tobacco (Picciotto 2003).

Psychological Aspects. In addition to the unique neurobiology of nicotine, the ready availability of tobacco influences the uptake of smoking as well as the development and maintenance of dependence. With illicit drugs, legal and social barriers constantly test a user's drive to consume the drug. In contrast, a smoker is presented with nearly ubiquitous opportunities and frequent cues to both purchase and use tobacco because of mass marketing and promotion of tobacco (Shiffman and West 2003). Young people, who are attracted to many risk behaviors, such as fast driving or binge drinking, do not "learn" from early smoking in the way that most young people become safer drivers and moderate drinkers as adults (Jha and others 2000; O'Malley, Bachman, and Johnston 1988).

Economics. The traditional economic formulation of costs and benefits tends not to take into account the unique properties of addiction (see Chaloupka, Tauras, and Grossman 2000 for a review). Newer models have begun to incorporate factors such as lack of information, regret, and addiction itself. One key innovation by Gruber and Koszegi (2001, 2002) permits smokers to be time inconsistent, meaning that, given preferences, smokers would make different decisions at different points in time. This approach, now widely used within the new field of behavioral economics, admits conflict between what smokers would like for themselves today and what they would like for themselves in the future.

Implications for Control Programs. These newer economic models have several implications for control programs. First is the need for much more aggressive tobacco taxation to deter the development of tobacco smoking. Estimates suggest that, in the United States, optimal taxation taking into account smoking initiation and nicotine addiction would be at least US$1 higher per pack (Gruber 2003; Gruber and Koszegi 2002; Gruber and Mullainathan 2002). The second implication is that the usual assumption that higher taxes reduce the welfare or satisfaction of continuing smokers may not be true. Higher taxes enhance welfare by acting like an external control device over the time-inconsistent preferences of smokers, which would reduce the likelihood of smoking initiation.

The third implication is that the overall economic benefits of tobacco control, taking into account addiction, are likely to be substantially positive. Earlier cost-benefit analyses have shown that if even modest costs are assigned to uninformed smoking choices, the net economic costs of tobacco are profoundly negative (Barnum 1994; Peck and others 2000). While some of the methods for such costing have been disputed, newer economic evidence supports the idea that widespread hazards of tobacco use lead to major economic costs. Jamison, Lau, and Wang (2005) have outlined that male survival explains income growth independent of changes in physical capital, education, fertility, economic openness, and technical progress. Thus, if adult male survival in the former socialist economies of Europe had been that of high-income countries, annual growth rates over the past three decades would have been about 1.4 percent rather than 1 percent, making 1990 per capita income about 12 percent higher, or an absolute value of US$140 billion. The chief determinant of the mortality gap between the former socialist economies and high-income countries from 1960 to 1990 is smoking (Peto and others 1994; Zatonski and Jha 2000). More recent economic studies that have put a value on "statistical life" suggest that smoking cessation generates huge benefits. For example, Murphy and Topel (2003) find that in the United States, the value of reduced mortality from all causes between 1970 and 1998 amounted to US$2.6 trillion per year, or half of gross domestic product (GDP) growth during the period. Fully US$1.1 trillion per year arose from reduced heart disease, of which at least one-third was from reduced smoking and saturated fat in diets (Cutler and Kadiyala 2003; see chapter 15 for a fuller discussion on the economic benefits of disease control).

INTERVENTIONS TO REDUCE DEMAND FOR TOBACCO

Numerous studies, mostly from high-income countries, have examined the effect of interventions aimed at reducing the demand for tobacco products on smoking and other kinds of tobacco use. The small but growing number of studies from low- and middle-income countries provide useful lessons about differences in the effect of these interventions between these countries and high-income countries. The following is a review of the effect of price and non-price interventions in reducing demand for smoking, including a discussion of each intervention's effect on initiation and cessation. A more complete study of the effectiveness of various interventions is available elsewhere (Jha and Chaloupka 2000b).

Tobacco Taxation

Nearly all governments tax tobacco products. However, significant differences exist across countries in levels of tobacco taxation. Some of these taxes are specific or per unit taxes; others are expressed as a percentage of wholesale or retail prices (ad valorem taxes). As illustrated in figure 46.4, taxes tend to be absolutely higher and account for a greater share of the retail price (two-thirds or more) in high-income countries. In

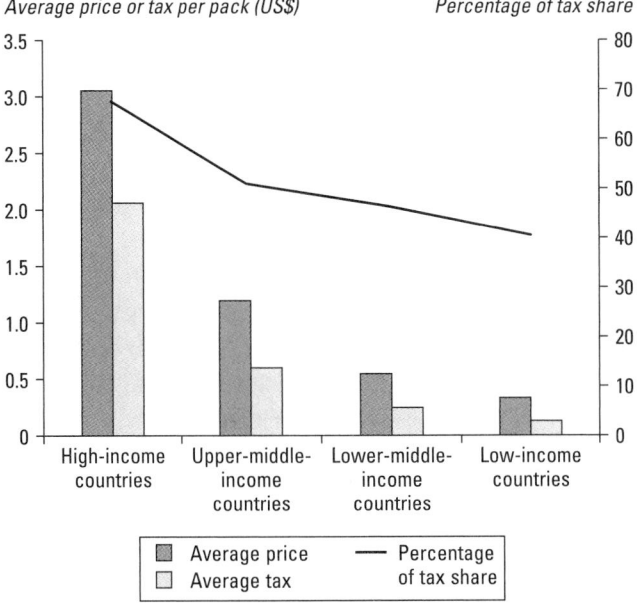

Source: Authors.

Figure 46.4 Average Cigarette Price, Tax, and Percentage of Tax Share per Pack, by Income Group, 1996

low- and middle-income countries, taxes are generally much lower and account for less than half of the final price of cigarettes. In the United States, federal and state excise taxes on cigarettes were one-third lower, in real terms, in 1995 than their peak level of the mid 1960s. However, taxes rose sharply over the next eight years and stood at US$1.12 per pack as of 2002.

Well over 100 studies from high-income countries clearly demonstrate that increases in taxes on cigarettes and other tobacco products lead to significant reductions in cigarette smoking and other tobacco use (Chaloupka, Hu, and others 2000). These reductions reflect the combination of increased smoking cessation, reduced relapse, lower smoking initiation, and decreased consumption among continuing tobacco users.

Studies from Canada, the United Kingdom, the United States, and many other high-income countries generally estimate that the price elasticity of cigarette demand ranges from −0.25 to −0.50, indicating that a 10 percent increase in cigarette prices will reduce overall cigarette smoking by 2.5 to 5.0 percent (Chaloupka, Hu, and others 2000; U.S. DHHS 2000). Estimates from a limited number of studies from low- and middle-income countries suggest a greater price elasticity of −0.8 in such countries. Recent studies using survey data have concluded that half or more of the effect of price on overall cigarette demand results from reducing the number of current smokers (CDC 1994; Wasserman and others 1991). Higher taxes increase both the number of attempts at quitting smoking and the success of those attempts (Tauras 1999; Tauras and Chaloupka 2003). A study in the United States (Taurus 1999) suggested that a 10 percent increase in price would result in 11

to 13 percent shorter smoking duration or a 3.4 percent higher probability of cessation.

Many recent studies from the United States have used individual-level data to explore differences in the price elasticity of cigarette demand by age, with a particular emphasis on youth and young adults (Chaloupka, Hu, and others 2000; U.S. DHHS 2000). Given that most smoking behavior becomes firmly established during teenage years and young adulthood, interventions that are effective in preventing smoking initiation and the transition to regular, addicted smoking will have significant long-term public health benefits. Estimates from these recent studies conclude that an inverse relationship exists between price elasticity and age, with estimates for youth price elasticity of demand up to three times those obtained for adults (Gruber 2003; Ross, Chaloupka, and Wakefield 2001). Several recent studies have begun to explore the differential effect of cigarette prices on youth smoking uptake, concluding that higher cigarette prices are particularly effective in preventing young smokers from moving beyond experimentation into regular, addicted smoking (Emery, White, and Pierce 2001; Ross, Chaloupka, and Wakefield 2001).

In the United Kingdom and the United States, increases in the price of cigarettes have had the greatest effect on smoking among the lowest-income and least educated populations (CDC 1994; Townsend, Roderick, and Cooper 1998). Furthermore, it was estimated that smokers in U.S. households below median income level are four times more responsive to price increases than smokers in households above median income level. In general, estimates of price elasticity for low- and middle-income countries are about double those estimated for high-income countries, implying that significant increases in tobacco taxes in these countries would be effective in reducing tobacco use.

Restrictions on Smoking

Over the past three decades, as the quantity and quality of information about the health consequences of exposure to passive smoking have increased, many governments, especially in high-income countries, have enacted legislation restricting smoking in a variety of public places and private worksites. In addition, increased awareness of the consequences of passive smoke exposure, particularly to children, has led many workplaces and households to adopt voluntary restrictions on smoking. Although the intent of those restrictions is to reduce nonsmokers' exposure to passive tobacco smoke, the policies also reduce smokers' opportunities to smoke. Additional reductions in smoking, especially among youths, will result from the changes in social norms that are introduced by adopting these policies (U.S. DHHS 1994).

In Western populations, comprehensive restrictions on cigarette smoking have been estimated to reduce population smoking rates by 5 to 15 percent (see review by Woolery, Asma, and Sharp 2000) and can also lead to changes in social norms regarding smoking behavior, especially among youths. As with higher taxes, these restrictions reduce both the prevalence of smoking and cigarette consumption among current smokers. Smoking bans in workplaces generally reduce the quantity of cigarettes smoked by 5 to 25 percent and reduce prevalence rates by up to 20 percent (Levy, Friend, and Polishchuk 2001). No-smoking policies were most effective when strong social norms against smoking helped make smoking restrictions self-enforcing.

Health Information and Counteradvertising

The 1962 report by the British Royal College of Physicians and the 1964 U.S. Surgeon General's Report were landmark tobacco-control events in high-income countries. These publications resulted in the first widespread press coverage of the scientific links between smoking and lung cancer. The reports were followed, in many countries, by policies requiring health warning labels on tobacco products, which were later extended to tobacco advertising.

Research from high-income countries indicates that these initial reports and the publicity that followed about the health consequences of smoking led to significant reductions in consumption, with initial declines of between 4 and 9 percent and longer-term cumulative declines of 15 to 30 percent (Kenkel and Chen 2000; Townsend 1993). Efforts to disseminate information about the risks of smoking and of other tobacco use in low- and middle-income countries have led to similar declines in tobacco use in those countries (Kenkel and Chen 2000). In addition, mass media antismoking campaigns, in many cases funded by earmarked tobacco taxes, have generated reductions in cigarette smoking and other tobacco use (Kenkel and Chen 2000; Saffer 2000). Decreases in smoking prevalence were largest in Western countries, where the public is constantly and consistently reminded of the dangers of smoking by extensive coverage of issues related to tobacco in the news media (Molarius and others 2001).

In many low- and middle-income countries, a lack of awareness continues to exist about the risks of mortality and disease posed by smoking. For example, a national survey in China in 1996 found that 61 percent of smokers thought that tobacco did them "little or no harm" (Chinese Academy of Preventive Medicine 1997). In high-income countries, smokers are aware of the risks, but a recent review of psychological studies found that few smokers judge the size of these risks to be higher and more established than do nonsmokers, and that smokers minimize the personal relevance of these risks (Weinstein 1998).

Bans on Advertising and Promotion

Cigarettes are among the most heavily advertised and promoted products in the world. In 2002, cigarette companies spent US\$12.5 billion on advertising and promotion in the United States alone, the highest spending level reported to date (U.S. Federal Trade Commission 2004). Tobacco advertising efforts worldwide include traditional forms of advertising on television, radio, and billboards and in magazines and newspapers as well as favorable product placement; price-related promotions, such as coupons and multipack discounts; and sponsorship of highly visible sporting and cultural events.

Numerous econometric studies, largely from the United Kingdom and the United States, have explored the relationship between cigarette advertising and promotional expenditure and cigarette demand. In general, these studies have resulted in mixed findings, with most studies concluding that advertising has a small positive effect on demand (Chaloupka, Hu, and others 2000; Townsend 1993). However, critics of these studies note that econometric methods, which estimate the effect of a marginal change in advertising expenditures on smoking, are ill suited for studying the effect of advertising (Chaloupka, Hu, and others 2000; U.S. Federal Trade Commission 2004; Townsend 1993). Approaches used by other disciplines, including survey research and experiments that assess reactions to and recall of cigarette advertising, do support the hypothesis that increases in cigarette advertising and promotion directly and indirectly increase cigarette demand and smoking initiation (U.S. DHHS 1994; U.K. Department of Health 1992). These studies conclude that cigarette advertising is effective in getting and retaining children's attention, with the strength of the association strongly correlated with current smoking behavior, smoking initiation, and smoking intentions.

Comprehensive advertising and promotion bans on cigarettes provide more direct evidence on the effect of advertising these products (Saffer 2000). One study using data from 22 high-income countries for the period 1970 through 1992 provides strong evidence that comprehensive bans on cigarette advertising and promotion led to significant reductions in cigarette smoking. The study predicts that a comprehensive set of tobacco advertising bans in high-income countries could reduce tobacco consumption by more than 6 percent, taking into account price and non-price control interventions (Saffer and Chaloupka 2000). However, the study concludes that partial bans have little effect on smoking behavior, given that the tobacco industry can shift its resources from banned media to other media that are not banned.

Smoking Cessation Treatments

Near-term reductions in smoking-related mortality depend heavily on smoking cessation. Numerous behavioral smoking cessation treatments are available, including self-help manuals, community-based programs, and minimal or intensive clinical interventions (U.S. DHHS 2000). In clinical settings, pharmacological treatments, including nicotine replacement therapies (NRT) and bupropion, have become much more widely available in recent years in high-income countries through deregulation of some NRT from prescription to over-the-counter status (Novotny and others 2000; U.S. DHHS 2000). The evidence is strong and consistent that pharmacological treatments significantly improve the likelihood of quitting, with success rates two to three times those when pharmacological treatments are not used (Novotny and others 2000; Raw, McNeill, and West 1999; U.S. DHHS 2000). The effectiveness of all commercially available NRT seems to be largely independent of the duration of therapy, the setting in which the therapy is provided, regulatory status (over-the-counter versus prescribed therapy), and the type of provider (Novotny and others 2000). Over-the-counter NRT without physician oversight have been used in many countries for a number of years with good success.

Although NRT are successful in treating nicotine addiction, the markets for NRT and other pharmacological therapies are more highly regulated and less affordable than are nicotine-containing tobacco products. Recent evidence indicates that the demand for NRT is related to economic factors, including price (Tauras and Chaloupka 2003). Policies that decrease the cost of NRT and increase availability—such as mandating private health insurance coverage of NRT, including such coverage in public health insurance programs, and subsidizing NRT for uninsured or underinsured individuals—would likely lead to substantial increases in the use of these products. Given the demonstrated efficacy of NRT in treating smoking, these policies could generate significant increases in smoking cessation.

INTERVENTIONS TO REDUCE THE SUPPLY OF TOBACCO

The key intervention on the supply side is the control of smuggling. Recent estimates suggest that 6 to 8 percent of cigarettes consumed globally are smuggled (Merriman, Yurekli, and Chaloupka 2000). Of note, the tobacco industry itself has an economic incentive to smuggle, in part to increase market share and decrease tax rates (Joossens and others 2000; Merriman, Yurekli, and Chaloupka 2000). Although differences in taxes and prices across countries create a motive for smuggling, a recent analysis comparing the degree of corruption in individual countries with price and tax levels found that corruption within countries is a stronger predictor of smuggling than is price (Merriman, Yurekli, and Chaloupka 2000). Several governments are adopting policies aimed at controlling smuggling. In addition to harmonizing price differentials between countries, effective measures include prominent tax stamps and warning labels in local languages, better methods for tracking cigarettes through the distribution chain, aggressive enforce-

ment of antismuggling laws, and stronger penalties for those caught violating these laws (Joossens and others 2000). Recent analysis suggests that, even in the presence of smuggling, tax increases will reduce consumption and increase revenue (Merriman, Yurekli, and Chaloupka 2000).

In contrast to the effectiveness of demand-side interventions, there is much less evidence that interventions aimed at reducing the supply of tobacco products are as effective in reducing cigarette smoking (Jha and Chaloupka 1999, 2000a). The U.S. experience provides mixed evidence about the effectiveness of limiting youth access to tobacco products in reducing youth tobacco use (U.S. DHHS 2000; Woolery, Asma, and Sharp 2000). In addition, the effective implementation and enforcement of these policies may require infrastructure and resources that do not exist in many low- and middle-income countries. A preliminary discussion is occurring in Canada about reducing its number of retail outlets for tobacco from the current 65,000. Neither the effect of such a move nor its enforcement costs are well known. Crop substitution and diversification programs are often proposed as a means of reducing the supply of tobacco. However, little evidence exists that such programs would significantly reduce the supply of tobacco, given that the incentives for growing tobacco tend to attract new farmers who would replace those who abandon tobacco farming (Jacobs and others 2000). Similarly, direct prohibition of tobacco production is not likely to be politically feasible, effective, or economically optimal. Finally, although trade liberalization has contributed to increases in tobacco use (particularly in low- and middle-income countries), restrictions on trade in tobacco and tobacco products that violate international trade agreements or draw retaliatory measures (or both) may be more harmful (Taylor and others 2000).

EFFECTIVENESS AND COST-EFFECTIVENESS OF TOBACCO-CONTROL INTERVENTIONS

Using a static model of the cohort of smokers alive in 2000, we estimate the number of deaths attributable to smoking over the next few decades that could be averted by (a) price increases, (b) NRT, and (c) a package of non-price interventions other than NRT. Cost-effectiveness of these policy interventions was calculated by weighing the approximate public sector costs against the years of healthy life saved, measured in DALYs. The details of an earlier version of this model have been published previously (Ranson and others 2002).

Results of Model Projections

The following is an updated analysis, using higher price increases and a greater effectiveness for NRT than did the

Table 46.3 Reductions in Future Tobacco Deaths among Smokers Alive in 2000 from Price Increases of 10 Percent, 33 Percent, 50 Percent, and 70 Percent by World Bank Region

	Baseline smoking-attributable deaths (millions)	Reduction in number of deaths (millions)							
		10 percent price increase		33 percent price increase		50 percent price increase		70 percent price increase	
World Bank region		Low	High	Low	High	Low	High	Low	High
East Asia and the Pacific	173	2.9	8.7	9.6	27.5	14.5	37.5	20.3	46.2
(percent)		(1.7)	(5.0)	(5.5)	(15.9)	(8.4)	(21.7)	(11.7)	(26.8)
Europe and Central Asia	51	0.9	2.6	2.8	8.1	4.3	11.2	6.0	13.8
(percent)		(1.7)	(5.1)	(5.6)	(16.0)	(8.5)	(22.0)	(11.8)	(27.2)
Latin America and the Caribbean	40	0.7	2.1	2.3	6.7	3.5	9.5	4.9	11.6
(percent)		(1.8)	(5.3)	(5.8)	(16.8)	(8.8)	(23.7)	(12.3)	(29.1)
Middle East and North Africa	13	0.2	0.7	0.8	2.2	1.2	3.1	1.6	3.8
(percent)		(1.7)	(5.2)	(5.8)	(16.6)	(8.7)	(23.2)	(12.2)	(28.5)
South Asia	62	0.9	2.6	2.9	8.5	4.4	12.5	6.2	16.0
(percent)		(2.4)	(8.6)	(9.5)	(27.7)	(14.3)	(40.6)	(20.1)	(52)
Sub-Saharan Africa	23	0.4	1.1	1.3	3.7	1.9	5.5	2.7	6.6
(percent)		(1.6)	(4.9)	(5.4)	(15.9)	(8.2)	(23.6)	(11.5)	(28.5)
Low- and middle-income countries	362	6.0	17.9	19.7	56.8	29.8	79.2	41.7	98.2
(percent)		(1.6)	(4.9)	(5.4)	(15.7)	(8.2)	(21.9)	(11.5)	(27.1)
High-income countries	81	0.6	2.6	2.1	8.5	3.2	12.2	4.5	16.2
(percent)		(0.8)	(3.2)	(2.6)	(10.6)	(4.0)	(15.1)	(5.6)	(20.0)
World	443	6.6	20.5	21.8	65.3	33.0	91.5	46.2	114.3
(percent)		(1.5)	(4.6)	(4.9)	(14.7)	(7.5)	(20.7)	(10.4)	(25.8)

Source: Authors' calculations.

original (Ranson and others 2002). This analysis is conservative in its assumptions about effectiveness and generous in its assumptions about the costs of tobacco control.

Potential Effect of Price Increases. With a price increase of 33 percent, the model predicts that 22 million to 65 million smoking-attributable deaths will be averted worldwide, which is approximately equivalent to 5 to 15 percent of all smoking-attributable deaths expected among those who smoke in 2000 (see table 46.3). Low- and middle-income countries account for about 90 percent of averted deaths. East Asia and the Pacific alone will account for roughly 40 percent of averted deaths. Total smoking-attributable deaths averted worldwide range from 33 million to 92 million for a 50 percent price increase and 46 million to 114 million for a 70 percent price increase. A 70 percent price increase would avert 10 to 26 percent of all smoking-attributable deaths worldwide.

Of the tobacco-related deaths that would be averted by a price increase, 80 percent would be male, reflecting the higher overall prevalence of smoking in men. The greatest relative effect of a price increase on deaths averted is among younger cohorts. Note that these projections use conservative price increases. In certain countries, such as Poland and South

Africa, recent tax increases have doubled the real price of cigarettes (Guindon, Tobin, and Yach 2002).

Potential Effect of Nicotine Replacement Therapies. Provision of NRT with an effectiveness of 1 percent is predicted to result in the avoidance of about 3.5 million smoking-attributable deaths (table 46.4). NRT of 5 percent effectiveness would have about five times the effect. Again, low- and middle-income countries would account for roughly 80 percent of the averted deaths. The relative effect of NRT (of 2.5 percent effectiveness) on deaths averted is 2 to 3 percent among individuals age 15 to 59 and lower among those age 60 and older (results not shown).

Potential Effect of Non-price Interventions Other Than NRT. A package of non-price interventions, other than NRT, that decreases the prevalence of smoking by 2 percent is predicted to prevent about 7 million smoking-attributable deaths (more than 1.6 percent of all smoking-attributable deaths among those who smoked in 2000; see table 46.4). A package of interventions that decreases the prevalence of smoking by 10 percent would have an effect five times greater. Low- and middle-income countries would account for approximately four-fifths

Table 46.4 Reductions in Future Tobacco Deaths among Smokers Alive in 2000 from Price Increases of 33 Percent, Increased NRT Use, and a Package of Non-price Measures by World Bank Region

| World Bank region | Baseline smoking-attributable deaths (millions) | Reduction in number of deaths (millions) | | | | | |
| | | 33 percent price increase | | NRT effectiveness | | Non-price intervention effectiveness | |
		Low elasticity	High elasticity	1 percent	5 percent	2 percent	10 percent
East Asia and the Pacific	173	9.6	27.5	1.4	6.9	2.8	13.8
(percent)		(5.5)	(15.9)	(0.8)	(4.0)	(1.6)	(8.0)
Europe and Central Asia	51	2.8	8.1	0.4	2.1	0.8	4.1
(percent)		(5.6)	(16.0)	(0.8)	(4.0)	(1.6)	(8.1)
Latin America and the Caribbean	40	2.3	6.7	0.3	1.7	0.7	3.4
(percent)		(5.8)	(16.8)	(0.8)	(4.2)	(1.7)	(8.5)
Middle East and North Africa	13	0.8	2.2	0.11	0.6	0.2	1.1
(percent)		(5.8)	(16.6)	(0.8)	(4.2)	(1.7)	(8.4)
South Asia	62	2.9	8.5	0.4	2.2	0.9	4.3
(percent)		(9.5)	(27.7)	(1.4)	(7.2)	(2.8)	(13.9)
Sub-Saharan Africa	23	1.3	3.7	0.2	0.9	0.4	1.8
(percent)		(5.4)	(15.9)	(0.8)	(4.0)	(1.6)	(7.9)
Low- and middle-income countries	362	19.7	56.8	2.9	14.3	5.7	28.6
(percent)		(5.4)	(15.7)	(0.8)	(4.0)	(1.6)	(7.9)
High-income countries	81	2.1	8.5	0.6	3.1	1.2	6.1
(percent)		(2.6)	(10.6)	(0.8)	(3.8)	(1.5)	(7.6)
World	443	21.8	65.3	3.5	17.4	6.9	34.7
(percent)		(4.9)	(14.8)	(0.8)	(3.9)	(1.6)	(7.8)

Source: Authors.

of quitters and averted deaths. The greatest relative effect of non-price interventions on deaths averted would be among younger cohorts.

Figure 46.5 summarizes the potential effect of a set of independent tobacco-control interventions, using 33 and 70 percent price increases (using a high elasticity of −1.2 for low- and middle-income regions and −0.8 for high-income regions), a 5 percent effectiveness of NRT, and a 10 percent reduction from non-price interventions other than NRT. In this cohort of smokers alive in 2000, approximately 443 million are expected to die in the next 50 years in the absence of interventions. A substantial fraction of these tobacco deaths are avoidable with interventions. Price increases have the greatest effect on tobacco mortality, with the most aggressive price increase of 70 percent having the potential to avert almost one-quarter of all tobacco deaths. Even a modest price increase of 33 percent could potentially prevent 66 million tobacco deaths over the course of the next 50 years. Although NRT and other non-price interventions are less effective than price increases, they can still avert a substantial number of tobacco deaths (18 million and 35 million deaths, respectively). The greatest effect of these tobacco-control interventions would occur after 2010, but a substantial number of deaths could be avoided even before then.

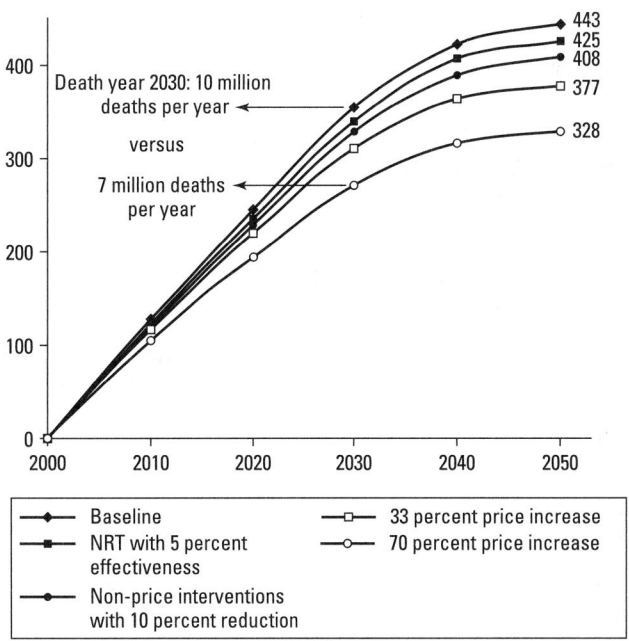

Source: Authors.

Note: Price increases assume a high price elasticity (−1.2 for low- and middle-income countries and −0.8 for high-income countries).

Figure 46.5 Potential Effect of Tax Increases, NRT, and Non-price Interventions on Tobacco Mortality, 2000–50

Note that no attempt has been made in this analysis to examine the effect of combining the various packages of interventions (for example, price increases with NRT, or NRT and other non-price interventions). A number of studies have compared the effect of price and non-price interventions; few empirical attempts have been made to assess how these interventions might interact. Although price increases have been found in this analysis to be the most cost-effective antismoking intervention, policy makers should use both price and non-price interventions to counter smoking. Non-price measures may be required to affect the most heavily dependent smokers, for whom medical and social support in stopping will be necessary. Furthermore, these non-price measures may be effective in increasing social acceptance and support of tobacco price increases.

Cost-Effectiveness of Antismoking Interventions. In general, price increases are found to be the most cost-effective antismoking intervention. A 33 percent price increase (our base case scenario) could be achieved for a cost of US$13 to US$195 per DALY saved globally, or US$3 to US$42 in low-income countries and US$85 to US$1,773 in high-income countries. Wider access to NRT could be achieved for between US$75 and US$1,250 per DALY saved, depending on which assumptions are used. Non-price interventions other than NRT could be implemented for between US$233 and US$2,916 per DALY saved (table 46.5). Thus, NRT and other non-price measures are slightly less cost-effective than price increases but remain cost-effective in many settings. The cost-effectiveness of NRT is highly sensitive to the actual price of the NRT. NRT with a price of US$25 have a cost-effectiveness of US$75 per DALY compared with US$329 for an NRT price of US$150 (data not shown).

For a given set of assumptions, the variation in the cost-effectiveness of each intervention between low- and middle-income regions is relatively small and sensitive to the discount rate (data not shown). All three interventions are most cost-effective in South Asia and Sub-Saharan Africa. The difference between low- and middle-income countries and high-income countries is more pronounced. For NRT, the cost per year of healthy life gained is 3 to 10 times higher in high-income countries than elsewhere. For non-price interventions other than NRT, the cost in high-income countries is 22 times higher, and for price increases, almost 42 times higher. Of note, the estimates of cost-effectiveness are given as wide ranges, which reflect the range of assumptions used.

For price increases, the high-end estimates are roughly 25 times the low-end estimates, and this difference is consistent among the regions. For NRT, the high-end estimates are 2.5 to 10 times the low-end estimates, varying among the regions. For non-price interventions other than NRT, the high-end estimates are 20 times the low-end estimates, and this difference is consistent among the regions.

The cost-effectiveness results can be compared against existing studies only for high-income countries because of a lack of studies situated elsewhere. Our estimates of deaths avoided for a 10 percent price increase are conservative compared with those of Moore (1996) and Warner (1986).

Table 46.5 Range of Cost-Effectiveness Values for Price Increase, NRT, and Non-price Interventions, 2000
(2002 U.S. dollars per DALY saved)

World Bank region	Baseline smoking-attributable deaths (millions)	33 percent price increase		NRT with effectiveness of 1 to 5 percent		Non-price interventions with effectiveness of 2 to 10 percent	
		Low-end estimate	High-end estimate	Low-end estimate	High-end estimate	Low-end estimate	High-end estimate
East Asia and the Pacific	173	2	30	65	864	40	498
Europe and Central Asia	51	3	42	45	633	55	685
Latin America and the Caribbean	40	6	85	53	812	109	1,361
Middle East and North Africa	13	6	89	47	750	115	1,432
South Asia	62	2	27	54	716	34	431
Sub-Saharan Africa	23	2	26	42	570	33	417
Low- and middle-income countries	362	3	42	55	761	54	674
High-income countries	81	85	1,773	175	3,781	1,166	14,572
World	443	13	195	75	1,250	233	2,916

Source: Authors.

COMPREHENSIVE TOBACCO-CONTROL PROGRAMS

In recent years, several governments, mostly in high-income countries, have adopted comprehensive programs to reduce tobacco use, often funded by earmarked tobacco tax revenues. The programs generally have similar goals for reducing tobacco use:

- preventing initiation among youths and young adults
- promoting cessation among all smokers
- reducing exposure to passive tobacco smoke
- identifying and eliminating disparities among population subgroups (U.S. DHHS 1994).

Furthermore, the programs have one or more of four key components: community interventions engaging a diverse set of local organizations; countermarketing and health information campaigns; program policies and regulations (such as taxes, restrictions on smoking, bans on tobacco advertising, and access to better cessation treatments); and surveillance and evaluation of potential issues, such as smuggling (U.S. DHHS 1994). Programs have placed differing emphasis on these four components, with substantial diversity among the types of activities supported within each component. Disaggregating current tobacco-control program spending reveals that the greatest effect can be achieved through a focus on macro-level changes, such as policy change. Recent analyses from the United Kingdom and United States clearly indicate that these comprehensive efforts have been successful in reducing tobacco use and in improving public health (Farrelly, Pechacek, and Chaloupka 2003; Townsend, Roderick, and Cooper 1998; U.S. DHHS 1994). In California, for example, the state's comprehensive tobacco-control program has produced a rate of decline in tobacco use double that seen in the rest of the United States.

The cost of implementing control programs is low. Table 46.6 provides the estimated total costs of implementing price and NRT interventions by World Bank region. Current estimates of the costs of implementing a comprehensive tobacco-control program range from US$2.50 to US$10 per capita in the United States. The U.S. Centers for Disease Control and Prevention recommends spending US$6 to US$16 per capita for a comprehensive tobacco-control program in the United States (CDC 1999). Canadian spending on tobacco-control programs was approximately US$1.70 per capita in 1996 (Pechmann, Dixon, and Layne 1998). At the highest recommended spending level (US$16 per capita) in the United States, annual funding for a comprehensive tobacco program would equal only 0.9 percent of U.S. public spending, per capita, on health.

Evidence from the United States demonstrates that states with the greatest prevalence of smoking have a greater marginal effect with their tobacco-control spending, suggesting that the potential gains from modest investments in comprehensive tobacco-control measures are large. Each US$10 spent per capita on tobacco control annually has resulted in a 55 percent reduction (variation of 20 to 70 percent) in per capita cigarette consumption (Tauras and others 2005). In the United States, US$10 translates into 0.03 percent of per capita GDP in 2003.

Table 46.6 Estimated Cost of Price Intervention and NRT Programs
(2002 U.S. dollars)

| World Bank region | GDP (billions) | Cost for price increase (millions) | | Cost of NRT (US$25 to US$150) (millions) | | | | | |
| | | Low-end estimate (0.02 percent GDP) | High-end estimate (0.05 percent GDP) | To treat 1 percent of current smokers | | | To treat 5 percent of current smokers | | |
				US$25	US$50	US$150	US$25	US$50	US$150
East Asia and the Pacific	1,802	360	901	1,079	2,158	6,474	5,395	10,791	32,372
Europe and Central Asia	1,136	227	568	318	635	1,906	1,588	3,176	9,529
Latin America and the Caribbean	1,673	335	836	250	500	1,500	1,250	2,500	7,499
Middle East and North Africa	694	139	347	84	169	506	422	843	2,530
South Asia	655	131	327	2,312	1,926	3,853	11,558	2,312	1,926
Sub-Saharan Africa	319	64	159	868	723	1,447	4,340	868	723
Low- and middle-income countries	6,279	1,256	3,138	4,911	6,111	15,686	24,553	20,490	54,579
High-income countries	25,992	5,198	12,996	3,034	2,529	10,114	15,172	3,034	2,529
World	32,271	6,454	16,134	7,945	8,640	25,800	39,725	23,524	57,108

Source: Authors.

CONSTRAINTS TO EFFECTIVE TOBACCO-CONTROL POLICIES

Although substantial evidence exists concerning the effectiveness of numerous policy interventions to reduce tobacco use, the use of these interventions globally is uneven and limited (see a more formal analysis in Chaloupka and others 2001). World Bank data reveal that ample room exists to increase tobacco taxes. In 1995, the average percentage of all government revenue derived from tobacco tax was 0.63 percent. Middle-income countries averaged 0.51 percent of government revenue from tobacco taxes, while lower-income countries averaged only 0.42 percent. An increase in cigarette taxes of 10 percent globally would raise cigarette tax revenues by nearly 7 percent, with relatively larger increases in revenues in high-income countries and smaller increases in revenues in low- and middle-income countries (Sunley, Yurekli, and Chaloupka 2000). Despite this evidence, price increases have been underused. Guindon, Tobin, and Yach (2002) studied 80 countries and found that the real price of tobacco, adjusted for purchasing power, fell in most developing countries from 1990 to 2000.

Why does so much variation exist in tobacco-control policies? The political economy of tobacco control has been inadequately studied. A few plausible areas of interest are outlined here. First, the recognition of tobacco as a major health hazard appears to be the impetus for most of the tobacco-control policies in many high-income countries. Some evidence shows that improved national capacity and local needs assessment could increase the likelihood that tobacco-control measures will be adopted. For example, econometric analyses in South Africa geared to local policy requirements substantially increased the willingness of the government to implement tobacco-control policies (Abedian and others 1998). Second, tobacco-control budgets are only a fraction of what is required. Funding is needed not so much to implement programs as to fight off tobacco industry tactics and to build popular support for control. Third, the most obvious constraint to tobacco control is political opposition, which is difficult to quantify. Opposition from the tobacco industry is well organized and well funded (Pollock 1996).

A key tool for addressing political opposition is earmarking tobacco taxes. Earmarking has been successfully used in several countries, including Australia, Finland, Nepal, and Thailand. Of the 48 countries currently in the World Health Organization's European region, 12 earmark taxes for tobacco control and other public health measures. The average level of allocation is less than 1 percent of total tax revenue (WHO 2002). Earmarking does introduce clear restrictions and inefficiencies on public finance, and for this reason alone most macroeconomists do not favor earmarking, no matter how worthy the cause. However, analysis suggests that the efficiency or "dead-weight losses" from earmarking tobacco taxes are minimal (Hu, Xu, and Keeler 1998). Furthermore, earmarking tobacco taxes can be justified if governments use the funds to benefit those who pay (the *benefits principle*), provide assured funding for tobacco-control policies and programs, and secure public support for new or higher tobacco taxes. Earmarked taxes also have a political function in that they help concentrate political winners of tobacco control and thus influence policy. Earmarked funds that support broad health and social services (such as other disease programs) broaden the political and civil society support base for tobacco control. In Australia, broad political support from the Ministries of Sports and Education helped convince the Ministry of Finance that raising tobacco taxes was possible. Indeed, after an earmarked tax was passed, the Ministry of Finance went on to raise tobacco taxes further without earmarking (Galbally 1997). Additionally, targeting revenue from tobacco taxes to other health programs for the poorest socioeconomic groups could produce double health gains—reduced tobacco consumption combined with increased access to and use of health services. In China, a 10 percent increase in cigarette taxes would decrease consumption by 5 percent and would increase government revenue by 5 percent. The increased earnings could finance a package of essential health services for one-third of China's poorest 100 million citizens in 1990 (Saxenian and McGreevey 1996).

Finally, a key pillar in tobacco control that can help overcome some of these constraints is the Framework Convention on Tobacco Control (FCTC). The World Health Assembly of the World Health Organization adopted the FCTC in May 2003. It consists of a series of negotiated protocols within a general framework. The first three protocols are negotiations covering smuggling, advertising, and treatment of tobacco addiction. Countries agreeing to the negotiated protocols are to adopt appropriate legislation and, if necessary, implement the appropriate measures. As of February 2005, 168 countries had signed the FCTC, 57 had ratified it, and it had come into force on February 27, 2005.

CONCLUSION

Worldwide, only two large and growing causes of death exist. One is HIV-1 infection, and the other is tobacco. On current consumption patterns, about 1 billion people in the 21st century will be killed by their addiction to tobacco. Strong evidence shows that tobacco tax increases, the dissemination of information about health risks from smoking, restrictions on smoking in public places and workplaces, comprehensive bans on advertising and promotion, and increased access to cessation therapies are effective both in reducing tobacco use and in improving the health of populations. Despite this evidence, these policies, especially higher taxes, have been applied aggressively only in a few high-income countries, covering a small proportion of the world's smokers. Limited implementation of effective tobacco control in developing countries is due to political constraints as well as the lack of awareness of the unique effectiveness and cost-effectiveness of these interventions.

ACKNOWLEDGMENTS

We thank Allison Gilbert for help with the cost-effectiveness analyses and Hellen Gelband, Andra Ghent, and Dhirendra Sinha for comments.

REFERENCES

Abedian, I., R. van der Merwe, N. Wilkins, and P. Jha, eds. 1998. *The Economics of Tobacco Control: Towards an Optimal Policy Mix*. Cape Town, South Africa: Applied Fiscal Research Centre, University of Cape Town.

Barnum, H. 1994. "The Economic Burden of the Global Trade in Tobacco." *Tobacco Control* 3 (4): 358–61.

CDC (U.S. Centers for Disease Control and Prevention). 1994. "Response to Increases in Cigarette Prices by Race/Ethnicity, Income, and Age Groups—United States, 1976–1993." *Morbidity and Mortality Weekly Report* 43 (26): 469–72.

———. 1999. "Best Practices for Comprehensive Tobacco Control Programs." Atlanta: U.S. Department of Health and Human Services, Centers for Disease Control and Prevention, National Center for Chronic Disease Prevention and Health Promotion, Office on Smoking and Health.

Chaloupka, F. J., T. W. Hu, K. E. Warner, R. Jacobs, and A. Yurekli. 2000. "The Taxation of Tobacco Products." In *Tobacco Control in Developing Countries*, ed. P. Jha and F. Chaloupka. Oxford, U.K.: Oxford University Press.

Chaloupka, F., J. P. Jha, M.A. Corrao, V. Costa e Silva, H. Ross, C. Czart, and D. Yach. 2001. "The Evidence Base for Reducing Mortality from Smoking in Low and Middle Income Countries." Commission on Macroeconomics and Health Working Paper Series. http://www.cmhealth.org/docs/wg5_paper7.pdf.

Chaloupka, F. J., J. A. Tauras, and M. Grossman. 2000. "The Economics of Addiction." In *Tobacco Control in Developing Countries*, ed. P. Jha and F. J. Chaloupka. Oxford, U.K.: Oxford University Press.

Chinese Academy of Preventive Medicine. 1997. *Smoking in China: 1996 National Prevalence Survey of Smoking Pattern*. Beijing: China Science and Technology Press.

Crispo, A., P. Brennan, K. H. Jockel, A. Schaffrath-Rosario, H. E. Wichmann, F. Nyberg, and others. 2004. "The Cumulative Risk of Lung Cancer among Current, Ex- and Never-Smokers in European Men." *British Journal of Cancer* 91 (7): 1280–86.

Cutler, D. M., and S. Kadiyala. 2003. "The Return to Biomedical Research: Treatment and Behavioral Effects." In *Measuring the Gains of Medical Research: An Economic Approach*, ed. K. M. Murphy and R. H. Topel. Chicago: University of Chicago.

Doll, R., R. Peto, J. Boreham, and I. Sutherland. 2004. "Mortality in Relation to Smoking: 50 Years' Observation on Male British Doctors." *British Medical Journal* 328 (7455): 1519–28.

Emery, S., M. M. White, and J. P. Pierce. 2001. "Does Cigarette Price Influence Adolescent Experimentation?" *Journal of Health Economics* 20 (2): 261–70.

Ezzati, M., and A. D. Lopez. 2003. "Estimates of Global Mortality Attributable to Smoking in 2000." *Lancet* 362 (9387): 847–52.

Farrelly, M. C., T. F. Pechacek, and F. J. Chaloupka. 2003. "The Impact of Tobacco Control Program Expenditures on Aggregate Cigarette Sales: 1981–2000." *Journal of Health Economics* 22 (5): 843–59.

Gajalakshmi, C. K., P. Jha, K. Ranson, and S. Nguyen. 2000. "Global Patterns of Smoking and Smoking-Attributable Mortality." In *Tobacco Control in Developing Countries*, ed. P. Jha and F. J. Chaloupka. Oxford, U.K.: Oxford University Press.

Gajalakshmi, V., R. Peto, T. S. Kanaka, and P. Jha. 2003. "Smoking and Mortality from Tuberculosis and Other Diseases in India: Retrospective Study of 43,000 Adult Male Deaths and 35,000 Controls." *Lancet* 362 (9883): 507–15.

Galbally, R. L. 1997. "Health-Promoting Environments: Who Will Miss Out?" *Australia and New Zealand Journal of Public Health* 21 (4 Spec. No.): 429–30.

Gruber, J. 2003. "Government Policy toward Smoking: A New View from Economics." Disease Control Priorities Project Working Paper Series. Paper presented at the Disease Control Priorities Project Nicotine Addiction Workshop, Mumbai, India, September 2003.

Gruber, J., and B. Koszegi. 2001. "Is Addiction Rational? Theory and Evidence." *Quarterly Journal of Economics* 116 (4): 1261–303.

———. 2002. "A Theory of Government Regulation of Addictive Bads: Optimal Tax Levels and Tax Incidence for Cigarette Taxation." NBER Working Paper 8777. Cambridge, MA: National Bureau of Economic Research.

Gruber, J., and S. Mullainathan. 2002. "Do Cigarette Taxes Make Smokers Happier?" NBER Working Paper 8872. Cambridge, MA: National Bureau of Economic Research.

Guindon, G. E., S. Tobin, and D. Yach. 2002. "Trends and Affordability of Cigarette Prices: Ample Room for Tax Increases and Related Health Gains." *Tobacco Control* 11 (1): 35–43.

Gupta, P. C., and H. C. Mehta. 2000. "Cohort Study of All-Cause Mortality amongst Tobacco Users in Mumbai, India." *Bulletin of the World Health Organization* 78 (7): 877–83.

Hu, T. W., X. Xu, and T. Keeler. 1998. "Earmarked Tobacco Taxes: Lessons Learned." In *The Economics of Tobacco Control*, ed. I. Abedian, R. van der Merwe, N. Wilkins, and P. Jha. Cape Town, South Africa: Applied Fiscal Research Centre, University of Cape Town.

Jacobs, R., H. F. Gale, T. C. Capehart, P. Zhang, and P. Jha. 2000. "The Supply-Side Effects of Tobacco-Control Policies." In *Tobacco Control in Developing Countries*, ed. P. Jha, and F. J. Chaloupka. Oxford, U.K.: Oxford University Press.

Jamison, D. T., L. J. Lau, and J. Wang. 2005. "Health's Contribution to Economic Growth in an Environment of Partially Endogenous Technical Progress." In *Health and Economic Growth: Findings and Policy Implications*, eds. G. Lopez-Casasnovas, B. Rivera, and L. Currais. Cambridge: MIT Press, 67–91.

Jarvis, M. J. 2004. "ABC of Smoking Cessation: Why People Smoke." *British Medical Journal* 328 (7434): 277–79.

Jha, P., and F. J. Chaloupka. 1999. *Curbing the Epidemic: Governments and the Economics of Tobacco Control*. Washington, DC: World Bank.

———. 2000a. "The Economics of Global Tobacco Control." *British Medical Journal* 321 (7257): 358–61.

———, eds. 2000b. *Tobacco Control in Developing Countries*. Oxford, U.K.: Oxford University Press.

Jha, P., P. Musgrove, F. J. Chaloupka, and A. Yurekli. 2000. "The Economic Rationale for Intervention in the Tobacco Market." In *Tobacco Control in Developing Countries*, ed. P. Jha and F. J. Chaloupka. Oxford, U.K.: Oxford University Press.

Jha, P., M. K. Ranson, S. N. Nguyen, and D. Yach. 2002. "Estimates of Global and Regional Smoking Prevalence in 1995 by Age and Sex." *American Journal of Public Health* 92 (6): 1002–6.

Joossens, L., F. J. Chaloupka, D. Merriman, and A.Yurekli. 2000. "Issues in the Smuggling of Tobacco Products." In *Tobacco Control in Developing Countries*, ed. P. Jha and F. J. Chaloupka. Oxford, U.K.: Oxford University Press.

Kenkel, D., and L. Chen. 2000. "Consumer Information and Tobacco Use." In *Tobacco Control in Developing Countries*, ed. P. Jha and F. J. Chaloupka. Oxford, U.K.: Oxford University Press.

Koop, C. E. 2003. "Tobacco Addiction: Accomplishments and Challenges in Science, Health, and Policy." *Nicotine and Tobacco Research* 5 (5): 613–19.

Lam, T. H., Y. He, Q. L. Shi, J. Y. Huang, F. Zhang, Z. H. Wan, and others. 2002. "Smoking, Quitting, and Mortality in a Chinese Cohort of Retired Men." *Annals of Epidemiology* 12 (5): 316–20.

Laviolette, S. R., and D. van der Kooy. 2004. "The Neurobiology of Nicotine Addiction: Bridging the Gap from Molecules to Behavior." *Nature Reviews* 5 (1): 55–65.

Levy, D. T., K. Friend, and E. Polishchuk. 2001. "Effect of Clean Indoor Air Laws on Smokers: The Clean Air Module of the SimSmoke Computer Simulation Model." *Tobacco Control* 10 (4): 345–51.

Lightwood, J., D. Collins, H. Lapsley, and T. E. Novotny. 2000. "Estimating the Costs of Tobacco Use." In *Tobacco Control in Developing Countries*, ed. P. Jha and F. J. Chaloupka. Oxford, U.K.: Oxford University Press.

Liu, B. Q., R. Peto, Z. M. Chen, J. Boreham, Y. P. Wu, J. Y. Li, and others. 1998. "Emerging Tobacco Hazards in China: 1. Retrospective Proportional Mortality Study of One Million Deaths." *British Medical Journal* 317 (7170): 1411–22.

Markou, A., and J. E. Henningfield. 2003. "Background Paper on the Neurobiology of Nicotine Addiction." Paper presented at the Disease Control Priorities Project Nicotine Addiction Workshop, Mumbai, India, September 2003.

Martinson, B. C., P. J. O'Connor, N. P. Pronk, and S. J. Rolnick. 2003. "Smoking Cessation Attempts in Relation to Prior Health Care Changes: The Effect of Antecedent Smoking-Related Symptoms?" *American Journal of Health Promotion* 18 (2): 125–32.

Merriman, D., A. Yurekli, and F. J. Chaloupka. 2000. "How Big Is the Worldwide Cigarette Smuggling Problem?" In *Tobacco Control in Developing Countries*, ed. P. Jha, and F. J. Chaloupka. Oxford, U.K.: Oxford University Press.

Molarius, A., R. W. Parsons, A. J. Dobson, A. Evans, S. P. Fortmann, K. Jamrozik, and others. 2001. "Trends in Cigarette Smoking in 36 Populations from the Early 1980s to the Mid-1990s: Findings from the WHO MONICA Project." *American Journal of Public Health* 91 (2): 206–12.

Moore, M. J. 1996. "Death and Tobacco Taxes." *RAND Journal of Economics* 27 (2): 415–28.

Murphy, K. M., and R. H. Topel. 2003. "The Economic Value of Medical Research." In *Measuring the Gains of Medical Research: An Economic Approach*, ed. K. M. Murphy and R. H. Topel, 41–73. Chicago: University of Chicago.

Niu, S. R., G. H. Yang, Z. M. Chen, J. L. Wang, G. H. Wang, X. Z. He, and others. 1998. "Emerging Tobacco Hazards in China: 2. Early Mortality Results from a Prospective Study." *British Medical Journal* 317 (7170): 1423–24.

Novotny, T. E., J. C. Cohen, A. Yurekli, D. Sweaner, and J. de Beyer. 2000. "Smoking Cessation and Nicotine-Replacement Therapies." In *Tobacco Control in Developing Countries*, ed. P. Jha and F. J. Chaloupka. Oxford, U.K.: Oxford University Press.

O'Malley, P. M., J. G. Bachman, and L. D. Johnston. 1988. "Period, Age, and Cohort Effects on Substance Use among Young Americans: A Decade of Change, 1976–86." *American Journal of Public Health* 78 (10): 1315–21.

Pechmann, C., P. Dixon, and N. Layne. 1998. "An Assessment of U.S. and Canadian Smoking Reduction Objectives for the Year 2000." *American Journal of Public Health* 88 (9): 1362–67.

Peck, R., F. J. Chaloupka, P. Jha, J. Lightwood. 2000. "Welfare Analyses of Tobacco." In *Tobacco Control in Developing Countries*, ed. P. Jha and F. J. Chaloupka, 131–52. Oxford, U.K.: Oxford University Press.

Peto, R., S. Darby, H. Deo, P. Silcocks, E. Whitley, and R. Doll. 2000. "Smoking, Smoking Cessation, and Lung Cancer in the U.K. since 1950: Combination of National Statistics with Two Case-Control Studies." *British Medical Journal* 321 (7257): 323–29.

Peto, R., and A. D. Lopez. 2001. "The Future Worldwide Health Effects of Current Smoking Patterns." In *Critical Issues in Global Health*, ed. C. E. Koop, C. E. Pearson, and M. R. Schwarz. New York: Jossey-Bass.

Peto, R., A. D. Lopez, J. Boreham, and M. Thun. 2003. *Mortality from Smoking in Developed Countries*. 2nd ed. Oxford, U.K.: Oxford University Press.

Peto, R., A. D. Lopez, J. Boreham, M. Thun, and C. Heath, Jr. 1994. *Mortality from Smoking in Developed Countries, 1950–2000*. Oxford, U.K.: Oxford University Press.

Picciotto, M. R. 2003. "Nicotine as a Modulator of Behavior: Beyond the Inverted U." *Trends in Pharmacological Sciences* 24 (9): 493–99.

Pollock, D. 1996. "Forty Years On: A War to Recognise and Win—How the Tobacco Industry Has Survived the Revelations on Smoking and Health." *British Medical Bulletin* 52 (1): 174–82.

Ranson, M. K., P. Jha, F. J. Chaloupka, and S. N. Nguyen. 2002. "Global and Regional Estimates of the Effectiveness and Cost-Effectiveness of Price Increases and Other Tobacco Control Policies." *Nicotine and Tobacco Research* 4 (3): 311–19.

Raw, M., A. McNeill, and R. West. 1999. "Smoking Cessation: Evidence-Based Recommendations for the Healthcare System." *British Medical Journal* 318 (7177): 182–85.

Ross, H., F. J. Chaloupka, and M. Wakefield. 2001. "Youth Smoking Uptake Progress: Price and Public Policy Effects." Research Paper 11. ImpacTeen, Health Research and Policy Centers, University of Illinois at Chicago.

Saffer, H. 2000. "Tobacco Advertising and Promotion." In *Tobacco Control in Developing Countries*, ed. P. Jha and F. J. Chaloupka. Oxford, U.K.: Oxford University Press.

Saffer, H., and F. Chaloupka. 2000. "Tobacco Advertising: Economic Theory and International Evidence." *Journal of Health Economics* 19 (6): 1117–37.

Saxenian, H., and B. McGreevey. 1996. "China: Issues and Options in Health Financing." Report 15278-CHA, World Bank, Washington, DC.

Shiffman, S., and R. West. 2003. "Background Paper on the Psychology of Nicotine Addiction." Paper presented at the Disease Control Priorities Project Nicotine Addiction Workshop, Mumbai, India, September 2003.

Sunley, E. M., A. Yurekli, and F. J. Chaloupka. 2000. "The Design, Administration and Potential Revenue of Tobacco Excises." In *Tobacco Control in Developing Countries*, ed. P. Jha and F. J. Chaloupka. Oxford, U.K.: Oxford University Press.

Tauras, J. A. 1999. "The Transition to Smoking Cessation: Evidence from Multiple Failure Duration Analysis." NBER Working Paper 7412. Cambridge, MA: National Bureau of Economic Research.

Tauras, J. A., and F. J. Chaloupka. 2003. "The Demand for Nicotine Replacement Therapies." *Nicotine and Tobacco Research* 5 (2): 237–43.

Tauras, J. A., F. J. Chaloupka, M. Farrelly, G. A. Giovino, M. Wakefield, L. D. Johnston, and others. 2005. "State Tobacco Control Spending and Youth Smoking." *American Journal of Public Health* 95 (2): 338–44.

Taylor, A. L., F. J. Chaloupka, E. Guindon, and M. Corbett. 2000. "The Impact of Trade Liberalization on Tobacco Consumption." In *Tobacco Control in Developing Countries*, ed. P. Jha and F. J. Chaloupka, 343–64. Oxford, U.K.: Oxford University Press.

Townsend, J. L. 1993. "Policies to Halve Smoking Deaths." *Addiction* 88 (1): 43–52.

Townsend, J. L., P. Roderick, and J. Cooper. 1998. "Cigarette Smoking by Socio-Economic Group, Sex, and Age: Effects of Price, Income, and Health Publicity." *British Medical Journal* 309 (6959): 923–26.

U.K. Department of Health. 1992. "Effect of Tobacco Advertising on Tobacco Consumption: A Discussion Document Reviewing the Evidence." London: U.K. Department of Health, Economics and Operational Research Division.

U.S. DHHS (United States Department of Health and Human Services). 1994. *Preventing Tobacco Use amongst Young People. A Report of the Surgeon General*. Atlanta: U.S. DHHS, Public Health Service, Centers for Disease Control, Center for Chronic Disease Prevention and Health Promotion, Office on Smoking and Health.

———. 2000. *Reducing Tobacco Use: A Report of the Surgeon General*. Atlanta: U.S. DHHS, Public Health Service, Centers for Disease Control, Center for Chronic Disease Prevention and Health Promotion, Office on Smoking and Health.

U.S. Federal Trade Commission. 2004. *Cigarette Report for 2002*. Washington, DC: U.S. Federal Trade Commission. http://www.ftc.gov/reports/cigarette/041022cigaretterpt.pdf.

Warner, K. E. 1986. "Smoking and Health Implications of a Change in the Federal Cigarette Excise Tax." *Journal of the American Medical Association* 255 (8): 1028–32.

———. 2003. "The Costs of Benefits: Smoking and Health Care Expenditures." *American Journal of Health Promotion* 18 (2): 123–24.

Warner, K. E., F. J. Chaloupka, P. J. Cook, W. G. Manning, J. P. Newhouse, T. E. Novotny, and others. 1995. "Criteria for Determining an Optimal Cigarette Tax: The Economist's Perspective." *Tobacco Control* 4: 380–86.

Wasserman, J., W. G. Manning, J. P. Newhouse, and J. D. Winkler. 1991. "The Effects of Excise Taxes and Regulations on Cigarette Smoking." *Journal of Health Economics* 10 (1): 43–64.

Weinstein, N. D. 1998. "Accuracy of Smokers' Risk Perceptions." *Annals of Behavioral Medicine* 20 (2): 135–40.

WHO (World Health Organization). 1997. *Tobacco or Heath: A Global Status Report*. Geneva: WHO.

———. 2002. "The European Report on Tobacco Control Policy." Paper presented at the WHO European Ministerial Conference for a Tobacco-free Europe, Warsaw. Document EUR/01/5020906/8, WHO Regional Office for Europe, Copenhagen.

Woolery, T., S. Asma, and D. Sharp. 2000. "Clean Indoor-Air Laws and Youth Access." In *Tobacco Control in Developing Countries*, ed. P. Jha and F. J. Chaloupka. Oxford, U.K.: Oxford University Press.

Zatonski, W., and P. Jha. 2000. "The Health Transformation in Eastern Europe after 1990: A Second Look." Warsaw: Marie Skeodowska-Curie Cancer Center and Institute of Oncology.

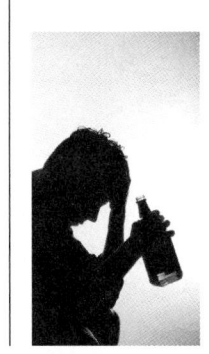

Chapter **47**

Alcohol

Jürgen Rehm, Dan Chisholm, Robin Room, and Alan D. Lopez

This chapter provides an overview of epidemiology of alcohol use and health consequences as well as introducing cost-effectiveness interventions to reduce alcohol-related harm.

EPIDEMIOLOGY OF ALCOHOL USE AND ALCOHOL-RELATED DISEASE CONDITIONS

Alcoholic beverages and the problems they engender have been familiar fixtures in human societies since the beginning of recorded history. Because alcohol is causally related to more than 60 International Classification of Diseases codes (Rehm, Room, Graham, and others 2003), disease outcomes are among the most important alcohol-related problems. Depending on the pattern of consumption, alcohol is also protective against diseases, most important among them, coronary heart disease (Rehm, Sempos, and Trevisan 2003). However, the net effect is negative, and 4 percent of the global burden of disease is attributable to alcohol, or about as much death and disability globally as is attributable to tobacco and hypertension (Ezzati and others 2002; WHO 2002). Alcohol thus constitutes a serious public health problem (Room, Babor, and Rehm 2005). Evidence-based preventive measures are available at both the individual and the population levels, with alcohol taxes, restrictions on alcohol availability, and drinking-and-driving countermeasures among the most effective policy options (Babor and others 2003). This chapter reviews the cost-effectiveness of different interventions in developing regions of the world.

Dimensions of Alcohol Related to Disease

The relationship between alcohol consumption and health and social outcomes is complex and multidimensional (Rehm and

others 2004). As figure 47.1 shows, alcohol consumption is linked to acute and long-term health and social consequences through three intermediate mechanisms—toxic and beneficial biochemical effects, intoxication, and dependence (Babor and others 2003; Rehm, Room, Graham, and others 2003)—as follows:

- *Toxic and beneficial biochemical effects.* These effects of alcohol consumption may influence chronic disease in either beneficial or harmful ways. Accepted beneficial effects include the influence of moderate drinking on coronary heart disease through reduction of plaque deposits in arteries, protection against blood clot formation, and promotion of blood clot dissolution (Zakhari 1997). Examples of harmful effects include increased risk for high blood pressure and for liver damage (Rehm, Room, Graham, and others 2003) and direct toxic effects on acinar cells triggering pancreatic damage (Apte, Wilson, and Korsten 1997) or hormonal disturbances (Emanuele and Emanuele 1997). These are just examples, because alcohol exposure is associated with a multitude of toxic effects on different organs.
- *Intoxication.* Alcohol intoxication is a powerful mediator for acute health outcomes, such as accidental or intentional injuries or deaths, although intoxication can also be implicated in chronic health and social problems and in certain forms of heart disease. The subjective feeling of intoxication is mainly caused by the effects of alcohol on the central nervous system, and these effects are felt and can be measured even at light to moderate consumption levels (Eckardt and others 1998).
- *Dependence.* Alcohol dependence is a clinical disorder in its own right, but it is also a powerful mechanism sustaining alcohol consumption and mediating its impact on both

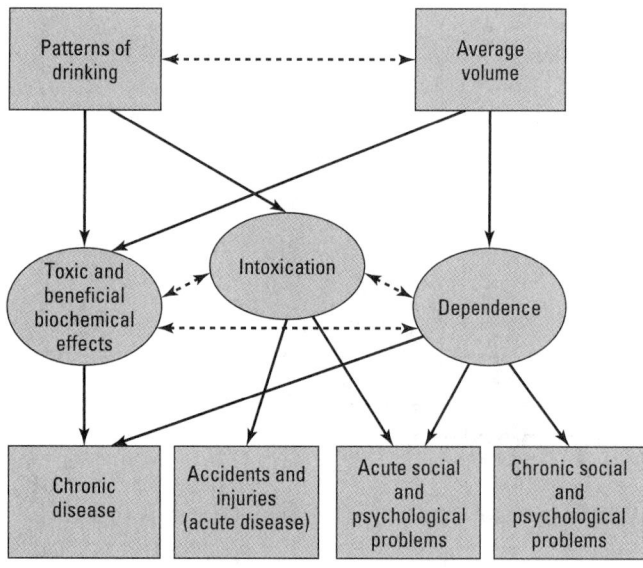

Source: Adapted from Babor and others 2003.

Figure 47.1 Model of Alcohol Consumption, Intermediate Outcomes, and Long-Term Consequences

chronic and acute physiological and social consequences of alcohol (Drummond 1990). In the quantitative analyses reported in this chapter, alcohol dependence—and alcohol-use disorders (AUDs) in general—will be considered only as a health outcome related to high-risk alcohol use.

This chapter, including the section on the cost-effectiveness of interventions, focuses primarily on health consequences, although later it briefly discusses the social consequences of high-risk drinking and recommended interventions. The epidemiological calculations are taken from Ezzati and others' (2002) comparative risk analysis (CRA) and the World Health Organization (WHO) assessment of the global burden of disease (WHO 2002). (For further information, see Mathers and others 2003; Rehm, Rehn, and others 2003; Rehm, Room, Graham, and others 2003; Rehm, Room, Monteiro and others 2003; Rehm and others 2004). The CRA defines alcohol exposure using two measures: the average volume of alcohol consumption and patterns of drinking (figure 47.1). It then relates these exposure measures to disease outcomes.

The average volume of consumption has been the conventional measure of exposure in alcohol epidemiology (Bruun and others 1975) and has been linked to many disease categories following the seminal work of English and others (1995; see also Rehm, Room, Graham, and others 2003). Patterns of drinking have been linked mainly to two categories of disease outcome: acute effects of alcohol (such as accidental and intentional injuries) and cardiovascular outcomes (mainly coronary heart disease). The CRA defines patterns of drinking primarily

in terms of high-risk drinking occasions and also in terms of drinking in public settings and the proportion of drinking that occurs outside of meals (for further details, see Rehm and others 2004).

Epidemiology of High-Risk Alcohol Use

The intervention analyses presented in this chapter focus on average high-risk drinking, although patterns of drinking were also incorporated into the disease burden calculations. High-risk drinking is defined in sex-specific terms as drinking 20 grams per day or more of pure alcohol on average for females and 40 grams per day or more of pure alcohol on average for males (a bottle of table wine contains about 70 grams of pure alcohol). This definition of high-risk drinking is fairly standard in alcohol epidemiology and was first introduced by English and others (1995) on the basis of Australian guidelines. Originally, English and others (1995) used two categories: *hazardous drinking* (defined as drinking between 20 and 40 grams per day of pure alcohol on average for females and between 40 and 60 grams per day of pure alcohol for males) and *harmful drinking* (defined as drinking 40 grams per day or more of pure alcohol on average for females and 60 grams per day or more of pure alcohol on average for males). These categories have been used in almost every comprehensive meta-analysis on alcohol and disease since 1995 (see Rehm, Room, Graham, and others 2003 for an overview). However, critics asserted that the terms *hazardous drinking* and *harmful drinking* were not neutral; thus, the CRA uses drinking categories II and III, referring to the term *high-risk drinking* when both categories are considered together. High-risk drinking thresholds differ by sex because the risk for chronic disease is related to lower volumes of drinking for women than for men; thus, the thresholds for high-risk drinking were set to reflect an approximately similar risk of chronic disease.

Table 47.1 shows the distribution of high-risk drinking by age and by World Bank region. The table excludes the Middle East and North Africa because prevalence rates of high-risk drinking are considerably lower than 1 percent and this situation is unlikely to change in the near future.

Calculating the burden of high-risk alcohol use that is avertable by means of effective interventions requires additional epidemiological data—in particular, rates of incidence to and remission from high-risk alcohol use and the relative fatality of high-risk alcohol users compared with non-high-risk alcohol users. We derived remission rates from studies of natural recovery from alcohol problems, which found an average of 10.9 years to remission (Sobell, Ellingstad, and Sobell 2000), with an adjustment of plus 20 percent for older age groups and minus 20 percent for younger age groups. We set the relative risk of mortality for high-risk alcohol users age 15 to 44 at 2.5 and the relative risk for older age groups at 1.3 for men and 1.4 for women (Gmel, Gutjahr, and Rehm 2003; Rehm, Gutjahr, and Gmel

Table 47.1 Prevalence of High-Risk Drinking by Gender, Age Group, and Region, 2000
(percentage of the population)

Region	Gender	Age group (years)				
		15–29	30–44	45–59	60–69	70+
Europe and Central Asia	Male	20.8	18.7	21.4	15.2	8.1
	Female	11.2	10.4	11.5	7.9	5.7
Latin America and the Caribbean	Male	9.7	11.1	10.6	7.9	3.4
	Female	6.8	7.5	6.5	5.8	3.1
Sub-Saharan Africa	Male	10.4	14.3	12.9	11.3	8.4
	Female	3.1	4.7	5.1	3.2	2.2
East Asia and the Pacific	Male	6.2	7.5	7.1	6.5	5.0
	Female	0.3	0.2	0.1	0.1	0.0
South Asia	Male	0.8	2.5	0.3	0.1	0.0
	Female	1.2	0.4	0.4	0.0	0.0
High-income countries	Male	18.0	17.9	16.2	10.9	7.6
	Female	10.9	8.7	9.8	6.8	5.4

Source: Authors' calculations based on Rehm, Rehn, and others 2003 and Rehm and others 2004.
Note: The criteria for high-risk drinking were set sex specific (for details see text).

2001). Using WHO disease-modeling software, we derived an internally consistent epidemiological profile of current high-risk alcohol use in each region, including specifications of incidence and the relative risk of mortality, with currently observed rates of prevalence, remission, and risk of mortality as inputs. A final input parameter is the disability level for high-risk alcohol use, which we estimated at 0.154 (where zero equals no disability); this is a weighted average based on the severity breakdown of high-risk drinkers from the CRA (80 percent category II, or hazardous; 20 percent category III, or harmful). The preference values for these health states of 0.11 and 0.33, respectively, are derived from Stouthard, Essink-Bot, and Bonsel (2000).

Relationship between High-Risk Drinking and AUDs

Assessing the relationship between high-risk drinking and AUDs is not a straightforward exercise. Even though high-risk drinking over a long period entails the risk of AUDs, that all people with AUDs are also high-risk drinkers does not automatically follow. First, neither the definition of alcohol dependence nor WHO's (1993) definition of harmful use includes actual consumption levels. An individual is considered dependent if at least three of the following criteria apply:

- strong desire or compulsion to take the substance
- impaired control and physiological withdrawal if the substance is reduced or ceased
- tolerance to the effects of the substance
- preoccupation with use of the substance
- persistent use despite clear evidence of harmful consequences.

By contrast, harmful alcohol use is defined as a pattern of use that is causing damage to physical or mental health. Thus,

whereas many of these criteria are associated with high-risk alcohol use, no strict classificatory rule indicates that people with AUDs are a subcategory of high-risk drinkers.

Second, the prevalence of AUDs is often derived from surveys, where the operationalization usually requires that three symptoms be present in a lifetime and at least one of these criteria be present within the past 12 months (see, for example, Demyttenaere and others 2004, table 2). Thus individuals may be categorized as alcohol dependent even if they are currently abstaining from alcohol.

Third, qualitative studies across a wide range of cultures have found that the criteria used for diagnosing AUDs often have different meanings and implications in different cultural settings (Room and others 1996; Schmidt and Room 1999). For instance, in the United States over the past decade, the level of reported AUDs increased despite decreases in high-risk drinking (Grant and others 2004). This fact has been explained in terms of changes in drinking norms and social attitudes during a period when the United States has become a "drier" culture. Thus, the measurement of AUDs is quite complex and culturally dependent. Moreover, AUDs are only one outcome of alcohol consumption and, in many parts of the world, not the most important one. As a result, we decided to focus on high-risk alcohol consumption rather than AUDs.

Relationship between Alcohol Use and Disease Categories

The exact procedures for quantifying the risk of disease attributable to alcohol are described in detail elsewhere (Rehm, Room, Graham, and others 2003; Rehm and others 2004). For most chronic disease categories, investigators have derived alcohol-attributable fractions of disease by combining prevalence and relative risk estimates based on meta-analyses (Corrao and others 2000; English and others 1995; Gutjahr, Gmel, and Rehm 2001; Ridolfo and Stevenson 2001; Single and others 1996, 1999). For depression, we drew alcohol-attributable fractions from mental health surveys, looking at the rates of comorbidity and the order of onset of depression and alcohol disorders. For coronary heart disease, we modeled the interaction of average volumes and patterns of drinking based on multilevel analyses that include temporal information as covariates (Gmel, Rehm, and Frick 2003; Rehm and others 2004). For the final estimates, we based alcohol-attributable fractions on these multilevel results for all countries, except for developed countries with relatively favorable drinking patterns (Australia, Japan, and countries in North America and Western Europe), which are not discussed here because the focus is on developing countries. For injuries, we took a similar multilevel approach to quantify the interaction of the average volume of consumption and patterns of drinking in determining alcohol-attributable fractions (Rehm and others 2004).

Thus the analysis includes the following major disease categories:

- chronic disease
  o cancer (mouth and oropharyngeal, esophageal, liver, female breast)
  o neuropsychiatric diseases (AUDs, unipolar major depression, epilepsy)
  o diabetes
  o cardiovascular diseases (hypertensive diseases, coronary heart disease, stroke)
  o gastrointestinal diseases (cirrhosis of the liver)
  o conditions arising during the perinatal period (low birthweight)
- injury
  o unintentional injury (motor vehicle accidents, drowning, falls, poisonings, other unintentional injuries)
  o intentional injury (self-inflicted injuries, homicide, other intentional injuries).

We did not include other disease categories that are clearly alcohol-related, such as fetal alcohol syndrome, because the current analysis was based on the CRA and was, thus, limited to the global burden-of-disease categories.

Social Determinants of Exposure and Risk

Alcohol-specific risks to health are in part determined and modified by social determinants. For example, Harrison and Gardiner (1999) find that for men age 25 to 69 in England and Wales in 1988–94, those in the lowest socioeconomic status category, unskilled labor, had a 15-fold greater risk for alcohol-related mortality than professionals in the highest category

had. These differences cannot be explained by the overall volume of drinking, which actually tended to be greater for those in higher socioeconomic groups. Rather, the differences can be explained by the fact that more of the drinking of those in lower socioeconomic status categories is in high-risk patterns; that is, depending on the use values for drinking in the culture, poor drinkers may see little point in wasting resources on drinking that is not to intoxication. Poorer drinkers are also likely to be less protected physically and socially from possible harm arising from drinking, such as injuries and chronic and infectious diseases. Mäkelä (1999) finds that multiple dimensions of socioeconomic status are required to capture all the adverse interactions of socioeconomic status with alcohol-related mortality.

A critical macroeconomic question is how a country's level of economic development is related to alcohol-related risks to health. The impact of alcohol on disease and mortality may be more potent in countries with greater poverty and nutritional deficiencies (Isichei, Ikwuagu, and Egbuta 1993; Room and others 2002, 119–30). However, most of the risk relationships between alcohol and disease have been derived from studies in established market economies, and the extent of systematic research is currently insufficient to allow quantification of this phenomenon. As a result, the estimated disease burden cited here may be considered as a lower-bound estimate of the actual alcohol-attributable disease burden in developing countries.

BURDEN OF DISEASE RELATED TO HIGH-RISK ALCOHOL USE

In the following sections, the procedures to estimate alcohol-related burden of disease are described, as well as the limitations of the used approach.

Determining the Alcohol-Related Burden of Disease

Table 47.2 breaks down alcohol-attributable disability-adjusted life years (DALYs) by disease category and World Bank region using a constant 3 percent per year discount rate, but with no age weighting. Results differ from those of the CRA (Ezzati and others 2002; Rehm and others 2004; WHO 2002) because of the use of non-age-weighted DALYs.[1]

Determining the Burden of Disease Related to High-Risk Alcohol Consumption

In determining the burden of disease related to high-risk alcohol consumption, we first divided the burden of disease between chronic and acute disease. For chronic disease, we assume that almost the entire disease burden reported in the CRA is associated with high-risk alcohol use. Indeed, the overall disease burden in the CRA is an underestimate, because drinking up to 20 grams per day of pure alcohol by females and

Table 47.2 Alcohol-Attributable DALYs by Disease Category and World Bank Region, 2001
(thousands of DALYs)

Disease category	Europe and Central Asia	Latin America and the Caribbean	Sub-Saharan Africa	Middle East and North Africa	East Asia and the Pacific	South Asia	High-income countries	World
Chronic disease								
Maternal and perinatal conditions	12	7	39	1	2	29	6	105
Cancer	526	296	635	25	2,820	189	1,103	5,594
Neuropsychiatric	2,159	3,315	1,035	89	4,726	1,444	4,752	17,600
Vascular	2,639	926	556	40	1,751	1,199	−2,488	5,209
Other noncommunicable diseases	1,175	739	504	27	997	306	1,153	5,126
Subtotal chronic disease	6,511	5,283	2,769	182	10,296	3,167	4,526	33,634
Injury								
Unintentional	4,127	1,984	2,308	135	3,613	2,222	1,753	15,619
Intentional	1,822	1,872	1,074	9	927	567	571	6,755
Subtotal injury	5,949	3,856	3,382	144	4,540	2,789	2,324	22,374
Total DALYs attributable to alcohol	12,460	9,139	6,151	326	14,836	5,956	6,850	56,008
Total DALYs from all diseases	116,502	104,287	344,754	65,570	346,225	408,655	149,161	1,535,871
Proportion of DALYs attributable to alcohol (percent)	10.7	8.8	1.8	0.5	4.3	1.5	4.6	3.6

Source: Authors' calculations based on Rehm and others 2004 and WHO 2002.
Note: Negative DALYs can occur because certain patterns of alcohol have cardio-protective effects.

up to 40 grams per day of pure alcohol by males is globally associated with a net beneficial effect in relation to chronic disease. However, this effect occurs mainly in countries with moderate drinking patterns (Rehm, Sempos, and Trevisan 2003), which tend to be high-income countries (Rehm, Rehn, and others 2003). Although high-risk but regular drinking patterns may also have some beneficial effects, such effects are not important in countries with binge drinking patterns. (For the association between alcohol and coronary heart disease, see McKee and Britton 1998; Puddey and others 1999; Rehm, Sempos, and Trevisan 2003; for consequences on modeling the regional burden of disease, see Rehm and others 2004.)

For injuries, which are considered to be acute outcomes, we started by separating out the proportion of injury not caused by high-risk drinking, which we accomplished by assuming that injuries are linearly related to per capita consumption (Rehm and others 2004).[2] This assumption is probably conservative, because high-risk drinkers in countries with binge drinking patterns are likely to have more frequent and intensive drinking occasions, and the risk of injury usually rises logarithmically with the amount of drinking on a specific occasion (see, for example, National Highway Traffic Safety Administration 1992). Following this initial calculation, we

could calculate the proportion of per capita consumption related to high-risk drinking in each region, thereby determining the proportion of injury caused by high-risk drinking (table 47.3). Together with our calculation of the chronic disease burden attributable to high-risk alcohol use, this percentage enabled us to estimate the overall disease burden attributable to high-risk alcohol use: whereas 3.6 percent of the global burden was attributable to alcohol drinking generally, 2.8 percent was attributable to high-risk drinking.

Limitations of the CRA Approach

The CRA's estimates of the global and regional alcohol-related burden of disease are based on a number of assumptions, of which the following are the most crucial:

- The estimates of per capita consumption and unrecorded consumption for different countries do not contain substantial measurement error.
- The distribution of consumption as derived from surveys is similar to actual distribution in the population.
- The relationships between alcohol and chronic disease derived from meta-analyses of cohort and case-control studies are stable among countries and regions.

Table 47.3 DALYs Attributable to High-Risk Average Alcohol Consumption by Disease Category and Region, 2001
(thousands of DALYs)

Disease category	Europe and Central Asia	Latin America and the Caribbean	Sub-Saharan Africa	East Asia and the Pacific	South Asia	High-income countries	World
Total chronic disease	6,510	5,283	2,770	10,296	3,167	4,526	33,634
Total injury	3,149	1,500	1,693	1,532	514	1,092	9,207
Total DALYs attributable to high-risk alcohol consumption	9,659	6,783	4,463	11,828	3,681	5,618	42,841
Total DALYs from all diseases	116,502	104,287	344,754	346,225	408,655	149,161	1,535,871
Proportion of DALYs attributable to high-risk alcohol consumption	8.3	6.5	1.3	3.4	0.9	3.8	2.8

Source: Authors' calculations based on Rehm and others 2004 and WHO 2002.

Some evidence indicates that per capita consumption can be reliably estimated, and information on this indicator is available for the vast majority of countries (Rehm, Rehn, and others 2003). With respect to survey information, reliability and worldwide coverage are lower. However, because the overall volume of consumption and, thus, the average volume per capita are based on production and sales estimates, the measure of the volume of drinking overall can be considered reliable. These factors leave the stability of relationships between alcohol and chronic disease as the most crucial part of our estimates. Some indications suggest that relative risks may not be the same in developing countries as in developed countries (for example, for tobacco and lung cancers, see Liu and others 1998). Thus, the CRA's estimates may be biased, most likely toward an overestimation of the impact of alcohol.

One additional problem pertains to the usual epidemiological approach as applied to alcohol. Most information about alcohol and chronic disease is derived from cohorts. Because cohorts are frequently not representative of the population as a whole, specific patterns of consumption such as binge drinking are often not represented, and thus their influence cannot be analyzed (Rehm, Gmel, and others 2003). Unfortunately, the patterns most often missing are those that are the most detrimental with respect to health; thus, the impact of alcohol on chronic diseases that are influenced by patterns of drinking other than average volumes is underestimated.

INTERVENTIONS FOR REDUCING HIGH-RISK DRINKING

The next two sections estimate the burden of disease attributable to high-risk alcohol consumption that is currently being averted or could be averted by a range of personal and nonpersonal intervention strategies and calculate the expected costs and cost-effectiveness of such interventions. Methods and analyses draw on Chisholm and others (2004), adjusted as necessary to conform to the analytical standards of this volume, including the specification of all costs in U.S. dollars rather than international dollars.

Population Model

We determined intervention effectiveness using a state transition population model (Lauer and others 2003), which traces the development of a regional population taking into account births, deaths, and the specified risk factor—in this case, high-risk alcohol use. In addition to population size and structure, the population model uses a number of epidemiological parameters (incidence and prevalence, remission, and cause-specific and residual rates of mortality) and assigns age- and gender-specific health state valuations to both the disease in question and to the nondiseased population. The output of the model is an estimate of the total healthy life years experienced by the population over a lifetime period (100 years).

We ran the model for a number of possible scenarios, including no intervention at all (natural history), current intervention coverage, and scaled-up coverage of current and possible new interventions. For the intervention scenarios, we used an implementation period of 10 years for an intervention program (after which epidemiological rates return to their natural history levels), from which we derived the number of additional DALYs averted each year compared with the case for no intervention at all. We discounted DALYs at 3 percent but did not age weight them.

Effectiveness

A number of interventions have been evaluated and shown to be effective in reducing alcohol use, yet their level of implementation remains low in all but a handful of countries and their potential effect on population-level health has rarely been assessed. By contrast, some interventions without clearly established effects continue to be widely used, including, for example, mass media public information campaigns and school-based education aimed at reducing alcohol consumption. Recent reviews of measures to reduce alcohol misuse have assessed the quality of the evidence for four types of interventions specifically aimed at reducing high-risk alcohol use (Babor and others 2003; Ludbrook and others 2002):

- policy and legislative interventions, including taxation of alcohol sales, laws on drunk driving, restrictions on retail outlets, and controls on advertising
- measures to better enforce these interventions, such as random breath testing of drivers
- mass media and other awareness campaigns
- brief interventions with individual high-risk drinkers.

On the basis of these reviews, we included the following strategies and intervention effects in our analysis: drinking-and-driving legislation and random breath testing, taxation of alcoholic beverages, reduced hours of sale in retail outlets, and advertising bans (included as population-based interventions) and so-called brief interventions (included as interventions aimed at personal behavior). We considered including one other intervention strategy—mass media or school-based awareness campaigns—but omitted it in the final analysis on the grounds that evidence for its effectiveness was weak, both in terms of methodological quality and in terms of its effect on consumption (as opposed to transfer of information or knowledge alone) (Babor and others 2003; Edwards and others 1994; Foxcroft and others 2003; Foxcroft, Lister-Sharp, and Lowe 1997; Ludbrook and others 2002).

Drunk-Driving Legislation and Random Breath Testing. Drunk-driving laws and reinforcement policies, such as random breath testing of drivers, influence fatal and nonfatal traffic injuries among both high-risk alcohol users and other members of the population, such as passengers and pedestrians. We assessed two independent effects on alcohol-related traffic injuries, but note that evidence for these effects comes from the developed countries, where road infrastructures and driving patterns may differ significantly from those in the developing world. The first intervention was drunk-driving laws, estimated to reduce traffic fatalities by 7 percent if widely implemented across a region. The second was enforcement by random breath testing, estimated to reduce fatalities by 6 to 10 percent in regions partially implementing such a strategy and by 18 percent with wide implementation. The effect on nonfatal injuries was estimated to be a reduction of 15 percent (Peek-Asa 1999; Shults and others 2001). In each region, we applied these estimated effects to the proportion of total deaths and of years lived with a disability attributed to alcohol-related traffic accidents (table 47.4).

Taxation on Alcoholic Beverages. Excise taxation on alcoholic beverages primarily affects the incidence of drinking through reduced consumption. Effects are measured in terms of price elasticity, which relates the change in consumption to the size of the price increase (table 47.5). We derived price elasticities, adjusted downward by one-third to reflect possible reduced price responsiveness among high-risk drinkers, with reference to preferred type of alcoholic beverage (beer, wine, or spirits) by region, built up from country-level data (WHO 2003b). This downward adjustment of price elasticities for high-risk drinkers is a conservative approach; most of the literature found similar effects on high-risk and dependent drinkers as on social users (Babor and others 2003; see also Farrell, Manning, and Finch 2003).

Price elasticities ranged from −0.3 for the most preferred beverage category to −1.5 for the least preferred (Babor and others 2003; Levy and Ornstein 1983). For a beer-drinking region where wine is the second-most preferred beverage type, for example, elasticities were set as follows: beer −0.3, wine −1.0, distilled spirits −1.5. We performed sensitivity analysis around these elasticities. We evaluated three rates of excise tax on alcoholic beverages: the current rate of tax, a 25 percent increase over the current rate, and a 50 percent increase over the current rate. We adjusted estimated reductions in the incidence of high-risk alcohol use by the observed or expected level of unrecorded consumption resulting from illicit production and smuggling (for instance, an estimated 35 percent of alcohol consumption in Eastern Europe and Central Asia is unrecorded, a proportion that was modeled to increase by 10 to 15 percent with the tax increases). In regions with rates of unrecorded consumption already greater than 50 percent (South Asia and Sub-Saharan Africa), tax increases can actually have a regressive impact on incidence if accompanied by a rise in the already high level of unrecorded (and therefore untaxed) consumption.

Reduced Hours of Sale in Retail Outlets. Access to and availability of alcohol can be dramatically reduced by prohibition or rationing, but implementing and sustaining such strategies without adverse effects, such as black markets and poisonings from home-produced alcohol, present considerable challenges. A more modest strategy is to reduce the hours of sale of retail outlets selling alcoholic beverages (for example, no sales for off-premise consumption for a 24-hour period at the weekend), which in Scandinavia has reduced consumption and alcohol-related harm (Leppänen 1979; Nordlund 1984; Norström and Skog 2003). On the basis of these studies, we modeled a modest reduction of 1.5 to 3.0 percent in the incidence of high-risk drinking and 1.5 to 4.0 percent in alcohol-related traffic

Table 47.4 Effectiveness of Drinking-and-Driving Legislation and Its Enforcement
(per 100,000 population)

World Bank region	WHO subregion	Sex	Attributable fractions (per 100,000 deaths)		Effectiveness of drinking-and-driving laws and random breath testing	
			Deaths attributed to traffic accidents[a]	Deaths attributed to alcohol-related traffic accidents[a]	Reduced deaths (per 100,000)	Reduced years lost due to disability (per 100,000)
Europe and Central Asia	Europe B	Male	1,473	657	141	77
		Female	542	74	16	6
	Europe C	Male	2,197	1,396	299	193
		Female	799	223	48	30
Latin America and the Caribbean	Americas B	Male	4,358	2,053	439	148
		Female	1,514	220	47	12
	Americas D	Male	2,599	861	184	64
		Female	1,093	101	22	6
Sub-Saharan Africa	Africa D	Male	2,159	417	89	43
		Female	1,079	90	19	9
	Africa E	Male	2,075	803	172	107
		Female	1,027	123	26	17
East Asia and the Pacific	Southeast Asia B	Male	7,809	1,993	427	164
		Female	2,343	127	27	8
	Western Pacific B	Male	3,629	723	155	66
		Female	1,790	157	34	12
South Asia	Southeast Asia D	Male	3,689	591	126	45
		Female	1,451	53	11	3

Source: Deaths attributed to traffic accidents: WHO 2003a; deaths attributed to alcohol-related traffic accidents: Rehm and others 2004.

B = low child mortality, low adult mortality; C = low child mortality, high adult mortality; D = high child mortality, high adult mortality; E = high child mortality, very high adult mortality.

a. Percentages for all age groups combined shown here.

fatalities, depending on the regional pattern of drinking, with the largest effects in regions with the highest levels of high-risk drinking occasions.

Advertising Bans. Public health specialists are becoming increasingly interested in the effect of a comprehensive ban on alcohol advertising, including advertising on television and through radio and billboards. However, available evidence from econometric studies suggests a modest effect on consumption at best, even for a comprehensive ban, arguably because of the continuing presence of other alcohol marketing strategies, such as product placement or event sponsorship (Grube and Agostinelli 2000; Saffer 2000; Saffer and Dave 2002). Here we consider the potential effects of a comprehensive advertising ban (television, radio, and billboards) by modeling a 2 to 4 percent reduction in the incidence of high-risk alcohol use, depending on regional drinking patterns.

Brief Interventions. We modeled brief interventions (such as physician advice provided in primary health care settings), which involve a small number of education sessions and psychosocial counseling, to influence the prevalence of high-risk drinking by increasing remission and reducing disability. Efficacy reviews of brief interventions reveal an estimated 13 to 34 percent net reduction in consumption among high-risk drinkers (Higgins-Biddle and Babor 1996; Moyer and others 2002; Whitlock and others 2004), which, if applied to the total population at risk, would reduce the overall prevalence of high-risk drinking by 35 to 50 percent, equivalent to a 14 to 18 percent improvement in the rate of recovery over no treatment at all. After taking into account adherence (70 percent) and potential treatment coverage in the population (50 percent of high-risk drinkers), however, we estimated remission rates to be between 4.9 and 6.4 percent higher than natural history rates.

Table 47.5 Effect of Taxation on the Incidence of High-Risk Alcohol Use

World Bank region	WHO subregion[a]	Prevalence by preferred beverage (percent)			Rate of taxation by preferred beverage (percent)				Price increases (percent)[b]			Nonrecorded or untaxed consumption (percent)		Effect (percent)[c]		
		Most preferred	Next preferred	Least preferred	Most preferred	Next preferred	Least preferred		Elasticity −0.3, most preferred	Elasticity −1.0, next preferred	Elasticity −1.5, least preferred			Baseline	Lower[d]	Upper[e]
Europe and Central Asia	Europe B	0.45 (spirits)	0.30 (beer)	0.25 (wine)	0.29	0.13	0.12	(current rate)	−0.04	−0.08	−0.11	0.34 (current rate)		−0.05	−0.03	−0.06
					0.36	0.16	0.15	(25 percent increase)	−0.05	−0.09	−0.13	0.37 (10 percent increase)		−0.05	−0.04	−0.07
					0.44	0.20	0.18	(50 percent increase)	−0.06	−0.11	−0.15	0.39 (15 percent increase)		−0.06	−0.04	−0.08
	Europe C	0.68 (spirits)	0.21 (beer)	0.11 (wine)	0.65	0.13	0.25	(current rate)	−0.08	−0.08	−0.20	0.36 (current rate)		−0.06	−0.04	−0.08
					0.81	0.16	0.31	(25 percent increase)	−0.09	−0.09	−0.24	0.40 (10 percent increase)		−0.06	−0.05	−0.09
					0.98	0.20	0.38	(50 percent increase)	−0.10	−0.11	−0.27	0.42 (15 percent increase)		−0.07	−0.05	−0.09
Latin America and the Caribbean	Americas B	0.53 (beer)	0.30 (spirits)	0.17 (wine)	0.16	0.49	0.22	(current rate)	−0.03	−0.22	−0.18	0.29 (current rate)		−0.08	−0.06	−0.10
					0.20	0.61	0.28	(25 percent increase)	−0.03	−0.25	−0.22	0.32 (10 percent increase)		−0.09	−0.06	−0.12
					0.24	0.74	0.33	(50 percent increase)	−0.04	−0.28	−0.25	0.34 (15 percent increase)		−0.10	−0.07	−0.13
	Americas D	0.58 (spirits)	0.39 (beer)	0.03 (wine)	0.26	0.21	0.25	(current rate)	−0.04	−0.12	−0.20	0.22 (current rate)		−0.06	−0.04	−0.08
					0.33	0.26	0.31	(25 percent increase)	−0.05	−0.14	−0.24	0.24 (10 percent increase)		−0.07	−0.05	−0.09
					0.39	0.32	0.38	(50 percent increase)	−0.06	−0.16	−0.27	0.25 (15 percent increase)		−0.08	−0.05	−0.10
Sub-Saharan Africa	Africa D	0.79 (beer)	0.16 (spirits)	0.05 (wine)	0.36	0.41	0.35	(current rate)	−0.05	−0.19	−0.26	0.77 (current rate)		−0.02	−0.01	−0.03
					0.45	0.51	0.44	(25 percent increase)	−0.06	−0.23	−0.30	0.85 (10 percent increase)		−0.01	−0.01	−0.02
					0.54	0.62	0.53	(50 percent increase)	−0.07	−0.25	−0.34	0.89 (15 percent increase)		−0.01	−0.01	−0.02
	Africa E	0.49 (beer)	0.30 (spirits)	0.21 (wine)	0.28	0.50	0.38	(current rate)	−0.04	−0.22	−0.28	0.47 (current rate)		−0.08	−0.06	−0.10
					0.35	0.63	0.48	(25 percent increase)	−0.05	−0.26	−0.32	0.52 (10 percent increase)		−0.08	−0.06	−0.11
					0.42	0.75	0.57	(50 percent increase)	−0.06	−0.29	−0.36	0.55 (15 percent increase)		−0.09	−0.06	−0.11
East Asia and the Pacific	Southeast Asia B	0.88 (spirits)	0.12 (beer)	0.00 (wine)	0.30	0.40	0.00	(current rate)	−0.05	−0.19	0.00	0.36 (current rate)		−0.04	−0.03	−0.05
					0.38	0.50	0.00	(25 percent increase)	−0.05	−0.22	0.00	0.39 (10 percent increase)		−0.05	−0.03	−0.06
					0.45	0.60	0.00	(50 percent increase)	−0.06	−0.25	0.00	0.41 (15 percent increase)		−0.05	−0.03	−0.07
	Western Pacific B	0.88 (spirits)	0.11 (beer)	0.01 (wine)	0.17	0.09	0.11	(current rate)	−0.03	−0.06	−0.10	0.27 (current rate)		−0.02	−0.02	−0.03
					0.21	0.11	0.14	(25 percent increase)	−0.04	−0.07	−0.12	0.32 (10 percent increase)		−0.03	−0.02	−0.04
					0.26	0.14	0.17	(50 percent increase)	−0.04	−0.08	−0.14	0.31 (15 percent increase)		−0.03	−0.02	−0.04
South Asia	Southeast Asia D	0.89 (spirits)	0.11 (beer)	0.00 (wine)	0.40	0.25	0.00	(current rate)	−0.06	−0.13	0.00	0.79 (current rate)		−0.01	−0.01	−0.02
					0.50	0.31	0.00	(25 percent increase)	−0.07	−0.16	0.00	0.87 (10 percent increase)		−0.01	−0.01	−0.01
					0.60	0.38	0.00	(50 percent increase)	−0.08	−0.18	0.00	0.91 (15 percent increase)		−0.01	−0.01	−0.01

Source: WHO 2003b.

a. B = low child mortality, low adult mortality; C = low child mortality, high adult mortality; D = high child mortality, high adult mortality; E = high child mortality, very high adult mortality.

b. Price rise caused by tax = [percentage of tax/(1 + percentage of tax)] × elasticity × 2/3 (high-risk drinkers less responsive).

c. Effect = sum of (prevalence × price increase) for each beverage × (1 − percentage of unrecorded consumption).

d. Lower-range elasticities = −0.2, −0.7, −1.2.

e. Upper-range elasticities = −0.4, −1.3, −2.0.

Costs

Costs covered in the analysis include program-level costs associated with running the intervention (such as administration, training, and media costs) and patient-level costs (such as costs of primary care visits). Program-level costs include resource inputs used in the production of an intervention at a level above that of the patient or providing facility, such as central planning, policy, and administration functions, as well as resources devoted to preventive programs, such as the enforcement of drunk-driving legislation by police officers (Johns and others 2003). We derived estimated quantities of resources required to implement each intervention for 10 years at the national, provincial, and district levels with reference to the region's prevailing characteristics—for example, the stability and efficiency of tax systems, the volume of traffic (for breath testing), and the strength of antidrinking sentiment as indicated by existing alcohol controls (advertising bans, restricted sales). In this analysis, patient-level resource inputs used in the provision of a given health care intervention (for example, hospital inpatient days, outpatient visits, medications, and laboratory tests) are relevant only to brief interventions. We estimated an average of four primary care visits per year for the intervention itself, plus an additional 0.33 outpatient visits (20 percent × 1.67 visits) and 0.25 inpatient days (5 percent × 5 days) (see, for example, Fleming and others 2000). We applied these patient-level resource inputs to the 50 percent of prevalent high-risk alcohol users in receipt of brief advice in year 1 and (because we model an enduring effect for 10 years) year 6 and to the 50 percent of incident cases in years 2 to 5 and 7 to 10. Note that, throughout, the costing does not include possible offsetting revenues for the government, for instance, from drunk-driving convictions and, in particular, from the revenues likely to result from increased alcohol taxes.

Unit costs and prices of program- and patient-level resource inputs include the salaries of central administrators; the capital costs of vehicles, offices, and furniture; and the cost per outpatient visit (see chapter 7 for an overview of the costing methodology, plus prices by World Bank region). All costs are expressed in U.S. dollars for 2001 and are discounted at an annual rate of 3 percent.

COST-EFFECTIVENESS OF INTERVENTIONS

In the following section, we provide results relating to the population-level health effects, costs, and cost-effectiveness of the evidence-based interventions previously reviewed.

Population-Level Effects

Except for random breath testing, two-thirds of the total population-level health gain from these interventions was among males (the proportion for random breath testing rises to 80 to 90 percent because of the higher proportion of deaths and injuries attributed to traffic accidents among men). A clear difference is also apparent between regions with relatively high rates of high-risk alcohol use (that is, prevalence in the total population greater than 5 percent) and regions with generally low levels of high-risk drinking (that is, less than 2 percent).

As shown in table 47.6, in the three regions with a higher prevalence of high-risk alcohol use—Europe and Central Asia, Latin America and the Caribbean, and Sub-Saharan Africa—the most effective interventions were taxation and brief physician advice to individual high-risk drinkers, with each averting more than 500 DALYs per million population per year. The remaining control strategies—random breath testing, reduced access to alcoholic beverage retail outlets, and a comprehensive advertising ban—mainly produced effects in the range of 200 to 400 DALYs averted per million population per year. In the two regions with lower rates of high-risk drinking (particularly among the female population), by contrast, the burden that is avertable through taxation is very much reduced (10 to 100 DALYs averted per million population per year). In South Asia, the most effective intervention is enforcement of drinking-and-driving laws by means of random breath testing, because of the higher rate of traffic-related injuries than elsewhere as well as the low levels of high-risk drinking.

Population-Level Costs

Table 47.7 summarizes the costs and cost-effectiveness of each intervention and of two combination strategies by region. The most costly interventions to implement in all regions were random breath testing and brief physician advice in primary care. The higher costs of brief advice stem from a combination of patient-level costs in the provision of the intervention itself (an average annual cost of US$7 to US$20 per treated case), plus program costs associated with administration and training primary care providers (15 to 40 percent of total costs). Random breath testing is also a relatively resource-intensive intervention to implement because of the need for regular sobriety checkpoints administered by law enforcement officers. Other interventions, including taxation, had a per capita cost in the range US$0.02 to US$0.13, depending in part on the efficiency of the tax collection system and the degree of antidrinking sentiment.

Population-Level Cost-Effectiveness

Compared with doing nothing, taxation is the most cost-effective population-level strategy in Europe and Central Asia, Latin America and the Caribbean, and Sub-Saharan Africa, the three regions with a relatively high prevalence of high-risk drinking (table 47.7). At the current rate of tax, for example, each DALY averted costs US$104 to US$225, equivalent to 4,435 to 9,633 DALYs averted per US$1 million expenditure.

Table 47.6 Population-Level Effects of Interventions to Reduce High-Risk Alcohol Use by World Bank Region

	Coverage[a] (percent)	Europe and Central Asia	Latin America and the Caribbean	Sub-Saharan Africa	East Asia and the Pacific	South Asia
Burden of disease (DALYs/million population)		20,241	12,894	6,685	6,263	2,652
Total effect (DALYs averted/ million population/year)						
Excise tax on alcoholic beverages (current situation)	*0.95*	685	586	697	83	13
Excise tax on alcoholic beverages (25 percent increase)	*0.95*	756	654	724	96	10
Excise tax on alcoholic beverages (50 percent increase)	*0.95*	828	719	764	109	8
Reduced access to alcoholic beverage retail outlets	*0.95*	441	287	386	203	32
Comprehensive advertising ban on alcohol	*0.95*	395	243	406	226	20
Random breath testing of motor vehicle drivers	*0.80*	284	307	197	181	125
Brief advice to heavy drinkers by a primary care physician	*0.50*	1,328	713	539	362	80
Combination: highest tax + brief advice		2,048	1,360	1,237	447	83
Combination: highest tax + advertising ban + random breath testing + brief advice		2,551	1,784	1,715	790	210
Reduction in current burden (percent)						
Excise tax on alcoholic beverages (current situation)	*0.95*	0.03	0.05	0.10	0.01	0.01
Excise tax on alcoholic beverages (25 percent increase)	*0.95*	0.04	0.05	0.11	0.02	0.00
Excise tax on alcoholic beverages (50 percent increase)	*0.95*	0.04	0.06	0.11	0.02	0.00
Reduced access to alcoholic beverage retail outlets	*0.95*	0.02	0.02	0.06	0.03	0.01
Comprehensive advertising ban on alcohol	*0.95*	0.02	0.02	0.06	0.04	0.01
Random breath testing of motor vehicle drivers	*0.80*	0.01	0.02	0.03	0.03	0.05
Brief advice to heavy drinkers by a primary care physician	*0.50*	0.07	0.06	0.08	0.06	0.03
Combination: highest tax + brief advice		0.10	0.11	0.19	0.07	0.03
Combination: highest tax + advertising ban + random breath testing + brief advice		0.13	0.14	0.26	0.13	0.08

Source: Chisholm and others 2004.
a. Refers to the modeled percentage of all high-risk drinkers exposed to the intervention.

Advertising bans had a cost per unit of effect similar to that of reduced access to sales outlets, US$134 to US$380, equivalent to 2,631 to 7,442 averted DALYs per US$1 million dollars expenditure, whereas random breath testing had the highest estimated cost per DALY averted: US$973 to US$1,856 per DALY, approximately 500 to 1,000 DALYs averted per US$1 million dollars expenditure. Brief physician advice provided in primary care settings had an average cost-effectiveness in the range of US$204 to US$502 per DALY averted, or close to 2,000 to 5,000 averted DALYs for every US$1 million expenditure.

Table 47.7 Costs and Cost-Effectiveness of Interventions to Reduce High-Risk Alcohol Use by World Bank Region

	Coverage[a] (percent)	Europe and Central Asia	Latin America and the Caribbean	Sub-Saharan Africa	East Asia and the Pacific	South Asia
Total cost (US$ million/year/million population)						
Excise tax on alcoholic beverages (current situation)	*0.95*	0.10	0.13	0.07	0.04	0.04
Excise tax on alcoholic beverages (25 percent increase)	*0.95*	0.10	0.13	0.07	0.04	0.04
Excise tax on alcoholic beverages (50 percent increase)	*0.95*	0.10	0.13	0.07	0.04	0.04
Reduced access to alcoholic beverage retail outlets	*0.95*	0.10	0.10	0.06	0.03	0.03
Comprehensive advertising ban on alcohol	*0.95*	0.07	0.09	0.05	0.03	0.02
Random breath testing of motor vehicle drivers	*0.80*	0.53	0.47	0.19	0.18	0.07
Brief advice to heavy drinkers by a primary care physician	*0.50*	0.36	0.36	0.11	0.08	0.04
Combination: highest tax + brief advice		0.44	0.48	0.18	0.12	0.07
Combination: highest tax + advertising ban + random breath testing + brief advice		0.97	0.97	0.39	0.30	0.15
Cost-effectiveness relative to no intervention (US$/DALY averted)						
Excise tax on alcoholic beverages (current situation)	*0.95*	141	225	104	516	2,671
Excise tax on alcoholic beverages (25 percent increase)	*0.95*	127	202	100	447	3,654
Excise tax on alcoholic beverages (50 percent increase)	*0.95*	116	184	95	394	4,641
Reduced access to alcoholic beverage retail outlets	*0.95*	216	340	152	146	827
Comprehensive advertising ban on alcohol	*0.95*	185	380	134	123	1,123
Random breath testing of motor vehicle drivers	*0.80*	1,856	1,542	973	984	531
Brief advice to heavy drinkers by a primary care physician	*0.50*	270	502	204	224	462
Combination: highest tax + brief advice		216	350	143	269	845
Combination: highest tax + advertising ban + random breath testing + brief advice		381	546	229	383	707
DALYs averted/US$ million expenditure						
Excise tax on alcoholic beverages (current situation)	*0.95*	7,107	4,435	9,633	1,937	374
Excise tax on alcoholic beverages (25 percent increase)	*0.95*	7,847	4,953	10,007	2,239	274
Excise tax on alcoholic beverages (50 percent increase)	*0.95*	8,590	5,442	10,553	2,536	215
Reduced access to alcoholic beverage retail outlets	*0.95*	4,638	2,940	6,580	6,856	1,209
Comprehensive advertising ban on alcohol	*0.95*	5,417	2,631	7,442	8,139	891
Random breath testing of motor vehicle drivers	*0.80*	539	648	1,027	1,016	1,882
Brief advice to heavy drinkers by a primary care physician	*0.50*	3,705	1,992	4,891	4,460	2,163
Combination: highest tax + brief advice		4,627	2,859	7,016	3,718	1,184
Combination: highest tax + advertising ban + random breath testing + brief advice		2,621	1,833	4,364	2,612	1,415

Source: Chisholm and others 2004.

a. Refers to the modeled percentage of all high-risk drinkers exposed to the intervention.

Starting from the current situation in these regions, the most efficient strategies for reducing high-risk alcohol use would be tax increases (additional gains are obtained at virtually no extra cost because the costs of tax administration and enforcement remain relatively constant whatever the rate of tax), followed by the introduction or escalation of comprehensive advertising bans on alcohol products, reduced access to retail outlets, and the provision of brief interventions such as physician advice in primary care. Even a multifaceted strategy made up of an increase in taxation plus full implementation of the other interventions considered here has a favorable ratio of costs to health benefits.

In East Asia and the Pacific and South Asia, the two regions with lower rates of high-risk alcohol use, a comparison of intervention costs and effects to a no-intervention scenario reveals that current practice—namely, excise taxes on alcoholic beverages—is not the most efficient response to the existing burden of alcohol use. The reduced efficiency of taxation in these lower-prevalence regions is related both to the distribution of the fixed costs of administering and enforcing alcohol tax legislation across a smaller target population of drinkers and to underlying drinking patterns: more than 85 percent of all alcohol consumption falls into a single preferred drink category, spirits, which therefore diminishes the scope for reducing the consumption of less preferred but more elastic categories of alcoholic beverages. In South Asia, targeted strategies such as brief physician advice and random breath testing have the lowest cost per DALY averted (around US$500), while taxation policies are the most expensive at more than US$2,500 per DALY averted. In East Asia and the Pacific, the most cost-effective interventions are brief physician advice, a comprehensive ban on advertising, and reduced access to retail outlets (below US$250 per DALY averted).

Implications and Limitations of Sectoral Cost-Effectiveness Analyses

This cost-effectiveness analysis offers a new approach to generating economic evidence that can inform public health policy on alcohol in a wide range of cultural and epidemiological settings (Chisholm and others 2004). Resulting estimates of cost-effectiveness can inform policy makers not only by determining the efficiency of existing resource allocation and practices, but also by identifying priorities for future alcohol control strategies. Furthermore, use of a common methodology enables comparison with cost per DALY estimates for other risk factors or disease entities, which may constitute an important argument when considering priorities for the allocation of scarce health care resources. However, the application of a broad sectoral approach using entire regions as the unit of analysis clearly limits the approach's use in specific country contexts, where demographic or epidemiological characteristics, as well as treatment costs and coverage, may not coincide with estimates for the region as a whole. In addition, extrapolation of the extent of intervention effects from relatively information-rich countries to other sociocultural settings lessens the precision of derived estimates of population-level health gains.

Although an ongoing analytical step is to calibrate results at the country level, the primary purpose and utility of the sectoral approach is to identify interventions that are clearly cost-effective as opposed to those that clearly do not seem to offer good value for money. In this respect, the primary conclusion to be drawn from the analysis is that in regions with high or moderate rates of high-risk alcohol use, a number of intervention strategies can have a notable effect on population health, including both individual-based interventions, such as brief physician advice at the primary care level, as well as population-wide measures, such as taxation of alcoholic beverages. Of these, taxation has the most sizable and least resource-intensive effect on reducing the avertable burden of high-risk alcohol use. In regions where high-risk alcohol use represents less of a public health burden, targeted approaches such as brief physician advice as well as other intervention strategies that restrict the supply or promotion of alcoholic beverages appear to be the most cost-effective mechanisms, although greater empirical support for the efficacy of these interventions in these localities is clearly needed before considering their widespread implementation.

Even though sectoral cost-effectiveness analysis pursues a societal perspective, considerable challenges remain in relation to the appropriate measurement of certain societal costs and effects that fall outside the boundaries of the health system. Therefore, this analysis has not been able to successfully capture potential reductions in workforce and household productivity losses among high-risk drinkers, nor does it incorporate the economic costs associated with alcohol-related crime, violence, and harm reduction. It also does not value the time spent by patients and informal caregivers in seeking or providing care and support. Including these modest additional costs and substantial incremental effects is likely to improve the cost-effectiveness ratios of all interventions, but to a variable and currently unknown extent.

ECONOMIC BENEFITS OF INTERVENTIONS

By design, estimates of the burden of alcohol do not include most social harm and harm to people other than the drinker; however, the burden of social problems from drinking can be at least as significant as the health burden. The burden attributable to alcohol in the CRA estimates is actually a substantial underestimate of the full harm alcohol imposes on human welfare. The estimates reported earlier reflect primarily the chronic disease and injury effects of drinking. Because the CRA focused on disease and disability, the estimates were not designed to take account of the social harm and problems that are particular to alcohol and that result for the drinker and for others as a consequence of a person's drinking (Klingemann and Gmel 2001). These problems are quite prevalent in many populations (Room and others 2003) and are also affected by the interventions listed earlier.

Some information on the relative burden of alcohol for social services versus health services is available for a handful of societies. In an estimate of the staffing and service costs attributable to alcohol in different service systems in Scotland for fiscal year 2001/02, for instance, health services accounted for only 21 percent of the estimated costs, whereas social services accounted for 19 percent, and criminal justice and fire services accounted for 60 percent (Catalyst Health Consultants 2001, 3).

If those estimates are used as a rough gauge of the burden to society, the illness and disability burden of alcohol may thus constitute half or less of the total burden when social problems are also taken into consideration.

Thus, policies that affect the levels of alcohol-related health and social harm not only are a matter of intervening to save people from the detrimental effects of their own behavior, but also potentially have a broader effect on the health and well-being of families and of associates of drinkers. This issue is especially relevant for women: even though men predominate among high-risk drinkers worldwide (Rehm and others 2004; Room and others 2002), women bear much of the burden of harm from others' drinking, not only in such forms as domestic violence, but also in such forms as diversion of family resources from greater needs.

IMPLEMENTATION OF CONTROL STRATEGIES: LESSONS OF EXPERIENCE

The following paragraphs provide a few concrete examples of interventions or policy changes that illustrate the actual implementation and effects of control strategies in developing societies (the examples are taken from Room and others 2002).

Tax Rate Reduction and the Resulting Disease Burden in Mauritius

Mauritius, an island nation in the Indian Ocean, has a population of about 1 million. These people are of Indian, African, European, and Chinese origin. By religious affiliation, 53 percent are Hindu, 29 percent are Christian, and 17 percent are Muslim. Tourism is the third-ranked industry in terms of hard currency earnings. In June 1994, the government drastically lowered customs duties on imported alcoholic beverages to 80 percent from rates that had ranged from 200 percent for wine to 600 percent for whisky and other spirits (Abdool 1998). The government made the change under pressure from the hotel industry, which claimed that tourists were not purchasing enough alcohol because of its high prices (Lee 2001). Other reasons given for the change were to reduce unofficial imports from abroad and to make better, more refined alcoholic beverages available to the local population. Despite little evidence to support the view, there were claims in the public discussion that better-quality alcohol would result in fewer health problems.

The effects of the change were felt mainly by Mauritians rather than tourists, as follows:

- Arrests for driving with blood alcohol over the legal limit made primarily in connection with traffic crashes increased by 23 percent between 1993 and 1997.
- Admissions of alcoholism cases to the island's psychiatric hospital shot up in 1994. The 1995 rate was more than twice the 1993 rate, and the rate rose again slightly in 1996 and 1997. Medical specialists in Mauritius agree that patients with alcohol problems account for an increasing portion of admissions in general medical wards and now represent between 40 and 50 percent of bed occupancy (Abdool 1998).
- Age-adjusted death rates per 100,000 population for chronic liver disease and cirrhosis rose from 32.8 for males and 4.0 for females in 1993 to 42.7 for males and 5.3 for females in 1996 (WHO 1999, 2000).

Even though available statistics are limited, the reduction in alcohol import taxes clearly had a substantial negative effect on the health of Mauritians. Thus, the government's 1997 call for control measures for alcohol—specifically, new permits for licensed premises, increased excise duties on alcohol, and limitations on bars' opening hours—was not surprising. Alcohol taxes were increased somewhat in the 1999/2000 budget (U.S. Department of State 1999). However, an analysis by World Bank staff that did not take health effects into account called for further reductions in maximum tariff rates, identifying Mauritius as having an antitrade bias on the basis of the structure of its alcohol and tobacco taxes (Hinkle and Herrou-Aragon 2001).

Wallace and Bird (2003) suggest the following general principles for setting and collecting alcohol taxes in the context of developing societies from the perspective of revenue generation rather than public health (see also Tax Policy Chief Directorate 2002):

- Countries around the world need revenues they can raise relatively efficiently, but this need is probably more critical in the case of developing nations. That said, alcohol taxes are probably a good bet for future revenues.
- Excise taxes on alcohol should be set by alcohol content, rather than as a percentage of the price.
- Tax rates should be logically defined so that alcoholic beverages with similar alcohol content are treated similarly, with stronger alcohol beverages taxed more heavily.
- Analyses of revenue-maximizing rates should be conducted to determine a range of tax rates that is likely to maximize government revenues.
- Tax systems should be designed to be as simple as possible to allow for the maximum efficiency of tax administration.

Reduced Access through Locational Prohibition in Brazil

The second example involves the institution of a new control on alcohol availability in an environment where it is likely to be combined with driving. Although we have modeled the effects of another, better studied availability control (namely, closing on a weekend day), a wide variety of possible measures is available to control the time and place of alcohol purchase or drinking (Babor and others 2003; Room and others 2002). Even though in this case the particular control was extremely limited in scope, it appears to have had measurable effects.

Traffic deaths are an important source of mortality in Brazil, amounting to 3.6 percent of overall mortality. The few available studies suggest that alcohol plays a significant role in traffic casualties. For instance, one study in São Paulo found positive blood alcohol levels in 72 percent of pedestrian deaths and 32 percent of driver and passenger deaths of persons age 13 and older (Carlini-Cotrim and Chasin 2000).

In 1985, motivated by concern about alcohol and impaired driving and about the lax enforcement of drinking and driving laws, a conservative party politician from the state of São Paulo introduced legislation to prohibit alcohol sales in commercial facilities that had access to state highways. Even though the bill passed in the legislature, its implementation was delayed by the state's alcohol producers and commercial and industrial federations, which claimed that the law would be a barrier to improved facilities for travelers, would encourage people to carry bottles in their cars, and would restrict individual freedoms. Discussion in the press was also generally unsympathetic. In August 1988, however, a new state governor from the same party implemented the law. At that time, the press was slightly more supportive. Since then, the law has been on the books, although site visits to restaurants and snack bars along a state highway in 1997 suggested a low level of compliance. In 1995, another legislator from the same party proposed repealing the law on the grounds that no studies proved that it lowered traffic accidents. The repeal passed the legislature without significant public debate, but the state governor vetoed it. Undaunted, the same legislator then proposed a law to criminalize buying as well as selling alcohol along state highways. That law passed but has not yet been implemented.

A study by Carlini-Cotrim, Pinsky, and Serrano Barbosa (1998) assesses the effects of the intervention. Finding data for a controlled study comparing traffic casualties on state highways with casualties on federal highways, which were unaffected by the law, proved impossible. The best data available were on crashes and crashes resulting in injuries per 10,000 vehicles traveling on three short highway systems administered by a private agency. Linear regressions on those data for 1983–93 showed that the law had made a significant difference in the number of accidents resulting in injuries on all three roads and a significant difference in all accidents on two of the roads. A separate analysis on estimated accidents and accidents with injuries per 10,000 vehicles in two geographic areas of the state did not show significant effects of the law. Overall, the analyses do provide some support for the law having a beneficial effect on the rate of traffic casualties.

Drunk-Driving Enforcement in South Africa

No published studies are available of the implementation of random breath testing in a developing country. However, some data are available on a campaign to increase drunk-driving enforcement in South Africa, a strategy that has often shown some effects, although weaker and less lasting than those of random breath testing.

The minister of finance launched a short-term campaign, ARRIVE ALIVE, for the period October 1997 to January 1998, in response to the high rate of traffic fatalities and injuries. The campaign's main aim was to mobilize all available traffic policing, control, and education resources to reduce traffic accidents on South African roads by at least 5 percent, especially in the Western Cape, Gauteng, and KwaZulu Natal provinces, because 75 percent of all accidents occurred in those provinces. The ARRIVE ALIVE campaign targeted, in turn, what were considered the three critical factors having the greatest impact on injuries: failing to wear seat belts, drinking and driving, and speeding. Unofficially, the campaign came to be called "belts, booze, and bats out of hell."

As many of the parties interested in road safety as possible were involved, with funding drawn from a variety of government and business sources. The campaign included a number of components particularly relevant to alcohol use. New equipment purchased by the provinces included alcohol screening devices, alcohol evidentiary units, and so-called booze buses (vehicles containing all the technology needed to check breath and blood alcohol levels). Sentences were increased to underline the point that traffic violations are serious offenses, with a three-month suspension of a driver's license and an increased maximum fine for a first conviction for drunk driving and with license suspension for one to five years for second offenders. Traffic supervisors underwent intensive training courses before the start of the campaign.

Because the aim of the campaign included educating road users, advertisements covering aspects of the campaign were run on the radio, on television, and in movie theaters throughout the country. Supplements were published in national and provincial newspapers. Private companies, such as a supermarket chain and an automobile manufacturer, also promoted the campaign. A national transportation center, established to collect and collate data from local and provincial authorities, operated for 12 hours every day throughout the campaign. Traffic authorities staffed an additional 80 roadside communications points, and at selected points on certain routes, road signs were erected and updated to display the percentage of speed limit and drinking-and-driving violations and the rate of seat belt use in that area.

A total of 776 enforcement points were set up on 195 strategic routes in the selected provinces. Posters, pamphlets, key rings, and license decals were produced for distribution and display at roadblocks in the three provinces. Between October 1, 1997, and January 17, 1998, 6,674 notices of prosecution were issued for alcohol-related traffic offenses, 83 percent of which were issued in the intervention provinces.

Comparison studies showed a decrease in the drinking rate of drivers in the three provinces, whereas the other six provinces, as a group, showed an increase. KwaZulu Natal had the lowest drinking rate of all drivers throughout the campaign (3 to 7 percent), and the Western Cape had the most dramatic decrease (from 12.0 to 9.3 percent in October). Except for in Gauteng, the drinking rates for pedestrians decreased from more than 15 percent to less than 7 percent. Overall, during the months targeted, drinking-and-driving rates decreased by 2 to 4 percent, as measured by breath testing. The total number of crashes decreased by 8 percent, and fatalities dropped by 9 percent. The ratio of benefits to costs for the intervention was estimated as 4 to 1, based on an investment in the campaign of R50 million, or about US$4.4 million at 2002 rates (ARRIVE ALIVE Campaign 2000).

Despite the potential inconvenience of roadblocks and other enforcement activities, the public generally perceived the campaign positively. The liquor retail and hospitality industries complained about decreased sales, and tow truck operators complained about reduced business.

Even though driver behavior improved during the focus months, violations often increased after the focus was changed, for example, from drunk driving to seat belt use. This finding emphasizes the need for sustained enforcement as opposed to ad hoc campaigns. (This example was summarized from ARRIVE ALIVE Campaign 2000 and Cerff and Plüddemann 1998.)

Implementation of Brief Interventions in Several Developing Countries

In the first phase of the WHO Collaborative Project on Identification and Management of Alcohol Related Problems (Saunders and Aasland 1987), a screening measure suitable for use in both developing and developed countries—the alcohol-use disorders identification test—was developed to identify people at risk for alcohol problems among those attending primary health care services. In the second phase, a multicenter clinical trial of brief intervention procedures designed to reduce the health risks associated with hazardous alcohol use was carried out in primary health care settings in Australia, Bulgaria, Costa Rica, Kenya, Mexico, Norway, the Soviet Union, the United Kingdom, the United States, and Zimbabwe (Babor and others 1994).

The project's aims were to study the influence of simple advice and brief counseling, to examine the moderating role of reduced consumption on the prevention of alcohol-related problems, and to evaluate the cross-national generalizability of

brief intervention techniques. The project's hypothesis was that the amount of change in alcohol consumption over a nine-month period would be proportional to the intensity of the intervention provided by a trained primary health care professional. The results showed a significant effect of interventions on both consumption and intensity of drinking among males, but the intensity of the intervention was not related to the amount of change in drinking behavior; 5 minutes of simple advice turned out to be as effective as 20 minutes of brief counseling (Babor and Grant 1992). The female sample was too small for the results to attain significance, and the intervention did not significantly affect men's frequency of dependence symptoms, problems related to alcohol, or concern expressed by others (WHO Brief Intervention Study Group 1996).

The findings suggest that in a population of high-risk drinkers, behavior change is more a function of motivational factors and social influence than of the moderation skills and social learning techniques that behavioral self-control training packages typically use. Changes in drinking were not attributable solely to the small number of patients who achieved an abstinence goal, nor to the small number who gave up daily or almost daily drinking. Rather, changes seem to have been distributed across a broad spectrum of the drinkers who reduced their consumption by small, but clinically meaningful, amounts.

RESEARCH AND DEVELOPMENT AGENDA

Research and development needs in the area of alcohol consumption are large and multidimensional. The work reported in this chapter represents best estimates from the available data, some of which were developed to fill the needs of the analysis; however, we cite few figures for the developing world for which we can say that the underlying data are so good that they could not usefully be improved. Nevertheless, more and better data are available on alcohol than on many other health topics.

The health and social burdens of alcohol are clearly extremely large in most developing societies. Thus, the most urgent focus should be on development and evaluation projects to study the outcomes of various policy and program interventions. The projects must necessarily be attuned to what is politically feasible in a particular time and place. They are likely to include natural experiment studies, where the research tracks the effects of changes that governments undertake, whether those changes are expected to increase or to decrease the extent of alcohol problems. Where possible, the projects should include experimental and quasi-experimental studies, whereby the effects of a change at intervention sites are studied in comparison to outcomes at control sites, with random assignment where possible. Costing data should be included to permit cost-effectiveness analysis.

Also important are process studies—that is, research on how policy makers decide on policy changes, how they implement them, and what the reactions and sequelae are. For example, deciding to introduce a new alcohol tax may be the easiest part of an initiative, but actually implementing it in a developing society with a great deal of unrecorded alcohol in the informal market and with poorly guarded borders may be much more difficult. Currently, no international mechanism or nexus exists for developing and disseminating practical knowledge about implementing effective alcohol control strategies between developing countries.

At this time, nearly all studies of alcohol interventions come from a limited range of developed countries. Extending knowledge and experience in and between developing societies is urgently needed.

A secondary need, but one that is also important, is to extend the epidemiological database in developing societies on levels and patterns of drinking and on the health and social consequences of drinking. To this end, better estimation of unrecorded alcohol consumption is needed. Which dimensions of drinking patterns matter for what kinds of outcomes needs to be studied in the context of different kinds of developing societies. Studies of the effects that the interaction of drinking levels and patterns with poverty and social exclusion have on the extent of alcohol-related problems are also necessary. Because most of our knowledge about the health effects of drinking concerns mortality, studies of alcohol's role in various kinds of morbidity should be emphasized. Another area where data are lacking is the social harm arising from drinking, for which we cannot presently make the kinds of estimates that are possible to make for harm to health. Developing and reaching consensus on ways to measure the social harm caused by drinking is a substantial agenda for both the developed and the developing world.

Developing the epidemiological database can provide clues to etiology to be pursued further by biomedical and social researchers and, thus, offers hope for the development of new treatments or preventive interventions. It can provide information on the distribution of drinking patterns and problems in subpopulations that can be used to guide targeting and prevention and treatment priorities. However, from a short-term policy perspective, the most important function of developing the epidemiological database in a particular country may be providing a base for creating political will for action. For example, the development of devices to measure blood and breath alcohol and the collection of data on drinking and driving that they made possible were prerequisites for developing the political will and support for implementing drinking-and-driving countermeasures in industrial countries.

CONCLUSION

The burden of disease attributable to alcohol in the developing world is considerable, and the social harm not accounted for in this analysis increases the costs. However, known interventions can reduce the burden by up to 25 percent, depending on the region of the world. Compared with other interventions in the health care field, these interventions are quite cost-effective, but given the nature of many of the interventions, caution is needed. In particular, the following recommendations can be given:

- Interventions and research about their effectiveness are based mostly on experiences from established market economies; thus, the levels of effectiveness estimated in our analysis should be treated as broad indications. Depending on actual methods of implementation, individual interventions could be more or less effective.
- Interventions should ideally be modeled on the basis of the specific environment (that is, countries or provinces) and on the harm distribution in the respective environment, including social harm.
- General principles, such as restricting access to alcohol, should be attuned to local cultures and traditions when interventions are formulated.
- Population measures must take into account the complex interplay of public opinion and balance the interests of different groups and stakeholders with conflicting values. One of these stakeholders is, of course, the alcohol industry.

If policy makers keep these principles in mind, reducing the alcohol-related health burden could be one of the most cost-effective targets of population-level health programs in developing countries. This target is even more attractive because the measures discussed will also reduce the alcohol-related social burden, thereby further contributing to development.

NOTES

1. The global burden of disease attributable to alcohol is 4.0 percent using age-weighted DALYs and 3.6 percent using non-age-weighted DALYs. This difference can be explained by the many alcohol-attributable outcomes occurring during adolescence and young adulthood, when age weights are higher.

2. The CRA defined *per capita consumption* as average consumption of pure alcohol per person 15 years old or older.

REFERENCES

Abdool, R. 1998. "Alcohol Policy and Problems in Mauritius." Paper prepared for the World Health Organization Alcohol Policy in Developing Societies Project, World Health Organization, Geneva.

Apte, M. V., J. S. Wilson, and M. A. Korsten. 1997. "Alcohol-Related Pancreatic Damage: Mechanisms and Treatment." *Alcohol Health and Research World* 21 (1): 13–20.

ARRIVE ALIVE Campaign. 2000. "ARRIVE ALIVE Safety Campaign." Pretoria: Department of Transport. http://www.transport.gov.za/projects/arrive/presentation/slide41.htm.

Babor, T., F. Caetano, S. Casswell, G. Edwards, N. Giesbrecht, K. Graham, and others. 2003. *Alcohol: No Ordinary Commodity—A Consumer's Guide to Public Policy*. Oxford, U.K.: Oxford University Press.

Babor, T. F., and M. Grant, eds. 1992. *Project on Identification and Management of Alcohol-Related Problems: Report on Phase II—A Randomized Clinical Trial of Brief Interventions in Primary Health Care*. Geneva: World Health Organization, Program on Substance Abuse.

Babor, T. F., M. Grant, W. Acuda, F. H. Burns, C. Campillo, F. K. Del Boco, and others. 1994. "Randomized Clinical Trial of Brief Interventions in Primary Health Care: Summary of a WHO Project (with Commentaries and a Response)." *Addiction* 89: 657–78.

Bruun, K., G. Edwards, M. Lumio, K. Mäkelä, L. Pan, R. E. Popham, and others. 1975. *Alcohol Control Policies in Public Health Perspective*. Helsinki: Finnish Foundation for Alcohol Studies.

Carlini-Cotrim, B., and A. A. da M. Chasin. 2000. "Blood Alcohol Content and Death from Fatal Injury: A Study in the Metropolitan Area of São Paulo, Brazil." *Journal of Psychoactive Drugs* 32: 269–75.

Carlini-Cotrim, B., I. Pinsky, and M. T. Serrano Barbosa. 1998. *Alcohol Availability Restrictions in Developing Societies: The Case of São Paulo Highways, Brazil*. Report prepared for the WHO Alcohol Policy in Developing Societies Project, World Health Organization, Geneva.

Catalyst Health Consultants. 2001. *Alcohol Misuse in Scotland: Trends and Costs—Final Report*. Northwort, U.K.: Catalyst Health Consultants. http://www.scotland.gov.uk/health/alcoholproblems/docs/trco.pdf.

Cerff, P., and A. Plüddemann. 1998. "Brief on the ARRIVE ALIVE Campaign." Prepared for the Alcohol Policy in Developing Societies project. Cape Town, South Africa: Medical Research Council, Urbanisation, and Health Research Programme.

Chisholm, D., J. Rehm, M. van Ommeren, and M. Monteiro. 2004. "Reducing the Global Burden of Hazardous Alcohol Use: A Comparative Cost-Effectiveness Analysis." *Journal of Studies on Alcohol* 65 (6): 782–93.

Corrao, G., L. Rubbiati, V. Bagnardi, A. Zambon, and K. Poikolainen. 2000. "Alcohol and Coronary Heart Disease: A Meta-Analysis." *Addiction* 94 (10):1501–23.

Demyttenaere, K., R. Bruffaerts, J. Posada-Villa, I. Gasquet, V. Kovess, J. P. Lepine, and others. 2004. "Prevalence, Severity, and Unmet Need for Treatment of Mental Disorders in the World Health Organization World Mental Health Surveys." *Journal of the American Medical Association* 291 (21): 2581–90.

Drummond, D. C. 1990. "The Relationship between Alcohol Dependence and Alcohol-Related Problems in a Clinical Population." *British Journal of Addiction* 85 (3): 357–66.

Eckardt, M. J., S. E. File, G. L. Gessa, K. A. Grant, C. Guerri, P. L. Hoffman, and others. 1998. "Effects of Moderate Alcohol Consumption in the Central Nervous System." *Alcoholism: Clinical and Experimental Research* 22 (5): 998–1040.

Edwards, G., P. Anderson, T. F. Babor, S. Casswell, R. Ferrence, N. Giesbrecht, and others. 1994. *Alcohol Policy and the Public Good*. Oxford, U.K.: Oxford University Press.

Emanuele, N., and M. A. Emanuele. 1997. "The Endocrine System: Alcohol Alters Critical Hormonal Balance." *Alcohol Health and Research World* 21 (1): 53–64.

English, D. R., C. D. J. Holman, E. Milne, M. Winter, G. K. Hulse, G. Codde, and others. 1995. *The Quantification of Drug Caused Morbidity and Morality in Australia*. Canberra: Commonwealth Department of Human Services and Health.

Ezzati, M., A. D. Lopez, A. Rodgers, S. Vander Horn, C. J. L. Murray, and the Comparative Risk Assessment Collaborating Group. 2002. "Selected Major Risk Factors and Global and Regional Burden of Disease." *Lancet* 360: 1347–60.

Farrell, S., W. G. Manning, and M. D. Finch. 2003. "Alcohol Dependence and the Price of Alcoholic Beverages." *Journal of Health Economics* 22 (1): 117–47.

Fleming, M. F., M. P. Mundt, M. T. French, L. B. Manwell, E. A. Stauffacher, K. L. Barry, and others. 2000. "Benefit-Cost Analysis of Brief Physician Advice with Problem Drinkers in Primary Care Settings." *Medical Care* 38: 7–18.

Foxcroft, D. R., D. Ireland, D. J. Lister-Sharp, G. Lowe, and R. Breen. 2003. "Longer-Term Primary Prevention for Alcohol Misuse in Young People: A Systematic Review." *Addiction* 98: 397–411.

Foxcroft, D. R., D. Lister-Sharp, and G. Lowe. 1997. "Alcohol Misuse Prevention for Young People: A Systematic Review Reveals Methodological Concerns and Lack of Reliable Evidence of Effectiveness." *Addiction* 92: 531–38.

Gmel, G., E. Gutjahr, and J. Rehm. 2003. "How Stable Is the Risk Curve between Alcohol and All-Cause Mortality and What Factors Influence the Shape? A Precision-Weighted Hierarchical Meta-Analysis." *European Journal of Epidemiology* 18 (7): 631–42.

Gmel, G., J. Rehm, and U. Frick. 2003. "Trinkmuster, Pro-Kopf-Konsum von Alkohol und koronare Mortalität." *Sucht* 49 (2): 95–104.

Grant, B. F., D. A. Dawson, F. S. Stinson, S. P. Chou, M. C. Dufour, R. P. Pickering, and others. 2004. "The 12-Month Prevalence and Trends in DSM-IV Alcohol Abuse and Dependence: United States, 1991–1992 and 2001–2002." *Drug and Alcohol Dependence* 11 (3): 223–34.

Grube, J., and G. Agostinelli. 2000. *Alcohol Advertising and Alcohol Consumption: A Review of Recent Research*. Berkeley, CA: Prevention Research Center.

Gutjahr, E., G. Gmel, and J. Rehm. 2001. "Relation between Average Alcohol Consumption and Disease: An Overview." *European Addiction Research* 7 (3): 117–27.

Harrison, L., and E. Gardiner. 1999. "Do the Rich Really Die Young? Alcohol-Related Mortality and Social Class in Great Britain, 1988–94." *Addiction* 94: 1871–80.

Higgins-Biddle, J. C., and T. F. Babor. 1996. *Reducing Risky Drinking*. Report prepared for the Robert Wood Johnson Foundation, University of Connecticut Health Center, Farmington.

Hinkle, L. E., and A. Herrou-Aragon. 2001. "How Far Did Africa's First Generation Trade Reforms Go?" World Bank, Washington, DC. http://www.uesiglo21.edu.ar/pdfs%20dpto%20economia/ES?002?ECO.pdf.

Isichei, H. U., P. U. Ikwuagu, and J. O. Egbuta. 1993. "Pattern of Alcoholism in Jos, Nigeria, and Castrop-Rauxel, West Germany: A Comparative Study." In *Epidemiology and Control of Substance Use in Nigeria*, ed. I. S. Obot, 123–27. Jos, Nigeria: Centre for Research and Information on Substance Abuse.

Johns, B., R. Baltussen, T. Adam, and R. Hutubessy. 2003. "Programme Costs in the Economic Evaluation of Health Interventions." *Cost-Effectiveness and Resource Allocation* 1: 1. http://www.resourceallocation.com.

Klingemann, H., and G. Gmel, eds. 2001. *Mapping the Social Consequences of Alcohol Consumption*. Dordrecht, Netherlands: Kluwer Academic Publishers.

Lauer, J. A., C. J. L. Murray, K. Roehrich, and H. Wirth. 2003. "PopMod: A Longitudinal Population Model with Two Interacting Disease States." *Cost Effectiveness and Resource Allocation* 1: 6. http://www.resourceallocation.com.

Lee, V. J. 2001. *Tourism and Alcohol in the Developing World: Potential Effects on Alcohol Policies and Local Drinking Problems*. Stockholm: Stockholm University, Centre for Social Research on Alcohol and Drugs.

Leppänen, K. 1979. "Valtakunnallisen lauantaisulkemiskokeilun vaiku-tuksista alkoholijuomien myyntiin" (Effects of National Saturday Closing Experiment on Alcohol Sales). *Alkoholipolitikka* 44: 20–21.

Levy, F., and S. I. Ornstein. 1983. "Price and Income Elasticities and the Demand for Alcoholic Beverages." In *Recent Developments in Alcoholism*, ed. M. Galanter, 303–45. New York: Plenum.

Liu, B. Q., R. Peto, Z. M. Chen, J. Boreham, Y. P. Wu, J. Y. Li, and others. 1998. "Emerging Tobacco Hazards in China: 1. Retrospective Proportional Mortality Study of One Million Deaths." *British Medical Journal* 317 (7170): 1411–22.

Ludbrook, A, C. Godfrey, L. Wyness, S. Parrot, S. Haw, M. Napper, and others. 2002. *Effective and Cost-Effective Measures to Reduce Alcohol Misuse in Scotland: A Literature Review.* Aberdeen, U.K.: Health Economics Research Unit.

Mäkelä, P. 1999. "Alcohol-Related Mortality as a Function of Socio-Economic Status." *Addiction* 94: 867–86.

Mathers, C. D., C. Bernard, K. Moesgaard Iburg, M. Inoue, D. Ma Fat, K. Shibuya, and others. 2003. "Global Burden of Disease in 2002: Data Sources, Methods and Results." Global Programme on Evidence for Health Policy Discussion Paper 54, Geneva, World Health Organization.

McKee, M., and A. Britton. 1998. "The Positive Relationship between Alcohol and Heart Disease in Eastern Europe: Potential Physiological Mechanisms." *Journal Royal Society Medicine* 91: 402–7.

Moyer, A., J. W. Finney, C. E. Swearingen, and P. Vergun. 2002. "Brief Interventions for Alcohol Problems: A Meta-Analytic Review of Controlled Investigations in Treatment-Seeking and Non-Treatment-Seeking Populations." *Addiction* 97: 279–92.

National Highway Traffic Safety Administration. 1992. "Driving under the Influence: A Report to Congress on Alcohol Limits." Washington, DC: U.S. Department of Transportation.

Nordlund, S. 1984. "Effekten av lørdagsstengningen ved Vinmonopolets butikker" (Effects of Saturday Closing of the Wine/Liquor Monopoly Outlets). *Alkoholpolitik—Tidsskrift for Nordisk Alkoholforskning* 1: 221–29.

Norström, T., and O. J. Skog. 2003. "Saturday Opening of Alcohol Retail Shops in Sweden: An Impact Analysis." *Journal of Studies on Alcohol* 64: 393–401.

Peek-Asa, C. 1999. "The Effect of Random Alcohol Screening in Reducing Motor Vehicle Crash Injuries." *American Journal of Preventive Medicine* 16 (1 Suppl.): 57–67.

Puddey, I. B., V. Rakic, S. B. Dimmitt, and L. J. Beilin. 1999. "Influence of Drinking on Cardiovascular Disease and Cardiovascular Risk Factors—A Review." *Addiction* 94: 649–63.

Rehm, J., G. Gmel, C. T. Sempos, and M. Trevisan. 2003. "Alcohol-Related Mortality and Morbidity." *Alcohol Research and Health* 27 (1): 39–51.

Rehm, J., E. Gutjahr, and G. Gmel. 2001. "Alcohol and All-Cause Mortality: A Pooled Analysis." *Contemporary Drug Problems* 28: 337–61.

Rehm, J., N. Rehn, R. Room, M. Monteiro, G. Gmel, D. Jernigan, and U. Frick. 2003. "The Global Distribution of Average Volume of Alcohol Consumption and Patterns of Drinking." *European Addiction Research* 9 (4): 147–56.

Rehm, J., R. Room, K. Graham, M. Monteiro, G. Gmel, and C. T. Sempos. 2003. "The Relationship of Average Volume of Alcohol Consumption and Patterns of Drinking to Burden of Disease: An Overview." *Addiction* 98 (10): 1209–28.

Rehm, J., R. Room, M. Monteiro, G. Gmel, K. Graham, N. Rehn, and others. 2003. "Alcohol as a Risk Factor for Global Burden of Disease." *European Addiction Research* 9 (4):157–64.

Rehm, J., R. Room, M. Monteiro, G. Gmel, K. Graham, T. Rehn, and others. 2004. "Alcohol." In *Comparative Quantification of Health Risks: Global and Regional Burden of Disease Due to Selected Major Risk Factors*, ed. M. Ezzati, A. D. Lopez, A. Rodgers, and C. J. L. Murray, 959–1108. Geneva: World Health Organization.

Rehm, J., C. T. Sempos, and M. Trevisan. 2003. "Average Volume of Alcohol Consumption, Patterns of Drinking, and Risk of Coronary Heart Disease: A Review." *Journal of Cardiovascular Risk* 10 (1): 15–20.

Ridolfo, B., and C. Stevenson. 2001. *The Quantification of Drug-Caused Mortality and Morbidity in Australia 1998.* Canberra: Australian Institute of Health and Welfare.

Room, R., T. Babor, and J. Rehm. 2005. "Alcohol and Public Health: A Review." *Lancet* 365 (February 5): 519–30.

Room, R., K. Graham, J. Rehm, D. Jernigan, and M. Monteiro. 2003. "Drinking and Its Burden in a Global Perspective: Policy Considerations and Options." *European Addiction Research* 9 (4): 165–75.

Room, R., A. Janca, L. A. Bennett, L. Schmidt, N. Sartorius, and others. 1996. "WHO Cross-Cultural Applicability Research on Diagnosis and Assessment of Substance Use Disorders: An Overview of Methods and Selected Results." *Addiction* 91 (2): 199–220.

Room, R., D. Jernigan, B. Carlini-Marlatt, O. Gureje, K. Mäkelä, M. Marshall, and others. 2002. *Alcohol in Developing Societies: A Public Health Approach.* Helsinki: Finnish Foundation for Alcohol Studies.

Saffer, H. 2000. "Alcohol Consumption and Alcohol Advertising Bans." NBER Working Paper 7758, National Bureau of Economic Research, Cambridge, MA.

Saffer, H., and D. Dave. 2002. "Alcohol Consumption and Alcohol Advertising Bans." *Applied Economics* 34 (11): 1325–34.

Saunders, J. B., and O. G. Aasland. 1987. *WHO Collaborative Project on Identification and Treatment of Persons with Harmful Alcohol Consumption.* WHO/MNH/DAT 86.3. Geneva: World Health Organization.

Schmidt, L., and R. Room. 1999. "Cross-Cultural Applicability in International Classifications and Research on Alcohol Dependence." *Journal of Studies on Alcohol* 60: 448–62.

Shults, R. A, R. W. Elder, D. A. Sleet, J. L. Nichols, M. O. Alao, V. G. Carande-Kulis, and others. 2001. "Reviews of Evidence Regarding Interventions to Reduce Alcohol-Impaired Driving." *American Journal of Preventive Medicine* 21 (Suppl. 4): 66–88.

Single, E., L. Robson, J. Rehm, and X. Xie. 1999. "Morbidity and Mortality Attributable to Alcohol, Tobacco, and Illicit Drug Use in Canada." *American Journal of Public Health* 89 (3): 385–90.

Single, E., L. Robson, X. Xie, and J. Rehm. 1996. *The Cost of Substance Abuse in Canada.* Ottawa: Canadian Centre on Substance Abuse.

Sobell, L. C., T. P. Ellingstad, and M. B. Sobell. 2000. "Natural Recovery from Alcohol and Drug Problems: Methodological Review of the Research with Suggestions for Future Directions." *Addiction* 95: 749–64.

Stouthard, M. E., M. L. Essink-Bot, and G. L. Bonsel. 2000. "On Behalf of the Dutch Disability Weights Group: Disability Weights for Diseases—A Modified Protocol and Results for a Western European Region." *European Journal of Public Health* 10: 24–30.

Tax Policy Chief Directorate. 2002. *The Taxation of Alcoholic Beverages in South Africa and Its Impact on the Consumption Levels of Alcoholic Beverages.* Pretoria: National Treasury.

U.S. Department of State. 1999. "Mauritius: 1999–2000 Budget Increased." U.S. Department of State, Washington, DC. http://www.tradeport.org/ts/countries/mauritius/mrr/mark0003.html.

Wallace, S., and R. Bird. 2003. "Taxing Alcohol in Africa: Reflections from International Experience." Paper presented at the South Africa Conference on Excise Taxation, June 11–13, Gauteng, South Africa. http://www.iticnet.org/030707-PRESENTATION_Bird.pdf.

Whitlock, E. P., M. R. Polen, C. A. Green, T. Orleans, and J. Klein. 2004. "Behavioral Counseling Interventions in Primary Care to Reduce

Risky/Harmful Alcohol Use by Adults: A Summary of the Evidence for the U.S. Preventive Services Task Force." *Annals of Internal Medicine* 140: 557–68.

WHO (World Health Organization). 1993. *The ICD-10 Classification of Mental and Behavioral Disorders: Diagnostic Criteria for Research.* Geneva: WHO.

———. 1999. *Global Status Report on Alcohol.* WHO/HSC/SAB/99.11. Geneva: WHO, Substance Abuse Department.

———. 2000. *1997–1999 World Health Statistics Annual.* Geneva: WHO. http://www.who.int/whosis/.

———. 2002. *World Health Report 2002: Reducing Risks, Promoting Healthy Life.* Geneva: WHO.

———. 2003a. "Burden of Disease Project." WHO, Geneva. http://www.who.int/evidence/bod.

———. 2003b. "WHO Global Alcohol Database." WHO, Geneva. http://www3.who.int/whosis/alcohol.

WHO Brief Intervention Study Group. 1996. "A Cross-National Trial of Brief Interventions with High Risk Drinkers." *American Journal of Public Health* 86: 948–55.

Zakhari, S. 1997. "Alcohol and the Cardiovascular System: Molecular Mechanisms for Beneficial and Harmful Action." *Alcohol Health and Research World* 21 (1): 21–29.

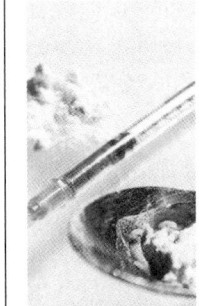

Chapter **48**

Illicit Opiate Abuse

Wayne Hall, Chris Doran, Louisa Degenhardt, and Donald Shepard

Illicit drugs are those banned by international drug control treaties. They include cannabis products (for example, marijuana, hashish, and bhang); stimulant drugs (such as cocaine and methamphetamine); so-called dance-party drugs (such as 3, 4-methylenedioxymethamphetamine, also known as *ecstasy* or *MDMA*); and illicit opioids (for instance, heroin and opium) and diverted pharmaceutical opioids (such as buprenorphine, methadone, and morphine) (see annex 48.A).

Worldwide, 185 million people were estimated to have used illicit drugs during 1998–2002 (UNODC 2004; UNODCCP 2002). Cannabis was the most widely used illicit drug, with 146.2 million users in 2002, or 3.7 percent of the global population over age 15. The stimulant drugs were the next most widely used illicit drugs: 29.6 million people worldwide used amphetamines; 13.3 million used cocaine; and 8.3 million used ecstasy. An estimated 15.3 million, or 0.4 percent of the world population age 15 to 64, used illicit opioids; more than half used heroin and the remainder used opium or diverted pharmaceutical opioids. Illicit opioids continue to be the major illicit drug problem in most regions of the world in terms of impact on public health and public order (UNODC 2004).

Even though cannabis use accounts for about 80 percent of illicit drug use worldwide, the mortality and morbidity attributable to its use are not well understood, even in developed countries (W. Hall and Pacula 2003; Macleod and others 2004; WHO Programme on Substance Abuse 1997). The same is true of the morbidity and mortality attributable to cocaine and amphetamine-type stimulants (Macleod and others 2004). Dance-party drugs have been used for too short a time in most developed societies to enable a good assessment of their potential for harm (Boot, McGregor, and Hall 2000; Macleod and others 2004). The remainder of this chapter is concerned with

disease control priorities for illicit opioid dependence, because dependent users account for most of the illicit opioids consumed and experience most of the harm such dependence causes (W. Hall, Degenhardt, and Lynskey 1999).

NATURE, CAUSES, AND HEALTH CONSEQUENCES OF ILLICIT OPIOID USE

Before considering interventions, we briefly summarize what is known about the antecedents, causes, and health consequences of illicit opioid use.

Antecedents of Heroin Use

Law enforcement efforts to reduce the availability of heroin aim to increase its price, deter illicit drug use, and promote social values that discourage heroin use (Fergusson, Horwood, and Lynskey 1998; Hawkins, Catalano, and Miller 1992; Newcomb and Bentler 1988). These gains may be at the cost of increasing harm among the minority who use opioids despite the prohibition—for example, by encouraging injecting use as the most efficient way to use an expensive drug and increasing needle sharing because clean injecting equipment is not freely available (Rhodes and others 2003; Strathdee and others 2003).

Two aspects of the family environment are associated with increased rates of both licit and illicit drug use in young people in developed countries. The first is exposure to a disadvantaged home environment, with parental conflict and poor discipline and supervision; the second is exposure to parents' and siblings' use of alcohol and other drugs (Hawkins, Catalano, and Miller 1992). In developed countries, children who perform poorly in school because of impulsive or problem behavior and those who are early users of alcohol and other drugs are most likely to use illicit opioids (Fergusson, Horwood, and Swain-Campbell 2002). Affiliation with drug-using peers is a risk factor for drug use that operates independently of individual and family risk factors (Fergusson, Horwood, and Lynskey 1998; Hawkins, Catalano, and Miller 1992).

Health Consequences of Heroin Use

The following sections describe the major health consequences of heroin use. They include dependence, increased mortality and morbidity attributable to drug overdoses, and bloodborne viruses.

Heroin Dependence. In household surveys, 1 to 2 percent of adults in Australia, the United States, and Europe report using heroin at some time in their lives (Australian Institute of Health and Welfare 1999; EMCDDA 2002; SAMHSA 2002). The highest rates are typically among adults age 20 to 29. Self-reported heroin use in population surveys probably underestimates rates of use because heroin users are undersampled and those who are sampled underreport their use (W. Hall, Lynskey, and Degenhardt 1999).

In developed countries, one in four of those who report heroin use become dependent on it (Anthony, Warner, and Kessler 1994). People who are heroin dependent continue to use heroin in the face of problems that they know (or believe) to be caused by its use. These problems include being arrested or imprisoned, having interpersonal and family problems, catching infectious diseases, and suffering from drug overdoses. Many heroin users who seek treatment have typically been daily heroin injectors, although in Europe (EMCDDA 2002), North America (Office of National Drug Control Policy 2001), and parts of Asia, illicit opioid users also smoke or "chase" the drug (inhale the fumes released when heroin is heated) (UNODC 2004).

The American Psychiatric Association defines *drug dependence* as "a cluster of cognitive, behavioral, and physiologic symptoms indicating that the individual continues use of the substance despite significant substance-related problems" (American Psychiatric Association 1994, 176). In the fourth edition of the association's *Diagnostic and Statistical Manual of Mental Disorders* (1994,), a diagnosis of substance dependence requires that three or more of the following occur together:

At any time in the same 12-month period:

1. tolerance, as defined by either of the following:
   a. need for markedly increased amounts of the substance to achieve intoxication or desired effect
   b. markedly diminished effect with continued use of the same amount of the substance;

2. withdrawal, as manifested by either of the following:
   a. the characteristic withdrawal syndrome for the substance
   b. the same (or closely related) substance is taken to relieve or avoid withdrawal symptoms;
3. the substance is often taken in larger amounts or over a longer period than was intended;
4. there is a persistent desire or unsuccessful efforts to cut down or control substance use;
5. a great deal of time is spent in activities necessary to obtain the substance (e.g., visiting multiple doctors, driving long distances), use the substance (e.g., chain smoking), or recover from its effects;
6. important social, occupational, or recreational activities are given up or reduced because of substance use;
7. the substance use is continued despite knowledge of having a persistent or recurrent physical or psychological problem that is likely to have been caused or exacerbated by the substance.

Indirect estimation methods suggest that in Australia, the United Kingdom, and the European Union fewer than 1 percent of adults age 15 to 54 are heroin dependent (EMCDDA 2002; W. Hall and others 2000). Research in the United States indicates that dependent heroin users who seek treatment or who come to the attention of the legal system may use heroin for decades (Goldstein and Herrera 1995; Hser, Anglin, and Powers 1993), with periods of use punctuated by abstinence (Bruneau and others 2004; Galai and others 2003), drug treatment, and imprisonment (Gerstein and Harwood 1990). When periods of abstinence are included, dependent heroin users use heroin daily for 40 to 60 percent of the 20 years that they typically are addicts (Ball, Shaffer, and Nurco 1983; Maddux and Desmond 1992).

Illicit opioid use increased in Asia, Europe, and Oceania and, to a lesser extent, in Africa and South America in the 1990s, but it has stabilized or declined since 2000 (UNODC 2004). Most illicit opioid users (7.8 million) live in Asian countries that surround the major opium-producing countries, Afghanistan and Myanmar. Europe accounts for about 25 percent of illicit opioid use (4 million users or 0.8 percent of the adult population age 15 to 64). Two-thirds of users are in Eastern Europe, which reported large increases in illicit opioid use during the second half of the 1990s (Atlani and others 2000; Hamers and Downs 2003; Kelly and Amirkhanian 2003; Rhodes and others 1999; Uuskula and others 2002).

Illicit opioid use stabilized in much of Asia between 2000 and 2002 (UNODC 2004) as a result of decreased opium production after the rapid expansion during the 1990s (Dorabjee and Samson 2000; Reid and Crofts 2000). After 2000, India and Pakistan reported stabilizing rates of illicit opioid use but increased injection of pharmaceutical opiates (Ahmed and others 2003; Dorabjee and Samson 2000; Strathdee and others

2003). China has reported a steady rate of growth in illicit opiate use in its southern and northern provinces (Beyrer 2003; Beyrer and others 2000; Yu and others 1998) and a 15-fold increase in the number of registered opioid addicts between 1990 and 2002, bringing the total to about 1 million (UNODC 2004).

Oceania experienced a marked rise in heroin use in the late 1990s, largely driven by a dramatic increase in the availability of heroin in Australia (Darke, Topp, and others 2002; W. Hall, Degenhardt, and Lynskey 1999). In late 2000, an abrupt heroin shortage resulted in a large reduction in fatal and nonfatal overdoses (Day and others 2004; Degenhardt, Day, and Hall 2004).

Mortality, Morbidity, and Heroin Dependence. In developed countries, dependent heroin users have an increased risk of premature death from drug overdoses, violence, suicide, and alcohol-related causes (Darke and Ross 2002; Goldstein and Herrera 1995; Vlahov and others 2004). Heroin users treated before the HIV epidemic were 13 times more likely to die prematurely than their peers (Hulse and others 1999), with opioid overdose the most frequent cause of death (W. Hall, Degenhardt, and Lynskey 1999). In countries with a high prevalence of HIV infection, AIDS is a major cause of premature death among drug users (EMCDDA 2002; UNAIDS and WHO 2002). Fatal opioid overdose deaths increased in many developed countries during the 1990s before declining after 2000 (UNODC 2004).

In parts of Asia, Eastern Europe, and the United States, the sharing of contaminated injecting equipment accounts for a substantial proportion of new HIV infections (EMCDDA 2002; UNAIDS and WHO 2002; UNODC 2004). Injecting opioid use has been a major driver of HIV epidemics in China (Yu and others 1998), Myanmar (Beyrer and others 2000), the Russian Federation and former Soviet republics (Hamers and Downs 2003), and Vietnam (Beyrer and others 2000; Hien and others 2001).

The prevalence of infection with hepatitis B and C viruses among injecting drug users is greater than 60 percent in Australia (National Centre in HIV Epidemiology and Clinical Research 1998), Canada (Fischer and others 2004), China (Ruan and others 2004), the United States (Fuller and others 2004), and the European Union (EMCDDA 2002). Chronic infection occurs in 75 percent of infections, and 3 to 11 percent of chronic hepatitis C virus carriers develop liver cirrhosis within 20 years (Hepatitis C Virus Projections Working Group 1998).

Heroin-related deaths primarily occur among young adults and account for a large number of life years lost in developed societies. In Australia in 1996, for example, such deaths accounted for 2.2 percent of life years lost, with each death accounting for 22 years of life lost (Mathers, Vos, and Stephenson 1999). In Scotland and Spain, opiate-related deaths

account for 25 to 33 percent of deaths of young adult males (EMCDDA 2002).

Economic Costs of Illicit Opioid Use. In Canada, Xie and others (1996) calculate the costs of illicit drugs as 0.2 percent of gross domestic product (GDP). In Australia, Collins and Lapsley (1996) estimate the economic costs of illicit drug abuse at 2 percent of GDP.

CONTRIBUTION OF OPIOID DEPENDENCE TO THE GLOBAL BURDEN OF DISEASE

Degenhardt, Hall, and others (2004) estimate the contribution of illicit opioid dependence to the global burden of disease using data on deaths caused by opioid and other drug overdoses, suicides and accidents, and HIV/AIDS. When estimates of morbidity attributable to illicit drug use were added in, illicit opioid use accounted for 0.7 percent of global disability-adjusted life years (DALYs) in 2000 (WHO 2003).

These estimates suggest that illicit opioid use is a significant global cause of premature mortality and disability among young adults. Even so, they probably underestimate the disease burden attributable to illicit opioids, because they omit differences across subregions in the quality of data on causes of mortality and estimates of mortality and morbidity attributable to hepatitis and violence (Degenhardt, Hall, and others 2004).

INTERVENTIONS FOR ILLICIT OPIOID DEPENDENCE

Methods adopted to control the problems arising from illicit opioid dependence include source-country control; interdiction of supply into end-use countries; enforcement by the police force and the criminal justice system of legal prohibitions on the supply, possession, and use of opioids; treatment of those who are opioid dependent, both voluntarily and under legal coercion from the criminal justice system; school-based and mass media preventive educational programs; and regulatory policies restricting the prescription of opioids (Manski, Pepper, and Petrie 2001).

Prevention of Heroin Use

Countries use a variety of interventions in attempts to prevent the initiation of use of illicit drugs such as cannabis (Manski, Pepper, and Petrie 2001; Spooner and Hall 2002), in the belief that early initiation of cannabis use leads to an increased risk of using illicit opioids (Fergusson, Horwood, and Swain-Campbell 2002). These interventions include legal prohibitions on the manufacture, sale, and use of opioid drugs for nonmedical purposes; enforcement of these sanctions by law enforcement officials by means of fines and imprisonment; and enforcement of restrictions on medically prescribed opioids to prevent their diversion (Manski, Pepper, and Petrie 2001). Preventive measures also include mass media and school-based educational campaigns about the health risks of opioid and other illicit drug use (Spooner and Hall 2002). It is unclear how effective these interventions are in preventing cannabis use and even less clear whether they reduce the initiation of opioids (Caulkins and others 1999; Manski, Pepper, and Petrie 2001).

The most popular interventions against illicit opioid use in many developed societies have been the interdiction of drug supply and the enforcement of legal sanctions against the possession, use, and sale of opioid drugs (Manski, Pepper, and Petrie 2001). As a consequence, imprisonment is the most common intervention to which many illicit opioid users have been exposed (Gerstein and Harwood 1990). In Asia and Eastern Europe, high rates of imprisonment of drug users have been a factor in HIV transmission, because drug users engage in high-risk injecting while imprisoned (Beyrer and others 2000).

Interventions to Reduce Heroin-Related Harm

The most effective intervention to reduce bloodborne virus infection arising from illicit injecting of opioids and other drugs is the provision of clean injecting equipment to reduce users' risks of contracting or transmitting bloodborne viruses. This intervention has been widely supported in most developed countries, but it has been incompletely adopted in developing countries that have problems with the concept of facilitating the injection of illicit drugs (UNAIDS and WHO 2002). Vaccinations are available against hepatitis B but not hepatitis C. These important interventions are covered in chapter 18.

A number of strategies can potentially reduce deaths from opioid overdoses (Darke and Hall 2003; Sporer 2003). First, injecting drug users can be educated about the dangers of combining the use of opioids with alcohol and benzodiazepines (McGregor and others 2001), both of which heighten the risk of a fatal opioid overdose (Darke and Zador 1996; Warner-Smith and others 2001). Heroin users also need to be discouraged from injecting in the streets or alone, thereby denying themselves assistance in the event of an overdose. These interventions have yet to be evaluated.

A second strategy is to encourage drug users who witness overdoses to seek medical assistance and to use simple resuscitation techniques until help arrives. A more controversial option is to distribute the opioid antagonist naloxone to high-risk heroin users (Darke and Hall 1997; Strang and others 1996). Neither of these interventions has been evaluated.

A third strategy is to provide supervised injecting facilities in areas with high rates of injecting opioid use (Dolan and others 2000; Kimber and others 2003). Supervised injecting facilities have been introduced in Germany, the Netherlands, and Switzerland (Dolan and others 2000; Kimber and others 2003), but their effect on overdose deaths has not been rigorously evaluated to date. A supervised injecting facility was evaluated in Australia, but the evaluation was limited by the concurrent onset of a heroin shortage that resulted in a 40 percent decline in overdose deaths (Kaldor and others 2003).

A fourth strategy is to increase methadone maintenance among older, high-risk opioid-dependent people, because individuals enrolled in methadone maintenance treatment (MMT) are substantially less likely to suffer from a fatal overdose (Caplehorn and others 1994; Gearing and Schweitzer 1974; Langendam and others 2001).

Treatment Interventions for Dependent Opioid Users

The range of treatment interventions includes voluntary programs such as detoxification, abstinence-oriented treatments, and oral Methadone maintenance treatment, as well as involuntary options imposed by criminal justice systems.

Detoxification. Detoxification is supervised withdrawal from a drug of dependence that attempts to minimize withdrawal symptoms. It is not a treatment for heroin dependence; it provides a respite from opioid use and may be a prelude to abstinence-based treatment (Mattick and Hall 1996).

Naltrexone is a longer-acting opiate antagonist than naloxone; it can be used to accelerate the opioid withdrawal process. Ultra-rapid opioid detoxification accelerates withdrawal by giving the patient naltrexone under general anesthetic. There is no evidence that accelerated withdrawal in itself reduces the high rate of relapse to heroin use in the absence of further treatment (W. Hall and Mattick 2000).

Abstinence-Oriented Treatments. Abstinence-oriented treatments aim to achieve enduring abstinence from all opioid drugs by providing some type of intervention after withdrawal to reduce the high rate of relapse to opioids (Mattick and Hall 1996). The interventions may include social and psychological support only or such support supplemented by pharmacological methods.

Residential treatment in therapeutic communities and outpatient drug counseling may entail encouraging patients to become involved in self-help groups such as Narcotics Anonymous. These approaches share a commitment to achieving abstinence from all opioids, using group and psychological interventions to help dependent heroin users remain abstinent. Therapeutic communities and drug counseling are usually provided through specialist addiction or mental health services. The former are residential, and the latter are provided on an outpatient basis.

No randomized controlled trials of therapeutic communities or outpatient drug counseling have been carried out. Observational studies in the United Kingdom (Gossop, Marsden, and Stewart 1998; Gossop and others 1997) and the United States (Hubbard and others 1989; Simpson and Sells 1982) have found that therapeutic communities and drug counseling were less successful than MMT in attracting and retaining dependent heroin users, but they substantially reduced heroin use and crime among those who remained in treatment for at least three months (Gerstein and Harwood 1990; Gossop, Marsden, and Stewart 1998; Gossop and others 1997). Some evidence indicated that therapeutic communities may be more effective if they are used in combination with legal coercion to ensure that heroin users are retained in treatment long enough to benefit from it (Gerstein and Harwood 1990).

Recovering drug users run Narcotics Anonymous groups using an adaptation of the 12-step philosophy of Alcoholics Anonymous. Some individuals use these groups as their sole form of support for abstinence, whereas for others these groups complement therapeutic communities that are based on the same principles. Such groups are usually not open to people who are in opioid substitution treatment programs.

The most extensive research on self-help has been in the treatment of alcohol dependence. Treated alcoholics who participate in Alcoholics Anonymous groups have higher rates of abstinence than those who do not (see, for example, Tonigan, Connors, and Miller 2003; Tonigan, Toscova, and Miller 1996). The good outcome in those who attend Alcoholics Anonymous meetings may reflect the self-selection of motivated participants into self-help groups. Recent studies that have attempted to control for this possibility using sophisticated statistical methods have produced mixed results, with some showing the persistence of an effect of self-help after correction (Tonigan, Connors, and Miller 2003) while others do not (Fortney and others 1998).

Shepard and others (forthcoming) evaluate the effect of self-help participation on substance abuse 24 months after treatment for members of a mixed population of substance abusers treated at two treatment facilities in the United States, some of whom had problems with heroin. They find that participation in self-help groups was associated with longer abstinence from all drugs. Correction for self-selection did not eliminate the association in one treatment setting, but it made the results much more equivocal in the other.

Oral Methadone Maintenance Treatment. This treatment substitutes a long-acting, orally administered opioid for the shorter-acting heroin, with the aim of stabilizing dependent heroin users so that they are amenable to rehabilitation (Marsh and others 1990; Ward, Hall, and Mattick 1998). When given in high or blockade doses, methadone blocks the euphoric effects of injected heroin, allowing the individual to take advantage of psychotherapeutic and rehabilitative services.

Every one of the small number of randomized controlled trials of MMT compared with placebo or no treatment has produced positive results (W. Hall, Ward, and Mattick 1998; Mattick and others 2003). Large observational studies show that MMT decreases heroin use and criminal activity and reduces HIV transmission while patients remain in treatment (Gerstein and Harwood 1990; Simpson and Sells 1990; Ward, Hall, and Mattick 1998). MMT is the best-supported form of opioid maintenance treatment (Farre and others 2002; Marsch 1998; Mattick and others 2003).

Buprenorphine is a mixed agonist-antagonist that also blocks the effects of heroin. When given in high doses, its effects can last for up to three days, while its antagonist effects substantially reduce overdose and abuse (Oliveto and Kosten 1997; Ward, Hall, and Mattick 1998). Meta-analyses have found that buprenorphine is effective in the treatment of heroin dependence (Mattick and others 2003) and is of equivalent efficacy to MMT when delivered in primary health care and specialist treatment settings in Australia (Gibson and others 2003).

Bammer and others (2003) have proposed injectable heroin maintenance as a way of attracting into treatment those heroin users who are not interested in or have failed to respond to MMT. This method has recently been evaluated in the Netherlands (Central Committee on the Treatment of Heroin Addicts 2002) and Switzerland (Perneger and others 1998; Uchtenhagen, Gutzwiller, and Dobler-Mikola 1998). Perneger and others (1998) report a randomized controlled trial of injectable heroin maintenance in people who had failed at MMT. Stabilizing and safely maintaining heroin addicts on injectable heroin (self-administered on-site in a comprehensive health and social service) proved feasible for six months and substantially improved their health and social well-being. The Swiss trials showed that it was possible to maintain opioid addicts on injectable heroin for up to two years (Rehm and others 2001; Uchtenhagen, Gutzwiller, and Dobler-Mikola 1998). A recent randomized controlled trial in the Netherlands (Central Committee on the Treatment of Heroin Addicts 2002) confirms the findings of Perneger and others (1998).

Criminal Justice Interventions for Dependent Illicit Opioid Users. The most common intervention for illicit opioid dependence in most developed societies is imprisonment (EMCDDA 2003; Gerstein and Harwood 1990). Imprisonment is not intended to be a health intervention. Nonetheless, it is an ineffective way of reducing opioid dependence, when judged by the high recidivism in longitudinal studies of dependent heroin users (see, for example, Hser, Anglin, and Powers 1993; Manski, Pepper, and Petrie 2001).

Legally coerced treatment is treatment that is legally forced on those who have been charged with or convicted of an offense to which their drug dependence has contributed (W. Hall 1997). It is most often provided as an alternative to imprisonment, under the threat of imprisonment if the person fails to comply with the treatment (W. Hall 1997; Manski, Pepper, and Petrie 2001; Spooner, Hall, and Mattick 2001). Its major justification is that it is an effective way of treating offenders' drug dependence that reduces the likelihood of their offending again (Gerstein and Harwood 1990). A consensus view prepared for the World Health Organization (WHO) (Porter, Arif, and Curran 1986) was that compulsory treatment was legally and ethically justified only if the rights of the individuals were protected by due process and if the treatment provided was effective and humane.

Research into the effectiveness of legally coerced treatment for opioid dependence has been limited to observational studies (W. Hall 1997; Manski, Pepper, and Petrie 2001; Wild, Roberts, and Cooper 2002). Anglin's (1988) quasi-experimental studies of the California Civil Addict Program provide the strongest evidence of efficacy. These studies compared heroin-dependent offenders who entered the program between 1962 and 1964 with a group of similar offenders who went through the criminal justice system during the same period. They found that compulsory hospital treatment followed by close supervision in the community substantially reduced heroin use and crime.

The effectiveness of less coercive forms of treatment has been supported by analyses of the effectiveness of community-based treatment provided while on probation or parole (Hubbard and others 1989; Simpson and others 1986). These studies showed that individuals who entered community-based therapeutic communities and drug-free outpatient counseling under legal pressure did as well as those who did so voluntarily (Hubbard and others 1988; Simpson and Friend 1988). The recent creation of specialized drug courts in the United States to process those arrested for drug-related offenses awaits rigorous evaluation (Belenko 2002; Manski, Pepper, and Petrie 2001).

Legally coerced MMT is also effective. The strongest evidence comes from a study in which drug offenders were randomly assigned to parole with and without community-based MMT (Dole and others 1969). This study showed a greater reduction in heroin use and lower rates of incarceration among those enrolled in MMT in the year following their release from prison. These findings are supported by observational studies that found no major differences in response to MMT between those who enrolled under legal coercion and those who did not (Anglin, Brecht, and Maddahain 1989; Brecht, Anglin, and Wang 1993; Hubbard and others 1988).

Economic Evaluations of Interventions for Illicit Opioid Dependence

The few published economic evaluations of treatment interventions for illicit opioid dependence indicate varying levels of cost-effectiveness.

Detoxification. The National Evaluation of Pharmacotherapies for Opioid Dependence Project in Australia conducted a cost-effectiveness analysis of five interventions:

- naltrexone-induced rapid opioid detoxification under anesthesia
- naltrexone-induced rapid opioid detoxification under sedation
- conventional inpatient detoxification
- conventional outpatient detoxification
- buprenorphine outpatient detoxification.

A successful outcome was defined as achieving abstinence from heroin for one week (Mattick and others 2001).

Rapid detoxification under sedation was the most cost-effective method of detoxification (US$2,355 for one week of abstinence) and conventional outpatient detoxification the least cost-effective (US$12,031). Rapid detoxification under anesthesia achieved high rates of abstinence in the first week, but its expense reduced its cost-effectiveness (Mattick and others 2001).

Doran and others (2003) compared the cost-effectiveness of detoxification from heroin using buprenorphine in a specialist Australian clinic and in a shared care setting. They conducted a randomized controlled trial with 115 heroin-dependent patients receiving a five-day treatment regime of buprenorphine. The specialist clinic was a community-based treatment agency in Sydney. Shared care involved treatment by a general practitioner, supplemented by weekend dispensing and some counseling at the specialist clinic. They estimate that buprenorphine detoxification in the shared care setting was US$17 more expensive per patient than the costs of treatment at the clinic (US$236 per patient).

Drug-Free Treatment. The limited economic evaluations of drug-free treatment have used data from observational studies of treatment outcomes in samples of patients who have mixed substance abuse problems that include opioids. For example, Shepard, Larson, and Hoffmann (1999) calculate a range of estimated costs for achieving an abstinent year in 408 patients at two different treatment facilities in the United States. The cost-effectiveness depended on the severity of the problem and the intensiveness and cost of the intervention. For outpatients with the least severe drug problems, the cost of an abstinent year was US$7,000, whereas the same outcome in patients with more severe problems who received long-term residential treatment cost US$20,000.

Shepard and others (forthcoming) use these data to estimate the cost-effectiveness of involvement in mutual self-help groups, such as Alcoholics Anonymous and Narcotics Anonymous, in sustaining abstinence for up to 24 months after treatment. They find a positive association between self-help involvement and abstinence 12 and 24 months after treatment. Applying statistical methods to correct for the effects of self-selection into self-help, they find that in a Veterans Administration hospital, the effects of self-help on abstinence persisted after the statistical correction, but at the other site, the results depended on the method of analysis that was used. They estimate the cost of achieving an abstinent year by means of self-help in the year following treatment at US$13,000, all of that due to the costs that participants incurred in attending a group.

Oral Opioid Maintenance Treatment. Goldschmidt's (1976) economic evaluation of MMT found that it was as effective as a therapeutic community intervention and twice as cost-effective. Cartwright's (2000) review of the literature since 1976 identified a number of studies, all of which reported positive benefit-cost ratios for MMT.

Gerstein, Harwood, and Suter's (1994) California Drug and Alcohol Treatment Assessment study is the most comprehensive cost-benefit analysis carried out to date. The authors examine the effects of treatment—residential programs, outpatient programs, and methadone programs—on alcohol and drug use, criminal activity, health and health care utilization, and source of income. For each treatment modality, they found that the benefits during the first year of treatment significantly exceeded the cost of delivering the care. The benefit-cost ratio was 4.8 for residential treatment and 11.0 and 12.6 for outpatients and discharged methadone participants, respectively.

Doran and others (2003) compared the cost-effectiveness of buprenorphine and methadone treatment for opioid dependence. In a randomized controlled trial, 405 subjects were randomly assigned to each treatment at one of three specialist outpatient drug treatment centers. The study found that treatment with methadone was less expensive and more effective than treatment with buprenorphine, but the difference in cost (US$143 per additional heroin-free day gained) had a wide range of uncertainty around it (−US$1,469 to US$1,284).

The National Evaluation of Pharmacotherapies for Opioid Dependence Project also provided a cost-effectiveness analysis of methadone, buprenorphine, LAAM (levo-alpha-acetyl-methadol), and naltrexone maintenance treatments (Mattick and others 2001). The daily costs of these maintenance treatments were similar for methadone and LAAM, but naltrexone was slightly more expensive. Buprenorphine maintenance treatment (BMT) was more expensive, but its cost-efficiency could have been improved to make its cost similar to that for the other treatments. MMT was the most cost-effective treatment for opioid dependence because it achieved one of the highest rates of retention in treatment among the four pharmacotherapies examined. Naltrexone treatment was the least cost-effective.

The costs of injectable heroin maintenance in the Dutch study was between US$18,015 and US$23,243 per patient per year (Bammer and others 2003). Most of the costs arose from the supervision of heroin use and the security required to prevent the diversion of heroin to the black market. Injectable heroin maintenance needs to produce substantially greater benefits for each participant than MMT to make it as cost-effective as MMT.

Economic Modeling of the Cost-Effectiveness of Opioid Maintenance Treatment. Barnett (1999), using data on the efficacy of MMT in reducing mortality derived from Gronbladh, Ohlund, and Gunne's (1990) Swedish study and U.S. cost data, estimated that MMT saved an additional year of life at a cost of US$5,900. Barnett, Zaric, and Brandeau (2001), using a similar approach, estimated that the use of buprenorphine by patients who would not use methadone would cost less than US$45,000 per quality-adjusted life year. Overall, however, they found that BMT was much less effective and more costly than MMT. Zaric, Barnett, and Brandeau (2000) assessed the economic benefits of using MMT to reduce HIV transmission in heroin users. They found that for heroin users living in a community with a high prevalence of HIV infection, expanding MMT use produced an additional year of quality-adjusted life at a cost of US$8,200.

Comparing the Cost-Effectiveness of Different Interventions

Comparative cost-effectiveness analyses of these interventions face major obstacles because the small number of published studies used different methods to cost interventions and different endpoints to assess the outcome of treatment. The following list, therefore, only ranks treatment interventions in the approximate order of their cost-effectiveness. We believe that estimates of their likely contribution to DALYs worldwide would be too speculative.

- *Detoxification.* Buprenorphine and supervised naltrexone-accelerated withdrawal delivered on an outpatient basis are the most efficient and effective ways to achieve withdrawal from opioids.
- *Self-help groups.* These groups provide the simplest form of postwithdrawal support for enduring abstinence and are also a low-cost intervention, because patients bear most of the costs; however, they have a low rate of uptake, and their effectiveness is only modest.
- *Oral opioid agonist maintenance treatment.* This form of treatment is the most widely used intervention for illicit opioid dependence in developed societies. It has a better uptake than other interventions, and it is moderately effective under the usual delivery conditions.
- *Drug-free residential treatment.* This form of treatment has a relatively low rate of treatment uptake and is costly because

of its residential character and the need for intensive staff-patient interaction. It is effective for the minority of people who are retained in treatment long enough to benefit from it (usually three months). Retention in treatment may be improved if patients enter treatment under some form of legal coercion.

- *Naltrexone maintenance treatment.* This form of treatment has not been rigorously evaluated.
- *Injectable opioid maintenance.* This intervention is a more expensive variant of agonist maintenance treatment that has been used for patients with more severe cases of dependency but for whom retention and treatment outcomes have been good.

Calculation of the Averted, Avertable, and Unavertable Burden

Assuming that the disease burden from opioid dependence is potentially avertable, we used the following approach to estimate the avoidable burden of opioid dependence. We initially modeled the avertable burden using MMT and used this model for BMT. The first step was to establish the base case for opioid dependence using 2002 as the baseline year. We established the model of the base case for opioid dependence for regions and subregions according to WHO country classifications. We used population estimates for each region for those age 15 to 59, the age range in which heroin dependence is most prevalent. We incorporated Degenhardt, Hall, and others' (2004, table 13.1) figures for the prevalence of opioid use by region, assuming that the prevalence was 30 percent higher among male users than female users.

We obtained population-attributable fractions related to opioid dependence from the editors of this volume. We used nine relevant WHO categories to estimate the burden of disease attributable to opioid dependence—namely HIV/AIDS, drug-use disorders, road traffic accidents, poisonings, falls, fires, drownings, other unintentional injuries, and self-inflicted injuries.

We calculated the mortality rate for opioid deaths by dividing the number of deaths by the estimated number of users. We took estimates of years of life lost (YLLs) and years lived with disability (YLDs), by gender, for each region from data obtained from the editors of this volume. We then used those estimates to calculate the DALYs for male users, female users, and all users (YLL + YLD = DALY). We discounted the YLLs, YLDs, and DALYs using a 3 percent discount rate.

The second step was to estimate the avertable burden by treatment with methadone or buprenorphine. Using the population and prevalence data, we assumed, in the first instance, that 50 percent of those dependent on opioids entered treatment. In the sensitivity analysis, we varied this proportion from 25 to 75 percent coverage. On the basis of Caplehorn and others' (1994) meta-analysis, we assumed that MMT reduced

mortality by 25 percent. In the sensitivity analysis, we varied the reduction from 15 to 35 percent (using the confidence intervals around the estimated reduction). We assumed that the reduction in mortality associated with BMT was 20 percent, which we varied in the sensitivity analysis from 10 to 30 percent. Finally, we assumed that those who were alive and in treatment experienced a 25 percent reduction in disability, consistent with the Dutch disability weights.

The third step was to estimate the burden for those not treated. For those users not in treatment, we calculated DALYs using the original mortality rates.

The fourth step was to estimate the total avertable burden from treatment with methadone or buprenorphine by (a) adding the results of the second and third steps, the revised DALYs for those in treatment, and the residual for those not in treatment and (b) subtracting those figures from the base case estimates.

The fifth step was to cost the interventions using data on MMT and BMT from Doran and others (2003). They estimated the cost of MMT at $A 1,415 and of BMT at $A 1,729 for six months of treatment. We converted these estimates into U.S. dollars and multiplied them by two to provide yearly estimates of treatment costs of US$1,732 for MMT and US$2,117 for BMT.

We applied relative price weights for each region using the Western Pacific as the reference case (1.00). We calculated the relative price weights for each cost type using data provided by the World Bank. The prices are a reflection of the public health systems in each region, and as far as possible they reflect the opportunity cost of health care resources in these regions.

Results. Our results are presented in table 48.1. We explored various combinations of coverage and reductions in mortality for MMT and BMT. For each intervention, as coverage and reductions in mortality increased, the number of DALYs averted increased. The wide discrepancies in DALYs averted within regions primarily reflect differences in population-attributable fractions for HIV/AIDS. Costs increased as a consequence of increased coverage for both interventions, whereas results for cost-effectiveness differ by both intervention and mortality.

The cost-effectiveness analysis suggests that for MMT (with a coverage of 25, 50, or 75 percent and reductions in mortality of 35 percent) the cost in international dollars per DALY averted ranges from a low of $128 in Africa, with high child and adult mortality where the prevalence of illicit opioid dependence is low (0.01 percent), to a high of $3,726 in Eastern Europe, with low child and adult mortality where the prevalence of illicit opioid dependence is high (0.55 percent). Across all the regions, the average cost-effectiveness ratio for MMT (with 25, 50, and 75 percent coverage and 35 percent reduction in mortality) is estimated at $2,236 per DALY averted.

Assessment. The results shown in table 48.1 provide a first approximation of the potential avertable burden in DALYs if

Table 48.1 Cost-Effectiveness Results

			Africa		The Americas			Eastern Mediterranean		Europe			Southeast Asia		Western Pacific	
Treatment	**Coverage (%)**	**Mortality (%)**	**AFR-D**	**AFR-E**	**AMR-A**	**AMR-B**	**AMR-D**	**EMR-A**	**EMR-D**	**EUR-A**	**EUR-B**	**EUR-C**	**SEAR-B**	**SEAR-D**	**WPR-A**	**WPR-B**

Total effect (DALYs averted per 1 million population)

Treatment	**Coverage (%)**	**Mortality (%)**	**AFR-D**	**AFR-E**	**AMR-A**	**AMR-B**	**AMR-D**	**EMR-A**	**EMR-D**	**EUR-A**	**EUR-B**	**EUR-C**	**SEAR-B**	**SEAR-D**	**WPR-A**	**WPR-B**
MMT	25	15	125	79	153	107	158	179	105	117	48	198	63	48	39	26
MMT	50	15	251	158	306	214	316	358	210	234	96	397	126	97	77	53
MMT	75	15	376	237	459	321	474	538	315	352	144	595	190	145	116	79
MMT	25	25	150	81	184	121	173	217	151	141	59	264	93	70	51	35
MMT	50	25	300	163	369	243	347	435	303	283	117	527	185	140	102	70
MMT	75	25	450	244	553	364	520	652	454	424	176	791	278	211	152	105
MMT	25	35	174	84	216	136	189	256	198	165	69	329	122	92	63	43
MMT	50	35	349	167	432	272	378	511	396	331	139	657	244	184	126	87
MMT	75	35	523	251	648	408	566	767	594	496	208	986	367	276	189	130
BMT	25	10	113	78	137	100	150	160	82	105	43	166	48	38	32	22
BMT	50	10	226	156	274	199	301	320	163	210	85	331	97	75	65	44
BMT	75	10	339	234	412	299	451	480	245	315	128	497	145	113	97	67
BMT	25	20	138	80	169	114	166	198	128	129	53	231	78	59	45	31
BMT	50	20	275	160	337	228	332	397	256	258	107	462	156	119	89	61
BMT	75	20	413	240	506	342	497	595	384	388	160	693	234	178	134	92
BMT	25	30	162	82	200	129	181	237	175	153	64	296	107	81	57	39
BMT	50	30	324	165	400	258	362	473	350	307	128	592	215	162	114	78
BMT	75	30	487	247	601	386	543	710	524	460	192	888	322	243	171	117

Total costs (US$ per 1 million population)

Treatment	**Coverage (%)**	**Mortality (%)**	**AFR-D**	**AFR-E**	**AMR-A**	**AMR-B**	**AMR-D**	**EMR-A**	**EMR-D**	**EUR-A**	**EUR-B**	**EUR-C**	**SEAR-B**	**SEAR-D**	**WPR-A**	**WPR-B**
MMT	25	15, 25, 35	0.10	0.01	0.25	0.06	0.12	0.95	0.65	0.20	0.16	0.35	0.06	0.19	0.07	0.03
MMT	50	15, 25, 35	0.19	0.02	0.50	0.11	0.24	1.90	1.30	0.40	0.32	0.71	0.11	0.39	0.13	0.07
MMT	75	15, 25, 35	0.29	0.03	0.74	0.17	0.36	2.86	1.95	0.60	0.49	1.06	0.17	0.58	0.20	0.10
BMT	25	10, 20, 30	0.12	0.01	0.30	0.07	0.15	1.16	0.80	0.24	0.20	0.43	0.07	0.24	0.08	0.04
BMT	50	10, 20, 30	0.24	0.03	0.60	0.14	0.29	2.33	1.59	0.49	0.40	0.86	0.14	0.47	0.16	0.08
BMT	75	10, 20, 30	0.35	0.04	0.91	0.20	0.44	3.49	2.39	0.73	0.59	1.29	0.20	0.71	0.24	0.12

Cost-effectiveness (US$ per DALY averted)

Treatment	**Coverage (%)**	**Mortality (%)**	**AFR-D**	**AFR-E**	**AMR-A**	**AMR-B**	**AMR-D**	**EMR-A**	**EMR-D**	**EUR-A**	**EUR-B**	**EUR-C**	**SEAR-B**	**SEAR-D**	**WPR-A**	**WPR-B**
MMT	25, 50, 75	15	768	136	1,618	520	755	5,315	6,213	1,711	3,379	1,782	875	3,984	1,716	1,284
MMT	25, 50, 75	25	643	132	1,342	458	688	4,381	4,300	1,419	2,764	1,341	597	2,749	1,301	974
MMT	25, 50, 75	35	552	128	1,146	408	632	3,726	3,288	1,212	2,339	1,074	453	2,099	1,048	784
BMT	25, 50, 75	10	1,041	168	2,204	682	969	7,269	9,764	2,329	4,646	2,606	1,396	6,277	2,493	1,867
BMT	25, 50, 75	20	855	164	1,793	595	880	5,869	6,210	1,895	3,716	1,869	867	3,975	1,809	1,354
BMT	25, 50, 75	30	726	159	1,510	527	805	4,921	4,553	1,598	3,096	1,458	629	2,909	1,419	1,062

DALYs averted per US$1 million spent

Treatment	**Coverage (%)**	**Mortality (%)**	**AFR-D**	**AFR-E**	**AMR-A**	**AMR-B**	**AMR-D**	**EMR-A**	**EMR-D**	**EUR-A**	**EUR-B**	**EUR-C**	**SEAR-B**	**SEAR-D**	**WPR-A**	**WPR-B**
MMT	25, 50, 75	15	1,302	7,363	618	1,922	1,325	188	161	585	296	561	1,142	251	583	779
MMT	25, 50, 75	25	1,556	7,575	745	2,185	1,453	228	233	705	362	746	1,676	364	768	1,027
MMT	25, 50, 75	35	1,811	7,787	873	2,448	1,582	268	304	825	428	931	2,210	476	954	1,275
BMT	25, 50, 75	10	961	5,939	454	1,465	1,032	138	102	429	215	384	717	159	401	536
BMT	25, 50, 75	15	1,170	6,112	558	1,681	1,137	170	161	528	269	535	1,153	252	553	739
BMT	25, 50, 75	20	1,378	6,286	662	1,896	1,242	203	220	626	323	686	1,590	344	705	942

MMT and BMT were applied to 50 percent of the opioid-dependent population in each region. Because the methods and data used to estimate avertable DALYs are subject to certain limitations, those results should be considered preliminary.

RELEVANCE TO DEVELOPING COUNTRIES

Much of the epidemiological research on illicit opioid dependence, its disease burden, and its societal harm comes from Australasia, Europe, and the United States. The major exception is research on the role of injecting drug use in HIV transmission in developing countries (see, for example, Beyrer and others 2000; Yu and others 1998). In addition, research on the effectiveness and cost-effectiveness of interventions for illicit opioid dependence has been conducted primarily in developed countries (Ward, Hall, and Mattick 1998), with the exception of studies of the effectiveness of methadone treatment in Hong Kong, China (see, for instance, Newman and Whitehill 1979), and in Thailand (Vanichseni and others 1991), both of which showed comparable effectiveness to that found in developed countries (W. Hall, Ward, and Mattick 1998).

Translating findings on interventions for opioid dependence in developed countries into disease control priorities for opioid dependence in developing countries presents three major challenges. First, countries differ in the scale of illicit opioid use and in the resulting disease burden. This variation reflects the effects of differences in the prevalence of injecting and noninjecting opioid users; the dependent opioid users' access to treatment and health services for overdoses, bloodborne viruses, and other complications of drug use; the access to needle and syringe programs; the extent to which illicit opioid use is concentrated in socially disadvantaged minority groups; and the capacity of public health services to monitor and respond to emerging infectious disease and drug-use epidemics. The burden is likely to be greatest in settings where the primary route of administration is injecting and where public and personal health services are poorly developed, as appears to be the case in Asia and in Eastern Europe.

Second, societal wealth and health care infrastructure affect the capacity of developing societies to treat illicit opioid dependence. A country's capacity to provide opioid substitution treatment will be affected by the cost of oral opioid drugs, such as methadone, LAAM, and buprenorphine, and the existence of specialist drug treatment centers; trained medical, nursing, and pharmacy staff; and a drug regulatory system, which are required so as to deliver opioid substitution treatment safely and effectively. Few developing countries possess this infrastructure. However, examples exist of apparently successful drug substitution programs, using such tools as sublingual buprenorphine, that have been conducted with minimal resources in extremely poor settings (Crofts and others 1998).

Third, in societies with a sizable illicit opioid dependence problem, cultural attitudes and beliefs will affect societal responses, especially attitudes toward illicit opioid use and dependence (Gerstein and Harwood 1990). A critical determinant of the social response will be the relative dominance of moral and medical understandings of drug dependence in general and opioid dependence in particular. A moral model of addiction sees addiction as largely a voluntary behavior, in which case it is seen as an excuse for bad behavior that allows drug users to continue to take drugs without assuming responsibility for their conduct (Szasz 1985). In this view, drug users who offend against the criminal code should be imprisoned (Szasz 1985). This model is the dominant one in many developed societies, which imprison drug users at high rates without any effect on the prevalence of drug abuse. Countries that adopt punitive policies toward drug users are reluctant to embrace harm reduction measures, such as needle and syringe programs and opioid maintenance treatment (Ainsworth, Beyrer, and Soucat 2003). A medical model of addiction, by contrast, recognizes that dependent opioid users require specific treatment if the sufferer is to become and remain abstinent (see, for example, Leshner 1997).

These competing views will affect the societal acceptability of opioid maintenance and abstinence-oriented approaches to the treatment of opioid dependence (Cohen 2003). Those who have a moral view of addiction will tend to prefer drug-free and self-help approaches toward treatment. Supporters of medical models of addiction will favor some form of opioid substitution treatment and the provision of clean needles and syringes to reduce the transmission of bloodborne viruses by injecting opioid and other drug users. Stronger advocacy by international organizations and agencies is needed for the adoption of such harm reduction measures as needle and syringe programs and agonist substitution programs.

RESEARCH AND DEVELOPMENT

Two main areas are important for research and development. First, better estimates are needed of the prevalence of illicit opioid dependence and prospective studies of the morbidity and mortality that it causes in both developed and developing countries. These estimates are especially needed in countries where illicit opioid use is high because of their proximity to source countries. Second, we need evaluations of the effectiveness and cost-effectiveness of self-help, drug-free, and oral opioid substitution treatment in developing countries. A priority should be the identification of safe, innovative, and less expensive ways of effectively delivering culturally acceptable forms of opioid maintenance treatments in developing countries. This effort may require experimentation with a range of substitute opioids, such as buprenorphine, and cheaper options, such as codeine and opium tincture.

CONCLUSIONS: PROMISES AND PITFALLS

Illicit opioid use, especially injecting use, contributes to premature mortality and morbidity in many developed and developing societies. Fatal overdoses and HIV/AIDS resulting from the sharing of dirty injecting equipment are major contributors to mortality and morbidity, and the economic costs of illicit opioid dependence are substantial. Illicit opioid dependence generates substantial externalities that are not included in burden-of-disease estimates, principally law enforcement costs incurred in handling drug dealing and property crime.

The most popular interventions for illicit opioid dependence in many developed societies have been law enforcement efforts to interdict the drug supply and enforce legal sanctions against the use of opioid drugs. One consequence of this strategy has been that most illicit opioid users have been exposed to the least effective intervention: imprisonment for drug or property offenses. Prisons rarely take the opportunity to treat dependence using opioid maintenance or to reduce the harm caused by illicit opioid use by providing access to clean injecting equipment.

In treatment settings, the most popular interventions have been detoxification (which is not a treatment but a prelude to treatment) and drug-free treatment (which is the least attractive and the least effective in retaining opioid-dependent people in treatment). Opioid agonist maintenance treatment has been ambivalently supported in many developed societies despite its being the treatment for which there is the best evidence of effectiveness, safety, and cost-effectiveness. The range of opioid agonists available for maintenance treatment is increasing. A number of developed countries have approved the use of BMT, which the limited data suggest may be approximately equivalent to MMT in efficacy and cost-effectiveness. Opioid antagonists have a niche role in the treatment of opioid dependence because of poor compliance and an increased risk of overdose on return to heroin use. Their efficacy may improve with the development of long-acting injectable forms of the drug.

ANNEX 48.A: PREVALENCE OF USE, ADVERSE HEALTH EFFECTS OF AND INTERVENTIONS FOR CANNABIS, COCAINE, AMPHETAMINES, AND MDMA USE AND DEPENDENCE

Cannabis

Cannabis is the most widely used illicit drug globally, with about 150 million users, or 3.7 percent of the world's population age 15 and older (UNODCCP 2003). Patterns of cannabis use have been most extensively studied in Australia, Canada, the United States, and Europe (W. Hall and Pacula 2003). Europe generally has lower rates of use than Australia, Canada, and the United States, with the highest rates in Denmark, France and the United Kingdom (EMCDDA 2002; W. Hall and Pacula 2003). The limited data from developing countries suggest that, with some exceptions (for example, Jamaica and South Africa), rates of cannabis use are lower in Africa, Asia, the Caribbean, and South America than they are in Europe and in English-speaking countries (W. Hall, Johnston, and Donnelly 1999).

Surveys in the United States have found long waves of cannabis use among young people since 1975. Cannabis use increased during the 1970s to peak in 1979, before declining steadily between 1980 and 1991. Use rose sharply in 1992 and increased throughout the 1990s, before leveling off in the late 1990s (Johnston, O'Malley, and Bachman 1994a, 1994b). There was also a rise in cannabis use during the early 1990s in Australia, Canada, and some European countries (W. Hall and Pacula 2003).

The natural history of cannabis use in the United States typically begins in the mid to late teens and reaches its maximum in the early 20s before declining in the mid to late 20s. Only a minority of young adults continue to use cannabis into their 30s (Bachman and others 1997; Chen and Kandel 1995). Getting married and having children substantially reduces rates of cannabis use (Bachman and others 1997).

Cannibis use can have several adverse health effects, as discussed below.

Acute Effects of Cannabis Use. The most frequent unpleasant effects of cannabis use are anxiety and panic reactions, which most often occur in users who are unfamiliar with the drug's effects. Psychotic symptoms such as delusions and hallucinations may be experienced following very high doses. There are no cases of fatal cannabis poisoning in the medical literature, and the fatal dose in humans is likely to exceed what recreational users are able to ingest (W. Hall and Pacula 2003).

Cannabis intoxication impairs a wide range of cognitive and behavioral functions that are involved in driving an automobile or operating machinery (Beardsley and Kelly 1999; Jaffe 1985). It has been difficult to determine whether these impairments increase the risk of being involved in motor vehicle accidents (Smiley 1999). Studies of the effect of cannabis on driving performance on the road have found only modest impairments, because cannabis-intoxicated drivers drive more slowly and take fewer risks than drivers intoxicated by alcohol (Smiley 1999).

Cannabinoids are found in the blood of substantial proportions of persons killed in motor vehicle accidents (Bates and Blakely 1999; Chesher 1995; Walsh and Mann 1999), but these findings have been difficult to evaluate because they have not distinguished between past and recent cannabis use (Ramaekers and others 2004). More recent research using better indicators of recent cannabis use has found a dose-response relationship between cannabis and risk of motor vehicle crashes (Ramaekers and others 2004). Cannabis used in combination with alcohol substantially increases risk of accidents (Bates and Blakely 1999; Ramaekers and others 2004).

Health Effects of Chronic Cannabis Use. Cannabis smoke is a potential cause of cancer because it contains many of the same carcinogenic substances as cigarette smoke (Marselos and Karamanakos 1999). Cancers have been reported in the aerodigestive tracts of young adults who were daily cannabis smokers (W. Hall and MacPhee 2002), and a case-control study has found an association between cannabis smoking and head and neck cancer (Zhang and others 1999). A prospective cohort study of 64,000 adults did not find any increase in rates of head and neck or respiratory cancers (Sidney and others 1997). Further studies are needed to clarify the issue.

Three studies of different types of cancer have reported an association with maternal cannabis use during pregnancy (W. Hall and MacPhee 2002). There have not been any increases in the rates of these cancers that parallel increases in rates of cannabis use (W. Hall and MacPhee 2002).

High doses of cannabinoids impair cell-mediated and humoral immunity and reduce resistance to infection by bacteria and viruses in rodents (Klein 1999). Cannabis smoke impairs the functioning of alveolar macrophages, the first line of the body's immune defense system in the lungs. The doses that produce these effects have been very high, and extrapolation to the doses used by humans is complicated by the fact that tolerance to these effects develops (Hollister 1992). There is as yet no epidemiological evidence that rates of infectious disease are higher among chronic heavy cannabis users. Several large prospective studies of HIV-positive homosexual men have not found that cannabis use makes it more likely that HIV-positive men develop AIDS (W. Hall and Pacula 2003).

Chronic administration of tetrahydrocannabinol (THC) disrupts male and female reproductive systems in animals, reducing testosterone secretion and sperm production, motility, and viability in males and disrupting ovulation in females (Brown and Dobs 2002). It is uncertain whether cannabis use has these effects in humans because of the limited research on human males and females (Murphy 1999).

The use of cannabis during pregnancy is associated with smaller birthweight (English and others 1997; Fergusson, Horwood, and Northstone 2002), but it does not appear to increase the risk of birth defects (W. Hall and Pacula 2003). In some studies, infants exposed to cannabis during pregnancy show behavioral and developmental effects during the first few months after birth; these effects are smaller than those seen after tobacco use during pregnancy (Fried and Smith 2001).

The changes that cannabis smoking causes in heart rate and blood pressure are unlikely to harm healthy young adults, but they may harm patients with hypertension, cerebrovascular disease, and coronary atherosclerosis (Chesher and Hall 1999; Sidney 2002). One controlled study suggests that cannabis use can precipitate heart attacks in middle-aged cannabis users who have atherosclerosis in the heart, brain, and peripheral blood vessels (Mittleman and others 2001).

Regular cannabis smoking impairs the functioning of the large airways and causes chronic bronchitis (Tashkin 1999; Taylor and others 2002). Given that tobacco and cannabis smoke contain similar carcinogenic substances, it is likely that chronic cannabis smoking increases the risks of respiratory cancer (Tashkin 1999).

Psychological Effects of Chronic Cannabis Use. Psychological effects of chronic cannabis use can include a dependence syndrome, cognitive effects, and psychotic disorders.

Dependence Syndrome A cannabis dependence syndrome occurs in heavy chronic users of cannabis (American Psychiatric Association 1994). Regular cannabis users develop tolerance to THC. Some experience withdrawal symptoms on cessation of use (Kouri and Pope 2000), and some report problems controlling their cannabis use (W. Hall and Pacula 2003). The risk of dependence is about 1 in 10 among those who ever use the drug, between 1 in 5 and 1 in 3 among those who use cannabis more than a few times, and about 1 in 2 among daily users (W. Hall and Pacula 2003).

Cognitive Effects Long-term daily cannabis use does not severely impair cognitive function, but it may more subtly impair memory, attention, and the ability to integrate complex information (Solowij 1998; Solowij and others 2002). It remains uncertain whether these effects are due to the cumulative effect of regular cannabis use on cannabinoid receptors in the brain or whether they are residual effects of THC that will disappear after an extended period of abstinence (W. Hall and Pacula 2003).

Psychotic Disorders There is now good evidence that chronic cannabis use may precipitate psychosis in vulnerable individuals (see, for example, Arseneault and others 2002; van Os and others 2002; Zammit and others 2002). It is less likely that cannabis use can cause psychosis de novo, because the incidence of schizophrenia has either remained stable or declined while cannabis use has increased among young adults (Degenhardt, Hall, and Lynskey 2003).

Effects of Cannabis Use on Adolescents. Cannabis use has a number of effects on adolescents.

Gateway Hypothesis Adolescents in developed societies typically use alcohol and tobacco before using cannabis, which in turn, they use before using hallucinogens, amphetamines, heroin, and cocaine (Kandel 2002). Generally, the earlier the age of first use and the greater the involvement with any drug in the sequence, the more likely a young person is to use the next drug in the sequence (Kandel 2002). The role played by cannabis in this sequence remains controversial (W. Hall and Lynskey forthcoming; W. Hall and Pacula 2003).

The simplest hypothesis is that cannabis use has a pharmacological effect that increases the risk of using drugs later in the sequence. Equally plausible hypotheses are that it is due to a combination of (a) early recruitment into cannabis use of nonconforming and deviant adolescents who are likely to use alcohol, tobacco, and illicit drugs; (b) a shared genetic vulnerability to dependence on alcohol, tobacco, and cannabis; and (c) socialization of cannabis users within an illicit drug–using subculture, which increases the opportunity, and encouragement to use other illicit drugs (W. Hall and Pacula 2003).

Adolescent Psychosocial Outcomes Cannabis use is associated with early withdrawal from high school, early family formation, poor mental health, and involvement in drug-related crime. In the case of each of these outcomes, the strong associations in cross-sectional data are more modest when account is taken of the fact that cannabis users show characteristics before they use cannabis that predict these outcomes. For example, they have lower academic aspirations and poorer school performance than peers who do not use cannabis (Lynskey and Hall 2000; Macleod and others 2004). Nonetheless, the evidence increasingly suggests that regular cannabis use adds to the risk of these outcomes in adolescents already at risk (W. Hall and Pacula 2003).

Interventions for Cannabis Dependence. Although many dependent cannabis users may succeed in quitting without professional help, some are unable to stop on their own and will need assistance to do so. There has not been a great deal of research on pharmacological treatments for cannabis dependence, although a recent study trialed divalproex sodium with promising results (Levin and others 2004). Limited research exists on the effectiveness of different types of psychosocial treatments for dependent cannabis use (Budney and others 2000; Copeland and others 2001; Stephens, Roffman, and Simpson 1994). These approaches have involved short-term cognitive behavioral treatments modeled on similar treatments for alcohol dependence, usually given in three to six sessions on an outpatient basis.

In all of these studies, rates of abstinence at the end of treatment have been modest (20 to 40 percent), and subsequent high rates of relapse mean that rates of abstinence after 12 months have been very modest (Budney and Moore 2002). Nonetheless, treatment does substantially reduce cannabis use and problems. These outcomes are not very different from those observed in the treatment for alcohol and other forms of drug dependence (Budney and Moore 2002). Much more research is needed before sensible advice can be given about the best ways to achieve abstinence from cannabis.

Cocaine

After cannabis, cocaine is one of the most widely used illicit drugs in developed and developing societies. Some 14 million people were estimated to have used cocaine globally in 2003, with demand for treatment second only to heroin (UNODCCP 2003). The highest rates of reported cocaine use—and the best data on trends in cocaine use—come from the United States, the world's largest cocaine market. Rates of cocaine use in the United States increased from the mid 1970s until 1985, when 5.7 million Americans age 12 and older reported using cocaine in the preceding month. Rates of cocaine use in the preceding month have declined steadily since 1985. In 2000, 11.2 percent of Americans over age 12 reported that they had used cocaine at some time in their lives, and 0.4 percent (800,000 people) reported weekly cocaine use (SAMHSA 2001). Among young U.S. adults age 18 to 25, lifetime prevalence was 14.9 percent in 2001, rising slightly to 15.4 percent in 2002 (SAMHSA 2003). In 2002, annual prevalence figures from student surveys were 15 percent lower than 1998 figures and 60 percent lower than 1985 figures (UNODCCP 2003). A more recent study of U.S. adults age 35 years found that 6 percent of men and 3 percent of women had used cocaine within the preceding 12 months (Merline and others 2004).

The reported prevalence of cocaine use in other developed societies is much lower than that in the United States. In Europe, for example, rates of lifetime cocaine use range from 0.5 percent to 5 percent (EMCDDA 2003), compared with 12.3 percent among American adults in 2001 (SAMHSA 2001). Rates of cocaine use in Australia resemble those in Europe, with 4.3 percent of adults reporting lifetime use (Darke and others 2000).

The prevalence of cocaine use is likely to be lower in developing societies, but the poor quality of the available data makes it difficult to be sure (UNDCP 1997). There probably has been an increase in cocaine use in some developing countries in recent years, but it is difficult to estimate the size of the increase (United Nations Commission on Narcotic Drugs 2000). The region with the highest rates of cocaine use among developing societies is likely to be Central and South America. The botanical source is indigenous to the region and has traditionally been used by local populations. Moreover, several nations in Central and South America have a history of production and export to global markets. Recent reports indicate that cocaine abuse is increasing in South America (UNODCCP 2003), and a recent household survey on drug abuse in São Paulo, Brazil, estimated cocaine prevalence at 2.1 percent (Galduroz and others 2003).

Adverse Health Effects of Cocaine. Most cocaine use is infrequent; regular cocaine use (monthly or more frequently) can be a major public health problem. Regular cocaine users who inject cocaine or smoke crack cocaine are especially likely to develop dependence and to experience problems related to their cocaine use (Platt 1997). In the United States, it has been estimated that one in six of those who ever use cocaine become dependent on the drug (Anthony, Warner, and Kessler 1994). High rates of cocaine dependence are found among people treated for alcohol and drug problems and among arrestees in the United States (Anglin and Perrochet 1998).

In large doses, cocaine may be harmful in both cocaine-naive and cocaine-tolerant individuals (Platt 1997; Vasica and Tennant 2002). The vasoconstrictor effects of cocaine in large doses place great strains on a number of the body's physiological systems (McCann and Ricaurte 2000). Effects on the cardiovascular system can result in a range of difficulties, from chest pain to fatal cardiac arrests (Lange and Hillis 2001). Neurological problems include cerebral vascular accidents such as strokes or seizures. Other effects of cocaine can include gastrointestinal problems such as vomiting, colitis, and bowel infarction and respiratory problems such as asthma, respiratory collapse, pulmonary edema, and bronchitis. Hyperthermia may occur because of the increased metabolism, peripheral vasoconstriction, and inability of the thalamus to control body temperature (Crandall, Vongpatanasin, and Victor 2002). Obstetric complications can include irregularities in placental blood flow, premature labor, and low neonate birthweight (Majewska 1996; Platt 1997; Vasica and Tennant 2002).

Adverse health effects from cocaine are potentially fatal and can occur among healthy users irrespective of cocaine dose and frequency of use (Lange and Hillis 2001; Vasica and Tennant 2002). Although the likelihood of health problems may increase with dosage and frequency of use, there is wide individual variation in reactions to cocaine and, therefore, no specific combination of conditions under which adverse health effects can be predicted. There is no antidote to cocaine overdose as there is for an overdose of heroin (Platt 1997).

The impact of cocaine on mental health is also complex. Although cocaine can produce feelings of pleasure, it may also result in negative psychological symptoms such as anxiety, depression, paranoia, hallucinations, and agitation (American Psychiatric Association 1994). Regular cocaine users experience high rates of psychiatric disorders. In the United States, regular cocaine users report high rates of anxiety and affective disorders (Gawin and Ellinwood 1988; Platt 1997). The repeated use of large doses of cocaine can also produce a paranoid psychosis (Majewska 1996; Manschreck and others 1988; Platt 1997; Satel and Edell 1991). People who are acutely intoxicated by cocaine can become violent, especially those who develop a paranoid psychosis (Platt 1997).

Animal studies suggest that cocaine use may be neurotoxic in large doses—that is, it can produce permanent changes in the brain and neurotransmitter systems (Majewska 1996; Platt 1997). It is unclear whether use is also neurotoxic in humans.

Previous studies have documented a variety of neuropsychological effects of cocaine use, including deficits in memory and problem solving (Beatty and others 1995; Hoff and others 1996; O'Malley and others 1992). More recently, a twin study indicated that cocaine may lead to impaired attention and motor skills up to one year after the conclusion of heavy use (Toomey and others 2003).

The method by which cocaine is administered can result in adverse health effects (Platt 1997). Snorting cocaine through the nose can lead to rhinitis, damage to the nasal septum, and loss of the sense of smell. Smoking cocaine can lead to respiratory problems, and injecting cocaine leads to the risks of infections and bloodborne viruses associated with all injecting drug use.

Users who inject cocaine, either on its own or in combination with heroin ("speedballs"), inject much more frequently than other injecting drug users and, as a consequence, engage in more needle sharing, take more sexual risks, and have higher rates of HIV infection (Chaisson and others 1989; Schoenbaum and others 1989; van Beek, Dwyer, and Malcolm 2001). Associations between cocaine use and HIV risk-taking have been reported in Europe (Torrens and others 1991), Australia (Darke and others 1992), and the United States (Chaisson and others 1989). Recent Australian research has indicated that injecting cocaine users report more problems related to injecting drug use—such as vascular problems, abscesses, and infections—than other injecting drug users (Darke, Kaye, and Topp 2002).

The link between cocaine use and HIV risk is not restricted to those who inject cocaine. Crack smoking has been linked to higher levels of needle risk, sexual risk taking, and HIV infection (Chaisson and others 1989; Chirgwin and others 1991; Desjalais and others 1992; Grella, Anglin, and Wugalter 1995). Two mechanisms probably underlie the relationship between cocaine use and HIV infection. First, the short half-life of cocaine promotes a much higher frequency of injecting by users than that seen in heroin injectors. Second, cocaine itself disinhibits and stimulates users, encouraging them to take greater risks with sexual activity and needle use (Darke and others 2000).

Cocaine is associated with a risk of intentional injuries and injuries in general. A recent review reported that 28.7 percent of people with intentional injuries and 4.5 percent of injured drivers tested positive for cocaine (Macdonald and others 2003). Users are also at risk of death from an accidental overdose of cocaine. A recent study of accidental deaths from drug overdose in New York between 1990 and 1998 found that 70 percent of deaths were caused by cocaine, often in combination with opiates (Coffin and others 2003). The causes of cocaine-related deaths are usually related to cardiovascular complications (Vasica and Tennant 2002), but death may also be due to brain hemorrhage, stroke, and kidney failure (Brands, Sproule, and

Marshman 1998). Injection of cocaine is most likely to cause an overdose, followed by smoking it, with intranasal use involving the least risk (Pottieger and others 1992).

Much less is known about nonfatal cocaine overdose. A study in Miami, Florida, found that 40 percent of users had overdosed on cocaine at least once (Pottieger and others 1992). More recently, a study in Brazil found that 20 percent of users had experienced an overdose, with 50 percent knowing someone who had died from an overdose (Mesquita and others 2001). A study in Sydney, Australia, found that 17 percent of injecting cocaine users and 6 percent of noninjecting cocaine users had ever overdosed, with 9 percent and 3 percent, respectively, overdosing in the preceding 12 months (Kaye and Darke 2003). Frequency of cocaine use, severity of dependence, and route of administration did not predict an overdose, supporting the view that cocaine overdose is an unpredictable event.

Interventions for Cocaine Dependence. Efforts at intervention have included pharmacological treatments as well as psychotherapy and cognitive behavioral therapy.

Pharmacological Interventions Despite much research effort there are no effective pharmacological treatments for cocaine dependence (Kreek 1997; McCance 1997; Mendelson and Mellon 1996; Nunes 1997; Silva de Lima and others 2002; van den Brink and van Ree 2003). Attempts have been made to develop longer-acting agonist drugs that act on the same molecular targets as cocaine without producing its euphoric effects (for example, methylphenidate) (Kreek 1997) or that block its rewarding and euphoric effects (McCance 1997). There has also been a search for drugs that indirectly change the effects that cocaine has on the brain by acting on other neurotransmitter systems, such as the serotonergic system (for example, fluoxetine) (McCance 1997). None of these approaches has produced an effective pharmacotherapy for cocaine dependence (Lima and others 2003; Platt 1997; Soares and others 2003).

Development of pharmacological therapies for cocaine dependence and their evaluation is complicated by the multiple interactive processes that may have contributed—for example, coexisting substance abuse or mental health issues (Mendelson and Mellon 1996). Many of the approaches to the treatment of cocaine dependence have also been used in treating patients with alcoholism and other substance abuse disorders.

A number of drugs have been used to treat cocaine based on their relevance to the symptoms of cocaine dependence (Silva de Lima and others 2002; van den Brink and van Ree 2003). The frequency of depressive symptoms has led to the exploration of the effectiveness of antidepressant drugs. Desipramine has been used with mixed effectiveness for cocaine detoxification and the maintenance of abstinence (Covi and others 1994; Gawin, Kleber, and Byck 1989), but it appears to be most effective when there is evidence of previous or consequent symptoms of depression. Other antidepressants have been used with mixed results: imipramine and trazodone have been found to have more adverse effects than desipramine, and fluoxetine has not been found to be effective (Mendelson and Mellon 1996). A recent systematic review found no current evidence to support the use of antidepressants in the treatment of cocaine dependence (Lima and others 2003).

Dopamimetic drugs have also been used to treat cocaine dependence; such treatments are based on the action of cocaine to block reuptake of dopamine. Unfortunately, although some of these drugs are relatively effective, they also result in quite severe adverse effects (Mendelson and Mellon 1996). Current evidence does not support the clinical use of dopamine agonists for cocaine dependence (Soares and others 2003). Opioid antagonists (for example, naltrexone) or opioid mixed agonist-antagonists (such as buprenorphine) have been explored, on the basis that cocaine dependence may be accompanied by dependence on opiates. Although there have been problems with compliance with naltrexone therapy (National Research Council Committee on Clinical Evaluation of Narcotic Antagonists 1978), buprenorphine has shown promising preclinical and clinical trial results (Kosten, Kleber, and Morgan 1989). Other promising directions include cannabinoid receptor antagonists and cortisol synthesis inhibitors (van den Brink and van Ree 2003) and vaccination against the effects of cocaine (Kantak 2003), but there is as yet no evidence on the effectiveness of any of these interventions.

Acupuncture has also been used to treat cocaine dependence. Auricular acupuncture is frequently used, but the small number of trials that have been conducted have not provided sufficient evidence of effectiveness (van den Brink and van Ree 2003).

Psychotherapy and Cognitive Behavioral Therapy The lack of evidence for pharmacological therapy means that treatment for cocaine dependence currently relies on cognitive behavior therapies combined with contingency management strategies. Unfortunately, psychosocial treatments for cocaine dependence are also of limited effectiveness. Treatments such as therapeutic communities, cognitive behavioral treatments, contingency management, and 12 step–based self-help approaches benefit cocaine-dependent people by reducing their rates of cocaine use and improving their health and well-being, but rates of relapse to cocaine use after treatment remain high (Platt 1997).

Mendelson and Mellon (1996) conclude that there are no specific cognitive or behavioral interventions that are uniquely effective in treating cocaine dependence. However, some success has been demonstrated with incentive-based programs in which rewards are provided for urine samples that are free of cocaine, although there is doubt about whether results are sustained (Roozen and others 2004). Such programs are generally more effective when the patient's family and friends are involved (Higgins and others 1994). Petry and others (2004) suggested that contingency management was effective in reducing cocaine use in a community-based treatment setting. They found that the benefits of treatment depended on the magnitude of reward, with those earning up to US$240 obtaining better results than those earning up to US$80. They suggested that this form of intervention may work best for people with more severe dependence on cocaine.

A multicenter investigation examining the efficacy of four psychosocial treatments for cocaine-dependent patients concluded that individual drug counseling in combination with group drug counseling showed the most promise for effective treatment of cocaine dependence over two forms of traditional psychotherapy (Crits-Christoph and others 1999). Community reinforcement involving an intensive, biopsychosocial, multifaceted approach to lifestyle change has shown positive effects over four to six weeks and has the advantage of being tailored to individual goals (Roozen and others 2004).

The few studies of the long-term effects of treatment have not shown particularly encouraging results. A one-year follow-up of the U.S. Drug Abuse Treatment Outcome Studies reported that reductions in the use of cocaine in the year following treatment were associated with longer duration of treatment, particularly six months or more in long-term residential or outpatient treatments (Hubbard, Craddock, and Anderson 2003). A five-year national follow-up study of 45 U.S. treatment programs found that only 33 percent of the sample had highly favorable outcomes (Flynn and others 2003).

Amphetamines

According to WHO, amphetamines and methamphetamines are the most widely abused illicit drugs after cannabis, with an estimated 35 million users worldwide (Rawson, Anglin, and Ling 2002).

In Australia, the lifetime prevalence of amphetamine use is between 6 and 8 percent in the general population, making amphetamines the most commonly used illicit drug after cannabis during that period (Makkai and McAllister 1998). In 1998, the lifetime prevalence of amphetamine use was highest (25 percent) among male users age 20 to 29.

The use of amphetamines is generally less frequent than that of opioids (Darke and Hall 1995; Darke, Kaye, and Ross 1999; W. Hall, Bell, and Carless 1993; Hando, Topp, and Hall 1997; Vincent and others 1998). This pattern is no doubt due to the physical and psychological toll taken by regular amphetamine use. Although such use is less frequent overall, however, there is widespread bingeing on amphetamines, with frequent use over several consecutive days, which may be followed by benzodiazepine use to "come down." Polydrug use is particularly common among amphetamine users, who show a marked preference

for stimulant drugs such as hallucinogens and cocaine (Darke and Hall 1995; Hando and Hall 1994; Vincent and others 1998).

Globally, Europe is the main center of amphetamine production, particularly Belgium, the Netherlands, and Poland, with production increasing in Eastern Europe (UNODCCP 2003). Half of all Western European countries reported an increase in amphetamine abuse in 2000, but in 2001 the figure fell to 33 percent (UNODCCP 2003). Lifetime use of amphetamines is reported to be between 0.5 percent and 6 percent among European Union countries, with the exception of the United Kingdom, where the figure is 11 percent. Denmark and Norway also have relatively higher rates of use (EMCDDA 2003).

Adverse Health Effects of Amphetamine Use. Amphetamine users who inject the drug are at high risk of bloodborne infections through needle sharing. Amphetamine users are as likely as opioid users to share injection equipment (Darke, Ross, Cohen, and others 1995; Darke, Ross, and Hall 1995; W. Hall, Bell, and Carless 1993; Hando and Hall 1994; Kaye and Darke 2000; Loxley and Marsh 1991). In addition, the youth of amphetamine users places them at risk of sexual transmission of diseases such as HIV and hepatitis B virus (although not hepatitis C). Primary amphetamine users have been demonstrated to be a sexually active group, and small proportions engage in paid sex to support their drug use (Darke, Ross, Cohen, and others 1995; Hando and Hall 1994). Among gay and bisexual men, amphetamines may be used to enhance sexual encounters, which may lead to unprotected anal intercourse and increased risk of HIV infection (Urbina and Jones 2004).

High-dose amphetamine use, especially by injection, can result in a schizophreniform paranoid psychosis, associated with loosening of associations, delusions, and hallucinations (Gawin and Ellinwood 1988; Jaffe 1985). The psychosis could be reproduced by the injection of large doses in addicts (Bell 1973) and by the repeated administration of large doses to normal volunteers (Angrist and others 1974).

High proportions of regular amphetamine injectors describe symptoms of anxiety, panic attacks, paranoia, and depression. The emergence of such symptoms is associated with injecting the drugs, greater frequency of use, and dependence on amphetamines (W. Hall and others 1996; McKetin and Mattick 1997, 1998). Recent evidence also suggests that women may experience more emotional effects of amphetamine intoxication than men and higher rates of anorexia nervosa than women without amphetamine disorders (Holdcraft and Iacono 2004).

In sufficiently high doses, amphetamines can be lethal (Derlet and others 1989). However, the risk is low compared with the high risks of overdose associated with central nervous system depressants such as heroin. Typically, amphetamine-related deaths are associated with the effects of amphetamines on the cardiovascular system—for example, cardiac failure and cerebral vascular accidents (Mattick and Darke 1995).

There is evidence that amphetamines are neurotoxic (Robinson and Becker 1986). Evidence from animal studies indicates that heavy amphetamine use results in dopaminergic depletion (Ellison 1992; Fields and others 1991). The few studies of the neuropsychological effects of amphetamine abuse report findings similar to those found with cocaine abuse. Deficits in memory and attention have been attributed to amphetamine use (McKetin and Mattick 1997, 1998). More recently, a twin study indicated that amphetamine abuse might lead to impaired attention and motor skills up to one year after the conclusion of heavy use (Toomey and others 2003).

Interventions for Amphetamine Dependence. Treatment for methamphetamine abuse has been a relatively recent development and has generally been based on previous treatments for cocaine abuse (Huber and others 1997). Cretzmeyer and others (2003) reviewed treatments for methamphetamine abuse, noting that there has been little research on the effectiveness of drug treatment, probably because many amphetamine users use multiple drugs. The combination of methamphetamine use with use of marijuana or other sedating drugs indicates that effective treatments need to address the use of multiple drugs. A Cochrane Review concluded that evidence for success in treatment of amphetamine dependence is very limited, with no pharmacological treatment demonstrated to be effective (Srisurapanont, Jarusuraisin, and Kittirattanapaiboon 2003).

An early study explored the use of aversion therapy in a multimodal treatment program using educational groups, individual counseling, occasional family counseling, and aftercare planning. The intervention paired an aversive stimulus (either chemical or electrical) with the act of using methamphetamines. Cocaine use was also treated in this way. After 12 months, 53 percent of patients were abstinent and the researchers noted that their results were promising, despite a number of limitations to the study (Frawley and Smith 1992).

An intervention combining imipramine, a tricyclic antidepressant, with intensive group counseling has been evaluated with cocaine and methamphetamine abusers. Patients received either a low or higher dose (as needed) of imipramine, as well as intensive group counseling and access to medical and psychiatric care. Those who received the higher dose stayed in treatment longer, but the results did not support the use of imipramine for methamphetamine abuse (Galloway and others 1994).

The Matrix Program for methamphetamine and cocaine abusers has also been evaluated. The Matrix Program uses a cognitive behavioral approach with an emphasis on relapse prevention (Huber and others 1997). The study evaluated the effectiveness of three conditions: Matrix treatment alone, Matrix treatment plus desipramine, and Matrix treatment plus placebo (Shoptaw and others 1994). The researchers concluded that those who received more Matrix treatment had better abstinence rates than those who had less treatment but that desipramine had no effect on treatment outcome.

J. Hall and others (1999) conducted an evaluation of the effectiveness of the Iowa Case Management Project. The project was designed to supplement interventions provided by a drug abuse treatment agency and is a comprehensive social work intervention, including outreach activities and provision of limited emergency funds. The results of the evaluation showed that comprehensive case management was effective in improving employment status among amphetamine users subsequent to treatment. There was an almost significant lower incidence of depression among those who received the program compared with controls. Drug use decreased significantly for clients in both control and program conditions.

More recently, an Australian study evaluated the effectiveness of brief cognitive-behavioral interventions among regular users of amphetamines (Baker, Boggs, and Lewin 2001). The researchers found a clinically significant reduction in daily amphetamine use among the intervention groups compared with controls and concluded that further studies of brief cognitive-behavioral interventions are feasible and warranted. Although some promising interventions have been identified to assist methamphetamine abusers, no single treatment option has yet been established as better than any other in a randomized controlled trial (Cretzmeyer and others 2003).

Methylenedioxymethamphetamine

Methylenedioxymethamphetamine is more widely known as *ecstasy* or *MDMA*. In Australia, the lifetime prevalence of MDMA use increased from 1 percent of the population in 1988 to 4.6 percent (about one in 20 persons) in 1998, with 2.3 percent reporting MDMA use in the preceding 12 months (Topp and others 1998). In 2001, 6.1 percent of Australians age 14 years or older reported lifetime use of MDMA, with 2.9 percent reporting use within the preceding year (Degenhardt, Barker, and Topp 2004). Rates of use are generally higher among males than females (3.1 percent versus 1.5 percent). MDMA use in the preceding 12 months is most common among those age 20 to 29 (5 percent of females and 12 percent of males) (Topp and others 1998).

The availability of MDMA has also increased, as indicated by the proportion of the population who have been offered MDMA (from 4 percent in 1988 to 7 percent in 1991) (Makkai and McAllister 1998), with 14 percent of those age 14 to 29 reporting that they had been offered MDMA in the preceding year.

Research suggests that the pattern of MDMA use changed during the 1990s (Topp and others 1998). Users of MDMA are commencing use at a younger age, and they appear to be using larger doses more frequently. The incidence of bingeing on MDMA appears to have increased, as does the prevalence of the parenteral use of this drug. The increase in the use of MDMA by injection has been noted among surveys of MDMA users and of injecting drug users generally.

An examination of trends in the United States suggested that, although the use of MDMA has increased over time, its prevalence is significantly less than that of other drugs of abuse (Yacoubian 2003b). A study of 14,520 U.S. college students indicated 6 percent lifetime use of MDMA, 3 percent within the preceding 12 months, and 1 percent within the preceding 30 days. Those who had used MDMA in the preceding 12 months were more likely to be white and a member of a fraternity or sorority and to have used a range of other drugs (Yacoubian 2003a). Rates of use are much higher in surveys of club attendees. A recent U.S. survey found 86 percent reporting lifetime use, 51 percent 30-day use, and 30 percent use within the preceding 2 days (Yacoubian and others 2003).

Abuse of MDMA had showed signs of decreasing in Western Europe but has recently shown signs of increase (UNODCCP 2003). Although MDMA use appears to be still diffusing, in 2003 only four countries (Ireland, the Netherlands, Spain, and the United Kingdom) reported a rate of more than 3 percent use among young adults in the preceding 12 months (EMCDDA 2003). In the United States, use declined in 2002 for the first time, but it increased in other regions, particularly the Caribbean, parts of South America, Oceania, Southeast Asia, the Near East, and southern Africa (UNODCCP 2003). Lifetime experience of MDMA is reported to range from 0.5 percent to 5 percent in European Union countries, with use more common in the Netherlands (EMCDDA 2003).

Population survey findings from New Zealand reported an increase in the preceding-year use of MDMA from 1.5 percent in 1998 to 3.4 percent in 2001. The increase was particularly evident among young men age 20 to 24 (from 4.3 percent to 12.5 percent) (Wilkins and others 2003).

Adverse Health Effects of MDMA. Early studies of MDMA use in Australia and the United States documented relatively few problems associated with the drug's use (Beck 1990; Beck and Rosenbaum 1994; Downing 1986; Solowij, Hall, and Lee 1992). A survey of 100 MDMA users (Solowij, Hall, and Lee 1992) found that the most common adverse effects were the side effects of acute use, such as appetite loss, dry mouth, palpitations, and bruxism (teeth grinding). Among the few heavy users in the study, only two reported feeling dependent on the drug.

With a change in the pattern of MDMA use in Australia, there has been an increase in the MDMA-related harms reported (Topp and others 1998). Some of the acute physical and psychological adverse effects that MDMA users have attributed to the use of this drug include energy loss, irritability, muscular aches, insomnia, and depression. More chronic adverse effects were also reported, including weight loss, depression, energy loss, insomnia, anxiety, and teeth problems.

A recent U.K. study of 430 regular users of MDMA reported that 83 percent of participants reported low mood and 80 percent experienced impaired concentration. Long-term effects of MDMA included the development of tolerance to MDMA (59 percent), impaired ability to concentrate (38 percent), and depression (37 percent) (Verheyden and others 2003).

Physical symptoms that were perceived as being due to MDMA use alone (Topp and others 1998) included an inability to urinate, blurred vision, vomiting, numbness or tingling, loss of sexual urge, and hot and cold flushes. As with amphetamines, the use of MDMA to facilitate sexual encounters may lead to risky sexual behavior and risk of sexually transmitted infections such as HIV. Studies of gay and bisexual men have found an association between MDMA use and high-risk sexual behavior (Urbina and Jones 2004).

MDMA has been implicated in a growing number of deaths, both in Australia and in other countries (Henry, Jeffreys, and Dawling 1992; Solowij 1993; White, Bochner, and Irvine 1997). Although the reasons for extreme reactions have yet to be clearly determined, deaths have most often been attributed to hyperthermia when MDMA was used at dance venues. A combination of sustained exertion, high ambient temperatures, and inadequate fluid replacement appears to compound the effect of MDMA on thermoregulatory mechanisms, causing a rapid and fatal rise in body temperature (Topp and others 1998). Some deaths have been attributed to excessive water consumption, which causes cerebral edema (Cook 1996; Matthai and others 1996).

REFERENCES

Ahmed, M. A., T. Zafar, H. Brahmbhatt, G. Imam, S. ul Hassan, J. C. Bareta, and S. A. Strathdee. 2003. "HIV/AIDS Risk Behaviors and Correlates of Injection Drug Use among Drug Users in Pakistan." *Journal of Urban Health* 80 (2): 321–29.

Ainsworth, M., C. Beyrer, and A. Soucat. 2003. "AIDS and Public Policy: The Lessons and Challenges of 'Success' in Thailand." *Health Policy* 64 (1): 13–37.

American Psychiatric Association. 1994. *Diagnostic and Statistical Manual of Mental Disorders.* 4th ed. Washington, DC: American Psychiatric Association.

Anglin, M. D. 1988. "The Efficacy of Civil Commitment in Treating Narcotic Drug Addiction." In *Compulsory Treatment of Drug Abuse: Research and Clinical Practice,* ed. C. G. Leukefeld and F. M. Tims, 8–34. Rockville, MD: National Institute on Drug Abuse.

Anglin, M. D., M. L. Brecht, and E. Maddahain. 1989. "Pre-treatment Characteristics and Treatment Performance of Legally Coerced versus Voluntary Methadone Maintenance Admissions." *Criminology* 27 (3): 537–57.

Anglin, M. D., and B. Perrochet. 1998. "Drug Use and Crime: A Historical Review of Research Conducted by the UCLA Drug Abuse Research Center." *Substance Use and Misuse* 33 (9): 1871–914.

Angrist, B., G. Sathananthan, S. Wilk, and S. Gershon. 1974. "Amphetamine Psychosis: Behavioural and Biochemical Aspects." *Journal of Psychiatric Research* 11: 13–23.

Anthony, J. C., L. Warner, and R. Kessler. 1994. "Comparative Epidemiology of Dependence on Tobacco, Alcohol, Controlled

Substances, and Inhalants: Basic Findings from the National Comorbidity Survey." *Experimental and Clinical Psychopharmacology* 2 (3): 244–68.

Arseneault, L., M. Cannon, R. Poulton, R. Murray, A. Caspi, and T. E. Moffitt. 2002. "Cannabis Use in Adolescence and Risk for Adult Psychosis: Longitudinal Prospective Study." *British Medical Journal* 325 (7374): 1212–13.

Atlani, L., M. Carael, J. B. Brunet, T. Frasca, and N. Chaika. 2000. "Social Change and HIV in the Former USSR: The Making of a New Epidemic." *Social Science and Medicine* 50 (11): 1547–56.

Australian Institute of Health and Welfare. 1999. "1998 National Drug Strategy Household Survey: First Results." Drug Statistics Series 1, Australian Institute of Health and Welfare, Canberra.

Bachman, J. G., K. N. Wadsworth, P. M. O'Malley, L. D. Johnston, and J. Schulenberg. 1997. *Smoking, Drinking, and Drug Use in Young Adulthood: The Impacts of New Freedoms and New Responsibilities.* Mahwah, NJ: Lawrence Erlbaum.

Baker, A., T. G. Boggs, and T. J. Lewin. 2001. "Randomized Controlled Trial of Brief Cognitive-Behavioral Interventions among Regular Users of Amphetamine." *Addiction* 96: 1279–87.

Ball, J. C., J. W. Shaffer, and D. N. Nurco. 1983. "The Day-to-Day Criminality of Heroin Addicts in Baltimore: A Study in the Continuity of Offence Rates." *Drug and Alcohol Dependence* 12 (2): 119–42.

Bammer, G., W. van den Brink, P. Gschwend, V. Hendriks, and J. Rehm. 2003. "What Can the Swiss and Dutch Trials Tell Us about the Potential Risks Associated with Heroin Prescribing?" *Drug and Alcohol Review* 22 (3): 363–71.

Barnett, P. G. 1999. "The Cost-Effectiveness of Methadone Maintenance as a Health Care Intervention." *Addiction* 94 (4): 479–88.

Barnett, P. G., G. S. Zaric, and M. L. Brandeau. 2001. "The Cost-Effectiveness of Buprenorphine Maintenance Therapy for Opiate Addiction in the United States." *Addiction* 96 (9): 1267–78.

Bates, M. N., and T. A. Blakely. 1999. "Role of Cannabis in Motor Vehicle Crashes." *Epidemiologic Reviews* 21: 222–32.

Beardsley, P., and T. Kelly. 1999. "Acute Effects of Cannabis on Human Behavior and Central Nervous System Functions." In *The Health Effects of Cannabis*, ed. H. Kalant, W. Corrigall, W. D. Hall, and R. Smart, 127–265. Toronto, ON: Centre for Addiction and Mental Health.

Beatty, W. W., V. M. Katzung, V. J. Moreland, and S. J. Nixon. 1995. "Neuropsychological Performance of Recently Abstinent Alcoholics and Cocaine Abusers." *Drug and Alcohol Dependence* 37: 247–53.

Beck, J. 1990. "The Public Health Implications of MDMA Use." In *Ecstasy: The Clinical, Pharmacological, and Neurotoxicological Effects of the Drug MDMA*, ed. S. J. Peroutka. Boston: Kluwer.

Beck, J., and M. Rosenbaum. 1994. *Pursuit of Ecstasy: The MDMA Experience.* Albany: State University of New York Press.

Belenko, S. 2002. "The Challenges of Conducting Research in Drug Treatment Court Settings." *Substance Use and Misuse* 37 (12–13): 1635–64.

Bell, D. S. 1973. "The Experimental Reproduction of Amphetamine Psychosis." *Archives of General Psychiatry* 29 (1): 35–40.

Beyrer, C. 2003. "Hidden Epidemic of Sexually Transmitted Diseases in China: Crisis and Opportunity." *Journal of the American Medical Association* 289 (10): 1303–5.

Beyrer, C., M. H. Razak, K. Lisam, J. Chen, W. Lui, and X. F. Yu. 2000. "Overland Heroin Trafficking Routes and HIV-1 Spread in South and South-East Asia." *AIDS* 14 (1): 75–83.

Boot, B., I. McGregor, and W. D. Hall. 2000. "MDMA (Ecstasy) Neurotoxicity: Assessing and Communicating the Risks." *Lancet* 355 (9217): 1818–21.

Brands, B., B. Sproule, and J. Marshman. 1998. *Drugs and Drug Abuse.* 3rd ed. Toronto, ON: Addiction Research Foundation.

Brecht, M. L., M. D. Anglin, and J. C. Wang. 1993. "Treatment Effectiveness for Legally Coerced versus Voluntary Methadone Maintenance Clients." *American Journal of Drug and Alcohol Abuse* 19 (1): 89–106.

Brown, T. T., and A. S. Dobs. 2002. "Endocrine Effects of Marijuana." *Journal of Clinical Pharmacology* 42 (Suppl. 11): 90S–96S.

Bruneau, J., S. B. Brogly, M. W. Tyndall, F. Lamothe, and E. L. Franco. 2004. "Intensity of Drug Injection as a Determinant of Sustained Injection Cessation among Chronic Drug Users: The Interface with Social Factors and Service Utilization." *Addiction* 99 (6): 727–37.

Budney, A. J., S. T. Higgins, K. J. Radonovich, and P. L. Novy. 2000. "Adding Voucher-Based Incentives to Coping Skills and Motivational Enhancement Improves Outcomes during Treatment for Marijuana Dependence." *Journal of Consulting and Clinical Psychology* 68 (6): 1051–61.

Budney, A. J., and B. A. Moore. 2002. "Development and Consequences of Cannabis Dependence." *Journal of Clinical Pharmacology* 42 (Suppl. 11): 28S–33S.

Caplehorn, J. R., S. Dalton, M. C. Cluff, and A. M. Petrenas. 1994. "Retention in Methadone Maintenance and Heroin Addicts' Risk of Death." *Addiction* 89 (2): 203–9.

Cartwright, W. S. 2000. "Cost-Benefit Analysis of Drug Treatment Services: Review of the Literature." *Journal of Mental Health Policy and Economics* 3 (1): 11–26.

Caulkins, J. P., C. P. Rydell, S. M. S. Everingham, J. R. Chiesa, and S. Bushway. 1999. *An Ounce of Prevention, a Pound of Uncertainty: The Cost-Effectiveness of School-Based Drug Prevention Programs.* Santa Monica, CA: Rand.

Central Committee on the Treatment of Heroin Addicts. 2002. *Medical Co-prescription of Heroin: Two Randomized Controlled Trials.* Utrecht, Netherlands: Central Committee on the Treatment of Heroin Addicts.

Chaisson, R. E., P. Bacchetti, D. Osmond, B. Brodie, M. A. Sande, and A. R. Moss. 1989. "Cocaine Use and HIV Infection in Intravenous Drug Users in San Francisco." *Journal of the American Medical Association* 261 (4): 561–65.

Chen, K., and D. B. Kandel. 1995. "The Natural History of Drug Use from Adolescence to the Mid-Thirties in a General Population Sample." *American Journal of Public Health* 85 (1): 41–47.

Chesher, G. 1995. "Cannabis and Road Safety: An Outline of Research Studies to Examine the Effects of Cannabis on Driving Skills and Actual Driving Performance." In *The Effects of Drugs (Other Than Alcohol) on Road Safety*, ed. Parliament of Victoria Road Safety Committee, 67–96. Melbourne, Australia: Road Safety Committee.

Chesher, G., and W. D. Hall. 1999. "Effects of Cannabis on the Cardiovascular and Gastrointestinal Systems." In *The Health Effects of Cannabis*, ed. H. Kalant, W. Corrigall, W. D. Hall, and R. Smart, 435–58. Toronto, ON: Centre for Addiction and Mental Health.

Chirgwin, K., J. A. DeHovitz, S. Dillon, and W. M. McCormack. 1991. "HIV Infection, Genital Ulcer Disease, and Crack Cocaine Use among Patients Attending a Clinic for Sexually Transmitted Diseases." *American Journal of Public Health* 81 (12): 1576–69.

Coffin, P. O., S. Galea, J. Ahern, A. C. Leon, D. Vlahov, and K. Tardiff. 2003. "Opiate, Cocaine and Alcohol Combinations in Accidental Drug Overdose Deaths in New York City, 1990–1998." *Addiction* 98: 739–47.

Cohen, J. 2003. "Asia: The Next Frontier for HIV/AIDS." *Science* 301 (5640): 1650–63.

Collins, D., and H. Lapsley. 1996. *The Social Costs of Drug Abuse in Australia in 1988 and 1992.* Canberra: Australian Government Publishing Service.

Cook, T. M. 1996. "Cerebral Oedema after MDMA ('Ecstasy') and Unrestricted Water Intake." *British Medical Journal* 313: 689.

Copeland, J., W. Swift, R. Roffman, and R. Stephens. 2001. "A Randomized Controlled Trial of Brief Cognitive-Behavioral Interventions for

Cannabis Use Disorder." *Journal of Substance Abuse Treatment* 21 (2): 55–64.

Covi, L., I. D. Montoya, J. Hess, and N. Kreiter. 1994. "Double-Blind Comparison of Desipramine and Placebo for Treatment of Cocaine Dependence." *Clinical Pharmacology and Therapeutics* 55: 132.

Crandall, C. G., W. Vongpatanasin, and R. G. Victor. 2002. "Mechanism of Cocaine-Induced Hyperthermia in Humans." *Annals of Internal Medicine* 136: 785–91.

Cretzmeyer, M., M. V. Sarrazin, D. L. Huber, R. I. Block, and J. A. Hall. 2003. "Treatment of Methamphetamine Abuse: Research Findings and Clinical Directions." *Journal of Substance Abuse Treatment* 24 (3): 267–77.

Crits-Christoph, P., L. Siqueland, J. Blaine, A. Frank, L. Luborsky, L. S. Onken, and others. 1999. "Psychosocial Treatments for Cocaine Dependence: National Institute on Drug Abuse Collaborative Cocaine Treatment Study." *Archives of General Psychiatry* 56 (6): 493–502.

Crofts, N., G. Costigan, P. Narayanan, J. Gray, J. Dorabjee, B. Langkham, and others. 1998. "Harm Reduction in Asia: A Successful Response to Hidden Epidemics—The Asian Harm Reduction Network." *AIDS* 12 (Suppl. B): S109–15.

Darke, S., A. Baker, J. Dixon, A. Wodak, and N. Heather. 1992. "Drug Use and HIV Risk-Taking Behaviour among Clients in Methadone Maintenance Treatment." *Drug and Alcohol Dependence* 29: 263–68.

Darke, S., and W. D. Hall. 1995. "Levels and Correlates of Polydrug Use among Heroin Users and Regular Amphetamine Users." *Drug and Alcohol Dependence* 39: 231–35.

———. 1997. "The Distribution of Naloxone to Heroin Users." *Addiction* 92 (9): 1195–99.

———. 2003. "Heroin Overdose: Research and Evidence-Based Intervention." *Journal of Urban Health* 80 (2): 189–200.

Darke, S., S. Kaye, and J. Ross. 1999. "Transitions between the Injection of Heroin and Amphetamines." *Addiction* 94: 1803–11.

Darke, S., S. Kaye, and L. Topp. 2002. "Cocaine Use in New South Wales, Australia, 1996–2000: 5-Year Monitoring of Trends in Price, Purity, Availability, and Use from the Illicit Drug Reporting System." *Drug and Alcohol Dependence* 6: 81–88.

Darke, S., and J. Ross. 2002. "Suicide among Heroin Users: Rates, Risk Factors, and Methods." *Addiction* 97 (11): 1383–94.

Darke, S., J. Ross, J. Cohen, J. Hando, and W. D. Hall. 1995. "Injecting and Sexual Risk-Taking Behavior among Regular Amphetamine Users." *AIDS Care* 7: 17–24.

Darke, S., J. Ross, and W. D. Hall. 1995. "Benzodiazepine Use among Injecting Heroin Users." *Medical Journal of Australia* 162: 645–47.

Darke, S., J. Ross, J. Hando, W. D. Hall, and L. Degenhardt. 2000. *Illicit Drug Use in Australia: Epidemiology, Use Patterns, and Associated Harm.* National Drug Strategy Monograph 43. Canberra: Department of Health and Aged Care.

Darke, S., I. Topp, H. Kaye, and W. Hall. 2002. "Heroin Use in New South Wales, Australia, 1996–2000: Five-Year Monitoring of Trends in Price, Purity, Availability, and Use from the Illicit Drug Reporting System (IDRS)." *Addiction* 97 (2): 179–86.

Darke, S., and D. Zador. 1996. "Fatal Heroin 'Overdose': A Review." *Addiction* 91 (12): 1765–72.

Day, C., L. Degenhardt, S. Gilmour, and W. D. Hall. 2004. "Effects of Reduction in Heroin Supply on Injecting Drug Use: Analysis of Data from Needle and Syringe Programmes." *British Medical Journal* 329 (7463): 428–29.

Degenhardt, L., B. Barker, and L. Topp. 2004. "Patterns of Ecstasy Use in Australia: Findings from a National Household Survey." *Addiction* 99 (2): 187–95.

Degenhardt, L., C. Day, and W. D. Hall, eds. 2004. *The Causes, Course, and Consequences of the Heroin Shortage in Australia.* Adelaide, Australia: National Drug Law Enforcement Research Fund.

Degenhardt, L., W. D. Hall, and M. Lynskey. 2003. "Testing Hypotheses about the Relationship between Cannabis Use and Psychosis." *Drug and Alcohol Dependence* 71 (1): 37–48.

Degenhardt, L., W. D. Hall, M. Warner-Smith, and M. Lynskey. 2004. "Illicit Drug Use." In *Comparative Risk Assessment,* vol. 1, ed. M. Ezzati, A. Lopez, and C. Murray, 1109–76. Geneva: World Health Organization.

Derlet, R. W., P. Rice, B. Z. Horowitz, and R. V. Lord. 1989. "Amphetamine Toxicity: Experience with 127 Cases." *Journal of Emergency Medicine* 7 (2): 157–61.

Desjalais, D. C., J. Wenston, S. R. Friedman, J. L. Sotheran, R. Maslansky, and M. Marmor. 1992. "Crack Cocaine Use in a Cohort of Methadone Maintenance Patients." *Journal of Substance Abuse Treatment* 9: 319–25.

Dolan, K., J. Kimber, C. Fry, J. Fitzgerald, D. MacDonald, and F. Trautmann. 2000. "Drug Consumption Facilities in Europe and the Establishment of Supervised Injecting Centres in Australia." *Drug and Alcohol Review* 19 (3): 337–46.

Dole, V. P., J. W. Robinson, J. Oracca, E. Towns, P. Searcy, and E. Caine. 1969. "Methadone Treatment of Randomly Selected Addicts." *New England Journal of Medicine* 280 (25): 1372–75.

Dorabjee, J., and L. Samson. 2000. "A Multi-Centre Rapid Assessment of Injecting Drug Use in India." *International Journal of Drug Policy* 11 (1–2): 99–112.

Doran, C. M., M. Shanahan, R. P. Mattick, R. Ali, J. White, and J. Bell. 2003. "Buprenorphine versus Methadone Maintenance: A Cost-Effectiveness Analysis." *Drug and Alcohol Dependence* 71 (3): 295–302.

Downing, J. 1986. "The Psychological and Physiological Effects of MDMA on Normal Volunteers." *Journal of Psychoactive Drugs* 18: 335–40.

Ellison, G. 1992. "Continuous Amphetamine and Cocaine Have Similar Neurotoxic Effects in Lateral Habenular and Fasciculus Retroflexus." *Brain Research* 598: 353–56.

EMCDDA (European Monitoring Centre for Drugs and Drug Addiction. 2002. *Annual Report on the State of the Drugs Problem in the European Union, 2001.* Lisbon: EMCDDA.

———. 2003. *Annual Report 2003: The State of the Drugs Problem in the European Union and Norway.* Lisbon: EMCDDA.

English, D., G. Hulse, E. Milne, C. Holman, and C. Bower. 1997. "Maternal Cannabis Use and Birth Weight: A Meta-Analysis." *Addiction* 92: 1553–60.

Farre, M., A. Mas, M. Torrens, V. Moreno, and J. Cami. 2002. "Retention Rate and Illicit Opioid Use during Methadone Maintenance Interventions: A Meta-Analysis." *Drug and Alcohol Dependence* 65 (3): 283–90.

Fergusson, D. M., L. J. Horwood, and M. Lynskey. 1998. "Child and Adolescent Psychiatric Disorders." In *Mental Health in New Zealand from a Public Health Perspective,* eds. P. Ellis and S. Collings, 136–63. Wellington: Ministry of Health.

Fergusson, D. M., L. J. Horwood, and K. Northstone. 2002. "Maternal Use of Cannabis and Pregnancy Outcome." *British Journal of Obstetrics and Gynaecology* 109 (1): 21–27.

Fergusson, D. M., L. J. Horwood, and N. Swain-Campbell. 2002. "Cannabis Use and Psychosocial Adjustment in Adolescence and Young Adulthood." *Addiction* 97 (9): 1123–35.

Fields, J. Z., L. Wichlinski, G. E. Drucker, K. Engh, and J. H. Gordon. 1991. "Long-Lasting Dopamine Receptor Up-Regulation in Amphetamine-Treated Rats Following Amphetamine Neurotoxicity." *Pharmacology, Biochemistry, and Behavior* 40 (4): 881–86.

Fischer, B., E. Haydon, J. Rehm, M. Krajden, and J. Reimer. 2004. "Injection Drug Use and the Hepatitis C Virus: Considerations for a Targeted Treatment Approach—The Case Study of Canada." *Journal of Urban Health* 81 (3): 428–47.

Flynn, P. M., G. W. Joe, K. M. Broome, D. D. Simpson, and B. S. Brown. 2003. "Looking Back on Cocaine Dependence: Reasons for Recovery." *American Journal on Addictions* 12 (5): 398–411.

Fortney, J., B. Booth, M. Zhang, J. Humphrey, and E. Wiseman. 1998. "Controlling for Selection Bias in the Evaluation of Alcoholics Anonymous as Aftercare Treatment." *Journal of Studies on Alcohol* 59 (6): 690–707.

Frawley, P., and J. L. Smith. 1992. "One-Year Follow-up after Multimodal Inpatient Treatment for Cocaine and Methamphetamine Dependencies." *Journal of Substance Abuse Treatment* 9: 271–86.

Fried, P. A., and A. R. Smith. 2001. "A Literature Review of the Consequences of Prenatal Marihuana Exposure: An Emerging Theme of a Deficiency in Aspects of Executive Function." *Neurotoxicology and Teratology* 23 (1): 1–11.

Fuller, C. M., D. C. Ompad, S. Galea, Y. Wu, B. Koblin, and D. Vlahov. 2004. "Hepatitis C Incidence: A Comparison between Injection and Noninjection Drug Users in New York City." *Journal of Urban Health* 81 (1): 20–24.

Galai, N., M. Safaeian, D. Vlahov, A. Bolotin, and D. D. Celentano. 2003. "Longitudinal Patterns of Drug Injection Behavior in the Alive Study Cohort, 1988–2000: Description and Determinants." *American Journal of Epidemiology* 158 (7): 695–704.

Galduroz, J. C., A. R. Noto, S. A. Nappo, and E. L. Carlini. 2003. "First Household Survey on Drug Abuse in São Paulo, Brazil, 1999: Principal Findings." *São Paulo Medical Journal* 121 (6): 231–37.

Galloway, G., J. A. Newmeyer, T. Knapp, S. Stalcup, and D. Smith. 1994. "Imipramine for the Treatment of Cocaine and Methamphetamine Dependence." *Journal of Addictive Diseases* 13 (4): 201–16.

Gawin, F. H., and E. H. Ellinwood Jr. 1988. "Cocaine and Other Stimulants. Actions, Abuse, and Treatment." *New England Journal of Medicine* 318 (18): 1173–82.

Gawin, F. H., H. D. Kleber, and R. Byck. 1989. "Desipramine Facilitation of Initial Cocaine Abstinence." *Archives of General Psychiatry* 46: 117–21.

Gearing, F. R., and M. D. Schweitzer. 1974. "An Epidemiologic Evaluation of Long-Term Methadone Maintenance Treatment for Heroin Addiction." *American Journal of Epidemiology* 100 (2): 101–12.

Gerstein, D., and H. Harwood. 1990. *Treating Drug Problems.* Vol. 1 of *A Study of Effectiveness and Financing of Public and Private Drug Treatment Systems.* Washington, DC: National Academy Press.

Gerstein, D., H. Harwood, and N. Suter. 1994. *Evaluating Recovery Services: The California Drug and Alcohol Treatment Assessment.* Sacramento: State of California Health and Welfare Agency, Department of Alcohol and Drug Programs.

Gibson, A. E., C. M. Doran, J. R. Bell, A. Ryan, and N. Lintzeris. 2003. "A Comparison of Buprenorphine Treatment in Clinic and Primary Care Settings: A Randomised Trial." *Medical Journal of Australia* 179 (1): 38–42.

Goldschmidt, P. G. 1976. "A Cost-Effectiveness Model for Evaluating Health Care Programs: Application to Drug Abuse Treatment." *Inquiry* 13 (1): 29–47.

Goldstein, A., and J. Herrera. 1995. "Heroin Addicts and Methadone Treatment in Albuquerque: A 22-Year Follow-up." *Drug and Alcohol Dependence* 40 (2): 139–50.

Gossop, M., J. Marsden, and D. Stewart. 1998. *NTORS at One Year: Changes in Substance Use, Health, and Criminal Behaviour One Year after Intake.* London: Department of Health.

Gossop, M., J. Marsden, D. Stewart, C. Edwards, P. Lehmann, A. Wilson, and G. Segar. 1997. "The National Treatment Outcome Research Study in the United Kingdom: Six-Month Follow-up Outcomes." *Psychology of Addictive Behaviors* 11 (4): 324–37.

Grella, C. E., M. D. Anglin, and S. E. Wugalter. 1995. "Cocaine and Crack Use and HIV Risk Behaviors among High-Risk Methadone Maintenance Clients." *Drug and Alcohol Dependence* 37 (1): 15–21.

Gronbladh, L., L. Ohlund, and L. Gunne. 1990. "Mortality in Heroin Addiction: Impact of Methadone Treatment." *Acta Psychiatrica Scandinavica* 82 (3): 223–27.

Hall, J., M. Vaughan, T. Vaughn, R. I. Block, D. L. Huber, and A. Schut. 1999. "Iowa Case Management for Rural Drug Abuse: Preliminary Results." *Case Management Journal* 1: 232–43.

Hall, W. D. 1997. "The Role of Legal Coercion in the Treatment of Offenders with Alcohol and Heroin Problems." *Australian and New Zealand Journal of Criminology* 30 (2): 103–20.

Hall, W. D., J. Bell, and J. Carless. 1993. "Crime and Drug Use among Applicants for Methadone Maintenance." *Drug and Alcohol Dependence* 31: 123–29.

Hall, W. D., L. J. Degenhardt, and M. T. Lynskey. 1999. "Opioid Overdose Mortality in Australia, 1964–1997: Birth-Cohort Trends." *Medical Journal of Australia* 171 (1): 34–37.

Hall, W. D., J. Hando, S. Darke, and J. Ross. 1996. "Psychological Morbidity and Route of Administration among Amphetamine Users in Sydney, Australia." *Addiction* 91 (1): 81–87.

Hall, W. D., L. Johnston, and N. Donnelly. 1999. "Epidemiology of Cannabis Use and Its Consequences." In *The Health Effects of Cannabis,* ed. H. Kalant, W. Corrigal, W. D. Hall, and R. Smart, 69–125. Toronto, ON: Centre for Addiction and Mental Health.

Hall, W. D., and M. Lynskey. Forthcoming. "Testing Hypotheses about the Relationship between Cannabis Use and the Use of Other Illicit Drugs." *Drug and Alcohol Review.*

Hall, W. D., M. Lynskey, and L. Degenhardt. 1999. *Heroin Use in Australia: Its Impact on Public Health and Public Order.* NDARC Monograph 42. Sydney, Australia: National Drug and Alcohol Research Centre.

Hall, W. D., and D. MacPhee. 2002. "Cannabis Use and Cancer." *Addiction* 97 (3): 243–47.

Hall, W. D., and R. P. Mattick. 2000. "Is Ultra-Rapid Opioid Detoxification a Viable Option in the Treatment of Opioid Dependence?" *CNS Drugs* 14 (4): 251–55.

Hall, W. D., and R. L. Pacula. 2003. *Cannabis Use and Dependence: Public Health and Public Policy.* Melbourne, Ausralia: Cambridge University Press.

Hall, W. D., J. E. Ross, M. T. Lynskey, M. G. Law, and L. J. Degenhardt. 2000. "How Many Dependent Heroin Users Are There in Australia?" *Medical Journal of Australia* 173 (10): 528–31.

Hall, W. D., J. Ward, and R. Mattick. 1998. "The Effectiveness of Methadone Maintenance Treatment 1: Heroin Use and Crime." In *Methadone Maintenance Treatment and Other Opioid Replacement Therapies,* ed. J. Ward, R. Mattick, and W. D. Hall, 17–57. Amsterdam: Harwood Academic.

Hamers, F. F., and A. M. Downs. 2003. "HIV in Central and Eastern Europe." *Lancet* 361 (9362): 1035–44.

Hando, J., and W. D. Hall. 1994. "HIV Risk-Taking Behavior among Amphetamine Users in Sydney, Australia." *Addiction* 89 (1): 79–85.

Hando, J., L. Topp, and W. D. Hall. 1997. "Amphetamine-Related Harms and Treatment Preferences of Regular Amphetamine Users in Sydney, Australia." *Drug and Alcohol Dependence* 46 (1-2): 105–13.

Hawkins, J. D., R. F. Catalano, and J. Y. Miller. 1992. "Risk and Protective Factors for Alcohol and Other Drug Problems in Adolescence and Early Adulthood: Implications for Substance Abuse Prevention." *Psychological Bulletin* 112 (1): 64–105.

Henry, J. A., K. L. Jeffreys, and S. Dawling. 1992. "Toxicity and Deaths from 3,4-Methylenedioxymethamphetamine ('Ecstasy')." *Lancet* 340: 384–87.

Hepatitis C Virus Projections Working Group. 1998. *Estimates and Projections of the Hepatitis C Virus Epidemic in Australia.* Sydney, Australia: National Centre in HIV Epidemiology and Clinical Research.

Hien, N. T., L. T. Giang, P. N. Binh, W. Deville, E. J. van Ameijden, and I. Wolffers. 2001. "Risk Factors of HIV Infection and Needle Sharing among Injecting Drug Users in Ho Chi Minh City, Vietnam." *Journal of Substance Abuse* 13 (1–2): 45–58.

Higgins, S. T., A. J. Budney, W. K. Bickel, F. E. Foerg, R. Donham, and G. J. Badger. 1994. "Incentives Improve Outcome in Outpatient Behavioral Treatment of Cocaine Dependence." *Archives of General Psychiatry* 51 (7): 568–76.

Hoff, A. L., H. Riordan, L. Morris, V. Cestaro, M. Wieneke, R. Alpert, and G. J. Wang. 1996. "Effects of Crack Cocaine on Neurocognitive Function." *Psychiatry Research* 60: 167–76.

Holdcraft, L. C., and W. G. Iacono. 2004. "Cross-Generational Effects on Gender Differences in Psychoactive Drug Abuse and Dependence." *Drug and Alcohol Dependence* 74 (2): 147–58.

Hollister, L. 1992. "Marijuana and Immunity." *Journal of Psychoactive Drugs* 24: 159–64.

Hser, Y. I., D. Anglin, and K. Powers. 1993. "A 24-Year Follow-up of California Narcotics Addicts." *Archives of General Psychiatry* 50 (7): 577–84.

Hubbard, R. L., J. J. Collins, J. V. Rachal, and E. R. Cavanaugh. 1988. "The Criminal Justice Client in Drug Abuse Treatment." In *Compulsory Treatment of Drug Abuse: Research and Clinical Practice*, ed. C. G. Leukefeld and F. M. Tims, 57–80. Rockville, MD: National Institute on Drug Abuse.

Hubbard, R. L., S. G. Craddock, and J. Anderson. 2003. "Overview of 5-Year Followup Outcomes in the Drug Abuse Treatment Outcome Studies (Datos)." *Journal of Substance Abuse Treatment* 25 (3): 125–34.

Hubbard, R. L., M. Marsden, J. V. Rachal, H. Harwood, E. Cavanaugh, and H. Ginzburg. 1989. *Drug Abuse Treatment: A National Study of Effectiveness*. Chapel Hill: University of North Carolina Press.

Huber, A., W. Ling, S. Shoptaw, V. Gulati, P. Brethen, and R. Rawson. 1997. "Integrating Treatments for Methamphetamine Abuse: A Psychosocial Perspective." *Journal of Addictive Diseases* 16 (4): 41–50.

Hulse, G. K., D. R. English, E. Milne, and C. D. Holman. 1999. "The Quantification of Mortality Resulting from the Regular Use of Illicit Opiates." *Addiction* 94 (2): 221–29.

Jaffe, J. 1985. "Drug Addiction and Drug Abuse." In *The Pharmacological Basis of Therapeutics*, eds. A. Gilman, L. Goodman and F. Murad, 532–81. New York: Macmillan.

Johnston, L. D., P. M. O'Malley, and J. G. Bachman. 1994a. *National Survey Results on Drug Use from the Monitoring the Future Study, 1975–1993: College Students and Young Adults*. Rockville, MD: National Institute on Drug Abuse.

———. 1994b. *National Survey Results on Drug Use from the Monitoring the Future Study, 1975–1993: Secondary School Students*. Rockville, MD: National Institute on Drug Abuse,.

Kaldor, J., H. Lapsley, R. P. Mattick, D. Weatherburn, and A. Wilson. 2003. *Final Report on the Evaluation of the Sydney Medically Supervised Injecting Centre*. Sydney, Australia: Medically Supervised Injecting Centre Evaluation Committee.

Kandel, D. B., ed. 2002. *Stages and Pathways of Drug Involvement: Examining the Gateway Hypothesis*. New York: Cambridge University Press.

Kantak, K. M. 2003. "Vaccines against Drugs of Abuse: A Viable Treatment Option?" *Drugs* 63 (4): 341–52.

Kaye, S., and S. Darke. 2000. "A Comparison of the Harms Associated with the Injection of Heroin and Amphetamines." *Drug and Alcohol Dependence* 58 (1–2): 189–95.

———. 2003. "Non-Fatal Cocaine Overdose and Other Adverse Events among Injecting and Non-Injecting Cocaine Users." NDARC Technical Report 170, National Drug and Alcohol Research Centre, University of New South Wales, Sydney, Australia.

Kelly, J. A., and Y. A. Amirkhanian. 2003. "The Newest Epidemic: A Review of HIV/AIDS in Central and Eastern Europe." *International Journal of STD and AIDS* 14 (6): 361–71.

Kimber, J., K. Dolan, I. van Beek, D. Hedrich, and H. Zurhold. 2003. "Drug Consumption Facilities: An Update since 2000." *Drug and Alcohol Review* 22 (2): 227–33.

Klein, T. 1999. "Cannabis and Immunity." In *The Health Effects of Cannabis*, ed. H. Kalant, W. Corrigall, W. D. Hall, and R. Smart, 347–73. Toronto, ON: Centre for Addiction and Mental Health.

Kosten, T. R., H. D. Kleber, and C. Morgan. 1989. "Role of Opioid Antagonists in Treating Intravenous Cocaine Abuse." *Life Science* 44: 887–92.

Kouri, E. M., and H. G. Pope. 2000. "Abstinence Symptoms during Withdrawal from Chronic Marijuana Use." *Experimental and Clinical Psychopharmacology* 8 (4): 483–92.

Kreek, M. J. 1997. "Opiate and Cocaine Addictions: Challenge for Pharmacotherapies." *Pharmacology, Biochemistry, and Behavior* 57 (3): 551–69.

Lange, R. A., and L. D. Hillis. 2001. "Cardiovascular Complications of Cocaine Use." *New England Journal of Medicine* 345: 351–58.

Langendam, M. W., G. H. van Brussel, R. A. Coutinho, and E. J. van Ameijden. 2001. "The Impact of Harm-Reduction-Based Methadone Treatment on Mortality among Heroin Users." *American Journal of Public Health* 91 (5): 774–80.

Leshner, A. I. 1997. "Addiction Is a Brain Disease, and It Matters." *Science* 278 (5335): 45–47.

Levin, F. R., D. McDowell, S. M. Evans, E. Nunes, E. Akerele, S. Donovan, and S. K. Vosburg. 2004. "Pharmacotherapy for Marijuana Dependence: A Double-Blind, Placebo-Controlled Pilot Study of Divalproex Sodium." *American Journal on Addictions* 13 (1): 21–32.

Lima, M. S., A. A. Reisser, B. G. Soares, and M. Farrell. 2003. "Antidepressants for Cocaine Dependence." *Cochrane Database of Systematic Reviews* (2): CD002950. [PMID: 12804445].

Loxley, W., and A. Marsh. 1991. "Nodding and Speeding: Age and Injecting Drug Use in Perth." National Centre for Research into the Prevention of Drug Abuse, Curtin University of Technology, Perth, Australia.

Lynskey, M., and W. D. Hall. 2000. "The Effects of Adolescent Cannabis Use on Educational Attainment: A Review." *Addiction* 96 (3): 433–43.

Macdonald, S., K. Anglin-Bodrug, R. E. Mann, P. Erickson, A. Hathaway, M. Chipman, and M. Rylett. 2003. "Injury Risk Associated with Cannabis and Cocaine Use." *Drug and Alcohol Dependence* 72 (2): 99–115.

Macleod, J., R. Oakes, A. Copello, I. Crome, M. Egger, M. Hickman, and others. 2004. "Psychological and Social Sequelae of Cannabis and Other Drug Use by Young People: A Systematic Review of Longitudinal, General Population Studies." *Lancet* 363 (9421): 1579–88.

Maddux, J. F., and D. P. Desmond. 1992. "Methadone Maintenance and Recovery from Opioid Dependence." *American Journal of Drug and Alcohol Abuse* 18 (1): 63–74.

Majewska, M. D., ed. 1996. *Neurotoxicity and Neuropathology Associated with Cocaine Abuse*. NIDA Research Monograph 163. Rockville, MD: U.S. Department of Health and Human Services.

Makkai, T., and I. McAllister. 1998. *Patterns of Drug Use in Australia, 1985–95*. Canberra: Australian Government Publishing Service.

Manschreck, T. C., J. A. Laughery, C. C. Weisstein, D. Allen, B. Humblestone, M. Neville, and others. 1988. "Characteristics of Freebase Cocaine Psychosis." *Yale Journal of Biology and Medicine* 61 (2): 115–22.

Manski, C. F., J. V. Pepper, and C. V. Petrie, eds. 2001. *Informing America's Policy on Illegal Drugs: What We Don't Know Keeps Hurting Us*. Washington, DC: National Academy Press.

Marsch, L. A. 1998. "The Efficacy of Methadone Maintenance Interventions in Reducing Illicit Opiate Use, HIV Risk Behavior, and Criminality: A Meta-Analysis." *Addiction* 93 (4): 515–32.

Marselos, M., and P. Karamanakos. 1999. "Mutagenicity, Developmental Toxicity and Carcinogeneity of Cannabis." *Addiction Biology* 4 (1): 5–12.

Marsh, K., G. Joe, D. Simpson, and W. Lehman. 1990. "Treatment History." In *Opioid Addiction and Treatment: A 12-Year Follow-Up*, eds. D. Simpson and S. Sells, 137–56. Malabar, FL: Krieger.

Mathers, C., T. Vos, and C. Stephenson. 1999. *The Burden of Disease and Injury in Australia*. Canberra: Australian Institute of Health and Welfare.

Matthai, S. M., J. A. Sills, D. C. Davidson, and D. Alexandrou. 1996. "Cerebral Oedema after Ingestion of MDMA ('Ecstasy') and Unrestricted Intake of Water." *British Medical Journal* 312: 1359.

Mattick, R. P., and S. Darke. 1995. "Drug Replacement Treatments: Is Amphetamine Substitution a Horse of a Different Color?" *Drug and Alcohol Review* 14: 389–94.

Mattick, R. P., E. Digiusto, C. M. Moran, S. O'Brien, M. Shanahan, J. Kimber, N. Henderson, C. Breen, J. Shearer, J. Gates, A. Shakeshaft, NEPOD Trial Investigators. 2001. "National Evaluation of Pharmacotherapies for Opioid Dependence (NEPOD)." Canberra: Commonwealth Department of Health and Ageing.

Mattick, R. P., and W. D. Hall. 1996. "Are Detoxification Programmes Effective?" *Lancet* 347 (8994): 97–100.

Mattick, R. P., J. Kimber, C. Breen, and M. Davoli. 2003. "Buprenorphine Maintenance versus Placebo or Methadone Maintenance for Opioid Dependence." Cochrane Database Systematic Review (2) CD002207 [PMID: 12804429].

McCance, E. F. 1997. "Overview of Potential Treatment Medications for Cocaine Dependence." In *Medication Development for the Treatment of Cocaine Dependence: Issues in Clinical Efficacy Trials*, NIDA Research Monograph 175, 36–72. Rockville, MD: U.S. Department of Health and Human Services.

McCann, U. D., and G. A. Ricaurte. 2000. "Drug Abuse and Dependence: Hazards and Consequences of Heroin, Cocaine, and Amphetamines." *Current Opinion in Psychiatry* 13: 321–25.

McGregor, C., R. Ali, P. Christie, and S. Darke. 2001. "Overdose among Heroin Users: Evaluation of an Intervention in South Australia." *Addiction Research* 9 (5): 481–501.

McKetin, R., and R. P. Mattick. 1997. "Attention and Memory in Illicit Amphetamine Users." *Drug and Alcohol Dependence* 48 (3): 235–42.

———. 1998. "Attention and Memory in Illicit Amphetamine Users: Comparison with Non-Drug-Using Controls." *Drug and Alcohol Dependence* 50 (2): 181–4.

Mendelson, J. H., and N. K. Mellon. 1996. "Management of Cocaine Abuse and Dependence." *New England Journal of Medicine* 334 (15): 965–72.

Merline, A. C., P. M. O'Malley, J. E. Schulenberg, J. G. Bachman, and L. D. Johnston. 2004. "Substance Use among Adults 35 Years of Age: Prevalence, Adulthood Predictors, and Impact of Adolescent Substance Use." *American Journal of Public Health* 94 (1): 96–102.

Mesquita, F., A. Kral, A. Reingold, I. Haddad, M. Sanches, G. Turienzo, and others. 2001. "Overdoses among Cocaine Users in Brazil." *Addiction* 96: 1809–13.

Mittleman, M. A., R. A. Lewis, M. Maclure, J. B. Sherwood, and J. E. Muller. 2001. "Triggering Myocardial Infarction by Marijuana." *Circulation* 103: 2805–9.

Murphy, L. 1999. "Cannabis Effects on Endocrine and Reproductive Function." In *The Health Effects of Cannabis*, ed. H. Kalant, W. Corrigall, W. D. Hall, and R. Smart, 375–400. Toronto, ON: Centre for Addiction and Mental Health.

National Centre in HIV Epidemiology and Clinical Research. 1998. *HIV/AIDS and Related Diseases in Australia: Annual Surveillance Report 1998*. Sydney, Australia: National Centre in HIV Epidemiology and Clinical Research.

National Research Council Committee on Clinical Evaluation of Narcotic Antagonists. 1978. "Clinical Evaluation of Naltrexone Treatment of Opiate-Dependent Individuals." *Archives of General Psychiatry* 35: 355–40.

Newcomb, M. D., and P. M. Bentler. 1988. *Consequences of Adolescent Drug Use: Impact on the Lives of Young Adults*. Thousand Oaks, CA: Sage.

Newman, R. G., and W. B. Whitehill. 1979. "Double-Blind Comparison of Methadone and Placebo Maintenance Treatments of Narcotic Addicts in Hong Kong." *Lancet* 2 (8141): 485–88.

Nunes, E. V. 1997. Methodologic Recommendations for Cocaine Abuse Clinical Trials: A Clinician-Researcher's Perspective. In *Medication Development for the Treatment of Cocaine Dependence: Issues in Clinical Efficacy Trials*, NIDA Research Monograph 175, 73–95. Rockville, MD: U.S. Department of Health and Human Services.

Office of National Drug Control Policy. 2001. *Pulse Check: Trends in Drug Abuse, November 2001*. Washington, DC: Executive Office of the President, Office of National Drug Control Policy.

Oliveto, A., and T. Kosten. 1997. "Buprenorphine." In *New Treatments for Opioid Dependence*, eds. S. Stine and T. Kosten, 25–67. New York: Guilford Press.

O'Malley, S., M. Adamse, R. K. Heaton, and F. H. Gawin. 1992. "Neuropsychological Impairment in Chronic Cocaine Abusers." *American Journal of Drug and Alcohol Abuse* 18: 131–44.

Perneger, T. V., F. Giner, M. del Rio, and A. Mino. 1998. "Randomised Trial of Heroin Maintenance Programme for Addicts Who Fail in Conventional Drug Treatments." *British Medical Journal* 317 (7150): 13–8.

Petry, N. M., J. Tedford, M. Austin, C. Nich, K. M. Carroll, and B. J. Rounsaville. 2004. "Prize Reinforcement Contingency Management for Treating Cocaine Users: How Low Can We Go, and with Whom?" *Addiction* 99 (3): 349–60.

Platt, J. J. 1997. *Cocaine Addiction: Theory, Research and Treatment*. Cambridge, MA: Harvard University Press.

Porter, L., A. Arif, and W. Curran. 1986. *The Law and the Treatment of Drug and Alcohol Dependent Persons: A Comparative Study of Existing Legislation*. Geneva: World Health Organization.

Pottieger, A. E., P. A. Tressell, J. A. Inciardi, and T. A. Rosales. 1992. "Cocaine Use Patterns and Overdose." *Journal of Psychoactive Drugs* 24: 399–410.

Ramaekers, J. G., G. Berghaus, M. van Laar, and O. H. Drummer. 2004. "Dose Related Risk of Motor Vehicle Crashes after Cannabis Use." *Drug and Alcohol Dependence* 73 (2): 109–19.

Rawson, R., M. Anglin, and W. Ling. 2002. "Will the Methamphetamine Problem Go Away?" *Journal of Addictive Diseases* 21: 5–19.

Rehm, J., P. Gschwend, T. Steffen, F. Gutzwiller, A. Dobler-Mikola, and A. Uchtenhagen. 2001. "Feasibility, Safety, and Efficacy of Injectable Heroin Prescription for Refractory Opioid Addicts: A Follow-Up Study." *Lancet* 358 (9291): 1417–23.

Reid, G., and N. Crofts. 2000. "Rapid Assessment of Drug Use and HIV Vulnerability in South-East and East Asia." *International Journal of Drug Policy* 11 (1–2): 113–24.

Rhodes, T., A. Ball, G. V. Stimson, Y. Kobyshcha, C. Fitch, V. Pokrovsky, and others. 1999. "HIV Infection Associated with Drug Injecting in the Newly Independent States, Eastern Europe: The Social and Economic Context of Epidemics." *Addiction* 94 (9): 1323–36.

Rhodes, T., L. Mikhailova, A. Sarang, C. M. Lowndes, A. Rylkov, M. Khutorskoy, and A. Renton. 2003. "Situational Factors Influencing Drug Injecting, Risk Reduction, and Syringe Exchange in Togliatti City, Russian Federation: A Qualitative Study of Micro Risk Environment." *Social Science and Medicine* 57 (1): 39–54.

Robinson, T. E., and J. B. Becker. 1986. "Enduring Changes in Brain and Behavior Produced by Chronic Amphetamine Administration: A Review and Evaluation of Animal Models of Amphetamine Psychosis." *Brain Research* 396 (2): 157–98.

Roozen, H. G., J. J. Boulogne, M. W. van Tulder, W. van den Brink, C. A. De Jong, and A. J. Kerkhof. 2004. "A Systematic Review of the Effectiveness of the Community Reinforcement Approach in Alcohol, Cocaine, and Opioid Addiction." *Drug and Alcohol Dependence* 74 (1): 1–13.

Ruan, Y. H., K. X. Hong, S. Z. Liu, Y. X. He, F. Zhou, G. M. Qin, and others. 2004. "Community-Based Survey of HCV and HIV Coinfection in Injection Drug Abusers in Sichuan Province of China." *World Journal of Gastroenterology* 10 (11): 1589–93.

SAMHSA (Substance Abuse and Mental Health Services Adminstration). 2001. *Summary of Findings from the 2000 National Household Survey on Drug Abuse*. Rockville, MD: Office of Applied Statistics, SAMHSA.

———. 2002. *Results from the 2001 Household Survey on Drug Abuse*. Vol. 1 of *Summary of National Findings*. Rockville, MD: Office of Applied Statistics, SAMHSA.

———. 2003. *Overview of Findings from the 2002 National Survey on Drug Use and Health Office*. Rockville, MD: Office of Applied Statistics, SAMHSA.

Satel, S. L., and W. S. Edell. 1991. "Cocaine-Induced Paranoia and Psychosis Proneness." *American Journal of Psychiatry* 148 (12): 1708–11.

Schoenbaum, E. E., D. Hartel, P. A. Selwyn, R. S. Klein, K. Davenny, M. Rogers, and others. 1989. "Risk Factors for Human Immunodeficiency Virus Infection in Intravenous Drug Users." *New England Journal of Medicine* 321 (13): 874–49.

Shepard, D., M. J. Larson, and N. G. Hoffmann. 1999. "Cost-Effectiveness of Substance Abuse Services: Implications for Public Policy." *Psychiatric Clinics of North America* 22 (2): 385–400.

Shepard, D., G. Strickler, J. McKay, D. Bury-Maynard, H. Yeom, C. Love, and others. Forthcoming. "Cost-Effectiveness of Self-Help for Controlling Substance Use: Controlling for Self-Selection."

Shoptaw, S., R. Rawson, M. McCann, and J. Obert. 1994. "The Matrix Model of Outpatient Stimulant Abuse Treatment: Evidence of Efficacy." In *Experimental Therapeutics in Addiction Medicine*, ed. S. Magura and S. Rosenblum, 129–41. Binghamton, NY: Haworth Press.

Sidney, S. 2002. "Cardiovascular Consequences of Marijuana Use." *Journal of Clinical Pharmacology* 42 (11 Suppl.): 64S–70S.

Sidney, S., J. E. Beck, I. S. Tekawa, C. P. Quesenberry, and G. D. Friedman. 1997. "Marijuana Use and Mortality." *American Journal of Public Health* 87 (4): 585–90.

Silva de Lima, M., B. Garcia de Oliveira Soares, A. Alves Pereira Reisser, and M. Farrell. 2002. "Pharmacological Treatment of Cocaine Dependence: A Systematic Review." *Addiction* 97: 931–49.

Simpson, D. S., and H. J. Friend. 1988. "Legal Status and Long-Term Outcomes for Addicts in the DARP Followup Project." In *Compulsory Treatment of Drug Abuse: Research and Clinical Practice*, ed. C. G. Leukefeld and F. M. Tims, 81–96. Rockville, MD: National Institute on Drug Abuse.

Simpson, D. S., G. W. Joe, W. E. K. Lehman, and S. B. Sells. 1986. "Addiction Careers: Etiology, Treatment, and 12-Year Follow-up Outcomes." *Journal of Drug Issues* 16 (1): 107–21.

Simpson, D. S., and S. Sells. 1982. "Effectiveness of Treatment for Drug Abuse: An Overview of the DARP Research Program." *Advances in Alcohol and Substance Abuse* 2 (1): 7–29.

———, eds. 1990. *Opioid Addiction and Treatment: A 12-Year Follow-up*. Malabar, FL: Krieger.

Smiley, A. 1999. "Marijuana: On Road and Driving Simulator Studies." In *The Health Effects of Cannabis*, ed. H. Kalant, W. Corrigall, W. D. Hall, and R. Smart, 171–91. Toronto, ON: Centre for Addiction and Mental Health.

Soares, B. G., M. S. Lima, A. A. Reisser, and M. Farrell. 2003. "Dopamine Agonists for Cocaine Dependence." Cochrane Database of Systematic Reviews (2): CD003352 [PMID: 12804461].

Solowij, N. 1993. "Ecstasy (3,4-Methalenedioxymethamphetamine)." *Current Opinion in Psychiatry* 6: 411–15.

———. 1998. *Cannabis and Cognitive Functioning*. Cambridge, U.K.: Cambridge University Press.

Solowij, N., W. D. Hall, and N. Lee. 1992. "Recreational MDMA Use in Sydney: A Profile of 'Ecstasy' Users and Their Experiences with the Drug." *British Journal of Addiction* 87: 1161–72.

Solowij, N., R. S. Stephens, R. A. Roffman, T. Babor, R. Kadden, M. Miller, and others. 2002. "Cognitive Functioning of Long-Term Heavy Cannabis Users Seeking Treatment." *Journal of the American Medical Association* 287 (9): 1123–31.

Spooner, C. and W. D. Hall. 2002. "Public Policy and the Prevention of Substance Use Disorders." *Current Opinion in Psychiatry* 15 (3): 235–39.

Spooner, C., W. D. Hall, and R. P. Mattick. 2001. "An Overview of Diversion Strategies for Australian Drug-Related Offenders." *Drug and Alcohol Review* 20 (3): 281–94.

Sporer, K. A. 2003. "Strategies for Preventing Heroin Overdose." *British Medical Journal* 326 (7386): 442–44.

Srisurapanont, M., N. Jarusuraisin, and P. Kittirattanapaiboon. 2003. "Treatment for Amphetamine Dependence and Abuse." Cochrane Database of Systematic Reviews (4): CD003022 [PMID: 11687171].

Stephens, R. S., R. A. Roffman, and E. E. Simpson. 1994. "Treating Adult Marijuana Dependence—A Test of the Relapse Prevention Model." *Journal of Consulting and Clinical Psychology* 62 (1): 92–99.

Strang, J., S. Darke, W. D. Hall, M. Farrell, and R. Ali. 1996. "Heroin Overdose: The Case for Take-Home Naloxone: Home-Based Supplies of Naloxone Would Save Lives." *British Medical Journal* 312 (7044): 1435–36.

Strathdee, S. A., T. Zafar, H. Brahmbhatt, A. Baksh, and S. ul Hassan. 2003. "Rise in Needle Sharing among Injection Drug Users in Pakistan during the Afghanistan War." *Drug and Alcohol Dependence* 71 (1): 17–24.

Szasz, T. 1985. *Ceremonial Chemistry: The Ritual Persecution of Drugs, Addicts, and Pushers*. Holmes Beach, FL: Learning Publications.

Tashkin, D. P. 1999. "Effects of Cannabis on the Respiratory System." In *The Health Effects of Cannabis*, ed. H. Kalant, W. Corrigall, W. D. Hall, and R. Smart, 311–45. Toronto, ON: Centre for Addiction and Mental Health.

Taylor, D. R., D. M. Fergusson, B. J. Milne, L. J. Horwood, T. E. Moffitt, M. R. Sears, and R. Poulton. 2002. "A Longitudinal Study of the Effects of Tobacco and Cannabis Exposure on Lung Function in Young Adults." *Addiction* 97 (8): 1055–61.

Tonigan, J., R. Toscova, and W. Miller. 1996. "Meta-Analysis of the Literature on Alcoholics Anonymous: Sample and Study Characteristics Moderate Findings." *Journal of Studies on Alcohol* 57 (1): 65–72.

Tonigan, J. S., G. J. Connors, and W. R. Miller. 2003. "Participation and Involvement in Alcoholics Anonymous." In *Treatment Matching in Alcoholism*, ed. T. F. Babor and F. K. Del Boca, 184–204. Cambridge, UK: Cambridge University Press.

Toomey, R., M. J. Lyons, S. A. Eisen, H. Xian, S. Chantarujikapong, L. J. Seidman, and others. 2003. "A Twin Study of the Neuropsychological Consequences of Stimulant Abuse." *Archives of General Psychiatry* 60 (3): 303–10.

Topp, L., J. Hando, L. Degenhardt, P. Dillon, A. Roche, and N. Solowij. 1998. *Ecstasy Use in Australia*. NDARC Monograph 39. Sydney, Australia: National Drug and Alcohol Research Centre, University of New South Wales.

Torrens, M., L. San, J. M. Peri, and J. M. Olle. 1991. "Cocaine Abuse among Heroin Addicts in Spain." *Drug and Alcohol Dependence* 27 (1): 29–34.

Uchtenhagen, A., F. Gutzwiller, and A. Dobler-Mikola. 1998. *Medical Prescription of Narcotics Research Programme: Final Report of the Principal Investigators*. Zurich, Switzerland: Institut für Sozial- und Präventivmedizin der Universität Zurich.

UNAIDS (Joint United Nations Programme on HIV/AIDS) and WHO (World Health Organization). 2002. *AIDS Epidemic Update December*

2002. Geneva: Joint United Nations Programme on HIV/AIDS and World Health Organization.

UNDCP (United Nations Drug Control Programme). 1997. *World Drug Report.* Oxford, U.K.: Oxford University Press.

United Nations Commission on Narcotic Drugs. 2000. "World Situation with Regard to Drug Abuse, in Particular among Children and Youth." Vienna, United Nations Commission on Narcotic Drugs.

UNODC (United Nations Office on Drugs and Crime). 2004. *World Drug Report.* Vienna: UNODC.

UNODCCP (United Nations Office for Drug Control and Crime Prevention). 2002. *Global Illicit Drug Trends, 2002.* New York: UNODCCP.

———. 2003. *Global Illicit Drug Trends, 2003.* New York: UNODCCP.

Urbina, A., and K. Jones. 2004. "Crystal Methamphetamine, Its Analogues, and HIV Infection: Medical and Psychiatric Aspects of a New Epidemic." *Clinical Infectious Diseases* 38 (6): 890–4.

Uuskula, A., A. Kalikova, K. Zilmer, L. Tammai, and J. DeHovitz. 2002. "The Role of Injection Drug Use in the Emergence of Human Immunodeficiency Virus Infection in Estonia." *International Journal of Infectious Diseases* 6 (1): 23–27.

van Beek, I., R. Dwyer, and A. Malcolm. 2001. "Cocaine Injecting: The Sharp End of Drug-Related Harm!" *Drug and Alcohol Review* 20: 333–42.

van den Brink, W., and J. M. van Ree. 2003. "Pharmacological Treatments for Heroin and Cocaine Addiction." *European Neuropsychopharmacology* 13 (6): 476–87.

Vanichseni, S., B. Wongsuwan, K. Choopanya, and K. Wongpanich. 1991. "A Controlled Trial of Methadone Maintenance in a Population of Intravenous Drug Users in Bangkok: Implications for Prevention of HIV." *International Journal of the Addictions* 26 (12): 1313–20.

van Os, J., M. Bak, M. Hanssen, R. V. Bijl, R. de Graaf, and H. Verdoux. 2002. "Cannabis Use and Psychosis: A Longitudinal Population-Based Study." *American Journal of Epidemiology* 156 (4): 319–27.

Vasica, G., and C. C. Tennant. 2002. "Cocaine Use and Cardiovascular Complications." *Medical Journal of Australia* 177 (5): 260–62.

Verheyden, S. L., J. A. Henry, and H. V. Curran. 2003. "Acute, Sub-Acute, and Long-Term Subjective Consequences of 'Ecstasy' (MDMA) Consumption in 430 Regular Users." *Human Psychopharmacology* 18 (7): 507–17.

Vincent, N., J. Shoobridge, A. Ask, S. Allsop, and R. Ali. 1998. "Physical and Mental Health Problems in Amphetamine Users from Metropolitan Adelaide, Australia." *Drug and Alcohol Review* 17: 187–95.

Vlahov, D., C. L. Wang, N. Galai, J. Bareta, S. H. Mehta, S. A. Strathdee, and K. E. Nelson. 2004. "Mortality Risk among New Onset Injection Drug Users." *Addiction* 99 (8): 946–54.

Walsh, G. W., and R. E. Mann. 1999. "On the High Road: Driving under the Influence of Cannabis in Ontario." *Canadian Journal of Public Health-Revue Canadienne De Santé Publique* 90 (4): 260–63.

Ward, J., W. D. Hall, and R. P. Mattick. 1998. *Methadone Maintenance Treatment and Other Opioid Replacement Therapies.* Amsterdam: Harwood Academic.

Warner-Smith, M., S. Darke, M. Lynskey, and W. D. Hall. 2001. "Heroin Overdose: Causes and Consequences." *Addiction* 96 (8): 1113–25.

White, J. M., F. Bochner, and R. J. Irvine. 1997. "The Agony of 'Ecstasy': How Can We Avoid More 'Ecstasy'-Related Deaths?" *Medical Journal of Australia* 166: 117–18.

WHO (World Health Organization). 2003. *The World Health Report 2003: Shaping the Future.* Geneva: WHO.

WHO (World Health Organization) Programme on Substance Abuse. 1997. *Cannabis: A Health Perspective and Research Agenda.* Geneva: WHO, Division of Mental Health and Prevention of Substance Abuse.

Wild, T. C., A. B. Roberts, and E. L. Cooper. 2002. "Compulsory Substance Abuse Treatment: An Overview of Recent Findings and Issues." *European Addiction Research* 8 (2): 84–93.

Wilkins, C., K. Bhatta, M. Pledger, and S. Casswell. 2003. "Ecstasy Use in New Zealand: Findings from the 1998 and 2001 National Drug Surveys." *New Zealand Medical Journal* 116 (1171): U383.

Xie, X., J. Rehm, E. Single, and L. Robson. 1996. *The Economic Costs of Alcohol, Tobacco, and Illicit Drug Abuse in Ontario: 1992.* Toronto, ON: Addiction Research Foundation.

Yacoubian, G. S. Jr. 2003a. "Correlates of Ecstasy Use among Students Surveyed through the 1997 College Alcohol Study." *Journal of Drug Education* 33 (1): 61–69.

———. 2003b. "Tracking Ecstasy Trends in the United States with Data from Three National Drug Surveillance Systems." *Journal of Drug Education* 33 (3): 245–58.

Yacoubian, G. S. Jr., C. Boyle, C. A. Harding, and E. A. Loftus. 2003. "It's a Rave New World: Estimating the Prevalence and Perceived Harm of Ecstasy and Other Drug Use among Club Rave Attendees." *Journal of Drug Education* 33(2): 187–96.

Yu, X. F., J. Chen, Y. Shao, C. Beyrer, and S. Lai. 1998. "Two Subtypes of HIV-1 among Injection-Drug Users in Southern China." *Lancet* 351 (9111): 1250.

Zammit, S., P. Allebeck, S. Andreasson, I. Lundberg, and G. Lewis. 2002. "Self Reported Cannabis Use as a Risk Factor for Schizophrenia in Swedish Conscripts of 1969: Historical Cohort Study." *British Medical Journal* 325 (7374): 1199–201.

Zaric, G. S., P. G. Barnett, and M. L. Brandeau. 2000. "HIV Transmission and the Cost-Effectiveness of Methadone Maintenance." *American Journal of Public Health* 90 (7): 1100–11.

Zhang, Z. F., H. Morgenstern, M. R. Spitz, D. P. Tashkin, G. P. Yu, J. R. Marshall, and others. 1999. "Marijuana Use and Increased Risk of Squamous Cell Carcinoma of the Head and Neck." *Cancer Epidemiology Biomarkers and Prevention* 8 (12): 1071–78.

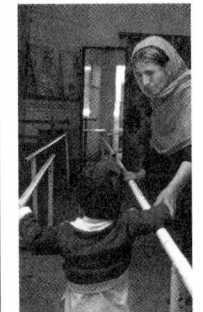

Chapter **49**

Learning and Developmental Disabilities

Maureen S. Durkin, Helen Schneider, Vikram S. Pathania, Karin B. Nelson, Geoffrey C. Solarsh, Nicole Bellows, Richard M. Scheffler, and Karen J. Hofman

Learning and developmental disabilities (LDDs) include functional limitations that manifest in infancy or childhood as a result of disorders of or injuries to the developing nervous system (Institute of Medicine Committee on Nervous System Disorders in Developing Countries 2001). These limitations range from mild to severe and can affect cognition, mobility, hearing, vision, speech, and behavior. The known causes of LDD are numerous and include genetic factors, nutritional factors, infections, toxic exposures, trauma, perinatal factors, and multifactorial conditions (table 49.1). Selected causes of LDD that are not addressed in detail in this chapter are described in box 49.1.

Although information on the prevalence and impact of disabilities in low- and middle-income countries (LMICs) is scarce, five considerations support the conclusion that LDDs are a public health priority in LMICs today:

- *Prevalence.* Although each individual cause is relatively rare, taken together, LDD affects a large proportion of children. In high-income countries, 10 to 20 percent of children have an LDD (Benedict and Farel 2003). With improvements in child survival in LMICs, it is not known whether the prevalence of disabilities among children is increasing, as has been seen in wealthier countries (Winter and others 2002), but the few data available from LMICs suggest that the prevalence of specific causes and types of LDD may be even higher than in high-income countries. Examples include cognitive disabilities associated with prenatal iodine deficiency, brain infections, and blindness associated with vitamin A deficiency (Durkin 2002). The prevalence of childhood disabilities in LMICs is not well established, but it is likely higher than in high-income countries.

- *Lifelong duration.* By definition, LDDs have an early onset, with the causes frequently occurring in the prenatal period. These effects are typically lifelong, affecting learning and other neurological functions, educational achievement, quality of life, earning potential, and productivity across the life span.

- *Costs.* The extensive costs include the direct costs of acute care, outpatient health care services, long-term care, rehabilitation, and special education, as well as the indirect costs of morbidity and increased mortality (Waitzman, Romano, and Scheffler 1994). Additionally, the costs and effects extend beyond the individuals affected to include entire families. Health, careers and employment of parents, family disposable income, health and adaptation of siblings, and family interaction are adversely affected when a family member has an LDD (Stein and Jessop 2003). It is difficult to comprehend the extent of these effects, just as it is difficult to measure them and develop economic models that account for them.

- *Education and work.* As societies and economies become increasingly information-oriented and dependent on educated and literate workers, the impact of disabilities affecting cognition and learning becomes greater (Institute of Medicine Committee on Nervous System Disorders in Developing Countries 2001).

- *Proven interventions.* The prospects for preventing LDD and for improving outcomes are considerable and can be achieved, to some extent, by implementing interventions that have been shown to be effective and cost-effective elsewhere but that are not being implemented in LMICs.

This chapter provides an overview of the range of interventions likely to improve child development and educational

933

Table 49.1 Categories of Causes of LDD

Category	Examples
Genetic	
Chromosomal	Down syndrome, chromosomal rearrangements
Segmental autosomal syndromes	Prader-Willi syndrome, Angelman syndrome
Sex-linked, single gene	Fragile X syndrome, Rett syndrome
Autosomal recessive	Phenylketonuria, Tay–Sachs disease
Autosomal dominant	Neurocutaneous syndromes, such as neurofibromatosis
Multifactorial	
Genetic and nutritional	Neural tube defects
Nutritional	
Prenatal: maternal iodine deficiency	Developmental iodine deficiency disorder
Childhood: vitamin A deficiency	Xerophthalmia, night blindness
Infections	
Prenatal or perinatal	Toxoplasmosis, rubella, cytomegalovirus, herpes, gonorrhea, syphilis, group B streptococcus, chlamydia, trichomonas vaginalis, bacterial vaginosis, herpes simplex virus, HIV
Postnatal or childhood	Encephalitis, meningitis, varicella, cerebral malaria, polio, trachoma, otitis media
Toxic exposures	
Prenatal	Alcohol, lead, mercury, antimicrobials (such as sulfonamides, isoniazid, ribavirin), anticonvulsants (such as phenytoin, carbamazepine), and other drugs (such as accutane, thalidomide)
Postnatal or childhood	Lead, mercury
Other maternal disorders	
Thyroid disease	Cerebral palsy
Other perinatal complications	
Brain injuries associated with premature birth, birth asphyxia	Cerebral palsy, cognitive disabilities, seizure disorders
Injury	
Traumatic brain injuries and other disabling injuries from vehicle crashes, child abuse and neglect, falls, burns, warfare, and so forth	Cognitive, motor, speech, vision, hearing, seizure, and behavioral disabilities
Poverty, economic disadvantage	
Social and cognitive deprivation	Mild mental retardation
Unknown	LDD of unknown cause

outcomes for children in LMICs. Evidence of cost-effectiveness is considered in some detail for three selected interventions. An overview of other key risk factors and conditions that result in LDD is provided. A research agenda is outlined for advancing knowledge of how to prioritize cost-effective interventions and how best to devote resources for the prevention of LDD in LMICs.

LDD AND THE GLOBAL BURDEN OF DISEASE

Estimates for disability-adjusted life years (DALYs) (Mathers 2006) are not available to convey the full range of LDDs or their risk factors. Attempts have been made to estimate the DALYs associated with specific causes of LDDs. For example, it is estimated that 9.8 million DALYs, or nearly 1 percent of the global burden of disease, are due to one relatively minor form of LDD, namely, mild mental retardation (MR) caused by lead ingestion from environmental sources (Fewtrell and others 2004). Since only a small fraction—probably much less than 10 percent—of LDD worldwide can be attributed to lead-induced mild MR, this estimate suggests that LDD as a whole must account for a large proportion, perhaps more than 10 percent of the global burden of disease. Where DALY estimates are available, we use them as a basis for economic analysis to estimate the costs of

Box 49.1

Interventions for the Prevention of Childhood Neurological Disabilities

Attention Deficit Hyperactivity Disorder

Attention deficit hyperactivity disorder (ADHD) is the most common neurological disorder in children in the United States, with an estimated prevalence of 3 to 11 percent. The prevalence is not known in LMICs, but as schooling increasingly becomes the norm, ADHD is likely to become more obvious. The burden of ADHD in settings of large class sizes will likely pose an increasing challenge. In addition to its major impact on school performance, ADHD affects family relationships and social competence, with lasting consequences. Children with ADHD are also at higher risk for injury, depression, and substance abuse. Worldwide, with the growing use in school settings of stimulants to control this chronic disorder, the impact on health care costs is potentially huge. Although there are a paucity of data on this topic, in one study, the cost of medicating children for ADHD was close to an average of US$500 or more per child per year, and this figure is considered a substantial underestimate (Chan, Zhan, and Homer 2002).

Autism Spectrum Disorders

All autism spectrum disorders (ASDs) are characterized by varying degrees of impairment in communication skills and social interactions and in restricted, repetitive patterns of behavior or interests. Although only 50 percent of children in the United States with ASDs are diagnosed before six years of age, this group of disorders can reliably be diagnosed by three years of age and in some cases by as early as 18 months. ASDs range from a severe form called *autistic disorder* to a milder form known as *Asperger syndrome*. Prevalence studies of ASDs in Asia, Europe, and North America estimate that 2 to 6 out of every 1,000 children have an ASD. Screening instruments using responses from children and parents are available. Evidence indicates that early intervention (ideally in optimal educational settings for at least two years during preschool) results in improved outcomes. Individuals with ASDs generally respond well to highly structured, specialized programs. A variety of medications is used to treat associated depression, anxiety, ADHD, seizures, and other behavioral symptoms. Adults with severe ASDs require intensive and constant supervision. Little information is available regarding the parental and service costs of ASDs. In a 2001 study in the United Kingdom, the lifetime cost for a person with autistic disorder exceeded UK £12.4 million, with most of the expense related to living support and daily activities.

Infection

Numerous prenatal, perinatal, and postnatal infections can damage the developing nervous system or sensory pathways and cause long-term disabilities in children. The relative contribution of these infections to the burden of LDD is likely to vary by country. It will be influenced by overall infant mortality, postneonatal contribution to infant mortality, and regional difference in the distribution of the infections known to be associated with neurological sequelae during different periods in the early life cycle. A few of the most important infections that may result in LDD include the following:

- *Congenital rubella (chapter 20).* This disease is a major global cause of preventable hearing impairment, blindness, and intellectual disability. The incidence of congenital rubella syndrome has been variably set at 0.5 to 2.2 out of every 1,000 live births in LMICs during epidemics, which occur every four to seven years (Cutts and others 1997). Though some LMICs have set elimination goals and vaccination has been noted to be cost-effective, only 28 percent of LMICs routinely vaccinate against rubella (Robertson and others 1997).
- *HIV/AIDS infection (chapter 18).* Neurological problems in HIV-infected children vary in different parts of the world but may be as high as 40 to 50 percent (Bobat and others 1998). The developmental trajectory of infected children is confounded by maternal, social, and biological risk factors during pregnancy and early childhood. Maternal substance and drug abuse, more common in HIV-infected women, have an independent adverse effect on brain growth and neurodevelopmental outcome. Low birthweight and prematurity, poverty, protein calorie malnutrition, and micronutrient deficiencies—more frequently seen in HIV-infected children and particularly in LMICs—may similarly compromise early child development (Brouwers and others 1996).
- *Malaria (chapter 21).* In Sub-Saharan Africa, malaria is the leading cause of childhood mortality and morbidity. Cerebral malaria is a well-known complication and

Box 49.1

(*Continued*)

may result in neurological sequelae in survivors, contributing significantly to the burden of LDD.

- *Bacterial meningitis (chapter 20).* This disease results in long-term sequelae for many children, including approximately 40 percent of children who survive *Haemophilus* influenza meningitis, 50 percent who survive pneumococcal meningitis, and 10 percent who survive meningococcal meningitis. Cost-effective immunization can prevent meningitis from all these causes.

Alcohol

Prenatal alcohol exposure resulting in fetal alcohol syndrome may be the most common single preventable cause of MR worldwide (Viljoen 1999), but substantial challenges remain in diagnosing and preventing this disorder (see chapter 47). In addition to growth retardation and congenital heart disease, effects include ADHD, memory deficits, and mood disorders. Adults continue to have attention and social difficulties and higher rates of alcohol, nicotine, and drug dependence. Children exposed to even small amounts of alcohol (half a drink per day) in utero have poor outcomes, suggesting that abstinence should be recommended during conception and throughout pregnancy (Sokol, Delaney-Black, and Nordstrom 2003).

Although tools are available to help providers identify women who consume alcohol, detection of maternal alcohol exposure is a challenge. The overall rate of fetal alcohol syndrome for LMICs has been placed at 1 to 4.8 out of every 1,000 population (Sampson and others 1997) and is higher among low socioeconomic populations and subpopulations with particularly high alcohol intakes. If individuals with the full spectrum of fetal alcohol syndrome–related effects are included, this rate may be as high as 1 in every 100 births. A prevalence rate of 40.5 to 46.4 out of every 1,000 children in South Africa, the highest rate worldwide, is attributable to particular historical and social conditions (May and others 2000).

Public health measures to prevent prenatal alcohol exposure have had limited success, and rates have not changed over the past decade in the United States (Floyd and Sidhu 2004). These measures include putting warning labels on alcoholic beverages and broadcasting public messages about alcohol dangers during pregnancy. Improved outcomes might result from targeting the use of

screening tools for high-risk drinkers, who include women in prisons, drug rehabilitation centers, hospital emergency facilities, and sexually transmitted disease clinics (Sokol, Delaney-Black, and Nordstrom 2003). Little is known about the costs around the world. Annual costs for all individuals with fetal alcohol syndrome in the United States during 1998 was estimated at US$4 billion, with lifetime care per person, for individuals requiring such care, at US$1.4 million (Lupton, Burd, and Harwood 2004).

Environmental Exposures

Children are more susceptible to environmental factors, including unsafe home environments, road traffic, and chemicals (see chapters 42 and 43). Even in high-income countries in Europe, mild MR resulting from lead exposure accounted for 4.4 percent of DALYs among children zero to four years of age. Legislative efforts are under way to eliminate lead from gasoline and other environmental sources of lead exposure in LMICs (Khan and Khan 1999; Alliance to End Childhood Lead Poisoning 2002). In the 0 to 19 years age group, injuries from all causes accounted for 19 percent of DALYs. The poor and vulnerable road users—pedestrians, cyclists, and motorcyclists—bear the greatest burden of road injuries. Nearly 25 percent of all nonfatally injured victims requiring hospitalization sustain a traumatic brain injury as a result of motor vehicle crashes (Peden and others 2004). Although the effectiveness of bicycle helmets for road safety is high, their use in LMICs is low (Thompson, Rivara, and Thompson 1999).

Interventions aimed at reducing children's exposure to environmental factors and injuries could result in substantial gains. Targeted action by region, even within a single country, is likely to prove most productive (Valent and others 2004).

Nutritional Deficiency

Iodine deficiency from inadequate quantities of iodine in soil, water, and food affects 13 percent of the world's population, and an additional 30 percent are at risk (see chapter 28). Maternal iodine deficiency during pregnancy may result in an average loss of 15 IQ points in offspring, making it a leading preventable cause of MR. Iodine deficiency can be prevented with adequate consumption of iodized salt, which is now consumed by about 70 percent of households worldwide.

prevention of LDD. In this chapter, we estimated only costs of the interventions for Down syndrome (DS), neural tube defects (NTDs), and congenital hypothyroidism.

IMPAIRMENT, DISABILITY, AND PARTICIPATION

Quantifying the impacts of LDD and their preventive interventions is complicated by the fact that these disorders can exist and be measured at multiple levels, including three levels distinguished by the World Health Organization (WHO) in *International Classification of Functioning, Disability, and Health* (WHO 2001):

- *impairment,* which refers to physiological or psychological defects or abnormalities, such as failure of the neural tube to close
- *function* or *disability,* which refers to the ability of an individual to perform a task, such as walking, seeing, hearing, learning language, and reading
- *participation,* which refers to the degree to which an individual participates in school, employment, social role, and recreational activities.

A given impairment may be associated with a range of functional outcomes. Some but not all of these may be recognized as disability. Disability is context specific and may vary from culture to culture. For example, conditions such as dyslexia, attention deficit and hyperactivity disorder (ADHD), and mild MR may be especially disabling in school but not as noticeable in nonacademic settings and environments where schooling is optional. Environmental factors and social stigma may determine the participation of people with disabilities more than do the functional deficits themselves. Some interventions may be designed to enhance participation (for example, ramps, accessible public toilets, inclusive education), whereas others may target impairment and disability (for example, nutritional fortification, surgery, rehabilitation, special education, newborn screening, and early treatment).

THREE LEVELS OF PREVENTION

Prevention of LDD involves primary, secondary, and tertiary prevention activities:

- *Primary prevention* includes efforts to control the underlying cause or condition that results in disability. Examples include (a) maternal antiretroviral therapy to reduce the risk of mother-to-child transmission of HIV and (b) fortification of the food supply to prevent birth defects such as spina bifida and iodine deficiency disorders.
- *Secondary prevention* aims at preventing an existing illness or injury from progressing to long-term disability. Examples include newborn screening for metabolic disorders followed by dietary restrictions to prevent damage to the nervous system and effective emergency medical care for head injury.
- *Tertiary prevention* refers to rehabilitation and special educational services to mitigate disability and improve functional and participatory or social outcomes once disability has occurred.

UNINTENDED CONSEQUENCES OF SUCCESSFUL OR PARTIALLY SUCCESSFUL INTERVENTIONS

Interventions to reduce mortality and morbidity may be followed by increases in the prevalence of LDD. Examples include the following:

- Improved survival of very low birthweight infants at high risk for LDD may cause the prevalence of disability in the population to increase at the same time that it increases the absolute number of survivors without disabilities.
- Rubella vaccination programs with less than optimal coverage will prevent infections in those vaccinated but leave unvaccinated girls at risk for acquiring rubella infection during their childbearing years (rather than during childhood, as might be expected in the absence of a vaccination program), thereby increasing the risk of congenital rubella infection and disability in the population.
- Newborn screening and treatment for phenylketonuria in infancy and childhood prevent MR, but phenylalanine dietary restriction for women with phenylketonuria during their childbearing years is essential to prevent prenatal neurological damage and MR in their offspring.

OTHER FACTORS LEADING TO INCREASES IN MEASURED PREVALENCE

Progress in the field of LDD may result in increases in the recognized prevalence of disability and in social and economic costs, as in the following examples:

- Increased availability of services may increase the number of children with recognized disabilities. Just as it is ethically problematic to screen for disorders for which no services can be offered, expansion of case finding becomes justified and ethically demanded as services become available, with the potential result of increasing the measured prevalence of disability.
- As educational expectations and awareness of LDD increase, the prevalence of recognized disability may increase.

In consideration of these trends and relationships between public health advances and increases in disability, it may not be realistic to expect short-term control of disability or cost savings following interventions that reduce mortality, even if those

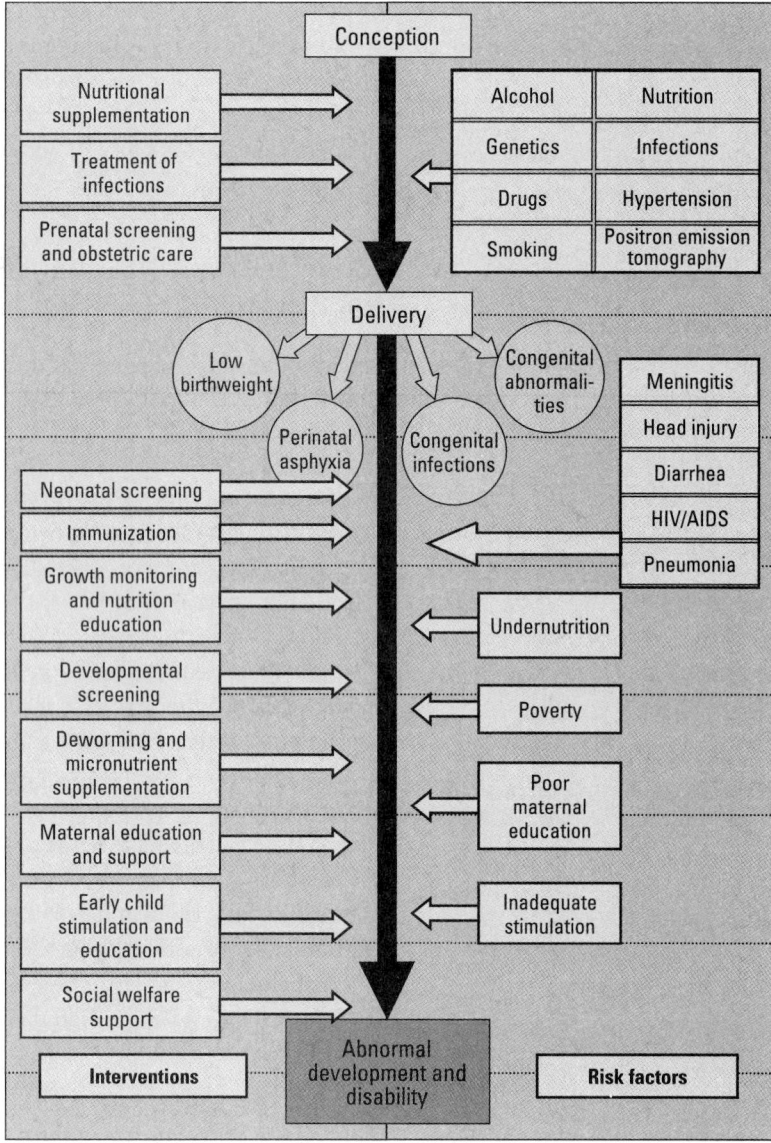

Source: Authors.

Figure 49.1 Causal Pathways for LDD

interventions have a net positive effect on public health. The costs of disability and its prevention may increase initially in the wake of interventions that successfully reduce mortality. Figure 49.1 summarizes the causal pathways and potential interventions for the prevention of LDD.

INTERVENTIONS IN LOW- AND MIDDLE-INCOME COUNTRIES

Numerous interventions are effective in preventing LDD. Table 49.2 provides a summary of these interventions classified on two axes. The horizontal axis distinguishes whether the intervention would accomplish primary, secondary, or tertiary

prevention of disability. The vertical axis distinguishes four levels of evidence for cost-effectiveness:

- evidence available for LMICs
- evidence available for high-income countries only
- evidence for cost-effectiveness not available, but cost-effectiveness can be estimated from existing data
- evidence not available, but potential for benefits exists.

The literature indicates that the economic outcomes of a given intervention may vary widely for two reasons:

- Variations exist across populations, even within the same country, in the prevalence of the disorder, the cost of health care, and the existing infrastructure available to implement the intervention.

Table 49.2 Classification of Interventions to Prevent LDD

	Primary (prevention of condition that can lead to disability)	Secondary (prevention of disability once condition has occurred)	Tertiary (rehabilitation or prevention of further disability once disability has occurred)
Evidence for cost-effectiveness available for LMICs	Food fortification (*folic acid* and iodine[a]) Rubella vaccine[a] Hemophilus vaccine Removal of lead from paint and fuel Vitamin A supplementation (vision) Measles vaccine		
Evidence for cost-effectiveness available for high-income countries only		*Prenatal screening for DS and prevention of DS births* *Newborn screening for metabolic disorders followed by interventions to prevent disability*	
Evidence for cost-effectiveness not available, but cost-effectiveness can be estimated from existing data	Malaria prevention[b]	Early detection and care of neonatal jaundice Management of malaria Treatment for otitis media Prevention and treatment of neonatal complications through emergency obstetric and pediatric services Eyeglasses Hearing aids Detection and treatment of maternal thyroid disorders	Special education Prosthetics Braille Sign language Occupational, physical, and speech therapies Surgery Residential care Assistive devices
Evidence for cost-effectiveness not available, but potential for benefits exists	Fetal alcoholism prevention Trauma prevention (bicycle helmets, burns) Prevention of shaken baby syndrome and child abuse	Dehydration/diarrhea treatment Postnatal combined cognitive stimulation and nutritional intervention Therapeutic stimulants for treatment of ADHD	*Community-based rehabilitation*

Note: Italicized text represents somewhat detailed consideration of cost-effectiveness included in this chapter.
a. Covered in chapter 56, but chapter emphasis is not on implications for preventing developmental disabilities.
b. Covered in detail in chapter 21.

• Differences between studies exist in analytical methods used, such as the willingness to pay versus the human capital approach to valuation, and in cost categories, such as whether to include parental time costs. Though these differences make cross-population comparisons difficult, the overall evidence of cost-effectiveness is demonstrated by repeated findings that the benefits of a particular intervention outweigh the costs in a number of different settings.

Current evidence suggests that three interventions are cost saving: folic acid fortification to prevent NTDs, prenatal screening and selective pregnancy termination to prevent DS, and neonatal screening and treatment for congenital hypothyroidism (CH).

Too little is known about the fourth type of intervention, community-based rehabilitation, to evaluate it. There is a paucity of knowledge and a history of failed interventions for the prevention of premature birth and the disabilities associated with premature birth.

Neural Tube Defects: Burden and Cost-Effectiveness of Folic Acid Fortification

NTDs, which are the most common malformation of the central nervous system, result from failure of the neural tube to close during the first month of pregnancy. Anencephaly typically results in pregnancy loss, stillbirth, or neonatal death. Spina bifida (open spine defect) is associated with a range of functional deficits (requiring multiple surgical and rehabilitative interventions), including paralysis of the lower extremities and often primary enuresis and cognitive disabilities. Large geographic variations in the prevalence of NTDs exist both within and between countries. The burden of disease is highest in South Asia and lowest in LMICs of Europe and Central Asia. Similarly, deaths from NTDs are high in South Asia but lowest in high-income countries. Estimates suggest that almost all NTD disease burden is concentrated in the age group zero to four years (Mathers 2006).

Folic Acid. Folate is a vitamin that occurs naturally in green leafy vegetables, legumes, citrus, and other foods. Folic acid (FA) is an easily absorbed synthetic form of folate that can be delivered as a dietary supplement or through FA fortification of flour or other common staple foods. NTDs can be reduced by 70 percent if women consume 400 μg of FA daily around the time of conception and until closure of the neural tube. At a population level, either supplementation or fortification of the food supply is necessary to ensure that 400 μg of FA is consumed at the critical period of fetal development, as this dose is higher than can reasonably be consumed by relying on naturally occurring folate in foods. Fortification is much more likely than supplementation to reach the population at risk because the benefit of enhanced FA intake occurs early, typically before the pregnancy is recognized. Fortification is of particular value to women who may not receive prenatal care until the third trimester.

This section considers only evidence of cost-effectiveness of FA fortification in LMICs with respect to the benefit of preventing NTDs. Additional health benefits can be expected with respect to stroke, heart disease, and cancer.

Cost-Effectiveness of Folic Acid Fortification A cost-benefit analysis of grain fortification in the United States (Romano and others 1995) included costs related to the addition of FA to food, to annual testing and surveillance, to a one-time packaging change, and to potential (though not substantiated) adverse health effects associated with undiagnosed vitamin B_{12} deficiency. Benefits included avoided costs of NTDs, such as mortality costs (particularly for anencephaly) and costs of caring for those with spina bifida. The benefits of fortification outweighed costs with cost-benefit ratios of 1 to 4.3 for low-level fortification and 1 to 6.1 for high-level fortification.

Cost-effectiveness relative to status quo of FA fortification depends on several factors:

- Costs of food fortification depend on the types and quantity of food that are fortified and the level of fortification.
- The proportion of the target population reached by the fortified food is important since, in most LMICs, many people consume food produced on their own farms or within their villages.

- Grains from large mills are relatively cheap to fortify; more resources are required to fortify grains milled in smaller neighborhood mills.
- The amount of folate consumed by different populations in the absence of fortification varies.
- Prevalence of NTDs varies across populations, and the cost-effectiveness increases with prevalence.

Costs of food fortification may be lower in high-income countries, where most people consume cereals processed in a few large mills, equipment for fortification is likely to be in place, and quality assurance is facilitated. In contrast, mills in LMICs lack fortification equipment and capital, and running costs are higher in the short run.

Costs of Food Fortification For optimal daily consumption, the actual level of food fortification (defined as μg of FA per 100 grams of the food item) should be adjusted for storage and other losses so that a daily dose of 400 μg is achieved. Food items that should be fortified depend on specific dietary habits. Staples such as rice and flour are obvious choices; salt, sugar, bread, milk, and edible oils are promising candidates. There are economies of scale in FA fortification. It can be and usually is carried out in conjunction with other forms of fortification, such as iron, iodine, and vitamin A fortification. Many food items are already fortified in high-income countries. Other factors to be considered in the choice of food for fortification are items that are centrally processed and allow for quality control. Soy sauce in China is an example: it is consumed on a daily basis by 70 percent of the population and is prepared in a few large factories.

The recommended fortification level is thus 240 μg per 100 grams of the staple food. This fortification rate is assumed for all regional strata where the per capita staple consumption per day is less than 300 grams. Wheat, rice, maize, or a combination of these foods is the staple in most countries. The recommended level of FA fortification varies from 150 μg to 240 μg per 100 grams of cereal. So that women receive a daily dose of 400 μg, the target cereals for fortification should be those for which daily per capita consumption is at least 200 grams. In Sub-Saharan Africa, daily per capita cereal consumption exceeds 200 grams only if wheat, rice, and maize are considered together.

Quality assurance is done through analytic testing of fortified products to confirm FA levels. Quality assurance costs in the United States are estimated at US$0.64 cents per ton of fortified grain in quality assurance costs.

The costs of FA fortification include the cost of FA, setup, and analytic testing. The analysis is done using two different cost estimates: US$0.15 and US$0.50 per ton of grain fortified. The cost of FA determines the cost of premix added to the flour. FA is almost never added alone; usually FA, iron, zinc, and niacin are added in combination. The material cost of FA alone is about US$0.10 to US$0.20 per metric ton of milled wheat. However, a more realistic cost for the premix (including other supplements) is about US$0.50 per metric ton of milled wheat. This higher estimate is conservative and does not account for the health benefits from the other supplements. Either way, the per capita costs are only a few cents in each region. The low per capita cost in high-income countries of US$0.009 assumes that 80 percent of the cereal supply is fortified. In South Asia, where NTDs have the highest burden, the per capita cost is estimated at US$0.067 (Bagriansky n.d.).

Benefits of Folic Acid Fortification The cost-effectiveness of FA fortification in terms of its cost per DALY and per death averted assumes that the fortification strategy will reduce the incidence of NTDs by 50 percent. The costs are relatively high because of the high cost of FA. Even a few cents per capita becomes expensive if the per capita prevalence of NTD is very low.

Other Costs and Benefits The benefits of FA fortification outweigh the costs. The benefits estimated here are conservative for three reasons:

- Strokes and coronary deaths are also prevented by FA fortification and occur more frequently than NTDs.
- The percentage of NTDs that can be prevented by FA fortification may be greater than 50 percent, because up to 70 percent of NTDs can be prevented by 400 μg of periconceptional FA daily.
- These estimates do not take account of the costs of clinical care and management for complications when NTDs are not prevented.

Interventions to Prevent Disability Caused by Down Syndrome

Screening programs are critical public health interventions that use universal or targeted screening tests to identify potential causes or cases of LDD, including DS.

Prenatal and Neonatal Screening. Prenatal screening for genetic abnormalities allows parents to determine whether to continue with an affected pregnancy, whereas neonatal screening's fundamental purpose is to improve the infant's prognosis through early diagnosis and treatment.

A number of LDDs have been screened for in high-income countries since the 1960s, and researchers have conducted economic evaluations of these screening programs, including those for Tay-Sachs disease carriers, DS (Cusick and others 2003), sickle cell disease (Panepinto and others 2000), phenylketonuria (Lord and others 1999), and several other inborn errors of metabolism (Insinga, Laessig, and Hoffman 2002).

Estimates for Prenatal Screening, Diagnosis, and Selective Pregnancy Termination for Down Syndrome. DS is the most common genetic cause of mental retardation. Identifying a fetus with DS before birth and giving parents the option to terminate the pregnancy early can help decrease the burden of the disease on families and society. During counseling, parents may receive information about the consequences of DS, which will allow them to make an informed decision about the best care for the newborn or about termination of the pregnancy. Prenatal screening services provide an opportunity to profoundly reduce the impact of MR. The cost-effectiveness of prenatal screening for DS is based on two parameters: efficacy (by assessing the false positive rate of screening procedures and the number of fetal losses caused by screening) and financial costs (costs of screening per DS pregnancy averted). On the basis of the evidence, the best screening method is proposed, and sensitivity of the parameters of interest to the LMIC is tested. No formal comparisons are made between the costs of screening and care for a person with DS. The purpose of this analysis is to suggest the most cost-effective way of screening that provides families with information about the health of the child; it is not a cost-benefit analysis of whether a couple should terminate a pregnancy.

Burden. DS is caused by trisomy of chromosome 21—an extra chromosome rather than the usual diploid form—and is a major cause of severe MR (IQ less than 50 with substantial deficits in adaptive behavior). The incidence of DS is higher than the birth prevalence because many fetuses are spontaneously miscarried and, in some cases, selectively terminated. In the absence of prenatal screening and intervention, most DS conceptions (71 percent) result in spontaneous abortion; another 3 percent result in stillbirth, and 26 percent result in live birth with subsequent LDD (Kline, Stein, and Susser 1989). Because the incidence of DS cannot be determined without doing surveillance of all conceptions, the frequency of DS is typically measured in terms of prevalence per 1,000 live births rather than in terms of incidence. Thus, the population prevalence of DS varies depending on the maternal age structure (steep increase after age 35 years) as well as the availability and use of prenatal diagnosis followed by selective termination. Estimates from 10 LMICs range widely, from 0.1 out of every 1,000 live births in Indonesia to 4.4 out of every 1,000 live births in Pakistan (Institute of Medicine 2003). Most studies, in both high-income countries and LMICs, show DS birth prevalence in the range of 1.0 to 1.6 out of every 1,000 births. The birth prevalence of DS is likely higher in LMICs because of a higher proportion of births among women over age 35 (11 to 15 percent) relative to that in high-income countries (5 to 9 percent) (Kline, Stein, and Susser 1989) and possibly because of differential access to prenatal screening for chromosomal abnormalities.

Life Expectancy and Quality of Life. Life expectancy for children with DS is substantially lower than that of the general

Table 49.3 Distribution of DALYs Lost to and Deaths Caused by Down Syndrome, by World Bank Region, 2002

Region	DALYs	Deaths
East Asia and the Pacific	4,101,694	1,328
Europe and Central Asia	507,723	652
High income countries	199,215	2,113
Latin America and the Caribbean	214,346	1,979
Middle East and North Africa	347,898	1,311
South Asia	2,005,766	11,336
Sub-Saharan Africa	478,851	4,967

Source: Mathers and others 2006.

population. Congenital heart disease occurs in 40 to 60 percent of children with DS and accounts for 30 to 35 percent of deaths. Survival and life expectancy of children with DS have increased dramatically: In a 1940–60 birth cohort in England, only 50 percent of infants with DS survived beyond age two. By comparison, in 1981–85, 90 percent survived beyond age five (McGrother and Marshall 1990). Table 49.3 describes the estimated total deaths caused by DS by region, as well as the estimated total DALYs lost.

DS is always associated with cognitive impairment. Disability can range from mild to profound, and most children are affected moderately (IQ 40–55). Early intervention and therapy can improve functional outcomes. Of children with DS, 60 to 80 percent have hearing loss, and approximately 70 percent have ophthalmologic problems. As life expectancy of DS individuals has increased, many grow to adulthood and face an increased risk of early onset Alzheimer's disease, cataracts, hearing loss, hypothyroidism, and degenerative vascular disease.

Costs of Care. Based on 1988 data, the estimated incremental lifetime economic costs of DS are US\$410,000 per case or US\$647,709 in 2004 dollars (Waitzman, Romano, and Scheffler 1994). In another study, the estimate of per capita incremental costs of DS, converted to 2004 dollars, include net medical costs of US\$168,567, developmental services costs of US\$80,530, special education costs of US\$171,593, and total costs of US\$420,690 (Waitzman, Romano, and Scheffler 1994).

An estimate of lifetime costs per live born baby with DS—including education, health, and lost productivity costs—ranged from US\$137,000 in 1990 to US\$515,000 in 1993 (Gilbert and others 2001). Net savings using the annual program of screening, diagnosis, and selective termination was estimated to be US\$885, with costs of US\$446,000 per 10,000 pregnancies for a program that detects and prevents 9.7 DS births per year and a lower bound estimate of US\$137,000 of potential lifetime costs per 9.7 births prevented.

The increased life span of individuals with DS and accompanying age-associated morbidity impose heavy demands on medical care and community services, as well as on sustained support from family members. It is also important to note that dollar costs of care for a DS child in LMICs would be much lower than such costs in high-income countries because of lower prices as well as lower treatment intensity. For example, in some countries, congenital heart disease, which affects 40 to 60 percent of DS children, cannot be treated effectively. This lack of treatment will lower costs of care as well as life expectancy, and cost estimates will vary for each individual area or region.

Cost-Effectiveness of Prenatal Screening, Diagnosis, and Selective Pregnancy Termination. Prenatal screening can be implemented to allow selective termination of DS pregnancies and prevention of disability related to DS in the population. This intervention raises ethical, social, and cultural concerns for some individuals and populations that may preclude its applicability.

A screening program incorporating maternal serum triple screening in all pregnant women, regardless of maternal age, yields an excellent DS detection rate and is associated with a low false-positive rate (Wald and others 2003). DS pregnancies yield lower levels of alpha-fetoprotein and unconjugated estriol but have elevated levels of human chorionic gonadotropin compared with other pregnancies. Ultrasound evaluation of the fetus neck thickness improves screening sensitivity. It is also useful when used in conjunction with serum screening (Wald and others 2003). A positive screening result is followed by diagnosis using amniocentesis or chorionic villus sampling (CVS).

Although both diagnostic procedures are guided by ultrasound to reduce risk, they are invasive, are more expensive than the screening procedure, and carry a small risk of miscarriage of an unaffected pregnancy. Thus, only a select group screening positive for possible trisomy 21 are offered the invasive diagnostic procedures. Amniocentesis, which involves the aspiration of amniotic fluid, is performed between the 14th and 16th weeks of pregnancy. CVS involves aspiration of villi and can be performed between the 10th and 12th weeks of pregnancy. Although CVS can be performed earlier in the pregnancy, amniocentesis is easier to perform and is more widely used in the second trimester. Following diagnostic confirmation of DS, parents are provided with genetic counseling and the option of terminating the pregnancy.

Although DS risk increases with maternal age, most births occur in younger women and, therefore, two-thirds of all DS births occur in younger mothers (Ross and Elias 1997). If prenatal diagnosis is available only for mothers 35 years or older, only 33 percent of DS births will be detected. Studies demonstrate that heavy reliance on maternal age to screen for DS may not be desirable in LMICs. Maternal age factor is not so useful in settings where early marriage and motherhood are the norm and most DS pregnancies involve mothers younger than 35 (Gupta and others 2001). Therefore, maternal serum screening of all pregnant women is important in preventing DS births and achieving cost-effectiveness (Wald and others 2003).

Procedure Costs Genetic screening and counseling services are expensive. Even after initial high fixed costs to establish prenatal screening services, provision of high-quality services requires staff training, equipment, and laboratory maintenance. A recent report suggests establishing genetic screening services when other public health interventions have reduced the infant mortality rate to the range of 20 to 40 out of every 1,000 live births (Institute of Medicine 2003). Above this level, other public health interventions may have greater benefits.

The breakdown of tasks is as follows:

- *screening costs,* which consist of laboratory expenses (consumables and staff); informing women of results (by mail if negative, by phone if positive); service costs (processing results and monitoring the service); training in ultrasound measurement of neck skin translucency; and overhead expenses
- *diagnostic costs,* which comprise counseling before CVS or amniocentesis, equipment and staff for these procedures, laboratory expenses (consumables and staff), and overhead expenses
- *costs of termination of selected pregnancies,* which include surgical dilation, evacuation (11 to 13 weeks), or medical termination with mifepristone (after 13 weeks).

We assume infrastructure exists for prenatal screening, diagnosis, and intervention. We use the following costs: triple serum test, US$70; amniocentesis, US$1,200; genetic counseling, US$100; and termination of pregnancy, US$2,000. These cost estimates have been widely used in the literature (Cusick and others 2003). However, the medical costs can be significantly lower in LMICs and will also vary across and within countries.

Cost-Effectiveness and Efficacy We assume that 100 percent of women attend a prenatal clinic between 10 and 14 weeks of gestation and are offered tests in the first trimester, or between 15 and 19 weeks for the tests in the second trimester. We discuss the effect of low uptake of prenatal care and its effect on cost-effectiveness of prenatal screening programs in our sensitivity analysis.

In terms of economic considerations, it is desirable to balance the probability of the birth of a DS child with the risk of procedure-related miscarriage. Sensitivity of prenatal screening and the false-positive rates vary widely, depending on the method used. The risk of procedure-related miscarriage can vary from 0.04 to 0.8 percent (Nyberg and others 1998). We use the conservative fetal loss rate of 0.9 percent (Gilbert and others 2001) for both procedures.

Efficacy of prenatal screening is defined as the number of unaffected fetuses lost due to prenatal testing per each DS birth averted (Institute of Medicine 2003). The goal is to minimize this ratio. The efficacy of prenatal screening varies with prevalence, and the primary determinant of variations in prevalence of DS is the age structure of women giving birth. The prevalence of DS and the efficacy of prenatal screening increase with the percentage of births to mothers over the age of 35. In this analysis, a 90 percent rate of selective termination is used (Waitzman, Romano, and Scheffler 1994). On this basis, the number of fetal losses per DS birth avoided varies from 7.13 (for 1 in 10,000 prevalence) to 0.16 (for 44 in 10,000 prevalence). Therefore, in countries with low prevalence of DS, such as Indonesia, more unaffected fetuses are lost than DS births averted because of screening. In areas where the ratio of unaffected fetal losses to DS births avoided is above 1, the efficacy of screening for DS is questionable.

Because of higher loss rates for CVS, we use a 1.5 percent fetal loss rate in our sensitivity analysis (Lippman and others 1992). Other costs not considered in this study are the psychological effects of a positive test on the parents, anxiety that may persist from a false-positive test, and potential complications resulting from pregnancy termination. Complications from termination may vary (Stray-Pedersen and others 1991) and may not be the same in LMICs, which should be taken into account. The sensitivity rate for the triple serum test followed by the amniocentesis is 62.3 percent in the clinical trials (Vintzileos and others 2000), and the uptake of amniocentesis is 90 percent for affected mothers and 80 percent for unaffected mothers (Waitzman, Romano, and Scheffler 1994). We assume the false-positive rate of 5 percent. The false-positive rate affects the probability of losing an unaffected fetus as a result of invasive testing that follows serum screening.

Financial cost-effectiveness is defined as the screening costs per DS birth averted. It is presented in table 49.4. Cost-effectiveness is the highest in countries with high birth prevalence of DS, given that women have access and receive prenatal care. Costs of prenatal screening and termination per DS birth averted vary from US$1,497,390 in Indonesia (for 1 in 10,000 prevalence) to US$37,185 in Pakistan (44 in 10,000 prevalence). A similar relationship is seen between prevalence and cost per DALY. In our analysis, we use costs data that are based on estimates from developed countries. Because costs of care will vary widely across and within countries, cost estimates should be done for individual regions. Lower costs of care will reduce cost-effectiveness of prenatal screening for DS. However, even after the cost adjustment, it is unlikely that the benefits will completely go away, because of the large difference between a relatively cheap screening program and high burden of disease of DS.

Sensitivity Analysis The results of the analysis above depend on assumptions that may not hold in some LMICs. For example, if many women accept screening but few decide to have an amniocentesis, cost-effectiveness will be adversely affected. The

Table 49.4 Financial Cost-Effectiveness and Efficacy of Prenatal Screening and Pregnancy Termination for the Prevention of Down Syndrome Births

Representative country	DS births per 100,000 population (birth prevalence)	DS births detected	Cost per 100,000 population (US$)	Cost per DS birth detected (US$)	DS births prevented	Cost of detection and termination (US$)	Cost per DS birth avoided (US$)	US$ per DALY	Unaffected fetal losses	Fetal losses per DS birth prevented
East Asia and the Pacific										
Indonesia	10	5.61	7,546,188	1,345,851	5.05	7,556,281	1,497,390	14.88	36.0	7.13
Europe and Central Asia										
Hungary	56	31.40	7,574,655	241,237	28.26	7,631,174	270,041	38.31	35.98	1.27
High-income countries										
Canada	120.79	67.73	7,614,750	112,433	60.95	7,736,658	126,926	36.09	35.96	0.59
Latin America and the Caribbean										
Argentina	160	89.71	7,639,014	85,150	80.74	7,800,496	96,612	22.50	35.94	0.45
Middle East and North Africa										
Israel	100	56.07	7,601,884	135,579	50.46	7,702,810	152,643	22.14	35.96	0.71
South Asia										
Pakistan	440	246.71	7,812,290	3,1666	222.04	8,256,364	37,185	4.12	35.84	0.16
Sub-Saharan Africa										
South Africa	210	117.75	7,669,956	65,139	105.9	7,881,901	74,377	16.46	35.92	0.34

public health benefits of screening for DS in socioeconomically deprived areas are small because of low uptake of amniocentesis (Ford and others 1998). With lower uptake rates of amniocentesis, both efficacy and financial cost-effectiveness are adversely affected as a result of low detection rates, and the number of unaffected fetal losses decreases. It is also important to note that, in some countries, many women may not have access to prenatal care or may not seek prenatal care and prenatal testing. In such areas, programs that try to reduce DS prevalence will have limited success, especially if a population at greater risk of DS is not tested.

Cost-effectiveness is often measured per DS birth averted since reduction in DS prevalence is the ultimate goal of prenatal testing. In many cultures, an abortion is not an acceptable option. Acceptance of elective termination of pregnancy may also vary across ethnicities and other subgroups within a given country. A study in California found the uptake of termination following the DS diagnosis varied from 47.5 percent for Hispanics to 65.8 percent for whites and 70.8 percent for Asians (Cunningham and Tompkinison 1999). If few families decide to terminate pregnancy to avoid having a child with severe disability, cost-effectiveness per DS birth averted will be adversely affected, and the screening program may fail to reduce the birth prevalence of DS. If a large percentage of families are opposed to induced abortion of fetal DS, the uptake of amniocentesis also will be low.

Because fetal losses following CVS are often higher than those for amniocentesis, efficacy analysis should be conducted assuming a 1.5 percent fetal loss risk attributable to invasive testing in the first trimester. With higher fetal losses, the efficacy of the prenatal screening is adversely affected, although the cost-effectiveness will not change.

In addition, assuming a higher false-positive rate of 8.3 percent increases the number of invasive tests on unaffected mothers and the number of unaffected fetal losses, thus adversely affecting the efficacy of the prenatal testing (Vintzileos and others 2000).

The analysis presented above is limited to an evaluation of the cost-effectiveness of prenatal screening for DS only. Some serum markers (for example, alpha-fetoprotein) will identify other abnormalities, the benefits of which are not included in this analysis.

Equity and Access The desirable policy is that women of similar risk for DS have equal access to diagnostic tests. With limited access to prenatal care, the introduction of the screening programs can have small public health effects. Although the approach used in cost-effectiveness analysis is optimization of societal net benefit, the policies to be recommended for the prevention of disability must also consider individuals' freedom in decision making at each step of the prenatal diagnosis. Successful policies need to be based on cost-effectiveness estimates that take into account the needs, sensitivities, and values of individuals and cultures (Institute of Medicine 2003).

Interventions to Prevent Disability Caused by Congenital Hypothyroidism

For CH, like DS, screening programs are critical public health interventions.

Neonatal Screening in Low- and Middle-Income Countries. When considering the costs and benefits associated with a CH screening program, one must first have an estimate of how prevalent CH is in the population so that the avoided costs associated with disability can be calculated. It is important to note that in high-income countries and in several middle-income countries screening is usually done for a series of conditions rather than for a single disorder. This fact is likely to affect the cost. In several of these conditions, the treatment includes dietary modification as well as costly prepared foods and formulas. Policies in countries where this type of screening occurs include labeling of food to alert potentially vulnerable consumers.

Several studies have examined the prevalence of CH in specific populations, with substantially varying results. A review of 13 studies reporting findings on CH prevalence identified through individual screening programs found the lowest rate to be 1 case of CH per over 6,000 screened in Thailand (Wasant, Liammongkolkul, and Srisawat 1999). Contrasting this is the highest rate reported: 1 case in 1,000 screened in Pakistan (Lakhani and others 1989). Prevalence can vary not only from one country to the next, but also within countries, depending on different analyses or subpopulations within one country. These variations demonstrate the need for identifying the appropriate population in order to conduct economic evaluations of screening interventions.

According to three cost-benefit analyses of CH screening (Layde, Von Allmen, and Oakley 1979; Barden and Kessel 1984), the benefits included savings from institutionalization, special education, medical care, lost parent and child productivity, and slightly decreased life expectancy. The costs included those of the screening program as well as the cost of treating detected cases. Overall, CH screening programs are substantially cost saving, with a cost-benefit ratio as high as 1 to 8.9 in high-income countries (Dhondt and others 1991). Such savings have not yet been evaluated in LMICs. Because the treatment is inexpensive and highly effective, it is anticipated that CH screening would also be substantially cost saving in LMICs.

Burden. Congenital hypothyroidism is a common cause of MR that can be prevented by newborn screening and treatment. By the end of the 1970s, neonatal screening programs had been established in many regions of Canada, Europe, Japan, and the United States. Thyroid hormone is required for normal brain development, and little or no thyroid hormone in the neonatal period results in damage to the nervous system. Various causes of anatomical maldevelopment of the thyroid gland are responsible for CH, and several genes have been implicated. With biochemical newborn screening (best conducted in centralized regional laboratories) using dried blood spots and diagnosis in the first few weeks of life, MR is avoidable. Without appropriate treatment, two-thirds of patients with CH have low IQ, and 30 percent experience severe or profound cognitive disability (Beaulieu 1994). Even with appropriate treatment, some subtle intellectual impairment and behavior deficits may still occur—the mean IQ may be approximately 10 points lower than that of the general population (Tillotson and others 1994). In the United States, infants are screened as newborns and again at two to six weeks of age to detect missed cases. For optimal outcomes, lifelong treatment with thyroid hormone is required, with subsequent monitoring and adjustments recommended every 3 to 12 months until growth and puberty are complete. Many females born with CH are now reaching childbearing age and require increased dosages of thyroid hormone during pregnancy for optimal neuropsychological outcome in their offspring.

Costs of Care. Estimated lifetime costs of care for the child with CH include the following (Barden and Kessel 1984):

- *Institutional care.* At the time of the study, 15 percent of congenital hypothyroid individuals were institutionalized from age 5 to 70.
- *Foster care.* About 25 percent of congenital hypothyroid cases received foster care from age 5 to 20.
- *Residential care.* Such care was provided for 40 percent of affected cases.
- *Special education expenditures.* Such expenses varied with the level of MR (15 percent severe, 25 percent moderate, and 40 percent mild).

In 2004, estimated lifetime costs of CH care is US$191,000, with a 6 percent discount rate. This estimate of the financial costs of care for an affected person is fairly conservative; it does not take into account lost productivity of the person with CH, a potential loss of income attributable to the time inputs of the family members who are taking care of the affected person, or effects on quality of life.

Cost-Effectiveness of Neonatal Screening. Table 49.5 presents cost-effectiveness analysis of neonatal screening for representative countries in the World Bank regions. Screening costs include blood sample collection, laboratory costs, discounted lifetime treatment cost, and costs of care for those missed by the screening. Specimen collection and laboratory costs (Barden and Kessel 1984; OTA 1988) constitute (in 2004 dollars) US$989,000 and US$969,000, respectively, per

Table 49.5 Cost-Effectiveness of Neonatal Screening for Congenital Hypothyroidism by World Bank Region

Representative country	CH births per 100,000 (birth prevalence)	CH births detected	Program costs for screening and treatment (US$)	Cost per disability averted (US$)	Cost without testing (US$)	Cost savings (US$)
East Asia and the Pacific						
Thailand	23.94	22.74	2,236,661	98,366	4,342,987	2,106,326
Europe and Central Asia						
Estonia	34.97	33.22	2,407,937	72,492	6,344,406	3,936,468
High-income countries						
United States	25.00	23.75	2,253,200	94,872	4,536,250	2,283,050
Latin America and the Caribbean						
Mexico	40.7	38.67	2,496,991	64,580	7,385,022	4,888,032
Middle East and North Africa						
Saudi Arabia	36.25	34.43	2,427,813	70,509	6,576,658	4,148,845
South Asia						
Pakistan	100.00	95.00	3,417,801	35,977	18,145,000	14,727,199
Sub-Saharan Africa						
South Africa	24.13	22.93	2,239,768	97,686	4,379,292	2,139,524

100,000 children tested. Lifetime discounted (at 6 percent) treatment costs are US$6,292.64 in 2004 dollars (Barden and Kessel 1984). Analysis of costs and benefits in table 49.5 shows that, although screening for the population as a whole requires considerable investment and infrastructure, the burden from the disorder is high and treatment is cheap. Screening all newborns is beneficial compared with the high costs of lifelong care for the affected individuals. Cost savings are positive for all representative countries despite high variance in the prevalence of CH. Even for a low birth prevalence estimate of 4 out of every 100,000 in Thailand (Wasant, Liammongkolkul, and Srisawat 1999), the cost savings would be US$106,326.

Effectiveness of the newborn screening in identifying the affected infants depends on the ability of the screening program to collect blood samples from all infants in the first week and to perform tests in time to initiate treatment. This effort may be difficult in some settings, where infants are born at home or released on the first day after birth and do not have contact with the health care system in the first month of their lives (Sack, Feldman, and Kaiserman 1998). The wider the coverage of the screening program, the higher will be the cost savings of screening. Also, follow-up screening for those infants who test as false negative will increase sensitivity to 100 percent and improve cost-effectiveness of the program.

In our cost-effectiveness analysis, we assumed the lifetime care and treatment costs to be similar to those estimated for the United States. However, medical costs may vary significantly among and within countries. Such variation is unlikely to alter

the cost-effectiveness analysis, because the difference between program and treatment expenditures and lifetime costs will remain even after we scale the medical costs.

The analysis presented above is limited to an evaluation of the cost-effectiveness of neonatal screening for CH. For minimal extra cost, collected blood samples for CH can also be used to identify other inherited disorders, including phenylketonuria, maple syrup urine disease, and other inborn errors of metabolism. Without the benefits of early detection and treatment for these conditions, the result is severe MR.

Community-Based Rehabilitation

Community-based rehabilitation is a set of low-cost approaches to providing rehabilitation services such as physical therapy, occupational therapy, prosthetics, and assistive devices for people with disabilities in developing countries. Such rehabilitation also aims to minimize stigmatization of people with disabilities and to support inclusive education and integration of people with disabilities into society. WHO and other organizations have actively promoted community-based models for providing rehabilitation services—including services for children with developmental disabilities—in resource-poor settings (Institute of Medicine Committee on Nervous System Disorders in Developing Countries 2001).

Although 80 percent or more of the world's people with disabilities live in developing countries, only 2 percent have access to rehabilitation services (WHO Community-Based

Rehabilitation 1982). If families of people with disabilities are taken into account, the number of people experiencing the effects of disability is estimated to be up to 25 percent of the world population. Community-based rehabilitation is designed to expand access to rehabilitation services in poor and rural areas by providing training in rehabilitation techniques to individuals with disabilities, their family members, and others in their communities. It also attempts to change negative attitudes toward disability and to remove barriers in the physical environment that prevent people with disabilities from fully participating in society.

Costs. In the community-based rehabilitation model, community interventions are shifted from institutions and centers to the homes and communities of people with disabilities and are carried out largely by family members and volunteers. By using volunteer workers and the existing infrastructure in the communities, this form of rehabilitation minimizes costs of delivering services and is assumed to be cost-effective relative to the alternative institution-based rehabilitation (Institute of Medicine Committee on Nervous System Disorders in Developing Countries 2001; WHO Community-Based Rehabilitation 1982; Lagerkvist 1992). Institutional care has higher costs because it relies on paid staff, medical equipment, building maintenance, and medical costs. Some advocate for provision of institutional, center-based, medical, and community-based approaches in a complementary fashion. In a Zimbabwean community-based rehabilitation project two-thirds of the patients were referred to hospitals or clinics (Rottier and others 1993). Annual costs for training workshops and salaries of rehabilitation workers amounted to US$60,000 to treat 1,614 individuals with disabilities.

Little information is available about the full costs of community-based rehabilitation and how they vary across disabilities, age groups, and societies. The cost-effectiveness of such rehabilitation or whether its costs are lower than alternative rehabilitation models is unknown. It is usually implemented in settings where no other rehabilitation models exist. The costs to consumers in terms of their efforts, time, and money may be substantial (Thomas and Thomas 1998). No formal estimates are available of time costs and opportunity costs to family members involved in community-based rehabilitation. Meeting the needs of a family member with a disability may prohibit or disrupt labor force participation of the caregiver and reduce family income. This need for caregiving may especially affect women (Giacaman 2001). The effectiveness of community-based rehabilitation in improving functional outcomes for children with cerebral palsy in Bangladesh showed no improvement, but researchers unexpectedly found a significant increase in reported stress and symptoms of depression in the mothers of children in the community-based rehabilitation intervention group (McConachie and others 2000).

Efficacy. Other attempts to evaluate community-based rehabilitation in different settings and for a range of outcomes include one for preschool children with disabilities in rural Guyana. The children showed significant improvement after six months in the program, and noticeable improvements in the attitudes of parents and others toward children with disabilities were seen (O'Toole 1988). Community-based rehabilitation programs in the Philippines and Zimbabwe found gains in activities of daily living and communication as well as higher rates of starting school and employment after six months in the program (Lagerkvist 1992). Similarly, people with disabilities participating in a community-based rehabilitation program in Botswana showed high levels of independence in activities of daily living; 20 percent of adults were working, and most school-age children were attending class (Lundgren-Lindquist and Nordholm 1996).

Some have questioned the efficacy of community-based rehabilitation and its ability to expand access for people with disabilities. Many people with disabilities do not patronize such programs, and many who do try leave dissatisfied (Kassah 1998). After initial diagnosis, only half of the identified individuals with disabilities continued (Rottier and others 1993). Community-based rehabilitation programs also face the difficulty of working in diverse communities with unique cultural, religious, economic, and social conditions, making it difficult for a single model to meet the needs for rehabilitation services in developing countries (Crishna 1999).

Prevention of Premature Birth

Premature birth—after 20 weeks but before 37 weeks—is a powerful predictor of death and disability. Infants born before 28 weeks of gestation have a 50-fold increased risk of cerebral palsy (Drummond and Colver 2002) and heightened risk of sensory, cognitive, and educational impairment (Taylor and others 2004). The rate of preterm births in the United State has increased steadily since 1990 (MacDorman and others 2002). Survival of infants born before 34 weeks requires intensive and expensive medical care (Gilbert, Nesbitt, and Danielsen 2003), and the global survival rate differs depending on neonatal care availability (Lorenz and others 2001). Infection or inflammation of the placenta is common in preterm pregnancies (Goldenberg and Culhane 2003), and many deaths attributed to asphyxia may be caused by maternal, placental, or neonatal infection. The cerebral palsy rate is significantly higher in premature infants whose births are monitored electronically (Shy and others 1990). With the exception of magnesium sulfate administered to women in preterm labor (Crowther and others 2003), no specific interventions result in decreased cerebral palsy among premature infants (Crowther and Henderson-Smart 2004).

Dietary supplements might decrease the frequency of low-birthweight births and perhaps the frequency of marked prematurity. In Bangladesh, where the rate of preterm labor was high, women who went into labor before term were older, shorter, thinner, less educated, and more disadvantaged economically, with closer spacing of births (Begum, Buckshe, and Pande 2003). Deaths attributable to prematurity in LMICs are seldom due to poor management and are largely related to poor health facilities (Pattinson 2004).

Electronic Fetal Monitoring in Labor

For decades most cerebral palsy and a major share of MR, epilepsy, and learning and behavioral disorders of childhood were considered to be due to deprivation of oxygen supply to the fetus during birth. Recent research confirms that only a minority of cerebral palsy cases, as well as associated MR and seizures, are related to markers of birth asphyxia (Nelson and Ellenberg 1986; Torfs and others 1990). Low Apgar scores, the need for respiratory support, and neonatal seizures are more commonly due to etiologies other than asphyxia, most notably intrauterine exposure to infection (Wu and others 2003). So that medical workers could recognize the onset of asphyxia and "rescue" the fetus, continuous electronic fetal monitoring (EFM) of the fetal heart rate during labor was introduced in the 1970s. This intervention was disseminated before being tested in randomized trials to compare continuous electronic monitoring with intermittent observation by stethoscope (auscultation). Since the introduction of EFM, fetal death in labor has decreased, the cesarean section rate has quadrupled (Natale and Dodman 2003), and the rate of cerebral palsy has remained steady. Accordingly, EFM cannot be recommended for use in LMICs. Intermittent auscultation with a stethoscope appears to be the appropriate way to monitor fetal status during labor.

RESEARCH AGENDA FOR PREVENTION OF DISABILITIES IN LOW- AND MIDDLE-INCOME COUNTRIES

Research needed as a basis for developing policies and interventions to prevent LDD in low- and middle-income countries includes basic research, epidemiology, and evaluations of early interventions, clinical treatments, prevention strategies, and health services that are culturally appropriate and feasible. Suggested research priorities include the following:

- etiology and prevention of adverse pregnancy outcomes associated with LDD, such as low birthweight, preterm birth, intrauterine growth retardation, and related factors
- community-based rehabilitation, including effectiveness, cost-effectiveness, and social effects of different models for providing rehabilitation services and special education to children with LDD in LMICs

- methodological and prevalence studies to ensure that the impacts of LDD are effectively measured by DALYs or other international indicators
- cost-effectiveness of interventions to prevent specific nutritional, infectious, genetic, and other causes of LDD
- impact on child development of multiple insults and risk factors especially common in LMICs, such as neurotoxic exposures, trauma, infectious disease or malnutrition, poverty, maternal illiteracy, and other social factors
- health services research related to access to prenatal care and prenatal and newborn screening and evaluation of components of the public health system that might impair or enhance integration of services for patients with LDD
- prevalence of ADHD and a cost-benefit analysis of the use of psychotropic medications
- prevalence and costs of autism spectrum disorders
- strategies to improve interventions for the prevention of fetal alcohol syndrome and to develop effective intervention programs for children affected by prenatal alcohol exposure
- evaluation of criteria for newborn screening and effects of new technology on measured incidence, costs, and system effectiveness
- evaluation of financing of successful newborn screening and treatment programs
- model systems of care for individuals diagnosed through newborn screening from infancy to adulthood.

SUMMARY

Many potential interventions exist for the prevention of LDDs, and relatively few are being implemented for the benefit of children in LMICs. The following three interventions are effective and cost-effective in preventing LDD:

- Folic acid fortification of the food supply can reduce the occurrence of NTDs by 50 percent or more. This intervention was found to be highly cost-effective in the United States; however, in low-income countries, high capital and running costs may compromise cost-effectiveness, at least in the short run.
- Prenatal screening and selective pregnancy termination to prevent DS are highly cost-effective under some conditions but raise ethical, social, and cultural concerns that may preclude their applicability in some LMICs. Screening is not only expensive; it also has negative health outcomes: the false-positive rates and the subsequent anxiety, a risk of miscarriage of an unaffected pregnancy, and the resulting potential complications from pregnancy termination. Another concern is that, where access to prenatal care is limited, the potential for public health benefits of prenatal screening will be small.

- Neonatal screening and treatment for CH is highly cost-effective in developed countries, where it provides a low-cost strategy for preventing MR. For minimal extra cost, collected blood samples from newborns can also be used to identify and prevent the disabling effects of other inborn errors of metabolism, such as phenylketonuria and maple syrup urine disease. However, when only a part of the newborn population is reached by screening, high costs will be incurred to care for those missed by the screening, thereby reducing the cost-benefit ratio.

For another type of intervention considered, community-based rehabilitation, costs and benefits have not been quantified sufficiently to allow evaluation. Such rehabilitation is designed to expand access to services in poor and rural areas, to change negative attitudes toward disability, to lower the costs of delivering services, and to enhance the participation of persons with disabilities in society. The benefits of community-based rehabilitation may come at a high cost in terms of time and financial resources of family members.

Another intervention, electronic fetal monitoring in labor, has been shown to be unsuccessful in preventing childhood neurological disability associated with premature birth: the risk of cerebral palsy was significantly higher in infants delivered using EFM. Consequently, this intervention is not recommended for use during labor.

DALY estimates are not available to convey the full range of LDDs or their risk factors. However, available data are consistent with the possibility that these disabilities account for a large proportion of the global burden of disease. Quantifying the impacts of LDDs and their preventive interventions is complicated by the fact that these disorders can exist at multiple levels and that disability is context-specific, with impacts that may vary across cultures. Several research priorities for improving knowledge and developing policies and interventions to prevent LDD in LMICs are suggested.

ACKNOWLEDGMENTS

The authors thank Emmy Cauthen at the Fogarty International Center for her support.

REFERENCES

Alliance to End Childhood Lead Poisoning. 2002. "The Global Lead Initiative: A Proposed Outcome for the World Summit on Sustainable Development." Alliance to End Childhood Lead Poisoning, Washington, DC. http://www.globalleadnet.org/pdf/GlobalLeadInitiative.pdf.

Bagriansky, J. No date. "What Are the Costs for the Premixes?" http://www.sph.emory.edu/wheatflour/Comm/Resource/CDs/Bali/Bali_files/v3_slide0089.htm.

Barden, H. S., and R. Kessel. 1984. "The Costs and Benefits of Screening for Congenital Hypothyroidism in Wisconsin." Social Biology 31 (3–4): 185–200.

Beaulieu, M. D. 1994. "Screening for Congenital Hypothyroidism." In Canadian Guide to Clinical Preventive Health Care, ed. Canadian Task Force on the Periodic Health Examination. Ottawa: Health Canada.

Begum, F., K. Buckshe, and J. N. Pande. 2003. "Risk Factors Associated with Preterm Labour." Bangladesh Medical Research Council Bulletin 29 (2): 59–66.

Benedict, R. E., and A. M. Farel. 2003. "Identifying Children in Need of Ancillary and Enabling Services: A Population Approach." Social Science and Medicine 57 (11): 2035–47.

Bobat, R., D. Moodley, A. Coutsoudis, H. Coovadia, and E. Gouws. 1998. "The Early Natural History of Vertically Transmitted HIV-1 Infection in African Children from Durban, South Africa." Annals of Tropical Paediatrics 18 (3): 187–96.

Brouwers, P., C. Decarli, M. P. Heyes, H. A. Moss, P. L. Wolters, G. Tudor-Williams, and others. 1996. "Neurobehavioral Manifestations of Symptomatic HIV-1 Disease in Children: Can Nutritional Factors Play a Role?" Journal of Nutrition 126 (Suppl. 10): S2651–62.

Chan, E., C. Zhan, and C. J. Homer. 2002. "Health Care Use and Costs for Children with Attention-Deficit/Hyperactivity Disorder: National Estimates from the Medical Expenditure Panel Survey." Archives of Pediatrics and Adolescent Medicine 156 (5): 504–11.

Crishna, B. 1999. "What Is Community-Based Rehabilitation? A View from Experience." Child: Care, Health, and Development 25 (1): 27–35.

Crowther, C. A., and D. J. Henderson-Smart. 2004. "Vitamin K Prior to Preterm Birth for Preventing Neonatal Periventricular Haemorrhage." Cochrane Database of Systematic Reviews (4).

Crowther, C. A., J. E. Hiller, L. W. Doyle, and R. R. Haslam. 2003. "Effect of Magnesium Sulfate Given for Neuroprotection before Preterm Birth: A Randomized Controlled Trial." Journal of the American Medical Association 290 (20): 2669–76.

Cunningham, G. C., and D. G. Tompkinison. 1999. "Cost and Effectiveness of the California Triple Marker Prenatal Screening Program." Genetics in Medicine 1 (5): 199–206.

Cusick, W., P. Buchanan, T. W. Hallahan, D. A. Krantz, J. W. Larsen Jr., and J. N. Macri. 2003. "Combined First-Trimester versus Second-Trimester Serum Screening for Down Syndrome: A Cost Analysis." American Journal of Obstetrics and Gynecology 188 (3): 745–51.

Cutts, F. T., S. E. Robertson, J. L. Diaz-Ortega, and R. Samuel. 1997. "Control of Rubella and Congenital Rubella Syndrome (CRS) in Developing Countries, Part 1: Burden of Disease from CRS." Bulletin of the World Health Organization 75 (1): 55–68.

Dhondt, J. L., J. P. Farriaux, J. C. Sailly, and T. Lebrun. 1991. "Economic Evaluation of Cost-Benefit Ratio of Neonatal Screening Procedure for Phenylketonuria and Hypothyroidism." Journal of Inherited Metabolic Disease 14 (4): 633–39.

Drummond, P. M., and A. F. Colver. 2002. "Analysis by Gestational Age of Cerebral Palsy in Singleton Births in North-East England 1970–94." Paediatric and Perinatal Epidemiology 16 (2): 172–80.

Durkin, M. 2002. "The Epidemiology of Developmental Disabilities in Low-Income Countries." Mental Retardation and Developmental Disabilities Research Reviews 8 (3): 206–11.

Fewtrell, L. J., A. Pruss-Ustun, P. Landrigan, and J. L. Ayuso-Mateos. 2004. "Estimating the Global Burden of Disease of Mild Mental Retardation and Cardiovascular Diseases from Environmental Lead Exposure." Environmental Research 94 (2): 120–33.

Floyd, R. L., and J. S. Sidhu. 2004. "Monitoring Prenatal Alcohol Exposure." American Journal of Medical Genetics 127C (1): 3–9.

Ford, C., A. J. Moore, P. A. Jordan, W. A. Bartlett, M. P. Wyldes, A. F. Jones, and W. E. MacKenzie. 1998. "The Value of Screening for Down's Syndrome in a Socioeconomically Deprived Area with a High Ethnic Population." *British Journal of Obstetrics and Gynaecology* 105 (8): 855–59.

Giacaman, R. 2001. "A Community of Citizens: Disability Rehabilitation in the Palestinian Transition to Statehood." *Disability and Rehabilitation* 23 (14): 639–44.

Gilbert, R. E., C. Augood, R. Gupta, A. E. Ades, S. Logan, M. Sculpher, and J. H. van der Meulen. 2001. "Screening for Down's Syndrome: Effects, Safety, and Cost Effectiveness of First and Second Trimester Strategies." *British Medical Journal* 323 (7310): 423–25.

Gilbert, W. M., T. S. Nesbitt, and B. Danielsen. 2003. "The Cost of Prematurity: Quantification by Gestational Age and Birth Weight." *Obstetrics and Gynecology* 102 (3): 488–92.

Goldenberg, R. L., and J. F. Culhane. 2003. "Infection as a Cause of Preterm Birth." *Clinics in Perinatology* 30 (4): 677–700.

Gupta, R., R. D. Thomas, V. Sreenivas, S. Walter, and J. M. Puliyel. 2001. "Ultrasonographic Femur-Tibial Length Ratio: A Marker of Down Syndrome from the Late Second Trimester." *American Journal of Perinatology* 18 (4): 217–24.

Insinga, R. P., R. H. Laessig, and G. L. Hoffman. 2002. "Newborn Screening with Tandem Mass Spectrometry: Examining Its Cost-Effectiveness in the Wisconsin Newborn Screening Panel." *Journal of Pediatrics* 141 (4): 524–31.

Institute of Medicine. 2003. *Reducing Birth Defects: Meeting the Challenge in the Developing World.* Washington, DC: National Academies Press.

Institute of Medicine Committee on Nervous System Disorders in Developing Countries. 2001. *Neurological, Psychiatric, and Developmental Disorders: Meeting the Challenges in the Developing World.* Washington, DC: National Academies Press.

Kassah, A. K. 1998. "Community-Based Rehabilitation and Stigma Management by Physically Disabled People in Ghana." *Disability and Rehabilitation* 20 (2): 66–73.

Khan, N. Z., and A. H. Khan. 1999. "Lead Poisoning and Psychomotor Delay in Bangladeshi Children." *Lancet* 353 (9154): 754.

Kline, J. K., Z. Stein, and M. Susser. 1989. *Conception to Birth: Epidemiology of Prenatal Development.* New York: Oxford University Press.

Lagerkvist, B. 1992. "Community-Based Rehabilitation—Outcome for the Disabled in the Philippines and Zimbabwe." *Disability and Rehabilitation* 14 (1): 44–50.

Lakhani, M., M. Khurshid, S. H. Naqvi, and M. Akber. 1989. "Neonatal Screening for Congenital Hypothyroidism in Pakistan." *Journal of the Pakistan Medical Association* 39 (11): 282–84.

Layde, P. M., S. D. Von Allmen, and G. P. Oakley Jr. 1979. "Congenital Hypothyroidism Control Programs: A Cost-Benefit Analysis." *Journal of the American Medical Association* 241 (21): 2290–92.

Lippman, A., D. J. Tomkins, J. Shime, and J. L. Hamerton. 1992. "Canadian Multicentre Randomized Clinical Trial of Chorion Villus Sampling and Amniocentesis: Final Report." *Prenatal Diagnosis* 12 (5): 385–408.

Lord, J., M. J. Thomason, P. Littlejohns, R. A. Chalmers, M. D. Bain, G. M. Addison, and others. 1999. "Secondary Analysis of Economic Data: A Review of Cost-Benefit Studies of Neonatal Screening for Phenylketonuria." *Journal of Epidemiology and Community Health* 53 (3): 179–86.

Lorenz, J. M., N. Paneth, J. R. Jetton, L. den Ouden, and J. E. Tyson. 2001. "Comparison of Management Strategies for Extreme Prematurity in New Jersey and the Netherlands: Outcomes and Resource Expenditure." *Pediatrics* 108 (6): 1269–74.

Lundgren-Lindquist, B., and L. A. Nordholm. 1996. "The Impact of Community-Based Rehabilitation as Perceived by Disabled People in a Village in Botswana." *Disability and Rehabilitation* 18 (7): 329–34.

Lupton, C., L. Burd, and R. Harwood. 2004. "Cost of Fetal Alcohol Spectrum Disorders." *American Journal of Medical Genetics* 127C (1): 42–50.

MacDorman, M. F., A. M. Minino, D. M. Strobino, and B. Guyer. 2002. "Annual Summary of Vital Statistics—2001." *Pediatrics* 110 (6): 1037–52.

Mathers, C. D., A. D. Lopez, and C. J. L. Murray. "The Burden of Disease and Mortality by Condition: Data, Methods, and Results for 2001." In *Global Burden of Disease and Risk Factors,* eds. A. D. Lopez, C. D. Mathers, M. Ezzati, D. T. Jamison, and C. J. L. Murray. New York: Oxford University Press.

May, P. A., L. Brooke, J. P. Gossage, J. Croxford, C. Adnams, K. L. Jones, and others. 2000. "Epidemiology of Fetal Alcohol Syndrome in a South African Community in the Western Cape Province." *American Journal of Public Health* 90 (12): 1905–12.

McConachie, H., S. Huq, S. Munir, S. Ferdous, S. Zaman, and N. Z. Khan. 2000. "A Randomized Controlled Trial of Alternative Modes of Service Provision to Young Children with Cerebral Palsy in Bangladesh." *Journal of Pediatrics* 137 (6): 769–76.

McGrother, C. W., and B. Marshall. 1990. "Recent Trends in Incidence, Morbidity and Survival in Down's Syndrome." *Journal of Mental Deficiency Research* 34 (Part 1): 49–57.

Natale, R., and N. Dodman. 2003. "Birth Can Be a Hazardous Journey: Electronic Fetal Monitoring Does Not Help." *Journal of Obstetrics and Gynaecology Canada* 25 (12): 1007–9.

Nelson, K. B., and J. H. Ellenberg. 1986. "Antecedents of Cerebral Palsy: Multivariate Analysis of Risk." *New England Journal of Medicine* 315 (2): 81–86.

Nyberg, D. A., D. A. Luthy, R. G. Resta, B. C. Nyberg, and M. A. Williams. 1998. "Age-Adjusted Ultrasound Risk Assessment for Fetal Down's Syndrome during the Second Trimester: Description of the Method and Analysis of 142 Cases." *Ultrasound Obstetrics and Gynecology* 12 (1): 8–14.

O'Toole, B. 1988. "A Community-Based Rehabilitation Programme for Pre-school Disabled Children in Guyana." *International Journal of Rehabilitation Research* 11 (4): 323–34.

Panepinto, J. A., D. Magid, M. J. Rewers, and P. A. Lane. 2000. "Universal versus Targeted Screening of Infants for Sickle Cell Disease: A Cost-Effectiveness Analysis." *Journal of Pediatrics* 136 (2): 201–8.

Pattinson, R. C. 2004. "Are Deaths Due to Prematurity Avoidable in Developing Countries?" *Tropical Doctor* 34 (1): 7–10.

Peden, M., R. Scurfiled, D. Sleet, D. Mohan, A. Hyder, E. Jarawan, and C. Mather, eds. 2004. *World Report on Road Traffic Injury Prevention.* Geneva: World Health Organization.

Robertson, S. E., F. T. Cutts, R. Samuel, and J. L. Diaz-Ortega. 1997. "Control of Rubella and Congenital Rubella Syndrome (CRS) in Developing Countries, Part 2: Vaccination against Rubella." *Bulletin of the World Health Organization* 75 (1): 69–80.

Romano, P. S., N. J. Waitzman, R. M. Scheffler, and R. D. Pi. 1995. "Folic Acid Fortification of Grain: An Economic Analysis." *American Journal of Public Health* 85 (5): 667–76.

Ross, H. L., and S. Elias. 1997. "Maternal Serum Screening for Fetal Genetic Disorders." *Obstetrics and Gynecology Clinics of North America* 24 (1): 33–47.

Rottier, M. J. N., R. W. Broer, A. Vermeer, and H. J. M. Finkenflügel. 1993. "A Study of Follow Up of Clients in Community-Based Rehabilitation Projects in Zimbabwe." *Journal of Rehabilitation Sciences* 6 (2): 35–41.

Sack, J., I. Feldman, and I. Kaiserman. 1998. "Congenital Hypothyroidism Screening in the West Bank: A Test Case for Screening in Developing Regions." *Hormone Research* 50 (3): 151–54.

Sampson, P. D., A. P. Streissguth, F. L. Bookstein, R. E. Little, S. K. Clarren, P. Dehaene, and others. 1997. "Incidence of Fetal Alcohol Syndrome and Prevalence of Alcohol-Related Neurodevelopmental Disorder." *Teratology* 56 (5): 317–26.

Shy, K. K., D. A. Luthy, F. C. Bennett, M. Whitfield, E. B. Larson, G. van Belle, and others. 1990. "Effects of Electronic Fetal-Heart-Rate Monitoring, as Compared with Periodic Auscultation, on the Neurologic Development of Premature Infants." *New England Journal of Medicine* 322 (9): 588–93.

Sokol, R. J., V. Delaney-Black, and B. Nordstrom. 2003. "Fetal Alcohol Spectrum Disorder." *Journal of the American Medical Association* 290 (22): 2996–99.

Stein, R. E., and D. J. Jessop. 2003. "The Impact on Family Scale Revisited: Further Psychometric Data." *Journal of Developmental and Behavioral Pediatrics* 24 (1): 9–16.

Stray-Pedersen, B., J. Biornstad, M. Dahl, T. Bergan, G. Aanestad, L. Kristiansen, and K. Hansen. 1991. "Induced Abortion: Microbiological Screening and Medical Complications." *Infection* 19 (5): 305–8.

Taylor, H. G., N. M. Minich, N. Klein, and M. Hack. 2004. "Longitudinal Outcomes of Very Low Birth Weight: Neuropsychological Findings." *Journal of the International Neuropsychological Society* 10 (2): 149–63.

Thomas, M., and M. J. Thomas. 1998. "Controversies on Some Conceptual issues in Community-Based Rehabilitation." *Asia Pacific Disability Rehabilitation Journal* 9 (1): 12–14.

Thompson, D. C., F. P. Rivara, and R. Thompson. 1999. "Helmets for Preventing Head and Facial Injuries in Bicyclists." Cochrane Database of Systematic Reviews (4) CD001855.

Tillotson, S. L., P. W. Fuggle, I. Smith, A. E. Ades, and D. B. Grant. 1994. "Relation between Biochemical Severity and Intelligence in Early Treated Congenital Hypothyroidism: A Threshold Effect." *British Medical Journal* 309 (6952): 440–45.

Torfs, C. P., B. van den Berg, F. W. Oechsli, and S. Cummins. 1990. "Prenatal and Perinatal Factors in the Etiology of Cerebral Palsy." *Journal of Pediatrics* 116 (4): 615–19.

Valent, F., D. Little, R. Bertollini, L. E. Nemer, F. Barbone, and G. Tamburlini. 2004. "Burden of Disease Attributable to Selected Environmental Factors and Injury among Children and Adolescents in Europe." *Lancet* 363 (9426): 2032–39.

Viljoen, D. 1999. "Fetal Alcohol Syndrome." *South African Medical Journal* 89 (9): 958–60.

Vintzileos, A. M., C. V. Ananth, J. C. Smulian, D. L. Day-Salvatore, T. Beazoglou, and R. A. Knuppel. 2000. "Cost-Benefit Analysis of Prenatal Diagnosis for Down Syndrome Using the British or the American Approach." *Obstetrics and Gynecology* 95 (4): 577–83.

Waitzman, N. J., P. S. Romano, and R. M. Scheffler. 1994. "Estimates of the Economic Costs of Birth Defects." *Inquiry* 31 (2): 188–205.

Wald, N. J., C. Rodeck, A. K. Hackshaw, J. Walters, L. Chitty, and A. M. Mackinson. 2003. "First and Second Trimester Screening for Down's Syndrome: The Results of the Serum, Urine and Ultrasound Screening Study (SURUSS)." *Health Technology Assessment* 7 (11): 1–77.

Wasant, P., S. Liammongkolkul, and C. Srisawat. 1999. "Neonatal Screening for Congenital Hypothyroidism and Phenylketonuria at Siriraj Hospital, Mahidol University, Bangkok, Thailand—A Pilot Study." *Southeast Asian Journal of Tropical Medicine and Public Health* 30 (Suppl. 2): 33–37.

WHO (World Health Organization). 2001. *International Classification of Functioning, Disability and Health.* Geneva: WHO. http://www3.who.int/icf/icftemplate.cfm?myurl=homepage.html&mytitle=Home%20Page.

WHO Community-Based Rehabilitation. 1982. "Report of a WHO Interregional Consultation." Colombo, Sri Lanka.

Winter, S., A. Autry, C. Boyle, and M. Yeargin-Allsopp. 2002. "Trends in the Prevalence of Cerebral Palsy in a Population-Based Study." *Pediatrics* 110 (6): 1220–25.

Wu, Y. W., G. J. Escobar, J. K. Grether, L. A. Croen, J. D. Greene, and T. B. Newman. 2003. "Chorioamnionitis and Cerebral Palsy in Term and Near-Term Infants." *Journal of the American Medical Association* 290 (20): 2677–84.

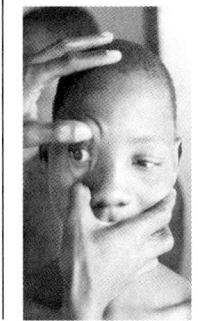

Chapter **50**

Loss of Vision and Hearing

Joseph Cook, Kevin D. Frick, Rob Baltussen, Serge Resnikoff, Andrew Smith, Jeffrey Mecaskey, and Peter Kilima

Although the loss of vision and hearing has multiple causes, and the burden of these diseases is complex, three major points emerge from the outset:

- Impairments of the essential senses of vision and hearing contribute to early demise and are important causes of morbidity for individuals who are blind or deaf.
- Cost-effective interventions are available to address several causes of these burdens now.
- The number of cost-effectiveness analyses of interventions to preserve hearing or vision in developing countries is quite limited.

Table 50.1 summarizes the conditions causing the sensory deficits, the proposed interventions and sites of delivery, and the cost and effectiveness of these interventions to the extent of current knowledge. Earlier work by Evans and others (1996) in Myanmar does not appear because the cost data are quite old and because the cost-effectiveness data were in dollars per case of blindness averted rather than dollars per disability-adjusted life year (DALY) averted, which the latest information provides.

NATURE, CAUSES, AND EPIDEMIOLOGY OF VISION LOSS

Table 50.2 provides definitions of visual impairment, blindness, and low vision according to the *International Classification of Diseases, Injuries, and Causes of Death* (WHO 1993). At this time, the World Health Organization (WHO) is considering changing the classification in order to take into

account uncorrected refractive errors, but this change has not yet been approved.

The major causes of adult-onset blindness are cataract (47.8 percent), glaucoma (12.3 percent), macular degeneration (8.7 percent), diabetic retinopathy (4.8 percent), trachoma (3.6 percent), and onchocerciasis (0.8 percent). Uncorrected refractive errors are also a major cause of morbidity related to vision, but this type of disability is not included in the global burden of disease by definition. It has been estimated to be on the order of 15 percent of the total blind population and could add 50 percent to the low-vision population. However, there are no published data to do more than speculate.

The major causes of childhood vision loss have marked regional variations. They include vitamin A deficiency (xerophthalmia) and ophthalmia neonatorum in low-income countries, retinopathy of prematurity and hereditary conditions in middle-income countries, and congenital cataract and glaucoma everywhere. Table 50.3 shows the estimated number of blind persons worldwide in 2002.

Vision loss is chronic and, almost invariably, without remission. The extent of morbidity is related to the level of alteration of vision function. However, 80 percent of cases are avoidable, either through treatment (cataract and refractive errors) or through primary prevention (onchocerciasis, trachoma, glaucoma, and diabetic retinopathy). Strictly speaking, blindness attributable to glaucoma and diabetic retinopathy can be prevented. However, prevention depends on the availability of a simple, cheap, and efficacious diagnostic test and rigorous treatment. These are not readily amenable to public health programs even in the most technologically advanced countries, especially in the case of glaucoma.

Table 50.1 Cost and Effectiveness Data for Vision and Hearing Care Interventions

Condition	Intervention	Cost data (2004 US$)	Effectiveness data	Incremental cost-effectiveness data (2004 US$/DALY averted)
Trachoma	Trichiasis surgery	7.14 per village-based surgery[a]	77 percent cure rate over two years[b]	4–82[c]
	Tetracycline	—	51 percent cure rate in children at six months following treatment[d]	>9,600[d]
	Azithromycin	—	88 percent cure rate in children at six months following treatment[e]	>4,100[d]
Cataract	Extracapsular surgery	—	—	<200 (low- and middle-income countries); <2,400 (high-income countries)[b]
Onchocerciasis	Ivermectin	—	—	40[f]

Source: Authors.
— = not available.
a. Frick, Keuffel, and Bowman 2001.
b. Baltussen, Sylla, and Mariotti 2004.
c. Baltussen and others (2005). Cost-effectiveness calculations are based on data from Frick and others (2001) for mass treatment of children only, not greater efficacy reported by Bowman and others (2000) and Solomon and others (2004) for mass treatment of entire communities. The greater efficacy reported in mass treatment of entire communities may lead to better cost-effectiveness.
d. Bowman and others 2000.
e. Reacher and others 1992.
f. Waters, Rehwinkel, and Burnham 2004.

Table 50.2 Definitions of Visual Impairment Levels

Degree of impairment	Definition	Visual impairment categories
Low vision	Visual acuity of less than 6/18 (Snellen 20/70) but equal to or better than 3/60 (20/400) in the better eye with best possible correction	1 and 2
Blindness	Visual acuity of less than 3/60 (20/400) or corresponding visual field loss of less than 10 degrees in the better eye with best possible correction	3, 4, and 5
Visual impairment	Blindness as well as low vision	1, 2, 3, 4, and 5

Source: Authors, based on current international definitions by WHO 1993.

Table 50.3 Number of Blind Worldwide in 2002 from Various Conditions

Condition	Number blind (millions)
Cataract	17.6
Glaucoma	4.5
Age-related macular degeneration	3.2
Corneal opacity	1.9
Diabetic retinopathy	1.8
Childhood blindness	1.4
Trachoma	1.3
Onchocerciasis	0.3
Other causes	4.8
Total	36.8

Sources: Pascolini and others 2004; Resnikoff and others 2004.

Burden of Loss for Vision and Risk Factors

The risk factors for loss of vision are age, gender, poverty, and poor access to health care. The overall prevalence of vision loss, which mainly affects the population above age 40, is a function of age. It is estimated that more than 82.2 percent of all blind individuals are 50 or older. Increasing life expectancy results in a growing number of cases of age-related blindness (for example, cataract, glaucoma, macular degeneration). Among the 50 and older age group, cigarette smoking is a clear risk factor for both cataract and macular degeneration. Childhood vision loss represents approximately 4 percent of the total number of visually impaired. However, it is the second largest cause of "blind-person years," following cataract. Retinopathy of prematurity

(ROP) is an important cause in middle-income countries (Gilbert and Foster 2001). Unfortunately, screening for ROP in preterm infants, as well as the organization and provision of low-vision services, is a tertiary-level function (requiring a well-equipped clinic or hospital with the most modern facilities), and no data on cost-effectiveness of interventions are available. More disease-specific factors are poor hygiene, overcrowding, ultraviolet radiation, diabetes mellitus, drugs, micronutrient deficiency, heredity and ethnic background, and consanguinity.

Estimates of the global burden of visual impairment in 2002 were updated using the most recent available data on blindness and low vision (Pascolini and others 2004). The global number of people who are visually impaired is in excess of 161 million, of whom 36.8 million are blind (Resnikoff and others 2004). Because the international definition refers to the best-corrected visual acuity (table 50.2), these figures actually underestimate the magnitude of the global burden of the visual impairment, especially in developing countries, where most of the refractive errors are not corrected (Dandona and Dandona 2003; Fotouhi and others 2004; Naidoo and others 2004). A WHO working group has recommended the use of the more accurate "presenting vision," recognizing that many people do not have their best-corrected vision. This recommendation is under review and, if approved, would substantially increase the estimates of the burden of disease attributable to impaired vision.

The number of women with visual impairment, as estimated from the available studies, is higher than that of men, even after adjustment for age. Female-to-male prevalence ratios indicate that women are more likely to have a visual impairment than men in every region of the world: the ratios from past studies range between 1.5 to 1 and 2.2 to 1. (Resnikoff and others 2004). The major reported reason is women's reduced access to eye care services. Higher exposure to risk factors also contributes in the case of trachoma. (Abou-Gareeb and others 2001; Nirmalan, Padmavathi, and Thulasiraj 2003).

Several population-based surveys reported higher risk of mortality among people with visual impairment. Relative risk of mortality among blind and low-vision people varied from 1.5 to 4.1 and from 1.1 to 1.6, respectively. In industrial countries, the relative risk of mortality varied from 1.6 to 2.0. The effect may vary by gender (Lee and others 2002; Taylor and others 1991). The link between visual impairment and mortality remains poorly understood and cannot be attributed to known associations with underlying disease.

The burden from visual impairment accounts for approximately 3 percent of the total global burden of disease and 9 percent of total years lived with disability in 2001. Table 50.4 shows the global burden by vision-related cause in DALYs. Globally, half of the burden from visual impairment is due to cataract.

The burden of visual impairment is not distributed uniformly throughout the world; the least developed regions carry the largest share, as shown by World Bank region in table 50.5. Local and in-country variations, as well as regional variations, are related to the following factors:

- Epidemiology of cause (for example, onchocerciasis, trachoma).

Table 50.4 Global Burden of Visual Impairment, by Major Cause, 2002

Condition	Blindness (thousands of DALYs)	Low vision (thousands of DALYs)	Visual impairment		
			Thousands of DALYs	Percentage of total YLDs	Percentage of total DALYs
Cataract	8,798	15,053	25,251	4.5	1.7
Glaucoma	1,202	2,442	3,866	0.7	0.3
Trachoma	1,403	772	2,329	0.4	0.2
Onchocerciasis	203	146	484	0.1	0.0
Other	4,657	8,814	14,191	2.5	1.0
Total	16,263	27,227	46,121	8.2	3.2

Source: Pascolini and others 2004; Resnikoff and others 2004.
YLDs = years of life lived with disability.

Table 50.5 Global Burden of Visual Impairment, by World Bank Region, 2002 (thousands of DALYs)

Condition	East Asia and the Pacific	Europe and Central Asia	Latin America and the Caribbean	Middle East and North Africa	South Asia	Sub-Saharan Africa	Worldwide
Cataract	6,141	239	956	934	10,259	5,369	23,898
Glaucoma	1,184	168	165	401	566	1,009	3,493
Trachoma	410	0	102	201	226	1,272	2,211
Onchocerciasis	0	0	1	23	0	458	482
Other	5,821	903	1,031	971	2,447	1,046	12,219
Total	13,556	1,310	2,255	2,530	13,458	9,154	42,303

Source: Pascolini and others 2004; calculated from Resnikoff and others 2004.

- Socioeconomic patterns (poverty and socioeconomic deprivation), an essential element in most causes.
- Access to adequate eye care. Uneven access to good-quality eye care (for example, for cataract, glaucoma, diabetic retinopathy) results from such factors as distance, affordability, and culture. Lack of resources is only part of the problem; existing facilities are sometimes underused.

Interventions

Not all causes of visual impairment can be addressed using public health types of interventions. Cataract, trachoma, childhood blindness, and onchocerciasis are discussed below.

Cataract. Surgery to remove the opacified lens is the only effective treatment for cataracts. Neither diet nor medications have been shown to stop cataract formation. There are several possible approaches for the surgical extraction of cataracts. Intracapsular cataract extraction using aphakic glasses is a technique by which the whole lens is removed from the eye. After surgery, special eyeglasses are provided to patients to restore sight. A disadvantage of this intervention is the noncompliance of people who need to wear glasses, which has been found to be between 18 and 73 percent. Although this behavior may be characterized as noncompliance, it must be said that some programs do not provide glasses or provide aphakic glasses of inferior quality. Also, replacing needed aphakic glasses is impossible for some patients. It is also true that aphakic glasses cause tremendous distortions in vision, thus impairing compliance.

In extracapsular cataract extraction with implantation of a posterior chamber intraocular lens, the lens and the front portion of the capsule are removed and then replaced with an artificial lens. Baltussen, Sylla, and Mariotti (2004) have evaluated work on the cost-effectiveness of cataract surgery. That work (done by WHO regions rather than by World Bank regions) showed that both intracapsular and extracapsular surgeries are cost-effective ways to reduce the impact of cataract blindness. However, extracapsular surgery is both less costly and more effective than intracapsular surgery and can therefore be considered the best choice for cataract control. Its cost-effectiveness ratios are below US$200 per DALY averted in low- and middle-income countries and below US$2,400 in high-income countries.

Trachoma. WHO recommends an integrative approach to trachoma control through its SAFE strategy (surgery, antibiotics to control the infection, facial cleanliness, and environmental improvements). The facial cleanliness and environmental improvements are preventive public health measures aimed at reducing the incidence of infection. Antibiotic treatment, especially when given on a mass or community basis, is both primary prevention (reducing transmission in the community) and secondary prevention (treating active infection to avoid

morbidity). Surgery is in fact tertiary prevention—that is, repairing (and halting further) damage. The SAFE strategy has not been subjected to a comprehensive economic evaluation, but some cost-effectiveness information is available regarding the antibiotic and surgery components.

The initial trachoma infection can be effectively treated with antibiotics, either through mass treatment of all children below 10 years of age or through targeted treatment of infected children and household members. A work by Baltussen and others (2005) for trachoma-endemic areas in the world—similar to studies of cataract control surgery—reveals that interventions using antibiotics cost between US$4,000 and US$220,000 per DALY averted for all regions studied. Targeted treatment with antibiotics (be it on the basis of azithromycin or tetracycline) is not cost-effective, and mass treatment of all children (not entire communities) is cost-effective only when azithromycin is donated. In Myanmar, tetracycline has been shown to be moderately cost-effective (Evans and others 1996). Cost-effectiveness studies are not available on mass treatment of entire communities, the approach now most commonly in use with donated azithromycin. Recent studies by Solomon and others (2004) report a 70 percent fall in prevalence in an area in Tanzania; moreover, the total community burden of ocular *Chlamydia trachomatis* infection (measured by polymerase chain reaction) fell to 8.7 percent of pretreatment levels at six months after treatment. Additionally, Chidambaram and others (2004) have demonstrated that, after mass azithromycin treatment of a population in Ethiopia, an indirect protective effect occurred among untreated children who resided in villages in which most individuals had been treated. As noted in table 50.1, greater efficacy of azithromycin than that used to calculate cost-effectiveness of mass treatment of children alone may lead to better cost-effectiveness than shown in the table. To date, if governments purchased the drug, mass distribution would be excessively expensive from a societal perspective. However, from the perspective of the governments of countries in which azithromycin (donated by Pfizer Inc. through the International Trachoma Initiative) is being distributed, mass distribution appears to be relatively cost-effective.

Trichiasis scarring is amenable to surgical repair. To date, the cost-effectiveness analyses that have been done suggest that surgery is not particularly expensive per case of blindness prevented, assuming that the eyelid correction prevents blindness and that the individuals with operated trichiasis are not more likely to be affected by other conditions (for example, dry eye) that might lead to corneal opacification. Baltussen and others (2005) suggest that trichiasis surgery—with cost-effectiveness ranging between approximately US$4 and US$82 per DALY averted across trachoma-endemic areas—would be even more cost-effective than cataract surgery.

From these cost-effectiveness evaluations, one could conclude that it is best simply to correct lid damage attributable to trachoma. Surgery (tertiary prevention) would then remain a low but continuing cost. These evaluations do not, of course, take into account the possibility of eliminating this blinding disease. The implementation of the full SAFE strategy includes primary, secondary, and tertiary prevention, and although more costly at the outset, it could eliminate infection, pain, and blindness (and the need and cost of lid surgery) into the future. The WHO Alliance for the Global Elimination of Trachoma (GET 2020) was established in 1997 to support the work of a broad spectrum of collaborating international organizations, nongovernmental development organizations, and foundations in implementing the SAFE strategy. Kumaresan and Mecaskey (2003) report that 10 countries have initiated trachoma elimination programs using donated azithromycin, and many more programs are expected. They make the point that the promise of elimination provides the justification for investing in trachoma control.

Childhood Blindness. In 1993, WHO estimated that as many as 13.8 million children have some degree of eye damage because of vitamin A deficiency; however, the number of children with actual blindness is much lower—less than 500,000 in 1992. Recent WHO studies (Resnikoff and others 2004) include vitamin A deficiency among causes of childhood blindness. Cost-effectiveness studies of vitamin A supplementation, discussed in chapter 56, focus only on deaths averted unrelated to blindness, but this public health intervention appears to be cost-effective.

Onchocerciasis. Onchocerciasis, or "river blindness," is endemic in 28 countries in tropical Africa, where 99 percent of infected people live. Isolated foci of infection also occur in Latin America (six countries) and Yemen. Although it accounts for only 0.8 percent of world blindness (Resnikoff and others 2004), the distribution of ivermectin, given at no cost by Merck, has so far proved successful in drastically reducing this cause of blindness. Additionally, patients suffer severe skin lesions and pruritus, also remedied by the annual dosing with ivermectin. Studies have shown that the cost per DALY averted is as little as US$40 when adjusted for inflation (Waters, Rehwinkel, and Burnham 2004).

During the past 25 years considerable progress has been made by the Onchocerciasis Control Program in West Africa, both through control of the black-fly vector (insecticide spraying) and through the distribution of ivermectin. This success, expressed in health, economic, and development terms, was the motivating rationale for the launching in December 1995 of a new program, the African Program for Onchocerciasis Control. The objective is to create, by 2007, sustainable community-directed distribution systems using ivermectin. In Latin America, the Onchocerciasis Elimination Program in the Americas is successfully using ivermectin distribution. A coordination group of nongovernmental organizations is working closely with all three onchocerciasis control programs and with national counterparts in virtually all endemic countries. If present efforts in endemic countries are successfully completed, the disease will be brought under control by 2010.

NATURE, CAUSES, AND EPIDEMIOLOGY OF HEARING LOSS

In this chapter, the term *hearing loss*, used by itself, denotes any or all levels of severity of hearing difficulty. These levels of hearing impairment comprise mild (26–40 decibel hearing level, dBHL), moderate (41–60 dBHL), severe (61–80 dBHL), and profound (81 dBHL or greater). The term *deafness* denotes profound hearing impairment (WHO 1991, 1997). Disabling hearing impairment in adults is defined as "a permanent unaided hearing threshold level for the better ear of 41 dB or greater; for this purpose, the hearing threshold level is to be taken as the better ear average hearing threshold level for the four frequencies 0.5, 1, 2, and 4 kHz." Disabling hearing impairment in children under the age of 15 years is defined as a permanent, unaided hearing threshold level for the better ear of 31 dB or greater; for this purpose, the hearing threshold level is to be taken as the better ear average hearing threshold level for the four frequencies 0.5, 1, 2, and 4 kHz.

Mathers and others (2003) estimate that in 2002, 255 million people worldwide had disabling hearing loss (moderate or worse hearing loss in the better ear). Those 192 million people with adult-onset loss (age 20 years and above) and 63 million people with childhood-onset loss make up almost 4.1 percent of the world's population and just over 40 percent of all people globally with hearing loss of any severity. The prevalence rates of adult-onset hearing loss were estimated by subtracting the prevalence rate for childhood onset (estimated in terms of prevalence in ages around 15 to 19). Numbers with childhood-onset hearing loss by cause have so far not been estimated separately but are included among sequelae of other diseases (for example, infectious diseases such as meningitis, otitis media, congenital conditions). It has been estimated that at least 50 percent of the burden of hearing loss could be prevented by primary, secondary, and tertiary preventive measures (Brobby 1989; WHO 1991).

Causes and Characteristics

Hearing loss is grouped according to *International Classification of Diseases and Related Health Problems*, 10th revision, version for 2003 (ICD-10) into conductive and sensorineural loss and other hearing loss, ICD-10 codes 90–91 (WHO 2003). The main causes are shown in table 50.6 according to the proportion that these contribute to the total burden (WHO 1986).

Table 50.6 Main Causes of Hearing Loss, by Proportion of Total Burden

High proportion	Moderate proportion	Low proportion
Genetic causes	Excessive noise	Nutritionally related
Otitis media	Ototoxic drugs and chemicals	Trauma related
Presbycusis	Prenatal and perinatal problems	Ménière's disease
	Infectious causes	Tumors
	Wax and foreign bodies	Cerebrovascular disease

Source: WHO 1986.

Chronic otitis media (COM, as in ICD-10 codes H65–H67) includes chronic suppurative otitis media and otitis media with effusion. These forms of otitis media, together with some other middle ear diseases, such as perforation of the tympanic membrane, cholesteatoma, and otosclerosis, are the major causes of conductive hearing loss. In most WHO estimates of the burden of otitis media, the data are not disaggregated into acute and chronic otitis media.

Hearing loss is a chronic and often lifelong disability that, depending on the severity and frequencies affected, can cause profound damage to the development of speech, language, and cognitive skills in children, especially if commencing prelingually. That damage, in turn, affects the child's progress in school and, later, his or her ability to obtain, keep, and perform an occupation. For all ages and for both sexes, it causes difficulties with interpersonal communication and leads to significant individual social problems, especially isolation and stigmatization. All these difficulties are much magnified in developing countries, where there are generally limited services, few trained staff members, and little awareness about how to deal with these difficulties.

In addition to its individual effects, hearing loss substantially affects social and economic development in communities and countries. Ruben (2000), taking into account rehabilitation, special education, and loss of employment, estimated the cost to the U.S. economy in 1999 of communication disorders (hearing, voice, speech, and language disorders) at between US$176 billion and US$212 billion (2004 dollars; 2.5–3 percent of the gross national product of the United States in that year). Hearing loss accounted for about one-third of the prevalence of these communication disorders.

Risk Factors

Occupations exposed to high levels of noise or ototoxic chemicals are also at risk, and noise exposure potentiates chemical ototoxicity in some cases (Fechter 1995; Morata 1998). Certain lifestyles (for example, use of personal stereos, noisy toys, firecrackers) and hobbies (for example, hunting) are also linked to levels of noise exposure that can cause hearing loss (Berglund and others 2000; Goelzer, Hansen, and Sehrndt 2001). Smoking may be a risk factor for high-frequency hearing loss, adding to the effect of noise (Mizoue, Miyamoto, and Shimizu 2003). Other risk factors include poverty, poor access to health care, poor hygiene, and overcrowding, all of which can lead to upper respiratory tract infections, otitis media, and other infections that may cause hearing loss, such as measles and meningitis. Detailed risk factors and indicators have been developed for neonates and infants (Joint Committee on Infant Hearing 2000); these include conditions that should require admission to a neonatal intensive care unit, stigmata of syndromes causing hearing loss, positive family history, craniofacial anomalies, certain in utero and post-natal infections (cytomegalovirus, herpes, rubella, syphilis, toxoplasmosis, meningitis), hyperbilirubinemia, conditions requiring prolonged mechanical ventilation or oxygenation, persistent otitis media with effusion, and others.

Ototoxic medications, low birth-weight, and low Apgar scores have also been cited as risk factors for neonates (Vohr and others 2000). Offspring of consanguineous marriages have a significantly higher incidence of autosomal recessive diseases, including hearing impairment. Such diseases are an important cause in communities where consanguinity is common (Shahin and others 2002; Zakzouk 2000). Certain ethnic groups (First Nations peoples such as Inuit and North American Indians, as well as Australian Aboriginal people) appear to be at higher risk of developing COM (WHO 1998).

Age, Geographic, and Gender Burdens

The prevalence of disabling hearing impairment that increases markedly with age is mainly related to the effect of presbycusis. The current shortage of data, particularly in developing countries, prevents accurate assessment of the global distribution of the burden and causes.

Male-to-female ratios of age-standardized adult-onset prevalence rates were found to be greater than 1 in most studies in all WHO regions (Mathers, Smith, and Concha 2005). This finding may be related to occupational noise-induced hearing loss, which differentially affects men.

Mortality

Barnett and Franks (1999) have found evidence that adults with postlingual onset of deafness have higher mortality than nondeaf adults. A 10-year longitudinal analysis of participants (age 55 to 74 years) in the U.S. National Health and Nutrition Examination Survey I found that, at baseline, hearing loss predicts mortality; relative risk = 1.17 (Mui and others 1998). Other studies have reported that the association disappears after controlling for age, and in any case, any relationship that may exist is too small to appear in published WHO estimates of deaths by cause (WHO 2004a, annex table 2) and by years of life lost, or YLLs (Mathers, Smith, and Concha 2005), in any region. A small number of deaths (4,000 globally in 2002) are recorded for otitis media (WHO 2004a), but these deaths are mainly due to infective complications and, hence, are not directly caused by hearing loss.

Years Lived with Disability and DALYs

Data on years of life lived with disability (YLDs) and DALYs are available only for adult-onset hearing loss. The disease model used, the assumptions and methods used for calculation, and the disability weights are described elsewhere (Mathers, Smith, and Concha 2005). Total global YLDs for adult-onset hearing loss in 2001 are estimated to be 25.87 million, or 4.7 percent of total YLDs attributable to all causes, which makes hearing loss a leading cause of YLDs. Because YLLs are taken to be zero for all regions, the DALY figures are identical to the YLD figures. The most comprehensive data available are for all adult-onset hearing loss (WHO 2004b; Mathers, Smith, and Concha 2003). Fewer data on the burden are available at present for childhood hearing loss and specific causes.

Interventions

Effective interventions include screening programs, education, surgery, medications, and assistive devices.

Population-Based Interventions. Neonatal or early infant hearing screening is important because early identification of hearing loss (before 6 months of age, with early intervention) is associated with significantly better language development and may lead to better school and occupational performance than that of children identified after 6 months with early intervention (Keren and others 2002; Yoshinaga-Itano and others 1998). Implementation of neonatal hearing screening raises from 20 to 80 percent the numbers of children with normal development of language, compared with children whose hearing loss is detected later (Yoshinaga-Itano and Gravel 2001). Early identification of hearing impairment can reduce the median age of identification of hearing impairment from between 12 and 18 months to 6 months or less. Universal neonatal hearing screening is highly sensitive, but depending on the test method used, it may result in many false positives (which may increase parental anxiety and lead to unnecessary follow-up tests and interventions). It has a low positive predictive value. Some screening protocols may decrease false-positive rates (Kennedy and others 2000). Universal neonatal hearing screening has been endorsed in developed countries (Joint Committee on Infant Hearing 2000), although some experts urge caution (Paradise 1999); however, it is expensive to implement and, for most developing countries, is not yet an option. Hearing screening targeted at high-risk neonates is generally used in developing countries that do any type of neonatal screening, but screening may fail to detect 50 percent or more of cases of impairment (Lutman and Grandori 1999). Neonatal screening programs will not detect the 10 to 20 percent of cases of permanent childhood hearing impairment that

starts later in life and for which later surveillance is needed (Grote 2000). No publications were found that have addressed the DALY burden that might be avoided by implementing neonatal hearing screening.

A recent WHO meeting of experts on noise-induced hearing loss (WHO 1998) concluded that exposure to excessive noise is the major avoidable cause of permanent hearing impairment worldwide. They agreed that, in developing countries, occupational noise and urban environmental noise are increasing risk factors for hearing impairment. Experts attending the meeting recommended that all countries implement national programs for prevention of noise-induced hearing loss, including effective hearing conservation. However, there are no published reports yet on the effectiveness of such programs in developing countries. The United States has produced a guide to hearing conservation programs in the workplace (Franks, Stephenson, and Merry 1996). It advises how to appraise programs by assessing the completeness of their components and by evaluating both the individual audiometric data for threshold shift and the group data for variability compared with a nonexposed population. Even in developed countries, there have been few, if any, clinical trials and little convincing evidence of the efficacy of occupational hearing conservation programs (Dobie 1995).

Personal Services. Chronic suppurative otitis media is one of the most common causes of hearing impairment in developing countries. Opportunities for prevention arise at all levels of national health systems, particularly in the community and at the primary level through primary ear and hearing care (PEHC) (WHO 1998). Appropriate health promotion measures include breastfeeding, immunization, adequate nutrition, personal hygiene, improved housing, reduced overcrowding, and adequate access to clean water. Primary health care workers can be given appropriate training and basic equipment for early detection and management of chronic suppurative otitis media, but the effectiveness and cost-effectiveness of this intervention in developing countries has not yet been assessed.

Although WHO does not currently recommend treating what is commonly called *chronic middle ear infection* with antibiotics at the primary level (WHO 2000), evidence suggests that antibiotics, especially topical quinolones, are more effective and cost-effective than ear toilet alone (Acuin, Smith, and Mackenzie 2000). WHO is reviewing these recommendations (WHO 2004b). New methods of delivery of effective but expensive topical antibiotics may lower the cost in poor communities, but treatment failure may be due to a high reinfection rate attributable to poor hygienic conditions. To be effective as public health measures, interventions need to be implemented on a large scale, with good coverage of the targeted population (van Hasselt and van Kregten 2002). Ear surgery plays an essential part in the prevention of further hearing impairment and, sometimes, in the improvement of hearing.

Services at the secondary level of intervention include provision of hearing aids in developing countries, which should assign priority to children with moderate or severe hearing loss, followed by adults (Arslan and Genovese 1996; WHO 2004c). However, even though globally about 6 million hearing aids are dispensed annually (WHO 1999), there have been no published randomized, controlled trials of the effectiveness of hearing aids in reducing hearing disability in developing countries and few trials in developed countries.

A randomized trial of amplification in 194 U.S. veterans showed significant improvements in communication, cognition, and social and emotional function, plus significant alleviation of depression, with hearing aids compared with controls (Mulrow and others 1990). No significant differences were observed in clinical effectiveness and cost-effectiveness between newer hearing aids that use digital signal processing and those that do not—in particular, analog-based aids (Parving 2003; Taylor, Paisley, and Davis 2001). Digital signal processing aids are not affordable for most people in developing countries. Over-the-counter hearing aids that can be purchased and used without prior training are commonly available in some developing countries. Those aids were found not to meet the prescription gain requirements of the majority of elderly clients who usually purchased them (Cheng and McPherson 2000).

Learning to use a hearing aid and developing "hearing tactics" are also important. Random assignment to a course for new hearing aid users significantly reduced the handicap compared with controls not assigned (Beynon, Thornton, and Poole 1997). Lack of compliance in use is a substantial problem everywhere among elderly and child users, including in developing countries (Furuta and Yoshino 1998; Sorri, Luotonen, and Laitakari 1984). Thus, measuring coverage without taking into account actual usage is not enough to assess alleviation of the burden.

Cochlear implants are provided to children and adults with severe and profound bilateral deafness on the basis that known short-term outcomes in auditory receptive skills (Richter and others 2002) will translate through various medium-term outcomes into greater social independence and quality of life (the social and quality outcomes have not yet been tested in a trial or observational study) (Summerfield and Marshall 1999). Cochlear implantation is beneficial in prelingually and postlingually deaf children (Makhdoum, Snik, and van den Broek 1997) and, when accompanied by aural (re)habilitation, leads to higher rates of mainstream placement in schools and lower dependence on special education support services (Francis and others 1999). Multichannel implants are superior to single-channel implants (Cohen, Waltzman, and Fisher 1993) and are more beneficial when implanted in young children (Richter and others 2002). There has been no economic analysis of cochlear implants in developing countries, and such interventions are currently not a priority in most parts of the developing world (Berruecos 2000; WHO 2004c; Zeng 1995).

Intervention Cost and Cost-Effectiveness. All the data on the costs and cost-effectiveness of interventions related to hearing loss (including school-age screening, treatment of COM, surgical interventions, hearing aids, and cochlear implants) come from developed countries. Although they can be summarized quite readily, it is not clear whether and how they relate to the costs that would be experienced in developing countries.

RESEARCH AND DEVELOPMENT AGENDA

The public health research and development agenda for controlling and reducing the burden of disease related to the loss of sight and hearing should include the following:

- further population-based studies on the magnitude, causes, and distribution of the burden
- economic analysis, especially on cost-effectiveness (for example, cost-effectiveness of each of the components of the SAFE strategy in trachoma control)
- research to develop eye and hearing care systems
- operational research on eye and hearing care delivery (particularly for cataract, diabetic retinopathy, and affordable hearing aids in underserved areas)
- clinical and field trials on interventions: pneumococcal and meningitis vaccines, treatment for chronic suppurative otitis media, primary care of ears and hearing, and prevention of noise damage.

Basic scientific research, particularly for age-related macular degeneration, must move forward, as it is doing in the industrial countries, where this disease constitutes a major burden and where highly developed research establishments exist.

CONCLUSIONS: PROMISES AND PITFALLS

With what we now know about some of the cost-effective interventions cited above, we could make significant reductions in the burden of disease related to loss of vision. Although waiting for someone to have a condition and then remedying the situation is not a particularly common "public health" recommendation, given the costs of and knowledge of prevention at this point, we can strongly recommend surgery both for cataract (the primary option) and for trachoma (apparently a better use of resources than mass treatment with antibiotics— even if not acceptable on a humanitarian basis). For example, clearing the backlog of cataract surgery globally could reduce the DALYs associated with vision loss by more than half.

Hearing loss interventions have only begun to demonstrate their potential effectiveness in developing countries, and no cost work has been done in these settings. Furthermore, although the means to reduce the burden of adult-onset hearing loss are not as straightforward nor as easily applied, eliminating adult hearing loss would avoid slightly more YLDs than eliminating the cataract surgery backlog. The data suggest that these interventions (particularly cataract surgery) are relatively cost-effective, but a lack of political will, a failure to recognize that steps can be taken now, insufficient capacity within ministries of health to carry out the known beneficial interventions, and, finally, a lack of equipment or funding for the programs still remain barriers to alleviating disabilities related to vision and hearing loss.

REFERENCES

Abou-Gareeb, I., S. Lewallen, K. Bassett, and P. Courtright. 2001. "Gender and Blindness: A Meta-Analysis of Population-Based Prevalence Surveys." *Ophthalmic Epidemiology* 8 (1): 39–56.

Acuin, J., A. Smith, and I. Mackenzie. 1998. "Interventions for Chronic Suppurative Otitis Media." *Cochrane Database of Systematic Reviews* (2): CD000473.http://www.cochrane.org/cochrane/revabstr/AB000473.htm.

Arslan E., and E. Genovese. 1996. "Hearing Aid Systems in Undeveloped, Developed, and Industrialized Countries. *Scandinavian Audiology* 42: (Suppl.) 35–39.

Baltussen, R., M. Sylla, K. Frick, and S. Mariotti. 2005. "Cost-Effectiveness of Trachoma Control in Seven World Regions." *Ophthalmic Epidemiology* 12 (2): 91–101.

Baltussen, R., M. Sylla, and S. Mariotti. 2004. "Cost-Effectiveness of Cataract Surgery: A Global and Regional Analysis." *Bulletin of the World Health Organization* 82 (5): 338–45.

Barnett, S., and P. Franks. 1999. "Deafness and Mortality: Analyses of Linked Data from the National Health Interview Survey and National Death Index." *Public Health Reports* 114 (4): 330–36.

Berglund, B., T. Lindvall, D. Schwela, and K.-T. Goh. 2000. *Guidelines for Community Noise*. Geneva: World Health Organization. http://www.who.int/docstore/peh/noise/guidelines2.html.

Berruecos, P. 2000. "Cochlear Implants: An International Perspective—Latin American Countries and Spain." *Audiology* 39 (4): 221–25.

Beynon, G. J., F. L. Thornton, and C. Poole. 1997. "A Randomized, Controlled Trial of the Efficacy of a Communication Course for First Time Hearing Aid Users." *British Journal of Audiology* 31 (5): 345–51.

Bowman, R. J., A. Sillah, C. Van Dehn, V. M. Goode, M. Muquit, G. J. Johnson, and others. 2000. "Operational Comparison of Single-Dose Azithromycin and Topical Tetracycline for Trachoma." *Investigative Ophthalmology and Visual Science* 41 (13): 4074–79.

Brobby, G. W. 1989. "Personal View . . . Strategy for Prevention of Deafness in the Third World." *Tropical Doctor* 19 (4): 152–54.

Cheng, C. M., and B. McPherson. 2000. "Over-the-Counter Hearing Aids: Electroacoustic Characteristics and Possible Target Client Groups." *Audiology* 39 (2): 110–16.

Chidambaram, J. D., M. Melese, W. Alemayehu, E. Yi, T. Prabriputaloong, D. C. Lee, and others. 2004. "Mass Antibiotic Treatment and Community Protection in Trachoma Control Programs." *Clinical Infectious Diseases* 39 (9): 95–97.

Cohen, N. L., S. B. Waltzman, and S. G. Fisher. 1993. "A Prospective, Randomized Study of Cochlear Implants." Department of Veterans Affairs Cochlear Implant Study Group. *New England Journal of Medicine* 328 (4): 233–37.

Dandona, R., and L. Dandona. 2003. "Childhood Blindness in India: A Population Based Perspective." *British Journal of Ophthalmology* 87 (3): 263–65.

Dobie, R. A. 1995. "Prevention of Noise-Induced Hearing Loss." *Archives of Otolaryngology—Head and Neck Surgery* 121 (4): 385–91.

Evans, T. G., M. K. Ranson, T. A. Kyaw, and C. K. Ko. 1996. "Cost Effectiveness and Cost Utility of Preventing Trachomatous Visual Impairment: Lessons from 30 Years of Trachoma Control in Burma. *British Journal of Ophthalmology* 80 (10): 880–89.

Fechter, L. D. 1995. "Combined Effects of Noise and Chemicals." *Occupational Medicine* 10 (3): 609–21.

Fotouhi, A., H. Hashemi, K. Mohammad, and K. H. Jalali. 2004. "The Prevalence and Causes of Visual Impairment in Tehran: The Tehran Eye Study." *British Journal of Ophthalmology* 88 (6): 740–45.

Francis, H. W., M. E. Koch, J. R. Wyatt, and J. K. Niparko. 1999. "Trends in Educational Placement and Cost-Benefit Considerations in Children with Cochlear Implants." *Archives of Otolaryngology—Head and Neck Surgery* 125 (5): 499–505.

Franks, J. R., M. R. Stephenson, and C. J. Merry, eds. 1996. *Preventing Occupational Hearing Loss*. NIOSH Publication 96-110. Cincinnati, OH: U.S. Department of Health and Human Services, National Institute for Occupational Safety and Health. http://www.cdc.gov/niosh/96-110.html.

Frick, K. D., E. L. Keuffel, and R. J. Bowman. 2001. "Epidemiological, Demographic, and Economic Analyses: Measurement of the Value of Trichiasis Surgery in The Gambia."*Ophthalmic Epidemiology* 8 (2–3): 191–201.

Frick, K. D., T. M. Lietman, S. O. Holm, H. C. Jha, J. S. Chaudhary, and R. C. Bhatta. 2001. "Cost-Effectiveness of Trachoma Control Measures: Comparing Targeted Household Treatment and Mass Treatment of Children." *Bulletin of the World Health Organization* 79 (3): 201–7.

Furuta, H., and T. Yoshino. 1998. "The Present Situation of the Use of Hearing Aids in Rural Areas of Sri Lanka: Problems and Future Prospects." *International Journal of Rehabilitation Research* 21 (1): 103–7.

Gilbert, C., and A. Foster. 2001. "Childhood Blindness in the Context of VISION 2020—The Right to Sight." *Bulletin of the World Health Organization* 79 (3): 227–32.

Goelzer, B., C. H. Hansen, and G. A. Sehrndt, eds. 2001. *Occupational Exposure to Noise: Evaluation, Prevention, and Control*. Special Report S 64. Dortmund and Berlin: Federal Institute for Occupational Safety and Health.

Grote J. 2000. "Neonatal Screening for Hearing Impairment." *Lancet* 355 (9203): 513–14.

Joint Committee on Infant Hearing. 2000. "Year 2000 Position Statement: Principles and Guidelines for Early Hearing Detection and Intervention Programs." *Pediatrics* 106 (4) (October): 798–817. http://www.jcih.org/jcih2000.pdf.

Kennedy, C., L. Kimm, R. Thornton, and A. Davis. 2000. "False Positives in Universal Neonatal Screening for Permanent Childhood Hearing Impairment." *Lancet* 356 (9245): 1903–4.

Keren, R., M. Helfand, C. Homer, H. McPhillips, and T. A. Lieu. 2002. "Projected Cost-Effectiveness of Statewide Universal Newborn Hearing Screening." *Pediatrics* 110 (5): 855–64.

Kumaresan, J. A., and J. W. Mecaskey. 2003. "The Global Elimination of Blinding Trachoma: Progress and Promise." *American Journal of Tropical Medicine and Hygiene* 69 (Suppl. 5): 24–28.

Lee, D. J., O. Gomez-Marin, B. L. Lam, and D. D. Zheng. 2002. "Visual Acuity Impairment and Mortality in U.S. Adults." *Archives of Ophthalmology* 120 (11): 1544–50.

Lutman, M. E., and F. Grandori. 1999. "Screening for Neonatal Hearing Defects: European Consensus Statement." *European Journal of Pediatrics* 158 (2): 95–96.

Makhdoum, M. J., A. F. Snik, and P. van den Broek. 1997. "Cochlear Implantation: A Review of the Literature and the Nijmegen Results." *Journal of Laryngology and Otology* 111 (11): 1008–17.

Mathers, C. D., K. Bernard, K. M. lburg, M. Inoue, D. Ma Fat, K, Shibuya, and others. 2003. "Global Burden of Disease in 2002: Data Sources, Methods and Results." GPP Discussion Paper No. 54. Geneva: World Health Organization.

Mathers, C., A. Smith, and M. Concha. 2005. "Global Burden of Adult-Onset Hearing Loss in the Year 2002." Paper in preparation, World Health Organization, Geneva. http://www3.who.int/whosis/burden/gbd2000docs/Hearing%20loss.zip.

Mizoue, T., T. Miyamoto, and T. Shimizu. 2003. "Combined Effect of Smoking and Occupational Exposure to Noise on Hearing Loss in Steel Factory Workers." *Occupational and Environmental Medicine* 60 (1): 56–59.

Morata, T. C. 1998. "Assessing Occupational Hearing Loss: Beyond Noise Exposures." *Scandinavian Audiology* 48 (Suppl.): 111–16.

Mui, S., D. Reuben, M. Damesyn, G. Greendale, and A. Moore. 1998. "Sensory Impairment as a Predictor of 10-Year Mortality and Functional Impairment." *Journal of the American Geriatric Society* 46 (9): 19–20.

Mulrow, C. D., C. Aguilar, J. E. Endicott, M. R. Tuley, R. Velez, W. S. Charlip, and others. 1990. "Quality-of-Life Changes and Hearing Impairment: A Randomized Trial." *Annals of Internal Medicine* 113 (3): 188–94.

Naidoo, K. S., A. Raghunandan, K. P. Mashige, P. Govender, B. A. Holden, G. P. Pokharel, and L. B. Ellwein. 2004. "Refractive Error and Visual Impairment in African Children in South Africa." *Investigative Ophthalmology and Visual Sciences* 44 (9): 3764–70.

Nirmalan, P. K., A. Padmavathi, and R. D. Thulasiraj. 2003. "Sex Inequalities in Cataract Blindness Burden and Surgical Services in South India." *British Journal of Ophthalmology* 87 (7): 847–49.

Paradise, J. L. 1999. "Universal Newborn Hearing Screening: Should We Leap before We Look?" *Pediatrics* 103 (3): 670–72.

Parving, A. 2003. "The Hearing Aid Revolution: Fact or Fiction?" *Acta Otolaryngologica* 123 (2): 245–48.

Pascolini, D., S. P. Mariotti, G. P. Pokharel, R. Pararajasegaram, D. Eya'ale, A.-D. Négrel, and S. Resnikoff. 2004. "Available Data on Visual Impairment: 2002 Global Update." *Ophthalmic Epidemiology* 11 (2): 67–115.

Reacher, M. H., B. Munoz, A. Alghassany, A. S. Daar, M. Elbualy, and H. R. Taylor. 1992. "A Controlled Trial of Surgery for Trachomatous Trichiasis of the Upper Lid." *Archives of Ophthalmology* 110 (5): 667–74.

Resnikoff, S., D. Pascolini, D. Etya'Alé, I. Kocur, R. Pararajasegaram, G. P. Pokharel, and S. P. Mariotti. 2004. "Global Data on Visual Impairment in the Year 2002." *Bulletin of the World Health Organization* 82: 844–51.

Richter, B., S. Eissele, R. Laszig, and E. Lohle. 2002. "Receptive and Expressive Language Skills of 106 Children with a Minimum of 2 Years' Experience in Hearing with a Cochlear Implant." *International Journal of Pediatric Otorhinolaryngoly* 64 (2): 111–25.

Ruben, R. J. 2000. "Redefining the Survival of the Fittest: Communication Disorders in the 21st Century." *Laryngoscope* 110 (2, part 1): 241–45.

Shahin, H., T. Walsh, T. Sobe, E. Lynch, M. C. King, K. B. Avraham, and M. Kanaan. 2002. "Genetics of Congenital Deafness in the Palestinian Population: Multiple Connexin 26 Alleles with Shared Origins in the Middle East." *Human Genetics* 110 (3): 284–89.

Solomon, A. W., M. J. Holland, N. D. Alexander, P. A. Massae, A. Aguirre, A. Natividad-Sancho, and others. 2004. "Mass Treatment with Single-Dose Azithromycin for Trachoma." *New England Journal of Medicine* 351 (19): 1962–71.

Sorri, M., M. Luotonen, and K. Laitakari. 1984. "Use and Non-Use of Hearing Aids." *British Journal of Audiology* 18 (3): 169–72.

Summerfield, A. Q., and D. H. Marshall. 1999. "Paediatric Cochlear Implantation and Health-Technology Assessment." *International Journal of Pediatric Otorhinolaryngoly* 47 (2): 141–51.

Taylor, H. R., S. Katala, B. Munoz, and V. Turner. 1991. "Increase in Mortality Associated with Blindness in Rural Africa." *Bulletin of the World Health Organization* 69 (3): 335–38.

Taylor, R. S., S. Paisley, and A. Davis. 2001. "Systematic Review of the Clinical and Cost Effectiveness of Digital Hearing Aids." *British Journal of Audiology* 35 (5): 271–88.

van Hasselt, P., and E. van Kregten. 2002. "Treatment of Chronic Suppurative Otitis Media with Ofloxacin in Hydroxypropyl Methylcellulose Ear Drops: A Clinical/Bacteriological Study in a Rural Area of Malawi." *International Journal of Pediatric Otorhinolaryngoly* 63 (1): 49–56.

Vohr, B. R., J. E. Widen, B. Cone-Wesson, Y. S. Sininger, M. P. Gorga, R. C. Folsom, and S. J. Norton. 2000. "Identification of Neonatal Hearing Impairment: Characteristics of Infants in the Neonatal Intensive Care Unit and Well-Baby Nursery." *Ear and Hearing* 21 (5): 373–82.

Waters, H. R., J. A. Rehwinkel, and G. Burnham. 2004. "Economic Evaluation of Mectizan Distribution." *Tropical Medicine and International Health* 9 (4): 16–25.

WHO (World Health Organization). 1986. *Prevention of Deafness and Hearing Impairment: Report by the Director General*. EB79/10. Geneva: WHO.

———. 1991. *Report of the Informal Working Group on Prevention of Deafness and Hearing Impairment Program Planning*. WHO/PDH/91.1. Geneva: WHO.

———. 1992. *International Statistical Classification of Diseases and Related Health Problems*. Rev. Geneva: WHO.

———. 1993. *International Classification of Disease, Injuries and Causes of Death*. 10th ed., rev. Geneva: WHO.

———. 1997. *Report of the First Informal Consultation on Future Program Developments for the Prevention of Deafness and Hearing Impairment*. WHO/PDH/97.3. Geneva: WHO.

———. 1998. *Prevention of Hearing Impairment from Chronic Otitis Media*. Report of a WHO/CIBA Foundation workshop, London, November 12–21, 1996. WHO/PDH/98.4. Geneva: WHO.

———. 1999. *Hearing Aids Services—Needs and Technology Assessment for Developing Countries*. Report of a WHO/CBM workshop, Bensheim, Germany, November 24–26, 1998. WHO/PDH/99.7. Geneva: WHO.

———. 2000. *Integrated Management of Childhood Illness: Handbook*. WHO/FCH/CAH/00.12. Geneva: WHO. http://www.who.int/child-adolescent-health/publications/IMCI/WHO_FCH_CAH_00.12.htm.

———. 2003. *International Statistical Classification of Diseases and Related Health Problems*, 10th rev. Geneva: WHO. http://www3.who. int/icd/vol1htm2003/fr-icd.htm.

———. 2004a. *Changing History: The World Health Report*. Geneva: WHO.

———. 2004b. *Chronic Suppurative Otitis Media: Burden of Illness and Management Options*. Geneva: WHO.

———. 2004c. *Guidelines for Hearing Aids and Services for Developing Countries*. 2nd ed. Geneva: WHO.

Yoshinaga-Itano, C., and J. S. Gravel. 2001. "The Evidence for Universal Newborn Hearing Screening." *American Journal of Audiology* 10 (2): 62–64.

Yoshinaga-Itano, C., A. Sedey, D. K. Coulter, and A. L. Mehl. 1998. "Language of Early- and Later- Identified Children with Hearing Loss." *Pediatrics* 102 (5): 1161–71.

Zakzouk, S. 2002. "Consanguinity and Hearing Impairment in Developing Countries: A Custom to Be Discouraged." *Journal of Laryngology and Otology* 116 (10): 811–16.

Zeng, F. G. 1995. "Cochlear Implants in China." *Audiology*. 34 (2): 61–75.

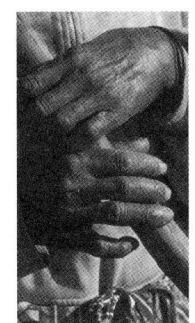

Chapter 51

Cost-Effectiveness of Interventions for Musculoskeletal Conditions

Luke B. Connelly, Anthony Woolf, and Peter Brooks

BURDEN OF MUSCULOSKELETAL DISEASE

Musculoskeletal conditions are the most common cause of chronic disability around the world. The importance of musculoskeletal conditions as a cause of mortality and morbidity has been recognized by the designation of 2000–10 as the Bone and Joint Decade (Hazes and Woolf 2000) by the United Nations, World Health Organization (WHO), and more than 60 countries around the world. WHO (2003, 2004) has highlighted the burden of musculoskeletal conditions. Estimates of the global burden of these conditions have increased 25 percent over the past decade (WHO 2000). Conditions considered under this rubric include osteoarthritis (OA); inflammatory arthritis (rheumatoid arthritis and the seronegative spondyloarthropathies); back pain; musculoskeletal injuries, including sports injuries; crystal arthritis (gout and calcium pyrophosphate disease), and metabolic bone disease, principally osteoporosis (OP).

Back pain is extremely common in both industrial and developing countries, with up to 50 percent of workers suffering an episode each year. Back pain causes 0.8 million disability-adjusted life years (DALYs) each year and is a major cause of absence from work and of correspondingly high economic losses. Nearly 40 percent of back pain is due to occupational risk factors, and many of these factors can be prevented with the cooperation of labor, management, industrial engineers, ergonomists, and health workers.

OA is increasing among the world's aging populations and is the sixth leading cause of years lost because of disability globally. It accounts for nearly 3 percent of the total global years lost to disability, and 10 percent of men and 18 percent of women over the age of 60 have OA. Table 51.1 provides an estimate of the contribution of musculoskeletal conditions to the global burden of disease, including a disaggregation by gender and between the developed and developing world. The proportions presented in the second and third panels are the most noteworthy data in table 51.1. First, the second panel shows that musculoskeletal conditions account for approximately 1.7 and 2.4 percent of the burden of disease experienced by males and females, respectively, or, across both genders, approximately 2 percent of the global burden of disease. The disaggregation by developing and developed regions, however, shows that while musculoskeletal conditions account for around 3.4 percent of the total burden of disease in the developed world, they account for 1.7 percent in the developing world. The data also show that, of the set of musculoskeletal conditions, OA accounts for the largest burden, approximately 52 percent of the total in developing regions and 61 percent in developed regions.

Table 51.2 provides a further disaggregation of the estimated burden of musculoskeletal conditions by developing region and mortality stratum. Note that the burden of disease caused by musculoskeletal conditions varies considerably by region: in Africa, mortality stratum D, musculoskeletal conditions account for less than 1 percent of the burden from all causes, while in the Western Pacific, mortality stratum B, they account for more than 3 percent of the total burden of disease. Similarly, the relative importance of rheumatoid arthritis (RA) and OA varies considerably by region. In the African regions, where the prevalence of RA is low, only 12 percent of the burden created by musculoskeletal diseases is due to RA; in the Americas, however, that proportion is approximately 24 to 27 percent.

Table 51.1 Estimated Burden of Musculoskeletal Diseases, by Gender and by Developed or Developing Regions, 2001

	Total	Males	Females	Developing regions (both genders)	Developed regions (both genders)
Numbers of DALYs (thousands)					
Rheumatoid arthritis	4,757	1,353	3,404	3,238	1,520
Osteoarthritis	16,372	6,621	9,750	11,049	5,323
Other musculoskeletal diseases	8,699	5,033	3,638	6,789	1,880
All musculoskeletal diseases	29,798	13,007	16,792	21,076	8,723
Percentage of total DALYs					
Rheumatoid arthritis	0.32	0.18	0.49	0.27	0.59
Osteoarthritis	1.12	0.86	1.39	0.91	2.05
Other musculoskeletal diseases	0.59	0.65	0.52	0.56	0.73
All musculoskeletal diseases	2.03	1.69	2.40	1.74	3.37
Percentage of musculoskeletal DALYs					
Rheumatoid arthritis	15.96	10.40	20.27	15.36	17.42
Osteoarthritis	54.94	50.91	58.07	52.43	61.02
Other musculoskeletal diseases	29.10	38.69	21.66	32.21	21.56

Source: Calculated from WHO (2004).
Note: Totals may not sum due to rounding.

Table 51.2 Estimated Burden of Musculoskeletal Conditions by Region and Mortality Stratum, Selected WHO Regions, 2001

	Africa		Americas		Southeast Asia		Eastern Mediterranean		Western Pacific
Condition	D	E	B	D	B	D	B	D	B
Numbers DALYs (thousands)									
Rheumatoid arthritis	127	141	532	83	117	855	99	218	1,065
Osteoarthritis	625	687	969	117	931	2,474	227	577	4,442
Other musculoskeletal diseases	285	316	677	107	516	1,756	159	408	2,590
All musculoskeletal diseases	1,037	1,144	2,178	307	1,564	5,085	485	1,203	8,097
Percentage of total DALYs									
Rheumatoid arthritis	0.09	0.07	0.66	0.47	0.19	0.24	0.43	0.19	0.44
Osteoarthritis	0.42	0.33	1.19	0.67	1.52	0.69	0.99	0.51	1.84
Other musculoskeletal diseases	0.19	0.15	0.83	0.60	0.84	0.49	0.69	0.36	1.06
All musculoskeletal diseases	0.70	0.55	2.68	1.74	2.55	1.42	2.11	1.06	3.34
Percentage of musculoskeletal DALYs									
Rheumatoid arthritis	12.28	12.29	24.45	27.23	7.50	16.82	20.38	18.11	13.19
Osteoarthritis	60.27	60.10	44.49	38.50	59.51	48.66	46.90	47.97	54.99
Other musculoskeletal diseases	27.44	27.61	31.06	34.27	32.99	34.53	32.71	33.92	31.82

Source: Calculated from WHO (2004).
Notes: The letters in the column heads refer to mortality strata. B = low child and low adult mortality, D = high child and high adult mortality, E = high child and very high adult mortality.

RA has a prevalence of 0.7 to 0.1 percent worldwide and results in significant work disability and long-term treatment costs. In addition, OP is increasing with the aging of populations: one in three people over the age of 50 suffers a fracture because of OP. Back pain, OA, trauma, and RA account for 32,948,765 DALYs, or 2.15 percent of the global total for 2000.

A recent review of the prevalence of rheumatic disorders in Sub-Saharan Africa suggests that the frequency of RA is increasing in East, Central, and South Africa but is rare in West Africa (McGill and Oyoo 2002). Gout is also prevalent throughout the continent, and the HIV epidemic has spawned a variety of associated spondyloarthropathies among the aging population. Countries such as Thailand are also recognizing an increasing burden of disease caused by arthritis and trauma (Jitapunkul and others 2003).

NATURE, CAUSES, AND EPIDEMIOLOGY OF MUSCULOSKELETAL CONDITIONS

Osteoarthritis is the most common condition affecting human joints and causes significant disability. The principal clinical features are pain, which varies in severity and character, and stiffness. Disability occurs as a result of pain, weakness, joint instability, and reduced range of motion.

The following are the major forms of inflammatory arthritis:

- rheumatoid arthritis
- seronegative spondyloarthropathies
  — ankylosing spondylitis
  — reactive arthritis
  — enteropathic arthritis
  — psoriatic arthritis
- juvenile chronic arthritis
  — systemic
  — pauciarticular
  — polyarticular
- arthritis associated with systemic connective tissue diseases
  — systemic lupus erythematosus
  — progressive systemic sclerosis
  — vasculitis
  — polydermatomyositis
- crystal arthritis
  — gout
  — calcium pyrophosphate deposition disease

RA has a prevalence of between 1 and 3 percent in most countries for which figures are available, but it may be slightly less common in tropical countries. The exact etiology of RA is unknown, but the evidence suggests an immune reaction, and it presents as an inflammation affecting joints and other tissues. Its clinical features can be divided into three groups: constitutional, articular, and extra-articular. Constitutional features involve tiredness, fatigue, weight loss, and fever, and articular features involve principally the synovial joints, producing pain and eventual deformity and disability.

The seronegative spondyloarthropathies are primarily inflammatory arthropathies and share several common features, including familial aggregation, asymmetric joint involvement, and mucocutaneous lesions. These conditions may follow gastrointestinal or sexually acquired infections and can be associated with HIV. Gout and other forms of crystal arthritis tend to present as an inflammatory response to the presence of uric acid (gout) or various calcium crystals (chondrocalcinosis).

Much of the pain that produces complaints and reduced function does not emanate from a frank arthropathy, but from the soft tissues in or around a joint. When these pains are confined to a particular area of the body's surface, they can be referred to as regional pain syndromes and may or may not be related to injury or overuse. If these pains are more widespread and are associated with specific tender points, the condition is known as fibromyalgia. Fibromyalgia is well recognized in the industrial world and has also been noted in China and Malaysia and among Tamil Indians.

The major causes of infectious arthritis can be viral, bacterial, fungal, or helminthic. Each can present as either a polyarticular presentation or a monarthritis. Many of the helminthic infections present with more generalized aches and pains and involvement of muscle tissues as well as joints. All the conditions have specific diagnostic features and treatments.

OP is characterized by low bone mass and deterioration in the microarchitecture of the bone, which leads to fracture after low or moderate trauma. The condition is defined by diagnostic criteria based on bone mineral density as follows: a bone mineral density of more than -2.5 standard deviations below the average bone mineral density of young adult women.

The clinical features of OP are primarily due to its major outcome: fracture. The most important fractures occur in the distal radius, vertebrae, or hip, often following minor trauma. Vertebral fractures lead to loss of height, kyphosis, and back pain. The incidence of fracture varies with country and with type of fracture. Hip fractures are low in African countries but high and increasingly reported in Australasia, Europe, and North America. Fracture risk increases with age and is beginning to have a significant impact on quality of life, mortality, and health care costs in many countries.

Rickets is caused by a mineralization defect of newly formed bone in the growing skeleton. This defect leads to an increase in the amount of nonmineralized bone tissue (osteoid) and a thinning of the growth plates. This condition produces bone pain, bone deformation, swelling of the joints, and growth retardation. Rickets is primarily caused by a lack of exposure to sunshine because of climate, pollution, or overuse of clothing or sunscreens. Rickets is relatively rare in industrial countries, but it does occur as a consequence of dietary deficiency or excess clothing.

Osteomalacia is the adult equivalent of rickets. It is similarly characterized by an increase in osteoid tissue and causes bone pain and fractures. It occurs primarily in the elderly in Europe and North America because of a lack of exposure to sunshine that is not compensated for by adequate vitamin D intake.

Osteomalacia may also occur in countries with abundant sunshine where clothing prevents sun exposure. Osteomalacia is commonly reported among migrants to Western Europe from India and the Middle East.

Back pain accounts for the majority of musculoskeletal disease presentations to health professionals, and its lifetime prevalence exceeds 80 percent in most industrial countries. *Spinal disorder* refers to a wide range of specific and nonspecific musculoskeletal disorders affecting the spinal column. These conditions include congenital lesions such as scoliosis, infective problems such as osteomyelitis and neoplastic disorder (myeloma or secondary cancers), and trauma and referred back pain.

The majority of individuals with acute back pain will improve significantly over a six-week period, although in many cases the pain may recur. Early diagnosis and treatment, particularly of pain, by means of a modified exercise program will reduce long-term morbidity and disability.

Musculoskeletal injuries are extremely common, whether in the workplace or associated with sporting activities or with daily living. Motor vehicle trauma, household accidents, and occupational accidents occur frequently and are a major cause of damage to the musculoskeletal system.

Table 51.3 shows the major genetic and environmental risk factors for musculoskeletal diseases. Lack of exercise and obesity are major contributors to soft tissue disorders, OA, and back pain. Infectious forms of musculoskeletal disease depend on the environment and on the types of organisms that are prevalent.

PREVENTIVE STRATEGIES

Obesity brought about by increases in sedentary lifestyles and changes in eating patterns is becoming a major problem worldwide. Weight reduction has been demonstrated to reduce pain and disability from OA of the knee and other forms of lower limb arthropathy. In OA of the knee, weight reduction will not only reduce pain and improve mobility, but it can put off the time when surgical replacement of the weight-bearing joint is necessary. Obesity can also be associated with back pain, and weight reduction is an important factor in reducing the recurrence of episodes of back pain and in reducing long-term disability and chronic pain.

Smoking and excessive alcohol use are also associated with OP. Adequate calcium intake (1,000 to 1,500 milligrams per day) has been shown to maintain bone density and reduce the risk of axial (vertebral) fractures. Smoking also increases the risk of developing RA.

Weight reduction and diet are also important considerations in the management of gout. Appropriate nutrition and exercise underpin many of the preventive and treatment strategies for musculoskeletal disease.

TREATMENTS

A range of treatment approaches is available to address the multiple aspects of musculoskeletal disorders.

Symptomatic Treatments

Symptomatic treatments for musculoskeletal disease principally involve pain reduction. Nonpharmacological treatments such as massage, heat, and ice, and physiotherapeutic techniques such as ultrasound may be useful in the short term. Pure analgesic agents such as acetaminophen should be tried initially; if no response occurs, compound analgesics or opioid derivatives, including codeine, may be useful. The side effects of the latter compounds are significant, particularly in the elderly, with constipation and disorientation being the most common. Table 51.4 shows the principal modalities of pain relief for arthritis and soft tissue rheumatism. In many countries, complementary medicines (traditional medicines) are also used extensively, particularly for the management of pain. These compounds remain unproven, and clinical studies to explore their worth should be encouraged.

Recent years have seen the introduction of a number of specific antiosteoarthritic agents, including glucosamine, chondroitin sulfate, soybean extract, and injectable hyaluronic acid derivatives. Clinical trials have demonstrated that glucosamine and chondroitin sulfate are beneficial in terms of pain reduction in patients with OA, but the effects are relatively small.

Table 51.3 Risk Factors for Musculoskeletal Disease

Condition	Genetic	Environmental
Rheumatoid arthritis	HLA DR	
Seronegative spondyloarthropathy	HLA B$_{27}$	
Osteoarthritis	Severe osteochondropathies	Obesity Lack of exercise
Soft tissue		Occupation Environment
Crystal arthritis	Congenital (Lesch Nyhan)	Obesity Nutrition
Infectious		Environment
Osteoporosis		Lack of exercise Nutrition
Metabolic bone disease		Environment Nutrition
Back pain		Obesity Occupation Lack of exercise
Trauma		Environment

Table 51.4 Treatment for Arthritis

Category	Analgesics	Specific antiosteoarthritis agents	Nonsteroidal anti-inflammatory drugs	Disease-modifying antirheumatic drugs

Pharmacological treatments	Acetaminophen
	Compound analgesics
	Codeine
	Opioid derivatives
		Glucosamine
		Avocado extract
		Soybean
		Chondroitin sulfate
		Diacerein
		Hyaluronic acid (injectable)
			Nonspecific NSAIDs
			Selective COX-1 sparing agents
				Chloroquine
				Hydroxychloroquine
				Sulfasalazine
				Gold
				D-penicillamine
				Methotrexate
				Azathioprine
				Cyclophosphamide
				Leflunomide
				Cyclosporine A
				Corticosteroids
				Minocycline
				Biologics:
				    Antitumor necrosis factor
				    Anti-interleukin-1 receptor antagonist

Nonpharmacological treatments	Massage Heat Ice Ultrasound	n.a.	n.a.	n.a.

Source: Authors.
n.a. = not applicable

Many cases of OA and soft-tissue rheumatism and most cases of the inflammatory forms of arthritis will require an anti-inflammatory drug as well as or instead of a pure analgesic. The nonsteroidal anti-inflammatory drugs (NSAIDs) have been the mainstay for treating arthritic conditions for nearly a century. More recently, concern about the adverse gastrointestinal side effects of NSAIDs led to the development of COX-1 (cyclo-oxygenase-1) sparing agents. These agents have similar effects on pain relief but a reduced incidence of gastrointestinal side effects, although they may produce adverse events in the renal and cardiovascular systems, such as hypertension, decreased renal function, and increased stroke and heart attacks.

Rheumatoid Arthritis

The medical community now appreciates the importance of early diagnosis and treatment of RA. All patients with RA should be started on a specific antirheumatic drug on diagnosis. These drugs have been shown to be efficacious in randomized controlled trials (Gabriel, Coyle, and Moreland 2001), but each has a quite different spectrum of adverse side effects. Even with the new biologic agents, few patients with RA actually go into complete remission, and disease activity continues despite a reduction in endpoints, such as the number of painful and swollen joints, function impairment, and pain. Most patients with RA now receive combinations of antirheumatic drugs, the

most common being methotrexate, hydroxychloroquine, and sulfasalazine. Corticosteroids are also used intermittently in many cases. Patients with RA also need to receive information about exercise programs and education on activities of daily living so that they can make informed choices in relation to their therapies.

Osteoporosis

A number of therapies are available for OP, including calcitonin, calcium, bisphosphonates, hormone replacement therapy (HRT), and selective estrogen receptor modifiers. Clinical trial data support the use of HRT, bisphosphonates, selective estrogen receptor modifiers, calcitonin, vitamin D and calcium supplementation, and calcitriol in reducing fracture rates in high-risk patients. Calcium and vitamin D supplementation are recommended to reduce hip fractures among the elderly living in assisted living accommodations and nursing homes. The recommended daily requirement for calcium varies significantly between countries—for example, from 1,000 milligrams per day in the United States to less than 500 milligrams per day in India. Recommended levels of vitamin D supplementation range from 500 to 1,000 international units per day, particularly for at-risk aging females. In addition to these pharmacological interventions, attention to risk factors for falling is also important.

Surgical treatments vary, from the use of external splints for fractures, to interventions such as arthroscopy, internal fixation for complicated fractures, and insertion of prosthetic devices, most commonly total hip and knee replacements. Biomaterials are increasingly being used to repair bone or cartilage defects in younger patients, particularly those with sporting or other traumatic injuries.

Rehabilitation treatments include a range of activities, from single discipline interventions such as physiotherapy to multi-disciplinary programs, particularly for complex problems such as back pain.

ECONOMIC ISSUES

An economic discussion of health policies designed to prevent, treat, and manage musculoskeletal conditions in developing countries is inherently difficult for a variety of reasons, but primarily because of the lack of both epidemiological and cost-effectiveness data for most developing countries. Some progress has been made by Symmons, Mathers, and Pfleger (2004a, 2004b), who provide incidence estimates for OA and RA from epidemiological data on prevalence and relative mortality risks, although data from many areas are scant.

Perhaps a more important constraint on economic evaluations in this field is the surprising number of interventions for which trial data on efficacy are inadequate. Another issue, currently the target of a concerted effort to improve practice in the field, is the lack of cross-study comparability of the results of economic evaluations of interventions for OA, RA, and OP. One of the most important variables is the choice of comparator used to assess the cost-effectiveness of interventions.

The Outcome Measures in Rheumatology Clinical Trials Economics Working Group, which was established in 1996, has made some progress toward redressing this problem. In principle, the relevant comparator is generally the next-best alternative or alternatives to the intervention of interest. The choice of comparator is especially important for cost-effectiveness analysis, because cost-effectiveness is a relative, not an absolute, concept; whether a particular intervention is considered efficient depends on the efficiency of other interventions and on budget constraints. This issue is a fundamental one, because a great many health sector innovations involve new ways of producing desirable effects with existing technology. The relevant consideration in such cases is the additional benefits that the innovation is expected to confer and the relative cost of achieving those benefits. In such circumstances, the computation of incremental cost-effectiveness ratios (ICERs) on the basis of a no-treatment alternative is of limited use, unless that scenario is genuinely under consideration. Unfortunately, the no-treatment (or, more accurately, the placebo treatment) option is precisely the comparator that much of the literature has used.

Another characteristic of economic evaluations in this field is that they have been performed almost entirely for developed countries. In the sections that follow, we discuss the steps we have taken in an attempt to minimize the adverse consequences of reliance on the literature for developed countries. Nevertheless, the pragmatic approach that we have adopted is subject to some important limitations and caveats.

Cost-effectiveness is a relative concept, in the sense that cost-effectiveness ratios (CERs) are useful only for comparing alternative ways of achieving a desired outcome—for instance, improving the quality and length of life. Assertions that an intervention is, in its own right, cost-effective are usually based on the notion that a particular CER represents a cutoff between those interventions that are efficient and those that are not. Thresholds of this kind involve an assumption about the value of life—for example, that a quality-adjusted life year (QALY) is worth US$30,000. Nevertheless, the literature routinely uses cost-effectiveness rules that are based on thresholds without the theoretically necessary explicit consideration of implicit budget constraints.

We have tried to avoid using a threshold type of approach in relation to the discussion of cost-effectiveness. Instead, we critically reviewed the cost-effectiveness literature in rheumatology to provide an indication of the relative costs and consequences of available interventions. In some cases, an intervention appears to be inefficient because it costs more and produces fewer benefits than a competing alternative or because two interventions produce identical effects but one costs less than the other. Nevertheless, we have provided a summary of our views—for ease of reference—as table 51.5. This table summarizes our thoughts on the weight of the current effectiveness and cost-effectiveness evidence and the likelihood that developing countries might realistically consider each intervention. For the reasons given above, though, we have articulated the evidence in more detail in the text.

Cross-country differences in the epidemiology of conditions of interest, the age structure of populations, and the access to health care, along with differences in relative prices, are liable to affect the cost-effectiveness of any given intervention. Some of the substantive gaps between the developed and developing worlds may compound the problem. For example, if the price of labor relative to that of capital is consistently lower in the developing countries, capital-intensive interventions may be relatively less attractive than they are in the developed countries, especially if labor-intensive alternatives exist.

To improve comparability across the literature, we adjusted reported CERs by converting them to 2001 U.S. dollar prices (therefore, those we report generally differ from those the original authors cite). Generally, we adjusted outcomes to U.S. dollars for studies outside the United States that reported CERs in local currencies using the official exchange rate in effect at that time, but wherever such studies reported only U.S. dollar

Table 51.5 Summary of the Economic Evaluation of Interventions for Musculoskeletal Conditions

Conditions and treatment options	Considered cost-effective in developed countries?[a]	Generally recommended for developing countries?[b]	References	Additional comments
Osteoporosis				
Primary prevention				
Physical activity	No	Yes (for low-cost interventions)	Katzmarzyk Gledhill, and Shephard 2000; Geelhoed, Harris, and Prince 1994; Patrick and others 2001	Based on consensus
Calcium plus vitamin D	Yes	Yes	Willis 2002	
HRT	Yes	—	Geelhoed, Harris, and Prince 1994; Armstrong and others 2001; Kanis and others 2002	
Raloxifene	No	No	Armstrong and others 2001; Kanis and others 2002	Based on evidence
Secondary prevention				
Screening	No	No	Norlund 1996	
Calcium and calcium plus vitamin D	Yes	Yes	Kanis and others 2002	
HRT	Yes	Yes	Fleurence, Torgerson, and Reid 2002; Kanis and others 2002	Differences in life expectancy and incidence of OP will affect age at which recommended
Raloxifene	No	No	Kanis and others 2002	
Calcitonin, alendronate, and biphosphonates	No	No	Coyle and others 2001; Kanis and others 2002	
Fluoride	No	No	Kanis and others 2002	
Alfacalcidol	No	No	Kanis and others 2002	More randomized clinic trials needed
Osteoarthritis				
Primary prevention	No evidence	Yes		Based on consensus
Secondary prevention				
Education program	No	Further research needed	Lord and others 1999	
Exercise program	No evidence	Low-cost programs may be useful	Patrick and others 2001	
Nonselective NSAIDs	No for nabumetone		McCabe and others 1998	
Gastroprotective agents	Yes, but several qualifiers		Van Dieten and others 2000; Gabriel, Campion, and O'Fallon 1994	
Synovial fluid replacement	Yes	No	Torrance and others 2002	Different comparators, relative price
Tertiary interventions				
Total hip arthroplasty	Yes	—	Chang, Pellissier, and Hazen 1996	
Knee replacement	Yes	—	Segal and others 2004	
Rheumatoid arthritis				
Inpatient or outpatient	No evidence	—		
Telephone help line	Yes	Yes	Nordstrom and others 1996; Hughes and others 2002	With good communications and low levels of access to medical care

(Continues on the following page.)

Table 51.5 Continued

Conditions and treatment options	Considered cost-effective in developed countries?[a]	Generally recommended for developing countries?[b]	References	Additional comments
Disease-modifying antirheumatic drugs				
Auranofin	Not effective	No	Thompson and others 1988	
Cyclosporine, azathioprine, D-penicillamine	Equal efficacy; cyclosporine should be used after cheaper, more effective drugs	No	Anis and others 1996	Cost, monitoring, and adverse events
Combination therapy	Yes, in some studies	Possibly	Verhoeven and others 1998	
Biologics	No data	No	—	Need trials in developing countries, but current costs are prohibitive
Corticosteroids	Yes	Possibly	Bae and others 2003	Side effects
Low back pain				
Back schools	No evidence	No	Van Tulder 2003	
Massage	Little evidence	Yes, if low cost	Furlan and others 2002	
Early interventions	Yes	Yes	Gatchel and others 2003	Depends on labor market conditions
Ankylosing spondylitis				
Spa exercise	Yes, but ICERs were sensitive to indirect costs	No	Van Tubergen and others 2002	Does not provide compelling evidence
Biologics	No	No	—	Unattractive because of their high price

Source: Authors.
n.a. = not available.
a. Based on a cost-effectiveness threshold value of approximately US$30,000 or other favorable quantitative data on costs and benefits.
b. Based on authors' judgment of generally favorable/unfavorable cost-effectiveness evidence. See text for precise cost-effectiveness (for example, cost per QALY) data.

equivalents, we took these as given. Finally, we used the U.S. Bureau of Labor Statistics consumer price index data for 2004 to inflate (deflate) the U.S. dollar CERs to 2001 prices. Thus, unless otherwise stated, all price data are expressed in 2001 U.S. dollars.

For clarity, we have classified cost-effectiveness results by condition and also according to whether the intervention constitutes a primary, secondary, or tertiary intervention. The exception is RA, for which the management protocols are less amenable to this type of abstraction. For RA, we found that categorizing the evidence according to a taxonomy that is problem or intervention based was more useful.

Primary Interventions

This section reviews the evidence on the cost-effectiveness of interventions designed to prevent the onset of OP. The works surveyed analyzed interventions in healthy people, primarily perimenopausal and postmenopausal women, with no established history of OP.

Physical Activity. The prophylactic effects of physical activity are generally well appreciated, and a large proportion of preventable disease is sometimes attributed to sedentary lifestyles. Katzmarzyk, Gledhill, and Shephard (2000) estimate the relative risks for those who are inactive compared with those who are physically active for a range of conditions, including OP. Their results for Canada suggest mean OP relative risk factors of 1.56 to 1.90 for sedentary versus active women, depending on race, and indicate that the population-attributable fraction of OP caused by inactivity was approximately 27 percent and accounted for more than 16 percent of the direct economic costs of physical inactivity.

The effectiveness and cost-effectiveness of programs intended to encourage lifestyle changes are generally not well established. Geelhoed, Harris, and Prince (1994) consider the effect of an intervention in Australia involving exercise and calcium supplements for healthy postmenopausal women to prevent osteoporotic fractures. They find that the cost of the intervention was US$96,119 per QALY; however, note that the authors assumed no toxic effect of the lifestyle regimen on diseases other than OP.

Calcium Plus Vitamin D. Willis (2002) analyzes the cost-effectiveness of administering calcium plus vitamin D_3 to healthy postmenopausal women in Sweden and demonstrates that this intervention is a cost-saving one for 50-, 60-, and 70-year-old women with a maternal family history of hip fracture and for 60- and 70-year-old women with either a history of fragility fractures or a smoking habit. In developing regions, calcium plus vitamin D therapy may be a cost-effective or cost-saving intervention if targeted at older, asymptomatic women with maternal histories of hip and other fragility fractures—especially those who smoke. A targeted strategy of this kind is likely to be the most cost-effective in regions where environmental uptake of these elements is limited for dietary or other reasons.

Hormone Replacement Therapy. Geelhoed, Harris, and Prince's (1994) cost-effectiveness analysis of interventions in a hypothetical cohort of 100,000 healthy postmenopausal women includes several HRT strategies: (a) estrogen from age 50 for life, (b) estrogen from age 50 for 15 years, and (c) estrogen from age 65 for life. Compared with a no-therapy alternative, the cost per QALY was US$8,609 for strategy c, US$13,268 for strategy a, and US$30,183 for strategy b.

Armstrong and others (2001) compare HRT with a no-therapy scenario in healthy postmenopausal women and examine how the risks of breast cancer and coronary heart disease (CHD) might influence the cost-effectiveness of the interventions over 5- and 10-year periods, as well as a lifetime intervention of approximately 31 years. They report a relatively low cost per QALY of US$2,238 to US$2,850 for women at a 10 to 15 percent risk of breast cancer. The cost-effectiveness of HRT fell as the risk of breast cancer increased.

Both the base cases in these studies assume that HRT reduces hip fracture rates, and Armstrong and others (2001) also assume reductions in CHD. These constitute important assumptions because, as Kanis and others (2002) point out, data from randomized clinical trials (RCTs) support the hypothesis of no effect of HRT on either appendicular fractures or CHD. Thus, the ICERs reported by both the studies may either understate or overstate the true cost per QALY produced by using HRT as a primary prevention.

Raloxifene. Armstrong and others' (2001) study also includes a cost-effectiveness analysis of raloxifene use (compared with HRT and no intervention) in healthy postmenopausal women. Their results indicate that, by comparison with raloxifene, HRT is a dominant long-term therapy for U.S. women at average risk (in this case, a 10 percent lifetime risk) of breast cancer: the 5- and 10-year period ICERs were US$37,620 and US$33,472 per QALY, respectively. For women at a 30 percent or higher risk of breast cancer, the ICER for raloxifene versus HRT was less than US$4,160, and decreased with risk.

Kanis and others (2002) argue that existing evidence on raloxifene suggests that it has no significant effect on either appendicular fractures or CHD. On the basis of the existing cost-effectiveness evidence, the use of raloxifene as a prophylactic intervention for OP in the developing regions has little to recommend it.

Secondary Interventions

The following studies were concerned with interventions in people with some indication of OP, either from a bone mineral density assessment or a fracture. Some of the general studies include Jönsson and others' (1999) study based on Swedish epidemiological data. The authors consider two different levels of intervention costs, those associated with HRT and those associated with HRT plus bisphosphonates, and find that the higher-cost intervention (HRT plus bisphosphonates therapy) was dominant for the 80-year-old group modeled. In the context of developing countries, note both the relatively higher incidence of osteoporotic fractures among 80-year-olds and the relatively larger size of this demographic group in Sweden.

Screening. Norlund (1996) conducted a cost-benefit analysis of fracture prevention in osteoporotic women age 50 to 54 in Sweden, assuming 70 percent participation in the screening program and an offer of HRT with 30 percent acceptance. The study provides evidence of a negative net benefit, indicating that the costs of a population screening program of this kind exceed its benefits. Thus, population-based bone mineral density screening programs aimed at perimenopausal or postmenopausal women are likely to be a poor use of health resources in the developing world.

Calcium and Calcium Plus Vitamin D. Citing trial evidence, Kanis and others (2002) assume that calcium supplements alone reduce only vertebral fracture risks in women with established OP. Assuming a compliance rate of 70 percent, the authors find that the intervention's cost per QALY for 50-, 60-, 70-, and 80-year-old cohorts were approximately US$64,995, US$31,548, US$10,271, and US$10,527, respectively. They also examine the cost-effectiveness of calcium plus vitamin D on the basis of trial evidence that this combination also reduces appendicular fractures. Assuming a 70 percent compliance rate, they find that calcium plus vitamin D was cost saving in 80-year-olds and either cost saving or a low-cost intervention (mean cost per QALY of US$584) in 70-year-olds. For 50- and

60-year-olds, the mean costs per QALY were US$29,357 and US$13,730, respectively. Thus, in developing regions, calcium plus vitamin D therapy may be an attractive investment for elderly women with established OP.

Hormone Replacement Therapy. Fleurence, Torgerson, and Reid (2002) demonstrate an ICER of US$12,800 to US$19,700 for HRT for their Scottish sample. Kanis and others (2002) show that while HRT was generally a dominant therapy for 80-year-olds, with a cost per QALY of US$4,527, it was an expensive therapy for 50-year-olds at a cost per QALY of US$42,940. These results suggest that HRT is likely to be an attractive intervention for established OP for some age groups in the developing regions. Differences in life expectancy and the underlying incidence of OP will, however, have a considerable bearing on the age at which HRT interventions may be considered desirable in each region.

Raloxifene. Kanis and others (2002) find that the cost per QALY associated with raloxifene was approximately US$835,622 in 50-year-olds, and although this cost generally fell with age, it remains an expensive intervention. Raloxifene therapy is not an attractive investment for the developing regions.

Calcitonin and Bisphosphonates. The cost-effectiveness evidence on nasal calcitonin is unambiguous. It is a particularly expensive intervention and represents an unattractive investment of health care resources even in wealthy developed countries. The most favorable cost-effectiveness results for nasal calcitonin come from a study by Coyle and others (2001), who find that both calcitonin and alendronate reduced wrist, hip, and vertebral fractures in postmenopausal women but that etidronate had no such effect on hip and wrist fractures. The ICERs for nasal calcitonin for 65-year-old women for five years of therapy were US$34,166 per QALY compared with no therapy and US$23,952 per QALY compared with etidronate. The results of this study were sensitive to the underlying fracture rate.

Kanis and others (2002, iv) also conclude that calcitonin is "not cost-effective at any age largely because of its costs." Indeed, their estimates of costs per QALY for 70- and 80-year-old women, the groups for which the intervention is most cost-effective, equate to approximately US$245,373 and US$181,109, respectively. By contrast, both alendronate and etidronate were dominating interventions for 80-year-olds. At current prices, calcitonin therapy is not an attractive investment for the developing regions.

Fluoride. Kanis and others (2002) find that fluoride was generally a dominant intervention in women with established OP, because it appears to decrease the risk of vertebral fracture but to increase the risk of hip fracture, although the latter result is

statistically insignificant. When they assume that fluoride has a neutral effect on hip fractures, the authors find that the cost per QALY was in the acceptable range for interventions in the United Kingdom—that is, less than US$46,684. Fluoride is unlikely to be a desirable intervention for preventing OP in developing countries.

Alfacalcidol. Kanis and others (2002) report wide confidence intervals on the cost per QALY of an alfacalcidol intervention. This result is largely due to substantial variation in the apparent vertebral, hip, and humeral fracture risk available from RCTs. Thus, alfacalcidol does not appear to be a good investment for developing economies; however, additional RCTs are required to reduce the uncertainty regarding the cost-effectiveness of this intervention.

COST-EFFECTIVENESS OF INTERVENTIONS FOR OA

Primary Interventions

Despite clear evidence of an association of OA with obesity and of a reduction in symptoms and progression of the disease with weight reduction, no formal studies of the cost-effectiveness of this intervention are available.

Secondary Interventions

Patient education programs, exercise programs, medications, and synovial fluid replacement have demonstrated varying levels of cost-effectiveness.

Education Programs. Lord and others (1999) evaluated the cost-effectiveness of a nurse-led education program for patients with OA of the knee in the United Kingdom, using usual care as the comparator. They found that the costs for the intervention group were greater than for the control group, but that the outcomes for the two groups were not statistically different.

The cost-effectiveness of education programs for OA patients in the developing countries is unknown. Education programs will be subject to diminishing returns, and their marginal effectiveness may depend directly on the basic level of education of those targeted. Though the scant evidence presented here suggests that education programs may not be cost-effective, further research on their effectiveness and cost-effectiveness in developing countries is required.

Exercise Programs. Patrick and others (2001) analyzed the cost-effectiveness of an aquatic exercise program for the management of OA and compare it with usual care. The study involved a 20-week randomized trial of aquatic classes for 249 adults age 55 to 75 with a confirmed diagnosis of OA. The results were generally unfavorable. In many cases (24 percent of the bootstrapped estimates), the exercise program was dominated by usual care, and the 95 percent confidence interval ranged from dominated to US$498,700 per QALY gained.

Evidence of the cost-effectiveness of exercise programs for established OA is currently meager. Nevertheless, as part of a diversified portfolio, low-cost exercise programs may still play a useful role in the aging populations of developing regions and confer some benefit on those with established OA, particularly if they are associated with weight reduction.

Nonselective NSAIDs. In a U.K. study, McCabe and others (1998) consider the cost-effectiveness of the use of five different NSAIDs (nabumetone, diclofenac, ibuprofen, piroxicam, and naproxen) in RA and OA. Taking the least and most expensive of the five NSAIDs—namely, ibuprofen and nabumetone, which were also at the high- and low-risk ends of the spectrum in terms of adverse gastrointestinal events—the authors conclude that nabumetone is not a cost-saving prescription.

Gastroprotective Agents. The most common side effects of NSAIDs are gastrointestinal; therefore, evaluating therapies to reduce these events is important. Van Dieten and others (2000) review the literature on the cost-effectiveness of misoprostol in reducing adverse gastrointestinal events in OA and RA patients who take NSAIDs. Unfortunately, the reviewed studies evidently reported CERs based on such nongeneralizable measures as cost per patient ratios. Nevertheless, van Dieten and others (2000) argue that strong evidence exists that gastroprotection is cost-effective for OA and RA patients taking NSAID therapy. This finding appears to be true in relation to several of the reviewed studies, which produced estimates of cost savings derived from prophylaxis. However, van Dieten and others' (2000) study is at variance with that of Gabriel, Campion, and O'Fallon (1994), who conclude that misoprostol was generally dominant in that it provided no greater quality-of-life improvement and cost more.

Synovial Fluid Replacement. In a Canadian study, Torrance and others (2002) analyzed the cost-effectiveness of synovial fluid replacement in a randomized, one-year, multicenter trial of 255 patients with OA of the knee. Patients were randomized to appropriate care with hylan G-F 20 or to appropriate care without hylan G-F 20. The mean QALY gain in the intervention group was 0.071, and the resulting ICER was US$5,233 per QALY (with similar results from sensitivity analyses). However, the relevant incremental comparators in developing regions are likely to be quite different from those used by the foregoing study. Also, the relative price of this product is likely to be higher. Thus, we cannot find strong grounds for recommending that developing regions adopt this intervention.

Tertiary Interventions

Total joint replacement for arthritis is one of the most commonly performed and cost-effective operations in developed countries. In developing countries, however, the availability of this intervention is constrained by the availability of surgeons able to perform the operation. If the surgical expertise is available, the cost-effectiveness of total joint replacement is likely to be as good as in Australia, Europe, and North America.

Total Hip Arthroplasty. Chang, Pellissier, and Hazen (1996) assess the cost-effectiveness of total hip arthroplasty in various age groups compared with nonsurgical management. Their analyses suggest that, in 60-year-old white women, total hip arthroplasty is dominant compared with nonsurgical management. For 85-year-old men, the cost per QALY is US$6,893. Generally, their results suggest that, when total hip arthroplasty is used as a treatment for OA of the hip with significant functional limitation, it is cost-effective.

Knee Replacement. Segal and others (2004) review a number of interventions for OA and suggest a cost per QALY of US$5,407 for knee replacement in Australia.

COST-EFFECTIVENESS OF INTERVENTIONS FOR RA

The result of a decade of vigorous debate about the appropriate treatment strategies for RA appears to be a consensus that patients with moderate or severe RA should be treated early and aggressively, if possible, by combining several disease-modifying antirheumatic drugs (DMARDs) (Maetzel and others 2002).

The complex medical management of RA can involve the use of a large number of agents, including NSAIDs, low-dose corticosteroids, and a long list of DMARDs. The economic literature for interventions in RA has, for good reason, tended to focus on the cost-effectiveness of the alternatives that arise when a particular management strategy fails. In that sense, the intervention-based taxonomy used in earlier sections of this chapter is a less helpful way to characterize some of the contributions to this field. Thus, the subsections used in this part of the chapter reflect at times a problem-based taxonomy and at other times an intervention-based classification.

Treatment Modalities

One of the challenges common to the developing world is that specialized medical expertise is often scarce. Thus, the consideration of a variety of treatment modalities is worthwhile, especially those that involve labor substitution between specialist and nonspecialist categories. Unfortunately, relatively few studies of this kind, let alone large randomized studies, are available for RA.

In a nonrandomized study of 26 patients in Finland, Nordstrom and others (1996) compare the costs of treating RA patients either as inpatients or as outpatients. Even though the authors find that the cost of treating patients as outpatients was approximately one-sixth the cost of inpatient treatment, the small sample size and possible bias associated with the nonrandomized design mean that the study's results cannot be generalized.

An interesting and possibly cost-effective strategy for managing RA involves the use of a telephone help line staffed by specialist nurses. Hughes and others (2002) examine the costs and benefits of such an intervention in the United Kingdom and conclude that it was cost saving. Their work was based on a sample of 87 RA patients who used the telephone help line in a given month. A large proportion of respondents indicated that they used the help line in place of a visit to a general practitioner, and on this basis, the authors computed that the service produced a net saving.

The existing evidence on the effectiveness and cost-effectiveness of a telephone help line for RA patients is based on a relatively small sample. Nevertheless, this type of intervention may be useful in developing regions with good communications but low levels of access to medical care. This type of intervention may be particularly worthy of consideration when direct access to a medical practitioner is associated with large travel costs.

Disease-Modifying Antirheumatic Drugs

DMARDs include cyclosporine, azathioprine, D-penicillamine, sulfasalazine, etanercept, hydroxychloroquine, methotrexate, leflunomide, and gold compounds. Gabriel, Coyle, and Moreland (2001) provide a comprehensive review of the effectiveness and cost-effectiveness of DMARDs, including a comprehensive literature search in which they retrieved 30 articles from 500 identified for possible relevance. Only six of those papers included economic evaluations, and of those six, only three included measures of both benefits and costs. Only one of the articles used a nonclinical outcome measure (QALYs). Thus, the cost-effectiveness evidence for the use of DMARDs to treat patients with RA is generally scant.

The three full economic evaluations of DMARDs that Gabriel, Coyle, and Moreland identified were studies of auranofin (oral gold) (Thompson and others 1988), cyclosporine (Anis and others 1996), and combined therapy (Verhoeven and others 1998).

Auranofin. Thompson and others (1988) compare the cost-effectiveness of auranofin with that of a placebo using data

from a six-month RCT of 311 patients with RA. The authors report that the cost of auranofin was approximately US$692 greater than for the placebo treatment, but the lack of efficacy of auranofin means that it is now rarely used in RA treatment.

Cyclosporine, Azathioprine, and D-penicillamine. In a Canadian study, Anis and others (1996) conduct a cost-effectiveness analysis of cyclosporine use in patients with RA based on the results of a meta-analysis of five RCTs. Their comparators included a placebo control, azathioprine, and D-penicillamine and analyses based on societal costs or third-party payer costs, but the ICERs were expressed as the cost per patient per year improved, so the results are difficult to interpret in the context of a general priority-setting exercise for health expenditures. For the purposes of this chapter, perhaps the study's most useful result was that it found no statistically significant differences between cyclosporine, azathioprine, and D-penicillamine.

Given that the existing evidence on cyclosporine, azathioprine, and D-penicillamine indicates similar levels of efficacy, cyclosporine should be used only after less expensive and more effective therapies for the management of RA, including azathioprine and D-penicillamine.

Combination Therapy. Verhoeven and others (1998) analyze the use of combination therapy using data from the Combinatietherapie Bij Reumatoide Artritis, or COBRA study, conducted in Europe between 1993 and 1995. The study was a 56-week trial that involved treating an intervention group with sulfasalazine, methotrexate, and prednisolone versus sulfasalazine alone as a control. Even though the authors conclude that combined therapy is cost-effective, they qualify the results by stating that the study was probably underpowered. Despite the lack of good cost-effective data, the standard approach to RA treatment is to use combination therapy with DMARDs and to maintain corticosteroids at 7.5 milligrams per day or less if possible.

Biologics. A number of trials have shown that the biologic agents (tumor necrosis factor inhibitors and others) are the most effective agents available for reducing inflammation in RA. Their cost (US$10,000 to US$15,000 per patient per year); mode of administration (intramuscular, subcutaneous, or by intravenous infusion); and potential side effects (particularly the reactivation of tuberculosis) preclude their use in developing countries. Until trials are carried out in developing environments and are combined with robust cost-effectiveness data, we cannot recommend their use.

Corticosteroids. Bae and others (2003) analyze the cost-effectiveness of low-dose corticosteroids for the long-term treatment of RA. They compare the results of corticosteroid treatment with treatment using any DMARDs plus a corticosteroid and with treatment using DMARDs and NSAIDs. Their modeling includes a consideration of the rates of relevant side effects of the treatments. They also look at NSAID-use scenarios that included Proton Pump Inhibitor prophylaxis and the use of COX-2–specific inhibitors rather than nonspecific NSAIDs.

The results generally showed that corticosteroids dominate nonselective NSAIDs in terms of their cost-effectiveness. The exceptions were when the adverse events rate for corticosteroids was assumed to be 1.5 times that of the base case and when the comparators' adverse events rates were assumed to be 0.5 to 1.0 times the base case rate. In the latter case, the cost per QALY was US$114,168, and in the former, NSAIDs were dominant. The comparison of COX-2–specific inhibitors with corticosteroids produced a higher-cost and higher-utility outcome: the resulting incremental cost per QALY was US$132,880.

The authors also produced useful age-specific estimates of the cost-effectiveness of the two alternative treatment approaches. Their ICERs show that corticosteroids dominate for the management of 50- and 60-year-olds with RA. For 40-, 30-, and 20-year-olds, the ICERs were US$11,258, US$30,938, and US$46,981, respectively.

The evidence suggests that a management strategy of DMARDs plus low-dose corticosteroids is a less costly and more effective strategy than DMARDs plus NSAIDs in older age groups, largely because of the higher risks of adverse gastrointestinal events in those groups. For developing countries, a relevant question to consider is the extent to which life expectancy and risk factors for adverse gastrointestinal events will differ from the age groups Bae and others (2003) studied. Corticosteroid-induced OP is also a long-term risk, but for women with RA starting corticosteroid therapy, watchful waiting is recommended as preferable to screening, as long as the steroid dose remains below 7 milligrams per day.

COST-EFFECTIVENESS OF INTERVENTIONS FOR OTHER MUSCULOSKELETAL CONDITIONS

Low Back Pain

Low back pain is as common in developing countries as it is in the developed world. Health professionals now generally agree that conservative care for acute lower back pain is the initial treatment of choice, unless there is structural evidence of pathology that is amenable to surgical intervention (Gatchel and others 2003). Evidence also indicates that programs that incorporate some physical activity may reduce the costs of both acute and chronic low back pain compared with those that do not involve activity.

For economic evaluations, one of the important complicating factors associated with low back pain is that the nonmeasurement of indirect costs may introduce substantial bias into estimates of the cost-effectiveness of interventions. This problem is potentially serious because, in some cases, investigators have estimated the indirect costs of low back pain at more than twice those of the direct medical costs (Bolten, Kempel-Waibel, and Pforringer 1998).

Back Schools. Van Tulder and others (2003) review 15 RCTs of back schools for patients with recurrent and chronic low back pain, but they consider only three of these to be of high quality. They conclude that the evidence is only moderate that back schools have better short-term effects than other treatments for chronic back pain. They also find some evidence that back schools are more effective than placebos or waiting list controls in occupational settings. However, the authors note that little is currently known about the cost-effectiveness of back schools. Thus, evidence is insufficient to provide a recommendation on the probable cost-effectiveness of back schools for low back pain in developing countries; however, early intervention, education, and exercise programs should be encouraged.

Massage. Furlan and others (2002) examine the effectiveness and cost-effectiveness of a variety of massage techniques for nonspecific low back pain by comparing them with (a) sham or placebo massage, (b) other medical treatments, or (c) no treatment. The authors conclude that massage might be beneficial for patients with subacute and chronic nonspecific low back pain, especially when combined with exercises and education. The evidence suggests that acupuncture massage is more effective than classic massage, but this finding needs to be confirmed.

Little is known about the cost-effectiveness of massage for low back pain. On the basis of the existing evidence, in countries or regions in which massage—especially acupunctural massage—is routinely available at low cost, the intervention may be cost-effective. Where acupunctural interventions are considered, the costs of bloodborne disease transmission must also be weighed against the expected benefits of the intervention. This consideration may be important in countries where the prevalence of bloodborne viruses is high, particularly if strict infection control measures are not routinely followed.

Early Interventions. The few studies of early intervention programs to reduce the progression of acute low back pain to chronic pain have tended to report considerable cost savings. Gatchel and others (2003) published a prospective trial of early interventions in individuals with acute low back pain and a high risk of the pain progressing to chronicity. The authors screened approximately 700 patients and designated them as being at either low or high risk. The patients were then assigned to early or nonintervention groups and followed for 12 months. The early intervention was generally conducted over a three-week period and involved an intensive, multidisciplinary approach that included exercise classes, biofeedback and pain management classes, group education sessions, case manager and occupational therapist sessions, and interdisciplinary team conferences.

The early intervention resulted in statistically significant differences in return-to-work outcomes, number of health care visits, and number of disability days caused by back pain. It also resulted in a variety of pain surrogates. Furthermore, the mean cost savings were approximately US$9,000 per patient. The direct costs for the intervention group were approximately US$2,500 higher than those for the intervention group, but this finding was largely the result of the up-front costs of the intervention program itself. The direct costs of health care visits and pharmaceuticals were considerably lower for the intervention group.

The evidence suggests that an intensive, multidisciplinary, early intervention program is cost saving for individuals with acute low back pain who are at high risk of having the pain progress to chronicity; however, the cost savings associated with this intervention are attributable to improved labor market outcomes and earnings for injured individuals. The intervention itself may increase costs in the short term, but it appears to be associated with medium and long-term net benefits. Labor market conditions, including wages, along with the age of low back pain sufferers, may have an important bearing on the viability of this type of intervention in developing countries.

Ankylosing Spondylitis

Although the direct costs associated with ankylosing spondylitis are relatively low, its impact on indirect costs, including pain and suffering, are substantial. To date, little work has been done on the economics of interventions for ankylosing spondylitis. Pharmaceutical interventions are currently typically limited to NSAIDs and DMARDs such as methotrexate and sulfasalazine. Van Tubergen and others (2002), however, analyze the cost-effectiveness of a spa exercise intervention. The intervention period was three weeks, and although the authors argue that the cost-effectiveness of the intervention was favorable, they also note that the ICERs were sensitive to variations in assumptions about indirect costs.

Although a spa exercise program is apparently beneficial and may even be considered cost-effective for ankylosing spondylitis sufferers in developed countries, the current cost-effectiveness evidence does not provide a compelling case for widespread adoption of the intervention in developing regions. Patients, however, should be encouraged to exercise—especially to swim. The cost-effectiveness of tumor necrosis factor–inhibiting drugs is not yet evident for ankylosing spondylitis, but the drugs are currently unattractive investments for developing countries because of their high price.

IMPLEMENTATION OF CONTROL STRATEGIES: LESSONS OF EXPERIENCE

Given the increasing burden of musculoskeletal conditions worldwide, addressing ways of preventing musculoskeletal conditions is an important step. Few examples are available of the implementation of strategies aimed specifically at preventing musculoskeletal conditions, but many recommendations are aimed at modifying determinants that affect other aspects of health in addition to musculoskeletal health. These recommendations include ensuring adequate physical activity to maintain physical fitness; maintaining an ideal body weight; ensuring a balanced diet that meets the recommended daily allowances for calcium and vitamin D; avoiding smoking; balancing the use of alcohol and avoiding alcohol abuse; and putting in place accident prevention programs to reduce musculoskeletal injuries related to road traffic accidents, leisure activities, and workplaces. Various programs involve changes in the behavior of individuals and control of environmental hazards (these programs are considered elsewhere in this volume). Personal behavior changes can be achieved by education but may require resources such as sports facilities. A safe environment will involve all sectors, and successful implementation may require legislation. The benefits of these interventions on musculoskeletal health are not quantified, but in any case they are probably small. Physical activity and an ideal weight will benefit the broadest range of musculoskeletal conditions.

Osteoarthritis

The strategy for managing OA is pain management with simple analgesics or NSAIDs, along with education to facilitate self-management and rehabilitative programs to improve function, activities, and participation. These strategies include general and specific exercise programs, devices such as walking sticks, and environmental modifications. Joint replacement surgery should be considered for end-stage joint damage. Simple analgesics can be accessible over the counter or through health clinics. Education and rehabilitative programs can also be delivered through health clinics. Joint replacement surgery requires resources in terms of physical facilities, financial resources, and expertise. The cost-effectiveness of arthroplasty is greatly affected by complications such as infection or failure of the prosthesis, both of which are related to inadequate resources.

Pain management should be available to those who have disabling symptoms and is dependent on access to drugs and education with respect to the benefits and risks. Access to arthroplasty will be the greatest challenge, given the increasing needs in the developing world brought about by aging populations and increases in other risk factors such as reduced physical activity and increasing obesity.

Rheumatoid Arthritis

The greatest successes in recent years include advances in managing RA and the ability to control disease activity; to prevent tissue damage; and to improve function, activities, and participation. Methotrexate is a readily accessible, effective antirheumatic drug. Monitoring full blood count and liver function is recommended, but the rarity of serious adverse events may necessitate a review of this recommendation if the costs and difficulties of monitoring would deny access to the drug. Symptomatic therapy with NSAIDs and multidisciplinary rehabilitation are also key components of the management of RA. Central to this approach is ensuring early and accurate diagnosis with long-term expert review, which requires public awareness about arthritis and adequate competency and facilities in the community and in health clinics for diagnosis and management. Education and rehabilitation can also be delivered in these settings. Paramedical workers can be trained to undertake much of this work. The problem is to ensure adequate training and experience of health care workers for a condition that affects 0.3 to 0.5 percent of adults in developing countries. Without treatment, the effects of RA can be great, so effective management can yield significant gains. The costs are relatively low, because paramedical workers can deliver much of the care and because the drugs are not new and are widely available.

Several established market economies have set up early arthritis clinics, but running such clinics effectively may be more difficult without a system to encourage and enable early access to specialist care. The management of established RA is usually undertaken by specialists in partnership with primary care. Programs for managing RA are usually self-sustaining and expandable because of the chronic incurable nature of the condition and the general public's gradual recognition of what can be achieved.

Osteoporosis

The prevention of fractures related to OP is based on a "bone-healthy" lifestyle of individuals who have adequate dietary calcium, vitamin D, and weight-bearing exercise and who avoid smoking and excessive alcohol consumption. Implementing such measures requires raising public awareness and educating primary care personnel. In addition, those at high risk of fracture who would benefit from a specific intervention need to be identified by the presence of risk factors, including low bone density. The limitation to this approach is a lack of access to bone densitometry, in which case the decision to treat may have to be made on clinical grounds alone. The occurrence of low-trauma fracture is a good indicator of OP and, in the presence of other clinical risk factors, may be reason enough to treat. In particular, multiple vertebral fractures are virtually diagnostic of OP.

Various local programs aim at identifying and treating those with OP. Their costs relate not only to diagnostic tests but also to treatment. The cost of bisphosphonates is high compared with the income levels in those countries likely to experience the greatest increase in the burden of OP. The speed of benefits of bisphosphonates is good, with clinical trials demonstrating fracture risk reduction within 12 to 18 months. The role of HRT is not clear at present, but because of the likely increased risk of cardiovascular disease and strokes outweighing the benefit of fracture prevention, it is not currently recommended for preventing OP in unselected women. However, the benefit-risk ratio will be favorable in those at increased risk of fracture and low risk of cardiovascular disease, and the costs of HRT are more feasible. Adherence to treatments for OP to prevent fracture is poor because of the silent nature of their effect, and patient education to modify expectations is important. The effectiveness of any fracture prevention program depends on adherence for as long as possible, given the long-term character of the condition.

RESEARCH AND DEVELOPMENT

Another important issue with musculoskeletal disease is the development of a research agenda.

Size and Nature of the Burden of Disease

Uncertainty about the epidemiology of some musculoskeletal conditions is still considerable, especially in developing countries (WHO 2003). Incidence estimates for OA and RA have recently been generated from available epidemiological data on prevalence, relative mortality risks, and so on, though for some regions even these basic epidemiological data are scant (Africa, Asia, and South America for RA and Africa, Eastern Europe, and South America for OA). Additional primary measurement is required to produce a more accurate picture of interregional and intraregional epidemiological variations. This deficiency limits estimates of the overall burdens of the various musculoskeletal conditions and the extent to which they might be reduced.

The studies of the Community-Oriented Program for Control of Rheumatic Disease (COPCORD) (Darmawan and others 1995) are, in part, meeting this need. The Bone and Joint Monitor Project is also undertaking initiatives to standardize data collection and reporting in epidemiological studies to improve the collation and comparison of needed epidemiological data. Global burden-of-disease data concentrate on specific diagnoses, but a far greater burden that has yet to be estimated relates to regional and generalized musculoskeletal problems characterized by pain with disability. More research is necessary in this area.

Evaluation of Existing Interventions

Few reliable economic evaluations of available interventions have been done. One reason is that a surprising number of interventions have inadequate trial data or efficacy measures, and many reasonably well-established interventions need to be tested in trials against appropriate comparators. The heterogeneity of comparators used in different economic evaluations and other methodological differences pose material risks to comparisons of the costs and consequences of different interventions for musculoskeletal conditions, and some standardization is needed.

Many studies have used only clinical outcomes and not life years saved or QALYs as outcome measures. Positive steps are being taken to correct the situation. The Outcome Measures in Rheumatology Clinical Trials Economics Working Group (Gabriel, Tugwell, and Drummond 2002) has made some progress toward redressing this problem in the rheumatology economics literature. Although work is not yet complete, this concerted approach to standardization holds promise for the literature.

Avertable Proportion of the Burden

New data are needed to estimate the burden that could be averted by implementing the proposed strategies. Available data are currently limited and relate predominantly to individual interventions in short-term clinical trials with outcomes that do not enable reliable estimates of the avertable burden. Interventions need to be evaluated, often in combination with outcome measures that enable the burden on individuals and society to be measured meaningfully and in more naturalistic circumstances. Concordance cannot be assumed, in particular for these largely chronic conditions, and it is influenced by many personal and environmental factors. The impact of musculoskeletal conditions is pervasive, underrecognized, and underestimated. Therefore, data are needed not only on what is theoretically avertable, but also on what is being averted and the reasons for any disparities.

Resource Requirements

The implementation of strategies for preventing and controlling musculoskeletal conditions is multisectoral, and the resource consequences of this need to be established. Different models for the delivery of a strategy may have different resource implications. These variations need to be explored to ensure appropriate investment and provision of resources.

Likely Effectiveness of Interventions on Both Health and Nonhealth Benefits

Musculoskeletal conditions are common and have a major impact on individuals and society; however, they are inadequately treated, and the success of simple interventions is not being achieved because of a lack of prioritization and resources. Strategies for preventing musculoskeletal conditions have a wide range of other health benefits; they need to be jointly promoted, and the additional benefits need to be better recognized. The various determinants of ill health—such as lack of physical activity or obesity—that pose a risk to musculoskeletal health need to be quantified along with their other detrimental effects. The benefits and cost-effectiveness of modifying these determinants of health, with regard to preventing or modifying the outcome of musculoskeletal conditions, need to be quantified and compared with strategies that focus on personal interventions.

Implementation

Improving musculoskeletal health requires implementing strategies for preventing and controlling certain diseases and environmental risk factors. Selected strategies must be in line with local needs, priorities, and resources. Informed decision making at the policy level requires data on the burden and the avertable burden of musculoskeletal conditions, plus the costs for particular populations by strategy. Changes in local demographics that are likely to increase the effect of musculoskeletal conditions also need to be considered before developing plans for implementation.

CONCLUSIONS: PROMISES AND PITFALLS

Musculoskeletal diseases are the most common cause of chronic disability worldwide and will become increasingly important as aging populations require relief from chronic pain and disability. One of the characteristics of musculoskeletal diseases is that they are not fatal and do not have the high profile of other conditions, such as cancer and heart disease. However, they are preventable in many cases, and simple interventions, such as maintaining ideal body weight and participating in an exercise program, may have a significant effect on long-term morbidity. However, the field of musculoskeletal disease is thwarted by a significant lack of epidemiological and outcome data across a broad spectrum of geography, condition, and treatments.

The designation of 2000–10 as the Bone and Joint Decade by the United Nations, WHO, and 60 countries will certainly help raise the profile of these diseases in local communities. All nations have a significant opportunity to embrace the decade, to ensure that their populations understand the importance of these diseases, and to encourage the training of a range of health professionals to deal with this burgeoning epidemic.

Improving knowledge among health workers at all levels about musculoskeletal conditions is important for early diagnosis and intervention, as is the provision of access to specialist services, such as orthopedic surgery. Simple programs that emphasize the importance of obesity and lack of exercise as predictors of poor musculoskeletal outcomes are low cost, but their implementation and their influence on health outcomes need to be assessed in properly conducted studies. Medications—particularly analgesic and anti-inflammatory drugs for arthritis and pain and vitamin D and calcium supplementation to prevent OP—need to be widely available.

Exciting advances in the treatment of inflammatory forms of arthritis with biologics need to be evaluated from an economic perspective, particularly in developing nations, where the risk of exacerbating underlining infections such as tuberculosis is much higher than in developed countries. Currently, biologic agents are not cost-effective in developing countries, but they may be in the future. Access to hip and knee replacements, probably the most cost-effective surgical intervention available, is important but depends on the availability of a qualified staff.

Musculoskeletal diseases will continue to present a challenge to the health systems of both developing and developed countries, but as we solve some of the issues related to communicable diseases, the hope is that more resources will become available for tackling the burgeoning epidemic of noncommunicable disease, including musculoskeletal conditions.

ACKNOWLEDGMENTS

We gratefully acknowledge the capable research assistance provided by Richard Supangan.

REFERENCES

Anis, A. H., P. X. Tugwell, G. A. Wells, and D. G. Stewart. 1996. "A Cost Effectiveness Analysis of Cyclosporine in Rheumatoid Arthritis." *Journal of Rheumatology* 23 (4): 609–16.

Armstrong, K., T.-M. Chen, D. Albert, T. C. Randall, and J. S. Schwartz. 2001. "Cost-Effectiveness of Raloxifene and Hormone Replacement Therapy in Postmenopausal Women: Impact of Breast Cancer Risk." *Obstetrics and Gynaecology* 98 (6): 996–1003.

Bae, S.-C., M. Corzillius, K. M. Kuntz, and M. H. Liang. 2003. "Cost-Effectiveness of Low Dose Corticosteroids versus Non-steroidal Anti-inflammatory Drugs and COX-2 Specific Inhibitors in the Long-Term Treatment of Rheumatoid Arthritis." *Rheumatology* 42 (1): 46–53.

Bolten, W., A. Kempel-Waibel, and W. Pforringer. 1998. "Analysis of the Cost of Illness in Backache." *Medizinische Klinik* 93 (6): 388–93.

Chang, R. W., J. M. Pellissier, and G. B. Hazen. 1996. "A Cost-Effectiveness Analysis of Total Hip Arthroplasty for Osteoarthritis of the Hip." *Journal of the American Medical Association* 275 (11): 858–65.

Coyle, D., A. Cranney, K. M. Lee, V. Welch, and P. Tugwell. 2001. "Cost Effectiveness of Nasal Calcitonin in Postmenopausal Women: Use of Cochrane Collaboration Methods for Meta-Analysis within Economic Evaluation." *Pharmacoeconomics* 19 (5, part 2): 565–75.

Darmawan, J., H. A. Valkenburg, K. D. Muirden, and R. D. Wigley. 1995. "The Prevalence of Soft Tissue Rheumatism in Indonesia: A WHO-ILAR COPCORD Study." *Rheumatology International* 15 (3): 121–24.

Fleurence, R., D. J. Torgerson, and D. M. Reid. 2002. "Cost-Effectiveness of Hormone Replacement Therapy for Fracture Prevention in Young Postmenopausal Women: An Economic Analysis Based on a Prospective Cohort Study." *Osteoporosis International* 13 (8): 637–43.

Furlan, A. D., L. Brosseau, M. Imamura, and E. Irvan. 2002. "Massage for Low-Back Pain: A Systematic Review within the Framework of the Cochrane Collaboration Back Review Group." *Spine* 27 (17): 1896–910.

Gabriel, S. E., M. E. Campion, and W. M. O'Fallon. 1994. "A Cost-Utility Analysis of Misoprostol Prophylaxis for Rheumatoid Arthritis Patients Receiving Nonsteroidal Antiinflammatory Drugs." *Arthritis and Rheumatology* 37 (3): 333–41.

Gabriel, S. E., D. Coyle, and L. W. Moreland. 2001 "A Clinical and Economic Review of Disease-Modifying Antirheumatic Drugs." *Pharmacoeconomics* 19 (7): 715–28.

Gabriel, S. E., P. Tugwell, and M. Drummond. 2002. "Progress towards an OMERACT-ILAR Guideline for Economic Evaluations in Rheumatology." *Annals of the Rheumatic Diseases* 61 (4): 370–73.

Gatchel, R. J., P. B. Polatin, C. Noe, M. Gardea, C. Pulliam, and J. Thompson. 2003. "Treatment- and Cost-Effectiveness of Early Intervention for Acute Low-Back Pain Patients: A One-Year Prospective Study." *Journal of Occupational Rehabilitation* 13 (1): 1–9.

Geelhoed, E., A. Harris, and R. Prince. 1994. "Cost-Effectiveness Analysis of Hormone Replacement Therapy and Lifestyle Intervention for Hip Fracture." *Australian Journal of Public Health* 18 (2): 153–60.

Hazes, M., and A. D. Woolf. 2000. The Bone and Joint Decade 2000–2010. *Journal of Rheumatology* 27:1–3.

Hughes, R. A., M. E. Carr, A. Huggett, and C. E. Thwaites. 2002. "Review of the Function of a Telephone Helpline in the Treatment of Outpatients with Rheumatoid Arthritis." *Annals of the Rheumatic Diseases* 61 (4): 341–45.

Jitapunkul, S., C. Kunanusont, W. Phoolcharoen, P. Suriyawongpaisal, and S. Ebrahim. 2003. "Determining Public Health Priorities for an Ageing Population: The Value of a Disability Survey." *Southeast Asian Journal of Tropical Medicine and Public Health* 34 (4): 929–36.

Jönsson, B., J. Kanis, A. Dawson, A. Oden, and O. Johnell. 1999. "Effect and Offset of Effect of Treatments for Hip Fracture on Health Outcomes." *Osteoporosis International* 10 (3): 193–99.

Kanis, J. A., J. E. Brazier, M. Stevenson, N. W. Calvert, and M. Lloyd Jones. 2002. "Treatment of Established Osteoporosis: A Systematic Review and Cost-Utility Analysis." *Health Technology Assessment* 6 (29): 1–146.

Katzmarzyk, P. T., N. Gledhill, and R. J. Shephard. 2000. "The Economic Burden of Physical Inactivity in Canada." *Canadian Medical Association Journal* 163 (11): 1435–40.

Lord, J., C. Victor, P. Littlejohns, F. M. Ross, and J. S. Axford. 1999. "Economic Evaluation of a Primary Care-Based Education Programme for Patients with Osteoarthritis of the Knee." *Health Technology Assessment* 3 (23): 1–55.

Maetzel, A., V. Strand, P. Tugwell, G. Wells, and C. Bombardier. 2002. "Cost-Effectiveness of Adding Leflunomide to a Five-Year Strategy of Conventional Disease-Modifying Antirheumatic Drugs in Patients with Rheumatoid Arthritis." *Arthritis and Rheumatism* 47 (6): 655–61.

McCabe, C. J., R. L. Akehurst, J. Kirsch, M. Whitfield, M. Backhouse, A. D. Woolf, and others. 1998. "Choice of NSAID and Management Strategy in Rheumatoid Arthritis and Osteoarthritis: The Impact on Costs and Outcomes in the U.K." *Pharmacoeconomics* 14 (2): 191–99.

McGill, P. E., and G. O. Oyoo. 2002. "Rheumatic Disorders in Sub-Saharan Africa." *East African Medical Journal* 79 (4): 214–16.

Nordstrom, D. C. E., Y. T. Kontinnen, S. Solovieva, C. Friman, and S. Santavirta. 1996. "In- and Out-Patient Rehabilitation in Rheumatoid Arthritis." *Scandinavian Journal of Rheumatology* 25 (4): 200–6.

Norlund, A. 1996. "Prevention of Osteoporosis: A Cost-Effectiveness Analysis Regarding Fractures." *Scandinavian Journal of Rheumatology* 25 (Suppl. 103): 42–45.

Patrick, D. L., S. D. Ramsey, A. C. Spencer, S. Kinne, B. Belza, and T. D. Topolski. 2001. "Economic Evaluation of Aquatic Exercise for Persons with Osteoarthritis." *Medical Care* 39 (5): 413–24.

Segal, L., S. E. Day, A. B. Chapman, and R. H. Osborne. 2004. "Can We Reduce Disease Burden from Osteoarthritis." *Medical Journal of Australia* 180 (Suppl. 5): S11–17.

Symmons D., C. Mathers, and B. Pfleger. 2004a. *Global Burden of Osteoarthritis in the Year 2000.* Geneva: World Health Organization.

———. 2004b. *The Global Burden of Rheumatoid Arthritis in the Year 2000.* Geneva: World Health Organization.

Thompson M. S., J. L. Read, H. C. Hutchings, M. Paterson, and E. D. J. Harris. 1988. "The Cost Effectiveness of Auranofin: Results of a Randomized Clinical Trial." *Journal of Rheumatology* 15 (1): 35–42.

Torrance, G. W., J. P. Raynauld, V. Walker, C. H. Goldsmith, N. Bellamy, and P. A. Band, and others. 2002. "A Prospective, Randomized, Pragmatic, Health Outcomes Trial Evaluating the Incorporation of Hylan G-F 20 into the Treatment Paradigm for Patients with Knee Osteoarthritis (Part 2 of 2): Economic Results." *Osteoarthritis and Cartilage* 10 (7): 518–27.

van Dieten, H. E. M., I. B. C. Korthals-De Bros, M. W. van Tulder, W. F. Lems, B. A. C. Dijkmans, and M. Boers. 2000. "Systematic Review of the Cost Effectiveness of Prophylactic Treatments in the Prevention of Gastropathy in Patients with Rheumatoid Arthritis or Osteoarthritis Taking Non-steroidal Anti-inflammatory Drugs." *Annals of the Rheumatic Diseases* 59 (10): 753–59.

van Tubergen, A., A. Boonen, R. Landewe, M. Rutten–van Molken, D. van der Heijde, A. Hidding, and S. van der Linden. 2002. "Cost Effectiveness of Combined Spa-Exercise Therapy in Ankylosing Spondylitis: A Randomized Controlled Trial." *Arthritis and Rheumatism* 47 (5): 459–67.

van Tulder, M. W., R. Esmail, C. Bombardier, and B. W. Koes. 2003. "Back Schools for Non-specific Low Back Pain." *Cochrane Library* (2), Update Software, Oxford, U.K.

Verhoeven, A. C., J. C. Bibo, M. Boers, G. L. Engel, and S. van der Linden. 1998. "Cost-Effectiveness and Cost-Utility of Combination Therapy in Early Rheumatoid Arthritis: Randomized Comparison of Combined Step-Down Prednisolone, Methotrexate, and Sulphasalazine with Sulphasalazine Alone." *British Journal of Rheumatology* 37 (10): 1102–9.

WHO (World Health Organization). 2000. "Global Burden of Disease." Global Programme on Evidence for Health Policy Discussion Paper 50, WHO, Geneva.

———. 2003. "The Burden of Musculoskeletal Conditions at the Start of the New Millennium." WHO Technical Report Series 919, WHO, Geneva.

———. 2004. *Annex 3: Burden of Disease in Disability-Adjusted Life-Years (DALYs), by Cause, Sex, and Mortality Stratum, in WHO Regions, Estimates for 2001.* Geneva: WHO. http://www.who.int/whr/2002/annex/en/print.html.

Willis, M. S. 2002. "The Health Economics of Calcium and Vitamin D₃ for the Prevention of Osteoporotic Hip Fractures in Sweden." *International Journal of Technology Assessment in Health Care* 18 (4): 791–807.

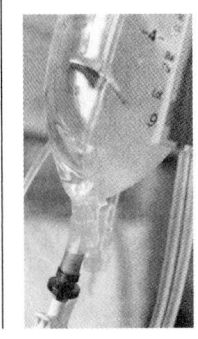

Chapter **52**

Pain Control for People with Cancer and AIDS

Kathleen M. Foley, Judith L. Wagner, David E. Joranson, and Hellen Gelband

The undertreatment of chronic pain is a global problem, especially for people in the final stages of cancer and, increasingly, AIDS. The pain of dying is often severe, but it can be controlled for most people by a simple and inexpensive intervention: oral analgesic drugs, including morphine and other opioids. Although it was long known that opioid drugs were essential for the relief of moderate to severe pain, even in the 1980s the amounts being used globally were so low that only a minority of those dying could have had adequate pain relief. Since then progress has been made, mainly in resource-rich countries, widening the gap between rich and poor. The absence of opioids in developing countries is not merely a problem of supply or costs, however. This chapter lays out the institutional and political barriers that restrict their availability in most low- and middle-income countries.

BURDEN OF PAIN FROM CANCER AND AIDS

Pain is "an unpleasant sensory and emotional experience associated with either actual or potential tissue damage or described in terms of such damage" (Task Force on Taxonomy 2004). Pain, in its various manifestations, is the most common symptom leading patients to seek medical assistance (box 52.1).

Measurement of Pain

Pain is a subjective experience, but it can be described by patients and assessed using validated questionnaires and scales (Cleeland 1990). In *categorical scales*, the patient describes the pain using specific words, for example, mild, moderate, severe,

or excruciating. With *numerical scales*, patients rate their pain by choosing a number—for example, from 0 (no pain) to 10 (worst pain). *Visual analog scales* often take the form of a ruled line, anchored on the left by the words *no pain* and on the right by *worst possible pain.*

Pain measurement instruments have been validated in clinical trials of analgesic therapies and subsequently used in national and international surveys, repeatedly demonstrating sensitivity and reliability for both cancer and AIDS patients. These instruments include the Brief Pain Inventory (Bernabei and others 1998; Cleeland and others 1996; Daut, Cleeland, and Flanery 1983), the Memorial Pain Assessment Card (Fishman and others 1987), the Memorial Symptom Assessment Scale (Portenoy and others 1994), and the Edmonton Symptom Assessment Scale (Chang, Hwang, and Feuerman 2000).

Effects of Pain

Pain dramatically affects quality of life. Patients with persistent serious pain cease participating in social activities and may be unable to work or care for their families (Daut, Cleeland, and Flanery 1983). Psychological effects, including depression and anxiety, increase with pain intensity (Rosenfeld and others 1996).

The suffering of an individual radiates throughout households, neighborhoods, and villages. Caregivers suffer distress, anxiety, and depression. They may have to give up their own employment to care for a dying relative. The loss of income of the patient and the caregiver may dramatically lower the family's social status (Murray and others 2003).

Box 52.1

Classification of Pain

Pain is classified according to two main characteristics: temporal and physiologic. *Temporal* categories are

- acute pain
  - characterized by a well-defined onset and self-limited end
  - allows clear description of location, character, and timing
  - shows signs of autonomic nervous system hyperactivity—for example, tachycardia, hypertension, profuse sweating (diaphoresis), dilated pupils (mydriasis), or pallor
- chronic or persistent pain
  - long lasting, usually defined as at least three months
  - characterized by a localization, character, and timing that is often more vague than with acute pain
  - characterized by adaptation of the autonomic nervous system, so signs of hyperactivity disappear

  - results in significant changes in psychological, functional, and social status.

Physiologic pain categories are

- somatic pain
  - originates in ligaments, tendons, bones, blood vessels, and nerves
  - sharp or dull, but typically well localized and intermittent
- visceral pain
  - originates in body organs and results from activation of nociceptive receptors and efferent nerves
  - characterized by deep aching and cramping, often referred to cutaneous sites
- neuropathic pain
  - results from direct injury to peripheral receptors, nerves, or the central nervous system
  - typically burning and dysesthetic (abnormal and unpleasant), often in area of sensory loss.

Source: Authors.

Pain in Patients with Cancer and AIDS

Several well-defined acute and chronic pain syndromes are associated with cancer, with HIV/AIDS, and with their treatment (Breitbart 2003; Foley 1979). In low-income countries, where patients usually present late in the course of illness, pain from the disease itself is more common than treatment-related pain.

Researchers consistently report that 60 to 90 percent of patients with advanced cancer experience moderate to severe pain, regardless of age and gender and whether ambulatory or hospitalized (Cleeland and others 1988; Cleeland and others 1996; Daut and Cleeland 1982; Foley 1979, 1999; Stjernsward and Clark 2003). The intensity, degree of pain relief, and effect of pain vary according to the type of cancer, treatment, and personal characteristics, but prevalence and severity of pain usually increase with disease progression. No population-based studies of AIDS-related pain have been published, but several researchers report that up to 80 percent of patients in the last phase of illness experience significant pain requiring analgesics (Larue, Fontaine, and Colleau 1997; Schofferman and Brody 1990; Singer and others 1993).

Pain Days

No standard metric has been developed to describe the pain burden for people at the end of life. We have adopted a transparent and direct measure—the *pain day*—defined as a

day of moderate or severe pain requiring an opioid drug for relief. The elements that determine the number of cancer and AIDS pain days in a population are the numbers dying from each condition and the average prevalence and duration of severe pain associated with dying.

Patterns of pain from specific cancers and from AIDS at given stages appear to be similar everywhere. However, because different cancers produce different symptoms, the mix of cancers in a country will influence the overall pattern and burden of pain reflected in the total number of pain days.

About 2.1 million deaths from cancer and about 3 million from AIDS occur annually in low- and middle-income countries (LMICs) worldwide, and these numbers are increasing. Using expert opinion, we estimate that about 80 percent of people dying from cancer and 50 percent of those dying from AIDS experience moderate or severe pain, lasting for an average of 90 days.

INTERVENTIONS FOR PAIN RELIEF

The goal of pain control is not to cure disease, but to allow patients to function as effectively as possible and to minimize pain. Interventions for pain relief include drugs, radiotherapy, and anesthetic, neurosurgical, psychological, and behavioral approaches (see table 52.1). However, analgesic drugs are the mainstay of treatment and the focus of this chapter. According

Table 52.1 Procedures Used to Control Specific Types of Cancer Pain

Type of procedure	Most common indications
Anesthetic	
Inhalation therapy with nitrous oxide	Breakthrough pain, incidental pain in patients with diffuse, poorly controlled pain
Intravenous barbiturates (for example, sodium pentobarbital)	Diffuse body pain and suffering inadequately controlled by systemic opioids
Local anesthetic by intravenous, subcutaneous, or transdermal application	Neuropathic pain in any site with local application to the area of hyperesthesia or allodynia
Trigger point injections	Focal muscle pain
Nerve block	
Peripheral	Pain in discrete dermatomes in chest and abdomen or in distal extremities
Epidural	Unilateral lumbar or sacral pain
	Midline perineal pain
	Bilateral lumbosacral pain
Intrathecal	Midline perineal pain
	Bilateral lumbosacral pain
Autonomic	
Stellate ganglion	Reflex sympathetic dystrophy
Lumbar sympathetic	Reflex sympathetic dystrophy of the lower extremities
	Lumbosacral plexopathy
	Vascular insufficiency of lower extremity
Celiac plexus	Midabdominal pain from tumor infiltration
Intermittent or continuous epidural infusion with local anesthetics	Unilateral and bilateral lumbosacral pain
	Midline perineal pain
	Neuropathic pain from the midthoracic region down
Intermittent or continuous epidural or intrathecal with local opioid analgesics	Unilateral and bilateral pain below the midthoracic region; often combined with local anesthetics
Intermittent or continuous intraventrical infusions with opioid analgesics	Head and neck pain and upper chest
Chemical hypophysectomy	Diffuse bone pain
Neuroablative	
Nerve root: rhizotomy	Somatic and neuropathic pain from tumor infiltration of the cranial and intercostal nerves
Spinal cord: dorsal root entry zone lesion	Unilateral neuropathic pain from brachial, intercostal, and lumbosacral plexopathy and postherpetic neuralgia
Spinal cord: cordotomy	Unilateral pain below the waist; often combined with local neurolytic blocks in perineal and bilateral lumbosacral plexopathy; may be performed bilaterally
Spinal cord: myelotomy	Midline pain below the waist, but rarely used because it involves extensive surgery
Brain stem: mesencephalic tractomy	Pain in the nasopharynx and trigeminal region
Thalamus: thalamotomy	Unilateral neuropathic pain in the chest and lower extremity
Cortex: cingulotomy	Useful through a stereotactic approach for diffuse pain
Pituitary: transsphenoidal hypophysectomy	Bone metastases in endocrine-dependent tumors, breast, and prostate
Neurostimulatory	
Peripheral nerve: transcutaneous and percutaneous electrical nerve stimulation	Dysesthesias from tumor infiltration of nerve or trauma
Spinal cord: dorsal column stimulation	Of limited use in neuropathic pain in the chest, midline, and lower extremities
Thalamus: thalamic stimulation	Of rare use in neuropathic pain in the chest, midline, or lower extremity
Radiotherapy	
External beam	Bone and brain metastases
	Nerve and spinal cord compression

(Continues on the following page.)

Table 52.1 Continued

Type of procedure	Most common indications
Physical	
Cutaneous stimulation (superficial heat, cold, massage)	Dysesthesias from tumor infiltration of nerve or trauma
Transcutaneous electrical nerve stimulation	Cutaneous nerve injury pain
Acupuncture	For focal or diffuse pain syndrome
Bed rest	Reduced movement–related pain syndrome
Psychological	
Hypnosis	Provides distraction and cognitive approach to reduce pain
Relaxation, imagery, biofeedback, distraction, reframing	Provides distraction and cognitive approach to reduce pain
Patient education	

Source: Breitbart 2003; Authors.

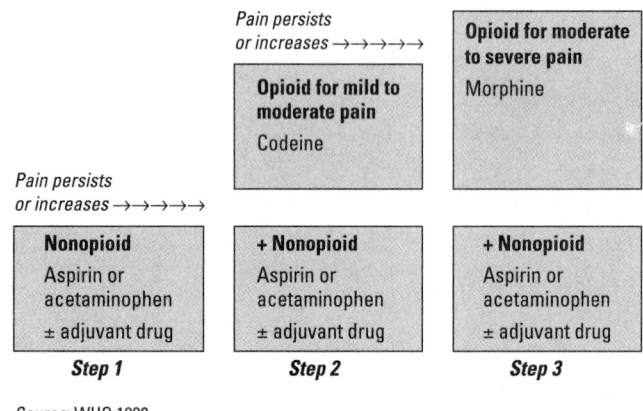

Source: WHO 1990.

Figure 52.1 The Three-Step Analgesic Ladder

to the World Health Organization (WHO), "A palliative care programme cannot exist unless it is based on a rational national drug policy," and this includes "regulations that allow ready access of suffering patients to opioids" (WHO 2002, 87).

WHO Three-Step Analgesic Ladder and Its Effectiveness

WHO has developed a "three-step analgesic ladder" (figure 52.1) for cancer pain and its treatment (WHO 1986), which includes a strong opioid (morphine) (table 52.2). The ladder is equally appropriate for patients with HIV/AIDS (O'Neill, Selwyn, and Schietinger 2003).

The steps in the ladder represent increasing pain severity and the drugs that should be used in each case:

- Step 1 is limited to nonopioids, including drugs that are widely available (for example, acetaminophen, aspirin, or nonsteroidal anti-inflammatory drugs, or NSAIDs).
- Step 2 describes moderate pain that requires a combination of a nonopioid and opioid for relief.

- Step 3 is for pain requiring a strong opioid. No specific dosages are recommended for opioid drugs because the concept of a standard dose does not apply: effective doses of oral morphine range from as little as 5 mg to more than 1,000 mg every four hours. Adjuvant drugs are also essential to treat side effects of analgesics or to provide additive analgesia (table 52.2).

Controlled field testing and clinical experience has demonstrated that 70 to 90 percent of cancer patients can achieve pain control using the ladder (Goudas, Carr, and Bloch 2001). Although the ladder has not been validated in formal studies for patients with AIDS, recent clinical reports describe its successful application (Anand, Carmosino, and Glatt 1994; Kimball and McCormick 1996; McCormack and others 1993; Newshan and Lefkowitz 2001; Newshan and Wainapel 1993; Schofferman and Brody 1990).

In an ideal world, a trained professional would prescribe pain medication throughout the course of illness, in accordance with the ladder. However, most patients self-medicate pain with analgesics and traditional medicines that they buy over the counter until they have late-stage disease and severe pain that can be treated only with a strong opioid. That is when they are most likely to seek formal medical care, which would start on step 3 of the ladder. Unfortunately, the opioid they need is unlikely to be unavailable in LMICs, even from health professionals.

Adequacy of and Barriers to Pain Control and Palliative Care in Developing Countries

The adequacy of pain control in populations is not easily measured. A useful and available surrogate is the per capita consumption of morphine (Joranson 1993), a figure based on mandatory annual reports by national governments to the International Narcotics Control Board (INCB). Of the 27 million grams of morphine used legally in 2002, 78 percent went to six countries—Australia, Canada, France, Germany,

Table 52.2 Basic Drug List for Cancer and AIDS Pain Relief: Analgesics and Adjuvant Drugs

Category Analgesics	Basic drugs	Alternatives
Nonopioids	Acetylsalicylic acid (aspirin)	Choline magnesium trisalicylate
	Acetaminophen	Diflunisal
	Ibuprofen	Naproxen
	Indomethacin	Diclofenac
Opioids for mild to moderate pain	Codeine	Dihydrocodeine
		Hydrocodone
		Tramadol
Opioids for moderate to severe pain	Morphine	Methadone
		Hydromorphone
		Oxycodone
		Pethidine
		Buprenorphine
		Fentanyl
Opioid antagonists	Naloxone	Nalorphine
Adjuvant drugs for analgesia and symptom control		
Antiemetics	Prochlorperazine	Metoclopramide
		Ondansetron
Laxatives	Senna	Cisacodyl
	Sodium docusate	Bran
	Mineral oil	Dantron
	Lactulose	Sorbitol
	Magnesium hydroxide	
Antidiarrheal agents	Loperamide	Paregoric
	Diphenoxylate hydrochloride and atropine sulfate	
Antidepressants (adjuvant analgesics)	Amitriptyline	Imipramine
		Paroxetine
Antipsychotic	Haloperidol	Thorazine
Anticonvulsants (adjuvant analgesics)	Gabapentin	Valproic acid
	Carbamazepine	
Corticosteroids	Prednisone	Prednisolone
	Dexamethasone	
Anxiolytics	Diazepam	Clonazepam
	Lorazepam	
	Midazolam	
Psychostimulants	Methylphenidate	Pemoline

Source: Foley, Aulino, and Stjernsward 2003.

the United Kingdom, and the United States. The rest went to the other 142 countries that reported. Morphine is largely unavailable in Africa, the eastern Mediterranean, and Southeast Asia (figure 52.2).

The major barriers to palliative care in LMICs are scarce resources, lack of national policies or low priority for pain relief, lack of awareness by health professionals and the public that cancer and AIDS pain can be relieved, concern that medical use of opioids will lead to drug abuse and addiction, and legal restrictions on opioids. Medical, religious, gender, social, and cultural factors also present barriers (see box 52.2). With AIDS, social and self-stigmatization work against adequate care of any kind. In addition, most of the emphasis in poor countries has been on prevention and, more recently, on antiretroviral drugs. In all cases, even less care is in place for children than for adults (Joranson, Rajagopal, and Gilson 2002).

Living with and Dying from Cancer in Scotland and Kenya

Physical suffering dominates the lives of people with advanced cancer in rural Kenya. In contrast, the concerns of cancer patients in Scotland, whose physical needs are met, focus on the prospect of death. A recent study compared these two groups.

The suffering in Kenya stems largely from poverty and the high cost of basic health care. Hospital care is limited, and patients feel happier at home. Families care for patients without drugs or supplies or even the knowledge of what to expect and how to help the patient. Patients are concerned about the physical and financial burden on

their families. They are comforted and inspired by religious beliefs and by the support of their communities. They accept their fate.

In Scotland, health care is free and of high quality. Patients are able to get primary treatment for the cancer and, when needed, palliative care. They are likely to be angry about their illness rather than accepting, and many feel isolated from family and friends. Although patients' physical needs are met routinely, psychosocial needs are met only for some.

Source: Murray and others 2003.

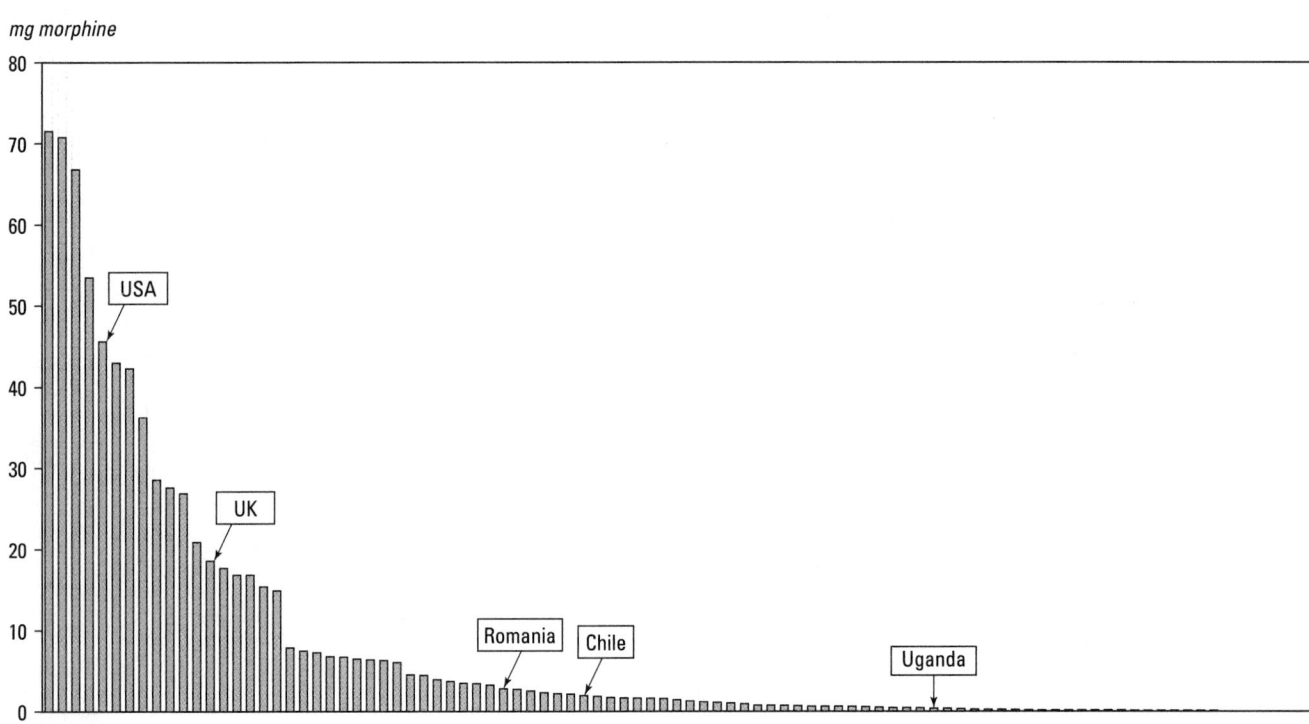

Source: INCB 2003 and authors' calculations.

Figure 52.2 Global Morphine Consumption, by Country (Per Capita, 2002)

Legal Controls on Opioid Drugs

The Single Convention on Narcotic Drugs of 1961, amended by the 1972 Protocol (United Nations 1961), is an international treaty that aims both to prevent the illicit production of, trafficking in, and use of narcotic drugs and to ensure their availability for medical and scientific needs. The INCB, established

in 1968 by the Single Convention, is the independent, quasi-judicial organization that implements the Single Convention.

The Single Convention requires that all countries (even nonsignatories) intending to make opioids available for medical use estimate national opioid needs and report annually on imports, exports, and distribution to the retail level. It also

Pain Control in Romania and Chile

Palliative care has developed in Romania since the early 1990s, largely through the Romanian Association for Palliative Care. Support has come predominantly from U.K. charities and from the Open Society Institute. Services are provided throughout the country by paid staff and volunteers in 10 hospital-based inpatient services, 9 hospice home care teams, 2 day care services, and 1 palliative care training center that provides services. Coverage is still low: only 15 percent of cancer patients are treated with opioid analgesics. Morphine is available (paid for by the government) only for terminally ill cancer patients. Prescription restrictions and extra authorization needed for releasing morphine to each patient are still so burdensome that patients may die before the paperwork is completed. The situation is improving gradually, however.

Palliative care has developed in Chile over the past 15 years, largely through nongovernmental organizations. The Ministry of Health's cancer program has also played a role by including palliative care in its National Cancer Control Program initiative and by moving to reform drug laws. As a result, morphine consumption increased from less than 5 kg in 1990 to 55 kg in 2000. Despite these efforts, only a minority of patients have access to oral morphine for chronic pain related to cancer or AIDS. The remaining barriers include inadequately trained clinicians, a lack of national standards and guidelines, cure-oriented cancer treatment policies, fear of addiction on the part of both professionals and the public, and a lack of resources to improve the health care infrastructure.

Sources: International Observatory on End of Life Care 2005.

sets out the following principles on which countries can develop their own policies and regulations:

- Individuals must be authorized to dispense opioids by virtue of their professional license or be specially licensed to do so.
- Opioids may be transferred only between authorized parties.
- Opioids may be dispensed only with a medical prescription.

Many governments have imposed even tighter restrictions, such as limiting the number of days for which an opioid prescription can be written.

COSTS AND COST-EFFECTIVENESS

This section describes the costs and benefits of providing oral morphine and essential adjuvant drugs to terminally ill cancer and AIDS patients who require it. It assumes the drugs are used according to the WHO analgesic ladder. We recognize that other analgesics can also contribute significantly to patients' costs and pain relief, but at least some such drugs (acetaminophen, for example) are available relatively cheaply in most places. Although not everyone has access to such drugs, we are unaware of any data that could be used to estimate that proportion. Costs are estimated for three countries at differing income levels and with different patterns of cancer and AIDS deaths: Chile, Romania, and Uganda (see box 52.3).

Costs Included in the Estimates

The quantitative analysis presented here is restricted to the costs, before such drugs reach the patient, of oral morphine and the adjuvant drugs needed to treat its side effects. We mention other costs associated with delivering oral morphine to terminal AIDS and cancer patients later in this section, but for reasons we discuss, we have not assigned dollar values to them.

Costs of Oral Morphine. The appropriate measure of drug cost is the sum of costs to all payers—governments, insurers, charities, and patients—for the drug itself, but that sum does not include the costs of personnel to administer the drug or otherwise care for the patient.

Oral morphine can be purchased in bulk powder or finished form and administered as a tablet or liquid (De Lima and others 2004; Rajagopal and Venkateswaran 2003). The cost to the final payer is influenced by import taxes, if any; requirements to document the chain of custody of the product; costs to local manufacturers of excipients, salts, diluents, and other materials required to produce finished forms; and price markups. The actual cost of oral morphine in LMICs is difficult to document because it is unavailable in so many places or is manufactured for finished use at different points in the distribution chain. The price of a 30-day supply of immediate-release oral morphine in 2003 ranged from US$10 in India to US$254 in Argentina, among the few countries for which prices were reported (De Lima and others 2004).

Morphine is likely to cost less where it is produced locally and used in easy-to-reach, urban locations. Liquid preparations made by mixing morphine powder will cost less than tablets. Even with these variations, if barriers to access to oral morphine are removed, a total drug cost of 1 cent per milligram or less for immediate-release oral morphine should be achievable for most countries. A realistic and conservative estimate of the cost of oral morphine is 0.5 cent to 1.0 cent per milligram in the countries in our analysis.

The cost of morphine per patient depends on the number of days that opioids are required and the average daily dose, recognizing that the required dosage typically increases with increasing pain nearer to death. An average daily dose in palliative care programs in developing countries is roughly 60 to 75 mg per day, and patients require this dose for an average of three months. (Merriman 2002; personal communication, L. De Lima, International Association for Hospice and Palliative Care, June 2004; personal communication, M. R. Rajagopal, Amrita Institute of Medical Sciences, Kochi, Kerala, India, June 2004).

Using the inputs above, we estimate the cost of oral morphine for a cancer or AIDS patient with severe pain near the end of life at about 30 to 75 cents per day, or US$9.00 to US$22.50 per month, which is needed for an average of three months.

Costs of Other Necessary Drugs. Morphine's most common side effects are constipation, nausea, and (less frequently) psychosis. Representative drugs to treat these conditions are senna, a laxative, available to some government purchasers for

Table 52.3 Background Data, Assumptions, and Results of Cost Analysis

Item	Uganda	Chile	Romania
Economic, demographic, and health characteristics			
Population, 2001	22,800,000	15,400,000	22,400,000
Gross national income per capita, 2001 (US$)	260	4,590	1,720
World Bank income designation	Low	Upper middle	Lower middle
Percentage of the population living in rural areas	85	14	45
Number of cancer deaths, 2000	10,504	18,315	38,360
Number of AIDS deaths, 2001	84,000	220	350
Prevalence of cancer and AIDS deaths (per million population)	4,145	1,204	1,728
Morphine use per capita, 2001 (mg)	0.1	2.1	2.2
Total morphine use, 2001 (mg millions)	2.191	31.770	48.809
Assumptions and estimates used to determine the costs of oral morphine			
Percentage of cancer patients requiring end-of-life care with oral morphine	80	80	80
Average number of days of oral morphine required for cancer patients	90	90	90
Average daily dose of oral morphine for cancer patients (mg)	60–75	60–75	60–75
Effectiveness of intervention, cancer (percentage of pain days averted per day of therapy)	80	80	80
Percentage of patients with cancer already receiving adequate end-of-life pain care	0.5	20.0	15.0
Percentage of AIDS patients requiring end-of-life care with oral morphine	50	50	50
Average number of days of oral morphine required for AIDS patients	90	90	90
Average daily dose of oral morphine for AIDS patients (mg)	60–75	60–75	60–75
Effectiveness of intervention, AIDS (percentage of pain days averted per day of therapy)	80	80	80
Percentage of patients with AIDS already receiving adequate end-of-life pain care	0.5	20.0	15.0
Average daily cost of related drugs for cancer and AIDS patients (US$)	0.18–0.33	0.18–0.33	0.18–0.33
Cost analysis results (all costs in 2002 US$)			
Total incremental annual cost of oral morphine (US$ millions)	2.2–4.9	0.6–1.2	1.1–2.6
Incremental annual cost per capita (US$)	0.10–0.21	0.03–0.07	0.05–0.11
Incremental number of pain days per year avoided with use of oral morphine (millions)	3.6	0.9	1.9
Incremental cost per person per day of pain avoided (US$)	0.60–1.35	0.60–1.35	0.60–1.35
Incremental cost per year of pain-free life added (US$)	216–420	216–420	216–420

Sources: Income and demographic data, World Bank 2003; cancer deaths, Ferlay and others 2001; AIDS deaths, UNAIDS and WHO 2002a, 2002b, 2002c; per capita morphine use, INCB 2003; authors' calculations.

about 3 cents per day; prochlorperazine, an antiemetic, about 8 cents per day; and haloperidol, an antipsychotic, about 15 cents per day (Management Sciences for Health 2003). Retail prices after markups would add 20 to 30 percent.

Under the assumptions of this analysis, oral morphine for all dying cancer and AIDS patients would cost between 3 cents and 21 cents per capita per year (table 52.3) in Chile, Romania, and Uganda. The cost per pain day avoided by oral morphine is the same in all three countries, assuming that each country can acquire and dispense morphine equally efficiently.

Cost-Effectiveness

The analysis indicates that the drug costs of oral morphine come to about US\$216 to US\$420 per year of pain-free life gained in the three sample countries. The next question is whether the pain relief that could be achieved would be worth the cost. We know that patients value pain-free days highly. A day lived with the certainty of experiencing severe pain is of very low value, perhaps even lower than death itself (Furlong and others 2001; Le Gales and others 2002). Bryce and others (2004) find that people are willing to give up several months of healthy life for access to good end-of-life care. Patients in low-income countries place as great or even greater value on pain relief as patients in high-income countries (Cleeland and others 1988; Murray and others 2003).

Costs Not Included in the Analysis

The analysis presented includes only the most basic costs—the costs of oral opioids and associated drugs—that would be incurred in a pain control program. Clearly, there are many other costs, ranging from the costs of services at the individual patient level to the costs of changing drug laws and policies at the national level. The most significant additional costs are discussed below.

Incremental Costs of Care Delivery. In addition to requiring the drugs themselves, implementation of the three-step ladder requires trained individuals to assess and monitor patients. Where health care systems are well developed, the incremental cost of adding oral morphine will be low. If it involved one additional health center visit, the cost per patient would increase by about US\$8 in Chile, US\$6 in Romania, and US\$4 in Uganda, amounting to less than 1 cent per capita in all three countries.

Where primary health care is weak, widespread access to oral opioids depends on the development of new systems, such as community- or hospital-based palliative care networks. Clearly, allocating the full cost of upgrading the health care system, or even the development of new palliative care programs, to oral morphine alone, would be inappropriate.

Other Costs. Security and recordkeeping related to stocking and distributing opioids, required by the Single Convention, entail additional fixed and ongoing costs. Because most hospitals handle injectable opioids (for example, pethidine), these costs would be less for hospital-based programs than for community-based programs.

Professional training and education is required for all personnel involved in the use of opioids for dying patients, in part to overcome fears and in part to ensure proper use. These costs are likely to be highest where the health care system is most deficient.

The costs of changing national policy toward opioids is substantial in terms of cost, time, expertise, and leadership (see, for example, Pain and Policy Studies Group 2003 and 2004 and other annual reports at http://www.medsch.wisc.edu/painpolicy/publicat/annrepts.htm). The time expended is an opportunity cost, but it may be amortized over a long time if the effort succeeds.

Potential Cost Savings. In some circumstances, making oral morphine available through a palliative care system could actually save money—for example, if it enabled some terminally ill patients who would otherwise be admitted to the hospital for pain control to die at home, or if it shortened their period of hospitalization. This outcome is more likely in places with good medical infrastructure, but even in low-income countries, patients in unbearable pain are often brought to hospitals by distressed relatives who are willing go into debt to ease the suffering.

IMPLEMENTATION OF STRATEGIES TO IMPROVE PAIN CONTROL

Providing adequate oral morphine involves medical, political, legal, and societal change. Model programs, such as Hospice Uganda and efforts in India, have demonstrated the feasibility of providing good palliative care, including oral morphine, even for poor rural dwellers. WHO and the INCB have supported these efforts.

WHO Guidance on Palliative Care and Pain Relief

WHO has affirmed the need for palliative care and has defined the elements of model programs in several reports. In 2002, WHO's executive board called for the integration of pain and palliative care into national cancer control programs (box 52.4; WHO 2002). The Joint United Nations Programme on HIV/AIDS and the WHO AIDS Program consider pain and palliative care to be essential and pain management to be integral to AIDS care (Foley, Aulino, and Stjernsward 2003). WHO, in collaboration with the INCB and the WHO

Collaborating Center (WHOCC), has developed guidelines for national authorities to self-diagnose their regulatory systems for problems that might lead to a lack of access to needed drugs (WHO 2000). These organizations also sponsor national and international workshops to help national authorities evaluate their policies, develop action plans, implement policy change, and evaluate outcomes. In addition to WHO and the INCB, a number of programs and organizations are making resources and expertise available to assist countries in various ways (box 52.5).

Hospice Uganda. Hospice Uganda began in 1993 with an old Land Rover, a grant to last three months, and a mandate to become Africa's model home-based hospice for dying cancer and AIDS patients (Ramsay 2001). By July 2004, the original Kampala location had served about 4,500 nearby patients. Two additional sites—Mobile Hospice Mbarara and Little Hospice Hoima—had served about 2,500 patients (Merriman 2004). Hospice Uganda's influence has spread across Africa through its reputation and the training programs it runs (Merriman 2004).

At the beginning, morphine was largely unavailable, and the law required that a physician prescribe it. Hospice Uganda's founder, Anne Merriman, convinced the government to amend the law to allow specialist palliative care nurses and clinical officers to prescribe morphine (Merriman 2003). Now, morphine, paid for by the government, is available for dying patients in about 15 of Uganda's 56 districts (Merriman 2003). In 1998, Uganda became the first nation in Africa to list palliative care as an essential clinical service.

The cost of treating a patient in Kampala and Mbarara is about US$7 per week, including one home visit. For patients who come to the hospice, the cost is about US$4 per week (personal communication, A. Merriman, Hospice Uganda, February 2003). Even at those prices, most patients cannot afford even the medicines, which are subsidized by contributions.

India. For decades, the only morphine available in India was injectable and used for postoperative pain. The enactment of a strict, national narcotics law caused morphine use to decline even further, from a high of 573 kilograms in 1985 to 18 kilograms in 1997, among the lowest per capita in the world. During the period of declining use, international efforts to promote pain control and palliative care programs began to reach India. In 1992, pain relief and the availability of morphine were designated priorities in the National Cancer Control Programme (Joranson, Rajagopal, and Gilson 2002; Rajagopal, Joranson, and Gilson 2001; Rajagopal and Venkateswaran 2003).

The Ministry of Health convened national workshops from 1992 to 1994 to ascertain why morphine use continued to decline. The following experience from a referral hospital, recounted by a former narcotics commissioner of India, is instructive:

the Institute has not been able to procure a single tablet [to] date, primarily due to the stringent state laws and multiplicity of licenses. After a lot of effort, the Institute had been able to obtain the licenses in 1994 and had approached [a manufacturer] for a supply of tablets . . . [but] by the time the tablets

Selected Resources for Developing National Palliative Care Programs

Resources available to countries include the following:

- The WHOCC for Policy and Communications in Cancer Care at the University of Wisconsin serves as a critical resource for palliative care education and country policy makers interested in assessing their opioid drug regulations and developing strategies for change. Its Web site links to WHO guidelines in several languages and provides articles and reports on efforts to improve national policy and opioid availability in Africa, Asia, Eastern Europe, and Latin America. See http://www.medsch.wisc.edu/painpolicy/.

- The WHOCC publishes *Cancer Pain Release* every quarter. The journal includes topical analysis of current issues in cancer pain management and palliative care and reviews recent international research and educational resources. See http://www.whocancerpain.wisc.edu/.

- The Open Society Institute sponsored workshops in cooperation with WHO's Essential Drug and Cancer units to bring together pain and palliative care experts and drug policy makers from Central and Eastern Europe and the former Soviet Union to develop strategies for implementing regulatory change to improve opioid availability. The Open Society Institute also supports the development of implementation strategies in 12 of these countries. That effort involves experts in pain and palliative care, cancer, and AIDS and representatives from ministries of health and financing and health insurance programs. See http://www.soros.org/initiatives/health/focus_areas/international.

- The *Journal of Pain and Symptom Management* has published three special supplements over the past nine years in association with the International Association for the Study of Pain. The supplements describe countries' efforts to advance opioid availability and palliative care. See http://www.elsevier.com/wps/find/journaldescription.cws_home/505775/description#description.

- The International Observatory on End of Life Care is a clearinghouse on palliative care in resource-poor countries that is aimed particularly at policy makers. The initial focus has been on Eastern and Central Europe, but the intent is to cover all resource-poor countries. See http://www.eolc-observatory.net/global_analysis/index.htm.

Source: Authors.

could be arranged, the licenses had expired. The doctors at the Institute and the associated pain clinic have stopped prescribing morphine tablets. (Joranson, Rajagopal, and Gilson 2002, 153).

In 1999, the INCB called on the government of India to take measures to make morphine available for medical uses. In 1994, an initiative begun by the WHOCC, the Indian Association of Palliative Care, and the Pain and Palliative Care Society systematically studied the reasons for the lack of morphine. In 1997, the WHOCC developed a proposal to reduce the number of licenses and extend their period of validity, and the following year all state governments were instructed to adopt a model rule based on the proposal. Gradually, rules have begun to change. By 2002, 7 of 28 states or territories had adopted the model rule, but it has been implemented successfully only in Kerala.

The success in Kerala can be attributed to three things: (a) the state government simplified the licensing process and stipulated that for oral morphine to be available from a center, it must have at least one doctor with at least one month of practical experience in palliative care; (b) the national drugs controller exempted palliative care programs from needing a drug license, thereby eliminating the need for a pharmacist; and (c) a palliative care network was established, which consists of about 50 small programs. Statewide, coverage has increased to about 20 percent of those needing palliative care.

RECOMMENDATIONS FOR RESEARCH AND DEVELOPMENT

Policy makers and program implementers need practical tools to improve pain control and palliative care. They need survey instruments, guidance on how to effect policy and legal changes, and palliative care models for resource-poor settings. Many tools exist, but those could be made more accessible through the use of toolkits, distance learning, Web sites, and so on. Each country also should gather information to assess its own capabilities and needs, such as the following:

- In relation to the national level:
  - Study the incidence and prevalence of pain related to major causes of illness and death using methodologies

adapted from developed countries (Breivik, Collett, and Ventafridda forthcoming).

- º Survey existing pain and palliative care programs to identify national and local leaders in pain control and palliative care and to catalog national guidelines and standards for acute and chronic pain. For hospice and palliative care services, assess the extent of available care, service delivery models, national and local policies, and professional and public knowledge about pain control and palliative care.
- º Assess national and local regulatory barriers to opioid availability using WHO (2000) guidelines and needs assessment protocols (Higginson 1997) to help countries identify the patient-related, physician-related, and institutional issues that impede drug distribution.
- º Study costs that affect opioid availability in several countries to document the costs of licensing, obtaining, storing, keeping records for, and dispensing opioid drugs.
- º Study the costs of alternative delivery models for pain control medications in LMICs.
- º Assess the offsetting savings achievable by reducing hospital days by means of better outpatient access to oral morphine, to document potential savings in representative countries, which might help reduce barriers to access.
- In relation to model programs:
  - º Construct an inventory of model programs for pain control and palliative care. Include their infrastructure and personnel needs, their operating costs, and so on, in easy-to-use formats such as toolkits and education and training programs for policy makers and implementers. Regularly add new information from ongoing and new initiatives.
  - º Devise additional models, particularly for poor rural communities, for providing palliative care and pain control practically, efficiently, and sustainably.

CONCLUSIONS

Unrelieved acute and chronic pain is a serious public health problem worldwide, and 80 percent of cancer patients and 50 percent of AIDS patients experience severe pain during the last months of life. Relief for these patients is possible only with oral morphine or another opioid, but developing countries face many barriers in this respect. Nevertheless, model pain and palliative care programs have demonstrated the feasibility of providing opioid treatment safely, effectively, and inexpensively in resource-poor settings. To this end, national governments must resolve the legal and regulatory barriers to opioid availability, but they need the expertise and support of the global community to make pain relief a reality.

REFERENCES

Anand, A., L. Carmosino, and A. E. Glatt. 1994. "Evaluation of Recalcitrant Pain in HIV-Infected Hospitalized Patients." *Journal of Acquired Immune Deficiency Syndromes* 7 (1): 52–56.

Bernabei, R., G. Gambassi, K. Lapane, F. Landi, C. Gatsonis, R. Dunlop, and others. 1998. "Management of Pain in Elderly Patients with Cancer." *Journal of the American Medical Association* 279 (23): 1877–82.

Breitbart, W. 2003. "Pain." In *A Clinical Guide to Supportive and Palliative Care for HIV/AIDS*, ed. J. F. O'Neill, P. Selwyn, and H. Schietinger, 85–122. Washington, DC: Health Resources and Services Administration.

Breivik, H., B. Collett, and V. Ventafridda. Forthcoming. "The Pain in Europe Survey: Detailed Results and Analysis." *European Journal of Pain*.

Bryce, C. L., G. Arnold, R. M. Schooler, J. Loewenstein, R. S. Wax, and D. C. Angus. 2004. "Quality of Death: Assessing the Importance Placed on End-of-Life Treatment in the Intensive-Care Unit." *Medical Care* 42 (5): 423–31.

Chang, V. T., S. S. Hwang, and M. Feuerman. 2000. "Validation of the Edmonton Symptom Assessment Scale." *Cancer* 88 (9): 2164–71.

Cleeland, C. S. 1990. "Assessment of Pain in Cancer: Measurement Issues." In *Advances in Pain Research and Therapy*, ed. K. M. Foley, J. J. Bonica, and V. Ventafridda, 47–55. New York: Raven Press.

Cleeland, C. S., J. L. Ladinsky, R. C. Serlin, and N. C. Thuy. 1988. "Multidimensional Measurement of Cancer Pain: Comparisons of U.S. and Vietnamese Patients." *Journal of Pain and Symptom Management* 3 (1): 23–27.

Cleeland, C. S., Y. Nakamura, T. R. Mendoza, K. R. Edwards, J. Douglas, and R. C. Serlin. 1996. "Dimensions of the Impact of Cancer Pain in a Four Country Sample: New Information from Multidimensional Scaling." *Pain* 67 (2–3): 267–73.

Daut, R. L., and C. S. Cleeland. 1982. "The Prevalence and Severity of Pain in Cancer." *Cancer* 50 (9): 1913–18.

Daut, R. L., C. S. Cleeland, and R. C. Flanery. 1983. "Development of the Wisconsin Brief Pain Questionnaire to Assess Pain in Cancer and Other Diseases." *Pain* 17 (2): 197–210.

De Lima, L., C. Sweeney, J. L. Palmer, and E. Bruera. 2004. "Potent Analgesics Are More Expensive for Patients in Developing Countries: A Comparative Study." *Journal of Pain and Palliative Care Pharmacotherapy* 18 (1): 59–70.

Ferlay, J., F. Bray, P. Pisani, and D. M. Parkin. 2001. *Globocan 2000: Cancer Incidence, Mortality, and Prevalence Worldwide*, Version 1.0, IARC CancerBase 5. Lyon, France: IARC Press.

Fishman, B., S. Pasternak, S. L. Wallenstein, R. W. Houde, J. C. Holland, and K. M. Foley. 1987. "The Memorial Pain Assessment Card. A Valid Instrument for the Evaluation of Cancer Pain." *Cancer* 60 (5): 1151–58.

Foley, K. M. 1979. "Pain Syndromes in Patients with Cancer." *Advances in Pain Research and Therapy*, ed. K. M. Foley, J. J. Bonica, and V. Ventafridda, 59–75. New York: Raven Press.

———. 1999. "Pain Assessment and Cancer Pain Syndromes." In *Oxford Textbook of Palliative Medicine*, 2nd ed., ed. D. Doyle, G. Hank, and N. MacDonald, 310–31. New York: Oxford University Press.

Foley, K. M., F. Aulino, and J. Stjernsward. 2003. "Palliative Care in Resource-Poor Settings." In *A Clinical Guide to Supportive and Palliative Care for HIV/AIDS*, ed. J. F. O'Neill, P. Selwyn, and H. Schietinger, 387–407. Washington, DC: Health Resources and Services Administration.

Furlong, W. J., D. H. Feeny, G. W. Torrance, and R. D. Barr. 2001. "The Health Utilities Index (HUI) System for Assessing Health-Related Quality of Life in Clinical Studies." *Annals of Medicine* 33 (5): 375–84.

Goudas, L., D. B. Carr, and R. Bloch. 2001. *Management of Cancer Pain.* Evidence Report/Technology Assessment 35, Publication 02-E002. Rockville, MD: Agency for Healthcare Research and Quality.

Higginson, I. 1997. *Palliative and Terminal Care.* Abingdon, England: Radcliffe Medical Press.

INCB (International Narcotics Control Board). 2003. *Report of the International Narcotics Control Board for 2003.* Geneva: INCB.

International Observatory on End of Life Care. 2005. "Hungary." http://www.eolc-observatory.net/global_analysis/hungary.htm.

Joranson, D. E. 1993. "Availability of Opioids for Cancer Pain: Recent Trends, Assessment of System Barriers: New World Health Organization Guidelines and the Risk of Diversion." *Journal of Pain and Symptom Management* 8 (6): 353–60.

Joranson, D. E., M. R. Rajagopal, and A. M. Gilson. 2002. "Improving Access to Opioid Analgesics for Palliative Care in India." *Journal of Pain and Symptom Management* 24 (2): 152–59.

Kimball, L. R., and W. C. McCormick. 1996. "The Pharmacologic Management of Pain and Discomfort in Persons with AIDS Near the End of Life: Use of Opioid Analgesia in the Hospice Setting." *Journal of Pain and Symptom Management* 11 (2): 88–94.

Larue, F., A. Fontaine, and S. M. Colleau. 1997. Underestimation and Undertreatment of Pain in HIV Disease: Multicentre Study." *British Medical Journal* 314 (7073): 23–28.

Le Gales, C., C. Buron, N. Costet, S. Rosman, and P. R. Slama. 2002. "Development of a Preference-Weighted Health Status Classification System in France: The Health Utilities Index 3." *Health Care Management Science* 5 (1): 41–51.

Management Sciences for Health. 2003. *International Drug Price Indicator Guide, 2003.* Boston: Management Sciences for Health.

McCormack, J. P., R. Li, D. Zarowny, and J. Singer. 1993. "Inadequate Treatment of Pain in Ambulatory HIV Patients." *Clinical Journal of Pain* 9 (4): 279–83.

Merriman, A. 2002. *Palliative Medicine: Pain and Symptom Control in the Cancer and/or AIDS Patient in Uganda and Other African Countries.* 3rd ed. Kampala: Hospice Africa Uganda.

———. 2003. "Model Programmes in Africa: Uganda 1993–2003." Background for presentation at White House Conference Center, February 25, 2003. [typescript]. Hospice Africa Uganda, Kampala.

———. 2004. "Some Facts about Hospice Uganda, July 2004." [typescript]. Hospice Africa Uganda, Kampala.

Murray, S. A., E. Grant, A. Grant, and M. Kendall. 2003. "Dying from Cancer in Developed and Developing Countries: Lessons from Two Qualitative Interview Studies of Patients and Their Carers." *British Medical Journal* 326 (7385): 368–71.

Newshan, G., and M. Lefkowitz. 2001. "Transdermal Fentanyl for Chronic Pain in AIDS: A Pilot Study." *Journal of Pain and Symptom Management* 21 (1): 69–77.

Newshan, G. T., and S. F. Wainapel. 1993. "Pain Characteristics and Their Management in Persons with AIDS." *Journal of the Association of Nurses in AIDS Care* 4 (2): 53–59.

O'Neill, J. F., P. A. Selwyn, and H. Schietinger. 2003. *A Clinical Guide to Supportive and Palliative Care for HIV/AIDS.* Washington, DC: Health Resources and Services Administration.

Pain and Policy Studies Group. 2003. *Improving Cancer Pain in the World, Report for 2002.* Madison, WI: World Health Organization Collaborating Center for Policy and Communications in Cancer Care.

———. 2004. *Improving Cancer Pain in the World, Report for 2003.* Madison, WI: World Health Organization Collaborating Center for Policy and Communications in Cancer Care.

Portenoy, R. K., H. T. Thaler, A. B. Kornblith, J. M. Lepore, H. Friedlander-Klar, N. Coyle, and others. 1994. "Symptom Prevalence, Characteristics, and Distress in a Cancer Population." *Quality of Life Research* 3 (3): 183–89.

Rajagopal, M. R., D. E. Joranson, and A. M. Gilson. 2001. "Medical Use, Misuse, and Diversion of Opioids in India." *Lancet* 358 (9276): 139–43.

Rajagopal, M. R., and C. Venkateswaran. 2003. "Palliative Care in India: Successes and Limitations." *Journal of Pain and Palliative Care Pharmacotherapy* 17 (3–4): 121–28.

Ramsay, S. 2001. "Raising the Profile of Palliative Care for Africa." *Lancet* 358 (9283): 734.

Rosenfeld, B., W. Breitbart, M. V. McDonald, S. D. Passik, H. Thaler, and R. K. Portenoy. 1996. "Pain in Ambulatory AIDS Patients. II: Impact of Pain on Psychological Functioning and Quality of Life." *Pain* 68 (2–3): 323–28.

Schofferman, J., and R. Brody. 1990. "Pain in Far Advanced AIDS." *Advances in Pain Research and Therapy,* ed. K. M. Foley, J. J. Bonica, and V. Ventafridda, 379–86. New York: Raven Press.

Singer, E. J., C. Zorilla, B. Fahy-Chandon, S. Chi, K. Syndulko, and W. W. Tourtellotte. 1993. "Painful Symptoms Reported by Ambulatory HIV-Infected Men in a Longitudinal Study." *Pain* 54 (1): 15–19.

Stjernsward, J., and D. Clark. 2003. "Palliative Medicine: A Global Perspective." In *Oxford Textbook of Palliative Medicine,* 3rd ed., ed. D. Doyle, G. W. C. Hanks, N. Cherny, and K. Calman, 1199–222. New York: Oxford University Press.

Task Force on Taxonomy. 2004. *Classification of Chronic Pain,* 2nd ed., ed. H. Merskey and N. Bogduk. Seattle: International Association for the Study of Pain Press.

UNAIDS (Joint United Nations Programme on HIV/AIDS) and WHO (World Health Organization). 2002a. *Epidemiological Fact Sheets on HIV/AIDS and Sexually Transmitted Infections, 2002 Update, Chile.* Geneva: UNAIDS and WHO.

———. 2002b. *Epidemiological Fact Sheets on HIV/AIDS and Sexually Transmitted Infections, 2002 Update, Romania.* Geneva: UNAIDS and WHO.

———. 2002c. *Epidemiological Fact Sheets on HIV/AIDS and Sexually Transmitted Infections, 2002 Update, Uganda.* Geneva: UNAIDS and WHO.

United Nations. 1961. "Single Convention on Narcotic Drugs." United Nations. http://www.incb.org/e/conv/1961/.

World Bank. 2003. *2003 World Development Indicators.* Washington, DC: World Bank.

WHO (World Health Organization). 1986. *Cancer Pain Relief.* Geneva: WHO.

———. 1990. *Cancer Pain Relief and Palliative Care.* Technical Report Series 804. Geneva: WHO.

———. 2000. *Achieving Balance in National Opioids Control Policy: Guidelines for Assessment.* Geneva: WHO.

———. 2002. *National Cancer Control Programmes: Policies and Managerial Guidelines.* 2nd ed. Geneva: WHO.

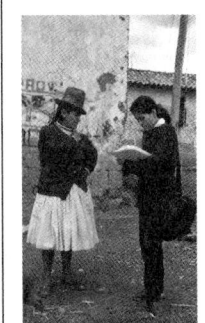

Chapter **53**

Public Health Surveillance: A Tool for Targeting and Monitoring Interventions

Peter Nsubuga, Mark E. White, Stephen B. Thacker, Mark A. Anderson, Stephen B. Blount, Claire V. Broome, Tom M. Chiller, Victoria Espitia, Rubina Imtiaz, Dan Sosin, Donna F. Stroup, Robert V. Tauxe, Maya Vijayaraghavan, and Murray Trostle

What gets measured gets done.
—Anonymous

Public health surveillance is the ongoing systematic collection, analysis, and interpretation of data, closely integrated with the timely dissemination of these data to those responsible for preventing and controlling disease and injury (Thacker and Berkelman 1988). Public health surveillance is a tool to estimate the health status and behavior of the populations served by ministries of health, ministries of finance, and donors. Because surveillance can directly measure what is going on in the population, it is useful both for measuring the need for interventions and for directly measuring the effects of interventions. The purpose of surveillance is to empower decision makers to lead and manage more effectively by providing timely, useful evidence.

Increasingly, top managers in ministries of health and finance in developing countries and donor agencies are recognizing that data from effective surveillance systems are useful for targeting resources and evaluating programs. The HIV and severe acute respiratory syndrome (SARS) epidemics underscored the critical role of surveillance in protecting individual nations and the global community. For example, in 2005, China rapidly began to expand its surveillance and response capacity through its Field Epidemiology Training Program (FETP); Brazil and Argentina chose to use World Bank loans to develop surveillance capacity; and the U.S. Agency for International Development (USAID) redesigned its surveillance strategy to focus on the use of data to improve public health interventions (USAID 2005). Additionally, the guidelines for implementing the 2004 draft revised International Health Regulations require World Health Organization (WHO) member states to have key persons and core capacities in surveillance (http://www.who.int/csr/ihr/howtheywork/faq/en/#draft).

Just as decision makers require competent, motivated economists to provide quality technical analyses, they also need competent staff members to provide scientifically valid surveillance information and communicate the results as information for action. Competent epidemiologists and surveillance staff members are not a luxury in developing countries; they are a necessity for rational planning, implementation, and intervention (Narasimhan and others 2004).

DEFINITIONS AND BASIC CONCEPTS

In this chapter, we use the following definitions:

- *Indicator:* a measurable factor that allows decision makers to estimate objectively the size of a health problem and monitor the processes, the products, or the effects of an intervention on the population (for example, the number of new cases of diarrhea, the proportion of children fully immunized in a district, or the percentage of high school students who report that they smoke at least one cigarette a day).

- *Active surveillance:* a system employing staff members to regularly contact heath care providers or the population to seek information about health conditions. Active surveillance provides the most accurate and timely information, but it is also expensive.

- *Passive surveillance:* a system by which a health jurisdiction receives reports submitted from hospitals, clinics, public health units, or other sources. Passive surveillance is a relatively inexpensive strategy to cover large areas, and it provides critical information for monitoring a community's health. However, because passive surveillance depends on people in different institutions to provide data, data quality and timeliness are difficult to control.

- *Routine health information system:* a passive system in which regular reports about diseases and programs are completed by public health staff members, hospitals, and clinics.

- *Health information and management system:* a passive system by which routine reports about financial, logistic, and other processes involved in the administration of the public health and clinical systems can be used for surveillance.

- *Categorical surveillance:* an active or passive system that focuses on one or more diseases or behaviors of interest to an intervention program. These systems are useful for program managers. However, they may be inefficient at the district or local level, at which staff may need to fill out multiple forms on the same patient (that is, the HIV program, the tuberculosis program, the sexually transmitted infections program, and the Routine Health Information System). At higher levels, allocating the few competent surveillance experts to one program may leave other programs underserved, and reconciling the results of different systems to establish the nation's official estimates may be difficult.

- *Integrated surveillance:* a combination of active and passive systems using a single infrastructure that gathers information about multiple diseases or behaviors of interest to several intervention programs (for example, a health facility–based system may gather information on multiple infectious diseases and injuries). Managers of disease-specific programs may be evaluated on the results of the integrated system and should be stakeholders. Even when an integrated system is functioning well, program managers may continue to maintain categorical systems to collect additional disease-specific data and control the quality of the information on which they are evaluated. This practice may lead to duplication and inefficiency.

- *Syndromic surveillance:* an active or passive system that uses case definitions that are based entirely on clinical features without any clinical or laboratory diagnosis (for example, collecting the number of cases of diarrhea rather than cases of cholera, or "rash illness" rather than measles). Because syndromic surveillance is inexpensive and is faster than systems that require laboratory confirmation, it is often the first kind of surveillance begun in a developing country. However, because of the lack of specificity (for example, a "rash illness" could be anything from the relatively minor rubella to devastating hemorrhagic fevers), reports require more investigation from higher levels. Also an increase in one disease causing a syndrome may mask an epidemic of another (for example, rotavirus diarrhea decreases at the same time cholera increases).

In the specialized area of surveillance for biologic terrorism, syndromic surveillance refers to active surveillance of syndromes that may be caused by potential agents used by biologic terrorists and sometimes refers to alternative measures such as increases in the use of over-the-counter drugs or increases in calls to emergency departments.

- *Behavioral risk factor surveillance system (BRFSS):* an active system of repeated surveys that measure behaviors that are known to cause disease or injury (for example, tobacco or alcohol use, unprotected sex, or lack of physical exercise). Because the aim of many intervention program strategies is to prevent disease by preventing unhealthy behavior, these surveys provide a direct measure of their effect in the population, often long before the anticipated health effects are expected. These surveys are useful for providing timely measures of program effectiveness for both communicable and noncommunicable disease interventions.

OBJECTIVES OF SURVEILLANCE SYSTEMS

Public health surveillance provides the scientific and factual database essential to informed decision making and appropriate public health action. The key objective of surveillance is to provide information to guide interventions. The public health objectives and actions needed to make successful interventions determine the design and implementation of surveillance systems. For example, if the objective is to prevent the spread of epidemics of acute infectious diseases, such as SARS, managers need to intervene quickly to stop the spread of disease. Therefore, they need a surveillance system that provides rapid early warning information from clinics and laboratories. In contrast, chronic diseases and health-related behaviors change slowly. Managers typically monitor the effect of programs to change risky behaviors such as tobacco smoking or chronic diseases once a year or even less often. A surveillance system to measure the population effects of a tuberculosis control program might provide information only every one to five years—for example, through a series of demographic and health surveys. The principle is that different public health objectives and the actions required to reach them require different information

Different Objectives, Different Data, Different Systems

Objective	*Action*	*Data*	*System*
Detect epidemics	Epidemic response	Early warning information	Active surveillance
Monitor intervention programs	Program monitoring	Program indicators	Health information
Monitor impact of policy change	Health policy	Health indicators	Health information
Monitor health system	Resource allocation	Administrative data	Health information and management

Source: Nsubuga, Eseko, and others 2002.

systems. The type of action that can be taken, when or how often that action needs to be taken, what information is needed to take or monitor the action, and when or how frequently the information is needed should determine the type of surveillance or health information system (box 53.1).

PRINCIPLES AND USES OF SURVEILLANCE

Foege, Hogan, and Newton (1976) state that "the reason for collecting, analyzing, and disseminating information on a disease is to control that disease. Collection and analysis should not be allowed to consume resources if action does not follow." The fundamental principle of public health surveillance is that the surveillance should be designed and implemented to provide valid (true) information to decision makers in a timely manner at the lowest possible cost. Because managers are unlikely to need to make interventions to address small differences between areas, sacrificing precision makes sense to improve timeliness and save resources that can be used for public health interventions. The utility of surveillance data can be viewed as immediate, annual, and archival, on the basis of the public health actions that can be taken (table 53.1; Thacker and Stroup 1998b).

ESTABLISHING AND MAINTAINING A SURVEILLANCE SYSTEM

What is worth doing is worth doing right. Managers who decide to use public health surveillance as a management tool must recognize that they will need to commit political support and human and financial resources. As with every health system, competent, motivated health workers need to be found or trained and provided with career paths and supervision. After a manager decides to create a surveillance system, there are six steps to establishing the system. Because the system must adapt constantly to changes in the population and the physical

Table 53.1 Utility of Surveillance Data

Immediate detection of	Epidemics
	Newly emerging health problems
	Changes in health practices
	Changes in antibiotic resistance
	Changes in distribution of population at risk for disease
Periodic dissemination for	Estimating magnitude of a health problem, including cost
	Assessing control activities
	Setting research priorities
	Determining risk factors for disease
	Facilitating planning
	Monitoring risk factors
	Monitoring changes in health practices
	Documenting distribution and spread of disease and injury
Stored information for	Describing natural history of diseases
	Facilitating epidemiologic and laboratory research
	Validating use of preliminary data
	Setting research priorities
	Documenting distribution and spread of disease and injury

Source: Adapted from Thacker and Stroup 1998b, 65.

and social environment, these steps are linked continuously (figure 53.1; Thacker and Stroup 1998a).

ANALYSIS AND DISSEMINATION OF SURVEILLANCE DATA

Surveillance information is analyzed by time, place, and person. Knowledgeable technical personnel should review data regularly to ensure their validity and to identify information

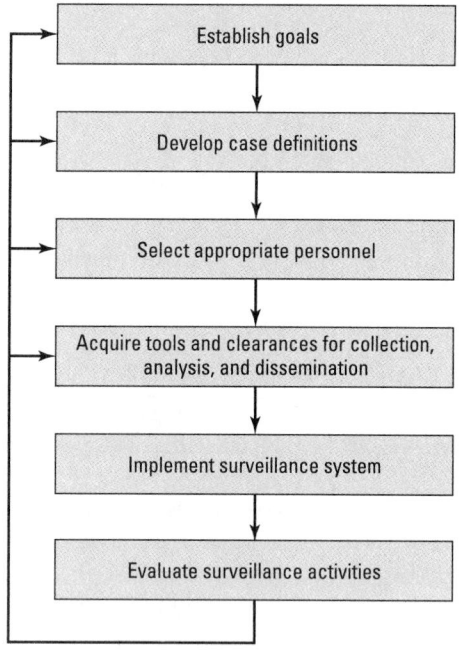

Source: Adapted from Thacker and Stroup 1998a, 119.

Figure 53.1 Elements in Establishing and Maintaining a Surveillance System

of use to top managers. Simple tables and graphs are most useful for summarizing and presenting data. Timely dissemination of data to those who make policy and implement intervention programs is critical to the usefulness of surveillance data.

The rapidly evolving field of public health informatics, which deals with collection, classification, storage, retrieval, analysis, and presentation of large amounts of health data, offers the potential for truly integrated public health surveillance based on data standardization, a communications infrastructure, and policies on data access and sharing. Surveillance will benefit by incorporating a systematic approach to standards for data content. For example, the U.S. Centers for Disease Control and Prevention (CDC) has used standards-based systems to support automatic electronic reporting of diagnostic laboratory results of notifiable diseases, thereby both increasing the number of cases reported and receiving results more rapidly (Effler and others 1999). Use of data standards facilitates comparability of surveillance information over time (for example, measurement of effect of program interventions), across different surveillance approaches (for example, facility-based reporting compared with sample surveys), and across countries and regions. To be credible, a standard should be developed through an open, participatory process, by an internationally recognized accredited standards-development organization that is also capable of long-term

maintenance and evolution of the standard. Public health data needs extend into multiple areas beyond clinical medicine (for example, environmental toxins, unintentional injury, and food safety).

One international standard computer program used in many countries' information systems is Epi Info, an epidemiology surveillance and biostatistics program widely used around the world for the analysis of surveillance data (http://www.cdc.gov/epiinfo). CDC created, maintains, and distributes Epi Info at no cost to users.

SURVEILLANCE AS A COMPONENT OF NATIONAL PUBLIC HEALTH SYSTEMS

WHO and the World Bank cite public health surveillance as an essential function of a public health system (World Bank 2001). When linked to policy and program units, surveillance information improves the efficiency and effectiveness of health services by targeting interventions and documenting their effect on the population.

A critical challenge in the health sector in developing countries is to ensure quality and effectiveness of surveillance and public health response in an environment of decentralization. National-level program and surveillance system managers may lose control of the quality and timeliness of locally collected data. This situation can be avoided by training local decision makers in how to use information to meet their needs and negotiating with them over the core information collected by each district local unit. National-level managers or donors can also improve information quality by sponsoring national surveillance scientific and quality assurance networks, linking funding to provision of adequate data, and performing periodic surveys to confirm the results of local reporting. If the responsibility for implementing programs is devolved to local managers, then national-level managers need only a few summary indicators, rather than the detailed information they may be used to. District or local managers tend to prefer integrated systems to minimize filling out redundant forms.

Donors need surveillance data to target and evaluate their investments. If they perceive weakness in the national system, they may create parallel nongovernmental surveillance systems to gather data directly to meet their needs. These systems invariably pay workers more than government jobs do, so the most competent people in the government system may leave to work for the parallel system. Although this system meets donors' short-term needs, it invariably weakens government systems. Parallel systems may weaken the very ministries that they are meant to help and may not be sustainable after external funding ends. Therefore, parallel systems are inherently inequitable and should be used only as a last resort.

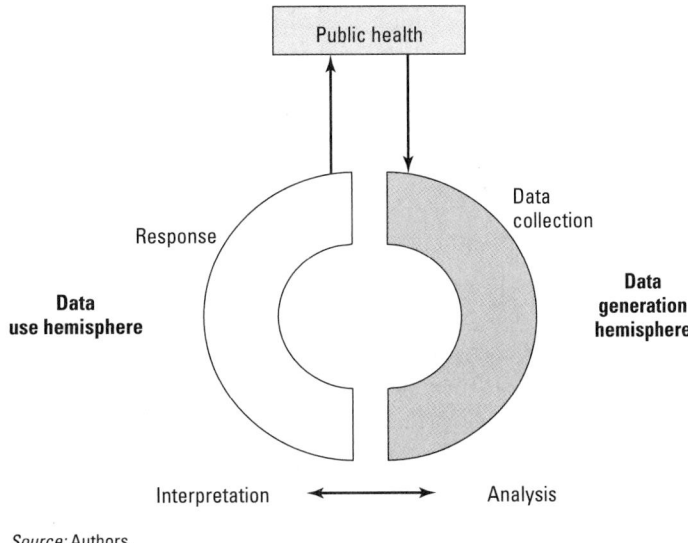

Source: Authors.

Figure 53.2 Surveillance and Response Conceptual Framework

SURVEILLANCE AS A TOOL TO IMPROVE PUBLIC HEALTH

Managers need focused, timely, scientifically sound information that provides evidence to make decisions on interventions for improving the health of the population in their jurisdiction. Simply collecting data and presenting them are not enough.

Using Surveillance Information for Evidence-Based Decisions

A major gap in promoting effective surveillance lies between the production of data and the ability to convert those data into usable information and then initiate the appropriate public health action. Surveillance and response can be described in terms of a *data generation hemisphere* and a *data use hemisphere* (USAID 2005). The data generation hemisphere is the traditional view of surveillance, whereas the data use hemisphere is the public health response that begins with interpretation of the data from the surveillance system (figure 53.2).

Substantial attention and the accompanying resources in surveillance have been devoted to the prompt and complete production of surveillance data. Although developing countries experience weaknesses in both hemispheres, more attention is needed to creating and strengthening the local capacity within developing countries to identify and manage effective responses to disease outbreaks and public health conditions of national and international concern. In some disease-specific programs, this capacity has to be imported through short-term expatriate assistance. Even when local capacity is developed, it is often specific to the disease program, making transfer of skills to other areas problematic. The failure to develop this indigenous capacity has limited the ability of developing countries to build national surveillance systems that respond to both international public health threats and local health concerns. This capability is essential to the sustained development of countries.

Role of Field Epidemiologists in Providing Evidence

Developed countries have constructed their public health and disease control strategies by using the principles of field epidemiology. Developing countries need to build and sustain human capacity in field epidemiology. Strengthened field epidemiologic capacity can serve a country in the following specific areas:

* providing a response to acute problems
* providing the scientific basis for program and policy decisions
* implementing disease surveillance systems
* supporting national health planning
* making resource allocation decisions
* allocating the human capacity base for national health priorities.

Specific competencies that should be developed include, but are not limited to, the ability to accomplish the following:

* design, implement, and evaluate surveillance for a health event
* identify and assess an actual public health problem
* design and conduct a scientific investigation
* analyze and interpret data from an investigation
* recommend logical and practical public health actions after the analysis and interpretation of data

- be proficient in all aspects of diseases of public health importance (for example, HIV and AIDS, sexually transmitted diseases, malaria, tuberculosis, and zoonoses).

These competencies need to be tailored to the various levels of the health care system.

Since 1975, CDC and WHO have collaborated with more than 30 countries to strengthen health systems and address training needs for disease detection and response in a country-specific, flexible, and sustainable manner. More than half of the world's population now lives in a country where surveillance, investigation, and response are carried out by staff members and trainees of FETPs and allied programs, which include the Epidemic Intelligence Service in the United States, the European Program for Intervention Epidemiology Training, and Public Health Schools without Walls (PHSWOWs). These programs generally function within central ministries of health and may not be visible outside the public health system. It can be argued that these programs provide most of the surveillance of and response to emerging infections in the world, in addition to training most of the public health workers who manage surveillance systems at the top level. FETPs are two-year courses designed to provide a ministry with a motivated, professional group of field epidemiologists with the expertise to respond to managers' needs for evidence, perform surveillance, respond to outbreaks, and train and supervise technical personnel at other levels (White and others 2001).

Other models have evolved. Guatemala's marriage of its FETP (part of a larger, Central American FETP) with the Data for Decision Making program (Pappaioanou and others 2003) exemplifies this successful local adaptation. Data for Decision Making recruits health workers from the community and sub-district levels to receive training in surveillance and outbreak investigation in the context of their daily work. This training is delivered as a series of linked workshops with practical field-based projects, providing short-term service at the local levels. The most promising graduates of the course are selected for further training in an FETP. India, with its decentralized system, complex cultural and population dynamics, and wide variance in the sophistication of public health institutions, provides another model for strengthening national surveillance. The World Bank initiated the Integrated Disease Surveillance Project, which develops the capacity of local and midlevel surveillance workers in India. Additionally, FETP graduates are recruited as the project's surveillance officers at the state level to coordinate the surveillance activities of the hundreds of local health workers throughout the states.

SELECTED SURVEILLANCE STRATEGIES

Surveillance systems need to be designed and implemented to meet top management's needs for focused, reliable, timely evidence gathered efficiently and presented effectively. Because these needs differ, depending on management's needs, a number of different strategies have been developed. Here are some of the most useful.

Sentinel Surveillance

In a sentinel surveillance system, a prearranged sample of reporting sources agrees to report all cases of defined conditions, which might indicate trends in the entire target population (Birkhead and Maylahn 2000). When properly implemented, these systems offer an effective method of using limited resources and enable prompt and flexible monitoring and investigation of suspected public health problems. Examples of sentinel surveillance are networks of private practitioners reporting cases of influenza or a laboratory-based sentinel system reporting cases of certain bacterial infections among children. Sentinel surveillance is excellent for detecting large public health problems, but it may be insensitive to rare events, such as the early emergence of a new disease, because these infections may emerge anywhere in the population.

Periodic Population-Based Surveys

Population-based surveys can be used for surveillance if they are repeated on a regular basis (Thacker and Berkelman 1988). Examples of population-based surveys in surveillance include the BRFSS in the United States, HIV-prevalence surveys, household surveys, and the demographic and health surveys that many developing countries conduct every five years (http://www.orcmacro.com). Population-based surveys require careful attention to the methodology, particularly the use of standard protocols, supervision of interviewers, comparable sampling strategy, and standard questionnaires. These surveys require a clear definition of the target population to which the results can be generalized, and they need careful attention to the sample size, based on efficiency and the epidemiologic characteristics of the health condition under surveillance (for example, rare conditions require substantial samples). Supervising interviewers and maintaining high response rates are critical to avoid bias. Because the surveys are repetitive, population changes (caused, for example, by mortality or mobility) might bias results.

Laboratory-Based Surveillance

The methods used for infectious disease surveillance form a spectrum that evolves with the economic development of a country. Foodborne disease (FBD) surveillance, for example, is divided into four distinct levels of surveillance. Each level is more complex and has greater capacity for controlling and detecting disease, but it also depends on more resources and infrastructure (figure 53.3).

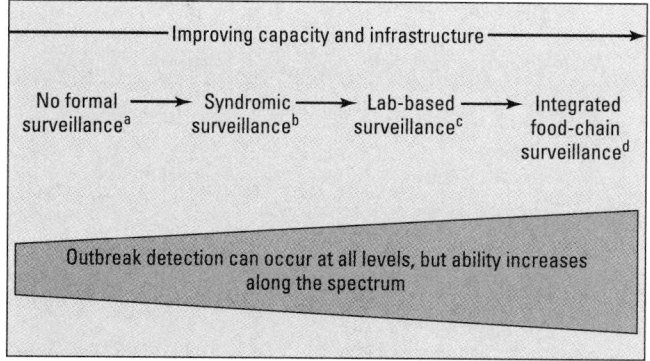

Source: Authors.

a. Without a formal surveillance, only large or unusual outbreaks can be detected.

b. Syndromic surveillance is based on groups of signs or symptoms indicative of a common diagnosis, such as acute gastroenteritis.

c. Laboratory-based surveillance relies on laboratory-confirmed pathogens, such as *Salmonella* or *Shigella*.

d. Integrated food-chain surveillance uses data from across the food chain.

Figure 53.3 Spectrum of Case-Based Foodborne Disease Surveillance

For FBD, surveillance for clinical syndromes is the most common method of surveillance in the developing world. Surveillance of FBD outbreaks that are investigated by public health authorities is often a useful means of monitoring both the safety of the food supply and the activities of the public health system. Although both surveillance for clinical syndromes and outbreak surveillance will remain important, the future in FBD is in laboratory-based surveillance. If microbiologic diagnosis is sought routinely for a sample of patients with acute gastroenteritis, then surveillance based on those diagnoses is possible. For enteric bacterial pathogens such as *Salmonella* or *Shigella,* determining the serotype of the strains in central reference laboratories allows more rapid and complete identification of epidemics, which may otherwise lead to preventable death and disability.

Laboratory-based surveillance systems require resources, facilities, and training. A central public health reference laboratory is essential for quality assurance and quality control and support. Such a laboratory-based system might begin with systematic referral of a sample of strains isolated at a sample of sentinel clinics, plus those strains that are part of outbreaks. A systematic sampling scheme provides better data than a more haphazard attempt at universal reporting. Regular sharing of information between the public health microbiology laboratory and epidemiologists is critical for the information to be used successfully.

The utility of serotyping as an international language for *Salmonella* subtypes has led to its widespread adoption. In a recent survey, 61 countries reported that they used *Salmonella* serotyping for public health surveillance (Herikstad, Motarjemi,

and Tauxe 2002). A collaborative WHO program called Global Salm-Surv promotes the use of *Salmonella* serotyping internationally among countries that wish to upgrade their national capacity for FBD surveillance (http://www.who.int/salmsurv/en).

Molecular subtyping is now expanding the power of laboratory-based surveillance to detect outbreaks in the background of sporadic cases by distinguishing the molecular "fingerprint" of an outbreak strain. CDC maintains PulseNet, an Internet-based network of all U.S. public health laboratories that uses a standardized genotyping method called pulsed-field-gel-electrophoresis (PFGE) as the basis for a national database of PFGE subtypes (Swaminathan and others 2001). Standardized subtyping protocols have now been developed for seven pathogens, and next-generation, gene-based technologies are under development for the future. Similar networks are developing around the world, with PulseNet Europe and PulseNet Canada already active and discussions rapidly advancing for PulseNet Asia Pacific and PulseNet Latin America. As with *Salmonella* serotyping itself, the global use of standard genotyping will facilitate the detection of multicontinent clusters.

Integrated Disease Surveillance and Response

The Integrated Disease Surveillance and Response (IDSR) strategy, first developed in Africa, links epidemiologic and laboratory data in communicable disease surveillance systems at all levels of the health system, with emphasis on integrating surveillance with response (WHO 1993, 1998). Districts were identified as a focus for strengthening efforts in collecting timely data, analyzing the collected data, and using the generated information for public health responses. The IDSR strategy is based on core activities, including case-patient detection, registration, and confirmation; reporting, analysis, use, and feedback of data; and epidemic preparedness and response (for example, outbreak investigations, contact tracing, and public health interventions). Support functions include coordination, supervision or performance evaluation, training, and resource provision for infrastructure, including communication (Nsubuga, Eseko, and others 2002).

Key steps in implementing the IDSR strategy include sensitizing key health authorities and stakeholders; conducting situational analysis; preparing a strategic IDSR plan; identifying and training a motivated, competent workforce; developing national IDSR technical guidelines; implementing the plan; and monitoring and evaluating implementation to improve performance (WHO 2000b). Assessment of the existing national surveillance and response activities provides baseline data to measure progress; to identify and build consensus on the national priority communicable diseases; to identify surveillance gaps of the selected priority diseases; to document

Table 53.2 Steps in the Development of the Philippine National Epidemic Sentinel Surveillance System

Steps	Data side	Human capacity side
1.	Identify the health problems thought to cause burden disease.	Consult top managers, donors, international agencies, and experts.
2.	Determine who will make interventions.	Involve users in design.
3.	Determine information users' need to make interventions.	Involve users in design.
4.	Decide how often decision makers need reports.	Involve users in design.
5.	Identify who collects, tabulates, and analyzes reports and who disseminates information.	Identify manager and staff to analyze, report, and enter data.
6.	Design report.	Involve users and staff in design.
7.	Make table shells.	Involve staff in design.
8.	Design questionnaire.	Involve staff in design.
9.	Pilot questionnaire.	Involve staff in implementation and evaluation.
10.	Pilot data flow and analysis.	Involve staff in implementation and evaluation.
11.	Pilot system.	Train staff in system and involve them in evaluation.
12.	Run system.	Involve staff in ongoing training and quality assurance monitoring.
13.	Evaluate system: Was information used? Are data and analysis of good quality?	Involve staff and users in design of external evaluation and in review of evaluator's report.

Source: Adapted from White and McDonnell 2000, 311.

the strengths, weaknesses, and opportunities of the existing systems; and to make appropriate recommendations. The WHO Regional Office for Africa, collaborating with its partners, has prepared tools and guidelines for implementation of IDSR at the country level. Indicators to monitor the performance of the surveillance and response systems have been prepared and field tested and are now in use in Africa.

Example: The Philippine National Epidemic Surveillance System

In the late 1980s, the Philippine Department of Health (PDOH), relying on its integrated management information system, detected less than one outbreak per year in a population of more than 60 million people. In 1989, the PDOH designed the National Epidemic Sentinel Surveillance System, a hospital-based sentinel surveillance system that encompasses both the flow of data and the personnel requirements needed to make the surveillance system work effectively (table 53.2). After the pilot study demonstrated promising results, the PDOH created personnel positions and a supervisory structure for sentinel physicians, nurses, and clerks in regional epidemiology and surveillance units (RESUs) integrated into the public health system. In 1995 alone, the system detected and formally investigated about 80 outbreaks, including 25 bacteriologically confirmed outbreaks of typhoid and 5 of cholera. As the Philippines developed HIV serological and behavioral risk surveillance, the RESU staff conducted surveys in their communities. By integrating surveillance functions that were based

on the skills of the workforce, PDOH was able to avoid the duplications, inefficiencies, and sustainability problems of multiple vertical systems (White and McDonnell 2000).

Informal Networks as Critical Elements of Surveillance Systems

WHO and other agencies frequently receive telephone calls or informal reports about urgent health events. WHO publishes an informal list of these "rumors," which allows public health workers to respond to health risks promptly rather than waiting for formal reports (http://www.who.int/csr/don/en/). The graduates of FETPs, PHSWOWs, and similar programs that provide competency-based on-the-job training in ministries of health make up one of the most important informal networks.

FETPs and allied programs both train epidemiologists and provide service to their ministries of health. For example, a student in the Brazilian FETP was assigned to review routine data on patients with leishmaniasis. She noted that some patients had symptoms of heavy metal poisoning, and further study indicated that a drug being used to treat leishmaniasis was contaminated with heavy metals. The drug was reformulated, and the problem was resolved. When this study was presented at a regional meeting of the Training Programs in Public Health Interventions Network (a network of FETPs and allied training programs), other countries banned the drug until it was reformulated (CDC 2004a).

Large categorical surveillance systems are expensive, and staff members might become complacent, especially if the disease under surveillance is rare. For example, the polio surveillance system for acute flaccid paralysis in the Western Hemisphere detected no cases in July 2000. A trainee from the FETP of the Dominican Republic, while investigating a case of suspected poisoning in a child, documented the first outbreak of circulating vaccine-type poliovirus in the Western Hemisphere since 1991. There were 13 confirmed cases in the Dominican Republic and 8 cases in Haiti. Her investigation led to national immunization days in both countries, which raised immunization levels and stopped the outbreak (Kew and others 2002).

THE ROLE OF SURVEILLANCE IN MAJOR OUTBREAKS

It seems incredible that a disease as devastating as AIDS could have spread silently to many countries over many years before it was detected and before effective control measures were implemented in the 1980s. In recent years, surveillance and response systems at all levels have been more effective at identifying and preventing spread of infectious diseases.

Example: Surveillance and Global Response to SARS

An epidemic of severe pneumonia of unknown etiology was detected in Guangdong province, China, in November 2002, and control measures were instituted on the basis of the way the disease spread from person to person. In February and March 2003, the disease spread to Hong Kong (China) and then to Vietnam, Singapore, Canada, and elsewhere (WHO 2003b). This new disease was named *severe acute respiratory syndrome*, and a preliminary case definition was established on the basis of initial epidemiologic investigations. A novel coronavirus (SARS-CoV) was identified as the causative agent in March, and mapping of the full genome was completed in April. This global pandemic ended in July 2003, as transmission was interrupted in Taiwan (China), after more than 8,000 patients in 26 countries and five continents were affected and 774 deaths were confirmed (Peiris and others 2003).

WHO spearheaded the global effort to control this pandemic, working with national and subnational health workers. In China, the FETP, which was initiated in October 2001 in the China Center for Disease Control, mobilized all 20 of its trainees, and they contributed substantially to the surveillance, investigation, and control of the SARS outbreak, working with local health officials (CDC 2003a). In Canada, which had the most cases of SARS outside Asia, 8 of the 10 FETP residents were involved in the SARS outbreak. They instituted surveillance, conducted epidemiologic investigations, designed prevention and control guidelines, responded to inquiries from the media and the public, and planned and implemented

epidemiologic studies (http://www.phac-aspc.gc.ca/cfep-pcet/outbreaks_e.html).

The success of this global effort to control the first new epidemic disease of the 21st century depended on a combination of open collaboration among scientists and politicians of many countries and the rapid and accurate communication of surveillance data within and among countries. Rapid global spread was recognized, and a global surveillance network was established on the basis of an agreed-upon case definition that was sufficiently specific to ensure effective reporting.

Public health surveillance is critical to recognizing new cases of SARS and differentiating this disease from other causes of severe respiratory illness, especially influenza (Heymann and Rodier 2004). Ongoing research into sources in the environment as well as clinical, laboratory, and epidemiologic concerns will improve surveillance for this critical public health problem. Notably, this highly contagious disease—for which there is neither a vaccine nor a cure—was controlled by competent, dedicated health workers with access to excellent communications. SARS presented a greater challenge than smallpox, for which long incubation periods and vaccine facilitate control (Mack 2005). Although it is reassuring that national, regional, and global systems were effective in controlling SARS, there is no reason to rest on our laurels. The only certainty is that there will be more new challenges, very possibly including further outbreaks of SARS.

Example: Avian Influenza in Thailand

The disastrous pandemic (worldwide epidemic) of influenza in 1918 is thought to have originated from epidemics in birds, as were the influenza pandemics of 1957 and 1968 (Ungchusak and others 2005). In early 2004, large epidemics of avian influenza were recognized in birds in eight Asian countries; by November, the disease had spread from birds to 44 humans, 73 percent of whom died (Ungchusak and others 2005). This contagion sparked fears that the highly lethal avian virus might be adapting to spread from person to person, which could cause extensive health and economic damage around the world. In Thailand, avian influenza was investigated by FETP graduates and others in the Thai Ministry of Health in partnership with CDC. By applying field epidemiologic techniques supported by laboratory studies, they detected that the virus was being spread from human to human in a family. It is likely that person-to-person transmission may have occurred in other countries, where field epidemiology was not used.

The Thai example is important for achieving the following: (a) raising global awareness of the potential of a global catastrophe early enough that plans can be made to avert or decrease harm and (b) demonstrating that, as with SARS, the disease could be controlled with proven field epidemiologic methods supplemented by good communications, without vaccines, drugs, or a high-technology laboratory or surveillance system (Mack 2005).

Example: Ebola in Uganda, the Role of the PHSWOW

On October 8, 2000, a second-year student in the Ugandan PHSWOW returned to Gulu district in northern Uganda for his field project. He found a hospital jammed with patients with high fevers, diarrhea, and bleeding. He diagnosed viral hemorrhagic fever. He called the Ministry of Health in Kampala, where that weekend a graduate of the PHSWOW was in charge of taking calls about epidemics. She agreed with his diagnosis and arranged for samples to be rushed to the National Institute for Virology in South Africa, the nearest WHO reference center for viral hemorrhagic fevers. When the minister of health arrived at his office the next day, the graduate briefed him. Recognizing the gravity of the situation, the minister sent the graduate to head the public health team surveillance and control team in Gulu, and the student headed the clinical team that established infection control in hospitals and treated patients.

Laboratory tests quickly confirmed that the illness was Ebola hemorrhagic fever, which usually kills more than 50 percent of those infected (Heymann 2004). Public health surveillance was difficult for several reasons. Because the disease was severe and rapidly fatal, rural villagers feared that they might be stigmatized if the government knew about cases in their area. Some sought out traditional healers; others fled as soon as they realized they had been exposed, which prompted outbreaks in two other districts. Gulu was a politically unstable area, and some villages were difficult to reach because of rebel or bandit activity. The Ugandan government mobilized its military to help with case finding and invited WHO, CDC, and other international teams to assist. Patients with Ebola infection require intense nursing and medical attention to control bleeding, diarrhea, and fevers. Some patients bleed easily, and all their secretions can be highly infectious. Hospitals in Gulu were desperately short of supplies to control the spread of infection from so many patients simultaneously. In spite of this situation, Ugandan health workers selflessly cared for the sick. By January 23, 2001, a total of 425 cases had occurred, the largest Ebola outbreak recorded. Only 53 percent of the patients had died, a proportion far less than the 88 percent reported in the 1976 Ebola outbreak in the Democratic Republic of Congo (formerly Zaire) and other previous epidemics (WHO Report of an International Commission 1978). Sadly, 22 health care workers were infected. Because the team from the Ugandan Ministry of Health set up active surveillance nationwide, the other two outbreaks, started when infected Gulu residents fled to distant villages, were quickly detected and controlled. International observers commented, "National notification and surveillance efforts led to the rapid identification of these foci and to effective containment" (CDC 2001).

The Ugandan Ministry of Health invested in developing competent, motivated health workers through the PHSWOW, an active partnership with Makerere University, the Rockefeller Foundation, CDC, and WHO. Both students and graduates contributed to the ministry's ability to rapidly identify and control this dangerous epidemic. Because the minister had timely evidence, he was able to notify other countries quickly and to bring in international teams before the disease spread further. Partially because of the lessons learned from this epidemic, Uganda has become one of the leading countries in implementing the IDSR program.

SURVEILLANCE FOR SPECIFIC CONDITIONS

Surveillance systems are important tools for targeting, monitoring, and evaluating many health risks and interventions. Because managers need a wide variety of information for specific interventions, systems have been developed and tested to meet those needs.

Environmental Public Health Surveillance

Surveillance for environmental public health practice requires the collection, analysis, and dissemination of data on hazards, exposures, and health outcomes (figure 53.4; Thacker and others 1996).

Health outcomes of relevance include death, disease, injury, and disability. However, relating those outcomes to specific environmental hazards and exposures is critical to

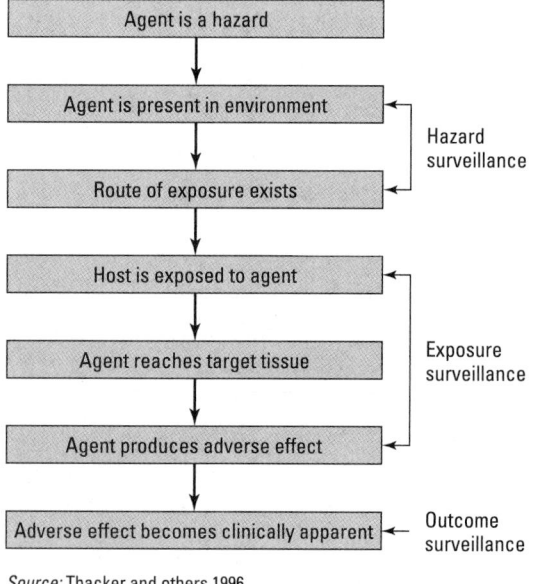

Source: Thacker and others 1996.

Figure 53.4 The Process of Adverse Effects and the Corresponding Surveillance

environmental public health surveillance. Hazards include toxic chemical agents, physical agents, biomechanical stressors, and biologic agents that are located in air, water, soil, food, and other environmental media. Exposure surveillance is the monitoring of members of the population for the presence of an environmental agent, its metabolites, or its clinically inapparent (for example, subclinical or preclinical) effects.

Four challenges complicate environmental public health surveillance. First, the ability to link specific environmental causes to adverse outcomes is limited by our poor understanding of disease processes, long lead times, inadequate measures of exposure, and multiple potential causes of disease. Second, data collected for other purposes rarely include sufficient information to meet a case definition for a condition caused by an environmental agent. Third, public alarm is often out of proportion to the hazard of concern, and sentiment will often influence public policy disproportionately to scientific information. Fourth, biologic markers will become increasingly critical elements of environmental exposure surveillance.

Obtaining data on exposure, which can include estimates derived from hazard data through sophisticated modeling or direct measurements of individual exposure obtained from use of personal monitors (for example, passive air samplers), is generally impractical in developing countries. Childhood blood lead levels are the only biomonitoring data that are collected routinely in several countries, either in national surveys or from screening programs for children at high risk.

Health outcome surveillance as applied to environmental public health is similar to traditional surveillance efforts. In the United States, the focus is on surveillance for birth defects; developmental disabilities (for example, cerebral palsy, autism, and mental retardation); asthma and other chronic respiratory diseases (for example, bronchitis and emphysema); cancer; and neurological diseases (for example, Parkinson's disease, multiple sclerosis, and Alzheimer's disease) (McGeehin, Qualters, and Niskar 2004). Other nations have different sets of priority conditions for surveillance. Disease registries, vital statistics data, annual health surveys, and administrative data systems (for example, hospital discharge data) are sources that have been used for monitoring health conditions. The challenges mentioned previously have constrained our ability in all nations, regardless of level of development, to establish and maintain effective and comprehensive environmental public health surveillance systems. As we invest in understanding the enlarging threats in the global environment, we must overcome these challenges and establish improved surveillance systems. The health of the global community depends on this investment.

Injury Surveillance

Injuries are a major public health problem and are among the 10 leading causes of death worldwide, killing an estimated 5 million persons each year and causing high rates of disability. People from all economic groups are at risk for injuries, but death rates caused by injury tend to be higher in developing countries (Peden, McGee, and Sharma 2002). Injury surveillance includes monitoring the incidence, causes, and circumstances of fatal and nonfatal injuries. Injuries are classified by the intention of the act into two groups: unintentional injuries and violence-related injuries. WHO (Holder, Peden, and Krug 2001) and the Pan American Health Organization (Concha-Eastman and Villveces 2001) have developed guidelines for establishing injury surveillance systems in developing countries.

If the range of fatal and nonfatal injuries, as well as the risk factors that can lead to injury, are to be fully captured, surveillance systems need to be established in multiple settings. Fatal injuries can be captured by using forensic or death certificate data. A far greater number of injuries are nonfatal and can be tracked through hospital- or primary care–based systems. Systematic information on nonfatal injuries, including prevalence, incidence, and related risk behaviors can also be obtained through ongoing population-based surveys.

Critical points should be addressed when planning an injury surveillance system in a developing country. First, data sources need to be clarified. In some developing countries, routine data on injuries are not always captured in health information systems. It is therefore necessary to consider other sources of data—for example, law enforcement agencies, coroners, or medical examiners. Next, the events and variables in an injury surveillance system should be defined according to the objectives of the system. Criteria such as the intentionality (violence-related injuries versus unintentional injuries); the outcome (fatal injuries versus nonfatal injuries); and the nature of violence-related injuries (physical, sexual, psychological, deprivation, or neglect) should be considered when establishing the system. Finally, case definitions and coding procedures should be defined before implementing the system.

For example, the Nicaraguan Ministry of Health, in collaboration with CDC and the Pan American Health Organization, began developing and implementing an injury surveillance system in 2001 (Clavel-Arcas, Chacon, and Concha-Eastman 2004). The system, based on the medical facility emergency department (ED), collects data on injuries in keeping with the *Injury Surveillance Guidelines* established by WHO (Holder, Peden, and Krug 2001). Under the system, a reportable case is defined as a patient who died from or was treated for an injury in the ED. Cases include patients with unintentional and violence-related injuries.

ED staff members identify cases and collect data in five hospitals in Nicaragua. Information used to complete the instrument is collected directly from the patients or their representatives. An ED admission clerk collects basic demographic data on the patient's arrival. ED medical staff members (physicians and nurses) collect the remaining information (for example, location, mechanism of injury, nature, severity, and circumstances surrounding the injury) during triage and assessment.

The hospital epidemiologist collects data collection forms daily from the ED, reviews the quality of data, and requests data from the ED staff if the forms are incomplete. The statistician reviews data daily. The country project coordinator also monitors the quality of the data periodically. Using Epi Info 2002 programs developed specifically for this project, the project coordinators analyze trends and identify potential risk factors (Noe and others 2004). The information is used to produce monthly reports for dissemination. Information is reported at both the regional and the country levels.

Injury prevention programs in Nicaragua use surveillance data to assess the need for new policies or programs and to evaluate the effectiveness of existing policies and programs. For example, the municipality of León is using the information from the hospital to monitor the increase in suicide attempts among youths abusing pesticides and to evaluate an intersectoral campaign to promote life that includes primary through tertiary prevention strategies.

Surveillance for Biologic Terrorism

Surveillance for biologic terrorism is conducted primarily for outbreak detection and management. Surveillance must support early detection of an incident of biologic terrorism and its characterization in the same manner as for the detection and control of naturally occurring outbreaks of infectious diseases. Early detection of outbreaks can be achieved by the following (Buehler and others 2004):

- timely and complete receipt, review, and investigation of disease case reports, including the prompt recognition and reporting to or consultation with health departments by physicians, health care facilities, and laboratories
- improvement of the ability to recognize patterns indicative of a possible outbreak early in its course (for example, by using analytic tools that improve the predictive value of data at an early stage of an outbreak or by lowering the threshold for investigating possible outbreaks)
- receipt of new types of data (such as purchases of health care products, absences from work or school, symptoms presented to a health care provider, or orders for laboratory tests) that can signify an outbreak earlier in its course.

Environmental detection systems for microbial pathogens and toxins of concern for biologic terrorism might also be categorized as new types of data early in the course of an outbreak, before infection (Meehan and others 2004). The primary surveillance tools for event detection and management are the traditional disease-reporting systems for notifiable diseases discussed elsewhere in this chapter. These core surveillance tools should be robust before new data types can be considered for supplementing public health surveillance.

Syndromic surveillance is an investigational approach by which health department staff members, assisted by automated data acquisition and generation of statistical signals (computerized algorithms), monitor disease indicators continually to detect outbreaks of disease earlier and more completely than might otherwise be possible with traditional reportable disease methods (Buehler and others 2004).

CDC's list of biologic terrorism agents and diseases can be found at http://www.bt.cdc.gov and an updated list of references dealing with syndromic surveillance is at http://www.cdc.gov/epo/dphsi/syndromic/.

Complex Emergency Surveillance

The key elements in planning a disaster surveillance system are establishing objectives, developing case definitions, determining data sources, developing simple data collection instruments, field testing the methods, developing and testing the analysis strategy, developing a dissemination plan for the report or results, and assessing the usefulness of the system. The surveillance needs are different in the preimpact, impact, and postimpact phases (Binder and Sanderson 1987).

The role of surveillance in disaster situations has included the following broad framework of activities:

- predisaster activities (for example, hazard mapping, provision of guidelines, and training for medical and rescue teams)
- continuous monitoring and surveillance for priority health problems in affected populations (for example, in the post-tsunami surveillance in Tamil Nadu, India, a one-page instrument was used for 10 priority health conditions for daily active surveillance in displaced populations at camps)
- prospective surveillance of affected populations focusing on the natural history of exposure and health effects and long-term effects of stress disorders among survivors.

Surveillance in Refugee Populations

Support of relief efforts following national and global disasters has been a relatively new application of epidemiologic practice for the public health professionals. Nevertheless, since the initial CDC involvement with the United Nations in a large-scale relief effort concerning approximately 20 million displaced people affected by the 1967–70 civil war in Nigeria, CDC staff members have participated in several assessments of the health needs, damage, and nutrition in refugee populations resulting from man-made and natural disasters. The more notable and extended actions were conducted in the 1979–82 Khmer

Thailand-Cambodia refugee-relief action, followed by long-term public health surveillance of Somalian refugees (1980–83), periodic but comprehensive health and nutritional assessments of Afghan refugees in Pakistan (1980–2002), and growth and nutritional assessments of internally displaced populations—especially children—in the Democratic People's Republic of Korea (1990s) and southern Sudan. Although these relief efforts occurred many years and many thousands of miles apart, they shared several important characteristics:

- Large numbers of people were in fixed camps or on the move searching for food and shelter. These needs were usually addressed by external aid agencies and many times caused local environmental degradation (fuel, temporary housing, water pollution, and so on).
- Refugees, after the initial phase, competed with indigenous populations for scarce jobs, leading to social strife and stress. Refugees were also exploited and suffered violence—additional factors leading to stress and social maladjustment.
- No administrative structure to provide and coordinate assistance of the necessary magnitude existed before the crisis, and thus, it had to be created after the fact.
- Assistance was complicated by the uncertainty associated with military activity, crime, and hostile governments.
- Data that were relatively simple to gather and analyze provided health workers and administrators information needed to plan and monitor assistance and its impact.
- Close collaboration with other local and international relief organizations (such as the United Nations High Commissioner for Refugees, the International Red Cross, the United Nations Children's Fund, WHO, and USAID) was essential to instituting and sustaining a meaningful surveillance system for refugees that led to interventions.

The major goal of these activities is to identify and eliminate preventable causes of morbidity and mortality. Planning requires effective use of existing knowledge about characteristic or predictable demographic patterns, easily applied health indicators, and avoidable errors of omission or commission. As in disasters, the principles of surveillance (data collection, data analysis, response to data, and assessment of response) and other public health techniques should be an integral part of relief efforts. Retrospective evaluation of these efforts has also proved useful (CDC 1983).

Chronic Disease Surveillance Systems

Development and evaluation of policies for health improvement require a reliable assessment of the burden of disease and injury, an inventory of the disposition of resources for health, assessment of the policy environment, and information on the cost effectiveness of interventions and strategies. In all these areas, consideration of noncommunicable (mostly chronic) conditions becomes critical. In 1999, noncommunicable diseases were estimated to cause approximately 60 percent of the deaths in the world and 43 percent of the global burden of disease (WHO 2000a). WHO forecasts that by 2020 the burden of disease from noncommunicable diseases for developing and newly industrialized countries will have increased more than 60 percent (Murray and Lopez 1996).

Some developing countries have found it difficult to acquire and analyze accurate mortality statistics regularly, let alone morbidity and quality-of-life information. Ensuring development, implementation, and widespread use of noncommunicable disease data for better decisions on resource allocation is critical to improving the quality of lives and promoting a more equitable future for health within and between countries.

Hypertension, elevated blood cholesterol, tobacco use, excessive alcohol consumption, obesity, and the multiple diseases linked to these risk factors are a global public health problem. In one study, smoking, high blood pressure, and high cholesterol alone explained approximately two-thirds to three-fourths of heart attacks and strokes (Vartiainen and others 1995). Until recently, surveillance for risk factors was an activity commonly associated with developed countries (Holtzman 2003). However, recently WHO has increased attention to noncommunicable disease surveillance by developing tools and working to achieve data comparability between countries (WHO 2003c). Data on key health behaviors, obesity, hypertension, lipids, and diabetes are collected inconsistently in developing countries, especially in Africa. Data on tobacco use are available through the Global Youth Tobacco Survey (http://www.cdc.gov/tobacco/global).

Incidence data (the number and proportion of new cases in a population) are limited in developing countries. However, India's National Cancer Registry program may serve as a notable exception (http://icmr.nic.in/ncrp/cancer_regoverview.htm). In 1981, the Indian Council of Medical Research, recognizing that there was a lack of information on follow-up of cancer patients to assess quality of care, instituted a cancer registry network. The network provides data on the magnitude and patterns of cancer in eight areas of India to enable studies of the histologic features correlating with prognosis and association studies (for example, whether a history of vasectomy is associated with cancer of the prostate). Another important example relates to the widespread use of folic acid in China and the resultant reduction in incidence of birth defects (Kelly and others 1996; Wald 2004).

Surveillance data have been critical in establishing the importance of obesity as a public health priority in the United States. Data for individual states provided by CDC's BRFSS have enabled individual health departments to document their obesity epidemic (Sturm 2003). These data provide a measure of the effectiveness of interventions to meet the control objectives. The BRFSS is a practical tool for developing and middle-income countries, as Jordan demonstrated when it implemented a BRFSS in 2002; the first survey documented substantial levels of obesity, especially among women, combined with low levels of physical activity (CDC 2003b).

ECONOMICS OF PUBLIC HEALTH SURVEILLANCE SYSTEMS

The outbreak of SARS in 2003 demonstrates the far-reaching economic impact of not having an effective global public health surveillance system in place, with an estimated reduction in real gross domestic product of more than US$1.0 billion in Canada (Darby 2003) and estimated income losses in the range of US$12.3 billion to US$28.4 billion for East and Southeast Asia as a whole (Fan 2003).

Public health surveillance is considered a global public good (Zacher 1999), particularly when it is used for eradication of such diseases as poliomyelitis. As eradication campaigns decrease the number of cases, maintaining systems to find the last few cases becomes more expensive. Often, the majority of the costs for these systems fall on hard-pressed developing countries. This factor raises questions of fairness and equity. For example, as poliomyelitis becomes rare, it ceases to be a significant risk to national populations, whereas other diseases, such as malaria and diarrhea, typically are major causes of morbidity and mortality. In such countries, it seems most fair and efficient for the global community to finance eradication campaigns, leaving national systems free to address the diseases that most affect their populations. The negative impact of globally mandated eradication surveillance systems can be mediated or reversed by leveraging on the eradication program's infrastructure to gather surveillance data for diseases of concern to local governments (Nsubuga, McDonnell, and others 2002). A similar case can be made for influenza early warning systems in countries that gather information that will be used to create vaccines that will benefit other populations but not their own. Equity demands that the countries that benefit from such systems finance them.

Public health surveillance systems serve an essential function in preventing and controlling disease spread within and across national borders. Although the private sector benefits, it lacks the incentive to invest in public health surveillance systems, and sovereign states depend on the contribution of others (WHO 2002); this situation has important implications for the financing of public health surveillance systems. Even within national borders, the difficulty of quantifying the benefits of surveillance systems for individual communities leads to neglect by local authorities, providing the economic rationale for funding by the national government. Developing countries

Table 53.3 Health Expenditures by National Income Level of Countries, 2001

Income group[a]	Government expenditures on health as a percentage of gross domestic product	Total expenditures on health as a percentage of gross domestic product
High income	6.30	10.74
Upper-middle income	3.68	6.41
Lower-middle income	2.58	5.63
Low income	1.22	4.78

Source: World Bank 2004.
a. All World Bank member economies with populations of more than 30,000 are classified into income groups, divided according to 2003 gross national income per capita, calculated using the World Bank Atlas method. The groups are low income, US$765 or less; lower-middle income, US$766 to US$3,035; upper-middle income, US$3,036 to US$9,385; and high income, US$9,386 or more.

are reportedly the weak link in the global surveillance framework, although they bear the greatest burden of disease, emerging and reemerging old pathogens, and drug-resistant pathogens (U.S. GAO 2001). The greatest need for surveillance systems is in these countries, but most lack both the resources and the political will to build human capacity and finance the systems (table 53.3). Resource constraints and intense pressure to provide care and treatment services lead public health authorities in the poorest countries to spend resources on surveillance (U.S. GAO 2001). Because the costs and benefits derive from surveillance systems spilling across national borders, donors should assist with capacity building in countries that have been unable to invest the human and material resources required.

An interesting and unresolved feature of these global public goods—the solution to their adequate provision and supply rests at local, national, and sometimes regional levels—has prompted the international health community to advocate for capacity building in developing countries rather than for consolidation of the fragmented systems at the global level (WHO 2002).

Standard tools of economic evaluation (Meltzer 2001) have been used to compare the benefits and costs of several public health interventions. The public good characteristics of surveillance systems, with benefits that are not easy to quantify, make the use of such tools difficult to implement in practice. However, economic evaluation of laboratory surveillance systems to detect specific disease-causing organisms have been undertaken in the developed world by comparing benefits and costs now and in the future (Elbasha, Fitzsimmons, and Meltzer 2000). These evaluations have not been done in developing countries and are needed. At best, an analysis of the benefits and costs of existing or proposed surveillance systems is feasible. This analysis requires an estimate of the cost of illness and answers the question of how many cases of a particular disease need to be prevented by the surveillance system to be exactly equal to the expenditure on the system.

Given expenditures on specific health interventions or programs, one can, by using traditional econometric tools, apply the data on health outcomes from the surveillance systems as inputs to economic analysis. Surveillance also clearly leads to a cost saving if it prevents the need for expenditure on treating patients.

FUTURE OF SURVEILLANCE

Public health agencies, ministries of finance, and international donors and organizations need to transform surveillance from dusty archives of laboriously collected after-the-fact statistics to meaningful measures that provide accountability for local health status or that deliver real-time early warnings for devastating outbreaks. This future depends in part on developing consensus on critical surveillance content and developing commitment on the part of countries, funding partners, and multilateral organizations to invest in surveillance system infrastructure and to use surveillance data as the basis for decision making. This vision of the future assumes a coherent, integrated approach to surveillance systems that is based on matching the surveillance objective with the right data source and modality and on paying attention to country-specific circumstances while maintaining global attention to data content needs.

Information technology and informatics can help in attaining this vision. Specifically, technology can facilitate the collection, analysis, and use of surveillance data, if data standards are developed and compatible systems are established. Data collection for surveillance would be an automatic by-product of any electronic systems used to support clinical care. Under this scenario, an automatic electronic message would be sent to the responsible public health jurisdiction with information about a health event (for example, death, disease, or injury), including all relevant information from the electronic health record about the patient, provider's name, patient's home address, risk factors, previous immunizations, and treatments. Even before this ideal capacity becomes widespread, technology such as cell phone–based systems could accelerate collection of key data (for example, occurrence of a viral hemorrhagic fever outbreak). The rapid penetration of cell phones in developing countries might obviate the need for prohibitively expensive landline-based systems. An accelerated system of wireless Internet access might also transform the capacities to which a local health post or a district health official might have access. These systems should also be considered as means for collecting information beyond traditional data. For example, telemedicine access can permit views of a rash illness to be shared with national or international medical specialists.

Analysis of surveillance data can also be transformed by using available technology. Software that is Web-enabled, together with the advances in geographic information system software and global positioning devices, means that anyone with Internet access can potentially apply the latest version of software running on a distant server in the national capital to local data to generate up-to-date maps and graphs describing health status in that jurisdiction.

Use of surveillance data can also be transformed. Sophisticated algorithms can be applied to data as it is collected to determine when (and how) an alert should be sent to local, national, or even international health officials to indicate a need for immediate investigation. Increasingly sophisticated visual display techniques and creation of custom channels with data of particular relevance to groups of data users are just some of the tools already being used to put public health content on the desktop of anyone with broadband, secure Internet access.

Realization of this future vision does not require technology beyond what is already feasible, but the following factors are needed:

- the organizational and political will to develop and coordinate the needed systems and standards that will enable those systems
- appropriate attention to individual privacy and system security
- removal of the financial and logistical barriers to broadband Internet access
- a strategic multisectoral approach to accelerating national infrastructure among the poorest developing nations.

GLOBAL SURVEILLANCE NETWORKS

Globally, infectious disease surveillance is implemented through a loose network that links parts of national health care systems with the media, health organizations, laboratories, and institutions focusing on particular disease conditions. WHO has described a "network of networks" (U.S. GAO 2001) that links existing regional, national, and international networks of laboratories and medical centers into a surveillance network (figure 53.5).

Government centers of excellence (for example, CDC, the French Pasteur Institutes, and FETPs) along with WHO country and regional offices also contribute to disease and health condition reporting. Military networks, such as the U.S. Department of Defense's Global Emerging Infectious Disease System, and Internet discussion sites, such as ProMed (http://www.promedmail.org) and Epi-X (http://www.cdc.gov/epix), also supplement the reporting networks. In 1997, WHO started the Global Outbreak Alert and Response Network, and

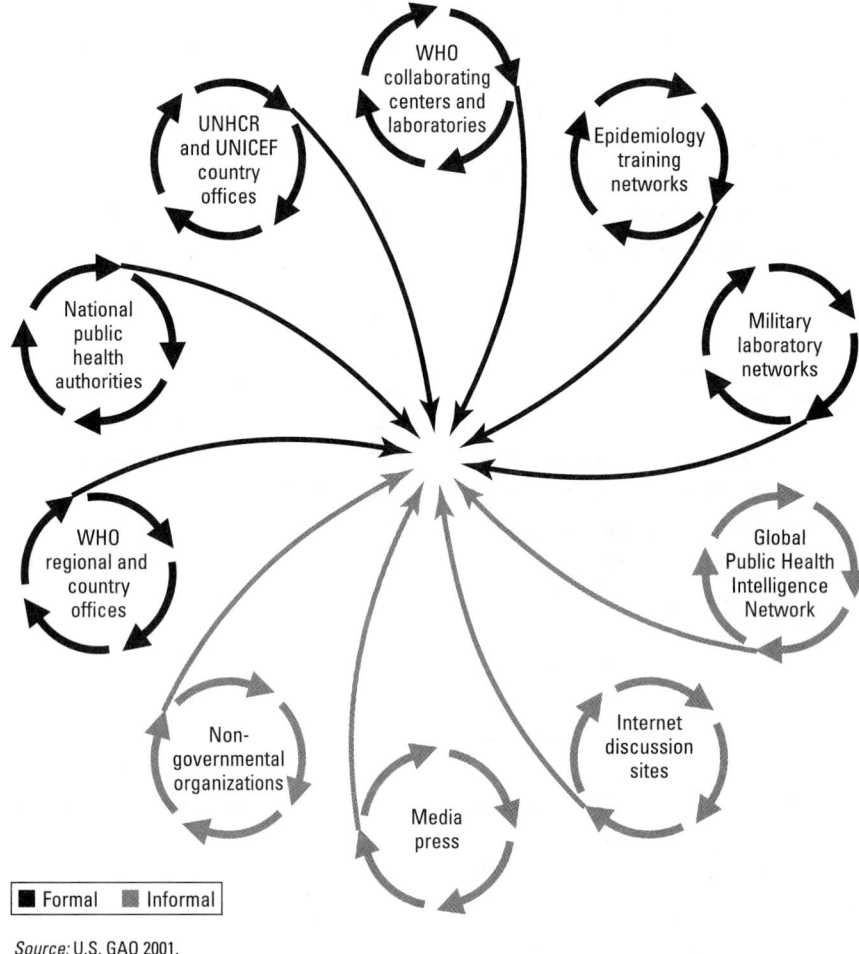

Source: U.S. GAO 2001.
a. UNHCR represents the United Nations High Commissioner for Refugees.
b. UNICEF represents the United Nations Children's Fund.

Figure 53.5 Global Infectious Disease Surveillance Frameworks

it was formally adopted by WHO member states in 2000. The network has more than 120 partners around the world and identifies and responds to more than 50 outbreaks in developing countries each year (Heymann and Rodier 2004).

The International Health Regulations are the only binding international agreements on disease control. The regulations provide a framework for preventing the international spread of disease through effective national surveillance coupled with the international coordination of response to public health emergencies of global concern by using the guiding principle of maximum protection, minimum restriction (WHO 2003a). The current regulations apply only to cholera, plague, and yellow fever; they require WHO member states to notify WHO of any cases of these diseases that occur in humans within their territories and then give further notification when the territory is free of infection. The regulations are being revised to include the development of national core capacities and national focal persons who have the competencies of graduates of FETPs and allied training programs. Programs established to improve the capacity of both epidemiologists and laboratorians to collect, use, and interpret surveillance and outbreak data (for example, the collaborative WHO program in foodborne diseases called the WHO Global Salm-Surv) are also important components in developing global surveillance networks.

RESEARCH AGENDA IN PUBLIC HEALTH SURVEILLANCE

Developing nations share surveillance needs with the rest of the world, yet they are challenged by economic limitations, weak public health infrastructure, and the overwhelming challenges of poverty and disease. As a result, countries in the developing world often depend on the research efforts of others, or they collaborate with others to conduct the research necessary for their surveillance needs. Within individual countries, surveillance systems are essential in measuring disease and injury burden as a first step in establishing public health priorities that lead to policies and programs.

The major research question for surveillance is how to develop and maintain a cadre of competent, motivated surveillance and response workers in developing countries. Other questions include how to design and maintain surveillance systems for these problems, especially morbidity systems for chronic diseases. Standard methods can be used to evaluate existing surveillance systems, which, in turn, will help define surveillance needs (Romaguera, German, and Klaucke 2000). Developing countries have used the IDSR strategy, which provides an efficient approach to data collection and analysis. Unfortunately, the majority of developing countries have limited surveillance systems for noninfectious diseases; instead, existing data systems (for example, vital records, motor vehicle crash records, or insurance claims data) are potential sources of surveillance data. In other settings, even these data sources are scarce, and approaches such as verbal autopsies and recurrent surveys might be alternatives (White and McDonnell 2000).

Surveillance for risk factors is another challenge, and BRFSSs need to be validated and applied more widely in developing countries. Surveillance for injuries, environmental hazards (such as traffic intersections that are associated with high rates of injuries), and exposures to chemical or biological agents is a key public health concern with few examples of effective application anywhere in the developed or less developed parts of the world. Rigorous research is required in this field (Thacker and others 1996).

The burgeoning use of electronic data systems and the almost universal availability of the Internet provide a tremendous opportunity for more timely and comprehensive surveillance in all parts of the world. Yet in this rapidly emerging field, critical needs exist, including the following:

- competent, motivated health workers
- data standards (Lober, Trigg, and Karras 2004)
- global policies and practices for international surveillance
- useful software (Dean 2000)
- evaluation of the effectiveness of all these applications.

New approaches that must be evaluated by using standard methods (Romaguera, German, and Klaucke 2000) include the following:

- IDSR for infectious diseases
- syndromic surveillance (CDC 2004b) for terrorism and emergency response
- laboratory-based surveillance methods to enhance diagnostic accuracy and increase timeliness of recognition of outbreaks and interventions (Swaminathan and others 2001).

Many research questions remain about surveillance methodology, including how to do the following:

- use data for forecasting or temporal and spatial analysis for aberration detection

- conduct surveillance for multiple competing risk factors that lead to a single condition (for example, smoking, cholesterol, hypertension, and overweight for heart disease)
- conduct surveillance for the adverse effects of drugs
- interpret ecologic data relative to data collected on individuals (Greenland 2004)
- measure cost-effectiveness of alternative approaches to surveillance (for example, integrated compared with categorical approaches)
- link data sources effectively (for example, hazard, exposure, and outcome data for environmental diseases)
- build and sustain human infrastructure in developing countries
- strengthen evidence-based decision-making cultures in ministries of health and finance.

CONCLUSION

Public health surveillance is an essential tool for ministries of finance, ministries of health, and donors to effectively and efficiently allocate resources and manage public health interventions. To be useful, public health surveillance must be approached as a scientific enterprise, applying rigorous methods to address critical concerns in this public health practice (Thacker, Berkelman, and Stroup 1989). Although the surveillance needs in the developing world appear to differ from those in the developed world, the basic problems are similar. In a time when we are confronted with SARS and avian influenza, the need to integrate global networks is undeniable, and research in how these concerns are addressed is essential. Collaboration among practitioners, researchers, nations, and international organizations is necessary to address the global needs of public health surveillance.

ACKNOWLEDGMENTS

The authors would like to acknowledge ORISE Fellow Danielle Backes of the Division of International Health, Coordinating Office for Global Health, U.S. Centers for Disease Control and Prevention, for her invaluable help in preparing this chapter.

REFERENCES

Binder, S., and L. M. Sanderson. 1987. "The Role of the Epidemiologist in Natural Disasters." *Annals of Emergency Medicine* 16 (9): 1081–84.

Birkhead, G. S., and C. M. Maylahn. 2000. "State and Local Public Health Surveillance." In *Principles and Practices of Public Health Surveillance*, ed. S. M. Teutsch and R. E. Churchill, 270. New York: Oxford University Press.

Buehler, J. W., R. S. Hopkins, J. M. Overhage, D. M. Sosin, and V. Tong. 2004. "Framework for Evaluating Public Health Surveillance Systems for Early Detection of Outbreaks: Recommendations from CDC Working Group." *MMWR Recommendations and Reports* 53 (RR-5): 1–11.

CDC (U.S. Centers for Disease Control and Prevention). 1983. "Surveillance of Health Status of Kampuchean Refugees—Khao I-Dang Holding Center, Thailand, December 1981–June 1983." *Morbidity and Mortality Weekly Report* 32 (31): 412–15.

———. 2001. "Outbreak of Ebola Hemorrhagic Fever, Uganda, August 2000–January 2001." *Morbidity and Mortality Weekly Report* 50 (5): 73–77.

———. 2003a. "Efficiency of Quarantine during an Epidemic of Severe Acute Respiratory Syndrome—Beijing, China, 2003." *Morbidity and Mortality Weekly Report* 52 (43): 1037–40.

———. 2003b. "Prevalence of Selected Risk Factors for Chronic Disease—Jordan, 2002." *Morbidity and Mortality Weekly Report* 52 (43): 1042–44.

———. 2004a. *Partnerships in Excellence: Charting the Future in Global Health.* Atlanta: CDC, Epidemiology Program Office, Division of International Health.

———. 2004b. "Syndromic Surveillance: Reports from a National Conference, 2003." *Morbidity and Mortality Weekly Report* 53 (Suppl.): 18–22.

Clavel-Arcas, C., R. Chacon, and A. Concha-Eastman. 2004. "Hospital Based Injury Surveillance Systems in Nicaragua and El Salvador, 2001–2002." Paper presented at the Seventh World Conference on Injury Prevention and Safety Promotion, Vienna, June 6–9.

Concha-Eastman, A., and A. Villveces. 2001. *Guidelines for the Design, Implementation and Evaluation of Epidemiological Surveillance Systems on Violence and Injuries.* Washington, DC: Pan American Health Organization.

Darby, Paul. 2003. "The Economic Impact of SARS." Publication 434-05, Conference Board of Canada, Ottawa.

Dean, A. D. 2000. "Computerizing Public Health Surveillance Systems." In *Principles and Practices of Public Health Surveillance*, ed. S. M. Teutsch and R. E. Churchill, 229–52. New York: Oxford University Press.

Effler, P., M. Ching-Lee, A. Bogard, M. C. Ieong, T. Nekomoto, and D. Jernigan. 1999. "Statewide System of Electronic Notifiable Disease Reporting from Clinical Laboratories: Comparing Automated Reporting with Conventional Methods." *Journal of the American Medical Association* 282: 1845–50.

Elbasha, E. H., T. D. Fitzsimmons, and M. I. Meltzer. 2000. "Costs and Benefits of a Subtype-Specific Surveillance System for Identifying *Escherichia coli* O157:H7 Outbreaks." *Emerging Infectious Diseases* 6 (3): 293–97.

Fan, E. X. 2003. *SARS: Economic Impacts and Implications.* ERD Policy Brief Series 15. Manila: Asian Development Bank.

Foege, W. H., R. C. Hogan, and L. H. Newton. 1976. "Surveillance Projects for Selected Diseases." *International Journal of Epidemiology* 5 (1): 29–37.

Greenland, S. 2004. "Ecologic Inference Problems in the Analysis of Surveillance Data." In *Monitoring the Health of Populations*, ed. R. Brookmeyer and D. F. Stroup, 315–40. New York: Oxford University Press.

Herikstad, H., Y. Motarjemi, and R. V. Tauxe. 2002. "Salmonella Surveillance: A Global Survey of Public Health Serotyping." *Epidemiology and Infection* 129 (1): 1–8.

Heymann, D. L. 2004. *Control of Communicable Diseases Manual.* Washington, DC: American Public Health Association.

Heymann, D. L., and G. Rodier. 2004. "Global Surveillance, National Surveillance, and SARS." *Emerging Infectious Diseases* 10 (2): 173–75.

Holder, Y., M. Peden, and E. Krug. 2001. *Injury Surveillance Guidelines.* Geneva: World Health Organization.

Holtzman, D. 2003. "Analysis and Interpretation of Data from the U.S. Behavioral Risk Factor Surveillance System (BRFSS)." In *Global Behavioral Risk Factor Surveillance*, ed. D. V. McQueen and P. Puska. New York: Kluwer Academic Press.

Kelly, A. E., A. C. Haddix, K. S. Scanlon, C. G. Helmick, and J. Mulinare. 1996. "Cost Effectiveness of Strategies to Prevent Neural Tube Defects." In *Cost-Effectiveness in Health and Medicine*, ed. M. R. Gold, J. E. Siegel, L. B. Russell, and M. C. Weinstein, 313–48. New York: Oxford University Press.

Kew, O., V. Morris-Glasgow, M. Landaverde, C. Burns, J. Shaw, Z. Garib, and others. 2002. "Outbreak of Poliomyelitis in Hispaniola Associated with Circulating Type 1 Vaccine-Derived Poliovirus." *Science* 296 (5566): 356–59.

Lober, W. B., L. Trigg, and B. Karras. 2004. "Information System Architectures for Syndromic Surveillance." *Morbidity and Mortality Weekly Report* 53 (Suppl.): 203–8.

Mack, T. M. 2005. "The Ghost of Pandemics Past." *Lancet* 365 (9468): 1370–72.

McGeehin, M. A., J. R. Qualters, and A. S. Niskar. 2004. "National Environmental Public Health Tracking Program: Bridging the Information Gap." *Environmental Health Perspectives* 112 (14): 1409–13.

Meehan, P. J., N. E. Rosenstein, M. Gillen, R. F. Meyer, M. J. Kiefer, S. Deitchman, and others. 2004. "Responding to Detection of Aerosolized Bacillus Anthracis by Autonomous Detection Systems in the Workplace." *MMWR Recommendations and Reports* 53 (RR-7): 1–12.

Meltzer, M. I. 2001. "Introduction to Health Economics for Physicians." *Lancet* 358 (9286): 993–98.

Murray C. J. L., and A. D. Lopez, eds. 1996. *Global Burden of Disease and Injury Series, Volume I: The Global Burden of Disease—A Comprehensive Assessment of Mortality and Disability from Diseases, Injuries, and Risk Factors in 1990 and Projected to 2020.* Cambridge, MA: Harvard University Press.

Narasimhan, V., H. Brown, A. Pablos-Mendez, O. Adams, G. Dussault, G. Elzinga, and others. 2004. "Responding to the Global Human Resources Crisis." *Lancet* 363 (9419): 1469–72.

Noe, R., J. Rocha, C. Clavel-Arcas, C. Aleman, M. E. Gonzales, and C. Mock. 2004. "Occupational Injuries Identified by an Emergency Department Based Injury Surveillance System in Nicaragua." *Injury Prevention* 10 (4): 227–32.

Nsubuga, P., N. Eseko, W. Tadesse, N. Ndayimirije, C. Stella, and S. McNabb. 2002. "Structure and Performance of Infectious Disease Surveillance and Response, United Republic of Tanzania, 1998." *Bulletin of the World Health Organization* 80 (3): 196–203.

Nsubuga, P., S. M. McDonnell, B. Perkins, R. Sutter, L. Quick, M. E. White, and others. 2002. "Polio Eradication Initiative in Africa: Influence on Other Infectious Disease Surveillance Development." *BMC Public Health* 2 (1): 27.

Pappaioanou, M., M. Malison, K. Wilkins, B. Otto, R. A. Goodman, R. E. Churchill, and others. 2003. "Strengthening Capacity in Developing Countries for Evidence-Based Public Health: The Data for Decision-Making Project." *Social Science and Medicine* 57 (10): 1925–37.

Peden, M., K. McGee, and G. Sharma. 2002. *The Injury Chartbook: A Graphical Overview of the Global Burden of Injuries.* Geneva: World Health Organization.

Peiris, J. S., K. Y. Yuen, A. D. Osterhaus, and K. Stohr. 2003. "The Severe Acute Respiratory Syndrome." *New England Journal of Medicine* 349 (25): 2431–41.

Romaguera, R., R. R. German, and D. N. Klaucke. 2000. "Evaluating Public Health Surveillance." In *Principles and Practices of Public Health Surveillance*, ed. S. M. Teutsch and R. E. Churchill, 176–93. New York: Oxford University Press.

Sturm, R. 2003. "Increases in Clinically Severe Obesity in the United States, 1986–2000." *Archives of Internal Medicine* 163 (18): 2146–48.

Swaminathan, B., T. J. Barrett, S. B. Hunter, and R. V. Tauxe. 2001. "PulseNet: The Molecular Subtyping Network for Foodborne Bacterial Disease Surveillance, United States." *Emerging Infectious Diseases* 7 (3): 382–89.

Thacker, S. B., and R. L. Berkelman. 1988. "Public Health Surveillance in the United States." *Epidemiologic Reviews* 10: 164–90.

Thacker, S. B., R. L. Berkelman, and D. F. Stroup. 1989. "The Science of Public Health Surveillance." *Journal of Public Health Policy* 10 (2): 187–203.

Thacker, S. B., and D. F. Stroup. 1998a. "Public Health Surveillance." In *Applied Epidemiology: Theory to Practice,* ed. R. C. Brownson and D. B. Petitti, 105–35. New York: Oxford University Press.

———. 1998b. "Public Health Surveillance and Health Services Research." In *Epidemiology and Health Services,* ed. H. K. Armenian and S. Shapiro, 61–82. New York: Oxford University Press.

Thacker, S. B., D. F. Stroup, R. G. Parrish, and H. A. Anderson. 1996. "Surveillance in Environmental Public Health: Issues, Systems, and Sources." *American Journal of Public Health* 86 (5): 633–38.

Ungchusak, K., P. Auewarakul, S. F. Dowell, R. Kitphati, W. Auwanit, P. Puthavathana, and others. 2005. "Probable Person-to-Person Transmission of Avian Influenza A (H5N1)." *New England Journal of Medicine* 352 (4): 333–40.

USAID (U.S. Agency for International Development). 2005. "Infectious Disease and Response Strategy 2005." USAID, Washington, DC.

U.S. GAO (U.S. General Accounting Office). 2001. *Challenges in Improving Infectious Disease Surveillance Systems.* GAO-01-722. Washington, DC: U.S. General Accounting Office.

Vartiainen, E., C. Sarti, J. Tuomilehto, and K. Kuulasmaa. 1995. "Do Changes in Cardiovascular Risk Factors Explain Changes in Mortality from Stroke in Finland?" *British Medical Journal* 310 (6984): 901–4.

Wald, N. J. 2004. "Folic Acid and the Prevention of Neural-Tube Defects." *New England Journal of Medicine* 350 (2): 101–3.

White, M. E., and S. M. McDonnell. 2000. "Public Health Surveillance in Low and Middle Income Countries." In *Principles and Practices of Public Health Surveillance,* ed. S. M. Teutsch and R. E. Churchill, 287–315. New York: Oxford University Press.

White, M. E., S. M. McDonnell, D. H. Werker, V. M. Cardenas, and S. B. Thacker. 2001. "Partnerships in International Applied Epidemiology Training and Service, 1975–2001." *American Journal of Epidemiology* 154 (11): 993–99.

WHO (World Health Organization). 1993. "Epidemiological Surveillance of Communicable Disease at the District Level." WHO Regional Committee for Africa, 43rd session, AFR/RC43/18. WHO, Geneva.

———. 1998. "Integrated Disease Surveillance: Regional Strategy for Communicable Diseases." WHO Regional Committee for Africa, 48th session. AFR/RC48/8. WHO, Geneva.

———. 2000a. *Global Strategy for the Prevention and Control of Noncommunicable Diseases.* Report by the Director-General, 53rd World Health Assembly. Provisional Agenda Items 2.11: A53/14. Geneva: WHO.

———. 2000b. "An Integrated Approach to Communicable Disease Surveillance." *Weekly Epidemiological Record* 75 (1): 1–7.

———. 2002. *Global Public Goods for Health: The Report of Working Group 2 of the Commission on Macroeconomics and Health.* Geneva: WHO.

———. 2003a. *Revision of the International Health Regulations World Health Assembly.* Resolution WHA 56.28. Geneva: WHO.

———. 2003b. "Severe Acute Respiratory Syndrome (SARS)." *Weekly Epidemiological Record* 78 (12): 81–83.

———. 2003c. *The SURF Report 1. Surveillance of Risk Factors Related to Noncommunicable Diseases: Current State of Global Data.* Geneva: WHO.

WHO Report of an International Commission. 1978. "Ebola Haemorrhagic Fever in Zaire, 1976." *Bulletin of the World Health Organization* 56 (2): 271–93.

World Bank. 2001. *World Development Report 2000–2001: Attacking Poverty.* New York: Oxford University Press.

———. 2004. *World Development Indicators 2004.* Washington, DC: World Bank. http://devdata.worldbank.org/hnpstats/query/default. html.

Zacher, M. 1999. *Global Epidemiological Surveillance: Global Public Goods.* New York: Oxford University Press.

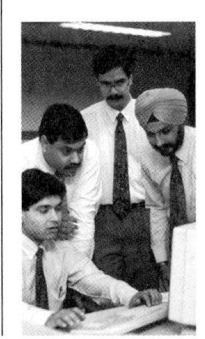

Chapter **54**

Information to Improve Decision Making for Health

Sally K. Stansfield, Julia Walsh, Ndola Prata, and Timothy Evans

The new source of power is not money in the hands of a few, but information in the hands of many.
—John Naisbitt and Patricia Aburdene, Megatrends 2000

This chapter focuses on the collection and management of public health information, in contrast to clinical information, which concerns individual patient care encounters. Even when aggregated, clinical data are necessary, but not sufficient, to inform efforts to improve the health of populations. While substantial attention has been focused on these facility-based clinical consultations and the health management information system (HMIS) used to track the relevant data, we focus here on the broader health information system (HIS) needed to inform decisions at individual, facility, district, and national levels. Considered here are the routine data collection systems upon which program management, planning, monitoring, and evaluation depend. Information needs for specific tasks, such as for research or for program evaluation, are discussed in the chapters on research (chapters 4 and 7). Other chapters in this volume refer to information needs to enable disease control or to evaluate programs and improve the delivery of interventions. Those interested in these issues should also pay special attention to chapter 53 and chapters 70–73. This chapter bridges the global and the local issues; it makes the case for strengthening the evidence base for action through comprehensive health information systems that include census, vital events, monitoring, public health surveillance, resource tracking, facility-based service statistics, and household surveys.

INTRODUCTION

From infancy on, we receive information that gives form to our thinking and problem solving. The method by which a phenomenon is measured shapes societal perceptions of it and the collective efforts to affect it. Likewise, the choices we make in the collection and use of information for health will determine our effectiveness in detecting problems, defining priorities, identifying innovative solutions, and allocating resources for improved health outcomes. Despite those fundamental realities, there has been little awareness to date of the ramifications that greater information use can have for advancing health, and even less attention has been given to systems needed to provide timely, accurate, and relevant information.

An example of the formative power of information for policy change lies in the history of the United Nations' Standard System of National Accounts, created by Richard Stone more than 50 years ago. The annual reporting of these accounts by most countries shapes our impressions of the relative position of nations, defines our views of the differential opportunities offered to their citizens, and drives the content of national and global political discourse (Jolly 2002). Another example is the measurement of disability-adjusted life years (DALYs), which has shaped priorities for investment in global health over the past decade.

1017

However, data or information alone will not transform outcomes. *Data,* which are simple measures of characteristics of people and things, have little inherent meaning or value. Analysis of the data enables the identification of patterns, thereby creating *information.* Finally, the use of information to generate recommendations, rules for action, and behavior change signifies the creation of *knowledge* that is used to make decisions and change human behavior.

Good decisions on effective policies, services, and behaviors require timely, accurate, and relevant information. Health information is required for strategic planning and the setting of priorities; clinical diagnosis and management of illness or injury; quality assurance and quality improvement for health services; detection and control of emerging and endemic disease; human resource management; procurement and management of health commodities (including drugs, vaccines, and diagnostics); regulation of toxic exposures; program evaluation; research; and other types of policies and programs (Walsh and Simonet 1995). Citizens require such information to choose healthy behaviors, to demand effective policies and services, and to hold their governments accountable for the allocation and use of resources for health. Internationally, information is required to meet transnational needs, such as for the detection and control of consequences of epidemics and infectious diseases, results-based management of development assistance programs, and advocacy for increased financing for health.

Several recent trends further enhance the pressures to deliver better health information. Global epidemics, such as of severe acute respiratory syndrome (SARS) and "bird flu," have amply demonstrated the need and potential benefits of sensitive and transparent systems for tracking health events. Donors, including the Global Fund and the Global Alliance for Vaccines and Immunization (GAVI), increasingly demand performance measures and detailed evidence to justify new requests for support. "Basket" funding and sectorwide approaches place further responsibilities on countries to define their own priorities. Decentralization and devolution of budgetary controls have shifted much of this growing burden to the periphery, requiring districts to provide local evidence as a basis for decisions. Tracking progress toward the Millennium Development Goals for health requires empowering countries to measure key indicators and produce evidence-based strategic plans to achieve and document that progress. Furthermore, nearly every chapter in this volume cites the need for better information, including through research dependent on a health information system, to accelerate improvements in health.[1]

Yet there is a striking disconnect between the need for information and the ability to respond to that need. To collect, collate, analyze, and communicate the necessary information in a timely and understandable fashion requires organized processes and procedures and a comprehensive HIS. However, donor-driven and disease-specific initiatives have actually undermined efforts to develop a comprehensive HIS by creating separate, parallel, and often duplicative systems to meet the need for each funding source.

Health information and the systems for its supply are a public good, meeting the defining criteria of being *nonexcludable* (in that, once the information is in the public domain, it is difficult to withhold from users) and *nonrival* (in that consumption of the information does not lessen its availability for use by others). As a public good, the supply of health information is the primary responsibility of governments: national governments for information within these jurisdictions, and international agencies and national governments together for international comparative information and global summary data.

Harmonizing the data collection, standards, best practices, and other elements of a national and global HIS has several advantages. Standardization enables economies of scale for training, hardware and software, and processes. Routine health information is a summative good in that the collation of each contribution produces a cumulative increase in the value of the public good, strengthening the credibility and importance of that information. Furthermore, standardization of systems improves the reliability and comparability of information, both within nations and across national and regional boundaries (Cibulskis and Hiawalyer 2002).

SYSTEMS AND SUPPLY OF HEALTH INFORMATION

To create an effective HIS, governments must finance the system, create the necessary policy environment (for example, through legislation and regulation), and develop systems and services for the collection, collation, dissemination, and use of health information. A substantial portion of the national health information is fully within the control of government health officials. However, information from the private health sector and other parts of the government is also required. Table 54.1 lists some of the data required and their sources. A principal challenge is the integration of these intra- and extrasectoral functions into a single, comprehensive HIS.

Direct Expenditures for Health Information

As for most public goods, the production of health information is mostly financed by government appropriation. Budget support for the HIS comes through both the ministry of health and a national statistics office (NSO) in most countries. The NSO is usually responsible for collecting information through the national census and most household surveys. For the least developed countries especially, bilateral and multilateral donors are essential sources of finance, particularly for HIS planning, infrastructure development, and training. In Africa, it has been estimated that grants or loans from donors account for between 20 and 70 percent of the financing for statistical

Table 54.1 Health Information from Sources Outside the Health Sector

Health information	Responsible agency
Census and national surveys: Income and poverty distribution Household expenditure for health Coverage with health interventions	National statistical office
National expenditures for health, economic development indicators, and industrial production and distribution data	Ministry of finance
Employment data: Human resources for health Occupational health information	Ministry of labor
Import data: Pharmaceuticals and vaccines Capital equipment and health commodities	Ministry of trade
Food production and security information and nutritional status data	Ministry of agriculture
Military health service statistics	Ministry of defense
Patterns of transportation injury (including motor vehicle accidents)	Ministry of transportation
Literacy rates and school health program information	Ministry of education

Source: Authors.

systems overall. Revenue generated by selling statistical products and services accounts for 10 to 20 percent of the financing for national statistical systems (Economic Commission for Africa 2003). User fees or taxes for use of information products and services can partially offset the costs of developing and maintaining the information system. In many countries, taxes and tariffs on computer equipment and government regulation of communications and Internet use remain barriers to public access to health information. Cost must not be a barrier to use of health information for the public good.

Information Policy

Sound information systems require a legislative and regulatory environment that encourages and supports effective HIS development. At the global level, many efforts have been made to establish international standards and policy frameworks for statistical data (United Nations Statistical Commission 1994). These policy frameworks are used to establish mandates for collection of basic health data (such as a decennial census or surveillance for reportable infectious diseases), to ensure the independence of official statistical agencies, to reinforce professional ethics, and to create norms for data quality and dissemination.

Another key policy intervention, less tangible though equally critical, is the creation of a culture of quality and transparency in the management of health information. There should be protection from political interference and full empowerment of the health statistics office to make public statements in response to criticisms of reports and the underlying methods. Ethical practices for protecting privacy and confidentiality must be well understood, and procedures should be in place to deal with breaches in these standards. Accuracy and reliability should be stated as expectations and ensured through periodic review of data collection methods and through benchmarking with internationally credible definitions of indicators. A client orientation should be instilled and users of data regularly consulted in defining outputs and formats for the presentation of data.

Systems for Collection, Management, and Analysis

Most developing countries have no comprehensive strategy for information management, reflecting the fractal nature of donor and national investments in these systems. Interventions to improve the HIS in the least developed countries, often donor driven, have often focused only on a specific subsystem, primarily for health service statistics, and have neglected other components of the HIS.

An effective HIS requires an overarching architecture that defines the data elements, processes, and procedures for collection, collation, presentation, and use of information for decision making throughout the health sector (see box 54.1). This information architecture promotes comparison and integration of data elements from a variety of subsystems. As O'Carroll (2003) points out, such a comprehensive design enables phased system development, reduces redundancy, increases efficiency, and improves interoperability. Interoperability is critical to ensuring, for example, that census data, vital statistics, and health facility data can be integrated to generate rates, ratios, cost-effectiveness estimates, and other information required to compare options for health investment.

The Pan American Health Organization (PAHO) has led the Regional Core Health Data Initiative "to facilitate speedy access to basic information on the health situation in the countries of the Region." This initiative has involved an international consultation and agreement on the priority data, collection methods, and indicators. The initiative has shown that it is possible to create a regional database of essential, consistent, valid, standardized, timely, and regular information. PAHO has used the information to set its priorities, whereas countries have applied the results to design health programs and to allocate resources to upgrade their information systems. In the future, the plan is to expand the systems to subnational districts (PAHO 2004).

Other WHO regions, including the Asia Pacific, are instituting similar initiatives with Web-based publication of core health indicators.

Data Collection. No single mechanism for data collection is adequate to meet the needs for public health decision making.

The Health Metrics Network: Harmonizing Investment in HIS Development

Developing countries, multilateral agencies, bilateral donors, and technical resource agencies have recently come together to form a global Health Metrics Network (HMN) that is designed to provide guidance for the development of the HIS, both in meeting national information needs and in producing the required indicators for tracking progress toward global goals. The HMN will provide the first consensus technical framework for HIS

architecture and a plan for development of national health information systems. This HMN Framework includes a blueprint for iterative improvements in the HIS; descriptions of core data collection subsystems (census, surveys, vital events monitoring, service statistics, and resource tracking); and procedures for management and dissemination of information.

Source: Authors.

These needs can be met using a combination of the six key health information subsystems: census, household surveys, public health surveillance, vital events monitoring, health service statistics, and resource tracking. Surveys are conducted on a sample in order to limit costs, whereas the other subsystems are more often designed to cover the entire population. In most developing countries, public health surveillance—except for certain disease-specific efforts—is conducted through passive reporting from health facilities. Especially where utilization rates are low, this facility-based surveillance may be considered a sample or "sentinel" surveillance strategy. Vital events monitoring is, ideally, universal; however, many countries use a phased introduction of vital events monitoring that makes it functionally a sentinel or sample-based data collection effort during the transition to universal coverage.

A *national census* every 10 years is an irreplaceable component of a national information system because it provides denominator data for so many indicators and sampling frames for subsequent sample surveys. The major costs of a census come from activities to establish the census maps, enumerate populations, enter data, and analyze the results. The cartographic costs can often be shared with other government departments, because the resulting updated maps can be instrumental in carrying out other critical public functions.

Sample surveys of households are a mainstay of health information collection in the developing world. They provide data on service utilization; coverage of health interventions (for example, immunization); morbidity (self-reported illness or disability); pregnancy outcomes; mortality levels, differentials, and trends; and causes of death (through associated *verbal autopsy;* that is, expanded interviews in the case of death to determine cause on the basis of signs and symptoms before death).

Surveys are, almost without exception, funded externally in the least developed countries and are not seen within the country as being part of a health information "system." They are, in

fact, generally undertaken to compensate for the lack of information available through routine systems (AbonZahr and Boerma 2005). The investment in surveys has thereby enabled donors and developing countries to sustain their neglect of the development of comprehensive and sustainable national health information systems. The United Nations Population and Statistics Divisions and the European Statistical Office (EUROSTAT) also support household survey work. Differences in methodologies among these surveys are currently a barrier to the comparison of results. The World Bank's Managing for Development Results Roundtable, held in Marrakech, Morocco, in 2004, recommended harmonization of these surveys to eliminate duplication.

Nonetheless, surveys offer an important source of information that transcends most of the selection bias that is inherent in service statistics. Especially in the least developed countries, where vital events registration systems and census taking are embryonic or nonexistent, surveys represent the only source of unbiased information about demography, socioeconomic status, coverage, morbidity, mortality, health expenditures, and other characteristics of the population. Where substantial proportions of the population use private health services, household surveys are particularly important. Even industrial countries rely on periodic community-based sample surveys for immunization coverage, for health service utilization rates, and for information on household health expenditures (Perrin, Kalsbeek, and Scanlan 2004).

The World Health Organization (WHO) recommends using periodic surveys to monitor coverage, such as for immunization programs, especially in view of the shortcomings of service statistics for obtaining these measures (Murray and others 2003). Some household surveys collect biological and clinical specimens, such as blood, saliva, urine, and self-collected vaginal swabs, or they check swabs for anemia, HIV, disease antibodies, vitamin A, and other conditions. However, the performance characteristics of most diagnostic technologies (for example, cost, ease of field use, sensitivity, and specificity) are designed for clinical use and do not lend themselves readily to use in population surveys, especially in remote areas of developing countries. Moreover, the collection of diagnostic information along with individual identifiers introduces complex ethical issues in the notification of people with treatable conditions, the financing of any required treatments, and the use of the specimens for other studies (Ties Boerma, Holt, and Black 2001).

Public health surveillance has been defined as the "ongoing systematic collection, analysis, and interpretation of data on specific health events affecting a population, closely integrated with the timely dissemination of these data to those responsible for prevention and control" (Thacker and others 1996). In developing countries, surveillance usually focuses primarily on a set of notifiable diseases, mainly infectious, which health care providers and laboratories are often required by law to report. Some nations also track risk factors for important diseases, injury events, adverse drug reactions, cancers, and pregnancy outcomes. Surveillance may be intensified over a period of years to enable targeting of special interventions for the control or elimination of diseases such as polio, tetanus, or measles. Active surveillance or screening of populations for target diseases may also be used in specific circumstances, such as during peak seasons for the disease or during natural disasters, when the potential for epidemics may be high.

Most passive surveillance data, however, are incomplete. Reliance on surveillance for reportable diseases diagnosed in health facilities omits diseases diagnosed among those who go to private providers or who are too poor to go to any health facilities. Even in health facilities, reportable diseases are often underrecognized or cannot be confirmed in laboratories that have inadequate resources. Sentinel surveillance methods and registries maintained in a few selected sites may be more representative of the entire population and more cost-effective in identifying and reporting the target diseases or health conditions; however, an outbreak may go undetected in a geographic area without a sentinel site. Special regional surveillance may also be used where populations are vulnerable to special health risks. The Vigisus project in Brazil, for example, has developed a system of epidemiologic and environmental surveillance for the prevention and control of disease among indigenous populations in the Amazon region (http://www.br.undp.org/propoor/BRA97028a.htm). Despite the methodological hazards, public health surveillance is essential for both national and global planning and preparedness, especially in view of the risks of regional expansion (for example, of meningitis and polio) or global spread of recent epidemics (for example, of SARS and bird flu).

Vital events monitoring is the continuous, compulsory, and (in most cases) universal civil registration of key vital events, such as births, deaths (sometimes including fetal deaths), marriages, divorces, and migrations. In many countries, vital events

monitoring systems function poorly and may be found only as remnants of past colonial administrations. In 2003, 115 of 192 WHO member states reported mortality data with causes of death, capturing about one-third of global deaths, or 18.6 million deaths per year. In South Asia, only 60 percent of births are registered (22.5 million), and in Africa, only 30 percent (17 million). Alternatives to universal registration include the sample registration systems used in China and India and the demographic surveillance sites in Tanzania. The International Network of Field Sites with Continuous Demographic Evaluation of Populations and Their Health in Developing Countries (INDEPTH), an association of longitudinal vital and health statistics surveillance sites in 17 countries, can provide technical support and training for development and management of these demographic surveillance sites (http://www.indepth-network.org/). The UN Statistics Division has developed principles and recommendations for vital statistics systems to guide countries in their development (http://unstats.un.org/unsd/demographic/sources/civilreg/civilreg methods.htm.)

Vital events monitoring systems may also be enhanced to determine causes of death, whether those deaths occur within health facilities or in the community. When deaths occur outside the health care system, a *verbal autopsy,* or structured interview of the relatives of the deceased, can assist in determining the cause of death. Verbal autopsies can, however, be used reliably to diagnose only those few conditions that have characteristic clinical signs or patterns of signs that can be recognized by family members or by the health workers who review the interview data. WHO is now developing standardized tools for verbal autopsy that will enhance the sensitivity and specificity of these instruments and permit comparisons over time and across geographics.

Health service statistics are critical management tools for both preventive and curative services. The statistics are collected at each level: community outreach service points, primary care facilities, and district and regional referral hospitals. Information from clients and providers documents the quantity and quality of services and enables managers to detect and solve problems in order to improve health outcomes and efficiencies. This health information subsystem must be "flexible and capable of adapting to local needs, while at the same time allowing for standardization of health care quality assurance indicators, and subsequent ability to measure and compare the quality performance of health facilities nationwide" (Duran-Arenas and others 1998). A principal barrier to improving service quality in many health care facilities is the lack of reliable systems for managing and retrieving individual patient records.

Service statistics are especially powerful when they can be compared with population-based measures from censuses and surveys to estimate rates and ratios, such as disease incidence or service coverage rates. Most service statistics subsystems track data only from public sector providers and facilities. Future improvements must implement systems and incentives to ensure reporting of service data from the private sector.

The *resource-tracking subsystem* must enable measurement and management of human resources; facilities; commodities (pharmaceuticals, vaccines, and other consumables); and finances. Human resource tracking provides a mechanism for licensing health service providers and accrediting health facilities. Licensure and accreditation can be paired with incentives to ensure service quality and private sector contributions to achieving public health goals.

The national health account (NHA) framework provides methods for measuring total national expenditures for health from household, public, private, and donor sources. NHA data document the sources of health financing, the amount spent for services, the distribution of funds across services and interventions, and the distribution of health benefits from those services and interventions. An NHA framework tracks the flow of funds, for example, from the ministry of health to health providers and government service programs or from households to pharmacies and private providers. These internationally comparable data enable benchmarking of performance among countries (Peters and others 2000).

Of the 68 countries that have implemented NHAs, only one-third have used the framework more than once. However, 19 of 21 countries studied can report at least one instance in which the NHA system has informed and shaped policies (De and others 2003). For example, South Africa's NHA analysis documented a higher per capita health expenditure in the richest districts, leading to intensified efforts to mitigate these inequities (Abt Associates 2003).

Information and Communications Technologies. The rapid evolution of information and communications technologies (ICT) over the past 30 years has immense implications for the potential speed, cost, and effectiveness of an HIS. But a "digital divide" persists, with poor countries failing to benefit fully from these ICT advances. Lack of access to reliable power sources, absence of Internet connectivity, inability to procure computer equipment and appropriate software, and inadequate technical support are some of the barriers. African users account for only 1 percent of the world's Internet traffic, 80 percent of which is in South Africa (http://www3.sn.apc.org/africa). Although less than 0.001 percent of the Internet use in Africa is among health professionals, this usage is growing rapidly.

Internet access in health facilities can make the HIS more effective and efficient by enabling instantaneous transmittal of data to central locations. Internet access in facilities can also speed data transmission and improve clinical outcomes by providing access to evidence-based decision support for clinical care (Godlee and others 2004; McLellan 2001). Even in remote areas where no telephone or cable access exists, satellite technology can provide access to e-mail. Several countries, such as Bolivia and Peru, have successfully used satellite telephone technologies to enable continuous Web-based updating of health databases. Because the effectiveness of epidemic control often depends on timely detection and reporting of outbreaks, e-mail and telephone technologies have shown particular promise for use in disease surveillance. In Peru, for example, 100 percent reporting was achieved and sustained within six months of rollout of a pilot surveillance system using cellular telephones (Lescano and others 2003). The system is to be expanded to national coverage this year.

Although individual citizens will not soon have equal access to ICT, these technologies can immediately be better used to improve public health. Automation of data entry and analysis can ease data capture, validation, analysis, and transmittal of health information. District managers can generate reports with tables and charts and transmit them to central levels, which can then apply this knowledge to improve local management. Special prompts and "exception reports" can alert managers to unexpected findings that require double-checking or immediate interventions (for example, outbreaks of infectious disease, low immunization coverage, or other management problems).

Use of free software, such as the U.S. Centers for Disease Control and Prevention's Epi Info, can lower costs, but often these software packages require substantial adaptation to local needs, along with additional training and technical support. Acquisition of computer equipment should be viewed not as a one-time capital expenditure but as a long-term commitment to buy periodic upgrades, maintenance, and technical support. Experience shows that purchase of inexpensive software and computers, such as in the Eastern Cape Province of South Africa, may actually increase overall costs when they require early replacement with more adequate alternatives.

Geographic information system (GIS) technologies have also been successfully used in districts in several countries to enable mapping and visual representation of the geographic distribution of risk factors, disease, and services. A desktop GIS viewer and mapping software are available in several shareware versions, including the WHO's "Health Mapper," so that maps can be produced at little cost. Other potentially promising technologies include electronic scanners and personal digital assistants for data capture (http://www.healthnet.org) and global positioning systems to facilitate the mapping process.

The principal barriers to improved information systems, however, are human, not technological. Substantial investment in training and technical support must accompany the introduction of any new technology. If the HIS is not functionally solid, introducing ICT will likely only worsen existing problems.

Dissemination and Use of Health Information

Information is a means to the end of improving health, but the availability of reliable information does not guarantee its use or improved decision making. Because decisions are often driven as much by politics as by evidence, it is critical to design information systems to meet the needs of decision makers and to create a culture of evidence that provides incentives and accountability for evidence-based decision making. Extensive dissemination promotes widespread use and accountability. The many users of information include the following:

- health ministries at national, regional, and district levels
- researchers and evaluators
- legislative and policy analysts
- nongovernmental organizations and consumer organizations
- advocacy groups
- private sector health providers and insurers
- communities, including groups of patients
- journalists
- donors and international agencies concerned with health
- individuals and families.

The literature on health information systems is replete with complaints of the neglect of existing information, yet remarkably little is known regarding the effectiveness of interventions to improve the use of information. The NHA experience (De and others 2003) suggests that policy makers are most likely to use information when it contributes to and informs a preferred government direction, especially if that information is not available to stakeholders outside the health ministry. But systems and dissemination patterns for information can be engineered to ensure that clients, providers, and managers will seek and use information to inform decisions. Standard procedures can be developed to ensure analysis and use of data at the level at which it is collected. Training of health workers can be designed to include both basic and refresher training in the analysis and interpretation of data that are relevant to each job. Expectations of information use can be built into routine job requirements, including use of evidence for planning, data requirements for periodic reporting to supervisors, and use of information during performance reviews. Groups of managers can be convened across districts or regions for benchmarking, in which each manager presents and compares performance data and is rewarded for transparency and learning. These practices will result only from intense training in analysis and use. For example, Loevinsohn (1994) demonstrated that fewer than half of midlevel managers were able to use the information system even to identify best- and worst-performing districts. Nonetheless, if managers use the information, and if improved efficiency and coverage with interventions is the result, the HIS becomes exceedingly cost-effective.

Information will "allow the public, their elected representatives, or donors to determine whether they are obtaining value for money" (Cibulskis and Hiawalyer 2002; see also Mackay 1998). Providing full access to the media will help to accelerate expectations of evidence-based decision making and accountability. Civil society, including nongovernmental organizations, should be the principal users of information to create and sustain citizen demand for quality services. The Healthy Communities Foundation's "dashboard" of lead indicators of health system performance exemplifies one promising example of the visual display of data (http://whatcom.healthycities.org/demo/aboutus.htm). Such dissemination and use of health information has enhanced government accountability for improved health in Papua New Guinea, where reports of local government performance in improving health systems transformed election results (G. Hiawalyer, personal communication).

BENEFITS, COSTS, AND COST-EFFECTIVENESS OF IMPROVED INFORMATION

There is broad agreement that information—plus the knowledge it enables—creates value. Yet it is challenging, indeed, to quantify the added value of information. Information, after all, is necessary but never sufficient to achieve improved outcomes. Other resources—human, material, and financial—are required for change. Nonetheless, it is possible to define the interventions necessary to improve health information and to draw on a few studies to estimate the cost and cost-effectiveness of these investments.

Strengthening of Systems

The steps involved in strengthening HIS include securing funding for a review of the current HIS and planning reforms and then using that plan to secure funding for implementing the reforms. The reforms depend on legislation and regulations that delineate the requirements, incentives, and disincentives for collecting the needed information. Finally, the review of the current HIS includes a situational analysis and outline of a plan that involves a comprehensive information architecture that is linked to both national and international needs.

The HMN Framework includes assessment and planning tools and HIS standards that will guide strengthening of systems. Full implementation will likely take at least 36 months, and the effects on decision making and health outcomes will be detectable only after approximately five years.

Benefits and Effectiveness of Improved Information

The value of health information can be characterized in terms of cost savings; system efficiencies (for example, increased coverage or quality of services); or improved health outcomes (for example, DALYs saved or improved health equity). Information can also be used to increase overall resources for health. Publications such as this volume, *World Development Report 1993: Investing in Health* (World Bank 1993), and the report of the Commission on Macroeconomics and Health (2000), are important examples of evidence that has been used to change health policies and increase resources for health.

The industrial world holds examples of the use of information to make service provision more effective and efficient. A quality improvement and evidence-based decision assistance program for diabetes patients in the United States created a net savings of US$510,133,[2] primarily by averting hospitalizations (Petrakos 1998). The U.S. Institute of Medicine estimates that a computerized system for managing physician orders for medications costing US$1 million to US$2 million could "pay for itself in three to five years" and prevent injury to hundreds of patients per year (Kohn, Corrigan, and Donaldson 2001).

There are also promising examples of the benefits and effectiveness of improved information from developing countries. Quality improvements driven by better information in Bolivia resulted in a 300 percent increase in hospital utilization rates (Pappaioanou and others 2003). In rural Mali, populations enrolled in a community-based information system calculated delivery costs for childhood immunization to be US$1.47 per child, compared with US$2.79 per child among populations not registered (Zayan, Berggren, and Doumbia 1992).

Better information can also improve efficiencies in the management of pharmaceutical resources. For example, implementing a subnational information system in the Eastern Cape province of South Africa led to improved access to pharmaceuticals, with a 39 percent reduction in stockouts of essential drugs. Such improvements undoubtedly lead to better health outcomes, which may result in increased productivity and consequently an increase in the growth rate of the gross domestic product (Jamison, Sachs, and Wang 2001; Nordhaus 2002).

Costs of Improved Health Information

Few studies have documented the costs of an HIS. Kleinau (2000) estimated the resource requirements for health service statistics, the most expensive of the six subsystems. Using similar assumptions, we have calculated updated costs.

This estimate includes only the public sector facilities, not private sector reporting systems. Reporting from private providers would likely include a more limited set of reported data: diseases, vaccinations, possibly staffing, and minimal utilization. Table 54.2 summarizes the total annual costs and per capita costs of the six health information subsystems.

The costs of a facility-based services statistics subsystem of the HIS (table 54.3) can be assumed in most developing countries to include routine public health surveillance, because these data are obtained at health facilities when ill patients are

Table 54.2 Cost of Essential HIS Subsystems

HIS subsystem	Total cost (US$ million)		Per capita cost (US$)	
	Low income	High income	Low income	High income
Health service statistics	4.8	25.9	0.16	1.66
Public health surveillance (included with health service statistics)	0	0	0	0
Census	7.5	30.0	0.25	1.0
Household surveys	0.6	1.0	0.02	0.03
Vital events surveillance	1.5	6.0	0.05	0.20
Resource tracking	1.5	3.0	0.05	0.10
Total	15.9	65.9	0.53	2.99

Source: Authors.

Note: Table is based on a population of 30 million. Household survey costs are based on the experience of the demographic and health surveys during 2001–2003 (Macro International, personal communication). Costs vary by sample size and by length of the survey instrument; Macro International estimates, an average cost of US$100 per survey participant. A sample of 6,000 is assumed for the low-income setting, and a sample size of 10,000 is assumed for the high-income setting. Cost estimates for vital events monitoring are based on demographic surveillance sites. In the high-income setting, the annual costs are assumed to quadruple. Resource-tracking costs are based on the experience of national health accounts (Abt Associates, personal communication), and the Egyptian Budget Tracking system. Similar costs are estimated for human resources and commodities.

brought for treatment. The additional costs of program-specific surveillance (for example, in support of polio eradication or tetanus elimination programs) could be assumed with a minor marginal investment in addition to facility-based and community-based information systems, including for vital events surveillance.

The calculated range for per capita annual costs of a comprehensive HIS—US$0.53 to US$2.99—compares closely to the estimates from a country setting in which those data have been obtained, including a low-resource country (Tanzania) with a per capita cost of approximately US$0.50 (Rommelmann and others 2004) and a high-resource country (Mexico) with a per capita cost of approximately US$1.00. The Health Metrics Network (HMN) Technical Task Force South Africa has also estimated costs of the HIS at approximately US$26 million (165 million rand) for a population of 43 million, yielding a per capita cost of US$0.60. The highest range of the estimate would apply in countries with higher salaries and a more comprehensive HIS.

Estimations of the Cost-Effectiveness of Interventions to Improve Health Information

The Tanzania Essential Health Interventions Program (TEHIP) is perhaps the best source of evidence for the cost-effectiveness of improved health information. The project was designed to

Table 54.3 Annual Costs of the Facility-Based Services Statistics Subsystem of an HIS

HIS cost	Low-resource setting	High-resource setting
Personnel		
Primary care facility	One person (salary US$4,514/year) spends 10 percent of time at each of 6,000 facilities (US$2,708,400)	Two people (salary US$10,351/year each) spend 20 percent of time at each of 6,000 facilities (US$24,842,400)
First referral level	One person (salary US$4,514/year) spends 25 percent of time at each of 1,000 facilities (US$1,128,500)	Two people (salary US$10,351/year each) spend 75 percent of time at each of 1,000 facilities (US$15,526,500)
District hospital	Two people (salary US$4,514/year each) spend 20 percent of time at each of 300 facilities (US$541,680)	Two people (salary US$10,351/year each) spend 100 percent of time at each of 300 facilities (US$6,210,600)
Regional level	Three people (salary US$10,962/year each) spend 50 percent of time at each of 15 facilities (US$246,645)	Three people (salary US$25,134/year each) spend 100 percent of time at each of 15 facilities (US$1,131,030)
National level	Six people (salary US$10,962/year each) spend 50 percent of time (US$32,886)	Ten people (salary US$25,134/year each) spend 100 percent of time (US$251,340)
Subtotal (personnel)	US$4,658,111	US$47,961,870
Data collection instruments and supplies		
Primary care facility	US$100/year	US$400/year
First referral level	US$250/year	US$1,000/year
District hospital	US$500/year	US$2,000/year
Regional	US$1,500/year	US$5,000/year
National	US$5,000/year	US$30,000/year
Subtotal (supplies)	US$7,350	US$38,400
Information technology: computers and software		
Primary care facility	0	0
First referral level	0	0
District hospital	0	20 percent use of each of two computers with software at US$1,100 at each of 300 facilities (US$132,000)
Regional level	0	Two dedicated computers with software at US$1,100 at each of 15 facilities (US$33,000)
National level	50 percent use of each of four computers with software at US$1,100 (US$2,200)	10 dedicated computers with software at US$1,100 (US$11,100)
Subtotal (information technology)	US$2,200	US$176,100
Training cost	US$180,000	US$1,730,000
Total cost	US$4,847,661	US$49,906,370
Per capita cost	US$0.16	US$1.66

Source: Authors.
Note: Based on a model country with a total population of 30 million.

test how evidence can be used to decentralize health sector planning at the district level and to what extent evidence-based priority setting would result in improved health outcomes. The project budgeted for a marginal investment of US$2.00 per capita for the information and for health interventions, although only US$0.80 per capita was actually spent. The slightly increased investment covered training in the use of the information to set priorities and to better manage the most

cost-effective interventions. The information systems included a district burden-of-disease intervention priority profile, district health accounts, a district cost information system, and district health service mapping. Management and technical support strengthened the district and regional health sector use of the information for management and administration. Communities participated in the ownership and management of health facilities. The cost-effectiveness estimates in this

The Tanzania Essential Health Interventions Program

TEHIP is a partnership between Tanzania's Ministry of Health and the International Development Research Centre. The project was established to determine the feasibility of an evidence-based approach to health planning at the district level. Testing the premise of the World Bank's (1993) *World Development Report 1993: Investing in Health,* TEHIP enabled district health planners in two of Tanzania's 117 districts to collect and use burden-of-disease and cost-effectiveness data to get the best value for

money from national investments in health. Interventions included door-to-door collection of data and training or technical support for managers in the analysis and use of the data for decision making. TEHIP districts allocated services to high-burden diseases, resulting in a tripling of clinic utilization rates and increased treatment effectiveness. With a per capita increase in spending of only US$0.80, district health managers achieved a 47 percent reduction in child mortality rates.

Source: Authors.

Table 54.4 The Effectiveness of Evidence-Based Resource Allocation in Improving Health

Year	Number of children < 5 years	Probability of dying (birth to 5 years)	Mortality rate (< 5 years)	Total deaths	Deaths averted	DALYs gained/ death	Total DALYs	DALYs discounted at 3 percent
1999	31,000	135.5	34	1,054	—	—	—	—
2000	31,500	119.0	25	791	263	41	10,850	11,511
2001	32,000	110.0	25	803	251	41	10,332	10,643
2002	32,661	114.0	26	853	202	41	8,303	8,304
Total DALYs gained							29,487	30,458

Source: Authors.
Note: 1999 is baseline year; therefore, no deaths were averted.

section are based solely on the declines in mortality of children under five years of age, even though adult mortality also decreased. To ensure a conservative estimate of the costs of the HIS, we used a per capita cost of US$2.00—higher than the actual investment for TEHIP and at the high end of the range of costs for a comprehensive HIS estimated in table 54.2— US$0.53 to US$2.99. All costs were ascribed to the information system, because there were no improvements in the interventions themselves. Expenditures and deaths before 2002 were discounted by 3 percent annually (see box 54.2).

The demographic and epidemiologic data were taken from the Rufiji district, where the most complete data were available. The estimate of the number of children under age five (32,661) is based on the 2002 census results. The Ministry of Health, census, and Rufiji Demographic Surveillance System estimates range from 31,000 to 36,000 children for 2003. Because of this discrepancy, the decline in the total fertility rate, from 5 to 4.7 (5 percent), is taken into account in estimating the number of children less than five years of age for 1999 to 2001. The probability of dying before five years of age declined by 15.6 percent, and because of declining fertility, each year has 1.5 percent

Table 54.5 Costs of Evidence-Based Resource Allocation for Improving Health

Year	Population	Total cost at US$2 per capita (US$)	Discounted cost (US$)
1998	186,809	373,618	420,510
1999	191,012	382,024	417,448
2000	196,515	393,030	416,966
2001	202,176	404,352	416,482
2002	208,000	416,000	416,000
Total costs		1,969,024	2,087,406

Source: Authors.

fewer children than the preceding year. DALYs saved from each child death averted is estimated at 41.2. The resulting calculations of effectiveness are summarized in table 54.4.

The estimates of cost are based on population size projected back from the 2002 census results, assuming an average annual growth rate of 2.8 percent. Costs incurred in 1998 are included because we assume that it takes at least two years (1998 to 2000) of improving the HIS before health benefits accrue.

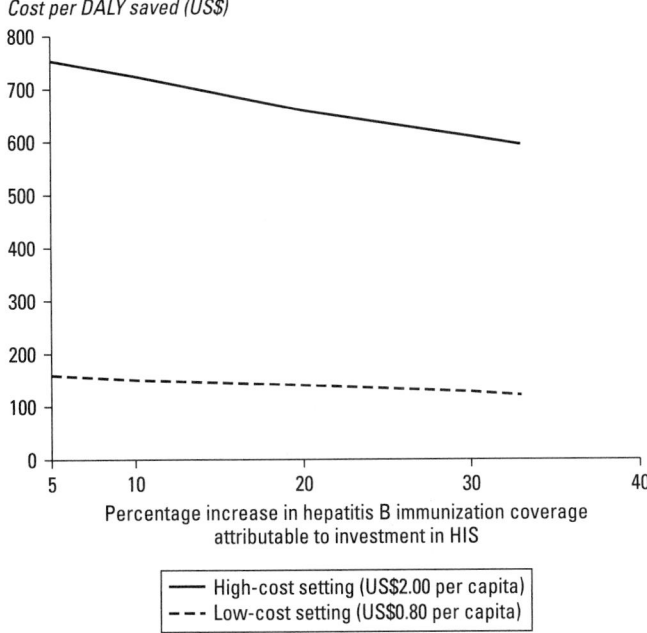

Cost per DALY saved (US$)

Percentage increase in hepatitis B immunization coverage attributable to investment in HIS

— High-cost setting (US$2.00 per capita)
--- Low-cost setting (US$0.80 per capita)

Source: Authors.

Figure 54.1 Cost-Effectiveness of Health Information Systems: Cost per DALY Saved Because of Increases in Coverage Attributable to HIS

Using these figures for effectiveness (table 54.4) and cost (table 54.5), we find that the cost-effectiveness of the HIS that results in improved evidence-based resource allocation and child health may be conservatively estimated at US$68.50 per DALY gained (US$2,087,406 to gain 30,457 DALYs). Even in the poorest countries, this is well below the gross national product (GNP) per capita benchmark for what is considered worthwhile for government investment in health.

This analysis for the TEHIP project is based solely on child deaths averted. But the improvement in health information would also yield substantial benefits for adult populations. For example, HIS-driven increases in coverage with hepatitis B vaccine have varied between 5 and 33 percent (Miller and McCann 2000). These increases in coverage with hepatitis B immunization will result in incremental reductions in death and disability among adults attributable to hepatitis B–induced cirrhosis and liver cancer, thereby averting the loss of substantial numbers of DALYs in low-income countries (World Bank 2002). Hepatitis B vaccine is a cost-effective addition to an existing immunization program, with a cost per death averted of US$11 to US$15 (US$193 to US$262 per DALY saved). But efficiency and coverage can be substantially improved with an additional investment in the HIS. The cost per DALY saved by incremental investment in the HIS can be calculated using estimates of costs of the HIS from table 54.2, plus the estimates of cost and deaths averted because of immunization from Miller and McCann (2000) for populations in all low-income countries (GNP per

capita less than US$997; World Bank 2002). Figure 54.1 shows that, for the high-prevalence countries (Miller and McCann 2000), the investment in a comprehensive HIS is highly cost-effective (US$159 to US$126 per DALY saved for low-cost settings and US$757 to US$597 per DALY saved for high-cost settings), even if the investment results in only minor increases in immunization coverage. A similar analysis for countries with a lower prevalence rate of hepatitis B demonstrates that the cost per DALY saved is higher, but the investment in an HIS still yields a savings of DALYs at a cost that is well below the GNP per capita for the majority of the low-income countries.

These calculations of the cost-effectiveness of investments in an HIS are highly conservative, because they consider health benefits within a single population group (children, in the case of TEHIP) or a single disease problem (hepatitis B). They therefore underestimate the true cost-effectiveness of investment in an HIS, which can drive improvements in program efficiency and effectiveness across a broader range of health interventions.

FINANCING OF IMPROVED HEALTH INFORMATION

The annual per capita cost, estimated earlier, of US$0.53 to US$2.99 for a comprehensive HIS, represents a substantial portion of the current per capita health expenditure for many developing countries. These figures include capital and recurrent costs, although they do not include the costs of any external technical assistance. Because most countries have already made a substantial investment in a HIS, the actual incremental costs to improve the existing HIS likely are much less. Salaries, which account for more than 90 percent of HIS costs, are expenditures that are already being made in most settings, so the marginal cost of HIS improvements would be primarily the initial development costs of planning, training, technical assistance, and information technology upgrades. Furthermore, the costs of HIS improvements may be fully offset or even exceeded by the savings from the resulting improvements in efficiencies in the health care system.

Existing funding is adequate to strengthen systems substantially in all low-income and lower-middle-income countries primarily through the major international initiatives (Global Fund to Fight AIDS, Tuberculosis, and Malaria; President's Emergency Plan for AIDS Relief; and Multi-country AIDS Program of the World Bank). All these funders recommend that 3 to 7 percent of grants and loans be allocated to monitoring and evaluation. Several bilateral development agencies and the multilateral development banks will provide financing for HIS reform, including the U.S. Agency for International Development (USAID) through the MEASURE (Monitoring and Evaluation to Assess and Use Results) Project, which is designed to improve and institutionalize the collection and use of data for health policy development and program monitoring. The HMN offers some financial assistance to countries that are preparing for and planning HIS reform and will assist countries in negotiating financing packages that blend loan funding with grants from bilateral donors to implement those reforms.

Several international agencies support strengthening systems for national statistics that extend beyond the health sector. STATCAP (Statistical Capacity Building), which is a new lending program offered by the Partnership in Statistics for Development in the 21st Century (PARIS21) through the World Bank, supports the development of national statistical systems. The separate Trust Fund for Statistical Capacity Building offers smaller amounts of grant funding to prepare the statistical master plan that is required for obtaining a STATCAP loan. Although short-term project funding can often be secured for system development, the resulting system and its recurrent costs must be within the country's capacity to sustain it, both technically and financially.

IMPLEMENTATION OF CHANGE: LESSONS OF EXPERIENCE

Underinvestment is the root cause of the nearly universal weaknesses in the HIS in developing countries. This failure is reflected in the poorly paid and undervalued HIS staff; in the irregular and unreliable transmittal of data from the periphery; in the underreporting of events, including births, deaths, and morbidity; and in the failures to base planning and decision making—at both the district and the central levels—on credible evidence (Azubuike and Ehiri 1999).

When the need for HIS improvement is identified, ministries of health should explicitly state the characteristics they need in a reformed system and quantify the expected benefits. A common mistake made in implementing HIS change is failing to recognize the associated need for change in management processes and organizational culture. In contrast, recent HIS reforms in Niger (Mock and others 1993) and Uganda (Gladwin, Dixon, and Wilson 2003) have had unprecedented success because they have been aligned with broader management reforms and changes in organizational culture. Failure to adjust management roles with HIS changes can constrain effectiveness, such as when HIS managers are not given the necessary increased status and authority to demand reports and trigger corrective actions (Gladwin, Dixon, and Wilson 2003). Failure to invest adequately in training, especially in skills for presentation and communication of results, may also inhibit the use of health information. The demand from international organizations and global programs, such as the Expanded Program on Immunization and Stop TB, for reports on vast numbers of indicators has retarded the smooth devel-

opment of the district-level HIS. The HMN will create an alliance of countries committed to a parsimonious consensus technical framework and encourage donors to cooperate with and strengthen the HMN-sanctioned HIS architecture in participating countries.

The predictors of success in developing and maintaining an HIS are as follows:

- high-level commitment to HIS development and the linked changes in management
- a champion of HIS reform who engages the stakeholders and can work across sectors
- an information architecture that is simple, is structured to drive decision making at the level that data are collected, provides incentives and accountability for performance, and links health information subsystems
- investment in training and increased status for the people who manage the HIS.

RESEARCH AND DEVELOPMENT

An effective HIS delivers routine information that enables informed policy making and management but also promotes health research. Routine information systems may serve as a research platform, but the HIS itself should also be a subject of research. Research should drive the continual refinement of HIS methods and tools, thereby ensuring expanding and well-documented returns on our investments in health.

The instruments and methods of the HIS must be continually refined to improve its effectiveness and reduce its costs. For the phased introduction of vital events monitoring, for example, there is a pressing need for the development and validation of methods for projecting subnational results to national rates of birth and death. More research is needed to develop and test new methods for rapid assessment in order to obtain timely and affordable information to solve management problems. As field-appropriate and cost-effective diagnostic technologies are developed, research should be performed to document the utility of obtaining biomarkers in household surveys.

Documenting improved outcomes and lower costs will provide evidence for policy makers on the effectiveness of HIS investments. To better decide how to improve the HIS, decision makers will need documentation of the costs and effects of introducing ICT in support of the HIS. Existing and emerging technologies should be tested for their cost and effectiveness in assisting field-based data capture, instantaneous data transmission, GIS-based mapping of indicators, and compelling presentation for decision making by policy makers, managers, and other stakeholders. Research and development efforts are needed to devise software—or preferably shareware—that is specifically tailored to support the consensus technical framework developed by the HMN.

Bailey and Pang (2004) point out the need for more research in the developing world to better understand users' information needs. In fact, research is needed to better document the entire information value chain, with special attention to improving the identification of information needs, to overcoming the natural disincentives to information sharing, and to enabling better use of information for constructive change. At present, there is still a need to improve the access to information and knowledge in the developing world. However, the future will bring the larger challenge of improving the management and use of information and the knowledge such information can bring. Research in the HIS will be instrumental in both accelerating equitable access to information and improving the management and use of knowledge for improved health.

CONCLUSIONS

More than ever before, it is in the mutual interest of the developing and industrial worlds to invest in strengthening systems for collection and management of health information (Stansfield 2005).

The trend toward "basket" funding for health and sector-wide approaches makes the need for priority setting all the more acute. Priority setting depends on accurate information. The success of efforts to reduce poverty and health inequity will depend on the existence of information systems to detect those problems, facilitate the design of solutions, and track progress toward eliminating the problems. Countries and donors must, therefore, accelerate and harmonize their investments in information systems.

Within countries, the trend toward decentralization of authority for management of health resources has led to further challenges for the HIS, as well as to greater reliance on the information it provides to inform decision making. It is clear from the instructive failures of underresourced systems that the accuracy and value of information reported to the national level will depend on that information's perceived value in the periphery. Information is relevant only if it is used to solve a local problem or if it helps to generate innovation that solves a local problem (Bailey and Pang 2004). Therefore, the decentralization of authority will be successful only with better information systems to support decisions at the periphery, and evidence-based decision making will be possible only if authority can be devolved to the periphery. This decentralization, along with increasing cooperation and collaboration across sectors to improve health outcomes, makes it all the more critical to present data in simpler ways that are understandable and compelling to a broader and nontechnical audience.

Although historically neglected, investments in comprehensive development of the HIS will clearly deliver good value for money. Improvements in the HIS can accelerate broad improvements in health if they are engineered to reflect, reinforce, and even drive health sector reforms. Even more compellingly, investments in the HIS can make health the "thin edge of the wedge," giving governments and politicians a positive experience with information sharing and overcoming the natural disincentives to transparency and accountability. HIS investments hold the promise, therefore, not only of transforming public health, but also of accelerating progress toward good governance in every sector.

NOTES

1. Sauerborn and Lippeveld (2000) have defined a *health information system* as the "set of components and procedures organized with the objective of generating information that will improve health management decisions at all levels of the health system."

2. The dollar amounts given are quoted from the references and are not adjusted for current dollar value.

REFERENCES

AbonZahr, C., and T. Boerma. 2005. "Health Information Systems: The Foundations of Public Health." *Bulletin of the World Health Organization* 83 (8): 578–83.

Abt Associates. 2003. *Primer for Policymakers—Understanding National Health Accounts: The Methodology and Implementation Process.* Bethesda, MD: Partners for Health Reform*plus* Project, Abt Associates.

Azubuike, M. C., and J. E. Ehiri. 1999. "Health Information Systems in Developing Countries: Benefits, Problems, and Prospects." *Journal of the Royal Society for the Promotion of Health* 119 (3): 180–84.

Bailey, C., and T. Pang. 2004. "Health Information for All by 2015?" *Lancet* 364 (9430): 223–24.

Boerma, Ties, J., E. Holt, and R. Black. 2001. "Measurement of Biomarkers in Surveys in Developing Countries: Opportunities and Problems." *Population and Development Review* 27 (2): 303–14.

Cibulskis, R. E., and G. Hiawalyer. 2002. "Information Systems for Health Sector Monitoring in Papua New Guinea." *Bulletin of the World Health Organization* 80 (9): 752–58.

Commission on Macroeconomics and Health. 2000.

De, S., T. Dmytraczenko, D. Brinkerhoff, and M. Tien. 2003. *Has Improved Availability of Health Expenditure Data Contributed to Evidence-Based Policymaking? Country Experiences with National Health Accounts.* Technical Report 022. Bethesda, MD: Partners for Health Reform*plus* Project, Abt Associates.

Duran-Arenas, L., C. C. Rivero, S. F. Canton, R. S. Rodriquez, F. Franco, R. W. Luna, and J. Catino. 1998. "The Development of a Quality Information System: A Case Study of Mexico." *Health Policy and Planning* 13 (4): 446–58.

Economic Commission for Africa. 2003. "Workshop on Organization and Management of Statistical Systems." Report on workshop in Addis Ababa, December 8–12. http://www.unstats.un.org/unscl/methods/statorg/workshops/AddisAbaba/presentation_session8b_financing.pdf.

Gladwin, J., R. A. Dixon, and T. D. Wilson. 2003. "Implementing a New Health Management Information System in Uganda." *Health Policy and Planning* 18 (2): 214–24.

Godlee, F., N. Pakenham-Walsh, D. Ncayiyana, B. Cohen, and A. Packer. 2004. "Can We Achieve Health Information for All by 2015?" *Lancet* 364 (9430): 295–300.

Jamison, D. T., J. Sachs, and J. Wang. 2001. "Mortality Changes and Economic Welfare in Sub-Saharan Africa, 1960–2000." Commission on Macroeconomics and Health, Background Paper for Working Group 1, World Health Organization, Geneva.

Jolly, R. 2002. "Statisticians of the World Unite: The Human Development Challenge Awaits." *Journal of Human Development* 3 (2): 263–72.

Kleinau, E. 2000. "Management of Health Information Systems." In *Design and Implementation of Health Information Systems*, ed. T. Lippeveld, R. Sauerborn, and C. Bodart. Geneva: World Health Organization.

Kohn, L., J. Corrigan, and M. Donaldson, eds. 2001. *To Err Is Human: Building a Safer Health System*. Washington, DC: National Academy Press.

Lescano, A. G., M. Ortiz, R. Elgegren, E. Gozzer, E. Saldarriaga, I. Soriano, and others. 2003. "Alerta DISAMAR: Innovative Disease Surveillance in Peru." Paper presented at the American Society of Tropical Medicine and Hygiene, Philadelphia, December 5.

Loevinsohn, B. P. 1994. "Data Utilization and Analytical Skills among Mid-Level Programme Managers in a Developing Country." *International Journal of Epidemiology* 23 (1): 194–200.

Mackay, K. 1998. "Public Sector Performance: The Critical Role of Evaluation." In *Public Sector Performance—The Critical Role of Evaluation: Selected Proceedings of a World Bank Seminar*, ed. K. Mackay, ix–xvi. Washington, DC: World Bank.

McLellan, F. 2001. "Information Technology Can Benefit Developing Countries." *Lancet* 358 (9278): 308.

Miller, M. A., and L. McCann. 2000. "Policy Analysis of the Use of Hepatitis B, *Haemophilus influenzae* type B, Streptococcus Pneumoniae-Conjugate and Rotavirus Vaccines in National Immunization Schedules." *Health Economics* 9: 19–35.

Mock, N., J. Setzer, I. Sliney, G. Hadizatou, and W. Bertrand. 1993. "Development of Information-Based Planning in Niger." *International Journal of Technology Assessment in Health Care* 9 (3): 360–68.

Murray, C. J. L., B. Shengelia, N. Gupta, S. Moussavi, A. Tanjon, and M. Thieren. 2003. "Validity of Reported Vaccination Coverage in 45 Countries." *Lancet* 362 (9389): 1022–27.

Nordhaus, W. 2002. "The Health of Nations: The Contribution of Improved Health to Living Standards." Cowles Foundation Discussion Paper 1355, Yale University, New Haven.

O'Carroll, P. W. 2003. "The Context for Public Health Informatics." In *Public Health Informatics and Information Systems*, ed. P. W. O'Carroll, W. Yasnoff, M. E. Ward, L. H. Ripp, and E. L. Martin. New York: Springer.

PAHO (Pan American Health Organization). 2004. "Ten Year Evaluation of the Regional Core Health Data Initiative." *Epidemiological Bulletin* 25 (3): 1–7.

Pappaioanou, M., M. Malison, K. Wilkens, B. Otto, R. A. Goodman, R. E. Churchill, and others. 2003. "Strengthening Capacity in Developing Countries for Evidence-Based Public Health: The Data for Decision Making Project." *Social Science and Medicine* 57: 1925–37.

PARIS21 (Partnership in Statistics for Development in the 21st Century). 2004. "Meeting the Data Challenge: A Funding Proposal for PARIS21 and the Trust Fund for Statistical Capacity Building for 2004 to 2006." PARIS21, Paris.

Perrin, E. B., W. D. Kalsbeek, and T. M. Scanlan, eds. 2004. *Toward a Health Statistics System for the 21st Century*. Summary of a workshop, Division of Behavioral and Social Sciences and Education, National Research Council and Committee on National Statistics, National Academy of Sciences. Washington, DC: National Academy Press.

Peters, D. H., A. E. Elmendorf, K. Kandola, and G. Chelleraj. 2000. "Benchmarks for Health Expenditures, Services, and Outcomes in Africa during the 1990s." *Bulletin of the World Health Organization* 78 (6): 761–68.

Petrakos, C. 1998. "Finding a Cure: Disease Management Aids the Search for Better Outcomes." *Modern Physician*, September 1, 2004. http://www.modernphysician.com.

Rommelmann, V., P. Setel, Y. Hemed, H. Mponezya, G. Angeles, and T. Boerma. 2004. "Costs and Results of Information Systems for Poverty Monitoring, Health Sector Reform, and Local Government Reform in Tanzania." MEASURE Evaluation, Adult Morbidity and Mortality Project, University of Newcastle upon Tyne, U.K., and University of North Carolina, Chapel Hill.

Sauerborn, R., and T. Lippeveld. 2000. "Why Health Information Systems?" In *Design and Implementation of Health Information Systems*, ed. T. Lippeveld, R. Sauerborn, and C. Bodart. Geneva: World Health Organization.

Stansfield, S. 2005. "Structuring Information Systems to Improve Health." *Bulletin of the World Health Organization* 83 (8): 562.

Thacker, S. B., D. F. Stroup, R. G. Parrish, and H. A. Anderson. 1996. "Surveillance in Environmental Public Health: Issues, Systems, and Sources." *American Journal of Public Health* 86 (5): 633–38.

Walsh, J. A., and M. Simonet. 1995. "Data and Data Needs for Health Sector Reform." *Health Policy* 32 (1–3): 295–306.

World Bank. 1993. *World Development Report 1993: Investing in Health*. Washington, DC: World Bank.

———. 2002. *World Development Indicators*. Washington, DC: World Bank.

Zayan, A., W. Berggren, and F. Doumbia. 1992. *The Price of Immunization and the Value of Information*. Westport, CT: Save the Children.

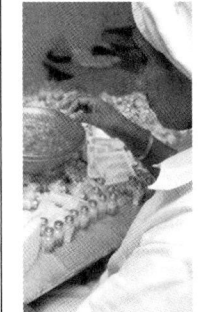

Chapter **55**

Drug Resistance

Ramanan Laxminarayan, Zulfiqar A. Bhutta, Adriano Duse, Philip Jenkins, Thomas O'Brien, Iruka N. Okeke, Ariel Pablo-Mendez, and Keith P. Klugman

The control of infectious diseases is seriously threatened by the steady increase in the number of micro-organisms that are resistant to antimicrobial agents—often to a wide range of these agents. Resistant infections lead to increased morbidity and prolonged hospital stays, as well as to prolonged periods during which individuals are infectious and can spread their infections to other individuals (Holmberg, Solomon, and Blake 1987; Rubin and others 1999). The problem is particularly severe in developing countries, where the burden of infectious diseases is relatively greater and where patients with a resistant infection are less likely to have access to or be able to afford expensive second-line treatments, which typically have more complex regimens than first-line drugs. Furthermore, the presence of exacerbating factors, such as poor hygiene, unreliable water supplies, civil conflicts, and increased numbers of immunocompromised patients attributable to the ongoing HIV epidemic, can further increase the burden of antimicrobial resistance by facilitating the spread of resistant pathogens. In this chapter, we discuss the causes and burden of drug resistance and evaluate interventions that address the resistance problem in developing countries. Although a number of the interventions we discuss are relevant to drug resistance in HIV/AIDS and other forms of antiviral resistance, chapter 18 includes a more in-depth discussion of this subject.

RISK FACTORS

Drug Use in Humans

The evolution of drug resistance is facilitated by a number of factors, including increasing use of antibiotics and antimalarials;

insufficient controls on drug prescribing; inadequate compliance with treatment regimens; poor dosing; lack of infection control; increasing frequency and speed of travel, which lead to the rapid spread of resistant organisms; and insufficient incentives for patients, physicians, or even governments to care about increasing resistance. It is important to distinguish between risk factors for the emergence of resistance (*de novo resistance*) and those for the spread of resistance (*primary resistance*).

The molecular basis of resistance may give a clue to the likelihood of resistance emerging. If a single DNA base pair mutation leads to the development of resistance, then its selection is likely to be widespread, especially if the biological fitness cost of the mutation is low. De novo or acquired resistance results in the appearance of a resistant strain in a single patient. Subsequent transmission of such resistant strains from an infectious case to other persons leads to disease that is drug resistant from the outset, a phenomenon known as primary resistance (IUATLD 1998). Independent, cumulative events result in multidrug-resistant bacteria or tuberculosis (MDR-TB). Both the creation and the transmission of drug resistance contribute to its prevalence in a given population. This mechanism also holds true in the case of antimalarials; that is, resistance develops when malaria parasites encounter drug concentrations that are strong enough to eradicate the susceptible parasite population, but they fail to inhibit the multiplication of naturally occurring resistant strains. Commonly used antimalarial drugs are not mutagenic.

In the case of tuberculosis, spontaneous mutations leading to drug resistance occur rarely in *Mycobacterium tuberculosis*, and multidrug regimens can prevent the emergence of clinical drug resistance (Cohn, Middlebrook, and Russell 1959). Resistance is thus an avertable phenomenon resulting from inadequate treatment, which, in turn, is often the result of an irregular drug supply, prescription of inappropriate regimens, or poor adherence resulting from a lack of supervision. In the case of malaria, the widespread misuse of chloroquine as prophylaxis is believed to be an important factor in the emergence and spread of resistance to this drug.

Despite conventional wisdom, the highest rates of antibiotic resistance in the pneumococcus bacterium globally are not for penicillins or macrolides, which usually require multiple DNA mutations or the import of foreign genes, respectively, but for sulfamethoxazole-trimethoprim, which can be selected from among a population of susceptible pneumococci by a single base change in the dihydrofolate reductase gene (Adrian and Klugman 1997). The direct selection of resistance following exposure of children carrying pneumococci has been shown in a prospective study in Malawi to occur in 42 percent of children exposed to sulfadoxine-pyremethamine for a week and in 38 percent of children a month after exposure to drug treatment for malaria (Feikin and others 2000).

Evolutionary biology suggests that drug selection pressure is an important factor in the emergence and spread of drug resistance. Although the relationship between antimicrobial use and drug resistance (in the pneumococcus, for example) is well established in developed countries (Bronzwaer and others 2002), direct evidence to support this hypothesis is less forthcoming in developing countries because of a lack of data on antibiotic use. Resistance to antimicrobials is less likely to arise in the poorest developing countries simply because of the lower levels of antibiotic use associated with poorer socioeconomic status. For instance, India—a large country with scant control over antibiotic prescribing—has very low rates of resistance among systemic isolates of pneumococci, at least in rural areas (INCLEN 1999). These low rates exist despite wide antibiotic availability, probably because extreme poverty limits the duration of antibiotic exposure for the treatment of acute pneumococcal infections. Rising incomes and increased affordability of antibiotics will likely change this low incidence of resistance; the same may be true of quinolones, which are widely available at relatively affordable prices, even in semirural and rural populations. This trend may be responsible for the emergence of nalidixic acid resistance to *Shigella* in Bangladesh and fluoroquinolone resistance to *Salmonella typhi* in India.

Recent evidence suggests that shorter courses of antibiotics may select for less resistance in the pneumococcus compared with longer courses (when patients comply with those courses) (Schrag and others 2001). Very low levels of resistance have also been found in isolated rural African communities (Mthwalo and others 1998). This observation, however, should not lead to complacency. Increased access to antibiotics in developing countries, without controls on over-the-counter use, has led to some of the highest rates of resistance in the world, as was seen with penicillin resistance in Vietnam. Relatively wealthy countries such as the Republic of Korea and Japan also have lax control and even greater access to funds to purchase antibiotics (Song and others 1999). Patterns of resistance differ by antimicrobial class, and resistance to several classes has been linked to particular patterns of use in developing countries. Macrolide use in children in China may be preferred to the use of beta-lactams, which are known to be associated in rare instances with serious anaphylactic reactions, and in Beijing and Shanghai, the highest global rates of macrolide resistance are encountered in nasopharyngeal isolates from children (Wang and others 1998; Yang, Zhang, and McGee 2001). Tetracycline use remains widespread in developing countries, and poor African countries, such as the Central African Republic, may have higher rates of resistance to tetracycline than to beta-lactams or macrolides (Rowe and others 2000).

The relationship between compliance and resistance emergence in the treatment of acute and largely self-limiting infections is less robust than in the case of chronic infections such as tuberculosis (TB). It is likely that resistance selection occurs more readily in the commensal flora (for example, the pneumococcal flora of the nasopharynx) than among the organisms causing the acute infection. Thus, shorter courses (and reduced compliance) may reduce the selection of resistance in commensal flora. In contrast, in TB, selection takes place in the infecting pathogen, and poor compliance is associated with the selection of resistant strains.

Antibiotic Use in Animals

Many developed countries use antibiotics for veterinary uses, both for improving feed efficiency and rate of weight gain (subtherapeutic use) and for disease prevention and treatment (therapeutic use) (Levy 1992). Although the extent of antibiotic use in animals in developing countries is unknown, one study from Kenya reported that tetracyclines, sulfonamides, and aminoglycosides were the most commonly used antimicrobials for veterinary purposes (Mitema and others 2001). Over 90 percent of the antibiotics used were for therapeutic purposes, and there was no evidence of use for growth promotion.

There is strong evidence that the use of antibiotics in farm animals promotes the development of drug-resistant bacteria in animals (Aarestrup and others 2001). Because routes for the movement of these resistant bacteria to humans are available, there is sufficient circumstantial evidence that drug resistance in bacteria associated with food animals can influence the level of resistance in bacteria that cause human diseases (Wegener and others 1999). Furthermore, mathematical models indicate that the effect of subtherapeutic use on resistance in humans is greatest when resistance levels are undetectable (Smith and others 2002). The appearance of drug-resistant strains of *Enterococcus faecium* in broiler meat products at retail outlets declined after the ban of antimicrobial growth promoters in Denmark (Emborg and others 2003). Salmonella has been recovered from chicken (35 percent), turkey (24 percent), and pork (16 percent) samples obtained from area supermarkets in Washington, D.C. (White and others 2001). There is evidence that dissemination of tetracycline-resistance-encoding plasmids between aquaculture and humans has already occurred in Europe (Rhodes and others 2000). The global nature of this problem became apparent in 2001, when authorities in some European countries found residues of chloramphenicol in tiger shrimp imported from China, Indonesia, and Vietnam (Holmstrom and others 2003).

Transmission of Resistant Pathogens

Once resistance has emerged in a population, it can spread both geographically and between age groups. Unsafe drinking water, unsanitary conditions, and poor infection control in hospitals are risk factors for the transmission of all infections, including resistant ones. The transmission of resistant strains from children to adults has been suggested by anecdotal reports as far back as the 1980s (Klugman and others 1986). That association is strongly supported by the role of conjugate pneumococcal vaccine in reducing antimicrobial resistance among adult pneumococcal bacteremic isolates in the United States (Whitney and others 2003). The association of HIV infection with pediatric serotypes and antimicrobial resistance in pneumococci suggests the potential utility of this approach in reducing the burden of antimicrobial resistance in pneumococci in developing countries where the burden of disease is overwhelmingly associated with HIV infection in both children (Madhi and others 2000) and adults (Jones and others 1998).

Disease Burden

Although no estimates of disease burden are currently available that are specific to drug resistance, the contribution of drug resistance to the burden of infectious diseases is believed to be large. Resistance has emerged in malaria, HIV, TB, and other bacterial infections that together constitute a significant proportion of the burden of disease in developing countries. An indication of the extent of the problem is provided by the burden of diseases for which drug resistance is a problem (table 55.1), as well as by the levels of drug resistance among these pathogens (table 55.2 and figures 55.1 and 55.2).

Pneumococci. Surveillance of drug resistance in pneumococci shows several general trends. The numbers of strains that are fully susceptible to penicillin-G, once nearly universal in most of the world, have declined by 30 to 50 percent in many countries and by 75 percent in some, as resistant clones have spread widely but irregularly throughout the world (Sa-Leao and others 2002). At the same time, percentages resistant to macrolides and to sulfamethoxazole-trimethoprim have increased, especially where those drugs have been widely used, and resistance to tetracycline or chloramphenicol has fluctuated widely. Linked resistance to these drugs results in a growing percentage of strains resistant to many or all of them. Resistance to fluoroquinolones is still rare but is beginning to be observed in many places (Ho and others 2001; Quale and others 2002).

Certain *Streptococcus pneumoniae* clones have been widely disseminated. A penicillin-, chloramphenicol-, and tetracycline-resistant clone (and sometimes erythromycin) of Spanish origin (Spain[23F]-1) has, since its original description, been isolated in other parts of Europe, the United States, South and Central America, South Africa, and East Asia (McGee and others 2001). It is likely that this clone is even more widespread and that the absence of reports from other areas reflects the absence of molecular testing techniques needed to delineate

Table 55.1 Estimated Burden of Disease in Disability-Adjusted Life Years, by Cause and Gender, 2001

Condition	Both sexes DALYs (Thousands)	Both sexes Percentage of total	Males DALYs (Thousands)	Males Percentage of total	Females DALYs (Thousands)	Females Percentage of total
Infectious and parasitic diseases	359,377	24.5	184,997	24.1	174,380	24.9
Respiratory infections	94,037	6.4	49,591	6.5	44,446	6.4
Diarrheal diseases	62,451	4.3	31,633	4.1	30,818	4.4
Gonorrhea	3,320	0.2	1,437	0.2	1,883	0.3
Tuberculosis	36,040	2.5	22,629	2.9	13,411	1.9
Malaria	42,280	2.9	20,024	2.6	22,256	3.2

Source: WHO 2002b, annex table 3, 194.

Table 55.2 Prevalence of *S. pneumoniae* Not Susceptible to Three or More Drug Classes, Alexander Project 1998–2000

Region and country	N	Percentage multiresistant defined as			
		Any three drug classes excluding penicillin	Any three drug classes including penicillin	Any four drug classes	Any five or more drug classes
Africa	540	14.3	24.8	13.5	3.3
Kenya	277	3.6	16.6	2.2	0.0
South Africa	263	25.5	33.5	25.5	6.8
Eastern Europe	1,109	10.1	11.7	6.0	1.0
Czech Rep.	275	0.7	1.1	0.4	0.0
Poland	453	13.0	15.2	6.4	1.1
Russian Fed.	161	10.6	12.4	3.7	1.2
Slovak Rep.	220	15.5	17.3	14.1	1.8
Western Europe	3,328	14.7	18.4	11.9	4.1
Austria	149	2.7	4.7	2.0	0.0
Belgium	230	13.9	15.7	7.0	2.6
France	444	35.6	49.1	34.9	11.7
Germany	321	4.7	5.9	1.6	0.0
Greece	431	18.6	19.5	13.9	2.1
Italy	304	19.7	22.4	9.9	1.0
Netherlands	185	0.0	1.1	0.0	0.0
Portugal	328	6.1	9.5	5.5	1.8
Ireland	54	9.3	14.8	9.3	1.9
Spain	295	27.8	32.9	25.4	15.3
Switzerland	349	5.7	7.7	4.9	2.3
United Kingdom	238	5.9	6.3	5.0	2.1
Far East	730	53.2	63.2	40.6	23.0
Hong Kong, China	193	76.2	79.3	70.5	60.1
Japan	404	48.3	63.1	29.2	6.4
Singapore	133	34.6	39.9	31.6	19.6
Middle East	314	11.2	18.2	10.5	4.1
Israel	148	8.8	12.2	8.8	2.0
Saudi Arabia	166	13.3	23.5	12.1	6.0
Latin America	2,861	13.3	20.1	12.1	1.9
Brazil	181	2.8	5.0	1.1	0.0
Mexico	248	21.0	31.1	20.2	3.2
United States	2,432	16.2	25.8	15.5	7.0
All isolates	8,882	17.5	23.7	14.6	5.9

Source: Jacobs and others 2003.
Note: Drug classes were defined as follows: β-lactams (penicillin MIC ≥ 0.12 mg/L), macrolides (erythromycin MIC ≥ 0.5 mg/L), tetracyclines (doxycycline MIC ≥ 0.5 mg/L), phenicols (chloramphenicol MIC ≥ 8 mg/L), folate pathway inhibitors (co-trimoxazole MICs ≥ 1 mg/L based on trimethoprim component), and quinolones (ofloxacin MIC ≥ 8 mg/L).

clones, rather than an absence of the organisms themselves. Other globally disseminated *S. pneumoniae* include specific clones of serotypes 19F, 14, 19A, 9N, 9V, 3, and 6 (McGee and others 2001). Spread of these pandemic clones has continued, even in areas where successful interventions have reduced selective pressure from antimicrobial use (Arason and others 2002). With increasing international travel, the potential of these strains to spread to areas where resistance is uncommon can no longer be considered remote.

Shigella. In many regions where *Shigella*, especially *Shigella dysenteriae*, is prevalent and an important cause of infant mortality, resistance first to sulfamethoxazole-trimethoprim, then to ampicillin, and commonly to tetracycline and

Percentage failure

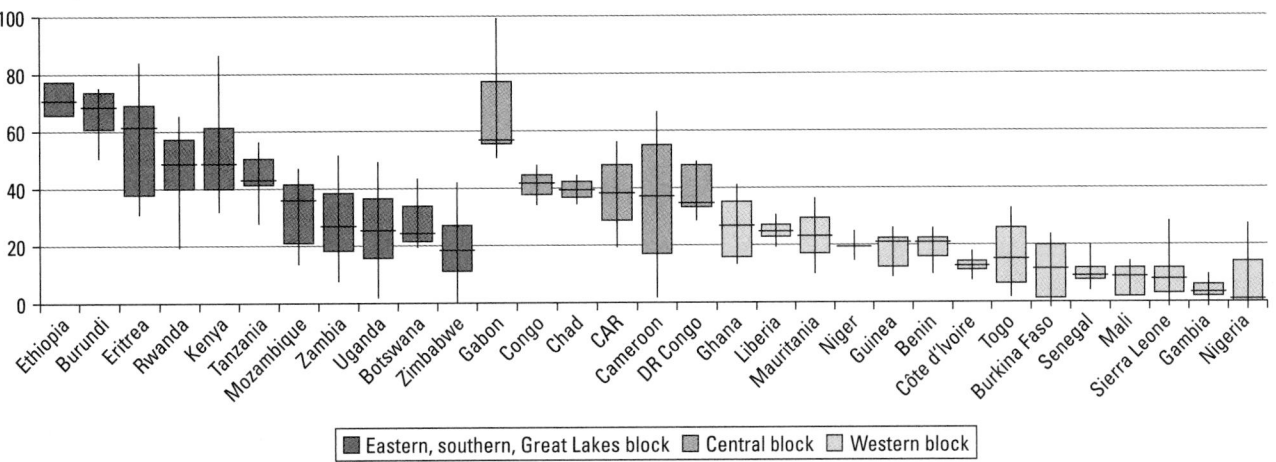

Source: WHO Regional Office for Africa, 1997–2002.

WHO has established 126 sentinel surveillance sites in 36 African countries that monitor the efficacy of locally used antimalarial drugs by following up patients in clinics. According to standard protocol (13, 14), results are expressed as I) early treatment failure (ETF); II) late clinical failure (LCF): in the future, late parasitological failure (LPF) will be considered as well. Treatment failure for policy change as shown here consists of the sum of ETF + LCF.

Note: The box indicates the 25th/75th percentile, the line limits lower/upper values, and where the lines cross, the median.

Figure 55.1 Chloroquine Treatment Failure in Africa

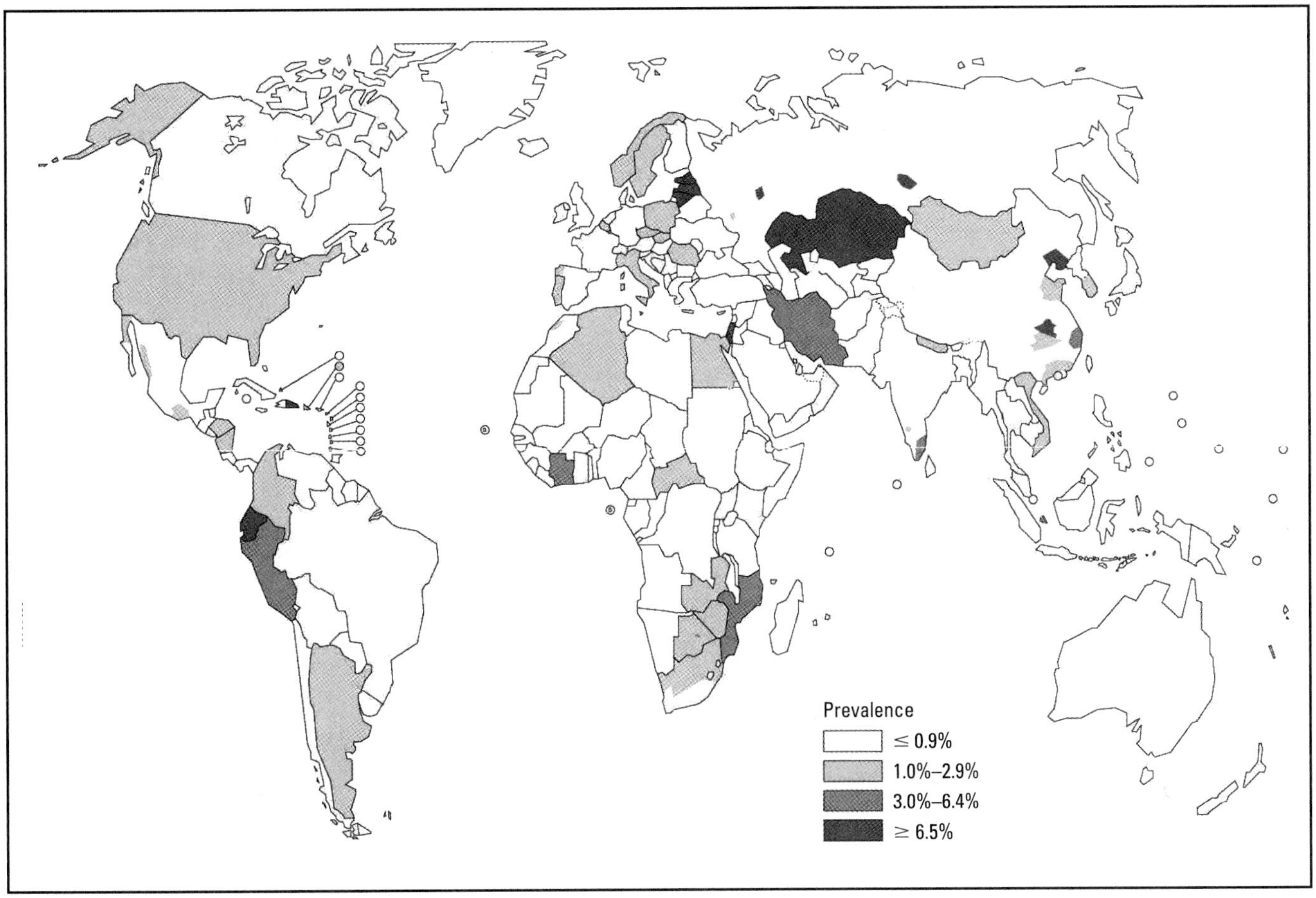

Source: WHO-IUATLD 2004.

Figure 55.2 Prevalence of MDR-TB among New TB Cases, 1994–2002

chloramphenicol has emerged and, over recent decades, spread to half or more of the strains sampled. In the 1990s, resistance has begun to emerge and spread to fluoroquinolones and third-generation cephalosporins, which in many places are the last effective oral drugs available (Ding and others 1999). In the past two decades, emergence and spread of *Shigella dysenteriae* type 1 resistant to sulfamethoxazole-trimethoprim, ampicillin, tetracycline, chloramphenicol, and—increasingly—nalidixic acid has reduced the effectiveness of these inexpensive and widely available antimicrobials in the empiric management of epidemic dysentery (Cunin and others 1999; Hoge and others 1995). The alternatives, ciprofloxacin and ceftriaxone, are relatively expensive and not always available. As a consequence, high fatality rates have been observed in a number of recent dysentery outbreaks (Legros and others 1998). The emergence of fluoroquinolone-resistant strains has quickly followed. The unchecked spread of these pathogens could pose a major public health challenge (Sarkar and others 1979).

Gonorrhea. Newly drug-resistant strains of gonococci tend to spread rapidly because of their peculiar epidemiology and the lack of control programs. Therefore, it is important to detect microepidemics of such strains, but this need is rarely met. The past half-century has witnessed the successive emergence and spread of gonococcal strains resistant to each new drug that becomes widely used to treat gonorrhea, including sulfonamides, penicillin, tetracycline, and sulfamethoxazole-trimethoprim (Tapsall 2002). Within less than a decade, such strains have commonly come to account for half or more of the isolates in many regions. The recent emergence of resistance to fluoroquinolones leaves only less available parenteral drugs, such as spectinomycin or ceftriaxone, as the reliable therapy (Ison and others 1998; Palmer, Leeming, and Turner 2001).

Tuberculosis. The emergence and spread of *multidrug-resistant tuberculosis,* which is defined as combined resistance to isoniazid and rifampicin, threaten the control of TB globally (Kochi, Vareldzis, and Styblo 1993). Patients infected with strains resistant to multiple drugs are very difficult to cure (Espinal and others 2000; Goble and others 1993), particularly if they are HIV-infected or malnourished (Fischl and others 1992), and alternative treatment is much more toxic and expensive (Drobniewski and Balabanova 2002). A patient with MDR-TB may remain infectious much longer than a patient with drug-susceptible organisms. Among new cases, prevalence of resistance to at least one TB drug ranges from 0 percent in some Western European countries to 57.1 percent in Kazakhstan, with a median of 10.2 percent. Multidrug resistance among untreated patients ranged from 0 percent in eight countries to 10.0 to 14.2 percent in six others. In previously treated cases, resistance to at least one drug ranged in different settings from 0 to 82.1 percent, with a median of 18.4 percent. Prevalence of

MDR-TB in previously treated cases ranged from 0 to 58.3 percent, with a median of 7.0 percent (WHO 2004).

An estimated 273,000 (at a 95 percent confidence interval [CI]; 185,000 to 414,000) new cases of MDR-TB occurred worldwide in 2000. By simple extrapolation, 70 million people could be latently infected with MDR-TB, and more than 1 million active MDR-TB cases could remain among previously treated patients. Despite its threatening potential, MDR-TB is—and will probably remain—generally rare. Decades after the introduction of TB drugs, the global prevalence of MDR-TB in new patients remains less than 2 percent (Dye and Espinal 2001). Old animal studies (Cohn and others 1954) and recent analyses using molecular epidemiology (Garcia-Garcia and others 2000) suggest that MDR-TB strains might be, on average, less infectious. And unlike most other bacteria, *M. tuberculosis* replicates rather slowly (low mutation rate) and shares little if any genetic material. Thus, even in the absence of widespread treatment of MDR-TB, its prevalence may not necessarily explode (Kam and Yip 2001).

Malaria. Chloroquine-resistant strains of *Plasmodium falciparum* malaria appeared a half-century ago in Southeast Asia and South America and spread across Africa, especially East Africa, in the past quarter-century (Wellems and Plowe 2001). The use of molecular markers testing indicates the wide geographical reach of *pfcrt* polymorphism for chloroquine resistance, and *dhfr* and *dhps* polymorphisms for sulfadoxine-pyrimethamine. Current levels of treatment failure of chloroquine are in figure 55.1. There is evidence that malaria mortality, especially in children under the age of five, is rising as a consequence of increasing resistance to chloroquine (Greenberg and others 1989; Trape 2001). In response to increasing treatment failure, many countries, including Malawi, South Africa, and Tanzania, adopted sulfadoxine-pyrimethamine as first-line treatment; however, resistance to this drug too is growing in many parts of Africa. In Southeast Asia, the emergence of multidrug resistance to sulfadoxine-pyrimethamine and mefloquine over the past decade and a half has prompted the use of combination treatments that include artemisinin (Wongsrichanalai and others 2001).

ECONOMIC BURDEN

Although few estimates have been made of the economic impact of drug resistance in developing countries, there is some indication that this burden is substantial. Estimates for costs associated with the loss of antibiotic effectiveness in outpatient prescriptions in the United States range from US$378 million to as high as US$18.6 billion (Elbasha 1999). A report by the Office of Technology Assessment to the U.S. Congress estimated the annual cost associated with antibiotic resistance in hospitals (attributable to five classes of hospital-acquired infections from six antibiotic-resistant bacteria) to be at least US$1.3 billion in 1992 dollars (Office of Technology Assessment 1995). The U.S. Centers for Disease Control and Prevention (CDC) estimated that the cost of all hospital-acquired infections, including both antibiotic-resistant and antibiotic-susceptible strains, was US$4.5 billion.

Patients infected with resistant strains are more likely to be sicker, to be hospitalized for longer periods of time, and to die of the infection (Carmeli and others 2002). Both the duration of hospitalization and the attributable cost of treating methicillin-resistant *Staphylococcus aureus* were found to be nearly three time as large as those for a susceptible infection (Abramson and Sexton 1999). One problem with estimating the attributable morbidity and mortality that is caused by resistant pathogens is that patients who are infected with resistant strains are more likely to have been sicker in the first place. Therefore, the ability to appropriately control for the underlying severity of the illness that causes hospitalization is a concern.

Another important cost of resistance comes from the need to move to second-line treatments, which are often much more expensive than the first-line treatment that is no longer effective. For instance, treating the roughly 300 million cases of malaria with artemisinin-based combinations would involve an excess burden of roughly US$200 million each year in drug costs. Periodically changing first-line treatment may also involve costs of assessing alternate treatment regimens, retraining health care providers, and restocking health care facilities. Though all these impose a significant economic burden, especially in poorer countries, they may be an inevitable consequence of past drug use. A focus on the cost of resistance alone may be misleading, because it is potentially possible to eliminate drug resistance by not using any drugs. To appropriately assess the net benefits of drug use, one must include the cost of increased resistance and the benefits of antibiotic or antimalarial use in treating infections and preventing their spread to uninfected individuals.

INTERVENTIONS

In this section, we discuss interventions to address the challenge of drug resistance (table 55.3). Many interventions to address the problem of resistance are the same as those that reduce the burden of disease (these are discussed in detail in the relevant disease-specific chapters in this volume). Reducing disease diminishes the need for drug treatment and, therefore, lowers the likelihood that resistant strains will emerge. Some interventions, such as the use of drug combinations, reduce the likelihood that resistance will emerge, whereas other interventions, such as improvements in drug prescribing and patient compliance with dosing, reduce the likelihood that a resistant pathogen will survive and proliferate. Prolonging the effective therapeutic life of existing drugs is not sufficient, however. Increasing incentives for pharmaceutical firms to bring new drugs to markets may also be called for.

Drug Treatment Strategies

The appropriate choice of drug treatment is an important step in delaying the evolution of drug resistance. Drug combinations that include drugs with different targets were first used in the treatment of tuberculosis and have now become routine practice in the treatment of cancer and HIV/AIDS. Combinations of artemisinin and its derivatives with other antimalarials, notably mefloquine, have accelerated recoveries, increased cure rates, and reduced transmissibility. In the refugee camps on the western border of Thailand, where most of the recent studies with artemisinin combinations have been conducted, the use of combinations delayed the development of resistance and reduced the incidence of disease (Nosten and others 2000). The rationale behind drug combinations is that, if resistance results from spontaneous genetic mutations, the chance that a parasite will emerge that is simultaneously resistant to two drugs with unrelated modes of action (that is, drug targets) is the mathematical product of the individual parasite mutation frequencies multiplied by the total number of parasites exposed to the drugs (White 1998, 1999). Combinations, therefore, reduce enormously the probability that a resistant mutant will arise. Sequential deployment of the drugs is much less effective, because it does not exploit the multiplicative reduction in selection risk.

In the context of antibiotics, combinations have typically been used to broaden the spectrum of antimicrobial coverage rather than to reduce the likelihood of the emergence of resistance. With the development of new penicillins and cephalosporins with broader spectra of activity a decade ago, most serious infections have been treated with monotherapy. The use of combination therapy to preserve new classes of antibiotics from the emergence of resistance at a societal level may be rational, but it has not been implemented because of cost concerns and the potential for enhanced toxicity associated with the use of more agents than necessary to effect a cure in an individual patient.

Other strategies include periodic withdrawal of a drug or rotation between different drugs. These strategies depend on the extent of the fitness cost of resistance[1] and the extent of multidrug resistance, which may vary with the specific combination of pathogen and drug. Withdrawal or drastic decline in antimicrobial use is occasionally but not always accompanied by the replacement of resistant strains with sensitive ones. The effects of antimicrobial removal have best been assessed for antibacterial drugs in northern Europe, where drug use is

Table 55.3 Potential Nonclinical Interventions: Evidence from Developing Countries

Strategy	Intervention	Reference	Description	Study location
Treatment strategies	Combination therapy for malaria	Nosten and others 2000	Use of an artesunate-mefloquine combination was found to reduce incidence of mefloquine resistance in *Plasmodium falciparum* malaria.	Thailand
	Cycling strategy	Kublin and others 2003	Replacement of chloroquine with sulfadoxine-pyrimethamine resulted in a decline in chloroquine-resistant strains over an eight-year period to levels that permit reintroduction of the drug.	Malawi
	Drug heterogeneity	Bonhoeffer, Lipsitch, and Levin 1997; Laxminarayan and Weitzman 2002	Modeling studies demonstrated the superiority and cost-effectiveness of policies involving use of different antibiotics on different patients compared with those using the same antibiotics on all patients.	n.a.
	Directly observed therapy short course	Balasubramanian, Oommen, and Samuel 2000	Directly observed therapy reduced the probability of treatment failure.	Kerala, India
		Dye and others 2002	Directly observed therapy for TB was 2.8 times cheaper to deliver and between 2.4 and 4.2 times more effective than conventional treatment.	South Africa
Reducing selection pressure	Training providers	Bexell and others 1996	Continuing education seminars for paramedical prescribers resulted in patients being prescribed antibiotics less frequently at intervention centers (34 percent) compared with control centers (42 percent). Drug choice and dosing were also improved.	Lusaka, Zambia
		Santoso, Suryawati, and Prawaitasari 1996	One-on-one educational interventions and seminars for medical and paramedical prescribers reduced antimicrobial prescription by 17 and 10 percent, respectively ($p < 0.001$).	Yogyakarta and Central Java provinces, Indonesia
	Training drug sellers	Agyepong and others 2002	Training drug dispensers on patient communication resulted in modest improvements in the proportion of patients showing strict, full adherence to antimalarial regimen.	Dangme West District, Ghana
	Treatment guidelines with education	Qingjun and others 1998	Blister packages increased compliance with chloroquine therapy to 97 percent, from 83 percent in the control group.	Hunan province, China
	Direct education of patients	Helitzer-Allen and others 1993	Introduction of a nonbitter antimalarial tablet and a new educational message were effective in improving antimalarial prophylaxis compliance among pregnant women by 57 to 91 percent.	Malawi
		Paredes and others 1996	Video, radio, and printed bulletins were used to educate women in an intervention community on the management of watery infantile diarrhea. The overuse of nonindicated medicines (antibiotics and antidiarrheals) dropped 11 percent in the intervention group and only 7 percent in the control group.	Lima, Peru
Reducing spread of resistance pathogens	Hand washing	Kurlat and others 1998	Training of nursing staff in hand washing, handling of infants, and care of intravenous lines resulted in 40 percent reduction in bacterimia rates.	Argentina
	Bednets (malaria)	Maxwell and others 2002	Use of netting resulted in a 55 to 75 percent reduction in malaria morbidity and consequent conservation of antimalarial drug use.	Tanzania
	Vaccination	Klugman 2001	Pneumococcal vaccines target the serotypes most commonly encountered clinically, which are more likely to be resistant to antimicrobials.	South Africa

Source: Authors.

tightly regulated and susceptibility patterns are closely monitored (Seppala and others 1997). A recent study demonstrated that after chloroquine was replaced by sulfadoxine-pyrimethamine in Malawi because of a loss of effectiveness attributable to resistance, chloroquine-susceptible *Plasmodium falciparum* strains appear to have returned (Kublin and others 2003). Though the results of this study offer promise for stopping or reversing resistance trends, if antimicrobials are more sparingly and less indiscriminately applied, little is known about the rate at which the resistance to chloroquine may reemerge with widespread use of this drug.

Rotating between two or more antibiotics has been proposed to address the problem of nosocomial drug resistance in the United States (Bergstrom, Lipsitch, and McGowan 2000; McGowan 1986), even though there is not much supporting empirical evidence to date. In one hospital-based study, switching from gentamicin to other aminoglycosides reduced resistance to gentamicin. However, when gentamicin was reintroduced, resistance developed rapidly (Gerding 2000). Modeling studies have indicated that a superior strategy may be to increase antimicrobial heterogeneity so that different patients are treated with drugs to which mechanisms of resistance are independent (Bonhoeffer, Lipsitch, and Levin 1997; Laxminarayan and Weitzman 2002). Although this may be difficult to implement in many developing countries, the approach incorporates an evolutionary perspective that may help deal with drug resistance.

Reducing Selection Pressure

Inappropriate antimicrobial use constitutes selective pressure without a corresponding benefit to individual or public health. (Eliminating all antibiotic use could, of course, eliminate the problem of drug resistance, but this strategy is clearly undesirable.) This multifaceted problem arises from behaviors of prescribers (not always physicians), dispensers (not always pharmacists), and consumers (not always infected). An important factor in overprescription is the issue of externalities; physicians, patients, and pharmacists have few incentives to consider the effects of their prescriptions or drug use on overall levels of resistance and the burden imposed on the rest of society. Physicians, both in private practice and in hospital settings, may also derive income from drugs sold and may, therefore, prescribe antibiotics more frequently than is desirable. In China, for instance, many hospitals rely on selling drugs for the bulk of their revenue (Hu and others 2001). Patient pressure demanding a prescription is known to influence prescribing in developed countries but could be less important in developing countries.

Interventions at the Provider Level

In this section, we discuss interventions directed at health care providers and local retail pharmacies, such as education and professional accountability.

Prescribing Patterns. Studies in developing countries have shown that as much as a third of drug prescriptions, accounting for 20 to 50 percent of drug costs, are irrational and that antimicrobials are among the most frequently prescribed medications (Bosu and Ofori-Adjei 2000). Although altering prescribing behavior is an important intervention to control drug resistance, the widespread availability of drugs without a prescription limits its effectiveness. The prescribing problem may be worse among private practitioners than among public practitioners (Siddiqi and others 2002). Continuing education for practicing health workers is one type of intervention that has been tested in several countries. In the United States, a decline in antimicrobial prescribing in pediatric ambulatory care has been attributed to educational programs directed at physicians as well as the public (McCaig, Besser, and Hughes 2002). In developing countries, successful educational programs for prescribers have improved diagnostic quality, dispelled perceptions of patient pressure, reduced unjustified antimicrobial prescription (Chuc and others 2002; Hadiyono and others 1996), and reduced polypharmacy (Hadiyono and others 1996) among private as well as public providers, including nonphysicians (Chakraborty, D'Souza, and Northrup 2000; Chuc and others 2002). In general, these measurable outcomes were improved by 5 to 20 percent by a single intervention—a modest but significant change that is best combined with parallel interventions. Although cost-effectiveness was not a focus of the studies, the resultant reduction in drug use would ultimately result in cost savings. Important components of educational interventions are long-term commitment and refresher courses, and complementary interventions are also desirable (le Grand, Hogerzeil, and Haaijer-Ruskamp 1999).

Prescription guidelines, essential drug lists, and formularies are essential for defining policy and provide a useful framework on which educational interventions can be based (Laing, Hogerzeil, and Ross-Degnan 2001). The World Health Organization (WHO) recommends standard treatment guidelines as one of several approaches for promoting rational drug use. Also, guidelines proposed by pharmacy and therapeutics committees or external advisers have been applied in developing countries, with mixed results. Although standard treatment guidelines reduced antibiotic use for respiratory infections by 50 percent in Fiji (le Grand, Hogerzeil, and Haaijer-Ruskamp 1999), they did not alter prescription patterns in a Ugandan study and produced a detectable but insignificant effect in Sri Lanka (Angunawela, Diwan, and Tomson 1991). In general, follow-up was essential for success, and the use of standard treatment guidelines was more effective with nonphysician prescribers (le Grand, Hogerzeil, and Haaijer-Ruskamp 1999). Education must form part of any treatment guideline intervention, and evidence suggests that, if anything, educational programs are more effective than simply formulating guidelines (Laing, Hogerzeil, and Ross-Degnan 2001). Rigid guidelines such as preprinted order forms or prepackaged drug kits for the management of community-acquired infections have been perceived as excessively prescriptive and have not been successful intervention tools (le Grand, Hogerzeil, and Haaijer-Ruskamp 1999). Devising incentives for compliance could potentially lower the higher prescription rates among private providers, where treatment guidelines by themselves are less likely to work.

Peer and supervisory monitoring increases professional accountability, thereby promoting the application of knowledge to practice. The requirement that antibiotic prescriptions for inpatients be countersigned by an infectious disease consultant was successful in reducing prescriptions by 50 percent, with a resultant cost savings of about US$350,000 over two years in a Panama hospital (Saez-Llorens and others 2000). Such a program would have limited applicability in other countries and settings where the number of trained medical professionals is small. A supervisory program in Vietnam, with medical equipment incentives, reduced the number of patients for whom antibiotics were prescribed and increased the number who received a correct dose regimen (Chalker 2001).

Diagnostic Tests. Bacterial culture and susceptibility testing, a necessary component of rational antimicrobial prescribing, is uncommon in many developing countries (Okeke, Lamikanra, and Edelman 1999). Furthermore, diagnostic tests to confirm or refute infections are also commonly unavailable or unreliable, so diagnoses are made largely on the strength of clinical signs and symptoms (Berkley and others 2001). Laboratory tests are expensive and routinely cost more than an empiric drug that could be effective. In contrast, malaria dipsticks can be an inexpensive tool for case detection and may be cost-effective in low transmission settings (Rimon and others 2003). Clinicians have been known to use chemotherapy as a diagnostic tool: a cure would confirm a diagnosis. Susceptibility testing of at least some specimens will provide much-needed surveillance data to support empiric prescribing, although efforts should be made to take into account spatial heterogeneity in resistance patterns.

Retail Pharmacies and Outlets. Drug distributors, including not only pharmacists but also pharmacy attendants, patent medicine stallkeepers, and itinerant drug sellers, often sell drugs without prescription and are an important source of primary care for people in many developing countries (Igun 1994; Indalo 1997). Patients in search of convenient and accessible health care often seek treatment at drug retail premises. Many drug sellers have not been formally trained in diagnosis and prescription but often have financial incentive to perform those tasks, with varying degrees of competence. Despite the potential loss of business to storekeepers, educational interventions have been successful in increasing prescription requirement demands and promoting referral advice, all steps in the right direction (Chuc and others 2002). Models for delivering

educational interventions in developing countries vary but can be broadly classified into focus group discussions (Hadiyono and others 1996) and large seminars (Bexell and others 1996). Both models have been found to be of comparable effectiveness; however, applicability and cost are situation-specific (Santoso, Suryawati, and Prawaitasari 1996).

Drug Quality. Ensuring drug quality is important, both to benefit the individual patient and to ensure that a patient is not subjected to suboptimal doses that would promote drug resistance. The few studies that have been conducted indicate that more than half of the antimicrobials marketed in developing countries do not match their labels. Hence, even when prescribers and consumers are using the drugs responsibly, therapeutic failure and subinhibitory levels of antimicrobials may occur. Substandard drugs are those that are degraded as a result of expiration or improper storage or that are counterfeit (Okeke and Lamikanra 2001; Prazuck and others 2002; Taylor and others 2001).

Interventions at the Patient Level

Improving communication between patients and providers could improve adherence to prescribed antimalarial regimens (Agyepong and others 2002). Compliance can also be positively affected by packaging. Blister packages, when combined with proper instruction about drug use, have been shown to produce modest increases in antimalarial compliance, particularly for long-term regimens, such as with primaquine (Qingjun and others 1998). Blister packages are also time-savers for primary health care workers, potentially allowing them more time to advise patients on drug use. However, the introduction of blister packages must be accompanied by clear directions to avoid injury following ingestion of blister packages.

Reducing patient self-medication may also desirable, although the effect on drug resistance remains to be precisely quantified. Enforcement of prescription-only regulations for most antimicrobials reduces self-medication in developed countries (Carey and Cryan 2003; Goff, Koff, and Geiling 2002; Pechere 2001) and may be desirable in developing countries as well. However, such a strategy may be difficult to implement in developing countries. There have been only rare reports of reduction in antibiotic use following blanket enforcement of prescription supply legislation in areas where antibiotics are freely available (Bavestrello, Cabello, and Casanova 2002). Opponents to enforcement demand a heavy financial and political investment, implying that a black market for medicines could emerge, particularly if the demand for these drugs is not lowered (Bhutta and Balchin 1996; le Grand, Hogerzeil, and Haaijer-Ruskamp 1999). The sale of antimicrobials is a lucrative business, even when illegal, because of high demand.

Educational interventions directed at consumers have been proposed to reduce self-medication and increase compliance, but evidence for the effectiveness of this strategy remains inconclusive, largely because so few studies have been conducted. Gonzalez Ochoa and others (1996) demonstrated that, although refresher training for health personnel managing acute respiratory infections reduced antibiotic prescribing by 9 to 19 percent in two intervention areas in Havana, no benefit was seen from community education programs when used alone or in conjunction with prescriber training. In contrast, Denis (1998) was able to show that a poster had 5 percent effectiveness alone and 20 percent effectiveness when used with a video to promote appropriate use of quinine and tetracycline regimens for malaria among Cambodian villagers. The best method to deliver information about the consequences of antibiotic resistance remains to be identified and will need to be modified to suit different cultures (Marin and others 1995).

In the case of tuberculosis, first-line directly observed therapy (DOT) remains one of the most cost-effective of all public health strategies (WHO 1994). The discovery that DOT can be administered successfully as a short course (DOTS) has been pivotal to successful implementation. Relatively simple, the DOTS approach can improve patient compliance, cure the vast majority of new TB patients, and prevent transmission of the disease and the emergence of MDR-TB (Balasubramanian, Oommen, and Samuel 2000; Dye and others 2002). Unfortunately, many countries have been slow to adopt and implement DOTS programs correctly, and only a minority of TB patients worldwide are managed according to this protocol (Dye and others 2002; Pungrassami and others 2002). Because many patients either are treated outside the DOTS regimen or do not adhere to the long-term chemotherapy necessary to eradicate the causative organism, MDR-TB is likely to emerge and treatment costs are likely to escalate to as high as 1,000 times the cost of conventional treatment of drug-sensitive infection.

A DOTS program requires good laboratory support for case identification and is highly employee intense, requiring health workers to observe the ingestion of every dose of antimicrobials over several months. However, the potential economic gains are immense because of the high costs of allowing the continued spread of the disease and of managing resistant patients and because of the benefit of reduced hospital admissions (Dye and others 2003). Several studies have investigated means for reducing the cost of conventional DOTS programs without compromising effectiveness. Lwilla and others (2003) demonstrated that both institutional and community-based DOTS programs are effective, permitting cost-effective implementation in remote areas. Furthermore, although DOTS involves supervised drug dosing, highly trained health workers are not essential. Studies in South Africa, Haiti, and Thailand have found that DOTS was effective when drug administration was supervised by appropriately trained volunteers, including

storekeepers and former TB patients (Barker, Millard, and Nthangeni 2002; Pungrassami and Chongsuvivatwong 2002).

Although DOTS was not designed to cure patients with MDR-TB, it succeeds in 50 percent of cases (Espinal and others 2000). Controversy has emerged about the best approach to MDR-TB in resource-constrained settings. Although some experts assert that standard TB control prevents the emergence of MDR-TB in a cost-effective way (Chaulet, Raviglione, and Bustreo 1996) and that expensive treatment of MDR-TB would divert scarce resources from struggling DOTS programs, others argue that it is unethical to abandon MDR-TB patients and maintain that, if untreated, MDR-TB strains will become dominant, undermining tuberculosis control in future generations (Farmer, Becerra, and Kim 1999). These arguments are of particular consequence for programs in poor countries.

Application of Antibiotics for Nonhumans

The use of antimicrobial agents in agriculture and aquaculture can contribute to the spread of antimicrobial resistance in humans, although the extent of this contribution has not been precisely quantified. It is believed that agricultural antibiotic use hastens the emergence of resistant pathogens in humans, and antibiotic use in humans contributes to the spread of resistance once it has emerged (Smith and others 2002). There are no reliable estimates of the extent to which antibiotics are being used for such nonhuman purposes even in developed countries. In developing countries, one would expect use to increase with rising incomes and greater industrialization of agriculture and food production.

WHO has recommended that antimicrobials normally prescribed for humans should no longer be used to promote growth in animals (WHO 2000). Some countries in Europe, including Denmark and Sweden, have already phased out such use, and under the current plan, the European Union will ban the use of antibiotics for growth promotion by 2006. Evidence of the effect of a ban on antibiotic use in swine production is available from Denmark. Although the ban significantly lowered the use of antibiotics in growth promotion and raised the cost of swine production by less than 1 percent, the resulting higher incidence of disease among swine increased the use of antibiotics used for veterinary therapeutic purposes (Hayes and Jensen 2003). A similar increase was noted in Sweden, where antibiotic use in animals was banned in 1986; however, this problem was temporary, and in the longer term, livestock producers were able to move to an effective production system with lower antibiotic use (Wierup 2001).

Containing the Spread of Resistant Micro-organisms

Although selection is a necessary component of the resistance archetype, the dissemination of resistant organisms may have a far greater effect on the current situation (Zaidi and others 2003).

Interventions that block this dissemination have the added benefit of improving health by interrupting disease transmission and reducing the need for antibiotics in the first place. A case in point is the reduction in drug-resistant *Streptococcus pneumoniae* infections in the United States following the introduction of a multivalent vaccine that protected against the serovars with which resistance is commonly associated (Whitney and others 2003). By contrast, a drop in antibiotic use had no detectable effect on resistance within a short period (Arason and others 2002). Because these types of interventions are easier to evaluate, and in many cases are cheaper to implement (Coast and others 2002), they are likely to be of great value to public health in developing countries.

Interventions that interfere with the spread of many infectious diseases will have a parallel effect on the dissemination of resistant micro-organisms. Because the potential health benefits are obvious, these types of interventions are likely to be sustained (Wilson and Chandler 1993). A simple, cost-effective example is hand washing, which could reduce diarrhea by 47 percent while also having beneficial effects on acute respiratory tract and other community-acquired infections (Curtis and Cairncross 2003) (see chapters 19 and 35). Similarly, insecticide-impregnated bednets are another important intervention for the control of malaria (see chapter 21).

The emergence, persistence, and intra- and interhospital spread of multidrug-resistant organisms have all been facilitated by inadequate infection control practices. Furthermore, the emergence and spread of drug-resistant nosocomial pathogens from hospitals to the community are also a concern, and a history of hospitalization has been identified as a significant risk factor for the acquisition of a resistant infection in family members (OR 4.5, $p = 0.007$) (Zaidi and others 2003). Unfortunately, we lack good clinical trials that compare the different approaches to infection control programs and their ability to control antimicrobial resistance in hospitals and other health care facilities (Duse and Smego 1999). It seems reasonable to assume, however, that if the overall frequency of nosocomial infections is decreased in a health care facility, then the need for antimicrobial agents may be reduced. Furthermore, well-structured and rational infection control strategies that balance resources with the magnitude of the local problem must surely play an important role in decreasing morbidity, mortality, and costs (direct and indirect) to the patient, his or her family, the hospital, and the health care sector in general. Hospital-acquired infections rank among the most important causes of death, either directly or indirectly, in the developing world (Duse and Smego 1999; Ponce-de-Leon and Rangel-Frausto 1993).

Global Coordination

Antimicrobial resistance is a global challenge that requires urgent global action, not just across national boundaries but also across the whole range of sectors involved. International travel and trade, particularly of food products, have facilitated the rapid globalization of resistance, and actions undertaken by any single nation have consequences for other countries. Drug resistance may threaten health gains made in other spheres of public health. Thus, coinfection with antimicrobial-resistant pathogens and HIV can lead to more rapid disease progression and enhanced dissemination of resistant pathogens. The emergence of antimicrobial resistance is considered a major threat to the future security and political stability of some regions (CIA 1999). Figure 55.3 shows the likely geography of the emergence, spread, and evolution of chloroquine resistance.

Concerted international action is needed to contain antimicrobial resistance. Failure of individual countries to act to contain resistance could lead to both national and international consequences. For instance, the use of artemisinin as monotherapy in any single country could potentially lead to the rapid evolution of resistant strains, which could threaten the use of this valuable drug in any other part of the world.

There is a considerable need for greater international collaboration on surveillance of antimicrobial resistance, both for routine surveillance and as an early warning system for unusual resistance events. Although existing laws at the international level require reporting of some infectious diseases, they do not include any systematic reporting of antimicrobial resistance. Certain multiresistant pathogens, such as methicillin-resistant *S. aureus,* are now notifiable at the national level in some countries, but the global nature of the resistance problem means that national legal measures alone are not enough. At the same time, the creation of new international duties would be undermined if they were not incorporated into national law (Fidler 1998).

To support such surveillance, the World Health Organization makes software (WHONET) available to enable clinical laboratories to enter their drug susceptibility test results into databases that can be analyzed for local management of resistance. Those results can also be merged, creating, thus far, approximately 80 national surveillance databases. Statutory notification about pathogens with new resistance phenotypes is under active discussion in several countries. Interpretation of existing surveillance data is hampered by the multiplicity of methods used to measure resistance and by the difficulties of assessing the quality of the data. Enhanced laboratory capacity is needed in many countries to provide effective diagnostic services and resistance surveillance. Multicountry external quality assurance schemes already exist but need to be extended to cover more resource-poor nations. WHO has begun establishing international surveillance standards by issuing antimicrobial resistance surveillance standards (WHO 2002a), guidelines for the management of drug-resistant tuberculosis (WHO 1997), and protocols for detection of antimicrobial drug resistance (WHO 1996). Monitoring the use of antimicrobial agents

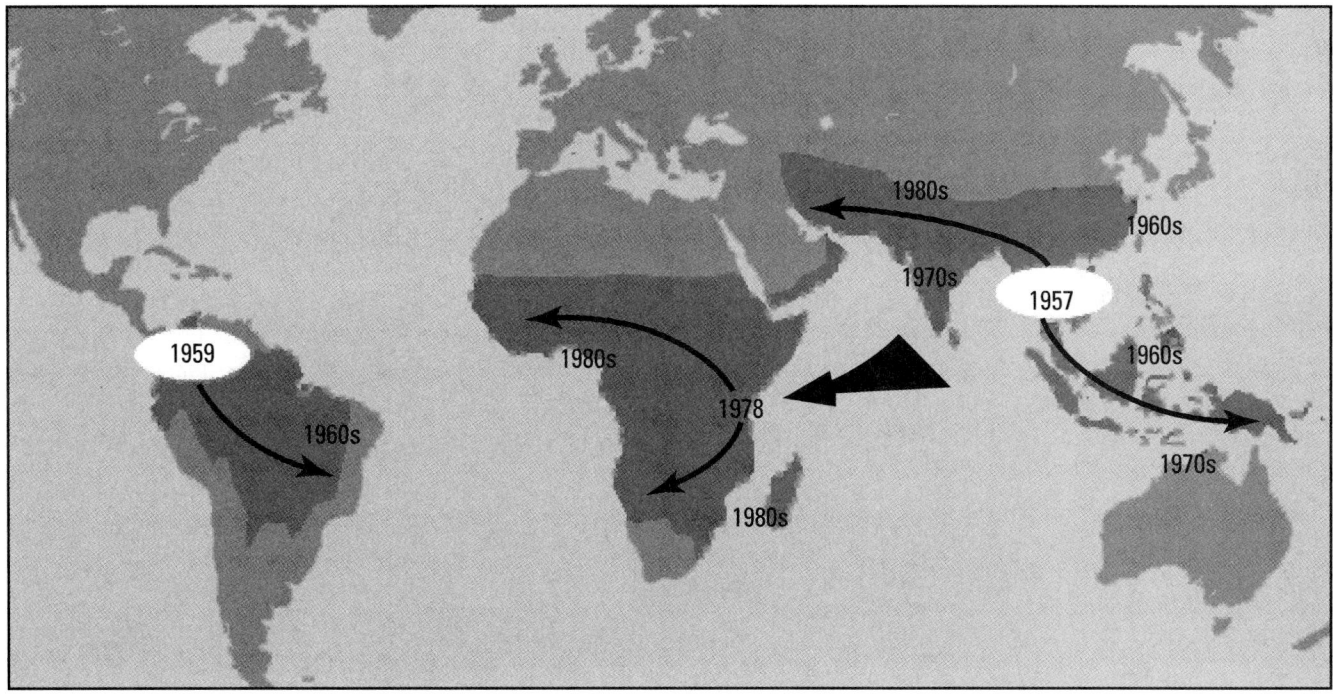

Source: Cell 1997.

Figure 55.3 Global Spread of Chloroquine-Resistant Strains of *P. falciparum*

is an important aspect of surveillance and needs to be strengthened internationally.

Coordinated surveillance for drug resistance to TB may be a useful prototype to follow. By 2003, a global network of 20 supranational reference laboratories and five regional subnetworks, known as the World Health Organization–International Union against Tuberculosis and Lung Disease (WHO–IUATLD) Global Project, was reporting data on representative cases of TB from 62 countries. The network has monitored participants' laboratory testing methods and developed uniform definitions, such as establishing clinical categories for new cases and previously treated cases. The WHO–IUATLD Global Project, which covers approximately 33 percent of the world's population and 28 percent of its reported cases of TB, and other surveillance efforts reveal great variations from place to place in the prevalence of resistance to antituberculosis drugs.

The WHO Global Strategy for Containment of Antimicrobial Resistance (WHO 2001) recommends more than 60 interventions that can slow the emergence and reduce the spread of resistance in diverse settings, and it provides a blueprint for global coordinated action. A recent report by the Institute of Medicine calls for such coordinated action at a global level to subsidize artemisinin-based combination treatments for malaria for deployment in developing countries to ensure that combination treatments are available at the same or lower price

than monotherapies. The underlying rationale is that this strategy would both save lives in the short term and delay the emergence of resistance in the long term, thereby benefiting all malarious countries (Arrow, Panosian, and Gelband 2004).

Encouraging the Development of New Drugs

The development of new products has not kept pace with the problem of addressing microbial resistance to drugs that are used to treat infections in human and veterinary medicine. In the context of drug resistance, it is not sufficient to design policies that will encourage only the development of new drugs. It is also important that such policies give pharmaceutical firms (a) an incentive to invest in new classes of drugs, rather than products that belong to existing drug classes and that are, therefore, more likely to be rendered obsolete by resistance, and (b) an incentive to care about drug resistance when making decisions about how to market and sell their product. (See chapter 6 for a discussion of product development not specific to drug resistance.)

Current public and private investment in drugs, vaccines, and other products to control major infectious diseases in developing countries has recently been less than 2 percent of total health research expenditures throughout the world. Of the 1,393 new chemical entities registered by Western health authorities between 1975 and 1999, only 13 (less than 1 percent) were intended for the treatment of tropical diseases, and half of those came from veterinary research.

Evidence suggests that in recent years, a steadily decreasing proportion of pharmaceutical company profits has been invested in antimicrobial research and development (R&D). One reason given for this decline is increased development costs, which result from more complex clinical trials, longer development times, and the relative attractiveness of returns from investing in drugs for chronic diseases, which must be taken continuously rather than just for the duration of an infection. Efforts to reduce inappropriate antibiotic use may paradoxically also reduce incentives for pharmaceutical firms to invest in developing new products (Monnet and Sorensen 2001; Philipson and Mechoulan 2003). The related issue, of using shorter treatment courses for many infections, may also affect R&D incentives (Pichichero and Cohen 1997).

Encouraging research into antimicrobial agents that will be used primarily in low-resource countries poses particular challenges, given the need for drug companies to make a profit. Various incentives to the industry, including both push and pull mechanisms, have been discussed (Kettler 2000). *Push mechanisms* consist of incentives to offset R&D costs, such as research grants, tax credits, public investment in applied research, cost-sharing between companies, and establishment of local development facilities. *Pull mechanisms* are designed to create a market, thereby improving the likelihood of a return on investments. They could include an international purchase fund for a new antimicrobial that meets specific criteria (United Kingdom Government 2001), tax credits on sales, and favorable patent policies, such as extension of patent terms or market exclusivity on new products. Time-limited exclusivities on new, clinically useful formulations might stimulate the additional pharmaceutical and clinical studies that are needed to support licensure. Better patent protection for new antimicrobial agents in areas of the world where patent laws are not enforced today would also help.

Patent policies to encourage investment in developing new antibiotics should also take into consideration the effect of those policies on incentives that would encourage pharmaceutical firms to conserve the effectiveness of their products. If effective patent lengths are too short, pharmaceutical companies will be less likely to care about growing drug resistance to their product and will be more interested in maximizing sales of their products during the period of patent production. Extending patent lengths may not solve the problem, however. If different firms make closely related antibiotics that have linked mechanisms of action, no single firm may have an incentive to care about drug resistance (Laxminarayan 2002). Increasing patent breadth, one solution to this problem, would have the added advantage of creating an incentive for firms to invest in developing new classes of drugs rather than introducing drugs that are closely related to existing products in modes of action.

IMPLEMENTATION OF STRATEGIES: TWO LESSONS FROM EXPERIENCE

Integrated Management of Childhood Illness

The program on the integrated management of infant and childhood illness (IMCI) was initiated by WHO, the United Nations Children's Fund, and other technical partners. The program, which provides a framework for stepwise assessment and management of sick children, has been successful in averting unnecessary antibiotic and antimalarial use and in reducing the cost of medications (Gove 1997). An underlying objective of IMCI is to detect, where present, conditions other than those responsible for the primary complaint. The result is that rational prescribing may actually increase, but because IMCI guidelines reduce irrational prescribing, the net effect is a reduction in drug use, including antimicrobials (Oluwole, Mason, and Costello 2000). Drug costs associated with treating children in Kenya were found to be reduced from an average of 44 cents per patient (U.S. currency) to between 16 and 39 cents per patient when IMCI guidelines were followed (Boulanger, Lee, and Odhacha 1999). A study that compared prescriptions arising from standard and IMCI-guided consultation with a health worker in Kaduna state, Nigeria, found a reduction in polypharmacy when IMCI guidelines were used, from a median of five drugs down to two drugs, and an 80 percent reduction in the cost of all medicines (Wammanda, Ejembi, and Iorliam 2003). This reduction represented savings of 93.4 and 68.6 percent for antibacterials and antimalarials, respectively, although part of the savings could be attributed to the substitution of tablets for more expensive syrup formulations.

The contribution of IMCI to promoting judicious drug use is worth noting. A study that compared four districts of Kenya—two districts that had IMCI programs (Morogoro and Rufiji) and two that did not (Ulanga and Kilombero)—found that in 73 percent (95 percent CI; 65–80) of consultations studied in the IMCI intervention districts, a child needing an oral antibiotic or antimalarial was prescribed correctly, compared with 35 percent (95 percent CI; 25–45) in the control districts (Armstrong Schellenberg and others 2004). Also, in the IMCI districts, 86 percent (95 percent CI; 80–92) of children who did not need antibiotics left the facility without an antibiotic, compared with 57 percent (95 percent CI; 48–66) in the control district.

Directly Observed Therapy

Strict compliance and cure verification make it possible to conduct directly observed therapy using shorter-term regimens (the DOTS program). Outpatient treatment of a single TB case in Pakistan, with complete compliance, was recently estimated at US$164 and increased to US$310 when an institution-based DOTS program was applied (Khan and others 2002). In Beijing, the cost of saving one disability-adjusted life year

(DALY) is 10 times higher when a DOTS TB program is not used (Xu, Jin, and Zhang 2000). Recent expansion of DOTS care in India has resulted in savings of about 0.2 million lives and US$400 million in indirect costs (Khatri and Frieden 2002). Progress with DOTS in India was initially slow, but following better implementation, recent findings suggest that huge successes have been made in the past five years. The successes can largely be attributed to improved management of the program, area-specific appraisals, infrastructure, personnel, and technical support as well as continuous supervision (Khatri and Frieden 2002). This model is one that may apply in other developing countries.

In New York city, individualized chemotherapy based on drug susceptibility testing was nearly as effective in new patients with MDR-TB as in those with drug-susceptible TB (Telzak and others 1995), and the number of MDR-TB cases decreased by more than 90 percent within the decade (Fujiwara and others 1997). The relatively large number of MDR-TB cases in high-income countries made second-line drugs more available and affordable, and experience in the management of MDR-TB grew considerably over the past decade (Mukherjee and others 2004). Yet questions remained about which interventions had led to the city's success. In 1999, WHO created a working group on DOTS-plus to assess the feasibility and cost-effectiveness of treating MDR-TB in low- and middle-income countries (Espinal and others 1999). DOTS-plus has already negotiated a 90 percent price reduction from the pharmaceutical industry (Gupta and others 2001), and experience from Peru suggests feasibility and a mean cost of US$211 per DALY gained (Suarez and others 2002).

AGENDA FOR ACTION

Although the evolution of resistance is a biological phenomenon, it is influenced strongly by the behavior of physicians, patients, and hospital administrators. In the language of economics, drug resistance is an *externality* associated with the use of antibiotics—a consequence not taken into consideration by those who use antibiotics or antimalarials. From a public policy perspective, there may be an economic case for societal intervention, because patients, physicians, and nations acting on self-interest alone may produce a higher degree of drug resistance than is ideal for society as a whole. From a global perspective, there is a case for international coordination to ensure that the actions of any single country or region do not increase the likelihood of emergence of resistance, which could then spread to other parts of the world.

Rising incomes in the developing world are likely to encourage greater use of Western medicine and, consequently, greater use of antibiotics. Moreover, the adoption of government-sponsored or employer-sponsored insurance plans in many parts of the developing world could further increase drug use. Because developing countries will be less able to bear the costs of increasing resistance, it is important that the patterns of overuse and misuse observed in high-income countries not be repeated. The right financial incentives must be in place for both patients and physicians to face the full cost of using antibiotics and antimalarials and to ensure that these drugs are not overused.

Recommended Interventions

Sets of interventions specific to the diseases discussed in this chapter are described below.

Pneumococci. A number of affordable interventions can be considered. Data suggest that hand washing can interrupt not only the spread of pathogens causing diarrhea but also the transmission of nosocomial pathogens, and it can reduce respiratory infection–related mortality and morbidity. The promotion of a culture of hand washing requires access to clean, sufficient water—an urgent goal. Patient education to reduce demand for antibiotics for viral infections, and alteration of perverse incentives for physicians to prescribe antibiotics excessively are recommended. Pneumococcal conjugate vaccine has been shown to reduce the burden of antibiotic-resistant invasive disease, reduce transmission of resistant strains, and reduce antibiotic use in vaccine recipients and their siblings. Strategies for introducing this type of vaccine into the high-risk populations of developing countries are urgently needed. Better diagnostics are a key to more appropriate and focused prescribing, but their application is likely to be delayed in poor countries. The long-term effects of blanket recommendations for antimicrobial prophylaxis among HIV-infected populations must be closely monitored.

Shigella. Interventions must include improved strategies for case definition, clinical recognition, and appropriate therapy of dysentery. These strategies require a focus on educating physicians and caregivers as well as restrictions on over-the-counter availability of antibiotics in developing countries. Recent strategies for reducing antimicrobial prescribing for diarrhea at the community level also include coadministration of zinc with oral rehydration therapy. This strategy has been shown to lead to significant reduction in antimicrobial prescribing for diarrhea in Bangladesh and may be a useful adjunctive strategy (Baqui and others 2002).

Tuberculosis. The top priority must be the expansion of DOTS (Iseman, Cohn, and Sbarbaro 1993), which itself can prevent the emergence of MDR-TB (Dye and others 2002). In individual countries or parts of countries, however, additional strategies may be appropriate. Pablos-Méndez, Gowda, and Frieden

(2002) have grouped countries according to the proportion of TB patients completing treatment successfully and the level of MDR-TB among previously untreated patients. The resulting matrix provides a reasonable framework for deciding whether to use second-line drugs in a national program. Countries with treatment success of less than 70 percent should introduce or improve the DOTS strategy as the top priority. In settings with primary MDR-TB of less than 1.5 percent, treating MDR-TB is not a public health priority, although individual cases could be referred to clinical experts. The hotspots—those areas with primary MDR levels above 5 percent—are international public health emergencies. Infection control practices must be emphasized in such settings. Intermediate situations are ideal for additional research comparing DOTS with various individualized regimens against MDR-TB.

Malaria. With declining effectiveness of chloroquine and rapidly emerging resistance to its replacement, sulfadoxine-pyrimethamine, it is imperative that significant attention be paid not just to the choice of an appropriate first-line treatment for malaria, but also to strategies to prolong the effective therapeutic life of the new treatment. WHO has recommended that new artemisinin derivatives be used only in combinations with other drugs. There is evidence that artemisinin has already found its way into shops as monotherapy; discouraging the use of this valuable drug in monotherapy through public subsidies for combinations, by mandate, or through a combination of measures is a necessary first step. Discouraging the use of artemisinin as monotherapy is not sufficient, however. It is also important to ensure that the partner drug in the combination used with the artemisinin derivative is effective and, hence, able to protect the artemisinin. Therefore, discouraging the use of the partner drug as monotherapy, except in cases in which no safe alternative exists, such as for sulfadoxine-pyrimethamine in intermittent preventive treatment of malaria in pregnant women, is an important step in ensuring the long-term sustainability of malaria treatment. Training shopkeepers and other purveyors of antimalarial treatments to recognize symptoms of malaria and to use diagnostics to detect malaria would help reduce malaria treatment to instances for which it is appropriate and would reduce the likelihood of the emergence of resistance. Finally, steps to reduce the burden of malaria through the use of insecticide-treated bednets and, in some areas, residual household spraying would help reduce the need for antimalarial treatment and thereby reduce treatment selection pressure.

Research Agenda

A description of a research agenda to explain the full range of issues related to drug resistance is outside the scope of this chapter and has been accomplished by other groups. Here, we restrict our focus to the following five priorities:

- accounting for attributable morbidity and mortality and the economic burden of drug resistance in the developing world
- measuring the cost-effectiveness of interventions to improve prescribing and patient compliance
- researching incentives for firms to invest both in developing new drugs and in maintaining the effectiveness of existing drugs
- identifying socioeconomic, demographic, and cultural factors that determine antibiotic use and misuse and projecting how antibiotic use will change in future years
- designing international coordinating mechanisms for surveillance to report resistance outbreaks and coordinate strategies for appropriate drug use, recognizing the global nature of drug resistance.

CONCLUSION

Modern medicine rests on the bedrock of effective anti-infective drugs. Unfortunately, the use of drugs creates selective pressure for resistance to arise, and thus, the growth of resistance may be an unavoidable consequence of our actions in treating disease. It is, however, important for governments to intervene to ensure that the effectiveness of our current arsenal of anti-infectives is not depleted at an excessively rapid rate. Given the potential for international spillovers of resistant pathogens and the ability of actions taken in one region or nation to affect other parts of the world where a disease is prevalent, a strong case can be made for coordinated international action—similar to another urgent global situation, the depletion of the ozone layer and the subsequent Montreal Protocol to phase out the use of chlorofluorocarbons—to manage the evolution of resistance.

Some interventions that we recommend, such as more restrictive prescribing policies and the use of combinations, could, in the absence of subsidies from the state, place a burden on the poorest patients. For instance, an overly restrictive policy on drug sales at the retail level could harm those who have less access to formal medical care and prescriptions. There may be similar effects from mandating that antimalarial drugs be sold in combinations that the poor cannot afford. Efforts to manage resistance should not be balanced on the backs of the poor, however, because the rationale for these efforts is that society as a whole gains from them. It is important that state subsidies be used to ensure that interventions to manage for resistance do not reduce patients' access to effective and affordable drugs.

Huge gains in life expectancy have come from the introduction of effective drugs to treat infectious diseases. Our history of treating infections successfully is brief, however, and dates back only 50 or 60 years. Sustaining this ability in the long term requires a willingness to invest in interventions both to extend the therapeutic life of existing drugs and to discover and develop new ones. Some of these interventions, such as better infection control, introduction of affordable vaccines, and proper dosing, would benefit patients immediately; others, such as using combination treatments for malaria and investing in new drugs, may not bear fruit in the near term. Without a sustainable, long-term vision of coexistence with harmful microbes and imaginative solutions to the problem of resistance, our ability to control infectious diseases stands in peril.

NOTE

1. The fitness cost of resistance is an evolutionary disadvantage placed on resistant pathogens. However, some argue that although most resistance-determining mutations engender some fitness cost, these costs are likely to be ameliorated by subsequent compensatory mutations.

REFERENCES

Aarestrup, F. M., A. M. Seyfarth, H. D. Emborg, K. Pedersen, R. S. Hendriksen, and F. Bager. 2001. "Effect of Abolishment of the Use of Antimicrobial Agents for Growth Promotion on Occurrence of Antimicrobial Resistance in Fecal Enterococci from Food Animals in Denmark." *Antimicrobial Agents and Chemotherapy* 45 (7): 2054–59.

Abramson, M. A., and D. J. Sexton. 1999. "Nosocomial Methicillin-Resistant and Methicillin-Susceptible Staphylococcus Aureus Primary Bacteremia: At What Costs?" *Infection Control and Hospital Epidemiology* 20 (6): 408–11.

Adrian, P. V., and K. P. Klugman. 1997. "Mutations in the Dihydrofolate Reductase Gene of Trimethoprim-Resistant Isolates of Streptococcus Pneumoniae." *Antimicrobial Agents and Chemotherapy* 41 (11): 2406–13.

Agyepong, I. A., E. Ansah, M. Gyapong, S. Adjei, G. Barnish, and D. Evans. 2002. "Strategies to Improve Adherence to Recommended Chloroquine Treatment Regimes: A Quasi-Experiment in the Context of Integrated Primary Health Care Delivery in Ghana." *Social Science and Medicine* 55 (12): 2215–26.

Angunawela, I. I., V. K. Diwan, and G. Tomson. 1991. "Experimental Evaluation of the Effects of Drug Information on Antibiotic Prescribing: A Study in Outpatient Care in an Area of Sri Lanka." *International Journal of Epidemiology* 20 (2): 558–64.

Arason, V. A., A. Gunnlaugsson, J. A. Sigurdsson, H. Erlendsdottir, S. Gudmundsson, and K. G. Kristinsson. 2002. "Clonal Spread of Resistant Pneumococci Despite Diminished Antimicrobial Use." *Microbial Drug Resistance* 8 (3): 187–92.

Armstrong Schellenberg, J., J. Bryce, D. de Savigny, T. Lambrechts, C. Mbuya, L. Mgalula, and others. 2004. "The Effect of Integrated Management of Childhood Illness on Observed Quality of Care of Under-Fives in Rural Tanzania." *Health Policy and Planning* 19 (1): 1–10.

Arrow, K., C. Panosian, and H. Gelband, eds. 2004. "Saving Lives, Buying Time: Economics of Malaria Drugs in an Age of Resistance." Washington, DC: Institute of Medicine.

Balasubramanian, V. N., K. Oommen, and R. Samuel. 2000. "DOT or Not? Direct Observation of Anti-Tuberculosis Treatment and Patient Outcomes, Kerala State, India." *International Journal of Tuberculosis and Lung Disease* 4 (5): 409–13.

Baqui, A. H., R. E. Black, S. El Arifeen, M. Yunus, J. Chakraborty, S. Ahmed, and P. Vaughan. 2002. "Effect of Zinc Supplementation Started during Diarrhoea on Morbidity and Mortality in Bangladeshi Children: Community Randomised Trial." *British Medical Journal* 325 (7372): 1059.

Barker, R. D., F. J. Millard, and M. E. Nthangeni. 2002. "Unpaid Community Volunteers—Effective Providers of Directly Observed Therapy (DOT) in Rural South Africa." *South African Medical Journal* 92 (4): 291–94.

Bavestrello, L., A. Cabello, and D. Casanova. 2002. "Impact of Regulatory Measures in the Trends of Community Consumption of Antibiotics in Chile" (in Spanish). *Revista Medica de Chile* 130 (11): 1265–72.

Bergstrom, C. T., M. Lipsitch, and J. E. McGowan Jr. 2000. "Nomenclature and Methods for Studies of Antimicrobial Switching (Cycling)." Paper prepared for the Conference on Antibiotic Resistance: Global Policies and Options, Harvard University, Cambridge, MA.

Berkley, J. A., I. Mwangi, C. J. Ngetsa, S. Mwarumba, B. S. Lowe, K. Marsh, and C. R. Newton. 2001. "Diagnosis of Acute Bacterial Meningitis in Children at a District Hospital in Sub-Saharan Africa." *Lancet* 357 (9270): 1753–57.

Bexell, A., E. Lwando, B. von Hofsten, S. Tembo, B. Eriksson, and V. K. Diwan. 1996. "Improving Drug Use through Continuing Education: A Randomized Controlled Trial in Zambia." *Journal of Clinical Epidemiology* 49 (3): 355–57.

Bhutta, T. I., and C. Balchin. 1996. "Assessing the Impact of a Regulatory Intervention in Pakistan." *Social Science and Medicine* 42 (8): 1195–202.

Bonhoeffer, S., M. Lipsitch, and B. R. Levin. 1997. "Evaluating Treatment Protocols to Prevent Antibiotic Resistance." *Proceedings of the National Academy of Sciences, U.S.A.* 94: 12106–11.

Bosu, W. K., and D. Ofori-Adjei. 2000. "An Audit of Prescribing Practices in Health Care Facilities of the Wassa West District of Ghana." *West African Journal of Medicine* 19 (4): 298–303.

Boulanger, L. L., L. A. Lee, and A. Odhacha. 1999. "Treatment in Kenyan Rural Health Facilities: Projected Drug Costs Using the WHO-UNICEF Integrated Management of Childhood Illness (IMCI) Guidelines." *Bulletin of the World Health Organization* 77 (10): 852–58.

Bronzwaer, S., O. Cars, U. Buchholz, S. Molstad, W. Goettsch, I. K. Veldhuijzen, and others. 2002. "A European Study on the Relationship between Antimicrobial Use and Antimicrobial Resistance." *Emerging Infectious Diseases* 8 (3): 278–82.

Carey, B., and B. Cryan. 2003. "Antibiotic Misuse in the Community—A Contributor to Resistance?" *Irish Medical Journal* 96 (2): 43–44, 46.

Carmeli, Y., G. Eliopoulos, E. Mozaffari, and M. Samore. 2002. "Health and Economic Outcomes of Vancomycin-Resistant Enterococci." *Archives of Internal Medicine* 162 (19): 2223–28.

Cell. 1997. Global spread of chloroquine-resistant strains of P. falciparum. [cover graph.] 91 (5).

Chakraborty, S., S. A. D'Souza, and R. S. Northrup. 2000. "Improving Private Practitioner Care of Sick Children: Testing New Approaches in Rural Bihar." *Health Policy and Planning* 15 (4): 400–7.

Chalker, J. 2001. "Improving Antibiotic Prescribing in Hai Phong Province, Viet Nam: The 'Antibiotic-Dose' Indicator." *Bulletin of the World Health Organization* 79 (4): 313–20.

Chan, F. K., J. J. Sung, P. Y. Tan, K. H. Khong, and J. W. Lau. 1997. "'Blister Pack'–Induced Gastrointestinal Hemorrhage." *American Journal of Gastroenterology* 92 (1): 172–73.

Chaulet, P., M. Raviglione, and F. Bustreo. 1996. "Epidemiology, Control and Treatment of Multidrug-Resistant Tuberculosis." *Drugs* 52 (Suppl. 2): 103–8.

Chuc, N. T., M. Larsson, N. T. Do, V. K. Diwan, G. B. Tomson, and T. Falkenberg. 2002. "Improving Private Pharmacy Practice: A Multi-Intervention Experiment in Hanoi, Vietnam." *Journal of Clinical Epidemiology* 55 (11): 1148–55.

CIA (U.S. Central Intelligence Agency). 1999. *The Global Infectious Disease Threat and Its Implications for the United States.* Washington, DC: Central Intelligence Agency.

Coast, J., R. Smith, A. M. Karcher, P. Wilton, and M. Millar. 2002. "Superbugs II: How Should Economic Evaluation Be Conducted for Interventions Which Aim to Contain Antimicrobial Resistance?" *Health Economics* 11 (7): 637–47.

Cohn, M. L., C. Kovitz, U. Oda, and G. Middlebrook. 1954. "Studies on Isoniazid and Tubercle Bacilli: II. The Growth Requirements, Catalase Activities, and Pathogenic Properties of Isoniazid-Resistant Mutants." *American Review of Tuberculosis* 70 (4): 641–64.

Cohn, M. L., G. Middlebrook, and W. F. Russell Jr. 1959. "Combined Drug Treatment of Tuberculosis: Prevention of Emergence of Mutant Populations of Tubercle Bacilli Resistant to Both Streptomycin and Isoniazid in Vitro." *Journal of Clinical Investigation* 38 (8): 1349–55.

Cunin, P., E. Tedjouka, Y. Germani, C. Ncharre, R. Bercion, J. Morvan, and P. M. V. Martin. 1999. "An Epidemic of Bloody Diarrhea: Escherichia Coli O157 Emerging in Cameroon?" *Emerging Infectious Diseases* 5 (2): 285–90.

Curtis, V., and S. Cairncross. 2003. "Effect of Washing Hands with Soap on Diarrhoea Risk in the Community: A Systematic Review." *Lancet Infectious Diseases* 3 (5): 275–81.

Denis, M. B. 1998. "Improving Compliance with Quinine + Tetracycline for Treatment of Malaria: Evaluation of Health Education Interventions in Cambodian Villages." *Bulletin of the World Health Organization* 76 (Suppl 1): 43–49.

Ding, J., Y. Ma, Z. Gong, and Y. Chen. 1999. "A Study on the Mechanism of the Resistance of Shigellae to Fluoroquinolones" (in Chinese). *Zhonghua Nei Ke Za Zhi* 38: 550–53.

Drobniewski, F. A., and Y. M. Balabanova. 2002. "The Diagnosis and Management of Multiple-Drug-Resistant-Tuberculosis at the Beginning of the New Millenium." *International Journal of Infectious Diseases* 6 (Suppl 1): S21–31.

Duse, A. G., and R. A. Smego. 1999. "Challenges Posed by Antimicrobial Resistance in Developing Countries." *Baillière's Clinical Infectious Diseases—Antibiotic Resistance,* 5 (2): 193–201.

Dye, C., and M. A. Espinal. 2001. "Will Tuberculosis Become Resistant to All Antibiotics?" *Proceedings of the Royal Society of London, Series B, Biological Science* 268 (1462): 45–52.

Dye, C., C. J. Watt, D. M. Bleed, and B. G. Williams. 2003. "What Is the Limit to Case Detection under the DOTS Strategy for Tuberculosis Control?" *Tuberculosis (Edinburgh)* 83 (1–3): 35–43.

Dye, C., B. G. Williams, M. A. Espinal, and M. C. Raviglione. 2002. "Erasing the World's Slow Stain: Strategies to Beat Multidrug-Resistant Tuberculosis." *Science* 295 (5562): 2042–46.

Elbasha, E. 1999. "Deadweight Loss of Bacterial Resistance Due to Overtreatment." U.S. Centers for Disease Control and Prevention, Atlanta.

Emborg, H. D., J. S. Andersen, A. M. Seyfarth, S. R. Andersen, J. Boel, and H. C. Wegener. 2003. "Relations between the Occurrence of Resistance to Antimicrobial Growth Promoters among Enterococcus Faecium Isolated from Broilers and Broiler Meat." *International Journal of Food Microbiology* 84 (3): 273–84.

Espinal, M. A., C. Dye, M. Raviglione, and A. Kochi. 1999. "Rational 'DOTS Plus' for the Control of MDR-TB." *International Journal of Tuberculosis and Lung Disease* 3 (7): 561–63.

Espinal, M. A., S. J. Kim, P. G. Suarez, K. M. Kam, A. G. Khomenko, G. B. Migliori, and others. 2000. "Standard Short-Course Chemotherapy for Drug-Resistant Tuberculosis: Treatment Outcome in Six Countries." *Journal of the American Medical Association* 283 (19): 2537–45.

Farmer, P., M. Becerra, and J. Kim, eds. 1999. *The Global Impact of Drug-Resistant Tuberculosis.* Boston: Harvard Medical School and Open Society Institute.

Feikin, D. R., S. F. Dowell, O. C. Nwanyanwu, K. P. Klugman, P. N. Kazembe, L. M. Barat, and others. 2000. "Increased Carriage of Trimethoprim/Sulfamethoxazole-Resistant *Streptococcus Pneumoniae* in Malawian Children after Treatment for Malaria with Sulfadoxine/Pyrimethamine." *Journal of Infectious Diseases* 181 (4): 1501–5.

Fidler, D. P. 1998. "Legal Issues Associated with Antimicrobial Drug Resistance." *Emerging Infectious Diseases* 4: 169–77.

Fischl, M. A., R. B. Uttamchandani, G. L. Daikos, R. B. Poblete, J. N. Moreno, R. R. Reyes, and others. 1992. "An Outbreak of Tuberculosis Caused by Multiple-Drug-Resistant Tubercle Bacilli among Patients with HIV Infection." *Annals of Internal Medicine* 117: 177–83.

Fujiwara, P. I., S. V. Cook, C. M. Rutherford, J. T. Crawford, S. E. Glickman, B. N. Kreiswirth, and others. 1997. "A Continuing Survey of Drug-Resistant Tuberculosis, New York City, April 1994." *Archives of Internal Medicine* 10 (157): 531–36.

Garcia-Garcia, M. L., A. Ponce-de-Leon, M. E. Jimenez-Corona, A. Jimenez-Corona, M. Palacios-Martinez, S. Balandrano-Campos, and others. 2000. "Clinical Consequences and Transmissibility of Drug-Resistant Tuberculosis in Southern Mexico." *Archives of Internal Medicine* 160: 630–36.

Gerding, D. N. 2000. "Antimicrobial Cycling: Lessons Learned from the Aminoglycoside Experience." *Infection Control and Hospital Epidemiology* 21 (Suppl.): S10–12.

Goble, M., M. D. Iseman, L. A. Madsen, D. Waite, L. Ackerson, and C. R. Horsburgh Jr. 1993. "Treatment of 171 Patients with Pulmonary Tuberculosis Resistant to Isoniazid and Rifampin." *New England Journal of Medicine* 328 (8): 527–32.

Goff, B. J., J. M. Koff, and J. A. Geiling. 2002. "Obtaining Antibiotics without a Prescription." *New England Journal of Medicine* 347 (3): 223.

Gonzalez Ochoa, E., L. Armas Perez, J. R. Bravo Gonzalez, J. Cabrales Escobar, R. Rosales Corrales, and G. Abreu Suarez. 1996. "Prescription of Antibiotics for Mild Acute Respiratory Infections in Children." *Bulletin of the Pan American Health Organization* 30 (2): 106–17.

Gove, S. 1997. "Integrated Management of Childhood Illness by Outpatient Health Workers: Technical Basis and Overview. The WHO Working Group on Guidelines for Integrated Management of the Sick Child." *Bulletin of the World Health Organization* 75 (Suppl. 1): 7–24.

Greenberg, A. E., M. Ntumbanzondo, N. Ntula, L. Mawa, J. Howell, and F. Davachi. 1989. "Hospital-Based Surveillance of Malaria-Related Paediatric Morbidity and Mortality in Kinshasa, Zaire." *Bulletin of the World Health Organization* 67 (2): 189–96.

Gupta, R., J. Y. Kim, M. A. Espinal, J. M. Cauldron, B. Pecoul, P. E. Farmer, and M. C. Raviglione. 2001. "Responding to Market Failures in Tuberculosis Control." *Science* 293 (5532): 1049–51.

Hadiyono, J. E., S. Suryawati, S. S. Danu, Sunartono, and B. Santoso. 1996. "Interactional Group Discussion: Results of a Controlled Trial Using a Behavioral Intervention to Reduce the Use of Injections in Public Health Facilities." *Social Science and Medicine* 42 (8): 1177–83.

Hayes, D. J., and H. H. Jensen. 2003. "Lessons from the Danish Ban on Feed-Grade Antibiotics." *Choices* (3rd quarter): 1–6.

Helitzer-Allen, D. L., D. A. McFarland, J. J. Wirima, and A. P. Macheso. 1993. "Malaria Chemoprophylaxis Compliance in Pregnant Women: A Cost-Effectiveness Analysis of Alternative Interventions." *Social Science & Medicine* 36 (4): 403–7.

Ho, P. L., W. C. Yam, T. K. Cheung, W. W. Ng, T. L. Que, D. N. Tsang, and others. 2001. "Fluoroquinolone Resistance among Streptococcus Pneumoniae in Hong Kong Linked to the Spanish 23F Clone." *Emerging Infectious Diseases* 7 (5): 906–8.

Hoge, C. W., L. Bodhidatta, C. Tungtaem, and P. Echeverria. 1995. "Emergence of Nalidixic Acid Resistant Shigella Dysenteriae Type 1 in Thailand: An Outbreak Associated with Consumption of a Coconut Milk Dessert." *International Journal of Epidemiology* 24 (6): 1228–32.

Holmberg, S. D., S. L. Solomon, and P. A. Blake. 1987. "Health and Economic Impacts of Antimicrobial Resistance." *Reviews of Infectious Diseases* 9 (6): 1065–78.

Holmstrom, K., S. Gräslund, A. Wahlström, S. Poungshompoo, B.-E. Bengtsson, and N. Kautsky. 2003. "Antibiotic Use in Shrimp Farming and Implications for Environmental Impacts and Human Health." *International Journal of Food Science and Technology* 38 (3): 255–66.

Hu, S., W. Chen, X. Cheng, K. Chen, H. Zhou, and L. Wang. 2001. "Pharmaceutical Cost-Containment Policy: Experiences in Shanghai, China." *Health Policy and Planning* 16 (Suppl. 2): 4–9.

Igun, U. A. 1994. "Reported and Actual Prescription of Oral Rehydration Therapy for Childhood Diarrhoeas by Retail Pharmacists in Nigeria." *Social Science and Medicine* 39 (6): 797–806.

INCLEN (International Clinical Epidemiology Network). 1999. "Prospective Multicentre Hospital Surveillance of Streptococcus Pneumoniae Disease in India. Invasive Bacterial Infection Surveillance (IBIS) Group, International Clinical Epidemiology Network (INCLEN)." *Lancet* 353 (9160): 1216–21.

Indalo, A. A. 1997. "Antibiotic Sale Behaviour in Nairobi: A Contributing Factor to Antimicrobial Drug Resistance." *East African Medical Journal* 74 (3): 171–3.

Iseman, M. D., D. L. Cohn, and J. A. Sbarbaro. 1993. "Directly Observed Treatment of Tuberculosis: We Can't Afford Not to Try It." *New England Journal of Medicine* 328 (8): 576–78.

Ison, C. A., P. J. Woodford, H. Madders, and E. Claydon. 1998. "Drift in Susceptibility of Neisseria Gonorrhoeae to Ciprofloxacin and Emergence of Therapeutic Failure." *Antimicrobial Agents and Chemotherapy* 42 (11): 2919–22.

IUATLD (International Union against Tuberculosis and Lung Disease). 1998. "Guidelines for Surveillance of Drug Resistance in Tuberculosis." *International Journal of Tuberculosis and Lung Diseases* 2: 72–89.

Jacobs, M. R., D. Felmingham, P. C. Appelbaum, R. N. Grünebera, and the Alexander Project Group. 2003. "The Alexander Project 1998–2000: Susceptibility of Pathogens Isolated from Community-Acquired Respiratory Tract Infection to Commonly Used Antimicrobial Agents." *Journal of Antimicrobial Chemotherapy* 52: 229–46.

Jones, N., R. Huebner, M. Khoosal, H. Crewe-Brown, and K. Klugman. 1998. "The Impact of HIV on Streptococcus Pneumoniae Bacteraemia in a South African Population." *AIDS* 12 (16): 2177–84.

Kam, K. M., and C. W. Yip. 2001. "Surveillance of *Mycobacterium Tuberculosis* Drug Resistance in Hong Kong, 1986–1999, after the Implementation of Directly Observed Treatment." *International Journal of Tuberculosis and Lung Diseases* 5 (9): 815–23.

Kettler, H. 2000. *Narrowing the Gap between Provision and Need for Medicines in Developing Countries.* London: Office of Health Economics.

Khan, M. A., J. D. Walley, S. N. Witter, A. Imran, and N. Safdar. 2002. "Costs and Cost-Effectiveness of Different DOT Strategies for the Treatment of Tuberculosis in Pakistan: Directly Observed Treatment." *Health Policy and Planning* 17 (2): 178–86.

Khatri, G. R., and T. R. Frieden. 2002. "Rapid DOTS Expansion in India." *Bulletin of the World Health Organization* 80 (6): 457–63.

Klugman, K. P. 2001. "Efficacy of Pneumococcal Conjugate Vaccines and Their Effect on Carriage and Antimicrobial Resistance." *Lancet Infectious Diseases* 1 (2): 85–91.

Klugman, K. P., H. J. Koornhof, V. Kuhnle, S. D. Miller, P. J. Ginsburg, and A. C. Mauff. 1986. "Meningitis and Pneumonia Due to Novel Multiply Resistant Pneumococci." *British Medical Journal (Clinical Research Ed.)* 292 (6522): 730.

Kochi, A., B. Vareldzis, and K. Styblo. 1993. "Multidrug-Resistant Tuberculosis and Its Control." *Research in Microbiology* 144 (2): 104–10.

Kublin, J. G., J. F. Cortese, E. M. Njunju, R. A. Mukadam, J. J. Wirima, P. N. Kazembe, and others. 2003. "Reemergence of Chloroquine-Sensitive *Plasmodium falciparum* Malaria after Cessation of Chloroquine Use in Malawi." *Journal of Infectious Diseases* 187 (12): 1870–5.

Kurlat, I., G. Corral, F. Oliveira, G. Farinella, and E. Alvarez. 1998. "Infection Control Strategies in a Neonatal Intensive Care Unit in Argentina." *Journal of Hospital Infection* 40 (2): 149–54.

Laing, R., H. Hogerzeil, and D. Ross-Degnan. 2001. "Ten Recommendations to Improve Use of Medicines in Developing Countries." *Health Policy and Planning* 16 (1): 13–20.

Laxminarayan, R. 2002. "How Broad Should the Scope of Antibiotics Patents Be?" *American Journal of Agricultural Economics* 84 (5): 1287–92.

Laxminarayan, R., and M. L. Weitzman. 2002. "On the Implications of Endogenous Resistance to Medications." *Journal of Health Economics* 21 (4): 709–18.

le Grand, A., H. V. Hogerzeil, and F. M. Haaijer-Ruskamp. 1999. "Intervention Research in Rational Use of Drugs: A Review." *Health Policy and Planning* 14 (2): 89–102.

Legros, D., D. Ochola, N. Lwanga, and G. Guma. 1998. "Antibiotic Sensitivity of Endemic Shigella in Mbarara, Uganda." *East African Medical Journal* 75 (3): 160–1.

Levy, S. B. 1992. *The Antibiotic Paradox: How Miracle Drugs Are Destroying the Miracle.* New York: Plenum Press.

Lwilla, F., D. Schellenberg, H. Masanja, C. Acosta, C. Galindo, J. Aponte, and others. 2003. "Evaluation of Efficacy of Community-Based vs. Institutional-Based Direct Observed Short-Course Treatment for the Control of Tuberculosis in Kilombero District, Tanzania." *Tropical Medicine and International Health* 8 (3): 204–10.

Madhi, S. A., K. Petersen, A. Madhi, M. Khoosal, and K. P. Klugman. 2000. "Increased Disease Burden and Antibiotic Resistance of Bacteria Causing Severe Community-Acquired Lower Respiratory Tract Infections in Human Immunodeficiency Virus Type 1-Infected Children." *Clinical Infectious Diseases* 31 (1): 170–6.

Marin, G., L. Burhansstipanov, C. M. Connell, A. C. Gielen, D. Helitzer-Allen, K. Lorig, and others. 1995. "A Research Agenda for Health Education Among Underserved Populations." *Health Education Quarterly* 22 (3): 346–63.

Maxwell, C. A., E. Msuya, M. Sudi, K. J. Njunwa, I. A. Carneiro, and C. F. Curtis. 2002. "Effect of Community-Wide Use of Insecticide-Treated Nets for 3–4 Years on Malarial Morbidity in Tanzania." *Tropical Medicine and International Health* 7 (12): 1003–8.

McCaig, L. F., R. E. Besser, and J. M. Hughes. 2002. "Trends in Antimicrobial Prescribing Rates for Children and Adolescents." *Journal of the American Medical Association* 287 (23): 3096–102.

McGee, L., L. McDougal, J. Zhou, B. G. Spratt, F. C. Tenover, R. George, and others. 2001. "Nomenclature of Major Antimicrobial-Resistant Clones of Streptococcus Pneumoniae Defined by the Pneumococcal Molecular Epidemiology Network." *Journal of Clinical Microbiology* 39 (7): 2565–71.

McGowan, J. E. 1986. "Minimizing Antimicrobial Resistance in Hospital Bacteria: Can Switching or Cycling Drugs Help?" *Infection Control* 7: 573–76.

Mitema, E. S., G. M. Kikuvi, H. C. Wegener, and K. Stohr. 2001. "An Assessment of Antimicrobial Consumption in Food Producing Animals in Kenya." *Journal of Veterinary Pharmacology and Therapeutics* 24 (6): 385–90.

Monnet, D. L., and T. L. Sorensen. 2001. "The Patient, Their Doctor, the Regulator, and the Profit Maker: Conflicts and Possible Solutions." *Clinical Microbiology and Infection* 7 (Suppl. 6): 27–30.

Mthwalo, M., A. Wasas, R. Huebner, H. J. Koornhof, and K. P. Klugman. 1998. "Antibiotic Resistance of Nasopharyngeal Isolates of Streptococcus Pneumoniae from Children in Lesotho." *Bulletin of the World Health Organization* 76 (6): 641–50.

Mukherjee, J. S., M. L. Rich, A. R. Socci, J. K. Joseph, F. A. Viru, S. S. Shin, and others. 2004. "Programmes and Principles in Treatment of Multidrug-Resistant Tuberculosis." *Lancet* 363 (9407): 474–81.

Nosten, F., M. van Vugt, R. Price, C. Luxemburger, K. L. Thway, A. Brockman, and others. 2000. "Effects of Artesunate–Mefloquine Combination on Incidence of *Plasmodium Falciparum* Malaria and Mefloquine Resistance in Western Thailand: A Prospective Study." *Lancet* 356 (9226): 297–302.

Office of Technology Assessment. 1995. *Impact of Antibiotic-Resistant Bacteria: A Report to the U.S. Congress.* Washington, DC: U.S. Government Printing Office.

Okeke, I., and A. Lamikanra. 2001. "Quality and Bioavailability of Ampicillin Capsules in a Nigerian Semi-Urban Community." *African Journal of Medicine and Medical Sciences* 30: 47–51.

Okeke, I. N., A. Lamikanra, and R. Edelman. 1999. "Socioeconomic and Behavioral Factors Leading to Acquired Bacterial Resistance to Antibiotics in Developing Countries." *Emerging Infectious Diseases* 5 (1): 18–27.

Oluwole, D., E. Mason, and A. Costello. 2000. "Management of Childhood Illness in Africa: Early Evaluations Show Promising Results." *British Medical Journal* 320 (7235): 594–95.

Pablos-Méndez, A., D. K. Gowda, and T. R. Frieden. 2002. "Controlling Multidrug-Resistant Tuberculosis and Access to Expensive Drugs: A Rational Framework." *Bulletin of the World Health Organization* 80 (6): 489–95.

Palmer, H. M., J. P. Leeming, and A. Turner. 2001. "Investigation of an Outbreak of Ciprofloxacin-Resistant Neisseria Gonorrhoeae Using a Simplified Opa-Typing Method." *Epidemiology and Infection* 126 (2): 219–24.

Paredes, P., M. de la Pena, E. Flores-Guerra, J. Diaz, and J. Trostle. 1996. "Factors Influencing Physicians' Prescribing Behaviour in the Treatment of Childhood Diarrhoea: Knowledge May Not Be the Clue." *Social Science and Medicine* 42 (8): 1141–53.

Pechere, J. C. 2001. "Patients' Interviews and Misuse of Antibiotics." *Clinical Infectious Diseases* 33 (Suppl. 3): S170–73.

Philipson, T., and S. Mechoulan. 2003. "Intellectual Property and External Consumption Effects: Generalizations from Pharmaceutical Markets." NBER Working Paper 9598, National Bureau of Economic Research, Cambridge, MA.

Pichichero, M. E., and R. Cohen. 1997. "Shortened Course of Antibiotic Therapy for Acute Otitis Media, Sinusitis and Tonsillopharyngitis." *Pediatric Infectious Disease Journal* 16: 680–95.

Ponce-de-Leon, R. S., and M. S. Rangel-Frausto. 1993. Organising for Infection Control with Limited Resources. In *Prevention and Control of Nosocomial Infections*, ed. R. P. Wenzel. Baltimore: Williams & Wilkins.

Prazuck, T., I. Falconi, G. Morineau, V. Bricard-Pacaud, A. Lecomte, and F. Ballereau. 2002. "Quality Control of Antibiotics before the Implementation of an STD Program in Northern Myanmar." *Sexually Transmitted Diseases* 29 (11): 624–27.

Pungrassami, P., and V. Chongsuvivatwong. 2002. "Are Health Personnel the Best Choice for Directly Observed Treatment in Southern Thailand? A Comparison of Treatment Outcomes among Different Types of Observers." *Transactions of the Royal Society of Tropical Medicine and Hygiene* 96 (6): 695–99.

Pungrassami, P., S. P. Johnsen, V. Chongsuvivatwong, and J. Olsen. 2002. "Has Directly Observed Treatment Improved Outcomes for Patients with Tuberculosis in Southern Thailand?" *Tropical Medicine and International Health* 7 (3): 271–79.

Qingjun, L., D. Jihui, T. Laiyi, Z. Xiangjun, L. Jun, A. Hay, and others. 1998. "The Effect of Drug Packaging on Patients' Compliance with Treatment for Plasmodium Vivax Malaria in China." *Bulletin of the World Health Organization* 76 (Suppl. 1): 21–27.

Quale, J., D. Landman, J. Ravishankar, C. Flores, and S. Bratu. 2002. "Streptococcus Pneumoniae, Brooklyn, New York: Fluoroquinolone Resistance at Our Doorstep." *Emerging Infectious Diseases* 8 (6): 594–97.

Rhodes, G., G. Huys, J. Swings, P. McGann, M. Hiney, P. Smith, and R. W. Pickup. 2000. "Distribution of Oxytetracycline Resistance Plasmids Between Aeromonads in Hospital and Aquaculture Environments: Implication of Tn1721 in Dissemination of the Tetracycline Resistance Determinant Tet A." *Applied and Environmental Microbiology* 66 (9): 3883–90.

Rimon, M. M., S. Kheng, S. Hoyer, V. Thach, S. Ly, A. E. Permin, and S. Pieche. 2003. "Malaria Dipsticks Beneficial for IMCI in Cambodia." *Tropical Medicine and International Health* 8 (6): 536–43.

Rowe, A. K., M. S. Deming, B. Schwartz, A. Wasas, D. Rolka, H. Rolka, and others. 2000. "Antimicrobial Resistance of Nasopharyngeal Isolates of Streptococcus Pneumoniae and Haemophilus Influenzae from Children in the Central African Republic." *Pediatric Infectious Disease Journal* 19 (5): 438–44.

Rubin, R. J., C. A. Harrington, A. Poon, K. Dietrich, J. A. Greene, and A. Moiduddin. 1999. "The Economic Impact of *Staphylococcus Aureus* in New York City Hospitals." *Emerging Infectious Diseases* 5 (1).

Saez-Llorens, X., M. M. Castrejon de Wong, E. Castano, O. de Suman, D. de Moros, and I. de Atencio. 2000. "Impact of an Antibiotic Restriction Policy on Hospital Expenditures and Bacterial Susceptibilities: A Lesson from a Pediatric Institution in a Developing Country." *Pediatric Infectious Disease Journal* 19 (3): 200–6.

Sa-Leao, R., S. E. Vilhelmsson, H. de Lencastre, K. G. Kristinsson, and A. Tomasz. 2002. "Diversity of Penicillin-Nonsusceptible Streptococcus Pneumoniae Circulating in Iceland after the Introduction of Penicillin-Resistant Clone Spain(6B)-2." *Journal of Infectious Diseases* 186 (7): 966–75.

Santoso, B., S. Suryawati, and J. E. Prawaitasari. 1996. "Small Group Intervention vs. Formal Seminar for Improving Appropriate Drug Use." *Social Science and Medicine* 42 (8): 1163–68.

Sarkar, R., A. N. Chowdhuri, J. K. Dutta, H. Sehgal, and M. Mohan. 1979. "Antibiotic Resistance Pattern of Enteropathogenic E. coli Isolated from Diarrhoeal Disease in Children in Delhi." *Indian Journal of Medical Research* 70: 908–15.

Schrag, S. J., C. Pena, J. Fernandez, J. Sanchez, V. Gomez, E. Perez, and others. 2001. "Effect of Short-Course, High-Dose Amoxicillin Therapy on Resistant Pneumococcal Carriage: A Randomized Trial." *Journal of the American Medical Association* 286 (1): 49–56.

Seppala, H., T. Klaukka, J. Vuopio-Varkila, A. Muotiala, H. Helenius, K. Lager, and P. Huovinen. 1997. "The Effect of Changes in the Consumption of Macrolide Antibiotics on Erythromycin Resistance in Group A Streptococci in Finland. Finnish Study Group for Antimicrobial Resistance." *New England Journal of Medicine* 337 (7): 441–46.

Siddiqi, S., S. Hamid, G. Rafique, S. A. Chaudhry, N. Ali, S. Shahab, and R. Sauerborn. 2002. "Prescription Practices of Public and Private Health Care Providers in Attock District of Pakistan." *International Journal of Health Planning and Management* 17 (1): 23–40.

Smith, D. L., A. D. Harris, J. A. Johnson, E. K. Silbergeld, and J. G. Morris Jr. 2002. "Animal Antibiotic Use Has an Early but Important Impact on the Emergence of Antibiotic Resistance in Human Commensal Bacteria." *Proceedings of the National Academy of Sciences, U.S.A.* 99 (9): 6434–39.

Song, J. H., N. Y. Lee, S. Ichiyama, R. Yoshida, Y. Hirakata, W. Fu, and others. 1999. "Spread of Drug-Resistant *Streptococcus pneumoniae* in Asian Countries: Asian Network for Surveillance of Resistant Pathogens (ANSORP) Study." *Clinical Infectious Diseases* 28 (6): 1206–11.

Su, Xin-Zhuan, L. A. Kirkman, H. Fuzioka, and T. E. Wellems. 1997. "Complex Polymorphisms in an 330 kDa Protein are Linked to

Chloroquine-Resistant P. Falciparum in Southeast Asia and Africa." *Cell* 91: 593–603.

Suarez, P. G., K. Floyd, J. Portocarrero, E. Alarcon, E. Rapiti, G. Ramos, and others. 2002. "Feasibility and Cost-Effectiveness of Standardised Second-Line Drug Treatment for Chronic Tuberculosis Patients: A National Cohort Study in Peru." *Lancet* 359 (9322): 1980–89.

Tapsall, J. 2002. Current Concepts in the Management of Gonorrhoea. *Expert Opinion on Pharmacotherapy* 3: 147–57.

Taylor, R. B., O. Shakoor, R. H. Behrens, M. Everard, A. S. Low, J. Wangboonskul, and others. 2001. "Pharmacopoeial Quality of Drugs Supplied by Nigerian Pharmacies." *Lancet* 357 (9272): 1933–36.

Telzak, E. E., K. Sepkowitz, P. Alpert, S. Mannheimer, F. Medard, W. el-Sadr, and others. 1995. "Multidrug-Resistant Tuberculosis in Patients without HIV Infection." *New England Journal of Medicine* 333 (14): 907–11.

Trape, J. F. 2001. "The Public Health Impact of Chloroquine Resistance in Africa." *American Journal of Tropical Medicine and Hygiene* 64 (Suppl. 1–2): 12–17.

United Kingdom Government. 2001. "International Action against Child Poverty—Meeting the 2015 Targets." *Proceedings of Conference on Elimination of Child Poverty*. London, February 26, 2001.

Wammanda, R. D., C. L. Ejembi, and T. Iorliam. 2003. "Drug Treatment Costs: Projected Impact of Using the Integrated Management of Childhood Illnesses." *Tropical Doctor* 33 (2): 86–88.

Wang, H., R. Huebner, M. Chen, and K. Klugman. 1998. "Antibiotic Susceptibility Patterns of *Streptococcus pneumoniae* in China and Comparison of MICs by Agar Dilution and E-Test Methods." *Antimicrobial Agents and Chemotherapy* 42 (10): 2633–36.

Wegener, H. C., F. M. Aarestrup, L. B. Jensen, A. M. Hammerum, and F. Bager. 1999. "Use of Antimicrobial Growth Promoters in Food Animals and *Enterococcus faecium* Resistance to Therapeutic Antimicrobial Drugs in Europe." *Emerging Infectious Diseases* 5 (3): 329–35.

Wellems, T. E., and C. V. Plowe. 2001. Chloroquine-Resistant Malaria. *Journal of Infectious Diseases*. 184: 770–76.

White, D. G., S. Zhao, R. Sudler, S. Ayers, S. Friedman, S. Chen, and others. 2001. "The Isolation of Antibiotic-Resistant Salmonella from Retail Ground Meats." *New England Journal of Medicine* 345 (16): 1147–54.

White, N. J. 1998. "Preventing Antimalarial Drug Resistance Through Combinations." *Drug Research, Updates* 1: 3–9.

———. 1999. "Antimalarial Drug Resistance and Combination Chemotherapy." *Philosophical Transactions of the Royal Society of London B Series* 354: 739–49.

Whitney, C. G., M. M. Farley, J. Hadler, L. H. Harrison, N. M. Bennett, R. Lynfield, and others. 2003. "Decline in Invasive Pneumococcal Disease after the Introduction of Protein-Polysaccharide Conjugate Vaccine." *New England Journal of Medicine* 348 (18): 1737–46.

WHO (World Health Organization). 1993. *WHO-RBM Africa Malaria Report*.

———. 1994. *Tuberculosis Program: Framework for Effective Tuberculosis Control*. Geneva: WHO.

———. 1996. *Assessment of Therapeutic Efficacy of Antimalarial Drugs for Uncomplicated Falciparum Malaria in Areas of Intense Transmission*. Geneva: WHO.

———. 1997. *Guidelines for the Management of Drug-Resistant Tuberculosis*. Geneva: WHO.

———. 2000. "WHO Global Principles for the Containment of Anti-microbial Resistance in Animals Intended for Food." Report of a WHO Consultation, Geneva, WHO.

———. 2001. *WHO Global Strategy for Containment of Antimicrobial Resistance*. Geneva: WHO.

———. 2002a. *Surveillance Standards for Antimicrobial Resistance*. Geneva: WHO.

———. 2002b. *The World Health Report 2002: Reducing Risks, Promoting Healthy Life*. Geneva: WHO.

———. 2004. *The WHO/IUATLD Global Project on Anti-Tuberculosis Drug Resistance Surveillance 1999–2002: Anti-Tuberculosis Drug Resistance in the World*. Report 3. Geneva: WHO.

Wierup, M. 2001. "The Swedish Experience of the 1986 Year Ban of Antimicrobial Growth Promoters, with Special Reference to Animal Health, Disease Prevention, Productivity, and Usage of Antimicrobials." *Microbial Drug Resistance* 7 (2): 183–90.

Wilson, J. M. and G. N. Chandler. 1993. "Sustained Improvements in Hygiene Behaviour amongst Village Women in Lombok, Indonesia." *Transactions of the Royal Society of Tropical Medicine and Hygiene* 87 (6): 615–16.

Wongsrichanalai, C., J. Sirichaisinthop, J. J. Karwacki, K. Congpuong, R. S. Miller, L. Pang, and K. Thimasarn. 2001. "Drug Resistant Malaria on the Thai-Myanmar and Thai-Cambodian Borders." *Southeast Asian Journal of Tropical Medicine and Public Health*. 32: 41–49.

Xu, Q., S. G. Jin, and L. X. Zhang. 2000. "Cost Effectiveness of DOTS and Non-DOTS Strategies for Smear-Positive Pulmonary Tuberculosis in Beijing." *Biomedical and Environmental Sciences* 13 (4): 307–13.

Yang, F., Y. Zhang, and L. McGee. 2001. "Population Biology of Streptococcus Pneumoniae Carried By Healthy Children in Shanghai"(in Chinese). *Zhonghua Yi Xue Za Zhi* 81 (10): 589–92.

Zaidi, M. B., E. Zamora, P. Diaz, L. Tollefson, P. J. Fedorka-Cray, and M. L. Headrick. 2003. "Risk Factors for Fecal Quinolone-Resistant Escherichia Coli in Mexican Children." *Antimicrobial Agents and Chemotherapy* 47 (6): 1999–2001.

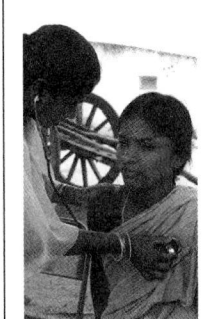

Chapter **56**

Community Health and Nutrition Programs

John B. Mason, David Sanders, Philip Musgrove, Soekirman, and Rae Galloway

Rapid improvements in health and nutrition in developing countries may be ascribed to specific, deliberate, health- and nutrition-related interventions and to changes in the underlying social, economic, and health environments. This chapter is concerned with the contribution of specific interventions, while recognizing that improved living standards in the long run provide the essential basis for improved health. Consideration of the environment as the context for interventions is crucial in determining their initiation and in modifying their effect, and it must be taken into account when assessing this effect.

Undoubtedly much change has stemmed from scientific advances, immunization being a prominent case. However, the organizational aspects of health and nutrition protection are equally critical. In the past several decades, people's contact with trained workers has been instrumental in improving health in developing countries. This factor applies particularly to poor people in poor countries but is relevant everywhere; indeed, it is a reason that social services have essentially eliminated almost all occurrences of child malnutrition in Europe (where, when malnourished children are seen, it is caused by neglect).

Community-based programs under many circumstances provide this crucial contact. Their role is partly in improving access to technology and resources, but it is also important in fostering behavior change and, more generally, in supporting caring practices (Engle, Bentley, and Pelto 2000; UNICEF 1990). Such programs may also play a part in mobilizing social demand for services and in generating pressure for policy change.

In community-based programs, workers—often volunteers and part-time workers—interact with households to protect

their health and nutrition and to facilitate access to treatment of sickness. Mothers and children are the primary focus, but others in the household should participate. Commonly, people go regularly to a central point in their community—for example, for growth monitoring and promotion—or are visited at home by a health and nutrition worker. The existence, training, support, and supervision of the community worker—based in the community or operating from a nearby health facility—are indispensable features of these programs. Thus community organizations are a key aspect of community-based health and nutrition programs (CHNPs).

This chapter focuses on large-scale (national or state) programs. Although these programs are primarily initiated and run at the local level, links with the national level and levels in between are necessary. Both horizontal and vertical organizations are needed. Local organizations make action happen, but they need input and resources, such as training, supervision, and supplies, from more central levels.

The experience on which this chapter is based comes from a considerable number of national and large-scale programs. Most of these programs include both nutrition and health activities, aimed particularly at the health and survival of reproductive-age women and children. We draw on these experiences as we try to put forward principles on which future programs can be based—programs that may have broader health objectives for other population groups and diseases.

As of 2001, some 19 percent of global deaths were among children—and 99 percent of all child deaths took place in low- and middle-income countries. The disability-adjusted life years (DALYs) lost attributed to zero- to four-year-olds—plus maternal and perinatal conditions, nutrition deficiencies, and endocrine disorders—amount to 42 percent of the total disease

Table 56.1 Estimated Contributions to the Disease Burden in Developing Countries

Factor	DALYs lost (percentage)		
	Direct effect	As risk factor	Total
General malnutrition	1.0	14.0	15.0
Micronutrient deficiencies	9.0	8.5	17.5
Total	10.0	22.5	32.5

Source: Mason, Musgrove, and Habicht 2003, table 10.

burden (all ages, both sexes) from all causes for developing regions. CHNPs address about 40 percent of the disease burden. In terms of prevention, Mason, Musgrove, and Habicht (2003) estimated that eliminating malnutrition would remove one-third of the global disease burden. Comparative studies by Ezzati, Lopez, and others (2002) and Ezzati, Vander Hoorn, and others (2003) have reemphasized malnutrition as the predominant risk factor and improvement of nutrition as playing a potentially major role in reducing the burden. Clinical deficiencies contribute directly to malnutrition, but even more, malnutrition is a risk factor for infectious diseases (table 56.1). Furthermore, changes in child malnutrition levels in developing countries are closely related to the countries' mortality trends (Pelletier and Frongillo 2003).

Dealing with women and children's health and nutrition addresses a substantial part of global health problems. Moreover, the experience of community-based programs linked to nutrition constitutes a significant part of the body of knowledge on ways of improving it. A number of large-scale, sustained health interventions, such as those described by Sanders and Chopra (2004), use a mix of improved access to facilities and community health workers. These interventions include the Comprehensive Rural Health Project, Jamkhed, India; community health projects in Brazil (Ceará, Pelotas); and the work of the Bangladesh Rural Advancement Committee (BRAC). Table 56.2 describes the program experiences drawn on.

The evidence is clear that significant differences occur between countries in the rates of change in health and nutritional status. Figure 56.1 shows a comparison of Indonesia, the Philippines, and Thailand. As is common, the indicator used is underweight children, which is likely to reflect broader conditions of health and survival. For Thailand, the figure shows the now-well-known rapid improvement in the 1980s and 1990s. For Indonesia, it shows slower but consistent improvement. The Philippines had little progress until recently, and the start of an improving trend coincided with increases in the number of village health workers and implementation of high-coverage interventions such as iodized salt and vitamin A supplementation (FNRI 2004). A crucial issue is how much of the improvements was caused by interventions that could be replicated—and within that issue is subsumed how much was because of

context, how much was programmatic, and what were the interactions. The contrasts between these three countries are instructive in part because they have several similar contextual factors; for instance, the status of women is relatively good, and social exclusion[1] is not extensive (compare both of these in, for example, South Asia). Thus programs may account for a significant part of the differences seen in improvement.

The benefits from CHNPs extend well beyond child nutrition (which is used as a summary measure). These benefits have not been quantified but would include improved educability (see chapter 49) and probably increased earning capacity associated with it and with physical fitness.

WHAT IS KNOWN ABOUT EFFICACY AND EFFECTIVENESS

The efficacy of health and nutrition interventions in developing countries has been established for decades (for example, Gwatkin, Wilcox, and Wray 1980). Prospective studies in several settings showed that health interventions with or without supplementary foods caused children to thrive and survive better: studies in Narangwal, India (Kielmann and others 1978; Taylor, Kielmann, and Parker 1978); by the Institute for Nutrition for Central America and Panama (Delgado and others 1982); in Jamaica (Waterlow 1992); and in The Gambia (Whitehead, Rowland, and Cole 1976) are examples.[2] These studies showed the effect of interventions on growth and (usually) mortality but did not generally factor out the relative contributions of health and nutrition. In fact, results from Narangwal showed similar mortality effects from food *or* health care; results from The Gambia indicated interaction such that sick children did not grow even with adequate food intake (appetite also playing an important role), and well children did not grow with inadequate food intake (Gillespie and Mason 1991, annex 2).

By the early 1980s, the conclusion, based on data at the experimental level (not from routine large-scale programs), was that better health and better nutrition are both required for child survival and development. This conclusion remains generally agreed on today; furthermore, concern exists that health interventions may become less effective unless nutrition is concurrently addressed (Measham and Chatterjee 1999; Pelletier and Frongillo 2003). In their chapter on malnutrition in the first edition of this book, Pinstrup-Andersen and colleagues (1993) drew largely on efficacy findings, with an emphasis on food supplementation. Those studies are not revisited here, but we can continue to build on their conclusions.

The efficacy studies were followed by a number of national or other large-scale programs in several countries. Some of those were a direct follow-on; for example, the World Bank Tamil Nadu Integrated Nutrition Program (TINP) followed the

Table 56.2 Country Experiences in Community-Based Programs

Country and program	Program experience
Africa	
Tanzania: Iringa	Area program with UNICEF and WHO inputs, 1984–91. After rapid initial drop in child malnutrition, moderate steady improvement. Program not sustained.
Tanzania: Child Survival and Development Program	1985–95, World Bank support. Results similar to Iringa.
Zimbabwe: Supplementary Feeding Programme	Wide-scale program following independence, 1980–90; infant mortality rate (IMR) dropped from 110 to 53 (1988). Not sustained.
Asia	
Bangladesh: Bangladesh Integrated Nutrition Program and national	BINP: area targeted covering 7 percent of population. Rapid improvement at start (1997); final evaluation not seen. National: program coverage expanding from 2000 on. Substantial improvement in anemia and child underweight seen in Bangladesh starting 1995.
Bangladesh: Bangladesh Rural Advancement Committee	Community-based health services with village health workers. Wide coverage since 1980s; particular focus on diarrhea.
India: Integrated Child Development Services	Implemented since 1976. Village program with community health (*anganwadi*) worker. Accelerated improvement reported in some states.
India: Tamil Nadu Integrated Nutrition Program	Implemented 1980 to mid 1990s. Village program in Tamil Nadu with World Bank support; growth monitoring, supplementary feeding, and so on. Substantial improvement in underweight reported.
Indonesia	Massive expansion of village programs 1975–90, covering all villages by 1990. Steady decrease in underweight during this time. Program not sustained in 1990s; now planned to restart.
Philippines: national	No wide CHNPs despite national decree in 1974. No significant improvement in child nutrition.
Thailand	National program from late 1970s; 600,000 village health volunteers trained (1 percent of population). Rapid improvement 1980–90; for example, 36 percent to 13 percent underweight children.
Americas	
Costa Rica	Expanding rural health services from 1970s following malaria control. Rapid fall in IMR, 1965–80; in stunting, 1979–89.
Jamaica	Expanded health services with community health aides from mid 1970s. Rapid fall in underweight, 1985–89.
Nicaragua	Community health movement, 1979–90, reduced IMR, eliminated polio; about 1 percent of population as village health volunteers.

Source: Authors, from data derived as follows: *Tanzania*—Gillespie and Mason 1991; Gillespie, Mason, and Martorell 1996; Jennings and others 1991, 117; Kavishe and Mushi 1993; Pelletier 1991; Sanders 1999; *Zimbabwe*—Sanders 1999; Tagwireyi and Greiner 1994; Werner and Sanders 1997; *Bangladesh*—BINP and UNICEF 1999; BRAC 2004; Chowdhury 2003; INFS and Department of Economics, University of Dhaka 1998; Mason and others 1999, 2001; Save the Children U.K. 2003; *India*—Administrative Staff College of India 1997; Mason and others 1999, 2001; Measham and Chatterjee 1999; Reddy and others 1992; Shekar 1989; *Indonesia*—Berg 1987; Jennings and others 1991, 108; Rohde 1993; Soekirman and others 1992; *the Philippines*—Guillermo-Tuazon and Briones 1997; Heaver and Hunt 1995; Heaver and Mason 2000; Mason 2003; *Thailand*—Kachondam, Winichagoon, and Tontisirin 1992; Tontisirin and Winichagoon 1999; Winichagoon and others 1992; *Costa Rica*—Horwitz 1987; Jennings and others 1991, 77–81; Muñoz and Scrimshaw 1995; *Honduras*—Fiedler 2003; *Jamaica*—ACC/SCN 1989, 1996; P. Samuda personal communication, 2004; Robinson personal communication, 2004; *Nicaragua*—Sanders 1985; Werner and Sanders 1997.

Narangwal study, which was supported by the U.S. Agency for International Development (USAID). A number of overviews and analyses of these programs have been conducted—for example, Allen and Gillespie (2001); Berg (1981, 1987); Gillespie, Mason, and Martorell (1996; includes a summary of overviews, 60); Gillespie, McLachlan, and Shrimpton (2003); Jennings and others (1991); Mason (2000); Sanders (1999); and Shrimpton (1989). These plus some newer examples provide case studies for this chapter, and the sources for the case studies are included in table 56.2.

Underweight prevalences are improving at about 0.5 percentage points (ppts) per year except in Sub-Saharan Africa, which is largely static (ACC/SCN 1989, 1992, 1996, 1998, 2004). Programs are needed to accelerate this trend. Cost data

from an earlier study (Gillespie and Mason 1991, 76), combined with the estimated improvements from large-scale programs, led to the assertion that "there seems to be some convergence on around $5 to $10 per head (beneficiary) per year being a workable, common level of expenditure in nutrition programmes, though not generally including supplementary food costs . . . effective programmes, with these levels of expenditure, seem to be associated with reducing underweight prevalences by around 1–2 percentage points per year" (Gillespie, Mason, and Martorell 1996, 69–70).

A further important consideration is that the effect is likely to be nonlinearly related to the expenditure, showing the familiar dose-response S-shaped curve. Thus, the first expenditures produce little effect on the outcome, and one needs a minimum

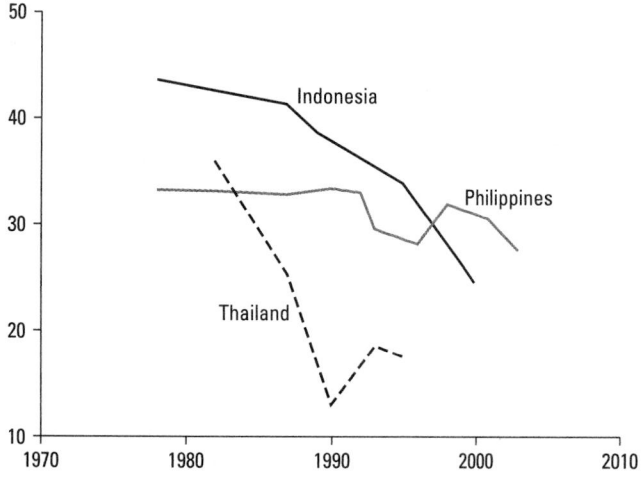

Prevalences of underweight children (percent)

Sources: ACC/SCN 2004; FNRI 2004; Mason, Rivers, and Helwig 2005.
Note: −2 standard deviations NCHS/WHO standards; ages 0–60 months.

Figure 56.1 Comparison of Trends in Underweight Children in Indonesia, the Philippines, and Thailand

input level of resource use before a worthwhile response is achieved (Habicht, Mason, and Tabatabai 1984). This factor generally applies to drawing inferences from cost-effectiveness ratios, which often assume linearity. If the relation *is* S-shaped, the implication is important: applying too few resources does not simply solve the problem more slowly but does not solve it at all and is a waste. Therefore, program intensity (resources per person) is a critical measure.

Effective interventions must include a range of activities relating to health and nutrition. They should be multifaceted, not just for effectiveness but also for organizational efficiency. The structure needed for community-based programs could never make sense or be sustainably set up for single interventions alone. One often-argued case (for example, by Save the Children U.K. 2003) concerns children's growth monitoring: evidently growth monitoring in isolation from activities that *improve* children's growth is not going to achieve anything (or worse, considering the opportunity cost); however, weighing children and charting their weight can be a useful part of broader programs (for example, as growth monitoring and promotion).

COMMUNITY- AND FACILITY-BASED PROGRAMS

Protecting and improving health, especially in poor communities, requires a combination of community- and facility-based activities, with support from central levels of organization, as well as some centrally run programs (for example, food fortification). The place of these activities in a strategy is likely to vary, depending on level of development (of infrastructure, health services, and socioeconomic status) and on many local factors. For the poorest societies, the first priorities are basic

preventive services, notably immunization, access to basic drugs, and management of the most serious threats to health, such as some access to emergency care. Moving up the development scale, starting community-based activities may soon become cost effective for prevention, referral, and management of some diseases (notably diarrhea) when coverage of health services is poor. Community-based programs continue to play a key role until health services, education, income, and communications have improved to the point that maternal and child mortality has fallen substantially and malnutrition is much reduced; at this intermediate development level, the needs are less felt, and health services again take on a more prominent role. In this scheme, the widely felt need for better access to emergency obstetric services is problematic, requiring a well-developed human and physical infrastructure, yet arguably being one of the highest priorities.

Facility-based programs can be seen either as linking with the community program (referrals, home visits from clinics, and so forth) or as actually being part of the same enterprise. A distinction is that community-based activities take place outside the health facility, in the home or at a community central point, even if they may be supported by health personnel based in health facilities. The local workers in community-based programs may be drawn from the community itself, may be home visitors from a health center or clinic, or may sometimes be volunteers supervised by these home visitors. Many community-based programs come under the health sector, whatever the exact arrangements with local health services. Regarding specific program components, we return to the relative role of community programs and facilities later.

The integrated management of infant and childhood illness (IMCI) program provides guidance mainly on the curative health aspects and contains a number of nutrition activities (for example, administration of vitamin A capsules). Links to local health facilities are essential for the maintenance of the community activities and for referral in cases of illness (see chapter 63). As the IMCI training and implementation progresses, it should integrate directly with CHNPs (in fact, become part of the same exercise), which will add treatment of additional diseases. IMCI addresses diarrhea, acute respiratory infection (ARI), malaria, nutrition, immunization, safe motherhood, and essential drugs (WHO 1997). The 16 key practices for child survival defined in the context of IMCI (Kelley and Black 2001, S115) are exactly those to be promoted within CHNPs, and most are already included (four are nutritional).

Decentralization should be considered in this context. Although decentralized systems might be thought to be more effective in supporting CHNPs, the evidence for this assumption is scarce. Decentralization can reduce resources available at the local level if it involves devolving responsibility without the concomitant budgetary resources (Mills 1994). For example, in Kenya, decentralization did not accompany devolving authority for raising revenue locally. In other cases (for example, the Philippines), decentralization has involved a shifting of resources, but with priorities set in the local government units by locally elected officials (municipal and city mayors), these resources may be used for shorter-term priorities than under previous, centrally decided, policies.

SUCCESS FACTORS

A number of useful concepts grew in the 1990s in relation to effective community-based programs. The concept of success factors helped sort out complex interactions: when numerous possibilities exist, understanding the successful pathway to effectiveness is more important than trying to disentangle what did not work. Focusing on successful programs helps simplify complexity and identify success factors, only some of which are

programmatic (directly under the influence of the intervention itself); others are contextual.

The importance of context, within which programs are initiated and run, thus emerged as crucial, and priority factors were proposed from studies of community-based programs in Asia (Gillespie, Mason, and Martorell 1996, 67; Jonsson 1997). Sanders (1999) described similar concepts under the headings of *community participation* and *political will*. This distinction and interplay between context and program factors is helpful in identifying required supporting policies to improve the context to make programs work. Details are in the later section titled "Contextual Factors."

An overall framework (figure 56.2) for causal links to child survival and nutrition, put forward by the United Nations Children's Fund (UNICEF 1990), gave a basis for a common language—even if the details might be questioned—revolving

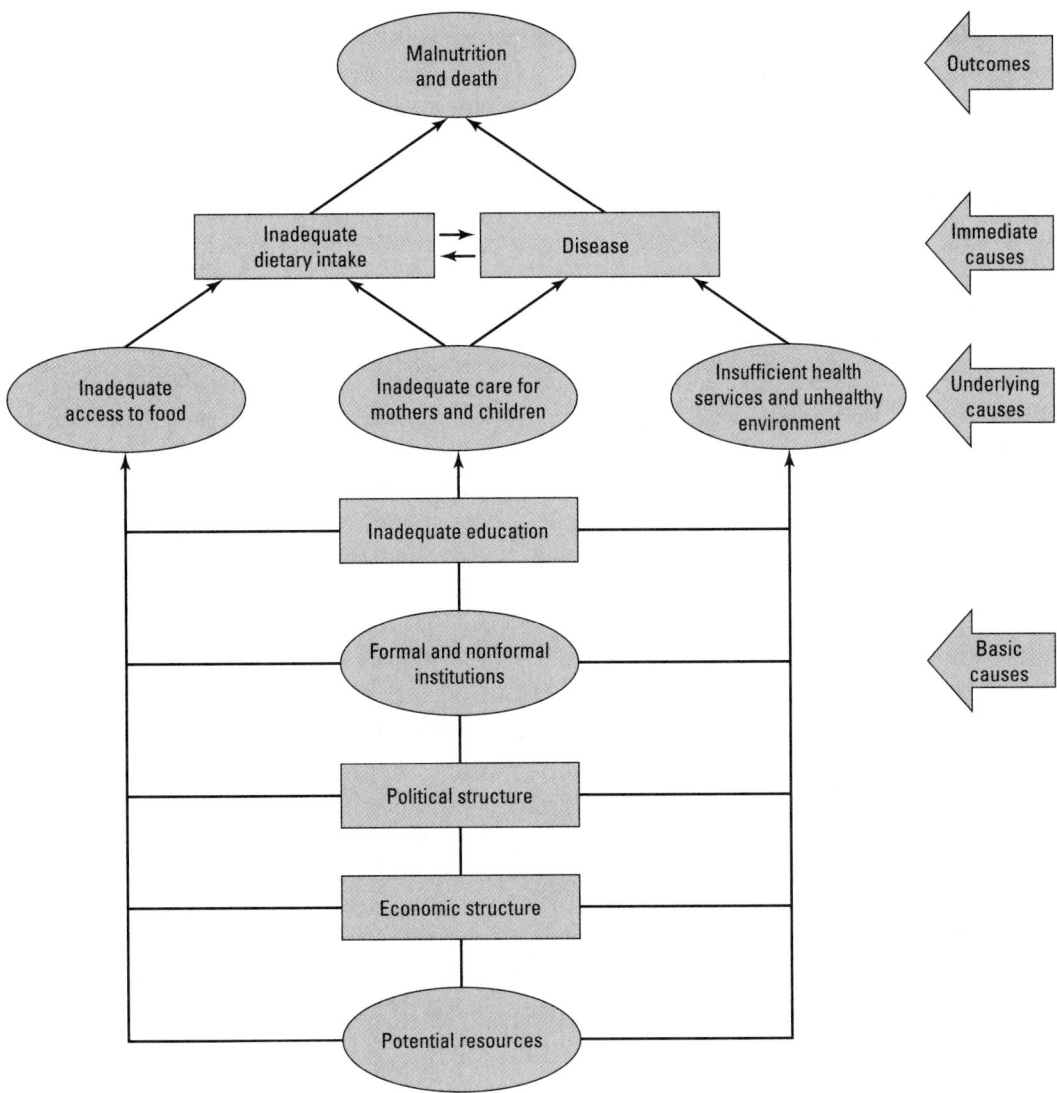

Source: Redrawn from UNICEF 1990.

Figure 56.2 Conceptual Framework for the Causes of Malnutrition in Society

around food, health, and care as proximal causes to be addressed through programs. Improving these factors attacks hunger, disease, and neglect, which are the converse of food, health, and care. Basic causes are, like context, open to influence through policy decisions and acting through directly influencing food, health, and care and by modifying the effect of programs. Here malnutrition is seen as the outcome of processes in society, and direct interventions are seen as both shortcutting the needed basic improvements in living conditions and being dependent on these improvements in the long run for sustainability.

COMMUNITY-BASED PROGRAMS—WHAT ARE THEY?

Community health and nutrition programs are often initiated and run by the health sector, but sometimes a separate ministry (for example, in India and Indonesia) or service (for example, in Bangladesh) is set up. Attempts to use a national coordinating body appear to be less effective in leading to widespread community programs; an example existed in the Philippines until approximately 2000 (Heaver and Mason 2000). This ineffectiveness stems from the tendency of the coordinating body not to have direct authority over fieldworkers or the budget to create a national program with sufficient coverage and intensity to have a measurable effect. In some other cases, the services linked to poverty alleviation and social welfare programs can play this role (for example, the Samurdhi program in Sri Lanka). Involvement of the health services remains crucial, sometimes as the operational agency responsible for the programs and certainly always for referral.

CHNPs have so far been much more relevant to communicable diseases than to noncommunicable diseases in conditions of poverty and where undernutrition is common. (An exception occurs if CHNPs help prevent intrauterine growth retardation with later risks of noncommunicable diseases.) However, in areas where diet-related chronic diseases are developing in conditions of poverty (for example, much of Latin America and the Caribbean) and obesity is rising rapidly, the promotion of behavior change through counseling in CHNPs may become increasingly important. Promoting healthier diets requires access to outlets for fruit and vegetables, often displaced by fast foods, which should be a concern of community activities, as should lifestyle improvements such as use of exercise and recreational facilities.

CHNPs often include activities well beyond direct prevention and behavior change. As envisaged with primary health care, water, sanitation, and other aspects of environmental health are frequently included, as well as agricultural interventions (for example, Zimbabwe in the 1980s). In Thailand, the village programs are part of the "Basic Minimum Needs" approach, which includes housing and environment, family planning, community participation, and spiritual and ethical development.

A diagram of the structure, derived from Thailand's program (figure 56.3), shows the relations between services that provide supervision and contacts with the community ("facilitators") and with community workers, referred to as "mobilizers."

The activities undertaken in CHNPs—the program content—are familiar and are described here only briefly. Program components, implemented by village workers or in facilities, come under the following headings, which form a menu, with the actual mix depending on local capabilities and conditions (UNICEF 1998, 84; see chapter 24):

- *Prenatal care* includes checking weight gain in pregnancy, prepregnancy weight, anemia, and blood pressure; providing multiple micronutrient supplementation and immunization (tetanus); counseling on diet, workload, breastfeeding; and predicting and arranging for delivery.
- *Women's health and nutrition* entails counseling on health and nutrition and checkups, promoting improved status and resource allocation in home and outside, promoting improved access to health services, and often offering family-planning services (these services may even be an initiating factor for CHNPs, for example, in Indonesia).
- *Breastfeeding* includes providing knowledge on practices (initial, exclusive, continued); arranging mutual support; building confidence; preventing misinformation and undermining factors; facilitating time for breastfeeding; and providing information along the lines of the infant formula code.
- *Complementary feeding* includes providing knowledge and counseling (timing of introduction, type, energy density, frequency, and so on); sometimes promoting village or urban area production of weaning foods; sometimes marketing inexpensive food; facilitating mother's time allocation; and promoting technology—storage, preservation, hygiene methods (fermentation, even refrigerators).
- *Growth monitoring and promotion* requires equipment (scales, charts, manuals); training and supervision; needs training of weigher to interpret charts and counsel mother; and a referral system for problems (for treatment, counseling, or other preventive intervention if growth is faltering). Weighing at birth and monthly weighing should be included, if possible, and adequate weight gain (rather than achieved weight or any gain) should be used for guidance on counseling or other intervention.
- *Micronutrient supplementation* should include vitamin A for nonpregnant and pregnant women (low dose weekly, preferably as part of multinutrients); for women within one month of delivery (massive dose to protect infant through breast milk); for infants and children (massive dose at nine months immunization contact and thereafter every six months and when medically indicated). It should also

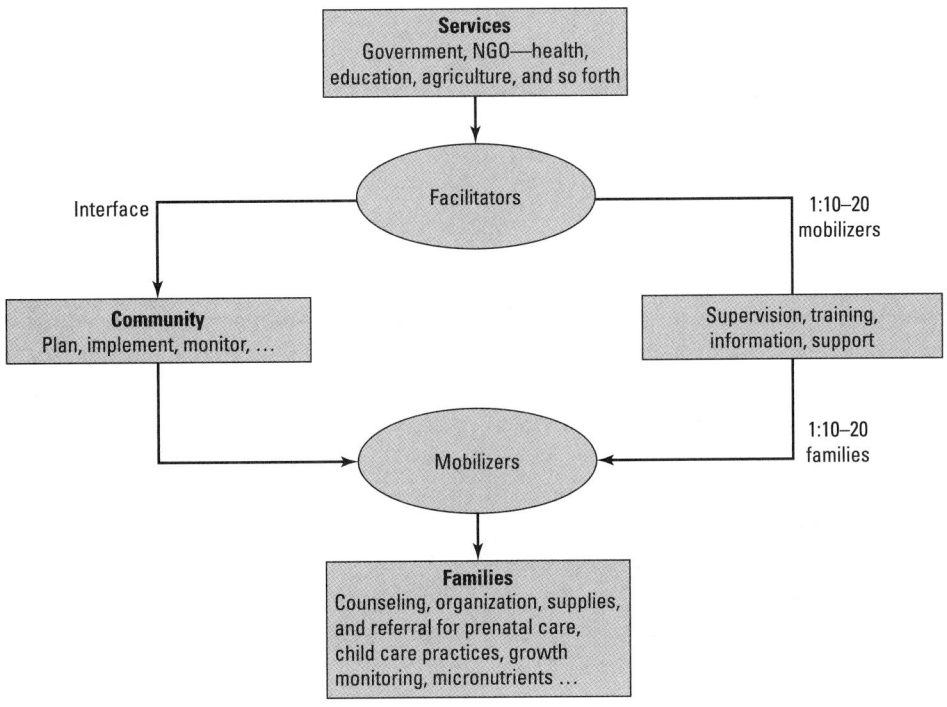

Source: Adapted from Tontisirin (1996, personal communication).

NGO = nongovernmental organization

Figure 56.3 General Structure for Community-Based Programs, Based on Thailand's Program

include vitamin A—daily or weekly, with immunization campaigns, and so forth—and iron—daily or weekly for women (especially during pregnancy) as well as for children and adolescents. Iron is usually provided together with folic acid and may also be provided as part of multiple micronutrient supplementation. Iodine is usually provided by fortification and can be an infrequent (six-monthly) oral supplement, if necessary, but it should be part of multiple micronutrients for pregnancy.

- *Micronutrient fortification* is not usually included locally, although it is an important central program, but local monitoring is a coming opportunity, especially of iodized salt testing kits.
- *Supplementary feeding, using external supplies* may sometimes be appropriate in emergencies and in conditions of extreme poverty (for example, the Bangladesh Integrated Nutrition Program, or BINP), providing 200 to 500 kilocalories per person per day, but otherwise it is to be avoided as costly, with high opportunity cost, and not very effective; moreover, it can distort programs, which come to be seen largely as a source of free food.
- *Supplementary feeding, using local supplies* can be useful for complementary feeding (weaning) if carefully organized (which requires some resources). Village community production and processing are useful, if feasible (for example, in Zimbabwe), and the system can move to coupon method (for example, in Thailand).

- *Oral rehydration* includes highly effective local preparations for dehydration in acute diarrhea, as well as (or better than) oral rehydration salts. These preparations require counseling of mothers and take a lot of parents' time. Persistent diarrhea requires other intervention, especially nutritional. Care of children during sickness—especially continued breastfeeding and other foods—needs to be stressed (applies also to other illnesses).
- *Immunization* includes informing, referring, and facilitating.
- *Deworming* requires distribution and dosage supervision of mebendazole every few months, a highly effective nutrition intervention. Distribution methods are an issue.

The relative suitability of community- and facility-based operations for the different components again depends on local conditions, and these operations should be complementary. Community activities are essential for infant and child feeding, other caring practices, environmental sanitation, and the like. Facilities have a key role in immunization, prenatal care, and—of course—referral for treatment. Growth monitoring, micronutrient interventions, oral rehydration, and similar activities may be focused in either. Because it has more regular contact with clients, a community-based program may be more effective in actually reaching mothers and children with the component interventions than one that is facility based. Box 56.1 compares two programs in Honduras that offered the same content but differed in where the programs were based.

PROGRAMMATIC FACTORS

Programmatic factors are considered first in terms of the characteristics of the activities—their population coverage and targeting, how much resources are applied per head (intensity), and the technologies used. Then the needs for initiating and sustaining these activities are discussed—the training needs, supervision methods, and (importantly) incentives and remuneration for field workers.

Coverage, Targeting, Resource Intensity, and Technology

Even effective programs improve the health and nutrition only of those they reach, so achieving as complete coverage as possible of those at risk is a major determinant of the effect. Although variations in the content of programs are seen in different circumstances, most activities are common to most programs. Variations in effect stem from factors such as coverage and adequacy of resources. How have CHNPs fared in reaching large sections of the population with adequate resources—and, indeed, what is the gap that would need to be filled? The achievements of the 14 programs drawn on here as case studies are summarized in table 56.3.

The programs expanded to include most of the communities within the areas targeted. The common evolution was to target select areas and specific biological groups within those areas—generally women and children—but not to give priority to any great extent to poorer or less healthy communities. Screening is sometimes done of individuals for admittance into the programs (a form of targeting), based on nutritional status, as in growth monitoring and promotion, as well as on a one-time basis (for example, thin children in Zimbabwe). Recent thinking suggests that because mortality risk, growth failure, and morbidity are concentrated in children less than two or three years of age, in contrast to an earlier focus on children under five, these younger children should increasingly be a focus of CHNPs. A common policy observed in practice, therefore, is to aim for complete coverage within the areas participating, adding new sites until the entire region is covered. Relatively untargeted expansion to universal coverage may have been at the expense of establishing adequate resources and quality in the areas initially covered. In at least one case (Thailand), having achieved broad coverage and reduced malnutrition, the program became more targeted to areas in which progress was lagging. The coverage figures in table 56.3, although approximate, demonstrate considerable success in initiating and implementing CHNPs on a large scale—usually enough to have a substantial effect if the other factors needed for success were met.

How complete a coverage of the population should one recommend? This factor relates to targeting, to the additional resource requirements to reach the nonparticipants, and to their level of risk. Usually risk is spread throughout the population, although the extent varies considerably—at least a doubling of indicators of risk is usually seen between better- and worse-off areas or groups (for example, see Mason and others 2001, figures 1.4–1.7, 1.10–1.13). The remoter areas—or

Table 56.3 Characteristics of Selected Programs

Country	Coverage, targeting	Resources, intensity
Africa		
Tanzania: Iringa F: (+)	Population served = 250,000 in 6 districts, 610 villages, 46,000 children, of which 33,700 participated (73 percent). Targeting: children < 5 years and women; no socioeconomic selection of communities. Progressed from 168 to 610 villages 1984–88.	US$8 to US$17/child/year (approximately US$30/child/year from total costs: approximately US$6 million) 2 village health workers/village = 1,220 total; approximately 1:40 children [Volunteers]
Tanzania: Child Survival and Development Program F: 0	9 of 20 regions (population total approximately 12 million; 2 million children). Aimed for complete coverage.	US$2 to US$3/child/year [Volunteers]
Zimbabwe: Supplementary Feeding Programme F: ++	Population served: 56,000–96,000 with supplementary feeding; up to 60 percent of all children in community-based growth monitoring.	External: US$3 million over 10 years For example, 1990, US$0.5 million, approximately US$0.50/child/year (Approximately 1:10–200, based on numbers per project) [Extension agents]
Asia		
Bangladesh: BINP F: +	BINP: in 6 *thanas*, or subdistricts (7 percent of population), children < 2 years, 8 million pregnant and lactating women.	US$14 million/year; approximately US$18/child/year 1 community worker per 1,000 population Approximately 1:200 children [Project supported]
Bangladesh: BRAC	Health coverage 25 percent. Nutrition with BINP, now expanding.	1 community health volunteer per 300 households; 1 community nutrition promoter per 200 households; community nutrition centers, 1:120 mothers and children; supervision of community nutrition promoters by community nutrition organizer, 1:10
India: ICDS F: ++/+	Children 0–6 years and pregnant and lactating women, in 3,900 of 5,300 blocks, or subdistricts; approximately 74 percent of population. Coverage expanded without targeting except by area.	Nonfood costs: approximately US$2/child/year. 1 community worker (*anganwadi* worker, or ANW) per 200 children; 1 supervisor per 20 ANWs [ANW paid, at low rate]
India: TINP F: +	Children 6–36 months, pregnant and lactating women. Children with growth failure selected. 40 percent of blocks in Tamil Nadu; 20 percent of children in 1990.	US$9/child/year, plus approximately US$3 on food. 1 community nutrition worker per 300 children; 1 supervisor per 10 community nutrition workers [Project supported]
Indonesia F: (+)	By 1990, 60,000 villages (of 65,000: 92 percent) had *posyandus* (village health/nutrition center). Women and young children.	US$2–11/child/year, depending on supplemental food; Rohde (1993) gives < US$1 recurrent. Village workers (approximately 3 million total), 1 per 60 people, approximately 1 per 10 children; supervision 1 per 200. [Volunteer]
Philippines: national F: 0	Several programs, all targeted (for example, to poorer areas), none with national coverage.	US$0.40/child/year in targeted areas. Village workers (*barangay* nutrition scholars) approximately 1:300 [Low allowance given]
Thailand: Primary Health Care + Poverty Alleviation Program + Basic Minimum Needs F: (+)	Expanded over about 5 years to cover 95 percent of villages. 600,000 village health communicators (1 percent of population) trained; 60,000 village health volunteers.	Ministry of Public Health; approximately US$11/head/year (1990) 1 village health communicator or volunteer per approximately 20 children; 1 supervision extension worker per 24 village health communicators and volunteers [Volunteer]

(Continues on the following page.)

Table 56.3 Continued

Country	Coverage, targeting	Resources, intensity
Americas		
Costa Rica F: ++ to 0	Expanded rural health program coverage 19–67 percent (1974–89).	Rural health program: US$1.70/child/year Food and Nutrition Program: US$12.50/child/year 2 health workers (full time) per 5,000 population; approximately 1:350 children [Health worker]
Honduras F: 0	With community health volunteers, AIN-C covers > 50 percent of health areas (expanded 1991 on), > 90 percent of children < 2 years in these; growth monitoring and home follow-up, plus referral and treatment.	Cost estimated as US$6/child/year Volunteer teams 3:25 children, about 3.5 hours/volunteer/week
Jamaica F: 0	Community health aides (CHAs), waged, cover most of country from health centers, with home visiting.	CHAs (full time) 1:500 households; approximately US$7/household/year [Health worker]
Nicaragua F: 0	Community health workers (*brigadistas*) with "multiplier" approach, training others; 1980 approximately 1 percent trained; many more for malaria control.	Volunteers, approximately 1:20 households

Source: See sources for table 56.2.
F = role of supplementary feeding in the program; F: ++ = mainly a feeding program, or primary role; F: + = significant but not main role, often to selected children; F: (+) = existed but relatively minor; F: 0 = none.
Note: The status of community workers is given in brackets in the last column.

groups that are hard to include for other reasons—may be more expensive to reach. Clearly the calculations depend on conditions and have to be made on a case-by-case basis. The principle is obvious: only those areas and people included in CHNPs are going to benefit; so wherever need exists, programs are indicated. The implementation strategy, in theory, may need to begin with the most urgent needs, although in practice, programs may expand from the easier, more accessible areas; this practice seems reasonable, provided that the expansion really occurs and leads to equitable use of resources.

The program content is a mix of the components described earlier, varying with local priorities. The most crucial difference is whether extensive supplementary feeding is included. In middle-income countries, supplementary feeding was less prominent, often considered unnecessary, and because expensive, perhaps counterproductive (for example, in Costa Rica; Mata 1991). At the other extreme, such as for the Integrated Child Development Services (ICDS) in India, food distribution became the raison d'être of the program but, alone, was again probably not worthwhile. For some of the intermediate cases, supplementary food played a supporting role, with varying results. Except in the very poorest societies, supplementary feeding seems unlikely to be cost-effective.

The resources used for the programs found in table 56.3 can be expressed per participant (referred to as *intensity*), as total expenditures, and in terms of personnel; the latter figures may be more generalizable. (The outcomes associated with these resources are shown in table 56.5.) Data such as these have been

the basis for estimating that US$5 to US$10 per child per year may be needed for effective programs. The dollar figures vary from less than US$1 to more than US$20. Probably the low end of this range (say, less than US$1 per child per year) does explain low or doubtful effect. Both low coverage and low intensity may explain the unchanged underweight prevalences in the Philippines until 2000. Fund levels in Indonesia are unsure; Rohde (1993) gave a figure of less than US$1, but others gave higher estimates. Most would reckon the intensity in India too low (Measham and Chatterjee 1999) at about US$2 per child per year. Looked at otherwise, the intensity planned for external funding (even if part of such funding is international costs) is in the US$10 to US$20 range (Bangladesh, India—Tamil Nadu, and Tanzania) and is the same as the estimate for Thailand. A level of US$10 to US$20 per participant per year is probably advisable for planning and sustaining effective programs.

The intensity measures of workers per mother-child and the supervision ratios are relevant in assessing needs. The suggested norms, originating from the Thai experience are 1:10–20 for both. Since then, it has emerged that the full-time equivalence of community workers must be taken into account; the Thai workers are local volunteers, probably devoting 10 to 20 percent of their time. In Honduras, Fiedler (2003) in a careful cost study estimated that each volunteer spent 3.5 hours per week (less than 10 percent of full-time equivalent, or FTE), with a ratio of 1 volunteer to 8 children. The ratio of community health and nutrition workers (CHNWs) to children may, therefore, be as low as 1:200 for FTEs and as high as 1:8 or 1:10

for part-time volunteers. In Jamaica, where the community health aides work full time, the ratio is 1:500 households; in the BRAC program in Bangladesh, it is 1:300, about half-time work (afternoons) (Chowdhury 2003). (An indication of the status of community workers is shown in brackets in the last column of table 56.3.) In any event, these ratios provide some basis for gauging the adequacy of personnel, and it seems that an effective ratio may be about 1:500 for community workers employed full time and 1:10 or 1:20 for local volunteers working part time.

In reality, the ratios of community workers to children are probably—not surprisingly—on the low side. Thailand, which trained 600,000 village workers (1 percent of the population), operated at about 1:20 for part-time volunteers, with similar supervision ratios. The Indonesian program was similar (or better) but had much less supervision. In contrast, the low resourcing of the ICDS in India shows up in a ratio of 1:200 (for part-time *anganwadi* workers, or ANWs), and in the Philippines, the ratio has until recently been 1:300 (for essentially voluntary workers).

Increased application of technology can contribute to the organization and running of community-based programs. Technology can be applied easily to methods of assessment and monitoring of children's progress; improved weighing scales (or in some circumstances, where rapid assessment in remote areas is important, using arm circumference) can simplify anthropometry. Modern computer technology for recordkeeping could be much more widely used, freeing staff time for home visits (for example, in Jamaica); e-mail, which is being rapidly adopted, has great potential for transferring information, troubleshooting, and consultation. Cell phone use is beginning to transform communications even in the poorest countries, where it is leapfrogging landline installation and use; as coverage expands, it will facilitate referral, for example, for emergency obstetric care, the need for which may first be identified by community workers. Coupled with improved transportation and procedures to allow the use of such transportation in cases of urgent need, modern communications can link communities to centers with advanced knowledge for information exchange and, by facilitating transportation when time is crucial, for referral. Modern communications may also provide more efficient ways of providing training, retraining, and supervision.

Application of current research and resulting technologies can improve many of the other interventions discussed earlier. In the micronutrient field, periodic supplementation (with vitamin A in high doses) can be extended through community programs, and fortified foods and micronutrient "sprinkles" can be promoted (see chapter 28). The prospect of enabling communities to test their salt for iodine content with simple and cheap test kits is intriguing and has often been recommended but has not yet been widely applied. Improved immunization technology should continue to protect health, for

which CHNPs' main role is to provide information and to ensure that children are taken for immunization (either to regular clinics or for National Immunization Days and the like). Periodic deworming can be conducted by community programs (and hookworm vaccines currently under development may soon contribute). Supporting the use of insecticide-treated bednets could be fostered through CHNPs. By far the most potentially important application of technology, certainly in Sub-Saharan Africa, will be the unprecedented effort to provide millions of people with antiretroviral therapy and associated care and support, as discussed later.

Training, Supervision, Incentives, and Remuneration

Community-based health and nutrition programs typically involve community workers, who may be entirely part-time volunteers (for example, in Honduras and Thailand) or may receive some remuneration financially or in kind (for example, in India). Community workers may be part of the health system, earning a wage and based in a local clinic (for example, in Jamaica) or in the community itself (for example, in Costa Rica); or they may be selected by and report to the community (for example, in Tanzania and Thailand). Table 56.3 indicates the status of community workers in the programs examined here. The training, supervision, and incentives for community workers are critical aspects of successful programs.

Inadequate training and supervisory support of community workers are common weaknesses. Considerable attention was given to training for the Iringa project (Tanzania), with village health workers trained for up to six months. In the Tamil Nadu Integrated Nutrition Program in India, community workers received three months of training and participated in annual refresher trainings. ICDS (India) initially trained the ANWs for three months, with two annual refresher courses, but this process declined. In Thailand, volunteers had two to five days of initial training, with annual refresher courses; Indonesian practice was similar. In Jamaica, where the community workers are employees of the health system, two months of initial training is provided to recruits with significant prior educational requirements. In Bangladesh, the BRAC community health volunteers have four weeks of training. The quality of the training has varied, poor training having been blamed for inadequate implementation in cases such as ICDS in India (Measham and Chatterjee 1999). Sanders (1985, 176–93) describes experiences in the 1980s of village health workers (and barefoot doctors) and their relation to the community.

Supervision of community workers is generally done by employees who are commonly in the sector. Training of supervisors (who often take on the role in addition to many other tasks) for these purposes is highly variable and not always adequate. Providing resources for visits to provide supervision to community workers is a further constraint. Supervision ratios in effective programs are about 1:20 (table 56.3, last column, when reported). Supervision and training of community workers are closely linked; indeed, supervision (which must be supportive rather than disciplinary) should include a substantial element of on-the-job training.

Remuneration and incentives for sustaining motivation are key issues in replicating the successful features of these programs, and the options vary with the culture. In Thailand, it is argued that village volunteers consider the prestige associated with the role of health worker preferable to getting a low wage. In many cases, some right of access to health care is part of the incentive. For the ICDS in India, in contrast, the ANW receives a small financial remuneration, but the government (as elsewhere) will not grant formal employment status (and attempts to form unions have been strongly discouraged). Direct comparisons of the options of paid remuneration and voluntary work are rare. One opportunity to study options for remuneration is in the Philippines, where under a World Bank Early Child Development project, the child development worker receives a wage, which could be compared to near-volunteers at the *barangay* (village) level.

When CHNWs are primarily voluntary, they are selected by the community and report to community committees in some form. CHNWs on government payrolls may come from the communities and thus may be known to and identify with the communities, but they may report to supervisors higher up in the system. Both models can work, depending on the culture. What probably works least well is when the community worker is paid little and receives inadequate support and recognition from the community or even comes from elsewhere. Furthermore, as development progresses, reliance on volunteerism may become less useful.

For planning CHNPs in terms of community workers, the total numbers and resource implications can be estimated as follows. A full-time equivalent CHNW might visit 5 to 10 households per day, averaging a visit to each household roughly every two months; a ratio of 1 CHNW to 200 households, therefore, seems to be in the range within which an effect in terms of improving child health and nutrition is expected. Calculations from salaries of community health aides (CHAs) in Jamaica work out to US$7 per household per year, within the usual range for expected effect. An important factor in regard to financial resources, however, concerns the substantial cadre of personnel who have training and job descriptions for community work, are based in health centers, and for administrative and financial reasons seldom leave the health facility. Moreover, funds may not be released to allow travel to nearby villages. An example is from Jamaica, where, because of clinic workloads, CHAs spend time helping in clinics rather than on home visits; in fact, technology could free staff time for community work by automating tasks, such as record keeping, that detain the CHAs. More effective deployment of existing personnel may frequently be an option. Hiring additional personnel as community health workers would consume a significant proportion of typical health budgets (at 1:200 households for FTEs, this would amount to US$1 to US$2 per person per year, or about 20 percent of public health budgets in low-income countries). A mix of redeployment of existing staff and new hiring from budget reallocations should, nonetheless, be cost-effective.

Organization

Effective, respected, and socially inclusive organization at the community level seems to have been a key feature of the success in launching, expanding, and sustaining CHNPs. Most of the successful CHNPs drew and built on established community procedures; where they did not, effect and sustainability were in doubt. In Thailand, the health services and the religious organization at village level were important. The health services themselves play a key role in Costa Rica, Honduras, and Jamaica. In Indonesia, it was the community organizations (and women's groups) together with (initially) the family-planning services. In Iringa, Tanzania, it was the local political party structure, with substantial input from UNICEF. In Zimbabwe, immediately after independence, it was the village organizations that had fought the war, later helped by a consortium of national and international nongovernmental organizations (NGOs). The major part of the still-expanding program in Bangladesh is run by BRAC, an NGO, and has built on its links to the community for development, food security, and educational activities, as well as for health. In contrast, CHNPs that either failed to launch a wide program (for example, in the Philippines) or had limited effect (in India, ICDS) probably lacked some of these features. Inclusiveness is probably hard to achieve if not inherent.

Support from the central government is also crucial: CHNPs need this support for training, supervision, wages, supplies, facilities, and the like. Where such support becomes a regular government budget item, activities tend to become embedded and are sustained, in contrast to where the support is from donors.

A further issue concerns maintaining the community program's preventive orientation. In Indonesia, for example, according to Rohde (1993), the health services co-opted (and medicalized) the *posyandu* (weighing post, or community health and nutrition center) system by adding a diagnostic and treatment module (in fact, a table in the meeting place). This module attracted most of the attention, to the disadvantage of the preventive aspects of the program. Thus, if the extension of IMCI into the community means treatment (by trained but not medically qualified people) in the community rather than referral to facilities, treatment could become the main or even sole focus, shifting attention from prevention. Some parallels exist to the experience of ICDS in India, where, as noted earlier, food became the raison d'être.

CONTEXTUAL FACTORS

Community-based programs *can* work usefully, bringing steady progress; whether they do depends on myriad factors relating to the context. Three different concerns are (a) factors affecting widespread initiation of CHNPs of potentially adequate coverage, intensity, and content; (b) factors that lead to sustainability; and (c) factors that allow activities to be effective in improving health and nutrition—at best, when they, themselves, also contribute to a rapid transitional improvement, as in Thailand, Costa Rica, and Jamaica.

Contextual factors may bring about improvements in health and nutrition without any additional direct action—through improving living conditions, education, and so forth. Often, the changes caused by such nonprogrammatic factors are diffi-cult to distinguish from program effects (current examples are in Bangladesh and Vietnam, both showing rapid improvement in nutrition). Moreover, the same factors (again, such as education) may both produce endogenous change and increase the effect of program activities.

Five contextual factors have been suggested as priorities (in Asia; Mason and others 2001):

- women's status and education
- lack of social exclusion
- community organization
- literacy
- political commitment.

Table 56.4 shows estimates of the positions of countries with case study programs in regard to these factors. The levels of

Table 56.4 Context in Which Selected CHNPs Start and Run

Country	Approximate period	Women's status and education[a]	Lack of social exclusion	Community organization	Literacy	Level of health and administrative infrastructure	Political commitment	Total minus political commitment	Total
Tanzania									
Iringa starts	1984–90	2	4	4	3	2	5	15	20
Iringa declines	1990–	2	4	2	3	2	2	13	15
Zimbabwe									
Supplementary Feeding Programme starts	1981–90	2	4	5	2	2	5	15	20
Supplementary Feeding Programme declines	1990–	2	2	2	2	2	2	10	12
Bangladesh									
BINP	1997–	1	3	2	2	3	3	11	14
India									
ICDS	1975–	1	1	2	2	2	3	8	11
TINP	1980–9	2	2	3	3	3	4	13	17
Indonesia									
UPGK starts	1975–	2	4	3	2	2	4	13	17
UPGK declines	1990–	2	4	2	2	3	2	13	15
Philippines[b]	1974–2000	4	4	3	4	3	1	18	19
Thailand	1982–	4	3	4	4	3	4	18	22
Costa Rica									
RHP	1973–	4	4	4	3	4	4	19	23
Jamaica	1985–	4	4	3	4	4	4	19	23
Nicaragua	1979–90	3	2	3	3	3	4	14	18

Source: Authors.

a. Women's status and education can be quantified by indicators such as adult literacy rates, females as percentage of males, and secondary school enrollment for girls.

b. Since 2000, the Philippines has begun a significantly improving trend, one factor being increased implementation of programs (CHNPs, as well as others, such as salt iodization); this increase is caused in part by increased political commitment, both as new legislation and resource allocations.

Note: 0: worst; 5: best.

health and administrative infrastructure have been added. The table also shows changes in these factors that may help explain why the CHNPs declined in three cases.

Political commitment can lead to initiating community programs and mobilizing resources. It may also respond to emerging community mobilization, as seems to be the case when programs start after political upheavals, as in Zimbabwe and Nicaragua. Declining political commitment accounts for loss of interest by the government in CHNPs; economic decline undermining resource availability may cause a shift away from financial support of CHNPs (for example, in Tanzania). In table 56.4, estimates of levels of contextual factors are totaled both without and including political commitment (last two columns). The total without commitment may indicate how favorable the context is if commitment is then made. Costa Rica, Jamaica, and Thailand had a favorable context and, with commitment, succeeded. The Philippines had comparable favorable conditions—the position of women is generally good, there is limited social division (exclusion), and so on. However, the necessary commitment (of resources, in particular) was made only recently, with new legislation, adherence to regulations (for example, iodized salt went from 25 to 65 percent coverage), and increased resource allocation and assignment of community workers. This new commitment may well explain the recently resumed decrease in child malnutrition (figure 56.2). In other examples—such as Indonesia and Tanzania—the conditions were moderately favorable, and while political support and finance existed, progress was made. In Tanzania, financial crisis denied the programs sustained support; in Indonesia and Zimbabwe, bureaucratization and centralization of the political process, followed by political turmoil, contributed to a similar outcome (Sanders 1993). The situations in India and Bangladesh have not been very favorable. The position of women and social rifts, amounting to exclusion, have probably inhibited effective programs, even with political commitment. This context may now be changing in Bangladesh, as seen in the activities of BRAC. Finally, this analysis demonstrates the relation of decline in programs to falling political commitment in Tanzania, Zimbabwe, and Indonesia.

If this analysis approximates the truth, the forward-looking policy implications may be important:

- First, investing initially in a favorable context makes sense (as does possibly committing resources preferentially to interventions in the more favorable contexts). Supporting policies can address social constraints—such as improving education for women—and (relatedly) seek to improve human rights. In many cases, human rights may be of overriding importance for health: Farmer (2003) has made a compelling case for rethinking health and human rights as a prerequisite for progress and as a responsibility for those working for health, especially of the poor and of the destitute sick. This investment may be long term and difficult—as in Kerala, India, for instance—but must be seen as integral to the struggle for health (Sanders 1985). Operationally, this commitment to human rights puts greater responsibility on advocates and investors in health to broaden the dialogue and scope for allocating resources and to avoid committing resources regardless of the prospect of success as influenced by the social and human rights context. In health and nutrition, as in other areas, adjustment of policies to support the success of interventions would be pragmatic as well as the right thing to do.

- Second, even if the context is more favorable, genuine political commitment is still essential. Excessive donor input may inhibit this commitment. It is striking that Thailand had to reject donor influence and make its internal decisions before its programs became successful (Tontisirin and Winichagoon 1999), Costa Rica had to fight and overcome a medicalized approach (Muñoz and Scrimshaw 1995), and Indonesia's *posyandu* system was undermined when treatment displaced prevention (Rohde 1993).

- Third, it is clear that severe economic stress, political pressure, or both have caused unsustainability (Indonesia, Nicaragua, Tanzania, and TINP).

- Fourth, if the context is unfavorable, it might be better to work on improving the context than to commit resources to programs that may not succeed—but, of course, success in improving context itself depends on circumstances, notably political commitment.

Considerations like these should contribute to identifying supporting policies needed for programs to be effective and modifications to interventions in particular conditions. For example, it is often observed that a particular factor—say, access to health services—is more strongly related to improvement among the better off (for example, the educated) population. This interaction of program with context leads to identifying new needs—in this example, perhaps facilitating access for the illiterate. In the longer run, resources or legislation (for example, to combat social exclusion or discrimination against women) may be highlighted as prerequisites before a program can be expected to work. Often failure to take account of context when trying to transfer experiences from a pilot trial ("scaling up") may explain why efficacious interventions prove ineffective in a larger population.

This analysis of contextual circumstances indicates that targeting the poor may not always be cost-effective, and some interventions may not be feasible in certain contexts. An example is when the health infrastructure and services are almost nonexistent; under those conditions, it can be argued that emergency treatment (especially for the diseases addressed by IMCI) should be established and reliable resources put in place first. A similar difficulty, often seen in food security, is that most interventions may not work for the poorest of the poor. For instance, supporting food (or cash crop) production in low-potential areas may not be realistic; nonagricultural employment may be better.

Thus, community-based programs work in a specific time and place: programs may start, work for a time, and then evolve or fade away. Even if they fade away, some useful effect may be achieved: sustainability need not be forever. At the same time, short project cycles (three years for many donors) can act against sustained programs. Some compromise in donor policies to allow assurance of continuity for reasonable periods (such as 10 years) could do a lot to increase the effectiveness of donor support to CHNPs.

The essence of time and place is not fully understood. Werner and Sanders (1997) give examples of favorable times, as when the old order is changing (for example, after internal conflict, as in Nicaragua and Zimbabwe) and when there is renewed vigor and some new organization is in place. Another generalization of a favorable context is when energy and interconnectedness exist in society. Thailand illustrates both: the Thais needed to change the approach, moving away from donor influence, in order to initiate the successful community programs that helped transform health and nutrition throughout the country, and that worked in part because of cohesive features of Thai society (Tontisirin and Winichagoon 1999).

In these examples, programs that continued on a large scale—either until the problem was largely resolved, as in Costa Rica, Jamaica, and Thailand, or as it was expanding, as in BRAC in Bangladesh or AIN-C (Atención Integral a la Niñez Comunitaria) in Honduras—clearly had supportive context, but their specific common features (and hence how they could be replicated) are elusive. Perhaps one crucial condition for success is that circumstances are such that people and communities begin to have the sense that they can take responsibility for—and control of—their health and quality of life. Responsibility comes with the emancipation of societies from colonial or other repressive conditions and possibly when grassroots attention becomes widespread, as it did in Bangladesh through an NGO that identified with the people. Evidence is growing that, among the poor in the United States, this sense of control is directly related to better health and reduced exposure to HIV and AIDS; Sampson, Raudenbusch, and Earls (1997) call the concept *collective efficacy*. Cohen and others (2000) show that health conditions improve when communities themselves fix up their environment—the "broken windows" theory. Such ideas may equally apply to poor communities, especially urban ones, in developing countries too.

RESULTS

Indicators of progress in implementation—*process indicators*—referring to coverage, intensity, and so on, are shown in table 56.3. As discussed earlier, most programs expanded population coverage without much targeting. But usually the level of resource application (intensity) was on the low side. More research is needed on the contribution of CHNPs to health process indicators, such as immunization coverage rates, as well as to nonhealth activities, for instance, in agriculture and community development.

Impact evaluation, which refers to the net effects of interventions on changing health outcomes, is sorely lacking. The efficacy of most of the component parts of CHNPs, when resources are adequate and the problems are correctly identified, is established, but in routinely administered large-scale programs, the changes in outcome that can be ascribed to program actions are less known. Although controlled trials by definition are not applicable, plausible evidence can be obtained by careful attention to research design, measurement, and analysis (Habicht, Victora, and Vaughan 1999). Some form of "with and without" and "before and after" comparisons is needed; for instance, such methods as staggered implementation, natural experiments, and selection of comparison groups with some statistical control can yield valuable information now lacking and should be more widely attempted. In this context, it should be noted that because of the timing and level of effort necessary for the evaluation, the impact evaluation results (changes in outcome ascribed to the program) may be more important for policy decisions on *future* programs than for the program that has been evaluated. Moreover, not all programs require detailed evaluation. Thus, financial support for such policy-relevant evaluations may come from budgets other than that of the program to be evaluated. The evaluations should also be prospective as far as possible, so decisions on evaluation design and finance are needed earlier rather than later.

Impact

For the examples used here, inferences were drawn from piecing together results either from ad hoc surveys or from program and administrative data; occasionally such inferences were made from the comparison of baseline estimates with midterm or final assessments, but the comparison groups, if any, were imperfectly matched. Thus, the conclusions on impact now put forward are tentative and based on judgments from available information. Some of these conclusions were drawn from trend assessments, details for which are in Mason (2000, annex 5).

The most widely available indicators are mortality rates (infant, child, and to a lesser extent, maternal; reliable data on age zero and cause-specific mortality rates are not usually available from most developing countries); prevalences of underweight in children from national surveys (often supported by demographic and health surveys or UNICEF Multi-Indicator Cluster Surveys); and indicators of health services (notably immunization coverage rates). Estimates of morbidity, even of the common diseases (such as diarrhea and ARI), are not available systematically enough to judge trends in relation to programs. Child underweight (or stunting) has a particular value, because it measures an attribute of all children (age and weight or height), rather than assessing a relatively rare event, as in mortality estimates. Moreover, experience is well established of how underweight prevalences behave as a robust indicator, having a useful degree of responsiveness but not being subject to wide fluctuations with transient events.

Under controlled conditions, improving health and nutrition allows rapid catch-up in bodyweight and fast rates of reduction in underweight prevalence (for example, Pinstrup-Andersen and others 1993, 405). But in the real-world conditions of CHNPs, the expected rate is slower. As examples, Thailand maintained a reduction in underweight of about 2.9 ppts per year in the 1980s (see figure 56.1); the 22 projects reviewed as reported by Jonsson (1997) ranged between about 1 and 3 ppts per year. A reduction rate of −2 ppts per year, suggested earlier as an expectation from successful programs, would lead to very significant improvement if achieved at national levels: for South Asia, it would mean going from a prevalence of underweight of about 60 percent in 1980 to 20 percent in 2000; for Africa, from 30 percent in 1990 to 10 percent in 2000.

Detecting this rate can be difficult with the noise of sampling and nonsampling errors and with the common seasonal changes, which can amount to 5 ppts fluctuations or more, certainly in Africa. The potential program-ascribed trend needs to be separated from the underlying secular trend for the country, roughly 0.5 ppts per year (from 1985 to 1995; ACC/SCN 1996). Clearly the longer the program and the observing periods, the easier it is to assess trends.

Where the data are detailed enough, an initial rapid fall is seen in severe malnutrition—and probably in mortality,—followed by a slower fall in mild to moderate malnutrition. The reasons for the initial rapid fall are presumed to be immediate effects of improved health care, immunization, and the use of oral rehydration therapy. The outcomes estimated for the programs considered here concentrate on the sustained trend—after a year or two of implementation—as summarized in table 56.5.

In Zimbabwe, from 1980 to 1988, the infant mortality rate (IMR) fell from 110 to 53 per 1,000 live births, and severe malnutrition fell from 17.7 to 1.3 percent. However, stunting fell only in 1982–88, from 35.6 to 29 percent (1.1 ppts per year). Tanzania shows a similar effect in Iringa, with severe and moderate malnutrition falling much faster for the first two years.

Interestingly, the Child Survival and Development Projects (supported by the World Bank, among others), which covered a much larger population (but with less intensity than in Iringa), appeared to show almost the same pattern as in Iringa: a rapid initial fall (as much as 8 ppts per year, for one to two years), continuing at 1 to 2 ppts per year.

In Costa Rica, the child mortality rate plummeted in the late 1960s, well before stunting fell in the 1970s (Saenz 1995, 129; Vargas 1995, 111). A lag was seen in Thailand, where the child mortality rate started to fall rapidly in 1977, and both severe and moderate malnutrition appeared to start their fall in 1983–84. Both these improvements preceded the major growth in gross national product, which began in 1987 (Kachondam, Winichagoon, and Tontisirin 1992, tables 8 and 33). In analyzing Indian experience, where the IMR has fallen faster than child malnutrition, Measham and Chatterjee (1999) suggest that further improvements in child survival may be constrained by the high rates of child malnutrition.

The sustained effects are generally of about an additional 1 ppt per year improvement (table 56.5). For Bangladesh (the BINP), Tanzania, and Thailand, it is possible to distinguish the sustained rate from the initial rapid fall. In Bangladesh, the BINP started during a period of rapid improvement overall, so extracting the underlying trend is especially important to give a plausible view of the "with-project" rate: about 1.6 ppts per year again seems a reasonable estimate. A similar extraction of likely with-project changes allowing for underlying trends was reported previously (Mason 2000, annex 5) for Tamil Nadu, Andhra Pradesh (ICDS), and Orissa, indicating plausible improvements for the first two states.

In sum, these results support the contention that after an initial rapid fall, the sustained rates of improvement in child underweight prevalence settle down to about an additional reduction of 1 or 2 ppts per year. This conclusion is the same as previously reached (Gillespie and Mason 1991), now supported by some new results.

Cost-Effectiveness

Therefore, if we use prevalences of underweight children as the basis for calculation, US$10 per child per year gives a reduction of 2 ppts per year. If we are to translate this cost into an implied effect on health and survival, underweight must be related to the measure of disease burden, DALYs lost. Then the resources needed per DALY saved—dollars per DALY—can be estimated. A 32.5 percent reduction in the loss of DALYs is associated with eliminating general plus micronutrient malnutrition as both direct effects and risk factors (see table 56.1, discussed earlier); as a first approximation, the average prevalence for developing countries of 30 percent underweight can be applied. We can calculate the associated DALYs gained from reducing malnutrition at this rate (and assume that loss of DALYs from *all*

Table 56.5 Outcomes and Resources in Selected Programs

Country	Outcomes	Resources
Africa		
Tanzania: Iringa	Underweight: 50 to 35 percent (1984–88)	US$8 to US$17/person/year (US$34/child/year from total costs);
	Immunization: 50 to 90 percent	2 village health workers/village = 1,220 total;
	Rates in underweight: initial 2 years, −8 ppts/year; first 4 years, −4.5 ppts/year; sustained (years 2–7), −0.8 ppts/year	Approximately 1:40 children
Tanzania: Child Survival and Development Program	Underweight reduction rates similar to Iringa	US$2 to US$3/child/year
Zimbabwe: Supplementary Feeding Programme	Stunting: 35.6 to 29 percent (1982–88) −1.1 ppts/year	External funds, approximately US$0.50/child/year
	IMR: 1980–88: 110 to 53	
Asia		
Bangladesh: BINP	BINP, first 6 *thanas*, initial effect (1997): approximately −11 ppts/year; then (to February 1999) approximately −1.6 ppts/year additional	1 community worker per 1,000 population; Approximately 1:200 children; US$14 million/year, approximately US$18/child/year
	Underlying (nonprogram) trend: national approximately −1.7 ppts/year, program area approximately −2.4 ppts/year	
Bangladesh: BRAC	No program-specific data, but child underweight and anemia in women have substantial falling trend in recent years.	Over all programs, US$196 million in 2003 (approximately US$8/household over all households); health program covered 31 million people, over 20 percent
India: ICDS	Overall underweight prevalence declining only slowly; some states reported faster, but link to ICDS not shown.	1 supervisor to 20 ANWs
India: TINP	1979–90: −1.4 ppts/year in TINP districts; −0.7 in non-TINP districts: increased improvement of approximately −0.7 ppts/year (Reddy and others 1992, 45). From other data, increased improvement of −1.0 ppts/year.	US$7–12/child/year
Indonesia	Probably about −1 ppt/year; underlying trend unknown	US$2 to US$11/child/year, depending on supplementary food. Rohde (1993) gives < US$1 recurrent.
	IMR: 1970, 1980, 1990: 118, 93, 61, respectively	Village workers (about 3 million total) 1:60 people; approximately 1:10 children; supervision 1:200
Philippines: national	No change found in underweight.	Low coverage and intensity
	IMR: 1960, 1996: 77, 32, respectively	
Thailand	Approximately −2.9 ppts/year improvement in child underweight. Breaks down to 1982–84: −7.8 ppts/year; 1985–90, −1.9 ppts/year.	Ministry of Public Health, approximately US$11/head/year (1990) Village health communicator or volunteer approximately 1:20 children; supervision by extension workers: village health communicators and volunteers approximately 1:24
	IMR: 1970, 1980, 1990: 73, 55, 27, respectively	
Americas		
Costa Rica	Stunting improved by approximately 1–1.5 ppts/year (estimated from Muñoz and Scrimshaw 1995, 111), 1979–89.	Rural health program: US$1.7/child/year Food and nutrition program: US$12.50/child/year 2 health workers (full time)/5,000 population, approximately 1:350 children
	IMR: 1970, 1980, 1988: 62, 19, 16, respectively	
Jamaica	−1.9 ppts/year 1985–89	
	IMR: 1960, 1996: 58, 10, respectively	
Nicaragua	IMR fell from (at least) 92 to 80	Large numbers community health volunteers trained and supported

Source: See sources for table 56.2.

malnutrition comes down at this rate; CHNPs include some attention to micronutrients). This reduction is then cumulated through time (five years here) and assumes a linear relation between cost, underweight reduction, and disease burden avoided. The calculation also assumes a persistent effect of reducing malnutrition.

Using these assumptions gives an estimate of US$200 to US$250 per DALY saved in sustained programs. This estimate does not include gains in DALYs from diseases that do not show up as underweight, which must be substantial. Moreover, if this calculation is applied just to the first rapid fall, typically (in the three cases examined) about 8 ppts per year, the ratio might fall by a factor of four, to US$50 to US$60 per DALY saved (but start-up costs are higher too). The sustained figure should be the more generalizable.

Many further provisos exist. Much of the effect here is on a risk factor—malnutrition—reducing which, in turn, makes other interventions more effective; hence, the comparison of CHNPs with more direct interventions may not be valid. But conversely (or perversely) improving nutrition could actually reduce the cost-effectiveness of other interventions—such as measles immunization—by reducing the mortality risk of children who are not immunized.

FUTURE APPLICATIONS

The experience so far in CHNPs can be applied more broadly, especially where community organizations can sustain support for CHNWs. CHNPs have worked best so far in Asia and Latin America. However, with the HIV/AIDS epidemic in Sub-Saharan Africa needing high-priority attention, application of CHNP experience to the HIV/AIDS crisis should be explored.

Extending CHNPs' Coverage and Intensity

In a project sponsored by the Asian Development Bank (ADB) and UNICEF that was aimed at identifying ways of investing in improved child nutrition, Mason and others (1999, 2001) have reviewed the extent of CHNPs in Asian countries. Resources were estimated in terms of annual expenditures per child and of ratios of population to community workers ("mobilizers"). The project addressed the needs of eight countries (Bangladesh, Cambodia, China, India, Pakistan, the Philippines, Sri Lanka, and Vietnam), and previous experience in Indonesia and Thailand provided additional guidance.

The population coverage of CHNPs was estimated as about 5 to 20 percent, except for India with the ICDS, which reports about 70 percent coverage. The next indicators refer to estimates *within* programs. The calculated intensity was commonly 200 children to 1 community worker (for example, Bangladesh, India, Sri Lanka); ratios of up to 100:1 were reported in Pakistan

and Vietnam and up to 60:1 in the Philippines. Further research has stressed the variation in time commitment of CHNWs in different places—hence the need to convert to FTEs. The ratio used as the norm, derived from experience in Thailand and Indonesia, of about 1:20 is probably equivalent to 1:200 in FTEs. In India, opinion has been that about a doubling of the ANW numbers in the ratios is needed to get more effect (Measham and Chatterjee 1999). From this perspective, these estimates indicate that both coverage and intensity are low, although intensity may be half that needed, whereas coverage (except in India) is far too small. Supervision ratios are estimated as about 1:20 and higher. Expanding the numbers of CHNWs also means increasing the number of supervisors (usually from the health system), with associated costs.

Calculations from scarce financial resource data show that most government programs cost about US$1 per participant child per year or less, whereas Bangladesh (BINP, with donor support and in line with other donor-supported programs) reached costs of US$15 to US$20 per child per year. By this calculation, too, the resources per head, as well as the coverage, were in most cases too low for widespread effect.

The estimates of coverage and intensity can be combined to calculate the extent of current programs in relation to that needed for full coverage at adequate intensity. The results based on a 1:20 ratio of CHNW to children suggest that less than 1 percent of the need was currently available; at 1:200 (which would cost more, because the CHNW would work full time) perhaps 10 percent of the need would be covered. Either way, a massive expansion would be called for if CHNPs were to be used as a means for widely improving health (but still calling for only about 20 percent of the public budget for health).

Expansion requires major resources, and not only financial ones. Thailand trained 1 percent of the population as community health workers (part time) and established an extensive supervision and support structure, including retraining. The estimates for the ADB-UNICEF project in financial terms were, for Bangladesh, Cambodia, Pakistan, Sri Lanka, and Vietnam, some US$190 million to US$280 million per year for improvement of underweight by an additional 1.5 ppts per year (Mason and others 2001, 64–68).

The Potential Role of CHNPs in Combating HIV and AIDS in Sub-Saharan Africa

Controlling the epidemic of HIV and AIDS in Sub-Saharan Africa will take an unprecedented effort. As antiretroviral therapy becomes available there will be new opportunities to turn the tide. Supply of antiretroviral therapy drugs, although essential and the cutting edge of new programs, is only part of the need. Food and income support, care for children (orphans and others affected), counseling, support to promote and sustain behavior change, and rehabilitation of people and communities are needed (see chapter 18). Many of these activities have precedents in the types of CHNPs run by community health workers that are discussed here. What lessons are transferable?

One concern is that CHNPs have a greater history of success in developing countries *outside* Africa. Those within Africa seem to have been sustained for limited periods, often linked to donor interests. Reasons may have to do with lower levels of administrative infrastructure, different existing community organization, and varying political commitment (see table 56.4). These factors may now be weakened as the AIDS epidemic reduces the numbers of qualified people and undermines community organizations. It will be urgent to work on such contextual factors to create conditions in which community organizations can be refurbished and built on.

Community organizations can work in Africa, as elsewhere, when they have a real function with activities perceived as useful to pursue and some resources (including mobilizing their own) to use. Some transferable lessons are that such local organizations are crucial; that in regard to supervision and access to certain resources, they need to work with the government structure—often through health system employees; and that they need sustained resource support, much of which must come from donors.

Treatment and rehabilitation of people with AIDS will be home based in most cases and will depend substantially on community support. Nutrition is an important component; improved food intake is likely to enhance the effect of antiretroviral therapy, and when treatment progresses, nutrition will help get sick people back on their feet and returned to a productive life. A village health worker could play a key role in this process. In much of Africa, HIV and AIDS affect many communities, and in southern Africa, where HIV prevalences reach 30 to 40 percent, almost all communities have chronically sick adults. This fact means that most communities need programs: the problem is not highly concentrated. On the positive side, the more developed and accessible communities are those most affected by AIDS (Mason and others forthcoming; UNICEF 2004), where establishing programs may be easier. HIV and AIDS are affecting children both directly, as pediatric AIDS, and indirectly, through the impoverishment and destitution of affected households. This effect is seen in worsening child malnutrition. Here, too, support through CHNPs could play a useful role.

The characteristics of CHNPs elsewhere—in terms of intensity, training, supervision, and so forth—may provide some guidance for establishing or extending them in Africa. Mechanisms for identifying, supporting, and training village or community health workers in this context can draw on experience with CHNPs; such issues as their identification in the community and links with community and facility programs will arise. A key issue will be the remuneration and incentives

for community workers, and this issue may need some research and testing of different approaches. The activities of community workers in dealing with treatment (and prevention) of HIV and AIDS have parallels to malnutrition and would probably include the following items:

- social support and facilitating access to resources (possibly including food aid)
- counseling
- treatment and referral for opportunistic infections
- promoting rehabilitation to productive life (which may benefit from improved nutrition) as antiretroviral therapy progresses.

Schools too have an extremely important role in the fight against HIV and AIDS and should be linked to, or part of, CHNPs. Schools provide a refuge and a means of providing help for orphans and vulnerable children, and they also provide a crucial opportunity for preempting and combating high-risk behavior.

RESEARCH NEEDS

The question of incentives, training, and support for community workers urgently needs research, both from current experience and with prospective designs. The issues include the following:

- What is the CHNW's status, relative to the community or to the government (or NGO) hierarchy?
- How are CHNWs selected and to whom do they report (for example, community health committees, supervisors employed in the health or other system)?
- What educational background and how much training and retraining—and by what methods—are needed for CHNWs?
- What ratios of CHNWs to households are effective (or most cost-effective), both as part-time workers (volunteer or otherwise) and as full-time employees?
- What supervision ratios work?
- What remuneration and incentives are effective?
- How can these efforts be financed?

Enough programs have been in operation for long enough that researchers could base on them much of the needed research on processes of implementation, launching new trials only for processes for which sufficient information does not exist. In contrast, impact evaluation requires new and preferably prospective studies.

A major gap in research is the application of community-based programs to urban areas. Urban communities are conceived differently from the rural areas of most CHNPs, organizations run along different lines, and so forth. Yet population growth is in urban areas, and some problems, notably HIV and AIDS, are worse there.

Finally, the cost-effectiveness analysis results given in an earlier section are based on rather few and approximate results. CHNPs may well provide a viable and cost-effective approach under many circumstances in poor countries, and it may be necessary to demonstrate this viability better and more quantitatively for support to CHNPs to compete with more traditional service delivery interventions. That, too, would constitute worthwhile research.

NOTES

1. Social exclusion refers to the exclusion of groups from the mainstream of public actions: lower castes in India, poorer groups in Pakistan, many indigenous ethnic groups throughout Asia and the Americas, and migrant workers in China and elsewhere; the result for public health is that excluded people do not participate in programs even if they are available.

2. Pinstrup-Andersen and others (1993) provide a more complete list.

REFERENCES

ACC/SCN (United Nations Administrative Committee on Coordination/Sub-Committee on Nutrition). 1989. *Update on the World Nutrition Situation: Recent Trends in Nutrition in 33 Countries.* Geneva: ACC/SCN.

———. 1992. *Global and Regional Results.* Vol. 1 of *Second Report on the World Nutrition Situation.* Geneva: ACC/SCN.

———. 1996. *Update on the Nutrition Situation, 1996.* Geneva: ACC/SCN.

———. 1998. *Third Report on the World Nutrition Situation.* Geneva: ACC/SCN.

———. 2004. *Fifth Report on the World Nutrition Situation.* Geneva: ACC/SCN.

Administrative Staff College of India. 1997. "National Strategy to Reduce Child Malnutrition; Investment Plan; Final Report." Asian Development Bank, Manila, December.

Allen, L. H., and S. R. Gillespie. 2001. "What Works? A Review of the Efficacy and Effectiveness of Nutrition Interventions." ACC/SCN Nutrition Policy Paper 19; Asian Development Bank (ADB) Nutrition and Development Series 5, United Nations Administrative Committee on Coordination/Sub-Committee on Nutrition, Geneva; ADB, Manila.

Berg, A. 1981. *Malnourished People: A Policy View.* Poverty and Basic Needs Series. Washington, DC: World Bank.

———. 1987. *Malnutrition: What Can Be Done?* Washington, DC: World Bank; Baltimore: Johns Hopkins University Press.

BINP and UNICEF (Bangladesh Integrated Nutrition Program and United Nations Children's Fund). 1999. "Preliminary Results." UNICEF.

BRAC (Bangladesh Rural Advancement Committee). 2004. "BRAC Health Programme," http://www.brac.net/health_programme.pdf, and "BRAC at a Glance," http://www.brac.net/aboutb.htm.

Chowdhury, M. 2003. "Health Workforce for TB Control by DOTS: The BRAC Case." Joint Learning Initiative Working Paper 5-2. http://www.globalhealthtrust.org/doc/JLI%20WG%20Paper%205-2.pdf.

Cohen, D, S. Spear, R. Scribner, P. Kissinger, K. Mason, and J. Wildgen. 2000. "'Broken Windows' and the Risk of Gonorrhea." *American Journal of Public Health* 90 (2): 230–36.

Delgado, H. L., V. E. Valverde, R. Martorell, and R. E. Klein. 1982. "Relationship of Maternal and Infant Nutrition to Infant Growth." *Early Human Development* 6 (3): 273–86.

Engle, P. L., M. Bentley, and G. Pelto. 2000. "The Role of Care in Nutrition Programmes: Current Research and a Research Agenda." *Proceedings of the Nutrition Society* 59 (1): 25–35.

Ezzati, M., A. Lopez, A. Rodgers, S. vander Hoorn, C. J. L. Murray, and the Comparative Risk Collaborating Group. 2002. "Selected Major Risk Factors and Global and Regional Burden of Disease." *Lancet* 360: 1347–60.

Ezzati, M., S. Vander Hoorn, A. Rodgers, A. Lopez, C. D. Mathers, C. J. L. Murray, and the Comparative Risk Collaborating Group. 2003. "Estimates of Global and Regional Potential Health Gains from Reducing Multiple Major Risk Factors." *Lancet* 362: 271–80.

Farmer, P. 2003. *Pathologies of Power: Health, Human Rights, and the New War on the Poor.* Berkeley and Los Angeles: University of California Press.

Fiedler, J. L. 2003. "A Cost Analysis of the Honduras Community-Based Integrated Child Care Program (Atención Integral a la Niñez-Comunitaria, AIN-C)." Health, Nutrition, and Population Discussion Paper, World Bank, Washington, DC.

FNRI (Food and Nutrition Research Institute). 2004. "Results of FNRI National Nutrition Surveys, 2001 and 2003." Department of Science and Technology, Food and Nutrition Research Institute, Government of the Philippines, Manila.

Gillespie, S., and J. Mason. 1991. "Nutrition-Relevant Actions—Some Experiences from the Eighties and Lessons for the Nineties." ACC/SCN State-of-the-Art Series Nutrition Policy Discussion Paper 10, United Nations Administrative Committee on Coordination/Sub-Committee on Nutrition, Geneva. http://www.unsystem.org/scn/archives/npp10/index.htm.

Gillespie, S., J. Mason, and R. Martorell. 1996. "How Nutrition Improves." ACC/SCN Nutrition Policy Discussion Paper 15, United Nations Administrative Committee on Coordination/Sub-Committee on Nutrition, Geneva. http://www.unsystem.org/scn/archives/npp15/index.htm.

Gillespie, S., M. McLachlan, and R. Shrimpton. 2003. *Combatting Malnutrition: Time to Act.* Washington, DC: World Bank.

Guillermo-Tuazon, A., and R. M. Briones. 1997. "Comprehensive Assessment of Nutrition Interventions." Report prepared for Asian Development Bank–UNICEF Regional Technical Assistance project. University of Philippines at Los Baños, Regional Training Programme on Food and Nutrition. UNICEF, Manila. Photocopy.

Gwatkin, D., J. Wilcox, and J. Wray. 1980. *Can Health and Nutrition Interventions Make a Difference?* Monograph 13, Overseas Development Council, Washington, DC.

Habicht, J.-P., J. Mason, and H. Tabatabai. 1984. "Basic Concepts for the Design of Evaluation during Programme Implementation." In *Methods for the Evaluation of the Impact of Food and Nutrition Programmes*, ed. D. Sahn, R. Lockwood, and N. Scrimshaw, 1–25. Tokyo: United Nations University.

Habicht, J.-P., C. G. Victora, and J. P. Vaughan. 1999. "Evaluation Designs for Adequacy, Plausibility, and Probability of Public Health Programme Performance and Impact." *International Journal of Epidemiology* 28 (1): 10–18.

Heaver, R. A., and J. M. Hunt. 1995. *Improving Early Child Development: An Integrated Program for the Philippines.* Washington, DC: World Bank and Asian Development Bank.

Heaver, R., and J. B. Mason. 2000. *Making a National Impact on Malnutrition in the Philippines: You Can't Get There from Here—A Case*

Study of Government Policies and Programs, and the Role of UNICEF and the World Bank. New York: UNICEF.

Horwitz, A. 1987. "Comparative Public Health: Costa Rica, Cuba, and Chile." *Food and Nutrition Bulletin* 9 (3): 19–29.

INFS (Institute of Nutrition and Food Science) and Department of Economics, University of Dhaka. 1998. "Strategies for Bangladesh." Dhaka Urban Community Health Program. Asian Development Bank, Manila.

Jennings, J., S. Gillespie, J. Mason, M. Lotfi, and T. Scialfa. 1991. "Managing Successful Nutrition Programmes." ACC/SCN State-of-the-Art Series, Nutrition Policy Discussion Paper 8, United Nations Administrative Committee on Coordination/Sub-Committee on Nutrition, Geneva. http://www.unsystem.org/scn/archives/npp08/index.htm.

Jonsson, U. 1997. "Success Factors in Community-Based Nutrition-Oriented Programmes and Projects." In *Malnutrition in South Asia: A Regional Profile*, ed. S Gillespie, 161–89. ROSA Publication 5. Kathmandu: UNICEF, Regional Office for South Asia.

Kachondam, Y., P. Winichagoon, and K. Tontisirin. 1992. "Nutrition and Health in Thailand: Trends and Actions." ACC/SCN case study, Institute of Nutrition at Mahidol University, Bangkok, and United Nations Administrative Committee on Coordination/Sub-Committee on Nutrition, Geneva.

Kavishe, F. P., and S. S. Mushi. 1993. *Nutrition-Relevant Actions in Tanzania.* ACC/SCN case study. Tanzania Food and Nutrition Centre, Monograph Series 1. Geneva: United Nations Administrative Committee on Coordination/Sub-Committee on Nutrition. http://www.unsystem.org/scn/archives/tanzania/index.htm.

Kelley, L. M., and R. E. Black. 2001. "Research to Support Household and Community IMCI. Report of a Meeting, 22–24 January 2001, Baltimore, Maryland, USA." *Journal of Health, Population, and Nutrition* 19 (Suppl. 2): S111–54.

Kielmann, A. A., C. E. Taylor, C. DeSweemer, I. S. Uberoi, H. S. Takulia, N. Masih, and S. Vohra. 1978. "The Narangwal Experiment: II. Morbidity and Mortality Effects." *Indian Journal of Medical Research* 68 (Suppl.): 42–54.

Mason, J. B. 2000. "How Nutrition Improves, and What That Implies for Policy Decisions." Paper prepared for World Bank–UNICEF Nutrition Assessment, UNICEF, New York, and World Bank, Washington, DC. http://www.tulane.edu/~internut/publications/WB_Bckgrd_Pprs/Narrative/NarrativethreeMason.doc.

———. 2003. "Philippines Case Study." In *Combating Malnutrition: Time to Act*, ed. G. Gillespie, M. McLachlan, and R. Shrimpton, 85–101. Washington, DC: World Bank.

Mason, J., A. Bailes, K. Mason, O. Yambi, U. Jonsson, C. Hudspeth, and others. Forthcoming. *AIDS, Drought, and Child Malnutrition in Southern Africa.* Public Health Nutrition.

Mason, J. B., J. Hunt, D. Parker, and U. Jonsson. 1999. "Investing in Child Nutrition in Asia." *Asian Development Review* 17 (1, 2): 1–32.

———. 2001. "Improving Child Nutrition in Asia." *Food and Nutrition Bulletin* 22 (3 Suppl.): 5–80.

Mason, J. B., P. Musgrove, and J.-P. Habicht. 2003. "At Least One-Third of Poor Countries' Disease Burden Is Due to Malnutrition." Disease Control Priorities Project Working Paper 1, Fogarty International Center/National Institutes of Health, Washington, DC. http://www.fic.nih.gov/dcpp/wps/wp1.pdf.

Mason, J., J. Rivera, and C. Helwig, eds. 2005. "Recent Trends in Malnutrition in Developing Regions: Vitamin A Deficiency, Anemia, Iodine Deficiency, and Child Underweight." *Food and Nutrition Bulletin* 26 (1) Special Issue: 1–110.

Mata, L. 1991. "National Nutrition and Holistic Care Programme (NNHCP), Costa Rica." In *Managing Successful Nutrition Programmes*, ed. J. Jennings, S. Gillespie, J. Mason, M. Lotfi, and T. Scialfa, 77–81.

ACC/SCN State-of-the-Art Series, Nutrition Policy Discussion Paper 8. Geneva: United Nations Administrative Committee on Coordination/Sub-Committee on Nutrition.

Measham, A. R., and M. Chatterjee. 1999. *Wasting Away: The Crisis of Malnutrition in India.* Washington, DC: World Bank.

Mills, A. 1994. "Decentralization and Accountability in the Health Sector from an International Perspective: What Are the Choices?" *Public Administration and Development* 14: 281–92.

Muñoz, C., and N. S. Scrimshaw. 1995. *The Nutrition and Health Transition of Democratic Costa Rica.* Boston: International Nutrition Foundation for Developing Countries.

Pelletier, D. L. 1991. "The Uses and Limitations of Information in the Iringa Nutrition Program, Tanzania." Cornell Food and Nutrition Policy Program, Working Paper 5, Cornell University, Ithaca, NY.

Pelletier, D. L., and E. A. Frongillo. 2003. "Changes in Child Survival Are Strongly Associated with Changes in Malnutrition in Developing Countries." *Journal of Nutrition* 133 (1): 107–19.

Pinstrup-Andersen, P., S. Burger, J.-P. Habicht, and K. Peterson. 1993. "Protein-Energy Malnutrition." In *Disease Control Priorities in Developing Countries*, ed. D. T. Jamison, W. H. Mosley, A. R. Measham, and J. L. Bobadilla, 391–420. New York: Oxford University Press.

Plowman, B., J. I. Picado, M. Griffiths, K. Van Roekel, and V. Vivas de Alvarado. 2002. *BASICS II Evaluation of the AIN Program in Honduras.* Arlington, VA: Basic Support for Institutionalizing Child Survival Project (BASICS II) for the U.S. Agency for International Development.

Reddy, V., M. Shekar, P. Rao, and S. Gillespie. 1992. "Nutrition in India." ACC/SCN case study. National Institute of Nutrition, Hyderabad, India. http://www.unsystem.org/scn/archives/india/index.htm.

Rohde, J. 1993. "Indonesia's Posyandus: Accomplishments and Future Challenges." In *Reaching Health for All*, ed. J. Rohde, M. Chatterjee, and D. Morley, 135–57. Oxford, U.K.: Oxford University Press.

Saenz, L. 1995. "Evolution of an Epidemiological Profile." In *The Nutrition and Health Transition of Democratic Costa Rica*, ed. C. Muñoz and N. S. Scrimshaw, 119–43. Boston: International Nutrition Foundation for Developing Countries.

Sampson, R. J., S. E. W. Raudenbusch, and F. Earls. 1997. "Neighborhoods and Violent Crime: A Multilevel Study of Collective Efficacy." *Science* 277: 918–24.

Sanders, D. 1985. With R. Carver. *The Struggle for Health.* London: Macmillan.

———. 1993. "The Potential and Limits of Health Sector Reform in Zimbabwe." In *Reaching Health for All*, ed. J. Rohde, M. Chatterjee, and D. Morley, 239–66. Oxford, U.K.: Oxford University Press.

———. 1999. "Success Factors in Community-Based Nutrition Programmes." *Food and Nutrition Bulletin* 20 (3): 307–14.

Sanders, D., and M. Chopra. 2004. "Child Health." Paper prepared for Save the Children U.K., London.

Save the Children U.K. 2003. *Thin on the Ground: Questioning the Evidence behind World Bank Funded Community Nutrition Projects in Bangladesh, Ethiopia, and Uganda.* London: Save the Children U.K. http://www.savethechildren.org.uk/temp/scuk/cache/cmsattach/666_ThinOnTheGround.pdf.

Shekar, M. 1989. "The Tamil Nadu Integrated Nutrition Programme: A Review of the Project with Special Emphasis on the Monitoring and Information System." Paper prepared for the Rockefeller Foundation and the Food and Nutrition Policy Programme, Cornell University, Ithaca, NY.

Shrimpton, R. 1989. "Community Participation in Food and Nutrition Programmes: An Analysis of Recent Governmental Experiences." Paper prepared for the Food and Nutrition Policy Programme, Cornell University, Ithaca, NY.

Soekirman, I. Tarwotjo, I. Jus'at, G. Sumodiningrat, and F. Jalal. 1992. *Economic Growth, Equity and Nutritional Improvement in Indonesia.* ACC/SCN case study. http://www.unsystem.org/scn/archives/indonesia/index.htm.

Tagwireyi, J., and T. Greiner. 1994. *Nutrition in Zimbabwe.* Washington, DC: World Bank.

Taylor, C. E., A. A. Kielmann, and R. L. Parker. 1978. "The Narangwal Nutrition Study: A Summary Review." *American Journal of Clinical Nutrition* 31: 1040–52.

Tontisirin, K., and P. Winichagoon. 1999. "Community-Based Programs: Success Factors for Public Nutrition Derived from Thailand's Experience." *Food and Nutrition Bulletin* 20 (3): 315–22.

UNICEF (United Nations Children's Fund). 1990. "Strategy for Improved Nutrition of Children and Women in Developing Countries." Policy Review Paper E/ICEF/1990/1.6, UNICEF, New York.

———. 1998. *State of the World's Children: Progress against Worms for Pennies.* New York: UNICEF.

———. 2004. *Drought, AIDS, and Child Malnutrition in Southern Africa: Preliminary Analysis of Nutritional Data on the Humanitarian Crisis.* Nairobi: UNICEF, Eastern and Southern Africa Regional Office.

Vargas, W. 1995. "Development and Characteristics of Health and Nutrition Services for Urban and Rural Communities of Costa Rica." In *The Nutrition and Health Transition of Democratic Costa Rica*, ed. C. Muñoz and N. S. Scrimshaw, 68–117. Boston: International Nutrition Foundation for Developing Countries.

Waterlow, J. C. 1992. *Protein Energy Malnutrition.* London: Edward Arnold.

Werner, D., and D. Sanders. 1997. *Questioning the Solution: The Politics of Primary Health Care and Child Survival.* Palo Alto, CA: HealthWrights.

Whitehead, R. G., M. G. Rowland, and T. J. Cole. 1976. "Infection, Nutrition, and Growth in a Rural African Environment." *Proceedings of the Nutrition Society* 35 (3): 369–75.

Winichagoon, P., Y. Kachondam, G. Attig, and K. Tontisirin. 1992. *Integrating Food and Nutrition into Development: Thailand's Experiences and Future Visions.* UNICEF/EAPRO and Institute of Nutrition at Mahidol University, Bangkok, Thailand.

WHO (World Health Organization). 1997. *Improving Child Health. IMCI: The Integrated Approach.* WHO/CHD/97.12 Rev 2. Geneva: WHO.

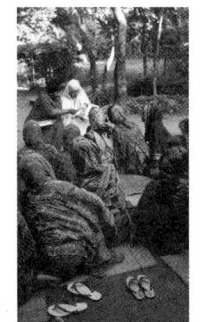

Chapter **57**

Contraception

Ruth Levine, Ana Langer, Nancy Birdsall, Gaverick Matheny, Merrick Wright, and Angela Bayer

The use of modern contraception to prevent pregnancies is a unique health intervention because, in many ways, it is not a health intervention at all. In general, couples in sexual relationships use contraception because, at the time the decision is made, one or both members do not wish to conceive a child, rather than because they wish to become healthier or to prevent a risk to health. Governments also may have an interest in promoting particular patterns of childbearing to meet social and economic objectives. This is most often the case when rapid population growth is seen as a drag on economic growth; in contrast, however, governments in low-fertility countries may promote pro-natalist policies to increase the labor supply. Thus, the effectiveness of contraception has to be seen, first and foremost, in terms of the effectiveness in permitting couples to achieve their desired family size.

Although contraception is rarely used to improve health, it does have health consequences. On the negative side, consequences may include the potential health risks of hormonal contraception or surgery. On the positive side, health may benefit from fewer pregnancies, lower exposure to sexually transmitted infections (STIs), and protection against ovarian cancer through the use of some types of contraception. Some of the consequences affect the users, some affect their sexual partners, and some affect their children. Contraceptives affect a user's sexuality by changing menstrual patterns and, therefore, particularly in some cultures, sexual activity. Also, by eliminating fear of unwanted pregnancy, contraceptives may enhance the quality of sexual experience. Finally, condoms may decrease sexual pleasure for men; true or not, this explanation is one of the most commonly cited to account for why some men (or couples) do not use condoms.

NATURE, CAUSES, AND BURDEN OF THE CONDITIONS THAT CAN BE ADDRESSED

Three rationales—each one involving controversy and touching on deeply held political and cultural perspectives—have underlain policy and programmatic interest in contraception, since the 1960s.

- The *demographic rationale*, typically framed around lowering the rate of population growth to achieve broad economic, social, and environmental aims, was most prominently applied in the 1960s and 1970s.
- The *fertility rationale*, which emerged in the 1980s, promoted lower fertility under the assumption that smaller families are better off in terms of economic and health conditions.
- The *human rights rationale*, which surfaced in 1994 at the International Conference on Population and Development in Cairo, served as a major force in the 1990s to focus attention on women's rights to autonomy and empowerment in childbearing and on female and male reproductive health. The Cairo Programme of Action stressed the political and cultural dimensions of contraception, including gender issues.

Population Growth and Fertility

In part because of the demand for and availability of modern contraception, the worldwide rate of annual population growth has declined from just over 2 percent in the late 1960s to 1.5 percent during 1980–2001. It is projected to decrease to 1 percent during 2001–15. Although the growth rate has slowed, population growth in absolute terms is unprecedented. World population increased from 2.5 billion people in 1950 to 6.3 billion in 2003 and is expected to rise to 7.1 billion by 2015 (UN 2003; World Bank 2003).

Fertility rates in developing countries have declined rapidly in the past 50 years, from more than 6.0 children per woman in the 1950s to about 2.8 children per woman today. Fertility rates remain high, however, in the 49 least developed countries, which had an average total fertility rate of 5.46 children per woman during 1995–2000 (UN 2003).

Fertility levels and trends vary greatly between regions. Fertility rates are lowest in low- and middle-income countries in East Asia and the Pacific, at 2.1 children per woman. Countries in Central Asia and Latin America and the Caribbean also have relatively low total fertility rates, at 2.5 and 2.6 children per woman, respectively. The Middle East and North Africa and South Asia follow, with average total fertility rates of 3.4 and 3.3 children per woman in 2001, respectively. Fertility rates are highest in Sub-Saharan Africa, at 5.2 children per woman (World Bank 2003).[1] Regional averages conceal substantial variation among and within countries.

Because of a legacy of high fertility and corresponding young population structures, population momentum ensures that many developing countries will continue to grow at a relatively high rate for many decades, even as fertility rates continue to decline. Population momentum alone will account for almost three-fourths of the population growth in developing countries in the next quarter-century. The largest growth at present is in Asia and Sub-Saharan Africa. Total population increase in these regions is now twice what it was in 1950. By 2015, population growth is expected to be substantially lower in all regions except Sub-Saharan Africa.

Demand for Contraception

If a woman wishes to postpone or avoid childbearing and is not using contraception (including use by her partners), she is said to have an unmet need for contraception. The most commonly reported reasons for unmet need are lack of knowledge, health concerns, and social disapproval (Casterline and Sinding 2000).

In 2003, an estimated 122.7 million women in developing countries had an unmet need for contraception, including 105.2 million married women, 8.4 million unmarried women, and 9.1 million women of all marital status in the states of the former Soviet Union. This figure represents 17 percent of all married women, a 2 percent decline from the late 1990s that is due to increasing contraceptive use.

Overall, the highest unmet need is in Sub-Saharan Africa, where 19.4 percent of all women have unmet need. About 13 percent of women in Asia, 10.6 percent of women in North Africa and the Middle East, and 8.5 percent of women in Latin America and the Caribbean and Central Asia have unmet need for contraception. Whereas women in the other regions of the world have an equally distributed unmet need for spacing and limiting births, the majority of unmet need in Sub-Saharan Africa is for spacing (Ross and Winfrey 2002). Unmet need is highest in countries where growing numbers of women want to avoid pregnancy but contraceptive prevalence is low. So, for example, among developing countries for which data are available from USAID's Demographic and Health Surveys, unmet need is currently highest in Haiti, where it nears 40 percent of all married women; it is more than 30 percent in Cambodia, Nepal, Pakistan, Rwanda, Senegal, Togo, Uganda, and the Republic of Yemen; and it is lowest, at less than 7 percent, in Brazil, Colombia, and Vietnam.

Total Potential Demand for Contraception. A rough measure of the total potential use of modern contraception in a country can be estimated by combining the measure of unmet need with the current proportion of women using contraception. Brazil, Colombia, and Vietnam all have demand for contraception greater than 80 percent of currently married women. They have satisfied most of this demand, with contraceptive prevalence rates above 75 percent, resulting in both low fertility rates and low unmet need (Westoff 2001). In contrast, in most Sub-Saharan African countries, the unmet need percentage exceeds the percentage of women currently using contraception (see table 57.1).

Health Consequences

Excess fertility is responsible for between 12 and 30 percent of the maternal burden of disease (see table 57.2)[2], although this is clearly an underestimate of the present and future burden of disease that can be prevented through investments in family planning. These estimates include only the direct health benefits of family planning for women by preventing unwanted births, decreasing the number of abortions, and increasing the length of birth intervals. Because of data limitations, these estimates exclude the potential effect of family-planning programs on children's long-term nutritional status and education; women's status and the household economy; and public savings from reduced fertility, AIDS, and other STIs through condom promotion and prevention of mother-to-child transmission (PMTCT). They also exclude the effect of such programs on environmentally related disease owing to population growth. Last, the estimates do not consider the disabling effects of unwanted pregnancies, despite the effect those pregnancies or their termination under unsafe conditions can have on women's welfare and productivity.

Each year, 585,000 women die and more than 54 million women suffer from diseases or complications caused by pregnancy and childbirth (WHO 1997).

Table 57.1 Total Potential Demand for Family Planning
(percentage of currently married women)

Country	Unmet need	Current contraceptive use	Total potential demand	Country	Unmet need	Current contraceptive use	Total potential demand
East Asia and the Pacific				*Sub-Saharan Africa*			
Cambodia	32.6	23.8	56.4	Benin	25.7	16.4	42.1
Indonesia	9.2	57.4	66.6	Burkina Faso	25.8	11.9	37.7
Philippines	18.8	47.8	66.6	Cameroon	19.7	19.3	39.0
Vietnam	6.9	75.3	82.2	Central African Rep.	16.2	14.8	31.0
Central Asian republics				Chad	9.7	4.1	13.8
Kazakhstan	8.7	66.1	74.8	Côte d'Ivoire	27.7	15.0	42.7
Kyrgyz Republic	11.6	59.5	71.1	Eritrea	27.5	8.0	35.5
Turkmenistan	10.1	61.8	71.9	Ethiopia	23.1	5.9	29.0
Uzbekistan	13.7	55.6	69.3	Gabon	28.0	32.7	60.7
Latin America and the Caribbean				Ghana	23.0	22.0	45.0
Argentina	—	—	—	Guinea	24.2	6.2	30.4
Belize	—	—	—	Kenya	23.9	39.0	62.9
Bolivia	26.1	48.3	74.4	Madagascar	25.6	19.4	45.0
Brazil	7.3	76.7	84.0	Malawi	29.7	30.6	60.3
Colombia	6.2	76.9	83.1	Mali	25.7	6.7	32.4
Dominican Republic	11.8	69.5	81.3	Mozambique	6.7	7.3	14.0
Guatemala	23.1	38.2	61.3	Namibia	21.9	28.9	50.8
Haiti	39.8	28.1	67.9	Niger	16.6	8.2	24.8
Nicaragua	14.7	60.3	75.0	Nigeria	17.5	15.3	32.8
Paraguay	15.0	48.4	63.4	Rwanda	35.6	13.2	48.8
Peru	10.2	68.9	79.1	Senegal	34.8	12.9	47.7
Middle East and North Africa				South Africa	15.0	56.3	71.3
Algeria	—	—	—	Tanzania	21.8	25.4	47.2
Egypt, Arab Rep. of	11.2	56.1	67.3	Togo	32.3	23.5	55.8
Jordan	14.2	52.6	66.8	Uganda	34.6	22.8	57.4
Morocco	16.1	50.3	66.4	Zambia	26.5	25.9	52.4
Yemen, Rep. of	38.6	20.8	59.4	Zimbabwe	12.9	53.5	66.4
South Asia							
Bangladesh	15.3	53.8	69.1				
India	15.8	48.2	64.0				
Nepal	31.4	28.5	59.9				
Pakistan	31.8	11.8	43.6				

Source: Demographic and Health Survey, various years.
— = not available.

Risks Associated with Unwanted Pregnancies. Unwanted pregnancies expose women to additional health risks by increasing the number of lifetime pregnancies and deliveries. Because the lifetime risk of maternal mortality is a function of the number of pregnancies and the quality and utilization of health care, reducing the number of pregnancies can lower maternal mortality rates (Koenig and others 1988).

Ambivalence toward pregnancy also is associated with less early and continuous prenatal care and lower use of professional delivery care (Gage 1998; Joyce and Grossman 1990; Weller, Eberstein, and Bailey 1987).

Many women who have unintended pregnancies turn to induced abortion, both in countries where abortion is legal and safe and in those where it is illegal and too often unsafe.

Table 57.2 Maternal Burden of Disease Associated with Unwanted Fertility and Unsafe Abortions

Region	Deaths	Years of life lost	Years lived with disability	Disability-adjusted life years (DALYs)	Percentage of all maternal DALYs
East Asia and the Pacific	3,637	107,795	380,255	420,030	17
Latin America and the Caribbean	6,323	190,544	298,390	429,399	30
Middle East and North Africa	8,428	244,461	256,742	395,368	12
South Asia	30,074	878,028	1,079,661	1,669,727	20
Sub-Saharan Africa	43,077	1,270,598	764,012	1,821,721	18

Sources: Adapted from WHO 2002a. Maternal morality related to unsafe abortions from WHO 1998. Percentage of infant disease preventable by family planning from Rutstein 2003.
Notes: Because of data limitations, estimates are not available for Eastern Europe and Central Asia. Burden-of-disease estimates include a 3 percent discount rate without age weighting. WHO regions are not identical to the World Bank Regions used here; however, a very close approximation was made by excluding WHO regions AMRO A, WPRO A, and EURO A. These estimates assume that 90 percent of abortion-related disease burden is preventable by family planning and that the percentage of other preventable maternal disease is equal to the percentage of all births that are unwanted.

Accurate measures of abortion are difficult to obtain in most parts of the world. In countries where abortion is illegal, data are lacking or incomplete, and even where it is legal, abortions may be underreported because of societal attitudes (Bongaarts 1997; Henshaw, Singh, and Haas 1999). It is estimated that about one-fourth of the 210 million pregnancies each year end in abortion.

In 1995, approximately 35.5 million abortions were performed in developing countries. The large majority of legal abortions, 10.6 million, occurred in China. Most of the remaining legal abortions took place in other parts of Asia (5.7 million) and in the Caribbean (0.2 million). Developing countries, which experienced an estimated 19 million illegal abortions in 1995, account for 95 percent of illegal abortions worldwide. Nearly 10 million illegal abortions occurred in Asia, followed by an estimated 5 million in Africa and 4 million in Latin America. These figures mark a particularly large increase for Africa, which was estimated to have only 1.5 million illegal abortions in 1987 (Henshaw, Singh, and Haas 1999).

Unsafe abortion, typically associated with illegality, has large impacts on both maternal mortality and maternal morbidity. Each year, unsafe abortion is believed to account for 80,000 maternal deaths, or 13 percent of the burden of disease in women of reproductive age (WHO 2002a). Deaths related to unsafe abortions are estimated at 100 to 600 death per 100,000 abortions, compared with the mortality rate from legal abortions of 0.6 deaths per 100,000 abortions (Salter, Johnston, and Hengen 1997). Survivors of unsafe abortions also experience consequences; unsafe abortion causes disability in an additional 5 million women (WHO 2002a). Treatment of complications from unsafe abortions constitutes a large proportion of emergency gynecological hospital admissions (Konje, Obisesan, and Ladipo 1992) and requires substantial resources (Kinoti and others 1995; Salter, Johnston, and Hengen 1997).

Legalizing abortion, improving the quality of abortion care, and increasing access to safe abortion can have profound impacts on the health consequences of abortion. When abortion was illegal in Romania in 1988, complications from unsafe abortion caused 86 percent of maternal deaths. After abortion was legalized in 1989, the frequency of abortion persisted because of contraceptive supply shortages, but the number of maternal deaths fell by 50 percent (Hord and others 1991).

Risks Associated with Pregnancy and Birth. All pregnancies and births involve some health risks to women, so preventing any pregnancy reduces women's health risks. Higher mortality and morbidity of women, infants, and children are positively associated with the risk factors of giving birth when a woman is too young or too old, the births are too close together, there are too many births, or a woman has a preexisting health condition. Births in most of these groups—women who are older (over age 35), births that are spaced too closely (24 months or less after the preceding birth), and births that are higher order (fifth or higher)—are also more likely to be reported as unintended, making their prevention doubly important (Tsui, Wasserheit, and Haaga 1997).

An estimated 15 million women under age 20 give birth each year. Women age 15 to 19 are twice as likely to die from childbearing as women in their 20s, and women under age 17 are at even greater risk (Starrs 1997). Adolescent mothers are more likely to suffer from obstetric complications if they lack physical maturity or are malnourished (Aitken and Walls 1986). They are also less likely to receive adequate prenatal or obstetric care, which may cause negative outcomes for them and for their infants (McDevitt and others 1996). In many contexts, negative social consequences are profound, including loss of school and employment opportunities.

Children born to adolescent mothers face a number of risks. Research has demonstrated that infants of teenage mothers are more likely than those born to mothers in their 20s to die before they reach their first birthday (Hobcraft 1992; McDevitt and others 1996; Ross and Frankenberg 1993; Starrs 1997; Sullivan, Rutstein, and Bicego 1994). Children of mothers under age 20 may have a 20 to 30 percent higher risk of death than children of older mothers (Hobcraft 1992; Sullivan, Rutstein, and Bicego 1994). Infants of teenage mothers are also at higher risk of being of low birthweight, small for gestational age, or premature. Finally, adolescent women are less likely to provide adequate care for their infants and children, because they often lack the maturity, education, and resources to do so (Geronimus 1987; Govindasamy and others 1993).

Women over age 35 face an increased risk of maternal mortality. Mothers age 40 to 44, for example, are five times more likely to die during pregnancy or childbirth than mothers in their 20s (Royston and Lopez 1987). Mothers in their late 30s and 40s may also face additional negative consequences, because they may have preexisting health problems owing to age or previous births.

As with children of adolescent mothers, children of women over age 35 also suffer negative consequences. Children born to mothers over age 40 are more likely than those born to younger mothers to die before age 5 (Bicego and Ahad 1996; Sullivan, Rutstein, and Bicego 1994). Older women are also more likely to have stillbirths or to bear children with congenital abnormalities who may not survive childhood (Cnattingius and others 1992; Fretts and Usher 1997).

Longer birth intervals reduce women's risks of death and ill health during pregnancy and childbirth. One study assessed the effects of birth spacing in 450,000 women on the basis of hospital records from 1985 to 1997 in 19 Latin American and Caribbean countries. The study found that women who have their babies 27 to 32 months after a preceding birth are more than two times more likely to survive pregnancy and childbirth than women who have short intervals of 9 to 14 months. Birth intervals of 27 to 32 months are also associated with lower incidence of third trimester bleeding, premature rupture of membranes, anemia, and other negative outcomes (Conde-Agudelo and Belizan 2000).

Recent research suggests that birth intervals of three to five years provide even greater benefits than the two-year intervals that were previously promoted. One study assessed the effect of this longer birth interval in more than 430,000 pregnancies in 18 countries and found that children who are born three to five years after the preceding birth are more likely to survive from the perinatal period through age five. Children born at intervals of three to five years are also 1.2 to 1.4 times less likely to be malnourished or underweight or to experience stunting than those born at intervals shorter than two years (Rutstein 2003).

Putting together a range of patchy data on the effect of family planning on child mortality can yield estimates of the total global impact, but those estimates are highly dependent on assumptions and have varied widely. The World Bank (1993) estimated that family-planning programs could prevent between 20 and 40 percent of all infant deaths by preventing mistimed and underspaced births. In a study of 25 countries, Hobcraft (1994) estimated that if all birth intervals of less than two years were prevented, child mortality levels would be reduced by an average of 17 percent and up to one-third in several countries. Rutstein (2003) found that birth spacing of three to five years alone could prevent up to 46 percent of infant mortality. Muhuri and Menken (1997) found that in rural Bangladesh poor spacing and timing accounted for 25 percent of child mortality. Trussell and Pebley (1984) estimated that spacing could decrease infant mortality by 10 percent and child (age 1 to 5) mortality by 21 percent. Another study found that, even in Latin America, which has lower child mortality rates, spacing could reduce perinatal mortality by 14 percent (Conde-Agudelo and Belizan 2000).

In a study of 19 African countries, Rafalimanana and Westoff (2001) found that median actual birth intervals in every country were shorter than the preferred birth intervals reported by women, reflecting the substantial unmet need for birth spacing. Achieving preferred intervals would decrease neonatal mortality by only 6 percent on average, and infant mortality by a comparable amount, whereas removing all short intervals would decrease both by 13 percent.

Women giving birth for the fourth or higher time are at much higher risk of maternal complications and death. Independent of a woman's age, her risk of dying when giving birth for the fourth or higher time is 1.5 to 3 times greater than during a second or third birth (Winikoff and Sullivan 1987). Women who have had at least three births are also more likely to experience hemorrhage, uterine rupture or prolapse, or kidney disease (Maymon and others 1998).

Children born to mothers who have had many births face risks similar to those of children born to older mothers; they are often the same women. Children born to mothers who have had three or more births are more likely than those born to younger mothers (those under age 20) to die before age 5 (Bicego and Ahad 1996; Sullivan, Rutstein, and Bicego 1994). Women who have had many births are also more likely to have stillbirths or to bear children with congenital abnormalities who may not survive childhood (Cnattingius and others 1992; Fretts and Usher 1997). Children from larger families often receive lower levels of education and health care than children from smaller families because of competition for finite family resources (Blake 1981).

Women with preexisting health conditions often face greater risks in pregnancy and childbirth. Pregnancy can aggravate conditions such as high blood pressure, heart disease, malaria, anemia, tuberculosis, hepatitis, and STIs, including HIV. Indirect causes, including these preexisting conditions, account for an estimated 20 percent of maternal deaths each year (WHO 1997).

INTERVENTIONS

The "intervention" of contraception can be considered as the method itself and as the means by which family-planning clients obtain services (including counseling) and contraceptive commodities. Both the methods and the types of services are diverse.

Contraceptive Methods

Contraceptive methods can be classified as permanent and long term—primarily for those women and couples who have completed childbearing—or temporary—primarily for those women and couples who wish to delay pregnancy.

Permanent and Long-Term Methods. Female sterilization, or tubal ligation, used by about 187 million women worldwide (WHO 2002a), is the most popular and effective contraceptive available. The most effective types of female sterilization have a 10-year cumulative pregnancy rate of 7.5 per 1,000 procedures (Peterson and others 1996).

Sterilization accounts for one-third of all contraceptive practice. Because sterilization is considered a permanent form of contraception, some women may regret their decision during ensuing years. Some dissatisfaction with sterilization is expected and is always observed among sterilized populations; in most cases, the proportion of women regretting sterilization falls below 10 percent. Regret is higher when sterilization was a woman's first and only contraceptive method, when a woman was sterilized at or under age 30, or when a woman has fewer than four living children (Loaiza 1995).

Between 40 million and 50 million men worldwide have undergone a vasectomy, a figure representing 8 percent of the world's couples of reproductive age. This method comes in fourth in contraceptive popularity, after female sterilization (19 percent), the intrauterine device (IUD; 13 percent), and oral contraceptives ("the pill"; 8 percent), and right ahead of the male condom (4 percent; WHO 2002a). The method is as effective as female sterilization (failure rate of less than 1 percent) and much simpler and safer than tubal ligation.

The IUD is now used by 150 million women worldwide, or about 13 percent of the world's women of reproductive age, because of its efficacy, safety, and convenience. After female sterilization, it is the most popular method of contraception. The 5-year life span of the IUD means fewer visits to health providers and less expenditure of money, time, and effort.

IUDs prevent pregnancy through several mechanisms: they alter sperm migrations, inhibit fertilization, and generate a foreign-body reaction in the endometrium. Progestogen-releasing IUDs cause changes in the amount and viscosity of cervical fluid, altering sperm penetration. In a small percentage of women, ovulation is inhibited in the first two years of use.

Failure rates for all copper-bearing IUDs are usually less than 1 per 100 women in the first year of use.

Temporary Methods. By far the most popular temporary contraceptive method is the oral contraceptive, commonly known as "the pill," which has a failure rate typical use of less than 10 percent over a year. Among 67 developing countries for which survey data are available (not including China or India), about 50 percent of married women who have ever used contraception have used the pill at some point. The pill has been most popular in Latin America; there, about 55 percent of all married women have used the pill. In the Near East and North Africa, about one-third of married women have used the pill, and in Sub-Saharan Africa, about 15 percent have used it at some time (Johns Hopkins Population Information Program 2000).

More than 20 million women use systemic contraceptives containing only progestins. These contraceptives include subdermal implants such as Norplant, injectable products, IUDs, and vaginal rings. These products have high rates of contraceptive efficacy (0.3 to 1.0 percent failure rate over 12 months). Their long duration of action allows for a relatively infrequent dose. Their main drawbacks are their tendencies to cause highly irregular endometrial bleeding and amenorrhea. Although altered bleeding does not have any ill health effects, it does pose a problem for women in societies that bar or restrict women from certain social and religious activities during menstruation. The World Health Organization estimates that between 10 and 30 percent of women abandon their progestin-only methods for this reason (WHO 2002a).

Barrier methods, although less effective than hormonal methods, IUDs, or sterilization, can offer effective contraception when used consistently and correctly. Barrier methods, and particularly condoms, are the only type of contraception that offers additional protection against STIs.

When used correctly during every act of sexual intercourse, the male latex condom is effective against both unwanted pregnancy and HIV infection and other STIs. Typical use results in pregnancy rates of 3 to 14 percent per year. If a condom breaks or tears during intercourse, emergency contraception can be used to reduce the risk of pregnancy.

The female condom, made of soft, pliable polyurethane and prelubricated with a silicone-based substance, is inserted into the vagina before sexual intercourse. The female condom is slightly less effective than the male condom, with a failure rate of 5 to 21 percent. Unlike the male condom, the female condom can be inserted up to eight hours before intercourse. The female condom adds to the arsenal of weapons in the fight against STIs; offers women more control in sexual negotiations; can be used in conjunction with the IUD, hormonal methods, and sterilization; and has no special storage requirements.

The diaphragm, although not a popular method in developing countries, is being studied as a means of preventing not only pregnancy but also bacterial STIs. Results from those randomized trials are pending.

Emergency Contraception. Since the mid 1960s, the use of certain oral contraceptives has been shown to be effective in preventing pregnancy. Two hormonal regimens have proved to be both safe and effective for emergency contraception: combined oral contraceptives and progestogen-only pills. Both can be taken for up to 120 hours after unprotected intercourse. Emergency contraception represents a second chance to prevent an unwanted pregnancy after unprotected sex, and it is particularly responsive to the needs of youths and of women who have been coerced into intercourse.

Despite the demonstrated safety and efficacy of emergency contraception, its acceptance by providers and the public, and its inclusion on the WHO's essential drug list, emergency contraception is not widely available in many developing countries (Langer and others 1999).

ORGANIZATION OF FAMILY-PLANNING PROGRAMS

Because of the variety of users and methods of contraception, a range of quite distinct ways to deliver needed goods and services has been developed and tried over the past several decades. Some programs are dedicated to providing only family-planning services, often referred to as *vertical programs;* some provide a range of reproductive and other health services, loosely termed *integrated programs;* and some try to reach current and potential clients through social marketing and community-based distribution methods.

Vertical versus Integrated Service Delivery

The original large-scale family-planning programs in developing countries, many of which were launched on the basis of the demographic rationale, tended to be organized around a vertical structure with central management and logistics. Family-planning workers based at fixed sites—whether run by government agencies or by nongovernmental organizations (NGOs)—were dedicated exclusively to providing information, services, and contraceptive commodities related to family planning. Funding, often from external donor agencies, was earmarked for family-planning activities. In many instances, the supervisory, budgeting, training, and logistics systems were all separate from those of other health services. Some of the largest vertical programs, such as the India program, promoted sterilization on a large scale, sometimes provided through rudimentary health facilities. Others, such as the Bangladesh program, relied on the provision of information and commodities through female outreach workers going house to house.

In the past two decades, increasing emphasis has been placed on integrating family-planning programs into other health services, particularly other types of reproductive health services. Under this arrangement, family-planning services are delivered in conjunction with routine primary care—a recognition that women's health needs are in no way confined to contraception and that a broad range of reproductive and other health services must be provided.

Social Marketing

Social marketing refers to a variety of strategies using traditional commercial-marketing techniques to promote socially beneficial behaviors, products, and services. In family planning, social marketing has focused on making supplies of methods of contraception widely available in existing commercial retail outlets and on promoting these contraceptives to consumers through mass media. In recent years, social-marketing programs have expanded their focus to behavior change and the delivery of clinical services through social franchises.

In countries with low contraceptive prevalence, social-marketing programs for contraceptives typically import donated contraceptives and then repackage and promote them with their own sales force. In higher-prevalence countries, programs may partner with commercial manufacturers to market existing brands, often subsidizing promotion in exchange for price guarantees. In the Dominican Republic, for instance, the oral contraceptive manufacturer Schering agreed to cut the price of its pills in half in exchange for advertising by a social-marketing organization.

Most social-marketing programs for contraceptives distribute commodities through existing commercial outlets, such as shops, pharmacies, and tobacco shops. Retailers make a small profit, which increases their incentive to stock and promote the products. Because such programs do not spend money building their own distribution network, they typically enjoy low costs per output.

Social-marketing programs have achieved dramatic contraceptive sales throughout the developing world, providing contraception to about 10 million couples in 60 countries, in addition to promoting a variety of other health products. However, evidence from cross-national studies suggests that social marketing's effect on contraceptive use is driven less by its brand sales—because users often switch brands—and more by its promotional activity (Bulatao 2002).

INTERVENTION COST AND COST-EFFECTIVENESS

Synthesizing data on family-planning costs, outputs, and outcomes to inform resource allocation has distinct challenges. First, nearly all existing studies have estimated average—not marginal—costs. The dearth of marginal cost data, general to most of the cost-effectiveness studies presented in this volume, severely weakens the ability to recommend interventions.

Second, cost data based on units of output that cannot be linked to health outcomes have limited use. Most studies on effectiveness have not included costs, and most studies on costs have not included effectiveness. In the family-planning literature, cost per output (such as the cost per couple-year of protection, or CYP) has often been called cost-effectiveness. Here, we reserve the term *cost-effectiveness* for measures of cost per unit of health impact (Gift, Haddix, and Corso 2003). Those studies that have measured cost-effectiveness typically come from mature programs, where both marginal costs and marginal effects are likely to be low.

Third, costs vary considerably according to the accounting method used, the program setting and scale, the level of latent demand among couples targeted, the method mix, the quality, and the existing supply and service infrastructure (Dayaratna and others 2000; Janowitz and Bratt 1992). Clinical costs are particularly sensitive to setting, given the broad differences in local salaries.

Finally, most evaluations of family planning estimate effects within a single generation. However, averting a birth also averts grandchildren, great-grandchildren, and so on. For economic cost-benefit analyses, the multigenerational effects of a single birth averted can be significant. However, this consideration can be addressed through the use of an appropriate discount rate.

Cost per Output

The most common measure of output in family-planning programs is the CYP. Stover and others (1996) estimated the number of contraceptives of various methods needed to provide 1 CYP, given typical use: 15 cycles of pills, 120 condoms, 120 foaming tablets, or 4 three-month or 12 one-month injectables. An IUD provides 3.5 CYPs; male and female sterilization, 11 CYPs; and an individual trained in natural methods, 2 CYPs.

IUDs and voluntary sterilization have the lowest cost per CYP, although they have a high up-front cost. Oral contraceptives are usually the least costly methods. Condoms and injectables are more expensive than the pill, and implants are often the most expensive method per CYP. Mauldin and Miller (1994) estimated that, based on the method mix in developing countries, the weighted average commodity cost of contraception was US$1.55 per CYP.[3]

Commodity costs are relatively constant across programs, although there is some variation owing to bulk procurement. When program costs are added, costs vary considerably by the program setting and mode of delivery. A review of programs in Africa, for instance, found method costs per CYP could vary by an order of magnitude, with the greatest variation in the cost of condoms.

Barberis and Harvey (1997) found considerable variation in costs per CYP by region and mode of service delivery in 14 developing countries. Across regions, costs per CYP were comparable in Asia, Latin America, and the Middle East, at US$4.00 to US$5.00. Costs were considerably greater in Africa, where the average cost per CYP was US$14.00.

The least expensive mode of service delivery was clinical provision of sterilization, with a weighted average cost of US$2.34 per CYP. The second most economical mode was social marketing of contraceptives, although those costs are highly dependent on setting. In African countries, where such programs were less developed, the costs were high—up to US$19.00 per CYP. The weighted average cost of social marketing of contraceptives was US$3.00.

Costs of community-based distribution programs ranged from US$4.85 to US$35.37 per CYP, with a weighted average of US$12.55. Costs of clinic-based services, excluding sterilization, ranged from US$4.44 to US$16.65 per CYP, with a weighted average of US$7.93. Clinic-based services supplemented with community-based distribution were the most expensive mode of service delivery, ranging from US$4.44 to US$19.38, with a weighted average of US$18.21. As noted above, these estimates have typically not included costs to users (see table 57.3).

Marginal Costs

Knowles and Wagman (1991) found that unit costs decline as the number of contraceptive users increases. Larger programs enjoy an economy of scale in procurement; average costs

Table 57.3 Weighted Average Program Costs per CYP, by Region and Mode of Delivery
(2001 U.S. dollars)

Region	Mode of service delivery	Cost per CYP
Africa	Social marketing	15.95
	Community-based distribution	20.32
	Clinics	16.65
	Clinics with community-based distribution	8.02
Asia	Social marketing	2.59
	Community-based distribution	6.50
	Clinics	5.07
	Clinics with community-based distribution	19.38
Latin America	Social marketing	−1.64
	Community-based distribution	35.37
	Clinics	6.40
	Clinics with community-based distribution	6.47
Middle East	Social marketing	3.82
	Community-based distribution	4.85
	Clinics	4.44
	Clinics with community-based distribution	9.03

Source: Adapted from Barberis and Harvey 1997.

decrease as fixed costs from training and from information, education, and communication (IEC) programs are distributed over more units; labor may be more efficiently used at higher volumes; and larger programs may be further ahead on the learning curve. However, as marginal costs diminish with size, so may marginal returns in mature programs (Haaga and Tsui 1995).

High rates of underutilization suggest marginal costs may be close to zero for many clinics. Knowles and Wagman (1991) and Janowitz and others (1996) found underutilization of clinical capacity in Morocco and Bangladesh. In Morocco, more than a third of all labor costs were spent waiting for patients. Foreit and others (1992) found that administrative costs accounted for 16 to 65 percent of fixed costs for a sample of clinics, whereas capacity utilization ranged from only 32 to 76 percent.

One study of a community-based distribution project in Bangladesh found that marginal costs represented 20 to 40 percent of average costs and decreased with scale (Attanayake, Fauveau, and Chakraborty 1993). In social-marketing programs, marginal costs are close to commodity costs less revenue (Bulatao 1993). A weighted average of current commodity costs based on the existing method mix in developing countries suggests a marginal cost of about US$1.55 per CYP (Mauldin and Miller 1994).

Cost-Effectiveness Outside of Programs

The estimates of cost-effectiveness included here show only the direct health benefits of family planning for women and children from increasing birth intervals and reducing teenage pregnancies. As noted earlier, these estimates ignore important benefits of family planning for the health of families. Because of data limitations, most of these omissions cannot be corrected here. Some are a general consequence of using the global burden-of-disease framework, which takes disease, rather than health interventions, as the starting point. This orientation makes results less useful for the purpose of setting priorities in health care, particularly for interventions, such as family planning, that affect a number of sequelae (Williams 1999).

Despite the abundance of cost-per-output data in family planning, these data cannot be used to set priorities in health funding because the protection offered by a unit of contraception is related to the behavior of a particular user. Several studies have sought to estimate a program's impact on fertility as a simple division of CYPs distributed in a population by the mean birth interval in the population (Cakir, Fabricant, and Kircalioglu 1996). However, such adjustments are not substitutes for actual measures of impact.

A considerable literature has developed around the problems of using CYP as a measure of protection (for reviews, see Fort 1996 and Shelton 1991). The typical calculation of CYPs does not account for use-failure rates, wastage, and client char-

acteristics such as fecundity, coital frequency, use effectiveness, or frequency of contraceptive use—one couple using condoms all the time has a greater effect on fertility than two couples using condoms half the time.

Most critically, even if CYP were an appropriate measure of protection, CYPs do not account for method substitution. Many clients who obtain contraceptives from a family-planning program, at some program expense, were buying or would otherwise have bought contraceptives from commercial providers or would have relied on natural methods. Community-based distribution programs, for instance, may be more expensive per CYP than social-marketing programs, but if such programs reach more nonusers than social-marketing programs, they may be more cost effective in preventing unwanted pregnancies. Similarly, sterilization is the cheapest method per CYP, but in many countries, it has a limited impact on fertility.

Three examples demonstrate the hazard of confusing output, or even intermediate outcomes, with impact. Jensen (1996) found that public providers in Indonesia, while more expensive per CYP than private providers, had a greater effect on fertility per unit output. Public programs may have reached more nonusers. Janowitz and others (1992) found that a Honduran social-marketing program distributed more than 40,000 CYPs but had no net effect on contraceptive prevalence. Users substituted one contraceptive brand or method for another. Bertrand and others (1986) found that a community-based distribution program in then Zaire increased modern contraceptive prevalence without affecting total contraceptive prevalence. Modern methods were substituted for traditional ones, such as prolonged lactation, periodic abstinence, or withdrawal. (Such substitution can be an improvement when the traditional method replaced is rhythm or withdrawal, but there is no more protective contraception than postpartum abstinence.)

Cost-effectiveness analysis thus requires true estimates of project effect—the difference between what happens in a project's presence and what happens in that project's absence. A number of studies have estimated effect, measuring births averted, total or unwanted pregnancies averted, unsafe abortions averted, maternal and child deaths averted, and measures of health utility, such as the disability-adjusted life year (DALY).

As table 57.4 shows, costs vary significantly within regions. In some regions, maximum and minimum costs differ by two orders of magnitude. Our sensitivity analysis found that the cost-effectiveness of programs was most sensitive (as a percentage of swing) to the existing level of unmet need for birth spacing and limiting.

Costs per Births Averted. In a review, Pritchett (1994) found that costs per birth averted ranged from US$37 in Jamaica, the Philippines, and Thailand to US$415 in Nepal, with the median value of 12 studies being US$82. Cochrane (1988) estimated US$78 per averted birth in a cross-national analysis.

Table 57.4 Average Costs per Benefit of Family Planning
(2001 U.S. dollars)

Region	Births averted	Infant deaths averted	Maternal deaths averted	Disability-adjusted life years saved	Years of life lost averted	Years lived with disability
East Asia and the Pacific	163	4,907	12,880	60	110	103
Latin America and the Caribbean	87	2,316	34,564	53	66	187
Middle East and North Africa	97	1,989	18,917	49	55	209
South Asia	113	1,577	5,172	30	37	98
Sub-Saharan Africa	131	1,367	10,231	34	37	194

Source: Authors, based on a model by AGI and others (2000).
Note: The model used country-level data for 68 developing countries. Output costs were based on Population Action International estimates in 1994 of the public sector cost per user. Estimates are not available for Eastern Europe and Central Asia.

Experimental studies in Bangladesh estimated the cost per averted birth at US$95 (Attanayake, Fauveau, and Chakraborty 1993), US$281 (Pritchett 1994), US$293 (Balk and others 1988), and US$296 (Simmons, Balk, and Faiz 1991), varying by the accounting method used. The Bangladesh experiment was likely more expensive than other programs, as it involved a frequent schedule of visitation for community-based distribution. The model we developed for the Disease Control Priorities Project produced costs between US$87 and US$163 per birth averted, with costs lowest in Latin America and the Caribbean and in the Middle East and North Africa.

Costs per Death Averted. Walsh and others (1993) estimated that in a typical high-mortality country with a 20 percent contraceptive prevalence rate, family-planning programs cost US$8,261 per maternal death averted and US$1,276 per perinatal infant death averted. In a setting with high mortality and low contraceptive prevalence rates, offering family planning alone was considerably more cost-effective in averting both maternal and infant deaths than offering an integrated program including prenatal care and birth attendant training. The model developed for the Disease Control Priorities Project produced regional average costs between US$5,172 and US$34,564 per maternal death averted and between US$1,367 and US$4,907 per infant death averted. Costs were lowest in South Asia and Sub-Saharan Africa. Costs within regions varied by as much as two orders of magnitude.

Stover (2003) estimated that by offering family-planning services at PMTCT and voluntary counseling and testing sites in countries with high HIV prevalence, child HIV infections could be averted at a cost of US$489, and child deaths could be averted at a cost of US$278 per event—well below the costs of averting these events using traditional PMTCT services. In addition, these family programs would avert orphans at a cost of US$278, and maternal deaths at a cost of US$1,824 per event.

Costs per DALY. The 1993 report on world development (World Bank 1993) estimated that family-planning programs in low-income countries cost from US$40 to US$60 per DALY. In the first edition of *Disease Control Priorities in Developing Countries,* Jamison (1993) estimated the costs of IEC or behavior-change communication (BCC) programs promoting condom use for family planning at between US$20 and US$100 per DALY, depending on child and maternal mortality rates.

Average costs for regions per YLL ranged from US$37 to US$110. Costs per DALY and year of life lost (YLL) were lowest in South Asia and Sub-Saharan Africa, whereas costs per year lived with disability (YLD) were lowest in South Asia and in East Asia and the Pacific. As with costs per death averted, costs per DALY varied within regions by as much as two orders of magnitude.

Family-planning programs that target HIV-positive women to prevent mother-to-child transmission may be even more cost-effective. According to an analysis of Stover's (2003) estimates, such programs cost about US$5 per DALY. In comparison, traditional PMTCT services, including antiretrovirals and replacement feeding, cost US$37 per DALY, and nevirapine regimens cost US$5 to US$12 per DALY (Marseille and others 1999; UNAIDS 1999). Kumar (2000) found that adding family-planning and abortion services to PMTCT programs increased their cost-effectiveness from US$124 per DALY for a short-course antiretroviral drug regimen to US$93 per DALY for an integrated strategy. Despite its cost-effectiveness, family planning is not currently included in most policies addressing mother-to-child transmission of HIV.

Cost-Effectiveness within Programs

Few studies compare the cost-effectiveness of program designs and elements—for instance, between social marketing and community-based distribution, or between price subsidies and promotional spending. Thus, although donors or government ministers may have enough information to justify funding family-planning programs, managers of such programs have much less information to use in deciding how best to spend money within their programs.

Program Inputs. Roughly half of program funds are spent subsidizing price (Sanderson and Tan 1996), but there is little evidence that price subsidies significantly affect contraceptive use, even among the poor (Matheny 2004). In every demographic and health survey over the past decade, price has been reported as a barrier to contraceptive use by fewer than 2 percent of women with unmet need. Several studies suggest that even the poorest urban users are typically willing to pay commercial contraceptive prices—once they intend to contracept. This finding is not entirely surprising, because the economic costs of childbearing dwarf those of contraception (Pritchett 1994). Particularly if profits are reinvested in a program's quality of services, higher prices may permit the provision of amenities that attract more clients (Foreit and Levine 1993; Litvack and Bodart 1993).

The most commonly reported barriers to contraceptive use are lack of knowledge, health concerns, and social disapproval (Casterline and Sinding 2000). It is likely, then, that the most cost-effective inputs are those that address these barriers—by increasing accurate knowledge about and social acceptance of contraception, as well as by improving the quality of and access to a variety of contraceptive methods.

Evidence suggests that quality has improved contraceptive use for birth spacing in Tunisia (Cochrane and Guilkey 1995). However, results are mixed in Peru (Mensch, Arends-Kuenning, and Jain 1996) and the Philippines (DeGraff, Bilsborrow, and Herrin 1993). Schultz (1994) found that, on average, improved quality does not affect the contraceptive prevalence rate at the national level.

Some improvements in quality require additional resources—expanding facilities, adding equipment and staff, and diversifying services. Quality improvements are necessary to respond to ethical imperatives. Beyond the ethical rationale, quality improvements can reduce the cost per unit of output—improving the flow of clients and shifting service delivery from physicians to paramedics. Improvements in quality can also increase utilization and allow higher prices to be charged.

Unfortunately, the relative cost-effectiveness of investments in these inputs has not been established. However, there is reason to believe that, among all inputs, investments in IEC and BCC activities are the most cost-effective—especially those that encourage users to purchase contraceptives or services from the private sector. Studies in many countries show that exposure to IEC and BCC messages through television, radio, and print increases the likelihood of contraceptive use (Dayaratna and others 2000; Westoff and Bankole 1997). Social-marketing programs appear to succeed in increasing contraceptive use principally through their promotional activities (Bulatao 2002). IEC and BCC activities can also increase the efficiency of clinic programs by increasing caseloads. Last, among all family-planning activities, IEC and BCC activities may be the most prone to market failure, providing a strong rationale for public investment.

Integration. Integrating family planning with other reproductive health services was a major goal of the 1994 International Conference on Population and Development. Although the logic of integration is compelling, little research has been done on the costs of integrated programs. In theory, integrated programs should be more efficient because they distribute joint costs across more services. In clinics, integration should increase cost-effectiveness if services such as Papanicolaou smears, ultrasounds, pregnancy testing, abortions, and post-abortion care are used to cross-subsidize less profitable contraceptive services. Mitchell, Littlefield, and Gutter (1999) found relatively low family-planning costs in two integrated clinics and concluded that adding clients has a larger effect on costs in a clinical setting than adding services does. Mancini, Stecklov, and Stewart (2003), however, found that vertical programs that focused exclusively on family planning offered contraceptive supplies and services at a significantly lower cost per CYP than integrated programs.

Delivering contraception services alongside abortion or postabortion care can be cost-effective. Few clinics and hospitals that treat women suffering from abortion complications offer contraceptive counseling and services as part of their postabortion care, yet these services are effective in increasing contraceptive use. The key obstacle is finding support from abortion providers—especially private providers, who may not see profit potential in providing family planning. The same is true of prenatal care. One study in Kenya showed that exposing women to information about family planning during prenatal care doubled the likelihood that they would use contraception (Ndhlovu 1997). A study of 27 countries found that two-thirds of women had an unmet need for contraception within one year of their last childbirth (Ross and Winfrey 2001). In fact, about one-third of all unmet need was among women postpartum. This need could be satisfied with greater integration of maternal and child health services and family planning, particularly during prenatal visits, delivery care, and six-week postpartum visits.

Finally, integrating STI services with family planning can help identify women with STIs who wish to avoid risky pregnancies and prevent fetal and neonatal complications. Integrating STI services may also draw more men to family-planning clinics.

EQUITY: DISTRIBUTING THE BENEFITS OF SUBSIDIES

It is the poorest whose health and prosperity are most threatened by unwanted pregnancies, and who are least able to pay for family-planning services. Yet a significant portion of public subsidies for family planning benefit the wealthy. This outcome is in part a natural consequence of the demand for family planning. Wealthier couples typically want smaller families than poorer couples. If subsidies follow demand rather than need, they will concentrate among the wealthy. However, because there is substantial unmet need for family planning among poor couples, an efficient segmentation of the market would have subsidized providers target poorer clients and unsubsidized providers target wealthier clients.

In a study of 10 countries, Sine (2002) found that nonpoor users obtained 45 percent of subsidized oral contraceptives and 56 percent of subsidized condoms supplied by governments and nonprofit organizations. An analysis in Indonesia found that only 16 percent of public subsidies for family planning accrued to the poorest quartile. In the Philippines, 64 percent of subsidies accrued to the richest half of households, whereas 17 percent accrued to the poorest quarter. In the Philippines, the distribution of subsidies varied widely by contraceptive method, with vasectomy subsidies concentrated among the poor and condom subsidies concentrated among the middle class (Haaga and Tsui 1995).

Behrman and Knowles (1998) found that the family-planning program in Vietnam was only weakly pro-poor. The main source of inefficiency stemmed from the greater use of more heavily subsidized government providers, particularly hospitals, by wealthier clients. One study in Bangladesh found that, although family-planning workers had the largest effect on the contraceptive behavior of uneducated women, the workers—who typically come from the educated class—were more likely to visit educated women (Arends-Kuenning 1997). For similar reasons, clinics are often located in wealthier areas.

Whereas a significant share of wealthier users obtain subsidized goods, a large share of poor users obtain goods from the commercial sector. In a study of 12 countries, more than half of even the poorest condom users purchased condoms from the commercial sector in all countries but the Philippines (Foreit 1999). Sine (2002), in turn, found that 20 percent of poor and near-poor users obtained their oral contraceptives from the commercial sector, even in countries where free or subsidized brands were available.

ECONOMIC BENEFITS OF INTERVENTION

Contraception or family planning can yield long-term economic benefits through three main routes. One is reasonably direct and easy to quantify; the others are more complex. First, contraception can produce economic benefits by reducing maternal mortality and morbidity and improving child health—benefits that can be captured through estimates of savings to the health system.

Second, contraception can have economic payoffs if it occurs in a setting where high fertility is constraining economic growth. Longstanding arguments in development economics have centered on whether rapid population growth acts as a drag on economic growth. Some camps argued that high fertility, in particular, would condemn a country to slow (or even negative) per capita income growth. Others argued that the negative effects would be mild and short lived, as households adapt to existing resource constraints by reducing childbearing and as technological changes, such as those that result in higher agricultural yields, alter the productivity equation. By the late 1990s, however, a consensus emerged from examination of more than 40 years of experience and data: rapid population growth, in general, and high fertility, in particular, typically lead to slower economic growth and higher levels of poverty than would otherwise be realized (Birdsall and Sinding 2003).

Third, when contraception reduces the rate of population growth, it can have multiple effects (economic and other) on the environment. High fertility, coupled with rural-to-urban migration, has led to rapid urban growth, often outpacing the provision of clean water and sanitation. In an analysis of 42 cities in Latin America, Asia, and Africa, Brockerhoff and Brennan (1998) found that urban growth rates were positively correlated with infant mortality rates, likely owing to crowding, a weakening of the public infrastructure, and increased air pollution. Ambient air pollution is now emerging as a serious threat to human health in virtually all the large cities in the world, responsible for 1 percent of global deaths and DALYs (WHO 2002b).[4]

Population growth is also responsible for much of the increase in carbon emissions that contribute to global climate change. Although developing countries account for only 20 percent of carbon emissions today, some researchers have estimated that these countries will account for 50 percent by 2050, given current rates of development (Bongaarts 1992). Bongaarts estimated that population growth would account for 48 percent of the growth in carbon emissions in developing countries between 1985 and 2100. Birdsall (1994) estimated that realistic reductions in fertility could reduce emissions in 2050 by as much as 15 percent in developing countries; more important, however, she estimated that by reducing fertility, family-planning programs could reduce emissions more cost-effectively than taxes on carbon emissions could. Similarly, Brinkley, Potts, and Walsh (2003) found that family-planning programs are likely more cost-effective than any emissions policy. (At the same time, it is important to note that the largest per capita consumption of nonrenewable natural resources occurs in the low-fertility settings of wealthy countries, where policies promoting conservation are overdue.)

RESEARCH AND DEVELOPMENT AGENDA

The agenda for research and development in the field of contraceptives and family planning is ample. It benefits from a strong tradition of data- and research-driven policy and programmatic decisions. Priorities suggested below fall into the realms of science, operations (or program), and policy.

On the scientific agenda, the top priority must be the development of contraceptive products that protect women and men against both pregnancy and HIV infection in ways that are more acceptable from a user perspective than male or female condoms. Two other high-priority topics are the development of male contraceptives and of microbicides, a female-controlled method that protects against both STIs (especially, HIV) and unwanted pregnancy.

With respect to operations research, high-priority questions include how to reach adolescents effectively and cost-effectively; what to do in settings where progress has stalled (for example, Bangladesh); and how to stimulate demand for family planning in Sub-Saharan African countries, where the demand is relatively low.

Another important and neglected topic is how to introduce the sexual health dimension into contraceptive services. In general, providers do not take into account sexuality and sexual health during counseling or service delivery, in spite of the mutual influence between sexual behavior and preferences and contraception. On the one hand, women and couples' sexual activities strongly influence the adoption of contraception, and the preference of these women and couples for a certain method, in turn, influences its effective use and continuity. On the other hand, particular characteristics of the different methods affect women's and couples' perceptions of their own sexuality (Bruce 1987). In spite of these obvious links, neither the family-planning literature nor family-planning services have yet paid enough attention to the matter (Dixon-Mueller 1993).

On the policy research agenda, further research is required to understand the relationship between fertility and other reproductive health outcomes and economic outcomes at microeconomic and macroeconomic levels. Such research includes, for example, a careful analysis of how access to contraception may affect women's productivity, as well as human capital investments in the next generation. In addition, better understanding of the distributional effect of family planning and other reproductive health services would inform policies about how best to target public resources.

NOTES

1. These are 2001 averages; country-by-country figures are 2000 and earlier.

2. One problem in applying the burden-of-disease framework to family planning is unique to interventions that affect the size of a population. In most effectiveness analyses, one compares the state of the world with a particular program to the state of the world without that program. However, effectiveness analyses using disabilty-adjusted life years (DALYs) are typically not conducted this way. The number of DALYs averted by family planning is not the number of DALYs without a family-planning program minus the total number of DALYs with a family-planning program. Given the negative nature of DALYs as a measure, such an exercise would lead to an absurd result. Nearly all lives have some number of DALYs attached to them. These DALYs may be averted most cost-effectively by preventing all births, reducing the burden of disease to zero. To avoid this result, we cannot measure the effect of family planning by comparison with a pure counterfactual. Rather, it is measured by ignoring the DALYs that would have been attributed to contingent persons. By the definition of DALYs, no individual can have any expectation of healthy life until the moment of live birth. This, however, is not an ideal solution. Both parents and health practitioners typically want to avoid perinatal deaths, even if doing so means preventing the birth of an infant. This fact suggests that one aim of health care is to prevent the ill health of contingent persons—in which case we ought, at least in some circumstances, to measure the potential DALYs averted by preventing a birth.

3. All dollar amounts are expressed in 2001 U.S. dollars. In a few cases, the year was not specified in the original source, and currency was converted from the year of publication.

4. Because of data limitations, these DALYs include no morbidity.

REFERENCES

AGI (Alan Guttmacher Institute), Futures Group International, Population Action International, Population Reference Bureau, and Population Council. 2000. *The Potential Impact of Increased Family Planning Funding on the Lives of Women and Their Families.* Washington, DC: AGI.

Aitken, I. W., and B. Walls. 1986. "Maternal Height and Cephalopelvic Disproportion in Sierra Leone." *Tropical Doctor* 16 (3): 132–4.

Arends-Kuenning, M. 1997. "The Equity and Efficiency of Doorstep Delivery of Contraceptives in Bangladesh." Policy Research Division Working Paper 101, Population Council, New York.

Attanayake, N., V. Fauveau, and J. Chakraborty. 1993. "Cost-Effectiveness of the Matlab MCH-FP Project in Bangladesh." *Health Policy and Planning* 8 (4): 327–38.

Balk, D., K. K. Faiz, U. Rob, J. Chakraborty, and G. Simmons. 1988. "An Analysis of Costs and Cost-Effectiveness of the Family Planning Health Services Project in Matlab, Bangladesh." International Centre for Diarrhoeal Disease Research, Dhaka.

Barberis, M., and P. D. Harvey. 1997. "Costs of Family Planning Programmes in Fourteen Developing Countries by Method of Service Delivery." *Journal of Biosocial Science* 29 (2): 219–33.

Behrman, J. R., and J. C. Knowles. 1998. "Population and Reproductive Health: An Economic Framework for Policy Evaluation." *Population and Development Review* 24 (4): 697–737.

Bertrand, J. T., N. Mangani, M. Mansilu, M. McBride, and J. Tharp. 1986. "Strategies for Family Planning Service Delivery in Bas Zaire. *International Family Planning Perspectives* 12 (4): 108–15.

Bicego, G., and O. B. Ahad. 1996. *Infant and Child Mortality.* Demographic and Health Surveys Comparative Studies 20. Calverton, MD: Macro International.

Birdsall, N. 1994. "Another Look at Population and Global Warming." In *Population, Environment, and Development,* ed. United Nations, 39–54. New York: United Nations.

Birdsall, N., and S. Sinding, eds. 2003. *Population Matters: Demographic Change, Economic Growth, and Poverty in the Developing World.* New York: Oxford University Press.

Blake, J. 1981. "Family Size and the Quality of Children." *Demography* 18 (4): 421–42.

Bongaarts, J. 1992. "Do Reproductive Intentions Matter?" *International Family Planning Perspectives* 18 (3): 102–8.

———. 1997. "Trends in Unwanted Childbearing in the Developing World." *Studies in Family Planning* 28 (4): 267–77.

Brinkley, G., M. Potts, and J. Walsh. 2003. "Reducing Global CO$_2$ Emissions through Family Planning Tradable Permits." School of Public Health, University of California, Berkeley.

Brockerhoff, M., and E. Brennan. 1998. "The Poverty of Cities in Developing Regions." *Population and Development Review* 24 (1): 75–114.

Bruce, J. 1987. "Users' Perspectives on Contraceptive Technology and Delivery Systems: Highlighting Some Feminist Issues." *Technology in Society* 9: 359–83.

Bula tao, R. 1993. *Effective Family Planning Programe.* Washington, DC: World Bank.

Cakir, H. V., S. J. Fabricant, and F. N. Kircalioglu. 1996. "Comparative Costs of Family Planning Services and Hospital-Based Maternity Care in Turkey." *Studies in Family Planning* 27 (5): 269–76.

Casterline, J. B., and S. W. Sinding. 2000. "Unmet Need for Family Planning in Developing Countries and Implications for Population Policy." *Population and Development Review* 26 (4): 691–723.

Cnattingius, S., M. R. Forman, H. W. Berendes, and L. Isotalo. 1992. "Delayed Childbearing and Risk of Adverse Perinatal Outcome. A Population-Based Study." *Journal of the American Medical Association* 268 (7): 886–90.

Cochrane, S. H. 1988. "The Effects of Education, Health, and Social Security on Fertility in Developing Countries." Policy, Planning, and Research Working Paper 93, World Bank, Washington, DC.

Cochrane, S. H., and D. K. Guilkey. 1995. "The Effects of Fertility Intentions and Access to Services on Contraceptive Use in Tunisia." *Economic Development and Cultural Change* 43: 779–804.

Conde-Agudelo, A., and J. M. Belizan. 2000. "Maternal Morbidity and Mortality Associated with Interpregnancy Interval: Cross Sectional Study." *British Medical Journal* (Clinical Research Ed.) 321 (7271): 1255–59.

Dayaratna, V., W. Winfrey, K. Hardee, J. Smith, E. Mumford, W. McGreevey, and others. 2000. "Reproductive Health Interventions: Which Ones Work and What Do They Cost?" Policy Project Occasional Paper 5, Futures Group International, Washington, DC.

DeGraff, D., R. Bilsborrow, and A. Herrin. 1993. "The Implications of High Fertility for Children's Time Use in the Philippines." In *Fertility, Family Size, and Structure: Consequences for Families and Children,* ed. C. Lloyd, 297–329. New York: Population Council.

Dixon-Mueller, R. 1993. "The Sexuality Connection in Reproductive Health." *Studies in Family Planning* 23 (5): 330–35.

Foreit, J. R., M. R. Garate, A. Brazzoduro, F. Guillen, M. C. Herrera, and F. C. Suarez. 1992. "A Comparison of the Performance of Male and Female CBD Distributors in Peru." *Studies in Family Planning* 23 (1): 58–62.

Foreit, K. G. 1999. "Use of Commercial and Government Sources of Family Planning and Maternal and Child Health Care." Policy Project Working Paper Series 4, Futures Group International, Washington, DC.

Foreit, K. G., and R. E. Levine. 1993. "Cost Recovery and User Fees in Family Planning." Options for Population Policy, Policy Paper Series 5, Futures Group International, Washington, DC.

Fort. A. L. 1996. "More Evils of CYP." *Studies in Family Planning* 27 (4): 228–31.

Fretts, R. C., and R. H. Usher. 1997. "Causes of Fetal Death in Women of Advanced Maternal Age." *Obstetrics and Gynecology* 89 (1): 40–45.

Gage, A. 1998. "Premarital Childbearing, Unwanted Fertility and Maternity Care in Kenya and Namibia." *Population Studies* 52 (1): 21–34.

Geronimus, A. T. 1987. "On Teenage Childbearing and Neonatal Mortality in the United States." *Population and Development Review* 13 (2): 245–79.

Gift, T. L., A. C. Haddix, and P. S. Corso. 2003. "Cost-Effectiveness Analysis." In *Prevention Effectiveness: A Guide to Decision Analysis and Economic Evaluation,* ed. A. C. Haddix, S. M. Teutsch, and P. S. Corso, New York: Oxford University Press.

Govindasamy, P., M. K. Stewart, S. O. Rutstein, J. T. Boerma, and A. E. Sommerfelt. 1993. *High-Risk Births and Maternity Care.* Columbia, MD: Macro International.

Haaga, J. G., and A. O. Tsui, eds. 1995. *Resource Allocation for Family Planning in Developing Countries.* Washington, DC: National Academy Press.

Henshaw, S. K., S. Singh, and T. Haas. 1999. "The Incidence of Abortion Worldwide." *International Family Planning Perspectives* 25 (Suppl.): S30–38.

Hobcraft, J. 1992. "Fertility Patterns and Child Survival: A Comparative Analysis." *Population Bulletin of the United Nations* 33: 1–31.

———. 1994. *The Health Rationale for Family Planning: Timing of Births and Child Survival.* New York: United Nations.

Hord, C., H. P. David, F. Donnay, and A. Koblinsky. 1991. "Reproductive Health in Romania: Reversing the Ceausescu Legacy." *Studies in Family Planning* 22 (4): 231–40.

Jamison, D. T. 1993. "Disease Control Priorities in Developing Countries." In *Disease Control Priorities in Developing Countries,* ed. D. T. Jamison, W. H. Mosley, A. R. Measham, and J. L. Bobadilla, 1–34. New York: Oxford University Press.

Janowitz, B., and J. Bratt. 1992. "Costs of Family Planning Services." *International Family Planning Perspectives* 18 (4): 137–44.

Janowitz, B., K. Jamil, J. Chowdhury, B. Rahman, and D. Hubacher. 1996. "Productivity and Costs for Family Planning Service Delivery in Bangladesh." Technical Report, Family Health International, Research Triangle Park, NC.

Janowitz, B., M. Suazo, D. B. Fried, J. Bratt, and P. Bailey. 1992. "Impact of Social Marketing on Contraceptive Prevalence and Cost in Honduras." *Studies in Family Planning* 23 (2): 110–7.

Jensen, E. R. 1996. "The Fertility Impact of Alternative Family Planning Distribution Channels in Indonesia." *Demography* 33 (2): 153–65.

Johns Hopkins Population Information Program. 2000. "Oral Contraceptives." *Population Reports* Series A-9, Johns Hopkins University, Baltimore.

Joyce, T. J., and M. Grossman. 1990. "Pregnancy Wantedness and the Initiation of Prenatal Care." *Demography* 27: 1–17.

Kinoti, S. N., L. Gaffikin, J. Benson, and L. A. Nicholson. 1995. *Monograph on Complications of Unsafe Abortion in Africa.* Arusha, Tanzania: Commonwealth Regional Health Community Secretariat.

Knowles, J. C., and A. Wagman. 1991. *The Relationship between Family Planning Costs and Contraceptive Prevalence: Will FP Costs per User Decline over Time?* Chapel Hill, NC: Futures Group International.

Koenig, M. A., V. Fauveau, A. I. Chowdhury, J. Chakraborty, and M. A. Khan. 1988. "Maternal Mortality in Matlab, Bangladesh, 1976–1985." *Studies in Family Planning* 19 (2): 69–80.

Konje, J. C., K. A. Obisesan, and O. A. Ladipo. 1992. "Health and Economic Consequences of Septic Induced Abortion." *International Journal of Gynecology and Obstetrics* 37 (3): 193–7.

Kumar, M. 2000. "Cost-Effectiveness of Prevention of Mother-to-Child HIV Transmission in Kerala, India." Paper presented at the International AIDS Economic Network Symposium, Durban, South Africa, July 7–8.

Langer, A., C. Harper, C. Garcia-Barrios, R. Schiavon, A. Heimburger, B. Elul, and others. 1999. "Emergency Contraception in Mexico City: What Do Health Care Providers and Potential Users Know and Think about It?" *Contraception* 60: 233–41.

Litvack, J. L., and C. Bodart. 1993. "User Fees plus Quality Equals Improved Access to Health Care: Results of a Field Experiment in Cameroon." *Social Science and Medicine* 37 (3): 369–83.

Loaiza, E. 1995. "Sterilization Regret in the Dominican Republic: Looking for Quality of Care Issues." *Studies in Family Planning* 26 (1): 39–48.

Mancini, D. J., G. Stecklov, and J. F. Stewart. 2003. "The Effect of Structural Characteristics on Family Planning Program Performance in Côte d'Ivoire and Nigeria." *Social Science and Medicine* 56 (10): 2123–37.

Marseille, E., J. G. Kahn, F. Mmiro, L. Guay, P. Musoke, M. G. Fowler, and J. B. Jackson. 1999. "Cost Effectiveness of Single-Dose Nevirapine Regimen for Mothers and Babies to Decrease Vertical HIV-1 Transmission in Sub-Saharan Africa." *Lancet* 354: 803–9.

Matheny, G. 2004. "Family Planning Programs: Getting the Most for the Money." *International Family Planning Perspectives* 30 (3): 134–8.

Mauldin, W. P., and V. C. Miller. 1994. *Contraceptive Use and Commodity Costs in Developing Countries, 1994–2005.* New York: United Nations Population Fund.

Maymon, E., F. Ghezzi, I. Shoham-Vardi, R. Hershkowitz, M. Franchi, M. Katz, and M. Mazor. 1998. "Peripartum Complications in Grand Multiparous Women." *European Journal of Obstetrics, Gynecology, and Reproductive Biology* 81 (1): 21–25.

McDevitt, T. M., A. Adlakha, T. B. Fowler, and V. Harris-Bourne. 1996. *Trends in Adolescent Fertility and Contraceptive Use in the Developing World.* Washington, DC: Bureau of the Census.

Mensch, B., M. Arends-Kuenning, and A. Jain. 1996. "The Impact of the Quality of Family Planning Services on Contraceptive Use in Peru." *Studies in Family Planning* 27 (N2): 59–75.

Mitchell, M. D., J. Littlefield, and A. Gutter. 1999. "Costing of Reproductive Health Services." *International Family Planning Perspectives* 25 (Suppl.): S17–21.

Muhuri, P. K., and J. Menken. 1997. "Adverse Effects of Next Birth, Gender, and Family Composition on Child Survival in Rural Bangladesh." *Population Studies* 51 (3): 279–94.

Ndhlovu, L. 1997. "The Route from MCH to Family Planning: Why Do Women Switch Health Facilities in the Kenyan MCH/FP Program?" Paper presented at the 125th annual meeting of the American Public Health Association, Indianapolis.

Peterson, H. B., Z. Xia, J. M. Hughes, L. S. Wilcox, L. R. Tylor, and J. Trussell. 1996. "The Risk of Pregnancy after Tubal Sterilization: Findings from the U.S. Collaborative Review of Sterilization." *American Journal of Obstetric Gynecology* 174 (4): 1161–68.

Pritchett, L. H. 1994. "Desired Fertility and the Impact of Population Policies." *Population and Development Review* 20 (1): 1–56.

Rafalimanana, H., and C. F. Westoff. 2001. *Gap between Preferred and Actual Birth Intervals in Sub-Saharan Africa: Implications for Fertility and Child Health.* Demographic and Health Surveys Analytical Studies 2. Calverton, MD: Macro International.

Ross, J. A., and E. Frankenberg. 1993. *Findings from Two Decades of Family Planning Research.* New York: Population Council.

Ross, J. A., and W. L. Winfrey. 2001. "Contraceptive Use, Intention to Use, and Unmet Need during the Extended Postpartum Period." *International Family Planning Perspectives* 27 (1): 20–27.

———. 2002. "Unmet Need for Contraception in the Developing World and the Former Soviet Union: An Updated Estimate." *International Family Planning Perspectives* 28 (3): 138–43.

Royston, E., and A. D. Lopez. 1987. "On the Assessment of Maternal Mortality." *World Health Statistics Quarterly* 40 (3): 214–24.

Rutstein, S. O. 2003. *Effect of Birth Intervals on Mortality and Health.* Calverton, MD: Measure/DHS+/Macro International.

Salter, C., H. B. Johnston, and N. Hengen. 1997. "Care for Postabortion Complications: Saving Women's Lives." *Population Reports* Series L-10, Johns Hopkins University, Baltimore.

Sanderson, E. C., and J. Tan. 1996. *Population in Asia.* Washington DC: World Bank.

Schultz, T. P. 1994. *Human Capital, Family Planning, and Their Effects on Population Growth.* New Haven, CT: Yale University.

Shelton, J. D. 1991. "What's Wrong with CYP?" *Studies in Family Planning* 22 (5): 332–35.

Simmons, G. B., D. Balk, and K. K. Faiz. 1991. "Cost Effectiveness Analysis of Family Planning Programs in Rural Bangladesh: Evidence from Matlab." *Studies in Family Planning* 22 (2): 83–101.

Sine, J. 2002. *How Much Is Enough? Estimating Requirements for Subsidized Contraceptives.* Washington, DC: Commercial Market Strategies.

Starrs, A. 1997. *The Safe Motherhood Action Agenda: Priorities for the Next Decade.* New York: Family Care International.

Stover, J. 2003. "Costs and Benefits of Providing Family Planning Services at PMTCT and VCT Sites." Futures Group International, Washington, DC.

Stover, J., J. Bertrand, S. Smith, N. Rutenberg, and K. Meyer-Ramirez. 1996. "Empirically Based Conversion Factors for Calculating Couple-Years of Protection." Futures Group, Chapel Hill, NC.

Sullivan, J. M., S. O. Rutstein, and G. T. Bicego. 1994. *Infant and Child Mortality.* Demographic and Health Surveys Comparative Studies 15. Calverton, MD: Macro International.

Trussell, J., and A. Pebley. 1984. "The Potential Impact of Changes in Fertility on Infant, Child, and Maternal Mortality." *Studies in Family Planning* 15 (6): 267–80.

Tsui, A. O., J. N. Wasserheit, and J. G. Haaga, eds. 1997. *Reproductive Health in Developing Countries: Expanding Dimensions, Building Solutions.* Washington, DC: Panel on Reproductive Health, Committee on Population, and Commission on Behavioral and Social Sciences and Education, National Research Council.

UN (United Nations). 2003. *State of the World's Population.* New York: UN.

UNAIDS (Joint United Nations Programme on HIV/AIDS). 1999. *Prevention of HIV Transmission from Mother to Child: Strategic Options.* Geneva: UNAIDS.

Walsh, J. A., C. N. Feifer, A. R. Measham, and P. J. Gertler. 1993. "Maternal and Perinatal Health." In *Disease Control Priorities in Developing Countries*, ed. D. T. Jamison, W. H. Mosley, A. R. Measham, and J. L. Bobadilla, 363–90. New York: Oxford University Press.

Weller, R. D., I. W. Eberstein, and M. Bailey. 1987. "Pregnancy Wantedness and Maternal Behavior during Pregnancy." *Demography* 24: 407–12.

Westoff, C. F. 2001. *Unmet Need at the End of the Century.* Demographic and Health Surveys Comparative Reports 1. Calverton, MD: ORC Macro International.

Westoff, C. F., and A. Bankole. 1995. *Unmet Need 1990–1994.* Demographic and Health Surveys Comparative Studies 16. Calverton, MD: ORC Macro.

———. 1997. *Mass Media and Reproductive Health.* Demographic and Health Surveys Analytical Reports 2. Calverton, MD: Macro International.

WHO (World Health Organization). 1997. "Maternal Health around the World." Wall Chart. Department of Reproductive Health and Research, Geneva.

———. 1998. *Abortion in the Developing World.* Geneva: WHO.

————. 2002a. *Research on Reproductive Health at WHO: Biennial Report 2000–2001*. Special Programme of Research, Development, and Research Training in Human Reproduction. Geneva: UNDP/UNFPA/WHO/World Bank.

————. 2002b. *World Health Report*. Geneva: WHO.

Williams, A. 1999. "Calculating the Global Burden of Disease: Time for a Strategic Reappraisal?" *Health Economics* 8 (1): 1–8.

Winikoff, B., and M. Sullivan. 1987. "Assessing the Role of Family Planning in Reducing Maternal Mortality." *Studies in Family Planning* 18 (3): 128–43.

World Bank. 1993. *Investing in Health: World Development Report 1993*. New York: Oxford University Press.

————. 2003. *World Development Indicators 2003*. New York: Oxford University Press.

Yun, S. H., D. L. Kincaid, Y. Yaser, and G. Ozler. 1990. "The National Family Planning IEC Campaign of Turkey." Population Communication Services, Johns Hopkins University, Baltimore.

Chapter **58**

School-Based Health and Nutrition Programs

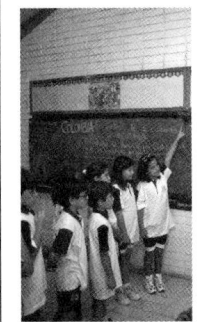

Donald A. P. Bundy, Sheldon Shaeffer, Matthew Jukes, Kathleen Beegle, Amaya Gillespie, Lesley Drake, Seung-hee Frances Lee, Anna-Maria Hoffman, Jack Jones, Arlene Mitchell, Delia Barcelona, Balla Camara, Chuck Golmar, Lorenzo Savioli, Malick Sembene, Tsutomu Takeuchi, and Cream Wright

The paradigmatic shift in the past decade in our understanding of the role of health and nutrition in school-age children has fundamental implications for the design of effective programs. Improving the health and nutrition of schoolchildren through school-based programs is not a new concept. School health programs are ubiquitous in high-income countries and most middle-income countries. In low-income countries, these programs were a common feature of early, particularly colonial, education systems, where they could be characterized as heavily focused on clinical diagnosis and treatment and on elite schools in urban centers. This situation is changing as new policies and partnerships are being formulated to help ensure that programs focus on promoting health and improving the educational outcomes of children, as well as being socially progressive and specifically targeting the poor, girls, and other disadvantaged children. This evolution reflects five key changes in our understanding of the role of these programs in child development.

- First, ensuring good health at school age requires a life cycle approach to intervention, starting in utero and continuing throughout child development. In programmatic terms this requirement implies a sequence of programs to promote maternal and reproductive health, management of childhood illness, and early childhood care and development. Promoting good health and nutrition before and during school age is essential to effective growth and development.

- Second, operations research shows that the preexisting infrastructure of the educational system can often offer a more cost-effective route for delivery of simple health interventions and health promotion than can the health system. Low-income countries typically have more teachers than nurses and more schools than clinics, often by an order of magnitude.

- Third, empirical evidence shows that good health and nutrition are prerequisites for effective learning. This finding is not simply the utopian aspiration for children to have healthy bodies and healthy minds, but also the demonstration of a systemic link between specific physical insults and specific cognitive and learning deficits, grounded in a new multisectoral approach to research involving public health and epidemiology, as well as cognitive and educational psychology.

- Fourth, the provision of quality schools, textbooks, and teachers can result in effective education only if the child is present, ready, and able to learn. This perception has additional political momentum as countries and agencies seek to achieve Education for All (EFA) by 2015 and address the Millennium Development Goals of universal basic education and gender equality in education access. If every girl and boy is to be able to complete a basic education of good quality, then ensuring that the poorest children, who suffer the most malnutrition and ill health, are able to attend and stay in school and to learn while there is essential.

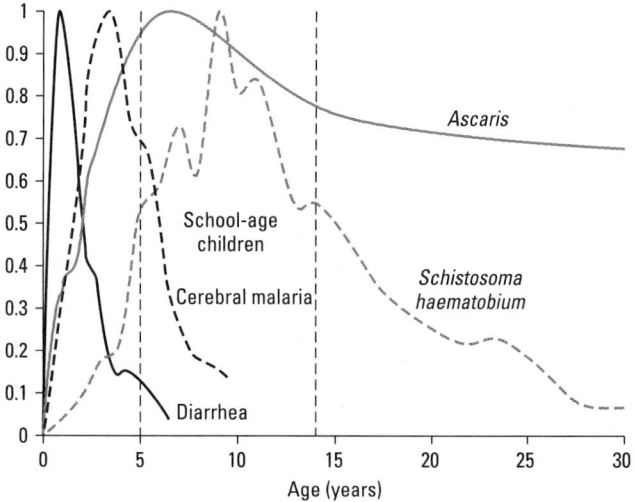

Ascaris

School-age
children

Cerebral malaria

Schistosoma
haematobium

Diarrhea

Age (years)

Source: Bundy and Guyatt 1996.

Figure 58.1 Age Distribution of Infection-Specific Morbidity

• Finally, education, including education that promotes positive health behaviors, contributes to the prevention of HIV/AIDS—the greatest challenge for generations to come. School health and nutrition programs that help children complete their education and develop knowledge, practices, and behaviors that protect them from HIV infection as they mature have been described as a "social vaccine" against the disease.

Because of the success of child survival programs, the number of children reaching school age (defined as 5 to 14 years of age) is increasing and is estimated to be 1.2 billion children, with 88 percent living in less developed countries (U.S. Census Bureau 2002). As figure 58.1 illustrates, the pattern of disease is age specific. A large body of evidence shows that these conditions affect cognition, learning, and educational achievement (see Jukes, Drake, and Bundy forthcoming; Pollitt 1990 for reviews of this extensive literature).

This chapter focuses on the health, nutrition, and education of the school-age child and on the programs that can be implemented at school age to promote positive outcomes.

INFECTIOUS DISEASE AND SCHOOL-AGE CHILDREN

A range of infectious diseases affect school-age children.

Helminth Infections

Between 25 and 35 percent of school-age children are estimated to be infected with one or more of the major species of worms (Bundy 1997; see also chapter 24). The most common

and important infections are caused by geohelminths (the roundworm *Ascaris,* the whipworm *Trichuris,* and the two species of hookworms *Ancylostoma* and *Necator*) and by the schistosomes (*Schistosoma* spp.), which give rise to a wide range of chronic but largely nonspecific symptoms. The most intense worm infections and related illnesses occur at school age (Partnership for Child Development 1998b, 1999) and account for some 12 percent of the total disease burden and 20 percent of the loss of disability-adjusted life years (DALYs) from communicable disease among schoolchildren (World Bank 1993).

Infected schoolchildren perform poorly in tests of cognitive function; when they are treated, immediate educational and cognitive benefits are apparent only for children with heavy worm burdens or with concurrent nutritional deficits. Treatment alone cannot reverse the cumulative effects of lifelong infection or compensate for years of missed learning, but studies suggest that children are more ready to learn after treatment for worm infections and may be able to catch up if this learning potential is exploited effectively in the classroom (Grigorenko and others forthcoming). In Kenya, treatment reduced absenteeism by one-fourth, with the largest gains for the youngest children who suffered the most ill health (Miguel and Kremer 2004).

Malaria

Up to 5 percent of children infected with malaria early in life have residual neurological sequelae (Snow 1999). In areas of unstable transmission, malaria accounts for 10 to 20 percent of all-cause mortality among school-age children (Bundy and others 2000), and those who have suffered repeated attacks have poorer cognitive abilities. In Kenya, primary school students miss 11 percent of school days because of malaria, equivalent to 4 million to 10 million days per year (Brooker and others 2000).

Oral antimalarial treatment reduced school absenteeism by 50 percent in Ghana (Colbourne 1955); the use of insecticide-treated bednets in Tanzania reduced malaria and increased attendance (Shiff and others 1996). Girls in The Gambia were more than twice as likely to enroll in primary school if they had received malaria prophylaxis in early childhood (Jukes and others submitted).

HIV/AIDS

Although school-age children have the lowest infection prevalence of any age group (figure 58.2), an estimated 3.8 million children under 15 years of age have been infected with HIV and more than two-thirds have died (UNAIDS 2002). Even uninfected children suffer physically, socially, and psychologically through death or illness in their family (World Bank 2002). The proportion of orphans, most of whom are of school age, has risen from 2 to 15 percent in some African countries, with

a. Male Cases

Percent infected in each age group, as a percentage of cases

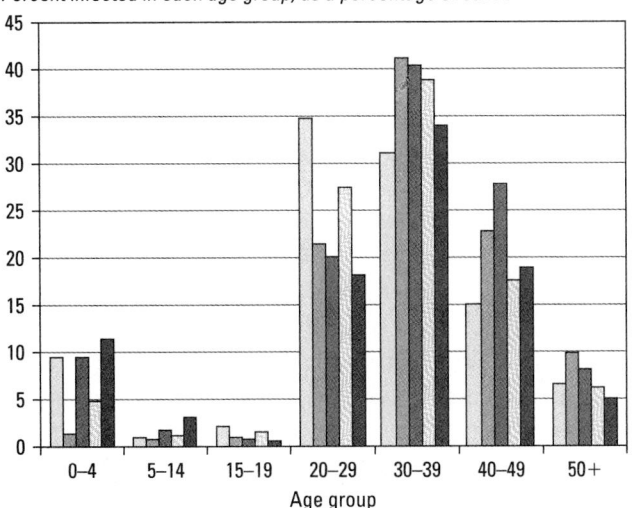

b. Female Cases

Percent infected in each age group, as a percentage of cases

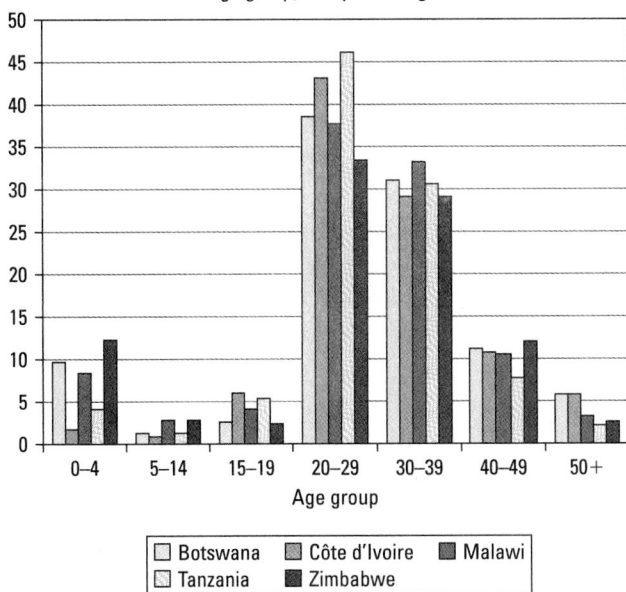

| □ Botswana | ▨ Côte d'Ivoire | ■ Malawi |
| ▨ Tanzania | ■ Zimbabwe | |

Source: UNAIDS epidemiological fact sheets 2000.

Note: Figure shows percentage of males (top) and females (bottom) infected with HIV in each age group (as a percentage of all HIV-infected males and females, respectively), for five countries in Africa. Infection peaks at a younger age in women than in men, and the lowest prevalence of infection occurs in school-age children.

Figure 58.2 Age Prevalence of HIV/AIDS

AIDS accounting for 50 percent of this increase. The number of orphans is expected to reach more than 25 million by 2010.

School-age children with HIV infections have lower IQ levels and poorer academic achievement, language, and visual motor functioning. These deficits can be reduced or reversed with antiretroviral therapy. The improvement is greater for children of school age than for younger children.

Acute Respiratory Infection

Acute respiratory infection, the most common acute infection in school-age children globally, is a significant cause of absenteeism. Research in industrial countries (Cohen and Smith 1996) finds that flu infection affects attention and reaction time; colds primarily affect hand-eye coordination, as well as reduce the ability to tolerate high levels of noise and other distractions common to the classroom.

MALNUTRITION, NONINFECTIOUS DISEASE, AND HEALTH AND EDUCATION

Malnutrition and noninfectious disease also affect school-age children.

Malnutrition

Stunting (low height for age) is a physical indicator of chronic or long-term malnutrition, whereas underweight (low weight for age) is an indicator of both chronic and acute malnutrition. Both are common in school-age children (figure 58.3).

Girls who are better nourished are more attentive and more involved during class, and boys have improved classroom behavior and increased activity levels. One Z-score increase in height for age is associated with an increase of 0.1 standard deviation (SD) in tests of arithmetic and language. Stunted children enroll in school later than other children. School food-service programs have been successful in improving school attendance.

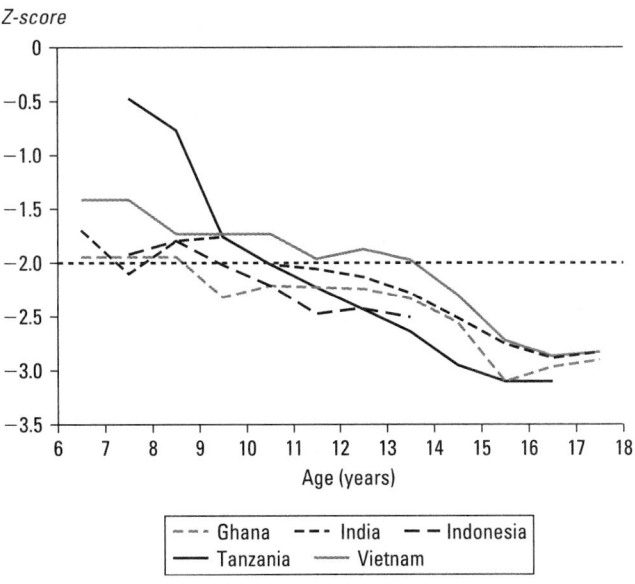

| ---- Ghana | - - - India | — — Indonesia |
| —— Tanzania | —— Vietnam | |

Source: Data from Partnership for Child Development 1998a.

Note: Z-scores of less than −2 indicate stunting.

Figure 58.3 Mean *Z*-Scores of Height-for-Age of Boys in Five Countries

Short-Term Hunger

Hunger, which reduces ability to perform school tasks, is readily reversed by feeding. Children age 11 to 13 years in Jamaica improved their scores on arithmetic tests after one semester of receiving breakfast at school because they attended more regularly and studied more effectively (Simeon 1998). Missing breakfast impairs performance to a greater extent for children of poor nutritional status, who also benefit most from food intervention (Pollitt, Cueto, and Jacoby 1998; Simeon and Grantham McGregor 1989).

Micronutrient Deficiency

Micronutrient deficiencies may take several different forms, each with negative impacts on children's ability to perform well in school.

Iron Deficiency. Iron deficiency, the most common form of micronutrient deficiency in school-age children, is caused by inadequate diet and infection, particularly by hookworm and malaria (Hall, Drake, and Bundy 2001). More than half the school-age children in low-income countries are estimated to suffer from iron deficiency anemia (Partnership for Child Development 2001). Children with iron deficiency score 1 to 3 SD worse on educational tests and are less likely to attend school. Iron supplementation reduces these deficits.

Iodine Deficiency. Iodine deficiency affects an estimated 60 million school-age children; studies indicate prevalence rates between 35 and 70 percent. Iodine deficiency is related to lowered general cognitive abilities and tests scores. No conclusive evidence shows that iodine supplementation improves cognitive abilities in this age group (Huda, Grantham-McGregor, and Tomkins 2001).

Vitamin A Deficiency. Vitamin A deficiency affects an estimated 85 million school-age children. The deficiency, which causes impaired immune function and increases risk of mortality from infectious disease, is an important cause of blindness. Recent studies suggest that this deficiency is also a major public health problem in school-age children. Multiple-micronutrient supplements have improved cognitive function and short-term memory in schoolchildren and have reduced absenteeism caused by diarrhea and respiratory infections.

Obesity

An estimated 17.6 million children worldwide are overweight. Obesity is associated with underperformance in education. In low-income countries obesity is still rare, but the prevalence in the children of many middle-income countries is similar to that in the United States.

ESTIMATING THE BURDEN OF DISEASE

The cost per DALY of school health programs has been estimated at US$20 to US$34, implying that the programs are at least as cost-effective as many other public health "best buys" (Bobadilla and others 1994). However, current methods of estimating the burden for school-age children result in a significant underestimation of both the developmental consequences of disease and malnutrition at school age and the overall benefits for health and development of school health and nutrition programs.

There are two key reasons for this underestimation. The first issue relates to time scales. Many serious diseases in adulthood, including heart disease and carcinomas, are a consequence of unhealthy practices established in early life. This later burden can be substantially and cost-effectively averted by early intervention, particularly by school-based life-skills programs. For example, in the United States (Del Rosso and Marek 1996), US$1 invested can avert US$18.80 spent on the later problems caused by tobacco and US$5.70 on problems of drug and alcohol abuse. DALY estimates cannot capture these downstream consequences of upstream intervention and instead attribute the disease burden to the adult age group in which it appears. This kind of estimate is particularly misleading in the case of HIV/AIDS, for which prevention education at school age is effective in averting later infection and disease (World Bank 2002), and in the case of estimates of intergenerational effects, in which ensuring the health of an adolescent girl may help secure the health of her baby born a few years later.

The second issue is illustrated by experience with helminth infections. In 1990, the burden was first estimated at 18 million DALYs, close to the value for tuberculosis, measles, and malaria. This estimate reflected the ubiquity of infection and the long-term consequences of cognitive impacts. In 2001, the estimate was only 4.7 million DALYs (WHO 2003), and during the intervening years one estimate put the value as low as 2.6 million.

This extraordinary variability is caused in part by different emphases on the cognitive and health impacts and illustrates how, for very common conditions, even minor changes in disability weight can affect the overall values. This variability also reflects the importance of a sectoral perspective, because the low estimates reflect a focus on health, whereas the higher estimates include impact on educational achievement and child development.

The scale of the burden of disease in terms of cognition is illustrated by estimating the impact of stunting, anemia, and helminths on the cognition of the estimated 562 million school-age children in developing countries. According to typical deficits in test scores attributable to these diseases, the total global loss of points ranges from 600 million to 1.8 billion IQ points, an additional 15 million to 45 million cases of mental retardation (defined here as IQ less than 70), and a loss of between 200 million and 524 million years of primary schooling (Jukes, Drake, and Bundy forthcoming). Although the precision of these striking figures may be open to debate, they clearly show that even minor cognitive deficits resulting from ubiquitous conditions can result in an extraordinarily large scale of effect.

INTERVENTIONS

In light of the significant effects of ill health and malnutrition on educational outcomes, the role of effective health promotion and simple school-based programs to deliver low-cost interventions becomes increasingly important (Bundy and others 1992). Other chapters provide information on the integrated management of childhood illness, early child development, and adolescent health (see chapters 63, 27, and 59, respectively). The focus here is on ill health and malnutrition at school age and the role of the formal and nonformal education sector in delivering interventions.

Developing a Programmatic Approach

The focus of school health and nutrition programs in low-income countries has shifted significantly over the past two decades away from a medical approach that favored elite schools in urban centers and toward an approach that improves health and nutrition for all children, particularly the poor and disadvantaged. This change began in the 1980s, when research showed not only that school health and nutrition programs were important contributors to health outcomes but also that they were essential elements of efforts to improve education access and completion, particularly for the poor.

In an effort to reconceptualize the relationship between health and education, the United Nations Education, Scientific, and Cultural Organization (UNESCO) hosted a series of workshops on this topic in the 1980s (Bundy 1989; Halloran, Bundy, and Pollitt 1989) and supported one of the first authoritative reviews of the area (Pollitt 1990). Similarly, the United Nations Development Programme, in conjunction with the Rockefeller, Edna McConnell Clark, and J. S. McDonnell Foundations supported the creation of the Partnership for Child Development to strengthen the evidence base across the education and health sectors and to support the dissemination of information (Berkley and Jamison 1990; Bundy and Guyatt 1996). This paradigm shift coincided with the World Conference on Education for All in Jomtien, Thailand, in 1990 and led to renewed efforts by countries and agencies to develop more effective programmatic approaches to school health and nutrition.

The United Nations Population Fund (UNFPA) has pioneered population and family life education (PopEd) as an intrinsic part of school curricula. In 1994, the International Conference on Population and Development placed specific emphasis on school health, including reproductive and sexual health. Efforts at country level have addressed PopEd both within the school system and outside, and the concept has evolved to include references to family life education, sex education, HIV/AIDS awareness and prevention, and life-skills programs. Today, approximately 84 countries have UNFPA-supported school health programs.

In 1995, the World Health Organization (WHO) launched its Global School Health Initiative to foster the development of health-promoting schools (HPSs) (WHO 1996). The concept started in Europe in the early 1990s, based on the Ottawa Charter of Health Promotion (WHO 1986; European Commission 1996), which recognized that health is created by caring for oneself and others, by being able to make decisions and have control over one's life and circumstances, and by creating conditions that support health for all. WHO's European Regional Office, the Council of Europe, and the Commission of the European Communities widely promoted the concept of HPSs to foster healthy lifestyles and develop environments conducive to health (European Commission, WHO Europe, and Council of Europe 1996). Although definitions vary among regions, countries, and schools, an HPS may be characterized as one that is constantly strengthening its capacity as a healthy setting for living, learning, and working. The initiative fosters the development of HPSs by the following:

- consolidating research and expert opinion to describe the nature and effectiveness of school health programs
- building capacity to advocate for the creation of HPSs and to apply the components to priority health issues
- strengthening collaboration and national capacities to assess the prevalence of important health-related behaviors and conditions and to plan and implement policies and programs that improve health through schools
- creating networks and alliances, including regional networks.

The key elements of how this approach is interpreted today are listed in table 58.1.

In the mid 1990s, the United Nations Children's Fund (UNICEF) began promoting the Child-Friendly Schools framework as a holistic way to promote children's rights as expressed in the Convention on the Rights of the Child (UNICEF 1990) and children's access to education as stated in the World Declaration of Education for All (UNESCO 1990). This approach included a gender-sensitive component, which was further strengthened when girls' education became the first priority in UNICEF's Medium Term Strategic Plan, 2002–5. Another key element is skills-based health education,

Table 58.1 Characteristics of Agency-Specific School Health and Nutrition Programs, within the FRESH framework

FRESH framework	Health-promoting schools (WHO)	Child-friendly schools (UNICEF)	PopEd (UNFPA)	Global school feeding campaign (World Food Program)
Policy	Respects an individual's well-being and dignity Provides multiple opportunities for success Acknowledges good efforts and intentions as well as personal achievements	Respects and realizes the rights of every child Acts to ensure inclusion, respect, and equality of opportunity for all children Is gender sensitive and girl friendly Is flexible and responds to diversity Sees and understands the whole child in a broad context Enhances teacher capacity, morale, commitment, and status	Creates a supportive and enabling policy environment for reproductive health and HIV prevention for young people	Focuses on the poorest and most food-insecure communities. Gives priority to girls and AIDS-affected children
School environment	Is healthy Provides opportunities for physical education and recreation	Is healthy, safe, and secure Is protective emotionally and psychologically	Protects young people from early and unwanted pregnancy, sexually transmitted diseases, sexual abuse, and violence	Serves as platform for essential package approach that includes water, sanitation, and environmental measures
Education	Provides skills-based health education Fosters health and learning	Promotes quality learning outcomes Provides education that is affordable and accessible Provides skills-based health education, including life skills relevant to children's lives	Strengthens HIV/AIDS and sexual and reproductive health education programs	Supports learning through good nutrition Promotes access to education
Services	Provides school health services Provides nutrition and food-safety programs Provides programs for counseling, social support, and mental health promotion Provides health promotion programs for staff Includes school and community projects and outreach	Promotes physical health Promotes mental health	Ensures access to youth-friendly sexual and reproductive health services	Provides food Promotes and supports deworming
Supportive partnerships	Engages health and education officials, teachers, teachers' unions, students, parents, health providers, and community leaders in efforts to make the school a healthy place	Is child centered Is family focused Is community based	Targets young people in school and out of school Ensures active participation of parents, youths, community leaders, and organizations	Promotes community and school partnerships

Source: Summarized from World Bank Fresh Toolkit (2000), WHO (1996), and personal communications from Arlene Mitchell and Sheldon Shaeffer (May 2005).

including life skills, which has been promoted through UNICEF with partner organizations as part of HPSs, child-friendly schools, and the framework for Focusing Resources on Effective School Health (FRESH). Research shows that this approach is more effective than traditional strategies, which tend to be didactic and to focus on scientific information alone. In contrast, skills-based health education uses the experiences of students as the starting point and explores the links between knowledge, attitudes, and the interpersonal skills required to promote health and learning (UNICEF, WHO, World Bank, UNFPA, UNESCO 2003). The approach is interactive, activity based, and flexible so that it can be used to address a range of health and social issues, including HIV/AIDS, sanitation, drug use, violence and bullying, nutrition, and cross-cutting issues such as gender and culture. Some key elements of how the child-friendly schools approach is interpreted currently, including its focus on healthy and protective learning environments, are listed in table 58.1.

Also during the 1990s, the World Bank Human Development Network sought to support countries in implementing school health and nutrition programs (Del Rosso and Marek 1996; World Bank 1993) and launched an International School Health Initiative with the aim of raising awareness among decision makers in the education sector.

Thus, the 1990s were characterized by the creation of a number of apparently separate programs to promote and support school health. However, analysis at the country level revealed that although the various agency initiatives used different "prisms" to view school health—public health for WHO, quality education for UNESCO, and child rights for UNICEF—the core activities for all the programmatic approaches were essentially the same.

FRESH Framework

A major step forward in international coordination and cohesion was achieved when the FRESH framework was launched at the World Education Forum in Dakar in April 2000 (World Bank FRESH Toolkit 2000). Among the early partners in this effort were the Education Development Centre, Education International, the Partnership for Child Development, UNESCO, UNICEF, the World Food Programme (WFP), WHO, and the World Bank. This partnership recognizes that the goal of universal education cannot be achieved while the health needs of children and adolescents remain unmet and that a core group of cost-effective activities can and must be implemented across the board to meet those needs and to deliver on the promise of EFA.

The expanded commentary on the Dakar Framework for Action reflects the recommendations of this partnership and describes three ways in which health relates to EFA: as an input and condition necessary for learning, as an outcome of effective quality education, and as a sector that must collaborate with education to achieve the goal of EFA. In the follow-up to the Dakar Forum, UNESCO designated FRESH as an interagency flagship program that will receive international support as a strategy to achieve EFA.

The FRESH framework, which is based on good practice recognized by all the partners, provides a consensus approach for the effective implementation of health and nutrition services within school health programs. The framework proposes four core components that should be considered in designing an effective school health and nutrition program and suggests that the program will be most equitable and cost-effective if all of these components are made available, together, in all schools:

- *Policy:* health- and nutrition-related school policies that are nondiscriminatory, protective, inclusive, and gender sensitive and that promote the nutrition and physical and psychosocial health of staff, teachers, and children

- *School environment:* access to safe water and provision of separate sanitation facilities for girls, boys, and teachers
- *Education:* skills-based education, including life skills, that addresses health, nutrition, HIV/AIDS prevention, and hygiene issues and that promotes positive behaviors
- *Services:* simple, safe, and familiar health and nutrition services that can be delivered cost-effectively in schools (such as deworming services, micronutrient supplements, and nutritious snacks that counter hunger) and increased access to youth-friendly clinics.

The FRESH framework further proposes that these four core components can be implemented effectively only if they are supported by strategic partnerships between the following groups:

- health and education sectors, especially teachers and health workers
- schools and the community
- children and others responsible for implementation.

Adopting this framework does not imply that these core components and strategies are the only important elements; rather, implementing all of these in all schools would provide a sound initial basis for any pro-poor school health program.

The common focus has encouraged concerted action by the participating agencies. It has also provided a common platform on which countries, agencies, donors, and civil society can support all programs, including agency-specific programs (table 58.1). Another important consequence of the FRESH consensus framework has been to offer a common point of entry for new efforts to improve health in schools, as illustrated by the three examples in box 58.1.

This consensus approach has increased significantly the number of countries implementing school health reforms. The simplicity of the approach, combined with the enhanced resources available from donor coordination, has helped ensure that these programs can go to scale. Annual external support from the World Bank for these actions approaches US$90 million, targeting some 100 million schoolchildren.

Common Interventions

Table 58.2 lists some specific interventions commonly combined within the school health intervention package, but it should be recognized that not all of these interventions will be needed or be appropriate for all locations. Some interventions are synergistic: for example, worm infection will be addressed by the provision of latrines, the promotion of hand washing, relevant health and hygiene education, and deworming services. Similarly, HIV/AIDS infection among youths will be addressed by ensuring girls' participation in school, offering

Three Efforts to Improve Health in Schools

The Multiagency Effort to Accelerate the Education Sector Response to HIV/AIDS in Africa

This effort, coordinated by a Working Group of the UNAIDS Inter-Agency Task Team on HIV/AIDS and Education, promotes the FRESH framework specifically and helps education systems do the following:

- adopt policies that avoid HIV/AIDS discrimination and stigmatization
- provide a safe and secure school environment
- provide skills-based health education, including life skills, in schools to promote positive behaviors and healthy lifestyles
- improve access to youth-friendly health services.

More than 36 countries and a similar number of agencies, bilateral donors, and nongovernmental organizations have collaborated in this effort since November 2002.

The Global School Feeding Campaign of the WFP

This campaign has gone beyond providing food aid to develop a programmatic link between nutrition and education. Working with partners, including national governments, parent-teacher and other community organizations,

UNICEF, WHO, the World Bank, UNESCO, and the Food and Agriculture Organization, the campaign promotes the following:

- policies that make food aid conditional on girls' participation in education
- an essential package that includes school sanitation and water and environmental improvement
- nutrition education that improves the quality of students' diets and HIV prevention education
- nutrition services that include food, deworming, and alleviation of short-term hunger.

Some 70 countries have begun to implement these principles and activities since 2002.

The Partnership for Parasite Control

Led by WHO and involving a broad range of development partners, this initiative promotes public and private efforts to include deworming in school health services, following a resolution of the 54th World Health Assembly to provide by 2010 regular deworming treatment to 75 percent of school-age children at risk (an estimated target population of 398 million). Of 41 target countries in Africa, 19 have begun school-based deworming programs since 2001.

Source: Authors.

skills-based health education (including life skills), offering peer education, providing access to health clubs, and providing access to treatment for sexually transmitted infections (STIs) at clinics. It is also apparent that whereas some interventions promote multiple outcomes—for example, skills-based health education and life-skills development can help promote positive behaviors that prevent STIs and substance abuse—other interventions may have a single focus, such as iron supplementation to avoid anemia.

Out-of-School Children

More than 100 million school-age children are out of school; 60 percent are girls (UNESCO 1993). School health programs in Guinea and Madagascar have demonstrated that many of these children will take advantage of simple services, such as deworming, provided in schools (Del Rosso and Marek 1996); the school acts essentially as a community center. It also has been demonstrated that deworming programs in schools benefit out-of-school children by reducing disease transmission in the community as a whole (Bundy and others 1990).

Nevertheless, it is apparent that out-of-school children cannot benefit from many of the important components of school-based programs, such as skills-based health education and life-skills development programs to prevent HIV/AIDS. Reaching these children requires more flexible approaches that combine the best of nonformal, informal, and community-based approaches (see chapter 59).

COST-EFFECTIVENESS OF INTERVENTION

A key issue in addressing the costs of the new approach to school health and nutrition programs is the significant savings offered by using the school system infrastructure rather than that of the health system as the key delivery mechanism. The school system provides not only a preexisting mechanism, so costs are at the margins, but also a system that aims at being pervasive and socially progressive. Some important interventions, especially in terms of health education, may be virtually cost free; they require only policy changes that result in doing things differently.

Table 58.2 Common Interventions within a School Health Program

FRESH category	Intervention	Expected outcome
Policy	1. Child rights, avoidance of discrimination and stigmatization, gender sensitive, child centered	1. Inclusion of all children
	2. Inclusion of pregnant girls and mothers in education	2. Specific inclusion of girls
	3. Enforcement of code of practice for teacher behavior zero tolerance policy	3. Avoidance of harassment and abuse
	4. Collaboration between health and education sectors	4. Effective implementation
Environment	1. Access to safe water	1,2,3,5. Reduced infection
	2. Hand washing	4. Reduced drop out of adolescent girls
	3. Provision of sanitation	
	4. Gender-separate sanitation	
	5. Garbage disposal	
Education	1. Curriculum addressing health, hygiene, and nutrition	1. Improved knowledge and skills to promote good health, hygiene, and nutrition
	2. Life-skills program	2. Lifelong positive behaviors such as avoidance of HIV/AIDS and substance abuse
	3. Peer education program	3, 4. Reinforcement of positive behaviors
	4. Health-promoting clubs	
Services	1. Deworming for intestinal worms and schistosomiasis	1. Reduction in worm infection
	2. Prompt recognition and treatment of malaria	2. Reduction in impact of malaria
	3. Insecticide-treated nets	3. Reduction in incidence of malaria
	4. Micronutrient supplements	4. Reduction in anemia and malnutrition
	5. Breakfast, snacks, and meals	5. Avoidance of hunger
	6. First-aid kits	6. Management of injuries
	7. Referral to youth-friendly clinics	7. Access to specific treatment
	8. Counseling and psychosocial support	8. Mental health

Source: Authors.

Table 58.3 Annual per Capita Costs of School-Based Health and Nutrition Interventions Delivered in Schools

Condition	Intervention	Cost (US$)
Intestinal worms	Albendazole or mebendazole	0.03–0.20
Schistosomiasis	Praziquantel	0.20–0.71
Vitamin A deficiency	Vitamin A supplementation	0.04
Iodine deficiency	Iodine supplementation	0.30–0.40
Iron deficiency and anemia	Iron folate supplementation	0.10
Refractive errors of vision	Spectacles	2.50–3.50
Clinically diagnosed conditions	Physical examination	11.50
Undernutrition, hunger	School feeding	21.60–151.20, 21.26–84.50[a]

Sources: Del Rosso and Marek 1996; Partnership for Child Development 1999; WHO 2000.
a. For South America and Africa, costs are standardized for 1,000 kilocalories for 180 days.

Annual costs of providing some common school-based interventions to students are given in table 58.3. This table illustrates two important points. First, some of the most widely needed interventions can be provided at remarkably low cost. Second, significant diversity exists in the cost of interventions, which is affected by factors such as local capacity, location and remoteness of communities, and community values and opinions; hence, these factors must be borne in mind when identifying a school health package. (See chapter 41 for details of the costs of sanitation provision.)

Not illustrated in the table is the cost advantage of using the existing school infrastructure for delivery. Estimates for delivery of simple interventions (such as anthelmintic pills or micronutrient supplements) suggest that the teacher-delivery approaches listed here may be one-tenth of the cost of the more traditional mobile health teams and yet equally effective (Guyatt 2003). As with all education innovations, however, the additional cost of teacher orientation and training (inservice as well as preservice) needs to be factored into the costs of using the education system for delivery of health services.

ECONOMIC BENEFITS OF INTERVENTION

The most obvious benefit of school health interventions is arguably through the economic returns of improved adult health outcomes. Studies have increasingly documented a causal effect of adult health (broadly defined) on labor force participation, wages, and productivity in developing countries; Strauss and Thomas (1995) present an overview of economic studies in this area. For example, height has been shown to affect wage-earning capacity as well as participation in the labor force for both women and men (Haddad and Bouis 1991). The effect of health on productivity and earnings may be strongest where low-cost health interventions produce large effects on health, such as low-income settings where physical endurance yields high returns in the labor market. For a 1 percent increase in height, Thomas and Strauss (1997) find a 7 percent increase in wages in Brazil compared with a 1 percent increase in the United States.

However, the apparent benefits of school health and nutrition programs will be underestimated when measured using only mortality or health-related disability metrics because these measures do not capture the impact of ill health on cognitive development or educational outcomes. Evidence over the past decade suggests these impacts have effect sizes in the range 0.25 to 0.4 SD and have implications for the child's education and for life beyond school, including future earning potential. We investigate those implications by considering the economic benefits in terms of IQ and school attendance and by comparing school health programs with traditional education interventions.

Economic Benefits of Long-Term Improvements in IQ

School health interventions can yield considerable economic benefits through returns to wages and productivity if they translate into improved cognitive functioning and IQ in adulthood.

For the United States, Zax and Rees (2002) estimate conservatively that an increase in IQ of 1 SD is associated with an increase in wages of more than 11 percent, falling to 6 percent when controlling for other covariates. Similar estimates for the relationship between IQ and earnings have been made for Indonesia (Behrman and Deolalikar 1995) and Pakistan (Alderman and others 1997) and in a review of developing countries (Glewwe 2002). In South Africa, an increase of 1 SD in literacy and numeracy scores was associated with a 35 percent increase in wages (Moll 1998). Extrapolating these results, a 0.25 SD increase in IQ, which is a conservative estimate of the benefit resulting from a school health intervention, would lead to an increase in wages of from 5 to 10 percent.

Economic Benefit of Improved School Attendance

School health interventions can raise adult productivity not only through higher levels of cognitive ability, but also through their effect on school participation and years of schooling attained. Healthier children are more likely to attend, and modest improvements in examination scores can be associated with continuation in schooling.

Malaria chemoprophylaxis given in early childhood in The Gambia led to an increase of more than one year in primary

schooling. In preschool children in Delhi, iron supplementation was associated with an increase of 5.8 percent in rates of participation at the preschool level (Bobonis, Miguel, and Sharma 2004). In western Kenya, deworming treatment improved primary school participation by 9.3 percent, with an estimated 0.14 additional years of education per pupil treated (Miguel and Kremer 2004). On the basis of crude estimates of returns to schooling, an increase of 9.3 percent in participation rates results in a return of US$44. Miguel and Kremer (2004) conclude that these benefits still outweigh the costs even if increased school participation leads to greater costs in teacher compensation through the need for additional teachers. They note that the benefit-cost ratio remains over 10 even if the rate of return to an additional year of schooling is as low as 1.5 percent. These results suggest that for realistic estimates of returns to schooling, the net present discounted value of lifetime earnings is likely to be high compared to the costs of treatment even for small gains in school participation.[1]

In the absence of studies estimating the direct link between school health interventions and school participation, the relationship can be estimated indirectly by considering the effect of interventions on test scores and the implications that improved test scores have for school participation. Improvements in cognitive function can be converted into an equivalent number of years of schooling. For example, Jukes and others (2002) found that heavy schistosomiasis was (nonsignificantly) associated with a decrease in arithmetic scores of 1.35 marks (0.25 SD). An extra year of schooling was associated with an increase in arithmetic scores of 2.24 marks (0.42 SD). Thus, the negative effect of heavy schistosomiasis was equivalent to missing just over half a year of schooling. The cognitive gains from an extra year of schooling can also be estimated retrospectively: in a study of adults in South Africa, each additional year of primary schooling was associated with a 0.1 SD increase in cognitive test scores (Moll 1998). According to these estimates, a typical increase of 0.25 SD associated with school health and nutrition programs is equivalent to an additional 2.5 years of schooling.

Liddell and Rae (2001) assessed the direct effect of test scores on grade progression in Africa. Each additional SD scored in first-grade exams resulted in children being 4.8 times as likely to reach seventh grade without repeating a year of schooling.[2] According to these estimates, an increase of 0.25 SD in examination scores, which is typically achieved by school health and nutrition programs, will make children 1.48 times[3] as likely to complete seventh grade, which implies that the extra cumulative years of schooling attributable to the school health intervention average 1.19 years per pupil. The previous estimates for added years of schooling owing to school health interventions range from seven months to two years. Increased years of schooling are associated with, among other outcomes, higher worker productivity and generally higher productivity in nonmarket production activities, including greater farmer efficiency and productivity (Jamison and Lau 1982; Psacharopoulos and Woodhall 1985; Strauss and Thomas 1995). Psacharopoulos and Patrinos (2002) summarize a wide range of studies that focus on individual wage earnings. For Sub-Saharan Africa, they find a 12 percent rate of return to one additional year in school, compared with 10 percent for Asian countries. These returns are very high, even allowing for a portion of the return to years of schooling to be capturing ability and factors other than schooling itself (Card 2001).

Education brings benefits beyond improved earnings. One year of extra education for girls can lead to a reduction of from 5 to 10 percent in infant mortality (Schultz 1993). Five extra years of education for women in Africa could reduce infant mortality by up to 40 percent (Summers 1994).

Economic Benefits of Programs

The educational gains from school health and nutrition programs should be considered in the context of alternative educational inputs, such as improving teacher salaries and qualifications, reducing class size, improving school facility infrastructure, and providing instructional materials. Many studies relate student outcomes to school characteristics, but few of these studies provide information on the relative or actual costs of the educational inputs. The costs, however, are substantially greater than for the school health interventions considered here. Despite the higher costs, the evidence from the few randomized evaluations that have been conducted suggests that the scale of effect of additional education inputs is typically low (see discussion in Miguel and Kremer 2004). A review of studies showed that instructional materials (such as additional textbooks) had the highest productivity, raising student test scores significantly more than other inputs for each dollar spent. However, even these interventions have only a weak effect. In a randomized experiment in Kenya, for example, providing textbooks had no effect on the bottom three quintiles of students and raised test scores by only 0.2 SD for the upper two quintiles. Relating these results to the findings in the previous section and to the annual per pupil costs, school health interventions appear very cost-effective compared to the highest-productivity, more traditional education inputs.

Recently, conditional cash-transfer programs have been viewed as potentially very cost-effective methods to increase school enrollment. These programs are generally large in scope, representing a commitment of between 0.1 and 0.2 percent of gross national income. The Progresa program in Mexico is estimated to have increased enrollment by 3.4 percent and to have increased schooling by 0.66 years, with an average cash transfer (for grades 3 to 8) of about US$136 per child per school year (assumed to be 180 days). Gains from a similar program in Nicaragua were estimated at 0.45 years of school at a cost of US$77 per year. If we compare these results with those presented for school health and nutrition programs, the condi-

tional cash-transfer approach is, in both cases, apparently at the lower end of effectiveness and the higher end of cost.

IMPLEMENTATION OF PROGRAMS AND LESSONS FROM EXPERIENCE

The FRESH framework provides strategic guidance, but the practical design of actual programs reflects differences in local needs and capacity. Successful and equitable programs in low- and middle-income countries are characterized by a focus on school-based delivery, on a public health paradigm that minimizes the need for clinical intervention and reliance on health service facilities, and on participation of the public sector and civil society locally.

Policy and Economic Issues in Defining Sectoral Roles in Intervention

A negative correlation between income level and both ill health and malnutrition is clearly demonstrated both in cross-country comparisons and within countries (see de Silva and others 2003), partly because poverty promotes both disease and an inadequate diet. Similarly, children who are not enrolled in school come from households with lower income levels (Filmer and Pritchett 2001). This fact suggests that school health services that are pro-poor and specifically linked to efforts to achieve universal participation in education will have a greater return.

Early school health programs, particularly in colonial Africa, were intended to serve the minority of children who had access to school in urban centers or elite boarding facilities. They relied on specific infrastructures and services—such as mobile health teams, school visits, school nurses, and in-school clinics—that were additional to the normal range of health service provision. This approach has proven difficult to make universally available, even in middle-income countries. A school nurse program in KwaZulu-Natal, for example, achieved inadequate coverage (18 percent of the target population) and little referral or follow-up treatment of cases of ill health detected, despite a relatively high investment of US$11.50 per student targeted per year (World Bank FRESH Toolkit 2000). As shown in the following examples, using the FRESH framework approach reduces costs significantly and enhances both coverage and outcomes.

An important element of the new approach to school health is a focus on minimizing the need for clinical diagnosis. Mass delivery of services, such as deworming and micronutrient supplementation, is preferable on efficacy, economic, and equity grounds to approaches that require diagnostic screening (Warren and others 1993).

Sectoral Roles in Implementation

Table 58.4 gives examples from low- and middle-income countries of how the four core components of FRESH are being supported by different approaches. In about 85 percent

Table 58.4 Nine Low- and Middle-Income Countries and How They Use FRESH

Program approach	Country examples	Policy	Environment	Health education	Health services	Outcomes (Costs per child per year)
Public sector: public sector—supported and —implemented	Guinea, Ghana, and Tanzania	In all three countries, the Ministry of Education (or in Ghana, its executive body, the Ghana Education Service) implements the program under the guidance of the Ministry of Health, on the basis of a formal policy agreement. In Tanzania, the Ministries of Community Development and of Local Government are also parties to the agreement. The existing in-service teacher training and supply-line infrastructures are used to prepare teachers and supply the necessary materials.	Separate sanitation facilities for girls and boys in all new schools; access to potable water in all schools.	Health, hygiene, and nutrition education as part of the formal curriculum.	Deworming (for both schistosomiasis and intestinal worms) provided by teachers twice a year; in Guinea, this service is followed by iron folate supplementation.	In three years, in Guinea—1.1 million students, in Ghana—577 schools and 83,000 students (US$0.54), in Tanzania—353 schools and 113,000 students (US$0.89).
Parastatal support for public sector intervention	Madagascar	The Community Nutrition Programme provides training and support to the Ministry of Education on the basis of a formally agreed-on health policy for the education sector. In all schools in the 43 poorest districts (44 percent of all districts), the program prepares teachers and provides materials. In addition, the program also provides Parent-Teacher Associations (PTAs) with access to a social fund to support construction of facilities. Each PTA can request up to US$500, with a 20 percent community contribution based on an annual parental contribution of US$0.16.	Access to potable water and hand-washing facilities, in all schools; where requested by PTAs, construction of latrines, wells, fences, and sports facilities.	A formal health education curriculum, supported by community information, education, and communication (IEC).	Twice-yearly deworming and iron folate (for three months) delivered by teachers; test kits to confirm iodization of local sources of salt; where requested by PTAs, provision of food preparation facilities.	In three years, 14,000 teachers trained in 4,585 schools, 430,000 students (US$0.78 to US$1.08 per capita per year).
Social fund: public sector support for community intervention	Tajikistan	The Ministry of Labor and Social Protection, with the Ministries of Education and of Health, have developed a memorandum of understanding that sets out health policies for the education sector. The program channels resources through PTAs, which identify and assist needy children. A training program, delivered by NGOs, prepares PTA members to develop proposals of up to US$5,000 for their school to support activities selected from a menu of items.	Provision of sanitation facilities, potable water, and sports facilities.	Training of teachers in health promotion.	Training of teachers to provide first aid, micronutrients, and deworming; provision of food preparation facilities.	The program targets the 100,000 neediest children in all 200 schools in the six poorest districts of Tajikistan (US$1 per capita per year).

Private sector: community payment for NGO-implemented intervention	Indonesia	The NGO Yayasan Kusuma Buana has a formal agreement with the education department in Jakarta and three other major cities to train teachers, perform diagnostic tests, and provide medicines and materials. The NGO offers Papanicolaou smear tests and referral services to teachers. Unit costs are low because parasite diagnosis involves mass screening in a central laboratory (approximately 2,500 diagnoses per day) and medicines are obtained at preferential rates from two commercial partners.	Not included in program.	Nutrition and hygiene education as part of the curriculum.	Stool examination by the laboratory and deworming by teachers as necessary twice a year; iron folate provided by teachers twice a year (for three months).	The program has been in existence for 17 years and currently reaches 627 schools and 161,000 students, at a cost to parents of US$0.10 annually.
NGO implementation with financial support from public sector	Burkina Faso, Malawi, and the Philippines	The international NGO Save the Children U.S.A. implements school health and nutrition activities in nonformal schools created with support from government, local communities, and private donations.	Separate sanitation facilities for girls and boys and access to potable water.	Health, hygiene, and nutrition education as part of the curriculum supported by extracurricular IEC activities	Deworming and micronutrient supplementation (vitamin A and iron) provided by teachers annually.	In three years, in Burkina Faso, 42,000 students plus nonenrolled children in 171 schools (US$2). In four years, in Malawi, 122,000 children in 181 schools (US$3). In four years in the Philippines, 23,000 children in 53 schools (US$6).

Source: Authors.

of programs reviewed, school health and nutrition programs are delivered and funded by the public education sector, with a formal role for the health sector in design and supervision.

Although this public sector "mainstream" model has proven the most popular approach, it is not the only successful one. In some cases, the public sector has identified appropriate options and developed operational manuals but then has used a social fund to provide direct support to communities and has used schools to select and implement the most relevant actions locally, often with the assistance of nongovernmental organizations (NGOs). In other cases, services have been contracted out by the public sector, and in some middle-income countries, the move toward a demand-led approach has resulted in a private sector service.

The private sector approach has proven sustainable over nearly two decades in urban Indonesia but may require a technical infrastructure and local market base that are inappropriate for predominantly rural low-income countries. The approach is modeled on a program initiated in Japan in 1948, which relied on private sector technicians, working independently at first but later formalized within the Japan Association of Parasite Control, who conducted stool examinations and then treated infected individuals for a per capita fee equivalent to approximately US$0.74 in 2004. At its peak, the private sector program conducted some 12 million examinations annually, implying a turnover of nearly US$9 million at today's prices. The prevalence of roundworm infection fell from a high of 73 percent in 1949 to less than 0.01 percent by 1985.

Although a private sector response is effective in some circumstances, overall the characteristics of school health and nutrition programs make a compelling case for public sector intervention. First, treatment externalities may create external benefits to others in addition to the benefit for the treated individual. This situation is clearly the case for communicable disease interventions, especially against worm infection. Second, some forms of intervention (such as vector control, health education campaigns, epidemiological surveillance, and interventions that have strong externalities) are almost pure public goods; that is, no one can be excluded from using the goods or service they deliver, and thus the private sector is unlikely to compete to deliver these goods. Finally, there is typically little private demand for general preventive measures, such as information on the value of washing hands. None of these factors is an argument against a private sector role in service delivery, but they do suggest that private sector demand is likely to be greater in middle-income populations and where public sector actions have created a demand.

Roles of Key Stakeholders in Implementation

There are many ways to approach the delivery of school health, but these diverse experiences suggest common features—in particular, the consistency in the roles played by government and nongovernmental agencies as well as other partners and stakeholders (table 58.5). In nearly every case, the Ministry of Education is the lead implementing agency, reflecting both the goal of school health programs in improving educational achievement and the fact that the education system provides the most complete existing infrastructure for reaching school-age children. However, the education sector must share this responsibility with the Ministry of Health, particularly because the latter has the ultimate responsibility for health of children. It is also apparent that the program's success depends on the effective participation of numerous other stakeholders, including civil society, and especially the beneficiaries and their parents or guardians. The children and their families are the clients of these programs, and their support for program implementation is critical to the program's success.

Key Issues in Designing Effective Programs

The diverse experiences of school health programming suggest some key elements that are common contributors to success in many programs.

- *Focus on education outcomes.* Making explicit links among school health programs and learning and education sector priorities (especially EFA and gender equity) helps ensure the commitment of the sector to program support and implementation.
- *Develop a formal, multisectoral policy.* Education sector actions in health require the explicit agreement of the health sector. This potential tension can be resolved by defining sectoral responsibilities at the outset; failure to enter into dialogue has led, in Africa and Central Asia, to some health sectors resisting teacher delivery of deworming drugs, despite WHO recommendations.
- *Initiate a process of wide dissemination and consultation.* Because there are multiple stakeholders, implementers, enablers, and gatekeepers, a process of consultation is necessary to establish ownership and to identify obstacles before they constrain progress. The process should involve at least community-based organizations, NGOs, faith-based organizations, pupils, and teacher associations. In one country in East Africa, lack of prior agreement on the content of sexuality education delayed implementation for more than three years.
- *Use the existing infrastructure as much as possible.* Building on existing curriculum opportunities and the network of formal and nonformal teachers will accelerate implementation and reduce costs. Programs that rely on the development of new delivery systems—mobile school health teams, a cadre of school nurses—take longer to establish and are expensive and complicated to sustain and take to scale.

Table 58.5 Roles of Agencies, Partners, and Stakeholders in School Health and Nutrition Programs

Partner	Roles	Comments
Ministry of Education	Lead implementing agency	Health and nutrition of schoolchildren is a priority for EFA.
	Lead financial resource	Education policy defines school environment, curriculum, duties of teachers.
	Education sector policy	Education system has a pervasive infrastructure for reaching teachers and school-age children.
Ministry of Health	Lead technical agency	Health of school-age children has lower priority than clinical services, infant health.
	Health sector policy	Health policy defines role of teachers in service delivery, procurement of health materials.
Other public sector agencies (for example, Welfare, Social Affairs, local government)	Support for education and health systems	Ministries of local government are often fund holders for teachers and schools and for clinics and health agents.
	Fund holder	Ministries of Welfare and Social Affairs provide mechanisms for providing social funds.
Private sector (for example, health service, pharmaceuticals, publications)	Specialist service delivery	Sector has major role in drug procurement and training materials production.
	Material provision	Sector has specialist roles in health diagnostics.
Civil society (for example, NGOs, faith-based organizations, PTAs)	Training and supervision	At the local level, organizations serve as gatekeepers and fund holders and may target implementation.
	Local resource provision	Organizations provide additional resource streams, particularly international NGOs.
Teacher associations	Definition of teachers' roles	School health programs demand an expanded role for teachers.
Community (children, teachers, parents)	Partners in implementation	Communities are gatekeepers for the content of health education (especially moral and sexual content) and for the role of nonhealth agents (especially teachers) in health service delivery; pupils are active participants in all aspects of the process at the school level.
	Definition of acceptability of curriculum and teachers' roles	
	Supplementation of resources	Communities supplement program finance at the margins.

- *Use simple, safe, and familiar health and nutrition interventions.* Success in rapidly reaching all schools depends on stakeholder acceptance, which is more likely if the interventions are already sanctioned by local and international agencies and are already in common use by the community.
- *Provide primary support from public resources.* Compelling arguments exist for public investment in school health programs: the contribution to economic growth, the high rate of return, the large externalities, and the fact that the majority of interventions are public goods.
- *Be inclusive and innovative in identifying implementation partners.* Although public resources are crucial for school health programs, contributions from outside the public sector can be vital. NGOs have proven effective in supporting public sector programs through training and supervision, particularly at local levels. Although market failure appears to have largely precluded the private sector from effectively implementing national programs in low-income countries, examples of successful contributions do occur, particularly in dense urban populations and in middle-income countries.

RESEARCH AND DEVELOPMENT AGENDA

Reliable evidence suggests that ill health and malnutrition affect education access, participation, completion, and achievement, and that school-based health and nutrition programs can provide a cost-effective and low-cost solution. This evidence does not imply, however, that no uncertainties exist.

Cost-Effectiveness of School-Based HIV/AIDS Prevention

Substantial evidence suggests that skills-based health education, including life-skills development programs, can promote positive behaviors and reduce the risks of exposure to HIV infection, and that girls' education programs have similar effects (Kirby 2002). Evidence also exists for a positive effect of completing education on HIV prevalence (de Walque 2004; World Bank 2002). What is lacking is direct evidence about the contribution that school-based prevention programs can make in reducing the incidence of HIV infection, as well as evidence for the relative cost-effectiveness of such programs compared with existing efforts to promote education completion and girls' education.

Cost-Effectiveness of Malaria Programs

Malaria occurs commonly in schoolchildren, particularly in areas of unstable transmission in Africa and Asia. It is a leading source of mortality in this age group and adversely affects education by reducing school attendance, cognition, learning, and school performance. Current school-based approaches focus on knowledge of the disease and the use of impregnated bednets but do not address the need for treatment of affected children. Yet presumptive treatment by teachers has been shown to significantly reduce mortality (Pasha and others 2003), and intermittent preventive treatment also shows considerable promise (Brooker and others 2000). There is a need to confirm the success of school-based treatment in different epidemiological settings and to address questions about the cost and sustainability of this approach.

Cost-Effectiveness of Targeting Food Aid

The high prevalence of malnutrition in children continues to be a major challenge for low-income countries. Providing food to children at school is often seen as an important part of the solution and is a major focus for food aid. However, the nutrition literature suggests that ensuring good nutrition earlier in life—certainly before 3 years of age, but perhaps earlier—is essential to ensuring an appropriate development trajectory throughout life (see chapter 27). Where food is limiting, it raises the question whether the first target should be preschool rather than school-age children. This debate has been blurred by admixing the nutrition outcomes with broader social and education issues. Clearly, providing a meal at school is socially desirable and can offer education benefits for children who otherwise would have to walk often long distances home to eat or remain hungry. It is also clear that schools represent an extensive and established network for providing nutrition interventions to very large numbers of children at a low cost per child. No comparable network exists to reach preschool children. However, from a nutritional perspective, it remains unclear whether ensuring good nutrition early in life has more effect on subsequent development—including educational achievement—than providing food at school age.

CONCLUSIONS

The rationale for school-based health and nutrition programs and the approach to their implementation have undergone a paradigm shift over the past two decades.

The traditional perception of these programs as seeking to improve the health of schoolchildren cannot be justified on the basis of mortality or public health statistics alone. Instead, it is increasingly recognized that a major—perhaps the major—impact of ill health and malnutrition on this age group is that on cognitive development, learning, and educational achievement.

In consequence, the clearest benefit of school health and nutrition programs is measurable in terms of education outcomes and their economic returns. The scale of benefit is significant: school health and nutrition interventions can add four to six points to IQ levels, 10 percent to participation in schooling, and one to two years of education. This scale of benefit can add 8 to 12 percent to labor returns and provide a rate of return that offers a strong argument for public sector investment.

Compelling evidence suggests that education qua education can help protect individuals from HIV infection. Achieving EFA goals and combining this outcome with school health programs that help establish lifelong positive behaviors are now recognized as essential to the multisectoral prevention response to HIV/AIDS.

The scale of the education benefit and the role of education in the fight against HIV/AIDS mean that school health and nutrition programs are today seen as a priority for both the education and the health sectors. This focus, in turn, has resulted in a shift toward public health rather than clinical intervention and toward school-based delivery rather than health system approaches. These policy changes enhance cost-effectiveness and social progressiveness, because delivery through the school system is an order of magnitude less costly than using health systems and in low-income countries is better targeted to the poor.

These changes in emphases have coincided with significant technical and political policy reform. Technical consensus around the FRESH framework has encouraged countries and agencies to develop programs around a common coordinating principle, while the political imperative has been strengthened by the recognition that school health and nutrition programs are essential to achieving EFA and the Millennium Development Goals and are at the center of the preventative response to the HIV/AIDS pandemic.

Although much of this change has evolved over the past two decades, significant acceleration has occurred since the World Education Forum in 2000. Today, a majority of low-income countries have recognized the need for school health and nutrition programs and are seeking to implement them.

NOTES

1. These calculations assume the following: a return to an additional year of school is 7 percent; wage gains are earned over 40 years in the workforce, discounted at 5 percent per year with no wage growth; annual wage earnings are US$400 per year, which is below the estimated agricultural and nonagricultural annual wages for low-income countries (World Bank 2003). The opportunity costs of the additional schooling (child labor) have not been considered but are likely to be negligible.

2. These calculations assume that a pupil's falling behind the equivalent of one year in test scores has the same effect on earnings as losing one year of schooling; that the advantage that third graders have over second graders, for example, is the same as the advantage someone who has studied for a total of three years has over someone who has studied for two years; and that the impact of first-grade examination scores on

the probability of transition from one class to the next is the same at each grade level.

3. If an increase of 1 SD in exam scores leads to children being 4.8 times as likely to reach seventh grade, the increased likelihood of reaching seventh grade because of a 0.25 SD increase can be calculated as EXP (0.25 $\times$ LN(4.8)).

REFERENCES

Alderman, H., J. R. Behrman, S. Khan, D. R. Ross, and R. Sabot. 1997. "The Income Gap in Cognitive Skills in Rural Pakistan." *Economic Development and Cultural Change* 46: 97–122.

Behrman, J. R., and A. B. Deolalikar. 1995. "Are There Differential Returns to Schooling by Gender? The Case of Indonesian Labor-Markets." *Oxford Bulletin of Economics and Statistics* 57: 97–117.

Berkley, S., and D. Jamison. 1990. *A Conference on the Health of School Age Children.* New York: United Nations Development Programme and Rockefeller Foundation. Processed.

Bobadilla, J. L., P. Cowley, P. Musgrove, and H. Saxenian. 1994. "Design, Content, and Financing of an Essential National Package of Health Services." *Bulletin of the World Health Organization* 72: 653–62.

Bobonis, G., E. Miguel, and C. Sharma. 2004. "Iron Deficiency Anemia and School Participation." Working paper, University of California at Berkeley.

Brooker, S., H. Guyatt, J. Omumbo, R. Shretta, L. Drake, and J. Ouma. 2000. "Situation Analysis of Malaria in School-Aged Children in Kenya: What Can Be Done?" *Parasitology Today* 16: 183–86.

Bundy, D. A. P. 1989. "New UNESCO International Project." *Parasitology Today* 5: 168.

———. 1997. "This Wormy World: Then and Now." *Parasitology Today* 13: 407–8.

Bundy, D. A. P., and H. L. Guyatt. 1996. "Schools for Health: Focus on Health, Education, and the School-Aged Child." *Parasitology Today* 12: 1–16.

Bundy, D. A. P., A. Hall, G. F. Medley, and L. Savioli. 1992. "Evaluating Measures to Control Intestinal Parasitic Infections." *World Health Statistics Quarterly* 45: 168–79.

Bundy, D. A. P., S. Lwin, J. S. Osika, J. McLaughline, and C. O. Pannenborg. 2000. "What Should Schools Do about Malaria?" *Parasitology Today* 16: 181–82.

Bundy, D. A. P., M. S. Wong, L. L. Lewis, and J. Horton. 1990. "Control of Geohelminths by Delivery of Targeted Chemotherapy through Schools." *Transactions of the Royal Society of Tropical Medicine and Hygiene* 84: 115–20.

Card, D. 2001. "Estimating the Return to Schooling: Progress on Some Persistent Econometric Problems." *Econometrica* 69: 1127–60.

Cohen, S., and A. Smith. 1996. "Psychology of Common Colds and Other Infections." In *Viral and Other Infections of the Human Respiratory Tract,* ed. S. Myint and D. Taylor-Robinson. London: Chapman and Hall.

Colbourne, M. J. 1955. "The Effect of Malaria Suppression in a Group of Accra School Children." *Transactions of the Royal Society of Tropical Medicine and Hygiene* 4: 356–69.

Del Rosso, J. M., and T. Marek. 1996. *Class Action: Improving School Performance in the Developing World through Better Health and Nutrition School.* Washington, DC: World Bank.

de Walque, D. 2004. "How Does the Impact of an HIV/AIDS Information Campaign Vary with Educational Attainment? Evidence from Rural Uganda." Working paper, World Bank, Washington, DC.

European Commission, WHO (World Health Organization) Europe, and Council of Europe. 1996. *Facts about the European Network of Health Promoting Schools.*

Filmer, D., and L. H. Pritchett. 2001. "Estimating Wealth Effects without Expenditure Data—or Tears: An Application to Educational Enrolments in States of India." *Demography* 38: 115–32.

Glewwe, P. 2002. "Schools and Skills in Developing Countries: Education Policies and Socioeconomic Outcomes." *Journal of Economic Literature* 40: 436–82.

Guyatt, H. L. 2003. "The Cost of Delivering and Sustaining a Control Program for Schistosomiasis and Soil-Transmitted Helminthiasis." *Acta Tropica* 86: 267–74.

Grigorenko, E., R. Sternberg, D. Ngorosho, C. Nokes, M. Jukes, K. Alcock, and D. Bundy. Forthcoming. "Effects of Antiparasitic Treatment on Dynamically-Assessed Cognitive Skills." *Journal of Applied Developmental Psychology.*

Haddad, L., and H. Bouis. 1991. "The Impact of Nutritional Status on Agricultural Productivity: Wage Evidence from the Philippines." *Oxford Bulletin of Economics and Statistics* 53: 45–68.

Hall, A., L. J. Drake, and D. A. P. Bundy. 2001. "Public Health Measures to Control Helminth Infections." In *Nutritional Anemias,* ed. U. Ramakrishnan. Boca Raton, FL: CRC Press.

Halloran, M. E., D. A. P. Bundy, and E. Pollitt. 1989. "Infectious Disease and the UNESCO Basic Education Inititative." *Parasitology Today* 5: 359–62.

Huda, S. N., S. M. Grantham-McGregor, and A. Tomkins. 2001. "Cognitive and Motor Functions of Iodine-Deficient but Euthyroid Children in Bangladesh Do Not Benefit from Iodized Poppy Seed Oil (Lipiodol)." *Journal of Nutrition* 131: 72–77.

Jamison, D., and L. J. Lau. 1982. *Farmer Education and Farm Efficiency.* Baltimore: Johns Hopkins University Press.

Jukes, M. C. H., L. L. Drake, and D. A. P. Bundy. Forthcoming. *Leveling the Playing Field: The Importance of School Health and Nutrition in Achieving Education for All.* Washington, DC: World Bank.

Jukes, M., C. A. Nokes, K. L. Alcock, J. Lambo, C. Kihamia, A. Mbise, and others. 2002. "Heavy Schistosomiasis Associated with Poor Short-Term Memory and Slower Reaction Times in Tanzanian School Children." *Tropical Medicine and International Health* 7: 104–17.

Jukes, M. C. H., M. Pinder, E. L. Grigorenko, H. Banos Smith, E. Bariau-Meier, G. Walraven, and others. Submitted. "The Impact of Malaria Chemoprophylaxis in Early Childhood on Cognitive Abilities and Educational Outcomes 14 Years Later: Follow-up of a Randomised Controlled Trial in The Gambia."

Kirby, D. 2002. "The Impact of Schools and School Programs upon Adolescent Sexual Behavior." *Journal of Sexual Research* 39: 27–33.

Liddell, C., and G. Rae. 2001. "Predicting Early Grade Retention: A Longitudinal Investigation of Primary School Progress in a Sample of Rural South African Children." *British Journal of Educational Psychology* 71: 413–28.

Miguel, E., and M. Kremer. 2004. "Worms: Identifying Impacts on Education and Health in the Presence of Treatment Externalities." *Econometrica* 72: 159–217.

Moll, P. G. 1998. "Primary Schooling, Cognitive Skills and Wages in South Africa. " *Economica* 65: 263–84.

Partnership for Child Development. 1998a. "The Anthropometric Status of School Children in Five Countries in the Partnership for Child Development." *Proceedings of the Nutrition Society* 57: 149–58.

———. 1998b: "The Health and Nutritional Status of School Children in Africa: Evidence from School-Based Health Programmes in Ghana and Tanzania." *Transactions of the Royal Society of Tropical Medicine and Hygiene* 92: 254–61.

———. 1999. "The Cost of Large-Scale School Health Programmes Which Deliver Anthelmintics to Children in Ghana and Tanzania." *Acta Tropica* 73: 183–204.

———. 2001. "Anaemia in Schoolchildren in Eight Countries in Africa and Asia." *Public Health Nutrition* 4: 749–56.

Pasha, O., J. Del Rosso, M. Mukaka, and D. Marsh. 2003. "The Effect of Providing Fansidar (Sulfadoxine-Pyrimethamine) in Schools on Mortality in School-Age Children in Malawi." *Lancet* 361: 577–78.

Pollitt, E. 1990. *Malnutrition and Infection in the Classroom*. Paris: United Nations Educational, Scientific, and Cultural Organization.

Pollitt, E., S. Cueto, and E. R. Jacoby. 1998. "Fasting and Cognition in Well- and Undernourished Schoolchildren: A Review of Three Experimental Studies." *American Journal of Clinical Nutrition* 67: 779S–84S.

Psacharopoulos, G., and H. Patrinos. 2002. *Returns to Investment in Education: A Further Update*. Vol. 2881. Washington, DC: World Bank.

Psacharopoulos, G., and M. Woodhall. 1985. *Education for Development: An Analysis of Investment Choices*. New York: Oxford University Press.

Schultz, T. P. 1993. "Returns to Women's Schooling." In *Women's Education in Developing Countries: Barriers, Benefits, and Policy*, eds. E. King and M. Anne Hill. Baltimore: Johns Hopkins University Press.

Shiff, C., W. Checkley, P. Winch, Z. Premji, J. Minjas,and P. Lubega. 1996. "Changes in Weight Gain and Anaemia Attributable to Malaria in Tanzanian Children Living under Holoendemic Conditions." *Transactions of the Royal Society of Tropical Medicine and Hygiene* 90: 262–65.

Simeon, D. T. 1998. "School Feeding in Jamaica: A Review of Its Evaluation." *American Journal of Clinical Nutrition* 67: 790S–94S.

Simeon, D. T., and S. Grantham McGregor. 1989. "Effects of Missing Breakfast on the Cognitive Functions of School Children of Differing Nutritional Status." *American Journal of Clinical Nutrition* 49: 646–53.

Snow, R. W. 1999. "Estimating Mortality, Morbidity, and Disability Due to Malaria among Africa's Non-Pregnant Population." *Bulletin of the World Health Organization* 77: 624–40.

Strauss, J., and D. Thomas. 1995. "Human Resources: Empirical Modeling of Household and Family Decisions." In *Handbook of Development Economics*, ed. J. Behrman and T. N. Srinivasan, vol. IIIA. Amsterdam: Elsevier.

Summers, L. H. 1994. *Investing in All the People: Educating Women in Developing Countries*. Vol. 45. Washington, DC: World Bank.

Thomas, D., and J. Strauss. 1997. "Health and Wages: Evidence on Men and Women in Urban Brazil." *Journal of Economics* 77: 159–85.

UNAIDS (Joint United Nations Programme on HIV/AIDS). 2000.

———. 2002. *Report on the Global HIV/AIDS Epidemic: The Barcelona Report*. Geneva: UNAIDS.

UNESCO (United Nations Educational, Scientific, and Cultural Organization). 1990. "World Declaration on Education for All." http://www.unesco.org/education/information/nfsunesco/pdf/JOMTIE_E.PDF.

———. 1993. *World Education Report*. Paris: UNESCO.

———. 2003. *EFA Global Monitoring Report 2003/4: Gender and Education for All: The Leap to Equality*. Paris: UNESCO.

UNICEF (United Nations Children's Fund). 1990. "Convention on the Rights of the Child." http://www.unicef.org/crc/crc.htm.

UNICEF, WHO (World Health Organization), World Bank, UNFPA (United Nations Population Fund), and UNESCO. 2003. *Skills for Health: Skills-Based Health Education, Including Life Skills—An Important Component of a Child Friendly/Health Promoting School*.

U.S. Census Bureau. 2002. "Global Population Profile." http://www.census.gov.

Warren, K. S., D. A. P. Bundy, R. M. Anderson, A. R. Davis, D. A. Henderson, D. T. Jamison, and others. 1993. "Helminth Infection." In *Disease Control Priorities in Developing Countries*, ed. D. T. Jamison, W. H. Mosley, A. R. Measham, and J. L. Bobadilla, 131–60. New York: Oxford University Press.

WHO (World Health Organization). 1986. *Ottawa Charter*. Geneva: WHO.

———. 1996. *Global School Health Initiative*. WHO/HPR/98.4. Geneva: WHO.

———. 2000. *Elimination of Avoidable Disability Due to Refractive Errors*. Report of an informal planning meeting. WHO/PBC/00.79. WHO: Geneva

———. 2003. *World Health Report*. http://www.who.int/whr/2003.

World Bank. 1993. *World Development Report: Investing in Health*. New York: Oxford University Press.

———. 2002. *Education and HIV/AIDS: A Window of Hope*. Washington, DC: World Bank.

———. 2003. *World Development Indicators*. Washington, DC: World Bank.

———, with the Partnership for Child Development. 2000. "FRESH: Focusing Resources on Education and School Health. A FRESH Start to Improving the Quality and Equity of Education." http://www.schoolsandhealth.org/FRESH.htm.

World Bank 2000. *The FRESH Framework: A Toolkit for Task Managers*. Human Development Network, World Bank, Washington, DC.

Zax, J. S., and D. I. Rees. 2002. "IQ, Academic Performance, Environment, and Earnings." *Review of Economics and Statistics* 84: 600–16.

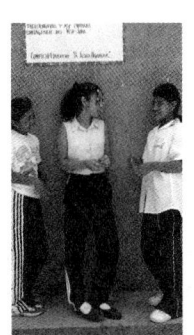

Chapter **59**

Adolescent Health Programs

Elizabeth Lule, James E. Rosen, Susheela Singh, James C. Knowles, and Jere R. Behrman

This chapter reviews the main direct causes of loss of productive life years among adolescents and the range of interventions to address these causes. It pays special attention to sexual and reproductive health because adolescence is when important transitions occur that can have a direct effect on young people's health as well as potential long-term consequences. In addition, a number of interventions have focused on this aspect of young people's behavior. The discussion centers on defined interventions that have some relatively rigorous evaluation component. There are some limitations to this chapter, however. First, it reviews existing research and does not carry out new research; however, it points to gaps in research and areas needing more work. Second, the chapter uses a focused definition of *health* that includes the most basic health outcomes (death, illness, timing of transitions, or specific risky or protective behaviors that research has attempted to measure). It does not attempt to cover aspects that would be included in a broad definition of health and well-being (for example, potential for growth, creativity, or participation) that are important but are poorly researched to date. Finally, although the broader environment in which adolescents live influences their behavior and responses to programs, this chapter does not attempt to review that important group of factors or the broader set of programs that have a more indirect effect on the health of young people (for example, school quality or public health promotion activities at the societal level).

NATURE AND CAUSES OF THE BURDEN OF DISEASE IN YOUNG PEOPLE

At first glance, adolescence appears to be a relatively healthy—although not hazard-free—period of life, given the relatively low mortality rates of young people.[1] Nevertheless, adolescents and young adults engage in a range of behaviors that can affect the quality of their health and the probability of their survival in the short term as well as affect their lifetime health and survival.

Health Challenges of Adolescents

If we look only at disability-adjusted life years (DALYs) for the adolescent age group, adolescents appear to be relatively healthy. Nonetheless, more than 33 percent of the disease burden and almost 60 percent of premature deaths among adults can be associated with behaviors or conditions that began or occurred during adolescence—for example, tobacco and alcohol use, poor eating habits, sexual abuse, and risky sex (WHO 2002). Adolescence-related risk factors are a greater problem in wealthier countries, largely because of the relatively greater impact of smoking and diet-related risks in those countries, though the prevalence of these risks is expanding rapidly in many low- and middle-income countries (LMICs). Thus, although adolescents are apparently healthy, they are practicing unhealthy behaviors that will ultimately result in much death and disability. This is an immense public health issue. Therefore, focusing attention both on diseases experienced during adolescence and on risk factors with their roots in adolescence makes sense. Adolescent health efforts should emphasize prevention because so much of the disease burden is preventable and because prevention is a particularly cost-effective strategy in relation to adolescents, given the long duration over which benefits will be reaped and adolescents' greater openness to change than adults.

Burden of Disease in Adolescence

The global burden-of-disease approach used to calculate DALYs is an imperfect representation of the prevalence, morbidity, and

Table 59.1 Worldwide Distribution of DALYs for Major Categories of Diseases and Conditions by Age Group and Sex, 2002 *(percent)*

Category	Women		Men	
	Age 5–14	Age 15–29	Age 5–14	Age 15–29
Sexual and reproductive causes	4.6	33.4	3.9	9.5
HIV/AIDS	3.8	11.9	3.7	8.6
Maternal conditions	0.4	16.3	0.0	0.0
Other sexual and reproductive conditions	0.4	5.2	0.2	0.9
Respiratory conditions	11.9	3.7	9.9	3.7
Cardiovascular conditions	2.2	2.9	2.0	3.3
Neuropsychiatric conditions	15.5	33.8	14.9	32.0
Unipolar depressive disorders	5.4	10.1	5.6	7.1
Bipolar disorders	0.6	4.1	0.7	4.2
Schizophrenia	0.7	4.4	2.3	4.2
Other mental health conditions	1.0	4.4	0.6	2.6
Alcohol use disorders	0.1	1.1	0.3	5.7
Drug use disorders	0.1	0.6	0.2	2.3
Other	7.6	9.1	5.2	5.9
Injuries	25.0	14.0	32.4	33.1
Unintentional, road traffic accidents	5.7	2.2	7.7	7.5
Unintentional, other	16.8	7.7	21.8	12.9
Intentional, self-inflicted	1.0	2.9	0.9	3.8
Intentional, not self-inflicted (war, violence)	1.5	1.2	2.0	8.9
Other communicable diseases	31.1	7.1	27.7	11.1
Tuberculosis	1.5	3.0	1.4	3.9
Other noncommunicable diseases	9.9	9.6	9.2	10.0
Total	100.2	104.5	100.0	102.7

Source: WHO 2004a.

mortality of conditions that adolescents face. DALYs fail to capture fully the complexity of adolescent health concerns. Nonetheless, no better comprehensive and comparative measure currently exists; thus, the discussion in this section will rely primarily on available DALY data.

The World Health Organization (WHO), in 1999, commissioned a special analysis of the burden of disease in adolescence, which examined the 10 to 14 and the 15 to 19 age groups. The study found that young people age 10 to 19, who constitute 19 percent of the world's population, account for 15 percent of the disease and injury burden worldwide. It also found that more than 1 million people in that age group die each year (WHO 1999). The top three causes of DALYs were found to be unipolar major depression, transportation accidents, and falls. The profile of disease burden was significantly different for younger and older adolescents. In the 10 to 14 age group, injuries and communicable diseases were prominent causes of DALYs. For the 15 to 19 age group, the disease burden shifted to outcomes of sexual behaviors and mental health.

Using 2002 data, WHO has made more detailed calculations of DALYs by sex for the 5 to 14 and 15 to 29 age groups (table 59.1). These age ranges overlap adolescence and are, thus, broadly indicative of the 10 to 19 age group. Notably, table 59.1 shows large differences by sex in the pattern and level of DALYs. These differences are important, because they relate to the different needs of young women and young men for interventions and services. Particular interventions also potentially have different costs and benefits because of the different proportions of females and males.

Worldwide, among young men age 15 to 29, injuries and neuropsychiatric illnesses account for a high proportion of DALYs (33 percent and 32 percent, respectively). By comparison, among young women age 15 to 29, injuries account for 14 percent of DALYs, and neuropsychiatric illnesses account for about the same percentage of DALYs as among young men. However, sexual and reproductive health conditions account for 33 percent of young women's DALYs, much higher than the 10 percent for young men. For both young men and young women, all other communicable and noncommunicable diseases account for moderate proportions of DALYs (7 to 11 percent, depending on sex and disease group).

The disease burden among 5- to 14-year-olds is markedly different from that for the 15- to 29-year-olds, and differences between males and females are quite small. Communicable diseases and respiratory illnesses account for much larger proportions of DALYs for this age group compared with the 15 to 29 age group, whereas neuropsychiatric and sexual and reproductive conditions account for much smaller proportions. HIV/AIDS accounts for less than 4 percent of DALYs for both males and females age 5 to 14.

Health Risk Behaviors among Adolescents and Young People

Young people's vulnerability to risky or unwanted sex and other unhealthy behaviors is tied to a host of individual, family, and community factors that influence their behavior and that are closely related to their economic and educational opportunities. Good health and other physical, moral, and intellectual development outcomes are often mutually reinforcing. For example, healthy children do better in school. Similarly, having more years of schooling provides essential information and skills that are linked to more protective and less risky behaviors.

Injuries. Violence and war account for more than a quarter of injury-related deaths among young men age 15 to 29. Adolescent boys and men in their 20s are an important part of the military forces in all countries that have such forces. As such, they are at high risk, particularly in areas where armed conflict is occurring. The United Nations Children's Fund estimates that approximately 300,000 soldiers under the age of 18 are involved in armed conflicts worldwide (National Research Council and Institute of Medicine 2005). Homicide is also an important cause of death for young men, in particular, and it is the leading cause of death for young men in some Latin American countries (WHO 2001b). In addition, road accidents account for significant proportions of injuries and deaths among young people. Self-inflicted injuries, including suicide, which are often related to mental illness, are also a major health problem for young people, accounting for 4 percent of DALYs in men age 15 to 29 and 3 percent of DALYs in women age 15 to 29.

Mental Health. Depression, schizophrenia, and other mental illnesses are important causes of illness and death among young men and women and account for a significant proportion of DALYs for both men (18 percent) and women (23 percent) age 15 to 29; for 5- to 14-year-olds, it is about 9 percent for boys and 8 percent for girls. The relative importance of mental illnesses is much greater in the high-income countries.

Smoking, Alcohol, and Drug Use. Most adult smokers worldwide begin smoking in adolescence or earlier (World Bank 1999a). An estimated 15 percent of young men and 7 percent of women age 13 to 15 are currently smoking cigarettes, according to more than 100 surveys that have been conducted since 1999 by the Global Youth Tobacco Survey Program and carried out under the auspices of WHO and the U.S. Centers for Disease Control and Prevention (National Research Council and Institute of Medicine 2005). Every day, worldwide, almost 100,000 young people start smoking, more than two-thirds of them in LMICs (World Bank 1999a). Of the 300 million young people smoking today, half will eventually die from tobacco use (WHO 2001b). By 2030, tobacco is expected to be the single biggest cause of death worldwide, accounting for about 10 million deaths per year (World Bank 1999a).

Although discouraging young people from starting to smoke and providing means for them to quit is extremely important, deaths caused by tobacco tend to occur many years later. Therefore, tobacco use as an underlying risk factor accounts for very few DALYs in the 5 to 29 age group (WHO 2002). Alcohol and drug use account for 8 percent of all DALYs for young men age 15 to 29 but for only 2 percent for young women. Evidence indicates that young people are starting to drink at earlier ages. Longitudinal studies have found that the earlier young people start drinking, the more likely they are to experience alcohol-related injuries and alcohol dependence later in life (WHO 2001a).

Nutrition and Exercise. Nutritional deficiencies such as anemia are widespread in both young men and women. Worldwide, these conditions account for almost 5 percent of DALYs among girls age 5 to 14 and almost 4 percent among boys of the same age, with anemia being an important component for both girls and boys. Although nutritional deficiencies are relatively less important among 15- to 29-year-olds (just over 1.0 percent among young men and about 1.5 percent among women), anemia accounts for the bulk of these deficiencies. Chronic undernutrition that causes stunting among young people delays growth and physical maturation, increases risks to pregnant mothers and their newborns, and decreases the capacity to learn and to work (Behrman and others 2004; Hoddinott and Quisumbing 2003). Malnutrition can take other forms, some of which lead to being overweight or obese, thereby increasing the risks for diseases such as diabetes. Such forms of malnutrition are of increasing relevance in middle-income countries such as Brazil, China, the Arab Republic of Egypt, Mexico, and South Africa and at times coexist with undernutrition (see, for example, Doak and others 2000).

Nutritional deficiencies increase the risks that girls and young women face during pregnancy and childbirth (Delisle, Chandra-Mouli, and de Benoist 2001), and evidence is emerging about the connection between poor maternal nutrition and greater risk of transmission of HIV from mothers to their infants (Piwoz and Greble 2000).

Diet and lifestyle-related chronic diseases—many with their roots in childhood and adolescence—are emerging as one of the most important health problems in LMICs. Cardiovascular diseases, which are responsible for 10 percent of DALYs lost in LMICs, typically occur in middle age or later; however, risk factors are determined to a great extent by behaviors learned during childhood and adolescence and continued into adulthood, such as dietary habits and smoking. Throughout the world, these risks are starting to appear earlier. Physical activity has decreased markedly in adolescence, particularly in girls, and obesity has increased substantially (MacKay and Mensah 2004).

Sexual and Reproductive Behaviors. Worldwide, the majority of young people initiate sexual activity during adolescence. Significant proportions—in some regions and countries, the majority—marry and become parents (table 59.2). Globally, the age of onset of puberty has been decreasing progressively for both boys and girls (National Research Council and Institute of Medicine 2005). The age at first marriage has also increased in most parts of the world over recent decades, except in Latin America (Mensch, Singh, and Casterline 2003). The decline in the age at puberty, combined with the general trend toward later marriage, increases the period of time during which adolescents may be sexually active before marriage and may result in sexual initiation at an earlier age (National Research Council and Institute of Medicine 2005).

Young women typically make the transition to marriage and parenthood at an earlier age than young men, and early marriage predisposes girls to HIV infection through unprotected sex, because the partner, by virtue of age, has an elevated risk of being HIV positive. In addition, marriage changes adolescent girls' support systems, thereby limiting their access to knowledge about HIV/AIDS (Bruce and Clark 2003).

All these key transitions to adulthood bring with them the potential for risks to health that may have both immediate and longer-term effects. Among young women age 15 to 29, illnesses related to pregnancy and childbearing account for 16 percent of their DALYs. Some have unwanted pregnancies, and in countries where abortion is legally restricted, unsafe abortion is an important source of mortality and morbidity for young women, with abortion complications accounting for almost 3 percent of DALYs worldwide among females age 15 to 29. (WHO 2004c).

Even though adolescent childbearing has declined in recent years, the proportion of young women who become mothers during adolescence remains high in most LMICs, and very early childbearing remains an issue in some regions (table 59.2). Childbearing before age 16 also brings with it a high risk of health consequences, both for the mother and for the newborn (Save the Children U.S.A. 2004; WHO forthcoming-b).

In the most recent surveys carried out in LMICs, high proportions of adolescents report that they have heard of contraceptive methods; however, little is known about the quality and accuracy of young people's knowledge of contraception. Moreover, substantial proportions of young women appear to have an unmet need for contraception; they are not using contraception even though they are sexually active and do not want to have a child (CDC and ORC Macro 2003; Westoff and Bankole 1995).

In addition to having a risk of early and unwanted pregnancy, adolescents are also at risk of acquiring sexually transmitted infections (STIs), including HIV. HIV/AIDS accounts for most of the sexual and reproductive health DALYs lost by young men age 15 to 29 (almost 9 percent). Among young women age 15 to 29, HIV/AIDS accounts for a higher proportion of DALYs than for young men (almost 12 percent) because of their higher levels of susceptibility. STIs and other sexual and reproductive health disorders together account for just over 5 percent of young women's DALYs, much more than among young men. About half of all HIV infections occur in people under age 25, and for biological, social, and economic reasons, young women are disproportionately affected, especially in Sub-Saharan Africa, where young women have twice the prevalence rate of young men (UNAIDS 2003).

Poverty and Adolescent Health

Poverty and inadequate health systems compound adolescents' vulnerability to sickness and early death. At the same time, poor health exacerbates poverty by disrupting and cutting short school opportunities, by weakening or killing young people in the prime of their working lives, or by placing heavy financial and social burdens on families.

Poor adolescents bear a disproportionate burden of the health problems in their age group. An analysis of data from demographic and health surveys (Macro International 1990–98, unpublished raw data) indicates a strong association between poverty and the health status of adolescents and between poverty and adolescents' use of health services. For example, the poorest 20 percent of young women are between 1.7 and 4.0 times as likely to have an early birth as the richest 20 percent of young women. Similar disparities between rich and poor adolescents are seen for indicators such as early marriage, skilled attendance at birth, use of contraception, and knowledge of HIV/AIDS transmission, and these disparities tend to be greater for adolescents than for older women. For example, surveys in 45 countries show that the poorest 20 percent of women age 15 to 49 have a total fertility rate almost double that of the richest 20 percent, whereas among adolescents age 15 to 19, total fertility among the poorest 20 percent is more than triple that of the richest 20 percent (Macro International 1990–98, unpublished raw data).

Table 59.2 Indicators of Sexual and Reproductive Behaviors among Adolescents and Youth by Gender and Age Group, Late 1990s to Early 2000s

a. Sexual Activity

	Percentage of females age 20–24 who became sexually active before age			Percentage of males age 20–24 who became sexually active before age		
Region	15	18	20	15	18	20
East and Southern Africa	17	57	77	14	45	65
West and Central Africa	21	59	77	12	40	61
Caribbean and Central America	13	44	62	31	70	84
South America	9	41	61	31	73	87
Former Soviet Asia	1	20	53	—	—	—
Middle East	—	—	—	—	—	—
South and Southeast Asia	—	—	—	—	—	—

b. Marriage

	Percentage of females age 20–24 who married before age		Percentage of males age 20–24 who married before age		Percentage of men age 20–24 ever married
Region	18	20	18	20	
East and Southern Africa	37	55		14	28
West and Central Africa	45	60		12	27
Caribbean and Central America	35	53		22	38
South America	23	38		14	29
Former Soviet Asia	16	50		—	24
Middle East	23	40		—	17
South and Southeast Asia	42	60		—	41

c. Childbearing

	Percentage of females age 20–24 whohad a child before age		Percentage of males who ever fathered a child at age	
Region	16	18	15–19	20–24
East and Southern Africa	9	27	2	24
West and Central Africa	13	31	2	13
Caribbean and Central America	7	22	2	27
South America	4	16	3	23
Former Soviet Asia	0	4	—	—
Middle East	3	11	—	—
South and Southeast Asia	9	24	—	—

d. Contraceptive Use

	Percentage of sexually active females age 15–19 using contraception		Percentage of sexually active females age 20–24 using contraception	
Region	All	Unmarried	All	Unmarried
East and Southern Africa	21	28	30	42
West and Central Africa	20	26	23	35
Caribbean and Central America	24	—	36	—
South America	28	38	33	59
Former Soviet Asia	25	—	43	—
Middle East	—	—	—	—
South and Southeast Asia	—	—	—	—

Source: National Research Council 2005.
— = not available.

INTERVENTIONS

Improving the health of young people is complex and difficult, arguably more so than for other age groups. Compared with children, adolescents are less protected by their families and communities and less amenable to simple solutions to their health problems, many of which are behavior based. Compared with adults, adolescents know less about how to stay healthy and have fewer resources to prevent or treat health problems. By contrast, their behaviors are less firmly entrenched, and they are often involved in institutional activities, such as schools, training programs, and the military, where programs with high coverage can be sustained. The influences on young people's behaviors are becoming better understood (Blum and Mmari 2004; Pitts and others 2004), but even given what is known about such influences, the challenge of designing interventions to reinforce protective factors and mitigate risk factors remains. Many of the factors associated with less risky health behaviors, such as family connectedness and academic performance, go far beyond the purview of health program managers.

Programs will have to seek multisectoral solutions that link health sector interventions with other types of interventions delivered through other sectors, either at the program level or at the policy level. The difficulty in attributing improvements in health outcomes among adolescents to interventions delivered in multiple settings or sectors reflects the challenges involved. Programs aimed at young people are relatively new and untested. Nevertheless, accumulated experience, backed by an increasing body of research, has created international consensus around a multi-intervention approach centered on the following (WHO 1999):

- Young people need information and skills to make the right decisions about behaviors that affect their health, such as whether and when to have sex and whether to use tobacco.
- Young people need access to a broad range of health services that give them the means to act on their knowledge, including access to condoms.
- Young people need a social, legal, and regulatory environment that supports healthy behaviors and protects them from harm.

Interventions to improve adolescent health have typically reflected this consensus and are echoed in goals that have been adopted internationally.

This section summarizes what is known about the effectiveness of such interventions. Note that the health community's consideration of adolescent health has only occasionally advocated attention to those health conditions that are of relatively greater importance to the adolescent age group, at least as measured by indicators such as DALYS. Much of the focus has been on sexual and reproductive health and on risky behaviors such as tobacco and drug abuse. The lack of age-specific data and traditional reliance on mortality and morbidity statistics contribute to the unbalanced attention. Another factor may be that such behaviors tend to have longer-term health consequences that are not reflected in standard DALY calculations. An additional reason for the imbalance in adolescent data may be the significant social impacts of sexual and reproductive behavior (for example, the contribution of high fertility to rapid population growth); the social and economic implications of large proportions of HIV-infected adolescents in many countries; the mortality implications of initiating tobacco use during adolescence; and the antisocial behavior associated with substance abuse. Public health systems' efforts to address health problems associated with road safety, malaria, and mental health have devoted inadequate attention to developing and implementing programs that target adolescents.

Evidence on Sexual and Reproductive Health Interventions

Two recent reviews summarize research on the effectiveness of adolescent sexual and reproductive health interventions. Table 59.3 presents the results of the FOCUS on Young Adults (2001) review. The FOCUS report looks at interventions in LMICs and is based on relatively rigorous evaluations of 40 programs. The general findings from the FOCUS review, supplemented by more recent research findings, are as follows:

- *Almost all programs are effective in promoting positive knowledge and attitudes.* Almost all the rigorously evaluated programs that FOCUS reviewed improved knowledge of reproductive health and selected attitudes.
- *Most programs effectively influence behaviors.* A majority of programs significantly changed at least one important adolescent behavior pertaining to reproductive health. Often, however, programs tried and failed to improve many important behaviors. Where research has found programs to be effective in changing behaviors, such changes have typically not been large.
- *All six categories of interventions studied proved effective at influencing reproductive behavior in at least one study.* However, maintaining that certain models are more effective than others is impossible because the period of observation and the behaviors that were influenced varied by study. Moreover, further replications in multiple settings are necessary to provide a basis for identifying the key features or elements of successful interventions.
- *The evidence base is limited in a number of ways.* Few studies look at the effects on ultimate health outcomes, such as pregnancy rates or rates of HIV infection. Furthermore, many promising approaches have not been rigorously evaluated. Only a few studies assessed effects on the use of health services, and none examined the effect of creating a

Table 59.3 Effectiveness of Adolescent Sexual and Reproductive Health Programs, LMICs

		Number of programs showing significant impact/Total number of programs studied						
			Impact on key behaviors					
Type of program	Number of studies[a]	Improved knowledge and attitudes	Delayed sex	Reduced number of partners	Increased contraceptive use	Increased service use	Improved at least one behavior
All programs	40	33/36	6/17	6/10	18/23	4/9	23/30
School	21	17/19	4/11	3/6	6/10	1/3	9/14
Mass media	6	5/6	1/4	2/3	5/5	1/2	5/5
Community	4	4/4	1/1	—	4/4	—	4/4
Youth development	(1)	1/1	—	—	1/1	1/1	1/1
Peer education	(3)	3/3	1/1	—	3/3	—	3/3
Workplace	4	4/4	—	—	2/2	—	2/2
Health facility	4	2/2	—	—	0/1	2/3	2/4
Youth-friendly services	(3)	1/1	—	—	—	2/3	2/3
Youth center	(1)	1/1	—	—	0/1	—	0/1
Multicomponent	1	1/1	0/1	1/1	1/1	0/1	1/1

Sources: Multicomponent program: AMREF, LSHTM, and NIMR 2003; all other programs: FOCUS on Young Adults 2001.
— = not available.
a. Numbers of studies in parentheses are subsets.

supportive environment on behaviors. Furthermore, much of the available evidence from strong studies is for small-scale programs that are carried out over short periods of time, and little evidence is available on long-term effects on behaviors (Speizer, Magnani, and Colvin 2003). A recent study in Tanzania provides the first rigorous evidence that the benefits of adolescent sexual and reproductive health programs in low-income countries can last for at least three years (AMREF, LSHTM, and NIMR 2003).

Kirby's (2001) review covers roughly 70 rigorously evaluated programs in Canada and the United States. The review divides programs into three categories: (a) programs that focus on sexual antecedents, such as sexuality and HIV education and clinical programs; (b) programs that focus on nonsexual antecedents; and (c) programs that incorporate both youth development and reproductive health components. Kirby finds that programs in all three categories proved effective in reducing sexual risk taking, pregnancy, and childbearing among teens. In relation to youth development programs, Kirby finds that a type of intervention known as *service learning,* in which students work on community projects, had the strongest evidence of effectiveness. By contrast, other types of youth development programs were not effective in improving reproductive health outcomes. Programs that incorporate both youth development and reproductive health components were effective over long periods.

In synthesizing U.S. and international data, Kirby (2003) finds that programs are effective with different groups of adolescents in different countries. Also, programs seem to be particularly effective for adolescents who are at especially high risk of negative sexual and reproductive behaviors. In addition, programs do not hasten or increase sexual activity—a common criticism of opponents of adolescent programs. Of all the programs that have been rigorously evaluated, none has reported a decrease in the age of sexual debut or an increase in sexual activity among young people. A recent effort to review the evidence on interventions for preventing HIV among young people has made tentative conclusions about the effectiveness of and subsequent support for wide-scale implementation (WHO 2004b).

On the basis of these international reviews, relatively strong evidence of effectiveness on a range of outcomes has emerged for the following interventions:

- *Life-skills and health and sexuality education in schools.* Well-designed, well-implemented sexuality and reproductive health education can provide young people with a solid foundation of knowledge and skills to enable them to engage in safe and responsible sexual behavior.
- *Peer education.* Peer education programs are especially appropriate for young people who are not in school and for hard-to-reach, at-risk subsets of the youth population, including sex workers and street children.

- *Mass media and community mobilization.* Mass media and community mobilization efforts that engage influential adults, such as parents, teachers, community and religious leaders, and music and sports stars, can help normalize positive adolescent behaviors and gender roles as well as direct young people to appropriate health services.
- *Youth development programs.* Youth development programs typically address a range of key adolescent needs, including life skills, education, jobs, and psychosocial needs. U.S. programs with a voluntary community service component have successfully improved key reproductive health behaviors, but no evidence is available for developing countries.
- *Clinical health services.* Although some young people seek care through the formal health system, many others are deterred by the often judgmental attitudes of health workers, particularly when seeking care and advice on matters related to sexuality.
- *Social marketing.* This approach involves the use of public health messages to promote healthy behaviors and the use of condoms and other health products and services. Effective programs bring products and services to places in the community that young people frequent, such as shops, kiosks, and pharmacies.
- *Workplace and private sector programs.* Programs that reach young people do so at their places of work and through private channels, such as pharmacies and for-profit medical services, where many young people prefer to seek care. Many successful U.S. youth development programs have a work component.

Evidence of Other Adolescent Health Interventions

Data on the effectiveness of other adolescent health interventions are more scattered, partly because some issues have not been recognized as adolescent-specific problems that require youth-focused interventions.

Nutrition. Because anemia is a critical health problem in many countries, many efforts have focused on improving the iron intake of adult women. Interventions aimed at adolescent girls have found that daily iron supplementation effectively lowers anemia and iron deficiency (Elder 2002; MotherCare 2000). Obesity is rapidly becoming a serious health problem among adolescents in many middle-income countries and is often also associated with loss of self-esteem among adolescents. A few studies show that preventing obesity is more successful among adolescents than among adults (Delisle, Chandra-Mouli, and de Benoist 2001).

Mass Deworming. In the Busia district of western Kenya, an ongoing World Bank study is evaluating the effect on learning outcomes of providing deworming treatment to all students in a school. After two years, observed effects of deworming treatment included fewer absences and lower dropout rates, but no effect on test scores (World Bank 2002a). The treatment also resulted in health and school participation benefits among untreated children in the same schools, as well as in neighboring schools, suggesting that the deworming had positive externalities.

Tobacco. Price increases are the most effective tool for reducing or deterring the use of tobacco products by young people. Studies in the United States have shown that price increases have a greater effect on tobacco use by young people than on use by older age groups (University of Illinois at Chicago Health Research and Policy Centers 2001). Other interventions have also reduced tobacco use among young people, such as comprehensive bans on all advertising, including bans on the promotion of tobacco products and trademarks (World Bank 2002c). Programs that give young people the skills to resist peer pressure and other social pressures to smoke have demonstrated consistent and significant reductions or delays in adolescent smoking. School-based programs are also more effective when combined with communitywide supportive efforts. Information campaigns that help young people see how the tobacco industry tries to manipulate their behavior through advertising have been highly effective in changing behavior and attitudes toward smoking among young people in the United States (American Legacy Foundation 2002).

Promising but Unproven Interventions

Many promising adolescent-focused interventions have not yet been rigorously evaluated. These interventions include programs aimed at providing young, newlywed couples with reproductive health information and services (Alauddin and MacLaren 1999); programs that combine livelihoods skills with reproductive health information and services (Rosen 2001b); voluntary counseling programs on and testing for HIV (YouthNet 2002); actions aimed at changing social norms such as gender roles (Horizons 2004); and interventions that address the political and social context (WHO forthcoming-a). A few studies of multipronged approaches are just becoming available and have shown mixed results. Findings from a four-country study found little or no effect of such an approach on key reproductive health behaviors among adolescents (Frontiers, Horizons, and YouthNet 2004). By contrast, a study in Tanzania found that a multicomponent approach had a significant effect on key reproductive health behaviors but no effect on health outcomes (AMREF, LSHTM, and NIMR 2003).

Other possibly promising efforts include suicide prevention programs, tuberculosis education linked with health education (interpersonally or through the mass media), and malaria treatment programs that focus on young people. Adequate evaluation is available on the efficacy of programs promoting the use of seat belts and crash helmets through enforcement of related laws and the support of intensive publicity and information campaigns, as well as on the efficacy of programs preventing alcohol use among adolescents. The evaluations are sufficient for building confidence for investment, and they serve as a basis for intervention design (National Research Council and Institute of Medicine 2004; WHO 2004d).

COSTS AND COST-EFFECTIVENESS OF INTERVENTIONS

Good cost studies of adolescent health programs in LMICs are rare. The reported cost of such programs varies greatly depending on the country, type of intervention, target group, and so on. For example, such programs cost between US$0.03 per adolescent reached in a family life education radio program in Kenya and US$71.00 per year per adolescent reached in a school-based HIV prevention program in Zimbabwe. Of the 32 programs studied, 12 have a unit cost of less than US$10 per year, and others have a unit cost of US$10 to US$25 (table 59.4). Cost estimates are available only for certain types of interventions, with most of the estimates being for reproductive health and HIV education programs. A few studies have tried to measure cost per DALY of adolescent sexual and reproductive health interventions; however, the estimates vary widely. For example, in India, a youth-focused HIV prevention program costs US$66.20 per DALY gained; in Honduras, the cost of a voluntary counseling and testing program aimed at youth is US$5,873 per DALY gained.

The estimates shown in table 59.4 should be interpreted with great caution. Comparing costs across types of programs and countries is difficult, but so is choosing comparable effectiveness measures.[3,4]

ECONOMIC ANALYSIS

Economic analysis of adolescent health programs can provide important information on their value relative to other interventions.

Economic Benefits of Interventions

The macro approach to measuring the economic benefits of interventions is to define the benefits of investing in youth in terms of the investments' effect on economic growth, which typically is measured in terms of growth in gross national product per capita. Some research suggests that investments in young people—whether in access to reproductive health care, in education, or in other key facets of their lives—have

synergistic effects that promote overall economic development (Birdsall, Kelley, and Sinding 2001). For example, shifts to smaller family size and slower rates of population growth in East Asia appear to have played a key role in the creation of an educated workforce, the accumulation of household and government savings, the rise in wages, and the spectacular growth of investment in manufacturing technology. The shift to smaller families that is taking place in many countries will open another window of opportunity as workers have proportionately fewer old and young dependents to support.

If societies invest in health, education, and job creation, the resulting economic gains will improve their overall quality of life. Education, particularly for girls, is strongly related to reproductive behavior. In most countries, girls who are educated are more likely to delay marriage and childbearing, whereas girls with less education are more likely to become mothers as adolescents. Unfortunately, the causal relationships involved are not clear. Are girls more likely to get married when they leave school, or do some girls prefer to terminate their schooling and marry early? The difference is critical. In the first case, the appropriate policy response would focus on improving schooling opportunities for girls. In the second case, research would need to be done first to determine the underlying reasons for girls'—and their parents'—preferences for early marriage instead of additional schooling. The next step would be to assess whether these reasons appear to reflect the girls' (and society's) best interests and, if not, to find interventions to address the root causes of this preference.

The micro approach to measuring the economic benefits of interventions is to build on microeconomic estimates of direct productivity effects that can be measured in monetary terms. For other effects that cannot readily be translated into monetary terms, analysts can use the cost of the most cost-effective alternative to achieve the same effects. Knowles and Behrman (2003a) use this approach to estimate the benefits of various youth-focused investments, including in health. They summarize the three types of effects: (a) those that can be directly valued in monetary terms, (b) those that may require indirect valuation, and (c) those that are particularly difficulty to monetize. Table 59.5 presents examples of these effects.

Cost-Benefit Analysis

Cost-benefit analysis is well suited to the economic analysis of projects aimed at youth, in part because many investments in young people yield multiple benefits, such as additional schooling and improved health. Finding any effectiveness measure that adequately reflects the wide range of benefits obtained from some types of investments in youth is difficult, but cost-benefit analysis has the advantage of allowing comparisons across a range of interventions that may vary considerably in terms of type and effects.

Table 59.4 Cost and Cost-Effectiveness of Adolescent Health Programs

Region and country	Program type (name)	Number served per year	Unit cost (US$)	Unit	Cost per DALY gained (US$)	Source
to be ignored						

Region and country	Program type (name)	Number served per year	Unit cost (US$)	Unit	Cost per DALY gained (US$)	Source
Sexual and reproductive health interventions						
Latin America						
Brazil	School-based HIV/AIDS prevention program	—	0.70	Per condom	—	Antunes and others 1997
Honduras	School-based reproductive health program to prevent HIV/AIDS	—	10.44	Per targeted adolescent	1,323	World Bank 2002b
Honduras	Social marketing of condoms to adolescents	904,612	10.20	Per targeted adolescent	3,292	World Bank 2002b
Honduras	Symptomatic treatment of STIs	—	48.97	Per adolescent treated	28,306	World Bank 2002b, as cited in Knowles and Behrman 2003b
Honduras	Voluntary counseling and testing for youth	1,000	18.29	Per adolescent undergoing voluntary counseling and testing	5,873	World Bank 2002b, as cited in Knowles and Behrman 2003b
Honduras	Workplace information, education, and communication	1,000	20.88	Per worker	2,623.77	World Bank 2002b
Mexico	Community peer educators	4,000	63.64	Per active user of contraception per year	—	Townsend and others 1987
Mexico	Youth center	4,000	203.47	Per active user of contraception per year	—	Townsend and others 1987
Peru	School-based sexuality and HIV/AIDS prevention education	604	3.00	Per student reached	—	Caceres and others 1994
Europe and Central Asia						
Hungary	School-based HIV/AIDS prevention program	41,250	1.40	Per student per year	—	Soderlund and others 1993
Newly independent states	School-based HIV/AIDS prevention program	—	1.33	Per student reached	—	Forrai, personal communication, 1992
Asia						
India	Information, education, and communication programs targeted to youth	—	1,324	Per HIV infection averted	66.20	World Bank 1999b
Sub-Saharan Africa						
Africa	School-based HIV/AIDS prevention program	—	75–200 (primary school); 121–241 (secondary school)	Average unit cost of teacher training and simple materials	—	UNECA 2000
Africa	School-based HIV/AIDS prevention program	—	1.40–7.90	Per student reached	—	Watts and others 2000
Africa	Peer education	—	8.00–10.81	Per out of school adolescent reached	—	Kumaranayake and Watts 2001
Cameroon	School-based HIV/AIDS prevention program	10,000	6.72	Per student reached	—	Kumaranayake and del Amo 1997
Kenya	Radio program delivering family life education (Youth Initiatives Project)	3,354,000	0.03	Per adolescent reached	—	Knowles and Behrman 2003b

Table 59.4 Continued

Region and country	Program type (name)	Number served per year	Unit cost (US$)	Unit	Cost per DALY gained (US$)	Source
Mozambique	Community based "stepping stones" approach (Action Aid)	500,000	0.30	Per person per year	—	World Bank 2003
Mozambique	Voluntary counseling and testing, peer education	11,726	18.40	Per person per year	—	World Bank 2003
Senegal	Mulitpronged school, clinic, and community interventions	—	68,215–111,714	Total intervention cost over a two-year period	—	RamaRao and Diop 2003
South Africa	Television show, mass media campaign (Soul Buddyz)	6 million	0.38	Per person per year	—	World Bank 2003
South Africa	Mass media campaign (LoveLife)	—	20 million	Annual budget	—	World Bank 2003
Tanzania	Primary school peer education (MEMA kwa Vijana)	2,850	1.37	Per person per year	—	World Bank 2003; Ross, personal communication. 2003
Tanzania	Secondary school peer education (School Health Education Program)	16,250 (over three years)	24.12	Per person per year	—	World Bank 2003
Uganda	Outreach program for street children (GOAL: Baaba Project)	5,000	18.50	Per person per year	—	World Bank 2003
Uganda	Newsletters, radio show (Straight Talk)	Nationwide program reaching all schools	630,000	Amount spent in 2001	—	World Bank 2003
Zambia	Life skills for teachers and pupils (AIDS Action Program for Schools)	—	0.16	Additional cost of one child-year of AIDS education	—	Knowles and Behrman 2003b
Zambia	School clubs, health clinics, peer education (Kafue Adolescent Reproductive Health Program)	53,000 (over five years)	2.26	Per person per year	—	World Bank 2003
Zimbabwe	Secondary school clubs, income generation, peer education (Africare)	35,200 (over two years)	8.89	Per person per year	—	World Bank 2003
Zimbabwe	Secondary school clubs, counseling, peer education (Midlands AIDS Service Organisation)	2,000	71.00	Per person per year	—	World Bank 2003
Other health interventions						
LMICs	Tax on tobacco products	—	—	—	5–17	World Bank 1999a
LMICs	Iron supplementation for 13- to 15-year-olds	—	0.18	Per child per year	—	Knowles and Berhman 2003a

Source: Authors.
— = not available.

One of the few cost-benefit analyses specific to adolescent health is Knowles and Behrman's (2003a) study that examines three interventions: a program to provide iron supplementation for secondary schoolchildren, a school-based program of health education to prevent HIV/AIDS, and a tobacco tax. The study estimates benefits and costs over a youth's life cycle, discounted back to the age of 18. The study uses direct estimates of benefits that could be readily estimated in monetary terms (such as gains in labor productivity) and indirect estimates of other benefits, such as reduced fertility and improved health, that could not be easily monetized. The latter were estimated as the least cost of investments currently made to obtain the same benefit; for example, the cost per birth averted in a family planning program was used to value reduced fertility. Table 59.6 summarizes the findings of these cost-benefit studies, together with estimates of the benefit-cost ratios for selected other youth-targeted interventions.

The examples of cost-benefit studies cited here and other calculations of benefit-cost ratios show that health interventions aimed at adolescents can be good public investments; however, the results must be interpreted with some caution. For example, the relatively low benefit-cost ratio of an HIV

Table 59.5 Types of Effects of Adolescent Health Interventions Categorized According to Ease of Monetization

Type of effect	Examples
Directly monetizable effects of investments in youth	Enhanced labor productivity
	Reduced underutilization of labor
	Increased or decreased work effort
	Expanded access to risk-pooling services
	Reduced age at which children achieve a given level of schooling
	Reduced cost of medical care
Indirectly monetizable broad effects of investments in youth	Increased education
	Averted teen pregnancy
	Averted HIV infection
	Averted tuberculosis infections
	Improved health
	Improved nutritional status
	Delayed marriage
	Averted abortion
	Reduced tobacco use
Effects that are particularly difficult to monetize	Increased social capital
	Averted infertility
	Averted social exclusion
	Improved self-esteem
	Enhanced national security (an effect of military training)

Source: Adapted from Knowles and Behrman 2003a.

Table 59.6 Estimated Benefit-Cost Ratios, Selected Investments in Youth

Investment	Estimated benefit-cost ratio (assuming 3 percent annual discount rate)	Plausible range of estimated benefit-cost ratio
Scholarship program (Colombia)	4.4	2.8–25.6
Adult basic education and literacy program (Colombia)	27.6	8.1–1,764.0
School-based reproductive health program to prevent HIV/AIDS (Honduras)	0.5	0.1–4.6
Iron supplementation administered to secondary schoolchildren (hypothetical low-income country)	45.2	25.8–45.2
Tobacco tax (hypothetical middle-income country)	20.2	7.0–38.6

Source: Adapted from Knowles and Behrman 2003a.

prevention program in Honduras was for a program in a country where HIV incidence among young people is relatively low (0.1 percent). Where the incidence is much higher, as in many of the hardest hit countries in Africa (1 percent or more), this ratio would be proportionately higher. In addition, in the Honduran study, the benefits included were limited to the prevention of HIV/AIDS and did not include other possible benefits, such as increased education, reduced STIs other than HIV, and reduced teen pregnancies and abortions. The Honduran study also assumed that the effects of the intervention would not continue beyond one year; however, if they were to continue at the same level to age 29 (assuming that any decrease in the effect of the intervention over time would be offset by increases in the incidence of HIV infection with age), the benefit-cost ratio would increase from 0.5 to 4.6. More than anything else, Knowles and Behrman's estimates demonstrate the sensitivity of the benefit-cost ratios of investments in youth to wide variations in key assumptions, which may be equally plausible because of the limited information available on the costs and effects of many investments in youth.

Beyond the question of how sensitive such estimates are to the underlying assumptions and the context, the basic question is what guidance they provide for public policy. High benefit-cost ratios certainly point to areas that merit further consideration for possible policy interventions, but they do not indicate whether using public resources for interventions has an efficiency rationale, because they generally do not identify differences between private and social benefit-cost ratios. If the purely private benefit-cost ratios for an investment are high, then presumably incentives to use private resources for this investment are high, but an efficiency rationale for using public resources does not exist unless the social benefit-cost ratio exceeds the private one because of factors such as spillovers or market imperfections. High benefit-cost ratios that do not distinguish between social and private returns, therefore, call for further investigation. Interventions may warrant the use of public resources on efficiency grounds, but they also must answer that important question of whether the benefits are social or private.

PROGRAM IMPLEMENTATION AND LESSONS OF EXPERIENCE

Relatively few adolescent-focused programs have been tried on a large scale. Sexual and reproductive health interventions and suicide prevention are some of the few that have gone to scale, and even in those areas, large-scale interventions are relatively infrequent. The vast majority of interventions have been in relatively small programs, often through nongovernmental organizations.

Perhaps the main lesson learned from the experience to date is an obvious one: programs to reach young people are not simply programs for adults applied to a younger population; they require different thinking and a different approach.

Determining Key Principles of Health Programming for Adolescents

Experience to date suggests that effective, youth-focused efforts share a set of common general principles. These principles include the following:

- *Recognize the diversity of the youth age group.* A sexually inexperienced 11-year-old has vastly different needs than a married 20-year-old. Programs should apply different strategies to reach youth, who vary by age, sex, employment, schooling, and marital status.
- *Involve young people.* Policies and programs are more effective when young people are involved in all aspects of their design, implementation, and evaluation. Involvement must go beyond tokenism and be genuine, meaningful, and sustained.
- *Make health services appealing to youth.* A key to rapidly expanding young people's access to health services is to make them more youth friendly by using specially trained health workers and by bolstering the privacy, confidentiality, and accessibility of care.
- *Address gender inequality.* Gender inequalities expose young girls to coerced sex, HIV infection, unwanted pregnancy, and poor nutrition. Efforts should focus on changing the factors that perpetuate gender inequalities.
- *Address the needs of boys.* Adolescence presents a unique opportunity to help boys form positive notions of gender relations and to raise their awareness of health issues. At the same time, boys seem to be disproportionately exposed to a number of adolescent health risks, including accidents and injuries, suicide, tobacco use, substance abuse, and violence. Program design should take into account the specific needs of boys and young men as well as of girls and young women.
- *Design comprehensive programs.* Comprehensive programs that provide information and services while addressing the social and political context are more effective than narrowly focused interventions.
- *Consider all important benefits.* Many adolescent health interventions focus on only one benefit. For example, a school-based sex education program may focus exclusively on HIV prevention and may neglect other possible benefits from the intervention, such as increased education, averted teen pregnancy and abortions, and other averted STIs.
- *Address the many nonhealth factors that influence adolescent health.* Linking school and livelihood opportunities to adolescent health programs, at either the policy or program level, is key to helping young people avoid risky behaviors.
- *Address underlying risk and protective factors.* Factors such as feelings of self-efficacy, attitudes and behaviors of friends, connectedness with parents and other influential adults, and

involvement in the community can either increase (risk factor) or decrease (protective factor) the chances that a young person will engage in unhealthy behaviors.

Making a Difference on a Large Scale

Adolescent health programs are complex and may not be easy to scale up because of technical, management, and political challenges. The following are examples of adolescent health programs that are national in scope. Unfortunately, little is known about the costs and effectiveness of such large-scale efforts.

National Suicide Prevention Program in New Zealand. Among industrial nations, New Zealand has one of the highest suicide rates for both males and females age 15 to 24 (New Zealand Ministry of Health 2002). In 1998, on the basis of international good practice, the government developed the National Youth Suicide Prevention Strategy. This strategy, which includes a component for the general population and one that focuses on the indigenous Maori community, provides a framework for understanding suicide prevention and signals the steps that government agencies, communities, and service providers must take to reduce suicide. Even though the national strategy has not been in place long enough to adequately gauge its effects, in 1999, the first year following the adoption of the strategy, youth suicide rates fell to their lowest levels since 1991.

Sexuality Education in Mongolia. Mongolia has implemented a locally developed and tested sexuality education curriculum in 60 percent of schools nationwide. Current challenges include increasing the number of hours allocated to sexuality education; developing more and better written resources for adolescents, including textbooks; developing materials that will help parents communicate better with their children on sexuality; expanding access to clinical services for adolescents through the public health system; reaching out-of-school youths and the broader community with sexuality education; and monitoring and evaluating the program regularly to assess its weaknesses and strengths and how it could be improved (Gerdts 2002).

Addressing the Health Needs of Poor Youth

The following strategies, based on what is known about services for poor people more generally and about the specific needs of young people, show promise for meeting the needs of poor youth:

- *Targeting out-of-school youth.* Out-of-school youth of a given age are likely to be more marginalized than those who are in school, and they are often those most in need of critical services, such as pregnancy prevention and prevention of HIV/AIDS and other STIs. A number of countries, including Paraguay, South Africa, and Zimbabwe, have launched effective programs targeting out-of-school youth that combine the use of mass media, peer education, and community-based efforts. For instance, the Arte y Parte project targeted out-of-school youth in three cities in Paraguay using a booklet about adolescent sexuality, street drama, radio programming, newspaper columns, and distribution of promotional items (Magnani and others 2000).

- *Focusing efforts on vulnerable youth.* Young people who have been orphaned or left vulnerable by AIDS typically rely first on their extended families and communities for support. Efforts to help vulnerable youth should strengthen those safety nets. One example is the COPE program in Malawi, where a nongovernmental organization–sponsored effort works through existing government structures to help orphans and other vulnerable children (Phiri, Foster, and Nzima 2001).
- *Tailoring subsidized programs to poor youth.* Social marketing of reproductive health products and services—such as contraceptives and condoms for pregnancy and disease prevention or promotion of iron supplementation—often targets young consumers, but such efforts should ensure that they reach the desired clients—namely, those who are poor and less likely to be able to afford market prices. The Social Marketing for Adolescent Sexual Health Project in four African countries combined the use of mass media with peer education to encourage young people to practice safer sex, including condom use (Agha 2000).

Improving Health Systems to Meet Adolescents' Health Needs

The shortcomings of health systems in LMICs are well known, and adolescents in particular would benefit from the following health system improvements:

- *Strengthening human resource capacities.* The poor quality of the interaction with health workers is one of the main barriers to adolescents' use of health care in public sector facilities. Through training, supervision, and other means, health systems should encourage health workers to adopt a more youth-friendly outlook. In addition, health systems should integrate such training into the curricula of medical, nursing, and nurse auxiliary schools.
- *Involving the private sector.* Many young people already seek care from private doctors, nurses, and nurse-midwives or from local pharmacies or other drug distribution outlets. Along with encouraging private for-profit health providers to serve youth, government policies should encourage efforts to tap into the private sector as a source of health care for adolescents by means of interventions such as social marketing, contracted services, youth-focused social franchising, and programs that serve young people at their place of work. (Carranza 2003; LaVake and Rosen 2003; Rosen 2001a; Senderowitz and Stevens 2001).

- *Strengthening the stewardship oversight function of governments.* Governments have a key role to play in developing supportive policies, both within the health sector and across sectors; in contributing to cross-sectoral policies such as national youth policies; and in providing input into policy making in other sectors, especially education and labor. Ideally, governments should have an overarching adolescent health policy with specific reference to adolescent health in policy documents for specific programs or diseases, such as for AIDS, tuberculosis, malaria, sexual and reproductive health, and population (WHO forthcoming-a; POLICY Project and YouthNet forthcoming).

RESEARCH AND DEVELOPMENT AGENDA

The striking lack of good research and evaluation of adolescent health interventions limits countries' ability to address serious health problems. At this juncture, research in the following broad areas is critical:

- *Refining estimates of DALYs for adolescents.* Available DALY information is inadequate to fully explore the burden of disease for adolescent age groups. Future DALY estimates should be made for five-year age groups in the 10 to 24 age range.
- *Documenting the effectiveness of current approaches.* This area includes better process evaluation to understand the functioning of successful programs. Such evaluation necessitates more rigorous research designs so that the effectiveness of programs can be better documented, both in terms of health outcomes and in terms of DALYs saved. Another area in which more research could help is better documentation of the nonhealth effects of adolescent health interventions. Greater investment is also needed to evaluate the effects of health promotion strategies on reducing smoking, including the smoke-free spaces prevalent in the Americas and life-skills education.
- *Testing new interventions.* This area includes more research on multicomponent programs and on new types of interventions. In relation to sexual and reproductive health, new interventions include approaches such as providing antiretroviral therapy to HIV-infected youth and voluntary counseling and testing for HIV, encouraging adolescents to have fewer sexual partners, reducing the trafficking of young people, preventing and addressing the health consequences of early marriage, and reaching young married women with information and services. Research must better inform interventions so that they reach groups at particularly high risk of poor health outcomes, such as child prostitutes, child workers, refugees, AIDS orphans, and street children. More research is also needed on a broad range of other adolescent

health interventions, especially for those health problems that are among the biggest killers and disablers of young people: HIV/AIDS and mental illnesses for both males and females, maternal conditions for females, and road accidents for males. In addition, research is needed on programs that attempt to influence gender roles and social norms and investments designed to avert drug and alcohol abuse and to improve mental health.

- *Enhancing understanding of the risk and protective factors influencing young people's behavior.* Even though our understanding of the major influences on youth behaviors has come far, more refinement of such understanding is needed, along with a better understanding of how to incorporate such knowledge into the design of programs and policies.

- *Improving cost and cost-benefit analysis.* Good cost estimates are rare, and more needs to be done to more fully estimate the costs of the range of adolescent health interventions. This effort means collecting more data on program costs and more accurate data that include programs' nonmonetary costs. Few full cost-benefit analyses of youth programs exist, and more need to be done to improve evaluations of the economic value of investments targeted at young people.

CONCLUSIONS

The health community has only recently recognized the importance of adolescent health problems. To address the unique health problems associated with the adolescent years, policy makers and the health community must expand the knowledge base on effectiveness, costs, and economic benefits and pay more attention to areas such as road safety, nutrition, mental health, and malaria. Well-documented implementation experiences from mostly small programs have produced a sound body of knowledge about how programs function. These experiences can provide the foundation for scaled-up efforts and can help the health community improve health systems in ways that will benefit adolescent health efforts.

ACKNOWLEDGMENTS

The authors acknowledge the generous help of the following people: Peju Olukoya for sharing materials and studies and for providing early feedback; Kimberly Switlick for preparing graphics and providing editorial assistance; and peer reviewers, including Maria Teresa Cinqueira, Jane Ferguson, Elena Nightingale, and Audrey Smith Rogers.

NOTES

1. The United Nations defines *youth* as those age 15 to 24. The World Health Organization defines *adolescence* as age 10 through 19 and uses the term *young people* to refer to those age 10 to 24.

2. Regional data cited from this report here and elsewhere in the chapter are based on nationally representative surveys carried out between the mid 1990s and 2001.

3. Knowles and Behrman (2003b) find that many cost estimates incorrectly treat income transfers as costs and frequently fail to include estimates of administrative and distortionary costs (for example, the distortionary cost of financing programs through taxes).

4. In cost-effectiveness analysis, as in cost-benefit analysis, estimates are needed not only of what has actually happened, but also of what would have happened in the absence of the program or intervention (that is, an estimate of the counterfactual). There are no exceptions to this rule.

REFERENCES

Agha, S. 2000. "An Evaluation of Adolescent Sexual Health Programs in Cameroon, Botswana, South Africa, and Guinea." Population Services International Research Division Working Paper 29, Population Services International, Washington, DC.

Alauddin, M., and L. MacLaren. 1999. *InFOCUS: Reaching Newlywed and Married Adolescents.* Washington, DC: FOCUS on Young Adults.

American Legacy Foundation. 2002. "New American Legacy Foundation Study Shows Truth® Campaign Helping to Drive Down Youth Smoking Rates." American Legacy Foundation, Washington, DC. http://www.americanlegacy.org.

AMREF (African Medical and Research Foundation), LSHTM (London School of Hygiene and Tropical Medicine), and NIMR (National Institute for Medical Research). 2003. "MEMA kwa Vijana: Randomised Controlled Trial of an Adolescent Sexual Health Programme in Rural Mwanza, Tanzania." Technical briefing document, LSHTM, London, August 11.

Antunes, M., R. Stall, V. Paiva, C. A. Peres, J. Paul, M. Hudes, and others. 1997. "Evaluating an AIDS Sexual Risk Reduction Program for Young Adults in Public Night Schools in São Paulo, Brazil." *AIDS* 11: S121–27.

Behrman, J. R., J. Hoddinott, J. A. Maluccio, A. Quisumbing, R. Martorell, and A. D. Stein. 2004. "The Impact of Experimental Nutritional Interventions on Education into Adulthood in Rural Guatemala: Preliminary Longitudinal Analysis." Paper presented to the 2004 Population Association of America Annual Meeting, Boston, April 1–3.

Birdsall, N., A. C. Kelley, and S. W. Sinding, eds. 2001. *Population Matters: Demographic Change, Economic Growth, and Poverty in the Developing World.* New York: Oxford University Press.

Blum, R., and K. Mmari. 2004. *Risk and Protective Factors Affecting Adolescent Reproductive Health in Developing Countries. An Analysis of the World's Literature 1990–2004. Summary.* Geneva: World Health Organization.

Bruce, J., and S. Clark. 2003. "Including Married Adolescents in Adolescent Reproductive Health and HIV/AIDS Policy." Paper prepared for technical consultation on married adolescents, World Health Organization, Geneva.

Caceres, C. F., A. M. Rosasco, J. S. Mandel, and N. Hearst. 1994. "Evaluating a School-Based Intervention for STD/AIDS Prevention in Peru." *Journal of Adolescent Health* 15 (7): 582–91.

Carranza, J. M. 2003. "What Do Salvadoran Teens Think? Determining the Feasibility of Youth-Friendly Pharmacies: A Focus Group Report." U.S. Agency for International Development and Commercial Market Strategies Project, Washington, DC. http://www.cmsproject.com/resources/PDF/CMS_ElSalvador_Youth.pdf.

CDC (U.S. Centers for Disease Control and Prevention) and ORC Macro. 2003. *Reproductive, Maternal, and Child Health in Eastern Europe and Eurasia: A Comparative Report.* Atlanta: U.S. Department of Health and Human Services.

Delisle, H., V. Chandra-Mouli, and B. de Benoist. 2001. "Should Adolescents Be Specifically Targeted for Nutrition in Developing

Countries? To Address Which Problems, and How?" http://www. who.int/child-adolescent-health/New_Publications/NUTRITION/ Adolescent_nutrition_paper.pdf.

Doak, C., L. Adair, C. Monteiro, and B. M. Popkin. 2000. "Overweight and Underweight Co-exists in Brazil, China, and Russia." *Journal of Nutrition* 130: 2965–80.

Elder, L. 2002. "Adolescent Nutrition: Issues and Interventions." Background paper prepared for the World Bank Learning Exchange on Exploring Strategies for Reaching and Working with Adolescents, Washington, DC, June 5.

FOCUS on Young Adults. 2001. *Advancing Young Adult Reproductive Health: Actions for the Next Decade.* Washington, DC: FOCUS on Young Adults.

Frontiers, Horizons, and YouthNet. 2004. "New Findings from Intervention Research: Youth Reproductive Health and HIV Prevention." Meeting report, Washington, DC, September 9, 2003.

Gerdts, C. 2002. "Universal Sexuality Education in Mongolia: Educating Today to Protect Tomorrow." Quality 12, Population Council, New York. http://www.popcouncil.org/publications/qcq/QCQ12.pdf.

Hoddinott, J., and A. Quisumbing. 2003. "Investing in Children and Youth for Poverty Reduction." Unpublished paper, International Food Policy Research Institute, Washington, DC.

Horizons. 2004. "Promoting Healthy Relationships and HIV/STI Prevention for Young Men: Positive Findings from an Intervention Study in Brazil." Population Council's Research Update series, Population Council and Horizons Communications Unit, Washington, DC. http://www.popcouncil.org/pdfs/horizons/brgndrnrmsru.pdf.

Kirby, D. 2001. *Emerging Answers: Research Findings on Programs to Reduce Teen Pregnancy.* Washington, DC: National Campaign to Prevent Teen Pregnancy.

———. 2003. "Changing Youth Behaviors: Findings from U.S. and Developing Country Research and Their Implications for A, B, and C." Paper presented at the meeting on HIV Prevention for Young People in Developing Countries, Washington, DC, July 24. http://www.fhi.org/en/Youth/YouthNet/NewsEvents/HIVprevenmeeting.htm.

Knowles, J. C., and J. R. Behrman. 2003a. "Assessing the Economic Benefits of Investing in Youth in Developing Countries." Health, Nutrition, and Population Discussion Paper, World Bank, Washington, DC.

———. 2003b. "The Economic Returns to Investing in Youth in Developing Countries: A Review of the Literature." Unpublished paper. World Bank, Washington, DC.

Kumaranayake, L., and J. del Amo. 1997. *Resource Allocation for HIV Prevention: Cost, Epidemiological, and Behavioural Analysis—HIV/AIDS Education in Schools.* London: London School of Hygiene and Tropical Medicine.

Kumaranayake, L., and C. Watts. 2001. *Scaling-Up Priority HIV/AIDS Interventions: A Problem of Constrained Optimisation.* London: London School of Hygiene and Tropical Medicine, Department of Public Health and Policy Publication.

LaVake, S., and J. Rosen. 2003. *Private Sector Country Assessment Manual, 2003: A Handbook for Assessing the Potential for Youth Reproductive Health and HIV/AIDS Interventions in the Private Sector.* Arlington, VA: YouthNet.

MacKay, J., and G. A. Mensah. 2004. *The Atlas of Heart Disease and Stroke.* Geneva: World Health Organization.

Magnani, R., A. Robinson, E. Seiber, and G. Avila. 2000. *Evaluation of "Arte y Parte": An Adolescent Reproductive Health Communications Project Implemented in Asunción, San Lorenzo, and Fernando de la Mora, Paraguay.* Washington, DC: FOCUS on Young Adults.

Mensch, B. S., S. Singh, and J. Casterline. 2003. "Trends in the Timing of First Marriage among Men and Women in the Developing World."

Paper presented at the Annual Meeting of the Population Association of America, Minneapolis, May 1–3.

MotherCare. 2000. "Anemia and Iron Deficiency in Adolescent Students in Lima, Peru: Causes, Consequences, and Prevention." *Reproductive Health Focus* 14. http://www.jsi.com/intl/mothercare/rhfocus.htm.

National Research Council and Institute of Medicine. 2004. *Reducing Underage Drinking: A Collective Responsibility.* Washington, DC: National Academies Press.

———. 2005. *Growing up Global: The Changing Transitions to Adulthood in Developing Countries.* Washington, DC: National Academies Press.

Phiri, S., G. Foster, and M. Nzima. 2001. *Expanding and Strengthening Community Action: A Study of Ways to Scale Up Community Mobilization Interventions to Mitigate the Effect of HIV/AIDS on Children and Families.* Washington, DC: Displaced Children and Orphans Fund. http://www.usaid.gov/pop_health/dcofwvf/reports/orphanreps/dcaction.html.

Pitts, M., G. Dowsett, M. Couch, D. Keys, and S. Dutertre. 2004. "Looking for More: A Review of Social and Contextual Factors Affecting Young People's Sexual Health." Document prepared for the World Health Organization, Department of Child and Adolescent Health and Development. La Trobe University, Melbourne, Australia.

Piwoz, E., and E. Greble. 2000. *HIV/AIDS and Nutrition: A Review of the Literature and Recommendations for Nutritional Care and Support in Sub-Saharan Africa.* Washington, DC: USAID Support for Analysis and Research in Africa (SARA) Project and the Academy for Educational Development.

POLICY Project and YouthNet. Forthcoming. *Guide to Key Elements of Youth Reproductive Health Policy.* Washington, DC: POLICY Project; Arlington, VA: YouthNet.

Rosen, J. 2001a. "A Dialogue on Social Marketing and Other Commercial Approaches to Improving Adolescent Reproductive Health." Meeting report. FOCUS on Young Adults, Washington, DC, February 15.

———. 2001b. *In FOCUS: Youth Livelihoods and HIV/AIDS.* Washington, DC: FOCUS on Young Adults.

RamaRao, S., and N. J. Diop. 2003. "Serving the Reproductive Health Needs of Adolescents in Senegal: Analysis of Costs." Frontiers Project Report. Population Council, Washington, DC.

Save the Children U.S.A. 2004. *Children Having Children: State of the World's Mothers 2004.* Westport, CT: Save the Children U.S.A.

Senderowitz, J., and C. Stevens. 2001. *Leveraging the For-Profit Sector in Support of Adolescent and Young Adult Reproductive Health Programming.* Washington, DC: Futures Institute for Sustainable Development.

Soderlund, N., J. Lavis, J. Broomberg, and A. Mills. 1993. "The Costs of HIV Prevention Strategies in Developing Countries." *Bulletin of the World Health Organization* 71 (5): 595–604.

Speizer, I. S., R. J. Magnani, and C. Colvin. 2003. "The Effectiveness of Adolescent Reproductive Health Interventions in Developing Countries: A Review of the Evidence." *Journal of Adolescent Health* 33 (5): 324–48.

Townsend, J. W., E. Dias de May, Y. Sepulveda Santos de Garza, and S. Rosenhouse. 1987. "Sex Education and Family Planning Services for Young Adults: Urban Strategies in Mexico." *Studies in Family Planning* 18 (2): 103–8.

UNAIDS (Joint United Nations Programme on HIV/AIDS). 2003. *AIDS Epidemic Update: December 2003.* Geneva: UNAIDS.

UNECA (United Nations Economic Commission for Africa). 2000. *Costs of Scaling HIV Programme Activities to a National Level in Sub-Saharan Africa: Methods and Estimates.* http://www.uneca.org/adf2000/costsofaids.htm.

University of Illinois at Chicago Health Research and Policy Centers. 2001. *Cigarette Taxes and Kids.* Policy Briefs, vol. 1, April. Chicago: Health Research and Policy Centers, University of Illinois at Chicago.

Watts, C., P. Vickerman, L. Kumaranayake, C. Cheta, C. C. Nama, G. Kwenthieu, and J. Del Amo. 2000. "Impact and Cost-Effectiveness Modelling of In-School Youth Programmes in Sub-Saharan Africa." Paper presented at the 13th International AIDS Conference, Durban, South Africa, July 9–14.

Westoff, C. F., and A. Bankole. 1995. *Unmet Need: 1990–1994*. Comparative Studies 16, Demographic and Health Surveys. Calverton, MD: Macro International.

WHO (World Health Organization). 1999. *Programming for Adolescent Health and Development: Report of a WHO/UNFPA/UNICEF Study Group on Programming for Adolescent Health*. Technical Report 886. Geneva: WHO.

———. 2001a. *Global Status Report: Alcohol and Young People*. WHO/MSD/MSB/01.1. Geneva: WHO.

———. 2001b. *The Second Decade: Improving Adolescent Health and Development*. Geneva: WHO.

———. 2002. *World Health Report*. Geneva: WHO.

———. 2004a. "Estimates of DALYs by Sex, Cause, and WHO Mortality Subregion, Estimates for 2002, 2003." WHO, Geneva. http://www3.who.int/whosis/menu.cfm?path=evidence,burden,burden_estimates_2002,burden_estimates_2002_subregion&language=english.

———. 2004b. "Steady, Ready GO!" Information brief on the Talloire consultation to review the evidence for policies and programmes to achieve the global goals on young people and HIV/AIDS. WHO, Geneva.

———. 2004c. *Unsafe Abortion: Global and Regional Estimates of Incidence of Unsafe Abortion and Associated Mortality in 2000*. 4th ed. Geneva: WHO.

———. 2004d. *World Report on Road Traffic Injury Prevention: Summary*. Geneva: WHO.

———. Forthcoming-a. *Making Policy Happen: Lessons from Countries on Developing National Adolescent Health and Development Policy*. Geneva: WHO, Department of Child and Adolescent Health and Development.

———. Forthcoming-b. *Pregnant Adolescents: Delivering on Global Promises of Hope*. Geneva: WHO.

World Bank. 1999a. *Curbing the Epidemic: Governments and the Economics of Tobacco Control*. Washington, DC: World Bank.

———. 1999b. *Project Appraisal Document on a Proposed Credit in the Amount of SDR 140.82 Million to India for a Second National HIV/AIDS Control Project*. Report 18918-IN, Washington, DC: World Bank.

———. 2002a. "The Impact of Deworming Treatment on Primary School Performance in Busia, Kenya." Abstract of Current Research. http://www.worldbank.org/research.

———. 2002b. *Optimizing the Allocation of Resources among HIV Prevention Interventions in Honduras*. Washington, DC: World Bank.

———. 2002c. *Tobacco at a Glance*. Washington, DC: World Bank.

———. 2003. *Education and HIV/AIDS: A Sourcebook of HIV/AIDS Prevention Programs*. Washington, DC: World Bank.

YouthNet. 2002. "VCT and Young People." *YouthLens*. http://www.fhi.org/en/youth/youthnet/publications/youthlens+english.htm.

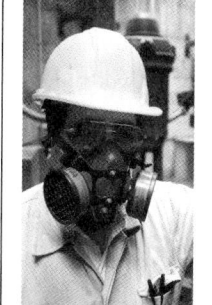

Chapter **60**

Occupational Health

Linda Rosenstock, Mark Cullen, and Marilyn Fingerhut

Workers around the world—despite vast differences in their physical, social, economic, and political environments—face virtually the same kinds of workplace hazards. These hazards are traditionally categorized into four broad types: chemical, biological, physical, and psychosocial. What emerges from our incomplete knowledge of their risk, however, is that the more than 80 percent of the world's workforce that resides in the developing world disproportionately shares in the global burden of occupational disease and injury. Several classic occupational diseases, such as silicosis and lead poisoning, that have been substantially eliminated in industrial countries remain endemic elsewhere in the world. Whether this high and preventable burden of ill health faced by workers in the developing world is the result of ignorance, inattention, or intent, compelling evidence indicates that work-related health conditions could be substantially reduced, often at modest cost.

NATURE AND CAUSES OF OCCUPATIONAL HEALTH CONDITIONS IN THE DEVELOPING WORLD

Despite country-to-country differences, some commonalities exist within the workforce of the developing world that are worth noting. Workforce distribution by economic sector is different from that in the industrial world. Compared with industrial countries, where single-digit percentages prevail—for example, approximately 2 percent in the United Kingdom—developing countries employ about 70 percent of their economically active population in the agricultural sector (World Bank 2003). For many of these workers, the distinction between health at work and health at home is blurred, because

health in the workplace is integrated into all aspects of daily life for these often subsistence agricultural workers. For example, pesticide poisoning is a hazard faced by workers and their families and communities.

The informal workforce, which in industrial countries is rarely larger than 10 percent of total employment, looms large in developing countries. This workforce includes self-employed, household-based unpaid labor (family members, for example) and independent service workers such as street vendors. In the developing world, employment in the informal sector may reach 70 percent, with the contribution to the gross domestic product (GDP) ranging from 10 to 60 percent (ILO 2002).

Informal economy workers are often unprotected in the regulatory arena even in the industrial world. This circumstance is exacerbated when the vulnerable employment status in the developing world is coupled with problems of poverty and ill health. Cottage-industry workers abound in the informal sector, and home-based work can fully blur distinctions between occupational and other environmental hazards. Not uncommon across the developing world are lead-poisoned adults who manufacture batteries in crude facilities at home and their lead-poisoned children, exposed to the lead while sleeping and playing in the next room.

The migrant workforce, which is increasing worldwide, is estimated to be 120 million (ILO 2000). In the industrial world, immigrant workers often perform work deemed unattractive (seasonal agricultural work in the United States, service sector work in the United Kingdom), but the issues of a migrant workforce in some parts of the developing world take on even greater import. In southern Africa, for example, migrant mining workers face the extraordinary burden of risk for the triad of silicosis, tuberculosis, and HIV/AIDS—diseases that are inextricably linked to interactive determinants of workplace, housing, and social and economic factors (Trapido and others 1996).

Workers in the developing world face different risks in the health transition than do their counterparts in the industrial world. They may be exposed to the combined and often synergistic risks of both traditional and emerging hazards. Workers may also face unregulated and unprotected exposures to known hazards just as those same hazards—silica and asbestos, for example—were faced decades ago by millions of workers in the industrial world. A significant difference, though, is that workers in the developing world are being exposed when widespread knowledge is available about the risks and effective preventive measures (Kjellstrom and Rosenstock 1990). Even as these workers are forced to replay history, despite the availability of information and knowledge transfer unthinkable just a generation ago, they face other hazards, including the production, marketing, and importation of environmental hazards such as cigarettes. In the instance of asbestos and tobacco, both products are being aggressively marketed and exported by the industrial world (especially asbestos from Canada and tobacco from the United States) to the developing world.

A real example of hazards faced by developing workers in what might be called the *risk transition* is that posed by dual exposure to asbestos and cigarette smoke and risk for lung cancer. This example is especially troubling not only because the risk is dauntingly high but also because exposures to both are occurring with full knowledge of their individual and cumulative effects. As shown in table 60.1, against a background of relative risk for lung cancer of 1 for a nonsmoking, nonasbestos-exposed population, a working population with significant asbestos exposure but no tobacco exposure may face a relative risk of lung cancer of 5; a smoking population not exposed to asbestos faces a relative risk of 10; and rather than these risks being additive (that is, 15) the smoking, asbestos-exposed population has the extraordinary relative risk of lung cancer of 50. Most important, in this well-recognized multiplicative-effect scenario, if the smoking exposure alone were eliminated among the asbestos-exposed workers, the overall risk of lung cancer

would be reduced by 90 percent; even if the smoking exposure continued, elimination of the asbestos exposure would reduce the overall risk by 80 percent. Those considerations are not theoretical but well supported by empirical data. In parts of China and elsewhere in the developing world, asbestos exposure abounds as cigarette smoking is rising. Effective intervention strategies will be those based on a comprehensive approach to the overall burden rather than those addressing the individual burdens of specific exposures, recognizing that organizational or institutional interventions (such as eliminating asbestos from the workplace) are far more effective than those targeting individual behaviors (such as smoking cessation).

GLOBAL BURDEN OF DISEASE FROM OCCUPATIONAL HEALTH RISKS

The overall picture that emerges from all parts of the developing world is one of increased health and safety risks in all occupations for which data are available.

Dramatic changes in the global labor force will occur as globalization and population growth continue to affect the global economy. For example, the labor force in Latin America and the Caribbean is one of the fastest growing in the world, with 217 million workers in 2000; the number of workers is expected to reach 270 million in 2010 (PAHO 2002). The burden of disease and injury attributable to workplace risks in the formal and informal sectors is grave and will continue to rise. Inadequate data and reporting systems make capturing the effect of workplace risks problematic. Nonetheless, several recent efforts by international bodies have shed some light on the staggering burden, although in general attempts to derive evidence-based estimates are likely to systematically and significantly underrepresent the extent of the problem.

The gravity of workplace risks is seen in the recent International Labour Organization (ILO) estimate that among the world's 2.7 billion workers, at least 2 million deaths per year are attributable to occupational diseases and injuries. The ILO estimates for fatalities are the tip of the iceberg because data for estimating nonfatal illness and injury are not available for most of the globe. The ILO also notes that about 4 percent of the GDP is lost because of work-related diseases and injuries (Takala 2002).

A recent effort of the World Health Organization (WHO) has provided insight into the global dimensions of several selected occupational health risks. WHO included five occupational risk factors in its comparative risk assessment in a unified framework of 26 major health risk factors contributing to the overall global burden of disease and injury (Ezzati and others 2004; WHO 2002). The WHO comparative approach used a common statistical model that allows a reader to compare the contribution (attributable fraction) of several risk

Table 60.1 Relationship between Asbestos, Smoking, and Risk for Lung Cancer

Smoking[b]	Asbestos exposure[a]	
	No	Yes
No	1	5
Yes	10	50

Source: Kjellstrom and Rosenstock 1990.
a. If asbestos exposure eliminated, eliminate 80 percent lung cancers in asbestos workers.
b. If smoking eliminated, eliminate 90 percent lung cancers in asbestos workers.

factors to a single outcome—lung cancer, for example. Stringent requirements for consistency in describing risk factors limited the number of occupational risk factors that could be included in the study. For all risk factors, it was necessary to estimate an exposed population and exposure levels for 224 age, sex, and country groups in the 14 WHO geographic regions of the world. Where possible, data could be extrapolated to age, sex, and country groups for which data were not available, based on similarities in demographic, socioeconomic, or other relevant indicators. Because knowing the existing burden of disease and injury globally was necessary, the only outcomes included were those for which WHO had rates of disease or injury for all regions calculated by International Classification of Disease (ICD) codes. Finally, estimates of the risk factor–burden relationships by age, sex, and WHO subregion were generated. Risk measures (relative risks or mortality rates) for the health outcomes resulting from exposure to the risk factors were determined primarily from studies published in peer-reviewed journals. Adjustments were made to account for differences in levels of exposure; exposure duration; and age, sex, and subregion, as appropriate. The information about each risk factor was entered into the WHO common model for comparative analysis. The resulting burden was described as the attributable fraction of disease or injury, using mortality and disability-adjusted life years (DALYs) lost, with one DALY being equal to the loss of one healthy life year—the common currency measure that includes mortality and morbidity.

Because of the requirements for global data, only five occupational risk factors could be described: risks for injuries, carcinogens, airborne particulates, ergonomic risks for back pain, and noise. The exposed worker populations were estimated using an approach based on the International Standard Industrial Classification of All Economic Activities (ISIC), an economic classification system of the United Nations that organizes all economic activities by economic sectors and relevant subgroupings (UN 2000). The ISIC system is used almost universally by national and international statistical services to categorize economic activity; therefore, it allows global comparisons. The ILO has developed economically active population (EAP) estimates by applying economic activity rates, by sex and by age group (older than age 15), to the population estimates and projections of the United Nations (ILO 1996). The EAP provides the most comprehensive global accounting of people who may be exposed to occupational risks because it includes people in paid employment, the self-employed, and people who work to produce goods and services for their own household consumption, both in the formal and in the informal sectors (ILO 2002). For the WHO comparative risk assessment, the EAP was further divided into nine economic subsectors (where people work) and seven occupational categories (what type of work people do), on the basis of country-level data for 31 countries (ILO 1995).

The absence of data in much of the developing world limited the range of occupational risk factors that WHO could measure, and the available data excluded children under age 15 who work. The WHO comparative risk assessment also excluded important occupational risks for reproductive disorders, dermatitis, infectious disease, coronary heart disease, intentional injuries, musculoskeletal disorders of the upper extremities, and most cancers. Psychosocial risk factors such as workplace stress could not be studied, nor could pesticide, heavy metal, or solvent exposures. The potential consequences of omitting just pesticides from the global burden analysis can be illustrated by the situation in Central America (PAHO 2002). The isthmus is primarily an agricultural and forested area of .5 million square kilometers, of which 40 percent is arable. Pesticide imports almost tripled from 15,000 metric tons in 1992 to 41,000 in 1998, and 35 percent of the pesticides were restricted in the exporting countries. In 2000, the subregion imported some 1.5 kilograms of pesticides per inhabitant per year, a quantity 2.5 times greater than the world average estimated by WHO. Exposures in the formal and informal sectors extend to the homes and families of the pesticide workers. Although this situation is common in developing nations, the WHO comparative risk assessment captured none of these exposures.

The ILO and WHO data provide the most current, yet still incomplete, picture of the overall problem of occupational health risks. Nonetheless, with just the few occupational risk factors studied in depth by WHO a picture emerges of the significant effect of largely preventable conditions (Ezzati and others 2004). WHO found that occupational injuries result in about 312,000 deaths per year for the world's 2.7 billion workers; this figure contrasts to the approximately 6,000 deaths per year caused by occupational injuries for the 150 million workers in the United States. As in the industrial world, high injury fatality rates in the developing world are clustered in certain sectors, including agriculture, construction, and mining. Using this metric, occupational injuries account for more than 10 million DALYs and 8 percent of unintentional injuries worldwide.

The second occupational factor WHO analyzed was the effect of exposure to workplace lung carcinogens (such as asbestos, diesel exhaust, and silica) and leukemogens (such as benzene, ionizing radiation, and ethylene oxide). WHO concluded that occupational exposures account for about 9 percent of all cancers of the lung, trachea, and bronchus and about 2 percent of all leukemias. Overall, about 102,000 deaths were attributable to these two occupational cancers and about 1 million DALYs.

Estimates of the global burden of chronic lung disease demonstrate the significant contribution of occupational exposures, which account for about 13 percent of all chronic obstructive pulmonary disease (COPD) and about 11 percent of asthma. In total, WHO found the annual worldwide burden of work-related COPD to be about 318,000 deaths per year and about 3.7 million DALYs. The occupational risk contribution to the worldwide asthma burden was about 38,000 deaths and about 1.6 million DALYs, reflecting the fact that a great deal of asthma occurs at younger ages and is not fatal. WHO found that 37 percent of all back pain worldwide is attributable to work, resulting in an estimated 800,000 DALYs, a significant loss of time from work, and a high economic loss. Worldwide, 16 percent of all hearing loss is attributable to workplace exposures, resulting in 4.2 million DALYs.

WHO made a special risk analysis of hepatitis B, hepatitis C, and HIV infections among health care workers caused by contaminated sharps, such as syringe needles, scalpels, and broken glass (WHO 2002). This analysis illustrates the general problem of high risks existing in the small worker population having exposure. WHO found that, among the 35 million health workers worldwide, there were 3 million percutaneous exposures to bloodborne pathogens in 2000. This finding is equivalent to between 0.1 and 4.7 sharps injuries per year per health worker. WHO concluded that of all the hepatitis B and hepatitis C present in health care workers, about 40 percent was caused by sharps injuries, with wide regional variation. WHO also found that between 1 and 12 percent of HIV infections in health care workers was caused by sharps injuries. The comparative risk assessment by region and type of infection indicates where special emphasis is needed (see figure 60.1). Clearly, solutions exist to these problems, as shown by the

countries that have engaged in serious prevention efforts. Proper needle handling and waste management, substitutions for sharps, hepatitis B virus (HBV) immunization, postexposure prophylaxis, training, and legislative measures have been successful. Beyond the personal and workplace consequences, the potentially devastating societal impact of loss of this critical worker group can be anticipated if prevention measures are not ensured in developing countries, where the proportion of health care workers in the population is already small.

In total, the few occupational risk factors considered here were responsible for about 800,000 deaths worldwide in 2000. Not considered by WHO because of lack of global data are the additional 1.2 million deaths that ILO estimated are attributable to work-related risks (Takala 2002). The leading occupational cause of death was unintentional injuries, followed by COPD and lung cancer. Workers who developed outcomes related to these occupational risk factors lost about 25 million years of healthy life. Among the occupational factors analyzed in this study, injuries, hearing loss, and COPD accounted for about 80 percent of years of healthy life lost. Low back pain and hearing do not directly produce premature mortality, but they do result in substantial disability. This feature differentiates these conditions from the others analyzed in the study. Figure 60.2 provides summary results for the occupational risk factors.

The WHO comparative risk assessment has accounted for only about 800,000 (40 percent) of the 2 million deaths estimated by ILO to occur each year because of occupational illness and injury. Deaths attributable to a wide range of occupational exposures could not be included because of the

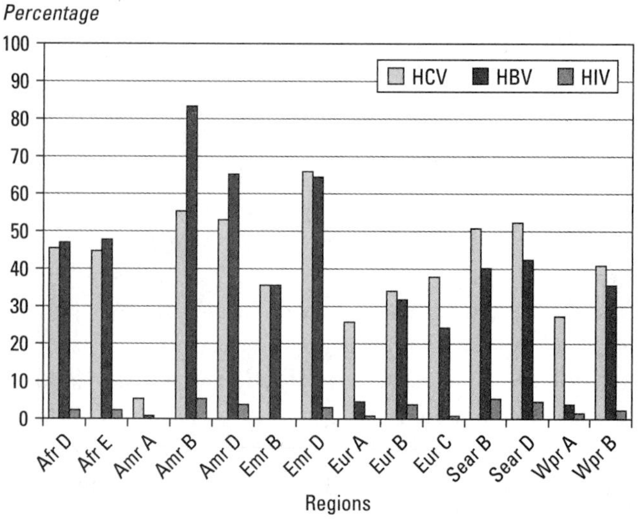

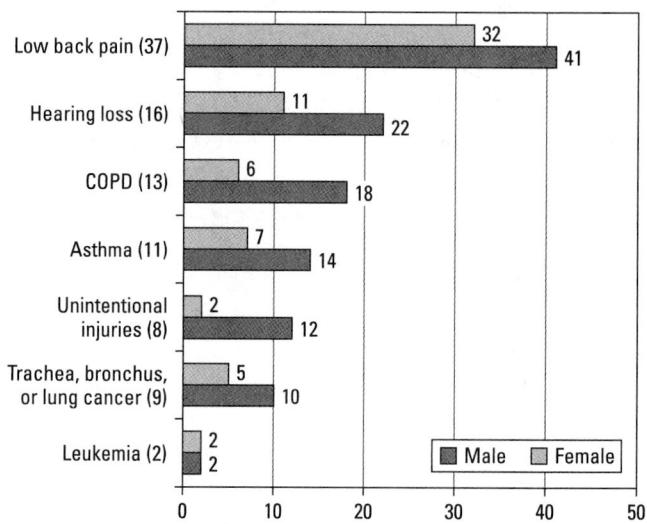

Percentage

Figure 60.1 Fraction of Hepatitis C Virus, Hepatitis B Virus, and HIV Infections in Health Care Workers Attributable to Injuries with Contaminated Sharps, Ages 20 to 65

Source: WHO 2002, 130.

HCV = hepatitis C virus; HBV = hepatitis B virus; HIV = human immunodeficiency virus; Afr = Africa; Amr = America; Emr = Eastern Mediterranean; Eur = Europe; Sear = Southeast Asia; Wpr = Western Pacific.

Figure 60.2 Fraction of Global Disease and Injury Attributable to Occupational Risk Factors
(percent)

Source: Adapted from Nelson and others 2005.

strict requirements for global data. Missing are deaths attributable to asbestosis, silicosis, and other dust diseases; infectious diseases; cardiovascular diseases; and violence. Deaths attributable to workplace exposures to pesticides, heavy metals, solvents, and other chemicals are not included. Outcomes such as dermatitis, psychological disorders, and upper-extremity musculoskeletal disorders that cause little mortality but substantial disability are also not captured by the WHO comparative risk analysis. Additionally, the consequences of underreporting in existing systems and the dearth of record-keeping systems in the developing nations lead to substantial undercounting by both the ILO and WHO. Nonetheless, the analyses provide important insights into the immense global burden of disease and injury attributable to occupational risk factors.

INTERVENTIONS

Strategies for controlling injury and occupational disease, developed by industrial hygienists and others over many decades in industrial countries, are as fully applicable in developing countries. The strategies include a hierarchy of controls in the following decreasing order of preference: substituting major hazards for less hazardous materials or processes; applying engineering controls to separate workers from hazards that remain; using administrative controls to minimize contact uncontrollable by engineering; and, as the last line of defense, using personal protective equipment such as respirators and protective garments. What differs in developing countries is the context in which the paradigm must be applied. Options are often sharply limited, and knowledge of them even more so; economic and political factors may impede otherwise obvious or desirable solutions; and the differing workplace context may demand that attention be paid to certain problems and concerns that would not be relevant in industrial countries in temperate climates.

The following generic factors associated with work in developing countries may alter industrial hygiene practice and must be considered in every effort to intervene to improve working conditions and occupational health:

- Access to industrial hygiene consultation is limited; professionals, sampling equipment, and laboratories are all in short supply.
- Knowledge level about occupational health among managers and workers is often limited.
- Markets for production materials as well as safety equipment may be limited and may include more hazardous materials or less effective protective equipment "dumped" from industrial countries where they are no longer marketable (Hecker 1991; Ives 1985; Jeyaratnam 1990).

- Regional conflict, economic pressures, climatologic factors, and lack of foreign exchange may make otherwise straightforward choices impractical.
- Supply of labor is often high, as is turnover, so economic incentives for investment in health capital are lower than in industrial countries.

Strategies for Improving Working Conditions

With these differences in context in mind, we now consider the major types of intervention: international, national, workplace, and individual.

International Interventions. The ILO–WHO Joint Committee on Occupational Health was formed in 1950 to provide guidance to the ILO and WHO regarding international occupational health issues. The committee meets periodically. At its 13th session, held in December 2003, the committee recommended that WHO and ILO pursue the following priorities (ILO and WHO 2003):

- Guide and support national occupational safety and health programs. Such guidance and support includes providing models for organizing at national or subnational levels; providing basic occupational health services; promoting management systems and tools, including control banding; developing national profiles and indicators; assessing the cost-effectiveness of interventions; and establishing effective enforcement agencies.
- Enhance regional collaboration and coordination, including the development and dissemination of models for cooperation, such as the African Joint Effort.
- Coordinate and enhance information and educational programs and materials (for example, by developing a joint Internet-based global portal) and statistics.
- Provide awareness-raising activities and instruments through campaigns, events, and special days.

State or Government Interventions. The major role the government can play is to establish workplace rules and provide a system of dissemination and enforcement. Evidence from industrial countries is overwhelming that conditions are substantially improved when both a strong regulatory framework and enforcement are achieved. An added benefit of government, rather than private sector, control is to "level the playing field": all employers in an economic sector carry the same burden. Conversely, improved health of the workforce, achieved by developing strategies beyond the minimum required, could be used to confer competitive advantages, a message to reluctant employers that has been used in different parts of the world with some success.

Regulatory decisions, such as the choice of exposure limits or allowable practices, often stimulate the biggest discussion—

for example, the debate about dust levels to be allowed in South African mines—but the larger issue for most countries is garnering resources to ensure compliance, to attract adequately trained personnel to conduct inspections, and to establish and monitor laboratories to support regulatory efforts. The most stringent exposure levels (often referred to as *threshold limit values*, or *TLVs*) are useless if the offending hazard cannot be routinely and accurately measured. Indeed, the South African experience, despite the presence of excellent regulations, is not encouraging in this regard (Joubert 2002).

Other forms of government intervention may indirectly improve working conditions. Among these are workers' compensation regulations and stipulations that employers of certain sizes must engage professionals in health and safety (most often nurses). Each of these interventions has the advantage of stimulating certain behaviors and practices without requiring the government to maintain the elaborate and technically complex machinery required for direct monitoring of workplace conditions.

Constraints on governmental regulatory and other interventions are many. Occupational and environmental regulations are often perceived as burdensome costs that impede investment and growth, perhaps creating what has been referred to as "the race to the bottom," in which threat of outmigration of industry from one jurisdiction enhances reluctance to regulate or enforce control strategies (Frumkin 1999). Moreover, the costs to the government itself, notwithstanding technical support from such agencies as the ILO, may be considerable in terms of personnel and equipment, and occupational health has to compete with other public health priorities for scarce resources. The result may be the promulgation of minimal standards or emasculated enforcement of those that already exist. The general impression of those working throughout the developing world is that the level of regulation and enforcement is woefully inadequate compared with that in industrial countries. Detailed case examples from Brazil (Bedrikow and others 1997); Kenya (Mbakaya and others 1999); Nigeria (Asuzu 1996); and Taiwan, China (Chen and Huang 1997), underscore the ubiquity of this problem.

Workplace-Based Interventions. Issues beyond the economic and legal ones impede application of the principles of industrial hygiene. A primary factor is ignorance; many employers may be uninformed about available controls and their value. Insurance agencies, local safety groups, and—in some regions of the world—trade unions may serve as facilitators of positive influence. In general, however, such resources fall short of the benefit of on-site industrial hygiene expertise that is lacking in many regions of the world.

Economic factors often impede efforts to institute voluntary controls. Materials used are frequently far cheaper than safer substitutes, often precisely because these materials no longer have markets in industrial countries that have banned or restricted their use—for example, solvent mixtures containing benzene and construction materials containing asbestos. Similarly, equipment such as machines that are well guarded to prevent injury or well baffled to limit noise may be prohibitively expensive in a marketplace geared to "hand-me-downs" compared with respirators or gloves. Unfortunately, even these last lines of defense may be difficult to obtain or relatively expensive unless local suppliers are available.

The single strategy for which no compelling economic disincentive exists—training—may also be difficult. Through the efforts of the ILO and numerous nongovernmental organizations and with widening access to the Internet, vast resources have become available. Ample documentation from the industrial and developing world indicates that even rudimentary knowledge by supervisors and workers about risks and risk-prevention measures is beneficial. Major impediments remain, however, such as educational proficiency, language barriers, and the applicability of training materials—often developed in other contexts—to local situations. Thus, for example, although the ILO has recently reported success with information programs in rural Thailand (Kawakami and Kogi 2001), a report from Ghana (Smith-Jackson and Essuman-Johnson 2002) suggests that workers and supervisors were unable to correctly interpret four of the most common warning signs used for hazard identification, despite having been trained in their use. Worker training appears, on the whole, widely underused.

Problems of infections in patients and health care workers from reused needles and needlestick injuries have prompted the international organizations to develop model interventions that can be transferred elsewhere. WHO initiated Project Focus: Ensuring Immunization Safety in Burkina Faso in July 2002 as a pilot project to use WHO materials in a focused effort to address all issues related to injection and immunization safety: availability of equipment and supplies (auto-disposable syringes, safety boxes, incinerators); safe injection practices; safe vaccine delivery; and safe waste management (WHO 2002). In 2000, WHO conducted a survey to assess the safety of injections in a study group of a random sample of 80 health centers. The situation was reassessed in June 2003 to evaluate the use of safety boxes (which had been provided in a WHO immunization campaign in Burkina Faso in 2001) and the impact of Project Focus. Table 60.2 shows results of the reassessment. Dramatic reductions were found in needle recapping, needlestick injuries, and misuse of safety boxes. Additionally, the number of clinics using safety boxes increased from fewer than half to 86 percent.

Small enterprises present special challenges because they lack resources and expertise to address health and safety problems. Thailand's National Institute for the Improvement of Working Conditions and Environment has used the ILO

Table 60.2 Prevalence of Risk Factors and Injuries at 80 Observed Health Centers
(percent)

Year	Needle recapping	Needlestick injuries	Lack of safety boxes	Misuse of safety boxes
2000	55	71	51	83
2003	17	32	14	18

Source: S. Khamassi, WHO Mediterranean Centre, personal communication 2003.

training approach called WISE (Work Improvement in Small Enterprises) with some success. In one example, six enterprises in the metal industry in Bangkok with between 15 and 115 workers participated in the WISE program, in which practical workshops involved workers and management in deciding on changes to be made in the workplaces. A wide range of inexpensive changes were put in place, and a booklet to illustrate good practices for others was prepared (Krungkraiwong 2000).

Individual Interventions. The general principle that, for most public health intervention, organization-level change is more effective than strategies targeting the individual is even more true when it comes to the workplace. With the exception of self-employed workers, such as those in the informal sector and subsistence farmers, occupational health and safety does not lend itself readily to individual solutions, with the same factors limiting employees more likely to limit individuals.

Improvement of Access to Health Care

In a few developing countries, workers enjoy broad access to high-quality health care. Chile, for example, has a system of nonprofit employer mutual associations that provide advice on reducing risks in workplaces and medical treatment and sick pay for work-related illness and injury (Contreras and Dummer 1997). In most countries, the role of on-site services is generally limited to emergency services for an injury or accidental overexposure and the conduct of medical surveillance examinations for workers at risk for chronic conditions such as noise-induced hearing loss, pneumoconiosis, or cancer.

In the developing world, access to health care is critical both for work-related and other health issues. In many areas, especially remote or rural areas, on-site service may be the only health care services available to workers and their families. Moreover, the blurred distinction between "general health" and "occupational health" in societies where people live and work in the same community and environment, and where children and spouses of workers may share common exposures and adverse conditions with workers, serves to confer some advantage to a more holistic approach to health services often best provided at or near the workplace itself.

Control of Nonoccupational Exposures

In industrial countries, a sharp demarcation exists between environmental risks associated with work and those associated with home life. This differentiation is not the case in many developing countries, especially at large, remote industrial complexes and farms. Workers—with or without their families—often cohabit with the workplace—and often with many or all of its risks, including noise, chemicals, and biohazards. The most dramatic examples of this situation were the industrial disasters at Chernobyl and Bhopal. It is not just in disaster, however, that risk occurs. Pesticides, for example, result in hundreds of thousands of cases of poisoning a year, a high fraction from the misuse of farm chemicals for nonwork applications, such as the appropriation of empty (but not clean) drums for transporting water or other household goods, a disturbingly common practice. In the industrial setting, carcinogens, neurotoxins, and other hazardous chemicals often pollute homes, drinking supplies, and common areas for recreation on a daily basis, adding to the exposure of workers and placing nonworking family members at risk from what would normally be seen as workplace hazards.

The remedy is often complex and beyond traditional industrial hygiene practice. Housing, which in any event may be substandard, needs to be modified to exclude the possibility of contamination by effluent from farm or factory under any foreseeable circumstances. Children and family members need to be apprised of the hazards of all materials used for work and prevented from even accidental access, a situation complicated by the fact that children are themselves often inappropriately engaged in the workplace. Food and water supplies need to be secure and protected from cross-contamination, a particular problem in the farm setting.

Surveillance and Reporting

Even in industrial countries, the strategies for recording any aspect of workplace harm beyond acute injury has been an issue; in most developing countries, even injury reports are largely nonexistent. Still, broad agreement exists on the value of statistical summaries of occurrences.

Unfortunately, a strong disincentive exists for such reporting unless it is required by law or by a parent company (as in the case of some multinationals). If reporting is required, as in the formal laws of many countries, successful implementation calls for resources for systematic review, verification, and maintenance of the information. Even records whose limitations are otherwise legion, such as workers' compensation records or regional reporting schemes, have proven highly advantageous to control efforts in industrial countries. These, too, have a role in developing countries, helping target even rudimentary and limited control efforts.

Capacity Building

Human capital in the form of professional capacity is critical to improving working conditions. Professional capacity varies greatly in developing nations but is higher where recognition of the field is high and the need for professionals and for workplace expertise is driven by occupational safety and health legislation and enforcement. In Malaysia, for example, four decades of rapid industrialization have included a series of legislative acts; development of federal agencies; and inclusion of training at various levels in occupational health in universities, the public sector, and the private sector (Rampal, Aw, and Jefferelli 2002). Key international events, such as joining the World Trade Organization, encourage the development of an economic culture that better recognizes the value of safe workplaces. Enforcement of national regulations, adoption of International Standards Organization standards, and establishment of management systems lead to broadening of training for workers and managers, although the scarcity of trained professionals is a major obstacle to adequately implementing regulations and policies and providing occupational health services (Christiani, Tan, and Wang 2002; Wang, Cheng, and Guo 2002).

In countries with some capacity, the expertise tends to be medical, rather than in other areas, such as industrial hygiene, engineering, or ergonomics. In most countries, ministries of health and of labor have jurisdiction over working conditions but often have too few experts and inadequate coordination. Moreover, the large percentage of work conducted in the informal sector presents a special challenge to these ministries. Because globalization has brought the need for professionals in occupational health to a crisis level, it is appropriate for international trade and development bodies to support national and international capacity-building programs.

In 1970, when the United States enacted the Occupational Safety and Health Act that established the National Institute for Occupational Safety and Health (NIOSH), the country had little professional capacity in that field. The new law charged NIOSH with ensuring an adequate number of trained professionals and accomplished this task successfully by funding graduate programs in U.S. universities. A follow-up 25 years later found that 90 percent of NIOSH-supported trainees pursued careers in the field, with more than 50 percent working in private organizations and the balance in government and academia (U.S. DHHS 1996). Similar results could be achieved by a determined, large-scale effort focused on assisting developing countries in achieving adequate professional capacity.

Both infrastructure and programs are necessary to build adequate capacity. In the international arena, a number of successful coalitions exist that provide experienced institutions and individuals. The WHO Global Network of Collaborating Centers in Occupational Health is a strong international coalition of 70 national, governmental, and academic centers of occupational health that work together with WHO and ILO headquarters and regional offices and three international nongovernmental organizations: the International Commission on Occupational Health, the International Occupational Hygiene Association, and the International Ergonomics Association (Fingerhut and Kortum-Margot 2002). These partners, located in approximately 40 countries, work together in 15 priority areas within a 2001–2005 Work Plan. More than 300 projects are under way, independently or jointly, to benefit workers in developing and industrializing nations in about 15 priority areas (WHO 2003).

Another strong regional coalition, coordinated with and benefiting from the Global Network of Collaborating Centers, is the WHO–ILO Joint Effort on Occupational Health and Safety in Africa (WHO and ILO 2002b). This partnering coalition—where centers outside Africa assist African partners—includes individual occupational safety and health professionals, employers, labor unions, and governmental and academic institutions in all countries in Africa.

Enlarging small but successful existing programs is one approach to capacity building. The U.S. National Institutes of Health Fogarty International Center, NIOSH, and the National Institute of Environmental Health Sciences sponsor a successful program, International Training and Research in Occupational and Environmental Health, which has developed small but strong programs between U.S. universities and institutions in more than 30 developing nations (NIH 2003).

Capacity building requires high-quality educational opportunities. Advances in information technology over the past decade are revolutionizing methods of education, and universities worldwide are developing large numbers of Internet-based courses. Fostering access of students from developing nations to these courses in leading universities is now feasible, but a national or international program is needed to address issues such as tuition, competition, intellectual property, and degree requirements. This effort might be called Access to Universities, following the model WHO program Access to Biomedical Journals, through which WHO and the world's largest medical journal publishers have provided about 100 developing countries with Internet access to journals at no cost or at deeply reduced rates (WHO 2001).

Professional associations have a long history of assisting in capacity building through training, research, and conferences. Recently, when the University of Witwatersrand in Johannesburg developed the first Diploma Occupational Hygiene program in South Africa, the country had too few industrial hygienists to provide mentors for the field research of the graduate students. The American Conference of Governmental Industrial Hygienists responded to a request of the International Occupational Hygiene Association, and 11 U.S. industrial hygienists volunteered to be occupational hygiene field practitioner long-distance mentors for the incoming students during the 2003 course year. This approach will continue until there are adequate industrial hygienists in country to serve as mentors to future classes (WHO and ILO 2002a).

The U.K. Health and Safety Executive developed a model program that provides clear solutions to chemical control problems in workplaces. This Web-based, user-friendly product was launched to enable small business owners in the United Kingdom to use information from the suppliers of chemicals to proceed through a series of simple steps to identify practical control solutions that reduce worker exposures to levels that present no danger to health (U.K. HSE 2002). This approach, which eliminates the need to measure exposures and meets the regulatory requirements of the United Kingdom, has immense potential value for employers in developing nations, who could devote scarce resources to controlling exposures rather than to measuring exposures. The approach has gained momentum through adoption by the International Program on Chemical Safety and through formation of an international workgroup to advance the approach in developing nations. To enable global use of this approach, the ILO has translated the U.K.-specific system into a product called the ILO Chemical Control Banding Toolkit (ILO 2003).

ECONOMIC ASPECTS OF INTERVENTION

Measures to prevent occupational risks are not cost-free, and where those costs ultimately come to rest affects the willingness of employers to implement the preventive measures.

Who Bears the Costs of Preventive Measures?

In industrial countries, compelling economic incentives exist for employers to control risks for injury and illness on the job, especially those that result in demonstrable near-term lost work or function. These include the high cost of medical care (especially in the United States), the burden of workers' compensation payments, high replacement costs for the labor, risk of litigation and liability, and negative business consequences of adverse publicity. Although these factors may differ by country and sector, they are less likely in the developing world to confer on employers a strong economic imperative for prevention—labor is plentiful, its replacement cost is low, and—most important—a high portion of the real cost of injury and illness will not be borne by the employer. The statistics in Latin America are staggering: although an estimated 2 to 4 percent of the GDP of the region is lost because of occupational fatalities alone, no evidence exists of private sector investment to reduce the risk (Giuffrida, Iunes, and Savedoff 2002). Multinational companies appear to be an exception. For many, the costs of injury and illness may accrue to the parent

country in terms of legal liability and adverse publicity, a lesson well taught by Union Carbide's experience in the aftermath of the Bhopal disaster in 1984.

One approach to align economic incentives is to use regulatory and legal reform to shift the existing cost burden to those in a position to remedy the situation—that is, to employers. Increasing workers' compensation benefits, especially those for long-term effects and disabilities, is an example of such an approach. Some evidence exists that, at least in southern Africa, this approach does stimulate preventive behavior by employers. An alternative is to critically reexamine the assumption that employers do not harbor substantial underrecognized costs of injury and illness even under the current situation, especially in terms of indirect costs such as lowered productivity and morale. Harari and his colleagues in Ecuador (Cullen and Harari 1995) have been studying the effect of such exposures as solvents and organophosphate pesticides on production levels. They are attempting to make the case that relatively inexpensive strategies for exposure control are economically advantageous to employers.

Intervention Costs and Cost-Effectiveness

Workplace illness and injury produce personal suffering and high economic costs. The ILO estimates that about 4 percent of GDP worldwide is lost because of work-related diseases and injuries (Takala 2002). The European Agency for Occupational Safety and Health at Work (1998) indicates that the costs to society in European countries ranged from 0.4 percent to 4 percent of gross national product.

Examining Industrial Countries. Identifying interventions to successfully reduce or prevent workplace injuries and illnesses will benefit society, employers, and workers. In 1996, stakeholders in the United States identified intervention effectiveness research as one of 21 priority areas in occupational health research for the next decade (U.S. DHHS 1996). From 1996 to 2002, research conducted or funded by NIOSH to develop and evaluate the effectiveness of solutions to prevent work-related injury and illness has increased nearly sixfold, from about US$5.5 million to US$33 million (U.S. DHHS 2003).

Research studies of workplace interventions often use surrogate or implied measures for economic evaluation. For example, economic benefit is assumed to occur following an intervention if symptoms of illness or injury in a workforce decrease while productivity remains constant. Intensive data-entry workplaces are increasing rapidly in both industrial and developing nations. Three studies of U.S. Internal Revenue Service data-entry clerks by NIOSH found that short, strategically placed rest breaks of 5 to 15 minutes during the regular daily schedule reliably reduced eyestrain, fatigue, and

Use of a Toolkit to Determine Return on Investment in Central American Garment Factories

The Regional Occupational Safety and Health Center (Centro Regional de Seguridad y Salud Ocupacional) Project in Central America developed an occupational safety and health toolkit to enable managers and line workers in garment factories to self-diagnose plant and workstation hazards and to estimate the costs and benefits of interventions (Amador and others 2003). Managers and employees at more than 100 Central American garment factories have been trained to use the toolkit. An in-depth evaluation of the use of the toolkit in three garment factories, each employing between 700 and 1,000 workers, in El Salvador, Guatemala, and Nicaragua found that within one year the factories generated savings that were four to eight times the costs of the interventions.

The overall investment by Confecciones La Palma in 2002 was US$6,360, and the savings attributed to that year were US$27,242 from reduced injury, illness, and absenteeism and an increase in productive days (see table).

Source: Amador and others 2003.

Change in Illness and Injury Indicators in the First Quarter of 2003 Compared with the First Quarter of 2002 at Confecciones La Palma

Indicator	2002	2003	Percent change
Number of accidents	63	36	−40
Days of absenteeism	200	149	−25
Sick days	822	426	−48
Visits to factory clinic	2,716	2,163	−20
Productive person-days	Not given	Not given	+12

Source: Data provided by Confecciones La Palma.

A CD-ROM version of the tool kit in Spanish and English also contains the guide "How to Design and Establish an Occupational Safety and Health Program in a Garment Factory" and can be found on the NIOSH Web site at http://www.cdc.gov/niosh.

musculoskeletal discomfort for video-display terminal operators without decreasing productivity (Galinsky and others 1999, 2000). Similar benefits of improved comfort and reduced stress from short rest breaks were observed among workers in a meat-processing plant without affecting productivity (Dababneh, Swanson, and Shell 2001).

Including economic costs of interventions is more difficult but is an important measure to allow employers to make decisions about interventions. A model intervention study, "Evaluation of a Best Practices Back Injury Prevention Program in Nursing Homes," received the 2003 National Occupational Research Agenda Partnering Award for Worker Safety and Health (APHA 2003; Collins and others 2004). Members of the partnership that carried out the intervention study included a large nonprofit U.S. health care system that owns nursing homes; manufacturers of lifting equipment; researchers at Washington University, West Virginia University, and NIOSH; and health care workers. The prevention program combined measures to reduce back injury by identifying the movements and postures that put nursing assistants at risk of back strain, stress, and injury in lifting and moving residents. Mechanical lifting devices for reducing those stresses and strains were evaluated in the laboratory and then in the nursing homes. A best-practices training and lifting program was put in place on the basis of researcher and employee input, and

rates for key measures of success were recorded for the three years before the intervention and for the three years after the intervention. The successful project reduced the frequency of back injuries in six nursing homes by 57 percent, lowered injury rates by 58 percent, and decreased workers' compensation expenses by 71 percent. Box 60.1 illustrates the value of evaluating costs of interventions in garment factories in Central America.

Reducing Risk for Back Pain. The WHO summary of a variety of cost-effectiveness studies for interventions addressing all aspects of global health illustrated that the cost-effectiveness of interventions in some areas of personal health has been well studied but that environmental and occupational topics have had relatively few studies. The WHO comparative risk assessment concluded that about 37 percent of back pain globally is attributable to occupational risk factors (WHO 2002). A cost-effectiveness study of interventions to reduce occupational back pain was also reported, using economic models developed to calculate costs of interventions in three WHO geographic regions that illustrate different levels of development. Intervention studies were obtained from the published and unpublished literature. All costs of running the interventions were measured in international dollars (not exchange rate dollars, as in the analysis reported later in this chapter) and

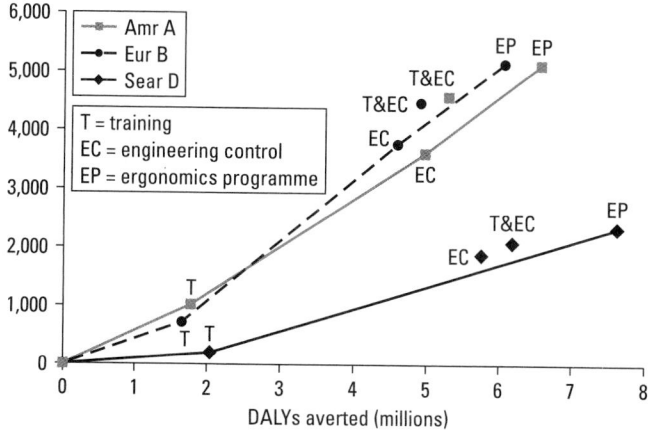

Cost (international dollars, millions)

Source: Reprinted from WHO 2002, 130.
Amr = Americas; Eur = Europe; Sear = Southeast Asia

Figure 60.3 Cost-Effectiveness of Interventions for Lower Back Pain

effectiveness was measured as age-weighted DALYs gained by the intervention. The interventions for the prevention of back pain were grouped into three major categories: worker training (awareness education and hazardous job training); engineering control (physical measures that control the exposure to the hazard, including equipment that assists lifting, pushing, and pulling); and the full ergonomics program (which includes both of the previous interventions and implementation procedures).

As shown in figure 60.3, the analysis found that the most effective intervention is the full ergonomics program, offering a 74 percent reduction in back-pain incidence. Lesser benefits are obtained by engineering control (56 percent reduction) and training (20 percent reduction). The total costs of worker training are largely labor related, the costs of engineering control are primarily capital costs, and the full ergonomics program costs are equally shared between the two. Training was found to be the most cost-effective intervention, as indicated by the lower slopes of the lines from 0 to T, and was recommended as the first choice when resources are scarce. However, the incremental cost-effectiveness ratios for the other options (indicated by higher slopes of the lines) demonstrated that both engineering control and the full ergonomics program are attractive alternatives. Thus, even the full ergonomics programs were found to be cost-effective in all three regions for their health effects alone, without even considering the possible increase in productivity that could be brought about by the interventions (WHO 2002). Recalculating these results according to Disease Control Priorities Project methods—using exchange rate dollars and removing the age weights from DALYs (see chapter 15)—would increase effectiveness somewhat because back pain is more common at later ages and would reduce the apparent costs in both Europe and Southeast Asia. It would have little effect on costs in the high-income countries of the

Americas. The relative cost-effectiveness of the three interventions would be unchanged in each region.

Reducing Risk for Silicosis. Silicosis is a disabling and often fatal workplace lung disease caused by inhalation of silica dust. The high-risk sectors of the economy include construction, mining and mineral processing, foundries, and manufacturing of pottery and glass. Large numbers of workers in both industrial and developing nations are exposed. Box 60.2 illustrates control of silica caused by grinding wheels in the agate cottage industry in India. In the United States, more than 3.2 million workers are exposed to silica dust, even though methods exist to eliminate exposure (Harley and Vallyathan 1996).

A study was conducted to evaluate the cost-effectiveness of alternative interventions to reduce silicosis in industrial and developing nations (Lahiri and others 2005). The authors used the limited published and unpublished data on costs of the various interventions and on the efficacy of exposure reduction. To analyze the cost-effectiveness of each intervention in reducing disease incidence, they used models developed for WHO (Murray and others 2000). The WHO DALY concept was used to combine mortality and morbidity resulting from silicosis. Two WHO regions were studied: the highly developed America A region, represented by the United States and Canada; and the developing Western Pacific B1 region, represented by China, the Democratic People's Republic of Korea, the Republic of Korea, and Mongolia. Exposure estimates were taken from the WHO comparative risk assessment study (Ezzati and others 2004).

The interventions included engineering control interventions that protect many workers (use of the wet method—that is, spraying a surface or wetting a blade to reduce dust; of local exhaust ventilation; and of total plant ventilation) and worker training plus personal protective equipment, an intervention that protects the individual worker. The training involved four types of personal protective equipment: comfort masks, dust masks, full-face respirators, and half-face respirators. Lahiri and others (2005) summarize the evidence of reduction in exposure through the use of selected interventions from the literature. The difference in the health life years gained with and without the intervention represented the effectiveness of the intervention and was used as the denominator for the cost-effectiveness ratio.

The engineering control interventions involve large capital expenditures, whereas the implementation of personal protective equipment requires ongoing large equipment costs (filters and cartridges) as well as labor costs for training the workers. Costs of interventions vary from region to region, depending on wage rates and raw material costs, but the costs of equipment seem not to vary. The authors found the least expensive alternative is training associated with use of a comfort mask. However, that intervention has a relatively low efficacy of

Economic Evaluation of an Engineering Control for Silica Dust in India

The agate industry is a cottage industry concentrated in residential settings in Khambhat and Dahegam, in the state of Gujarat, India, where 15,000 grinders and 60,000 other workers, family members, and neighbors are exposed to silica dust. The making of key chains, necklaces, and art pieces involves baking, chipping, grinding, and polishing agate stones. The grinding-machine wheels are driven at speeds of 1,440 rpm, generating large amounts of dust containing respirable silica. The table shows the extraordinary prevalence in the total exposed populations (noted above) of silicosis and tuberculosis caused by silica exposure.

Prevalence of Diseases in Agate-Dominated Areas of Khambat and Dahegam

Category	Silicosis		Tuberculosis[a]	
	Percent	Number	Percent	Number
Grinders	30	4,500	36	5,400
Nongrinding workers, family, and neighbors	8	4,800	16	9,600

Source: Bhagia, Ramnath, and Saiyed 2003.
a. National tuberculosis prevalence in India of 4 percent and resulting cases have been subtracted.

The National Institute of Occupational Health in India designed and distributed 10 dust control devices for the grinding machines to employers, who generally employ 5 to 10 workers (see figure). The efficacy of the devices was found to be 93 percent, and dust was greatly reduced

(Bhagia, Ramnath, and Saiyed 2003). Economic analysis was based on 600 dust control devices that could be installed in the communities. The total costs include the initial one-time cost of the devices (Rs 8,000, or approximately US$92); depreciation (10 percent per year); maintenance of machines (equivalent to the costs saved by recycling the dust to be used in polishing); and the cost of treating the diseases (about Rs 4,000, or approximately US$184 per year per case). The gains included annual income per avoided case of silicosis. Total savings per year were estimated to be between Rs 23 million and Rs 29 million (US$527,039 to US$664,528). The conclusion is that installation of dust control devices in all the agate-grinding units of Gujarat would reduce silicosis and tuberculosis as well as yield financial and health benefits to the workers, families, and the greater society that bears the cost of illness.

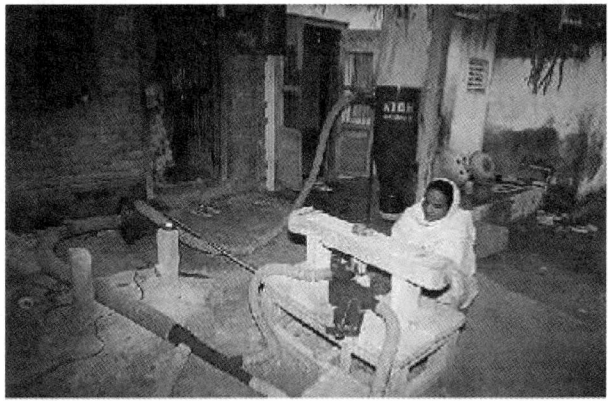

Traditional Grinding Machine with Dust Control System

30 percent exposure reduction. Although the initial capital expenditures are high for engineering controls, the annualized costs based on a 10-year horizon are encouraging, with exposure reduction of about 70 to 85 percent. The greatest exposure reduction of 95 percent was achieved at the highest cost, with training plus use of a full-face respirator, but an 80 percent reduction was achieved at half this cost when training was combined with a dust mask.

Table 60.3 shows that engineering controls in both industrial and developing regions are the most cost-effective

Table 60.3 Average Cost-Effectiveness Ratio *(US$/DALY gained)*

	America A region	Western Pacific B1 region
Engineering control	105.89	109.35
Comfort mask	111.04	117.19
Dust mask	191.38	173.90
Half-face respirator	299.82	272.45
Full-face respirator	304.87	265.74

Source: Lahiri and others 2005.

interventions, with expenditures of between US$105 and US$109 per healthy year saved in the two regions. Although exposure reductions with respect to each intervention type are identical in both regions and the cost of interventions is somewhat higher in the America A region, it might seem perplexing that the cost per unit of health gain is relatively lower in the America A region than in the Western Pacific B1 region. The reason for this result is that effectiveness (the denominator of the average cost-effectiveness ratio) is represented by health outcomes that are higher for this region because life expectancy in the America A region is higher than in the Western Pacific B1 region. Therefore, lives saved through interventions in industrial regions contribute more toward the healthy years generated by the model.

The study concluded that engineering controls are the most cost-effective interventions in both regions and should be considered as the first choice in cases in which resources are scarce. The results underestimate the health gains because other silica-related diseases such as tuberculosis and cancer are not considered.

IMPLEMENTATION

The health of a country's workforce, even more than the health of the country's overall population, is critical to its economic and national security. No country has become a successful economic power without sustained attention to the health of workers, who create the successful economy. Responsibility for the safety and health of workers lies with the government, the employers, and the workers themselves. However, it is the governmental framework, whether at a national or local level or both, that is the linchpin on which other efforts rest.

Institutions and Programs

The potential to continually improve work-related health status, as measured by morbidity and mortality data across multiple economic sectors and across many countries, has been compellingly demonstrated. Not surprisingly, because these conditions are inherently preventable, what may be the lowest achievable level of risk is debated in industrial countries. In the United States, for example, occupational injury fatality rates have been steadily declining, now approaching 3.8 per 100,000 workers, down from 7.5 just 20 years earlier (NIOSH 2000).

Key elements in improving worker health and safety, regardless of the level of development, include regulatory and enforcement framework; worker, employer, and health professional education; surveillance and reporting systems; and dissemination and implementation of best practices. Often these elements overlap in multifaceted approaches to addressing complex and disparate work settings.

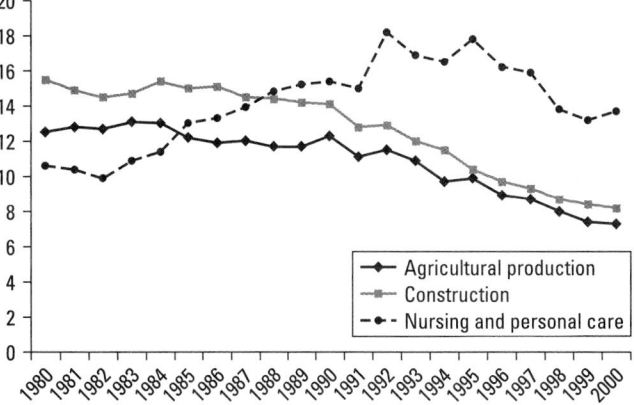

Injury rate per 100 full-time workers

Source: BLS 2002.

Figure 60.4 Incidence Rates of Nonfatal Occupational Injuries (Total Recordable Cases) by Selected Industry Sectors, 1980–2000

In the developing world, a patchwork of some of these approaches has brought success: in Vietnam by reducing silicosis through industrial hygiene practices of wetting the process and through surveillance (effective but much less so than protective equipment or, better yet, substitution of a safer product), and in Nicaragua by efforts to reduce pesticide poisoning through worker and health professional education and reporting systems. Even in highly developed countries, the continued need for a responsive and broadly based framework, with government involvement at the center, is evident.

An example recently identified in the United States is the comparison of injury indicators for workers across three prominent sectors: construction, agriculture, and health care (figure 60.4). Two decades of data demonstrate improving nonfatal injury rates for construction and agricultural workers (falling steadily from about 16 and 12 per 100 full-time workers, respectively). This rate is in contrast to injury rates for health care workers, which have risen by about one-third from a starting point of about 10 per 100 workers (BLS 2002). Why the difference? Although the reason is not fully delineated, major efforts (including government regulation, research investment and policy setting, education, and best-practice efforts)—plus, in the case of construction workers, active trade union involvement—in the two industrial sectors clearly were under way in this time period. In contrast, in the health care worker sector, no such national program existed in the period, and industry pressures resulted in a number of potential workforce problems, such as increasing work demands on a stressed and ill-prepared workforce.

Lessons Learned

As countries undergo rapid economic development, industrialization, and the effects of globalization, leaders can examine available occupational health system models as they develop their national occupational health systems. The Republic of Korea has experienced major economic and societal changes since it emerged from the Korean War in the 1950s with a need to establish occupational safety and health programs without any historical experience. The system directed by the Industrial Safety and Health Act of Korea is modeled after the specialist-based system of Japan, which relies on medical screening and specialists outside the workplace to deliver health and safety services (Paek and Hisanaga 2002). Paek and Hisanaga note that national traditions and culture strongly influence the choice of system when developing countries examine models from which to choose—for example, from the code-based system of the United States, the performance-based system of the United Kingdom, and the management system of the Nordic countries.

Government involvement is necessary but not sufficient, regardless of the level of development. Because national and local legislation and policies create the framework within which a society functions, international influence, assistance, and requirements play a key role in encouraging developing and industrializing nations to create appropriate laws and policies to support healthy workers. International trade, development, and funding organizations have immense power, which is not fully exercised to date, to influence countries on working conditions. The large multinational trade agreements have also failed to ensure that worker health and safety is adequately addressed, and multinational corporations have generally not transferred the safety and health systems of the industrial world to developing nations. The consequences are grave, as seen in the deaths of 2 million workers each year from occupational injuries and illness. Great power lies in these institutions and trade agreements to produce direct changes in the health of workers globally.

The ILO provides strong guidance internationally for industrial and developing nations through its tripartite conventions and recommendations. Each year the ministers of labor of all member nations, employer representatives, and worker representatives agree on policies in conventions, which the member states are asked to ratify. The models provided by the ILO are regularly used by some countries as they create their national systems. Brazil, for example, has been a member country of the ILO since 1919 and has ratified 75 ILO conventions. Set in place by legislation in the 1970s, the Brazilian model for occupational health services followed the ILO's Recommendation 112 (1959) as a paradigm (Dias, Mendes, and Schwartz 2002). Although few countries ratify most conventions, more than 150 countries have ratified Convention 182, which was passed in 1999 and addresses the worst forms of child labor. A current critical need is assistance to developing nations to meet the obligations required by ratification. WHO sets international policies on health, including worker health, at its annual meeting of health ministers of all member nations. Both ILO and WHO regional offices provide technical assistance and training. An unfortunate gap exists, however, because often the national ministries of labor relate to the ILO and the ministries of health to the WHO. Because working people are influenced by the national ministries of both labor and health, the international organizations have been advised to correct the situation (WHO and ILO 1995). A promising WHO/ILO Joint Effort on Occupational Safety and Health in Africa has embraced partners across ministries and broadly within and outside Africa to work together to assist countries, workers, and employers in the formal and informal sectors (WHO and ILO 2002b).

Several coalitions of organizations have successfully assisted developing countries to increase professional capacity and to improve worker health and safety. A regional illustration is the Association of Southeast Asian Nations Occupational Safety and Health Network, which was established to promote regional cooperation in training and research as well as harmonization of standards in safety and health. The primary international coalition is the WHO Global Network of Collaborating Centers in Occupational Health, described previously. The U.S. Fogarty International Training and Research Program in Occupational and Environmental Health is another stable and experienced network, consisting of U.S. universities working with universities in more than 30 developing nations to increase professional capacity. Some of the institutions are also WHO Collaborating Centers, and others are partners in Africa. The relationships have provided opportunities for synergy and streamlining of training and technical assistance (WHO and ILO 2002b).

Globalization has brought work-related hazards to developing countries lacking the infrastructure and professional capacity to handle them adequately. It is incumbent on the national and international bodies responsible for globalization to assist the recipient nations. Organizations with proven track records in occupational health could play key roles if international and national laws provide the appropriate context and funding.

Globalization

Increased globalization has caused important changes for many developing countries. Dias, Mendes, and Schwartz (2002) identify the series of developmental stages through which a country passes: underdevelopment and poverty, industrial revolution and accelerated economic development, internal adjustments to strengthen national competitive power to enter globalized markets, adjustments to foreign policy to integrate globalized markets, and aims toward long-term sustainable human development. These authors also analyze the positive and negative effects on occupational health conditions in countries such as Brazil, where crises and opportunities are experienced simultaneously. On the risk side, for example, free trade agreements have intensified rapid industrialization and the export of industry and materials—many hazardous—to regions with poor occupational infrastructure. These effects are likely increasing risk and rates of injury and occupational disease.

Globalization has also engendered major occupational health and safety development projects, most notably sponsored by Scandinavian governments (Partanen and others 1999). These initiatives have infused developing countries with expertise, training programs, and equipment and have provided much-needed (external) economic incentives for adoption of change on national, regional, and local levels. The major concern is sustainability, because the incentives are external.

Globalization has resulted in a rapid increase in the number of multinational companies operating outside industrial countries. Indeed, this outcome was the underlying economic intent of recent free trade agreements such as the North American Free Trade Agreement (NAFTA). In general, these companies bring with them a highly developed infrastructure in occupational health practice from their base countries. Unfortunately, although these model companies undoubtedly upgrade the availability of high-quality services and training, enhance workers' awareness, and create pressure on other industries in the region to conform, the pressure likely goes in both directions. The competitive advantage of lowered investment in health and safety, as long as the labor markets are plentiful and the direct costs to employers of illness and injury low, results in strong pressure to minimize—or at least reduce—the intensity and quality of services.

Even at their best, multinationals may inadvertently create an occupational health and safety "caste system." Many provide extremely high levels of care and service for their international managers and for technical support staff members, while offering local resources to indigenous workers. More broadly, occupational clinics, industrial hygiene services, and the like are often developed but available for the exclusive use of the multinationals, creating communities inside which modern occupational health exists but outside which nothing changes except the incorrect perception that progress has occurred. Often the reverse of progress has actually occurred because the limited numbers of trained physicians, occupational health nurses, industrial hygienists, and safety professionals are siphoned off to the higher-paying, more prestigious positions.

Free trade zones, established by treaties such as NAFTA, create special considerations. Although the agreements offer the potential to incorporate strong industrial world rules regarding labor, environment, and health in underdeveloped zones, the host countries often resist such changes, perceiving these rules as trade restrictions. The final language regarding health and safety in NAFTA, for example, is significantly less stringent than rules in the United States. Moreover, some multinationals resist even these rules, seeking broad economic relief as a foundation of moving across the border (Frumkin 1999).

Nonetheless, globalization does offer potential solutions. One is the link provided by international lending agencies such as the World Bank and International Monetary Fund of health and safety considerations to development loans. As a condition of receiving the development funds, control of health and safety conditions could be mandated and enforced. A second opportunity is voluntary initiatives, as were recently developed in the Apparel Industry Partnership, wherein a consortium of European and U.S. garment manufacturers agreed to control labor and safety practices in their facilities in developing countries by joint consent.

Implications for Health System Development

Workers' health and safety in most of the developing world may fall under the jurisdictions of both the ministry of labor and the ministry of health, with little collaboration and coordination between the two. The ministry of labor most commonly is the governmental focus of any regulatory and enforcement efforts, even though without requisite expertise and access to follow-up care, it may mandate services falling squarely within the traditional health system (for example, pulmonary function testing as ongoing screening for individual response to exposure to pulmonary toxicants). Whatever the country-specific organizational and structural constraints, the following set of principles can be applied in providing health services to workers:

- *Coordination between occupational health services and overall health services.* Occupational health services, consisting of efforts to prevent work-related disease and disability as well as to recognize and treat them once they occur, must be coordinated with overall health services. The separation between work-related and other health conditions, often driven by regulatory and liability concerns, insurance, and other external constructs (workers' compensation system or the disability system, for example), is not only clinically challenging but inefficient in optimizing individual health status. Although many work-related injuries and a few specific illnesses, such as asbestosis, can be readily pinpointed as stemming from work alone, most health problems result from multiple causes. This fact is as true in the developing world as in the industrial one—whether it be cumulative pesticide exposure from work and community sources, the interaction of poverty and poor health status with chemical work exposures, or the cumulative psychosocial stressors of life both inside and outside work. A holistic approach to the individual, recognizing the multisectoral, multiple determinants of health on overall health status, should be the goal in the provision of health services.
- *Attribution of causality and access to health services.* In parts of the developing world, as in the industrial world, a phenomenon exists wherein some threshold of causality (such

as "more probably than not work related") is the trigger to workers' compensation or other employer responsibility for taking care of the illness or injury. All too often in this setting, the incentive for the employer to disclaim responsibility leaves the worker, whatever the cause or causes of the condition under question, falling through the cracks of occupational health care and traditional health care. Universal access to health care, unfortunately not available in the United States or in much of the developing world, can mitigate this problem.

• *Health professional workforce expertise in occupational health.* As discussed in the section on capacity building, adequate expertise does not exist in the developing world to address traditional and emerging occupational health problems. Occupational health services are multidisciplinary, including nonmedical (industrial hygiene and engineering expertise, for example) in addition to health (nursing and physician) expertise. Without being prescriptive, health systems need to ensure the existence of an adequately prepared workforce (whether through broadly based training for all health personnel, training for occupational health specialists, or most likely some combination of the two) if they are to grapple even minimally successfully with reducing the human and economic burden of work-related injuries and illnesses.

Unifying the three principles identified above is the need to recognize that occupational health should be in the mainstream of both health education (at the professional, employer, and individual level) and health care. An argument against this approach is the perception that doing so will result in an untenable burden on already underfunded health care. We suggest that not so doing will create a greater burden, in both financial and human terms.

RESEARCH AGENDA

Before 1996, there was no known national effort to identify and promote an occupational health research agenda. That changed with NIOSH taking the lead to launch the National Occupational Research Agenda (NORA) (U.S. DHHS 1996). Since then, a number of other countries in the industrial world have launched similar efforts (for example, Italy, Sweden, and the United Kingdom). Although all these efforts are relevant to the developing world, the reality is that country-specific research, even at the risk of reinventing the wheel, is often needed to strengthen political will to effect policy. Moreover, although traditional epidemiological etiologic research in occupational health is not a priority or even feasible for much of the developing world, research targeted at local conditions and institutions is often what is most needed. Six areas are identified, with appropriate modifications for local conditions, as ongoing research priorities to address injury and disease

control strategies in the developing world. This research need not be undertaken solely—and sometimes not even in part—in the countries of concern, but rather is likely to be aided by the capacity building derived from partnership between academic institutions and government agencies across countries of different levels of development.

Public Health Systems Research

Although health services research has emerged as an important area of inquiry in the health field in the industrial world over the past few decades, scant attention has been paid to public health systems research (Institute of Medicine 2003). Given that occupational health sits at the interface between individual and population health, this area of inquiry is particularly germane to research in the field. This research would examine the effectiveness of government systems working in coordination with other sectors (academic institutions, employers, unions, voluntary agencies) in promoting occupational health status.

Occupational Health Policy Research

Public policy to address improving occupational health in the developing world should rest on a sound scientific base (that is, be evidence based) and should be coupled with an understanding of the local and national frameworks for policy (whether through legislative, regulatory, or other means). Adequate research has not been undertaken to evaluate policy development and implementation in public health in general and occupational health specifically. As with the need for new health systems research, this area of inquiry would undoubtedly benefit from partnerships among countries in the industrial world and in the developing and industrializing world.

Intervention Effectiveness Research

Intervention effectiveness research, a cornerstone of the U.S. NORA initiative, is critical to advancing occupational health in the developing world. The absence of data in this chapter to demonstrate cost-effectiveness of occupational health measures is indicative of the need for more such information to target what will always be a demand for limited resources. Recognizing the relative dearth of intervention effectiveness research in countries with high research investments, this recommendation is made cautiously for countries with fewer resources. However, it is assumed all too often that an accepted intervention in a country with higher economic productivity might not be viable in one with fewer resources. The research agenda for the developing world in this arena needs to be tailored to what is known and proven coupled with local and national conditions and needs.

Control Technology and Protective Equipment Research

Investigation of control technology and protective equipment, another NORA priority, is critical for developing effective and feasible control strategies in the developing world. Much of the primary research in this category can be done in the industrial world, but along with investments in intervention effectiveness research, new technologies may still need to be tested in real situations in developing countries. Simplified approaches to management of chemicals suitable to the local work settings have been developed in Indonesia and are being evaluated, and the International Program for Chemical Safety is helping other countries modify, implement, and evaluate the U.K. system, which was originally designed for use by small enterprises in the United Kingdom (ILO 2003).

Disease and Injury Research

Many questions of epidemiologic importance to improving the health of all workers can best be answered in settings in the developing world. This situation is not unique to occupational health, but in the occupational health arena, it is important to recognize that workers are often the first exposed and are exposed to the highest levels of potential hazards (as compared with their community counterparts). So, too, are levels of exposure to many hazards far greater in the developing world than elsewhere, and undertaking studies becomes efficient and feasible in these settings that would prove difficult if not impossible in settings where exposures are lower and larger numbers of study participants are needed to detect meaningful differences in risk. Not surprisingly, then, sentinel studies of health effects of interest to the industrial world have been undertaken in other countries—for example, studies in Latin America identifying the potential for acute pesticide intoxication to cause chronic neurological effects (Rosenstock and others 1991).

Surveillance Research

Surveillance is a critical component of all effective occupational health programs; thus, continuing research is needed into the most effective ways to gather and interpret this information. Surveillance systems are often limited at best in many developing countries, and evaluation research needs to be undertaken to determine the benefits of investing in gathering both generic (absences from work, for example) and specific (blood lead levels, for example) information on which to target public health action.

CONCLUSIONS

The burden of occupational health problems is staggering in both human and economic costs, and workers in the developing world bear this burden disproportionately. Moreover, the most vulnerable—children and the poor—are also disproportionately at risk. Compounding this tragedy is that many effective and economically feasible interventions are available to address these largely preventable health conditions.

Despite relatively little systemic data on cost and cost-effectiveness, even this "tip of the iceberg" picture demonstrates work-related conditions contributing significantly to overall mortality and morbidity and demonstrates the overall societal benefit of their prevention and treatment. Externalization of costs by employers—to the society as a whole—often obscures the actual overall benefit of a framework that relies on government regulation and enforcement, education, and best practices. Effectively addressing these problems takes active involvement from national and local government, employers, and workers and their representatives. The challenges to reducing the burden are heightened to the degree that public health and health care delivery systems isolate occupational health from the mainstream of health and health care.

Despite structural and political barriers to overcoming this high burden of disease and injury, evidence exists of enormous progress in the industrial world and of isolated progress in parts of the developing world. Targeted future investments in research and public health and health systems are critical to ensuring that progress continues and is more equitably distributed.

REFERENCES

Amador, R., C. Maldonado, R. Venezia, and C. Rivera. 2003. "Return on Investment in Prevention via the CERRSO Tool Kit." Central American Regional Occupational Safety and Health (CERSSO) Project, San Salvador, El Salvador.

APHA (American Public Health Association). 2003. "Recent Conference on Protecting the Nation's Workforce. *Nation's Health*." http://www.apha.org/journal/nation/tnhfullstories.htm.

Asuzu, M. C. 1996. "The Development and State of Health and Safety in the Workplace in West Africa: Perspectives from Nigeria." *West African Journal of Medicine* 15 (1): 36–44.

Bedrikow, B., E. Algranti, J. T. Buschinelli, and L. C. Morrone. 1997. "Occupational Health in Brazil." *International Archives of Occupational and Environmental Health* 70 (4): 215–21.

Bhagia, L. J., T. Ramnath, and H. Saiyed. 2003. "Cost Benefit Analysis of Engineering Control Devices in the Agate Industry." National Institute of Occupational Health, Ahmedabad, India.

BLS (Bureau of Labor Statistics). 2002. "Survey of Occupational Injuries and Illnesses." Washington, DC: U.S. Department of Labor, Bureau of Labor Statistics, Safety and Health Statistics Program.

Chen, M-S., and C-L. Huang. 1997. "Industrial Workers' Health and Environmental Pollution under the New International Division of Labor: The Taiwan Experience." *American Journal of Public Health* 87 (7): 1223–31.

Christiani, D., X. Tan, and X. Wang. 2002. "Occupational Health in China." *Occupational Medicine* 17: 355–70.

Collins, J., L. Wolf, J. Bell, and B. Evanoff. 2004. "An Evaluation of a 'Best Practices' Musculoskeletal Injury Prevention Program in Nursing Homes." *Injury Prevention* 10: 206–11.

Contreras, R., and W. Dummer. 1997. "Occupational Medicine in Chile." *International Archives of Occupational and Environmental Health* 69 (5): 301–5.

Cullen, M. R., and R. Harari. 1995. "Occupational Health Research in Developing Countries: The Experience in Ecuador." *International Journal of Occupational and Environmental Health* 1 (1): 39–46.

Dababneh, A. J., N. G. Swanson, and R. L. Shell. 2001. "Impact of Added Rest Breaks on the Productivity and Well Being of Workers." *Ergonomics* 44 (2): 164–74.

Dias, E. C., R. Mendes, and B. Schwartz. 2002. "Occupational Health in Brazil." *Occupational Medicine* 17: 523–27.

European Agency for Occupational Safety and Health at Work. 1998. *Annual Report*. Bilbao, Spain: European Agency for Occupational Safety and Health at Work.

Ezzati, M., A. D. Lopez, A. Rodgers, and C. J. L. Murray, eds. 2004. *Comparative Quantification of Health Risks: Global and Regional Burden of Disease Attributable to Selected Major Risk Factors*. Geneva: World Health Organization.

Ezzati, M., A. Lopez, A. Rodgers, S. Vander Hoorn, C. Murray, and the Comparative Risk Assessment Collaborating Group. 2002. "Selected Major Risk Factors and Global and Regional Burden of Disease." *Lancet* 360 (9343): 1342–43. http://image.thelancet.com/extras/02art9066web.pdf.

Fingerhut, M., and E. Kortum-Margot. 2002. "Network of WHO Collaborating Centres in Occupational Health, Communication and Information Dissemination." *Asian-Pacific Newsletter on Occupational Health and Safety* 9 (2): 28–30.

Frumkin, H. 1999. "Across the Water and Down the Ladder: Occupational Health in the Global Economy." *Occupational Medicine* 14 (3): 637–63.

Galinsky, T. L., N. G. Swanson, S. L. Sauter, J. J. Hurrell, and L. M. Schleifer. 2000. "A Field Study of Supplementary Rest Breaks for Data-Entry Operators." *Ergonomics* 43 (5): 622–38.

Galinsky, T. L., N. G. Swanson, S. L. Sauter, J. J. Hurrell, L. M. Schleifer, J. Martin, and others. 1999. "Three Studies of Rest Break Interventions for IRS Data Transcribers." Abstract of paper prepared for "Work, Stress and Health 99: Organization of Work in a Global Economy," a meeting of the American Psychological Association, Washington, DC, March.

Giuffrida, A., R. F. Iunes, and W. D. Savedoff. 2002. "Occupational Risks in Latin America and the Caribbean: Economic and Health Dimensions." *Health Policy and Planning* 17 (3): 235–46.

Harley, R., and V. Vallyathan. 1996. "History of Silicosis." In *Silica and Silica-induced Lung Disease*, ed. V. Castranova, V. Vallyathan, and W. Wallace. Boca Raton, FL: CRC Press.

Hecker, S. 1991. *Labor in a Global Economy*. Eugene, OR: University of Oregon Books.

ILO (International Labour Organization). 1995. *Economically Active Population, by Industry and by Occupation: Year Book of Labour Statistics*. 54th ed. Geneva: ILO.

———. 1996. *Year Book of Labour Statistics*. 55th ed. Geneva: ILO.

———. 2000.

———. 2002a. *Decent Work and the Informal Economy*. Report VI of the International Labour Conference, 90th Session, Geneva: ILO. http://www.ilo.org/public/english/employment/infeco/ilc2002.htm.

———. 2003. "ILO Chemical Control Banding Toolkit." ILO, Geneva. www.ilo.org/public/english/protection/safework/ctrl_banding/index.htm.

ILO and WHO. 2003. "SafeWork: Thirteenth Session of the Joint Committee on Occupational Health." ILO, Geneva. www.ilo.org/public/english/protection/safework/health/session13/.

Institute of Medicine. 2003. *Who Will Keep the Public Healthy? Educating Health Professionals for the 21st Century*. Washington, DC: Institute of Medicine.

Ives, J. H. 1985. *The Export of Hazard: Transnational Corporations and Environmental Control Issues*. Boston: Routledge & Kegan Paul.

Jeyaratnam, J. 1990. "The Transfer of Hazardous Industries." *Journal of the Society of Occupational Medicine* 40 (4): 123–26.

Joubert, D. M. 2002. "Occupational Health Challenges and Success in Developing Countries: A South African Perspective." *International Journal of Occupational and Environmental Health* 8 (2): 119–24.

Kawakami, T., and K. Kogi. 2001. "Action-Oriented Support for Occupational Safety and Health Programs in Some Developing Countries in Asia." *International Journal of Occupational Safety and Ergonomics* 7 (4): 421–34.

Kjellstrom, T., and L. Rosenstock. 1990. "The Role of Occupational and Environmental Hazards in the Adult Health Transition." *World Health Statistics Quarterly* 43: 188–96.

Krungkraiwong, S. 2000. "Occupational Safety and Health Improvement and Productivity in Small and Medium-Sized Enterprises Program in Thailand, Case Studies in Safety and Productivity." National Safety Council, Itasca, IL.

Lahiri, S., C. Levenstein, D. Imel Nelson, and B. J. Rosenberg. 2005. "The Cost Effectiveness of Occupational Health Interventions: Prevention of Silicosis." *Amer J Ind Med* 48 (6): 503–14.

Mbakaya, C. F., H. A. Onyoyo, S. A. Lwaki, and O. J. Omondi.1999. "A Survey of Management Perspectives of the State of Workplace Health and Safety Practices in Kenya." *Accident Analysis Prevention* 31 (4): 305–12.

Murray, C., D. B. Evans, A. Acharya, and R. M. P. M. Baltussen. 2000. "Development of WHO Guidelines on Generalized Cost-Effectiveness Analysis." *Health Economics* 9 (3): 235–51.

Nelson, D. I., M. Concha-Barrientos, T. Driscoll, K. Steenland, M. Fingerhut, L. Punnett, A. Prüss-Üstün, J. Leigh, and C. Corvalan. 2005. "The Global Burden of Selected Occupational Diseases and Injury Risks: Methodology and Summary." *Amer J Ind Med* 48 (6): 400–18.

NIH (National Institutes of Health). 2003. "Fogarty International Training and Research in Occupational and Environmental Health (ITREOH) Program." Bethesda, MD, NIH. http://www.fic.nih.gov/.

NIOSH (National Institute for Occupational Safety and Health). 2000. *Worker Health Chartbook, 2000*. Publication 2000-127. Washington, DC: U.S. Department of Health and Human Services.

Paek, D., and N. Hisanaga. 2002. "Occupational Health in South Korea." *Occupational Medicine* 17 (3): 39–408.

PAHO (Pan American Health Organization). 2002. "The Environment and Public Health." In *Health in the Americas*. Vol. 2. Washington, DC: PAHO and WHO.

Partanen, T. J., C. Hogstedt, R. Ahasan, A. Aragon, M. Arroyave, J. Jeyaratnam, and others. 1999. "Collaboration between Developing and Developed Countries and between Developing Countries in Occupational Health Research and Surveillance." *Scandinavian Journal of Work and Environmental Health* 25 (3): 296–300.

Rampal, K. G., T. C. Aw, and S. B. Jefferelli. 2002. "Occupational Health in Malaysia." *Occupational Medicine* 17 (3): 409–25.

Rosenstock, L., M. Kiefer, W. E. Daniell, R. McConnell, K. Claypoole, and the Pesticide Health Effects Study Group. 1991. "Chronic Central Nervous System Effects of Acute Organophosphate Pesticide Intoxication." *Lancet* 338 (8761): 223–27.

Smith-Jackson, T. L., and A. Essuman-Johnson. 2002. "Cultural Ergonomics in Ghana, West Africa: A Descriptive Survey of Industry and Trade Workers' Interpretation of Safety Symbols." *International Journal of Occupational Safety and Ergonomics* 8 (1): 37–50.

Takala, J. 2002. "Introductory Report: Decent Work—Safe Work." Paper presented at the 16th World Congress on Safety and Health, Vienna, May 27.

Trapido, A. S. M., N. P. Mqoqi, C. M. Macheke, B. G. Williams, J. C. A. Davies, and C. Panter. 1996. "Occupational Lung Disease in Ex-Mineworkers—Sound a Further Alarm" (letter). *South African Medical Journal* 86 (4): 559.

U.K. HSE (Health and Safety Executive). 2002. "COSHH Essentials—Easy Steps to Control Chemicals." London, HSE. http://www.coshh-essentials.org.uk.

UN (United Nations). 2000. *International Standard Industrial Classification of All Economic Activities (ISIC).* 3rd Revision. St/ESA/SER.M/4/Rev3. New York: United Nations.

U.S. DHHS (Department of Health and Human Services). 1996a. "National Occupational Research Agenda (NORA)." DHHS (NIOSH) Publication 96-115. Washington, DC, U.S. DHHS.

———. 2003. "National Occupational Research Agenda (NORA) Update." DHHS (NIOSH) Publication 2003-148. Washington, DC, U.S. DHHS.

Wang, J. D., T. J. Cheng, and Y. L. Guo. 2002. "Occupational Health in Taiwan." *Occupational Medicine* 17: 427–35.

WHO (World Health Organization). 2001. "Access to Biomedical Journals." WHO, Geneva. http://www.who.int/inf-pr-2001-32.html.

———. 2002. *The World Health Report 2002—Reducing Risks, Promoting Healthy Life.* Geneva: WHO.

———. 2003. *WHO Compendium of Activities of the Network of Collaborating Centers in Occupational Health.* Geneva: WHO.

WHO and ILO (World Health Organization and International Labour Organization). 1995. *Report of the 12th Meeting of the WHO/ILO Joint Advisory Board on Occupational Safety and Health.* Geneva: WHO.

———. 2002a. "Long-Distance Occupational Hygiene Mentoring Program." WHO, Geneva. http://www.sheafrica.info/en/About/who_cc.htm.

———. 2002b. "The WHO/ILO Joint Effort on Occupational Safety and Health in Africa." WHO, Geneva. http://www.sheafrica.info/en/About.htm.

World Bank. 2003. *World Development Indicators.* Washington, DC: World Bank.

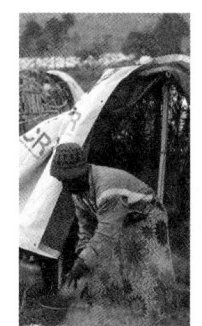

Chapter **61**

Natural Disaster Mitigation and Relief

Claude de Ville de Goyet, Ricardo Zapata Marti, and Claudio Osorio

Sudden-onset natural and technological disasters impose a substantial health burden, either directly on the population or indirectly on the capacity of the health services to address primary health care needs. The relationship between communicable diseases and disasters merits special attention. This chapter does not address epidemics of emerging or reemerging diseases, chronic degradation of the environment, progressive climatic change, or health problems associated with famine and temporary settlements.

In line with the definition of *health* adopted in the constitution of the World Health Organization (WHO), the chapter treats disasters as a health condition or risk, which, as any other "disease," should be the subject of epidemiological analysis, systematic control, and prevention, rather than merely as an emergency medicine or humanitarian matter. The chapter stresses the interdependency between long-term sustainable development and catastrophic events, leading to the conclusion that neither can be addressed in isolation.

DISASTERS AS A PUBLIC HEALTH CONDITION

According to the International Federation of Red Cross and Red Crescent Societies, internationally reported disasters in 2002 affected 608 million people worldwide and killed 24,532—well below the preceding decade's annual average mortality of 62,000 (IFRC 2003). Many more were affected by myriad local disasters that escaped international notice.

Disaster has multiple and changing definitions. The essential common element of those definitions is that disasters are unusual public health events that overwhelm the coping capacity of the affected community. This concept precludes the universal adoption of a threshold number of casualties or vic-

tims. What would be a minor incident in a large country may constitute a major disaster in a small isolated island state. Not only are "quantitative definitions of disasters unworkably simplistic" as noted by Alexander (1997, 289), but when based on the economic toll or the number of deaths, they are also misleading with regard to the immediate health needs of the survivors or their long-term impact on the affected country.

Classification of Disasters

In the early 1970s, a series of well-publicized disasters (the civil war and resulting famine in Biafra, the cyclone in Bangladesh, and the earthquake in Peru) triggered the scientific interest of the international public health community.

Disasters can be classified as *natural disasters, technological disasters,* or *complex emergencies.* The latter include civil wars and conflicts. These classifications are arbitrary and refer to the immediate trigger—a natural phenomenon or hazard (biological, geological, or climatic); a technologically originated problem; or a conflict. In reality, all disasters are complex events stemming from the interaction of external phenomena and the vulnerability of man and society.

The human responsibility in so-called natural disasters is well acknowledged. The term *natural disaster* remains commonly used and should not be understood as denying a major human responsibility for the consequences.

Disaster Terminology

The following definitions are adapted from those proposed by the Secretariat of the International Strategy for Disaster Reduction (ISDR), a United Nations (UN) body established to sustain the efforts of the International Decade for Natural

Disaster Reduction (UN/ISDR 2004) and the WHO *World Health Report 2002* (WHO 2002):

- *Hazards* are potentially damaging physical events, which may cause loss of life, injury, or property damage. Each hazard is characterized by its location, intensity, frequency, and probability.
- *Vulnerability* is a set of conditions resulting from physical, social, economic, and environmental factors that increase the susceptibility of a community to the effects of hazards. A strong coping capacity—that is, the combination of all the strengths and resources available within a community—will reduce its vulnerability.
- *Risk* is the probability of harmful consequences (health burden) or economic losses resulting from the interactions between natural or human-induced hazards and vulnerable or capable conditions. In a simplified manner, risk is expressed by the following function:

$$Risk = f\ (Hazards \times Vulnerability)$$

A public health approach to disaster risk management will aim to decrease the vulnerability by adopting prevention and mitigation measures to reduce the physical impact and to increase the coping capacity and preparedness of the health sector and community, in addition to providing traditional emergency care (response) once the disaster has occurred.

Distribution and Risk Factors

Health and relative economic losses of natural disasters disproportionately affect developing countries (Alexander 1997; UN/ISDR 2004). More than 90 percent of natural disaster–related deaths occur in developing countries. Even though the economic losses are far greater in industrial countries, the percentage of losses in relation to gross national product (GNP) in developing countries far exceeds that percentage in industrial countries (figure 61.1). At an individual level, a sudden reduction of US$5,000 from an annual income of US$50,000 is worrisome; however, the ongoing loss of US$50 from a monthly income of US$100 may be catastrophic.

For this reason, statistics of economic damage and mortality alone are not true indicators of the effect of disasters on the health and development of people and communities.

Disaster impact statistics show a global trend: more disasters occur, but fewer people die; larger populations are affected, and economic losses are increasing (IFRC 2000).

Geographic Distribution of Risk. Natural disasters do not occur at random. Geological hazards (earthquakes and volcanic eruptions) occur only along the fault lines between two tectonic plates on land or on the ocean floor. However, the local population often does not recognize the implications (the risks), as shown in the December 2004 tsunami in the Indian Ocean.

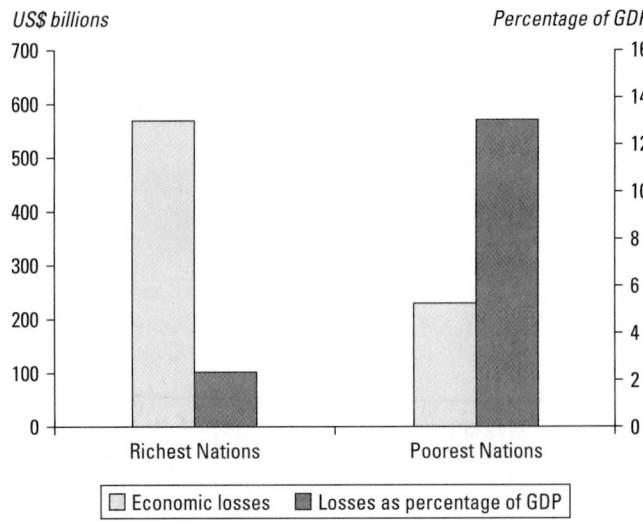

Source: UN/ISDR, 2004.

Figure 61.1 Disaster Losses, Total and as Share of Gross Domestic Product, in the Richest and Poorest Nations, 1985–99

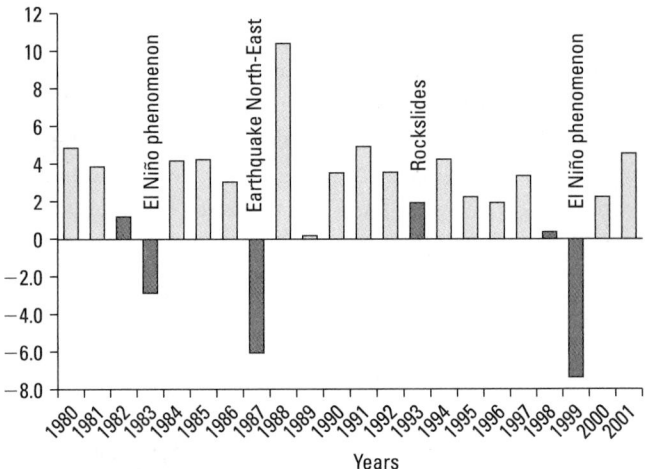

Source: UN/ISDR, 2004.

Figure 61.2 Annual Growth of Gross Domestic Product and Occurrence of Major Natural Disasters in Ecuador, 1980–2001

Hydrometeorological hazards do not follow a well-established distribution. Although the areas subject to seasonal flood, drought, or tropical storms (cyclones, hurricanes, or typhoons) are well known locally, global warming may possibly redraw the map of climatic disasters. As the National Research Council (1999, 34–35) notes, "This change is far from uniform. A pattern of response 'modes' appears to be involved, in which warming is concentrated in northern Asia . . . while large regions of the northern Pacific and North Atlantic Oceans and their neighboring shores have actually cooled." El Niño–related fluctuations in relation to the gross domestic product (GDP) of Ecuador are shown in figure 61.2.

The risk of massive technological disasters, such as the catastrophic release of chemicals in Bhopal, India (methyl isocyanate), in December 1984, is serious in countries with significant industry (WHO 1992, 1996). Very few countries are immune to public health risks from hazardous chemical substances (from insecticides to industrial by-products) or discarded radioactive material from therapeutic or diagnostic use. Technological hazards increase rapidly with the unregulated industrialization of developing countries and the globalization of the chemical industry, suggesting that chemical emergencies may become a major source of disasters in the 21st century.

Factors Affecting Vulnerability. Vulnerability to all types of disasters—and to poverty—is linked to demographic growth, rapid urbanization, settlement in unsafe areas, environmental degradation, climate change, and unplanned development.

Age The importance of age as a factor of vulnerability can be significant in situations where physical fitness is necessary for survival. The higher fatality among children, elderly, or sick adults following the 1970 tidal wave in Bangladesh (250,000 fatalities) and the 2004 tsunami in Asia (more than 180,000 dead or missing) illustrates this point.

Gender Reports on immediate morbidity and mortality according to gender are not as conclusive. An Inter-American Development Bank paper indicated that 54 percent of the 3,045 people who died as a result of Hurricane Mitch in Nicaragua were male (IDB 1999). Stereotypes of gender vulnerability at the time of impact often do not apply. Depending on the type of disaster, far more significant vulnerability factors than gender or age are the time of day of the impact (and, therefore, the occupational activity of each group) and the structural vulnerability of housing, factories, and public buildings, including the location of the victims within the buildings. Following disasters, increased vulnerability of women is commonly noted in temporary settlements, where violence and sexual abuse are common. Specialized health care also may not be available (Armenian and others 1997).

Poverty Economic vulnerability might play a much greater role than age and gender. What has been noted regarding the greater vulnerability of poor countries also holds true at the community and family levels. Disasters predominantly affect the poor. Poverty increases vulnerability because of the unequal opportunity for healthy and safe environments, poor education and risk awareness, and limited coping capacity. A notable exception was the 2004 tsunami in Banda Aceh, Indonesia, where the middle- and upper-class neighborhood close to the shore was particularly affected.

A major example is the settlement of a large number of economically disadvantaged populations in highly vulnerable locations, particularly urban areas. Following Hurricane Mitch in Tegucigalpa, Honduras, families that were relocated from flooded areas to safer (but inconveniently remote) ground were rapidly replaced by new illegal settlers. In 2003, families killed by a landslide in Guatemala had been warned about their vulnerability but were unable to afford resettlement in safer (and more costly) areas. Subsidies alone may not have prevented this effect, given the overarching issue of land ownership by a few in Central America.

Short-Term Health Burden

Losses fall under three categories, which may have both direct and indirect components:

- lives and disabilities (both direct damage and an indirect consequence)
- direct losses in infrastructure and supplies (direct impact)
- loss or disruption in the delivery of health care, both curative and preventive (indirect impact).

The immediate health burden is directly dependent on the nature of the hazard. National health budgets of developing countries are, in normal times, insufficient to meet the basic health needs of the population. In the aftermath of a major disaster, authorities need to meet extraordinary rehabilitation demands with resources that often have been drained by the emergency response (as distinct from the resources destroyed by the event). Beyond the immediate response, decision making in the allocation of resources among sectors is mostly influenced by the magnitude of the economic losses rather than by the health statistics (principally the disability-adjusted life year, or DALY, losses) or social costs.

Earthquakes. As noted by Buist and Bernstein (1986), in the past five centuries, earthquakes caused more than 5 million deaths—20 times the number caused by volcanic eruptions. In a matter of seconds or minutes, a large number of injuries (most of which are not life-threatening) require immediate medical care from health facilities, which are often unprepared, damaged, or totally destroyed, as was the case in the earthquake in Bam, Iran, in 2003. In the aftermath of that earthquake, which resulted in 26,271 deaths, the entire health infrastructure of the city was destroyed. All traumas were evacuated by air to the 13 Iranian provinces long before the arrival of the first foreign mobile hospitals. Table 61.1 illustrates the accelerated pace with which priorities evolve and overlap in the first week following an earthquake.

After a few weeks, national political solidarity and external assistance wane, and the local budgetary resources are drained. At the same time, health authorities face the overwhelming task of providing services to a displaced population, rehabilitating

Table 61.1 Health Priorities Following Earthquakes

Priority	Time period	Comments
Search and rescue	0 to 48+ hours	Returns are rapidly diminishing. Most effective work is done by local teams.
Trauma care	0 to 48 hours: initial lifesaving care[a] 48 hours to 6 months: secondary care	External assistance generally arrives too late for initial care. Traumas may include burns and crush syndrome, especially in urban areas. Paraplegics and amputees require long-term care.
Routine medical emergencies and primary health care	Resumes as soon as the need for acute lifesaving care subsides (within 24 hours)	Emergencies include earthquake-related cardiovascular emergencies and premature births.
Attention to the dead	Varies. Not a public health issue but a social and political one	Priorities are identification and ritual burial.
Disease surveillance	Urgent—within 48 hours, unsubstantiated rumors of impending epidemics will be circulating	Surveillance is a sensitive public information and education issue. A simple, syndrome-based system is needed that will involve humanitarian organizations.
Provision of safe water	A predominant issue within 48 hours	The challenge is to provide a sufficient quantity of reasonably safe water.
Temporary shelter	48 hours to several months	Sanitation and provision of health services is a main issue. Accommodating families near their residence is preferable to setting up camps.
Provision of food	3 days to 6 weeks	Food provision is a social or economic issue. Food stocks and agricultural output are not affected by earthquakes.
Psychosocial care	7 days to 6 months	Mental health assistance is best provided by local personnel, if available.

Source: de Ville de Goyet 2001.

a. Following the earthquake in Mexico City in 1985 (10,000 deaths), bed occupancy rates did not exceed 95 percent despite the loss of 5,829 hospital beds.

health facilities, restoring normal services, strengthening communicable disease surveillance and control, and attending to the long-term consequences, such as permanent disabilities, mental health problems, and possibly long-term increases in rates of heart disease and chronic disease morbidity (Armenian, Melkonian, and Hovanesian 1998).

Tsunamis. Earthquakes on the ocean floor may cause catastrophic tidal waves (*tsunamis*) on faraway shores. Waves caused by the seismic event crest at less than a meter in open seas, but they are travel several hundred kilometers per hour, so when they reach shallow waters, they can be 10 meters high. Damage on the coast can be extensive. Usually, the number of survivors presenting severe injuries is small in proportion to the number of deaths.

Volcanic Eruptions. Volcanoes persist as a serious public health concern, though they are often overlooked by authorities and communities lulled by long periods of inactivity. Eruptions are preceded by a period of volcanic activity, which provides an opportunity for scientific monitoring, warning, and timely evacuation.

Some issues, such as ash fall, lethal gases, lava flow, and projectiles, although of concern to the public, are of minimal health significance: Ash fall causes a significant burden on medical services but is unlikely to result in excess mortality or significant permanent problems. However, ash fall affects transportation, communications, water sources, treatment plants, and reservoirs. Studies by Bernstein, Baxter, and Buist (1986) following the 1980 eruption of Mount St. Helens (United States) reviewed the transient, acute irritant effects of volcanic ash and gases on the mucous membranes of the eyes and upper respiratory tract as well as the exacerbation of chronic lung diseases with heavy ash fall. Concentrations of volcanic gases are rapidly diluted to nonlethal levels, which lead to inconvenience but negligible morbidity for the general public. Lava flows present little health risk because of their very slow speed of progression. Mortality caused by ballistic projectiles from a volcanic eruption is minimal.

Attention to these public concerns may distract the authorities from preparing for the greatest factors of mortality: the pyroclastic flows (Mount Pelé in Martinique, in 1902, with 29,000 deaths) and lahars. *Lahars* are mud flows or mud and ash flows caused by the rapid melting of a volcano's snowcap, as in Colombia in 1985 (23,000 deaths), or caused by heavy rains on unstable accumulations of ash, as in the Philippines in 1991. Historically, pyroclastic explosions or lahars have caused about 90 percent of the casualties from volcanic eruptions.

Potential contamination of water supplies by minerals from ash; displacement of large populations for an undetermined period of time (over five years in Montserrat, a small island in the Caribbean); accompanying sanitation problems; and mental health needs are of great public health significance (PAHO 2002a). Among the long-term problems, the risk of developing silicate pneumoconiosis requires further investigation.[1]

Climatic Disasters. Many communities and health services have learned to live with seasonal floods of moderate intensity. Periodically, the magnitude of the phenomenon exceeds the local coping capacity and overwhelms the resources of the health systems. The health burden associated with seasonal floods is well known locally: increased incidence of diarrheal diseases, respiratory infections, dermatitis, and snake bites. The actual risk of compromised water supplies depends on the level of contamination of the community's water supply before the disaster, compared with contamination after the flooding. Saline contamination is a long-term issue following sea surges and tsunamis. Prolonged flooding endangers local agriculture and occasionally requires food assistance on a large scale. The primary factors of morbidity remain overcrowded living conditions and poor water and sanitation in temporary settlements and other areas where water and sanitation services have deteriorated or are suspended.

Mortality and morbidity caused by tropical storms (hurricanes in the Atlantic Ocean and typhoons in the Pacific Ocean) result from, in increasing order of importance, high winds, heavy rainfall, and storm surge. When Hurricanes Mitch and George hit the Caribbean in 1998, traumatic injuries (lacerations or electrocution) caused by high winds of up to 150 miles per hour were relatively few; deaths from extensive rainfall (leading to flash floods and landslides) constituted the bulk of the more than 13,000 fatalities (PAHO 1999). In the Bangladesh delta, storm surges up to 6 meters traveled unimpeded over hundreds of kilometers and claimed between 250,000 and 500,000 lives in 1970 and up to 140,000 lives during five cyclones in the 1990s—primarily during one storm in 1991. Another cost is the need for specialized psychosocial assistance to large numbers of the population who survive the sustained violence of nature.

Cumulative mortality caused by small, undocumented mudslides and rockslides from water-saturated, unstable slopes probably approach the toll from well-known landslides (earthquakes in Peru in 1970 and in El Salvador in 2001, and the rains in Caracas, Venezuela, in 1999). Morbidity problems are often minimal, as survivors in the path of the landslide are few.

Impact on Communicable Diseases

Disasters related to natural events may affect the transmission of preexisting infectious diseases. However, the imminent risk of large outbreaks in the aftermath of natural disasters is overstated. Among the factors erroneously mentioned is the presence of corpses of victims, many buried beneath rubble. Dead bodies from a predominantly healthy population do not pose a risk of increased incidence of diseases (Morgan 2004). Catastrophic incidence of infectious diseases seems to be confined to famine and conflicts that have resulted in the total failure of the health system.

In the short term, an increased number of hospital visits and admissions from common diarrheal diseases, acute respiratory infections, dermatitis, and other causes should be expected following most disasters (Howard, Brillman, and Burkle 1996; Malilay and others 1996). This increase may reflect duplicate reporting (diarrhea cases were reported through both the emergency and the routine surveillance systems in Maldives after the 2004 tsunami), a temporary surge in surveillance, and medical attention available to an otherwise underserved population rather than representing a genuine change in the epidemiological situation.

In the medium term, heavy rainfalls may affect the transmission of vectorborne diseases. Following an initial reduction as mosquito-breeding sites wash away, residual waters may contribute to an explosive rise in the vector reservoir. When associated with a breakdown of normal control programs, this rise in the vector reservoir may lead to epidemic recrudescence of malaria or dengue. Retrospective studies (Bouma and Dye 1997; PAHO 1998; UN/ISDR 2004, 156) all confirm a direct but delayed relationship between the intensity of rainfall (regardless of the existence of flooding) caused by the El Niño phenomenon and the incidence of malaria. Flooding has contributed to local outbreaks of leptospirosis (in Brazil and Jamaica, for example; PAHO 1982) and hepatitis A in Latin America and Africa (WHO 1994).

In summary, what can be expected and prevented is a local surge in problems that the health services are normally used to handling.

Long-Term Impact and Economic Valuation

In addition to the delayed impact on transmission and control of endemic diseases and the burden of disabilities (paraplegia, amputation, burns, or chronic or delayed effects of chemical or radiological exposure), the health sector bears a significant share of the economic burden. Disasters must be seen in a systemic (that is, intersectoral) manner: what affects the economy will affect the health sector—and vice versa. After the emotional response of the first few days, decision makers in a crisis react primarily to political and economic realities, not to health indicators. Economic valuation of the social burden—that is, placing a monetary value on the cost—becomes a critical tool as the various sectors compete for scarce resources. The health sector, in particular, must learn how to use this tool in spite of being absorbed by its immediate relief responsibilities.

Valuation of Disasters. The Economic Commission for Latin America and the Caribbean (ECLAC) has developed over the decades a methodology for the valuation of disasters (ECLAC 2003). This tool, intended for reconstruction, has also proved its usefulness by developing historical records of major events, particularly of the health burden expressed in economic terms.

Valuation is made using all possible sources of information, from georeferenced satellite mapping and remote sensing to more conventional statistical data, direct observation, and surveys, with a reliance on information gathered immediately after the event. Economic valuation rests on the basic concepts of direct damage and indirect losses.

Direct damage is defined as the material losses that occur as an immediate consequence of a disaster.[2] Direct damage is measured first in physical terms. The physical loss includes assets, capital, and material things that can be counted: hospital beds lost, equipment and medicines destroyed, damaged or affected health service installations (number and type of installations, stocks of medicines, laboratory facilities, operating rooms, and so on), and pipes and water plants destroyed.

The physical plant then is valued both in terms of discounted present value and estimated replacement cost. Reconstructing facilities with the same vulnerability and level of service as before would be unacceptable; the affected health infrastructure must be replaced by more resilient and efficient installations to ensure better and sustainable service. This need is most evident in developing countries where impacts tend to be concentrated in those most at risk (the poor, marginalized, and less resilient sectors of the population).

Indirect effects refer to production of goods and services that will not occur as an outcome of the disaster, reduced income associated with those activities not occurring, and increased costs to provide those goods and services.

In the case of health services, indirect effects encompass both the income losses associated with the diminished supply of health care services and the increased costs of providing the services following the disaster. Indirect effects are valued at the current market value of goods or services not produced and the costs associated with the necessary provision of services under emergency, disaster-related conditions. Both components of the cost of illness—the cost of treatment and the cost of lost opportunities (lost income and employment, loss of time and productivity)—are sharply increased. The social burden is heavier on the poorest, who are unable to adjust their willingness to pay to absorb the additional expenses of alternative (private) providers of care.

The same approach applies to the economic valuation of lives lost. Kirigia and others (2004) found a statistically significant impact of disaster-related mortality on the GDP of African countries. One single disaster death reduced the GDP per capita by US$0.01828. Lost lives are given a higher economic value in places where productivity is high.

Because economic valuation uses standard sectored procedures that allow comparability of results, it can be used in the decision-making process and for policy formulation since it identifies sectors, geographical areas, and vulnerable groups that are more severely affected economically. Over the years, a number of conceptual improvements have been made to allow for the measurement of aspects not included in national accounting systems—to bring attention to environmental losses as a cross-cutting issue; to highlight the contribution of specific groups, namely women, as agents for change; and to focus on the better management of both the emergency and the reconstruction processes. It is also a valuable tool for preparedness and mitigation of future damage.

Table 61.2 summarizes the valuations made by ECLAC over the years for Latin America and the Caribbean in terms of deaths, affected populations, and economic losses (2003 values). Of interest are the decrease in the number of deaths and the increase in total damage (in particular, indirect damage) over time.

The distribution of direct and indirect damage in the health sector also varies. According to ECLAC (2003), direct damage between 1998 and 2003 in Latin America ranged from 44.6 percent to 77.2 percent of total damage.

Table 61.2 Impact of Disasters in Latin America and the Caribbean

Date	Population		Damage (2003 US$ millions)		
	Deaths	Affected	Total	Direct	Indirect
1972–80	38,042	4,229,260	9,376	5,420	3,956
1981–90	33,638	5,442,500	19,603	13,916	5,687
1991–2000	11,086	2,318,508	20,902	10,401	10,501
2001–2002	120	4,828,470	4,498	2,270	2,228
Total of major events 1972–2002	82,886	16,818,738	54,379	32,007	22,372
Overall estimate including small disasters[a]	103,608	21,023,422	67,974	40,009	27,965
Average per year	3,454	700,781	2,266	1,334	932

Source: ECLAC 2003.

a. The full image should include the recurrent small disasters that do not make the headlines but have a cumulative negative effect. Such disasters can be more pervasive and damaging to the development process because their economic, social, psychological, and political effects are hardly perceived. An estimate of the average losses of small disasters would be at least 25 percent greater than those of large disasters.

Specific Damage to the Health Infrastructure. Damage to housing, schools, channels of communication, industry, and so on contributes to the health burden. However, the following analysis focuses on the health infrastructure (understood as health care facilities, including hospitals, health centers, laboratories, and blood banks) and the drinking water and sanitation infrastructure.

Damage to Hospitals and Health Installations Most data and examples presented here come from Latin America and the Caribbean because of the disaster reduction programs in the health sectors of those regions. In the past two decades, damage to approximately 260 hospitals and 2,600 health centers resulted in interruption of services at a direct cost of US$1.2 billion. In the 1985 earthquake in central Mexico, 5,829 beds were destroyed or evacuated (PAHO 1985), at a direct cost of US$550 million (ECLAC 1998). Hurricane Gilbert (1988) damaged 24 of the 26 hospitals on Jamaica, and the El Salvador earthquake (2001) resulted in the loss of 2,000 beds—40 percent of the country's hospital capacity (PAHO 2002b). The health burden is not limited to the loss of medical care. The control of communicable diseases and other public health programs suffer from loss of laboratory support and diagnostic capabilities of hospitals. Further research on the actual impact of these losses, in terms of DALYs, is essential.

A common misperception is that damage to critical health facilities is promptly repaired. Experience shows that damaged health infrastructure recovers at a slower pace than infrastructure in other service sectors, such as trade, roads, bridges, telecommunications, and even housing. For example, as a result of the earthquake that affected El Salvador in 1986, renovation of the general hospital, the most sophisticated referral hospital in the capital, was completed 15 years after the earthquake. The only national pediatric facility was fully rehabilitated and strengthened six years after the earthquake. Two years after the earthquake of 2001 in El Salvador, several key hospitals still remained vacated or services were transferred to unsuitable temporary facilities. The factors are many: low priority assigned to a nonproductive sector, the sector's inexperience in developing comprehensive proposals for funding, conflicting attempts to use the reconstruction process to influence the ongoing reform and decentralization processes, the novelty of the engineering and design issues for safe hospital construction, the complicated negotiation process for loans, and the administrative inexperience of the health sector in executing large investment projects. Indeed, few large health installations have been built directly by developing countries in the past decades.

Damage to Water and Sewage Systems The primary goal of water and sewage systems is to safeguard the public health of the population. For that reason, these systems are considered part of the health infrastructure.

The developmental burden is significant. In the past 30 years in Latin America and the Caribbean alone, an estimated 400 urban water supply systems and 1,300 rural systems (in addition to 25,000 wells and 120,000 latrines) were severely damaged, at an estimated cost of almost US$1 billion—a major setback to efforts to expand coverage and improve those services. In severe flooding, the sudden interruption of these basic services coincides with the direct effect on the transmission of waterborne or vectorborne diseases. In the case of earthquakes, the number of people who are adversely affected by water shortage may far exceed those injured or suffering direct material loss.

As in the case of health care facilities, the rehabilitation of public water systems is slow, particularly for community-owned or community-operated rural systems, which may not be repaired for decades. The foregoing demonstrates the need for water authorities to harmonize their short-term objectives, which are oriented almost exclusively to increasing the coverage of these services, with the long-term objective of reducing vulnerability to extreme natural hazards.

INTERVENTIONS: FROM RESPONSE TO PREVENTION

The immediate lifesaving response time is much shorter than humanitarian organizations recognize. In a matter of weeks, if not days, the concerns of both the population and authorities shift from search and rescue and trauma care to the rehabilitation of infrastructure (temporary restoration of basic services and reconstruction). In Banda Aceh, Indonesia, after the December 2004 tsunami, victims were eager to return to normalcy while external medical relief workers were still arriving in large numbers.

Response and Rehabilitation

Immediate emergency response is provided under a highly political and emotional climate. The public demands visible, albeit perhaps unnecessary, measures at the expense of proven low-key approaches. The international community, eager to demonstrate its solidarity or to exercise its "right of humanitarian intervention," undertakes its own relief effort on the basis of the belief that local health services are unwilling or unable to respond. Donations of useless medical supplies and medicines and the belated arrival of medical or fact-finding teams add to the stress of local staff members who may be personally affected by the disaster. The cultural disregard of the humanitarian community to cost-effective approaches in times of disaster and the tendency to base decisions on perceptions and myths rather than on facts and lessons learned in past disasters contribute to making disaster relief one of the least cost-effective health activities.

The responsibilities of the national or local health authorities are significant.

Assessment of the Health Situation. A country's ministry of health is expected to assess the health situation. To influence the course of humanitarian response, this assessment must be rapid and, therefore, simple; transparent in collaboration with the main actors—nongovernmental organizations (NGOs) and donors; and technically credible. The input of WHO, as the lead agency in health matters, is most valuable. Confusion should be avoided between assessing emergency needs and inventorying or valuating the damage. In the first hours or days, relief actors base their decision making on the ministry of health's assessment of what is required and, more importantly, what is not required for emergency response. Later, the international community will request detailed data, such as the number of persons affected, buildings damaged, and monetary valuation.

Mass Casualties Treatment. Following natural disasters, hospital capacity may be considerably reduced by actual damage to the facility or, in the case of a seismic event, an often unnecessary—but hard to reverse—evacuation. Triage of patients is required in order to first treat those likely to benefit most, rather than the terminally injured or those whose care can be delayed. Lifesaving primary care takes place in the first six hours (the golden rule of emergency medicine), making most of the foreign field hospitals irrelevant for intensive acute care of traumas (WHO and PAHO 2003). Effectiveness of immediate care will depend on local preparedness before the disaster, not on faraway resources.

Strengthened Surveillance, Prevention, and Control of Communicable Diseases. Because the surveillance, prevention, and control of communicable diseases are strengthened, the anticipated massive outbreaks generally do not actually occur.

Traditional surveillance systems that are based on periodic notification of diseases by the health services are inadequate in a crisis situation. Early warning requires flexible and simple syndrome-based monitoring in temporary settlements and health centers, with information collected not only by the official health services but also by the medical humanitarian organizations. Systems that do not include consultation with NGOs are unlikely to succeed.

Disease control programs in place before the disaster are the fruit of local experience and external technical advice. In a disaster situation, there is generally no need to resort to new and expensive control measures. The key is to quickly resume, strengthen, and better monitor the routine control programs. No public health concerns justify the hurried disposal of corpses through mass burial or unceremonious incineration. This practice is socially and culturally damaging. In addition, improvised mass immunization campaigns, especially by external relief groups, should be discouraged in favor of opportunistically strengthening national routine immunization coverage, especially in temporary settlements.

Environmental Health. Typical interventions in the aftermath of disasters include strengthening the monitoring and surveillance of water quality, vector control, excreta disposal, solid waste management, health education, and food safety.

A first priority is water supply. It is often preferable to have a large quantity of reasonably potable water than a smaller amount of high-quality water (UNHCR 1998). Massive distribution of water purification disinfectants can be effective if the public is already familiar with their use and not confused by the availability of many different brands and concentrations of donated chemicals.

Health education and hygiene promotion efforts target populations in shelters, temporary camps, collective kitchens, or prepared food distribution centers.

The cost-effectiveness of the external relief effort could often be increased by shifting resources from the overattended medical response to the improvement of environmental health in temporary settlements.

Transparent Management of Donations and Supplies. If donations and supplies are managed transparently during the emergency, the flow of assistance to the intended beneficiaries will be improved. Unsolicited and often inappropriate medical donations compete with valuable relief supplies for scarce logistical resources. Good governance is critical, and effective logistics cannot be improvised following a disaster. A humanitarian supply management system developed by PAHO and WHO successfully helped developing countries improve transparency and accountability in managing humanitarian supplies and donations (de Ville de Goyet, Acosta, and others 1996).

Coordination of the Humanitarian Health Effort. Coordination of the humanitarian health effort is essential to maximize the benefit of the response effort and ensure its compatibility with the public health development priorities of the affected country. Effective coordination in the health sector must do the following:

- Be comprehensive and include all external health actors.
- Be based on mutual respect rather than regulatory authority alone. Dialogue and consultation are more effective than enforcement.
- Benefit all parties, starting with the victims. It should aim to support and facilitate the activities of other partners.
- Be evidence-based and transparent. Information is made to be shared and used, not jealously guarded.

Coordination cannot be improvised in the aftermath of a disaster. Preparedness before the occurrence of the hazard is essential.

Emergency Preparedness of the Health Sector

Effective response by national health authorities cannot be impromptu. Ministries of health that neglected to invest in capacity building before emergencies have generally experienced serious difficulties in exercising their technical and political leadership in the immediate aftermath of a disaster. Disaster preparedness is primarily a matter of building institutional capacity and human resources, not one of investing heavily in advanced technology and equipment.

Building local coping capacity is one of the most cost-effective ways to improve the quality of the national response and the external interventions.

Disaster preparedness is not merely having a disaster plan written by experts. It must involve the following:

- Identifying vulnerability to natural or other hazards. The health sector should seek information and collaborate with other sectors and institutions (civil protection, meteorology, environment, geology) that have the primary responsibility for collecting and analyzing this information.
- Building simple and realistic health scenarios of a possible and probable occurrence. It is challenging enough to prepare for a moderate-size disaster; building and sustaining a culture of fear based on unrealistic worst-case scenarios may serve the corporate interests of the disaster community but not the interests of the public at large.
- Initiating a participative process among the main actors to develop a basic plan that outlines the responsibilities of each actor in the health sector (key departments of the ministry of health, medical corps of the armed forces, private sector, NGOs, UN agencies, and donors). What matters is the process of identifying possible overlaps or gaps and building a consensus—not the paper plan itself. Disasters often present problems that are unforeseen in the most detailed plans.
- Maintaining a close collaboration with these main actors. A good coordinator is one who appreciates and adapts to the strengths and weaknesses of other institutions. Stability is essential. Changes of key emergency staff members during a disaster situation or when a new administration or minister take over have occasionally complicated the tasks.
- Sensitizing and training the first health responders and managers to face the special challenges of responding to disasters. Participation of external actors (UN agencies, donors, or NGOs) in designing and implementing the training is critical. The incorporation of disaster management in the academic curriculum of medical, nursing, and public health schools should complement the on-the-job training programs of the ministry of health, UN agencies, and NGOs. Well-designed disaster management training programs will improve the management of daily medical emergencies and accidents as well.

Prevention and Mitigation

The slogan "prevention is better than cure" was invented by the health sector. However, this sector has been slow to adopt the concept of preventing deaths and injuries from disasters through the mitigation (that is, reduction) of damage to its own facilities. As is unfortunately often the case, political action is often triggered only by a major disaster, such as the collapse of Hospital Juarez in Mexico in the earthquake of 1985; in that disaster 561 patients and employees died, (Poncelet 1997). Evaluating the damage (the past vulnerability) helps establish mitigation criteria for the future.

The level of protection required for each health installation must be negotiated—from life protection, which prevents an immediate structural collapse to permit the evacuation of people; to investment protection, which minimized the economic losses; to operational protection, which guarantees the sustainability of services under any extreme circumstances. Though a commercial or office building may be structurally designed only to prevent loss of lives, key hospitals must remain operational during the times they are most needed.

Local engineering and architectural experts play a key role in developing the knowledge, technical abilities, and cost-effectiveness analysis to establish mitigation priorities. Technical mitigation guidelines prepared at a global level (PAHO, WHO, World Bank, and ProVention Consortium 2004) need to be adapted to local culture, conditions, and resources.

Reducing the physical vulnerability of infrastructure can take place on three different occasions (UN/ISDR 2004, 324):

- *When reconstructing the infrastructure destroyed by a disaster.* At that time, risk awareness is high, political will is present, and resources are available.
- *When planning new infrastructure.* Reducing vulnerability is most cost-effective and politically acceptable when it is included at the earliest planning and negotiation stage, whether it involves a 1 to 2 percent additional cost for wind resistance or a 4 to 6 percent additional cost for earthquake resilience. Full resistance to any damage is prohibitively expensive.
- *Strengthening of existing facilities (retrofitting).* This most expensive measure has been adopted by several developing countries (Chile, Colombia, Costa Rica, Mexico, Peru, and others) to protect their most critical health facilities. In the earthquake in Colombia in 1999, partial retrofitting of the main hospital is credited for saving the installation. Costs vary greatly (see table 61.3).

Mitigation of Damage to Hospitals. Mitigation does not pretend to eliminate all possible damage from hazards but aims to ensure the continuing operation of the health facility at a level previously defined by the health authority. Hospitals

Table 61.3 Retrofitting of Hospitals in Costa Rica

Hospital	Number of beds	Duration of retrofitting (months)	Cost of retrofitting (US$)	Percentage of total value of the hospital
Hospital Mexico	600	31	2,350,000	7.8
Children's Hospital	375	25	1,100,000	4.2
Hospital Monseñor Sanabria	289	34	1,270,000	7.5

Source: PAHO and WHO 2000.

should be subject to stricter norms than other less critical facilities that are designed to prevent only total collapse and loss of life.

Hospital mitigation interventions fall into three categories:

- *Functional mitigation* to ensure that the necessary supporting infrastructure services permit continuing operation: water, electricity, road access, communications, and so forth. Improving routine maintenance will facilitate operations under normal circumstances and in the event of extreme hazards.
- *Nonstructural mitigation* to reduce losses and health injuries from falling or moving objects. Measures include, for instance, proper anchoring of equipment for earthquakes or strong winds or the location of only noncritical services on flood-prone floors.
- *Structural mitigation* to ensure the safety of the structure itself (columns, beams, load-bearing walls).

Given the high economic, health, and political costs represented by the avoidable loss of critical health facilities, health authorities and funding agencies should require that, in all new health infrastructure projects, natural hazards be a decisive factor for selecting the facility's location and for formulating the specifications at the earliest stage of the process.

Mitigation of Damage to Water Systems. Unlike hospitals, water supply systems are geographically extensive and thus are exposed to different types of hazards. The search for technical solutions is more complex, given the diversity of the water system's components. Finally, in many countries, the health authorities have no jurisdiction over the construction or operation of those services owned or administered by many local or municipal agencies.

Even a short disruption of water services may have serious and direct implications for the health of individuals, the operation of health services, and the community at large through its impact on business. A probabilistic model studied the disruptive potential of a water outage in the event of an earthquake in Los Angeles county in the United States. As noted by the authors, "water outage is more likely to be disruptive for businesses in some industries, such as health services, than for others" (Chang and Chamberlin 2004, 89).

The health sector should, therefore, coordinate with the institutions in charge of constructing, operating, and maintaining water and sanitation services, both urban and rural, to promote reduction of the vulnerability of existing systems. The health sector should also ensure that health aspects and mitigation of damage be included in the regulatory framework and operating procedures of water and sanitation services.

Protecting the water supply is feasible in developing countries. The Costa Rican Institute of Aqueducts and Sewage Systems reduced the vulnerability of one of the main aqueducts of the country, the Orosi Aqueduct. Over 10 years, Costa Rica invested almost US$1.5 million in studies and reinforcements, an amount equivalent to 2.3 percent of the total cost of the aqueduct. This investment would prevent a loss of nearly US$7.3 million in direct damages alone (FEMICA 2003).

INTERVENTION COST, COST-EFFECTIVENESS, AND ECONOMIC BENEFITS

The highly emotional and sensationalized climate of disaster response has long prevented the adoption of a cost-effectiveness approach in decision making. When survival of both people and political institutions is threatened, perceptions and visibility tend to prevail over facts and analysis, resulting in a lack of evidence-based studies on costs and benefits.

The willingness to spend hundreds of thousand of dollars per victim rescued from a collapsed building in a foreign country is a credit to the solidarity of the international community, but it also presents an ethical issue when, once the attention has shifted away, modest funding is unavailable for the mid-term survival of tens of thousands of victims.

Cost-Effectiveness of Selected Humanitarian Interventions

Emergency health interventions are more costly and less effective than time-tested health activities. Improvisation and rush inevitably come with a high price. The preferential use of expatriate health professionals; the emergency procurement and airlifting of food, water, and supplies that often are available locally or that remain in storage for long periods of time; and the tendency to adopt dramatic measures contribute to making disaster relief one of the least cost-effective health activities.

Search and Rescue. Few developing countries have established the technical capacity to search for and attend to victims trapped in confined spaces in the event of the collapse of multistory buildings. Industrial nations routinely dispatch search and rescue (SAR) teams. Costs are high and effectiveness is reduced by delayed arrival and quickly diminishing returns. Following the 1988 earthquake in Armenia, in the former Soviet Union, the U.S. SAR team extracted alive only two victims at a cost of over US$500,000. In Turkey in 1999, 98 percent of the 50,000 people pulled alive from the rubble were salvaged by relatives and neighbors. In Bam in 2003, the absence of high-rise and reinforced concrete buildings ruled out the need for specialized teams. Nevertheless, according to UN statistics, at least US$2.8 million was spent on SAR teams. An alternative solution consists of investing these resources in building the capacity of local or regional SAR teams—the only ones able to be effective within hours—and training local hospitals to dispatch their emergency medical services to the disaster site.

Field Hospitals. The limited lifesaving usefulness of foreign field hospitals has been discussed. Again, the lessons learned from the Bam earthquake are clear. The international community spent an estimated US$10.5 million to dispatch approximately 10 mobile hospitals,[3] which arrived from two to five days after the impact, long after the last casualty had been evacuated to other Iranian provinces. This delay alone, hard to reduce further, rules out any significant contribution to immediate trauma care and led the hospitals to compete for routine outpatient care with the teams of Iranian volunteers from across the country. A few of the mobile hospitals, better prepared to meet nontrauma needs and to stay much longer than the usual two to three weeks, have been invaluable. No data are available on the number of lives actually saved by mobile hospitals (that is, lives that would not have been saved by local means). Less understood are the negative effects of such hospitals on local health services, which are often marginalized and discredited for their lack of technology and sophistication but which must cope once the external facility leaves.

The cost of mobilizing a mobile hospital for a few weeks often exceeds US$1 million, funds that would be more productive in the construction and equipping of a simple but sturdy temporary facility. Such an approach was adopted by the U.S. Army Southern Command in Wiwili, Nicaragua, in the aftermath of Hurricane Mitch. In the case of Bam, Iran, the cost of rebuilding the entire primary and secondary health care facilities and teaching institutions was estimated by the government of Iran to be US$10.75 million, an amount very similar to that expended for the dispatch of field hospitals

from the international community. Guidelines for the use of foreign field hospitals are available from WHO and PAHO (2003).

In-Kind Donations. Unsolicited donations of inappropriate medical supplies not only are of limited use, but often cause serious logistic, economic, and political problems in the recipient country. Warehousing those supplies and, in many instances, building facilities (incinerators, for example) for the safe disposal of pharmaceutical donations diverts humanitarian funds from more effective uses. Recipient countries collectively share part of the responsibility by not clearly indicating what they do not want to receive and by not speaking out once inappropriate items arrived.

Disease Prevention and Control. Postdisaster interventions in surveillance and control of communicable diseases should focus on strengthening existing programs. Benefits will outlive the crisis. Improvised mass immunizations (instead of improved sanitation and public awareness) and vector control by aerial spraying or fogging (instead of breeding-site reduction or waste disposal) are just two examples of wasteful managerial decisions.

Shelters. Tent cities should be a last resort. Family-size tents may be expensive and do not last long. Establishing large settlements is easy, but such settlements are difficult to sustain and nearly impossible to terminate. They come with their own sanitation problems and social shortcomings (lack of privacy, loss of family identity, and loss of empowerment). Distributing construction material (or, preferably, cash subsidies) is more cost-effective and tailored to the needs and priorities of end users.

Cash Assistance. Developed societies long ago abandoned the distribution of in-kind relief goods and services to their nationals in favor of direct financial assistance in the form of subsidies, grants, or tax relief. The individual is free to determine actual priorities and to seek the most cost-effective source of services (shelter, medical, food, or other). It is therefore surprising that external assistance from these same countries remains focused on the costly delivery of predetermined services or commodities.

The most immediate lifesaving needs can be addressed only locally with existing resources and capacity. No cash contribution will meet those immediate needs. Beyond the acute phase, in many countries with market economies, most other services and goods are easily procured by those with financial means, suggesting that income availability is often the single limiting factor in rehabilitation.

Undoubtedly, this approach would affect considerably the type (and number) of humanitarian actors by transferring power and decision making to the local beneficiaries and relying on local economic forces for delivery to the end user. It may also bring its own set of problems (and abuses), though perhaps that is a small cost, considering the economic and social benefits of the most interested party—the victim—being in charge.

Cost-Effectiveness of Prevention and Mitigation

The social benefits of making hospitals and water systems more resilient to the effects of natural hazards are recognized but too rarely applied. On the economic side, mitigation also increases the investment capacity in the health sector by preventing losses and the need for reconstruction (PAHO and UN/ISDR 1996; Bitrán 1996).

The most compelling case for the cost-effectiveness of mitigation can be made during the planning phase for new installations, when costs of additional structural safety are minimal. Although the social benefits of prevention and risk management are more evident in the health sector than in others, further studies are needed to provide decision makers with quantified parameters of the economic benefits brought about by investment in risk management and disaster reduction.

PAHO and UN/ISDR (1996) studies indicate that such increased investment fluctuates between 4 and 8 percent of a hospital's local construction cost. When the value of services lost is added to the infrastructure loss, the additional investment is reduced to between 2 and 4 percent of direct and indirect losses observed. Even though this is a gross estimate that requires further research in other regions and types of health facilities, the figure is ratified by the estimated cost of reinforcement, which fluctuates but averages between US$2,000 and US$5,000 per bed, compared with the average cost of a new hospital bed of between US$100,000 and US$150,000 (at 1996 prices).

Prevention of chemical and radiation accidents can be a highly cost-effective expense that is normally absorbed by the respective industries. Respect for existing norms in the use of radiotherapy and diagnostic equipment and, once such equipment is decommissioned, its proper disposal reduces DALYs from accidents at a modest cost.

Mobilization of Resources

Funding for preparedness and response programs follows rules and procedures that are distinct from those applicable to development projects. Most donors maintain a specific office or department for humanitarian affairs with a separate budget line. Procedures are also streamlined for quick response to unexpected situations. Processing a request takes a matter of days in emergencies and takes months for preparedness or mitigation projects, but it can take years in typical development projects negotiated with donors or financial institutions.

From a ministry of health point of view, competition for disaster resources is with other sectors or humanitarian organizations, not within the sector (as it would be, for instance, with malaria or tuberculosis control projects).

Funding for Preparedness. "By strengthening our public health planning for natural disasters and disease outbreaks, we will be in a better position to care for our populations, regardless of the type of hazard that confronts our health departments" (Rottman 2003, 1). This message, addressed to the public health community in the United States, is even more pertinent for developing countries. Most humanitarian offices in more developed countries allocate a modest but increasing proportion of their funds for predisaster capacity building. The capacity of the ministries of health to secure directly nonreimbursable funding depends on the following:

- The existence of an established disaster program within the ministry, demonstrating a long-term commitment to health disaster preparedness.
- An ongoing dialogue with local representatives of donors and their prior involvement in disaster-related activities or meetings of the health sector.
- A realistic projection of concrete activities, taking into consideration the efforts of others, especially NGOs. One- or two-year training or capacity-building projects are more likely to be supported than those of longer duration that have recurrent costs or involve the purchase of equipment (radios, vehicles).
- The technical endorsement and support of WHO and other UN agencies.

A multisectoral preparedness component is also increasingly included in loans negotiated in the aftermath of disasters. Intended to strengthen the capacity of the civil protection agency, the funding is no substitute for local political commitment to assume recurrent expenses, the only guarantee of sustainability.

Resources for Emergency Response. The amount of external resources available for response, financial or material, is influenced by the type of hazard, geopolitical considerations, and the number of deaths (rather than that of survivors in need of assistance). Funding is channeled mostly through humanitarian NGOs, the Red Cross system, or multilateral organizations, rather than through national governments. Consequently, the priority of the health authorities, rather than to seek direct contributions to the ministry, should be to ensure that health needs are properly identified and adequately covered by those agencies benefiting from the donations. Ministries of health often can obtain indirect financial support for their own activities through UN projects.

Concentrating on several key factors will improve the flow of external resources toward health priorities:

- Issuing a rapid and reliable assessment of what is needed and what is not needed for the emergency response, rather than waiting for a detailed assessment of the physical damage.
- Focusing on tomorrow's emergency health problems. External response is unable to address today's short-lived problems.
- Keeping a long-term view. Funding for emergency response is limited to a few months, whereas the health problems caused by the disaster will stay much longer. Projects should offer sustained benefits beyond their conclusion.
- Recognizing shortcomings in governance when in contact with the many bilateral fact-finding or assessment missions coming to the disaster site.

Funding for Reconstruction. Funding for reconstruction is multisectoral and is often coordinated by an international financing institution (global or regional), together with a consortium of large donor countries. The health sector will compete with other social priorities and the "productive" sectors in an arena where the health burden (measured in DALYs) does not carry the same weight as economic factors. Success will depend on an exhaustive monetary valuation of the health damage, rapid formulation of projects, political support from the country's highest authorities, and technical support and endorsement of specialized UN agencies and larger NGOs.

Funding for Mitigation of Damage. Protecting the national capital investment of the health sector is primarily the responsibility of the country at risk. Development agencies or financial institutions may contribute only marginally to the actual cost of retrofitting installations or improving the design of new facilities.

Modest funding for pilot or demonstration prevention programs may be available from both the humanitarian and the development sources of donor countries. Humanitarian offices may support promotion of the concept, development of guidelines or studies on vulnerabilities, and training.

The health sector will benefit from close contacts with financial institutions, the ministry of foreign affairs, and other national ministries. Negotiations to ensure that new installations are able to withstand disasters must be initiated at the earliest opportunity, and the corresponding additional costs should be considered in the earliest stages of the project.

IMPLEMENTATION OF CONTROL STRATEGIES: LESSONS OF EXPERIENCE AND CHALLENGES FACED

All countries in Latin America and the Caribbean have established programs and structures for disaster risk management

within their ministries of health. Some lessons can be learned from this process:

- The occurrence of a major disaster in the country or its neighbor is the initial catalyst for health authorities to recognize that disasters represent public health risks that must be addressed in an institutionalized manner.
- Access to and support from the political level has determined the success or failure in coordinating the external and domestic health response.
- A multihazard program covering the entire health sector is most effective. Assigning responsibility for coordination and management among different technical departments according to the type of hazard (chemical or natural, for instance) does not work.
- A risk management program should cut across departments (medical care, epidemiology, water supply, sanitation, nutrition, and so forth) of the ministry of health and become sector wide.
- The synergy between normal development, preparedness, and disaster response activities should be recognized. Poor development practices increase vulnerability, whereas preparedness improves the attention to daily health challenges. Programs narrowly focused on operational response have generally failed.

In Asia, the Asian Disaster Preparedness Center also has documented some interesting experiences (http://www.adpc. ait.ac.th/).

THE RESEARCH AND DEVELOPMENT AGENDA

Disasters in any one country are relatively infrequent. In addition to being a dangerous temptation for the authorities to postpone preventive actions, this infrequency is an impediment for research and institutional memory. On one hand, the humanitarian culture tends to raise ethical questions on the role of observers at a time when action at all costs is expected. On the other hand, few health academicians wish to embark on projects when control groups and time for advance planning are unavailable.

Particularly encouraging are the increased numbers of publications and guidelines by UN organizations and NGOs and the trend toward organizing workshops on lessons learned a few months after a major disaster. These meetings of national experts and officials together with representatives from external actors are invaluable for identifying and sharing operational or institutional successes and failures for the collective benefit of other countries at risk.

Epidemiological Research

Most of the DALYs attributable to disasters occur immediately at the time of the disaster. Epidemiological research should, therefore, complement engineering studies to design better facilities and preparedness measures. After the initial disaster, basic questions need to be answered: How many secondary deaths and disabilities can actually be prevented by improving search and rescue and trauma care? How critical is the time factor in reducing DALY losses and assessing the effectiveness of foreign SAR and field hospitals teams? How can researchers objectively assess the risk of outbreak following disasters? In particular, how can they better differentiate between cases attributable to increased transmission and those resulting from improved surveillance and medical attention provided to the victims? What is needed are data to put to rest unquestioned assumptions and clichés. The alternative is to continue to divert scarce resources away from routine disease control programs and toward costly measures of doubtful effectiveness.

Strategic Research

Research is required that will compare the effectiveness of preparedness and response strategies and approaches:

- With respect to preparedness, how should researchers assess the effectiveness of training and coordination versus that of investing in hardware and stockpiles? For instance, will the accreditation of hospitals based on their safety and readiness improve their disaster performance?
- With respect to mitigation, how should limited funding for retrofitting health facilities be allocated? Is nonstructural mitigation a workable alternative in the absence of structural measures?
- With respect to response, what is the effect of international assistance in terms of reductions in DALY losses that could not be achieved locally? Is it contributing to strengthening the capacity of the developing countries? What type of humanitarian assistance has proven to be development friendly?
- Finally, how should researchers measure the effectiveness of preparedness or mitigation given the unpredictability of disasters?

Economic Research

Humanitarian response is resistant to concepts of cost-effectiveness. Economists should contribute to the comparative study of the immediate and long-term effects of external interventions versus less costly alternatives such as relying on local resources and building local capacity. A cost-benefit analysis of international medical interventions prior to and during a disaster situation is also overdue.

Economic assessment of the damage to the health sector remains focused on physical losses and fails to sufficiently consider the broader burden on a society caused by the loss of health services over a sustained period. Refining the existing methodology and developing quantitative indicators to estimate those indirect costs should be a research priority.

CONCLUSIONS

Natural hazards are not likely to decrease in the foreseeable future. Though geological events may occur independently of any human control, available data suggest that mankind plays a role in global climate. Technological hazards may also increase rapidly as a result of the unregulated development of industries in most countries and possibly the use of weapons-grade hazardous substances against civilian populations. An increase in the number of hazards should not mean that the resulting health burden will also increase. A sustained effort is needed to minimize risk, both by reducing vulnerability through prevention and mitigation and by increasing capacity through preparedness measures.

A Strategic Approach

The prime objective of a developing country is to develop. Emergencies and disasters have proven to be major obstacles and setbacks in the path toward sustainable development. Conversely, the shortcomings in development programs and institutions reduce the effectiveness of the health response in times of crisis. Development and disaster risk management cannot be addressed separately. Reducing risk is not a luxury reserved for more developed societies; it is a necessity in countries with fragile economies and health systems. It is clearly a public health priority.

Disasters, as any other public health problem, need to be addressed on a long-term and institutionalized basis through the establishment in the ministry of health of a program or department for prevention, mitigation, preparedness, and response for all types of disasters. Trends in Latin America suggest that such an approach in the context of sustainable development contributes to narrowing the gap in disaster-related deaths and disabilities (as measured by DALYs) between industrial and developing countries.

Disaster risk reduction is not merely a health issue. The economic and political dimensions should not, however, be allowed to overshadow the fundamental fact that disasters are, above all, human tragedies incompatible with the definition of *health* adopted by the WHO constitution. On one hand, the health sector should adapt and use the methodology of economic valuation of disaster impact as developed by ECLAC; on the other hand, the financial world should also learn to give equal consideration to the health burden (DALYs) in its decision making for development or reconstruction. For this to take place, health and humanitarian actors need to dramatically improve the availability of data.

Disaster risk reduction is not the exclusive domain of a few experts or officials. It is the collective responsibility of all disciplines and programs in the health sector, as well as a remarkable tool or gateway for collaboration with other sectors. Alone, the ministry of health cannot reduce the health burden or play its coordinating role in the response.

Disaster risk reduction is unlikely to produce immediate results. It requires sustained commitment over the years.

Learning from Errors

Learning from past disasters is difficult. At a national level, the relatively long periods between major disasters result in few decision makers having prior disaster management experience. At an international level, the frequent turnover of relief workers ensures that many of the actors are relatively inexperienced and susceptible to adopting myths and clichés, which are rarely challenged by the media and the academic world. It is time for an international initiative to identify the best practices, and it is time for affected countries and scientists to point out the inadequacies of responses.

Humanitarian health interventions, as any other health intervention, should be subject to cost-benefit reviews that compare their benefits in terms of DALY loss reduction to other alternatives, including a possible shift of international emphasis from immediate medical response to preparedness or rehabilitation projects.

Local health services are best situated to address the health consequences of disasters. They should be better prepared to do so. A formalized mechanism to transmit and share those lessons learned from past errors and to build the response capacity is required in the health sector.

Finally, the greatest potential for saving lives is in reducing the risks and the vulnerability through better infrastructure, land-use management, public awareness, and training.

The challenge in risk reduction is to sustain public support and political will in periods of calm. International organizations—WHO in particular—have a unique and critical role to play as advocates for a long-term approach to disaster risk management in the context of sustainable development.

ACKNOWLEDGMENTS

The field of disaster epidemiology, a concept first introduced in the early 1970s by M. F. Lechat of the University of Louvain in Belgium, is now calling on many disciplines and fields of knowledge. The authors express their gratitude to Caridad Borras for her contribution on radiological disasters and to Jean-Luc Poncelet, Karl Western, Guy Arcuri, Steve Devriendt, and Roberto Jovel for their advice, comments, and suggestions.

This chapter relies heavily on the successes and failures of the health sectors in Latin America and the Caribbean, a region where a sustained effort over 25 years, with the support of PAHO, WHO, and donor countries, traced the way to the reduction of risks from extreme events. This chapter owes greatly to a large number of experts and professionals in the health sector of those countries.

NOTES

1. In a nonnatural phenomenon, such as the attacks in New York on September 11, 2001, a similar risk has been detected and is perceived as a remnant potential long-term health risk similar to the effect of air contamination from ash from volcanoes.

2. Evidently these direct losses are not easy to determine in long-developing events (such as the ones associated with slow processes or climatic variability), because over time there will be overlapping damage, in contrast to the damage that occurs in sudden events such as hurricanes or earthquakes.

3. Data came from reports of the UN Office of Coordinator for Humanitarian Affairs (http://www.reliefweb.org), supplemented by authors' estimated costs for donors that did not report actual costs.

REFERENCES

Alexander, D. 1997. "The Study of Natural Disasters 1977–1997: Some Reflections on a Changing Field of Knowledge." *Disasters* 21 (4): 284–304.

Armenian, H. K., A. K. Melkonian, and A. P. Hovanesian. 1998. "Long-Term Mortality and Morbidity Related to Degree of Damage Following the Earthquake in Armenia." *American Journal of Epidemiology* 148 (11): 1077–84.

Armenian, H. K., A. Melkonian, E. Noji, and A. P. Hovanesian. 1997. "Deaths and Injuries Due to the Earthquake in Armenia: A Cohort Approach." *International Journal of Epidemiology* 26 (4): 806–13.

Bernstein, R. S., P. J. Baxter, and A. S. Buist. 1986. "Introduction to the Epidemiological Aspects of Explosive Volcanism." *American Journal of Public Health* 76 (Suppl.): 3–9.

Bitrán, D. 1996. "Impacto económico de los desastres naturales en la infraestructura de salud." Paper presented to the PAHO International Conference on Disaster Mitigation in Health Facilities, Mexico City, January. Document LC/MEX/L.2911. ECLAC, Mexico City.

Bouma, M. J., and C. Dye. 1997. "Cycles of Malaria Associated with El Niño in Venezuela." *Journal of the American Medical Association* 278 (21): 1772–74.

Buist, A. S., and R. S. Bernstein. 1986. "Health Effects of Volcanoes: An Approach to Evaluating the Health Effects of an Environmental Hazard." *American Journal of Public Health* 76 (Suppl.):1–2.

Chang, S. E., and C. Chamberlin. 2004. "Assessing the Role of Lifeline Systems in Community Disaster Resilience." In *Research Progress and Accomplishments 2003–2004, Multidisciplinary Center for Earthquake Engineering Research.* Buffalo, NY: 87–94.

de Ville de Goyet, C. 2001. "Earthquakes in El Salvador." *Revista Panamericana de Salud Publica* 9 (2): 107–13.

de Ville de Goyet, C., E. Acosta, P. Sabbat, and E. Pluut. 1996. "SUMA: A Management Tool for Post-Disaster Relief Supplies." *World Health Statistics Quarterly* 49 (3–4): 189–94.

ECLAC (Economic Commission for Latin America and the Caribbean). 1998. *Análisis Costo-Efectividad en la Mitigación de Daños de Desastres Naturales sobre Infraestructura Social.* Document LC/MEX/R.643. Mexico City: ECLAC.

————. 2003. *Handbook for Estimating the Socio-economic and Environmental Effects of Disaster.* LC/MEX/G.5. Mexico City: ECLAC.

FEMICA (Federación de Municipios del Itsmo Centro Americano). 2003. "Acueducto Orosi: Una experiencia regional sobre implementación de medidas de prevención y mitigación," Paper presented at the 10th meeting of the Network for Decentralization and Municipal Development on the topic Local Risk Management: A Challenge for the Development of Municipalities in Central America. Antigua, Guatemala, October 21–24.

Howard, M. J., J. C. Brillman, and F. M. Burkle. 1996. "Infectious Disease Emergencies in Disasters." *Emergency Medicine Clinics in North America* 14 (2): 413–28.

IDB (Inter-American Development Bank). 1999. "Hurricane Mitch: Women's Needs and Contributions." Document SOC-115, IDB, Washington, DC.

IFRC (International Federation of Red Cross and Red Crescent Societies). 2000. *World Disasters Report 2000: Focus on Public Health.* Geneva: IFRC.

————. 2003. *World Disasters Report 2003: Focus on Ethics in Aid.* Geneva: IFRC.

Kirigia, J. M., L. G. Sambo, W. Aldis, and G. Mwabu. 2004. "Impact of Disaster-Related Mortality on Gross Domestic Product in the WHO African Region." *BMC Emergency Medicine* 4 (1): 1. http://www.biomedicalcentral.com/1471-227x/4/1.

Malilay, J., M. G. Real, A. Ramirez Vanegas, E. Noji, and T. Sinks. 1996. "Public Health Surveillance after a Volcanic Eruption: Lessons from Cerro Negro, Nicaragua, 1992." *Bulletin of the Pan American Health Organization* 30 (3): 218–25.

Morgan, O. 2004. "Infectious Disease Risks from Dead Bodies Following Natural Disasters." *Revista Panamericana de Salud Publica* 15 (5): 307–12.

National Research Council. 1999. *From Monsoons to Microbes: Understanding the Ocean's Role in Human Health.* Washington, DC: National Academy Press.

PAHO (Pan American Health Organization). 1982. *Disaster Reports Number 2: Jamaica, St. Vincent, and Dominica.* Washington, DC: PAHO.

————. 1985. "Earthquake in Mexico." In *Disaster Chronicles No. 3.* Washington, DC: PAHO.

————. 1998. "El Niño and Its Impact on Health." Official document CE/122/10. PAHO, Washington, DC.

————. 1999. "Huracanes Georges y Mitch, 1998." In *Cronicas de Desastres No. 7.* Washington, DC: PAHO.

————. 2002a. "Protección de la salud mental en situaciones de desastres y emergencias." In *Serie de Manuales y Guías sobre Desastres No. 1.* Washington, DC: PAHO.

————. 2002b "Terremotos en El Salvador 2001." In *Crónicas de Desastres No. 11.* Washington, DC: PAHO.

PAHO and UN/ISDR (Pan American Health Organization and United Nations/International Strategy for Disaster Reduction). 1996. *Lecciones aprendidas en América Latina de mitigación de desastres en instalaciones de salud: Aspectos de costo-efectividad.* Washington, DC: PAHO.

PAHO and WHO (Pan American Health Organization and World Health Organization). 2000. "Mitigación de desastres en instalaciones de salud: Aspectos estructurales." In *Mitigación de desastres en instalaciones de salud—Material técnico y de capacitacion* (CD-ROM). Washington, DC: PAHO and WHO.

PAHO (Pan American Health Organization), WHO (World Health Organization), World Bank, and ProVention Consortium. 2004. *Guidelines for Vulnerability Reduction in the Design of New Health Facilities.* Washington, DC: PAHO and World Bank.

Poncelet, J.-L. 1997. "Earthquakes in Latin America: The Role of Cities in Disaster Management." In *Earthquakes and People's Health: Proceeding of a WHO Symposium, Kobe, Japan, January 27–30.* Geneva: WHO. http://www.helid.desastres.net.

Rottman, S. 2003. "Director's Message." *UCLA Center for Public Health and Disasters Newsletter* 9 (Fall): 1.

UNHCR (United Nations High Commissioner for Refugees). 1998. *Handbook for Emergency Situations.* Geneva: UNHCR.

UN/ISDR (United Nations/International Strategy for Disaster Reduction). 2004. *Living with Risk: A Global Review of Disaster Reduction Initiatives.* Vol 1. Geneva: UN/ISDR.

WHO (World Health Organization). 1992. *Assessing the Health Consequences of Major Chemical Incidents—Epidemiological Approaches.* Geneva: WHO.

————. 1994. *Health Laboratory Facilities in Emergencies and Disaster Situations.* Geneva: WHO. http://www.helid.desastres.net.

————. 1996. *Health Consequences of the Chernobyl Accident: Results of the IPHECA Pilot Projects and Related National Programmes.* Geneva: WHO.

————. 2002. *Reducing Risks, Promoting Healthy Life: World Health Report 2002.* Geneva: WHO.

WHO and PAHO (World Health Organization and Pan American Health Organization). 2003. *Guidelines for the Use of Foreign Field Hospitals Following Sudden-Impact Natural Disasters.* Washington, DC: WHO and PAHO. http://www.paho.org/English/DD/PED/FieldH.htm.

Chapter **62**

Control and Eradication

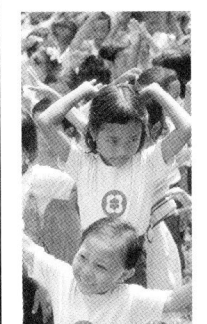

Mark Miller, Scott Barrett, and D. A. Henderson

The Controversy: Control or Eradication?

We cannot refrain altogether from examining the roots of this controversy if only because the extreme views for and against eradication have exerted and are still exerting a . . . highly detrimental influence on public health practice.

—P. Yekutiel, *Eradication of Infectious Diseases: A Critical Study*

Eradication of an infectious disease is an extraordinary goal. Its possibility became apparent as soon as Edward Jenner demonstrated an ability to provide immunity to smallpox. Writing in 1801, Jenner observed that, through broad application of vaccination, "it now becomes too manifest to admit of controversy that the annihilation of the Small Pox, the most dreadful scourge of the human species, must be the result of this practice" (Jenner 1801). Louis Pasteur claimed that it was "within the power of man to eradicate infection from the earth" (Dubos and Dubos 1953). And yet, by and large, public health has proceeded with more modest goals of local and regional disease control. Notable successes have occurred. Indeed, some diseases now thought of as "tropical" were previously endemic in temperate climates. Systematic application of hygiene, sanitation, environmental modification, vector control, and vaccines have led, in many countries, to the interruption of transmission of microbes causing such diseases as cholera, malaria, and yellow fever.

Intensive efforts to eliminate breeding sites of the yellow fever mosquito vector, *Aedes aegypti*, interrupted transmission of this disease in Havana in 1901 and throughout Cuba soon thereafter. Subsequently, yellow fever and malaria were able to be controlled in Panama, thus permitting construction of the Panama Canal. In 1915, the Rockefeller Foundation launched an effort to eradicate the disease worldwide. Transmission appeared to have ceased in the Americas by 1928, but then cases reappeared, and by 1932, it became clear that a nonhuman

endemic focus was serving to reinfect areas otherwise free of yellow fever. In the 1930s, F. L. Soper set out to eradicate the *Aedes aegypti* vector from the Americas. By 1961, Soper reported that he had largely succeeded except for the United States, where the program received little support. By the 1980s, *Aedes aegypti* had become reestablished in Central and South America.

In 1953, Brock Chisholm, the first director-general of the World Health Organization (WHO), tried to persuade the World Health Assembly (WHA) to undertake smallpox eradication, but a number of countries objected on the grounds that eradication was not technically feasible. Instead, in 1955, under the leadership of his successor, Marcolino Candau, WHO began a global effort to eradicate malaria primarily by means of household spraying of DDT. The relatively sophisticated science of malaria control was abandoned in favor of this simplistic technology (Jeffrey 1976). Despite an expenditure of more than US$2 billion, the effort failed.

Even while the malaria eradication effort was under way, the Soviet Union, in 1958, proposed to the WHA that smallpox be eradicated. A resolution to this effect was offered in 1959 and passed unanimously. However, the resolution provided little international funding or support. Over the next seven years, disease transmission was interrupted in some 30 countries in Africa, Asia, and South America, but endemic smallpox persisted in the Indian subcontinent, Indonesia, most of Sub-Saharan Africa, and Brazil. WHO launched an intensified effort in 1967 to eradicate the disease within a decade. This new resolution included an annual budget of US$2.4 million, to be paid according to the WHO scale of assessments. The resolution passed by the narrowest of margins, but a reinvigorated effort was soon under way and paved the way for a historic public health achievement (Henderson 1988). Following an extraordinary worldwide effort, the last case of smallpox was isolated in October 1977, and the disease was certified as being eradicated in 1979, 170 years after Edward Jenner first dreamed of that possibility. Understanding how and why smallpox eradication succeeded is essential to the study of control and eradication.

The smallpox success was inspirational, even though the leaders of WHO's smallpox eradication effort cautioned that, among all the diseases that might be considered candidates for eradication, smallpox was unique (Fenner and others 1988) and that they foresaw no other disease as a candidate for eradication (Henderson 1982). At a meeting convened by the Fogarty International Center of the National Institutes of Health in 1980, scientists, public health officials, and policy makers discussed the merits of eradicating other diseases, with schistosomiasis, dracunculiasis, poliomyelitis, and measles identified as possible candidates (Henderson 1998a). However, no consensus was reached at that time on moving forward with any of those diseases.

Poliomyelitis became the next principal target when mass vaccination campaigns, proposed by Albert Sabin (1991), proved remarkably successfully in Cuba and Brazil. In 1985, an American Health Organization coordinated campaign was launched to interrupt poliovirus transmission in the Americas by 1991, and this effort succeeded. Some believed that global eradication might be possible, although others were concerned that the far less developed infrastructure of health, transportation, and communications services in many parts of Asia and Africa would make it an unachievable task. In 1988, the WHA adopted a resolution to eradicate polio, but at that time, a longer-term strategy for ending polio vaccination was neither formulated nor agreed on by the public health and scientific community.

The WHA has adopted only one other resolution to eradicate a disease—guinea worm, or dracunculiasis. The eradication of this disease can be achieved by applying simple technologies for providing water that is free of the vector copepod and parasite and for treatment of patients with the disease. This eradication program has made steady progress but has been hampered in part by civil and political unrest and lack of program priority because of low mortality and low incidence in some remaining endemic areas. However, given the environmental restriction of the parasite to rural tropical areas and its relatively low transmissibility, eventual global eradication seems within reach.

One other case—that of measles—is worth noting. A number of public health authorities have raised the possibility of eradicating that disease. In the Americas, spurred on by the success of regional cessation of transmission of wild poliovirus, eventual consensus was reached to intensify measles control efforts, primarily through surveillance and periodic pulse application of measles vaccine in national campaigns. As a consequence, transmission of measles virus was temporarily interrupted in the Americas on several occasions but reestablished again by importations (CDC 1998a). Although the U.S. Centers for Disease Control and Prevention (CDC) and WHO have advocated extending measles "elimination" through vaccination campaigns and second-dose opportunities to other regions (Biellik and others 2002; CDC 1998a, 1998b, 1999a, 1999b, 2003d, 2004b, 2004d, 2004f), the intensive control efforts required to break transmission of this highly infectious agent make global eradication unlikely at this time.

DEFINITIONS

Yekutiel (1980, 5–8) provides an excellent treatise on the concept of *eradication*, which includes a summary of the multiple definitions that have been formulated (Andrews and Langmuir 1963; Cockburn 1961, 1963; Payne 1963a, 1963b; Spînu and Biberi-Moroianu 1969). A conference devoted to eradication held in Dahlem, Germany, in 1997 (Dowdle and Hopkins 1998) set out to provide precise definitions for *control, elimination, eradication,* and *extinction* in a biological, economic, and political context (Dowdle 1998, 1999; Ottesen and others 1998); however, a number of eminent public health officials (Cochi and others 1998; de Quadros 2001; Goodman and others 1998b; Henderson 1998b; Salisbury 1998) challenged these definitions at two subsequent meetings at the CDC (Goodman and others 1998a, 1998b) and the U.S. Institute of Medicine (Knobler, Lederberg, and Pray 2001).

Unfortunately, broadly accepted, standard definitions for key concepts pertaining to disease control and eradication do not exist in the literature. Making matters more confusing, certain of the concepts have been given names that are part of our everyday language and so are easily misinterpreted by nonspecialists as meaning something different from the meanings understood by those who are preoccupied with eradication programs. Most unfortunate is the all too casual use of the words *elimination* and *eradication* to promote programs that cannot reasonably be expected to achieve the promise implicit in these words. Moreover, the two words themselves are commonly used interchangeably.

Control

Two concepts are central to this chapter: control and eradication. By *control*, we mean a public policy intervention that restricts the circulation of an infectious agent beyond the level that would result from spontaneous, individual behaviors to protect against infection (Barrett 2004).

Although control is a range rather then a level, a particular level of control may be an aim of policy. Because every choice entails consequences, choice of the "optimal" level of control requires economic analysis. *Optimal* here is defined in relation to the model that gives rise to the result. Control is local and so needs to be looked at from the local perspective. Because one country's (or region's) control may affect other countries (regions), a global perspective exists as well. The level of control that is optimal for one country (region) may not be optimal from the perspective of the world as a whole. Thus, a need exists to distinguish between, say, a locally optimal level of control and one that is globally optimal.

Finally, control requires ongoing intervention. Sustaining a given level of control requires an annual expenditure.

Eradication

Eradication differs from control in that it is global. The term denotes the certified total absence of human cases, the absence of a reservoir for the organism in nature, and absolute containment of any infectious source. Eradication permits control interventions to stop or at least to be curtailed significantly. Finally, eradication is binary. Control levels can vary, but a disease is either certified as eradicated or not.

Every disease can be controlled, even if only by using simple measures, such as quarantine. The ultimate achievement of control is eradication. But not every disease that can be controlled can be eradicated. Very few diseases, in fact, are potential candidates for eradication. The criteria for the feasibility for eradication as a preference over control are discussed in the section titled "Economic Considerations."

Elimination

Control and eradication are the essential concepts, but two other terms bear mention. The first is *elimination*. Some who are concerned with eradication programs have explicitly defined this term to denote the cessation of transmission of an organism throughout a country or region. In contrast, *eradication* is defined as a global achievement. Like control, elimination is location-specific and would require ongoing interventions to be sustained in order to prevent reemergence of the disease from microbe importations.

Two problems exist with the term *elimination*. First, it has been used to describe different phenomena, not just that described in the definition given above. For example, some public health officials have promoted programs aimed at "eliminating a disease as a public health threat," which is interpreted to mean reducing incidence to an "acceptable" level but not necessarily to zero. This usage is very different from the one outlined above and is almost certain to be misunderstood. Second, the definition of the word *elimination* in common use, as applied to disease control, is indistinguishable from eradica-

tion. The 1993 edition of the *New Shorter Oxford English Dictionary,* for example, defines *eliminate* as to "remove, get rid of, do away with, cause to exist no longer." This same dictionary defines *eradicate* as "pull up or out by the roots, uproot, remove or destroy completely, extirpate, get rid of." This ambiguity invites misunderstanding among those not intimately involved in an eradication effort. For purposes of clarity, we seldom use the term *elimination* in this chapter and then only to signify control measures sufficient to interrupt microbe transmission in a specified area.

Extinction

Finally, the literature sometimes refers to *extinction* as a possible policy goal. In the context of infectious disease control, the concept is problematic for two reasons. First, proving that an organism has become extinct is impossible. To do so would require demonstrating not only that the organism no longer exists in nature but also that it no longer exists in any controlled environment—a practical impossibility. Second, de novo synthesis of viral agents from published genomes (Cello, Paul, and Wimmer 2002) now put the concept in peril, although much research remains to be done in this area. Extinction, in the context of infectious diseases, may no longer be irreversible.

Clearly, policy making will be improved by stating the goal of any particular intervention in precise language.

FRAMEWORKS FOR ERADICATION

Numerous issues need to be considered in planning expanded control measures that lead, possibly, to regional cessation of transmission or global eradication of disease. These complex issues will be further examined in the chapter.

Scientific Considerations

Scientific considerations include the nature of potential reservoirs for disease-causing microbes or their vectors, technologies available for interrupting disease transmission, changes in host capabilities to deter infections and disease, and satisfactory containment of organisms in laboratories.

Geographic and Environmental Controls. The limit of endemicity for microbes and their associated diseases is determined in part by their ability to exist in nature outside the human host. Both geographic and temporal variations determine the ecological niche of microbes, resulting in variable annual incidence rates throughout the world. This niche limitation is further extended to intermediary vectors and hosts in complex biological systems. Natural environmental barriers also may isolate the habitats of helminths. Infectious agents that are not limited to an environmentally restricted intermediary host or those that have longer latent periods, thereby allowing translocation, may have a global pattern of distribution. Examples include the highly transmissible viral agents such as measles, rubella, influenza, and varicella. Although these agents are not geographically constrained, their transmission patterns are directly and indirectly influenced by seasonal environmental factors and population-based immunity.

Potential Reservoirs. A microbe and associated disease can not be eradicated if the microbe is capable of persisting and multiplying in a reservoir. Microbes that thrive in nonhuman species may reemerge if control efforts cease, thus leaving human populations susceptible. Similarly, if the infectiousness of a human is long lived or could lead to potential recrudescence, surveillance efforts would have to continue as long as the last individual remained potentially capable of transmitting infection, as would be the case with tuberculosis or hepatitis B infection.

Transmissibility. The inherent rate of a microbe's ability to cause secondary infections is defined by an organism's reproductive rate in a fully susceptible (R_0) and partially susceptible (R) population. The reproductive rate of organisms that infect individuals only once because of durable immunity is inversely proportional to the average age of infection in an endemic area. Agents that cause childhood infections, such as viral respiratory agents, are far more transmissible than helminths and subsequently require more intensive control efforts to interrupt transmission.

Natural Resistance to Reinfection. Many natural infections induce long-lived immunity to reinfection. Although the most commonly used vaccines have been available for fewer than 50 years—less than the lifetime of an individual—they, too, are assumed to offer long-lasting immunity. Because eradication depends on reducing susceptible populations in potentially endemic areas, long-lived protection through immunization or natural disease is important to successful programs.

Laboratory Containment. Laboratory specimens containing the organism targeted for eradication could serve as reservoirs. Considerable effort may be necessary to ensure their maximum security. That these microbes may be inconspicuous in specimens collected for other purposes poses special challenges. This situation is especially true for the poliomyelitis virus, which may be found in many stool specimens collected for studies completely unrelated to current poliomyelitis eradication efforts.

Operational Considerations

Optimization of control requires a fundamental appreciation of the biological systems that govern the ecology of microbes and their intermediary and human hosts. The reproductive rate, R, is influenced by many local factors, including population density (of vectors, intermediary hosts, and humans) and other environmentally determined conditions, all highly variable throughout the world. For a disease to be controlled to stop transmission, the intervention-altered reproductive rate must be maintained below 1.0. At the same time, all reservoirs of the responsible microbe must be controlled.

Three main components of possible eradication programs are

- surveillance, including environmental sampling where appropriate and clinical testing
- interventions, including vaccination and chemotherapy or chemoprophylaxis or both
- environmental controls and certification of eradication.

Each of these components must be undertaken at local, community, national, regional, and global levels. Eradication differs from control in that it is expected to be permanent. Success depends on having adequate surveillance to identify potentially infectious persons and on stopping transmission before infection of a new cohort of susceptible persons arises as a result of births, migration, or the waning effectiveness of prophylactic measures.

Disease Surveillance. Effective surveillance requires a sensitive system to detect the presence of microbes within the environment, intermediary hosts, and clinical cases. Surveillance and response systems need to be more efficient than the rate of transmission of the targeted agent. As eradication progresses, the sensitivity of detection systems must be steadily enhanced to detect all existing foci. Nonclinical or latent infections pose formidable barriers to eradication efforts. Operationally, the need for near-perfect sensitivity comes at the expense of lower specificity. Thousands of skin lesions from suspected smallpox patients were tested in reference laboratories during confirmation of smallpox eradication, and tens of thousands of stool specimens are being examined for poliovirus. Highly sensitive systems used to detect measles cases in the Americas began to identify a greater proportion of rubella and parvovirus infections because of the nonspecific surveillance of rash illness. Such findings are important because the identification of other diseases that mimic the targeted disease can lead to a misdirection of resources. However, the ability to detect such similar clinical cases can serve as a proxy measure for the adequacy of surveillance. For example, identification of a minimum incidence of cases of acute flaccid paralysis that is not related to polio has served as an indicator of adequate efforts of case finding for polio.

Interventions. Interventions to block transmission of the targeted infectious agent should be easy to deploy and adaptable to diverse conditions, given the global goal of eradication. Cost considerations and local acceptance of the required sacrifices (both short and long term) are crucial for success. Interventions may be designed for environmental control of microbes, isolation (quarantine) of clinically infectious individuals to limit their contacts with susceptible persons, treatment of clinical cases to limit the duration of infectiousness, or reduction in the infected pool of individuals through immuno- or chemoprophylaxis.

Certification. The last tool for eradication is a certification process whereby independent, respected parties certify the absence of disease transmission or the existence of any specific microbe in an uncontrolled reservoir, including laboratories (Breman and Arita 1980). Although certification can be implemented on a regional basis, it must ultimately be done globally. Certification is one of the greatest challenges in any eradication effort, given the exceedingly great difficulty of verifying a negative finding in a reasonably short period of time. When certification is completed, curtailment of control measures should be possible.

Strengthening control efforts sufficiently to achieve eradication is a difficult and expensive task. It requires that scaling up of such efforts occur over a wide area—at the community, national, regional, and global levels. Its efficacy depends heavily on the adequacy of local financial and human resources, as well as on a broad range of logistical factors.

Economic Considerations

Control and eradication programs have many economic dimensions: private versus social net benefits, short-term versus long-term net benefits, and local versus international net benefits. Such interventions also have implications for existing public health programs.

Private versus Social Net Benefits. Individuals have private incentives to protect themselves from disease—by means of vaccination, for example. But when individuals protect themselves—when they elect to be vaccinated—they offer a measure of protection to others by helping limit the spread of infection. In brief, the social benefit of vaccination is greater than the private benefit alone. As more people become vaccinated, the *marginal* private and social benefit of vaccination— that is, the benefit of vaccinating an additional susceptible person—declines. The marginal private benefit is likely to fall because, as more people are vaccinated, the probability of a susceptible person becoming infected falls. The marginal social benefit is likely to fall for the same reason and for one other: as more people become protected, the total number of susceptible persons falls. The marginal social benefit of vaccination falls sharply at the *critical* level of immunization—the level at which

herd immunity is conferred on all susceptible persons. When a population is immunized to this level, a disease ceases to be endemic, and imported infections cannot spark an epidemic.

This level is determined by the epidemiology of a disease, but whether it pays to vaccinate to this level depends on the economics, and the economics depend in turn on the social costs and not only the social benefits of vaccination. These costs consist of the direct costs of producing, distributing, and administering a vaccine. The economics depend also on the costs borne by the individuals who are vaccinated, such as those incurred by individuals who experience vaccine complications. The proportionate costs of reaching people who live in remote areas and those who are at special risk, such as migrants and the homeless, increase as the fraction of the population vaccinated increases.

The economics of varying levels of disease control depend on the relationship between the marginal social benefits and the marginal social costs of vaccination. As vaccination levels increase, the marginal social benefits of vaccination fall, whereas the marginal social costs rise. Social welfare is maximized where these two relations intersect, which might be called the "optimal" level of vaccination—a level that may or may not achieve cessation of transmission or eradication.

Short-Term versus Long-Term Net Benefits. Control programs require ongoing intervention. Sustaining a given level of protection requires that, over time, a certain proportion of new susceptible persons be vaccinated. Eradication differs from control in being permanent. The economics of eradication must therefore take account of long-term benefits as well as short-term costs.

The long-term benefits of eradication consist of avoided future infections and vaccination costs—a dividend. To calculate this benefit, one projects future infection and vaccination levels in the absence of eradication, attaches values to these, and discounts them. If this sum exceeds the costs of eradication, then eradication enhances social well-being, and it therefore should be undertaken.

In deciding on the benefits of eradication, the cost of future infections and vaccination should ideally be compared with the best alternative to eradication: the level of optimal control (Barrett and Hoel 2003).

The costs of eradication must also take into account ongoing surveillance requirements, laboratory containment, and perhaps the maintenance of stockpiles of vaccine in the chance event of disease reemergence. From an economic perspective, attractive candidates for eradication are those diseases that some countries have themselves targeted for interruption of transmission nationally or regionally.

Local versus International Net Benefits. Control differs from eradication in another important way. Control refers to location-specific interventions. Eradication, by contrast, is global. In economic terms, eradication is a global public good. No country can be excluded from the benefit of eradication, and no country's consumption of that benefit diminishes the amounts available to other countries. Control, by contrast, supplies only a local public good.

Eradication requires a global effort. A disease can be eradicated only if microbe transmission ceases everywhere. This spatial dimension to eradication is of fundamental importance because no world government can implement an eradication policy; the WHA can declare its support for eradication, but WHO does not have the power to enforce the execution of a national program in support of that goal. The outcome experienced by any country depends not only on whether the country itself eliminates the disease within its borders but also on whether all other countries do so. Indeed, eradication is a weakest-link public good.

Whether eradication is achieved depends on the level of control adopted by the country that undertakes the least control. In practical terms, any country in which disease is endemic can prevent eradication from being achieved. In 2004, the global polio eradication initiative, after investing more than US$3 billion and involving some 20 million volunteers over a period of 16 years, was placed at risk of failure by the actions of one local administration. In the Kano state of Nigeria, local leaders claimed that the polio vaccine was tainted with the AIDS virus and sterility drugs and declined to participate in a national immunization day program. The European Union then declined to pay for the national program in Nigeria, believing the money would be wasted (Roberts 2004). One consequence was the subsequent spread of polio to nine formerly polio-free countries. Concerted efforts by WHO later persuaded local leaders in Nigeria to rejoin global efforts, but special vaccination programs had to be launched over a population area of more than 300 million persons. This situation dramatically illustrated the vulnerabilities inherent in a weakest-link public good.

What are the incentives for states to participate in an eradication effort? To begin, assume that countries are symmetric, meaning that all countries have the same benefits and costs of control. Assume as well that eradication is feasible. Four possible situations then exist (Barrett 2003):

- First, the global net benefit of eradication may be negative—the cumulative programmatic costs outweigh the net present value of the cumulative benefits. In this case, elimination would also yield a negative net benefit to every country, and so no country would eliminate the disease.
- Second, the global net benefit of eradication may be so large that each country would choose to eliminate the disease even if others did not. In this case, all countries would eliminate the disease, and the disease would therefore be

eradicated. In these two cases, no need exists for an international policy.

- Third, each country may have an incentive to eliminate a disease only if all other countries have eliminated it. In this case, achieving global eradication requires coordination. Here a role exists for international policy, but all that is required is for each country to be assured that all others will eliminate the disease.
- Finally, and noting that the "last" country to eliminate a disease would get just a fraction of the global dividend from eradication, under some circumstances no incentive may exists for this country to eliminate the disease—even if all other countries have done so and even if the entire world would be better off if it did. This case is the most worrisome, because implementation of the efficient outcome would likely require enforcement.

All this hypothesizing assumes that countries are symmetric, and of course they are not. Some countries gain less from control and would gain less from eradication than others. Some are unable to implement an elimination program, even if they would very much like it to succeed. In these situations, achieving an eradication goal will require international financing and technical assistance, with the countries that benefit most from eradication compensating the other countries for the costs of eradicating the disease. National and international reproach are often expressed if a country lags in its eradication efforts. International financing has been a key element in all eradication programs.

We have thus far looked at eradication from the perspective of only the self-interests of states. But eradication also has implications for development. In particular, eradication has two advantages over control programs. The first is that the rich countries may gain directly if the goal is achieved, giving them a vested interest in ensuring that the goal is achieved. The second is that eradication is permanent, making an investment in eradication financially sustainable. This second advantage is important because financial sustainability has proved to be a key problem for disease control programs in developing countries (Kremer and Miguel 2004).

Vertical versus Horizontal Programs. Control and eradication programs cannot be viewed in isolation. All programs have implications for the delivery of comprehensive primary care services. An important question is whether targeted, or so-called vertical, programs draw critical resources away from other health care programs or whether they serve instead to augment competence and capacity. The evidence is mixed.

Evidence suggests that disease-specific systems can serve to expand polyvalent services (Aylward and others 1998). Smallpox eradication, for example, gave many national governments the confidence to introduce the Expanded Program on

Immunization, with the ability to deliver vaccines and micronutrients in routine schedules and through national campaigns. However, other evidence suggests that some vaccination programs have adversely affected primary health services (Steinglass 2001; Taylor, Cutts, and Taylor 1997) and may have even increased costs. Implementation of international initiatives can also expose conflicts of priorities. The polio eradication initiative, for example, has successfully vaccinated children in the poorest of countries against this disease, but in some of these countries it has failed to timely include the co-administration of measles and other common childhood vaccines, which would have had a much greater effect on child mortality.

DISEASE-SPECIFIC CASE STUDIES

In this section, we apply the reasoning developed previously to provide an empirical analysis of the three most recent eradication programs—smallpox and the two ongoing programs, poliomyelitis and dracunculiasis.

Smallpox

As noted before, smallpox eradication was achieved in October 1977, 11 years after the intensified program began. Following implementation of a rigorous certification procedure, the WHA declared smallpox eradicated in 1980.

Fenner and others (1988) have estimated the annual benefits of smallpox eradication to developing and industrial countries (see table 62.1). These aggregate estimates, obtained by prorating estimates of the benefits of eradication for India and the United States to all developing and industrial countries, respectively, suggest that developing countries benefited more from smallpox eradication than industrial countries. Qualitatively, a consistent picture emerges: smallpox eradication was not only an extraordinary investment for the world; it was also an investment that benefited every country, rich and poor alike.

When the eradication effort began, smallpox was no longer endemic in most industrial countries. Nonetheless, these countries needed to maintain populationwide immunity under the threat of possible imported cases from endemic countries. They would gain from eradication not only through the cessation of vaccination and its associated costs but also by being able to decrease the number of quarantine inspectors at ports of entry and by averting costs of care related to the adverse events from this live vaccine.

The still-endemic countries would also save vaccination costs, although most were vaccinating only a comparatively small proportion of their populations. The greater benefit to them was the avoided cost of disease, including the extraordinary death toll. A number of developing countries had accorded smallpox prevention a high priority, as was evidenced by the number that succeeded in interrupting transmission without international assistance. This list includes China, which was not a member of WHO at the time the eradication effort commenced.

Indeed, and as shown in table 62.1, the still-endemic countries contributed an estimated two-thirds of the US$298 million cost of eradication. International sources funded the balance. If the latter cost is interpreted as the incremental cost of achieving eradication, the benefit-cost ratio of global smallpox eradication was over 450:1, a singularly high figure. Even including the expenditure by endemic countries, the benefit of eradication exceeded the cost by an unusually large amount.

Brilliant (1985) calculated the annual costs of the smallpox eradication campaign for India to be about US$17 million per year, including indirect costs (lost productivity caused by adverse reactions to vaccination) and opportunity costs (health workers being diverted from other programs). These costs were only a fraction of the annual benefits of eradication to India, which, by Brilliant's calculations, were US$150 million. The benefit estimates by Fenner and others (1988) are much larger, and those of Ramaiah (1976) are smaller, but all three studies draw the same (qualitative) conclusion: smallpox eradication was a good investment for India. Basu, Ježek, and Ward (1979, 312) present estimates identical to those in Ramaiah (1976), but without giving attribution.

Originally, India had decided to undertake a smallpox program just one month after the WHA voted to eradicate the disease globally in 1959. The attempt failed, however, largely for administrative reasons (Basu, Ježek, and Ward 1979; Brilliant

Table 62.1 Benefits and Costs of Smallpox Eradication
(Millions of U.S. dollars)

	Annual amount
Beneficiary	
India	722
United States	150
All developing countries	1,070
All industrial countries	350
Total annual benefit	1,420
Expenditure	
Total international, on eradication	98
Total national, by endemic countries	200
Combined total, on eradication	298
Benefit-cost ratio	
International expenditure	483:1
Combined total expenditure	159:1

Source: Adapted from Fenner and others 1988.

1985; Fenner and others 1988). Essentially, India had an economic incentive to control smallpox on its own (Brilliant 1985, 33) but lacked organizational capacity and an effective strategy for achieving this goal. Note, however, that India had other health priorities, including family planning. According to Brilliant (1985, 33), "for India's health planners, occupied then by emergencies and competing political demands on scarce resources, the long-term benefits from disease eradication were not a great motivation. Health planners are sensitive to immediate political realities, and the benefits of smallpox eradication would be realized only at some future time when the $3 million annual expenditures for smallpox could be applied to other health problems. In the meantime, however, the cost of putting so many scarce resources into one program rather than into many health needs was high."

Table 62.2 provides estimates of the benefits of smallpox eradication to the United States. The total benefit of eradication to the United States is about the same order of magnitude as India's, but the breakdown is different. Whereas India benefited mainly from avoided infections, the United States benefited mainly from avoided vaccinations. By the time the eradication program was launched, the United States had already interrupted smallpox transmission, but vaccination was costly, both in economic and human health terms (a small number of people died every year from infections arising from the live vaccine). Defending the nation from imported infections imposed additional costs.

In health terms, smallpox eradication saved millions of lives; in economic terms, it yielded a benefit many times greater than the cost. Identifying another investment that has yielded comparable returns and has benefited every country is difficult. One reason that the economics of smallpox eradication were so favorable is that all countries had strong incentives to join in

the eradication of the disease. A huge organizational effort, but only a relatively small incremental cost, was needed to achieve eradication. The specter of global terrorism has recently caused some countries to prepare themselves for a possible smallpox attack by stockpiling vaccine. Although such actions reduce the benefits of eradication, the economics remain favorable.

Smallpox, however, was a special case. Many attributes of the disease and the vaccine favored eradication. The vaccine was heat stable and required only a single dose to protect a person for a period of at least 5 to 10 years. Vaccination was easily performed and protected immediately on application. Every individual who became infected exhibited a typical, easily recognized rash, thus permitting accurate surveillance without recourse to laboratory diagnosis. The disease spread slowly so that transmission could readily be stopped by isolating the patient and vaccinating contacts within the area.

Poliomyelitis

The polio eradication program, launched by the WHA in 1988, has made substantial progress (CDC 2003a, 2003b, 2003c, 2004a, 2004c, 2004e, 2004g, 2005). The incidence of paralytic poliomyelitis in children fell by more than 99 percent, from an estimated 1,000 cases per day worldwide in 1988 to fewer than 4 cases per day in 2003. The number of poliomyelitis-endemic countries also fell, from 125 in 1988 to just 6 by 2003 (Afghanistan, the Arab Republic of Egypt, India, Niger, Nigeria, and Pakistan). This laudable reduction was the result of repetitive vaccination campaigns with easily administered oral polio vaccine to whole regions, to nations, and to large subpopulations.

During 2004, however, polio immunization activities in northern Nigeria were halted for an extended period for fear of tainted vaccines, and this permitted the development of epidemics extending throughout the country. The disease spread as well to 10 other African countries and to Saudi Arabia, Yemen, and Indonesia. Transmission has again been reestablished in several African countries (Burkina Faso, Central African Republic, Chad, Côte d'Ivoire, and Sudan). Heroic efforts are being made to control these outbreaks by large-scale immunization, but in countries such as these, where health services are stressed and the health, communication, and transportation infrastructures are weak, disease transmission is difficult to interrupt. Meanwhile, other countries throughout the world that appear to be polio free are continuing their vaccination programs but finding it increasingly difficult to maintain a momentum of interest, effort, and financing.

The difficulties of maintaining credible surveillance systems throughout the developing countries were vividly demonstrated by the discovery of polio in Sudan in May 2004, more than three years after the last case had been reported (CDC 2005). In the interim, specimens from 75 to 90 percent of such

Table 62.2 Benefits of Smallpox Eradication to the United States, 1968
(Millions of U.S. dollars)

	Amount
Direct costs for medical services	
Vaccination	92.8
Treatment of complications	0.7
Indirect costs, loss of productivity	
Work losses attributable to vaccination and reactions	41.7
Permanent disability attributable to complications	0.4
Premature death	0.1
Cost of international traffic surveillance and delays in clearance of vessels	14.5
Total	150.2

Source: Sencer and Axnick 1973; see also Fenner and others 1988, table 31.2.

cases were processed in the laboratory, and measures of surveillance for acute flaccid paralysis cases were reported to have been entirely satisfactory. At first, the Sudanese cases were considered to have resulted from importations from Nigeria, and, indeed, some cases were. However, from more detailed laboratory studies, it was determined that type 1 wild virus had been circulating undetected for more than three years and type 3 virus for nearly five years.

Clearly, stopping the continuing transmission of wild poliovirus is itself a formidable challenge, the success of which is by no means certain. A problematic discovery since the global eradication program began was the finding that individuals with particular immunologic disorders shed polio vaccine virus for many months to years, thus serving as a reservoir for this virus. The virus, in turn, can revert to a neurovirulent form, which is capable of causing outbreaks of disease (Bellmunt and others 1999). Such individuals may be wholly without symptoms and impossible to identify except through fecal cultures. Moreover, no treatment is known to stop them from shedding virus. They pose an all but insurmountable challenge to the current poliomyelitis eradication effort.

The program is further hampered by the tool that has provided so much success—oral poliovirus vaccine (OPV). In resource-poor environments, poliomyelitis is best controlled with the inexpensive, live, and easily administered oral vaccine. The live vaccine is excreted and can infect other susceptible contacts. The ability of OPV to immunize others indirectly makes it an ideal vaccine for achieving high levels of population-based immunity, especially in lower socioeconomic populations that are the most difficult to reach. However, the excreted virus occasionally reverts to a pathologic state, causing not only cases but outbreaks of vaccine-associated paralytic polio, which may not emerge until months or even years after the vaccine has been administered (Kew and others 2004). Unfortunately, the alternative inactivated polio vaccine (IPV) is not immediately an option in many nations, not least because global manufacturing capacity could not begin to meet demand. Other problems include the current cost differential between OPV and IPV, the increased difficulty of administering the vaccine by syringe and needle, and the need to achieve higher coverage rates with IPV because it does not spread from person to person as does OPV.

Tragically, if OPV use were discontinued, in the absence of alternative immunity, polioviruses would likely circulate silently (Eichner and Dietz 1996) and reemerge. Preliminary results from a model presented by WHO indicate a greater than 60 percent chance of an outbreak within two years of the possible global cessation of OPV (WHO 2004) because of continuous circulation of undetected live vaccine viruses that can revert. Outbreaks have already been observed in several regions where decreasing use of live vaccine has left pockets of susceptible persons who eventually have been exposed to vaccine-

derived pathogenic viruses (Kew and others 2002). Such an outbreak could occur with disastrous speed because the polio virus is far more contagious than that of smallpox. In developing countries, virtually all cases of polio occurred among those under five years of age, older persons having been protected by the natural immunity of earlier infection. Within five years after vaccination ceased, therefore, the population immunity level in the developing countries would be no better than it was before vaccination was introduced. With this is mind, it seems questionable as to whether all health ministers could be persuaded to call for a country-wide cessation of poliomyelitis vaccination itself, given the uncertainties of virus detection in so many remote and inaccessible areas of the world.

By definition, eradication implies certifying cessation of virus transmission and the absence of reservoirs so that control interventions can cease. As noted earlier in this chapter, it is only for this reason that eradication yields a dividend. Although the interruption of wild poliomyelitis virus transmission is theoretically feasible, the obstacles to achieving and maintaining this goal are formidable. At this time, it is difficult to foresee a future that does not envisage a continuing vaccination program, perhaps with IPV use in countries that can afford the substantial additional costs entailed and with OPV use in all other countries.

The polio eradication initiative, like that for smallpox, has had to rely primarily on voluntary donations provided both to WHO and bilaterally. Playing an especially important role have been the Rotary International Foundation and the Bill & Melinda Gates Foundation. From 1988 to 2004, more than US$3 billion was spent on the effort (WHO 2003).

What are the economics of polio eradication? Bart, Foulds, and Patriarca (1996) developed the first global cost-benefit analysis of polio eradication, beginning with the costs incurred since 1986, the year that the Pan American Health Organization launched a regional eradication effort, and extending to 2040. They assumed that eradication would be achieved in 2005, using OPV, and that vaccination would cease after eradication had been certified. Benefits (like costs, discounted at 6 percent) reflect the avoided costs of acute care and avoided vaccination costs after certification. Their analysis showed that the initiative would break even by 2007 and yield a net benefit to the world of more than US$13 billion by 2040—an encouraging result, but it was based on the assumption that all vaccination would stop abruptly in 2005.

Khan and Ehreth (2003) developed a similar analysis but provided regional detail. They estimated the costs and medical costs avoided of polio immunization and eradication over the period 1970 to 2050, assuming that vaccination could cease after 2010. As table 62.3 shows, Khan and Ehreth estimated that polio immunization and eradication would entail a negative net cost overall, with Europe and the Americas saving the most and with other regions incurring a positive net cost. Compared

Table 62.3 Net Costs of Polio Immunization and Eradication
(Millions of U.S. dollars)

WHO region	Medical care cost savings	Immuni-zation costs	Net costs	Cost/DALY saved
Africa	1,100	3,942	2,842	442
Americas	76,900	25,460	−51,440	−4,983
Eastern Mediterranean	1,930	3,512	1,582	426
Europe	38,250	17,249	−21,001	−2,780
Southeast Asia	1,270	6,519	5,249	1,041
Western Pacific	8,670	10,327	1,657	356
World	128,120	67,009	−61,111	−1,457

Source: Khan and Ehreth 2003.
Note: Cost savings, immunization costs, and net costs are present values for 2000 in millions of U.S. dollars, calculated for the period 1970–2050 and discounted at 5 percent. These estimates assume that immunization by OPV can cease after 2010.

Table 62.4 Postpolio Eradication Costs
(Millions of U.S. dollars)

	Continue OPV	Stop OPV	Universal IPV
Low-income countries	1,364	487	4,418
Middle-income countries	12,196	12,196	12,196
High-income countries	6,409	6,409	6,409
Subtotal	19,969	19,092	23,023
Global response capacity	1,120	1,320	1,120
Total	21,089	20,412	24,143

Source: Sangrujee, Cáceres, and Cochi 2004.
Note: Costs are expressed in present value terms, calculated over the period 2005 to 2020, and discounted at 3 percent.

with other health interventions, this cost to developing countries may still be comparatively cost-effective. However, Khan and Ehreth comment that the cost per disability-adjusted life year (DALY) saved is high for developing countries (see table 62.3). As they explain (Khan and Ehreth 2003, 705), "This implies that without the financial support from developed countries of the world many developing countries would not have opted for polio interventions for implementation. From the developed countries' point of view, providing support for the polio program is not simply helping the poor and the disadvantaged, it actually represents a good economic investment."

Unfortunately, both of these cost-benefit studies have substantial limitations. First, both show that eradication is economically attractive if one incorporates all costs and benefits from the inception of this program. Because eradication has not yet been achieved, this approach mixes retrospective evaluation and prospective analysis (historical expenditures and benefits are sunk and so are irrelevant to the current situation). Second, benefits and costs are calculated in both studies relative to a world without immunization. A better approach would be to calculate the net benefits of eradication compared with the alternative of an optimal control program. The choice is not between doing nothing and eradication. It is between an optimal level of control and eradication. Finally, both studies assume that vaccination can cease in 2005 or 2010. As explained previously, this possibility is highly unlikely.

A more recent analysis by Sangrujee, Cáceres, and Cochi (2004) calculates the costs for 15 years following the goal of certification of eradication in 2005 for three different scenarios: continued use of OPV, OPV cessation with optional use of the killed or inactivated polio vaccine, and OPV cessation with universal IPV. Table 62.4 shows their results.

The respective cost to middle- and high-income countries is the same for all three scenarios, reflecting the assumption that the high-income countries will switch to IPV by 2005 and middle-income countries will do so between 2006 and 2008. The scenarios differ only for the low-income countries. In the first scenario, these countries are expected to continue routine immunization using OPV; in the second, immunization ceases in 2011, followed by a system of surveillance and response. In the third scenario, the low-income countries join the others in switching to IPV between 2008 and 2010. Of these three scenarios, the second comes closest to the 2005 post-eradication strategy now advocated by the polio eradication program leadership.

Unfortunately, this analysis is also deficient. First, interruption of transmission will not occur before 2006, and certification will take an additional three years. Hence, analysis of post-eradication costs should begin in 2009 at the earliest, with the costs of continuing immunization needing to be borne up until that time. Second, the analysis assumes a capacity to supply IPV that exceeds current estimates. It is not obvious that this scenario is feasible or, if it were, if the costs of scaling up production are adequately reflected in the calculations. Third, and most importantly, table 62.4 indicates that only low-income countries would benefit from polio eradication over this 15-year time scale—and yet the table does not include any estimate of the risk these countries would bear of a possible outbreak.

Although this analysis suggests that the discontinued use of OPV promises the greatest return to eradication, this assumes that circulating vaccine-derived polioviruses could be contained if and when they emerged. However, preparing for this possibility would require a far more effective global surveillance system than now exists, maintenance of a laboratory infrastructure, and stockpiles of OPV. In addition, controlling outbreaks with OPV without the risk of viruses reverting to virulence will be exceedingly difficult in the setting of an accelerating proportion of immunologic-naive individuals. The use of OPV in this scenario could very well cause poliomyelitis to again become endemic. In any case, the estimated cost of any of the strategies exceeds $20 billion.

The economics of polio eradication are thus not as favorable as concluded by either Bart, Foulds, and Patriarca (1996) or Khan and Ehreth (2003). Both studies assume that vaccination can cease without IPV being used as a substitute anywhere, both exclude the costs of maintaining a response capacity, and neither accounts for the real threat of reemergence. Sangrujee, Cáceres, and Cochi (2004) take account of two of these considerations, but their analysis calculates only the costs for 15 years, ignoring both the risk of reemergence and the benefits of eradication. Hence, each study provides only a partial glimpse of the economics of polio eradication and does not adequately address the fundamental difficulty (inability) of stopping vaccination and maintaining eradication.

In conclusion, although the economics of polio eradication may have been thought to be favorable by some (Aylward and others 2003), they are far less favorable than were the economics of smallpox eradication, even assuming that polio vaccination could cease.

Dracunculiasis

Dracunculiasis, or guinea worm disease, is a nematode infection, which is controlled not by vaccination but by education of the affected population, provision of nematode-free water through wells or filtration, and treatment of cases. It is not a global disease but found only in the rural areas of a few very poor tropical countries. This last difference is especially important from an economics perspective. It means that international financing of a guinea worm eradication program needs to rely more heavily on development assistance rather than on the self-interest of donor countries.

Thus far, the eradication program has been successful in reducing the number of cases of guinea worm 99 percent from the 1986 level (Carter Center 2004). The geographic range of the disease has also been reduced from 20 to just 12 countries. Although this achievement is important, eradication remains elusive many years beyond 1995, the year that the WHA set for eradication in 1991 (Cairncross, Muller, and Zagaria 2002, 232).

Only one cost-benefit study of the guinea worm eradication program has been published (Kim, Tandon, and Ruiz-Tiben 1997), and it is unfortunately flawed in a number of respects. First, as indicated previously, eradication costs should be compared with those associated with an alternative optimal control program. Second, the cost-benefit analysis applies to the period 1987 to 1998 and thus is backward looking. The analysis can reveal whether the money spent previously yielded a benefit in excess of the cost (it did), but it cannot reveal whether eradication was worth pursuing at the time that this study was undertaken. Finally, it takes no account of the investment decision of eradication—the main reason for pursuing the eradication goal in the first place.

This last omission is especially relevant to the study's analysis of the eradication program in Sudan. The study projected that, by 1998, infections would cease everywhere except Sudan. (Plainly, this prediction was wrong, although Sudan is the largest problem for the program, mainly because of the ongoing civil war, which has limited accessibility to endemic areas; see Hopkins and others 2002.) It then calculates the net present value of eliminating the disease there. The results are not promising. They show that eradication is attractive only if the disease can be eliminated in Sudan within five years. However, this analysis ignores the dividend that eradication would earn Sudan. It also disregards the most important feature of eradication—that if the disease were certified to have been eliminated from its last stronghold, it would yield a benefit to *all* potentially vulnerable countries. Thus, the economics of eliminating dracunculiasis from Sudan, if that is where the disease makes its last stand, will be much more attractive than suggested by this analysis.

CONCLUSIONS

Of the several attempts to eradicate diseases, all but one has failed. Even the exception, smallpox, barely succeeded despite the many factors favorable to eradication. Whether any eradication effort will ultimately succeed or fail cannot be known with certainty at the time it is launched. Eradication entails risk. Money spent on eradication may not ultimately pay a dividend. Health risks may also exist. If eradication fails and vaccination levels drop after the eradication goal is abandoned, susceptible persons who were previously shielded from infection may become infected at a later age, when the disease can cause greater harm. The risk also exists that, even if eradication succeeds, the disease may be reintroduced by accidental or deliberate release.

The reasons for potential failure of an eradication effort are many. A nonhuman host may not be discovered until the number of infected humans drops to a very low level (as happened with yellow fever). The tools of eradication may be vulnerable to resistance (insecticides and drugs in the case of malaria). Political problems and civil strife may prevent an eradication program from being executed in critical areas where the disease makes its last stand (a problem today for guinea worm). Termination of vaccination may leave populations vulnerable to microbe reintroduction from an unforeseen reservoir or vaccine strain reversion (a risk now facing the poliomyelitis initiative). Another potential reason for failure is the inability to raise the financial resources needed to complete programs that extend beyond expected targets. All eradication programs have experienced serious financial stringencies during the course of their execution.

Most eradication programs to date have been launched as visionary, far-reaching efforts but with vastly incomplete information. Basic epidemiological information and knowledge of the effectiveness and operational constraints of interventions and costs in different settings are often inadequate, and the required monitoring, evaluation, training, and research components of the program may be absent. If a program's administrators lack a careful, probing analysis of the epidemiology of the various candidate diseases or of the technologies available, and if their comprehension of the potential costs and who would bear them is limited, a program is likely to founder, causing a dispirited staff, confused beneficiaries, and donor fatigue and ambivalence. It is crucial that the eradication methodologies and assumptions in those regions of the world that would be most likely to pose the most significant problems be tested and addressed before launching an eradication program and that evaluation and research continue during the program.

Proposals for disease eradication have seldom been brought to the WHA with specific plans, costs, and uncertainties fully laid out. Nor have the expected sources of fiscal support and needed country support been addressed with specific commitments requested of the members. The WHA has only a limited deliberative capacity, and too much cannot be expected of its members in session. However, designated special committees of the WHA can and should be appointed, consisting of both visionary eradicationists and field-experienced public health and social science personnel. The WHA should take up the question of eradication only after the subject has been thoroughly vetted and sufficiently large-scale pilot programs in the most problematic areas have clarified that an adequate understanding of the epidemiology exists and that the appropriate technologies are available.

In the past, members have not voted for a specific program for which all the uncertainties have been laid out and the benefits and costs associated with different outcomes have also been calculated. Nor, with one exception, have they voted for a resolution imposing responsibilities, including financing obligations, on individual states. The next time a proposal to eradicate a disease is presented to the WHA, it should be comprehensive. It should demonstrate why the effort is worth taking, even if the final outcome is uncertain; it should bind states, morally if not legally, to fulfill the pledges needed to see the program through to its completion; and it should prepare contingencies should the eradication effort fail.

ACKNOWLEDGMENTS

We would like to acknowledge Walter Dowdle and Maria Teresa Valenzuela for their critical review of our manuscript; Joel Breman and Philip Musgrove for providing editorial guidance; John Sentz for his numerous hours devoted to research and editorial assistance; and Cherice Holloway for her preparation of various versions of this manuscript.

REFERENCES

Anderson, R. M., and R. May. 1991. *Infectious Diseases of Humans: Dynamics and Control.* Oxford, U.K.: Oxford University Press.

Andrews, J. M., and A. D. Langmuir. 1963. "The Philosophy of Disease Eradication." *American Journal of Public Health* 53: 1–6.

Aylward, R. B., A. Acharya, S. England, M. Agocs, and J. Linkins. 2003. "Polio Eradication." In *Global Public Goods for Health: Health Economic and Public Health Perspectives,* eds. R. Smith, R. Beaglehole, D. Woodward, and N. Drager, 33–53. Oxford, U.K.: Oxford University Press.

Aylward, R. B., J. M. Olive, H. F. Hull, C. A. De Quadros, and B. Melgaard. 1998. "Ensuring Common Principles Lead to Mutual Benefits: Disease Eradication Initiatives and General Health Services." In *The Eradication of Infectious Diseases,* eds. W. R. Dowdle and D. R. Hopkins. New York: John Wiley and Sons.

Barrett, S. 2003. "Global Disease Eradication." *Journal of the European Economic Association* 1: 591–600.

———. 2004. "Eradication vs. Control: The Economics of Global Infectious Disease Policy." *Bulletin of the World Health Organization* 82 (9): 683–88.

Barrett, S., and M. Hoel. 2003. "Optimal Disease Eradication." Disease Control Priorities Project Working Paper 22.

Bart, K. J., J. Foulds, and P. Patriarca. 1996. "Global Eradication of Poliomyelitis: Benefit-Cost Analysis." *Bulletin of the World Health Organization* 74 (1): 35–45.

Basu, R. N., Z. Ježek, and N. A. Ward. 1979. *The Eradication of Smallpox from India.* New Delhi: World Health Organization.

Bellmunt, A., G. May, R. Zell, P. Pring-Akerblom, W. Verhagen, and A. Heim. 1999. "Evolution of Poliovirus Type I during 5.5 Years of Prolonged Enteral Replication in an Immunodeficient Patient." *Virology* 265: 178–84.

Biellik, R., S. Madema, A. Taole, A. Kutsulukuta, E. Allies, R. Eggers, and others. 2002. "First 5 Years of Measles Elimination in Southern Africa: 1996–2000." *Lancet* 359 (9317): 1564–68.

Breman, J. G., and I. Arita. 1980. "The Confirmation and Maintenance of Smallpox Eradication." *New England Journal of Medicine* 303 (22): 1263–73.

Brilliant, L. B. 1985. *The Management of Smallpox Eradication in India.* Ann Arbor: University of Michigan Press.

Cairncross, S., R. Muller, and N. Zagaria. 2002. "Dracunculiasis (Guinea Worm Disease) and the Eradication Initiative." *Clinical Microbiology Reviews* 15 (2): 223–46.

Carter Center. 2004. "Guinea Worm Eradication: Review, June 1, 2003." Carter Center, Atlanta. http://www.cartercenter.org/printdoc.asp?docID=1785andsubmenu=news.

CDC (U.S. Centers for Disease Control and Prevention). 1998a. "Progress toward Elimination of Measles from the Americas." *Morbidity and Mortality Weekly Report* 47 (10): 189–93.

———. 1998b. "Progress toward Global Measles Control and Regional Elimination, 1990–1997." *Morbidity and Mortality Weekly Report* 47 (48): 104.

———. 1999a. "Global Measles Control and Regional Elimination, 1998–1999." *Morbidity and Mortality Weekly Report* 48 (49): 1124.

———. 1999b. "Progress toward Measles Elimination—Southern Africa, 1996–1998." *Morbidity and Mortality Weekly Report* 48 (27): 585.

———. 2003a. "Global Progress toward Certifying Polio Eradication and Laboratory Containment of Wild Polioviruses—August 2002–August 2003." *Morbidity and Mortality Weekly Report* 52 (47):1158.

———. 2003b. "Progress toward Poliomyelitis Eradication—Angola and the Democratic Republic of Congo, January 2002–June 2003." *Morbidity and Mortality Weekly Report* 52 (34): 816.

———. 2003c. "Progress toward Poliomyelitis Eradication—Southern Africa, 2001—March 2003." *Morbidity and Mortality Weekly Report* 52 (22): 521.

———. 2003d. "Update: Global Measles Control and Mortality Reduction—Worldwide, 1991–2001." *Morbidity and Mortality Weekly Report* 52 (20): 471.

———. 2004a. "Brief Report: Global Polio Eradication Initiative Strategic Plan, 2004." *Morbidity and Mortality Weekly Report* 53 (05): 107.

———. 2004b. "Measles Mortality Reduction—West Africa, 1996–2002." *Morbidity and Mortality Weekly Report* 53 (02): 28.

———. 2004c. "Progress toward Global Eradication of Poliomyelitis, January 2003–April 2004." *Morbidity and Mortality Weekly Report* 53 (24): 532.

———. 2004d. "Progress toward Measles Elimination—Region of the Americas, 2002–2003." *Morbidity and Mortality Weekly Report* 53 (14): 304.

———. 2004e. "Progress toward Poliomyelitis Eradication—Nigeria, January 2003–March 2004." *Morbidity and Mortality Weekly Report* 53 (16): 343.

———. 2004f. "Progress toward Sustainable Measles Mortality Reduction—South-East Asia Region, 1999–2002." *Morbidity and Mortality Weekly Report* 53 (25): 559.

———. 2004g. "Wild Poliovirus Importations—West and Central Africa, January 2003–March 2004." *Morbidity and Mortality Weekly Report* 53 (20): 433.

———. 2005. "Progress toward Poliomyelitis Eradication—Poliomyelitis Outbreak in Sudan, 2004." *Morbidity and Mortality Weekly Report* 54 (4): 97–99.

Cello, J., A. V. Paul, and E. Wimmer. 2002. "Chemical Synthesis of Poliovirus cDNA: Generation of Infectious Virus in the Absence of Natural Template." *Science* 297 (5583): 1016–18.

Cochi, S., C. de Quadros, W. Dowdle, R. Goodman, P. Ndumbe, D. Salisbury, and others. 1998. "Post-Conference Small Group Report." In *Global Disease Elimination and Eradication as Public Health Strategies*, eds. R. A. Goodman, K. L. Foster, F. L. Trowbridge, and J. P. Figueroa. *Bulletin of the World Health Organization* 76 (Suppl. 2): 113.

Cockburn, A. 1961. "Eradication of Infectious Diseases." *Science* 133: 1050–58.

———. 1963. *The Evolution and Eradication of Infectious Diseases.* Baltimore: Johns Hopkins University Press.

de Quadros, C. 2001. "Introduction." In *Considerations for Viral Disease Eradication Lessons Learned and Future Strategies*, eds. S. Knobler, J. Lederberg, and L. A. Pray, 22–32. Washington, DC: National Academy Press.

Dowdle, W. R. 1998. "The Principles of Disease Elimination and Eradication." *Bulletin of the World Health Organization* 76 (Suppl. 2): 22–25.

———. 1999. "The Principles of Disease Elimination and Eradication." *Morbidity and Mortality Weekly Report* 48 (Suppl.): 23–27.

Dowdle, W. R., and D. R. Hopkins, eds. 1998. *The Eradication of Infectious Diseases.* New York: John Wiley and Sons.

Dubos, R., and J. Dubos. 1953. *The White Plague: Tuberculosis, Man and Society.* London: Gollancz. Quoted in Fenner, Hall, and Dowdle 1998.

Eichner, M., and K. Dietz. 1996. "Eradication of Poliomyelitis: When Can One Be Sure That Polio Virus Transmission Has Been Terminated?" *American Journal of Epidemiology* 143 (8): 816–22.

Fenner, F., A. J. Hall, and W. R. Dowdle. 1998. "What Is Eradication?" In *The Eradication of Infectious Diseases*, eds. W. R. Dowdle and D. R. Hopkins, 3–17. New York: John Wiley and Sons.

Fenner, F., D. A. Henderson, I. Arita, Z. Ježek, and I. D. Ladnyi. 1988. *Smallpox and Its Eradication.* Geneva: World Health Organization.

Goodman, R. A., K. L. Foster, F. L. Trowbridge, and J. P. Figueroa, eds. 1998a. "Comments and Discussion Following Work Group Reports." In "Global Disease Elimination and Eradication as Public Health Strategies," *Bulletin of the World Health Organization* 76 (Suppl. 2): 104–8.

———. 1998b. "Global Disease Elimination and Eradication as Public Health Strategies: Proceedings of a Conference. Atlanta, Georgia, February 23–25, 1998." *Bulletin of the World Health Organization* 76 (Suppl.) 2: 5–162.

Henderson, D. A. 1982. "The Deliberate Extinction of a Species." *Proceedings of the American Philosophical Society* 126: 461–71.

———. 1988. "Development of the Global Smallpox Eradication Programme, 1958–1966." In *Smallpox and Its Eradication*, eds. F. Fenner, D. A. Henderson, I. Arita, Z. Ježek, and I. D. Ladnyi, 365–419. Geneva: World Health Organization.

———. 1998a. "Eradication: Lessons from the Past." *Bulletin of the World Health Organization* 76 (Suppl. 2): 17–21.

———. 1998b. "The Siren Song of Eradication." *Journal of the Royal College of Physicians of London* 32 (6): 580–84.

Hopkins, D. R., E. Ruiz-Tiben, N. Diallo, P. C. Withers Jr., and J. H. Maguire. 2002. "Dracunculiasis Eradication: And Now, Sudan." *American Journal of Tropical Medicine and Hygiene* 67 (4): 415–22.

Jeffrey, G. M. 1976. "Malaria Control in the Twentieth Century." *American Journal of Tropical Medicine and Hygiene* 25: 361–71.

Jenner, E. 1801. *The Origin of Vaccine Inoculation.* London: Shury. Quoted in Fenner, Hall, and Dowdle 1998.

Kew, O. M., V. Morris-Glasgow, M. Landaverde, C. Burns, J. Shaw, Z. Garib, and others. 2002. "Outbreak of Poliomyelitis in Hispaniola Associated with Circulating Type 1 Vaccine-Derived Poliovirus." *Science* 296 (5566): 356–59.

Kew, O. M., P. F. Wright, V. I. Agol, F. Delpeyroux, H. Shimizu, N. Nathanson, and M. A. Pallansch. 2004. "Circulating Vaccine-Derived Polioviruses: Current State of Knowledge." *Bulletin of the World Health Organization* 82 (1): 16–23.

Khan, M., and J. Ehreth. 2003. "Costs and Benefits of Polio Eradication: A Long-Run Global Perspective." *Vaccine* 21: 702–5.

Kim, A., A. Tandon, and E. Ruiz-Tiben. 1997. "Cost-Benefit Analysis of the Global Dracunculiasis Eradication Campaign." Policy Research Working Paper 1835, World Bank, Washington, DC.

Knobler, S., J. Lederberg, and L. A. Pray, eds. 2001. *Considerations for Viral Disease Eradication Lessons Learned and Future Strategies.* Washington, DC: National Academy Press.

Kremer, M., and E. Miguel. 2004. "The Illusion of Sustainability." NBER Working Paper W10324, National Bureau of Economic Research, Cambridge, MA.

New Shorter Oxford English Dictionary. 1993.

Ottesen, E. A., W. R. Dowdle, F. Fenner, K. O. Habermehl, T. J. John, M. A. Koch, and others. 1998. "Group Report: How Is Eradication to Be Defined and What Are the Biological Criteria?" In *The Eradication of Infectious Diseases*, eds. W. R. Dowdle and D. R. Hopkins. New York: John Wiley and Sons.

Payne, A. M.-M. 1963a. "Basic Concepts of Eradication." *American Review of Respiratory Disease* 88: 449–55.

———. 1963b. "Disease Eradication as an Economic Factor." *American Journal of Public Health* 53: 369–75.

Ramaiah, T. J. 1976. "Cost-Benefit Analysis of the Intensified Campaign against Smallpox in India." *National Institute of Health Administration and Education Bulletin* 9 (3): 169–203.

Roberts, L. 2004. "Polio Endgame. Polio: The Final Assault?" *Science* 303 (5666): 1960–68.

Sabin, A. B. 1991. "Measles, Killer of Millions in Developing Countries: Strategy for Rapid Elimination and Continuing Control." *European Journal of Epidemiology* 7 (1): 1–22.

Salisbury, D. 1998. "Report of the Work Group on Disease Elimination/Eradication and Sustainable Health Development." In *Global Disease Elimination and Eradication as Public Health Strategies,* eds. R. A. Goodman, K. L. Foster, F. L. Trowbridge, and J. P. Figueroa. *Bulletin of the World Health Organization* 76 (Suppl. 2): 72–79.

Sangrujee, N., V. M. Cáceres, and S. L. Cochi. 2004. "Cost Analysis of Post-Polio Certification Immunization Policies." *Bulletin of the World Health Organization* 82 (1): 9–15.

Sencer, D. J., and N. W. Axnick. 1973. "Cost Benefit Analysis." In *International Symposium on Vaccination against Communicable Diseases, Monaco 1973,* 22: 37–46. Symposia Series in Immunobiological Standardization. Basel, Switzerland: Karger.

Spînu, I., and S. Biberi-Moroianu. 1969. "Theoretical and Practical Problems Concerning the Eradication of Communicable Diseases." *Archives roumaines de pathologie experimentales et de microbiologie* 28: 725–42.

Steinglass, P. 2001. *Thematic Evaluations in 2001 Eradication of Poliomyelitis.* Report by the director general, Programme Development Committee of the Executive Board Eight Meeting, December 13, 2001. Document EBPDC8/3. Geneva: World Health Organization.

Taylor, C. E., F. Cutts, and M. E. Taylor. 1997. "Ethical Dilemmas in Current Planning for Polio Eradication." *American Journal of Public Health* 87 (6): 922–25.

WHO (World Health Organization). 2003. *Global Polio Eradication Initiative: Estimated External Financial Resource Requirements 2004–2008.* Geneva: WHO.

———. 2004. *Report of the Strategic Advisory Group of Experts (SAGE).* Geneva: WHO. http://www.who.int/vaccines-documents/DocsPDF05/Sage_Report_2004.pdf.

Yekutiel, P. 1980. *Eradication of Infectious Diseases: A Critical Study.* New York: Karger.

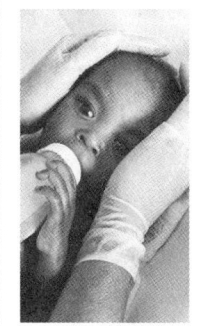

Chapter **63**

Integrated Management of the Sick Child

Cesar G. Victora, Taghreed Adam, Jennifer Bryce,
and David B. Evans

NATURE, CAUSES, AND BURDEN OF CHILD MORTALITY

Every year, over 10 million children under five years of age die. Most of those deaths are due to a small number of causes. In the mid 1990s, it was estimated that 70 percent of all global child deaths were due to five conditions: diarrhea, pneumonia, malaria, measles, and malnutrition (Gove 1997; Tulloch 1999). The World Health Organization (WHO) has since conducted a comprehensive review of under-five deaths using additional data and improved methods (Bryce and others 2005), and now estimates that six causes accounted for 73 percent of these deaths in 2000–2003: pneumonia (19 percent), diarrhea (18 percent), malaria (8 percent), neonatal pneumonia or sepsis (10 percent), preterm delivery (10 percent), and asphyxia at birth (8 percent). Undernutrition is an underlying cause in at least half of all under-five deaths. Few conditions, therefore, account for a large proportion of all deaths.

These deaths are not randomly distributed. They tend to occur in the poorest countries of the world, mostly in Sub-Saharan Africa and South Asia (Black, Morris, and Bryce 2003), and within any country they affect mostly the poorest families (Victora and others 2003). Fortunately, cost-effective interventions are available to prevent most of these deaths. Chapters 19, 21, 24–28, and 56 in this volume, as well as the next section in this chapter, describe these interventions in greater detail. Achieving universal coverage with these interventions would likely prevent 60 percent of those deaths (Jones and others 2003). Yet coverage levels for nearly all of these interventions remain below 50 percent (Bryce and others 2003), and children from the poorest families are least likely to be reached (Victora and others 2003).

In addition, comorbidity is common. Among children who die, a large proportion present with two or more diagnoses (Black, Morris, and Bryce 2003). Comorbidity is also highly prevalent at the community level and among children seeking health care. Nutritional factors—including underweight, micronutrient deficiencies, and inadequate infant feeding practices (see chapter 28)—play a major role in morbidity and mortality, and yet these are often overlooked by practitioners. Also, there are many missed opportunities for preventive interventions during outpatient visits—for example, immunizations and promotion of insecticide-treated mosquito nets.

POLICY SHIFT TO INTEGRATED MANAGEMENT

Until the mid 1990s, actions aimed at improving child health were organized as vertical programs, each addressing a specific disease or providing a given intervention or set of interventions (Claeson and Waldman 2000). Typical examples of these programs are the Expanded Program on Immunizations (EPI), Control of Diarrhoeal Diseases (CDD), acute respiratory infection (ARI) programs, malaria control programs, and nutrition programs that include growth monitoring, breastfeeding promotion and support, and micronutrient supplementation.

The need for an integrated approach to improve child health became evident in the mid 1990s for a number of reasons. From the perspective of epidemiology, a small number of diseases accounted for a high proportion of deaths, and those diseases were often present in the same children and had overlapping clinical signs. Integrated management was expected to increase the probability that children would receive treatment for all major diseases and to decrease the possibility that children would receive correct treatment for one disease and die from another unrecognized illness. The important role played by nutrition across these major diseases also suggested that an integrated approach to case management was needed to ensure that health workers addressed children's nutritional needs throughout the clinical encounter.

A second set of reasons for the policy shift to an integrated approach was based on the need to promote managerial efficiency. The vertical approach required countries to appoint managers at national, provincial, and district levels to run each program. It also led to separate training activities; for example, health workers might be required to leave their posts on a number of occasions to be trained for the programs. Similar examples of duplication of effort were often found in supervision and provision of essential drugs. There was a strong logical basis for believing that integrating the management structure of child health programs would lead to improved efficiency.

A third group of reasons for the shift to integrated case management related to the need to improve the quality of case management provided by health workers. Vertical programs trained health workers to manage one disease at a time, and decisions about how best to assess and treat those diseases, as well as how to promote nutrition and educate caretakers, were often left to individual health workers. An integrated set of guidelines for managing sick children ensured that health workers, including those with low levels of training, applied the best available knowledge of case management systematically and in correct sequence.

The realization that a few diseases were responsible for most child deaths, that comorbidity was highly prevalent, that effective interventions were available, and that there were many missed opportunities for prevention led to the recognition that an integrated approach was needed. Thus, WHO and United Nations Children's Fund (UNICEF) launched the Integrated Management of Childhood Illness (IMCI) strategy in the mid 1990s (Tulloch 1999). Tanzania and Uganda began implementing IMCI in 1996. By 2003, more than 100 countries had adopted the strategy (http://www.who.int/child-adolescent-health).

INTERVENTIONS

A key aspect of IMCI was the integration of effective interventions to improve child health and nutrition into a coordinated strategy. IMCI has three components, each of which was meant to be adapted at the country level according to local epidemiology, health system characteristics, and culture.

Improving Health Worker Performance

The first component of IMCI includes health worker training and the reinforcement of correct performance. Training is based on a set of adapted algorithms (Gove 1997) that guide health workers through a process of assessing signs and symptoms, classifying the illness according to treatment needs, and providing appropriate treatment and education to the child's caregiver. Figure 63.1 shows a general outline of the approach for children age two months to five years (WHO and UNICEF 2001). Sick children attending a first-level health facility are initially checked for danger signs and for the main symptoms of the key IMCI diseases: diarrhea, malaria, pneumonia, measles, and other severe infections. Next, all children are assessed for malnutrition and anemia, and vaccination status is verified. Children under two years of age, as well as older children presenting low weight for age, receive nutrition counseling. Other health problems related by caretakers are then assessed, and children are classified according to a color code: pink (immediate referral), yellow (management in the outpatient facility), or green (home management). Separate case-management algorithms are available for children under two months of age. IMCI health worker training emphasizes the integration of curative care with preventive measures, including nutrition and vaccinations. A special training module addresses how to communicate effectively with mothers. The training course was originally designed to last 11 days, including a large amount of hands-on experience.

Improving Health Systems

The second component of IMCI is aimed at providing support for child health service delivery, including drug availability, effective supervision, referral services, and health information systems. Tools were developed for implementing specific system-strengthening interventions, including a planning guide for national and district managers, an integrated health facility assessment tool, and a tool for improving referral level care. In particular, several countries—beginning in Latin America through the Pan American Health Organization (PAHO) and more recently in Africa with WHO's Regional Office for Africa—made substantial efforts to improve the management and availability of the specific drugs required for IMCI (A. Bartlett, personal communication).

Improving Family and Community Practices

The third component, known as *community IMCI*, focuses on 12 key family practices relevant to child health and development (see http://www.who.int/child-adolescent-health/PREVENTION/12_key.htm). Community IMCI supports the development and implementation of community- and household-based messages and interventions to increase the proportions of children exposed to these practices. These behaviors address breastfeeding, complementary feeding, micronutrients, personal hygiene, immunizations, insecticide-treated nets, mental and social development, continued feeding

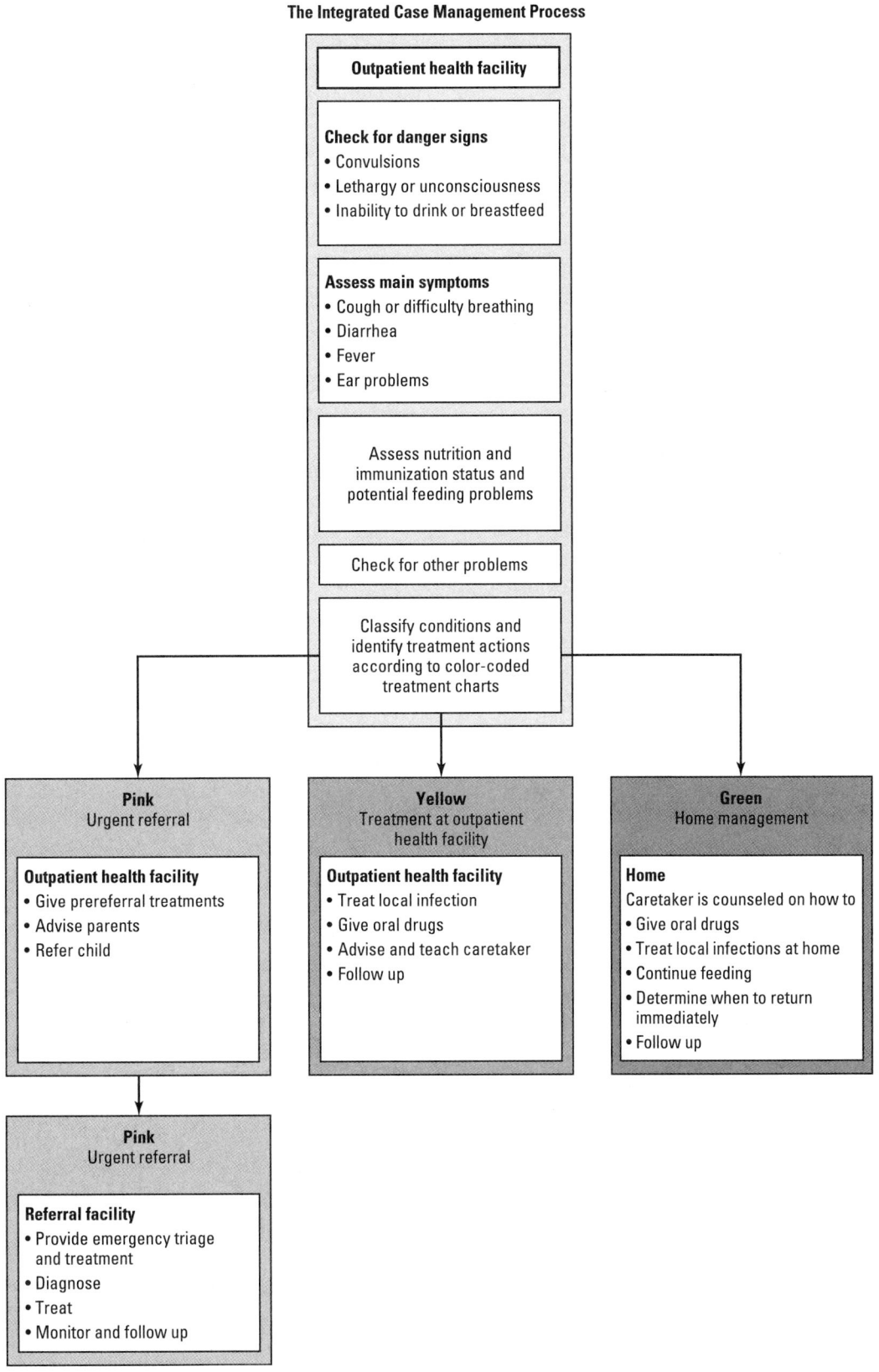

The Integrated Case Management Process

Outpatient health facility

Check for danger signs
- Convulsions
- Lethargy or unconsciousness
- Inability to drink or breastfeed

Assess main symptoms
- Cough or difficulty breathing
- Diarrhea
- Fever
- Ear problems

Assess nutrition and immunization status and potential feeding problems

Check for other problems

Classify conditions and identify treatment actions according to color-coded treatment charts

Pink
Urgent referral

Outpatient health facility
- Give prereferral treatments
- Advise parents
- Refer child

Yellow
Treatment at outpatient health facility

Outpatient health facility
- Treat local infection
- Give oral drugs
- Advise and teach caretaker
- Follow up

Green
Home management

Home
Caretaker is counseled on how to
- Give oral drugs
- Treat local infections at home
- Continue feeding
- Determine when to return immediately
- Follow up

Pink
Urgent referral

Referral facility
- Provide emergency triage and treatment
- Diagnose
- Treat
- Monitor and follow up

Source: WHO and UNICEF 2001.

Figure 63.1 Schematic Outline of IMCI Case Management for Children Age Two Months to Five Years

and increased fluids during illness, home treatment of infections, care-seeking practices, compliance with health worker recommendations, and prenatal care.

This chapter addresses issues related to the integrated delivery of these interventions, most of which are covered in greater detail in other chapters in this book. These include case management of ARI (chapter 25), diarrhea (chapter 19), malaria (chapter 21), and malnutrition (chapter 28); community interventions to improve nutrition, including breastfeeding promotion and complementary feeding (chapter 56); insecticide-impregnated bednets (chapter 21); anthelmintic treatment (chapter 24); vaccinations (chapter 20); and micronutrient supplementation (chapter 28).

INTERVENTION COST AND COST-EFFECTIVENESS

One of the rationales for developing the IMCI strategy was the belief that treating the sick child in an integrated manner, by building on interventions that had already been shown to be cost-effective, would result in gains in efficiency. Two types of questions can be asked from an economic perspective. First, is treating children on the basis of the IMCI strategy cost-effective? Second, do the additional health benefits gained by switching from routine practice to IMCI justify the additional costs (if any)?

Only one publication has reported the cost-effectiveness of the IMCI strategy as a whole. Using a modeling exercise, the *World Development Report 1993* identified IMCI as being able to avert 14 percent of the global burden of disease in children under age five in resource-poor countries at a cost of only US$1.60 per capita per year, with a cost-effectiveness of US$30 to US$100 per disability-adjusted life year (DALY) averted. No details of the methods used to derive those estimates are available (World Bank 1993). It is not clear if the costs are the additional costs of moving from current practice to IMCI or the costs of undertaking care for children under age five using IMCI, nor is it clear if the effectiveness is the additional effectiveness of changing current practice or the total effect of the package.

Detailed studies of the cost-effectiveness of some of the components of IMCI are available. For example, oral rehydration therapy for diarrhea, case management for pneumonia, and childhood vaccinations have been shown to be very cost-effective when evaluated as separate interventions (see chapters 19, 25, and 26). It is likely that the combination of different sets of childhood interventions, as proposed by IMCI, would also be cost-effective, although this depends on the relationship between costs and effects when the interventions are undertaken at the same time in the same population.

No published studies of the extent and nature of efficiency gains through integration were found. WHO has recently explored some of these gains for slightly different combina-

tions of childhood interventions in different parts of the world (see http://www.who.int/evidence/cea). This research resulted in estimates of the cost-effectiveness of single or combined interventions compared with doing nothing or with incremental intervention or current practice. Because large-scale trials on the effects of joint interventions have not yet been undertaken, the joint effects were modeled using the effectiveness of the individual interventions taken from systematic reviews. The interventions included vitamin A and zinc fortification and supplementation, oral rehydration therapy, case management for pneumonia, and supplementary feeding and growth monitoring. Costs and effects were estimated at various levels of population coverage and in various combinations.

The results showed that a childhood package consisting of vitamin A and zinc supplementation, oral rehydration therapy, and case management of pneumonia was cost-effective compared with doing nothing in most settings but that including supplementary feeding and growth monitoring was not cost-effective. Implementation of this combination at 50 percent coverage was estimated to cost, in 2000 prices, approximately US$4.10 per child (US$0.60 per capita) in poor African countries such as Tanzania. The cost-effectiveness was US$38 per DALY averted. Costs increase faster than the increase in coverage. In Tanzania, it was estimated to cost an additional US$12.10 per child under age five (US$1.80 per capita) to reach 95 percent coverage, with a resulting incremental cost-effectiveness ratio of US$60 per DALY averted.

This study is important because it is one of the few that has specifically explored the cost-effectiveness of undertaking combined interventions in the same population, and the effect of increasing coverage on costs. These absolutely critical questions for policy makers considering different intervention strategies are also critical to IMCI. However, the WHO study did not analyze the same interventions included in the IMCI package, nor did it evaluate the effect of moving from current practice to IMCI-based care.

Some information on the effect of moving from current practice is available from two studies in Kenya and Nigeria. Those studies compared the cost to the provider of traditional prescribing patterns with the costs of pharmaceuticals that would have resulted if the IMCI guidelines had been followed strictly. In Nigeria, the traditional prescribing method was five times more expensive: US$1.44 per child visit for pharmaceuticals compared with US$0.29, using 1996 estimates (Wammanda, Ejembi, and Iorliam 2003). In Kenya, also in 1996, the traditional method was almost three times costlier per child visit if the low-cost combination of drugs was assumed (US$0.44) and similar if the high-cost combination was assumed (US$0.16) (Boulanger, Lee, and Odhacha 1999). In Bangladesh, it was estimated that strict adherence to the IMCI protocol could result in US$7 million in savings at the national level simply from more rational use of drugs—almost 3 percent of the total health budget of the government of Bangladesh (Khan, Ahmed, and Saha 2000; Khan, Saha, and Ahmed 2002).

These estimates were based on models and assumptions, sometimes using evidence from separate systematic reviews addressing the costs and effects of an intervention. It would be valuable if information on relative cost-effectiveness of different combinations of interventions at variable levels of coverage could be derived from field studies rather than developed solely by modeling. Such an approach would allow the use of comparable methods and counterfactuals across the evaluation sites to make the results more useful and generalizable to other settings. In addition to answering questions related to the cost-effectiveness of IMCI, it would clarify gains that can be obtained from delivering interventions at the same time as part of an integrated package rather than delivering them in a vertical manner. This is one of the reasons the Multi-Country Evaluation of IMCI Effectiveness, Cost, and Impact (MCE) was launched (Bryce and others 2004). Five countries are currently participating in in-depth studies—Bangladesh (in 20 catchment areas), Brazil (in 46 municipalities), Peru (in all 24 departments in the country), Tanzania (in 4 districts), and Uganda (in 10 districts). Seven other countries—Bolivia, Cambodia, Kazakhstan, the Kyrgyz Republic, Morocco, Niger, and Zambia—were assessed for the evaluation but could not be included, mostly because of insufficient implementation of IMCI.

The overall objective of the MCE is to evaluate the actual changes associated with IMCI as it is implemented in different settings. All studies measured an identical set of indicators and, with minor exceptions, used identical data collection tools (Bryce and others 2004). The remainder of this section presents the main findings from two MCE countries, Tanzania and Brazil, for which evaluation results are currently available.

MCE in Tanzania

The MCE in Tanzania uses an observational design to compare two districts where IMCI has been implemented since late 1997 (IMCI districts) with two districts where implementation began in 2002 (comparison districts). The four districts had reasonably well-functioning health services, comparable levels of per capita health expenditure, high utilization rates of government health facilities, and high coverage of selected interventions (for example, EPI). Large numbers of governmental and nongovernmental health actors were also active in the districts, many of which were involved in health worker training and community activities, although their coverage was patchy. The two IMCI districts had engaged in activities designed to strengthen district management skills; the districts also had authority for priority setting and control over their health budgets. These activities of national health sector reform had not started in the comparison districts at the time of the study. In the comparison districts, a high level of coverage of IMCI

training for health workers had been achieved, but there had been no increase in the provision of under-five interventions at the community level, as opposed to the facility level.

Cost data were collected for the start-up period of implementing IMCI (from 1996 to 1997)—defined as the time from the national decision to implement IMCI to the time when IMCI started to be provided in health facilities—and for the maintenance of child health services in both types of districts. Costs were estimated from the societal perspective and were collected from the national, district, hospital, health facility, and household levels. Costs at all these levels were summed to obtain the total cost to the district of providing care for children under age five. So that comparison could be made across districts, cost estimates were standardized to a hypothetical district with a population of 50,000 children under age five. This figure corresponds to a total population of around 300,000, which is roughly the average district population for Tanzania. Estimates of the additional cost to the district of implementing IMCI were based on the difference in cost of under-five care between the IMCI districts and the comparison districts, which, at the time of the study, had not yet implemented IMCI (Adam and others 2004b).

For 1999, the cost per child of caring for children under age five in IMCI districts was US$11.19, 44 percent lower than in the comparison districts (US$16.09) (Adam and others 2004b). The lower cost per child in IMCI districts was due to lower hospitalization and administrative costs at the district level. There was no statistically significant difference in costs incurred to treat children at primary care facilities and at the household level (figure 63.2).

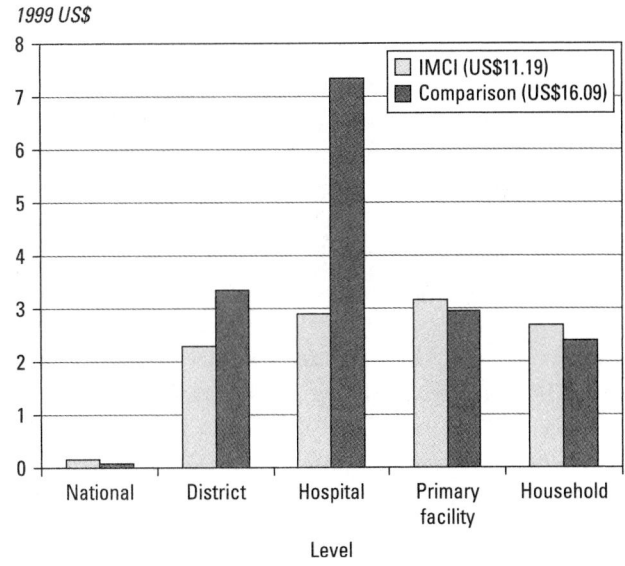

1999 US$

Source: Adam and others 2004b.

Note: Standard district with 50,000 children under age five.

Figure 63.2 Cost Components of Under-Five Care per Child in a Standard District

Hospital costs were 2.5 times higher in the comparison districts, not because of differences in the cost per under-five admission, but because more children under age five were hospitalized in those districts relative to IMCI districts (6 percent in IMCI districts compared with 15 percent in comparison districts; t–test: $p < 0.001$). There are two possible explanations: (a) improved quality of care and drug availability for children under age five at IMCI primary facilities reduced the need for referral and subsequent admission to hospitals, or (b) factors other than IMCI, such as differences in quality or geographical access to the hospitals in the different settings, meant that children in non-IMCI districts were more likely to seek care at hospitals. Given that IMCI training had only started one year before data collection of hospital admissions, the second possibility may have played a bigger role in this finding. Even if one takes the most conservative assumption—that all the difference was due to other factors—and excludes the hospital component from the analysis, the total cost per under-five child in IMCI districts was still lower than in comparison districts (6 percent).

The other important difference in costs between both types of districts was found in costs incurred at the district level, which were 50 percent higher in the comparison districts. These costs were mainly linked to more frequent trips for drug distribution and general purpose supervision in comparison districts than in IMCI districts.

Similar costs of training were observed in both types of districts during the study period. This finding was unexpected given the emphasis of IMCI on training, but a wide variety of training courses were performed in comparison districts for preventive, curative, and administrative issues during the study period. These courses included training for immunization, for use of insecticide-treated bednets, and for use of district Health Management Information System forms.

At the facility level, univariate comparison between IMCI and comparison district health facilities showed a 16 percent difference in the average cost per under-five visit (including vaccination visits) at government health centers and dispensaries (US$1.40 and US$1.60 in IMCI and comparison districts, respectively; t-test: $p = 0.5$). The average number of visits per child per year was 30 percent higher in the IMCI districts (3.28) compared with comparison districts (2.49). Taken together, the lower cost per visit but higher number of visits per child per year in IMCI facilities resulted in similar overall costs per child under age five for treatment in the two types of districts. Multivariate regression analysis, however, led to a different conclusion. Taking into account differences in other determinants across facilities, in particular the number of visits per facility, the cost per visit was at least 30 percent lower in IMCI facilities (t-test: $p < 0.001$).

Sensitivity analysis showed the importance of hospitalization costs in interpreting total district costs—the difference between IMCI and comparison districts was not sensitive to variation in the other parameters, only to the assumption about rates of hospitalization. Therefore, if one assumes that hospital admission rates were not related to IMCI, there is no difference in the cost of under-five care in the two types of districts. Otherwise, the costs in IMCI districts are lower than in the comparison districts.

In the IMCI districts, IMCI was implemented concurrently with measures designed to strengthen district management, such as evidence-based planning and expenditure mapping at district level (http://web.idrc.ca/en/ev-3170-201-1-DO_TOPIC.html). In fact, it has been argued that the decision to implement IMCI in the study districts was a result of the introduction of the evidence-based planning. It is not possible to separate the effects of IMCI from district-strengthening measures. The findings of the MCE study in Tanzania, therefore, can be interpreted as the costs of IMCI in the presence of a strong health system with adequate managerial capacity.

The US$11.20 cost per child of treating children under age five using IMCI in Tanzania translates into a per capita cost of US$1.70, compared with US$2.30 for routine care. This finding is similar to previous per capita estimates of the cost of IMCI in resource-poor countries (World Bank 1993). In addition, the Tanzania evaluation had similar findings with respect to savings from drug costs to those expected based on previous studies (Khan, Saha, and Ahmed 2002; Wammanda, Ejembi, and Iorliam 2003; World Bank 1993).

The effects of IMCI can be assessed in terms of changes in intermediate outcomes, such as improved quality of care at health facilities, or in terms of final outcomes, such as changes in under-five mortality or DALYs averted. In the Tanzania evaluation, a health facility survey was carried out in 2000 to compare the quality of case management and health systems support in IMCI and comparison districts. The results indicate that children in IMCI facilities received better care than children in comparison districts. Their health problems were more thoroughly assessed, they were more likely to be diagnosed and treated correctly as determined through a gold-standard reexamination, and the caretakers of the children were more likely to receive appropriate counseling and reported higher levels of knowledge about how to care for their sick children (Tanzania IMCI Multi-Country Evaluation Health Facility Survey Study Group 2004).

Estimating the effectiveness of IMCI training in improving health workers' performance required measuring the proportion of children correctly managed in IMCI and comparison facilities. *Correct management* is defined as the correct drug being provided in the correct formulation (amount, times per day, number of days) and the health worker explaining correctly to the caretaker how the drug should be administered at home. Not prescribing an antibiotic or antidiarrheal drug for a child who did not need one was also considered to be correct performance. In Tanzania, 65 percent of children under age five

Impact of IMCI on Mortality and Nutrition in Tanzania

Tanzania is the only MCE site where the evaluation has been completed. Its design included a comparison of mortality in four districts—two with and two without IMCI—over the two-year period starting in mid 2000. Demographic surveillance systems were used to compare under-five mortality rates in areas of the IMCI and control districts. Adjustments for age (zero to one and one to four years) and rainfall were made using Poisson regression models. During the IMCI phase-in period (July 1999 to June 2000), under-five mortality levels were almost identical in IMCI and comparison districts, at about 27 deaths

per 1,000 child-years or approximately 120 deaths per 1,000 children between birth and the age of less than five years. The quality of health care provided in the IMCI districts was substantially higher than in the control districts (see box 63.2). Over the following two years, mortality levels became 13 percent lower in IMCI districts than in the comparison areas, corresponding to a rate difference of 3.8 fewer deaths per 1,000 children per year. Stunting rates also became significantly lower in the IMCI districts. Contextual factors, such as mosquito net use, all favored the comparison districts.

Source: Armstrong Schellenberg and others 2004.

presenting to the surveyed IMCI facilities were correctly managed, compared with 16 percent in the comparison facilities. When the information on costs and effectiveness are taken together, the cost per child correctly managed is six times less in IMCI districts (US$4.02) than in the comparison districts (US$25.70) (Bryce and others forthcoming).

Some of the differences in costs might be due to factors other than IMCI, so these ratios have to be interpreted with care. What is clear, however, is that treating children using IMCI in Tanzania was no more costly—and probably less costly—than treating children using routine care. At the same time, it resulted in higher quality of care. To the extent that this higher quality of care leads to better health outcomes, IMCI is cost-effective—it costs less (or at least no more) and results in better outcomes (see box 63.1).

MCE in Brazil

Brazil is another MCE site where IMCI is being implemented in the context of an ambitious family health program (FHP), which is supported by the Ministry of Health and the World Bank and based at first-level government facilities. IMCI implementation started in 1996 and is moving ahead in the whole country, particularly in the northeast regions. IMCI training is targeted at FHP team members.

The MCE in Brazil was carried out in four states, all in northeast Brazil, the poorest area of the country. In total, 23 municipalities with both FHP and IMCI were compared with matched municipalities with FHP but without IMCI. Early results from one component of the evaluation—the time and motion study—provide useful insights. After controlling for possible confounding factors using regression analysis, the

evaluation found that IMCI-trained providers spent 1 minute and 26 seconds longer per consultation with under-five children than untrained providers did. The difference was much greater when patient load was low but decreased as the number of patients a provider saw per day increased. This finding suggests that the system's ability to absorb IMCI depends on current capacity utilization. In terms of the assessment of quality of care in the surveyed facilities, IMCI-trained health workers were shown to provide significantly better care than those who had not been trained (Amaral and others 2004; Gouws and others 2004). (See "Lessons about Implementation Success and Failure" later in this chapter for additional results on quality of care.)

These results are important for policy development relating to child health. Where current caseloads are relatively low, providers spend additional time to provide better child health services, using IMCI as the basis of part of their current activities. In this study, the mean number of consultations per provider per day was 34, and 95 percent of the providers had caseloads of fewer than 50 patients per day. If this finding is representative of the rest of Brazil, it would be possible to introduce IMCI relatively easily throughout the country without encountering capacity constraints in terms of provider time. In areas with high patient loads, however, it would be important to explore whether it is possible to maintain high quality of care under IMCI in those areas and what the alternatives should be (Adam and others, forthcoming).

Summary of MCE Results

The available results from the MCE so far show that costs of child health care in Tanzania were comparable or lower in districts with IMCI than with routine case management. Quality of care was higher, and a 13 percent reduction in mortality was also found in the IMCI districts in the study period. This finding strongly suggests that IMCI is a cost-effective intervention compared with routine care, as it costs less and is more effective in saving children's lives.

In Brazil, the MCE study also showed improved quality of care for children under age five after health workers were trained in IMCI. The results also showed that staff time constraints were unlikely to limit the application of IMCI, because, in settings with low caseloads, health workers could be expected to use the available excess capacity to provide better care for children under age five. Assuming that primary health facilities will experience savings on drug costs similar to those observed in Tanzania and previous modeling studies, one could also argue that IMCI is a good value for money in the Brazilian setting.

Equity Issues

Some of the equity implications related to care seeking and treatment have also been evaluated in the four rural districts included in the IMCI evaluation in Tanzania (Schellenberg and others 2003; Victora and others 2003). The MCE analysis found no association between sex and any indicator of morbidity, care seeking, case management, or compliance with treatment or follow-up instructions, suggesting that mothers and health workers treat boys and girls similarly (Schellenberg and others 2003). This finding is in accordance with that of Gwatkin and others (2000). Similarly, there were no statistically significant associations between socioeconomic status and reported prevalence of fever, diarrhea, severe diarrhea, or pneumonia. However, hospital admissions were almost half as common in the lowest socioeconomic status quintile as in the highest (t-test: $p = 0.0093$), suggesting that referral care is more readily accessible to the wealthy.

Positive associations were observed between socioeconomic status and care seeking from an appropriate provider (a qualified health worker practicing allopathic medicine) for fever without cough or diarrhea, for care seeking for episodes perceived as severe, and for using an appropriate provider as the first source of care. This finding is illustrated in figure 63.3, which puts households into five wealth categories. The poorest group was at least 25 percent less likely to have sought care than the least poor. Among the children who sought care, antibiotic use for probable pneumonia was less than half as common among the poorest than among the least poor. Also, children in the lowest socioeconomic group were half as likely to have been given antimalarials as those in the highest category (t-test: $p < 0.0001$).

These findings suggest that, although the prevalence of disease (self-reported) does not differ by socioeconomic status, care seeking and the probability of receiving appropriate care

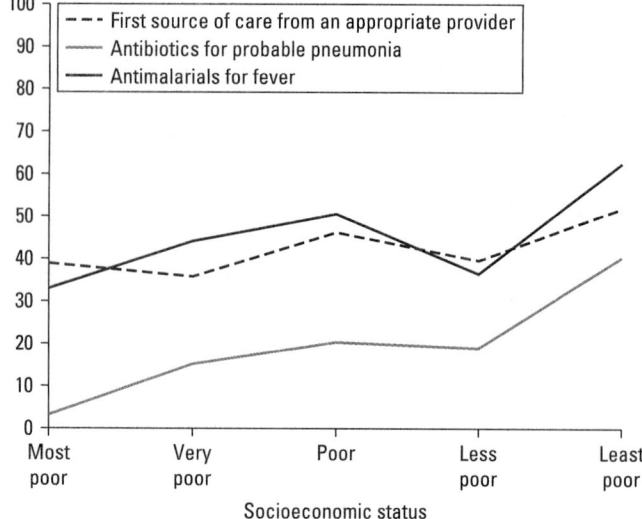

Proportion of children (percent)

- - - First source of care from an appropriate provider
—— Antibiotics for probable pneumonia
—— Antimalarials for fever

Socioeconomic status

Most poor / Very poor / Poor / Less poor / Least poor

Source: Victora and others 2003, based on data taken from Schellenberg and others 2003.

Figure 63.3 Proportions of Children, by Socioeconomic Quintiles, Who Were Brought to an Appropriate Provider and Who Received Correct Care, in Rural Tanzania

vary markedly, even within an apparently homogeneous rural population. This observation agrees with data on mortality and nutritional status inequalities for Tanzania (Schellenberg and others 2003). There is no evidence yet showing whether the introduction of IMCI has reduced or increased this type of inequality.

IMPLEMENTATION OF PROGRAMS: LESSONS OF EXPERIENCE

The IMCI strategy was thoroughly evaluated from its onset. Only two years after the first health worker training course took place, the MCE was launched (Bryce and others 2004). MCE researchers visited 12 countries and carried out in-depth studies in five of those. The MCE and the more recent Analytic Review of IMCI (DFID and others 2003), which included visits to six countries, provide the background for this section.

Institutions and Programs

IMCI introduction was highly successful. As of December 2002, WHO's global monitoring team reported that IMCI had been introduced in 109 countries (see http://www.who.int/child-adolescent-health/overview/child_health/map12_02.jpg). Twelve countries were included in the introduction phase, in which the strategy was officially endorsed, a national IMCI coordination group was appointed, and key ministry of health staff members were trained in the IMCI clinical guidelines. Another 50 countries were in the early implementation phase, which included development of a national plan, selection of initial districts for implementation, adaptation of the IMCI clinical guidelines and materials, training of course facilitators, and planning at the district level. Finally, 47 countries were in the expansion phase, which included scaling up IMCI activities in districts already covered and expanding to cover additional districts (WHO and UNICEF 1999).

The fact that a country has adopted the IMCI strategy, however, does not mean that a high population coverage has been reached. The best available estimates of IMCI coverage are provided by the percentage of health workers who underwent IMCI training and are managing sick children. For example, the Brazil MCE (Amaral and others 2004) has shown that IMCI is being implemented in all 27 states, but in some of those states only a few health professionals were trained. In the three states selected for the evaluation because of reportedly strong IMCI implementation, there was at least one IMCI-trained health worker in 239 out of 443 municipalities (54.0 percent), but only 23 municipalities (5.2 percent) had at least 50 percent of health workers trained after three years. In Peru, also a leading country in IMCI training, approximately 10 percent of all doctors and nurses providing child care were trained after seven years of IMCI implementation (Huicho and others 2005). Therefore, levels of training coverage in most countries appear to be low.

Lessons about Implementation Success and Failure

Both the MCE (Bryce and others 2004) and the Analytic Review of IMCI that were carried out in 2002–3 (DFID and others 2003) confirm that IMCI has been highly successful in motivating managers and health workers. The training program is highly regarded, and trainees are pleased with its logical, consistent approach to child health problems. Innovative clinical skills, such as the use of palmar pallor to diagnose anemia and the use of breathing rate for pneumonia, are often praised. Nutritional counseling, an area in which most health workers receive little formal training in school, is also greatly appreciated. When asked about the limitations of IMCI, health workers often mention the increased time required for a consultation and the difficulty of following the IMCI guidelines when there is a high patient load.

Several studies have shown that health workers trained in IMCI do perform better than those not trained. Health facility surveys carried out in Tanzania (Schellenberg and others 2003), Brazil (Amaral and others 2004), and Uganda show that IMCI training substantially improves health worker performance in assessing and managing sick children, and in counseling their caretakers. Box 63.2 summarizes MCE findings on antibiotic prescribing patterns, a critical area for managing sick children (Gouws and others 2004).

Important constraints to IMCI implementation were also identified through visits to 17 countries by the MCE and Analytic Review teams. Using the framework developed by the Commission on Macroeconomics and Health (Hanson and others 2001), the teams described shortcomings in three areas: community and household issues, health service delivery issues, and issues related to health sector policy and strategic management.

Community and Household Issues. Coverage levels for effective interventions to improve child survival are remarkably low in most developing countries. A review of the 42 countries that account for 90 percent of global child deaths showed that only two out of nine key interventions reached more than half of all children (Bryce and others 2003). This finding agrees with

---

| Box 63.2 |

Improving the Use of Antimicrobials through IMCI Case-Management: Findings from the MCE

Antimicrobial drugs, including antibiotics and antimalarials, are an essential child survival intervention. Prompt and correct provision of drugs to children under age five who need them can save lives. Ensuring that these drugs are not prescribed unnecessarily and that those who receive them complete the full course can slow the development of antimicrobial resistance. Analysis of data collected through observation-based surveys at randomly selected first-level health facilities in Brazil, Tanzania, and Uganda shows that children receiving care from health workers trained in IMCI are significantly more likely than those receiving care from workers not yet trained in IMCI to receive correct prescriptions for antimicrobial drugs, to receive the first dose of the drug before leaving the health facility, to have their caregivers advised on how to administer the drug, and to have caregivers who are able to describe correctly how to give the drug at home as they leave the health facility. IMCI training is an effective intervention to improve the rational use of antimicrobial drugs for sick children visiting first-level health facilities in low- and middle-income countries.

Source: Gouws and others 2004.

those of the MCE, showing that the third component of IMCI—improving family and community practices—was poorly implemented. At the global level, UNICEF was primarily in charge of developing this component (see http://www.childinfo.org/eddb/imci/practices.htm), and at the country level, UNICEF often acted through nongovernmental organizations (NGOs). Coverage with these community-based programs tended to be patchy. In Peru (Huicho and others 2005) and Tanzania, the districts that were selected for implementation of the community component were not the same as those prioritized for health worker training, which were chosen by the ministry of health with WHO support. This precluded any possible synergy at the district level between improved quality of care in health facilities and community interventions, including those aimed at improving care seeking and compliance with health workers' advice.

All the countries that were visited, however, have a number of programs and projects that deliver child survival interventions at the community level. Many of these interventions are part of the key IMCI family practices, but they are being delivered in an uncoordinated manner by national, international, and nongovernmental organizations in limited geographical areas. The low population coverage of these projects makes it unlikely that they will ever result in a substantial effect on a larger scale. The notable exceptions are the EPI programs, which, despite some recent evidence of falling coverage (Bryce and others 2003), still reach the vast majority of children in developing countries.

On the basis of the experience obtained in these countries, it appears that those key family practices that are most likely to be synergistic with facility-based IMCI—improved care seeking, home management of disease, and compliance with health worker advice—are among those least likely to be supported by existing programs. Existing programs seem to favor biological interventions such as vaccines, micronutrient supplementation, and insecticide-treated materials.

The present criticism of community IMCI should not be extrapolated to community-level child health interventions in general, which can often be highly successful. These interventions are covered in chapter 56.

Health Service Delivery Issues. Given the difficulties in implementing the community component, IMCI was largely restricted in nearly all countries to training health workers in the improved management of care for young children. Even there, some difficulties were apparent.

In countries such as Peru, Brazil, and Uganda, after an initial sharp increase in the number of health workers who were trained, budgetary and other restrictions led to a decrease in the number of training courses being offered. In Peru, about 10 percent of all eligible health workers in the public sector were trained after seven years of implementation. At the

current rate of training, several decades will be needed before full coverage is reached (Huicho and others 2005). Similar results were observed in Uganda (J. Nsungwa-Sabiti, personal communication).

Staff turnover is also a major problem. In Peru, between 1996 and 2001, 43 percent of IMCI-trained health workers had already been rotated since their training (Huicho and others 2005). In Tanzania, where staffing patterns appear to be quite stable in comparison with the situation in other countries, 23 percent of trained staff had moved within three years of initial training (C. Mbuyia, personal communication). Problems with turnover were also observed in Bolivia, Brazil, and Niger. These health workers did not necessarily leave government employment, but high rotation means that IMCI may not be continually delivered to the same target population over time.

Another relevant issue mentioned in several countries was that of low staff motivation, which was often associated with low salary levels. In Uganda, the performance of health workers fell dramatically in 2001 after the government discontinued cost-sharing schemes that were used to supplement drug supplies and health worker salaries at the facility level (Burnham and others 2004). In Cambodia and Tanzania, salary levels are so low that health workers need other sources of income to maintain their families. Issues related to human resources are addressed in greater detail in chapter 71.

Poor supervision was a major issue in all countries that were visited. IMCI recommends regular supervisory visits that should include systematic observation and feedback on case management. In Peru, the average number of supervisory visits was 0.19 per facility per year (Huicho and others 2005). In Bangladesh, a baseline (pre-IMCI) health facility survey conducted in 2000 found that none of the facilities in the study area had received a supervisory visit, including observation of case management, within the previous six months (S. E. Arifeen, personal communication). Common reasons given by health workers for erratic supervision activities are shortages of vehicles, fuel, and staff members.

Problems with referral were also common. The Urgent Referral category in figure 63.1 requires immediate referral to a hospital. In several countries (Bangladesh, Cambodia, Niger, Uganda, and Tanzania), it was reported that children in this category are often not taken to a hospital because of distance or lack of funds for travel and hospitalization-related expenses. For example, in a Tanzania survey, only 5 of 13 children who had been referred were actually taken to a hospital (Schellenberg and others 2003). Also, in some countries hospital staff members who had not been trained in IMCI were reluctant to admit children with danger signs identified through the IMCI algorithm. This situation highlights the need for reinforcing training of referral-level health workers using IMCI guidelines.

Another important limitation, observed in Bangladesh, Cambodia, Niger, and Uganda, is the low use of public sector health care for a variety of reasons (accessibility, official or under-the-table user fees, perceived poor quality, lack of drugs, and so on). For example, using Ministry of Health documents in Niger, the authors estimated that the average annual number of attendances by children under age five was 0.5. In Bangladesh, only 8 percent of children who were ill were taken to a qualified provider (S. E. Arifeen, personal communication). In the presence of such low utilization rates, it is unlikely that health worker training can have an effect on mortality rates, unless simultaneous community activities improve care-seeking practices.

Although equipment and vaccines that are needed for IMCI delivery were available in most countries visited, availability of drug supplies varied from country to country. Shortages were reported in Cambodia and Zambia, and other countries, such as Peru and Tanzania, reported that essential IMCI drugs were mostly available.

Health Sector Policy and Strategic Management Issues. Several of the problems described in the preceding section are directly related to health sector issues. In addition, issues related to higher-level policy and management may also represent constraints to successful IMCI implementation.

In some countries, IMCI was not fully institutionalized at national or subnational levels. For example, a national coordinator was not appointed or was appointed on a part-time basis. In Peru, IMCI was implemented side by side with CDD and ARI programs, which it was expected to replace, and in several districts the ARI coordinator's tasks were expanded to also encompass IMCI. In several countries, IMCI activities did not have a separate budget line, or they were not included in district health plans, or neither. A report on the Analytic Review of IMCI (DFID and others 2003, 39) states, "IMCI was generally introduced as a strategy, not as a program. If this was not a barrier in the pilot phase, it seemed to generate problems for rapid scaling up. In five of the six Analytic Review countries, IMCI focal persons did not have the rank or the responsibility of previous disease specific program managers within their Ministry of Health, and IMCI did not have a budget line and a strong management structure." The report also argued that decentralization, as part of health sector reform, reduced managerial capacity at the central level and had, at least in the short term, a negative effect on IMCI implementation.

Conflict between IMCI guidelines and existing policies and regulations was present in some countries, particularly the former Soviet republics of Kazakhstan and the Kyrgyz Republic, where policies for hospital admission—requiring, for example, that all children with diarrhea be hospitalized—were in conflict with IMCI guidelines. Another regrettable example comes from Brazil, where both doctors and nurses were being trained in IMCI until medical associations threatened legal action to prevent nurses from being trained in using antibiotics for life-threatening conditions. This obstruction succeeded despite an MCE health facility survey that showed that IMCI-trained nurses performed as well as doctors in managing sick children (Amaral and others 2004). In Morocco, IMCI-trained nurses are also unable to prescribe antibiotics because of central regulations.

A particular challenge came to light when the MCE team visited Cambodia and Niger and the Analytic Review team visited Mali. These countries have high levels of under-five mortality and thus the greatest need for IMCI. They also have weak health systems and low utilization rates and are therefore having difficulty implementing IMCI successfully. Just as for individuals, the *inverse care law*—which suggests that those who most need high quality care are the least likely to get it—seems to also apply to countries (Hart 1971).

However, there is a possibility that IMCI (or other approaches to managing sick children) might help strengthen selected health system functions through specific approaches, as the Analytic Review team observed in regard to drug and commodity availability, service management, and health worker motivation through IMCI in the Arab Republic of Egypt (DFID and others 2003).

Implications for Health System Development

The first component of IMCI, which involves training of health care workers, has been implemented in many developing countries and has resulted in important improvements in the quality of care delivered to children in first-level facilities in limited geographic areas. The potential population-level effect of IMCI case-management training has not been realized, however, for three reasons:

- Sufficient resources were not available for full implementation.
- Few health systems in low-income countries are capable of providing the policy, personnel, and managerial support needed to expand and sustain high levels of IMCI training coverage.
- At the time of this writing, not one country had succeeded in mounting a behavior-change program capable of improving care seeking, home management of illness, and nutrition-related practices to coverage levels that will result in population-level changes in service utilization or health status.

One implication for health system development is that support should be continued and expanded for integrated case management in first-level facilities as an essential component of an effective child survival strategy. A second implication, however, is that greatly expanded efforts must be directed simultaneously to the development of new and innovative approaches to strengthening health systems and to reaching families and communities with known and affordable child survival interventions.

An important distinction can be made between interventions and delivery strategies (Bryce and others 2003). The same intervention (vitamin A capsules, perhaps) can be delivered through different strategies—for example, to children attending health facilities, on National Immunization Days, or directly at the household level through community networks. In spite of its community component—which in most countries has not been operational anyway—IMCI, as implemented to mid 2004, relies on health facilities as its key delivery strategy.

The first component of the IMCI strategy—a focus on improving health worker skills—was innovative to the extent that it provided clear technical guidelines and yet required country-level adaptation. Similar levels of technical clarity and country-level flexibility did not exist for the second and third components of the IMCI strategy, which focused on improving health systems to support IMCI and improving family and community practices. Within these two components, the IMCI strategy has been criticized for attempting to become a uniform global strategy, with guidelines for implementation that do not allow room for country-level modifications, especially the incremental approaches to implementation needed by weak health systems (Bryce and others 2003). The first component of IMCI can serve as a model for the types of development work that must now move forward in the health systems and family practice areas; however, in these areas, key decisions about how best to deliver interventions will need to be made at the country level and below.

One example of progress is that WHO and its partners have now developed a process for assessing country-level opportunities and requirements for achieving population-level behavior change in relation to key family practices and for developing feasible and collaborative work plans for effectively implementing child health activities at the community level (A. Bartlett, personal communication).

As the MCE and Analytic Review have shown, IMCI requires a functional health system with managerial capacity; an ability to train health workers and to keep them on the job; an efficient means of supplying drugs, vaccines, and equipment; and the capacity to maintain regular supervisory activities. It also requires appropriate care-seeking practices, leading to a reasonable level of health services utilization by children under age five. In most countries, appropriate health services utilization is unlikely to be achieved without strong family and household-level interventions such as those promoted by community IMCI.

These problems, however, are not specific to IMCI; they affect every other delivery strategy that relies heavily on health facilities, including the predecessors of IMCI, namely the CDD

and ARI programs. In fact, at least in theory, the efficiency gains represented by the integration promoted by IMCI should make it easier for developing countries to implement as the key child health strategy, so a return to vertical programs is not the answer.

Given these difficulties, however, there may be a temptation to bypass health services altogether in the poorest countries by promoting the delivery of child health interventions directly to families and households. There are successful examples of such community delivery schemes—for example, projects dispensing antimalarials (Pagnoni and others 1997; Kidane and Morrow 2000) and antibiotics for pneumonia (Sazawal and Black 1992). This approach may, in fact, be the most viable short-term solution for countries with weak health services, but it should not be forgotten that most success stories represent small-scale pilot projects with strong managerial backup. In countries with weak systems, the managerial support for implementing and sustaining high-quality, community-based interventions is also likely to be lacking, so it may be naive to assume that such programs will have the effects that health services have failed to deliver. Also, just as first-level health facility care depends on referral services for backup, community delivery schemes will require operational first-level health facilities to handle complications and treatment failures.

There is no substitute for strengthening health systems in the poorest countries. In the long run, strengthening these systems will be the key intervention for reducing child mortality as well as for promoting healthy growth and development. Delivery strategies that reach communities either directly or through other mechanisms are needed in the short term, but the long-term goal of improving health services is paramount.

THE RESEARCH AND DEVELOPMENT AGENDA

This section starts by addressing health systems research issues related to scaling up child health interventions effectively. Key issues on the research agenda are how to make the best possible use of integrated case management in settings where health systems are weak and how to design alternative delivery strategies to improve child survival in such settings.

Specific issues relate to how to counteract the main constraints to scaling up IMCI that were described earlier in "Implementation of Programs: Lessons of Experience." For example, research is needed in the following areas:

- how to increase utilization in the public sector (and the role of user fees in this respect)
- how to develop viable public sector–private sector partnerships
- how to reduce staff turnover

- how to improve supervision and make it sustainable
- how to institutionalize IMCI case-management training and supervision at the district level.

In addition, research is needed on how to strengthen health systems and improve family and community practices for child survival in ways that take into account and build on features of the country context. These features include the epidemiologic profile and the characteristics of the health system. Country-level assessments and planning and support for longer-term implementation are required to achieve high and equitable coverage and population effect in different epidemiologic, health system, and cultural settings (Bellagio Study Group on Child Survival 2003). Innovative research is needed involving country-level investigators and program staff members, with international partnerships if required, to develop and evaluate different combinations of health facility–based and household-based delivery schemes. In particular, research should address how to go to scale with interventions that have been proven effective in pilot studies. From the costing perspective, research should address the issue of how to estimate the cost of scaling up using different scenarios of resource availability and constraints.

Monitoring and evaluation are key components of the required research. Tools must be developed for use at the district and national levels, and capacity to use them must be strengthened.

CONCLUSIONS: PROMISES AND PITFALLS

IMCI was introduced in the mid 1990s as an ambitious global strategy that held many promises. Cost-effective vertical interventions against the main causes of under-five mortality in the world were integrated into a single, facility-based health worker training program. The program was accompanied by efforts to improve health systems support for child health care and to promote key family practices at the community level. Integration was expected to further improve coverage levels and the cost-effectiveness of child survival interventions relative to their delivery through separate vertical programs.

IMCI case-management training was repeatedly shown to improve the quality of care delivered in first-level health facilities, and the costing data reviewed above suggest that it can do so at similar or lower costs than those of existing health services. IMCI, therefore, is able to deliver better child health care at no increase in costs.

Nevertheless, community IMCI interventions only reached meager population coverage in the countries studied, and even health worker training was never effectively scaled up in most countries as a result of health system constraints. The major effect on child survival that was initially expected as a result of

IMCI implementation has not yet materialized, and country reports of the barriers to achieving and maintaining high coverage levels suggest that effects will not be seen unless IMCI in first-level facilities is buttressed by equally strong or stronger efforts to develop health system capacity and reach families and communities. In fact, progress in child survival in the late 1990s and early 21st century has been slower than in earlier decades (Bellagio Study Group on Child Survival 2003), and current trends suggest that the Millennium Development Goals are unlikely to be achieved for most countries unless major new investments are made very soon.

The Tanzania results suggest that, in a setting where IMCI was implemented in conjunction with health system strengthening and where utilization of health facilities is high, an effect on mortality and nutritional status is likely. However, experience from other countries showed that reaching high and sustained implementation was difficult.

Although IMCI has only partially lived up to initial expectations, it has many positive aspects that must be fostered. A return to isolated vertical programs for child survival will not solve the difficulties faced by scaling up IMCI effectively, and integration should continue to be a key goal of child survival strategies in the future. In fact, much of the frustration associated with reported underperformance of IMCI arises from the fact that sufficient resources—financial, human, and organizational—were not planned for or available to support its full implementation, either at national or at international levels. The meager training coverage levels observed in most of the MCE countries are clear evidence of insufficient implementation, and it is thus not surprising that coverage and effect were also less than expected.

Renewed and expanded efforts to reduce child mortality should build on the proven effectiveness of IMCI case management in first-level facilities, but they also should incorporate new knowledge. Country-specific planning is needed to reach families and communities and to build on the existing health system to achieve and sustain population-level coverage. Countries with weak health systems will require creative approaches to intervention delivery in the short term at the same time that health systems are strengthened as a long-term strategy. The poorest strata of the population are also the neediest in terms of health care and the hardest to reach. The challenge of improving equity is not unique to IMCI or to child survival; it affects virtually every intervention and delivery strategy. Unless equity considerations become a key part of policy making and of monitoring outcomes, interventions may widen instead of narrow inequity gaps (Victora and others 2003).

A continuing challenge is how to raise and sustain the standing of child survival in the international agenda. The more than 10 million annual deaths of children under age five—more than 20 deaths per minute—represent twice the number of deaths attributable to AIDS, malaria, and tuberculosis combined (Black, Morris, and Bryce 2003). Putting child survival back on the public health and development agenda is an essential developmental step in the process of refining country-level and global child health strategies. Only through taking stock of the lessons learned in early IMCI implementation can a flexible, integrated program be developed that will improve child survival in particular and child health in general.

ACKNOWLEDGMENTS

A substantial portion of this chapter is based on early results from the Multi-Country Evaluation of IMCI Effectiveness, Cost, and Impact. The MCE is funded by the Bill & Melinda Gates Foundation and is supported by technical assistance from the World Health Organization and a technical advisory group representing global expertise in cost-effectiveness analysis, measurement, research design, and child health.

REFERENCES

Adam, T., D. G. Amorim, S. Edwards, J. Amaral, and D. B. Evans. Forthcoming. "Capacity Constraints to the Adoption of New Interventions: Consultation Time and the Integrated Management of Childhood Illness in Brazil."

Adam, T., D. Bishai, M. Khan, and D. Evans. 2004a. *Methods for the Costing Component of the Multi-Country Evaluation of IMCI.* Geneva: World Health Organization. http://www.who.int/imci-mce.

Adam, T., F. Manzi, C. Kakundwa, J. Schellenberg, L. Mgalula, D. de Savigny, and others. 2004b. *Analysis Report on the Costs of IMCI in Tanzania.* Geneva: World Health Organization. http://www.who.int/imci-mce.

Amaral, J., E. Gouws, J. Bryce, A. J. M. Leite, A. L. A. Cunha, and C. G. Victora. 2004. "Effect of Integrated Management of Childhood Illness (IMCI) on Health Worker Performance in Northeast Brazil." *Cadernos de Saude Publica 2004.* 20 (suppl. 2): 209–12.

Armstrong Schellenberg, J. R. M., T. Adam, H. Mshinda, H. Masanja, G. Kabadi, O. Mukasa, and others. 2004. "Effectiveness and Costs of Facility-Based Integrated Management of Childhood Illness (IMCI) in Tanzania." *Lancet* 364 (9445):1583–94.

Bellagio Study Group on Child Survival. 2003. "Knowledge into Action for Child Survival." *Lancet* 362 (9380): 323–27.

Black, R. E., S. S. Morris, and J. Bryce. 2003. "Where and Why Are 10 Million Children Dying Every Year?" *Lancet* 361 (9376): 2226–34.

Boulanger, L. L., L. A. Lee, and A. Odhacha. 1999. "Treatment in Kenyan Rural Health Facilities: Projected Drug Costs Using the WHO-UNICEF Integrated Management of Childhood Illness (IMCI) Guidelines." *Bulletin of the World Health Organization* 77(10): 852–58.

Bryce, J., S. Arifeen, G. Pariyo, C. F. Lanata, D. Gwatkin, J. P. Habicht, and the Multi-Country Evaluation of IMCI Study Group. 2003. "Reducing Child Mortality: Can Public Health Deliver?" *Lancet* 362 (9378): 159–64.

Bryce, J. C., Boschi-Pinto, K. Shibuya, R. E. Black, and the WHO Child Health Epidemiology Reference Group. 2005. "WHO Estimates of the Causes of Death in Children." *Lancet* 365 (9465): 1147–52.

Bryce J., E. Gouws, T. Adam, R. Black, J. A. Schellenberg, C. Victora, and J-P. Habicht. Forthcoming. "Improving the Efficiency of Facility-Based Child Health Care: A Success Story from Tanzania."

Bryce, J., C. G. Victora, J-P. Habicht, J. P. Vaughan, and R. E. Black. 2004. "The Multi-Country Evaluation of the Integrated Management of Childhood Illness Strategy: Lessons for the Evaluation of Public Health Interventions." *American Journal of Public Health* 94 (3): 406–15.

Burnham, G. M., G. W. Pariyo, E. Galiwango, and F. Wabwire-Mangen. 2004. "Discontinuation of Cost-Sharing in Uganda." *Bulletin of the World Health Organization* 82 (3): 187–95.

Claeson, M., and R. J. Waldman. 2000. "The Evolution of Child Health Programmes in Developing Countries: From Targeting Diseases to Targeting People." *Bulletin of the World Health Organization* 78 (10): 1234–45.

DFID (U.K. Department for International Development), UNICEF (United Nations Children's Fund), World Bank, USAID (U.S. Agency for International Development), and WHO (World Health Organization). 2003. *The Analytic Review of Integrated Management of Childhood Illness Strategy (Final Report).* Geneva: World Health Organization. http://www.who.int/child-adolescent-health/New_Publications/IMCI/ISBN_92_4_159173_0.pdf.

Gouws, E., J. Bryce, J. P. Habicht, J. Amaral, G. Pariyo, J. A. Schellenberg, and O. Fontaine. 2004. "Improving Antimicrobial Use among Health Workers in First-Level Facilities: Results from the Multi-Country Evaluation of the Integrated Management of Childhood Illness Strategy." *Bulletin of the World Health Organization* 82 (7): 509–15.

Gove, S. 1997. "Integrated Management of Childhood Illness by Outpatient Health Workers: Technical Basis and Overview." *Bulletin of the World Health Organization* 75 (Suppl. 1): 7–24.

Gwatkin, D. R., S. Rustein, K. Johnson, R. P. Pande, and A. Wagstaff. 2000. "Socio-Economic Differences in Health, Nutrition, and Population in Tanzania." World Bank, Washington, DC. http://www.worldbank.org/poverty/health/data/tanzania/tanzania.pdf.

Hanson, K., K. Ranson, V. Oliveira-Cruz, and A. Mills. 2001. "Constraints to Scaling up Health Interventions: A Conceptual Framework and Empirical Analysis." Working Group 5 Paper 14, WHO Commission on Macroeconomics and Health, Geneva. http://www.cmhealth.org/docs/wg5_paper14.pdf.

Hart, J. T. 1971. "The Inverse Care Law." *Lancet* 1 (7696): 405–12.

Huicho, L., M. Dávila, M. Campos, C. Drasbeck, J. Bryce, and C. G. Victora. 2005. "Scaling up IMCI to the National Level: Achievements and Challenges in Peru." *Health Policy and Planning* 20 (1): 14–24.

Jones, G., R. Steketee, R. E. Black, Z. A. Bhutta, S. S. Morris, and the Bellagio Study Group on Child Survival. 2003. "How Many Child Deaths Can We Prevent This Year?" *Lancet* 62 (9377): 65–71.

Khan, M. M., S. Ahmed, and K. K. Saha. 2000. "Implementing IMCI in a Developing Country: Estimating the Need for Additional Health Workers in Bangladesh." *Human Resources for Health Development Journal* 4: 73–82.

Khan, M. M., K. K. Saha, and S. Ahmed. 2002. "Adopting Integrated Management of Childhood Illness Module at Local Level in Bangladesh: Implications for Recurrent Costs." *Journal of Health and Population Nutrition* 20 (1): 42–50.

Kidane, G., and R. H. Morrow. 2000. "Teaching Mothers to Provide Home Treatment of Malaria in Tigray, Ethiopia: A Randomised Trial." *Lancet* 356 (9229): 550–55.

Mathers, C. D., C. J. L. Murray, and A. D. Lopez. 2006. "The Burden of Disease and Mortality by Condition: Data, Methods, and Results for the Year 2001." In *Global Burden of Disease and Risk Factors,* eds. Alan D. Lopez, Colin D. Mathers, Majid Ezzati, Dean T. Jamison, and Christopher J. L. Murray. New York: Oxford University Press.

Pagnoni, F., N. Convelbo, J. Tiendrebeogo, S. Cousens, and F. Esposito. 1997. "A Community-Based Programme to Provide Prompt and

Adequate Treatment of Presumptive Malaria in Children." *Transactions of the Royal Society of Tropical Medicine and Hygiene* 91 (5): 512–17.

Sazawal, S., and R. E. Black. 1992. "Meta-Analysis of Intervention Trials on Case-Management of Pneumonia in Community Settings." *Lancet* 340 (8818): 528–33.

Schellenberg, J. A., C. G. Victora, A. Mushi, D. de Savigny, D. Schellenberg, H. Mshinda, and J. Bryce. 2003. "Inequities among the Very Poor: Health Care for Children in Rural Southern Tanzania." *Lancet* 361 (9357): 561–66.

Tanzania IMCI Multi-Country Evaluation Health Facility Survey Study Group. 2004. "Health Care for Under-Fives in Rural Tanzania: Effect of Integrated Management of Childhood Illness on Observed Quality of Care." *Health Policy and Planning* 19 (1): 1–10.

Tulloch, J. 1999. "Integrated Approach to Child Health in Developing Countries." *Lancet* 354 (Suppl. 2): SII16–20.

Victora, C. G., A. Wagstaff, J. A. Schellenberg, D. Gwatkin, M. Claeson, and J. P. Habicht. 2003. "Applying an Equity Lens to Child Health and Mortality: More of the Same Is Not Enough." *Lancet* 362 (9379): 233–41.

Wammanda, R. D., C. L. Ejembi, and T. Iorliam. 2003. "Drug Treatment Costs: Projected Impact of Using the Integrated Management of Childhood Illnesses." *Tropical Doctor* 33 (2): 86–88.

WHO (World Health Organization) and UNICEF (United Nations Children's Fund). 1999. *IMCI Planning Guide: Gaining Experience with the IMCI Strategy in a Country.* WHO/CHS/CAH/99.1. Geneva: WHO. http://www.who.int/child-adolescent-health/New_Publications/ IMCI/WHO_CHS_CAH_99.1.pdf.

———. 2001. *Model Chapter for Textbooks: Integrated Management of Childhood Illness.* WHO/CAH/00.40. Geneva: WHO.

World Bank. 1993. *World Development Report 1993: Investing in Health.* New York: Oxford University Press.

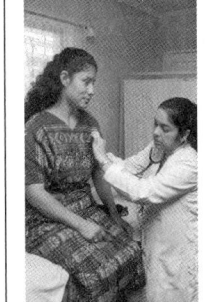

Chapter **64**

General Primary Care

Stephen Tollman, Jane Doherty, and Jo-Ann Mulligan

Primary health care has always been a feature of health care systems and—from a modern perspective—involves four interrelated aspects: a set of activities, a level of care, a strategy for organizing health care, and a philosophy that permeates health care provision. At full stretch, then, the "primary health care approach" can affect the configuration and focus of the entire health system and extend to the development of communities (Vuori 1985).

It is not always easy to see how information on the cost-effectiveness of individual interventions—the focus of part 2 of this volume—contributes to the achievement of the wider features of primary health care. Indeed, Starfield (1998) points out that the importance of particular services or interventions is overrated, in part because of limited appreciation of the "essential and unique functions" of primary care. These functions are mutually reinforcing and include first-contact care; continuity in care (in Starfield's words, "person-focused over time"); comprehensiveness of available services; and coordination with specialized services and other levels of care. The functions point to the centrality of how primary care is organized and delivered, something with which the cost-effectiveness approach has hitherto not been greatly concerned. This chapter attempts to identify some of the common ground between the primary health care approach and the cost-effectiveness approach. We propose that resource constraints simultaneously require (a) the targeting of services toward burdens of disease that are amenable to highly cost-effective interventions and (b) the general strengthening of the health system, particularly at the primary care and district levels.

THE SCOPE OF GENERAL PRIMARY CARE PRACTICE

General primary care can be defined as the immediate—and often continuing—medical and health management of a child, adult, or family when the patient first presents to the formal health system. In low- and middle-income countries, such care is often provided from publicly funded health posts and health centers by nurses or other midlevel health workers, with medical doctors expected to play a support, training, and referral role.

Comprehensive versus Selective Care

The 1978 Alma Ata declaration on primary health care (WHO and UNICEF 1978) was informed by a number of well-described, small-scale health and development efforts in a range of settings (Newell 1975; Tollman 1991). It focused international health care efforts on low-cost, potentially high-impact interventions, both medical and social, at both the primary and community levels. In particular, the declaration emphasized the importance of health promotion and community development through, for example, the supply of water and sanitation and the involvement of communities in decision making.

Before long, the extent of resources and capacities needed to implement such comprehensive activities led to the emergence of the concept of "selective primary health care" (Walsh and Warren 1979). This concept advocated a focus on a limited number of priority conditions, such as children's health and particular tropical diseases. Selective interventions, often centrally planned, and managed and operated by a dedicated staff, were intended as entry points into the health care system. Such an approach, when fully operationalized as a "vertical program," proved especially useful in implementing control and eradication campaigns and in dealing with epidemics following natural disasters (Unger, de Paepe, and Green 2003; World Bank 1994).

The selective approach attracted strong criticism for not acknowledging that primary care practice needs to take account of the range of conditions that present, many of which—by definition—were excluded from the selective agenda (World Bank 1993). In addition, administrators responsible for vertical programs tended to have little contact with local health officers and seldom coordinated well with other vertical efforts, leading to duplication of training, supervision, and logistics management (Briggs, Capdegelle, and Garner 2003). Other inefficiencies resulted from the need for specialized personnel, which led to growing numbers of dedicated staff members as well as excessive demand on service users' time if they needed multiple services. Verticalization can also lead to competition between programs, favoring of some conditions at the expense of others, weaknesses in continuity of care, disruption of routine health services, and erosion of country-level delivery capacity (Coker, Atun, and McKee 2004).

Concerns about the appropriateness of individual vertical programs were matched at that time by concerns about the continuing misallocation of resources toward expensive, cost-ineffective care, culminating in the publication of *Investing in Health: World Development Report 1993* (World Bank 1993). The report identified highly cost-effective interventions targeted at the major causes of the prevailing burden of disease in low- and middle-income settings. These interventions were grouped into a "minimum package of health services," which, it was argued, governments and donors should prioritize for funding (World Bank 1993). The delivery vehicle for most of these services was the primary care system.

The definition and costing of intervention packages has evolved over time, and this evolution is reflected in the World Bank's *Better Health in Africa* (1994), the World Health Organization's *World Health Report 2000* (WHO 2000), and the report of Working Group 5 of the Commission on Macroeconomics and Health (Jha and Mills 2002). Although some services have been added and others have been described more specifically (partly informed by new research), the essential components of the package have remained remarkably constant. Another World Health Organization (WHO) publication (2002), *World Health Report 2002*, which focused solely on interventions against risk factors, corroborated several of the interventions in the package (Doherty and Govender 2004; see annex 64.A). Thus, a broad consensus appears to exist on the nucleus

of activities that is appropriate at the primary care level (see table 64.1). In many ways, this consensus existed before the publication of *Investing in Health* (World Bank 1993), but economic evaluation has subjected conventional wisdom to empirical validation and considerations of affordability; it has also scrutinized the components of particular interventions (frequency of prenatal health care visits, for example). This evaluation has served the purpose of providing a basis for consensus that is more convincing to key constituencies, such as national treasuries and donors. Consequently, several low- and middle-income countries have delineated minimum or essential packages for their own national contexts.

The notion of such packages is not without controversy, however. Whereas some criticisms relate to methodological issues—and hence to the advisability of generalizing the findings of local studies and using them to establish priority services on a global scale—others relate to the disease-oriented basis of essential packages (Doherty and Govender 2004). The authors of essential packages are not necessarily proponents of verticalization (in some instances, they have argued strongly for the cost-effectiveness that a horizontally well-integrated service can achieve). However, the reality of activity by international agencies, donors, and even governments means that, in many instances, the implementation of narrowly defined programs continues to be favored (with HAART—highly active antiretroviral therapy for the treatment of HIV/AIDS—having the potential to follow suit). Continuing verticalization also reflects the resource constraints faced by countries that are unable to mount a comprehensive set of services and suggests that services in developing countries are chronically underfunded (Jha and Mills 2002).

The disease-based construction of packages may have reinforced this tendency to verticalization, as may have incentives for program managers to monitor program activities in terms of their effect on specific diseases. This factor accounts partly for the suspicion that sometimes greets efforts at cost-effectiveness-based planning, and it signals the need to continually promote the effective integration of activities at the health facility level.

General Primary Care at a Key Interface

Although the primary care level constitutes the first point of patient or family contact, it is also a critical base for extending care to communities and vulnerable groups. These outreach services may focus on individual preventive measures (such as immunization, vitamin A, or oral rehydration therapy) or communitywide health-promoting efforts (such as education on child nutrition or adult diets and exercise; see chapter 56). Increasingly, home-based care for chronic conditions, such as HIV and AIDS and poststroke rehabilitation, can be expected to feature in outreach services. These services depend substantially

Table 64.1 Selected Sets of Interventions Used in the Cost Analysis of the Commission on Macroeconomics and Health, 2002

Disease area	Nature of interventions
Maternity-related interventions	Prenatal care
	Treatment of complications during pregnancy
	Skilled birth attendance
	Emergency obstetric care
	Postpartum care (including family planning)
Childhood disease–related interventions (immunization)	Vaccinations (Bacillus Calmette-Guérin, oral polio vaccine, diphtheria-pertussis-tetanus, measles, hepatitis B, *Haemophilus influenzae* type B)
Childhood disease–related interventions (treatment of childhood illnesses)	Treatment of various conditions (acute respiratory infections, diarrhea, causes of fever, malnutrition, anemia), now increasingly combined as integrated management of childhood illness
Malaria prevention	Insecticide-treated nets
	Residual indoor spraying
Malaria treatment	Treatment for malaria
Tuberculosis treatment	Directly observed short-course treatment for smear-positive patients
	Directly observed short-course treatment for smear-negative patients
HIV/AIDS prevention	Youth-focused interventions
	Interventions working with sex workers and clients
	Condom social marketing and distribution
	Workplace interventions
	Strengthening of blood transfusion systems
	Voluntary counseling and testing
	Prevention of mother-to-child transmission
	Mass media campaigns
	Treatment for sexually transmitted infections
HIV/AIDS care	Palliative care
	Clinical management of opportunistic illnesses
	Prevention of opportunistic illnesses
	Home-based care
HIV/AIDS treatment	Provision of highly active antiretroviral therapy

Source: Jha and Mills 2002.
Note: Smoking cessation interventions, although considered a priority, were not included in this cost analysis because it was assumed that they would be financed by tobacco taxes.

on community support and mechanisms for identifying, training, and supporting village or community health workers.

At the same time, primary care facilities mediate patient access to hospital care, particularly at the district level. General primary care, as a level of care, is thus located at a key interface that links, on the one hand, ambulatory care with hospital and specialty services and, on the other, individual clinical care with community-wide or population-wide health, nutrition, and family planning programs. Acting as the fulcrum of a comprehensive care and support system, development of general primary care requires that local management teams plan services for their defined catchment communities (Jha and Mills 2002)—recognizing that catchment populations can be more difficult to define in urban (particularly high-density) settings. Delineating the community for which a local health system is responsible—and thereby making explicit the population under the care of providers—makes it feasible to undertake ongoing monitoring and evaluation of the performance of local primary care services (quality of care and extent of coverage, for example) and contributes to the assessment of health systems more broadly.

Given the pivotal position of general primary care, distinguishing sharply the cutoff between activities that occur at this level and those that occur elsewhere is difficult. The balance of services provided at the primary level rather than other health service levels is, in fact, a moving target, affected by an array of factors. For example, diagnostic and technological innovation can influence substantially the level at which interventions are delivered. In many middle-income countries, great potential exists to move elements of surgical, psychiatric, and medical care upstream to the primary care level, provided that the necessary competencies, equipment, and technical or managerial support exist. However, the converse also holds: no matter how appropriate in theory, if service delivery is ineffective, the downstream momentum to district and secondary hospital levels (and into the private sector) is almost unstoppable, with serious implications for the accessibility of care. In practice, therefore, factors such as geographic and financial inaccessibility, limited resources, poor capacity, and erratic drug supply and faulty equipment often mean that the services offered at the primary care level are disappointingly limited in their range, coverage, and effect.

"Fitting" of Interventions to the Health System

Recognition is growing that focusing simply on selecting cost-effective interventions as the basis for services development is inappropriate. Paying close attention to the qualities of the delivery system that are required to support the introduction of these interventions and, in time, provide support to their scale-up is essential. The Multi-Country Evaluation of IMCI Study Group (Bryce and others 2003, 159) highlights the "importance of separating biological or behavioural interventions from the delivery systems required to put them in place, and the need to tailor delivery strategies to the stage of health-system development."

Thus, seeking and evaluating the goodness of fit between interventions with the potential to be highly cost-effective and the health system responsible for their effective delivery are critical. A major challenge in focusing on the primary care level is to establish the most effective combinations or clusters of interventions that can target multiple conditions and risk factors affecting key community groups (children, women, and older adults, for example) and that are appropriately adapted to local epidemiologic, economic, and sociocultural contexts. Clustering interventions appears to be a pragmatic approach that achieves a degree of comprehensiveness while at the same time acknowledging resource constraints. It also provides opportunities to intensify training, improve the quality of care provided, and assess community health impact (see chapter 63). If clusters, such as integrated management of infant and childhood illness (IMCI) or reproductive health services, can be fully integrated into health service planning, management, and operations, the health system will be provided with some focus while the shortcomings of vertical disease programs can be potentially avoided. Thus, clustering may allow for broader horizontal strengthening of local health system inputs. As stated earlier, persistent efforts to achieve such integration are essential, given that, as expressed by the Bellagio Study Group on Child Survival (2003, 324), "in today's environment of disease-specific initiatives, cross-disease planning, implementation, and monitoring are hard to establish and maintain."

However, clustering does not entirely address concerns that interventions based solely on cost-effectiveness assessments, which seldom examine indirect and nonhealth benefits (Doherty and Govender 2004), might deplete some of primary care's unique features, including responsiveness to the expressed needs of local communities. Indeed, Gilson (2003,) writes that "future analysis and policy development must recognise that health systems are complex socio-political institutions and not merely delivery points for bio-medical interventions." Community expectations of the services provided at a health center or health post tend to be holistic and may well depart from selected priority intervention categories. The exclusion of services from clusters, or the exclusion of whole clusters, can lead to inequity. Failure to manage this situation adequately can undermine clients' confidence in the public health system and affect provider behavior negatively. WHO (2000, 59) notes that providers "usually react to this . . . by cross-subsidizing the excluded activities through the budget received to pay for the defined benefit package; or by charging extra for the additional services."

These considerations need to be taken into account when identifying clusters of interventions to be provided in local contexts. Nonetheless, likely intervention clusters, with potentially high goodness of fit at the primary care level, will generally include IMCI; maternal and reproductive health services; clinic and community-based management of tuberculosis,

HIV and AIDS, and sexually transmitted infections; malaria management; management of hypertension, other cardiovascular risk factors, and—increasingly—stroke and cardiovascular disease; and mental illness and substance abuse. In all cases, a systematic approach must be taken to establish explicit criteria, guidelines, or regulations regarding the appropriate treatment level (primary, secondary, and so on) for key conditions and the interventions suitable for these conditions at different levels of severity, according to a country's stage of health system development. Broadly categorizing countries according to their income status and the general features of their health system is too blunt an approach to allow the detailed mapping of interventions to the health system capability that is required, and it fails to recognize the wide disparities in health system organization and effectiveness that exist within national boundaries.

THE EFFECTIVENESS OF GENERAL PRIMARY CARE

Whereas it can be argued that highly cost-effective interventions deserve to be implemented, no matter the level for which they are designed, unique reasons exist for giving priority to those based at the primary level. As implied earlier, these reasons relate to the extent of the burden of disease that is potentially avertable through primary-level care (the health effect), the welfare benefits that accrue to households spared the experience of disease (the nonhealth effect), and the potential to provide widely accessible services (an equity effect based on degree of need).

Unfortunately, although many small-scale projects and assessments of single interventions have been able to measure such effects (see part 2 of this volume), the empirical evidence with regard to large-scale and routine primary care programs—whether in industrial or low- and middle-income settings—is scant (Doherty and Govender 2004; Starfield 1998). The key problem is to demonstrate the causal link between provision of general primary care services and positive health outcomes—and especially to disentangle the influences of socioeconomic conditions. This difficulty is compounded by other factors, ranging from the complexity of the study design required to convincingly evaluate routine programs (as opposed to field trials) to the difficulties faced by health ministries in ensuring that monies targeted at primary care are translated into the delivery of quality health services.

Thus, we are able to comment only in broad terms on the positive contributions of general primary care services, recognizing that, although these contributions are potentially enormous, the gains made by such services over the past two decades have been mixed. Importantly, Almeida and others (2001) caution against ascribing the failures of primary care to inherent weaknesses in the concept. In commenting on analyses of the effectiveness of primary care, they point to "the cataclysmic effect on public health systems in less-developed countries of the global economic recession of the 1980s and the application of policies stressing privatisation and decreased public spending in that decade and the next; [this] resulted in rising poverty and under-funding of health services in many less-developed countries, to the point of near-collapse in the poorest countries" (Almeida and others 2001,).

Health Effects

Investing in Health reported that in countries with moderate to high mortality only a few conditions accounted for the majority of the burden of ill health (World Bank 1993). Thus, in 1990, 55 percent of the global burden of disease was concentrated in children under 15, and 75 percent of this burden was caused by 10 disease conditions or clusters (Bobadilla and others 1994). Except for congenital malformations, all these causes could be aligned with highly cost-effective interventions, many of which are classic components of general primary care (labeled the "clinical services" component of the package). Indeed, almost all of the activities included in the "public health" component of the package also involve some element of individual service delivery in the primary care setting. Together, it was estimated, these interventions could eliminate 21 to 28 percent of the burden of ill health in children.

With respect to adults, the World Bank (1993) found the burden of disease to be less concentrated: here the 10 main causes of disease and injury accounted for some 50 percent of the burden.[1] Most interventions against these problems were found to be quite cost-effective, but their overall estimated effect was moderate because they prevent or treat only part of the problems. Such interventions could thus eliminate 10 to 18 percent of the adult disease burden.

These figures give some sense of the potential effect of interventions at the primary level when they are targeted at common, high-burden conditions in the population. Subsequent work by the World Bank estimated that the primary care level could potentially deal with up to 90 percent of health care demands (World Bank 1994) and that only 10 percent of care needs require the services and skills typically associated with hospitals.

Shifting from estimates to empirical evidence, we find that some studies have been able to demonstrate large-scale success in the sphere of child health. For example, using data from a national survey in Niger, Magnani and others (1996) showed that children living in villages near health dispensaries were 32 percent less likely to die than children without access to modern primary care services (differential access resulted from the phased implementation of services, which produced a natural quasi-experiment). Drawing on earlier work, Ewbank

(1993,) concluded that the results of surveys in Zaire and Liberia "suggest that child survival programmes in Africa can reduce mortality substantially in populations living in different environments at very different initial levels of child mortality. . . . In both countries, it appears that the programme reduced mortality under age 5 by about 20% or more." More generally, many examples of successful health programs clearly depend on the existence of a strong primary health care system (see chapter 8).

Given the paucity of evidence from developing countries, turning to the experience of high-income countries is useful, although the configuration of primary care services in such settings may be quite different. Following a detailed comparative study of 11 industrial nations (which involved the methodologically complex—and at times controversial—assigning of primary care and health system scores by country and then associating these scores with a range of health status indicators and total health care costs per capita), Starfield (1994,) concluded that "countries with a stronger orientation to primary care indeed are more likely to have better health levels and lower costs." Shi (1994,) found that, in the United States, availability of primary care was "by far the most significant variable related to better health status, correlating to lower overall mortality, lower death rates due to diseases of the heart and cancer, longer life expectancy, lower neonatal death rate, and less frequent low birth weight." Although working largely at the level of health output rather than outcome, Blumenthal, Mort, and Edwards (1995), in reviewing a number of studies in the United States, found considerable evidence of the positive effect of primary care services (see box 64.1). They argue that the literature does not adequately address the issue of whether primary care reduces the cost of providing care for underserved populations, but they conclude that "a commitment to primary care should be made for its potential to improve the satisfaction and health status of the American public, not for its potential to save money" (Blumenthal, Mort, and Edwards 1995,).

Nonhealth Effects

Although most of the recent literature on primary care packages places value on primary care services because of their ability to reduce the burden of disease considerably and at low cost, such services potentially bring other benefits to society. Among the most striking may be the welfare benefits that accrue to households as a result of the prevention of illness. Severe disease can limit the ability of patients and caregivers to work, leading to the consumption of household assets in the purchasing of care. Russell (2003) found that such costs amounted to just over 10 percent of household income in three developing countries, a proportion that can have a catastrophic impact on the sustainability of poor households. Through

Evidence of the Effectiveness of Primary Care Services

The effectiveness of primary care services is illustrated as follows:

1. Community-based interventions improve access to services, reduce the use of emergency and outpatient departments at hospitals, increase the use of noninstitutional ambulatory care, and reduce the use of hospital care (especially with respect to preventable hospitalizations).
2. Primary care is associated with improved control of routine illnesses that have serious consequences if untreated.

3. The availability of primary care services is associated with improvement in patients' self-perceived health status.
4. The longitudinal care afforded by primary care services is independently associated with improved patient satisfaction, reduced use of ancillary and laboratory tests, improved patient compliance, shorter length of stay, and improved recognition of patients' behavioral problems.

Source: Blumenthal, Mort, and Edwards (1995).

prevention and early treatment, geographically accessible and financially affordable primary care services can reduce the negative economic consequences of ill health for households, reduce absenteeism, and enhance children's performance at school.

Serving of Equity Goals

Primary care services have the advantage over hospital care of tending to be more physically, financially, and culturally accessible to local communities. Because of their staffing and organization, they are less costly and more easily able to provide comprehensive, integrated, personalized, and continuous care (World Bank 1993). Because that part of the burden of disease that is addressed by primary care services disproportionately affects the poor, primary care services are theoretically well placed to improve equity in health and health care. Again, few data exist to demonstrate the equity effects of primary care delivered on a large scale in middle- and low-income countries. This gap is compounded by the fact that cost-effectiveness analyses seldom take into account the costs incurred by patients in seeking care (Doherty and Govender 2004).

However, in studies by Shi and Starfield (2000, 2001) examining income inequality and primary care in the United States, a significant association between higher primary physician supply and good health status was established, even in a context of high income inequality: "The finding of a significant association between primary care and self-rated health contributes to the mounting evidence that specific aspects of health services

have an independent [of income levels] effect in improving population health—in particular, the beneficial effects of primary care" (Shi and Starfield 2000,). The authors suggest that, at least within the particular settings studied, strengthening the primary care aspects of health services could mitigate some of the adverse impacts that income inequality has on individuals' health status.

Primary-level services are also potentially responsive to patients' nonhealth needs. These include a need for the range and quality of health services to meet community expectations and a need for services to treat patients in a helpful and dignified manner. In addition, primary-level facilities can act as community resources (providing communal meeting places, for example), and primary care services can contribute support to neighborhood sports and community development activities. All in all, well-functioning primary-level services represent the face of the health system and have the potential to inspire trust in the system as a whole.

Another source of suspicion regarding the cost-effectiveness approach is the fear that efficiency concerns will override these positive features of primary care. Paalman and others (1998,) note that "the fact that the most efficient interventions . . . tend to specifically benefit the poor is more a result of coincidence than of principle." Indeed, the cost-effectiveness approach does not intrinsically protect equity and could, for example, count against the extension of services to populations living in remote areas. Governments will, at times, need to make explicit choices between serving equity goals and responding to efficiency concerns when determining service priorities. This tradeoff is easier to manage in wealthier countries, where resources are less constrained.

Table 64.2 Cost-Effectiveness of the Health Interventions Included in the *Investing in Health* Minimum Package of Health Services for Low- and Middle-Income Countries *(2002 US$, 2001 prices)*

Interventions	Cost per DALY	
	Low-income countries	Middle-income countries
Public health		
Expanded program of immunization, including vaccine against hepatitis B and vitamin A supplementation	15–22	32–38
School health program	25–32	48–54
Tobacco and alcohol control program	44–70	57–70
AIDS prevention program	4–6[a]	16–23[a]
Other public health interventions (includes information, communication, and education on selected risk factors and health behaviors, plus vector control and disease surveillance)	—	—
Total	18	—
Clinical services		
Chemotherapy against tuberculosis	4–6	6–9
Integrated management of the sick child	38–63	63–127
Family planning	25–38	127–190
Sexually transmitted disease treatment	1–4	13–19
Prenatal and delivery care	38–63	76–139
Limited care (includes treatment of infection and minor trauma; for more complicated condition, includes diagnosis, advice, and pain relief, and treatment as resources permit)	253–380	507–760
Total	—	168

Source: Bobadilla and others 1994; World Bank 1993.

Note: — = not available, presumably because the authors were not able to aggregate data to country level.

a. Understates cost-effectiveness because the analysis examined the probability of transmission to others in the first year only.

THE COST-EFFECTIVENESS OF PRIMARY CARE INTERVENTIONS

Part 2 of this book details our best understanding of the cost-effectiveness of many of the individual interventions that have been clustered into "essential packages." According to *Investing in Health*, most of these interventions are highly cost-effective, costing less than US$100 per disability-adjusted life year (DALY) averted (see table 64.2; World Bank 1993).

Subsequent packages have expanded the *Investing in Health* list somewhat, yet the primary-level interventions put forward in 1993 remain among the most cost-effective available, especially when combined with population-based interventions (Commission on Health Research for Development 1990; Jha and Mills 2002; WHO 2000). It is important to appreciate that, because of the added costs of extending service delivery to people living in more rural and peripheral areas, achieving universal coverage would probably raise marginal costs considerably above the average figures normally quoted. Bobadilla and others (1994,) note that, in these instances, "the relative importance of cost-effectiveness versus equity will then determine whether to modify the package by leaving out some interventions, providing mobile services rather than fixed facilities, concentrating on public health rather than clinical interventions for the high-cost population, or sacrificing some efficiency in order to preserve equity." The need to redress gender imbalances or respond to cultural preferences and other factors, as well as the choice of interventions, also might affect costs.

SCALING UP

Adequate delivery of services (and health care more broadly) at the primary care level is, we believe, fundamental to effective functioning of health systems. However, for the most part, primary care systems in low- and middle-income countries have yet to receive the sustained attention and resources that their importance warrants. Early efforts at primary care expansion in the late 1970s and early 1980s were overtaken in many parts of the developing world by economic crisis, sharp reductions in public spending, political instability, and emerging disease. Although essential packages based on cost-effectiveness criteria have been criticized for their largely disease-oriented and vertical approach, in most poor countries even these limited versions of general primary care remain incompletely applied and largely unaffordable in relation to current per capita health care expenditure. At the same time, renewed awareness of the centrality of the primary level in responding to the consequences of the HIV/AIDS epidemic or to rapidly rising cardiovascular risk means that increasing demands will be placed on primary care services. This section examines critical elements of any strategy to scale up primary care efforts; a prerequisite, however, is an adequate understanding on the part of policy makers and planners of the position and role of primary care in the national health system (Travis and others 2004).

Committing More Financial Resources

In the mid 1980s, Drummond and Mills (1987) found the best estimate of the cost of effective primary health care (including

Table 64.3 Comparison of Per Capita Total Annual Health Expenditure Required to Provide Minimum Packages (*2002 U.S.$, 2001 prices*)

Report	Low-income countries	Middle-income countries
Investing in Health (World Bank 1993)	15	27
Better Health in Africa (World Bank 1994)	16–20	—[a]
Commission on Macroeconomics and Health (Jha and Mills 2002)	Least developed: 40	Lower-middle income: 39
	Other low income: 36	Upper-middle income: 331[b]

Source: Doherty and Govender 2004.
a. Estimate not provided.
b. Higher figure because of range of services provided (beyond minimum package) and higher input costs; applies to a small subgroup of countries.

the recurrent and capital costs of basic and village-level health services but not of water and sanitation) to be 2 percent of the annual per capita gross national product (GNP). This amount, they noted, is considerable, given that many governments in developing countries do not spend even 2 percent of annual per capita GNP on their entire health sector.

More recently, the Commission on Macroeconomics and Health (CMH) estimated that an additional US$40 billion to US$52 billion annual expenditure would be required by 2015 to scale up 49 priority health interventions—not all at the primary care level—to reach high levels of coverage in 83 deserving countries (that is, countries with a GNP per capita below US$1,200, plus all countries of Sub-Saharan Africa) (Jha and Mills 2002). Apart from the recurrent and capital costs of the interventions themselves, this estimate included management costs generated at levels above "close-to-client" services, expenditure to improve absorptive capacity, expenditure on improvements in the quality of care, and 100 percent increases in staff salaries to address the problems of staff recruitment and retention. The inclusion of these costs accounts largely for the greatly increased per capita estimates of the CMH package relative to earlier estimates by the World Bank (see table 64.3), and probably provides a better estimate of what is needed, given the enormous challenges facing primary care service delivery.

The CMH has placed great emphasis on donor funding of services to adequate levels (see chapter 12 for a more extensive discussion of sources of financing). Other avenues of funding include reprioritizing government budgets or recovering costs through health insurance schemes and user fees, although these all remain difficult options within low-income settings. In particular the experience of user fee schemes, which proliferated in the 1990s, suggests that such schemes have negative impacts on equity, especially at the primary care level, and

should be applied with great caution in poor communities (Gilson 1998). Yet the fact remains that an injection of additional resources is clearly one prerequisite for the successful scaling up of general primary care in the 21st century, backed up by political commitment to the centrality of general primary care (and primary health care more broadly) as a fundamental strategy for tackling the highest-burden diseases and their causes.

Developing Human Resources

Although increased financial resources are imperative, Kurowski and others (2003) emphasize that "human resource availability is likely to determine the capacity to absorb additional financial resources and thus the pace of scaling up." These authors warn that human resource availability is likely to be grossly insufficient to meet the scaling-up needs envisioned by the CMH.

The skills and competencies necessary to deliver and support effective primary care are in some respects similar to those required at other levels of the health system (see chapter 71), but certain competencies warrant special emphasis at the primary care level (see box 64.2). Above all, if local services are to meet community health needs, leaders at the primary care level will have to be freed from the constraints of stifling, rule-bound bureaucracies and encouraged to develop innovative and at times unorthodox responses to the demanding challenges they face. As expressed in the *World Health Report 2000* (WHO 2000, 64), "a key challenge in health service delivery is to balance the need for broad policy oversight with sufficient flexibility so that managers and providers can innovate and adapt polices to local needs and contexts in a dynamic way."

The creation of dynamic health teams at the primary level is one of the greatest requirements for scaling up effective primary care. The role of community health workers in such teams remains unresolved and bears further investigation. At the same time, one of the most challenging constraints is to overcome the loss of motivation and sense of resignation of the great body of primary care workers who work in understaffed settings; who lack consistent, quality support; and who have grown accustomed to a norm of inadequate service delivery (Narasimhan and others 2004). As Hongoro and Normand assert in chapter 71, the extent to which countries can improve access to good quality primary care will depend in large part on a "better matches of skills to needs . . . and clearer understanding of how improved structures and incentives will work."

Harnessing Private Sector Resources

Private sector health care provision is widespread and growing. It extends from local supply of drugs and equipment to fee-for-service and insurance-based medical care to the many forms of traditional practice. Although general primary care in most African, Asian, and Latin American settings is a major feature of publicly financed services that are provided by the public sector, private providers clearly play a significant role in many low- and middle-income countries with respect to the provision of primary care services (Berman and Rose 1996; Palmer and others 2003). Governments have thus viewed private sector providers as contributing additional human and related resources that can be deployed in the service of at least a portion of the population (usually those with means, including employees with access to reasonable health insurance coverage). By alleviating the workloads faced by public providers, private sector providers have allowed the public services to focus more directly on poorer communities and patients without means. Out-of-pocket payments, health insurance, and donations (as opposed to government contracts) that fund private sector services thus result in additional financing for the health sector.

Patients often prefer the private sector for a number of reasons. These reasons include geographic accessibility, convenient opening hours, and more favorable staff attitudes, as well as perceived better quality in terms of shorter waiting times, greater privacy, higher standards of diagnosis, better (perceived) treatment, and counseling (Doherty and Govender 2004). Although private providers are generally thought of in relation to curative care, interest is growing in the role they could play in meeting public health objectives, especially with respect to the scaling up of primary care services (Palmer and others 2003).

It is important that the potential contribution of private sector resources be optimized through appropriate use of public-private partnership mechanisms, public sector contracts, and government regulation. These mechanisms are generally easier for not-for-profit providers to contemplate, because they have often been instrumental in bringing primary care to poor communities. Some nongovernmental organizations (NGOs) are able to offer services that can fill notable gaps, home-based care to HIV and AIDS sufferers being but one example.

The potential of for-profit providers to contribute to the care of the poor is less obvious, especially given the incentives to overservice that are inherent in the fee-for-service reimbursement system. Mills and others (2002) find that consumers of private sector primary care are often unable to assess the technical quality of services, tending to place more weight on aspects of perceived quality, such as interpersonal skills of providers and the comfort of the environment in which treatment occurs, than on technical competence. Mills and others (2002,) argue that the effectiveness of private services is by and large rather low: "poor treatment practices have been reported for diseases such as tuberculosis and sexually transmitted infections, with implications not only for the individuals treated but also for disease transmission and the development of drug resistance."

Palmer and others (2003, 292) have reviewed a "new model of private primary care provision" that has emerged in South Africa. This innovation involves commercial companies providing "standardized primary care services at relatively low cost" that are targeted at the low-income employed rather than the very poor (Palmer and others 2003,). Regarding the growing popularity of these private clinics, the authors find that they maintain excellent standards with respect to the quality of services. The clinics also run at a cost per visit that is comparable with public sector primary care clinics, demonstrating that the acceptability of services to users and low-cost service delivery are not incompatible objectives.

Palmer and others (2003, 295) suggest that the increasing popularity of these (affordable) private clinics may provide an opportunity to encourage employed but low-income workers (who historically have used public sector health services at little or no charge) to make use of these clinic networks, which would enable the public sector to better tend to its "role as regulator and providing services to the poorest." Potentially, this redirection of care could remove some of the burden on the public sector, and the task of regulation might be made easier by the strong hierarchical control exercised within these clinic chains. To some extent, this shift has been the experience in Sri Lanka, where government services have been designed with the explicit assumption that certain forms of care will be provided through the private sector (Rannan-Eliya 2001).

However, Palmer and others (2003) point out that the model has potential drawbacks. The comprehensiveness and continuity of services provided by these private clinics fall short of that available in the public sector. Furthermore, how the behavior of private clinics would change under a system of contractual arrangements with the public sector is not clear. Whereas contracting with the not-for-profit sector tends to accommodate government objectives fairly easily (Gilson and others 1997), the experience of contracting with the for-profit sector has had mixed results. These and other concerns imply that, although the for-profit sector is an important resource, arrangements for the delivery of care through this sector should be developed with caution. It also bears mention that, where public sector systems are weak, private sector services gain ground to the extent of unbalancing the public-private mix, with potentially serious consequences for costs and continuity in patient care and for coverage and equity more generally.

Setting Population Health and Clinical Care Priorities

Along with securing additional resources for primary care delivery, country capacity to generate the information necessary for setting and reviewing public health and clinical care priorities must be strengthened as a fundamental measure (Commission on Health Research for Development 1990). This principle lies at the heart of influential pilot work—at times referred to as *community-oriented primary care*—that emerged in the first half of the 20th century and now underpins the Tanzanian Essential Health Interventions Program (TEHIP), 1997–2004. TEHIP, through a research and development arm tasked with devising practical tools for decentralized health planning, has tested "how and to what extent evidence can guide planning of the health sector at district level . . . [in order to] improve technical and allocative efficiency with regard to local choices for resource allocation and services offered" (de Savigny and others 2002,).[2] A dynamic process of using high-

quality local information, coupled with local problem solving, planning, and ownership, was central to appropriate decision making and consequent implementation.

Because local data on intervention costs and coverage are generally not available to district planners and managers, local cost-effectiveness analysis is difficult to incorporate into decentralized priority setting. With TEHIP, priority setting was driven more by the shares of the burden of disease that known cost-effective interventions could address. New analytic tools were devised that would help focus resource allocations on the major "intervention-addressable" disease burdens; targeted sets of cost-effective interventions were then applied—in place of embarking on a disease-by-disease or detailed cost-effectiveness approach (D. de Savigny, personal communication,). Available understanding on cost-effectiveness was used to eliminate interventions known to be grossly cost-ineffective; it was not used to prioritize or rank interventions generally considered to be highly cost-effective.

TEHIP indicates that gross technical and allocative efficiencies are relatively easy to address when incremental funding is available. As described by de Savigny and others (2002), the net effect of decentralized funding, together with a mutually reinforcing series of planning, management, and capacity-development inputs, was a proportional and absolute increase in resources for more efficient delivery of prioritized, cost-effective interventions addressing the largest shares of the preventable local burden of disease; an increase in the use of government health services; and a decrease in mortality in infants, children under five, adolescents, and adults. This effect was achieved with relatively limited resources.

TEHIP and related experience make clear that delivery of effective primary care requires a greatly stepped-up capacity to provide an evidence base that is founded on current and evolving local disease and risk factor burdens, the performance of local health services, client use of public as well as private and traditional services, and (where appropriate) the costs of providing care. Effective use of such information can profoundly enhance the ability of the health system to deliver on its core service functions, target high-risk and vulnerable groups, assess coverage in service provision, and gauge health effects. Moreover, such information is vital to establishing the dimensions of the local disease burden that should be managed at the primary care level (Kahn and others 1999). As cogently stated by the Bellagio Study Group on Child Survival (2003, 324), "the capacity of countries to obtain and use information to support child-health programmes will be a determining factor in reducing child mortality."

Developing a District Health System

Drawing from theory and experience in other branches of the public sector (Mills and others 1990)—and often as part of wider public sector developments—the health sector introduced decentralization widely in low- and middle-income countries throughout the 1980s and 1990s (WHO 2000). Positive justification for this method of delivering health care and primary care in particular lay, first, in its intended benefits—for patients and communities—through the provision of context-appropriate services of steadily improving quality. This service delivery was rightly seen as also conferring substantial financial benefit on households. Second, decentralization was expected to lead to the strengthening of local responsibility and accountability, with growing authority of district management teams over local cost centers. Third, it was presumed that the more central management levels would invest in enhanced support systems, including management support, further training, financial management and administration, laboratory services, and drug supply systems (World Bank 1994).

In developing settings, few health systems did not decentralize in some form or another over this period, and most based services development on a so-called district (or subdistrict) health system model. Considerable effort was devoted to achieving a balance between primary care service delivery and referral to the first-level (or district) hospital. Incentives as well as penalties were invoked to encourage first use of primary care facilities.

Notwithstanding the theoretical appeal of health system decentralization, numerous difficulties in implementation were encountered, with the consequence that the performance of decentralized, primary care–oriented systems and national-level support to these systems have fallen way below expectations (Bellagio Study Group on Child Survival 2003). Although various factors can account for this outcome—and although these factors will differ according to local and regional circumstances—common difficulties include inadequate or insufficient primary care skills and competencies, which result in poor-quality care; breakdown in referral systems for emergencies and more complex cases (McCord and Chowdhury 2003; Snow and others 1994); delegation of responsibilities without the concomitant delegation of authority, especially in relation to budgeting; authoritarian or strictly hierarchical managerial styles that are not conducive to local health services support and development; and weak or absent measures to develop workable cost-management systems appropriate to different service levels.

These problems in achieving successful delivery need to be addressed if decentralization is to achieve its intended benefits. Again, greater appreciation of the role of decentralized systems in the broader health care architecture, the support needed to ensure their effectiveness, and the time required to build the necessary capability are all necessary. As Bryce and others (2003, 160) put it, "although research on interventions is plentiful, little is known about the characteristics of delivery strategies capable of achieving and maintaining high coverage for specific interventions in various epidemiological, health system, and cultural contexts." From this perspective, a too-narrow preoccupation with the cost-effectiveness of interventions cannot but have shortcomings: "whatever package of services is delivered, the resulting effectiveness and equity will almost certainly depend on how the services are delivered, [in other words] the strategy for organizing the care" (B. Starfield, personal communication,).

Primary care is delivered through a system of facilities, equipment, and personnel; tackling inefficiencies in the system may have major positive benefits for quality of care, program coverage, and cost-effectiveness. In many settings a real opportunity exists to increase the efficiency of general primary care teams by giving attention to working conditions, ensuring functional equipment, and maintaining a stable drug supply. Meaningful step-ups in care, workable referral and communication systems, gatekeeper functions where indicated, and effectively aligned management and support are all needed. Achieving such efficiencies should result in many more patients being assessed and managed properly. Significant cost savings may accrue to the health service (through patients being managed at the primary care level rather than the first or specialist referral level) and to patients, families, and households (through care being delivered more rapidly and nearer to home).

Demanding Services: Relationships with Local Communities

Among poor and vulnerable communities, the need for care is demonstrably high, and the effectiveness of primary care services is likely to substantially influence demand on the public sector. In relation to infectious as well as noncommunicable disease, outreach services have a major role to play in promoting positive health and health-seeking behaviors and in supporting community-level preventive and promotive efforts. More generally, renewed efforts to enhance community relationships with primary care workers and the health system as a whole—and to ensure that community voices actively and appropriately bear on local service development and decision making—can help bring clients and communities into constructive public health care partnerships.

A RESEARCH AND DEVELOPMENT AGENDA FOR GENERAL PRIMARY CARE

Throughout this chapter, we have emphasized the challenges and constraints to the effective delivery of general primary care services. In this section, we single out a few areas that warrant concerted research and development in the effort to establish a high-functioning primary care platform to support the implementation of cost-effective interventions.

Evolving Health Transitions

A critical consequence of fast-changing economic and social conditions is the rapid transition in health profiles in essentially all low- and middle-income settings. This shift has already led or is leading to the coexistence of persisting infectious disease; nutrition and reproductive health problems; emerging noncommunicable disease and related risk factors (such as hypertension, obesity, diabetes, stroke, and cardiovascular disease); and a growing burden from accidents and intentional injury. The challenge this transition poses to primary care systems is considerable. For the most part, these systems are oriented to maternal and child health and the management of acute illness. An accelerating health transition will require extending the reach and capacity of widely established primary acute care systems (oriented to episodic care) to accommodate the need for effective systems of chronic and long-term care (including continuing, medium- to longer-term, patient or client management and monitoring).

Introduction of Antiretroviral Therapy for HIV and AIDS

Many countries, particularly those in southern Africa and East Africa, are moving to the rapid introduction and scale-up of antiretroviral therapies for HIV and AIDS. Substantial and rapidly increasing financial investments are envisaged (indeed are under way); a necessary accompaniment to such scale-up should be improved drug supplies, strengthened laboratory services, clinical training of primary care staff, and reassertion of the importance of health service relationships with local communities. Such measures—which can succeed only with sustained public sector commitment—have the potential to invigorate and motivate all facets of primary care delivery but, equally, could undermine existing services. The challenge is how to realize the positive potential of antiretroviral therapies in meeting the needs of HIV and AIDS sufferers and their communities, while ensuring a major contribution to strengthening primary care provision more generally. In other words, the challenge is to strengthen a particular service (HIV and AIDS treatment and care) and primary care services simultaneously—through building more effective health teams, improving drug supplies, strengthening service monitoring and evaluation, enhancing supervision and support systems, extending service coverage, and so forth. Such systemwide strengthening can be expected to greatly improve the technical efficiency of key elements of the general primary care system.

Effective Support and Networking for Community and Home-Based Care

Along with the reorientation of primary care systems to support chronic and long-term care are needs for "home-based" care—taking place in rural households, urban residences, or newer community-based facilities such as hospices. Although home-based care of people living with AIDS is most prominent, care and support for clients post-stroke or with other forms of physical or mental disability are as important. Primary care outreach services, working with community health initiatives, NGOs, and communities, are well placed to contribute expertise, training, and resources toward supporting such efforts, which are growing rapidly in importance.

Research to Strengthen General Primary Care in the Public Sector

An abiding need exists for experimental and quasi-experimental evaluation of innovation in general primary care services (whether delivered comprehensively or as clusters of interventions), providing greater insight into the enabling and constraining factors (which may be systemwide) and a more robust understanding of the effects, costs, and cost-effectiveness of modifications to these services in different settings. To maximize the likelihood of success in efforts to scale up effective interventions or system innovations, such initiatives should be carefully designed, implemented, and assessed in partnership with senior health ministry officers (Berwick 2004). Such evaluations are required to assess new forms of organizing primary care services (in particular, balancing persisting acute needs with the growing need for chronic and long-term care, or establishing the skills mix that is most effective in particular settings); similarly, they are necessary when assessing delivery of interventions—such as the cost-effectiveness of multi-disease intervention clusters in different epidemiological and social contexts, or the extent of uptake by vulnerable groups (such as children or the elderly) or marginal populations. Operational research efforts are needed in a range of spheres: to evaluate factors that facilitate or hinder effective performance by service providers or to develop easily managed monitoring systems to assist, for example, in assessments of intervention coverage.

CONCLUSIONS

Clearly, a great many of the most cost-effective interventions detailed in this volume depend on a high-functioning primary care system for their effective implementation. This system comprises the elements of the primary level of care (including facilities, equipment, drugs, personnel, and associated management support); their combination to form a competent delivery capability; and the services that are thereby delivered. Because cost-effectiveness estimates are based on the presumed effective delivery of primary care services, it can be argued that implicit in the estimates have been overly optimistic assumptions regarding key constituents (staff, drugs, equipment, monitoring and evaluation, and so forth) of the primary care level and their functioning. Great efforts to render such systems as effective as possible, subject to the constraints of particular environments, are therefore justified.

More generally, decisions on the best and most appropriate sites for delivery of interventions are not always straightforward, will benefit from expert discussion, and will often be context specific. Moreover, many interventions can be delivered from multiple sites—although a hierarchy of preference will usually exist, influenced by issues such as cost-effectiveness, ease of service provision, need for monitoring, access, and coverage. Careful review of the extensive range of interventions presented in part 2 of this volume and their likely site of delivery reveals the following:

- The interfaces between (a) community and primary care levels and (b) primary care and district levels are critical sites that profoundly affect the effectiveness of service delivery.
- No substitute exists for a well-functioning district health system comprising community, primary care, and first-referral (district) hospital levels. This organizational and service unit is fundamental to effective health care provision, and failure to recognize the interrelationship between component levels has had high health costs and resulted in great inefficiency.

The health and development cost of weak or inadequate primary care systems to high-risk or vulnerable groups—and to communities more generally—is demonstrably high. However, effective general primary care that responds to the rapid health transitions under way in all socioeconomic contexts offers the potential for major health and, hence, development gains that provide good value for money and enhance equity. Critical make-or-break points include upscaled financial investments paralleled by major and sustained investment in human resources (principally the strengthening of local staff capacity, the building up of key skill sets—including supportive management—and the encouragement of innovation in services development); far greater attention to improving delivery and service quality, monitoring service coverage, improving access by vulnerable groups and taking account of equity considerations in general; and establishment of a trusting and constructive partnership with local communities.

Annex 64.A Comparison of Proposed Basic Packages of Interventions

Intervention	Alma Ata Declaration (WHO and UNICEF 1978)	Investing in Health (World Bank 1993)	Better Health in Africa (World Bank 1994)	World Health Report 2000 (WHO 2000)	Commission on Macroeconomics and Health Working Group 5 (Jha and Mills 2002)	World Health Report 2002 (WHO 2002)[a]
Maternity-related interventions	+	+	+	+	+	
Prenatal care		+	+	+	+	
Treatment of complications during pregnancy		+	+	+	+	
Skilled birth attendants		+	+	+	+	
Emergency obstetric care		+	+	+	+	
Postpartum care		+	+	+	+	
Family planning		+	+	+	+	
Nutrition: pregnant and lactating women			+			
Tetanus toxoid				+		
Childhood disease–related interventions (prevention)	+	+	+		+	
Bacillus Calmette-Guérin	+	+	+	+	+	
Polio	+	+	+	+	+	
Diphtheria-pertussis-tetanus	+	+	+	+	+	
Measles	+	+	+	+	+	
Hepatitis B		+	+	+	+	
Haemophilus influenzae type B		+	+		+	
Vitamin A supplementation		+	+	+	+	+
Iodine supplementation			+	+	+	+
Zinc supplementation						+
Anthelmintic treatment				+		
School health program (incorporating micronutrient supplementation, school meals, anthelmintic treatment, health education)		+	+	+		
Childhood disease–related interventions (treatment)	+	+ (as part of IMCI)	+	+ (as part of IMCI)		
Acute respiratory infections				+	+	+
Diarrhea			+	+	+	+
Causes of fever			+	+	+	
Malnutrition			+ (including nutrition and supplementary feeding)	+	+	
Anemia				+	+	
Feeding and breastfeeding counseling				+		
Malaria prevention	[b]	+		+	+	
Insecticide-treated nets				+	+	
Residual indoor spraying					+	
Malaria treatment	[b]		+		+	

Annex 64.A Continued

Intervention	Alma Ata Declaration (WHO and UNICEF 1978)	Investing in Health (World Bank 1993)	Better Health in Africa (World Bank 1994)	World Health Report 2000 (WHO 2000)	Commission on Macroeconomics and Health Working Group 5 (Jha and Mills 2002)	World Health Report 2002 (WHO 2002)[a]
Tuberculosis treatment	b	+	+	+	+	
Directly observed treatment short course (DOTS) for smear-positive patients				+	+	
DOTS for smear-negative patients					+	
HIV/AIDS prevention		+ (more limited than later packages?)		+	+	+
Youth-focused interventions					+	
Interventions working with sex workers and clients				+	+	
Condom social marketing and distribution					+	
Workplace interventions					+	
Strengthening of blood transfusions systems				+	+	
Voluntary counseling and testing				+	+	
Prevention of mother-to-child transmission					+	
Mass media campaigns				+	+	
Treatment for sexually transmitted infections		+	+	+	+	
HIV/AIDS care					+	
Palliative care		+ (see under limited care)			+	
Clinical management of opportunistic illnesses			+		+	
Prevention of opportunistic illnesses					+	
Home-based care					+	
HIV/AIDS HAART provision						+
Tobacco control program (taxes, legal action, information, nicotine replacement)		+		+	+	
Alcohol control program		+				
Other public health interventions (includes information, education, and communication on selected risk factors and health behaviors, plus vector control and disease surveillance)	+	+	+ (information, education, and communication)			
Limited care (includes treatment of infection and minor trauma; for more complicated conditions includes diagnosis, advice, and pain relief, and treatment as resources permit)	+	+	+			
Noncommunicable diseases and injuries (selected early screening and prevention)				+		+
Populationwide interventions to reduce the risks of cardiovascular disease (salt- and cholesterol-lowering strategies)						+
Water and sanitation	+		+			+ (disinfection at point of use)

Sources: Jha and Mills 2002; WHO 2000, 2002; WHO and UNICEF 1978; World Bank 1993, 1994.

HAART = highly active antiretroviral therapy for the treatment of HIV/AIDS; IMCI = integrated management of infant and childhood illness.

Note: A "+" that appears in a shaded cell but not in the white cells beneath this area means that no details of the exact interventions were provided in the report.

a. Addressed only interventions against risk factors.

b. These and other disease prevention and control initiatives fell under a general item termed *prevention and control of locally endemic diseases* (HIV/AIDS was not an issue at the time).

ACKNOWLEDGMENTS

This chapter draws considerably on the background paper by Doherty and Govender (2004) titled "The Cost-Effectiveness of Primary Care Services in Developing Countries: A Review of the International Literature," commissioned by the Disease Control Priorities Project. It draws on productive discussions during the workshop "Integrating Interventions and Health Systems" held in July 2004 in Johannesburg; the workshop was supported by the project and convened by the School of Public Health, University of the Witwatersrand, South Africa, and the Health Policy Unit, London School of Hygiene and Tropical Medicine, United Kingdom. The authors acknowledge with pleasure the critique, insights, and support provided by the editors and chapter reviewers.

NOTES

1. Bobadilla and others (1994) comment that separating interventions according to age group is artificial because benefits may accrue in later life, as in the case of hepatitis vaccine, and may improve well-being, such as cognitive abilities. Adult interventions, such as HIV prevention and pre-natal care, also benefit children.

2. TEHIP has functioned in a "high mortality" setting. Relevant evidence is related to mortality levels and trends, including cause-specific mortality, as well as to district-level financial allocations and changes over time.

REFERENCES

Almeida, C., P. Braveman, M. R. Gold, C. L. Szwarcwald, J. Mendes Ribeiro, A. Miglionico, and others. 2001. "Methodological Concerns and Recommendations on Policy Consequences of the *World Health Report 2000.*" *Lancet* 357: 1692–97.

Bellagio Study Group on Child Survival. 2003. "Knowledge into Action for Child Survival." *Lancet* 362 (9380): 323–27.

Berman, P., and L. Rose. 1996. "The Role of Private Providers in Maternal and Child Health and Family Planning Services in Developing Countries." *Health Policy and Planning* 11 (2): 142–55.

Berwick, D. M. 2004. "Lessons from Developing Nations on Improving Health Care." *British Medical Journal* 328: 1124–29.

Blumenthal, D., E. Mort, and J. Edwards. 1995. "The Efficacy of Primary Care for Vulnerable Population Groups." *Health Services Research* 30 (1): 253–73.

Bobadilla, J. L., P. Cowley, P. Musgrove, and H. Saxenian. 1994. "Design, Content, and Financing of an Essential National Package of Health Services." *Bulletin of the World Health Organization* 72 (4): 653–62.

Briggs, C. J., P. Capdegelle, and P. Garner. 2003. "Strategies for Integrating Primary Health Services in Middle- and Low-Income Countries: Effects on Performance, Costs and Patient Outcomes" (Cochrane Review). In *The Cochrane Library,* Issue 4. Chichester, U.K.: John Wiley and Sons.

Bryce, J., S. el Arifeen, G. Pariyo, C. F. Lanata, D. Gwatkin, J.-P. Habicht, and the Multi-Country Evaluation of IMCI Study Group. 2003. "Reducing Child Mortality: Can Public Health Deliver?" *Lancet* 362 (9378): 159–64.

Coker, R. J., R. A. Atun, and M. McKee. 2004. "Health-Care System Frailties and Public Health Control of Communicable Disease on the European Union's New Eastern Border." *Lancet* 363 (9418): 1389–92.

Commission on Health Research for Development. 1990. *Health Research: Essential Link to Equity in Development.* New York: Oxford University Press.

de Savigny, D., H. Kasale, C. Mbuya, G. Munna, L. Mgalula, A. Mzige, and G. Reid. 2002. "Tanzania Essential Health Interventions Project: TEHIP Interventions—An Overview." Ministry of Health, Dar es Salaam, Tanzania.

Doherty, J., and R. Govender. 2004. "The Cost-Effectiveness of Primary Care Services in Developing Countries: A Review of the International Literature." Background paper for the Disease Control Priorities Project.

Drummond, M. F., and A. Mills. 1987. *Cost Effectiveness of Primary Health Care: A Review of Evidence.* London: Commonwealth Secretariat.

Ewbank, D. C. 1993. "Impact of Health Programmes on Child Mortality in Africa: Evidence from Zaire and Liberia." *International Journal of Epidemiology* 22 (Suppl. 5): S64–72.

Gilson, L. 1998. "The Lessons of User Fee Experience in Africa." In *Sustainable Health Care Financing in Southern Africa,* ed. A. Beattie, J. Doherty, L. Gilson, E. Lambo, and P. Shaw,. Washington, DC: World Bank.

———. 2003. "Trust and the Development of Health Care as a Social Institution." *Social Science and Medicine* 56: 1453–68.

Gilson, L., J. Adusei, D. Arhin, C. Hongoro, S. K. Mujinja. 1997. "Should African Governments Contract Out Clinical Health Services to Church Providers?" In *Private Health Providers in Developing Countries: Serving the Public Interest?*, ed. S. Bennett, B. McPake, and A. Mills, 276–302. London: Zed Press.

Jha, P., and A. Mills. 2002. "Improving Health Outcomes of the Poor: The Report of Working Group 5 of the Commission on Macroeconomics and Health." Geneva: World Health Organization.

Kahn, K., S. M. Tollman, M. Garenne, and J. S. S. Gear. 1999. "Who Dies from What? Establishing Cause of Death in South Africa's Rural Northeast." *Tropical Medicine and International Health* 4: 433–41.

Kurowski, C., K. Wyss, S. Abdulla, N. Yemadji, and A. Mills. 2003. "Human Resources for Health: Requirements and Availability in the Context of Scaling Up Priority Interventions in Low-Income Countries." Health Economics and Financing Programme, London School of Hygiene and Tropical Medicine, London.

Magnani, R. J., J. C. Rice, N. B. Mock, A. A. Abdoh, D. M. Mercer, and K. Tankari. 1996. "The Impact of Primary Health Care Services on Under-Five Mortality in Rural Niger." *International Journal of Epidemiology* 25 (3): 568–77.

McCord, C., and Q. Chowdhury. 2003. "A Cost Effective Small Hospital in Bangladesh: What It Can Mean for Emergency Obstetric Care." *International Journal of Gynecology and Obstetrics* 81: 83–92.

Mills, A., R. Brugha, K. Hanson, and B. McPake. 2002. "What Can Be Done about the Private Health Sector in Low-Income Countries?" *Bulletin of the World Health Organization* 80: 325–30.

Mills, A., J. P. Vaughan, D. L. Smith, and I. Tabibzadeh. 1990. *Health System Decentralization: Concepts, Issues and Country Experience.* Geneva: World Health Organization.

Narasimhan, V., H. Brown, A. Pablos-Mendez, O. Adams, G. Dussault, G. Elzinga, and others. 2004. "Responding to the Global Human Resources Crisis." *Lancet* 363 (9419): 1469–72.

Newell, K. 1975. "Health by the People." World Health Organization, Geneva.

Paalman, M., H. Bekedam, L. Hawken, and D. Nyheim. 1998. "A Critical Review of Priority Setting in the Health Sector: The Methodology of the 1993 World Development Report." *Health Policy and Planning* 13 (1): 13–31.

Palmer, N., A. Mills, H. Wadee, L. Gilson, and H. Schneider. 2003. "A New Face for Private Providers in Developing Countries: What Implications for Public Health?" *Bulletin of the World Health Organization* 81 (4): 292–97.

Rannan-Eliya, R. P. 2001. "Strategies for Improving the Health of the Poor: The Sri Lankan Experience." Paper prepared for Health Systems Resource Centre, Department for International Development. Health Policy Programme, Institute of Policy Studies of Sri Lanka, Colombo.

Russell, F. 2003. "The Economic Burden of Illness for Households: A Review of Cost of Illness and Coping Strategy Studies Focusing on Malaria, Tuberculosis and HIV/AIDS." Paper presented at the Disease Control Priorities Project Workshop, Johannesburg, South Africa, July 1–4.

Shi, L. 1994. "Primary Care, Specialty Care, and Life Chances." *International Journal of Health Services* 24 (3): 431–58.

Shi, L., and B. Starfield. 2000. "Primary Care, Income Inequality, and Self-Rated Health in the United States: A Mixed-Level Analysis." *International Journal of Health Services* 30 (3): 541–55.

———. 2001. "The Effect of Primary Care Physician Supply and Income Inequality on Mortality among Blacks and Whites in U.S. Metropolitan Areas." *American Journal of Public Health* 91 (8): 1246–50.

Snow, R. W., V. O. Mung'ala, D. Forster, and K. Marsh. 1994. "The Role of the District Hospital in Child Survival at the Kenyan Coast." *African Journal of Health Sciences* 1 (2): 71–75.

Starfield, B. 1994. "Primary Care: Is It Essential?" *Lancet* 344: 1129–33.

———. 1998. *Primary Care: Balancing Health Needs, Services, and Technology.* New York: Oxford University Press.

Tollman, S. M. 1991. "Community Oriented Primary Care: Origins, Evolution, Applications." *Social Science and Medicine* 32: 633–42.

Travis, P., S. Bennett, A. Haines, T. Pang, Z. Bhutta, A. A. Hyder, and others. 2004. "Overcoming Health-Systems Constraints to Achieve the Millennium Development Goals." *Lancet* 364: 900–906.

Unger, J.-P., P. de Paepe, and A. Green. 2003. "A Code of Best Practice for Disease Control Programmes to Avoid Damaging Health Care Services in Developing Countries." *International Journal of Health Planning and Management* 18: S27–39.

Vuori, H. 1985. "The Role of Schools of Public Health in the Development of Primary Health Care." *Health Policy* 4: 221–30.

Walsh, J. A., and K. Warren. 1979. "Selective Primary Health Care: An Interim Strategy for Disease Control in Developing Countries." *New England Journal of Medicine* 301: 967–74.

WHO (World Health Organization). 2000. *The World Health Report 2000. Health Systems: Improving Performance.* Geneva: WHO.

———. 2002. *The World Health Report 2002: Reducing Risks, Promoting Healthy Life.* Geneva: WHO.

WHO (World Health Organization) and UNICEF (United Nations Children's Fund). 1978. "Primary Health Care: A Joint Report by the Director-General of the World Health Organization and the Executive Director of the United Nations Children's Fund." WHO, Geneva.

World Bank. 1993. *Investing in Health: World Development Report 1993.* New York: Oxford University Press.

———. 1994. *Better Health in Africa: Experience and Lessons Learned.* Washington, DC: World Bank.

Chapter **65**

The District Hospital

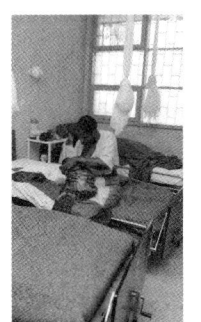

Mike English, Claudio F. Lanata, Isaac Ngugi, and Peter C. Smith

Health care comprises a continuum from home-based, self-administered treatment to highly specialized intervention dependent on professionals with many years of training and a heavy capital investment. In principle, the role of the health system planner is to balance the many separate components of the system to optimize the magnitude and distribution of health benefits, subject to a variety of constraints such as budgetary levels, geography, and human resources capacity. While recognizing that other paradigms are possible and valid, we generally adopt this optimization perspective in our discussions because it combines broad social (including user) and political dimensions with systematic economic principles when decisions are made in a competitive, resource-constrained environment. Following such logic, it should be possible to define the place, purpose, and size of the district hospital sector within a balanced system of care for any particular setting.

Although this view is theoretically appealing, the world of real health systems that have evolved under different historical and political pressures is somewhat different. This perspective does, nevertheless, suggest some common principles involved in defining the optimum balance of care even within groupings as diverse as "developing countries." Two further points are worth considering:

- First, although the focus of this chapter is the district hospital, crucial links exist with many other aspects of the health system. Choices made in relation to hospitals are likely to affect the whole health system and vice versa. For example, programs to improve peripheral clinic referrals of women with high-risk pregnancies may result in a paradoxical decline in the quality of care if critical human and other resources are inadequate at the hospital level. Thus, the

picture of public district hospitals as underused, inefficient, and providing poor quality care (Barnum and Kutzin 1993) may reflect deficiencies in the entire health system as well as at the hospital level.

- Second, optimizing the health system configuration is an active, continuing process that must often proceed incrementally, ideally tackling problems in order of priority. An optimal balance is not likely to be achieved naturally through neglect or reliance on market mechanisms.

Hospitals are major consumers of health budgets. However, there is a paucity of good evidence—even in industrial countries—on their effect (McKee and Healy 2002), whereas the body of theory and opinion on their role is wide. This chapter can serve as only an introduction to topics that include, among others, the political and social value of hospitals and their essential role in integrated health systems (Sachs 2001; Van Leberghe, de Bethune, and de Brouwere 1997; WHO 1999; World Bank 1993). The chapter first introduces basic concepts relevant to district hospitals that may affect their role and performance and a description of possible core services (see figure 65.1). For discussions of the evidence justifying inclusion of an intervention or process as a core service at this level of care, the reader is referred to disease- and service-specific chapters. Although recently attempts have been made to refine definitions of *performance* (WHO 2000b), the term is used in a general sense, referring to processes and outcomes that contribute to improved levels and distribution of health. The chapter then summarizes currently available economic data on hospital care, focusing where possible on the district level and acknowledging the difficulty in generalizing findings from one setting to another. An illustration follows of some of

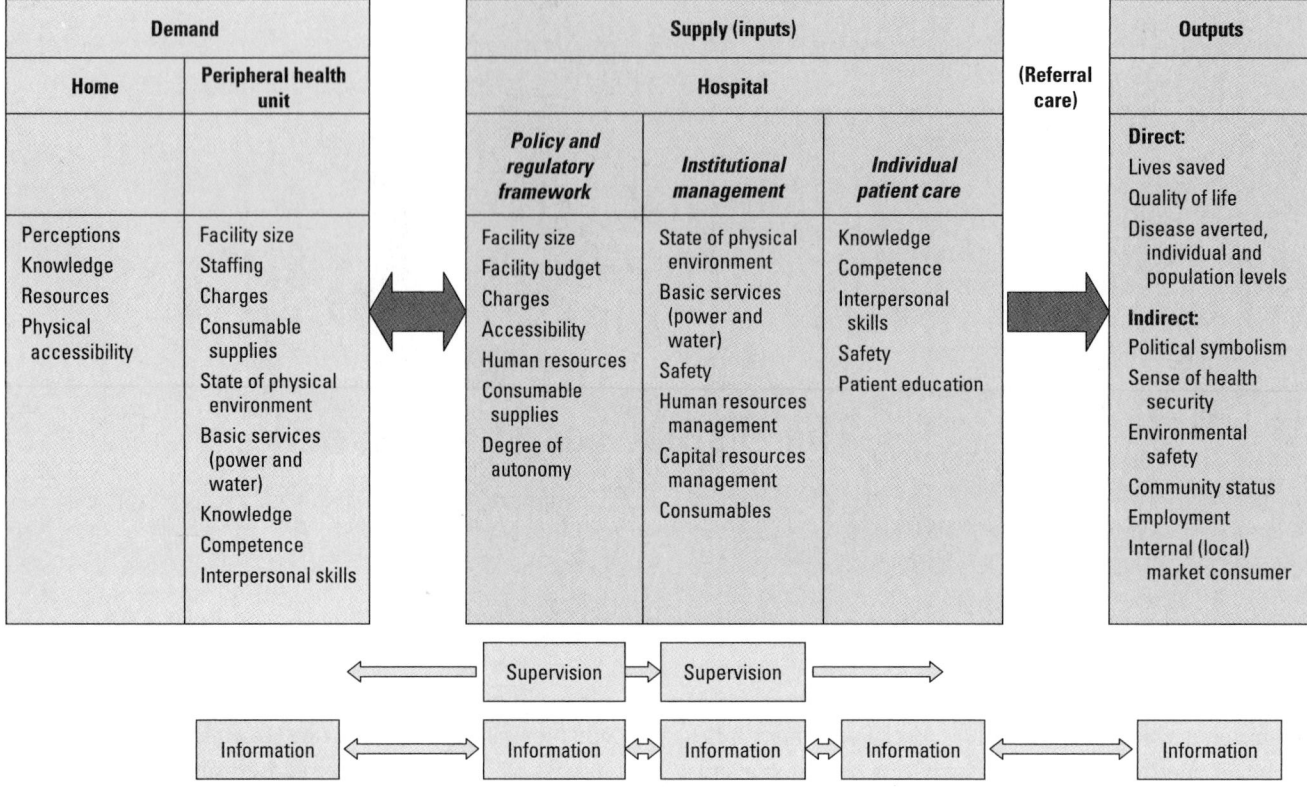

Demand		Supply (inputs)			(Referral care)	Outputs
Home	**Peripheral health unit**	**Hospital**				
		Policy and regulatory framework	*Institutional management*	*Individual patient care*		
Perceptions Knowledge Resources Physical accessibility	Facility size Staffing Charges Consumable supplies State of physical environment Basic services (power and water) Knowledge Competence Interpersonal skills	Facility size Facility budget Charges Accessibility Human resources Consumable supplies Degree of autonomy	State of physical environment Basic services (power and water) Safety Human resources management Capital resources management Consumables	Knowledge Competence Interpersonal skills Safety Patient education		**Direct:** Lives saved Quality of life Disease averted, individual and population levels **Indirect:** Political symbolism Sense of health security Environmental safety Community status Employment Internal (local) market consumer

	Supervision	Supervision		
Information	Information	Information	Information	Information

Source: Authors.

Note: Some of the factors that may influence a hospital's performance and its products or outputs, the value of which depends on one's perspective, are illustrated. The intrinsic roles of supervision and information flow are emphasized.

Figure 65.1 Conceptual Framework for Delivery of Health Services at the District Hospital

the factors that threaten district hospitals' performance, indicating the broad range of influences to which they are subject. Finally, possible strategies for improving performance are proposed, focusing on cross-cutting interventions, and highlight areas where current knowledge is inadequate and research is urgently needed.

DEFINITIONS, BASIC CONCEPTS, AND FRAMEWORK

The evolution of a hierarchical system of health care is readily explained if one assumes the perspective of the provider, although less obvious if one's perspective is that of the community using the hospital or a government seeking to create political capital. Concentrating skills and resources in one place for conditions that are often relatively uncommon or that cannot easily be treated closer to the home environment is intuitively attractive. Such concentration also offers the prospect of continued accumulation of experience and, thus, skill and potentially benefits from system resources that may serve a variety of needs.

What Is a District Hospital?

Health systems are often organized in a "hub-and-spoke" arrangement, with a large district hospital (the hub) having more and better-trained personnel and better equipment than more peripheral clinics (the spokes). Although variations frequently occur in practice (for example, a large district may have several relatively similar hospitals), this simple model of service provision is assumed throughout this chapter, with the district hospital supplying first referral-level care for both outpatients and inpatients. District hospitals also, in theory, may serve a gatekeeping role for those patients with less common problems, for whom skills and resources are most effectively concentrated at even higher levels of care provided at a regional or national level. Thus, from the perspective of provider efficiency, economies of scale and economies of scope are important basic concepts in considering district and referral hospital functions.

Such hierarchical health systems frequently overlap with wider political and administrative hierarchies that are based on geographically defined units. The district is, therefore, used in this chapter as a generic term for an administrative unit often comprising a population of 100,000 to 1 million people for whom one tier of local government is typically responsible. The shared administrative boundaries and frequent proximity of district hospitals to district political administrations often result in the district hospital's involvement in the much wider tasks of district health management and public health. The performance of these functions may be critical to the success of the health system as a whole, but this role is easily forgotten.

Efficiency. Allocative efficiency deals with the desire to allocate resources to secure the maximum health benefit from the inputs available (Hensher 2001). Within this paradigm planners search for the balance between community care, primary care, and facility-based care that results in the greatest health benefit at the least cost. At the level of an individual hospital, the issue of allocative efficiency arises when decisions must be made to allocate resources to different services. In theory, cost-effectiveness studies with a global health status outcome measure such as the disability-adjusted life year (DALY) should inform debate on allocative efficiency, because such studies provide a direct means of comparing alternative strategies.

Technical efficiency deals with the extent to which specific institutions are getting the most out of the resources available. For example, is a district hospital deploying its given resources in the most effective manner to achieve the desired output? Technical efficiency is often measured using partial indicators such as cost per procedure. Interpreting such data often requires great care, but most fundamentally it requires some comparator, because a way of knowing the resources needed to produce the desired output rarely exists. Thus, *technical efficiency* is usually a relative term, and performance indicators—carefully interpreted—can be used to identify best current practice. New technology or a change in the availability or price of resources may result in continual improvements in what is achievable, so a process that was technically efficient can become relatively inefficient over time. Data on technical efficiency often provide the basis for benchmarking hospital service providers and may identify poorly performing services for targeted improvement strategies.

Economies of Scale and Scope and Hospital Size. A central policy question is whether it is more efficient to concentrate resources in a small number of large centers, where the planned number of procedures can be high, or to have a greater number of smaller centers. The issue of economies of scale determines the most efficient size hospital. Where the average costs of care can be shown to depend on hospital (or unit) size, economies of scale exist (see figure 65.2). Recent evidence suggests that, at least for industrial countries, large centers may eventually suffer from diseconomies of scale, when the inefficiencies introduced in administering a very large facility begin to outweigh any advantages (Posnett 2002). The potential for diseconomies of scale in developing countries, where the mixture of cases, the costs of inputs (particularly the relative costs

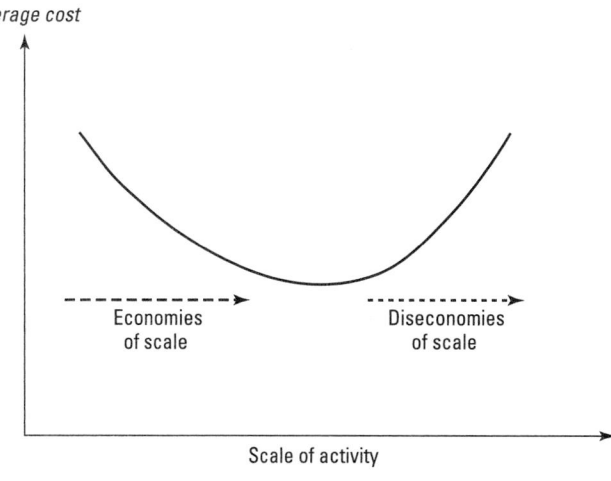

Source: Adapted from Posnett (2002).

Figure 65.2 Theoretical Long-Term Average Cost Curve

of staff salaries and technology), and the pattern of diseases vary widely, has not been examined.

In discussing economies of scale, we must consider two further issues. First, considerable evidence suggests that the ability to specialize and the experience gained with high volumes of patients can lead to better outcomes for physicians practicing in larger hospitals. Second, although reducing the number (and increasing the size) of hospitals may reduce health system costs and improve outcomes, it may shift some costs to patients in the form of increased travel time or even a reduction in the ability to reach the hospital and secure care. Thus, excessive concentration of hospital services may compromise health and equity objectives, particularly in rural areas. The planner may need to balance direct health system costs against the broader population costs of securing access. In many circumstances, this effort may give rise to an intermediate solution, such as medium-sized hospitals, smaller local hospitals equipped to deal with common procedures, or dispersed clinics staffed by peripatetic specialist teams.

The hospital also offers the potential for improving efficiency if different services use some of the same inputs. Although the hospital might not be able to justify paying the salary of a laboratory technician to perform hemoglobin measures and blood cross-matching only for the maternity unit, the fact that such a person also contributes to the work of the surgical, medical, and pediatric services makes that technician's presence more cost-effective. This laboratory service, therefore, offers an economy of scope. The concentration of inputs, both human and technological, evident at the district hospital offers major opportunities for unit-cost reductions and, therefore, economies of scope. Considering the mix of services provided as hospitals are planned or augmented is important to anticipate or account for economies of scope.

Equity. Equity is a fundamental principle guiding most public health systems. It can embrace concepts such as equality of provision or equality of access (for equal need), equality of benefit from health services, or equality of outcome. Although often not defined explicitly, many pro-poor policies, such as the Poverty Reduction Strategy Papers that encompass health, are based on some principle of equity. Loosely speaking, such policies aim to reduce disparities in access or overall health status observed between different sections of a population, most obviously the differences between rich and poor sections of a community.

For health planners, however, equity principles pose some hard challenges. For example, if an urban district has a public hospital with adequate staff and resources providing a range of acute services reasonably efficiently, should not every district hospital provide the same range of services? In practice, ensuring that a hospital in a poor, inaccessible rural district with a highly dispersed, smaller population provides a similar level and breadth of service may be difficult and considerably more expensive. The result can be a hospital with apparently high unit costs of treatment that, because of late presentation or resource constraints, secures poorer outcomes. The central policy question is: To what extent is society prepared to see resources deployed to address such equity concerns at the expense of pure efficiency?

Issues of efficiency, economies of scale and scope, and equity have contributed in part to the development of strategies defining an essential package of services that should be provided for an entire population (Bobadilla and others 1994). These packages are often targeted at the most important causes of mortality and morbidity, so the inefficiencies in providing an equitable service may be reduced. Nevertheless, the unit costs of reaching disadvantaged populations are often likely to be higher than average unit costs, and planners need to recognize this fact when designing packages and set budgets accordingly.

What Essential Services Should a District Hospital Provide?

The World Health Organization (WHO 1992) envisages that a district hospital should be able to offer diagnostic, treatment, care, counseling, and rehabilitation services provided by predominantly generalist practitioners spanning the following disciplines:

- family medicine and primary health care
- medicine
- obstetrics
- mental health
- eye care
- rehabilitation
- surgery (including trauma and orthopedics)
- pediatrics
- geriatrics.

Such hospitals will usually provide 24-hour care and be integrated into the district health system at a wider level to provide or support a range of services:

- districtwide health information
- implementation of peripheral primary health care policies
- administrative and logistics support to primary health care efforts
- communication with the community
- curative and chronic care for patients referred from peripheral units
- district laboratory services
- training and continuing medical education of health workers and students
- links between health and other development agendas
- development of local solutions to local health problems.

This menu of recommended services at the district hospital level does not represent a rigorous attempt to optimize the health system configuration to maximize its cost-effectiveness. Indeed, the logic of the earlier discussion is that the precise mix of services provided should be informed by overall health system design. Rather, the list represents what is perceived to be a fair minimum level of health provision for all, based on accumulated knowledge and experience of the common demands for hospital care (the visible burden), the availability and simplicity of interventions, the perceived effectiveness of interventions, and their acceptability in an environment constrained by limited information and limited availability of human and financial resources (Van Leberghe, de Bethune, and de Brouwere 1997).

An obvious logic supports the inclusion of many of these core functions, sometimes supported by evidence of their value. WHO's Commission on Macroeconomics and Health has attempted to define the services that small hospitals should offer as part of the close-to-client package on the basis of burden and likely cost-effectiveness (Sachs 2001). However, although useful for suggesting service priorities, the report considers primarily infectious diseases and maternal health. In addition, it is not clear whether recommended services were included on the basis of data on condition-specific burden and intervention cost-effectiveness or of the potential effect of the combined package of services considering potential economies of scale and scope. Future studies should perhaps address more clearly the issues of the incremental cost-effectiveness of new or additional interventions at the district hospital level when exploring the appropriateness of services.

Clinical Services

The initial drive to implement primary health care (PHC) left district hospitals sidelined. They were often grouped with expensive tertiary units; were labeled high cost, inequitable, and relatively ineffective; and were rarely protected by powerful professional groups based in the tertiary centers. Their position as an integral part of PHC was reestablished during the 1980s (Canadian International Development Agency and the Aga Khan Foundation 1981; WHO 1987). Currently the district hospital is envisaged as the apex of the pyramid of primary health care, most obviously in such programs as Safe Motherhood and Integrated Management of Childhood Illness. In programs such as Integrated Management of Childhood Illness, the expected role of district hospital–level care is explicit (WHO 2000a), with priority conditions reflecting burden-of-disease estimates (Black, Morris, and Bryce 2003). Although the effectiveness of this approach has yet to be established, evidence at the hospital level suggests that delivering a basic package of care may, in principle, cover the majority of admitted cases and improve service delivery (Ngoc Anh and Tram 1995). However, without tackling current difficulties at the hospital level, effectiveness cannot be assumed (see "Information and Integration" later in this chapter).

Other basic approaches to delivery of services at the district hospital level, such as triage of new outpatient attendees and a basic package of neonatal care, also show promise (Duke, Willie, and Mgone 2000; Robertson and Molyneux 2001). Interventions such as the provision of basic trauma care can effectively be offered only at this level of the health system (see chapter 68), while in other areas (for example, chapters 26, 31, and 67) hospital inpatient care should be considered together with alternative means of delivering services if cost-effectiveness is to be maximized. These examples all serve to emphasize that close-to-client health services must be tightly integrated with district hospital–level care and demonstrate strong dependency on the referral system. Thus, cases too complex or serious to be managed in the periphery are sent for care where skills and resources are more highly concentrated, in the expectation that health outcomes will be better. This attractively simple idea presupposes that the district hospital is able to provide the care desired; although some evidence supports the likely effectiveness of this approach (Van Leberghe and Pangu 1988), clearly numerous potential obstacles exist along this pathway (discussed in the later section "Factors Influencing District Hospitals' Performance").

Additionally, although the focus has often been on district hospitals as recipients of referrals, a much more dynamic relationship has been proposed (WHO 1987): for many PHC activities such as immunization programs the district hospital is both a provider of services and a coordinating center for information and supplies. To permit early discharge, enhance treatment compliance, and make home-based care possible— all of which may improve cost-effectiveness—hospitals need to play an active role in providing outreach services, supervision, and support.

Cross-Cutting Services at the District Hospital

Some medical services provide support to a range of departments or users and are referred to as cross-cutting services. Such services include those aimed at recuperation and rehabilitation (physiotherapy, occupational therapy, and so forth; see chapter XX; laboratory services, and diagnostic imaging. Whether and to what degree these services are provided may be major determinants of the overall range of services that can be offered, the fixed costs of providing care at district hospitals, and their cost-effectiveness. Their provision should, therefore, be planned as part of the portfolio of care to be offered, taking into account expected use and estimates of the value added. This strategy suggests a degree of flexibility that may conflict with historical perspectives about what is important and "one size fits all" national policies. Health information systems are also a critical cross-cutting service; they are discussed in the "Health Information Systems" section of this chapter.

It is worth noting here that the concentration in hospitals of cross-cutting resources used by different activities often gives rise to many accounting complications, such as allocating overhead costs, which bedevil attempts to secure meaningful cost comparisons across hospitals.

Wider Role in the District Health System

District hospitals often house the technical expertise and professional authority essential for local implementation of national policy, making them potentially key players in managing, monitoring, and supervising district health plans. They should also act as advocates for plans that address local health needs. This section examines this wider role of the district hospital, the value of which is often hard to quantify, but which may be critical to the effectiveness of the local health system as a whole.

Integration with Other Local Health-Related Services. A district hospital should, in most cases, be an integral part of a wider district health system. Although not specifically discussed here, part of the broader remit is often to link up with other governmental and nongovernmental actors in health and health-related programs, which may include water and sanitation, education, and social services. (A more specific discussion can be found in WHO 1990.) Those important coordination functions are hard to value in traditional examinations of cost and cost-effectiveness but may be critical in sustaining a coordinated health care approach, especially if greater autonomy is devolved to district administrations.

Training. District hospitals often have a direct role in the primary training of health workers, particularly clinical assistants, nurses, and health aides, as well as an ongoing role in providing continuing medical education. Their role in building human resources capacity among those actively participating in health care delivery and in ensuring that training and experience reflect the real health needs of the community is potentially of great value. Additionally, as the focal point of outreach for many programs that aim to disseminate knowledge through the cascade mechanism, district hospitals are often relied on to transmit knowledge to more peripheral levels of care.

Supervision. Together with their training function, district hospital staff members are often supposed to provide supervision and support to health workers at more peripheral levels of care and to act as part of the regulatory mechanism, sometimes in both the public and the private sectors. Although this function is likely to be an important means of developing and refining the referral system through two-way exchange of information and of seeing that policy decisions are implemented, the ability of the health staff to fulfill this function is often extremely limited. Because resources are scarce, activities with the least tangible benefit—such as supervision and monitoring—are frequently abandoned, breaking important chains of communication.

Health Information Systems. Many national health information systems rely on district hospitals to coordinate data collection in the district. In theory, for a number of diseases the district hospital may be the only source of information, for example, for severe diseases such as neonatal tetanus, acute flaccid paralysis, or operative deliveries. The district hospital is, thus, a core data source supposedly providing burden-of-disease data at greater resolution than is commonly available and at a meaningful administrative level if action is required. However, in many developing countries health information systems are inadequate and inaccurate; staff members are not equipped with the skills necessary to interpret data (Loevinsohn 1993) and are often unaware of their local value, thus depriving the local staff of essential planning and monitoring tools. Introducing an information culture and the necessary skills and infrastructure to support such a transition, although of potentially enormous value, presents significant challenges even for middle-income countries.

Formulating a Package of Services to Maximize Cost-Effectiveness

Interventions identified as being cost-effective in particular service areas or necessary to preserve the integrity of an effective and equitable health system should be a part of a basic package of services and responsibilities at the district hospital level. However, the way in which these individual components are combined and integrated is also critical. Factors, including economies of scale and scope, whether gains or losses in efficiency result from integration, and the influence of use and resource availability, will all have a profound influence on whether the district hospital itself is as cost-effective as the sum of its parts suggests it should be.

ECONOMICS OF DISTRICT HOSPITALS: A SUMMARY OF REPORTED EXPERIENCE

The previous sections outline the suggested functions and extended role of a district hospital. Although some countries have adopted the principle of essential packages of services and defined detailed norms and standards for care at this level as part of long-term health sector strategies, many countries lack any specific hospital strategy (WHO 1994). Even where a well-articulated strategy exists, decades of different political, social, economic, and historical influences on health system development result in great variability of district hospitals, both between and within developing countries. Thus, some district hospitals of 500 beds have a full complement of specialist consultants and access to a wide range of diagnostic and therapeutic services, while other hospitals of as few as 30 beds, but more often 80 to 150 beds, are run almost entirely by medical assistants and nurses, sometimes lack reliable power or water supplies, and often offer few or no high-quality modern diagnostic services. This variability makes it daunting to extrapolate findings from one setting to another and may seriously undermine the value of attempts to provide useful general descriptions of hospitals. In particular, when interpreting calculated costs of care at a national or individual level, we must remember several critical points:

- Relevant data may often be missing or inadequately defined at a country level.
- Because a number of accepted ways of calculating costs exist, particularly at the level of individual interventions, different methods are likely to lead to different estimates. The particular design used to estimate costs should be considered when interpreting any results.
- In particular, a central feature of the hospital is that many of its resources are used for more than one activity, so unit cost estimates depend crucially on how the costs of these resources are allocated among activities.
- The relative prices of inputs can vary substantially between regions and countries.
- In the majority of cases, only the cost of care is reported without reference to outcomes so that the cost per unit of health benefit (however defined) is unknown.
- Calculated costs usually reflect the care offered; it may not be the same as the care that is necessary, of an acceptable quality, or most effective.
- Cost estimates cannot indicate the extent of unmet need or other sources of inequity.
- The costs of care will depend to some extent on the severity of illness of the patients and, for average costs per bed day, on the variety and relative proportions of different illnesses (the *case mix*). These areas are rarely commented on or adjusted for.

Levels of Provision of Hospital Care

Data on the levels of service provision for many developing countries are crude. In the absence of any more meaningful data, the number of beds is most often used as a (poor) substitute. Bearing this weakness in mind, sources estimate the average number of total hospital beds to be 1.3 per 1,000 population in developing countries (World Bank 2002), a figure probably declining in many developing countries (Hensher and others 1999), with varying estimates of the average number of doctors from 0.5 per 1,000 population in low-income countries generally (World Bank 2002) to 0.09 doctors per 1,000 population in Sub-Saharan Africa (Peters and others 2000). These estimates are considerably lower than the averages for beds and doctors of 7.2 per 1,000 and 2.9 per 1,000, respectively, in high-income countries (World Bank 2002). Although these estimates provide some indication of the major disparities in service provision between rich and poor countries, their value is limited. Lack of information on the relative distribution of beds and staff by geographic zone, or between district and higher referral levels of care in a single country, and the fact that bed and staff numbers are probably a poor reflection of activity make these figures a poor substitute for data on patient throughput and outcomes, statistics rarely available for district hospitals. Furthermore, with the concentration on provision of service, the demand for services may often be ignored. It is still true in many countries that most deaths, presumably many preventable, occur at home and that many chronic diseases are inadequately treated. The need for hospital care is largely undetermined, but some have argued that the lack of provision of district hospital care, in Sub-Saharan Africa at least, is a significant impediment to improving overall health status (Van Leberghe, de Bethune, and de Brouwere 1997).

What Do District Hospitals Cost at a National Level?

Although it has been argued for some time that hospitals consume too much of health sector budgets, thereby depriving primary care of adequate resources, it is surprisingly difficult to identify how much hospitals cost in low- and middle-income countries. Even where data exist on health expenditure, such data are often at a highly aggregated national level and the functions that are included (clean water and sanitation, for example) are not always clear (World Bank 2002). Furthermore, whether private or nongovernmental expenditure, capital expenditure, or the value of noncash inputs—such as donations of equipment or volunteers' time—are included is rarely apparent. Add to this ambiguity the nearly impossible problem of separating what is spent at different levels of the health or hospital system—for example, to distinguish between district and referral hospitals—and it should be clear that we currently have only a crude understanding of the costs of district hospitals as a unit of service provision (Mills 1990a).

If just government health expenditure is considered, the available data suggest that hospitals at every level taken together consume 50 to 60 percent of recurrent national health budgets, with the proportion appearing to increase as countries become richer (Barnum and Kutzin 1993). If private expenditure on health care (insurance and out of pocket) is included, the proportion of total health expenditure consumed by all hospitals falls to 30 to 50 percent of the total in developing countries (excluding South America) (Mills 1990a). Whereas these figures reflect total hospital sector expenditure, the limited data available suggest that district hospitals may receive less than 50 percent of this total in many countries, consuming fewer resources than secondary and tertiary referral facilities (Mills 1990a).

The Nongovernmental and Private Sectors

In many countries (especially in Africa) nongovernmental institutions, often religious organizations, are major health service providers, and private physicians are often as numerous as those in the public sector. In Kenya, for instance, the number of private and nongovernmental hospitals is equal to the number of public hospitals (Government of Kenya 2001), while in Indonesia, 32 percent of hospital beds are private (Gani 1996). This potentially important contribution to the hospital sector may also be underrecognized, particularly in urban settings, where multiple, small facilities may operate without registration, resulting in inaccurate local, regional, and national data on levels of overall service provision. Although few data exist on the effectiveness and quality of these hospitals, the belief is widespread that they may be more efficient than public sector hospitals. This belief is not necessarily borne out by the limited data available (Bitran 1996), and concerns exist about the quality of care provided by private as well as public providers (Brugha and Zwi 1998).

District Hospital Efficiency

Data on hospital efficiency in developing countries are scant. Considerable variability has been observed in the technical efficiency with which surgical services were provided in a small number of Indian hospitals, with differences in total salary costs being the main explanatory variable (Purohit and Rai 1992). Also in India, some evidence has been provided that nongovernmental hospitals may be more efficient, on average, than public hospitals, although considerable variability existed within both groups (Bhat, Verma, and Reuben 2001). In Kenya, public hospitals were found to have an average inefficiency level of 30 percent (that is, the same resources could have achieved a 30 percent increase in output) with significant contributing factors including shortage of appropriate professional staff members, poor combinations of inputs (resources), nonfunctioning theaters and laboratories, lack of transportation, irregular distribution of drugs and supplies, and frequent breakdowns in medical equipment (Owino and Korir 1997). All these data highlight the critical role of human resources, often a hospital's principal recurrent input cost (see the next section). Underinvestment in or absence of staff or inadequate flexibility in reallocating roles between different health worker groups may prevent hospitals from functioning efficiently (Hensher 2001).

What Are the Costs of Providing Care in District Hospitals?

In a detailed review of actual hospital expenditure, Mills (1990b) identified two input categories that together accounted for two-thirds or more of recurrent expenditure in almost all settings. Salaries varied between 20 and 80 percent and medical supplies between 15 and 58 percent of reported hospital expenditure. These and other data also suggest that, in many countries, costs of referral hospital care are often more than double the cost of equivalent care at district hospitals, although without knowledge on case mix or illness severity such data are hard to interpret (Barnum and Kutzin 1993; Mills 1990b). More recent data collected from seven church-supported hospitals in Tanzania also demonstrate considerable variability in the proportion of costs attributable to salaries and supplies even within a single organization in the same country (Flessa 1998). The strong dependence of hospital costs on salaries particularly cautions against generalizations across countries.

In the following analysis, all original U.S. dollar costs have been adjusted to represent the U.S. dollar cost in 2004. The Tanzanian nongovernmental hospital data indicate that the average cost per inpatient day derived from 1995 reports (including expenditure on maintenance and expatriate salaries) would equate now to approximately US$3.60 (range US$2.60 to US$6.00) in district hospitals (Flessa 1998). However, if care had actually been provided according to the standards defined by the provider (including recommended staffing levels, building maintenance, and equipment), the estimated cost per day would have risen to the equivalent of US$11.60 (range US$9.20 to US$15.90) (Flessa 1998). This cost compares with costs reported in Kenya in 1993–94 (Kirigia, Fox-Rushby, and Mills 1998), adjusted to 2004 prices of actual inpatient costs per day from two district hospitals of US$8.30 to US$10.10, and adjusted 1995 data from a district hospital in Bangladesh of US$15.90 (McCord and Chowdury 2003). In a middle-income country, South Africa, the cost per inpatient day calculated between 1996 and 1998 and adjusted to 2004 prices in five district hospitals ranged from US$37.80 to US$96.30 (Daviaud and others 2000). These data do not necessarily reflect the cost of optimal care, and the Tanzanian study demonstrates that even in externally supported hospitals actual expenditure may be insufficient to provide good-quality care and cover essential maintenance, resulting in steady deterioration of capital stock and worsening efficiency in the long term.

Data describing costs of treating some specific conditions in district hospitals are summarized in table 65.1. Given the difficulties in extrapolating data across contexts and the potentially significant effect of exchange rate fluctuations, great caution

Table 65.1 Costs of Delivering Care at the District Hospital Level

Country and year	Item costed	Cost (original data adjusted to 2004 US$)	Comment
Kenya, 1993–94, two district hospitals, research study	Treatment of inpatient severe malaria in children	US$41.50 to US$132.00 per case treated	Step-down approach to allocate all costs, including capital costs
Zimbabwe, 1994–95, three district hospitals,[a] research study	Medical inpatient stay; HIV/AIDS care	Non-HIV: US$49.20 to US$110.00; HIV: US$133.00 to US$217.00 per inpatient stay	Bottom-up and step-down approaches used, including capital costs
Zimbabwe, 1999, six provincial hospitals, research study	Severe malaria inpatient care; Pulmonary tuberculosis inpatient care[b]	Severe malaria, mean costs per case US$26.60 to US$49.90; tuberculosis, median costs per case US$22.20 to US$61.00	Overhead costs purposefully omitted; 1999 exchange rates
Uganda, modeling based on 1997–99 data factoring in program expansion	Aspects of safe motherhood delivered at hospital[c]; actual and recommended practices	Eclampsia: actual US$63.40; recommended US$127.00; Cesarean: actual US$53.20; recommended US$57.80; Prenatal care: actual US$2.90; recommended US$8.30	Attempt to estimate current program costs and costs if program implemented as recommended; excludes facility costs

Sources: Kenya—Kirigia and others 1998; Zimbabwe 1994–95—Hansen and others 2000; Zimbabwe 1999—Hongoro and McPake 2003; Uganda—Weissman and others 1999.
Note: Shaded rows provide data from studies that did not include overhead or facility costs.
a. Only data from district hospitals are shown.
b. All hospitals had a median length of stay for tuberculosis cases of 10 days or less.
c. Only selected items are shown.

Table 65.2 Estimate of the Effectiveness of a Kenyan District Hospital in Preventing Childhood Deaths in a Rural Community with Good Access to the Hospital

Study site and population: Kenyan rural community with access to basic primary health care services provided by five clinics, three private	Population 51,183; 52 percent younger than age 15
Surveillance period	1991–93
Service provider	Kenyan Ministry of Health district hospital supplemented by research unit
Mortality rates:	
Neonatal	31.5 per 1,000 live births
Infant	58.3 per 1,000 live births
Child	12.4 per 1,000 children ages one to four years
Observed number of admissions	2,223
Admission rate	45 per 1,000 children ages 1 to 59 months per year
Proportion of deaths occurring in the hospital:	
Neonatal	28 percent
Ages 1 to 59 months	30 percent
Observed number of deaths	134
Expected number of deaths without inpatient care based on expert estimates for case fatality rates	349
Lives saved	215
Estimated cost per life saved[a]	US$104.40

Source: Snow and others 1994.
a. 2004 US$ equivalent, using admission cost data from Kirigia and others 1998. The estimated cost of the admissions in 2004 US$ would be 2,223 × 10.1 = US$22,452.30. This expenditure prevented 215 deaths; average cost of life saved therefore = 22,452.30/215 = US$104.40.

should be used in interpreting these data, which, it should be noted, derive in all cases from specific research rather than routine sources.

Measuring the Effect and Cost-Effectiveness of District Hospitals

In the previous section, some limited data on the costs associated with provision of care at the district hospital were presented. What of a hospital's cost-effectiveness? Ideally we would like to know the aggregate health output of a hospital in terms of improved health compared with a situation in which there is no hospital. Such data do not exist, even from industrial countries, where the hospital has been the subject of intense academic study.

However, some attempts have been made to estimate the effect of a hospital by comparing the observed outcome of illness treated with hospital care to consensus expert opinion on the likely outcome of illness in the absence of hospital care. Using this approach in Kenya, Snow and others (1994) estimated that a well-functioning rural district hospital might reduce all-cause child mortality by 44 percent in a population with reasonable access to the hospital (see table 65.2). Extending this approach, researchers in a small rural hospital in Bangladesh calculated the benefit of hospital admission for patients of all ages suffering from life-threatening conditions

using a slightly modified DALY (McCord and Chowdury 2003). Over a three-month period, the total costs (including all staff, capital, and hotel costs) of running the hospital were calculated and divided by the estimated total number of DALYs gained attributable to inpatient care over the same three months. The authors report an average cost per DALY of approximately US$11.00 in 1995, or US$13.30 in 2004 dollars (McCord and Chowdury 2003; see table 65.3). This figure compares favorably with costs per DALY of many primary care interventions regarded as highly cost-effective (World Bank 1993). To what extent these results depend on the quality of primary care, the referral system, the inpatient care, the hospital administration, and the commitment of health personnel working for a small independent nongovernmental organization will remain uncertain until more such data become available.

FACTORS INFLUENCING DISTRICT HOSPITALS' PERFORMANCE

The overall macroeconomic policy framework, as illustrated here with reference to financing mechanisms, may often be overlooked as a considerable influence on hospital performance. For the sake of simplicity, other factors (not exhaustively described and illustrated in figure 65.1) are discussed as primarily affecting the demand for hospital services or their supply and may

Table 65.3 Estimate of the Cost-Effectiveness of a Nongovernmental District Hospital in Rural Bangladesh

Study site and population: Rural Bangladesh, with community served by four peripheral clinics	Population 160,000
Surveillance period	July through October 1995
Service provider	Independent nongovernmental organization
Major causes of death	74 percent under-five mortality attributable to perinatal deaths; maternal mortality ratio high
Admissions analyzed	541 (33 percent obstetric/gynecological problems)
DALYs gained by hospital services:	
Adult medical	177.0 life years; 6.5 disability years
Surgical	459.4 life years; 236.3 disability years
Pediatric	371.5 life years; 10.8 disability years
Obstetric/gynecological	897.5 life years; 125.4 disability years
Newborn (resulting from ob/gyn interventions)	1,024.3 life years
Total DALYs gained	3,308.7
Cost per DALY	US$10.93 in 1995 ($13.30 in 2004 US$)

Source: McCord and Chowdury 2003.

operate at both national and local levels. The way some of these diverse factors affect people's daily lives is illustrated in box 65.1. What is clear is that failure to tackle these many challenges all too often results in facilities that fail their communities.

Central Financing Mechanisms

Three broad methods of government financing of public district hospitals are generally used: prospective with a fixed budget, prospective with revenue depending on activity, and retrospective in proportion to actual costs. The fixed budget is widely used, often based on historical spending levels, with a (frequently inadequate) provision for price changes. Such a system clearly can secure good expenditure control and is administratively undemanding. However, it can often perpetuate historical inequities and fail to respond to new demands and priorities. Moreover, fixed budgets offer few incentives to maximize the effectiveness, quality, or quantity of care offered by hospitals (Barnum, Kutzin, and Saxenian 1995).

Indeed, many budget systems continue to finance hospitals through line-item budgets directly from the ministry of health or finance. Such mechanisms allow central bureaucracies to exert the maximum level of control over peripheral spending with little or no capacity at peripheral levels for flexible use of funds in response to local needs. Thus, centralized budget systems can contribute to technical inefficiency by preventing local managers from optimizing the deployment of inputs. In contrast, global fixed budgets provide for central control of total spending but may permit increased independence when allocating funds at a local level. Fixed budgets based on capitation payments can be more sensitive to local needs than incremental budgeting and can contribute toward equity objectives.

However, they demand technical skill and accurate data at the central level, especially if capitation payments are adjusted for differences in population health status or other needs.

Financing based on activity levels (such as the diagnosis-related group methods in widespread use in high-income countries) are similarly demanding of central-level capacity and also require considerable competence and probity at more peripheral levels of the administration. However, such financing might be an essential prerequisite of insurance-based mechanisms. In contrast to fixed budgets, it has the potential for encouraging supplier-induced demand—the greater the hospital's income, the more services it provides. It produces some incentive to reduce unit costs. Expenditure control may be difficult unless a cap is put on the aggregate hospital sector budget.

Retrospective reimbursement of actual costs is a discredited system of financing hospitals because it offers no incentive to control costs or manage demand. In its favor, it may stimulate higher-quality care. In practice, many health systems use a mixture of all three payment mechanisms, with broadly fixed budgets, sometimes adjusted for changes in demand, and some element of retrospective reimbursement for unplanned activity. In general, no one strategy is perfect. However, the considerable demands on management for some schemes imply that a global budget, ideally based on population needs, in conjunction with some form of quality-monitoring system may be the most appropriate way forward for many developing countries (Barnum, Kutzin, and Saxenian 1995).

Mechanisms permitting local income generation (cost recovery, cost sharing, facility improvement funds, and local taxes) may be superimposed on any of these schemes. Such devices can help countries shift toward a local, more needs-based allocation of financing and help promote accountability

Hospital Performance: Perspectives from a Sub-Saharan African Country

Caretaker (C) and health worker (HW) experiences of hospital care:

"When the doctor realized my child was breathless he quickly called us into the office even though I was at the back in the queue." (C)

"The [nursing] sister came and talked to me and asked if I had a problem, and I felt good and cared for." (C)

"Things here have greatly improved; the ward is clean and the treatment prompt. We are happy and hope that this will continue." (C)

"I admitted a patient in very poor condition with malaria and anemia and I managed to remove blood for cross-match and fix a line, start on oxygen, and get the doctor. Blood was started quickly, and the child rapidly improved." (HW)

"I resuscitated a baby with severe asphyxia, and it successfully came up. The success was because I had attended a course in basic life support skills for neonates." (HW)

Caretaker and healthworker descriptions of referral to hospital:

"If you do not have the money, you have to look for it first. Sometimes you may even have to spend a day or two looking for the money for the treatment. If you have coffee,

then you sell it before you go." (C) (Peterson and others 2004).

"I spent a long time in MCH [Maternal and Child Health]; the doctor wanted money before he would see me, and I did not have any." (C)

"There is a lot of suffering when it comes to drugs because they are usually not enough and most of the time the mothers do not have money." (C)

"I want to know everything about the illness; I asked the nurses, but they refused to explain, so I got disheartened from asking anyone." (C)

"I had a patient with anemia and mild marasmus, and the mother waited for three hours in the lab for an Hb only to be turned away as she had no money. Then I went to get the child some milk, and I was turned away as the storeman said it was too late. The child had to wait until the next day." (HW)

"A child with severe LRTI [lower respiratory tract infection] was very dyspneic on admission. Only one cylinder of oxygen was available, but we started giving it to the child, and the condition improved. The condition became worse when the oxygen ran out, and there was none left; he started gasping and died." (HW)

Source: English and others 2004a, unless otherwise noted.

by focusing local attention on the efficiency and quality of local services. This flexibility presupposes that those empowered with authority have the skills and freedom to make and execute plans. The experience of such a decentralized policy on district hospital or district health system performance is mixed, with a lack of real transfer of authority reducing effectiveness in some areas (Blas and Limbambala 2001), while more balanced and carefully implemented mechanisms of decentralization may be productive (Bossert and others 2003).

The specific effects of requiring out-of-pocket payments to access health care are a matter of fierce debate. Although some data suggest an improvement in allocative or technical efficiency, other data do not (Arhin-Tenkorang 2000; Van der Geest and others 2000). It has been suggested that an improved quality of service may overcome the cost barrier to access (Van der Geest and others 2000). However, the likelihood that the poor will be excluded from hospital care is a major concern. There is also an increasing tendency to encourage district hospitals to provide some beds with an enhanced level of professional

attention and hotel services (sometimes referred to as *amenity beds*) as a means of generating profit; reports indicate that the fees levied may not even cover the cost of the enhanced service, let alone generate extra revenue with which to cross-subsidize services for the poor (Flessa 1998; Suwandono and others 2001).

Demand for Services

Patients' demand for services may be influenced by a wide variety of factors, many of which have little to do with the hospitals themselves. Patients' perceptions of the severity of their illness, cultural beliefs, physical accessibility, and financial and opportunity costs together with the performance of the peripheral health unit screening process all potentially limit the effectiveness of the referral mechanism and thus the hospital (Font and others 2002; Siddiqui and others 2001). Recent data highlighting the inability of many families to meet the financial costs of hospital referral (Peterson and others 2004) and the potentially catastrophic consequences of severe illness (Xu and others 2003) underscore the importance of financial barriers, especially for the poor. Not only are there obvious implications for health generally, but underusing service capacity also reduces efficiency and increases the costs per case of hospital care. Improving the efficiency and effect of a hospital may, therefore, be best achieved by tackling factors that influence demand—for example, providing emergency transport and limiting out-of-pocket expenses. However, often a concern exists that the provision of free high-quality services may itself promote unnecessary demand—the so-called moral hazard. In addition, the relative importance of demand factors may vary considerably in different settings, for example, in urban and rural areas, making universal rules unhelpful.

In the context of PHC, it is suggested that high demand for services provided by hospitals rather than peripheral clinics, driven by a perception that hospitals provide higher-quality service and resulting in bypassing of the PHC level of care, is inefficient. It has been proposed that hospitals be specifically prevented from delivering PHC services (WHO 1990). However, the view that patients who bypass PHC increase the costs to the provider may not always be true (Siddiqui and others 2001). Patients may also choose to bypass the district hospital and proceed directly to referral hospitals, often increasing the costs of care if the condition could have been treated in the lower-level facility. The perceived quality of care at the district level may be a major determinant of this behavior, with some data suggesting that improved district services increase use rates (Barnum and Kutzin 1993), potentially making district hospitals more cost-effective but more costly.

The Supply of Services

A fundamental role of policy makers is to determine the geographical distribution of hospitals and the functions they should undertake. These decisions are often severely circumscribed by topography, historical accident, and political imperatives, as well as by the level and quality of resources that are available. Often, changes can be made only incrementally, building on an existing structure of administration and capital that may not be in any sense optimal.

Nevertheless, many of the factors determining the quality of supply are theoretically under the influence of local management personnel, who are in a potentially powerful position to significantly affect a hospital's function. Lack of resources, low morale, inability to attract staff members to hardship areas, poor training, and inadequate supervision among many other factors may all conspire to prevent health workers from executing their duties effectively or even at all. Those factors may, in turn, result in less demand for services from consumers, who opt to avoid the hospital or go elsewhere for treatment. The paradox resulting from this decline is that the hospital may

continue to operate within a fixed budget, thereby satisfying finance ministries but having little or no effect on health. Long-term underinvestment in facilities and skilled, motivated staff may then condemn a health system to many years of underperformance, given the time necessary to address these issues. This is the fundamental reason for seeking to measure system outputs and quality as well as costs.

On a regional or national scale, the actual distribution of hospitals and personnel may work for or against effective service delivery. For political reasons (to reward a community or to honor a powerful politician, for instance), hospitals may be situated in areas that would not be chosen if purely rational plans had been followed. Nongovernmental providers or philanthropists may build or alter hospitals without regard to the overall function of a health system or achieving either equity or efficiency. Public, private, and nongovernmental hospitals may compete for patients, potentially reducing efficiency in some or all sectors. The crisis of inadequate personnel in low-income countries, which limits the range, quality, and quantity of services that can be offered, has been described (Narasimhan and others 2004). However, imbalances in the within-country distribution of staff members are less well publicized and equally damaging. All the factors mentioned and others are commonly encountered in health systems of developing countries and are major barriers to implementing potentially valuable interventions at an operational level (Oliveira-Cruz, Hanson, and Mills 2001). New interventions must therefore often be considered in the light of existing (rather than optimal) levels of service provision and performance. Little literature is available on these public choice features of decision making.

EFFECTING CHANGE WITH CROSS-CUTTING INTERVENTIONS

So far this chapter has outlined concepts fundamental to understanding the position, functions, and performance of the district hospital and has presented some of the existing (though limited) data on costs and cost-effectiveness. Operating at the interface between primary care—aimed often at the poor—and the more Western biotechnological model of care at secondary and tertiary levels—often more accessible to the better off—district hospitals are easy to ignore because they lack any advocates for their role. However, optimizing their role to maximize health benefits and promote equity does demand the following:

- explicit policy decisions about the services that should be offered at this level and about the balance between primary care, district hospital care, and higher-level care services provided

- national strategies on the distribution of services that encompass all providers
- commitment to provision and equitable distribution of essential human resources and supplies
- systems for monitoring hospital performance in terms of efficiency and quality and for intervention when performance is poor.

When a framework defining the district hospital is available, interventions that might improve performance can be considered. The focus here is on cross-cutting interventions rather than condition-specific or service area–specific interventions described elsewhere. Cross-cutting interventions seem to be rarely prioritized but have the ability to add value in many areas and are perhaps critical when thinking of developing an improved health system.

Human Resources

Key issues that affect district hospitals are the quantity and quality of personnel and their range of skills. Staff members should be appropriate to the tasks they are asked to perform. This approach may mean continuing to use nursing or auxiliary staff members with more limited training in district hospitals because they may be more cost-effective, running against the tide of rising academic requirements often demanded by professional associations (AED 2003). Similarly, devolving some tasks to lower cadres of staff may be practical and much more efficient—for example, training and licensing clinical assistants to perform emergency surgery including cesarean section. Such initiatives, too, may face opposition from powerful professional vested interests. Although some tasks may be transferred downward, a problem often faced by district hospitals is an absence of high-quality senior staff members or leaders. Traditionally, running a district hospital has commanded less respect and remuneration than work at a secondary or tertiary facility and has been regarded as a stage to be moved through as rapidly as possible. Arguably, the challenges to a district hospital professional are at least as great as those of a tertiary consultant specialist, and the development of appropriate skills-training programs, and parity of postgraduate qualifications and pay, might help foster the development of a professional group that improves performance and fills a much needed advocacy role.

Improving Clinical Management

For more than a decade, industrial countries have increasingly promoted the use of the best evidence in clinical management. Clinical guidelines, means to implement them, feedback on their use and value, clinical audit, and performance review are all now the subject of considerable research, with some evidence of benefit particularly when part of a broadly based approach (Grol and Grimshaw 2003). District hospitals in developing countries have largely missed out on this revolution, which may be of particular value in settings where care by nonspecialists with little or no access to recent information is the norm.

Information and Integration

Although much focus is given to technological development in the fields of diagnosis, treatment, and imaging, relatively little attention is paid to the potential for technology to change the collection and use of information, despite the possibly major effect on improving administrative and clinical management. As at the primary care level, where many of the interventions are currently available to achieve significant reductions in mortality (Claesen and others 2003), many of the tools that could be used to improve health are well known at the district hospital level. Making better use of these tools through more reliable provision, better training, improved information collection, on-the-spot analysis of data, and real-time use of the results for service planning might be both possible and of considerable benefit (Cibulskis and Hiawalyer 2002). Clearly, how a hospital is performing as part of an integrated primary care system is also vital. Local information on population health, on use and referral patterns, and on success and the reasons underlying successes and failures is invaluable if the hospital is to respond to the particular needs of its locality.

Quality Improvement and Accreditation

Quality improvement is a generic technique adapted from industry that involves a rolling approach to identifying problems, solving them, and assessing the results of change (see figure 65.3) and that has been institutionalized in hospital care in many developed countries (DiPrete-Brown and others 1993). An essential first step is defining standards for service provision, which can span all areas, including the technical content of care, the physical environment in which care takes place, and interpersonal relations between patients and health workers. This approach is often linked to formal systems for external assessment of hospitals' performance and accreditation. Accreditation may serve as a goal for participating hospitals, a means of promoting positive competition, and a means of identifying poorly performing institutions. Potential advantages of such initiatives are empowerment of local service providers to solve problems they feel are important and the overall aim of working toward a systemwide standard of care. However, although an obvious need exists for quality improvement in hospitals in developing countries (English and others 2004b; Nolan and others 2000), few examples exist of hospital-level interventions in industrial or developing countries that

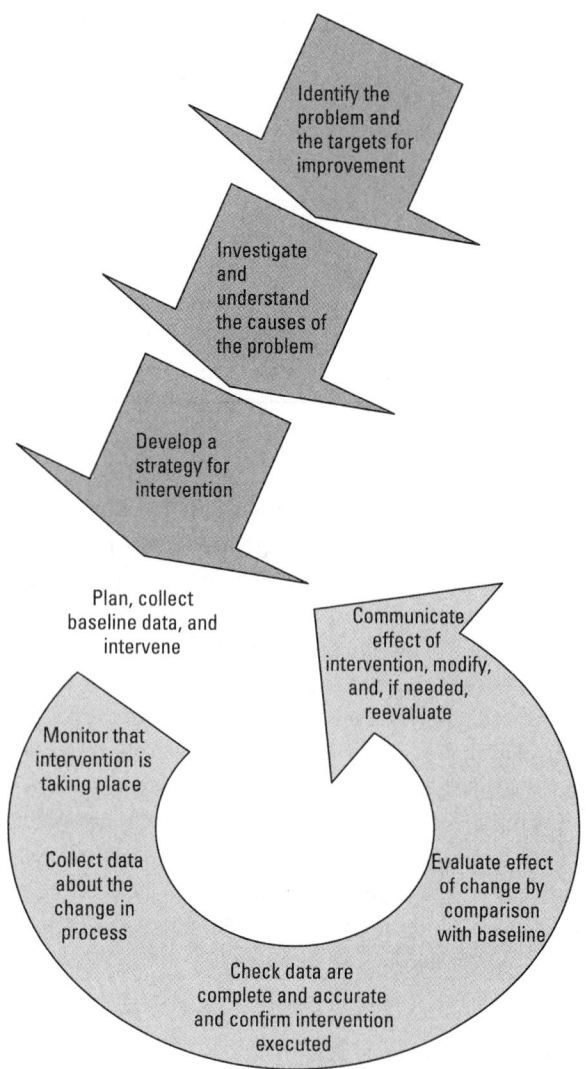

Identify the problem and the targets for improvement

Investigate and understand the causes of the problem

Develop a strategy for intervention

Plan, collect baseline data, and intervene

Communicate effect of intervention, modify, and, if needed, reevaluate

Monitor that intervention is taking place

Evaluate effect of change by comparison with baseline

Collect data about the change in process

Check data are complete and accurate and confirm intervention executed

Source: Adapted from Massoud and others (2001).

Figure 65.3 Quality Improvement Process

provide evidence of effect on major outcomes. One exception is a broadly based quality improvement intervention targeting maternal and child health in Peru that focused on the entire system of care. This project was associated with a 25 percent decrease in maternal deaths in program areas (see box 65.2 for details). However, the relatively poor progress of an operational-level quality improvement and accreditation program in Zambia's hospitals highlights the significant problems of intervening in countries with poorly functioning health systems that are severely constrained by lack of resources (Bukonda and others 2002).

Hospital-Acquired Disease

Probably the most important infection in developing countries that can be acquired as a result of hospital care is HIV, espe-

cially in Sub-Saharan Africa. Reuse of needles and blood transfusion are the main sources of infection and also carry the risk of hepatitis B and C and other viral infections important in their own right. It has been estimated that effective measures to improve blood safety in particular are a highly cost-effective intervention at approximately US$8 or less per DALY (Creese and others 2002).

Nosocomial infection, another major adverse consequence of admission to hospital, is common in some settings in industrial countries, contributing significantly to hospital costs. Historically, relatively simple approaches to prevention have proven reasonably effective with additional effect from dedicated prevention services (Ayliffe and English 2003). The potential effect of intervention in district hospitals in developing countries is largely unknown, although in China nosocomial infection rates of between 8 and 13 percent have been reported (Barnum and Kutzin 1993). Because overcrowding and lack of basic resources, even water, are common in some districts, the potential for simple cost-effective interventions to prevent such infections seems high.

Other Managerial Initiatives

In high-income countries, numerous other initiatives are being tested to promote improved efficiency and quality. They often rely heavily on having in place appropriate institutional arrangements, managerial capacity, and information systems, so their feasibility for local implementation is highly dependent on local circumstances. One of the most widely tested arrangements within public national health systems has been the experiment with internal markets, in which a range of public hospitals compete for contracts from separate public service purchasers, such as local governments. The split of purchaser and provider of public services is recognized as a potentially powerful instrument for securing efficiency improvements but can be demanding in terms of managerial skills (Le Grand, Mays, and Mulligan 1998).

A less direct way of introducing some form of competition into the hospital market is to require hospitals to publish performance reports that allow direct comparisons to be made between hospitals.

An alternative to relying on indirect methods of influencing behavior is to give physicians incentives or instructions to deliver care in line with guidelines reflecting best practice. In the United States, numerous experiments have been carried out under the general banner of managed care (Glied 2000), and other systems have attempted analogous approaches to hospital regulation. At one extreme is the centralized U.K. system of performance management, under which hospitals are given challenging and immediate targets and are rated according to measured outcomes (Smee 2002). At the other extreme is the system of guided self-regulation practiced in the Netherlands, under

Box 65.2

Prevention of Maternal and Child Deaths from Improvements in the Quality of Health Services: An Example from Peru

Recognizing the failure of previous training attempts to improve the quality of health services, the Ministry of Health, with support from the U.S. Agency for International Development and the participation of local institutions, developed an innovative program in Peru. Aiming to reduce maternal and perinatal deaths, the program expected to increase use of health services by improving quality and by strengthening links between the health services and their communities by working with midwives and community health workers. Multidisciplinary teams implemented a quality improvement program in approximately 2,500 health facilities, focusing on

- standardizing care
- ensuring the availability at all times of essential supplies and equipment
- making use of existing information systems and doing small operational studies to generate data at the local level to facilitate decision making
- promoting the participation of all personnel in a concerted and agreed-on plan of action
- measuring patients' satisfaction over time and addressing the causes of complaint.

Training activity mainly involved use of a participatory problem-solving technique. In parallel, health networks in each health region participated in a program to work with 1,143 midwives and 2,549 community health workers, under the coordination of a health facility member who was part of the multidisciplinary team.

Supervision and evaluation at each facility occurred three and six months after training and before accreditation visits. A tiered accreditation system was developed to promote participation and provide an incentive for improving quality. Results of each evaluation were presented to the Ministry of Health, which made accreditation decisions through an independent institution to generate political support. Quality in five areas (corresponding to the program aims) was assessed. Significant improvements were observed in the proportion of indicators achieved in all five aspects of quality evaluated (box figure). An evaluation one year after the end of the program found that performance had declined but remained at 60 to 80 percent of the levels achieved at accreditation.

Proportion of quality indicators achieved by Peruvian health facilities

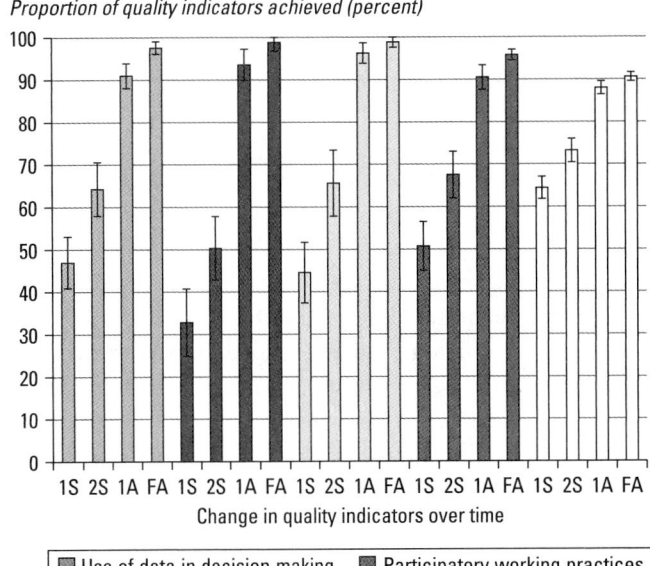

Proportion of quality indicators achieved (percent)

Change in quality indicators over time

- ▨ Use of data in decision making
- ◼ Patient satisfaction
- ▢ Essential supplies
- ◼ Participatory working practices
- ▢ Implementation of standardized care

Note: Proportion of quality indicators (with 95 percent Confidence Index) measured in the five domains achieved by health facilities at first supervision visit (1S), second supervision visit (2S), first accreditation visit (1A), and final accreditation visit (FA).

By the end of the three-year program (1996–99), demand for health services had increased considerably, the success itself creating managerial problems in many instances. Motivation and satisfaction of patients and health workers had also increased, and revenue collected (through fee-for-service payment) at the facilities rose. Maternal mortality in the regions included in the program was 60 percent higher than in other regions at the start of the intervention period and fell 25 percent after the intervention, while no change was observed in the other health regions. The inequitable distribution of maternal mortality was narrowed to a 20 percent excess in intervention areas. A national demographic and health survey examining Peru between 1995 and 2000 found a significant overall reduction of maternal mortality, increases in prenatal care coverage, and a higher proportion of deliveries in health facilities or attended by health professionals.

Sources: Lanata, Butron, and Espino 2002; Ministerio de Salud, Peru 2001.

which hospitals are required to engage in quality improvement but are given no prescription as to what format that effort might take (Klazinga, Delnoij, and Kulu-Glasgow 2002).

THE FUTURE: RESEARCH AND INFORMATION NEEDS

A few fundamental and urgent needs must be met as a prerequisite to improving understanding of district hospitals in low- and middle-income countries, although tackling these issues may be far from simple:

- developing and accepting meaningful performance indicators in conjunction with developing appropriate standards of care
- collecting higher-quality routine data from district hospitals
- improving understanding of the costs and health consequences of different, evidence-based, service provision portfolios proposed for district hospitals and improving understanding of the marginal benefits of incremental additions and their implications for planning infrastructure and estimating human resources and technology needs.

A solution to the first issue would perhaps pave the way for and enhance the value of further focused research in a number of areas.

Implications of a Changing Disease Spectrum

In many middle-income and some low-income countries, the demographic transition to noncommunicable diseases—notably cardiovascular, smoking-related, and malignant diseases—will have considerable implications for the hospital sector. Thus, hospital costs likely will rise as older patients with chronic diseases become an increasing proportion of inpatients (Barnum and Kutzin 1993). In some cases, the relative cost-effectiveness of hospital care will improve compared with further expansion of primary or preventive services that incur increasing marginal costs (Barnum and Kutzin 1993).

More immediately, in low-income countries in Africa, the massive impact of the HIV pandemic is most easily seen in the continent's hospitals. Bed occupancy is rising, and hospital stays appear to be lengthening, as an increasing proportion of hospital admissions, now over 50 percent in some countries' medical wards, have HIV-related disease (Mpundu 2000). Those diseases associated with HIV infection, notably tuberculosis, and changing demands for care, such as the need for palliation, may change not only the workload but also the nature of the demands placed on the service. The advent of antiretroviral therapy, which might ameliorate some of these problems, will itself place great demands on the hospital service provision mechanisms. With or without new drugs, HIV will continue to tax both planners, who have to respond to a rapid change in needs, and health care financing. Research that permits hospitals to tackle these new challenges and develop efficient and cost-effective strategies to provide care for HIV-related disease while preventing a decline in care standards for HIV-uninfected patients is a high priority.

Accounting for Case Mix and Case Severity When Measuring Hospital Performance

Overall inpatient-fatality rates and case-fatality rates of different common diseases are often included in district hospital performance measures. These are crude measures unless some adjustment is made for case mix when describing inpatient fatality and for severity of illness when describing case fatality. Alternatively, hospital outcomes should perhaps be replaced as key indicators of performance by carefully chosen process indicators, which are likely to be more generalizable tools of performance monitoring that offer the advantage of specifically identifying areas that require improvement (Lilford and others 2004).

Implications of Emerging and Existing Technologies

Technology has had an enormous effect on the amount of information available to clinicians and managers in industrial countries, from new rapid diagnostic tests to automated stock-checking and ordering procedures. A particularly exciting potential in developing countries may be the ability to undertake and interpret many diagnostic tests remotely, thereby enabling district hospitals to operate without a skilled diagnostic staff on site. It also seems probable that appropriately targeted technology could have a major effect, not least in the generation, communication, and analysis of hospital use, cost, and outcome data, without which the health system cannot identify and respond to needs.

Interventions That Improve Performance

Interventions aimed at improving hospital administration and clinical management at the district hospital level warrant investigation. For clinical management, interventions such as clinical guidelines, supervision, and feedback; audit and continuing professional development; quality improvement strategies and accreditation; and improvements in referral and integration with PHC may improve district hospital performance and be relatively cost-effective. Such interventions deserve attention, along with more traditional research aimed at optimizing treatment of specific diseases.

REFERENCES

AED (Academy for Educational Development). 2003. "The Health Sector Human Resource Crisis in Africa: An Issues Paper." Support for Research in Africa, U.S. Agency for International Development, Washington, DC.

Arhin-Tenkorang, D. 2000. "Mobilizing Resources for Health: The Case for User Fees Revisited." Commission on Macroeconomics and Health, World Health Organization, Geneva.

Ayliffe, G., and M. English. 2003. *Hospital Infection—from Miasmas to MRSA*. Cambridge, U.K.: Cambridge University Press.

Barnum, H., and J. Kutzin. 1993. *Public Hospitals in Developing Countries*. Baltimore, MD: Johns Hopkins University Press.

Barnum, H., J. Kutzin, and H. Saxenian. 1995. "Incentives and Provider Payment Methods." *International Journal of Health Planning and Management* 10 (1): 23–45.

Bhat, R., B. Verma, and E. Reuben. 2001. *Hospital Efficiency: An Empirical Analysis of District and Grant in Aid Hospitals in Gujarat*. Ahmedabad: Indian Institute of Management.

Bitran, R. 1996. "Efficiency and Quality in the Public and Private Sectors in Senegal." *Health Policy and Planning* 10 (3): 271–83.

Black, R., S. Morris, and J. Bryce. 2003. "Where and Why Are 10 Million Children Dying Every Year?" *Lancet* 361 (9376): 2226–34.

Blas, E., and M. Limbambala. 2001. "The Challenge of Hospitals in Health Sector Reform: The Case of Zambia." *Health Policy and Planning* 16 (Suppl. 2): 29–43.

Bobadilla, J. L., P. Cowley, P. Musgrove, and H. Saxenian. 1994. "Design, Content and Financing of an Essential National Package of Health Services." *Bulletin of the World Health Organization* 72 (4): 653–62.

Bossert, T., O. Larranaga, U. Giedion, J. Arbelaez, and D. Bower. 2003. "Decentralization and Equity of Resource Allocation: Evidence From Columbia and Chile." *Bulletin of the World Health Organization* 81 (2): 95–100.

Brugha, R., and A. Zwi. 1998. "Improving the Quality of Private Sector Delivery of Public Health Services: Challenges and Strategies." *Health Policy and Planning* 13 (2): 107–20.

Bukonda, N., P. Tavrow, H. Abdallah, K. Hoffner, and J. Tembo. 2002. "Implementing a National Hospital Accreditation Program: The Zambian Experience." *International Journal for Quality in Health Care* 14 (Suppl. 1): 7–16.

Canadian International Development Agency and the Aga Khan Foundation. 1981. *The Role of Hospitals in Primary Health Care*. Karachi: Canadian International Development Agency and the Aga Khan Foundation Canada.

Cibulskis, R., and G. Hiawalyer. 2002. "Information Systems for Health Sector Monitoring in Papua New Guinea." *Bulletin of the World Health Organization* 80 (90): 752–58.

Claeson, M., D. Gillespie, H. Mshinda, H. Troedsson, C. G. Victoria, and Bellagio Study Group on Child Survival. 2003. "Knowledge into Action for Child Survival." *Lancet* 362 (9380): 323–27.

Creese, A., K. Floyd, A. Alban, and L. Guinness. 2002. "Cost-Effectiveness of HIV/AIDS Interventions in Africa: A Systematic Review of the Evidence." *Lancet* 359 (9318): 1635–42.

Daviaud, E., B. Engelbrecht, P. Molefakgotia, G. Crisp, D. Collins, and P. Barron. 2000. "South African Health Report—District Health Expenditure Reviews." South African Ministry of Health, Pretoria.

DiPrete-Brown, L., L. Franco, N. Rafeh, and T. Hatzell. 1993. *Quality Assurance of Health Care in Developing Countries*. Bethesda, MD: Quality Assurance Project.

Duke, T., L. Willie, and J. Mgone. 2000. "The Effect of Introduction of Minimal Standards of Neonatal Care on In-Hospital Mortality." *Papua and New Guinea Medical Journal* 43 (1–2): 127–36.

English, M., F. Esamai, A. Wasunna, F. Were, B. Ogutu, A. Wamae, and others. 2004a. "Delivery of Paediatric Care at the First Referral Level in Kenya." *Lancet* 364 (9445): 1622–29.

———. 2004b. "An Evaluation of Inpatient Paediatric Care in First Referral Level Hospitals in 13 Districts in Kenya." *Lancet* 363 (9425): 1948–53.

Flessa, S. 1998. "The Costs of Hospital Services: A Case Study of Evangelical Lutheran Church Hospitals in Tanzania." *Health Policy and Planning* 13 (4): 397–407.

Font, F., L. Quinto, H. Masanja, R. Nathan, C. Ascaso, C. Menendez, and others. 2002. "Paediatric Referrals in Rural Tanzania: the Kilombero District Study: A Case Series." *BMC International Health and Human Rights* 2: 4.

Gani, A. 1996. "Improving Quality in Public Sector Hospitals in Indonesia." *International Journal of Health Planning and Management* 11 (3): 275–96.

Glied, S. 2000. "Managed Care." In *Handbook of Health Economics*, ed. J. P. Newhouse and A. J. Culyer. Amsterdam: Elsevier.

Government of Kenya. 2001. "Health Management Information Systems Report for the 1996 to 1999 Period." Ministry of Health, Republic of Kenya, Nairobi.

Grol, R., and J. Grimshaw. 2003. "From Best Evidence to Best Practice: Effective Implementation of Change in Patients' Care." *Lancet* 362 (9391): 1225–30.

Hansen, K., G. Chapman, I. Chitsike, O. Kasilo, and G. Mwaluko. 2000. "The Costs of HIV/AIDS Care at Government Hospitals in Zimbabwe." *Health Policy and Planning* 15 (4): 432–40.

Hensher, M. 2001. "Financing Health Systems through Efficiency Gains." Commission on Macroeconomics and Health Working Paper WG3:2, World Health Organization, Geneva.

Hensher, M., N. Fulop, J. Coast, and E. Jefferys. 1999. "The Hospital of the Future: Better out Than in? Alternatives to Acute Hospital Care." *British Medical Journal* 319 (7217): 1127–30.

Hongoro, C., and B. McPake. 2003. "Hospital Costs of High Burden Diseases: Malaria and Pulmonary Tuberculosis in a HIV High Prevalence Context in Zimbabwe." *Tropical Medicine and International Health* 8 (3): 242–50.

Kirigia, J., J. Fox-Rushby, and A. Mills. 1998. "A Cost Analysis of Kilifi and Malindi Public Hospitals in Kenya." *African Journal of Health Sciences* 5 (2): 79–84.

Kirigia, J., R. Snow, J. Fox-Rushby, and A. Mills. 1998. "The Cost of Treating Paediatric Malaria Admissions and the Potential Impact of Insecticide Treated Mosquito Nets on Hospital Expenditure." *Tropical Medicine and International Health* 3 (2): 145–50.

Klazinga, N., D. Delnoij, and I. Kulu-Glasgow. 2002. "Can a Tulip Become a Rose? The Dutch Route of Guided Self-Regulation toward a Community Based Integrated Health Care System." In *Measuring Up: Improving Health Systems Performance in OECD Countries*, ed. P. Smith. Paris: Organisation for Economic Co-operation and Development.

Lanata, C. F., B. Butron, and S. Espino. 2002. *Mejorando la calidad de la atención de salud en el Perú—El Programa de Capacitación Materno Infantil (PCMI) en su primera etapa: Cómo se hizo y a qué se debió su éxito?* Lima: Instituto de Investigación Nutricional.

Le Grand, J., N. Mays, and J. Mulligan, eds. 1998. *Learning from the NHS Internal Market*. London: King's Fund Institute.

Lilford, R., M. Mohammed, D. Spiegelhalter, and R. Thompson. 2004. "Use and Misuse of Process and Outcome Data in Managing Performance of Acute Medical Care: Avoiding Institutional Stigma." *Lancet* 363 (9415): 1147–54.

Loevinsohn, B. 1993. "Data Utilization and Analytical Skills among Mid-Level Health Programme Managers in a Developing Country." *International Journal of Epidemiology* 23 (1): 194–99.

Massoud, R., K. Askov, J. Reinke, L. Franco, T. Bornstein, E. Knebel, and C. MacAuley. 2001. *A Modern Paradigm for Improving Healthcare Quality*. Bethesda, MD: Quality Assurance Project.

McCord, C., and Q. Chowdury. 2003. "A Cost Effective Small Hospital in Bangladesh: What It Can Mean for Emergency Obstetric Care." *International Journal of Gynecology and Obstetrics* 81 (1): 83–92.

McKee, M., and J. Healy. 2002. "The Significance of Hospitals." In *Hospitals in a Changing Europe*, ed. M. McKee and J. Healy. Buckingham, U.K., and Philadelphia: Open University Press.

Mills, A. 1990a. "The Economics of Hospitals in Developing Countries— Part 1: Expenditure Patterns." *Health Policy and Planning* 5 (2): 107–17.

Mills, A. 1990b. "The Economics of Hospitals in Developing Countries— Part 2: Costs and Sources of Income." *Health Policy and Planning* 5 (3): 203–18.

Ministerio de Salud, Peru. 2001. "La Experiencia del PCMI." Ministerio de Salud, Lima.

Mpundu, M. 2000. "The Burden of HIV/AIDS on the Zambian Health System." *AIDS Analysis Africa* 10 (5): 6.

Narasimhan, V., H. Brown, A. Pablos-Menedez, O. Adams, G. Dussault, G. Elzinga, and others. 2004. "Responding to the Global Human Resources Crisis." *Lancet* 363 (9419): 1469–72.

Ngoc Anh, N., and T. Tram. 1995. "Integration of Primary Health Care Concepts in a Children's Hospital with Limited Resources." *Lancet* 346 (8972): 421–24.

Nolan, T., P. Angos, A. Cunha, L. Muhe, S. Qazi, E. A. Simoes, and others. 2000. "Quality of Hospital Care for Seriously Ill Children in Less-Developed Countries." *Lancet* 357 (9250): 106–10.

Oliveira-Cruz, V., K. Hanson, and A. Mills. 2001. "Approaches to Overcoming Health System Constraints at the Peripheral Level: Review of the Evidence." Commission on Macroeconomics and Health, World Health Organization, Geneva.

Owino, W., and J. Korir. 1997. *Public Health Sector Efficiency in Kenya: Estimation and Policy Implications.* Nairobi: Institute of Policy Analysis and Research.

Peters, D., A. Elmendorf, K. Kandola, and G. Chellaraj. 2000. "Benchmarks for Health Expenditures, Services and Outcomes in Africa during the 1990s." *Bulletin of the World Health Organization* 78 (6): 761–69.

Peterson, S., J. Nsugwa-Sabiti, W. Were, X. Nsabagasani, G. Magumba, J. Nambooze, and G. Mukasa. 2004. "Coping with Paediatric Referral— Ugandan Parents' Experience." *Lancet* 363 (9425): 1955–56.

Posnett, J. 2002. "Hospitals in a Changing Europe." In *European Observatory on Health Care Systems*, ed. M. McKee and J. Healy. Buckingham, U.K., and Philadelphia: Open University Press.

Purohit, B., and V. Rai. 1992. "Operating Efficiency in Inpatient Care: An Exploratory Analysis of Teaching Hospitals in Rajasthan, India." *International Journal of Health Planning and Management* 7: 149–62.

Robertson, M., and E. Molyneux. 2001. "Triage in the Developing World— Can It Be Done?" *Archives of Disease in Childhood* 85 (3): 208–13.

Sachs, J. D. 2001. "Macroeconomics and Health: Investing in Health for Economic Development." Commission on Macroeconomics and Health, World Health Organization, Geneva.

Siddiqui, S., A. Kielmann, M. Khan, N. Ali, A. Ghaffar, U. Sheikh, and Z. Mumtaz. 2001. "The Effectiveness of Patient Referral in Pakistan." *Health Policy and Planning* 16 (2): 193–98.

Smee, C. 2002. "Improving Value for Money in the United Kingdom National Health Service: Performance Measurement and Improvement in a Centralised System." In *Measuring Up: Improving Health Systems Performance in OECD Countries*, ed. P. Smith. Paris: Organisation for Economic Co-operation and Development.

Snow, R., V. Mungala, D. Forster, and K. Marsh. 1994. "The Role of the District Hospital in Child Survival at the Kenyan Coast." *African Journal of Health Sciences* 1 (2): 11–15.

Suwandono, A., A. Gani, S. Purwani, E. Blas, and R. Brugha. 2001. "Cost Recovery Beds in Public Hospitals in Indonesia." *Health Policy and Planning* 16 (Suppl. 2): 10–18.

Van der Geest, S., M. Macwan'gi, J. Kamwanga, D. Mulikelela, A. Mazimba, and M. Mwangelwa. 2000. "User Fees and Drugs: What Did the Health Sector Reforms in Zambia Achieve?" *Health Policy and Planning* 15 (1): 59–65.

Van Lerberghe, W., X. de Bethune, and V. de Brouwere. 1997. "Hospitals in Sub-Saharan Africa: Why We Need More of What Does Not Work as It Should." *Tropical Medicine and International Health* 2 (8): 799–808.

Van Lerberghe, W., and K. Pangu. 1988. "Comprehensive Can Be Effective: The Influence of Coverage with a Health Centre Network on the Hospitalisation Patterns in the Rural Area of Kasongo, Zaire." *Social Science and Medicine* 26 (9): 949–55.

Weissman, E., O. Sentumbwe-Mugisa, A. Mbonye, E. Kayaga, S. Kihuguru, and C. Lissner. 1999. *Uganda Safe Motherhood Programme Costing Study.* Geneva: Ministry of Health Uganda and World Health Organization.

WHO (World Health Organization). 1987. "Hospitals and Health for All." Report of the WHO Expert Committee on the Role of Hospitals at the First Referral Level, WHO, Geneva.

———. 1990. *The Role of the Hospital in the District—Delivering or Supporting Primary Health Care.* Geneva: WHO.

———. 1992. "The Hospital in Rural and Urban Districts." Report of a WHO Study Group on the Functions of Hospitals at the First Referral Level, WHO, Geneva.

———. 1994. *A Review of Determinants of Hospital Performance.* Geneva: WHO.

———. 1999. *The World Health Report—Making a Difference.* Geneva: WHO.

———. 2000a. *Management of the Child with a Serious Infection or Severe Malnutrition.* Geneva: WHO.

———. 2000b. *The World Health Report: Health Systems: Improving Performance.* Geneva: WHO.

World Bank. 1993. *World Development Report 1993.* Oxford, U.K.: Oxford University Press.

———. 2002. *World Development Indicators.* Washington, DC: World Bank.

Xu, K., D. Evans, K. Kawabata, R. Zeramdini, J. Klavus, and J. Murray. 2003. "Household Catastrophic Health Expenditure: A Multicountry Analysis." *Lancet* 362 (9378): 111–17.

Chapter **66**

Referral Hospitals

Martin Hensher, Max Price, and Sarah Adomakoh

The appropriate allocation of resources to referral hospitals within a national health system has long been a controversial issue in health system planning in developing countries. Consensus appears to be widespread that referral hospitals consume an excessive share of health budgets and that their contribution to improving health and welfare is low relative to the expenditure on these facilities, but the literature does not indicate what percentage of budgets should ideally be allocated to referral hospitals. Presumably, except in the poorest countries, some referral facility is needed, but how much is required, and how should the proportion allocated to referral facilities vary with increasing levels of health expenditure and health system sophistication?

One approach would be to review how much countries at different levels of gross domestic product (GDP) currently spend on referral hospitals. However, as explained later, the definition of *referral hospital* varies widely; therefore, analyses of national health accounts and studies of expenditure are rarely comparable. Thus, although the chapter summarizes the literature on expenditure on referral hospitals, this evidence cannot provide guidelines for policy makers.

A second approach might be to undertake a detailed analysis of the role of referral hospitals in treating disease to derive their contribution to total disability-adjusted life years (DALYs). A simple analysis of the cost-effectiveness of specific interventions offered by referral hospitals might allow the selection of those interventions that are justified given their marginal cost per DALY gained. Those interventions, multiplied by expected demand, would then be aggregated to give a total optimal allocation for referral hospital services. This approach is precisely the one used for evaluating and prioritizing disease-specific interventions throughout this volume. However, when this kind

of "pure" cost-effectiveness analysis is used to determine an appropriate or optimal resource allocation for referral hospital services, several problems arise. To begin with, hospitals have complex economies of scope and scale. At the point when hospitals offer a range of cost-effective interventions, the marginal cost-effectiveness of additional interventions may be much greater than would be the case if these other interventions were evaluated in isolation. Yet a standard disease-specific analysis of interventions would rarely be able to calculate the marginal costs of referral hospital–based interventions. Similarly, important and complex interdependencies exist between services and specialties within referral hospitals that may be almost impossible to capture adequately using a cost-effectiveness analysis.

A further limitation to a cost per DALY approach arises because referral hospitals produce multiple outputs, many of which contribute so indirectly to DALYs that they cannot be compared directly to individual health interventions, but which are critical to the functioning of the health system. For example, referral hospitals are arguably essential to the training of doctors, particularly specialists. If a country can justify training its own doctors, then it must have a referral hospital. Yet the value of this output in terms of DALYs probably cannot be calculated. Indeed, many of the functions of a referral hospital occur outside the hospital itself and involve enabling and facilitating the effective functioning of lower-level health services. Although the referral hospital's contribution may constitute only a small fraction of the total cost of an intervention provided at a lower level of care (which may perhaps be viewed as a fixed cost of the health system), the referral hospital's role may nevertheless be essential, thereby justifying a considerable premium on its valuation above and beyond the cost per DALY of the care directly provided within the hospital's own walls.

Finally, strong arguments can be made that cost-effectiveness analysis fails to capture important dimensions of the individual utility—and thus the social welfare—that accrues from the provision of health services, especially those relating to high-cost and low-frequency conditions.

We are, therefore, highly skeptical about the feasibility of proposing a formulaic and purely quantitative response to the question of how to achieve an appropriate allocation of resources to the referral hospital level. Although perhaps unsatisfying for some readers, this chapter attempts instead to provide an overview of the critical features of and challenges relating to referral hospital care in developing countries and a guide to the many issues that decision makers face in setting policy for this level of care. We suggest that planners need to adopt a far more qualitative and intuitive approach to deciding on the appropriate allocation of resources for referral hospitals than for other health care interventions. Such an approach is informed by a more extensive listing of the roles of referral hospitals and their direct and indirect benefits and costs to society. We acknowledge that analysis of the value of referral hospitals is bedeviled by the fact that, when judged empirically, they do not work as they are supposed to. The chapter, therefore, considers the key problems faced in the real environment in which referral hospitals operate in poor countries before reviewing what needs to be done to improve their functioning, drawing in particular on the authors' knowledge of South Africa and the Caribbean.

DEFINITION AND CHARACTERISTICS

Any hospital, including a district hospital, will receive referrals from lower levels of care. Indeed, *referral* can be defined as any process in which health care providers at lower levels of the health system, who lack the skills, the facilities, or both to manage a given clinical condition, seek the assistance of providers who are better equipped or specially trained to guide them in managing or to take over responsibility for a particular episode of a clinical condition in a patient (Al-Mazrou, Al-Shehri, and Rao 1990). Furthermore, higher-level hospitals in developing countries do not treat only referred patients; tertiary hospitals are frequently the first point of contact with health services for many patients.

Differentiating referral hospitals from district hospitals, therefore, requires consideration of the different resources used by different levels of hospital. Such a differentiation will tend to revolve around three features—the availability of increasingly specialized personnel, of more sophisticated diagnostic technologies, and of more advanced therapeutic technologies—that permit the diagnosis and treatment of increasingly complex conditions.

This volume, including this chapter, uses a standard definition of hospital levels (Mulligan and others 2003). Table 66.1 presents some of the commonly used alternative terminology for different levels of hospitals. Note that this chapter deals only with general—that is, multispecialty—secondary and tertiary hospitals. Specialized hospitals, such as psychiatric, substance abuse, tuberculosis, infectious diseases, and rehabilitation hospitals, clearly have important roles to play in a well-functioning referral system. However, they are attended by specific features and challenges, account for a relatively small share of overall resources, and operate in a significantly different manner than general hospitals do.

FUNCTIONS AND BENEFITS

The functions of referral hospitals may broadly be categorized into (a) the direct clinical services provided to individual patients within the hospital and the community and (b) a set of broader functions only indirectly related to patient care.

Table 66.1 Definitions and Terms for Different Levels of Hospital

Disease Control Priorities Project: terminology and definitions	Alternative terms commonly found in the literature
Primary-level hospital: few specialties—mainly internal medicine, obstetrics and gynecology, pediatrics, and general surgery, or just general practice; limited laboratory services available for general but not specialized pathological analysis	District hospital Rural hospital Community hospital General hospital
Secondary-level hospital: highly differentiated by function with 5 to 10 clinical specialties; size ranges from 200 to 800 beds; often referred to as a *provincial hospital*	Regional hospital Provincial hospital (or equivalent administrative area such as county) General hospital
Tertiary-level hospital: highly specialized staff and technical equipment—for example, cardiology, intensive care unit, and specialized imaging units; clinical services highly differentiated by function; could have teaching activities; size ranges from 300 to 1,500 beds	National hospital Central hospital Academic or teaching or university hospital

Source: Definitions from Mulligan and others 2003, 59.

Range of Clinical Services Provided

The primary function of the referral hospital is to provide complex clinical care to patients referred from lower levels; however, no agreed international definition exists of which specific services should be provided in secondary or tertiary hospitals in developing countries. The exact range of services offered tends to vary substantially, even between tertiary hospitals within the same country, as much because of historical accident as deliberate design.

In South Africa, the National Department of Health is attempting to improve the quality and accessibility of referral hospital services through development plans that will try to ensure that hospitals at each level move toward providing a comprehensive set of clinical services (National Department of Health, South Africa 2003). The department has developed a target template of services (table 66.2) for regional (secondary) hospitals, tertiary hospitals, and so-called national referral services (which will be offered at only a small number of the

Table 66.2 Target Service Configurations by Level of Referral Hospital, South Africa

Specialist services available on site	Components explicitly included	Specialist services available on site	Components explicitly included
Regional (secondary) hospitals			
Anesthetics	—	Mental health (psychiatry and psychology)	Acute inpatient and outpatient treatment
Diagnostic radiology	X-ray, CT scan, ultrasound, fluoroscopy		Child and adolescent psychiatry
General medicine	Echocardiography, stress electrocardiogram		Electroconvulsive therapy
	Specialist immunology nurse		Liaison psychiatry
	Regional intensive care unit		Satellite clinics
	Diabetes, endocrine clinic	Obstetrics and gynecology	Emergency obstetrics and gynecology
	Gastroenterology, including endoscopy, proctoscopy, sigmoidoscopy, colonoscopy (with general surgery)		Ultrasound, prenatal diagnosis
			Kangaroo mother care
	Geriatric care		Basic urogynecology
	Genetic nurse and counseling	Orthopedic surgery	General orthopedic surgery
	Oncology palliation and basic care		24-hour trauma service, accident and emergency
	Neurology basic care	Pediatrics	Neonatal low and high care
	Spirometry and oximetry		General pediatric medicine service
	Basic rheumatology		General pediatric surgery (general surgeon)
General surgery	Regional burns service	Rehabilitation center	Physiotherapy, occupational therapy, orthotics and prosthetics, speech therapy, dietetics, podiatry
	24-hour trauma service, accident and emergency		Acute rehabilitation team
Tertiary hospitals			
Anesthetics	—	General medicine	As regional plus:
Burns unit	Specialized burns intensive care unit and operating theater		Angiography
			Coronary care
Clinical pharmacology specialist	—		Echocardiography, stress electrocardiogram
Critical care and intensive care unit	Full intensive care unit service		Endoscopy, proctoscopy, sigmoidoscopy, colonoscopy (with general surgery)
Dermatology	Inpatient and ambulatory treatment		Genetic nurse and counseling
Diagnostic radiology	X-ray, multislice CT scan, ultrasound, fluoroscopy, mammography, color Doppler ultrasound		Oncology palliation and basic care
		General surgery	Complex and high-acuity care
Ear, nose, and throat surgery	—	Infectious diseases	—
Gastroenterology	—	Mental health (psychiatry and psychology)	Child and adolescent psychiatry, old-age psychiatry, forensic psychiatry, substance abuse treatment, liaison psychiatry, treatment for eating disorders, inpatient psychotherapy, social psychiatry, acute psychotic (complicated) care, acute nonpsychotic (complicated) care

(Continues on the following page.)

Table 66.2 Continued

Specialist services available on site	Components explicitly included	Specialist services available on site	Components explicitly included
Tertiary hospitals (continued)			
Neonatology	Neonatal intensive care unit	Rehabilitation center	Physiotherapy, occupational therapy, orthotics and prosthetics, speech therapy, dietetics, podiatry, audiology
Nephrology	Tertiary dialysis and nephrology service		
Obstetrics and gynecology service	As regional plus: Fetal and maternal medicine		Acute rehabilitation team, including spinal beds
Ophthalmology	—		Stroke unit
Orthopedic surgery	Subspecialty orthopedics	Respiratory medicine	—
Pediatric intensive care unit	Full pediatric intensive care unit	Trauma	Tertiary major trauma center (protocol-based transfer only, no walk-in accident and emergency service)
Pediatric medicine	Specialist general pediatricians		
Pediatric surgery	Specialist pediatric surgery service		
Plastic and reconstructive surgery	—	Urology	—
		Vascular surgery	—
National referral services			
Cardiology	Echocardiography, ultrasound, electrocardiography, stress testing, Holter pacemaker follow-up, catheterization laboratory, electrophysiology, ablation	Obstetrics and gynecology service	Oncology
			Urogynecology
			Reproductive medicine
Cardiothoracic surgery	—	Orthopedic surgery	Orthopedic oncology
Clinical immunology	—	Pediatric cardiology	—
Cranio-maxillofacial surgery	—	Pediatric endocrinology	—
		Pediatric gastroenterology	—
Critical care and intensive care unit	Additional intensive care unit capacity	Pediatric hematology and oncology	—
Diagnostic radiology	MRI	Pediatric infectious diseases	—
Endocrinology	—	Pediatric intensive care unit	Additional pediatric intensive care unit capacity
Genetics	—		
Geriatrics	—	Pediatric nephrology	Dialysis and renal transplant
Hematology	—	Pediatric neurology	—
Medical and radiation oncology	—	Pediatric respiratory medicine and allergology	—
Neurology	—	Renal transplant	Renal transplant unit
Neurosurgery	—	Rheumatology	—
Nuclear medicine	—	Urology	—

Source: National Department of Health, South Africa 2003.
— = not available.

largest tertiary hospitals). Although certainly not directly applicable to all developing countries, the template does give a helpful picture of how services "build up" from one level of care to another, and it can be used as a starting point for considering the situation in different countries.

Clinical Services within the Community

Referral hospitals may perform a number of functions that provide population-level health benefits through direct involvement in public health interventions. Responding to the HIV/AIDS epidemic in Latin America and the Caribbean has heightened awareness about the important role of the hospital in reducing incidence and preventing disease outbreaks. For example, hospitals scaled up services to prevent mother-to-child transmission and initiated follow-up clinics for mothers and babies. In Barbados, the main hospital scaled up voluntary counseling and testing services to address the prevention of horizontal transmission from mothers to their partners, with positive outcomes. The program also served to increase access to obstetric services at the primary health care level because of the screening campaign initiated through the hospital's prevention of mother-to-child transmission program (Adomakoh, St. John, and Kumar 2002).

Referral hospitals often prove to be a highly effective focal point for disease-specific health promotion and education activities. Bermuda's diabetes education program serves all levels of care and provides a strong link between the primary, secondary, and tertiary health care levels. The program is centered in the main referral hospital and serves not only diagnosed patients but also families at risk. Overall, hospitals in the Caribbean are recognizing that central coordination of public health programs within hospitals can provide benefits by strengthening coordination with other services.

Valuing the Benefit of Clinical Services

Measuring the improvement in an individual's health status produced by the combined activities of a referral hospital, whether for patient care in the hospital or for population-based programs, would theoretically be possible, although practically and methodologically demanding. To our knowledge, such an effort has not been attempted at the referral hospital level, though two studies have attempted to proxy the effect of hospital interventions on health outcomes for small district hospitals, focusing on survival only (McCord and Chowdhury 2003; Snow and others 1994). Both studies indicate that district hospitals appear to have a significant positive effect on health outcomes.

Large numbers of patients receive care in referral hospitals, and most survive with their suffering alleviated, having gained substantial benefit from the care they receive. Therefore, the aggregate direct personal health benefits from referral hospital care will almost certainly be high. The question of whether referral hospital care is cost-effective relative to other interventions delivered at lower levels of care is less easy to answer in aggregate. By its nature, appropriate care in a referral hospital will tend to require more complex input mixes and higher skill levels and, hence, will be relatively expensive. Analysis of the costs and cost-effectiveness of individual interventions offered at different levels is tackled directly by the disease-specific chapters in this volume.

Wider Activities and Functions

Aside from direct patient care, referral hospitals serve other functions within the health system, some of which are offered within the facility, such as teaching and research, while others reach out to the lower levels of the health services, such as technical support and quality assurance.

Advice and Support to Lower Levels. The referral process does not simply entail transferring a patient from a lower to a higher level of care, nor does it end when a patient is discharged from a referral hospital. An effective referral system requires good communication and coordination between levels of care and support from higher to lower levels to help

manage patients at the lowest level of care possible. Too often, personnel in referral hospitals adopt an insular and inward-looking perspective, focusing exclusively on the patients directly under their care. However, referral hospitals should offer significant support to personnel in lower-level facilities, and specialist staff members should ideally spend a significant portion of their time providing advice and support beyond the walls of their own hospital, either in person or through various modes of telecommunication. Even in poor countries, a steady improvement in communications infrastructure means that such support functions should become easier to provide over time. Key dimensions of this support function include the following:

- availability by telephone or e-mail to advise referring practitioners on whether referral is required
- specialist advice to the patient's local practitioner on post-discharge care
- specialist advice on the long-term management of chronic conditions
- specialist attendance at lower-level facilities to provide regular outreach clinics
- provision of expert diagnosis or consultation through telemedicine
- coordination of discharge planning between levels of care
- coordination of the development of and training in the use of shared care protocols and referral protocols
- provision of technology support by skilled technicians and scientists.

Quality Assurance and Quality Improvement. Referral hospitals can and do play a pivotal role in quality assurance and improvement. The most important mechanism for quality assurance and improvement is through the training that referral hospitals provide. The other key mechanism is through the setting of standards for treatment. For example, experts at referral hospitals should review evidence of effectiveness and cost-effectiveness applicable to the local context, determine the formularies to be used at each level of the health system, and develop and amend treatment protocols. Referral hospitals can improve the quality of peripheral services by giving advice, offering on-site training, providing clinical services alongside local practitioners, and monitoring the quality of the referrals they receive.

Education and Training. Many tertiary referral hospitals in developing countries are associated with universities and medical schools and may, therefore, also be regarded as teaching hospitals. Any country wishing to train its own doctors will need one or more teaching hospitals. The number of doctors a country needs will be influenced by its level of development, resources, and personnel structure. Many will aim for a ratio of at least

How Many Medical Students Should Be Trained Per 1 Million Population?

In a steady state (that is, the number of doctors being produced is equal to the number retiring from practice), and if we assume that doctors practice, on average, for 40 years after qualifying, the total number practicing will equal the number graduating in 1 year multiplied by 40 years. If a population of 1 million needs 1,000 doctors,

the number needing to be trained is $1,000/40 = 25$ per year. If 30 percent of doctors leave the country or leave medical practice within 8 years of qualifying, then each graduate, on average, contributes 30 years of service, and 1,000 practicing doctors $(1,000/30) = 33$ must qualify each year.

Source: Authors.

---

2 per 1,000 population, though most developing countries have 0.05 to 1.0 per 1,000 (Puzin 1996; WHOSIS 2004). If we assume a 40-year working life and loss through brain drain or other attrition of 25 percent, the number of doctors that must be produced each year is between 16 and 67 per 1 million population, resulting in 0.5 to 2.0 doctors per 1,000 population (box 66.1). A population of 40 million would, thus, need medical schools able to graduate between 640 and 2,680 doctors per year. Medical schools possess economies of scale, and although some extremely small schools train 50 or so students a year, agreement is widespread that a class size of about 150 to 200 is optimal (see, for example, Harden and Davis 1998). A country with fewer than 3 million population would really need to consider whether training doctors locally is justified on economic and other grounds, but for larger countries, the arguments for training doctors locally are strong, and a teaching hospital would, therefore, be required.

Basic generalist doctors should be trained in a range of facilities across all levels of care, reflecting the facilities in which they will work after graduation. Traditional approaches toward medical education have been widely criticized by educationalists and health planners for being dominated by training in tertiary settings by specialists. Not only is this setting inappropriate, but typical content and clinical experience do not reflect what the doctors will be doing or what they will need to know after qualification. Nevertheless, the university teaching hospital cannot be omitted from the basic training of doctors. If students and faculty were involved only in district-based services, they would miss many important advances in biomedical science and the care of complex problems (Husain 1996). Moreover, doctors need to know enough about what the various tertiary specialties do to be able to refer patients appropriately and to make personal career choices.

The training of specialists, of course, depends far more on the existence and proper functioning of referral hospitals. Again, a particular country will need to decide how many specialists it needs in which specialties and whether it should send its doctors abroad to specialize or train them internally. In

developed countries, 60 to 90 percent of doctors are specialists, whereas in developing countries the range is wider (for example, 76 percent of Indian doctors are specialists, 45 percent are specialists in Tanzania, and 31 percent are specialists in Morocco). A World Health Organization expert workshop agreed on a figure of 50 percent (Puzin 1996). Therefore, a country of 40 million would aim to train approximately 300 to 1,300 specialists per year. On average, such training lasts four years. Thus, at any time the academic referral hospital system would need to supply 1,200 to 5,200 residents. A guideline many countries use requires a ratio of postgraduate specialist supervision of not more than two residents per qualified specialist. This ratio can be used to get some idea of the referral hospital capacity required to train specialists.

Although basic doctors could spend most of their training time in primary care and district hospital facilities, with limited exposure to tertiary care hospitals, the training of specialists—as well as of other specialized allied staff members such as nurses for intensive care or specialized psychiatry, physiotherapists specializing in back injuries or burns, and pharmacists specializing in oncology—can take place only in referral hospitals.

In recent years, continuing medical education has grown in importance as the need for professionals to continually update their knowledge and acquire new skills has been more clearly appreciated. The coordination and provision of appropriate continuing medical education depends heavily on the specialists and academics associated with referral and academic hospitals.

Management and Administration. Referral hospitals in many developing countries play important roles in providing managerial and administrative support to other elements of the health system. These roles may include managing laboratory services on behalf of the whole health system; serving as the location for drug and medical supply depots and distribution systems and managing procurement systems; hosting and managing health information systems, often including epidemiological surveillance systems; managing centralized transport fleets; and, on occasion, providing financial management, payroll, and human resource management services to other health units. Our intent is not to consider whether such arrangements are "right" or "wrong"—complex factors would have to be taken into account in every individual circumstance—but to note that making changes to the functioning of referral hospitals may have unintended consequences. For example, moving referral hospitals from funding based on a global budget to reimbursement systems based on patient activity may unintentionally cause hospitals to cease to provide these wider support functions if explicit alternative funding mechanisms are not established.

Research and Innovation. Referral hospitals tend to be where most health research is undertaken. Whereas in developed countries they may often be associated with the development of new technologies, in developing countries they are more often the site of research for the initial piloting and introduction of new technologies developed elsewhere and for the evaluation of their local suitability and field efficacy. Referral hospitals are also the vehicle for disseminating such technologies through the exposure of staff during training as well as through the role that referral hospitals frequently play in continuing professional education.

Research activities are vital in attracting and retaining specialist staff members who are required not just for the treatment of complex patients, but also for the training of new specialists. Research that is responsive to local conditions—that is, local disease burdens and technology constraints—fills a critical gap because researchers in developed countries and pharmaceutical companies do not generally pursue such research questions if they do not foresee sufficient returns to their investments.

Valuing the Indirect Contribution to the Health System. From the enumeration of the many roles of referral hospitals and their indirect effect on health through their contribution to the health system by way of supervision, administration, training, research, and quality improvement, it is immediately evident that these benefits cannot readily be translated into DALYs or any other metric to be used in a relative cost-benefit analysis.

Externalities and Intangible Benefits

The previous sections reviewed the various functions of referral hospitals within the health system, all of which contributed directly or indirectly to the health status of individuals. This section addresses other ways in which referral hospitals contribute to welfare and well-being, and comments on how they complicate the issue of valuing the contribution of referral hospitals in society.

Referral hospitals have a broader effect on overall societal welfare than can be captured by measures of health outcomes.

Utility, or welfare, includes health as one of many important outcomes, such as financial security, risk alleviation, and psychological reassurance. However, as Hammer and Berman (1995) note, health policy is typically conducted as if it has a unidimensional objective—namely the maximization of health (DALY) outcomes. Determining the appropriate resource allocation to referral hospitals purely on the basis of the cost of generating health (DALYs) may, therefore, seriously underestimate the optimum level of resources, because such measures will fail to capture the full welfare gains from the availability of higher-level health services. An example will highlight the difference between valuing hospitals on the basis of their contribution to health status alone compared with including wider concepts of welfare in the valuation.

Renal failure leading to the need for dialysis is relatively rare, and certainly rare in comparison to many other infectious and chronic diseases in lower- or middle-income countries. Treatment is lifesaving, but must continue indefinitely (involving visits two or three times every week) and is, therefore, extremely expensive. In many cases, dialysis can be justified only if it is linked to a renal transplant program, which terminates the need for dialysis and frees the equipment for someone else. The proportion of the total population who will benefit from such a referral hospital program is small; therefore, the DALYs generated are low, and the program would not rank high among the priorities given a limited budget. However, every member of the population is at risk of renal failure and, if affected, would find that, in the absence of a publicly funded program, he or she would either die or face extremely high costs to secure treatment in the private sector or abroad.

Even in poor countries, patients' price elasticity of demand is low when faced with life-threatening illnesses, particularly when treatment can change the outcome. Studies on poverty have shown that a significant proportion of households that have become poor did so as a result of serious illness, which resulted in their liquidating assets to pay for health care (see, for example, Liu, Rao, and Hsiao 2003). Thus, people seek the peace of mind of knowing that they can obtain lifesaving treatment should they need it without the risk of incurring catastrophic costs of care. This additional welfare derives both from the financial security of not having to spend more than people can afford to save their lives and from the direct health benefits of treatment itself. The utility from the former (financial security) increases with the cost of the intervention required, whereas the utility derived from the latter (direct health benefits) is unrelated to the cost of the intervention. Paradoxically, one could, therefore, argue that the rarer a particular illness is—and the more costly the intervention required—the greater will be the welfare gain from public spending on that intervention.

This argument, of course, is likely to stand in direct contrast to the conclusions drawn from prioritization based on cost-effectiveness. For most individuals, willingness to pay is far less than the costs of the procedure to them; however, because the whole population benefits from the security of knowing that each individual would be entitled to referral hospital care should he or she need it, in the aggregate the welfare value generated by public provision or funding may be many times greater than the value of the DALYs generated directly for those few patients who do receive treatment. This literature review did not find evidence of studies on national willingness to pay for referral hospital care in developing countries, but this area could be of interest for future research.

In practice, too, the public—particularly an urban, middle-income public—expects the government to provide care of last resort for complex trauma or diseases, especially for natural and man-made disasters. Thus, even though referral hospitals may provide care to a small number of people, often with limited health benefits, politicians and the public alike may value and prioritize them simply because they meet the public's expectations for what the government must provide. In addition, politicians and the public often regard a country's ability to provide the kind of complex, high-tech care offered in a referral hospital as a measure of that country's level of development and sophistication, and it is a source of national pride. Whether economically rational or not, this nonhealth benefit appears to drive public choices to some extent.

Negative Impacts

The "negative" impact of referral hospitals is largely attributable to their potential to exert distortionary effects on the health system by diverting resources from peripheral areas and from lower levels of care (Fiedler, Schmidt, and Wight 1998; Filmer, Hammer, and Pritchett 1997) for the following reasons:

- Tertiary hospitals and specialists have a high political and public profile.
- Urban and political elites are more likely to use referral hospitals than rural primary care facilities or district hospitals.
- Harmful competition with lower levels of care may result from the maintenance of higher-level referral hospitals in many poor countries, lowering use of the former.
- Referral hospitals can be entry points for the introduction into the health system of inappropriate and unaffordable technologies.
- Skilled personnel frequently find referral hospitals far more attractive to work at than rural and district hospitals for such reasons as preferences for a metropolitan location, better hospital resources allowing for a more rewarding professional experience, and better opportunities for private practice (official or unofficial). However, given the huge problem of global migration of health workers from poor to rich countries (Bundred and Levitt 2000), one could argue that well-functioning referral hospitals might

provide local health professionals with a good incentive to remain at home, whereas the absence of referral hospitals would increase the propensity of local professionals to emigrate.

DETERMINANTS OF AN APPROPRIATE BALANCE OF REFERRAL-LEVEL CARE

When one considers the ideal level of resources to be provided for referral hospital care and the appropriate balance between resources for referral hospitals and for other levels of the health care system, no simple formula is available that can be applied to different countries and contexts. However, certain key factors have an important influence on the need and demand for referral-level care, the resources that may be available to the health sector, and the ability of the health sector to provide adequate and effective care in different settings.

General Determinants

Arguably the most important determinant of demand for and ability to pay for referral hospital care is a society's level of economic development and wealth, captured (albeit imprecisely) by measures of GDP per capita. Extensive international evidence indicates that national health expenditure displays an unambiguously positive income elasticity both across countries and over time; that is, as a country gets richer, it spends relatively more on health (see, for example, Getzen 2000; Schieber 1990). Studies in developed countries indicate that in the United States, every 1 percent long-run increase in GDP leads to a 1.6 percent increase in health expenditure, and in other countries the increase is between 1.2 and 1.4 percent (Getzen 2000). Therefore, expecting developing countries to spend a higher proportion of their GDP on health care as they become wealthier seems to be reasonable. If the poorest countries were to focus their limited resources on highly cost-effective interventions in primary health care, somewhat better-off countries might be expected to spend progressively more on the referral hospital level as resources became available.

An overlapping set of demographic and geographical factors also plays an important role in determining the balance of referral care—namely, population size, population density, terrain, distances between main urban centers, and access. Populations of some millions are required to justify a major tertiary hospital with a full range of tertiary services. Small countries with populations of less than 1 million will certainly not be able to provide a full range of tertiary hospital services because of the need to achieve minimum volumes to ensure service viability and to attract a critical mass of specialized personnel. Countries with fewer than 100,000 inhabitants (generally island states) may find even secondary hospital services beyond their means and capabilities. Supranational referral, reliance on larger neighbors, or regional collaboration may be unavoidable for smaller countries, especially for tertiary care provision, with the Caribbean and southern Africa providing clear examples of many smaller states relying on referral facilities in larger or wealthier neighbors. Within larger countries, population density can complicate the planning of referral services. Compact countries or regions with dense populations can typically provide high levels of access to referral care at a relatively small number of sites, whereas countries or regions with more dispersed populations face more complex tradeoffs regarding number of sites, volume thresholds, and transportation systems.

The other main influence on the appropriate balance of referral services for a given country is its particular pattern and burden of disease. Although referral-level services will always be needed, as a society passes through epidemiologic and demographic transitions, it is likely to require more of those services typically found at referral hospitals. For example, rapidly increasing rates of heart disease and cancers are typically encountered in industrializing nations and aging populations, and these are diseases whose effective management requires access to the interventions, skills, and equipment that will typically be concentrated at the referral hospital level.

Health System Determinants

A number of factors specific to the particular context of a country's health system will also influence the appropriate balance between referral hospitals and lower levels of care. These factors are especially important in considering the appropriateness of plans to change the balance of care between levels. Broadly, they can be summarized as follows:

- capabilities of lower levels
- availability of specialized personnel
- training capacity, organization, and needs
- cultural issues, political issues, and traditions.

The first three factors are closely interrelated. If primary health care and district hospital services are weak, cutting resources for referral hospitals without destabilizing the system will be more difficult. In such circumstances, rapid rebalancing of resources is unlikely to be possible because careful efforts will be required to develop lower-level services first, while still maintaining the referral service. Where lower-level services are strong, devoting relatively fewer resources to referral hospitals may well be possible. However, even though an effective district health system will be able to treat a large proportion of patients at lower levels of care, it will also be better able to identify patients who require referral for more complex care and, thus, may generate a greater appropriate demand for referral hospital care.

Referral hospital services require a specialized staff to fulfill their mission. If specialized personnel are not available in a country, then attempting to develop referral hospitals on a large scale will clearly be infeasible. However, many countries arguably have too many specialized staff persons and too few well-trained generalists. Where large numbers of specialists exist, their presence will likely tend to draw resources disproportionately toward the referral level and away from district health systems. Wherever such imbalances exist, positive changes will require a substantial training or retraining agenda. The feasibility of such efforts is closely linked to the professional and social status of different professional groups and subgroups—for example, whether medical specialists are viewed as having a higher status than general practitioners—and to the premium a society places on having access to "advanced" medical care.

CURRENT BALANCE OF CARE IN PRACTICE

In this section, we summarize data on the current balance between referral and lower levels of care. We first look at the share of total health expenditure going to these different levels, but given that referral care normally has much higher unit costs, we recognize that the balance also needs to be viewed in terms of volume of cases and access and equity.

Share of Health Expenditure

Different health systems categorize hospitals and services rendered differently. Methodologies in national health accounts in developing countries during the 1990s and early 2000s have tended to use a simple, catch-all category of "hospitals" or "acute hospitals" (for example, WHO 2002). Even high-income countries following the Organisation for Economic Co-operation and Development's system of health accounts provider classification (OECD 2000, 136) distinguish only between "general" hospitals and "mental health and substance abuse" and other "specialty" hospitals in their national health accounts. Consequently, making valid cross-country comparisons of spending by levels of hospital care remains extremely difficult.

Mills (1990a) reviews published data on hospital expenditure patterns in developing countries, and Barnum and Kutzin (1993) provide a comprehensive survey of expenditure on hospital services in a number of developing countries, drawing their information largely from World Bank sector reviews. These analyses remain the most authoritative assessment of the proportion of public health expenditure absorbed by secondary and tertiary hospitals, even though their data represent only a handful of countries at different points in time.

Overall, Mills (1990a) finds that hospitals in developing countries appear to absorb from 30 to 50 percent of total health expenditure. Public hospitals of all types absorb some 50 to 60 percent of public health expenditure, and secondary and tertiary hospitals absorb about 60 to 80 percent of public hospital expenditure, with the remainder going to district hospitals. Her results are broadly similar to those of Barnum and Kutzin (1993, 26–33), who find that public hospitals at all levels absorb a mean of approximately 60 percent of recurrent public health expenditures. Across five countries (Belize, Indonesia, Kenya, Zambia, and Zimbabwe), they find that tertiary hospitals account for between 45 and 69 percent of total public expenditure on hospitals. In South Africa, Thomas and Muirhead (2000) find that tertiary hospitals account for 28 percent of hospital expenditure and 17 percent of total public health expenditure, but when taken together with regional referral hospitals, constitute 59 percent of hospital expenditure.

Unit Costs of Care

One of the explanations for the high share of expenditure that flows through higher-level referral hospitals is, of course, that the unit costs of a referral hospital are necessarily higher than the unit costs of a district hospital. This difference results from the more complex case mix they treat, their more expensive inputs, and the additional costs of their teaching functions (Barnum and Kutzin 1993, 26). Mills (1990b) reports that her analysis of available data indicated that secondary-level hospitals were typically twice as expensive per bed day as district hospitals and that tertiary hospitals were typically between twice and five times as expensive per bed day as district hospitals. Barnum and Kutzin (1993) find similar relationships between unit costs by level of hospital in a variety of different countries. This upward gradient in unit costs has also been found in econometric studies of hospital costs (Adam, Evans, and Murray 2003) and has been explicitly incorporated into the regression-based unit cost estimates used in other chapters in this volume.

Table 66.3 shows data on unit costs by level of care from Mauritius and highlights a commonly encountered contradiction of the preceding paragraph—namely, that costs appear

Table 66.4 Cost Per Bed Day for Selected Specialties, Tertiary Hospitals, Mauritius, 1995 *(2001 U.S. dollars)*

Specialty	Minimum	Maximum
Medicine	16	20
Orthopedics	18	23
Pediatrics	29	43
Cardiothoracic surgery	36	39
Burns	37	37
Intensive care unit	106	120

Source: Murray and others 1996.

similar at all levels. This phenomenon is explained by average bed occupancy in Mauritian district hospitals of around 45 percent in 1995, compared with average bed occupancies of 90 percent or more in tertiary hospitals. Thus, the high cost of district hospital care in this case reflects not inputs, which are much less extensive than in a tertiary hospital, but the effect of low levels of utilization. Such a difference in utilization between levels of hospital tends to be the norm in many developing countries (Barnum and Kutzin 1993, 91–96). Note that the regression-based unit costs of district hospitals used in the cost analysis for this volume reflect an "optimized" bed occupancy of 80 percent (Mulligan and others 2003, 29). This assumption is entirely defensible from a long-run perspective, assuming cost-minimizing behavior is necessary and appropriate. It does, however, reflect quite a substantial shift from the levels of utilization and productivity commonly seen in rural district hospitals in most developing countries.

The use of a simple unit cost hides important cost differences between services and specialties within the same hospital, as demonstrated by the breakdown for Mauritian tertiary hospitals in table 66.4. Differences in length of stay for different specialties and conditions also obviously contribute to radically different costs per admission or patient; however, these differences should be captured by the condition and procedure costs used in the disease chapters in this volume.

Table 66.3 Cost Per Bed Day in a Medical Ward by Level of Hospital, Mauritius, 1995 *(2001 U.S. dollars)*

Level of hospital	Cost
District	17
Regional	21
Tertiary	20

Source: Murray and others 1996.

Appropriateness of Utilization of Referral Hospitals

Perhaps the most frequent theme in the research literature on referral hospitals in developing countries is the inappropriate utilization of higher-level facilities and the apparent failure of most referral systems in developing countries to function as intended. Broadly speaking, hospitals of all levels, up to and including national tertiary centers—especially in their outpatients departments—are overwhelmed by patients who could have been treated successfully at lower-level facilities, many of whom have self-referred, bypassing primary health care or district hospitals in the process (Holdsworth, Garner, and Harpham 1993; London and Bachmann 1997; Omaha and others 1998; Sanders and others 2001).

Atkinson and others (1999) describe an extreme manifestation of this phenomenon, whereby the University Teaching Hospital is actually the only public hospital in Lusaka. Combined with the bypassing of primary health clinics in the city, this situation results in the University Teaching Hospital's functioning primarily as a glorified health center and first-contact provider for most of Lusaka's population. The problem of bypassing typically seems to be driven by a number of factors, including patients' perception of superior quality of care and resource availability at referral hospitals, which often may be entirely well founded and rational (see, for example, London and Bachmann 1997; Nolan and others 2001); the desire to avoid delays in care if referral to a higher-level facility proves to be necessary; and the fact that for many urban populations a referral hospital may simply be the closest health facility. Grodos and Tonglet (2002) argue that many countries' failure to develop an adequate urban equivalent of the district health concept greatly exacerbates inappropriate utilization of hospitals. The urban phenomenon of widespread bypassing and self-referral is frequently accompanied by low rates of formal referral from rural and outlying facilities (see, for example, Nordberg, Holmberg, and Kiugu 1996; Omaha and others 1998).

These problems have a number of negative impacts and consequences. Simple conditions are unnecessarily treated in a high-cost environment; outpatient departments are congested by patients requiring primary care, thus causing long waiting times; scarce staff time is diverted from specialized areas and into inappropriate care; and more complex cases requiring specialized care are crowded out by more urgent but less technically demanding cases that could be cared for at lower levels. The latter has been a particular concern in those countries with more serious HIV/AIDS epidemics. As the number of patients falling sick with AIDS increases rapidly, they start to occupy a significant proportion of beds in hospitals at all levels (Gilks and others 1998), inevitably crowding out patients requiring other forms of care. Although AIDS cases may well require hospitalization, only a small proportion of cases require specialized or tertiary care. Gilks and others (1998) find that this crowding-out effect may fall over time as the health system adjusts to the pressures of AIDS, but countries facing impending AIDS epidemics should be prepared for its initial appearance.

Taken together, this complex of problems undermines the effective delivery of both specialized care and appropriate primary health care. Specialized care is pushed to the background by the human wave of demand for primary care, while hospitals unwittingly further undermine the credibility of the primary health care system through one-sided competition

(Stefanini 1994), which reinforces the cycle and ensures that primary health care facilities remain underused and inefficient.

Access and Equity

By their nature, referral hospitals must be limited in number and will inevitably be sited in major towns and cities. As a result, a significant portion of the population, especially people living in rural areas, will tend to live at some distance from the nearest referral hospital. Studies of the accessibility of referral hospital care in countries such as Ethiopia (Kloos 1990) and Nigeria (Lyun 1983; Okafor 1983) have repeatedly confirmed the existence of a steep distance-decay function, indicating that—other things being equal—individuals with a given need for a clinical service will be less likely to access that service the farther away from the referral center they live.

Compounding the impact of distance, investigators find that problems relating to the availability, regularity, and cost of transportation to referral centers also affect service utilization (Kloos 1990; Martey and others 1998). The same authors indicate that prohibitive hospital fees are often a significant barrier to utilization, especially among poorer patients. Other important barriers included perceived lack of drugs and essential supplies, even at referral centers; negative staff attitudes; and cultural and linguistic differences (for example, where the staff at a referral center does not speak the language of a patient from a remote area). As noted earlier, peripheral district hospitals also tend to have low rates of referral. These barriers, which all disproportionately affect rural patients, must be contrasted with the phenomenon noted earlier of excessive and inappropriate use of referral hospitals for primary care by urban residents.

In addition to finding that public hospitals favor urban residents over rural dwellers, a number of studies have indicated that public hospitals in many poor countries disproportionately benefit the better off, leading their authors to argue that diverting public funds from hospitals and toward primary health care would be pro-poor (see, for instance, Castro-Leal and others 2000; Filmer, Hammer, and Pritchett 1997; Mahal and others 2002). Other studies find this tendency in some countries but not in others (Makinen and others 2000). By contrast, in Latin American countries, Barnum and Kutzin (1993) find strong evidence that public hospitals are pro-poor in their distributional effect. Even if referral hospital services are not currently pro-poor, policy makers face two contradictory alternatives: either to retarget public funds toward primary health care for the poor, hence greatly reducing or abandoning public funding for referral hospitals, or to attempt to remove the barriers that prevent the poor from using higher-level services, which would probably require increased spending on all levels of care.

GETTING BETTER VALUE FOR MONEY FROM THE HOSPITAL SYSTEM

Although prescribing how resources should be allocated across levels of care is hard, at least they should be efficiently used, wherever they are spent within the hospital system. The preceding analysis has highlighted how deficiencies at the lower levels of the hospital system render referral hospitals less efficient and how factors that affect access lead to skewed benefits and inequity. Here we look more specifically at three areas for improving the efficiency of the hospital system: interventions within the referral hospital, the use of public-private partnerships, and strengthening of the referral chain.

Improving the Efficiency of Referral Hospitals

Although space does not permit a lengthy discussion of approaches to improve efficiency in the context of referral hospitals, this aspect is nonetheless important in planning and system strengthening (for a more detailed discussion see Barnum and Kutzin 1993; Hensher 2001; Walford and Grant 1998). In summary, the key areas on which planners and managers should focus are as follows:

- reducing inappropriate outpatient and inpatient use of referral
- improving systems to allow early discharge from the hospital
- ensuring that bed occupancy rates can be maintained as close as possible to optimal rates—namely, 85 percent for referral hospitals
- developing systems for booked outpatient appointments, admissions, and procedures to permit better planning of activity and staffing
- undertaking as much activity as possible on an ambulatory rather than an inpatient basis, supported by the use of "step-down" beds and patient hotels
- evaluating the staff skill mix and the potential for skill substitution, as well as efficient remuneration strategies, on a continuous basis
- evaluating and improving processes and systems, including cost-effective clinical guidelines for patient treatment, on a continuous basis
- ensuring that new or replacement referral hospitals conform as much as possible to available evidence on economies of scale—that is, that hospitals with fewer than 200 beds are likely to be scale inefficient and that diseconomies of scale are likely to become increasingly evident in hospitals with more than 600 beds
- adopting intelligent procurement processes and engaging in effective negotiations with suppliers in relation to prices and service levels

- ensuring effective ordering, stock control, and distribution systems to minimize theft and wastage of key supplies
- undertaking planned preventive maintenance and programmed replacement of equipment and buildings.

Can Public-Private Interactions Improve Efficiency?

In the context of this discussion, privately owned hospitals that provide subsidized care to public patients, such as nongovernmental organization and mission hospitals, are regarded as public hospitals. *Private* refers to for-profit hospitals that are generally funded by paying patients and are minimally subsidized. Few studies have been undertaken of how private hospitals operate in developing countries (see, for example, Muraleedharan 1999). Although the exact balance of and relationship between the public and private health sectors varies greatly from country to country at all levels of the health system, a common theme in almost all low- and middle-income countries is that private hospitals do not follow the pyramidal referral form that public hospital systems have adopted almost universally. Most private health sectors do not clearly delineate district, secondary, or tertiary hospitals. Different private hospitals may offer different services and facilities on a more or less idiosyncratic basis, with independent medical specialists practicing and admitting patients at various different hospitals.

In most systems, scope exists for both positive collaboration and competition between public and private hospitals, especially for secondary and tertiary services. Competition between public and private sectors obviously has the potential to be beneficial by driving quality up and costs down, but it may also have negative effects by encouraging a duplication of services and resulting in the underutilization of fixed capital by creating perverse incentives for physicians and patients and by competing with the public sector for scarce human resources. In some settings, the private sector may be able to offer services that the public purse cannot afford to provide, thus allowing patients who could not afford private care some chance of accessing sophisticated treatments through the government's paying private providers or by some pro bono provision of treatment for poor patients.

In many countries, government hospitals are establishing private wards as a vehicle for income generation. The fees for such units are lower than those at private hospitals, offering access to private facilities to patients who may not be able to afford private hospitals. The link with academic medicine often adds to the appeal of such facilities. However, as is the case in South Africa, effectively only tertiary hospitals and a handful of secondary hospitals are felt to be attractive enough to private patients to offer genuine opportunities as preferred providers. The mass of district and regional hospitals are unlikely to be attractive to private patients; therefore, the positive spinoffs of these initiatives may be limited in their scale and reach.

Contracting out services to private providers, particularly high-cost, low-volume services, may be an efficient way to offer such services to public patients. For example, the government of Barbados contracts out surplus demand for dialysis to a private facility on the island. In some provinces of South Africa, expensive imaging such as MRI has been contracted out to private radiology practices. South Africa is also experimenting with contracting out the management of some academic referral hospitals to a private hospital group that is assumed to have greater management expertise and is free from certain public sector constraints, such as salary scales for senior managers. It is too early to judge the success of this arrangement, but in all cases it is imperative that contracts be carefully regulated, monitored, and enforced. For a comprehensive review of contracting, see Bennet, McPake, and Mills (1997).

Particular problems may arise where the same doctors provide care in both public and private hospitals. Under fee-for-service arrangements, physicians may focus on their more lucrative private patients to the disadvantage of public hospital patients, refer patients with adequate insurance to their private practices and private hospitals, and transfer patients with expensive diseases or inadequate insurance to public hospitals.

Improving the Functionality of Referral Systems

An ideal referral system would ensure that patients can receive appropriate, high-quality care for their condition in the lowest-cost and closest facility possible, given the resources available to the health system, with seamless transfer of information and responsibility as that patient is required to move up or down the referral chain. Although few referral systems anywhere in the world live up to this ideal fully, it does provide a target in relation to improving the current situation. Improving the effective functioning of referral systems broadly requires progress in three areas: referral system design, facilitation of the smooth transfer of patients and information between levels, and what Walford and Grant (1998, 38) refer to as effective "referral discipline."

Improving referral system design must start with a detailed attempt to assess which services should be provided at which level of care, encompassing community- and home-based care, primary health care, district hospitals, secondary hospitals, tertiary hospitals, and specialized hospitals. Such an assessment must take local circumstances into account, requires a significant analytical and consultative effort by planners and clinicians if it is to be credible, and must explicitly be open to revision in light of practical experience. After such an exercise has identified which services can appropriately be provided at each level of care, adequate resources must be dedicated to strengthening lower levels of care to make them attractive and credible in the eyes of patients. This effort will require significant

investment and funding to ensure the availability of appropriate staff members and supervision, to ensure continuous drug supplies, and to provide basic laboratory tests (Walford and Grant 1998, 38). Given the pervasiveness of inappropriate use of referral hospitals for primary health care problems by urban residents, both urban and rural primary health care and district health systems must be adequately strengthened. Financing strategies that redistribute funds from urban to rural regions may unwittingly hamper such strengthening of the referral system by failing to allow for the development of appropriate lower-level facilities for urban residents. This risk is especially high when a country is pursuing a redistributive agenda against a background of limited or zero overall growth in expenditure.

From a physical planning perspective, planners should consider providing primary health care and district hospital walk-in ambulatory services (emergency and general outpatients) in a physically distinct facility sited immediately next to the referral hospital. This arrangement not only enables triage and filtering of less severe cases (while proximity ensures that severe emergency cases can be transferred rapidly) but also enables rigorous enforcement of a referral-only policy within the referral hospital.

The development of effective patient transportation arrangements is also critical, not only to ensure that patients from remote areas have a fair chance of being successfully referred to a center of excellence (bearing in mind that most referral systems will almost certainly need to increase referral rates from rural areas), but also to ensure that patients can be discharged in a timely and well-planned fashion.

Perhaps more challenging is the concurrent need to align the incentives of referral hospitals, district hospitals, and primary health care services. This goal may or may not be achievable by means of an integrated management structure, but it certainly requires a good deal of communication, collaborative planning, and collaborative development of shared care protocols, and senior personnel need to be given responsibility for coordination and liaison across key interfaces of the referral network. A single, global budget controlled by an authority that is concerned with optimizing the cost-effectiveness of health care delivery would seem to be a necessary condition to achieve alignment across service levels; however, a consideration of financing mechanisms is beyond the scope of this chapter.

At the patient level, a number of mechanisms to improve referral discipline can be considered. In situations in which eliminating nonreferred patients entirely from the referral hospital is impossible, queuing systems should be redesigned to separate referred patients from nonreferred patients so that referrals can be fast-tracked. Explaining to nonreferred patients why other patients are being fast-tracked past them is important to encourage them to seek referral in future. Ideally, they should be diverted to an on-site primary health care facility where they can be treated more quickly than in the referral hospital. Another possibility may be to institute bypass fees for nonreferred patients, charging them a penalty fee for failing to use the referral system. Such a decision requires careful consideration and planning. Credible lower-level care must be readily available, and substantial efforts to communicate the new policy to the public will be required if this approach is to be seen as fair. More broadly, intensive public communication and education will be essential to inform the public how, where, and when they should seek health care at different levels and to build their confidence that lower-level facilities really will be able to offer acceptable quality care when they need it.

CONCLUDING COMMENTS

This review of the available evidence indicates that referral hospitals frequently do command a large share of health sector resources and expenditure, yet no simple way exists of assessing what an appropriate share would be. Strong referral hospitals can distort priorities and undermine basic services, but they also provide important health benefits to large numbers of patients whom they treat successfully. Referral hospitals provide essential support to lower levels of the system, which cannot function effectively without access to upward referral, and they are frequently the most functional component of the health system, paying greatest attention to quality of care.

Overall, we have argued that both national and international policy makers should be cautious before demanding the reallocation of resources away from referral hospitals and should be still more cautious in allowing themselves to believe that such a reallocation is likely to be achievable in practice. In particular, this chapter has made the case that a unidimensional focus on cost-effectiveness analysis and cost per DALY gained will fail to capture the importance of referral hospital services adequately. In reality, in most developing countries, the scope for reallocation of resources from referral hospitals to lower levels of care is limited, and the managerial demands of achieving a successful reallocation are great. Lower levels of care certainly require strengthening, but this need is more likely to reflect inadequate financing of the entire public health system than a grossly excessive allocation to referral hospitals. Instead, referral hospitals should perhaps be seen as the capstone of the referral pyramid: they should not be too heavy, but if they are too light, the levels below them will lose cohesion. A restructuring of referral hospital services is certainly called for to improve appropriate referral and utilization, especially by remote and rural populations; to transform the inappropriate use of referral hospitals as primary health care providers; to improve efficiency; and to provide much better outreach and support to lower levels of care.

This restructuring should not be confused with wholesale demolition. Undermining referral services will be far more likely to undermine and destabilize the entire health system than to liberate resources for primary health care. Clearly, countries must critically evaluate their health priorities and their balance of care and resources between levels, but they should do so carefully and thoroughly, with a clear understanding of the analytical effort required to draw meaningful conclusions, of the planning and managerial capacity that they will require to bring about successful change, and of the long time frames required to develop and implement robust plans for major system changes.

ACKNOWLEDGMENTS

The authors gratefully acknowledge the crucial assistance of Etienne Yemek in undertaking literature reviews.

REFERENCES

Adam T., D. B. Evans, and C. J. Murray. 2003. "Econometric Estimation of Country-Specific Hospital Costs." *Cost Effectiveness and Resource Allocation* 1:3.

Adomakoh, S., A. St. John, and A. Kumar. 2002. "Reducing Mother to Child Transmission of HIV-1 in Barbados. Cost-Effectiveness of the PACTG 076 Protocol in a Middle Income, Low Prevalence Setting." Paper presented at the 14th International AIDS Conference, July 7–12, Barcelona, Spain.

Al-Mazrou, Y., S. Al-Shehri, and M. Rao. 1990. *Principles and Practice of Primary Health Care.* Riyadh: Al-Helal Press.

Atkinson, S., A. Ngwengwe, M. Macwan'gi, T. J. Ngulube, T. Harpham, and A. O'Connell. 1999. "The Referral Process and Urban Health Care in Sub-Saharan Africa: The Case of Lusaka, Zambia." *Social Science and Medicine* 49: 27–38.

Barnum, H., and J. Kutzin. 1993. *Public Hospitals in Developing Countries: Resource Use, Cost, Financing.* Baltimore: Johns Hopkins University Press.

Bennet, S., B. McPake, and A. Mills, eds. 1997. *Private Health Providers in Developing Countries.* London: Zed Books.

Bundred, P., and C. Levitt. 2000. "Medical Migration: Who Are the Real Losers?" *Lancet* 356: 245–46.

Castro-Leal, F., J. Dayton, L. Demery, and K. Mehra. 2000. "Public Spending on Health Care in Africa: Do the Poor Benefit?" *Bulletin of the World Health Organization* 78: 66–74.

Fiedler, J., R. Schmidt, and J. Wight. 1998. "Public Hospital Resource Allocations in El Salvador: Accounting for the Case Mix of Patients." *Health Policy and Planning* 13 (3): 296–310.

Filmer, D., J. Hammer, and L. Pritchett. 1997. "Health Policy in Poor Countries: Weak Links in the Chain." Policy Research Working Paper 1874, World Bank, Washington, DC.

Getzen, T. E. 2000. "Health Care Is an Individual Necessity and a National Luxury: Applying Multilevel Decision Models to the Analysis of Health Care Expenditures." *Journal of Health Economics* 19: 259–70.

Gilks, C., K. Floyd, L. Otieno, A. Adam, S. Bhatt, and D. Warrell. 1998. "Some Effects of the Rising Case Load of Adult HIV-Related Disease on a Hospital in Nairobi." *Journal of Acquired Immune Deficiency Syndrome and Human Retrovirology* 18 (3): 234–40.

Grodos, D., and R. Tonglet. 2002. "Maîtriser un espace sanitaire cohérent et performant dans les villes d'Afrique subsaharienne: Le district de santé à l'épreuve" (in French). *Tropical Medicine and International Health* 7 (11): 977–92.

Hammer, J., and P. Berman. 1995. "Ends and Means in Public Health Policy in Developing Countries." *Health Policy* 32 (1–3): 29–45.

Harden, R. M., and M. H. Davis. 1998. "Educating More Doctors in the U.K.: Painting the Tiger." *Medical Teacher* 20 (4): 306.

Hensher, M. 2001. "Financing Health Systems through Efficiency Gains." Working Paper WG3:5, Commission on Macroeconomics and Health Working Group 3. http://www.cmhealth.org/docs/wg3_paper2.pdf.

Holdsworth, G., P. Garner, and T. Harpham. 1993. "Crowded Outpatient Departments in City Hospitals of Developing Countries: A Case Study from Lesotho." *International Journal of Health Planning and Management* 8 (4): 315–24.

Husain, M. 1996. "The University Hospitals in Pakistan: The Case of the Aga Khan University Hospital." In *The Proper Functioning of Teaching Hospitals within Health Systems*, ed. D. Puzin, 73–80. Geneva: World Health Organization.

Kloos, H. 1990. "Utilization of Selected Hospital, Health Centers, and Health Stations in Central, Southern, and Western Ethiopia." *Social Science and Medicine* 31 (2): 101–14.

Liu, Y., K. Rao, and W. C. Hsiao. 2003. "Medical Expenditure and Rural Impoverishment in China." *Journal of Health and Population Nutrition* 21 (3): 216–22.

London, L., and O. Bachmann. 1997. "Paediatric Utilisation of a Teaching Hospital and a Community Health Centre." *South African Medical Journal* 87 (1): 31–36.

Lyun, F. 1983. "Hospital Services Areas in Ibadan City." *Social Science and Medicine* 17: 601–16.

Mahal, A., J. Singh, F. Afridi, V. Lamba, A. Gumber, and V. Selvaraju. 2002. *Who "Benefits" from Public Sector Health Spending in India?* New Delhi: National Council for Applied Economic Research.

Makinen, M., H. Waters, M. Rauch, N. Almagambetova, R. Bitran, L. Gilson, and others. 2000. "Inequalities in Health Care Use and Expenditure: Empirical Data from Eight Developing Countries and Countries in Transition." *Bulletin of the World Health Organization* 78: 55–65.

Martey, J., J. Djan, S. Twum, E. Browne, and S. Opoku. 1998. "Referrals for Obstetric Complications from Ejisu District, Ghana." *West African Journal of Medicine* 17: 58–63.

McCord, C., and Q. Chowdhury. 2003. "A Cost Effective Small Hospital in Bangladesh: What It Can Mean for Emergency Obstetric Care." *International Journal of Gynaecology and Obstetrics* 81: 83–92.

Mills, A. 1990a. "The Economics of Hospitals in Developing Countries—Part I: Expenditure Patterns." *Health Policy and Planning* 5 (2): 107–17.

———. 1990b. "The Economics of Hospitals in Developing Countries—Part II: Costs and Sources of Income." *Health Policy and Planning* 5 (3): 203–18.

Mulligan, J., J. Fox-Rushby, T. Adam, B. Johns, and A. Mills. 2003. "Unit Costs of Health Care Inputs in Low and Middle Income Regions." Working Paper 9, Disease Control Priorities Project, Fogarty International Center, National Institutes of Health, Bethesda, MD. http://www.fic.nih.gov/dcpp/wps/wp9.pdf.

Muraleedharan, V. R. 1999. "Characteristics and Structure of the Private Hospital Sector in Urban India: A Study of Madras City." Small Applied Research Paper 5, Abt Associates, Partnerships for Health Reform Project, Bethesda, MD.

Murray, C., P. Mahapatra, R. Ashley, C. Michaud, A. George, P. Hrobon, and others. 1996. *The Health Sector in Mauritius: Resource Use, Intervention Cost, and Options for Efficiency Enhancement.* Cambridge, MA: Harvard Center for Population and Development Studies, Burden of Disease Unit.

National Department of Health, South Africa. 2003. "Strategic Framework for the Modernisation of Tertiary Hospital Services". National Department of Health, South Africa, Pretoria. http://www.doh.gov.za/mts/docs/framework.html.

Nolan, T., P. Angos, A. Cunha, L. Muhe, S. Qazi, E. Simoes, and others. 2001. "Quality of Hospital Care for Seriously Ill Children in Less-Developed Countries." *Lancet* 357 (9250): 106–10.

Nordberg, E., S. Holmberg, and S. Kiugu. 1996. "Exploring the Interface between First and Second Level Care: Referrals in Rural Africa." *Tropical Medicine and International Health* 1 (1): 101–11.

OECD (Organisation for Economic Co-operation and Development). 2000. *A System of Health Accounts: Version 1.0.* Paris: OECD.

Okafor, S. 1983. "Factors Affecting the Frequency of Hospital Trips among a Predominantly Rural Population." *Social Science and Medicine* 17: 591–95.

Omaha, K., V. Melendez, N. Uehara, and G. Ohi. 1998. "Study of a Patient Referral System in the Republic of Honduras." *Health Policy and Planning* 13 (4): 433–45.

Puzin, D., ed. 1996. *The Proper Functioning of Teaching Hospitals within Health Systems.* Geneva: World Health Organization.

Sanders, D., J. Kravitz, S. Lewin, and M. McKee. 2001 "Zimbabwe's Hospital Referral System: Does It Work?" *Health Policy and Planning* 13 (4): 359–70.

Schieber, G. J. 1990. "Health Expenditures in Major Industrialized Countries, 1960–87." *Health Care Financing Review* 11: 159–68.

Snow, R., V. Mung'ala, D. Forester, and K. Marsh. 1994. "The Role of the District Hospital in Child Survival at the Kenyan Coast." *African Journal of Health Sciences* 1 (2): 71–75.

Stefanini, A. 1994. "District Hospitals and Strengthening Referral Systems in Developing Countries." *World Hospitals* 30 (2): 14–19.

Thomas, S., and D. Muirhead. 2000. *National Health Accounts Project: The Public Sector Report.* Cape Town, South Africa: University of Cape Town.

Walford, V., and K. Grant. 1998. "Health Sector Reform: Improving Hospital Efficiency." London: Department for International Development, Health Sector Resource Centre.

WHO (World Health Organization). 2002. *WHO National Health Accounts 2002: Enhancing Country Templates-in-the-Making: Guidelines.* Geneva: WHO, National Health Accounts Unit.

WHOSIS (World Health Organization Statistical Information System). 2004. "Physicians per 100,000 Population." World Health Organization, Geneva. http://www.who.int/GlobalAtlas/DataQuery/geoSelection.asp.

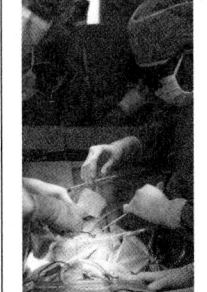

Chapter **67**

Surgery

Haile T. Debas, Richard Gosselin, Colin McCord, and Amardeep Thind

Countries with developing economies have not considered surgical care to be a public health priority, yet surgically treatable conditions—such as cataracts (Javitt 1993); obstructed labor (Neilson and others 2003); symptomatic hernias (Olumide, Adedeji, and Adesola 1976; Rahman and Mungadi 2000); osteomyelitis (Bickler and Rode 2002; Hilton 2003); otitis media (Smith and Hatcher 1992; Whitney and Pickering 2002); and a variety of inflammatory conditions—add a chronic burden of ill health to populations. These acute and chronic conditions take a serious human and economic toll and at times lead to acute, life-threatening complications.

Inadequacies in the initial care of injured patients (Hyder and Peden 2003; Jat and others 2004; Mock 2003; Mock and others 1995); of women with obstructed labor; and of children with treatable congenital anomalies, such as clubfoot (Ponseti 1999; Turco 1994) lead to preventable deaths or to chronic disabilities that make productive employment impossible and impose dependency on family members and society.

The role of surgery as a preventive strategy in public health needs to be studied and measured far more extensively than is currently the case. Another key reason for this study is that virtually all countries are developing their economies, and as a result, developing nations are increasingly facing a double burden—that is, the infectious diseases that have historically been so relevant and the conditions that emerge with economic development (for example, trauma from motorcycle, truck, and car accidents). The inclusion of a surgery chapter in this book recognizes that surgical services may have a cost-effective role in population-based health care. Recent studies (for instance, McCord and Chowdhury 2003) show that basic hospital service, which requires no sophisticated care, can be cost-

effective, with a cost per disability-adjusted life year (DALY) that is much lower than might have been expected, and can be on a par with other well-accepted preventive procedures, such as immunization for measles and tetanus and home care for lower respiratory infections (Armandola 2003; Dayan and others 2004; Moalosi and others 2003; Ruff 1999).

We have identified four types of surgically significant interventions with a potential public health dimension: (a) the provision of competent, initial surgical care to injury victims, not only to reduce preventable deaths but also to decrease the number of survivable injuries that result in personal dysfunction and impose a significant burden on families and communities; (b) the handling of obstetrical complications (obstructed labor, hemorrhage); (c) the timely and competent surgical management of a variety of abdominal and extra-abdominal emergent and life-threatening conditions; and (d) the elective care of simple surgical conditions such as hernias, clubfoot, cataract, hydroceles, and otitis media.

NATURE, CAUSES, AND BURDEN OF SURGICAL CONDITIONS

Surgery is at the end of the spectrum of the classic curative medical model and, as such, has not been routinely considered as part of the traditional public health model. However, no matter how successful prevention strategies are, surgical conditions will always account for a significant portion of a population's disease burden, particularly in developing countries where conservative treatment is not readily available, where the incidence of trauma and obstetrical complications is high, and where there is a huge backlog of untreated surgical diseases (Murray and Lopez 1996). Some surgical procedures can certainly be perceived as forms of secondary or tertiary prevention. Since the publication of the first edition of this book, which did not have a chapter on surgery, the health care community has recognized that the surgical management of some common conditions can indeed be a cost-effective intervention (Javitt 1993; McCord and Chowdhury 2003). The purpose of this chapter is to explore this hypothesis in more depth.

Methods for Determining Burden of Surgical Disease

We have arbitrarily decided to define a *surgical condition* as any condition that requires suture, incision, excision, manipulation, or other invasive procedure that usually, but not always, requires local, regional, or general anesthesia. We prefer this definition for two main reasons, to one that would define *surgery* as procedures performed by trained surgeons. First, surgery does not have to be performed by qualified surgeons. Indeed, in developing countries with few doctors, nondoctors can be trained to perform several types of operations satisfactorily. Second, we believe that the concept of surgery should include minor surgical procedures that nurses or general practitioners could perform along with nonoperative management of surgical diseases (for example, certain types of abdominal, thoracic, or head trauma and burns and infections). Any definition of surgery will have limitations, as has ours, and those limitations must be kept in mind when making interpretations, extrapolations, or estimates. Our broad definition is compatible with the concept of regionalized, coordinated, and interdependent services provided at the community clinic level and at the district and tertiary hospital levels. The most difficult task we then face is trying to determine the burden of surgical conditions as measured in DALYs. To our knowledge, this measurement has never been attempted. What we provide here is a starting point, with the understanding that the calculations will change as data are developed.

Our methodology was based on data from the *World Health Report 2002: Reducing Risks, Promoting Healthy Life* (WHO 2002) and the global burden of disease study (Murray and Lopez 1996). We began by listing all the conditions for which surgery might be indicated into three groups, with group I being communicable diseases, group II being noncommunicable diseases, and group III being injuries. We then undertook a comprehensive literature review for each condition to determine the proportion of the total burden of disease attributable to it and the proportion of the burden that could be prevented or treated by surgery. Essentially, we found no data of value except maybe for cataracts (group II-F), for which a single intervention (intraocular lens removal with or without implant) is or should ultimately be indicated for nearly 100 percent of patients (Dandona and others 1999; Javitt 1993).

The *World Health Report 2002* attributes 8,269, of a total 1,467,257,000 DALYs, to cataracts (0.56 percent), and all those DALYs are considered potentially surgical. Maternal conditions (group I-C), perinatal conditions (group I-D), diabetes (group II-C), intentional injuries (group III-B), and unintentional injuries (group III-A), to name a few, are much broader categories of conditions for which the demarcation between the surgical and nonsurgical burden is not as clear as for cataracts.

Faced with a near total lack of pertinent data, we decided that the next best approach was to try to obtain consensus on a "best educated guess" for the surgical burden of each condition. We developed a survey instrument that listed all the possible surgical conditions (all potential surgical DALYs representing the maximum imaginable DALYs that could conceivably be surgical). We sent the questionnaire to 32 surgeons in various parts of the world, asking them what was, in their opinion, the proportion of each condition that would require surgery, which we have referred to as *estimated surgical DALYs* or the *conservative minimum*. For each of the 18 completed questionnaires, we discarded the two lowest and two highest values for each condition, leaving a sample of 14 surveys. The lowest value of this sample was consistently chosen so as to err systematically on the conservative side. Note that more than 90 percent of all retained values were within 10 percent of the chosen value. We then applied this value to the DALY numbers provided by the *World Health Report 2002* for each category of potentially surgical conditions.

Findings

Table 67.1 presents our estimates of the actual surgical burden for each category of potential surgical conditions for the world as a whole and by region. The table indicates that conditions requiring surgery account for a significant proportion of DALYs. Developing more refined, region-specific information to help policy makers will require more detailed data on the burden of surgical diseases (diseases requiring surgical treatment) and on the cost-effectiveness of surgical therapy. To this end, an extremely helpful step would be for international surgical associations to regularly monitor the disease burden attributable to surgical conditions throughout the world.

A few salient points about the burden of surgical diseases can be made from data provided in table 67.1. We estimate very conservatively that 11 percent of the world's DALYs are from conditions that are very likely to require surgery. Our estimated figures are as high as 15 percent for Europe and as low as 7 percent for Africa. Estimated surgical DALYs for the world are 27 per 1,000 population. The estimated figure is about twice as much for Africa (38 per 1,000) as for the Americas (21 per 1,000).

Table 67.2 summarizes the burden of common surgical conditions based on *World Health Report 2002* data. A more

Table 67.1 Estimated Surgical DALYs by Region

Region	Total DALYs (millions)	Estimated surgical DALYs (millions)	Estimated surgical DALYs as a percentage of total DALYs	Estimated surgical DALYs per 1,000 population
World	1,468	164	11	27
Africa	358	25	7	38
Americas	145	18	12	21
Eastern Mediterranean	137	15	11	30
Europe	151	22	15	25
Southeast Asia	419	48	12	31
Western Pacific	258	37	15	22

Source: WHO 2002 and authors' estimates.

Table 67.2 Burden of Common Surgical Conditions

Condition	Surgical DALYs		Estimated surgical DALYs as a percentage of total DALYs	Estimated surgical DALYs per 1,000 population
	Estimated (millions)[a]	Percentage		
Injuries	63	38	4.3	10
Malignancies	31	19	2.1	5
Congenital anomalies	14	9	1.0	2
Obstetrical complications	10	6	0.7	2
Cataracts and glaucoma	8	5	0.5	1
Perinatal conditions	7	4	0.5	1
Other	31	19	2.1	5

Source: WHO 2002 and authors' estimates.
a. *Estimated surgical DALYs* refers to our conservative estimate of DALYs averted by surgical treatment in the most likely diseases for the most likely indications.

detailed look at these data allows us to make the following observations:

- Injuries account for 63 million DALYs, or about 4 percent of all DALYs and 38 percent of the world's estimated surgical DALYs.
- Surgical infections, including infected wounds, superficial and deep abscesses, septic arthritis, and osteomyelitis, undoubtedly account for a significant portion of surgical DALYs, but the available data do not permit quantification.
- Surgical DALYs pertaining to acute abdominal conditions, including appendicitis, intestinal obstruction, gastrointestinal bleeding, hernias, and blunt or penetrating injuries also cannot be calculated because of the lack of data.
- Approximately one-third of maternal conditions, including hemorrhage, obstructed labor, and obstetrical fistulas, are surgical, and these represent 10 million DALYs, or 0.7 percent of all DALYs.

- *Congenital anomalies* refer to an ill-defined grouping of disparate pathologies that includes congenital malformations such as cleft lip and palate, hernias, anorectal malformations, and clubfoot. We estimate that some 50 percent of congenital anomalies are surgical, representing about 14 million DALYs, or 1 percent of all DALYs.
- Malignancies account for 31 million surgical DALYs, or slightly more than 2 percent of all DALYs.

Table 67.3 breaks down the burden of common surgical conditions by region, also showing rates per 1,000 population. The absolute burden of injuries is highest in Southeast Asia, followed by the Western Pacific and Africa. In terms of population rates, whereas injuries account for 10 DALYs per 1,000 population for the world, the estimated figure is almost twice as much for Africa (15 per 1,000) as for Europe (8 per 1,000). Similarly, rates of obstetrical complications are far higher in Africa than elsewhere, at 6 DALYs per 1,000 population. In

Table 67.3 Estimated Surgical DALYs by Condition and Region
(DALYs in millions followed by DALYs per 1,000 population in parentheses)

Condition	Africa	Americas	Eastern Mediterranean	Europe	Southeast Asia	Western Pacific
Injuries	10 (15)	7 (8)	6 (12)	7 (8)	20 (13)	13 (8)
Obstetrical complications	4 (6)	1 (1)	1 (2)	(<0.5)	3 (2)	1 (1)
Cataracts and glaucoma	1 (2)	(<0.5)	1 (2)	1 (1)	3 (2)	2 (1)
Malignancies	2 (3)	4 (5)	1 (2)	8 (9)	6 (4)	10 (6)
Perinatal conditions	2 (3)	1 (1)	1 (2)	(<0.5)	3 (2)	1 (1)
Congenital anomalies	2 (3)	2 (2)	2 (4)	1 (1)	4 (3)	3 (2)
Other	4 (6)	3 (4)	3 (6)	5 (6)	9 (6)	7 (4)

Source: WHO 2002 and authors' estimates.

contrast, Europe has the highest rate of surgical DALYS related to malignancies—9 per 1,000 population.

All these estimates are debatable. Work is needed to obtain more valid, accurate, and reliable data, but in the meantime, we believe that our results represent a conservative and acceptable baseline estimate of the burden of surgical conditions against which prospectively gathered data for given interventions can be compared in order to assess the extent to which they address the burden. In addition, the burden needs to be monitored over time. Evidence suggests that the burden of intentional and unintentional injuries is rising, particularly in Sub-Saharan Africa and the Middle East. Some of the important contributing risk factors include (a) aging populations; (b) increased access to and use of mechanized vehicles and tools without commensurate improvements in roads, traffic control systems, or capacity for trauma care; and (c) persistent armed conflicts (Kaya and others 1999; Krug, Sharma, and Lozano 2000; Meyer 1998; Mock and others 1995, 1999; Nantulya and Reich 2002; Peden and Hyder 2002).

INTERVENTIONS

Both population-based strategies and personal sevices provided in community clinic, district, and tertiary hospitals are considered in this section.

Population-Based Strategies

Population-based approaches to the prevention of unintentional and intentional injuries are discussed in the chapters on those topics. A population-based approach to injury should not, however, be limited to injury prevention. Patients may survive their primary injuries only to become chronically disabled and a burden to their families and to society (Krug, Sharma, and Lozano 2000; Mock and others 1999; Nantulya and Reich 2002; Peden and Hyder 2002). The incidence and severity of the complications of survivable injury may be significantly lessened by the provision of adequate surgical care during prehospital care and initial hospitalization. No published data from developing countries are available, however, either to prove this plausible contention or to quantify the benefits of adequate initial surgical treatment. A strategy to prevent chronic disability arising from survivable injury requires well-coordinated services for resuscitation, evacuation, and early and expert operative management of the initial injury.

Many other surgical conditions that can be treated electively, such as hernias, hydroceles, and otitis media, are treated when they present with complications requiring emergency surgery. Thus, a pertinent question is whether treating such conditions electively would be more cost-effective, but no reliable data are available to answer this question positively or negatively.

Population-based strategies could also be applied to prevent or treat some musculoskeletal conditions. For example, the incidence of clubfoot is estimated at 1 or 2 per 1,000 live births, but in developing countries these children are typically brought in for orthopedic care when it is too late for effective nonsurgical conservative management (Ponseti 1999; Turco 1994). Because we have no baseline data for the burden of clubfoot and other musculoskeletal conditions, we are unable to quantify the DALYs that could be averted by comprehensive surgical care.

The following sections describe the organization of surgical services that we think would begin to provide coordinated surgical care in developing countries. The provision of surgical services in developing countries requires organizational structure and capacity at the level of community-based clinics, district hospitals, and tertiary care hospitals. Our concept of minimally adequate modules of surgical care is informed by our personal experiences, the experiences of others, and a recent World Health Organization report (WHO 2003). We recognize that to accommodate local needs and reality on the ground, any proposed plan to develop surgical services must be flexible. Table 67.4 presents our estimates of the needs for infrastructure, equipment and supplies, and workforce for the three levels of surgical care: community clinic, district hospital, and tertiary hospital.

Community Clinics

Table 67.4 shows resource and workforce requirements and types of surgical services a community clinic could provide for a population of around 20,000. We assume that surgical services in community clinics would be provided at no cost to patients. A cost-recovery system would be unlikely to succeed everywhere but, if implemented, should be equitable, with payments adjusted to patients' ability to pay. A mechanism for accountability and monitoring should be established to avoid the misuse of drugs and supplies. Simple patient records should be maintained, including outcomes of treatment and use of supplies. Even though the community clinic described here is what we think it should be as opposed to what we know it to be, our model may serve the needs of rural areas in developing countries and could provide a starting point for estimating costs.

District Hospitals

The next level of organization of surgical services is the district hospital, which in addition to providing primary care for the local population would also provide secondary-level surgical services and serve as a referral center for a number of community clinics in a defined region. In turn, the district hospital would ideally refer patients requiring complex surgical care to a tertiary-level hospital, but we recognize that such referral cannot always be achieved in practice because of transportation limitations, economic constraints, and prevalent social and cultural contexts. District hospitals vary in size from as small as 10 to 20 beds to as large as 200 to 300 beds and vary in their degree of sophistication in relation to diagnostic and therapeutic capabilities. For this discussion, we have arbitrarily chosen to focus on district hospitals with 100 beds or fewer.

Table 67.4 shows the infrastructure requirements for this type of hospital. Patients requiring more complex imaging studies and laboratory tests would be referred to the tertiary hospital.

To the extent possible, all equipment and supplies (table 67.4) should be standardized, and an efficient and reliable system for maintenance and replacement should be ensured. Operating room instruments and supplies should be available to enable the performance of laparotomy, thoracotomy, obstetrical and gynecological procedures, treatment of extremity fractures, skin grafting, and emergency burr hole of the skull. These instruments should be available at least in duplicate. Table 67.4 also shows workforce needs and the types of surgical procedures that may be performed in a district hospital.

The district hospital is assumed not only to serve as the referral hospital for community clinics, but also to coordinate the community clinics in its own region as a single operating unit, assuming responsibility for wireless communication, training the workforce, providing continuing medical education, and monitoring the quality and outcome of care. It would also provide primary care to its contiguous population.

Tertiary Hospitals

The tertiary hospital would function as the referral center for all complex surgical care in a region, country, or group of countries. Ideally, but depending on the country's resource constraints, it would provide the full range of care shown in table 67.4. The tertiary hospital would also provide primary surgical care for its local population and could take on the role of a teaching hospital for doctors, nurses, and other health care workers.

In the proposed organizational structure, the tertiary hospital is viewed as the top of a pyramid of surgical services, with several district hospitals referring patients requiring complex surgical care to the tertiary hospital. As such, it should also take the primary responsibility for coordinating and collaborating with all the district hospitals and community clinics in its area of responsibility to ensure that surgical care is available throughout the region and that well-functioning wireless communication and ambulance systems are available. If a regionalized system of separate ambulance services is not available, the tertiary hospital can provide the ambulance services required. Specialists in the tertiary hospital should provide telephone and electronic consultation for doctors and nurses in district hospitals. The tertiary hospital should also coordinate and monitor the quality of care in the region that serves as its referral base, undertake clinical outcome studies, and provide continuing medical education. In addition, it should be the main teaching hospital for medical students, nurses, and technicians, with the district hospitals and even the community clinics serving as clinical rotation sites for trainees. This organizational

Table 67.4 Resource Requirements for Surgical Services and Surgical Procedures by Level of Care

Category of requirement	Community clinic	100-bed district hospital	Tertiary hospital
Infrastructure	Weatherproof building (100 square meters) Storage space Clean water supply Power supply	Inpatient facility of 100 beds including several wards and an isolation ward Outpatient facility including an emergency room Operating rooms (at least two: one clean, one contaminated) Labor and delivery rooms Recovery room or intensive care unit Blood bank Pharmacy Clinical laboratory Radiology and ultrasonography suite	A major facility providing: • Full emergency services with advanced diagnostic services; • Inpatient wards for complex general medical and surgical care • Various types of specialty services • Several delivery rooms and operating rooms • One or more recovery rooms and intensive care units • Rehabilitation and occupational therapy facilities
Equipment and supplies	Furniture Refrigerator Blood pressure machine Minor surgical trays Sterile and burn dressings Autoclave Intravenous sets and solutions Bandages and splints Drugs: local anesthetics, nonsteroidal anti-inflammatory drugs, antibiotics, tetanus toxoid, silver nitrate ointment, oxytocin, magnesium sulfate Wireless communication equipment Materials for recordkeeping	Anesthetic machines and inhalation gases Monitors (electrocardiogram, blood pressure, pulse oximetry) Fully equipped operating room Fully equipped delivery room Fully equipped recovery room or intensive care unit Respirators and oxygen supply Blood products and intravenous fluids Basic microbiology equipment Pharmaceuticals (anesthetics, analgesics, antibiotics) Surgical materials (drapes, gowns, dressings, gloves) and other consumables (disposable equipment and devices)	All required equipment and supplies to undertake the range of routine and complex services provided
Human resources[a]	Nurse or nurse equivalent Skilled birth attendant Orderly	Nurses (20) Midwives (2–3) Anesthetists (2–3) Anesthesiologist (1)[b] Primary care physicians (4)[c] Obstetrician/gynecologist (1–2) General surgeons (2) Pharmacy assistants (2) Pharmacist (1)[b] Radiology technician (1) Radiologist (1) Physiotherapist (1)	Nurses (50) Midwives (5) Anesthetists (5) Anesthesiologists (3) Primary care physicians (10) Obstetricians/gynecologists (5) General surgeons (5) Orthopedic surgeon (1) Pharmacy assistants (2) Pharmacist (1) Radiology technicians (5) Radiologists (2) Physiotherapists (5) Neurosurgeon (1)[b] Cardiac surgeon[b] Reconstructive surgeon[b]

Table 67.4 Continued

Category of requirement	Community clinic	100-bed district hospital	Tertiary hospital
Services provided	Simple suturing and dressing of wounds	Emergency abdominal, thoracic, head injury	Full emergency service
	Incision and drainage of abscesses		Management of all complex general surgery
	Care of simple burns	Uncomplicated general surgical operations for hernias, anorectal conditions, and biliary tract disease	Full range of services in orthopedics, trauma, urology, otolaryngology, ophthalmology, and obstetrics and gynecology
	Control of hemorrhage	Surgical infection treatment and control	Basic (and, if resources permit, advanced) neurosurgery and cardiovascular surgery
	Splinting	Obstetrical (including surgery for complications)	Intensive care services
	Deliveries	Simple orthopedic care: extremity fractures, dislocations, and amputations	Major burn service
	Vacuum extraction and manual vacuum aspiration	Burn care	Radiology services including CT and MRI imaging and angiography
		Physiotherapy and occupational therapy	Full service clinical laboratory
		Education and training	Physiotherapy
			Occupational therapy
			Training of doctors, nurses, and midwives

Source: Authors.

a. Because of the variability in size and the complexity of services provided by tertiary hospitals, it is difficult to describe a standard tertiary hospital; the human resource needs given in the table represent what we think are minimally adequate.

b. Desirable, but not absolutely necessary.

c. Can be a general internist, general practitioner, or general pediatrician.

structure is ideally suited for the tertiary hospital to serve as the backbone of community-based surgical education. The extent to which this ideal function of a tertiary hospital can be implemented will depend on the financial and other resources available to the country.

Coordinated Model System for Surgical Care

The proposed system for surgical services requires the coordination and integration of the following:

- wireless communication
- continuing education programs
- regionalized supply system for equipment, essential drugs, and surgical materials
- ambulance service
- uniform data collection system
- coordinated and ongoing monitoring of quality and outcomes of care.

A wireless system of communication could render costly wired systems unnecessary and could connect community clinics, district hospitals, and tertiary hospitals in a dependable way that facilitates consultation and referral. A Web-based system of communication could be particularly important for mentoring and for providing continuing medical education. The Web can also be used to enhance contributions by volunteer surgeons, anesthesiologists, surgical specialists, nurses, and technicians

from around the world. Associations such as the International Surgical Association could develop a Web portal tied to national surgical associations to ensure greater success in this regard.

A regionalized system for the purchase and delivery of equipment and supplies is highly desirable. Such a system could ensure that all equipment and supplies were standardized and made available on demand in an efficient and predictable manner.

Ground ambulance services are essential for patient transfer. In some areas, collaboration with local taxi or bus services might offer the needed support. In some more economically advanced countries, tertiary hospitals might be able to provide ambulance services using fixed-wing aircraft or helicopters.

If the proposed model for a surgical system is to be developed, systems for ongoing data acquisition and for evaluation and monitoring should be built into the model. In this way, not only could information be captured, but also the quality and outcomes of care could be monitored on an ongoing basis.

COSTS AND COST-EFFECTIVENESS OF INTERVENTIONS

In today's resource-constrained world, policy makers increasingly need to be aware of the value of selective health care interventions. Cost-effectiveness analysis is one method that links inputs (costs) with the resulting health care gains measured along a common metric, usually using DALYs.

Even though an extensive body of literature examines the cost-effectiveness of a range of nonsurgical interventions in developing countries (Jha, Bangoura, and Ranson 1998), the literature examining surgical interventions in these countries is more sparse. Moreover, most of the available studies examine surgical interventions for specific conditions (Marseille 1996; Singh, Garner, and Floyd 2000). A common criticism of such studies is that they do not fully capture the choices policy makers face in real life. For example, policy makers must often choose between allocating resources for constructing several community clinics or a single district hospital, both of which provide a mix of surgical and nonsurgical services. Generally, the surgical ward in a district hospital will provide care for a wide range of conditions, such as trauma, childbirth, and abdominal conditions. We assume that for policy makers, knowing the cost-effectiveness of the surgical service, ward, or clinic (as an intervention) is more useful than information about the cost-effectiveness of each condition-specific surgical intervention. Unfortunately, no literature exists that examines the cost-effectiveness of a surgical service or ward. This section attempts to fill that void with respect to district hospitals and community clinics but not in relation to tertiary-level hospitals, which vary in size, available resources, and role from region to region, making it difficult to describe the cost-effectiveness of a prototypical tertiary hospital.

Method for Estimating Costs and DALYs

On the basis of the resource requirements listed in table 67.4, we developed cost estimates for each of the six regions defined by the World Bank. Table 67.5 details the assumptions and table 67.6 provides the regional costs. We defined the standard hospital in such a way as to facilitate comparisons across regions, conceptualizing it as a 100-bed hospital with a male ward and a female ward; two operating rooms; a recovery room, an intensive care unit, or both; an x-ray unit and an ultrasound machine; and a laboratory that can carry out basic blood chemistry tests, examine urine, and cross-match blood. This hospital also has an on-site laundry and kitchen and two vehicles to serve as ambulances. The staff consists of 6 doctors (4 primary care physicians, 1 obstetrician and gynecologist, and 1 general surgeon); 20 nurses; 6 midwives; 2 physiotherapists; and 6 orderlies. The costs of an anesthetist and x-ray technician have been included in the operating costs of the operating rooms and radiology area, respectively. The model assumes that the hospital averages 80 percent occupancy and that two-thirds of inpatients will be surgical cases.[1]

We defined a standard community clinic (see table 67.4) as a facility of 100 square meters serving a population of approximately 20,000, staffed by a nurse or nurse-substitute, a skilled birth attendant, and an orderly. Such a clinic treats approximately 4,000 surgical cases per year, with a *surgical case* being

defined as treatment of bruises, simple cuts requiring suturing, foreign body removal, drainage of abscesses, basic burn treatment, normal deliveries, and simple trauma.

As far as possible, we used standardized regional cost estimates provided to the authors. When such information was unavailable, we used our consensus judgment. Given the wide variation in costs between and within regions, we conducted sensitivity analyses to capture the range of possible outcomes. When more than one source of cost estimates was available, the mean of the estimates for that region were used as the best estimate and a high-low range was noted. However, in many cases, only a single cost estimate could be obtained, in which case the data provide a point estimate,[2] and we vary the cost estimate by ±20 percent to obtain a high-low range.

Our calculation of the number of DALYs averted was based on the work of McCord and Chowdhury (2003), who calculate the DALYs averted by a 50-bed hospital in Bangladesh, as described in box 67.1. We adjusted this figure to reflect the bed size of our standard district hospital. In the absence of region-specific data, we applied this figure to all six regions after making suitable adjustments. For the community clinic, we estimated that such a clinic averts approximately 200 DALYs per year as a result of surgical treatment, primarily from the incision and drainage of abscesses and the preliminary treatment of burns. Because these DALY estimates are based on a single source, we vary the estimate by ±20 percent to obtain a high-low range and apply these estimates across the six regions.

Results

Figure 67.1 presents the results of the cost per DALY averted calculations for a district hospital and community clinic. The low estimate represents the scenario in which the costs are the lowest and the DALYs averted are the highest—that is, the best-case scenario. In a similar vein, the high estimate is the worst-case scenario: the costs are highest and the DALY averted is the lowest.

The best estimates for cost per surgical DALY averted at a community health center (panel a of figure 67.1) hover in a narrow range between US$212 and US$241. The cost per surgical DALY gained at a district hospital is cheapest for Sub-Saharan Africa at US$33 (range of US$19 to US$102) and most expensive for Latin America and the Caribbean at US$94 (range of US$47 to US$164).

Standard economic costs can differ from costs actually incurred in service delivery, both because in practice not all time may need to be paid for (for example, hospitals may be able to economize on staff because relatives help care for patients) and because low-cost solutions may be found (for example, use of paramedical staff members in place of professionals). Box 67.2 describes some of these strategies and compares the standard economic cost presented above with the much lower financial cost of a nongovernmental organization (NGO) hospital.

Table 67.5 Costing Assumptions for District Hospital and Community Clinic

Category	Assumptions and comments
100-bed district hospital	
Inpatient hospital bed days	The estimate includes "hotel" costs (capital, salaries, overhead, building, equipment, and food) for a hospital running at 80 percent occupancy. Assumption: two-thirds of all cases seen are surgical and costs are adjusted accordingly.
Operating rooms	The estimate includes all operating room–related costs (surgeon, nurses, equipment, and so on). Assumption: the operating room is running for 8 hours/day, 5 days/week, 52 weeks/year.
Laboratory	Assumption: 16 new admissions/day, all of whom will require a laboratory test once during their hospital stay. Yearly costs have been adjusted to reflect the percentage of surgical cases.
X-ray	Assumption: 16 new admissions/day, of whom half will undergo an x-ray examination once during their hospital stay. Yearly costs have been adjusted to reflect the percentage of surgical cases.
Pharmacy	Assumption: all admitted patients will use US$10 worth of drugs during their stay. Yearly costs have been adjusted to reflect the percentage of surgical cases.
Blood transfusion	Assumption: 400 units of blood transfused/year.
Ambulance	The estimate includes 2 ambulances; 15 percent markup for freight, insurance, and distribution; US$500/year running costs added; ambulance depreciated over 9 years.
Staff	
Nurses	Assumption: nurses devote two-thirds of their time to surgical patients and costs have been adjusted accordingly.
Midwives	Assumption: midwives devote 100 percent of their time to surgical patients.
Doctors	These are the four doctors whose costs have not been included in the operating room costs listed above. Because they provide ward coverage, two-thirds of their costs are attributed to surgical patients.
Physiotherapists	Assumption: physiotherapists devote two-thirds of their time to surgery patients.
Orderlies	Assumption: six orderlies, each devoting two-thirds of their time to surgical activities.
Community clinic	
Building costs	The estimate includes costs of lighting and power. Assumption: building size is 100 square meters, 20-year straight-line depreciation is used; 25 percent of costs are attributed to surgical patients.
Water supply	Assumption: US$20 for water supply, of which 25 percent attributed to surgery.
Supplies	The estimate includes surgical trays, sterile and burn dressings, intravenous sets and cannulas, bandages, splints, and plaster of Paris for 4,000 patients. Assumption: local costs of US$5/patient.
Drugs	The estimate includes local anesthetics, nonsteroidal anti-inflammatory drugs, tetanus toxoid, silver nitrate, and basic antibiotics. Assumption: 4,000 patients, US$5/patient.
Furniture	The estimate includes autoclave, surgical light, examination table, and beds. Assumption: total cost US$2,000, straight-line depreciated for 10 years.
Refrigerator	The estimate includes locally manufactured refrigerator, straight-line depreciated for 5 years; surgical cost attribution only.
Wireless telephone	Assumption: US$200 cost; 25 percent attributed to surgery.
Staff	
Nurses and nurse-substitutes	Assumption: nurses devote 25 percent of time to surgical duties and costs adjusted accordingly.
Skilled birth attendants	Assumption: attendants devote 25 percent of time to surgical duties and costs adjusted accordingly.
Orderlies	Assumption: orderlies devote 25 percent of time to surgical duties and costs adjusted accordingly.

Sources: Authors.

Note: The figures for the district hospital should be viewed with particular caution. First, we used a single source of data for our assumptions. Had we used other data sources, the results could conceivably be different. Second, as a prototype we used a Sub-Saharan Africa district hospital that provides basic, low-tech surgical services. The provision of more sophisticated care can be expected to drive up the costs of care significantly.

Discussion

The data in figure 67.1, when compared with similar data for other services presented in this book, indicate providing basic surgical services is relatively cost-effective. Figure 67.1 also indicates that, from a surgical perspective, the costs per DALY averted at a community clinic tend to be higher than those averted at a district hospital despite the lower costs of a community clinic. Although these observations may be taken as evidence that surgical services are best provided at the district hospital level, this goal may be impossible to put into practice.

Table 67.6 Annual Costs Attributable to Surgical Patients in a District Hospital and a Community Clinic, Best Estimates *(2001 U.S. dollars)*

Category	East Asia and the Pacific	Europe and Central Asia	Latin America and the Caribbean	Middle East and North Africa	South Asia	Sub-Saharan Africa
100-bed district hospital						
Inpatient hospital bed days	204,042	363,277	640,071	498,904	156,826	148,635
Operating rooms	778,752	1,130,688	1,163,136	896,064	526,656	419,328
Laboratory	34,304	44,403	45,251	37,619	27,058	23,974
X-ray	18,578	26,788	27,501	21,276	12,700	10,195
Pharmacy	38,544	38,544	38,544	38,544	38,544	38,544
Blood transfusion	7,572	8,548	8,632	7,892	6,872	6,572
Ambulance	7,389	7,389	7,389	7,389	7,389	7,389
Staff						
Nurses	24,652	29,808	58,591	95,227	21,973	30,390
Midwives	11,100	13,422	26,382	42,870	9,894	13,680
Doctors	11,856	14,340	28,187	45,807	10,571	14,618
Physiotherapists	3,522	4,258	8,370	13,604	3,139	4,341
Orderlies	5,714	6,914	13,587	22,081	5,097	7,045
Total	1,146,026	1,688,380	2,065,641	1,727,277	826,718	874,551
Community clinic						
Building costs	1,280	1,321	601	1,324	569	574
Water supply	5	5	5	5	5	5
Supplies	20,000	20,000	20,000	20,000	20,000	20,000
Drugs	20,000	20,000	20,000	20,000	20,000	20,000
Furniture	200	200	200	200	200	200
Refrigerator	10	10	10	10	10	10
Wireless telephone	50	50	50	50	50	50
Staff						
Nurses and nurse-substitutes	667	807	1,585	2,577	595	822
Skilled birth attendants	667	807	1,585	2,577	595	822
Orderlies	361	437	858	1,394	322	445
Total	43,240	43,635	44,895	48,136	42,345	42,928

Sources: All district hospital costs and community clinic building and staff costs: DCPP guidelines; other community clinic costs: authors' estimates.

The type of surgical care provided at the community clinic level, though not resulting in a very large DALY gain, is nevertheless important. It is inconceivable to think of a community clinic that does not have facilities for minor foreign body removal, simple suturing of cuts and wounds, or splinting of simple fractures. Furthermore, community clinics' referral and primary treatment functions, which are hard to evaluate separately from the delivery of final treatment, are critical for many conditions, notably trauma.

Costs per surgical DALY averted at the district hospital level seem to fall into three groups. Sub-Saharan Africa and South Asia are the cheapest, with the best estimates of cost per surgical DALY averted ranging between US$33 and $US38; Europe and Central Asia, Middle East and North Africa, and Latin America and the Caribbean seem to be the most expensive, with the cost per surgical DALY averted ranging between US$77 and US$94; and East Asia and the Pacific falls in the middle. This finding indicates that, from the perspective of providing surgical care, a district hospital is an exceptional "buy" in Sub-Saharan Africa and South Asia, both areas with high disease burdens. Coupled with evidence that district hospitals are comparatively underfunded compared with national (tertiary) hospitals (Fiedler, Wight, and Schmidt 1999), a prima facie case exists for increasing support for

---

Box 67.1

Estimation of the DALYs Averted by a Small Hospital in a Developing Country

The DALY estimates in this chapter are based on a report from a 40-bed nongovernmental hospital in rural Bangladesh in 1995 (McCord and Chowdhury 2003). Obviously this experience was localized from one hospital, in one country, at one time, but it is the only analysis available from such a hospital that estimates effectiveness using DALYs or any other measure of the effect of a hospital on the disease burden. The hope is that other similar studies done in a variety of hospital situations will permit generalizing with more confidence, but our personal experience leads us to believe that the disease pattern presented to small district hospitals in poor countries is remarkably constant, especially for surgical conditions.

McCord and Chowdhury (2003) present the methods for calculating DALYs in detail. They reviewed all discharges and deaths every week for three months, confirmed the discharge diagnosis by means of a chart review, and estimated the percentage chance that the hospital stay had prevented death or disability. The review covered all patients discharged, classifying them as medical, surgical, obstetrical and gynecological, or pediatric. Of the discharges, 62 percent were of surgical and obstetrical and gynecological patients. Of the DALYs, 21 percent of those averted were for surgical patients and 61 percent from obstetrical and gynecological patients. Eighty-nine percent of the estimated DALYs averted were generated by averting premature death, and only 11 percent by preventing serious disability. Of the 192 surgical operations, 118 were emergencies. Of 137 obstetrical patients, 81 had complicated deliveries, complications of abortion, or ectopic pregnancies.

Source: Authors.

Our estimates of the risk of death or serious disability were based on tables McCord and Chowdhury created and were necessarily arbitrary, but we believe they are extremely conservative. For example

- If the chance of death or disability was less than 5 percent, it was considered to be 0 percent. Because normal out-of-hospital deliveries had less than a 5 percent chance of death or disability, normal deliveries in the hospital made no contribution to the estimated DALYs averted.
- A cesarean section for obstructed labor was estimated at 10 percent averted risk for the infant and 0 percent for the mother.
- A cesarean for transverse lie was estimated at 90 percent averted risk for the infant and 90 percent for the mother.
- An appendectomy for nonruptured appendicitis was estimated at 10 percent averted risk, because many cases of appendicitis respond to antibiotics outside the hospital setting.
- An appendectomy for a ruptured appendix with generalized peritonitis was estimated at 90 percent averted risk.
- An elective herniorrhaphy for a small hernia was estimated at 0 percent averted risk.
- A herniorrhaphy for a large, disabling hernia was estimated at 80 percent averted risk.
- A herniorrhaphy for a strangulated hernia that did not reduce with conservative management was estimated at 80 percent averted risk.

---

district hospitals in developing countries. However, those providing such support have to be cognizant of realities on the ground, especially political realities, because they have a significant effect on the direction of change (Blas and Limbambala 2001).

Data on the cost-effectiveness of surgical interventions for specific conditions in developing countries are scarce. One notable exception is for the surgical treatment of cataracts (removal of the opaque lens with or without the insertion of an intraocular implant). Blindness from cataracts is a significant public health problem in many developing countries, and as their populations age, estimates indicate that by 2020 more

than 40 million people will be blind or almost blind because of cataracts (Brian and Taylor 2001). Box 67.3 describes a successful program in India.

RESEARCH AND DEVELOPMENT AGENDA

The literature on surgical care in developing countries is so meager that insufficient data are available to formulate an agenda for research and development. Hence, of necessity, the research that needs to be done is extremely basic, much of it

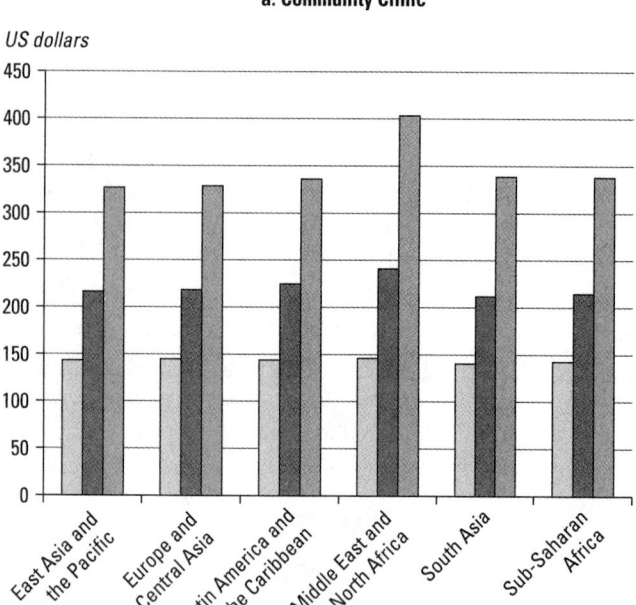

a. Community Clinic

US dollars

Legend: Low estimate | Best estimate | High estimate

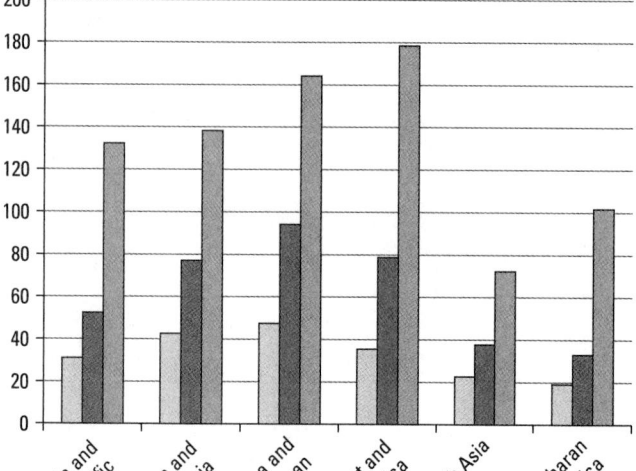

b. District Hospital

US dollars

Legend: Low estimate | Best estimate | High estimate

Source: Authors' calculations using costs in table 67.6 and methods for estimating DALYs averted described in box 67.1.

Figure 67.1 Cost per Surgical DALY Averted for a Community Clinic and a District Hospital

information gathering. The following are some of the areas that require investment in research and development:

- Estimates are needed of the burden of disease that requires surgical intervention along with a determination of region-

specific DALYs that can be averted by means of surgical intervention. We have applied the DALYs averted from a single study in a developing country (McCord and Chowdhury 2003) to other regions, a procedure that negates regional differences in disease incidence, health care–seeking behavior, case mix, and clinical practice variations. In addition, the calculation of DALYs averted should ideally be adjusted for region-specific life expectancy and disability weights.

- Estimation of costs, both at a facility and regional level, is needed, including reducing variability in estimation methods (Adam and Koopmanschap 2003). In addition, multiple estimates of costs are needed. For example, Mulligan and others (2003) derive their operating room costs from a single study of ambulatory surgery in Colombia (Shephard and others 1993). Even though they made adjustments to reflect regional characteristics, further research is required to validate their results, especially as they apply to different settings in different countries.

- Better surgical data collection and analysis tools critical to needs assessment should be designed.

- Development of appropriate surgical care models for all levels of care based on local and regional characteristics and surgical needs would be useful.

- Cost-effectiveness and cost-benefit analyses of health systems implementation need to be determined, as do the policy implications of creating the surgical care model proposed in this chapter. The evaluation of surgery as a prevention strategy in public health should include cost-effectiveness analysis of adequate, prompt, initial surgical treatment of injury to prevent chronic disability from poorly diagnosed and treated survivable injuries and of elective treatment of hernia, hydrocele, otitis media, cataract, and clubfoot to prevent complications and disability.

- The surgical workforce in developing countries requires more in-depth study to look at the mixes of workers needed, the level of training required for the widely varying local situations of district hospitals, and the role for part-time surgical talent. The thesis is that volunteer doctors, nurses, and anesthesiologists who now contribute considerably to surgical care in developing countries in a relatively unstructured fashion could do so more effectively and in a manner that could help create sustainable local surgical workforces if a well-coordinated system with extensive information and communication support could be developed. This concept merits in-depth study. If a well-planned, Web-coordinated, global, highly integrated system could be developed, health care volunteers around the world could be organized strategically so as to deliver not only surgical care, but also training of local surgical workforces. The emphasis on training is crucial and would mitigate the complaints often heard that surgical volunteers too often contribute to the care of individual patients but fail to leave behind a

Surgical Cost in a Bare-Bones Hospital

The estimated economic costs in this chapter assume staffing and service levels generally derived from World Health Organization recommendations for developing countries (Mulligan and others 2003), but in many places, surgical services are delivered in much simpler and less expensive facilities. Independent project hospitals (NGO hospitals) often operate on remarkably tight budgets. Private hospitals, often set up in private houses by individual surgeons, use locally trained staff with minimal "hotel" service. Extremely poor countries operate hospitals with a cost per patient per day of US$10 or less simply because they cannot afford more. Such hospitals achieve financial savings in several ways:

- Unpaid family members provide personal nursing care and food, eliminating the need for a kitchen and many trained nurses.
- Locally trained staff members substitute for professionally trained personnel.
- Many staff members have duplicate functions. In the operating room the same person may work as surgical assistant, scrub nurse, and orderly who cleans instruments or transports patients.
- Day staff members cover night calls for emergencies.

- Specialized services are provided by general physicians or technicians trained to do surgery or give anesthesia.
- Laboratory tests and x-rays are used sparingly. The only laboratory procedure for an obstetrical patient could be a hemoglobin determination.
- Only basic medicines are provided. More expensive or complicated supplies are purchased outside the hospital by the family.

For one independent, nongovernmental hospital in Bangladesh, we were able to obtain the actual financial cost of all aspects of hospital operations during a three-month period. These costs included salaries, supplies, hotel costs, and depreciated cost of equipment and buildings, as well as an overhead estimate to allocate a share of the total project cost for administration, electricity, transportation, and so on. Separating the surgical service costs for 3 months, extrapolated to 12 months and a 100-bed hospital, we come up with a much lower total cost than the low estimate in this chapter for the economic costs of a model district hospital, as shown in the table below. Part of the difference is caused by differing cost definitions (financial versus economic), but a good part is owing to the use of low-cost approaches to the delivery of surgical care.

Category	NGO hospital (2001 US$)	District Hospital in South Asia (2001 US$)
Inpatient bed days	110,936	156,826
Operating time	178,508	526,656
Laboratory	11,788	27,058
X-Ray	6,676	12,700
Pharmacy	n.a[a]	38,544
Blood transfusion	3,858	6,872
Ambulance	n.a.[a]	7,389
Staff	n.a.[b]	50,673
Total	311,766	826,718

Source: NGO hospital: McCord and Chowdhury 2003; district hospital: table 67.6.
n.a. = not available.
a. Included in overhead, which is added to each cost center.
b. Included in total cost of ward and operating room.

mechanism for sustaining surgical care when they have left. Those volunteers who come from the high-tech world of modern surgery should realize that the latest technology is often more of a burden and diversion than a help in poor countries. Convincing demonstrations of how much can be done without recourse to CT scans, ultrasound, and video-assisted surgery could be the most useful contribution a visitor could make.

Box 67.3

Success Story: Cataract Surgery in India

Prevention strategies aimed at known risk factors, such as tobacco use and exposure to the sun, are unlikely to have a significant effect on the need for surgical treatment of cataracts in the foreseeable future (Ellwein and Kupfer 1995). The benefits of cataract surgery have been well documented in many developing countries.

In 1993–94, with a World Bank credit of US$118 million, India expanded cataract surgery coverage to the disadvantaged with the goal of reducing the prevalence of blindness. District blindness control societies were set up and given the flexibility of financing different providers of cataract surgery services to low-income groups at the district level (Rose 1997). Mobile camps were a strategy adopted for providing cheap and efficient cataract surgery in rural districts. Because of these efforts, cataract surgery nationally increased from 1.2 million surgeries in 1991–92 to 2.7 million in 1996–97. Singh, Garner, and Floyd (2000) analyze the cost-effectiveness of publicly funded options

for delivering cataract surgery in Mysore, India, by assessing outcomes in a systematic sample of patients operated on in 1996–97. Patient satisfaction was 51 percent among those operated on in government mobile camps, 82 percent among those treated at the medical college hospital, and 85 percent among those treated in nongovernmental hospitals. Cost-effectiveness was US$97 per patient treated for the mobile camps, US$176 for the state medical college hospital, and US$54 for nongovernmental hospitals. Javitt (1993) estimates the cost of cataract surgery in India at less than US$25 per DALY averted.

As the World Health Organization (Brian and Taylor 2001) has stressed, successful and sustainable surgical treatment of cataracts is linked to a spectrum of other equally important activities, including ongoing training of surgeons, nurses, and administrators; reliable and affordable supply chains; and equipment purchase and maintenance.

Source: Authors.

CONCLUSIONS

The inclusion of this chapter indicates the evolving appreciation that surgery has a role to play in public health strategies. Previous concerns that surgery is a curative intervention performed in expensive, high-tech hospitals precluded appreciation of the potential role of surgery in public health. Public health specialists now recognize not only that surgery has a preventive role, but also that surgical treatment provided in low-tech community hospitals is cost-effective. In addition, a significant number of surgical procedures, including cesarean sections and other abdominal operations, can be successfully performed by surgical technicians (Jamisse and others 2004; Pereira and others 1996).

Surgery has an important role as a public health strategy in at least four areas:

- in the prevention of death and chronic disability in injured patients by the provision of timely, expert, and complete initial surgical treatment
- in the timely surgical intervention in obstructed labor, in pre- and postpartum hemorrhage, and in other obstetrical complications
- in the provision of competent surgery to treat a wide range of emergency abdominal and nonabdominal conditions

- in the surgical care of several elective conditions that have a significant effect on the quality of life, such as cataract, otitis media, clubfoot, hernias, and hydroceles.

Few published data are available to enable reliable estimates of either the burden of surgical diseases or the cost-effectiveness of surgical treatments in a region-specific manner to help policy makers and voluntary groups. This area merits a great deal of attention in relation to research and development. Nevertheless, the clear conclusion is that surgery must be considered a public health priority.

NOTES

1. This structure is based on the authors' personal experiences of practicing in developing countries. We have defined *surgical cases* to include deliveries and cesarean sections.
2. For example, operating room costs are based on the results of a single study by Shepard and others (1993).

REFERENCES

Adam, T., and M. A. Koopmanschap. 2003. "Cost-Effectiveness Analysis: Can We Reduce Variability in Costing Methods?" *International Journal of Technological Assessment of Health Care* 19 (2): 407–20.

Armandola, E. 2003. "Conference Report: Global Vaccines—What Are the Challenges? Highlights from the Viral Vaccine Meeting, October 25–28, 2003, Barcelona, Spain." *Medscape General Medicine* 5 (4): 29.

Bickler, S. W., and H. Rode. 2002. "Surgical Services for Children in Developing Countries." *Bulletin of the World Health Organization* 80 (10): 829–35.

Blas, E., and M. Limbambala. 2001. "The Challenge of Hospitals in Health Sector Reform: The Case of Zambia." *Health Policy and Planning* 16 (Suppl. 2): 29–43.

Brian, G., and H. Taylor. 2001. "Cataract Blindness: Challenges for the 21st Century." *Bulletin of the World Health Organization* 79 (3): 249–56.

Dandona, L., R. Dandona, T. J. Naduvilath, C. A. McCarty, P. Mandel, M. Srinivas, and others. 1999. "Population-Based Assessment of the Outcome of Cataract Surgery in an Urban Population in Southern India." *American Journal of Ophthalmology* 127 (6): 650–58.

Dayan, G. H., L. Cairns, A. Mtonga, V. Nguyen, and P. Strebel. 2004. "Cost-Effectiveness of Three Different Vaccination Strategies against Measles in Zambian Children." *Vaccine* 22 (3–4): 475–84.

Ellwein, L. B., and C. Kupfer. 1995. "Strategic Issues in Preventing Cataract Blindness in Developing Countries." *Bulletin of the World Health Organization* 73 (5): 681–89.

Fiedler, J. L., J. B. Wight, and R. M. Schmidt. 1999. "Risk Adjustment and Hospital Cost-Based Resource Allocation, with an Application to El Salvador." *Social Science Medicine* 48 (2): 197–212.

Hilton, P. 2003 "Vesico-Vaginal Fistulas in Developing Countries." *International Journal of Gynecology and Obstetrics* 82 (3): 285–95.

Hyder, A. A., and M. Peden. 2003. "Inequality and Road Traffic Injuries: Call for Action." *Lancet* 362 (9401): 2034–35.

Jamisse, L., and F. Songane, and others. 2004. "Reducing Maternal Mortality in Mozambique: Challenges, Failures, Successes and Lessons Learned." *Int J Gynaecol Obstet* 85 (2): 203–12.

Jat, A. A., M. R. Khan, H. Zafar, A. J. Raja, Q. Hoda, R. Rehmani, and others. 2004. "Peer Review Audit of Trauma Deaths in a Developing Country." *Asian Journal of Surgery* 27 (1): 58–64.

Javitt, J. C. 1993. "The Cost-Effectiveness of Restoring Sight." *Archives of Ophthalmology* 111(12): 1615.

Jha, P., O. Bangoura, and K. Ranson. 1998. "The Cost-Effectiveness of Forty Health Interventions in Guinea." *Health Policy Planning* 13 (3): 249–62.

Kaya, E., H. Ozguc, R. Tokyay, and O. Yunuk. 1999. "Financial Burden of Trauma Care on a University Hospital in a Developing Country." *Journal of Trauma* 47 (3): 572–75.

Krug, E. G., G. K. Sharma, and Q. Lozano. 2000. "The Global Burden of Injuries." *American Journal of Public Health* 90 (4): 523–26.

Marseille, E. 1996. "Cost-Effectiveness of Cataract Surgery in a Public Health Eye Care Programme in Nepal." *Bulletin of the World Health Organization* 74 (3): 319–24.

McCord, C., and Q. Chowdhury. 2003. "A Cost-Effective Small Hospital in Bangladesh: What It Can Mean for Emergency Obstetric Care." *International Journal of Gynaecology and Obstetrics* 81 (1): 83–92.

Meyer, A. 1998. "Death and Disability from Injury: A Global Challenge." *Journal of Trauma* 44 (1): 1–12.

Moalosi, G., K. Floyd, J. Phatshwane, T. Moeti, N. Binkin, and T. Kenyon. 2003. "Cost-Effectiveness of Home-Based Versus Hospital Care for Chronically Ill Tuberculosis Patients, Francistown, Botswana." *International Journal of Tuberculosis and Lung Diseases* 7 (9 Suppl. 1): S80–85.

Mock, C. N. 2003. "Improving Prehospital Trauma Care in Rural Areas of Low Income Countries." *Trauma* 54 (6): 1197–98.

Mock, C. N., F. Abantanga, P. Cummings, and T. D. Koepsell. 1999. "Incidence and Outcome of Injury in Ghana: A Community-Based Survey." *Bulletin of the World Health Organization* 77 (12): 955–62.

Mock, C. N., E. Adzotor, D. Denno, E. Conklin, and F. Rivara. 1995. "Admissions for Injury at a Rural Hospital in Ghana: Implications for Prevention in the Developing World." *American Journal of Public Health* 85 (7): 927–31.

Mulligan, J., J. A. Fox-Rushby, T. Adam, B. Johns, and A. Mills. 2003. *Unit Costs of Health Care Inputs in Low and Middle Income Regions*. Working Paper 9, Disease Control Priorities Project. Bethesda, MD.

Murray, C. J. L., and A. D. Lopez, eds. 1996. *The Global Burden of Disease: A Comprehensive Assessment of Mortality and Disability from Diseases, Injuries, and Risk Factors in 1990 and Projected to 2020*. Cambridge, MA: Harvard University Press.

Nantulya, V. M., and M. R. Reich. 2002. "The Neglected Epidemic: Road Traffic Injuries in Developing Countries." *British Medical Journal* 324: 1139–41.

Neilson, J. P., T. Lavender, S. Quenby, S. Wray. 2003. "Obstructed Labor." *British Medical Bulletin* 67: 191–204.

Olumide, F., A. Adedeji, and A. O. Adesola. 1976. "Intestinal Obstruction in Nigerian Children." *Journal of Pediatric Surgery* 11 (2): 195–204.

Peden, M., and A. A. Hyder. 2002. "Road Traffic Injuries Are a Global Health Problem." *British Medical Journal* 324 (7346): 1153–54.

Pereira C., A. Bugalho, S. Bergstrom, F. Vaz, and M. Cotiro. 1996. "A Comparative Study of Caesarian Deliveries by Assistant Medical Officers and Obstetricians in Mozambique." *British Journal of Obstetrics and Gynecology* 103 (6): 508–12.

Ponseti, I. V. 1999. *Idiopathic Clubfoot*. New York: Oxford University Press.

Rahman, G. A., and I. A. Mungadi. 2000. "Gangrenous Bowel in Nigerians." *Central African Journal of Medicine* 46 (12): 321–24.

Rose, J. 1997. "National Program for Control of Blindness." *Indian Journal of Community Health* 3: 5–9.

Ruff, T. A. 1999. "Immunization Strategies for Viral Diseases in Developing Countries." *Review of Medical Virology* 9 (2): 121–38.

Shepard, D. S., J. Walsh, W. Munar, L. Rose, R. Guerrero, L. F. Cruz, and others. 1993. "Cost-Effectiveness of Ambulatory Surgery in Cali, Colombia." *Health Policy Plan* 8 (2): 136–42.

Singh, A. J., P. Garner, and K. Floyd. 2000. "Cost-Effectiveness of Public-Funded Options for Cataract Surgery in Mysore, India." *Lancet* 355 (9199): 180–84.

Smith, A., and S. Hatcher. 1992. "Preventing Deafness in Africa's Children." *African Health* 15 (1): 33–35.

Turco, V. 1994. "Present Management of Idiopathic Clubfoot." *Journal of Paediatric Orthopedics. Part B* 3: 149–54.

Whitney, C. G., and L. K. Pickering. 2002. "The Potential of Pneumococcal Conjugate Vaccines for Children." *Pediatric Infectious Diseases Journal* 21 (10): 961–70.

WHO (World Health Organization). 2002. *World Health Report 2002: Reducing Risks, Promoting Healthy Life*. Geneva: WHO.

———. 2003. *Surgical Care in a District Hospital*. Geneva: WHO.

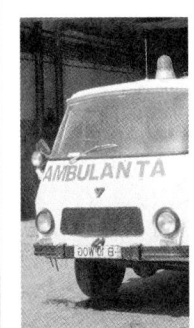

Chapter **68**

Emergency Medical Services

Olive C. Kobusingye, Adnan A. Hyder, David Bishai, Manjul
Joshipura, Eduardo Romero Hicks, and Charles Mock

INTRODUCTION

Emergency medical conditions typically occur through a sudden insult to the body or mind, often through injury, infection, obstetric complications, or chemical imbalance; they may occur as the result of persistent neglect of chronic conditions. Emergency medical services (EMS) to treat these conditions include rapid assessment, timely provision of appropriate interventions, and prompt transportation to the nearest appropriate health facility by the best possible means to enhance survival, control morbidity, and prevent disability (see table 68.1). The goal of effective EMS is to provide emergency medical care to all who need it. Advances in medical care and technology in recent decades have expanded the parameters of what had been the traditional domain of emergency services. These services, no longer limited to actual in-hospital treatment from arrival to stabilization, now include prehospital care and transportation.

Despite the best efforts of primary care providers and public health planners, not every emergency is preventable. Emergency medical care is needed in diverse circumstances: prospective patients range from rural farmers or fishers whose most common mode of transportation may be canoes or animal-drawn carts, to factory workers living in densely populated urban slums, to residents of high-income cities and suburbs. Actual provision of emergency care may range from delivery using trained emergency professionals to delivery by laypeople and taxi drivers. Developing strategies to meet the range of needs posed by such diverse circumstances will require innovation and a reorientation of public health planning.

A number of misconceptions about emergency care are often used as a rationale for giving it low priority in the health sector, especially in low-income countries. These ideas include equating emergency care with ambulance transportation, neglecting the role of the community and facility care provided, and assuming that emergency departments and physicians are the only acute care resources. Such a narrow view ignores the important contributions of other disciplines, skills, and personnel. Perhaps the most common misperception is that emergency medical care is inherently expensive and requires high-technology interventions as opposed to simple and effective strategies.

Emergency care, which may be delivered in crisis situations with poor planning and ineffective use of resources, may be inefficient. In many countries, few resources are set aside for possible emergencies, and when situations that demand emergency care arise, they precipitate hurried and costly resource deployment. Efforts to improve emergency care, however, do not necessarily increase costs. This chapter shows that improved organization and planning for emergency care can be done at a reasonable cost and lead to more appropriate use of resources, improved care, and better outcomes (White, Williams, and Greenberg 1996). This chapter does not address nonacute conditions, even though emergency care is often the only recourse for people with nonemergency conditions because of the failure of these other components of the system (see figure 68.1).

Table 68.1 Overview of Emergency Medical Services

	Acute event	On-site management	Transportation	Health facility care
Role of EMS	Recognition	Triage, stabilization, or both	Safe and efficient transportation	Prompt, appropriate, and quality care
Key issues	Surveillance and identification	Trained personnel, equipment	Safe transportation, equipment, referral system	Personnel, equipment, organization of services

Source: Authors.

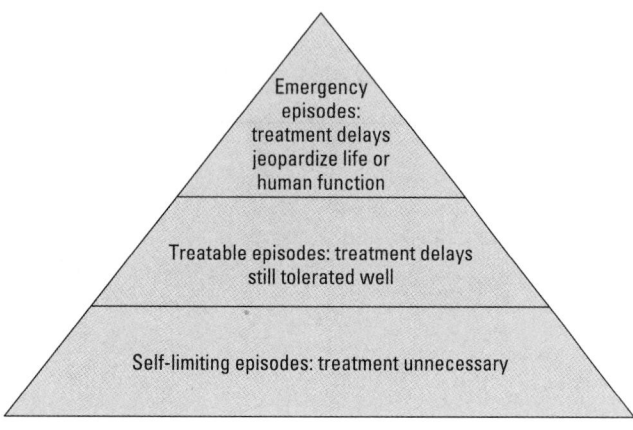

Source: Authors.

Figure 68.1 The Emergency Medical Care Pyramid

Definitions

The current literature is often inconsistent in the use and interpretation of terminology. Accordingly, the specific terms used in this chapter are defined as follows:

- *Emergency care.* Emergency medical care is that care delivered in the first few hours after the onset of an acute medical or obstetric problem or the occurrence of an injury, including care delivered inside a fixed facility.
- *Paramedical personnel.* Paramedical personnel refers to all persons with medical training who are involved in the care and transportation of patients in need of emergency medical care. The length and quality of training vary, from highly specialized personnel with capabilities for advanced life support to those with simple first-aid training and limited field experience.
- *Hospital.* A hospital is a geographically fixed facility in which personnel with some acceptable level of training deliver emergency medical care. The distinctions between a clinic, health center, and hospital are unclear, and the presence or absence of a doctor is not a determining factor in this distinction. A range of facilities from small, basic units up to tertiary care hospitals provides an increasing level of capability for emergency and other care.
- *Triage.* Triage is the screening of patients in the field or in the receiving area of a fixed facility to determine their relative priority for treatment. Triage, which is usually necessary

in the occurrence of mass casualties, may be necessary whenever a large number of patients requiring emergency care present at the same time. It typically entails categorizing patients into three groups: those very unlikely to survive, even with treatment; those whose conditions are minor and who will recover without emergency care; and those with potentially lethal conditions who are likely to survive if they receive timely emergency care. Patients in the last category form the highest priority for emergency care.

- *Stabilization.* A distinction is often made between initial emergency care and stabilization on one hand and definitive medical care on the other. Initial emergency care and stabilization are usually considered the domain of mobile EMS; lower levels of the health care system (for example, clinics and smaller hospitals); and the emergency departments of any fixed facility. Definitive care is usually considered the domain of the hospital and of larger facilities and implies the resolution of the condition needing treatment. However, the distinction is somewhat arbitrary; a more accurate approach is to view care as a continuum. Many of the elements of early care delivered in the course of emergency treatment, whether in the field or in fixed facilities, can be considered definitive (McCord and Chowdhury 2003; McCord and others 2001).

Burden of Disease

Investing in emergency medical care should become a priority. Emergency medical systems address a diverse set of diseases that span the spectrum of communicable infections, noncommunicable conditions, obstetrics, and injuries. All of these conditions may present to the EMS in their acute stages (for example, diabetic hypoglycemia, septicemia, premature labor, or asthma), or they are acute in their natural presentation (for example, myocardial infarction, acute hemorrhage, or injuries). Accordingly, defining the burden of disease addressed by EMS can be problematic.

Malaria causes 300 to 500 million acute episodes worldwide annually and results in an estimated 1 million deaths, mostly in Sub-Saharan Africa. Effective emergency care can avert these deaths, as well as those from acute respiratory and diarrheal diseases in children and from noncommunicable diseases such as diabetes, hypertension, and other cardiovascular diseases. In addition to the acute presentation of chronic conditions, the lack of access to medical care and lack of sustained effective treatment means that subacute episodes and flare-ups may be life threatening. Early recognition can prevent the emergency precipitated by infectious disease and many other medical conditions or can limit the effects.

More than 500,000 maternal deaths occur each year; 95 percent of these deaths are in low-income countries where emergency care is often lacking. It is estimated that 15 percent of all pregnant women experience a potentially life-threatening condition and will need emergency care. Prenatal screening methods alone may not be effective in reducing this risk ratio. Although identifying risk factors for acute complications is easy, identifying which of the at-risk women will actually develop a life-threatening condition is not possible (Graham 1997). The only way to prevent the deaths is by ensuring access to emergency obstetric care for all pregnant women.

Injuries were responsible for 21.7 percent of global deaths and 31.1 percent of disability-adjusted life years (DALYs) lost in 2001 (WHO 2002). Because both unintentional injuries (chapter 39) and injuries caused by interpersonal violence (chapter 40) are by definition acute events, nearly all require emergency care (see table 68.2). In 2001, more than 80 percent of all deaths attributable to injury were in low-income countries. Most injuries attributable to violence involve a predominantly young and productive population (WHO 2002) that is resilient and can respond well to appropriate emergency care.

The conditions listed in table 68.2 represent 45 percent of all deaths and 36 percent of the disease burden (including disability) that occur in low-income countries. The numbers represent a conservative estimate of the potential burden, because they do not include all the conditions that could benefit from emergency care and they do not include data from high-income countries.

INTERVENTIONS FOR EMERGENCY CARE: SYSTEMS, STRUCTURES, AND ORGANIZATION

Emergency care must be appreciated as an entire system with interdependent components. These components include prehospital care, transportation, and hospital care. Each component is important, but all of them must work together to make a lasting effect on the health of a population. The organization and operation of the prehospital care system will vary by country, but it should be linked to the local hospitals or facilities where patients are taken. When prehospital transportation is poor or absent, deaths occur that could have been prevented even by inexpensive procedures (Mock and others 1998). For example, the majority of maternal deaths may fall into this category. Poor quality of care at the hospitals will lead to inhospital deaths and may eventually discourage communities that might have the capacity to promptly transfer patients to such facilities (Leigh and others 1997; Prevention of Maternal Mortality Network 1995). Skilled and motivated personnel, appropriate supplies, pharmaceuticals, equipment, coordination, and management oriented to the needs of the critically ill

Table 68.2 Burden of Diseases Potentially Addressed by EMS in Low- and Middle-Income Countries
(2001, all ages, both sexes)

Group	Disease	Deaths (thousands)	DALYs (thousands)	DALY rates/1,000 population	YLL (thousands)	YLD (thousands)
I: Communicable	Diarrheal diseases	1,777	58,697	11.25	50,883	7,835
	Childhood cluster[a]	1,362	43,131	8.26	40,506	2,624
	Maternal conditions	507	26,383	5.05	13,363	13,020
	Meningitis	169	5,475	1.05	4,343	1,131
	Malaria	1,207	39,961	7.66	35,461	4,438
II: Chronic	Diabetes	757	15,804	3.03	10,140	5,661
	Hypertensive heart	760	9,969	1.91	9,077	888
	Ischemic heart	5,699	71,882	13.77	67,925	3,921
	Cerebrovascular	4,608	62,669	12.01	51,539	11,100
	Asthma	205	11,514	2.21	3,799	7,714
III: Injuries	Unintentional	3,214	113,235	21.70	73,140	40,104
	Intentional	1,501	42,615	8.16	34,374	8,242
	Total EMS related	**21,766**	**501,335**	**96.06**	**394,550**	**106,678**
	Percentage of LMIC total	45	36		43	22

Source: Global Burden of Disease Project 2001.
YLL = years of life lost to premature mortality; YLD = years lived with disability; LMICs = low- and middle-income countries.
a. Pertussis, poliomyelitis, diphtheria, measles, and tetanus.

all contribute to make emergency care effective in reducing death and disability.

Prehospital Care

Prehospital care encompasses the care provided from the community (scene of injury, home, school, or other location) until the patient arrives at a formal health care facility capable of giving definitive care. This care should comprise basic and proven strategies and the most appropriate personnel, equipment, and supplies needed to assess, prioritize, and institute interventions to minimize the probability of death or disability. Most effective strategies are basic and inexpensive, and the lack of high-tech interventions should not deter efforts to provide good care. Even where resources allow them, the more-invasive procedures performed by physicians in some prehospital settings, such as intravenous access and fluid infusion or intubations, do not appear to improve outcomes, and evidence suggests that they may, in fact, be detrimental to outcomes (Liberman and others 2003; Sampalis and others 1994, 1995, 1997).

Prehospital care should be simple, sustainable, and efficient. Because resource availability varies greatly among and within countries, different tiers of care are recognized. Where no formal prehospital system exists, the first tier of prehospital care may be composed of laypeople in the community who have been taught basic techniques of first aid. Recruiting and training particularly motivated citizens who often confront emergencies, such as drivers of public transportation, to function as prehospital care providers can add to this resource.

The second tier comprises paramedical personnel who use dedicated vehicles and equipment and are usually able to get to patients and take them to hospitals within the shortest possible time. This second tier may involve the performance of advanced procedures, the administration of intravenous and other medications by physician or nonphysician providers, or both. This care is not always available in low-income countries; few trained personnel and inadequate funding make round-the-clock coverage impossible. Although providing advanced life-saving measures in the prehospital environment may be beneficial in some cases, these benefits may be negated if such measures divert scarce resources from more basic interventions that can benefit far larger numbers of patients (Hauswald and Yeoh 1997). In most low- and middle-income countries of Africa, Asia, and Latin America, high maternal and child mortality are linked to inadequate emergency care, especially poor access to quality hospital care. In these settings, it is imperative that resources be integrated, instead of one system for injuries and another for obstetric emergencies.

Personnel. Most of the world's population does not have access to formal prehospital care. No personnel are employed for the sole purpose of dealing with medical emergencies outside of hospitals, and no transportation is dedicated to the task of getting patients in need of emergency care into hospitals. There is a paucity of literature on the effect of first responders, except for one study that evaluated a program to train a core group of paramedics, who then trained thousands of lay first responders in northern Iraq and Cambodia. No data are available on the effectiveness of lay responders compared with the more trained paramedics.

The following discussion introduces a scenario in which the observed mortality rate reduction could be achieved in a developing country's health system by a small group of paramedics working together with a large group of trained lay responders. The scenario uses only emergencies caused by trauma, although it is expected that both the paramedics and the lay first responders would also save lives from medical or obstetric emergencies. Existing studies have not been large enough to document these effects, and they are not included in the estimates of cost-effectiveness.

Trained Lay Responders A case is made for training lay persons able to recognize threatening conditions—whether obstetric, traumatic, or medical. Cultural reasons may require that those responding to obstetric emergencies be traditional birth attendants or similar persons in the community. Husum and colleagues demonstrated that lay people who are given first-aid skills could effectively respond to emergencies in a community with a high trauma burden (Husum, Gilbert, and Wisborg 2003; Husum, Gilbert, Wisborg, and others 2003). In Ghana, it was demonstrated that commercial taxi and minibus drivers trained in first aid could provide effective prehospital care (Mock and others 2002). Lay responders are likely to be successful where the burden of injuries and other emergencies is high. Attrition of both the responders and the skills is a concern unless they are put to frequent use.

Paramedical Personnel In most middle-income countries and some cities of low-income countries, trained paramedical personnel render prehospital care (Mock and others 1998; Tannebaum and others 2001). As for lay responders, coverage varies by country. In most of Sub-Saharan Africa and Asia, paramedical personnel and ambulances transfer patients between health facilities and not from the scenes of injury or from homes (Joshipura and others 2003). In middle-income countries, though, they are a major component of existing emergency medical systems (Arreola-Risa and others 2000; Mock 2002). Their presence (coupled with vehicle ambulances) reduces the interval between the recognition of an emergency and the arrival at the hospital, and some evidence suggests that training them in basic life-saving skills improves patient outcomes (Ali and others 1997, 1998; Arreola-Risa and others 2000).

Effectiveness has also been demonstrated for well-placed dispatch sites in urban populations, where the vehicles and personnel can be optimized. There is no evidence, however, for the effectiveness of training prehospital care paramedical personnel in advanced life-saving skills (Sethi and others 2003). Shorter prehospital times, in general, are considered an important parameter of the quality of prehospital care. These times have the following components:

- *Notification time* is the time elapsed from occurrence of injury or recognition of severe illness until the EMS system is notified.
- *Response time* is the time elapsed from notification until arrival of an ambulance to the site of the ill or injured person.
- *Scene time* is the time taken by prehospital providers from arrival at until departure from the scene.
- *Transport time* is the time elapsed from leaving the scene until arrival at the hospital or other treatment facility.

Notification time is influenced by the availability of telecommunications. Response time is influenced by the capabilities of a dispatch center to handle emergency calls and especially by the geographic distribution of sites of ambulance dispatch. The greater in number and the more widely distributed the number of ambulance stations are, the shorter the response times are.

Geographic distribution and associated response times can be improved in some circumstances by using a tiered or layered response system. This system requires having a relatively larger number of basically trained and equipped first responders with wider geographic distribution and a smaller number of centrally located, more highly trained and equipped second responders. This system allows the first responders to respond more rapidly, with second responder involvement only if needed (Arreola-Risa and others 1995).

Accordingly, paramedical personnel should be introduced in large urban areas where they do not function at present and should be stationed at dispatch sites with dedicated vehicles, fast communications with the hospitals in the area, and links with other emergency services such as the fire and police departments. The communities served by the system should have a well-known and rapid method of calling the paramedical teams when an emergency arises. Because skills depreciate with time, these personnel require refresher courses. Where paramedical personnel already exist as part of the EMS, their numbers and organization (location, training, deployment, and monitoring) should be enhanced to improve response times and, hence, patient outcomes, especially for cardiac and obstetric emergencies. Availability of EMS for a given population can be looked at either as number of units on duty or number of sites of ambulance dispatch. They are usually closely related, with one or two units per site, but not in systems where a large number of units are on duty from one central dispatch station.

The recommended ratio of one unit for 50,000 people suggested by McSwain (1991) results in response times as low as four to six minutes. The ratio does not distinguish between basic life-support and advanced life-support capabilities. Traffic congestion, poor maps, and poor road signs may all increase this response time in cities with poor infrastructure. In Monterrey, Mexico, one unit per 100,000 people manages an average response time of 10 minutes. Hanoi, Vietnam, with one unit for 3 million people, has an average response time of 30 minutes (Mock and others 1998).

Where paramedical services exist alongside lay responder services, these two could be managed by the same organizational unit. The paramedical staff will be more successful in urban areas, where distances between dispatch sites, communities served, and hospitals are short. Other enabling factors are good telecommunications; rapid and dedicated transportation; and coordinating capacity among the community, hospitals, and other emergency services.

Intervention Cost and Effectiveness Training lay responders is an intervention potentially available in low-income countries. Projections for costs and effectiveness have been made based on the following assumptions:

- Serving a population of 1 million requires 7,500 trainees. Sensitivity analysis ranges from 5,000 to 10,000 trained lay responders.
- Trained lay responders can be trained in half a day (St. John Ambulance 1996).
- Training would have to be repeated every three years to maintain efficacy.
- Annually, 2,500 laypeople would be trained on a rolling basis.

Using these assumptions (see annex 68.A for technical details on costing guidelines) would require the following:

- 1,250 days of trainees' time (0.5 days each) valued at salary level 1
- 62.5 trainer days of time, with a ratio of 20 trainees per trainer, valued at wages for salary level 3
- one training facility with a classroom (100 square meters) valued at rent for basic space for 62.5 days
- 2,500 copies of photocopied curricula annually valued at US$1 each.

The costs of providing trained paramedics can be estimated using the following assumptions:

- Trained paramedic responders can be trained in 25 days (St. John Ambulance 1996).
- Serving a population of 1 million requires 7,500 trainees. Sensitivity analysis ranges from 100 to 200.

- Training would have to be repeated every three years to maintain efficacy.
- Annually, 50 paramedics would be trained.

As a result, the following would be required:

- 25 × 50 = 1,250 days of paramedic trainee time (salary level 1)
- 125 trainer days, with a ratio of 10 trainees per trainer valued at salary level 3
- one training facility offering a classroom (100 square meters) valued at basic building values
- 50 photocopied curricula annually, valued at US$1 each
- one paramedic kit with stethoscope, gloves, bandages, and splint material for each trainee (kits would be renewed by patient contributions).

The trainees would offer volunteer services after training. We assume that volunteers are highly motivated individuals who consider emergency medical service to their community as the most rewarding use of their leisure time (Fiedler 2000). The opportunity cost of their recurrent emergency service is assumed to be zero. Communities or cultures that have a shortage of individuals with an ethic of volunteer service may have to devote funds toward maintaining incentives for "volunteer" paramedics to serve. In such cases, this strategy may not be cost-effective.

Table 68.3 shows the estimated costs of the lay first responders and paramedics intervention, drawing on the Disease Control Priorities Project's standardized input prices by region for low, best, and high estimates.

Outcomes According to the World Health Organization burden-of-disease estimates, the global incidence of trauma is 410 per 100,000 or 4,100 per million. Husum, Gilbert, and Wisborg (2003) indicate that first-level responders and trained paramedics can lower mortality in trauma by 9 percent; thus, in 4,100 traumas, 370 lives can be saved. Dividing the sum of the costs in table 68.3 by the 370 deaths averted provides a rough estimate of costs per death averted. These costs per death averted are divided by the regional life expectancy at age 20 (LE 20), with the assumption that the average age of trauma is 20, to give the cost per life year saved. LE 20 is roughly 50 years in every region except Sub-Saharan Africa, where it is only 37 years. Shortages of equipment and supplies may reduce the effectiveness of the prehospital personnel.

It is possible to offer more refined "regional" estimates of the numbers of deaths averted by using local estimates of the burden of injuries instead of the global estimate of 4,100 injuries per million people. Yet given the uncertainty about regional variation in the effectiveness of the intervention based on administrative, infrastructure, and human resource capacity, it would perhaps give a false impression that a firm and universal basis exists to speculate quantitatively on the relative effectiveness of the intervention in various regions. As a result, the above estimates, as used in table 68.4, serve to inform global dialogue rather than offer specific empirical numbers.

Equipment and Supplies. Equipment and supplies should match the knowledge and skills of the personnel available to use them. Even teams with the least resources should have the following:

- protective wear, especially gloves and aprons
- a stretcher or the equivalent
- pressure dressings (bandages—elastic, if possible—and cotton or gauze dressings)
- splints—various sizes, made out of local materials
- radio, telephone, or other mode of rapid communication.

Annex 68.A provides a comprehensive list for better-resourced communities. Intervention cost and effectiveness

Table 68.3 Cost of Using Trained Lay First Responders Together with Trained Paramedics
(local currency converted to 2001 U.S. dollars using exchange rates)

Region	Low	Best	High
East Asia and the Pacific	27,539	48,050	75,232
Europe and Central Asia	30,209	52,339	79,605
Latin America and the Caribbean	32,777	74,589	110,453
Middle East and North Africa	33,050	104,585	261,935
South Asia	27,183	45,637	116,456
Sub-Saharan Africa	30,765	52,339	115,171
Unweighted average	30,254	62,923	126,475

Source: Authors.
Note: Cost of treating community of 1 million.

Table 68.4 Cost-Effectiveness of Combining Paramedics with Lay Responders
(local currency converted to 2001 U.S. dollars using exchange rates)

Region	Low	Best	High
Cost per death averted with trained lay first responders together with volunteer paramedics			
East Asia and the Pacific	74	130	203
Europe and Central Asia	82	141	215
Latin America and the Caribbean	89	202	299
Middle East and North Africa	89	283	708
South Asia	73	123	315
Sub-Saharan Africa	83	141	311
Unweighted average	82	170	342
Cost per life year saved with trained lay first responders together with volunteer paramedics			
East Asia and the Pacific	3	5	8
Europe and Central Asia	3	5	8
Latin America and the Caribbean	3	8	11
Middle East and North Africa	3	11	27
South Asia	3	5	12
Sub-Saharan Africa	4	6	14
Unweighted average	3	7	13

Source: Authors.
Note: Cost of treating community of 1 million.

cannot be estimated because no studies are available on this issue from low-income countries.

Traditional and Innovative Communications Systems. Nowhere is the demand for efficient communication and rapid transportation more critical than in emergency medical care. The best teams equipped with state-of-the-art technology and supplies will be wasted if they cannot be reached quickly or if they have no contact with the hospitals where patients are to be taken. Most of the world's population lives in areas where there is no telecommunications infrastructure, and this situation may not change significantly in the near future. Innovation is needed so that these populations can be enabled to access effective emergency care interventions that already exist without waiting for traditional telephone lines to get to their rural homes. Radio communication is one solution in such settings. Equipping traditional birth attendants and remote health units with radio receiver sets linked to local hospitals has been used to shorten the response time and reduce maternal deaths (Samai and Sengeh 1997). Cellular telephones may offer communities that are remote from standard communications infrastructure an opportunity to leap into a more modern and efficient mode.

Intervention Costs and Effectiveness There are no studies from low-income countries on which to base intervention cost and effectiveness estimates. The costs will depend on whether the community adopts traditional communication or more modern communication systems. If radio communication were introduced, the purchase and maintenance of radio receivers, supplies, and government licensing costs would need to be estimated. If cellular telephones options were being explored, then the purchase of telephones, plans, licenses, and maintenance costs would need to be included. Where satellite towers need to be installed, however, this cost will be much higher than for all other components. Finally, if traditional landline installation is being considered, the lines, equipment, and telephone bills will need to be taken into account. The health sector may be able to share the costs of such interventions, especially traditional telephone lines, with other development and infrastructure units of a national government.

Basic and Advanced Transportation Systems. Transporting a patient from the location of the acute event to a hospital facility is a critical element of the prehospital component. Lack of transportation is often a major barrier to accessing emergency care (Lungu and others 2001; Samai and Sengeh 1997). In devising a prehospital system of transportation, one should consider locally available resources and the range of viable alternatives for transportation. In some countries such transportation may be part of a formal EMS system, whereas in other cases it is entirely informal. For example, commercial vehicles, the police, and relatives using private motorized or nonmotorized forms of transportation may bring seriously ill and injured patients to medical facilities (Andrews, Kobusingye, and Lett 1999; Joshipura and others 2003; Kobusingye and others 2002). A bicycle ambulance in Malawi set up to improve emergency obstetric care was actually used more often for injuries and medical emergencies (Lungu and others 2001).

Transportation should be accessible at short notice. A vehicle with a stretcher is ideal, but almost any transportation that will get a patient to a facility where definitive care can be obtained is acceptable. Although a fully fitted and equipped ambulance vehicle complete with trained paramedics delivers better outcomes, ethical and equity considerations dictate that before this vehicle is made available to an elite population in the urban areas, basic transportation must be assured for all who need emergency transportation and care.

In a city setting, a vehicle ambulance can make as many as 20 trips per day. On average this schedule will require salaries for an administrator and two crews, each comprising a driver and two paramedics or nurses, as well as expenses for communication, supplies, pharmaceuticals, and the costs of operating the vehicle. A study of a decision to develop an EMS in Kuala Lumpur (1.1 million people, 243 square kilometers) estimated that the purchase and staffing of 48 ambulances at US$53,000 each per year would be required, totaling US$2.5 million per year (Hauswald and Yeoh 1997). The authors noted that, despite the paucity of ambulances, severely injured or ill patients did get to a hospital with only minor delays by using taxis, family transportation, or the police. Ambulances need accurate maps, house numbers, and street or road signs, all of which might not be in place in low-income cities. It was estimated that ambulances were unable to locate patients in 20 percent of calls in Kuala Lumpur because of mapping and signage problems (Hauswald and Yeoh 1997).

A study conducted in Turkey found that ambulance vehicle costs were the leading component of capital costs (Altintas, Bilir, and Tuleylioglu 1999). The cost per trip was US$163, and the cost per patient transported was US$180.50, which the authors thought were beyond the means of the private sector. In state-run ambulance services in New Delhi, India, the cost per trip was approximately US$40, yet one in three of the ambulances served only to transport patients, with no paramedic staff on board (India, Government of Delhi 2001).

The debates in high-income countries about helicopter ambulances provide lessons for low-income countries. In some cases, helicopter services have been discontinued because they were not considered cost-effective (Hutton 1995). A study conducted in the United States, which concluded that helicopters were cost-effective, found that the cost per patient transported was US$2,214 and that for every 100 flights there were six survivors more than was predicted on the basis of injury severity indices (Gearhart, Wuerz, and Localio 1997). Each additional

survivor cost an average of US$15,883, and the authors acknowledged that the helicopter had to be used fully to spread the high fixed costs across many patients and trips. A review of civilian helicopter ambulance programs in the United States concluded that the primary factor in the reduction of trauma mortality was not the speed at which the patient was transported but the administration of life-saving care by the helicopter medical crew at the scene or at the outlying hospital (Moylan 1988). In low-income countries, for the very few who benefit from such a high-end intervention, there are likely to be thousands who cannot access care even using the most basic means.

Intervention Costs and Effectiveness Costing transportation systems requires the following assumptions:

- In an urban population, one ambulance unit can serve a population of 30,000 people. Thus, 1 million people would require 33 ambulance units (1 million/30,000).
- Each ambulance unit requires staffing of a rotation of six paramedic-drivers and a seventh paramedic-driver to cover vacation times and sick leaves.
- A supervisor oversees three ambulance units per year.
- A garage for the ambulance and communications equipment would be 100 square meters but would entail rental of office-style accommodations.
- A vehicle to be outfitted as an ambulance can be purchased for as much as an off-road vehicle with a useful life of nine years.
- The cost to modify the vehicle into a basic ambulance is US$5,000 for a useful life of nine years.
- The ambulance will require fuel and maintenance based on usage of 20,000 kilometers per year.

Given the preceding assumptions,

- The 231-member ambulance staff (33 ambulance units of 7 persons each) would be paid at salary level 2.
- The 10 administrators would be paid at salary level 2.

We ignore the additional burden on the health system from additional visits. Quite possibly, hospital costs will rise as more patients now get to the hospital with the help of ambulances. It is also possible that patients currently arrive in less desperate condition, so that the cost of care is lessened. No studies are available on which to base cost estimates to address those issues.

Table 68.5 shows the estimated costs of the ambulance intervention, drawing on the Disease Control Priorities Project's standardized input prices by region for low, best, and high estimates.

Outcome Based on the World Health Organization's 2001 burden of disease estimates on epidemiology of trauma, ischemic heart disease, and obstetric emergencies, we estimate that for each 10,000 population there will be 9 deaths from trauma,[1]

Table 68.5 Cost and Effectiveness of Ambulances
(U.S. dollars)

Region	Low	Best	High
Cost of treating community of 1 million with urban ambulances			
East Asia and the Pacific	691,603	871,208	1,090,032
Europe and Central Asia	839,468	1,024,235	1,220,888
Latin America and the Caribbean	849,556	1,550,521	1,747,630
Middle East and North Africa	894,379	2,435,000	4,960,705
South Asia	676,111	803,361	1,973,093
Sub-Saharan Africa	781,568	951,906	1,905,417
Unweighted average	788,781	1,272,705	2,149,628
Cost per death averted of treating community of 1 million with urban ambulances			
East Asia and the Pacific	988	1,245	1,557
Europe and Central Asia	1,199	1,463	1,744
Latin America and the Caribbean	1,214	2,215	2,497
Middle East and North Africa	1,278	3,479	7,087
South Asia	966	1,148	2,819
Sub-Saharan Africa	1,117	1,360	2,722
Unweighted average	1,127	1,818	3,071
Cost per life year saved of treating community of 1 million with urban ambulances			
East Asia and the Pacific	50	63	79
Europe and Central Asia	62	75	90
Latin America and the Caribbean	61	111	126
Middle East and North Africa	65	176	359
South Asia	50	60	147
Sub-Saharan Africa	67	81	163
Unweighted average	59	95	161
Cost per death averted of treating community of 1 million with rural ambulances			
East Asia and the Pacific	2,978	3,748	4,686
Europe and Central Asia	3,613	4,405	5,248
Latin America and the Caribbean	3,652	6,656	7,500
Middle East and North Africa	3,847	10,449	21,274
South Asia	2,911	3,457	8,470
Sub-Saharan Africa	3,361	4,092	8,178
Unweighted average	3,394	5,468	9,226

Source: Authors.

11 deaths from ischemic heart disease,[2] and 2 deaths from lethal obstetric emergencies.[3] For modeling purposes, we confine our attention to trauma, ischemic heart disease, and obstetric cases. Although many possible lethal emergencies may present, such as sepsis, malaria, snakebites, and asthma, by confining attention to the major emergency conditions we locate 2,200 (900 + 1,100 + 200) potentially savable lives in a population of 1 million. The savings are outlined as follows:

- *Savings from trauma reductions.* Saving lives from trauma depends on the quality of trauma care at the destination facility. In one year for 1 million people, there will be 4,100

trauma cases and 900 trauma deaths. With rapid resuscitation and oxygen available through use of ambulances, we assume we can save 300 lives.

- *Savings from myocardial infarction management.* In one year for 1 million people in low-income countries, 1,100 deaths will typically result from myocardial infarction. Low-dose aspirin provided to myocardial infarction victims lowers mortality by 18 percent (Weisman and Graham 2002). In a population without ambulance services, rapid aspirin administration cannot be ensured; with EMS, aspirin use can potentially be increased from about 0 percent to 100 percent for heart myocardial infarction. Therefore, instead of 1,100 deaths, there will be $1,100 \times (1 - 0.18)$ deaths, saving 200 lives, but with only an average of five life years per life saved.

- *Savings from emergency obstetrics management.* Obstetric deaths for medically attended patients are approximately 100 times lower than for patients who do not receive medical care. Accordingly, an ambulance system essentially saves all of the obstetric emergencies from death; this saving would amount to 200 deaths averted in the case described previously. As a result, in the hypothetical population of 1 million people in low-income countries, 700 lives can be saved by an ambulance system focusing on three causes only: ischemic heart disease (200), obstetric (200), and trauma (300).

The middle section of table 68.6 displays the cost per death averted. To compute life years saved in the last section of the table, we assume that the 500 deaths averted from obstetric emergencies and trauma occur at age 20, but the 200 deaths averted from ischemic heart disease save only five additional life years per case. Regional life expectancy at age 20 years (estimated) is used as before.

Costs for a Rural Ambulance Service The key difference determining higher costs for rural ambulances is that more ambulance units are necessary to cover the population. We assume that in rural areas one ambulance unit can cover a population of 10,000, although variation will occur, depending on population density and geographical topography. On the basis of this assumption, all of the cost estimates for rural ambulances are essentially three times higher for a population of 1 million, as are the costs per death averted and per life year gained. They are assumed to have the same effectiveness as the urban services because the increase in units aims at delivering the same quality

Table 68.6 Summary of Cost and Effectiveness
(U.S. dollars)

Region	Trained lay first responders and paramedic responders	Staffed community ambulance, urban	Staffed community ambulance, rural
Costs for a population of 1 million			
East Asia and the Pacific	48,050	871,208	2,623,392
Europe and Central Asia	52,339	1,024,235	3,083,637
Latin America and the Caribbean	74,589	1,550,521	4,659,017
Middle East and North Africa	104,585	2,435,000	7,314,544
South Asia	45,637	803,361	2,419,607
Sub-Saharan Africa	52,339	951,906	2,864,062
Unweighted average	62,923	1,272,705	3,827,376
Cost per death averted for a population of 1 million[a]			
East Asia and the Pacific	130	1,245	3,748
Europe and Central Asia	141	1,463	4,405
Latin America and the Caribbean	202	2,215	6,656
Middle East and North Africa	283	3,479	10,449
South Asia	123	1,148	3,457
Sub-Saharan Africa	141	1,360	4,092
Unweighted average	170	1,818	5,468
Cost per life year gained for a population of 1 million[a]			
East Asia and the Pacific	5	63	190
Europe and Central Asia	5	75	227
Latin America and the Caribbean	8	111	335
Middle East and North Africa	11	176	530
South Asia	5	60	180
Sub-Saharan Africa	6	81	245
Unweighted average	7	94	284

Source: Authors.
a. Personnel consist of lay first responders together with paramedics.

of care as in the urban centers. This assumption may not hold true if the quality of care at the receiving facilities is lower than that in the urban areas.

Uncertainty of Estimates Substantial uncertainty remains over the actual effectiveness of the interventions in emergency medicine. The tables in this chapter should be approached with due caution because ultimately the projections of the effectiveness of interventions have been patched together from a handful of intervention trials whose success may or may not be similar in other contexts. The projections include the following:

- Ambulance services can and do save lives by performing field stabilization and by hastening the arrival of critical patients when time makes a difference in the outcome.
- Only several dozen ambulance runs per year for a unit serving a population of 10,000 will actually have the potential to save lives.
- Ambulance services are more cost-effective in denser populations and when roads are more passable, making trips shorter.
- Training lay responders and paramedics can be relatively cost-effective.

The financial support of an ambulance unit may rely on the value perceived by the hundreds of patients who are comforted by having rapid access to care or by knowing ambulances are there if needed, even though their lives and health are not actually improved by ambulances.

Table 68.6 summarizes the best estimates of cost, cost per death averted, and cost per life year.

Health Facility–Based Subsystem

This subsystem refers to a level within the health care system where appropriate definitive care is delivered. Formal health facilities vary immensely between and within countries. In some countries, this subsystem may be a regional hospital with specialists; in others, a district hospital with general practitioners or nonspecialist doctors; and in still others, a health center with competent nonphysician clinicians. In some low-income countries, some types of emergency medical care, for conditions such as acute diarrhea or severe malaria, may be effectively delivered at a health center staffed by nondoctor clinicians. However, such a facility will be grossly inadequate for the management of a severe multiple injury or obstructed labor. The triage process in the prehospital subsystem should determine which patients receive transportation to which facility, instead of merely transportation to the nearest facility. Precious time and lives may be lost when patients are taken to facilities where the desired definitive care is not available.

Because the goal of an effective EMS is the provision of emergency care to all who need it—*universal emergency care*—the following section presents guidelines on the necessary inputs at different levels. Two of the components in hospital emergency care are discussed in more detail: (a) training and (b) equipment and supplies. The first level of formal health care is often staffed by nonphysician clinicians; the second level is staffed by at least one physician and other trained health care professionals; and the third is staffed by specialists in addition to other health care professionals. Some middle-income countries have additional levels (major emergency care centers), and some hospitals are specialized (chapters 65 and 66).

Training. Most in-service training for emergency care professionals working in hospitals is designed to address a particular problem, such as severe injuries, emergency pediatrics, or obstetric emergencies. Yet because of the resource constraints of low-income countries, the same personnel will be confronted with all these problems. Few courses in emergency care have been rigorously evaluated (Black and Brocklehurst 2003; Sethi and others 2003). The Advanced Trauma Life Support (ATLS) course for doctors has resulted in improved patient outcomes in some settings, although it may be too expensive for most low-income countries and inappropriate in settings where doctors do not see the majority of patients. In a tertiary hospital in Trinidad and Tobago, injury mortality was reduced by 50 percent following ATLS training (Ali and others 1993).

Life-saving obstetric skills training was found to contribute to a reduction in maternal deaths. In Kebbi state in Nigeria, this training led to a drop in case-fatality rates among women with obstetric complications from 22 percent to 5 percent. Similar trends were observed in other sites where the intervention was implemented (Oyesola and others 1997; Prevention of Maternal Mortality Network 1995). Emergency Triage Assessment and Treatment has been used in many countries to improve pediatric emergency care (WHO 2000). Other examples are Primary Trauma Care, which is a trauma management course to train doctors and other health workers in district hospitals and remote locations (Wilkinson and Skinner 2000), and Advanced Life Support in Obstetrics (see http://www.aafp.org/also). These courses have been beneficial in standardizing protocol-based emergency care, but their outcome evaluations are still awaited. Low-income countries need to identify training models for their versatile emergency care personnel, especially those working at middle-level facilities, who respond to different types of emergencies.

The costs of this intervention are not available in the literature and will require an estimation of trainer costs, space, materials, and refresher courses.

Equipment and Supplies. A specimen list of resources for emergency care required at different levels of facilities is provided in annex 68.A. This template is flexible, and countries can customize it to suit local conditions, such as existing facility levels and prevailing burden of emergency disease conditions. Equipment and supplies at each level should match the knowledge and skills of the personnel available to use them.

Systems Organization

Emergency care needs to be planned and implemented carefully. The various components that make up the EMS should be linked to ensure that the entire system operates as a unit. A coordinator should be responsible for monitoring and coordinating all emergency medical care in the community or district and should work with a committee to which the other components send representation. A community representative should be a key member of this committee.

Coordination costs are very important and should not be overlooked in the development of a new EMS. Such costs include the salary of the coordinator, an efficient telephone or communication system, a vehicle, fuel, and a budget to organize meetings of stakeholders at least twice a year (Bazzoli, Harmata, and Chan 1998; Nurok 2001).

Health Financing for Emergency Care

Emergency medical systems in low-income countries must be pro-poor in their orientation, which requires explicit consideration of how the poor interact with an EMS and how barriers to acute care for the poor can be overcome. Issues of access to an EMS become critical because the lack of money often keeps people from using emergency services. Direct payment of costs for transportation, medical treatment, and drugs makes lack of money a major barrier to EMS for the poor in every country. As a result, emergencies frequently cripple individuals and families financially in poor communities, often for many years in the future.

Financial protection for emergency health care is a necessity in low-income countries and has not received adequate attention. The goal of such protection is to ensure that individuals and families do not spiral down the pathway to abject poverty as a result of interaction with the national health system. Such financial protection may be achieved by a number of different means, including community financing (Ande and others 1997; Desmet, Chowdhury, and Islam 1999; Macintyre and Hotchkiss 1999). Community loan funds to cover transportation and other requirements for emergencies, especially for obstetrics, have been explored with mixed results (Essien and others 1997; Shehu, Ikeh, and Kuna 1997). Some experience seems to indicate that these approaches can indeed overcome several of the barriers to accessing emergency medical services and should be explored further.

Documentation and Quality Assurance

Quality of care is critical to the interaction of the poor with the EMS. Lack of funds, lower-paid jobs, social class distinctions, ethnicity, and other affiliations make the already vulnerable poor susceptible to receiving poor-quality care. For an EMS to maintain and improve the care of patients, systematic documentation and periodic audits, or other processes to ensure quality of care, need to be incorporated. Quality management systems that are simple, are continuous, and allow for rapid changes in the system need to be implemented.

Because of scarcity of resources, expensive machines and elite specialists should not be advocated for the urban privileged at the expense of the majority of the rural poor. The most difficult decisions concern balancing funds invested in the emergency care capacity of secondary and primary care centers with support for referral and transportation networks to feed tertiary care centers. These decisions are too variable and too system specific to yield to a uniform policy prescription. Two principles are advocated to inform these difficult decisions:

- Collect data on costs, capacities, and outcomes.
- Tighten the integration of the emergency care system to improve function and lead to wiser decisions on where to invest.

Legislative Instruments to Ensure Emergency Care

The issues discussed in the preceding sections supply the rationale for countries to have specific legislation addressing the provision of emergency care. This area requires major cooperation between public health and law, which together provide the legal framework for ensuring that all individuals who deserve emergency care can receive it, irrespective of their personal characteristics or their ability to pay. Having laws that protect trained individuals and laypeople as they provide such care is also important.

IMPLEMENTATION OF CONTROL STRATEGIES: LESSONS OF EXPERIENCE

A large proportion of trauma patients in developing countries do not have access to formal emergency medical services. Boxes 68.1 and 68.2 contain examples of interventions to provide appropriate emergency care in such countries.

THE RESEARCH AND DEVELOPMENT AGENDA

The research and development priorities for emergency care are challenging to define because emergency care is a neglected area of research in low-income countries and the needs are

Box 68.1

Improving Trauma Care in the Absence of a Formal Ambulance System

Background: The efficacy of a program that builds on the existing, although informal, system of prehospital transportation in Ghana was assessed. In Ghana, the majority of injured persons are transported to the hospital by some type of commercial vehicle, such as a taxi or bus.

Methods: A total of 335 commercial drivers were trained using a six-hour basic first-aid course. The efficacy of this course was assessed by comparing the process of prehospital trauma care provided before and after the course, as determined by self-reporting from the drivers.

The course was conducted with moderate amounts of volunteer labor and gifts in kind, such as transportation to the course. The actual cost of the course amounted to US$3 per participant.

Results: Follow-up interviews were conducted on 71 of the drivers a mean of 10.6 months after the course. In the interviews, 61 percent indicated that they had provided

first aid since taking the course. There was considerable improvement in the provision of the components of first aid in comparison to what was reported before the course:

Component of first aid	Before (percent)	After (percent)
Crash scene management	7	35
Airway management	2	35
Bleeding control	4	42
Splint application	1	16
Triage	7	21

Conclusions: Even in the absence of a formal EMS, improvements in the process of prehospital trauma care are possible by building on existing, although informal, prehospital transportation.

Source: Mock and others 2002.

Box 68.2

Training for Emergency Care in India

The training of personnel working in emergency medical services is crucial to the success of efficient delivery of care. Evidence exists to support usefulness of life-support training for emergency caregivers in low- and middle-income countries. Courses such as the ATLS are available and well established in some high- and middle-income countries. In most low-income countries, such training is not available, mainly because of prohibitive costs. The three-day ATLS course costs on average US$700 per trainee and is taught by six trainers to a group of 20 trainees at a time. The National Trauma Management

Course is an indigenous two-day course developed in India by the Academy of Traumatology (India) with the help of international peers. The curriculum takes into account local conditions and capabilities. The cost is US$50 per trainee, and the course is taught by local trainers to a group of 100 trainees at a time. Animal specimens are used to teach life-saving procedures instead of expensive commercially produced manikins. More than 2,000 health professionals have been trained in less than three years. The course has now become a national training standard for immediate trauma care in India.

Source: Authors.

great. As a neglected topic, emergency care is part of the "10-90" gap of health research: less than 10 percent of global research investments are for problems affecting 90 percent of the world's population (Global Forum 2000).

Approach to Research and Development for EMS

The spectrum of research required is diverse and may be easily understood with the help of the schematic shown in

figure 68.2. The rectangle is a schematic representation of the totality of the global burden of disease that can be potentially addressed by EMS (see "Burden of Disease"). A portion of this potential burden is being addressed (or reduced) by those existing interventions that have been implemented, defined by box A. If the efficiency of current interventions were to be enhanced and their coverage increased, then another portion of the burden defined by box B could be addressed; this increase

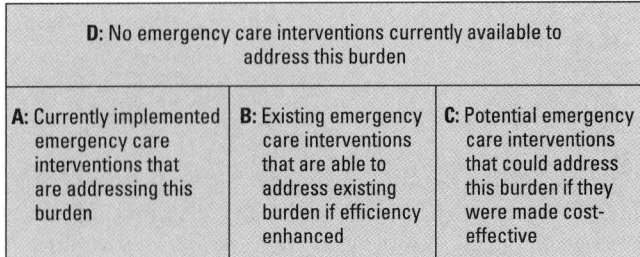

Figure 68.2 Schematic Illustration of the Burden of Disease Potentially Addressed by EMS

in efficiency will require operations research, policy research, and social science research. If existing interventions, which have not been implemented because of their high costs, were made more cost-effective, then another portion of the burden defined by box C could be reduced. This process of making interventions more cost-effective will require economic analysis and clinical research in many instances. Finally, a portion of the burden exists for which we do not have existing interventions, defined by box D; it requires basic and clinical research to develop and pilot interventions that can address other determinants of the emergency care–related burden in the future.

This schematic representation is thus useful to demonstrate two critical needs:

- essential research on emergency care in low-income countries
- a diverse set of research studies and approaches to reduce the burden that can be addressed by EMS.

Priority Setting for Research and Development of Emergency Care

Setting priorities for research and development on EMS needs to be a region-specific, if not country-specific, process. No current list exists of global research and development priorities for EMS, again reflecting the need for more attention and investments in this area. This chapter does not intend to prescribe a list of issues or topics for global research and development efforts, but rather to highlight the gap in global research and development and to suggest possible issues and topics that may be broadly relevant to low-income countries for these efforts in the short to middle term.

A number of methods exist for setting research priorities in the health sector, such as the Combined Approach Matrix promoted by the Global Forum for Health Research (Global Forum 2002) and the Essential National Health Research process promoted by the Council for Health Research for Development. Countries and regions can use these approaches to help develop their research agenda for EMS.

The review of evidence available in the field of emergency care as applicable to low-income countries reveals many gaps

in global knowledge. Following on the illustration of figure 68.2, there is a need to better understand the epidemiology of those conditions that can be addressed by an EMS in a low-income country and which interventions currently in place are addressing them. We have little knowledge of how to enhance the efficiency of these existing interventions and reduce their costs. Most important, the lack of intervention trials done in low-income countries creates a major research priority for the field of EMS. Well-designed, locally appropriate interventions that establish their effectiveness are urgently needed and should include both interventions that may be available in high-income countries and new ones. Economic analysis is another area for major research input in the field of EMS, where cost and cost-effectiveness information from low-income countries is scant. These gaps only reflect the need for a more systematic analysis of where research investments should be directed in the next five years for EMS.

CONCLUSIONS: PROMISES AND PITFALLS

Emergency medical systems are a critical component of national health systems in low-income countries. Governments and ministries of health in low-income countries need to pay specific attention to the development of EMS in their countries and to ensure that the evolution of any EMS is both evidence based and appropriate to their national needs. More important, the context and implementation of EMS should help health equity and not widen existing health disparities.

This chapter highlights not only the urgent need for more attention to EMS in low-income countries but also points out an opportunity for these countries in defining better EMS for their needs. In promoting the systematic development of an evidence-based EMS, low-income countries could help define more effective and cost-effective emergency systems than currently exist in high-income countries. This opportunity should not be lost as a result of political inattention or lack of funds; the international and national stakeholders must move forward to stem the preventable loss of life from the lack of an EMS.

Emergency care needs to be planned as an integral component of public health systems in low-income countries. Too little is known about the true extent of the need for emergency care, the designs of EMS that would work well for different communities and populations, and the costs and benefits of delivering emergency care in low-income countries. These gaps are a call for more investments in the research, development, and implementation of EMS, especially in these countries. Universal emergency care is consistent with the right to health care because, by definition, emergency care is a matter of life and death. Society should endeavor to ensure that prompt appropriate care is available in critical moments when a delay in care—or the delivery of inappropriate care—could mean loss of lives.

Annex 68.A Essential Resources for the Delivery of Emergency Care in Hospitals

Resources	Major emergency care center	Regional emergency care center	District emergency care center	Primary emergency care center
Organization and administration				
Multidisciplinary emergency care team	✓	✓		
Maintenance of statistical data	✓	✓	✓	
Resources				
Immediate access to radiology or CT and ultrasound scan facility on site	✓	✓		
Blood bank on site	✓			
Access to blood bank		✓	✓	
Radiological technician on site 24 hours a day	✓	✓		
Radiological services available promptly			✓	
Clinical laboratory services				
Laboratory services on site available 24 hours a day (including, but not limited to, the following tests)	✓	✓		
Hemoglobin, glucose, gram stain, blood slide test	✓	✓	✓	
Bacterial cultures	✓	✓		
Quality improvement				
Evidence of quality improvement program in accident and emergency department	✓	✓	✓	
Monthly morbidity and mortality review	✓	✓		
Medical nursing audit and utilization review	✓	✓		
Personnel				
Designated doctor in charge, member of the emergency care team, with special competence in care of critically ill and injured patients, present in the emergency care unit 24 hours a day	✓	✓		
Designated doctor in charge, member of the emergency care team, with special competence in care of critically ill and injured patients, available on call			✓	
Nursing personnel with special competence in the care of the critically ill and injured patients, designated member of the emergency care team, present in the emergency unit 24 hours a day	✓	✓	✓	
All personnel trained in airway, breathing, and circulatory support techniques	✓	✓	✓	✓
Equipment required for resuscitation per station shall include but not be limited to				
Bag valve resuscitator with reservoir	✓	✓	✓	
Sphygmomanometer (blood pressure cuff)	✓	✓	✓	
Cervical collars	✓	✓	✓	✓
Chest decompression set	✓	✓	✓	

(Continues on the following page.)

Annex 68.A Continued

Resources	Major emergency care center	Regional emergency care center	District emergency care center	Primary emergency care center
Cut down set	✓	✓	✓	
Delivery pack	✓	✓	✓	✓
Diagnostic peritoneal lavage set open (1)	✓	✓		
Dressing trolley	✓	✓	✓	✓
Drip stand	✓	✓	✓	
Laryngoscope and blades (adult)	✓	✓	✓	
Laryngoscope and blades (pediatric)	✓	✓	✓	
McGills forceps (adult and pediatric)	✓	✓	✓	
Ophthalmoscope	✓	✓	✓	
Overhead x-ray gantry (full access to all beds)	✓			
Portable ventilator capable of pediatric vent	✓			
Resuscitation patient trolley	✓	✓	✓	
Scissors to cut clothing	✓	✓	✓	✓
Scoop stretcher (1)	✓	✓	✓	✓
Spine board (1)	✓	✓	✓	✓
Spot lamp (1)	✓	✓		
Sterile basic packs (2 per station)	✓	✓	✓	
Stethoscope	✓	✓	✓	✓
Suction apparatus	✓	✓	✓	✓
Wheelchair (1)	✓	✓	✓	✓
X-ray gowns (staff)	✓	✓		
X-ray viewing box	✓	✓	✓	
Consumables (adult and pediatric)				
Catheters (all sizes)	✓	✓	✓	
Central lines	✓	✓		
Chest drains	✓	✓	✓	
Diathermy	✓			
Endotracheal tubes	✓	✓	✓	
Eye protection for staff	✓	✓	✓	✓
Gloves	✓	✓	✓	✓
Humidification filters	✓	✓	✓	
Intraosseous needles	✓	✓		
Intravenous cannulas, fluids, lines	✓	✓	✓	
Introducers and endotracheal tubes (all sizes)	✓	✓		
Lumbar puncture set	✓	✓	✓	

Resources	Major emergency care center	Regional emergency care center	District emergency care center	Primary emergency care center
Malaria test kits	✓	✓	✓	✓
Masks	✓	✓	✓	✓
Medical waste disposal systems	✓	✓	✓	✓
Nasal cannula	✓	✓	✓	✓
Nasogastric tubes (all sizes)	✓	✓	✓	✓
Nebulization masks	✓	✓	✓	
Oropharyngeal airways	✓	✓	✓	
Oxygen mask	✓	✓	✓	✓
Suction catheters	✓	✓	✓	✓
Syringes (assorted)	✓	✓	✓	✓
Tracheotomy tubes	✓	✓		
Urine dipstick				✓
Wound care products	✓	✓	✓	✓
Drugs shall include but not be limited to the following				
Activated charcoal	✓	✓	✓	✓
Adrenaline	✓	✓		
Flumazenil (or similar benzodiazepine)	✓	✓	✓	
Antihistamine (such as diphenhidramine)	✓	✓	✓	✓
Atropine	✓	✓	✓	✓
Ciprofloxacin or equivalent	✓	✓	✓	
Beta-2 antagonist (such as propranolol)	✓	✓	✓	✓
Calcium chloride	✓	✓	✓	✓
Calcium gluconate	✓	✓	✓	✓
Dextrose, 50 percent	✓	✓	✓	✓
Diazepam	✓	✓	✓	
Dopamine	✓	✓		
Emetic (ipecac)	✓	✓	✓	✓
Metronidazole IV	✓	✓	✓	
Furosemide or equivalent	✓	✓	✓	
Heparin, 1,000 μg/ml	✓	✓	✓	
Hydrocortisone	✓	✓	✓	✓
Lidocaine IV	✓	✓	✓	✓
Magnesium sulfate IV	✓	✓	✓	
Midazolam	✓	✓	✓	
Morphine	✓	✓	✓	

(Continues on the following page.)

Resources	Major emergency care center	Regional emergency care center	District emergency care center	Primary emergency care center
Naloxone	✓	✓	✓	
Nitroglycerin	✓	✓	✓	✓
Crystalloids (such as normal saline)	✓	✓	✓	✓
Phenytoin	✓	✓	✓	
Polyvalent snake venom	✓	✓		
Potassium chloride	✓	✓	✓	
Scoline (suxamethonium chloride)	✓	✓		
Sodium bicarbonate	✓	✓	✓	✓
Streptokinase	✓	✓		
Tetanus toxoid	✓	✓	✓	✓
Vitamin K	✓	✓	✓	✓

Note: Additional information on recommended drugs is available in the *Model List of Essential Medicines* (WHO 2002) and the WHO's *Complementary Model List.*

NOTES

1. There are 4,715,000 trauma deaths in low- and middle-income countries per population of 5,219,401,000; thus, there are 9.033 trauma deaths per 10,000 people.

2. There are 5,699,000 ischemic heart disease deaths per 5,219,401,000 population; thus, there are 10.9 ischemic heart disease deaths per 10,000 people.

3. There are 2,000 to 4,000 births among 10,000 people based on crude birth rates of 26 (South Asia), 39 (Sub-Saharan Africa), 22 (Latin America), and 17 (East Asia). Maternal mortality runs at 1 per 1,000 people.

REFERENCES

Ali, J., R. Adam, A. K. Butler, H. Chang, M. Howard, D. Gonsalves, and others. 1993. "Trauma Outcome Improves Following Advanced Trauma Life Support (ATLS) Program in a Developing Country." *Journal of Trauma* 34: 890–99.

Ali, J., R. Adam, T. J. Gana, and J. I. Williams. 1997. "Trauma Patient Outcome after the Pre-hospital Trauma Life Support Program." *Journal of Trauma* 42 (6): 1018–21; discussion: 1021–22.

Ali, J., R. Adam, D. Josa, I. Pierre, H. Bedsaysie, U. West, and others. 1998. "Effect of Basic Pre-hospital Trauma Life Support Program on Cognitive and Trauma Management Skills." *World Journal of Surgery* 22 (12): 1192–96.

Altintas, K. H., N. Bilir, and M. Tuleylioglu. 1999. "Costing of an Ambulance System in a Developing Country, Turkey: Costs of Ankara Emergency Aid and Rescue Services' (EARS) Ambulance System." *European Journal of Emergency Medicine* 6: 355–62.

Ande, B., J. Chiwuzie, W. Akpala, A. Oronsaye, O. Okojie, C. Okolocha, and others. 1997. "Improving Obstetric Care at the District Hospital, Ekpoma, Nigeria." *International Journal of Gynecology and Obstetrics* 59 (Suppl.): S47–53.

Andrews, C. N., O. C. Kobusingye, and R. R. Lett. 1999. "Road Traffic Accident Injuries in Kampala." *East African Medical Journal* 76 (3): 189–94.

Arreola-Risa, C., C. N. Mock, L. Lojero-Wheatly, O. de la Cruz, C. Garcia, F. Canavati-Ayub, and G. J. Jurkovich. 2000. "Low-Cost Improvements in Prehospital Trauma Care in a Latin American City." *Journal of Trauma* 48 (1): 119–24.

Bazzoli G. J., R. Harmata, and C. Chan. 1998. "Community Based Trauma Systems in the United States: An Examination of Structural Development." *Social Science and Medicine* 46 (9): 1137–49.

Black, R. S., and P. Brocklehurst. 2003. "A Systematic Review of Training in Acute Obstetric Emergencies." *International Journal of Gynecology and Obstetrics* 110 (9): 837–41.

Desmet, M., A. Q. Chowdhury, and M. K. Islam. 1999. "The Potential for Social Mobilization in Bangladesh: The Organization and Functioning of Two Health Insurance Schemes." *Social Science and Medicine* 48: 925–38.

Essien E., D. Ifenne, K. Sabitu, A. Musa, M. Alti-Mu'azu, V. Adidu, and others. 1997. "Community Loan Funds and Transport Services for Obstetric Emergencies in Northern Nigeria." *International Journal of Gynecology and Obstetrics* 59 (Suppl. 2): S237–44.

Fiedler, J. L. 2000. "The Nepal National Vitamin A Program: Prototype to Emulate or Donor Enclave?" *Health Policy and Planning* 15 (2): 145–56.

Gearhart, P. A., R. Wuerz, and A. R. Localio. 1997. "Cost-Effectiveness Analysis of Helicopter EMS for Trauma Patients." *Annals of Emergency Medicine* 30: 500–6.

Global Forum for Health Research. 2002. *The 10/90 Report on Health 1700–2100.* Geneva: Global Forum for Health Resarch.

Graham, W. 1997. "Every Pregnancy Faces Risk." Presentation at a Safe Motherhood Technical Consultation, Sri Lanka, October 18–23.

Hauswald, M., and E. Yeoh. 1997. "Designing a Pre-hospital System for a Developing Country: Estimated Cost and Benefits." *American Journal of Emergency Medicine* 15: 600–3.

Husum, H., M. Gilbert, and T. Wisborg. 2003. "Training Pre-hospital Trauma Care in Low-Income Countries: The 'Village University' Experience." *Medical Teacher* 25 (2): 142–48.

Husum, H., M. Gilbert, T. Wisborg, Y. Van Heng, and M. Murad. 2003. "Rural Pre-hospital Trauma Systems Improve Trauma Outcome in Low-Income Countries: A Prospective Study from North Iraq and Cambodia." *Journal of Trauma* 54 (6): 1188–96.

Hutton, K. C. 1995. "The End of an Era: The Demise of Life Flight San Diego." *Air Medical Journal* 10: 11–13.

India, Government of Delhi. 2001. "Report of Evaluation Study on CATS." Evaluation Unit, Planning Department, New Delhi.

Joshipura, M. K., H. S. Shah, P. R. Patel, P. A. Divatia, and P. M. Desai. 2003. "Trauma Care Systems in India." *Injury* 34 (9): 686–92.

Kobusingye, O., D. Guwatudde, G. Owor, and R. Lett. 2002. "Citywide Trauma Experience in Kampala, Uganda: A Call for Intervention." *Injury Prevention* 8: 133–36.

Leigh, B., H. B. S. Kandeh, M. S. Kanu, M. Kuteh, I. S. Palmer, K. S. Daoh, and F. Moseray. 1997. "Improving Emergency Obstetric Care at a District Hospital, Makeni, Sierra Leone." *International Journal of Gynecology and Obstetrics* 59 (Suppl. 2): S55–65.

Liberman, M., D. Mulder, A. Lavoie, R. Denis, and J. S. Sampalis. 2003. "Multicenter Canadian Study of Prehospital Trauma Care." *Annals of Surgery* 237 (2): 153–60; comment: 161–62.

Lungu, K., V. Kamfose, J. Hussein, and H. Ashwood-Smith. 2001. "Are Bicycle Ambulances and Community Transport Plans Effective in Strengthening Obstetric Referral Systems in Southern Malawi?" *Malawi Medical Journal* 12 (2): 16–18.

Macintyre, K., and D. Hotchkiss. 1999. "Referral Revised: Community Financing Schemes and Emergency Transport in Rural Africa." *Social Science and Medicine* 49: 1473–87.

McCord, C., and Q. Chowdhury. 2003. "A Cost Effective Small Hospital in Bangladesh: What It Can Mean for Emergency Care." *International Journal of Gynecology and Obstetrics* 81 (1): 83–92.

McCord, C., S. Premkumar, S. Arole, and R. Arole. 2001. "Efficient and Effective Emergency Obstetric Care in a Rural Indian Community Where Most Deliveries Are at Home." *International Journal of Gynecology and Obstetrics* 75 (3): 297–307.

McSwain, N. E. 1991. "Prehospital Emergency Medical Systems and Cardiopulmonary Resuscitation." In *Trauma*, 2nd ed., ed. E. E. Moore, K. L. Mattox, and D. V. Feliciano, 99–107. Norwalk: Appleton & Lange.

Mock, C. N., G. J. Jurkovich, D. nii-Amon-Kotei, C. Arreola-Risa, and R. V. Maier. 1998. "Trauma Mortality Patterns in Three Nations at Different Economic Levels: Implications for Global Trauma System Development." *Journal of Trauma* 44 (5): 804–12.

Mock, C. N., M. Tiska, M. Adu-Ampofo, and G. Boakye. 2002. "Improvements in Prehospital Trauma Care in an African Country with No Formal Emergency Medical Services." *Journal of Trauma* 53 (1): 90–97.

Moylan, J. A. 1988. "Impact of Helicopters on Trauma Care and Clinical Results." *Annals of Surgery* 208 (6): 673–78.

Nurok, M. 2001. "The Death of a Princess and the Formulation of Medical Competence." *Social Science and Medicine* 53 (11): 1427–38.

Oyesola, R., D. Shehu, A. T. Ikeh, and I. Maru. 1997. "Improving Emergency Obstetric Care at a State Referral Hospital, Kebbi State, Nigeria." *International Journal of Gynecology and Obstetrics* 59 (Suppl. 2): S75–81.

Prevention of Maternal Mortality Network. 1995. "Situation Analysis of Emergency Obstetric Care: Examples from Eleven Operations Research Projects in West Africa." *Social Science and Medicine* 40 (5): 657–67.

Samai, O., and P. Sengeh. 1997. "Facilitating Emergency Obstetric Care through Transportation and Communication, Bo, Sierra Leone." *Int J Gynecol Obstet* 59 (Suppli. 2): S157–64.

Sampalis, J. S., S. Boukas, A. Lavoie, A. Nikolis, P. Frechette, R. Brown, and others. 1995. "Preventable Death Evaluation of the Appropriateness of the On-site Trauma Care Provided by Urgences-Sante Physicians." *Journal of Trauma* 39 (6): 1029–35; comment: 1027–28.

Sampalis, J. S., A. Lavoie, M. Salas, A. Nikolis, and J. I. Williams. 1994. "Determinants of On-scene Time in Injured Patients Treated by Physicians at the Site." *Prehospital and Disaster Medicine* 9 (3): 178–89.

Sampalis, J. S., H. Tamim, R. Denis, S. Boukas, S. A. Ruest, A. Nikolis, and others. 1997. "Ineffectiveness of On-site Intravenous Lines: Is Prehospital Time the Culprit?" *Journal of Trauma* 43 (4): 608–15; discussion: 615–17.

Sethi, D., I. Kwan, A. M. Kelly, I. Roberts, and F. Bunn. 2003. "Advanced Trauma Life Support Training for Ambulance Crews." *Cochrane Library* 2, Oxford, U.K.: Update Software.

Shehu, D., A. T. Ikeh, and M. J. Kuna. 1997. "Mobilising Transport for Obstetric Emergencies in Northwestern Nigeria." *International Journal of Gynecology and Obstetrics* 59 (Suppl. 2): S17–80.

St. John Ambulance. 1996. *First on the Scene: Emergency and Standard Levels.* Instructor's Guide, 2nd ed. Ottawa: St. John Ambulance Canada.

Tannebaum R. D., J. L. Arnold, A. De Negri Filho, and V. S. Spadoni. 2001. "Emergency Medicine in Southern Brazil." *Annals of Emergency Medicine* 37 (2): 223–28.

Weisman, S. M. and D. Y. Graham. 2002. "Evaluation of the Benefits and Risks of Low-Dose Aspirin in the Secondary Prevention of Cardiovascular and Cerebrovascular Events." *Arch Intern Med.* 162: 2197–2202.

White, K. L., T. F. Williams, and B. G. Greenberg. 1996. "The Ecology of Medical Care. 1961." *Bulletin of the New York Academy of Medicine* 73 (1): 187–205; discussion: 6–12.

Wilkinson, D. A., and M. W. Skinner. 2000. *Primary Trauma Care Manual: A Manual for Trauma Management in District and Remote Locations.* Oxford, U.K.: Primary Trauma Care Foundation.

WHO (World Health Organization). 2000. "Management of the Child with Serious Infection or Severe Malnutrition: Guidelines for Care at the First Referral Level in Developing Countries." Integrated Management of Childhood Illness, Department of Child and Adolescent Health and Development, WHO, Geneva.

———. 2002. *World Health Report 2002: Reducing Risks, Promoting Healthy Life.* Geneva: WHO.

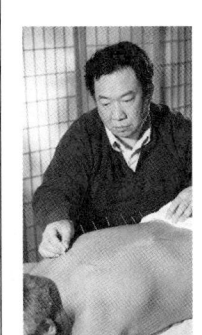

Chapter **69**

Complementary and Alternative Medicine

Haile T. Debas, Ramanan Laxminarayan, and Stephen E. Straus

The objective of medicine is to address people's unavoidable needs for emotional and physical healing. The discipline has evolved over millennia by drawing on the religious beliefs and social structures of numerous indigenous peoples, by exploiting natural products in their environments, and more recently by developing and validating therapeutic and preventive approaches using the scientific method. Public health and medical practices have now advanced to a point at which people can anticipate—and even feel entitled to—lives that are longer and of better quality than ever before in human history.

Yet despite the pervasiveness, power, and promise of contemporary medical science, large segments of humanity either cannot access its benefits or choose not to do so. More than 80 percent of people in developing nations can barely afford the most basic medical procedures, drugs, and vaccines. In the industrial nations, a surprisingly large proportion of people opt for practices and products for which proof as to their safety and efficacy is modest at best, practices that in the aggregate are known as *complementary and alternative medicine* (CAM) or as *traditional medicine* (TM).

Much of this book considers the formidable challenges to advancing human health through the further dispersion of effective and economical medical practices. This chapter considers both proven and unproven but popular CAM and TM approaches and attempts to portray their current and potential place in the overall practice of medicine.

With globalization, the pattern of disease in developing countries is changing. Unlike in the past, when communicable diseases dominated, now 50 percent of the health burden in developing nations is due to noncommunicable diseases,

such as cardiovascular diseases, diabetes, hypertension, depression, and use of tobacco and other addictive substances. Because lifestyle, diet, obesity, lack of exercise, and stress are important contributing factors in the causation of these noncommunicable diseases, CAM and TM approaches to these factors in particular will be increasingly important for the development of future health care strategies for the developing world.

DEFINITIONS AND DOMAINS OF COMPLEMENTARY AND ALTERNATIVE MEDICINE AND TRADITIONAL MEDICINE

We refer to medical practices that evolved with indigenous peoples and that they have introduced to other countries through emigration as traditional medicine. We refer to approaches that emerged primarily in Western, industrial countries during the past two centuries as scientific or Western medicine, although we acknowledge that not all Western medicine is based on scientifically proven knowledge. The terms *complementary* and *alternative* describe practices and products that people choose as adjuncts to or as alternatives to Western medical approaches. Increasingly, the terms *CAM* and *TM* are being used interchangeably (Kaptchuk and Eisenberg 2001; Straus 2004).

Endless varieties of practices are scientifically unproven and poorly accepted by medical authorities. For the sake of organizing an agenda for research into these approaches, the U.S. National Institutes of Health has grouped them into five somewhat overlapping domains (http://nccam.nih.gov/health/whatiscam) as follows:

- *Biologically based practices.* These include use of a vast array of vitamins and mineral supplements, natural products such as chondroitin sulfate, which is derived from bovine or shark cartilage; herbals, such as ginkgo biloba and echinacea; and unconventional diets, such as the low-carbohydrate approach to weight loss espoused by the late Robert Atkins.
- *Manipulative and body-based approaches.* These kinds of approaches, which include massage, have been used throughout history. In the 19th century, additional formal manipulative disciplines emerged in the United States: chiropractic medicine and osteopathic medicine. Both originated in an attempt to relieve structural forces on vertebrae and spinal nerve roots that practitioners perceived as evoking a panoply of illnesses beyond mere musculoskeletal pain.
- *Mind-body medicine.* Many ancient cultures assumed that the mind exerts powerful influences on bodily functions and vice versa. Attempts to reassert proper harmony between these bodily systems led to the development of mind-body medicine, an array of approaches that incorporate spiritual, meditative, and relaxation techniques.
- *Alternative medical systems.* Whereas the ancient Greeks postulated that health requires a balance of vital humors, Asian cultures considered that health depends on the balance and flow of vital energies through the body. This latter theory underlies the practice of acupuncture, for example, which asserts that vital energy flow can be restored by placing needles at critical body points.
- *Energy medicine.* This approach uses therapies that involve the use of energy—either biofield- or bioelectromagnetic-based interventions. An example of the former is Reiki therapy, which aims to realign and strengthen healthful energies through the intervention of energies radiating from the hands of a master healer.

Alternative systems of medicine use elements from each of these CAM and TM domains. For example, traditional Chinese medicine incorporates acupuncture, herbal medicines, special diets, and meditative exercises such as tai chi. Ayurveda in India similarly uses the meditative exercises of yoga, purifying diets, and natural products. In the West, homeopathic medicine and naturopathic medicine each arose in the late 19th century as reactions to the largely ineffectual and toxic conventional approaches of the day: purging, bleeding, and treatments with heavy metals such as mercury and arsenicals.

DEMOGRAPHY, USE, TOXICITY, AND EFFICACY

The use of CAM and TM varies widely between and within countries. The World Health Organization (WHO) has published and

Table 69.1 Estimated Use of CAM and TM by Patients and Practitioners Worldwide

Region or country	Extent of use
Africa	Used by 80 percent of the population for primary health care
Australia	Used by 49 percent of adults
China	Accounts for 30 to 50 percent of total health care
	Fully integrated into the health system
	95 percent of Chinese hospitals have TM units
India	Widely used
	2,860 hospitals provide TM
Indonesia	Used by 40 percent of the entire population
	Used by 70 percent of the rural population
Japan	72 percent of physicians practice TM
Thailand	TM integrated into 1,120 health centers
Vietnam	Fully integrated into the health care system
	30 percent of the population is treated with TM
Western countries	CAM and TM not strongly integrated into the health care system
	France: at least 75 percent of the population has used CAM at least once
	Germany: 77 percent of pain clinics provide acupuncture
	United States: 29 to 42 percent of population uses CAM

Source: WHO 2002.

summarized numerous surveys of use (table 69.1). In developing nations, TM is the sole source of health care for all but the privileged few. By contrast, in affluent countries individuals select CAM approaches according to their specific beliefs. For example, as many as 60 percent of those living in France, Germany, and the United Kingdom consume homeopathic or herbal products. Only 1 to 2 percent of Americans use homeopathy, but 10 percent of adults use herbal medicines, 8 percent visit chiropractors, and 1 to 2 percent undergo acupuncture every year (Ni, Simile, and Hardy 2002). Use of CAM and TM among patients with chronic, painful, debilitating, or fatal conditions, such as HIV/AIDS and cancer, is far higher, ranging from 50 to 90 percent (Richardson and Straus 2002).

There is remarkably little correlation between the use of CAM and TM approaches and scientific evidence that they are safe or effective. For many CAM and TM practices, the only evidence of their safety and efficacy is embodied in folklore. Beginning more than 1,500 years ago, data on the use of thousands of natural products were assembled into impressive monographs in China, India, and Korea, but these compendiums—and similar texts from Arabic, Egyptian, Greek, and Persian sources and their major European derivatives—are merely catalogs of products and their use rather than formal analyses of safety and efficacy.

Table 69.2 Some Natural Products That May Alter Drug Actions

Herbal product	Class of drug
Ephedra (*ma huang*)	Alpha and beta adrenergics
Garlic	Anticoagulants; some HIV protease inhibitors
Ginkgo biloba extract	Anticoagulants
Glucosamine	Antidiabetics
Saw palmetto	Androgens
St. John's wort	HIV protease inhibitors; some chemotherapy drugs; cyclosporine A; birth control
Valerian	Sedatives

Source: Niggemann and Gruber 2003.

Many people who today choose herbal products in lieu of prescription medications assume that because these products are natural, they must be safe, even when the evidence for this assertion is essentially anecdotal. Recent studies have shown that herbals are highly variable in quality and composition, with many marketed products containing little of the intended ingredients and containing unintended contaminants, such as heavy metals and prescription drugs. A few herbals are banned outright in several countries. Comfrey and kava have been associated with liver failure, aristolochia with genitourinary cancer (De Smet 2002), and ephedra with heart attacks and strokes (Shekelle and others 2003). More important, herbals contain ingredients that can accelerate or inhibit the metabolism of prescription drugs (table 69.2). The most notorious of these is St. John's wort, which affects the metabolism of nearly 50 percent of all prescription drugs (Markowitz and others 2003). The cumulative data on the pharmacological and potential adverse effects of herbal supplements now dictate that patients discuss their use of supplements with knowledgeable practitioners before initiating treatment.

As to evidence of the efficacy of CAM and TM approaches, thousands of small studies and case series have been reported over the past 50 years. Few were rigorous enough to be at all compelling, but they are sufficient to generate hypotheses that are now being tested in robust clinical trials. The existing body of data already shows that some approaches are useless, that for many the evidence is positive but weak, and that a few are highly encouraging (table 69.3).

ECONOMICS OF COMPLEMENTARY AND ALTERNATIVE MEDICINE AND TRADITIONAL MEDICINE

Although social, medical, and cultural reasons may account for why people in a given country prefer CAM and TM to conventional (Western) medicine, economic forces are also at play.

This section describes the socioeconomic determinants of seeking treatment from traditional healers and providers of CAM; reviews the evidence on the cost-effectiveness of CAM and TM; and discusses cost-effective approaches to regulating, improving, and expanding the use of CAM and TM. Much of this evidence is from industrial countries; few studies have been conducted in or are applicable to low- and middle-income countries. This caveat is important for two reasons. First, the CAM and TM modalities discussed in this section may not be used in many developing countries. Second, the limited data on cost-effectiveness may not be applicable in the case of those countries. Nevertheless, the data give a rough picture of the relative cost-effectiveness of a number of CAM and TM practices.

Economic Factors That Influence the Use of Complementary and Alternative Medicine and Traditional Medicine

Users of CAM and TM approaches choose health practices that resonate with their beliefs about health (Astin 1998). Although economic factors play a role in this choice, the underlying incentives are not always predictable. For instance, a common misconception is that patients opt for CAM and TM services because they are cheaper alternatives to conventional medical care. Even though there are certainly instances when the cost of treatment using CAM or TM is much cheaper than the cost of accessing a conventional medical service, several studies have found that CAM and TM cost the same or more than conventional treatments for the same conditions (see, for example, Muela, Mushi, and Ribera 2000).

At least one study has shown that financial considerations are rarely the primary factor in choosing a traditional healer, ranking behind such reasons as confidence in the treatment, ease of access, and convenience (Winston and Patel 1995). In the United States, the average cost of a single visit to a Navajo healer was US$388, and the average annual cost of using a traditional healer represented roughly a fifth of the reported annual income of respondents in a survey (Kim and Kwok 1998). The high cost of using a healer was cited as the most common barrier to seeking care from this source. In Kenya, the average charge per patient per visit to a TM practitioner was K Sh 46 (US$4 in 1981), which was significantly greater than the average charge per visit even in private health care facilities (Mwabu, Ainsworth and Nyamete 1993). Finally, a survey in Zimbabwe reported that the median cost of consulting an herbalist was Z$23 per visit, compared with Z$1 for a government clinic and Z$29 for a private doctor (Winston and Patel 1995). The same survey found that outcomes tended to be better when patients went to government clinics (67.3 percent of visits resulted in a good outcome) than when patients consulted herbalists (50 percent of visits resulted in a good outcome).

TM is not always more expensive than conventional medicine, however. Survey respondents in Ghana reported that the

Table 69.3 Levels of Evidence for the Efficacy of Selected CAM and TM Approaches

CAM or TM approach	Potential use	Study outcome	Level of evidence	Source
Artemisia annua	Treating drug-resistant malaria	Positive	A	van Agtmael, Eggelte, and van Boxtel 1999
Black cohosh	Controlling menopausal symptoms	Mixed	B	Kronenberg and Fugh-Berman 2003
Cranberry	Preventing urinary tract infection	Positive	B	Jepson, Mihaljevic, and Craig 2000
Echinacea	Preventing or treating viral colds	Mixed	B	Barrett 2003; Taylor and others 2003
Garlic	Lowering blood cholesterol	Positive	C	Le Bars and others 1997
Ginkgo biloba extract	Preventing or treating dementia	Mixed	B	Kanowski and Hoerr 2003
Ginseng	Improving energy and immunity against infection	Mixed	C	Richy and others 2003
Glucosamine	Relieving osteoarthritis	Positive	A	Reginster, Deroisy, and Rovalty 2001
Hawthorn	Improving cardiac function	Mixed	B	Pittler, Schmidt, and Ernst 2003
Milk thistle	Improving liver function	Positive	C	Jacobs and others 2002
St. John's wort	Treating moderate to severe depression	Negative	A	Hypericum Depression Trial Study Group 2002
	Treating mild depression	Positive	B	Di Carlo and others 2001
Saw palmetto	Relieving symptoms of benign prostatic hypertrophy	Positive	B	Gerber and others 2001
Acupuncture	Relieving arthritis pain	Positive	B	Berman and others 1999
	Relieving the pain of tooth extraction	Positive	B	Lao and others 1995
	Treating hypertension	Mixed	C	Chiu, Chi, and Reid 1995
	Relieving nausea from chemotherapy	Positive	A	Shen and others 2000
	Relieving addiction withdrawal	Mixed	B	Margolin and others 2002
	Treating asthma	Negative	B	Linde, Jobst, and Panton 2000
Meditation	Decreasing anxiety	Positive	B	Speca and others 2000
	Decreasing blood pressure	Mixed	B	Schneider and others 1995
Biofeedback	Preventing migraine	Positive	B	Holroyd and Penzien 1990
Homeopathy	Treating asthma	Mixed	B	White and others 2003
	Treating gastroenteritis	Positive	C	Jacobs and others 2003
Magnet therapy	Treating plantar fasciitis	Negative	B	Winemiller and others 2003
Chiropractic	Treating lower back pain	Positive	B	Cherkin and others 2003

Source: Authors.

A = multiple high-quality, randomized, controlled trials; B = single high-quality trials or smaller, less rigorous trials; C = weaker clinical trials; Mixed = conflicting results among studies of similar quality.

cost of malaria treatment at a health clinic ranged from ¢1,900 to ¢3,000 (US$1.30 to US$2.00 in 1997), treatment at home using drugs bought from pharmacies or health care workers ranged between ¢200 and ¢1,000 (US$0.10 to US$0.70), and treatment by an herbalist was virtually free (Ahorlu and others 1997).

Another common misconception is that the poor are more likely to use TM. At least one study shows that this may not be true. In Zimbabwe, the mean monthly income of households visiting an herbalist, Z$877, was greater than the mean monthly income of households using government clinics, Z$718 (Winston and Patel 1995).

Although some traditional healers charge more than conventional practitioners, their fees may be negotiable, the method of payment may be flexible (often on credit or in exchange for labor), and payment may be contingent on outcome. The availability of an outcome-contingent contract favors TM over Western medicine when the disease condition requires providers to both exert effort in curing patients and induce patients to comply with their recommendations. Nonetheless, this strategy may be difficult to apply to the larger health care system.

Furthermore, patients tend to seek care from traditional healers for conditions such as mental illness, impotence, and chronic disorders, which they perceive as requiring greater involvement by the extended family and kinship group. Accordingly, the availability of financial support for seeking treatments for these disorders is greater than it is for illnesses such as malaria or diarrhea, for which patients more often seek conventional treatment.

Few published data are available on the financial costs of TM in low- and middle-income countries. The data presented here on the use of traditional healers are extracted from the World Bank's living standards surveys in Vietnam to provide one nationally representative snapshot of the situation. Of 28,254 individuals in the sample, 10,033 had consulted a health care provider in the four weeks preceding the survey. These consultations included both home visits and visits to a provider. Of the 10,033, 1,829 had been to a public provider, 1,431 to a private provider, 7,650 to a pharmacy, and 259 to a traditional healer.[1] The most common reasons for visiting a traditional provider were headache, followed by cough and fever. The per visit drug cost for consulting a traditional healer was D 46, and the total cost per visit was D 51, compared with drug costs of D 38 and total costs of D 41 for going to a private clinic.

One commonly cited motivation for using CAM and TM is that their use might lower the incidence and costs of side effects associated with conventional treatments, but the published evidence on this point remains mixed. There is some evidence that CAM is used in addition to conventional treatments (Thomas and others 1991), but CAM may also have the effect of displacing conventional treatments. An outpatient survey found that, of 246 patients who had been receiving conventional treatment from the Royal London Homeopathic Hospital since the onset of care, a third had halted their conventional treatment and another third had reduced their intake of conventional medication (van Haselen 2000).[2] The extent to which homeopathic treatment displaced conventional treatment varied by indication. The use of homeopathic treatment often replaced conventional treatments in patients with skin and respiratory infections; in patients with cancer, its use was purely complementary and therefore added to overall health care costs.

Thomas and others (1991) observe that patients who use CAM and TM also commonly access conventional medical care. In industrial countries, most CAM usage complements conventional care, but this is also common in developing nations. For instance, Mwabu (1986) provides evidence from Kenya that patients are likely to use more than one type of provider from the range of those available, such as government facilities, mission clinics, private clinics, pharmacies, and traditional healers. Furthermore, the choice of provider depends on patients' illness, condition, socioeconomic status, and education. If an initial visit to one kind of provider did not resolve the disease satisfactorily, a follow-up visit was made to a different kind of provider. Finally, the quality of care—including efficiency of service and waiting time at government and private clinics—is an important determinant of whether patients choose to go to traditional healers. Most traditional healers surveyed in a second study referred patients to Western practices for treatment when necessary (Mwabu, Ainsworth, and Nyamete 1993).

Economic Evidence

Although most studies tend to focus on a specific CAM or TM practice, Sommer, Burgi, and Theiss (1999) looked more broadly at whether the provision of CAM and TM services through prepaid health plans or government insurance reduces the overall costs of health care and found that it does not. A possible reason is that few individuals who are offered access to CAM use them, and those who do might access those services in addition to, not in place of, more conventional health services.

Studies that compare the cost-effectiveness of different CAM and TM approaches using the same analytical framework are rare. One such study in Peru looked at the costs and cost-effectiveness of treatment using conventional medicine and TM (EsSalud andOPS 2000). Complementary medical practices evaluated included acupuncture, homeopathy, tai chi, meditation, reflexology, hydrotherapy, naturopathy, and massage. Patients were enrolled in either the Western medicine group or the CAM group. Patients were not randomized between the two treatment groups, but they were matched by disease pathology and severity, age, and sex. Furthermore, selected patients had completed at least one year in the health system, as the investigators reasoned that this would enable them to evaluate their follow-up. Overall, the investigators found that complementary medicine was between 53 and 63 percent less expensive than conventional medicine for achieving equivalent levels of effectiveness. Complementary medicine was especially cost-effective for osteoarthritis, hypertension, facial paralysis, and peptic ulcers.

The rest of this section looks at the economic evidence on specific forms of CAM or TM.

Acupuncture. Lindall's (1999) study finds that an acupuncture referral for musculoskeletal conditions costs a mean of US$422, roughly 60 percent less than the cost of referral to a Western practitioner. However, this study was not randomized, and patients had to have failed first-line drug treatment before being offered the choice of second line-treatment, either with acupuncture or with Western medicine.

Homeopathy. Evidence indicates that the cost of homeopathic medication is lower than the average cost of allopathic products, which would be an economic factor in favor of its use if homeopathy were proven to be effective. A study by the National Health Service in the United Kingdom found that the drug costs associated with homeopathy were lower than those of allopathic practitioners (Swayne 1992). A four-year study of 100 patients that compared homeopathic drug costs with those of conventional drugs found an average cost saving of US$96 during the study period for those using homeopathic drugs (Jain 2003).[3]

Ayurveda. A study that compared medical expenditures over a four-year period for participants in a comprehensive program of ayurvedic-based natural medicine (which included antioxidant strategies, mind-body medicine, and other techniques) with participants whose expenditures were covered through a BlueCross BlueShield health insurance plan found that the expenditures for the ayurvedic group were 50 percent lower per person (Orme-Johnson and Herron 1997). However, the study was not randomized and failed to control for the inclination of only a subset of people to accept and remain compliant with ayurvedic approaches.

Chiropractic. Some studies found that spinal manipulation is less expensive than conventional treatments for episodes of back pain. One nonrandomized study found that the cost of chiropractic treatment over a five-year period, including both provider costs and equipment costs (US$28,902), was 24 percent less than the cost of Western pain therapy (US$38,029) (Kumar, Malik, and Demeria 2002). Moreover, 15 percent of patients in the chiropractic group were able to return to work, compared with none in the control group.

However, other larger and better-controlled studies failed to find a difference between chiropractic and physical therapy in terms of either outcomes or costs (Cherkin and others 1998; Skargren and others 1997; Skargren, Carlsson, and Oberg 1998). A study of adults with low back pain who were randomly assigned to physical therapy or chiropractic manipulation or were just given an educational booklet found no significant differences in either the mean costs of care or the outcomes between the physical therapy and chiropractic groups (Cherkin and others 1998). Three-quarters of the participants in these groups—who incurred costs of roughly US$430 over the two-year period of the study—reported that their outcome was either good or excellent, compared with a third of those who were assigned booklets; however, the mean cost of care for the booklet group was only US$153 for the two-year period.

Mind-Body Treatments. Little evidence is available on the cost-effectiveness of practices such as meditation and yoga, but the cost of acquiring the skills required for these practices, as well as the time costs of practicing them, are so low relative to conventional medicine that evidence of their clinical effectiveness might suffice to justify their use on economic grounds. Available evidence from clinical studies suggests that mind-body treatments can be cost-effective (Caudill and others 1991; Friedman and others 1995; Hellman and others 1990; Sobel 1995). Blumenthal and others (2002) find significant declines in coronary events and in predicted costs of care for patients who were assigned to a one-and-a-half-hour long weekly class on stress management, relative to usual care for each of the first two years of follow-up and after five years.

Beyond Cost-Effectiveness: Ancillary Benefits and Costs of CAM and TM

Although cost-effectiveness is one guiding rationale for determining resource allocations for expanding (or restricting) access to CAM and TM, additional societal benefits and costs, such as effects on biodiversity, must also be considered. CAM and TM could provide a rationale for conserving species, but overharvesting of endangered species for medicinal purposes is also a concern. According to WHO, 85 percent of the world's population (principally those in developing countries) depends on plants for medicine, and 25 percent of prescription drugs have an active ingredient derived from a flowering plant (Cox 2001). The possible extinction of medicinal plants is of concern not only to developing countries but also to industrial countries, as in the cases of poaching of American ginseng and overharvesting of native saw palmetto. Similarly, the reliance of Chinese TM on tiger genitals, bear gallbladders, and black rhinoceros horns has played an important role in poaching and threatens to wipe out these mega fauna.

Local knowledge and culture regarding the uses of medicinal plants may be important determinants of whether a certain species will survive (Etkin 1998). In addition to the biodiversity value of these saved species, scientists may be able to analyze these plants for potential clinical application on a broader scale than TM permits. Although preserving traditional knowledge of healing practices helps preserve the culture and identity of indigenous populations, CAM and TM may impose significant costs. In such instances, promoting conventional treatments that do not depend on endangered species may bring important benefits to society.

EXPANDING THE BENEFICIAL USE OF COMPLEMENTARY AND ALTERNATIVE MEDICINE AND TRADITIONAL MEDICINE

Despite the uncertainty about the clinical efficacy and cost-effectiveness of certain CAM and TM practices, expansion of their use in instances in which moderate evidence of their efficacy and good evidence of their safety exists could yield health, social, and economic benefits. A number of surveys show that local pharmacies are the primary source of treatment for many ailments, especially in rural areas where government or private clinics are less accessible. In these situations, improving the quality of TM might serve as an effective substitute for allowing the unregulated use of conventional medical treatments. Training traditional healers is substantially less expensive than training doctors or nurses. A study of 52 traditional healers interviewed as part of a survey in Kenya estimated that the average out-of-pocket (cash) costs of training to be a traditional healer were K Sh 418 (US$40 in 1981) (Mwabu, Ainsworth, and Nyamete 1993).

Traditional healers can also be recruited into a more broadly based system for delivering public health; for example, with additional training, traditional healers can serve as primary health care workers (Hoff 1997) and provide advice on such matters as sexually transmitted diseases and oral rehydration therapy (Nations and de Souza 1997; Nations and others 1988; Ndubani and Hojer 1999). In addition, permitting access to CAM and TM within the context of the conventional health care system would facilitate access to multiple health services at one location.

Comprehensive policy on CAM and TM is lacking in most countries, including the United States. According to the 1994 Dietary Supplement, Health, and Education Act, the U.S. Food and Drug Administration cannot require proof that dietary supplements and herbal products are safe and effective before they are sold, although it is charged with requiring good manufacturing practices. The quality of herbal products is not regulated, and herbal products typically differ from source to source and from batch to batch in terms of their component ingredients and respective amounts and in terms of whether they contain contaminants. In the United States, no single entity is responsible for all aspects of CAM and TM control, education, information, and research, and no national, voluntary system of self-regulation exists. National nongovernmental organizations, such as the Accreditation Commission for Acupuncture and Oriental Medicine, the American Board of Medical Acupuncture, the Council of Chiropractic Education, the Council of Homeopathic Education, and the Commission on Massage Therapy Accreditation, accredit education in some CAM and TM fields, but such accreditation bodies do not exist in many developing countries. Nearly all countries lack rigorous research training programs in CAM and TM.

A common misperception is that in the developing world CAM and TM is used primarily by poorer, uneducated populations, while in industrial countries it is used more by affluent and better-educated segments of the population (Eisenberg and others 1998). In both settings, relatively little evidence supports this view. Many investigators have failed to critically assess the use of CAM and TM by minority and immigrant populations in Western nations. In Africa, nearly 85 percent of the population uses TM, often as the only way to obtain primary health care, and wealthier people in developing countries often use TM (WHO 2002). Investments in improving the quality and consistency of TM could reduce the cost of health care delivery, especially for chronic conditions such as arthritic pain and AIDS, where TM interventions may improve patients' sense of well-being, appetite, and energy. At the same time, in the absence of resources to extend the public health infrastructure, a network of certified CAM and TM providers could provide the infrastructure for delivering other care, such as immunizations and maternal-child health programs.

Recognizing the redistributive nature of investment in TM is important. Indigenous people will seek the help of traditional healers because of proximity, familiarity, and trust. Investments in TM could therefore be used strategically to increase access to conventional preventive and therapeutic care. Including the traditional healer as part of the health care team may thus be an important strategy both to attract patients and to upgrade the skills and training of traditional healers.

How equity is affected by the proportions in which different condition-specific interventions are combined and how other interventions (regulations, tax policy, managerial changes) are likely to affect equity need to be studied. Given that the majority of indigenous populations in developing countries use TM for their primary health care, the availability, safety, and affordability of TM, including herbal medicines, should be ensured as a matter of equity. One way to do this is by supporting local production of safe and effective herbals such as artemisia at affordable prices. In addition, rigorous research on TM should be supported. WHO is currently conducting collaborative studies on herbal treatments for HIV/AIDS, malaria, sickle cell anemia, and diabetes. Ineffective or unsafe herbal products identified by such studies should be removed from use, while those with proven efficacy and safety should be made available for therapeutic use.

LESSONS LEARNED AND IMPLEMENTATION

The pervasiveness of different modalities of TM and CAM varies greatly from country to country. For example, in China, where traditional Chinese medicine is well integrated into the health system, many different modalities may be used to treat a given condition. In the United States, by contrast, CAM programs are slowly being integrated with conventional medicine. Several medical schools have nascent CAM programs and have integrated them into medical school curricula to differing degrees. One of the more acclaimed programs of this kind in the United States is that developed by Andrew Weil at the University of Arizona Health Sciences Center. His Integrative Medicine Fellowship Program trains physicians in CAM and TM and strives to produce a new delivery model whereby physicians, patients, and nurses form a healing team for the care of the patient. However, this program needs to be critically evaluated before its adoption by more institutions can be urged.

Despite the complexity, diversity, and controversy surrounding CAM/TM approaches, some notable success stories reveal the influence of globalization, whereby modalities discovered in the developing world have been adopted in the West, with or without modifications, and vice versa.

Artemisinin

Artemisinin is a recently developed, active metabolite of artemisia, an herbal extract that has been used in China for centuries to treat fever. Chinese scientists determined the active ingredient of the herbal in the 1970s, and Western pharmaceutical companies have developed several derivatives as drugs for use against resistant *Plasmodium* malaria (Li and others 2000). Randomized clinical trials have shown that one such drug, dihydroartemisinin-piperaquine, is effective against drug-resistant *Plasmodium falciparum* malaria (Hien and Dolecek 2004). Another artemisinin derivative, artesunate, was shown to increase parasite clearance and reduce the gametocyte count when added to existing drugs to combat malaria (Adjuik and others 2004).

Acupuncture

Another CAM and TM modality that has considerable acceptance is acupuncture. Many pain management clinics, hospitals, and academic centers in the West now provide acupuncture services, and some insurance companies reimburse for acupuncture services. Rigorous clinical trials have demonstrative positive efficacy in two areas: (a) management of postoperative nausea and emesis (Shen and others 2000) and (b) amelioration of the pain of chronic osteoarthritis (Ezzo and others 2001; Soeken 2004; Tukmachi and others 2004). Studies providing rational explanations of the mechanisms whereby acupuncture might be achieving its effects complement the evidence about its efficacy; for example, one mechanism of action appears to involve opioid-dependent brain pathways. This kind of two-step process—that is, initial demonstration of clinical efficacy followed by scientific research into the mechanism of action—is one way that CAM and TM will gain scientific acceptance and integration into conventional medicine.

Chiropractic Medicine and Osteopathy

Chiropractic medicine was invented in the American heartland during the waning years of the 19th century. It uses spinal manipulation to treat an array of conditions thought to arise because of abnormal alignment of or stresses on vertebrae, most often in patients with musculoskeletal complaints. Two aspects of chiropractic medicine are success stories. First, even though practitioners of conventional medicine ostracized practitioners of chiropractic medicine in the late 19th century and the first half of the 20th century, it has gradually evolved into a viable healing discipline that is increasingly accepted by the conventional medicine community. The evolution of chiropractic can be compared with that of osteopathy. Osteopathy was developed in the United States in parallel with chiropractic, but the field elected to accommodate rather than reject allopathic techniques.

The second success story is research showing that chiropractic manipulation for low back pain is superior to bed rest, physical therapy, or provision of an educational booklet (Cherkin and others 1998). Chiropractic manipulation has also shown results comparable to those achieved with nonsteroidal, anti-inflammatory drugs in alleviating back pain (Straus 2004).

Homeopathy

Homeopathy is a success in terms of its broad appeal and use, not because of the strength of evidence supporting it. Indeed, few conventional scientists and physicians find homeopathy to be plausible. According to the "principle of similars" underlying homeopathy, practitioners choose remedies that, when given in high concentrations, produce symptoms similar to those that the patient presents with. The substance is then put in solution and serially diluted by as much as 10^{60}, well beyond the point defined by Avogadro's number (at which a single molecule of the original substance could remain in the solution). Homeopathy claims that the acts of serial diluting and vigorous shaking imprint information into water so that medicinal properties are retained even when no or few molecules of the starting medicine are present.

As implausible as this claim may seem, homeopathy is used worldwide with reported success (Jonas, Kaptchuk, and Linda 2003). Randomized controlled trials have suggested that it might be effective for treating influenza (Vickers and Smith 2000), allergies (Taylor and others 2000), and postoperative ileus (Barnes, Resch, and Ernst 1997). However, critics have questioned the quality and analyses of these trials. Some have questioned the validity of pooling data from trials of different populations, interventions, and outcome measures, as several reviews of homeopathy have done. Jonas, Kaptchuk, and Linda (2003, 393) assert that "there is a lack of conclusive evidence on the effectiveness of homeopathy for most conditions. Homeopathy deserves an open-minded opportunity to demonstrate its value by using evidence-based principles, but it should not be substituted for proven therapies."

Mind-Body Intervention

The work of David Spiegel at Stanford University on group support for breast cancer patients excited wide interest in the potential value of mind-body interventions (Spiegel and others 1989). The study was a randomized controlled trial with a 10-year follow-up involving 86 women with metastasized breast cancer. A one-year psychosocial intervention consisting of weekly supportive group therapy with self-hypnosis for pain showed that the mean survival time in the treated group was 37 months, compared with 19 months for the control group. Moreover, Spiegel (1994) notes that appropriate psychotherapy (both group and individual) not only reduced depression and anxiety and improved coping skills, but also saved money by reducing the number of office visits, diagnostic tests, medical procedures, and hospital admittances. Although Spiegel's findings have not been replicated, they do illustrate the potential benefits of mind-body intervention and have led to studies of possible mechanisms through which such interventions may operate.

THE RESEARCH AND DEVELOPMENT AGENDA

The lack of product quality and consistency and the absence of compelling data on the safety and efficacy of most CAM and TM approaches present major challenges to any effort to optimize the distribution of precious health resources. These difficulties also pose opportunities for research. Other formidable challenges include the variability in training, credentialing, and licensing CAM and TM practitioners. Increasingly, efforts are being made in several countries to regulate both products and practitioners. Ultimately, stringent controls on training, practices, and products must be complemented by rigorous research to ascertain which approaches are safe and effective—and for which indications.

The global use and potential effect of CAM and TM practices, the lack of adequate data validating their safety and efficacy, and the existence of highly effective conventional alternatives for many of them dictate that resources should be devoted to fuller characterization and standardization of CAM and TM approaches. Investing precious resources in integrating such approaches further into health care infrastructures can be justified only on the basis of compelling data. This point leads to the question of what constitutes a rational agenda for this work.

For resource-rich industrial nations, one model for CAM and TM research is that being implemented by the National Center for Complementary and Alternative Medicine (NCCAM) of the U.S. National Institutes of Health (http://nccam.nih.gov). In 2004, NCCAM planned to invest US$117 million in research and research training. It is supporting some 800 individual projects at present, including studies of the composition of natural products and their pharmacological effects, studies of the neurobiological mechanisms of acupuncture and the placebo effect, and clinical trials with 30 to 30,000 participants. NCCAM now has a strategic plan for its international programs that emphasizes research, training, and efforts to learn about the rich, indigenous TM heritage. Australia, through a government agency similar to NCCAM, is conducting research and training programs in collaboration with its indigenous people. Although the scope of NCCAM's research agenda is larger than what most other nations could accommodate, its underlying philosophy should be universal. That is, the standards for research into CAM and TM approaches

should be no different from those used in conventional biomedical research.

Both CAM and TM and biomedical practitioners need to understand the strengths, limitations, and contributions of their particular approaches so that they can work together in ways that ensure the best possible care for their patients and the achievement of their shared goals of improved individual and public health. Once these issues have been addressed, countries could devote additional resources to studying those CAM and TM approaches that appear to be the most promising in relation to their most pressing public health problems. Some priority areas for CAM and TM research are widely applicable, including studies of approaches to palliate chronic pain and suffering, relieve depression, help release the grip of addictive substances, and slow the progression of degenerative disorders such as arthritis and dementia.

NOTES

1. Because some individuals had gone to more than one provider during the four-week period, the total comes to more than 10,033.

2. The median duration of current treatment at the Royal London Homeopathic Hospital was three years.

3. This study did not take into account the costs of physician time, the costs of laboratory tests, or patients' costs.

REFERENCES

Adjuik, M., A. Babiker, P. Garner, P. Olliaro, W. Taylor, and N. White. 2004. "Artesunate Combinations for Treatment of Malaria: Meta-Analysis." *Lancet* 363 (9402): 9–17.

Ahorlu, C. K., S. K. Dunyo, E. A. Afari, K. A. Koran, and F. K. Nkrumah. 1997. "Malaria-Related Beliefs and Behavior in Southern Ghana: Implications for Treatment, Prevention, and Control." *Tropical Medicine and International Health* 2 (5): 488–99.

Astin, J. A. 1998. "Why Patients Use Alternative Medicine: Results of a National Study." *Journal of the American Medical Association* 279 (19): 1549–53.

Barnes, J., K. L. Resch, and E. Ernst. 1997. "Homeopathy for Postoperative Ileus? A Meta-Analysis." *Journal of Clinical Gastroenterology* 25: 628–33.

Barrett, B. 2003. "Medicinal Properties of Echinacea: A Critical Review." *Phytomedicine* 10: 66–86.

Berman, B. M., B. B. Singh, L. Lao, P. Langenberg, H. Li, V. Hadhazy, and others. 1999. "A Randomized Trial of Acupuncture as an Adjunctive Therapy in Osteoarthritis of the Knee." *Rheumatology* 38: 346–54.

Blumenthal, J. A., M. Babyak, J. Wei, C. O'Connor, R. Waugh, E. Eisenstein, and others. 2002. "Usefulness of Psychosocial Treatment of Mental Stress-Induced Myocardial Ischemia in Men." *American Journal of Cardiology* 89 (2): 164–68.

Caudill, M., R. Schnable, P. Zuttermeister, H. Benson, and R. Friedman. 1991. "Decreased Clinic Use by Chronic Pain Patients: Response to Behavioral Medicine Interventions." *Clinical Journal of Pain* 7: 305–10.

Cherkin, D. C., R. A. Deyo, M. Battie, J. Street, and W. Barlow. 1998. "A Comparison of Physical Therapy, Chiropractic Manipulation, and Provision of an Educational Booklet for the Treatment of Patients with Low Back Pain." *New England Journal of Medicine* 339 (15): 1021–29.

Cherkin, D. C., K. J. Sherman, R. A. Deyo, and P. G. Shekelle. 2003. "A Review of the Evidence for the Effectiveness, Safety, and Cost of Acupuncture, Massage Therapy, and Spinal Manipulation for Back Pain." *Annals of Internal Medicine* 138: 898–906.

Chiu, Y. J., A. Chi, and I. A. Reid. 1995. "Cardiovascular and Endocrine Effects of Acupuncture in Hypertensive Patients." *Clinical and Experimental Hypertension* 19: 1047–63.

Cox, P. A. 2001. "Biodiversity and Pharmacology." In *Encyclopedia of Biodiversity*, vol. 4, ed. S. A. Levin. San Diego, CA: Academic Press.

De Smet, P. A. 2002. "Herbal Remedies." *New England Journal of Medicine* 347: 2046–56.

Di Carlo, G., F. Borrelli, E. Ernst, and A. A. Izzo. 2001. "St. John's Wort: Prozac from the Plant Kingdom." *Trends in Pharmacologic Science* 22: 292–97.

Eisenberg, D. M., R. B. Davis, S. G. Ettner, and S. Appel. 1998. "Trends in Alternative Medicine Use in the United States, 1990–1997: Results of a Follow-Up National Survey." *Journal of the American Medical Association* 28 (18): 1569–75.

EsSalud and OPS (Organización Panamericana de Salud [Pan American Health Organization]). 2000. "Estudio costo-efectividad: Programa Nacional de Medicina Complementaria." Seguro Social de EsSalud. Lima: EsSalud and OPS.

Etkin, N. L. 1998. "Indigenous Patterns of Conserving Biodiversity: Pharmacologic Implications." *Journal of Ethnopharmacology* 63 (3): 233–45.

Ezzo, J., V. Hadhazi, H. Birch, L. Lao, G. Kaplan, and M. Hochberg. 2001. "Acupuncture for Osteoarthritis of the Knee: A Systematic Review." *Arthritis and Rheumatism* 44 (4): 819–825.

Friedman, R., D. Sobel, P. Myers, M. Caudill, and H. Benson. 1995. "Behavioral Medicine, Clinical Health Psychology, and Cost Offset." *Health Psychology* 14: 509–18.

Gerber, G. S., D. Kuznetsov, B. C. Johnson, and J. D. Burstein. 2001. "Randomized, Double-Blind, Placebo-Controlled Trial of Saw Palmetto in Men with Lower Urinary Tract Symptoms." *Urology* 58: 860–64.

Hien, T. T., and C. Dolecek. 2004. "Piperaquine against Multidrug-Resistant *Plasmodium falciparum* Malaria." *Lancet* 363: 18–22.

Hellman, C. J., M. Budd, J. Borysenko, D. C. McClelland, and H. Benson. 1990. "The Study of the Effectiveness of Two Group Behavioral Medicine Interventions for Patients with Psychosomatic Complaints." *Behavioral Medicine* 16: 165–73.

Hoff, W. 1997. "Traditional Health Practitioners as Primary Health Care Workers." *Tropical Doctor* 27 (Suppl. 1): 52–55.

Holroyd, K. A., and D. B. Penzien. 1990. "Pharmacological versus Non-Pharmacological Prophylaxis of Recurrent Migraine Headache: A Meta-Analytic Review of Clinical Trials." *Pain* 42: 1–13.

Hypericum Depression Trial Study Group. 2002. "Effect of *Hypericum perforatum* (St. John's Wort) in Major Depressive Disorder: A Randomized Controlled Trial." *Journal of the American Medical Association* 287: 1807–14.

Jacobs, B. P., C. Dennehy, G. Ramirez, J. Sapp, and V. A. Lawrence. 2002. "Milk Thistle for the Treatment of Liver Disease: A Systematic Review and Meta-Analysis." *American Journal of Medicine* 113: 506–13.

Jain, A. 2003. "Does Homeopathy Reduce the Cost of Conventional Drug Prescribing? A Study of Comparative Prescribing Costs in General Practice." *Homeopathy* 92 (2): 71–76.

Jepson, R. G., L. Mihaljevic, and J. Craig. 2000. "Cranberries for Preventing Urinary Tract Infections." Cochrane Database Systematic Review CD001321 [PMID:15106157].

Jonas, W. B., T. J. Kaptchuk, and K. Linda. 2003. "Critical Overview of Homeopathy." *Annals of Internal Medicine* 138: 393–99.

Kanowski, S., and R. Hoerr. 2003. "Ginkgo Biloba Extract EGb 761® in Dementia: Intent-to-Treat Analyses of a 24-Week, Multicenter, Double-Blind, Placebo-Controlled, Randomized Trial." *Pharmacopsychiatry* 36: 297–303.

Kaptchuk, T. J., and D. M. Eisenberg. 2001. "Varieties of Healing. 2: A Taxonomy of Unconventional Practices." *Annals of Internal Medicine* 135: 196–204.

Kim, C., and Y. S. Kwok. 1998. "Navajo Use of Native Healers." *Archives of Internal Medicine* 158 (20): 2245–49.

Kronenberg, F., and A. Fugh-Berman. 2003. "Complementary and Alternative Approach for Menopause: A Review of Randomized, Controlled Trials." *Reproductive Toxicology* 17: 137–52.

Kumar, K., S. Malik, and D. Demeria. 2002. "Treatment of Chronic Pain with Spinal Cord Stimulation versus Alternative Therapies: Cost-Effectiveness Analysis." *Neurosurgery* 51 (1): 106–15.

Lao, L., S. Bergman, P. Langenberg, R. H. Wong, and B. Berman. 1995. "Efficacy of Chinese Acupuncture on Postoperative Oral Surgery." *Oral Surgery, Oral Medicine, Oral Pathology, Oral Radiology, and Endodontics* 79: 423–28.

Le Bars, P. L., M. M. Katz, N. Berman, T. M. Itil, A. M. Freedman, and A. F. Shatzberg. 1997. "A Placebo-Controlled, Double-Blind, Randomized Trial of an Extract of Ginkgo Biloba for Dementia, North American EGb Study Group." *Journal of the American Medical Association* 278: 1327–32.

Li, Y., Y. M. Zhu, H. J. Jiang, J. P. Pan, G. S. Wu, J. M. Wu, and others. 2000. "Synthesis of Antimalarial Activity of Artemisinin Derivatives Containing an Amino Group." *Journal of Medical Chemistry* 43 (8): 1635–40.

Lindall, S. 1999. "Is Acupuncture for Pain Relief in General Practice Cost-Effective?" *Acupuncture Medicine* 17: 97–100.

Linde, K., K. Jobst, and J. Panton. 2000. "Acupuncture for Chronic Asthma." Cochrane Database Systematic Review CD000008 [PMID:11416076].

Margolin, A., H. D. Kleber, S. K. Avants, J. Konefal, F. Gawin, E. Stark, and others. 2002. "Acupuncture for the Treatment of Cocaine Addiction: A Randomized Controlled Trial." *Journal of the American Medical Association* 287: 55–63.

Markowitz, J. S., J. L. Donovan, C. L. DeVane, R. M. Taylor, Y. Ruan, J. S. Wang, and K. D. Chavin. 2003. "Effect of St. John's Wort on Drug Metabolism by Induction of Cytochrome P450 3A4 Enzyme." *Journal of the American Medical Association* 290: 1500–4.

Muela, S. H., A. K. Mushi, and J. M. Ribera. 2000. "The Paradox of the Cost and Affordability of Traditional and Government Health Services in Tanzania." *Health Policy Planning* 15 (3): 296–302.

Mwabu, G. 1986. "Health Care Decisions at the Household Level: Results of a Rural Health Survey in Kenya." *Social Science and Medicine* 22 (3): 315–19.

Mwabu, G., M. Ainsworth, and A. Nyamete. 1993. "Quality of Medical Care and Choice of Medical Treatment in Kenya." *Journal of Human Resources* 28 (4): 838–62.

Nations, M. K., and M. A. de Souza. 1997. "Umbanda Healers as Effective AIDS Educators: Case Control Study in Brazilian Urban Slums (Favelas)." *Tropical Doctor* 27 (Suppl. 1): 60–66.

Nations, M. K., M. A. de Sousa, L. L. Correia, and D. M. da Silva. 1988. "Brazilian Popular Healers as Effective Promoters of Oral Rehydration Therapy (ORT) and Related Child Survival Strategies." *Bulletin of the Pan American Health Organization* 22 (4): 335–54.

Ndubani, P., and B. Hojer. 1999. "Traditional Healers as a Source of Information and Advice for People with Sexually Transmitted Diseases in Rural Zambia." *Tropical Doctor* 29 (1): 36–38.

Ni, H., C. Simile, and A. M. Hardy. 2002. "Utilization of Complementary and Alternative Medicine by United States Adults: Results from the 1999 National Health Interview Survey." *Medical Care* 40: 353–58.

Niggemann, B., and C. Gruber. 2003. "Side Effects of Complementary and Alternative Medicine." *Allergy* 58: 707–16.

Orme-Johnson, D. W., and R. E. Herron. 1997. "An Innovative Approach to Reducing Medical Care Utilization and Expenditures." *American Journal of Managed Care* 3 (1): 135–44.

Pittler, M. H., K. Schmidt, and E. Ernst. 2003. "Hawthorn Extract for Treating Chronic Heart Failure: A Meta-Analysis of Randomized Trials." *American Journal of Medicine* 114: 665–74.

Reginster, J. Y., R. Deroisy, and L. Rovalty. 2001. "Long-Term Effects of Glucosamine Sulphate on Osteoarthritis Progression: A Randomised, Placebo-Controlled Clinical Trial." *Lancet* 357: 251–56.

Richardson, M. A., and S. E. Straus. 2002. "Complementary and Alternative Medicine: Opportunities and Challenges for Cancer Management and Research." *Seminars in Oncology* 29: 531–45.

Richy, F., O. Bruyere, O. Ethgen, M. Cucherat, Y. Henrotin, and J. Y. Reginster. 2003. "Structural and Symptomatic Efficacy of Glucosamine and Chondroitin in Knee Osteoarthritis: A Comprehensive Meta-Analysis." *Archives of Internal Medicine* 163: 1514–22.

Schneider, R. H., F. Staggers, C. N. Alexander, W. Sheppard, M. Rainforth, K. Kondwani, and others. 1995. "A Randomized Controlled Trial of Stress Reduction for Hypertension in Older African Americans." *Hypertension* 26: 820–27.

Shekelle, P. G., M. L. Hardy, S. Morton, M. Maglione, W. A. Mojica, M. J. Suttorp, and others. 2003. "Efficacy and Safety of Ephedra and Ephedrine for Weight Loss and Athletic Performance: A Meta-Analysis." *Journal of the American Medical Association* 289: 1537–45.

Shen, J., N. Wenger, J. Glaspy, R. D. Hays, P. S. Albert, C. Choi, and P. G. Shekelle. 2000. "Electroacupuncture for Control of Myeloablative Chemotherapy-Induced Emesis: A Randomized Controlled Trial." *Journal of the American Medical Association* 284: 2755–61.

Skargren, E. I., P. G. Carlsson, and B. E. Oberg. 1998. "One-Year Follow-Up Comparison of the Cost and Effectiveness of Chiropractic and Physiotherapy as Primary Management for Back Pain: Subgroup Analysis, Recurrence, and Additional Health Care Utilization." *Spine* 23 (17): 1875–84.

Skargren, E. I., B. E. Oberg, P. G. Carlsson, and M. Gade. 1997. "Cost and Effectiveness Analysis of Chiropractic and Physiotherapy Treatment for Low Back and Neck Pain: Six-Month Follow-Up." *Spine* 22 (18): 2167–77.

Sobel, D. S. 1995. "Rethinking Medicine: Improving Health Outcomes with Cost-Effective Psychosocial Interventions." *Psychosomatic Medicine* 57: 234–44.

Soeken, K. L. 2004. "Selected CAM Therapies for Arthritis-Related Pain: The Evidence from Systematic Reviews." *Clinical Journal of Pain* 20 (1): 13–18.

Sommer, J. H., M. Burgi, and R. Theiss. 1999. "A Randomized Experiment of the Effects of Including Alternative Medicine in the Mandatory Benefit Package of Health Insurance Funds in Switzerland." *Complementary Therapeutic Medicine* 7 (2): 54–61.

Speca, M., L. E. Carlson, E. Goodey, and M. Angen. 2000. "A Randomized, Wait-List Controlled Clinical Trial: The Effect of a Mindfulness-Based Stress Reduction Program on Mood and Symptoms of Stress in Cancer Patients." *Psychosomatic Medicine* 62: 2613–22.

Spiegel, D. 1994. "Health Caring, Psychosocial Support for Patients with Cancer." *Cancer* 74 (4): 1453–56.

Spiegel, D., J. R. Bloom, H. C. Kraemer, and E. Gottheil. 1989. "Effect of Psychosocial Treatment on Survival of Patients with Metastatic Breast Cancer." *Lancet* 2 (8668): 888–91.

Straus, S. E. 2004. "Complementary and Alternative Medicine." In *Cecil Textbook of Medicine*, 22nd ed., ed. L. Goldman and D. Ausiello, Philadelphia: Saunders.

Swayne, J. 1992. "The Cost and Effectiveness of Homeopathy." *British Homeopathic Journal* 81: 148–50.

Taylor, J. A., W. Weber, L. Standish, H. Quinn, J. Goesling, M. McGann, and C. Calabrese. 2003. "Efficacy and Safety of Echinacea in Treating Upper Respiratory Tract Infections in Children: A Randomized Controlled Trial." *Journal of the American Medical Association* 290: 2824–30.

Taylor, M. A., D. Reilly, R. H. Llewellyn-Jones, C. McSharry, and T. C. Aitchison. 2000. "Randomised Controlled Trial of Homeopathy versus Placebo in Perennial Allergic Rhinitis with Overview of Four Trial Series." *British Medical Journal* 321: 471–76.

Thomas, K. J., J. Carr, L. Westlake, and B. T. William. 1991. "Use of Nonorthodox and Conventional Health Care in Great Britain." *British Medical Journal* 302 (6770): 207–10.

Tukmachi, E., R. Jubb, E. Dempsy, and P. Jones. 2004. "The Effect of Acupuncture on Symptoms of Knee Osteoarthritis: An Open Randomized Controlled Study." *Acupuncture Medicine* 22 (1): 14–22.

van Agtmael, M. A., T. A. Eggelte, and C. J. van Boxtel. 1999. "Artemisinin Drugs in the Treatment of Malaria: From Medicinal Herb to Registered Medication." *Trends in Pharmacologic Science* 20: 199–205.

van Haselen, R. 2000. "The Economic Evaluation of Complementary Medicine: A Staged Approach at the Royal London Homoeopathic Hospital." *British Homeopathic Journal* 89 (Suppl. 1): S23–26.

Vickers, A. J., and C. Smith. 2000. "Homeopathic Oscillococcinum for Preventing and Treating Influenza and Influenza-Like Symptoms." Cochrane Database Systematic Review CD001957 [PMID:10796675].

White, A., P. Slade, C. Hunt, A. Hart, and E. Ernst. 2003. "Individualized Homeopathy as an Adjunct in the Treatment of Childhood Asthma: A Randomized Placebo Controlled Trial." *Thorax* 58: 317–21.

WHO (World Health Organization). 2002. "Fact Sheet No. 271" (June). WHO, Geneva.

Winemiller, M. H., R. G. Billow, E. R. Laskowski, and W. S. Harmsen. 2003. "Effect of Magnetic versus Sham-Magnetic Insoles on Plantar Heel Pain: A Randomized Controlled Trial." *Journal of the American Medical Association* 290: 1474–78.

Winston, C. M., and V. Patel. 1995. "Use of Traditional and Orthodox Health Services in Urban Zimbabwe." *International Journal of Epidemiology* 24 (5): 1006–12.

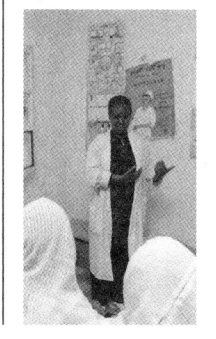

Chapter **70**

Improving the Quality of Care in Developing Countries

John W. Peabody, Mario M. Taguiwalo, David A. Robalino, and Julio Frenk

Although the quantity rather than quality of health services has been the focus historically in developing countries, ample evidence suggests that quality of care (or the lack of it) must be at the center of every discussion about better health. The following examples are illustrative: In one study evaluating pediatric care in Papua New Guinea, 69 percent of health center workers reported that they checked for only two of the four examination criteria for pneumonia cases. Only 24 percent of these workers were able to indicate correct treatment for malaria. When clinical encounters were observed at aid posts, providers met minimal examination criteria in only 1 percent of cases (Beracochea and others 1995). In a study in Pakistan, only 56 percent of providers met an acceptable diagnostic standard for viral diarrhea, and only 35 percent met the acceptable standard for treatment (Thaver and others 1998).

QUALITY DEFINITION AND POPULATION FRAMEWORK

These deficiencies in quality of care represent neither the failure of professional compassion nor necessarily a lack of resources (Institute of Medicine 2001). Rather, they result from gaps in knowledge, inappropriate applications of available technology (Murray and Frenk 2000), or the inability of organizations to change (Berwick 1989). Local health care systems may have failed to align practitioner incentives and objectives, to measure clinical practice, or to link quality improvement to better health outcomes.

Increasing evidence, much of it developed since the mid 1990s, shows that quality can be improved rapidly. However, to improve clinical practice—and thus quality of care—quality must be defined and measured, and appropriate steps must be taken (Silimper and others 2002). This chapter highlights approaches to improving clinical practice and quality of care that take place over months instead of years. Indeed, better quality can improve health much more rapidly than can other drivers of health, such as economic growth, educational advancement, or new technology.

Definition and Framework

Health systems provide health actions—activities to improve or maintain health. These actions take place in the context of and are influenced by political, cultural, social, and institutional factors (shown along the edges of figure 70.1). Demographic and socioeconomic makeup, including genetics and personal resources, affect the health status of individuals seeking care. Access to the health care system is required to obtain the care that maintains or improves health, but simple access is not enough; the system's capacities must be applied skillfully. Thus, *quality* means optimizing material inputs and practitioner skill to produce health. As the Institute of Medicine defines it, quality is "the degree to which health services for individuals and populations increase the likelihood of desired health outcomes and are consistent with current professional knowledge" (Institute of Medicine 2001, 244).

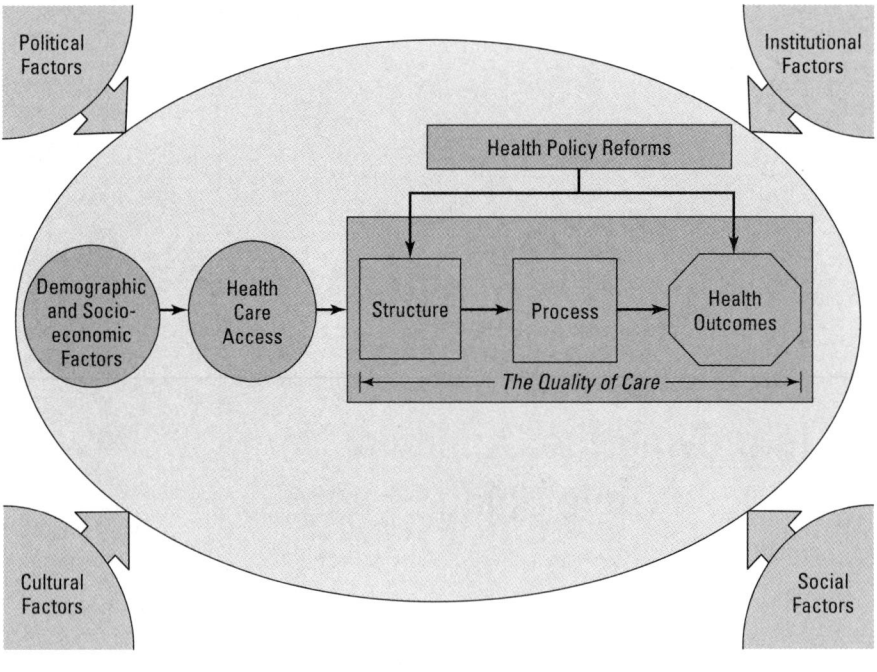

Source: Peabody and others 1999.

Figure 70.1 Quality-of-Care Framework

Elements of Quality. Quality comprises three elements:

- *Structure* refers to stable, material characteristics (infrastructure, tools, technology) and the resources of the organizations that provide care and the financing of care (levels of funding, staffing, payment schemes, incentives).
- *Process* is the interaction between caregivers and patients during which structural inputs from the health care system are transformed into health outcomes.
- *Outcomes* can be measured in terms of health status, deaths, or disability-adjusted life years—a measure that encompasses the morbidity and mortality of patients or groups of patients. Outcomes also include patient satisfaction or patient responsiveness to the health care system (WHO 2000).

Structural measures are the easiest to obtain and most commonly used in studies of quality in developing countries. Many evaluations have revealed shortages in medical staff, medications and other important supplies, and facilities, but material measures of structure, perhaps surprisingly, are not causally related to better health outcomes (Donabedian 1980). Although higher technology or a more pleasant environment may be conducive to better-quality care, the evidence indicates only a weak link between such structural elements and better health outcomes (Donabedian 1988). The notable exceptions are cases in which physical improvements either increase access to primary care in very poor settings or increase the volume of a clinical procedure, such as cataract surgery, that is specifically linked to

better health outcomes (Javitt, Venkataswamy, and Sommer 1983). At best, however, structure is a blunt approximation of process or outcomes; structural improvements by themselves rarely improve the health of a population.

Process, by contrast, can be measured with every visit to a provider. Measuring process is difficult, however, particularly in developing countries. The private nature of the doctor-patient consultation, a lack of measurement criteria, and the absence of reliable measurement tools have limited the ability to assess process (Peabody, Tozija, and others 2004). However, new methods are being developed that can provide valid measurements of clinical practice (Thaver and others 1998). In addition, evidence-based clinical studies have steadily revealed which process measures lead to better health outcomes. This combination of ubiquity, measurability, and linkage to health outcomes makes the measurement of process the preferred way to assess quality.

Although good outcomes are the objective of all health actions, outcomes alone are not an efficient way to measure quality for two reasons. The first is the quality conundrum. A patient may receive poor-quality care but may recover fully, or a patient may receive high-quality care for an illness such as cerebral malaria and still not recover. Second, adverse health outcomes are relatively rare and obviously do not occur with every encounter.

The classic framework of structure-process-outcome is well established. However, in recent years the concept of quality has been expanded to include specific aims for improvement. For example, the Institute of Medicine's (2001) landmark report,

Crossing the Quality Chasm, broadens the concept to include other, more contextual elements to illuminate how process changes can improve care. It focuses on six aims: patient safety, effectiveness, patient centeredness, timeliness, efficiency, and equity (see box 70.1).

Quality Assessment Perspectives. We can look at the Institute of Medicine's aims from two perspectives: patient perception, and technical or professional assessment. Patients' perceptions of quality depend on their individual characteristics and affect their compliance, follow-up decisions, and long-term lifestyle changes (Zaslavsky and others 2000). Interpersonal relationships, cultural appropriateness, and gender sensitivity—long thought to be luxuries of wealthier countries—are also major determinants of patient access and utilization in developing countries. These findings have led to the inclusion of patient satisfaction and patient responsiveness as outcome measures.

Technical assessment concerns whether providers meet normative standards for appropriateness of care or adherence to explicit evidence-based criteria. Although patient perception or satisfaction is important, researchers increasingly rely on objective, evidence-based quality criteria that can be more readily linked to better health outcomes at both the individual and the population levels.

Population-Level Considerations. Quality is typically assessed through the interaction between individual doctors and patients. However, emerging evidence shows that the average quality of care given by groups of doctors and other providers is an important determinant of overall community health status. For example, in a cross-sectional analysis in the former Yugoslav Republic of Macedonia, researchers found not only that patients' heath status was significantly higher in areas where quality was higher but also that the overall self-reported health status of those members of the general population who had not recently received care was higher (Peabody, Tozija, and others 2004).

Our quality-of-care framework supports these findings. When process is improved among groups of providers, the aggregate improvement in quality leads to better health outcomes for the entire patient population. In addition, resources can be allocated among clinical interventions based on actual effectiveness and the overall impact of care on the population. For example, cancer chemotherapy may be available and may prolong the lives of cancer patients. However, it may result in fewer lives saved than the expansion of coverage of directly observed treatment short-course coverage for tuberculosis patients.

QUALITY OF CARE IN DEVELOPING COUNTRIES

The process of providing care in developing countries is often poor and varies widely. A large body of evidence from industrial countries consistently shows variations in process, and these findings have transformed how quality of care is perceived (McGlynn and others 2003). A 2002 study found that physicians complied with evidence-based guidelines for at least 80 percent of patients in only 8 of 306 U.S. hospital regions (Wennberg, Fisher, and Skinner 2002). It is important to note that these variations appear to be independent of access to care or cost of care: Neither greater supply nor higher spending resulted in better care or better survival. Studies from developing countries show similar results. For example, care in tertiary and teaching hospitals and care provided by specialists may be better than care for the same cases in primary care facilities and by generalists (Walker, Ashley, and Hayes 1988).

One explanation for variation and low-quality care in the developing world is lack of resources. Limited data indicate, however, that high-quality care can be provided even in environments with severely constrained resources. A study in Jamaica, which used a cross-sectional analysis of government-run primary care clinics, showed that better process alone was linked to significantly greater birthweight (Peabody, Gertler, and Liebowitz 1998). A study in Indonesia attributed 60 percent of all perinatal deaths to poor process and only 37 percent to economic constraints (Supratikto and others 2002).

Cross-system or cross-national comparisons provide the best examples of the great variation in clinical practice in developing countries. In one seven-country study, researchers directly observing clinical practice found that 75 percent of cases were not adequately diagnosed, treated, or monitored and that inappropriate treatment with antibiotics, fluids, feeding, or oxygen occurred in 61 percent of cases (Nolan and others 2001). Another study compared providers' knowledge and practice in California and FYR Macedonia, using vignettes to adjust for case-mix severity. Although the quality of the overall or aggregate process was lower in FYR Macedonia, a poor country, the top 5 percent of Macedonian doctors performed as well as or better than the average Californian doctor (Peabody, Tozija, and others 2004).

In a study commissioned for this chapter, an international team measured quality in five developing countries (China, El Salvador, India, Mexico, and the Philippines), using the same clinical vignettes at each site. The team evaluated the process for common diseases according to international, evidence-based criteria. Quality varied only slightly among countries. The within-country range of quality of doctors was 10 times as great as the between-country range. Such wide variation strongly suggests that efforts to improve health status must involve policies that change the quality of clinical care.

POLICY INTERVENTIONS TO IMPROVE QUALITY

The success of quality improvement policies can be measured by their ability to raise the average level of health and reduce variation in quality. Two types of policies are intended to improve quality and thus health outcomes:

- those that influence provider behavior by altering the structural conditions of organization and finance or that involve the design and redesign of health care systems
- those that directly target provider behavior at the individual or the group level.

Within each category, the evidence is examined to see the effect of the policy on the health outcomes of populations.

Interventions Affecting Provider Practice by Changing Structural Conditions

Although structural components such as materials and staff are not strongly linked to outcomes, other components of structure—organization and finance—can influence process

by changing the socioeconomic, legal and administrative, cultural, and information context of the health care system.

Legal Mandates, Accreditation, and Administrative Regulations. Legal mandates, accreditation, and administrative regulations affect quality by controlling entry into the practice of health care. These policies include the licensing of professionals and facilities, their accreditation or certification to perform certain procedures, and the formal delineation of functions that various types of health workers can legally perform. Although these policies assume that providers' prior qualifications are good predictors of actual performance in health care delivery, there is little evidence that such policies have a positive effect on process or outcomes. They are more successful at barring unqualified persons from practicing than at ensuring quality among those who are allowed to practice. A review of health sector regulations in Tanzania and Zimbabwe, for example, revealed that the regulations primarily control entry into the market and ensure a minimum standard of quality (Kumaranayake and others 2000).

Hospital accreditation, with its periodic reviews of health facility performance standards, can potentially provide ongoing regulatory pressure for improvement. To date, research has not demonstrated that hospital accreditation programs are linked to improvements in health outcomes. In a randomized controlled trial of a hospital accreditation program in the KwaZulu-Natal province of South Africa, researchers showed a conclusive link between the implementation of the program and improvements in the accreditation standard indicators. However, they were unable to link those indicators to improvements in health outcomes (Salmon and others 2003).

Malpractice Litigation to Enforce Legal Mandates To be effective in promoting quality, malpractice litigation must rely on adequate legal and judicial systems, which are deficient in most developing countries. In India, one of the few developing countries with the appropriate legal structure in place, inclusion of the medical sector under the Consumer Protection Act of 1986 allows victims to receive redress for negligent medical practice. Although improvements have resulted, some argue that the system needs greater involvement of professional organizations to be effective (Bhat 1996).

Professional Oversight Peer review is as old as professional societies. The power and the influence of such societies vary widely among countries (Heaton 2000). Large provider organizations, such as hospitals or public health institutions, often routinely collect information on provider practices and patient outcomes and use those data to guide, educate, supervise, discipline, or recognize providers. In the Philippines, public health managers used a checklist of 20 observable behaviors against which health workers in remote provinces were rated. The performance of providers in facilities where workers were reviewed was significantly better than in comparable facilities that did not adopt the reviews (Loevinsohn, Guerrero, and Gregorio 1995). Others, however, assert that the "quality by inspection" environment engendered by oversight leads to an antagonistic relationship between workers and managers and precludes cooperative problem solving and continuous improvement (Berwick 1989). A qualitative study evaluating supervisor-provider interactions in health care facilities in Zimbabwe found that supervisors were adept at giving technical feedback but were not as proficient at making suggestions for improvement or at working with providers and patients to solve problems (Tavrow, Kim, and Malianga 2002).

National and Local Clinical Guidelines In many industrial countries, evidence-based clinical guidelines are used to ensure high-quality care, better health outcomes, and cost-effective treatments. (Examples of institutions supporting this approach are the U.K. National Institute for Clinical Excellence, the U.S. Agency for Healthcare Research and Quality, and the Dutch College of General Practitioners.) Guidelines are typically developed for a clinical disease or symptom. They should be derived from evidence-based criteria resulting from well-designed clinical investigations or expert opinion. Because they are derived from empirical studies, guidelines in developing countries can, in principle, be identical to those in industrial countries. When resource constraints limit transferability, diagnostic and treatment guidelines may have to be modified. Technologies such as x-ray studies have gained widest acceptance in preventive and primary care services, such as integrated management of childhood illness, where they serve both as clinical standards and as educational guides. Including physicians in the development and review of guidelines has proved particularly effective in the challenging process of implementing guidelines.

Sharing Information on Quality Improvement Technology.
Worldwide interest in quality has given rise to new professional bodies, scientific publications, and institutions dedicated to sharing ideas and innovations in quality improvement. Organizations such as the Robert Wood Johnson Foundation, the Nuffield Trust, and the Institute for Healthcare Improvement cultivate ideas for improvement, bring people and organizations together to learn from each other, and take action to achieve results. Although the sharing of information on quality health care practices has long been an established part of provider education and training networks, the sharing of information on successful systemwide policies for process improvements could potentially accelerate the scale-up of quality practice.

One organization active in developing countries is the Council on Health Research for Development (COHRED), which promotes, facilitates, and evaluates the Essential National Health Research strategy in such countries as Benin, the Arab Republic of Egypt, and Indonesia. COHRED aims to develop a system of effective health research to improve health services, including quality of care. The Quality Assurance project funded by the U.S. Agency for International Development has studied and shared information about quality in the developing world since 1990. Under the Quality Assurance project umbrella, researchers have studied and implemented quality measurement and improvement interventions and have used these case studies to develop a library of tools and articles to promote global quality improvement.

Public-Private Provision of Care.
In most health care systems, a professional regulatory framework governs the network of civil servants delivering health care. These civil servants operate alongside autonomous, self-governed, private providers—independent for-profit physicians and health clinics and nonprofit nongovernmental organizations (NGOs). Two conclusions arise from the often heated debate about the right balance between public and private services. First, private practitioners provide a significant amount of care in developing countries. Second, though there is no one prescription for striking the right public-private mix, in some cases the public regulatory framework has led to private provision of higher-quality care. The government of Senegal successfully contracted with community-based groups for preventive nutrition services. Eighteen months after nutrition services were implemented, severe malnutrition disappeared among children age 6 to 11 months (Marek and others 1999). The success of the program has led to its expansion nationwide.

Targeted Education and Professional Retraining.
Continuing medical education is a common approach to improving clinical practice, but it neither changes clinical practice nor advances health outcomes (Davis and others 1995). Newer techniques—targeted education, case-based learning, and interactive and multimodel teaching techniques—have had some success. In Guatemala, distance education targeting diarrhea and cholera case management increased accurate assessment and classification of diarrhea cases by 25 percent. Rehydration did not improve, however, and improvements in counseling were insignificant (Flores, Robles, and Burkhalter 2002). In Tanzania, training staff in the control of acute respiratory infections of young children yielded reductions in under-five mortality within two years (Mtango and Neuvians 1986).

Organizational Change.
In recent years, organizational change in the health care system has been shown to influence quality of care and to further the six aims of the Institute of Medicine by focusing on the continual design and redesign of

systems. The emphasis is on developing organizational and individual capabilities where they most profoundly affect the process of care. Design and redesign interventions assume that simply adding a new resource or a new process in isolation will not improve care because better care is the product of many processes working together. Although change interventions have not been widely used in the developing world because they require large investments to plan and implement, four related models of organizational change have been successful in changing provider practice in developing nations:

- *Total Quality Management in health care* Advances in business management practices to continually design and redesign systems for quality improvement have been effectively adapted for health systems. In Total Quality Management, also known as *Continuous Quality Improvement,* teams use mutually reinforcing techniques in a cycle of planning, implementing, evaluating, and revising to improve the quality of clinical and administrative processes. These techniques include process mapping, statistical quality control, and structured team activities. In rural Bihar, India, private practitioners who treat sick children were provided with standard case-management information, were given feedback on their performance, and were tracked and monitored over time. This strategy produced significant improvements in practitioners' case-management skills (Chakraborty, D'Souza, and Northrup 2000). In Malaysia, anesthesia safety has been improved through the implementation of consensus-based protocols that emphasize (a) communication among the operating, recovery, and ward team members; (b) individual feedback; and (c) frequent monitoring to identify areas for improvement (Tan 1999).
- *Collaborative Improvement Model* The early success of Total Quality Management techniques has given rise to a related model, the Collaborative Improvement Model. It addresses broad and complex systemic processes within health care systems and has facilitated the scale-up of quality improvements. This model, designed to continuously improve organizational and individual performance, comprises four elements: definition of an aim, measurement, innovation, and testing to see whether the innovation meets the original aim. This approach strikes a pragmatic balance between the need for action and the need to be scientifically grounded. It has been used with success in Peru and the Russian Federation. In Peru, the collaborative improvement model was used by multidisciplinary teams in 41 clinics to design changes aimed at achieving world-class tuberculosis care. The preliminary results have led to impressive changes in the process of care, but it is too early to determine whether they have been effective in improving quality (Berwick 2004).
- *Plan-Do-Study-Act cycle* The Plan-Do-Study-Act (PDSA) cycle calls for action-oriented learning in quality improve-

ment. Team members using the PDSA model design a quality-improvement intervention (plan), implement it on a small scale (do), evaluate the results (study), and implement or alter the intervention accordingly (act). Often multiple PDSA cycles are necessary before the appropriate improvement method can be identified. All improvement techniques that involve the design and redesign of systems use some form of the PDSA cycle. Successful scale-up of a PDSA prototype is possible with careful leadership oversight. A team of investigators in Russia's Tula province developed a series of successful interventions for adults who have poorly controlled hypertension. The interventions, which were started in 20 clinics, were expanded to 500 clinics within 18 months. The scale-up resulted in a sevenfold increase in patients receiving hypertension management at the primary care level and an 85 percent reduction in admissions for hypertension. In Tver province, the same group addressed problems related to prenatal care. They began with 5 hospitals and scaled up to cover all 42 hospitals and all maternity clinics in the province. The result was a 99 percent reduction in newborns with hypothermia and a reduction in pregnancy-induced hypertension from 44 percent to 6 percent (Berwick 2004). Although the experience of researchers implementing interventions that are based on system redesign in the developing world has been largely positive, it is not clear whether the resources and leadership exist to bring these interventions to scale through country or regional policies. Further evidence is needed concerning the real-world feasibility and cost-effectiveness of system redesign.

- *Internal enabling environment* Creating the right environment for change involves leadership and leadership training, clinicians empowered to make quality improvement decisions, and resources for quality improvement planning activities (Silimper and others 2002). The internal enabling environment in Costa Rica promoted strong leadership that led to the adoption of structural adjustment loans in the early stages of health sector reforms. The loans were used to maintain such public health programs as mother and child nutrition, even though public spending dropped and prices increased dramatically (Peabody 1996). An enabling environment can also be created by teams of individuals, each representing different stakeholder groups (physicians, nurses, staff members, patients, and so forth) or simply by a strong leader with an interest in teamwork and the resources to support a discrete quality improvement function for team members.

Interventions Directly Affecting Provider Practice

Practitioners are often forced to provide care in uncertain settings. Technical limitations may reduce the ability to diagnose or predict outcomes, or they may have only probabilistic knowledge about the efficacy of their proposed treatment for a particular patient. The nature of clinical practice is often solitary, and physicians have few available ways to gauge their clinical acumen and skills. Performance-based feedback, however, can reward high-quality care and increase knowledge about appropriate actions. If the feedback mechanism is effective, it can also serve as the basis for establishing systemwide incentives for improving quality of care.

Training with Peer Review Feedback. In Mexico City, physician retraining on treatment of diarrhea, combined with the concurrent creation of a peer-review structure, decreased the use of antibiotics and increased the use of oral rehydration therapy (ORT). These improvements continued to be seen in a follow-up evaluation 18 months later (Gutierrez and others 1994). The approach has been effectively expanded to prescribing practices for rhinopharyngitis among primary care physicians, using an interactive training workshop and a managerial peer-review committee (Perez-Cuevas and others 1996).

Performance-Based Remuneration. A potentially powerful instrument for accelerating quality improvements involves making payments directly to providers who meet quality standards that are based on process indicators associated with favorable patient outcomes. Systems that tie performance to remuneration use relatively small incentives—equivalent to 3 to 10 percent of the provider's total compensation. Performance-based remuneration has been successfully used in the United States to compensate both private and public providers (McBride, Neiman, and Johnson 2000).

Examples of performance-based incentives come from developing countries too. The Nicaraguan Ministry of Health has implemented a pilot program in six hospitals that offers an incentive bonus (a maximum average of 17 percent of hospital revenue) for facilities that achieve performance targets that include quality measures (Jack 2003). In Haiti, a performance-based payment scheme was set up for NGOs that provided services to the population. The scheme resulted in all three participating NGOs reaching target immunization coverage rates (Eichler, Auxila, and Pollock 2001). Thus, payment for specified and observable performance (in terms of provider effort, client coverage, or health impact on the population) can be usefully applied to NGOs and private providers.

The specific features of performance-based remuneration are crucial. A study evaluating the South African government's experience in contracting with private organizations to operate district hospitals found no cost savings—in fact, the government was spending more than if it provided the services itself. The contracting may have failed because remuneration was not based on specific process or outcome measures. Instead, the

contractor's obligation, the methods of monitoring performance, and the sanctions for nonperformance were only minimally specified (Broomberg, Masobe, and Mills 1997).

High Volume of Care. Evidence exists that a high volume of care by individuals or institutions leads to better health outcomes (Habib and others 2004). Physician experience (learning) and practice (repetition) lead to fewer complications, less resource use, and better quality for a variety of procedures, such as cataract surgery and laparoscopy (Brian and Taylor 2001). More complex procedures, including endarterectomy, cancer surgery, and coronary bypass surgery, have shown similar effects.

Volume effects leading to better health outcomes are not confined to surgical procedures (Zgibor and Orchard 2004). Facilities specializing in the care of chronic diseases such as diabetes, myocardial infarction, and heart failure are also associated with better outcomes. Debate exists over how much of the volume effect is due to specialist care. The benefits of high-volume care persist, however, even after controlling for referral and case-mix biases. When carefully trained nonphysicians are substituted for physicians, volume effects persist but can be accomplished at significantly lower costs. In one study, nurse practitioners and physician's assistants were able to provide high-quality care for common outpatient conditions such as hypertension, diabetes, asthma, otitis media, pharyngitis, and back pain at substantially lower costs than that of physicians (Douglas and others 2004).

Performance-Based Professional Recognition. Providers work in a community of peers in which professional status, prestige, and recognition are often as valuable as material rewards. Nonmonetary incentives, such as public recognition or disclosure, administrative privileges, and awards from professional organizations, can promote improvements in quality. Uganda, for example, implemented the Yellow Star Program as part of a broader health services improvement project. This program evaluated health facilities on a quarterly basis, using 35 indicators of technical and interpersonal quality, and awarded a large yellow star to facilities that scored 100 percent in two consecutive quarters. The star was then prominently displayed outside the facility.

The Mexican Ministry of Health has implemented a strategy that combines the accreditation and the training strategies discussed earlier with nonmonetary incentives. The National Crusade for Quality in Health Care introduces quality-oriented incentives to health facilities and medical schools. It also includes public recognition in an effort to encourage learning and to change practice. The National Crusade has already generated measurable improvements in the responsiveness of state-level health systems (Secretaría de Salud de Mexico 2003).

Both types of policies examined in this section are associated with better quality and better health outcomes—lower premature mortality and avoidable morbidity, increased patient satisfaction, and more health-seeking behaviors. When effective, these policies result in increased coverage rates, better prescribing patterns, and increased adherence to clinical guidelines. They can spell the difference between an individual's survival or death, between an individual benefiting from the encounter with the health sector or being harmed by it, and between an individual and society rising from poverty or sinking deeper into it.

MEASURING QUALITY

Improving quality requires that we measure it accurately. The successful outcomes discussed in the previous section rely on the links between policy and changes in clinical practice. Such links, however, can be created and demonstrated only when valid and reliable measures of process are easily understood, inexpensive to obtain, resistant to manipulation, and related to better health outcomes.

Measuring Structure

Material measures of structure abound. Numerous facility-based surveys in developing countries have cataloged capital equipment and staffing levels, and financial reports track budgets and expenditures (but rarely production costs). Facility inventories of drugs and supplies are generally available; service utilization figures are routinely reported to national-level authorities. Such measurements, however, are often beside the point. Even when material structural deficiencies are corrected, they are not reliably linked to changes in health outcomes. Measuring the organization and financing of health care is more difficult. Although descriptions of the organization and financing of health systems exist, objective functional assessments of systems (such as patient flows, the patient referral system, or details of the relative pricing of services) are less often available.

Measuring Process

Technical advances have mitigated longstanding difficulties in measuring process. Five approaches and their strengths and weaknesses merit consideration: chart abstraction, direct observation and recording of visits, administrative data, standardized patients, and clinical vignettes.

Chart Abstraction. Chart abstraction, or review of the medical record, has long been used to measure technical quality. Such familiar quality evaluations as clinical audits, physician report cards, and profiles are based on chart abstraction. The core strength of the medical record is that it is ubiquitous and can generally be obtained after each encounter. Chart reviews, however, suffer from problems of legibility when notes are handwritten. Often they are generated for reasons other than recording the actual events of the clinical visit (legal protection

or obtaining payments, for example) and thus lack crucial clinical details. One prospective study showed that charts identified only 70 percent of items performed during the clinical encounter (Luck and others 2000). In a related analysis, 6.4 percent of the items recorded in the chart were false and had never really occurred.

Where resources and infrastructure are sufficient, the electronic medical record (EMR) is becoming a priority for health systems worldwide. EMR technology promotes uniformity, legibility, and communication, which can lead to guideline use and reduce prescription errors. It also holds the promise of managing populations rather than individuals by aggregating patients into groups. However, the EMR has not always lived up to its potential. In many countries, some impressive successes have occurred—as have spectacular failures, costing billions of dollars (McConnell 2004). The great heterogeneity in record-keeping practices, problems with medical records (both paper and electronic), and costs of trained medical abstractors have led to a search for other reliable ways to measure quality.

Direct Observation and Recording of Visits. Direct observation and recording of visits is a commonly used approach in developing countries (Nolan and others 2001). Ethically, the provider and the patient must be informed of the observation or recording, which introduces participation bias because provider behavior may change as a result of being evaluated. In addition, trained observers are costly, and variation between observers is difficult to remedy.

Administrative Data. Administrative data, collected for purposes of managing the delivery of care, are available in all but the poorest settings. A data collection system, once established, is ubiquitous and can provide information on charges and many cost inputs. Administrative data, however, lack sufficient clinical detail to be useful in evaluating process. In a 2003 study, an incorrect diagnosis was recorded in the data 30 percent of the time (although the diagnosis was made correctly). Overall, these data reflected the actual clinical diagnosis only 57 percent of the time (Peabody, Luck, Jain, and others 2004). As information systems advance, accuracy problems may be mitigated, although the lack of adequate clinical detail will continue to limit the use of administrative data.

Standardized Patients. Standardized patients can be a gold standard for process measurement (Luck and Peabody 2002). Trained to simulate illness, standardized patients present themselves unannounced into a clinical setting to providers who have previously given their consent to participate in the study. At the conclusion of the visit, the standardized patient reports on the technical and interpersonal elements of process. Standardized patients are reliable over a range of conditions and provide valid measurements that accurately capture variation in clinical practice among providers over time. However, they are expensive and useful only for adult conditions and only those conditions that can be simulated. Thus, they are not practical for routinely evaluating quality.

Clinical Vignettes. Clinical vignettes were developed explicitly for measuring quality within a group of providers and evaluating quality at the population level. Vignettes are responsive to variation in quality, and providers readily accept them if they are given anonymously (Peabody, Luck, Glassman, and others 2004). More than 20 vignettes have been used in 13 countries around the world. They can be administered on paper, by computer, or over the Internet. Providers are typically presented with several cases. When process is being measured for many providers, each provider is presented with the same case or set of cases, thus eliminating the need for case-mix adjustment. The provider completing the vignette is asked to take a history, do an examination, order the necessary tests, make a diagnosis, and specify a treatment plan. The questions are open ended and include interactive responses that simulate the visit and evaluate the physician's knowledge. In two separate, prospective validation studies among randomly selected providers, vignettes consistently demonstrated greater predictive validity of process than did the abstracted medical record. Vignettes have been validated against the gold standard of standardized patient visits, and they reflect actual clinical practice, not just physicians' knowledge. Vignettes have several other advantages. Because exactly the same case can be given to many providers, vignettes are useful for comparison studies. They are also useful for pre- and postevaluations of policy interventions designed to improve quality. Finally, they are inexpensive to administer and straightforward to score, making them particularly useful in developing countries.

ECONOMIC BENEFITS AND COSTS OF QUALITY CARE

Policy interventions can lead to higher-quality process of care and can rapidly improve a population's health outcomes, but is quality improvement cost-effective? This section shows that it is. We compare the economic benefits of better quality of care at the individual and population levels with the costs of implementing quality improvement interventions. We then discuss why these interventions not only increase individual and social welfare but also are cost-effective in the long run.

Individual Economic Benefits

Individuals benefit from better quality of care because they are physically, emotionally, and mentally healthier. These benefits can be quantified subjectively by self-report, objectively by physiological assessments (such as blood pressure), and monetarily by measuring income. Other things being equal, a healthy individual generates more income than one who is often sick. This benefit goes beyond the period of illness. Research on early childhood development has shown that higher-quality prenatal and postnatal care not only decreases mortality but also improves subsequent school performance, which is critical to future labor productivity (Van der Gaag 2000). The monetary benefits of better individual health can be assessed by examining the individuals' expected income in the context of a life cycle model. Expected income depends on the risk of death at various points in time and the corresponding opportunities for educational attainment. This scenario can be simulated by improving quality and then estimating how much the higher quality lowers mortality and increases education attainment, both of which increase an individual's future income (see figure 70.2).

Social Macroeconomic Benefits

Societies that have healthier populations also have higher levels of human capital and a greater capacity to generate wealth. Higher quality of care for the individual increases society's human capital by reducing both the number of premature deaths (thus increasing the labor force) and the amount of temporary or permanent disability (thus improving worker productivity). Providers and insurers also benefit from lower costs by avoiding unnecessary or inappropriate care. Thus, society benefits from both better health and lower public expenditures for treatment, which can then be reallocated to other productive uses. Interventions that improve quality have an especially high social value when they have large positive externalities (for instance, when better process reduces the incidence of a communicable disease). Sometimes, however, society benefits but some stakeholders do not. For example, physicians who provide better preventive care may experience less demand for their curative services and associated resources.

Several attempts have been made to estimate the correlation between health outcomes and long-term economic growth. The high prevalence of such diseases as malaria has been linked in some studies to a slowing of economic growth by one to two percentage points per year. These studies were severely limited by the number of countries and by the many unobserved factors excluded from the models (Sachs 2001). These limitations suggest another way to estimate the benefits of higher quality on health outcomes and long-term economic growth. Because diagnostic accuracy and treatment of malaria can be improved with better-quality care, improving quality should increase national income through reductions in mortality rates.

Indeed, cross-country data suggest that a one-year increase in life expectancy is associated with an increase in the gross domestic product (GDP) growth rate of 1 to 4 percentage points (Bloom, Canning, and Sevilla 2001). Our own simulations show

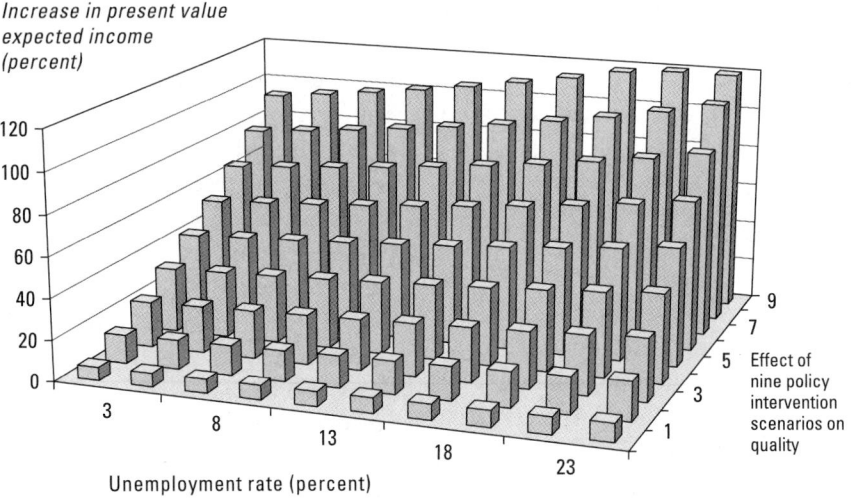

Increase in present value expected income (percent)

Unemployment rate (percent)

Effect of nine policy intervention scenarios on quality

Source: Authors' calculations.

Note: These results model the effect on income of a policy intervention that leads to higher quality. The effect is determined as an increase in the present value of income for varying rates of unemployment. Higher quality is based on nine different scenarios of quality improvement. For each successive scenario, infant mortality rates are reduced by 1 percent and educational attainment is increased by 5 percent. The baseline possibilities are for the Islamic Republic of Iran.

Figure 70.2 Economic Benefits of a Quality Intervention That Reduces Child Mortality Rates and Leads to Higher Educational Attainment

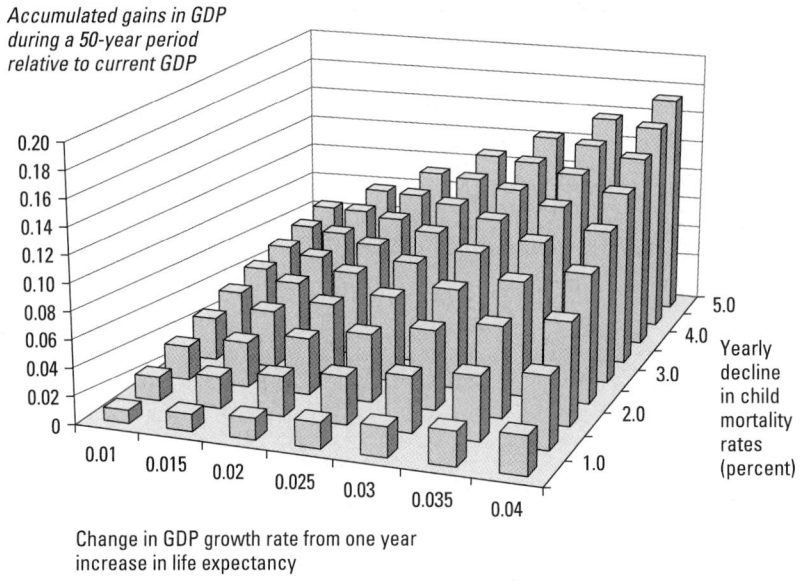

Accumulated gains in GDP during a 50-year period relative to current GDP

Yearly decline in child mortality rates (percent)

Change in GDP growth rate from one year increase in life expectancy

Source: Authors' calculations.

Figure 70.3 Gains in GDP Resulting from Reductions in Child Mortality Rates

that quality improvements can result in as much as a 5 percent annual reduction in child mortality rates, which can generate, over 50 years, economic gains equivalent to 18 percent of current GDP (see figure 70.3). Similar results would be obtained if the effect of better quality on morbidity and disability were simulated.

Economic Costs

Policies that improve the quality of care have both direct and indirect costs. Direct costs relate to the human and physical resources needed to implement the intervention. Indirect costs come from more subtle changes, including alterations in the quantity of health services provided, in provider demand for various inputs (such as equipment and medication), in the market prices of heath care, in government health budgets, and ultimately in the macroeconomy. For interventions at the local level, such as training doctors in a particular region, it is usually sufficient to measure direct costs. Although the level of detail required can be overwhelming when the interventions are complex, the calculations are usually straightforward. The costs of local interventions depend on local prices of such inputs as labor, transportation, training kits, food, space rental, and accommodations. The cost of training providers in the appropriate treatment of childhood illnesses ranges from a low of US\$1 to a high of US\$430 (Santoso, Suryawati, and Prawaitasari 1996).

The direct and indirect costs of interventions at the central or local government level are harder to quantify. Expanding training programs to all public providers, enforcing standards for private and public providers, changing payment systems, and developing policies to protect consumers against malpractice are macro-level interventions that have direct program-level costs. They affect the economy as a whole by changing the allocation of public resources and the relative prices of goods and services. Macroevaluations of health policy interventions are seldom conducted, even though systemwide interventions are likely to have the highest effect on quality and health-related benefits.

Cost-Effectiveness of Improved Process

Two interventions that vividly illustrate the cost-effectiveness of improvements in clinical practice and outcomes have been chosen: detection and treatment of acute respiratory illnesses and appropriate drug use and treatment for diarrhea.

Better Treatment of Pneumonia in Children. Part of the high mortality from childhood pneumonia in the developing world can be explained by poor-quality care, which is defined as the inability either to accurately diagnose or to treat the disease. Our prototype intervention has two cost components: the cost of implementing an educational activity for providers and the cost of treating nonsevere and severe childhood pneumonia. The former component is based on a study and uses conservative high-end cost estimations (Kelley and others 2001); the latter is the midpoint from another study (Stansfield and Shepard 1990). The number of lives saved depends on the effect of the intervention—that is, the change in the percentage of cases diagnosed and treated; the prevalence rate of both types of pneumonia; the population covered by each provider; the case-fatality ratio; and the effectiveness of the treatment. Both the case-fatality ratio and the effectiveness ratio were fixed at middle values suggested by earlier work (Stansfield and Shepard 1990). For the other parameters, a large range of variation was considered, producing 450 scenarios. Finally, six

impact levels were considered, which were based on two previous studies (Chakraborty, D'Souza, and Northrup 2000; Mtango and Neuvians 1986).

The analysis showed that, under average conditions, improving quality of care for conditions of acute respiratory illness can be very cost-effective. When the baseline quality is low and the disease prevalence is high, an intervention that raises quality has a cost-effectiveness ratio of US\$132 to US\$800 per life saved; if the policy intervention is ineffective or the prevalence of pneumonia is low, the average cost of saving a life could be more than US\$2,000. When 60 percent of cases are already appropriately diagnosed and treated, the cost-effectiveness ratio rises to US\$5,000 per life saved.[1]

Better Treatment of Diarrhea. Diarrhea remains one of the leading causes of childhood morbidity and mortality in the developing world. The diarrhea incidence rate among children in resource-constrained countries can reach six to seven episodes per year (Thapar and Sanderson 2004). ORT is the accepted standard of care for acute diarrhea. Unfortunately, a large proportion of cases are still treated with nonrehydration medication, including antibiotics and antidiarrheals. Improved diagnosis of dehydration and reduced use of unnecessary medications, however, lead to better outcomes.

Various interventions can make sizable changes in the diagnostic and prescribing patterns of providers. Verbal case review, combined with a package of additional intervention referred to as INFECTOM (Information, Feedback, Contracting with Providers to Adhere to Practice Guidelines, and Ongoing Monitoring), increased the proportion of cases treated correctly from 16 percent to 48 percent (Bloom, Canning, and Sevilla 2001). One study reports that small group, face-to-face interventions reduced antimicrobial prescriptions by 16 percent and antidiarrheal prescriptions by 7 percent among a group of providers treating acute diarrhea in Indonesia (Santoso, Suryawati, and Prawaitasari 1996). The same study showed that formal seminars reduced antimicrobial use by 10 percent and antidiarrheal use by 7 percent. On the basis of these studies, an average cost per intervention was used, ranging from US\$25 to US\$125.

The savings from switching to a less costly treatment (instead of antibiotics, for example) were subtracted from the direct costs that are related to implementing the training activity. Because other savings, such as those related to a lower use of inpatient services, were ignored, the estimates are conservative. Savings could be greater: Two years after an ORT unit was established at the Kamuza Central Hospital in Malawi, 50 percent fewer children with diarrhea were admitted to the pediatric ward, and those admitted required 56 percent less intravenous fluid for rehydration (Martines, Phillips, and Feachem 1990).

Again, the number of lives saved depends on the disease prevalence; the effect of the policy on treatment quality; the population covered by each provider; the average case-fatality ratio, which was set at 6 per 1,000 on the basis of Snyder and Merson (1982); and the effectiveness of the treatment. For the latter parameter, reductions in mortality rates following ORT treatment of 40 to 60 percent and reductions in effectiveness ratios of 5 to 100 percent have been reported (Shepard, Brenzel, and Nemeth 1986). Accordingly, the effectiveness ratio was set at 80 percent. As before, alternative values for the other parameters were adopted, generating 450 scenarios.

Educational interventions to improve the quality of care for treatment of diarrheal diseases are also highly cost-effective. In general, the cost of saving a life through educational interventions is less than US$500 and could be as low as US$14. Scenarios with high cost per life saved (more than US$6,000) are when prevalence rates are low or when implementation costs for quality-related interventions are high.

Although the data available to estimate the costs and benefits of health outcomes and process are limited, these simulations, combined with published reports of successful policy interventions, clearly show the cost-effectiveness of interventions that improve health outcomes through better quality of care. However, reliable measures of quality are necessary to design and evaluate these interventions.

RESEARCH AGENDA ON QUALITY

Most of the issues discussed throughout this chapter represent important topics for research. Establishing a research agenda requires prioritizing both the type of research and the topics to be studied. Quality-of-care research must also strike a balance between relevance to decision making and excellence in scientific rigor (Frenk 1992).

Observational studies are needed to document the extent and correlates of quality at various levels: individual providers, institutional providers, health care systems, and whole populations. Apart from offering much-needed basic descriptions (especially in developing countries), these studies can test specific indicators of the dimensions of quality and can compare the measurement approaches discussed earlier.

Intervention studies introduce planned changes into health care settings and assess their consequences. It is fundamentally important that intervention studies compare one provider group or policy alternative with another. In addition, control groups must be used so that any observed change can be attributed to the intervention itself rather than to another source of variation. The external validity of studies is often undermined by the choice of highly specific sites, making it difficult to generalize the findings and to build a body of sound evidence. If randomized trials cannot be conducted, the preferred option is quasi-experimental studies with clear control groups and longitudinal designs (Peabody and others 1999).

Such studies should be complemented by cost-benefit and cost-effectiveness analyses. Sometimes, in public health emergencies, for example, control groups may not be practical or ethical, in which case real-time operations research is an acceptable substitute.

In the area of research topics, top priority should be given to quality monitoring and assurance strategies to gain an understanding of exactly what the health system is contributing to society and at what cost. Quantifying the associated costs of different variants of quality monitoring and assurance strategies should also be a high-priority item on the quality research agenda. The second priority should be to increase the evidence base regarding the effects on provider behavior of public policies concerning quality of care and whether they lead to better health outcomes. We need to learn more about the long-term effects of different contracting and remuneration policies on providers' practices and the consequent results of such policies for health outcomes. Finally, we need to understand how contracting and remuneration policies affect problems unique to the developing world, such as the use of doctor substitutes and the migration of skilled providers to wealthier countries.

CONCLUSION

Good quality means that providers are able to manage an individual's or a population's health care by timely, skillful application of medical technology in a culturally sensitive manner within the available resource constraints. Eliminating poor quality involves not only giving better care but also eliminating underprovision of essential clinical services (systemwide microscopy for diagnosing tuberculosis, for example); stopping overuse of some care (prenatal ultrasonography or unnecessary injections, for example); and ending misuse of unneeded services (such as unnecessary hysterectomies or antibiotics for viral infections). A sadly unique feature of quality is that poor quality can obviate all the implied benefits of good access and effective treatment. At its best, poor quality is wasteful—a tragedy in severely resource-constrained health care systems. At its worst, it causes actual harm.

Despite the urgency of improving health in developing countries, quality of care has been largely ignored. Both providers and patients agree this must change, but how can this goal be reached? From the information marshaled for this chapter, we can draw five conclusions:

- Better quality leads to better health outcomes in developing countries.
- Process, the proximate determinant of health outcomes, can be measured in valid and reliable ways, such as clinical vignettes and electronic medical records.

- Measured in the above ways, the process of care in developing countries is poor.
- The process of care can be improved in the short term.
- Policies affecting structural conditions, including the actual process of care or the continual design and redesign of the health care system, have been shown to be effective in developing countries.

We believe that two broad strategies would help to rapidly improve health care quality in developing countries:

- encouraging explicit comparative research on outcomes and process
- disseminating empirical findings on quality variation.

Encouraging Explicit Comparative Research on Outcomes and Process

Comparisons highlighting different outcomes can be compelling. For example, when 30-day mortality rates for coronary artery bypass surgery at various facilities were disclosed in the United States, care started to shift from many low-volume hospitals to high-volume hospitals (Chassin 2002). In developing countries, comparisons show that the insured are more likely to have cesarean sections than are the uninsured (Barros and others 1991). Although critics of comparative analysis are justified in saying that systems and populations vary, such criticism misses an important point: Differences in outcome highlight possibilities that help in the search for the underlying causes of poor quality. Although poor quality may have many causes, one of them is almost always poor clinical practice, which can be remedied. We also favor a league or summary table approach to making comparisons. In this approach, the providers being compared agree on criteria before prospective assessments are done. The data for the comparison should be of the highest quality; the league tables themselves should be easy to interpret; and the findings should be rapidly available (Devers, Pham, and Liu 2004). The league table itself should be set up at the regional, national, and international levels so that a variety of benchmarks are available.

Implementing quality comparisons will greatly facilitate the process of policy evaluation and cost-benefit analysis and help indicate directions for future research. Access to accurate, consistent quality-of-care data will compel external funders, such as the World Bank, to build quality assurance into their lending and development programs. As major health programs such as the Global Fund to Fight AIDS, Tuberculosis, and Malaria are scaled up around the world, mechanisms to measure and improve care quality will grow more important.

Disseminating Empirical Findings on Quality Variation

Public dissemination of information on quality, particularly in low-literacy countries, does not seem to create the individual-based choice market that many have envisaged. Instead, it motivates managers and providers to undertake changes that improve the delivery of care (Schneider and Lieberman 2001). Outside pressure—perceived or real—appears to extend the quality debate beyond traditional boundaries, allowing for innovative collaborations and "out of the box" thinking (Devers, Pham, and Liu 2004). Nongovernmental and private organizations involved in health care delivery should also be required to report basic quality measures, perhaps as a condition for funding, thus ensuring that similar pressure to improve quality is exerted outside the public sector.

Public dissemination can create shock waves when poor quality is "discovered," leading to popular demand to increase quality. For example, findings of widespread medical errors in the United States, estimated to have resulted in as many as 98,000 deaths per year, launched the medical safety revolution (Institue of Medicine 2001). Dissemination among physicians and surgeons by means of report cards and ratings has been effective at changing clinical practice. One advantage of dissemination among providers is that the results can be more refined and technical than ratings meant for wider audiences. Dissemination is the responsibility of public research and public initiative. Because dissemination is inherently controversial, it requires public financing—even more than other public goods (Jamison, Frenk, and Knaul 1998).

Ultimately, improving quality is about value. In health care, price is not a reliable proxy for quality and cannot be used as a guide. Because patients and consumers cannot directly observe quality, their ability to demand high-quality services is limited, and they are often left to settle for a market that has suboptimal equilibrium and poor quality of care. In addition, providers often lack knowledge of optimal treatments and technologies and thus are not aware of how they can produce higher-quality care. Because the provider-patient interaction is so private and personal, quality of care is hard to observe and to measure. New measurement tools, however—such as clinical vignettes and the electronic medical record—are being developed and improved. As research links care with outcomes and cost inputs, we can expect to have more accurate and reliable data about clinical practice for use in making quality assessments.

Investments in quality, however, must be judged critically as well. When we invest in quality, an investment can be beneficial but can come at a cost. So while quality goes up, value can go up or down—or costs can go up while quality actually goes down or stays the same, thus pushing the value of care down and undermining other efforts to improve quality. Finally, as we showed for acute respiratory illness and diarrhea, quality can go up and costs go down, thus increasing overall value. Examples of this optimal outcome must be actively sought out and reported, because the success of a given investment cannot be known in advance (Berwick 2004).

Improving health status does not have to rely solely on macroeconomic growth or other long-term development indicators. Health outcomes can be rapidly improved in the short term by ensuring the appropriateness of the circumstances or setting under which the health care encounter occurs (structural improvement) or by increasing the likelihood that health care providers behave in ways most beneficial to patients under the prevailing circumstances (process improvement). However, this improvement will not occur spontaneously or routinely, despite the best intentions of beneficiaries, providers, and governments. Quality improvement tools and technologies and information on successful quality improvement policies must be consistently shared among developing countries to build local capacity. Funding and incentives must also be consistent with high quality. Finally, the political will to ensure that quality becomes a top priority on the health reform agenda must be sustained.

NOTE

1. As a reference, if the average expected value of a life is close to US$30,000, even the highest cost-effectiveness ratio found in the analysis (US$12,000 per life saved), would imply a cost-benefit ratio below 50 percent, assuming an initial average wage of US$1,000 growing at 2 percent per year, a 5 percent discount rate, and unchanged mortality rates.

REFERENCES

Barros, F. C., J. P. Vaughan, C. G. Victora, and S. R. Huttly. 1991. "Epidemic of Caesarean Sections in Brazil." *Lancet* 338 (8760): 167–69.

Beracochea, E., R. Dickson, P. Freemand, and J. Thomason. 1995. "Case Management Quality Assessment in Rural Areas of Papua New Guinea." *Tropical Doctor* 25 (2): 69–74.

Berwick, D. 1989. "Continuous Improvement as an Ideal in Health Care." *New England Journal of Medicine* 320 (1): 53–56.

———. 2004. "Lessons from Developing Nations on Improving Health Care." *British Medical Journal* 328 (7448): 1124–29.

Bhat, R. 1996. "Regulating the Private Health Care Sector: The Case of the Indian Consumer Protection Act." *Health Policy and Planning* 11 (3): 265–79.

Bloom, D. E., D. Canning, and J. Sevilla. 2001. "The Effect of Health on Economic Growth: Theory and Evidence." NBER Working Paper 8587, National Bureau of Economic Research, Cambridge, MA.

Brian, G., and H. Taylor. 2001. "Restoring Sight to the Millions: The Aravind Way." *Bulletin of the World Health Organization* 79 (3): 270–71.

Broomberg, J., P. Masobe, and A. Mills. 1997. "To Purchase or to Provide? The Relative Efficiency of Contracting-Out versus Direct Public Provision of Hospital Services in South Africa." In *Private Health Providers in Developing Countries: Serving the Public Interest?*, ed. S. Bennett, B. McPake, and A. Mills. London: Zed Press.

Chakraborty, S., S. A. D'Souza, and R. S. Northrup. 2000. "Improving Private Practitioner Care of Sick Children: Testing New Approaches in Rural Bihar." *Health Policy and Planning* 15 (4): 400–7.

Chassin, M. R. 2002. "Achieving and Sustaining Improved Quality: Lessons from New York State and Cardiac Surgery." *Health Affairs* 21 (4): 40.

Davis, D. A., M. A. Thomson, A. D. Oxman, and R. B. Haynes. 1995. "Changing Physician Performance: A Systematic Review of the Effect of Continuing Medical Education Strategies." *Journal of the American Medical Association* 274 (9): 700–5.

Devers, K. J., H. H. Pham, and G. Liu. 2004. "What Is Driving Hospitals' Patient-Safety Efforts?" *Health Affairs* 23 (2): 103–16.

Donabedian, A. 1980. *The Definition of Quality and Approaches to Its Assessment*. Ann Arbor, MI: Health Administration Press.

———. 1988. "The Quality of Care: How Can It Be Assessed?" *Journal of the American Medical Association* 260 (12): 1743–48.

Douglas W. R., D. H. Howard, E. R. Becker, E. K. Adams, and M. H. Roberts. 2004. "Use of Midlevel Practitioners to Achieve Labor Cost Savings in the Primary Care Practice of an MCO." *Health Care Economics* 39 (3): 607–25.

Eichler, R., P. Auxila, and J. Pollock. 2001. "Performance-Based Payment to Improve the Impact of Health Services: Evidence from Haiti." *World Bank Institute Online Journal*.

Flores, R., J. Robles, and B. R. Burkhalter. 2002. "Distance Education with Tutoring Improves Diarrhea Case Management in Guatemala." *International Journal of Quality in Health Care* 14 (Suppl. 1): 47–56.

Frenk, J. 1992. "Balancing Relevance and Excellence: Organizational Responses to Link Research with Decision Making." *Social Science and Medicine* 35 (11): 1397–404.

Gutierrez, G., H. Guiscafre, M. Bronfman, J. Walsh, H. Martinez, and O. Munoz. 1994. "Changing Physician Prescribing Patterns: Evaluation of an Educational Strategy for Acute Diarrhea in Mexico City." *Medical Care* 32 (5): 436–46.

Habib, M., K. Mandal, C. V. Bunce, and S. G. Fraser. 2004. "The Relation of Volume with Outcome in Pachoemulsification Surgery." *British Journal of Ophthalmology* 88: 643–46.

Heaton, C. 2000. "External Peer Review in Europe: An Overview from the ExPeRT Project. External Peer Review Techniques." *International Journal of Quality in Health Care* 12 (3): 177–82.

Institute of Medicine. 2001. *Crossing the Quality Chasm*. Washington, DC: National Academy Press.

Jack, W. 2003. "Contracting for Health Services: An Evaluation of Recent Reforms in Nicaragua." *Health Policy and Planning* 18 (2): 195–204.

Jamison, D. T., J. Frenk, and F. Knaul. 1998. "International Collective Action in Health: Objectives, Functions, and Rationale." *Lancet* 351 (9101): 514–17.

Javitt, J., G. Venkataswamy, and A. Sommer. 1983. "The Economic and Social Aspects of Restoring Sight." In *24th International Congress of Ophthalmology*, ed. P. Henkind, New York: J. B. Lippincott.

Kelley, E., C. Geslin, S. Djibrina, and M. Boucar. 2001. "Improving Performance with Clinical Standards: The Impact of Feedback on Compliance with the Integrated Management of Childhood Illness Algorithm in Niger, West Africa." *International Journal of Health Planning Management* 16 (3): 195–205.

Kumaranayake, L., P. Mujinja, C. Hongoro, and R. Mpembeni. 2000. "How Do Countries Regulate the Health Sector? Evidence from Tanzania and Zimbabwe." *Health Policy and Planning* 15 (4): 357–67.

Loevinsohn, B. P., E. T. Guerrero, and S. P. Gregorio. 1995. "Improving Primary Health Care through Systematic Supervision: A Controlled Field Trial." *Health Policy and Planning* 10 (2): 144–53.

Luck, J., and J. Peabody. 2002. "Using Standardised Patients to Measure Physicians' Practice: Validation Study Using Audio Recordings." *British Medical Journal* 325 (7366): 679.

Luck, J., J. Peabody, T. R. Dresselhaus, M. Lee, and P. Glassman. 2000. "How Well Does Chart Abstraction Measure Quality? A Prospective Comparison of Standardized Patients with the Medical Record." *American Journal of Medicine* 108 (8): 642–49.

Marek, T., I. Diallo, B. Ndiaye, and J. Rakotosalama. 1999. "Successful Contracting of Prevention Services: Fighting Malnutrition in Senegal and Madagascar." *Health Policy and Planning* 14 (4): 382–89.

Martines, J., M. Phillips, and R. G. Feacham. 1993. "Diarrheal Diseases." In *Disease Control Priorities in Developing Countries,* ed. D. Jamison, W. H. Mosley, A. R. Measham, and J. L. Bobadilla, New York: Oxford University Press.

McBride, A. B., S. Neiman, and J. Johnson. 2000. "Responsibility-Centered Management: A 10-Year Nursing Assessment." *Journal of Professional Nursing* 16 (4): 201–9.

McConnell, H. 2004. "International Efforts in Implementing National Health Information Infrastructure and Electronic Health Records." *World Hospitals and Health Services* 40 (1): 33–37, 39–40, 50–52.

McGlynn, E. A., S. M. Asch, J. Adams, J. Keesey, J. Hicks, A. DeCristofaro, and E. A. Kerr. 2003. "The Quality of Health Care Delivered to Adults in the United States." *New England Journal of Medicine* 348 (26): 2635–45.

Mtango, F. D., and D. Neuvians. 1986. "Acute Respiratory Infections in Children under Five Years: Control Project in Bagamoyo District, Tanzania." *Transactions of the Royal Society of Tropical Medicine and Hygiene* 80 (6): 851–58.

Murray, C. J., and J. Frenk. 2000. "A Framework for Assessing the Performance of Health Systems." *Bulletin of the World Health Organization* 78 (6): 717–31.

Nolan, T., P. Angos, A. J. Cunha, L. Muhe, S. Qazi, E. A. Simoes, and others. 2001. "Quality of Hospital Care for Seriously Ill Children in Less-Developed Countries." *Lancet* 357 (9250): 106–10.

Peabody, J. 1996. "Economic Reform and Health Sector Policy: Lessons from Structural Adjustment Programs." *Social Science and Medicine* 43 (5): 823–35.

Peabody, J., P. Gertler, and A. Liebowitz. 1998. "The Policy Implications of Better Structure and Process on Birth Outcomes in Jamaica." *Health Policy* 43 (1): 1–13.

Peabody, J., J. Luck, P. Glassman, S. Jain, J. Hansen, M. Spell, and M. Lee. 2004. "Measuring the Quality of Physician Practice by Using Clinical Vignettes: A Prospective Validation Study." *Annals of Internal Medicine* 141 (10): 771–80.

Peabody, J., J. Luck, S. Jain, D. Bertenthal, and P. Glassman. 2004. "Assessing the Accuracy of Administrative Data in Health Information Systems." *Medical Care* 42 (11): 1066–72.

Peabody, J., M. Rahman, P. J. Gertler, J. Mann, D. O. Farley, and G. M. Carter. 1999. *Policy and Health: Implications for Development in Asia.* Cambridge, UK: Cambridge University Press.

Peabody, J., F. Tozija, J. Muñoz, R. J. Mordyke, and J. Luck. 2004. "Using Vignettes to Compare the Quality of Care Variation in Economically Divergent Countries." *Health Services Research* 39: 1937–56.

Perez-Cuevas, R., H. Guiscafre, O. Munoz, H. Reyes, P. Tome, V. Libreros, and G. Gutierrez. 1996. "Improving Physician Prescribing Patterns to Treat Rhinopharyngitis: Intervention Strategies in Two Health Systems of Mexico." *Social Science and Medicine* 42 (8): 1185–94.

Sachs, J. D. 2001. *Macroeconomics and Health: Investing in Health for Economic Development.* Report of the Commission on Macroeconomics and Health. Geneva: World Health Organization.

Salmon, J., J. Heavens, C. Lombard, and P. Tavrow. 2003. "The Impact of Accreditation on the Quality of Hospital Care: KwaZulu-Natal Province, Republic of South Africa." *Operations Research Results* 2 (17). Published for the U.S. Agency for International Development (USAID) by the Quality Assurance Project, University Research Co., Bethesda, MD.

Santoso, B., S. Suryawati, and J. E. Prawaitasari. 1996. "Small Group Intervention vs. Formal Seminar for Improving Appropriate Drug Use." *Social Science and Medicine* 42 (8): 1163–68.

Schneider, E. C., and T. Lieberman. 2001. "Publicly Disclosed Information about the Quality of Health Care: Response of the U.S. Public." *Quality in Health Care* 10 (2): 96–103.

Secretaría de Salud de Mexico. 2003. *Salud: México 2002.* Mexico City: Secretaría de Salud.

Shepard, D. S., L. E. Brenzel, and K. T. Nemeth. 1986. "Cost-Effectiveness of Oral Rehydration Therapy for Diarrhoeal Diseases." PHN Technical Note 86-26, Population, Health, and Nutrition Development, World Bank, Washington, DC.

Silimper, D. R., L. M. Franco, T. Veldhuyzen van Zanten, and C. MacAulay. 2002. "A Framework for Institutionalizing Quality Assurance." *International Journal for Quality in Health Care* 14 (Suppl. 1): 67–73.

Snyder, J. D., and M. H. Merson. 1982. "The Magnitude of the Global Problem of Acute Diarrhoeal Disease: A Review of Active Surveillance Data." *Bulletin of the World Health Organization* 60 (4): 605–13.

Stansfield, S. K., and D. S. Shepard. 1990. "Acute Respiratory Infection." In *Disease Control Priorities in Developing Countries,* ed. D. Jamison, W. H. Mosley, A. R. Measham, and J. L. Bobadilla. New York: Oxford University Press.

Supratikto, G., M. E. Wirth, E. Achadi, S. Cohen, and C. Ronsmans. 2002. "A District-Based Audit of the Causes and Circumstances of Maternal Deaths in South Kalimantan, Indonesia." *Bulletin of the World Health Organization* 80 (3): 228–34.

Tan, S. K. P. 1999. "Safety with Anaesthesia—The Paradigm of Continuous Improvement." *Medical Journal of Malaysia* 54 (1): 1–3.

Tavrow, P., Y.-M. Kim, and L. Malianga. 2002. "Measuring the Quality of Supervisor-Provider Interactions in Health Care Facilities in Zimbabwe." *International Journal of Quality in Health Care* 14 (Suppl. 1): 57–66.

Thapar, N., and I. Sanderson. 2004. "Diarrhoea in Children: an Interface between Developing and Developed Countries." *Lancet* 363 (9409): 641–53.

Thaver, I. H., T. Harpham, B. McPake, and T. Garner. 1998. "Private Practitioners in the Slums of Karachi: What Quality of Care Do They Offer?" *Social Science and Medicine* 46 (11): 1441–49.

Van der Gaag, J. 2000. "From Child Development to Human Development." In *From Early Child Development to Human Development,* ed. M. E. Young, Washington, DC: World Bank.

Walker, G. J., D. E. Ashley, and R. J. Hayes. 1988. "The Quality of Care Is Related to Death Rates: Hospital Inpatient Management of Infants with Acute Gastroenteritis in Jamaica." *American Journal of Public Health* 78 (2): 149–52.

Wennberg, J. E., E. S. Fisher, and J. S. Skinner. 2002. "Geography and the Debate over Medicare Reform." *Health Affairs* (Millwood) Suppl. Web Exclusives: W96–114.

WHO (World Health Organization). 2000. *World Health Report 2000 Health Systems: Improving Performance.* Geneva: WHO.

Zaslavsky, A. M., J. N. Hochheimer, E. C. Schneider, P. D. Cleary, J. J. Seidman, E. A. McGlynn, and others. 2000. "Impact of Socio-demographic Case Mix on the HEDIS Measures of Health Plan Quality." *Medical Care* 38 (10): 981–92.

Zgibor, J. C., and T. J. Orchard. 2004. "Specialist and Generalist Care for Type 1 Diabetes Mellitus—Differential Impact on Processes and Outcomes." *Disease Management and Health Outcomes* 12 (4): 229–38.

Chapter **71**

Health Workers: Building and Motivating the Workforce

Charles Hongoro and Charles Normand

Policy on human resources for health should support health policy objectives and be a means for achieving policy goals. The implication of such a focus is that health systems development should start by identifying the tasks that must be carried out and the skills needed to perform them. Meeting policy goals depends on being able to recruit, train, and retain staff with the necessary bundles of skills. Traditionally, skills are defined by membership of a profession, especially medicine, nursing, midwifery, and the allied health professions. Low- and middle-income countries (LMICs), often from necessity, have widened the range of health care workers to meet the service needs, with some people trained in extremely basic skills and others receiving enhanced training, such as nurses trained in emergency obstetrics. What is meant by a doctor or nurse also varies.

Even though structures and institutions vary widely, some problems are common to most LMICs. First, persuading doctors to work in remote rural areas is difficult, and they typically do not remain long in such posts. Second, emigration of doctors and nurses is extensive. Third, it is common for doctors to work in both the public and the private sectors (referred to as *dual practice*), sometimes harming public services. Dual practice may encourage doctors to skimp on their public health efforts, to pilfer supplies, and to induce demand for their private services (Bir and Eggleston 2003).

Many health sector human resource (HR) problems are predictable from a simple labor market perspective, given the combinations of incentives confronting health care workers and the constraints policy makers face. Experience in LMICs shows how problems have arisen and what policies have succeeded.

Economics predicts that employers will employ workers as long as the additional value of their services is at least as great as the cost of employing them, and workers will work if the rewards are of greater value than those accruing to other uses of their time. If key professionals are in short supply, higher salaries will be needed to attract them. Workers will invest in training if they value higher future incomes and more interesting work above the costs of income lost during training and of fees paid for training programs. This chapter focuses on how health systems might build and improve HR capacity.

Appropriate HR capacity is critical for the effective implementation of disease control interventions. Salaries account for 50 to 80 percent of health sectors' recurrent costs (Bach 2000). Table 71.1 shows the number of physicians and nurses per 100,000 population in selected countries. The number of health workers is related to the level of development because of the tight resource constraints facing LMICs and because of supply constraints, often exacerbated by migration of skilled workers (Awases, Gbary, and Chatora 2003) and prevalence of AIDS. In Africa, where the disease burden is high and increasing rapidly, the number of health workers is particularly low. Most African countries export health professionals to high-income countries.

A study in six African countries showed that most health workers intend to migrate for higher salaries. In Ghana, 70 percent of 1995 medical graduates had emigrated by 1999 (Awase, Gbary, and Chatora 2003). Pay differentials provide strong incentives to migrate. For example, a junior doctor in the United Kingdom averages a monthly salary of US$3,029 and a registered nurse averages US$1,500, compared with US$300

Table 71.1 Numbers of Physicians and Nurses, Selected Countries and Country Groups, 1998

Country	Physicians per 100,000 population	Nurses per 100,000 population	Physician-nurse ratio
Angola	5	100	0.05
Bangladesh	19	11	1.7
Bolivia[a]	29	14	2.1
Botswana	20	100	0.2
Brazil	136	44	3.1
Burkina Faso	<3	20	0.15
Central African Republic	<3	<10	0.3
Equatorial Guinea	20	50	0.4
India	106	94	1.1
Nepal	4	5	0.8
Pakistan	57	34	1.7
Papua New Guinea	7	67	0.1
Peru[b]	10	7	1.4
South Africa	20	100	0.2
Sri Lanka	37	103	0.4
Low-income countries	73	132	0.6
Middle-income countries	142	278	0.5
High-income countries	286	750	0.4
Global average	146	334	0.4
Global median	114	233	0.5

Sources: PAHO 2003; Support for Analysis and Research in Africa 2003.
a. 1999 data.
b. 1996 data.

per month for a Ugandan medical officer and US$180 for a registered nurse.

Scaling up service provision using current provision models would require large increases in resources and could require a change in strategy by development partners toward supporting recurrent costs (Jha and Mills 2002). The labor market model indicates that higher salaries would be needed to attract additional staff members, so funding would have to increase more than in proportion to the number of staff members employed.

Many LMICs pay health workers on civil service scales, which they control to contain overall government spending. This practice further widens the gap between salaries for professionals at home and abroad.

Although improved economic performance and increased development assistance may allow some increases in health spending, in most LMICs it is not plausible that such increases would be sufficient to make the necessary skills available without a range of strategies, including better regulation, stronger incentives, and initiatives to make key skills available at lower cost.

HEALTH CARE PROVISION AND ASSOCIATED HUMAN RESOURCE NEEDS

Studies on developing services to meet the Millennium Development Goals emphasize the importance of making health workers with the appropriate skills available and motivating them (Jha and Mills 2002). The problems include lack of technical skills, low motivation, and poor support networks (Kurowski and others 2003). This chapter, therefore, focuses on HR planning, training and professional development, incentives for workers to accept and stay in posts and to deliver services, and alternatives to conventional professional groups.

Incentives and Motivation

The labor market model outlined earlier provides a framework for analyzing the role of incentives. A health worker will accept a job if the benefits of doing so outweigh the opportunity cost. Improving recruitment and retention requires either offering higher rewards that make alternative employment less attractive or making qualifications less "portable"—that is, less likely to be recognized in other countries. The development of new health professions in many countries is a way of reducing the portability of qualifications, thereby reducing the opportunity cost of jobs at home. Another advantage is that training can be more specific to local health system needs, but ensuring quality and safety are important issues.

Health workers will choose to train and increase their skills if the rewards of doing so exceed the cost. In general, the supply of skilled professionals rises as rewards increase, because more will seek training, more will return to the workforce, and fewer will move to other jobs or other countries. Because health workers value both financial and nonfinancial rewards, they will work for lower salaries if other job characteristics are attractive.

The causes of health HR problems in developing countries are complex, and attempts to address them must reflect this complexity. Table 71.2 suggests a framework for exploring links between factors at individual, organizational, and health system levels. The framework is inspired by a systems approach, which gives prominence to the roles of and relationships between different component parts in influencing the whole.

The individual health worker level serves as a starting point for exploring the determinants of health worker behavior and performance (Kyaddondo and White 2003). *Performance* here means productivity and quality of services. Individuals respond to individual concerns through coping strategies, such as informal and dual practices, with associated consequences. There are multiple links between individual health worker behavior and organizational and systemic factors. Organizational and system arrangements define

Table 71.2 Framework for Diagnosing HR Issues
in the Health Sector

Level	Issue
Individual health worker	
Internal capacity	Knowledge, skills, competencies, attitude
Remuneration	Salary and perquisites, payment methods
Work environment	
Immediate environment	See organizational-level issues
Distant environment	See systemic-level issues
Productivity	Outputs or outcomes per given unit of time or per individual or group of individuals
Responses to organizational and systemic constraints	Low motivation, morale, productivity, and quality of services
	Informal practices, for example, unofficial fees, dual practice, misuse of public resources, and unethical practices
	Emergence of unskilled informal practitioners
Organizational level	Presence or absence of an appropriate physical and operational context—that is, availability of materials and facilities to deliver services of acceptable quality, workload management, and organizational norms and practices (organizational culture, management and leadership styles)
	Organizational autonomy across key strategic and functional issues
Systemic level	Level of bureaucracy and decentralization in the health system, and funding and regulatory arrangements
	Policy context—for example, pro-market policies and diversification of the health care market in the spirit of a public-private mix
	Socioeconomic and political context
	Medico-legal policy and enforcement

Source: Authors.
Note: This chapter uses a narrow definition of *health system* that considers socioeconomic and political issues as part of a wider context.

the incentive context for health workers and influence both organizational and individual performance.

Therefore, the configuration of the health system must create incentives for appropriate supply and deployment of health workers. HR development experts tend to focus more on problems encountered in the lower tiers of this framework. Political pressure for short-term solutions partly explains why many countries do not address HR problems comprehensively. The wider context can also be important. Good governance at the national level is necessary to make policy interventions at the health system level or below effective.

Financial Incentives

Most of the comparatively scarce evidence on the relative importance of financial and other incentives for health workers at the individual level comes from developed countries. Two findings emerge from recruitment and turnover studies. First, at extremely low salaries, financial incentives are particularly important (Normand and Thompson 2000). Second, at least half of the variation in turnover can be attributed to financial incentives (Gray and Phillips 1996). These findings leave considerable scope for improving retention using organizational changes, but such changes will be only partially successful if much better financial rewards are available elsewhere.

International migration has increased as restrictions on moves to high-income countries have been eased (Bach 2000). Many developed countries have shortages of health professionals and actively recruit from low-income countries, thereby raising the opportunity cost of remaining at home.

Health Care Systems' Responses to Health Worker Issues

Health sector reforms have been widespread in recent years, often with international support. These reforms tended to focus more on structures and financing and less on resource issues (Martineau and Buchan 2000). Other government reforms aimed mainly at improving efficiency and reducing the cost of government administration have often had large effects on the health workforce (Adams and Hicks 2000; Corkery 2000). Some changes have attempted to introduce better incentives, such as performance-related pay and renewable contracts, and to remove underperformers and ghost workers. Evidence on the effects of these reforms suggests that more emphasis should have been placed on designing incentives to improve performance and retention and on moving further away from workforce quotas and norms. Using the three levels of analysis, the following sections consider policies, management, and incentives and how they can help match skills to needs.

HEALTH CARE STAFF

Workforce planning should be dynamic and should link policy goals to staff members' skills and numbers and to performance-enhancing incentives.

Workforce Planning to Meet Policy Goals

Several factors make workforce planning in health particularly difficult, including changing needs as service models change, long training time for some professions, and lack of direct government control over the number of professionals being trained, for example, because of the growth of private medical schools, such as in Bangladesh, or because of people going overseas for training (although Singapore has addressed this problem by restricting the colleges that the government recognizes for registering doctors). The greatest difficulty comes from the unpredictable loss of skilled staff members to private health sector jobs, jobs abroad, and jobs outside health. Thus, a close link exists between HR planning and incentives and regulation. In Ghana, nurse training has often been the only available form of tertiary education for women, and many of those who are trained do not practice.

A key to more rational workforce planning is better coordination between health planning and planning for training and education. Powerful interest groups can oppose the expansion of training. Training establishments often oppose change because it may disrupt existing arrangements and threaten current staff members. The development of new professional groups faces particular resistance from existing professional groups, which, quite correctly, perceive the new groups as posing a threat to their interests. For example, some dentists in South Africa expressed concern over training of dental technicians who carry out a wide range of preventive and restorative dentistry at lower fees (Matomela 2004).

Models for HR needs are easy to devise, but determining the appropriate model parameters is difficult. For example, health planners must estimate the length of a nursing career—potentially up to 45 years but often much less, especially if nurses are willing to work outside nursing (Phillips and others 1994). Good data are needed on dropout rates from training. HR sections of health ministries are usually poorly resourced, have low status, and work with poor-quality data, and this situation must be changed if planning is to improve.

Basic Skills Training and Continuing Skill Development

Whereas the quality of basic training of health professionals varies widely in LMICs, the provision of continuing education and development is almost universally inadequate. Hence, skill levels of staff members fall over time. Evidence indicates that good-quality continuing professional development is a positive incentive and helps to retain staff members. Requirements to undertake continuing education can be made a condition of continued professional registration and can thereby provide some guarantee of competence.

Good basic education includes development of both professional skills and learning skills. Basic training and continuing development should be planned together. In many cases, the large investment in basic training is lost because of lack of maintenance, so that shifting some resources to updating and renewing skills is efficient.

A further challenge is to align the content of training to the skills professionals need. Many training programs in LMICs provide skills oriented toward service needs in developed

countries, although there have been attempts to change this balance. For example, more than 25 percent of Malawi's curriculum for medical students focuses on community health. Given that any training program can cover only a portion of relevant knowledge, focusing on locally relevant topics is increasingly important. Educational reforms in many medical schools in Africa and elsewhere are based on the community-based educational model (Jinadu, Olofeitime, and Oribador 2002).

Numbers and Types of Health Professionals

Categories of workers result from combinations of previous and current needs, national traditions, interest group pressures, and historical accidents. Doctors, nurses, and some paramedical professions have wide international recognition but vary in definition. Professional traditions and professional bodies bring some safeguards for quality and safety, and at best, professionals champion the needs of patients. Membership of a recognized profession can bring desirable independence from management. However, internationally recognized qualifications make it easy for professionals to migrate to countries offering higher incomes and better careers.

Most developing countries have new categories of staff that do not match internationally recognized professions (Buchan and Dal Poz 2003). Examples include nurses with extended training and roles and people working at subnurse levels with training of a few weeks to three years. Bangladesh has family welfare visitors, health assistants, and medical assistants who might elsewhere be classified as nurses or auxiliary nurses; in Uganda, clinical officers have three years of training and work as subdoctors; and nursing aids in Uganda have three months of training. Training is for specific roles without the generic training in conventional professions. Typically, such employees are mobile nationally, but they do not transfer easily across countries.

In the labor market model, employers want to employ staff members if their contribution to service provision is of greater value than the cost of their employment. Because those with portable qualifications can work in other countries, salary levels needed to retain workers reflect that possibility. Theory suggests that staff members will develop new skills if such an investment of their time and money produces significantly increased salary or benefits. Many countries cannot fulfill their requirements for health workers, but normally this difficulty reflects salaries that are too low to attract staff. However, raising salaries may make employment of the full complement of staff members unaffordable.

Staffing norms serve little useful role if the salaries needed to fill the posts are unaffordable. Decisions about how many people should be employed and in what capacities should be based on the contributions those employees will make and the costs of employing them. Staffing norms can be useful for planning, but they require careful analysis of affordability of care, the skills needed, and the way to provide those skills most efficiently. Several countries have of necessity turned to new models of provision using staff skilled in the delivery of key elements of high-priority services, such as immunization and emergency obstetric care.

Safety and Effectiveness of New Health Professions

Research on the new professions is limited, and much of the material is anecdotal (Buchan and Dal Poz 2003). A growing literature from developed countries indicates that nurses can be safe and effective in place of doctors in primary care (Venning and others 2000). The fear is that the absence of a formal profession and the lack of internationally recognized training could damage quality and safety. This issue is important, but even if new professionals are less safe than doctors, they may be much safer than the absence of a service such as emergency obstetric care. In some countries, new professions play a major part in the provision of services. A good example is Malawi, where clinical officers with extensive training (but much less than that of doctors) are a major resource, carrying out surgical procedures and administering anesthetics as well as providing medical care. In some countries, regulations govern such extended roles (McAuliffe and Henry 1995).

Fenton, Whitty, and Reynolds's (2003) study of emergency cesarean sections carried out by clinical officers in Malawi found that the overall maternal death rate was 1.3 percent, which is high, but much lower than if services had not existed. Perinatal deaths were 13.6 percent. None of the anesthetists was medically qualified, but outcomes were better when these practitioners had received anesthetics training (maternal deaths were 0.9 percent compared with 2.4 percent). The researchers found no significant difference in outcome between medically qualified surgeons and those trained as clinical officers. Care should be taken in interpreting the results of one study, but it does suggest that well-trained clinical officers can safely substitute for doctors in providing some important procedures.

Human Resource Policy and New Staff Groups

New staff groups are increasingly providing essential services in LMICs. In Zimbabwe, a new cadre called primary health care nurses, whose qualifications are lower than general nurses, was introduced in 2003 to curb external migration by nurses (Chimbari 2003). At the system level, such a development requires regulation and standard setting; at the service provision level, appropriate supervision and management is needed; and at the individual level, incentives and training need to be considered. Employing fully qualified doctors and nurses might be the safest option, but failing to provide services because of staffing constraints is unlikely to be the next best option.

HEALTH WORKER INCENTIVES

The World Health Report 2000 defines *incentives for health workers* as "all the rewards and punishments that providers face as a consequence of the organizations in which they work, the institutions under which they operate, and the specific interventions they provide" (WHO 2000, p. 61). Health workers face a hierarchy of incentives or disincentives generated by the work they do, the way they are paid, and the organizational and system context in which they work. Incentives are generally designed to accomplish the following:

- to encourage providers to furnish specific services
- to encourage cost containment
- to support staff recruitment and retention
- to enhance the productivity and quality of services
- to allow for effective management.

Responses of providers to incentives depend on context and on the stage of their career. Incentives that induce productivity vary with experience, stage in a career path, and changes in providers' social responsibilities. Ideally, incentive structures should recognize the evolutionary nature of work expectations.

Typically, incentives vary by type of employer: nongovernmental organization, public, or private. Public sector incentives tend to be the weakest because resource constraints and bureaucratic rules on civil servant employment constrain the use of both financial and nonfinancial incentives.

Typology of Incentives

Extrinsic incentives can be individual and organizational, monetary and nonmonetary (table 71.3). Discussions of provider behavior in LMICs have focused mainly on financial incentives, partly because of their low income levels compared with industrial countries. The challenge is to establish an optimal mix of financial and nonfinancial incentives that generate the desired behavior of health workers.

Experience from vertical programs for priority diseases or services—for example, poliomyelitis, malaria, family planning, and sexually transmitted diseases—provide evidence about different incentives. Programs often offered staff members better pay and incentive packages than those other public health workers received (Beith and others 2001). The exact effects of stronger incentives are unknown, but these programs generally succeeded, as evidenced by the eradication of leprosy, the near eradication of poliomyelitis in many countries, and the large drop in average fertility in developing countries in the 1990s.

Successful vertical programs used combinations of incentives, including better salaries, field and transportation allowances, streamlined management, specialized training, better facilities and material resources, and results-oriented

Table 71.3 Typology of Incentives

Individual incentives	Organizational incentives	Environmental incentives
Financial	*Internal*	Amenities
Salary	Autonomy	Transportation
Pensions	Accountability	Job for spouse
Illness, health, accident, and life insurance	Market exposure	School for children
Travel and transport allowances	Financial responsibility	
Child care allowance	*External*	
Rural location allowance	Governance	
Heat allowance	Public finance policy	
Retention and professional allowances	Regulatory mechanisms	
Subsidized meals, clothing, and accommodation		
Nonfinancial		
Vacation days		
Flexible working hours		
Access to training and education		
Sabbatical and study leave		
Planned career breaks		
Occupational health		
Functional and professional autonomy		
Technical support and feedback systems		
Transparent reward systems		
Valued by the organization		

Source: Adapted from Zurn 2003.
Note: These are mostly extrinsic incentives.

management to support improved health worker productivity and program performance. Goals were clearly specified, were understood and shared by the staff, and were often linked to incentives. The choice of vertical structures also reflects the perceived difficulties of using existing health systems, with their excessive bureaucracy, underfunding, and lack of capacity to implement integrated disease control.

Vertical programs must eventually be reintegrated into the system. The HIV/AIDS pandemic is a good example of a disease that might require targeted interventions until the capacity of health systems in LMICs improves to a level that allows the disease to be managed like other diseases. The success in integrating vertical programs depends on the parallel development of health system capacity, which depends in part on the alignment of health workers' objectives with policy and with system goals.

Aligning health worker and system objectives is difficult. The aim is to have satisfied health workers who are motivated to work harder (Hicks and Adams 2001). Evidence is limited, but financial and nonfinancial incentives are mutually reinforcing, and changing the culture of the health system to make goals more readily understood and shared can make financial incentives more powerful. Such change in the organization of health care can be politically sensitive because it can give health sector workers advantages over other public employees.

Incentives may have conflicting effects. For example, decentralization might create the autonomy needed for effective management, but without transparent management and career structures and job security, providers might view such a change as a threat (Kyaddondo and White 2003). Getting the balance right requires understanding the socioeconomic and political circumstances and may be helped by using participatory approaches to policy making and implementation.

Context

Context is defined here from an individual or an organizational provider's perspective. It constitutes what Adams and Hicks (2000) refer to as *external incentives*—that is, methods used by health systems to control the activities of health organizations or funders.

The power of incentives depends on context. Health systems in developing countries have varying cultural and economic histories that shape providers' expectations and responses to incentives. Financial incentives are strong when health workers' incomes are low, as in most developing countries. Nevertheless, examples of strong nonfinancial incentives exist in countries such as Thailand, where family ties and kinship affect health workers' decisions on where to work. Such nonfinancial incentives affect the size of the financial incentives needed to change where people choose to work.

History and experience determine a country's working culture and norms. In developing countries, most health systems are large bureaucracies whose management is driven centrally by guidelines, standards, and reporting systems. Incentives in such systems work against innovation, risk taking, and improved efficiency. A possible approach is to introduce changes that are based on the ideas of so-called new public management. New public management replaces line management with contracts or agreements between funders and policy makers on the one hand and providers on the other. Providers are given more managerial autonomy and are controlled by means of contracts and regulation. This approach can more easily embody new financial incentives, and autonomous providers can develop cultures that are more innovating. Such a radical change in managerial context can, in principle, make other incentives easier to use.

Other dimensions of context are the regulatory framework and its enforcement. Most developing countries have regulations governing the activities of the health sector. These regulations tend to be outdated or poorly enforced (Bloom, Han, and Li 2001). The main reason for regulatory ineffectiveness is low institutional capacity and widespread corruption. The symptoms of regulatory failure are widespread informal activities, dual practice, malpractice and medical negligence, and the presence of unqualified drug sellers (for example, in Bangladesh and Tanzania) and practitioners (as in India) (Bhat 1996; Killingsworth and others 1999; McPake and others 1999). Where the regulatory system is dysfunctional, providers tend to pursue their individual interests, often in private practice, to the detriment of organizational and system performance. Effective incentive systems that are based on performance require regulation and governance structures that minimize the common problems of patronage and corruption (Rasheed 1995).

Health system organization factors include governance and the degree of decentralization. Links exist between working culture and norms and the structural aspects of health system organization. The locus of control and decision making play an important part in health worker behavior. In theory, designing incentive schemes that are responsive to health workers' needs is much easier in a decentralized system. This theory is based on the belief that subnational units are better placed to make effective decisions on funding, regulating, and organizing frontline activities than are centralized units. However, experience in developing countries shows that lack of capacity at subnational levels has constrained decentralization, sometimes leading to unintended effects such as wrong priorities (Bloom, Han, and Li 2001). Any move toward decentralization requires investment in new management skills and capacities.

Incentives in Practice

Many countries have attempted to reform their economies and health sectors to improve general economic and health system performance. For example, Cambodia, the Arab Republic of Egypt, Uganda, and Zambia have attempted civil service reforms (Corkery 2000). These reforms include attempts to reduce the size of the civil service to lower costs and to improve productivity using incentives such as formal employment contracts and performance-based pay and promotion. Such reforms have been largely unsuccessful in developing countries because of the political difficulties in reducing the size of the civil service. Structural and organizational changes are typically unpopular with labor unions, especially if union members perceive them as threatening their well-being. Experience also underscores the difficulties of aligning system and organizational objectives with individual providers' objectives (Martineau and Buchan 2000).

The effect of incentives can be assessed in terms of their objectives (Adams and Hicks 2000). Table 71.4 summarizes incentive packages used in selected countries. The results shown should be interpreted with caution, because of problems of attribution and poor data. Adams and Hicks (2000) argue that economic incentives in payment mechanisms for physicians conform to economic logic, but little is known about the response of other categories of health workers to such incentives.

Experience in Thailand illustrates the labor market model outlined earlier. In general, public doctors prefer to practice in urban areas, where conditions are usually more attractive and opportunities for private practice are better. Thailand pays public doctors who work in rural and remote areas significantly more than those working in urban areas, and this incentive has persuaded some to move (Wibulpolprasert and Pengpaiboon 2003). The government also added nonfinancial incentives, such as changing physicians' employment status from civil servants to contracted public employees, providing housing, and introducing a system of peer review and recognition. These initiatives were coupled with significant environmental changes, including sustained rural development. In most developing countries, providers in rural areas are paid less than those in cities, and it is hard to recruit and retain health workers in rural areas.

China provides another example of how changes in the environment—for example, the introduction of pro-market policies—can change provider behavior, in this case from relying on government salaries alone to the use of "red packages" (Bloom, Han, and Li 2001). These red packages were gifts that were traditionally exchanged as an expression of mutual appreciation, but they have now evolved into informal cash payments from patients to health workers.

Health systems have a spectrum of workers with different skills and expectations, and incentives for one group can have negative effects on others (Adams and Hicks 2000). Policy makers must strike a balance between competing interests of professional groups and system goals. The unionization of labor and the growth of professional associations or councils can give health workers considerable bargaining power.

Solving one problem can create others. This situation often occurs when governments respond to the grievances of the most vocal professional groups, usually doctors, and neglect other groups. This piecemeal approach has caused HR crises, such as strikes and go-slows. Although health workers are normally somewhat motivated to pursue health policy goals, their own interests can conflict with those goals. Providing higher salaries to health workers, by increasing costs, can reduce access to services by some social groups (Bloom, Han, and Li 2001).

Compensation

Provider payment systems transfer resources from payers (governments, insurers, and patients) to providers (Maceira 1998)

Table 71.4 Incentive Packages for Health Workers, Selected Countries

Objectives	Incentives	Complementary measures	Constraints	Results
Recruiting and retaining staff in the country	Pay competitive salaries Include seniority awards in pay scales	Fiscal policies that increase the after-tax marginal value of salaries	Budget limitations Low public service salaries Policies to reduce salaries as a share of operating costs	Helped retain physicians in Bahrain
	Allow after-hours private practice in public institutions	Service standards and controls to prevent reduced work effort in the public system	Work effort that may be concentrated in private practice, leading to a deterioration of quality in public practice	Considered successful in Bahrain In some countries, resulted in deterioration of public systems where providers also engage in independent private practice (McPake and others 1999)
	Tolerate informal payments	Not applicable	Informal charges that limit access and may impede reforms that involve formal user fees and exemptions	Resulted in widespread use of informal payments in Eastern and Central Europe, Sub-Saharan Africa, and some East Asian and Pacific countries (Balabanova and McKee 2003; Chakraborty and others 2002; Thompson and Witter 2000)
Recruiting and retaining staff in rural areas	Provide higher salaries or location allowances (Wibulpolprasert and Pengpaiboon 2003) Base remuneration on workload	Decentralized administration Freedom to allocate institutional revenues or savings from operational efficiency to fund incentives Improved infrastructure and staff competence	Overall staff shortages Budget limitations Professional and lifestyle disadvantages Smaller potential for earnings from private practice than in urban areas Conflicting financial incentives (for example, loss of housing allowance in Bangladesh) Risks posed by internal conflicts and civil wars (for example, Colombia and Uganda)	Premium payments for working in rural areas found successful in Thailand (Wibulpolprasert and Pengpaiboon 2003)
	Require service in defined areas as condition of licensing or specialty training Provide opportunities for government-sponsored further education	Consistent application of policies on transfers and tenure	Loss of confidence if health workers perceive the selection process as arbitrary Providers' concerns that a temporary posting may become indefinite	Aided retention of professionals in Ghana and Zimbabwe (Chimbari 2003)
	Provide housing and good-quality educational opportunities for health workers' families	Adequate salary	Budget limitations	Found successful for nurses but not doctors in Nepal
	Recruit trainees from rural areas	Emphasis on public health and family practice in training curricula	Traditionally, overrepresentation of urban area students in student populations	Found successful in Thailand

Table 71.4 Continued

Objectives	Incentives	Complementary measures	Constraints	Results
Enhancing the quality and availability of primary care	Provide training and promotion opportunities for nurses and medical auxiliaries Train multifunctional health workers Mobilize women volunteers from communities, traditional birth assistants, and local leaders	Clear job descriptions and criteria for promotion	Opposition by professional associations to expanded roles for multifunction health workers in Nepal Limited training capacity in Uganda	Resulted in successful retraining of health assistants and other health workers in rural areas in Nepal to make them eligible for promotion Resulted in regrading of state-certified nurses to state-registered nurses in Zimbabwe (Chimbari 2003; Pannarunothai, Boonpadung, and Kittidilokkul 2001)
Encouraging teaching and research and reducing the internal brain drain	Pay health workers more if they do not practice privately	None	Allowances perhaps uncompetitive with private practice earnings	In Nepal, found successful in basic medical sciences but resulted in massive resignations in clinical departments Uncommon incentive, although a few countries (for example, Thailand) do pay professional allowances or nonpractice allowances
Improving the quality of care	Specify clinical guidelines in provider contracts	Leadership role by professional organizations Inclusion in the curricula of medical schools	Vested interests of professional associations Weak peer review systems Low consumerism and weak advocacy	Uncommon in developing countries Some success recorded in Cambodia's contracting experiment
	License institutions and professionals based on defined standards Pass laws requiring the registration of drugs and other potentially dangerous substances	Tradition of professional self-regulation Acceptance of civil and legal authority	Regulatory capture and a culture of self-protection Low capacity to enforce laws and regulations	Reduced number of hospitals and unqualified doctors in Estonia Resulted in limited success according to evidence from most developing countries (Bhat 1996)

Source: Adapted from Adams and Hicks 2000.

and can be structured to provide financial incentives. Most studies focus on payment mechanisms for doctors and their effect on productivity, costs, and quality of services (Bitran and Yip 1998). Table 71.5 summarizes common payment mechanisms and the desired incentives. The evidence shows that the operation of payment mechanisms is sensitive to the payment structure and how it is implemented (Berman and others 1997; Bitran and Yip 1998; Chomitz and others 1998).

Payment systems are more successful when built on existing traditions and culture (that is, when they take into account gift systems or, indeed, levels of corruption). It is normally best to use a combination of payment methods. For instance, if there is a shortage of public providers, they might be paid a basic salary for normal working hours and fees for service for after-

hours work. This method creates incentives for providers to do extra work and increase throughput, but providers may divert patients to after-hours services, and the method's feasibility depends in part on monitoring and governance standards. The challenge is to find payment combinations that motivate providers to provide desired volume and quality of services while containing costs.

Empirical Evidence on Payment Methods

Evidence of provider payment systems that have successfully aligned system and provider incentives is still limited (Bitran and Yip 1998). Interesting findings come from small-scale experiments such as Cambodia's New Deal (box 71.1). Health

Table 71.5 Major Payment Mechanisms

Payment mechanism	Key incentives for providers
Fees for service	Increase the number of cases seen
	Increase service intensity
	Provide more expensive services
Case payment (for example, diagnosis-related groups)	Increase the number of cases seen
	Decrease service intensity
	Provide less expensive services
Daily charge	Increase the number of bed days through longer stays or more cases
Flat rate (bonus payment)	Provide specific bonus services and neglect other services
Capitation	Attract more patients to register while minimizing the number of contacts with each and minimizing service intensity
Salary	Reduce the number of patients and the number of services provided
Global budget	Reduce the number of patients and the number of services provided

Source: Bennett, McPake, and Mills 1997.

workers' salaries were considered by many to be below the minimum required for a decent life, and workload is increasing because of HIV/AIDS.

The Cambodian experiment attempted to align individual health workers' and system goals through performance-based bonus payments and a set of internal regulations. Regulations can alter the working and organizational culture in a way that allows individual-based incentives to work. There were problems in enforcing penalties for violating regulations. Failure to enforce regulations may lead providers to lose confidence in the system. Countries with limited administrative and institutional capacity should use simple payment mechanisms that are enforceable within their capacity constraints (Barnum, Kutzin, and Saxexian 1995). A lesson from the experiment is that the context matters, and any strategy for offering incentives to workers must be embedded in traditions and cultural practices.

In a competitive environment, contracts are a useful tool for aligning health workers' behavior with organizational and system objectives. In the Cambodian example, contracts between the purchaser and district-level facilities—and between district-level facilities and management committees—were an attempt to establish accountability structures that specify targeted activities. More interesting was the attempt to transfer some management risk and responsibilities to individual health workers using subcontracts that permitted management committees to monitor their activities and pay them accordingly, though whether the contracts were well specified is not clear, and the administrative and transaction costs are unknown. The use of contracts requires management and monitoring capacity.

Introducing financial incentives for health workers is costly. Policy makers in governments and development partners need to ensure that adequate funding is available and sustainable. Resources are also needed to improve working environments and system capacities. Both financial incentives and other incentives are important, but services are likely to improve only if financial incentives are strengthened.

Group Incentives

Health workers typically work in teams. This system weakens financial incentives because the efforts of individuals may have little influence on overall performance. Indeed, individual incentives can worsen team cooperation. For example, if promotion is competitive and depends on measures of individual productivity, this approach can be a disadvantage for those who work for system goals in cooperative ways.

Designing effective group incentives is difficult. Paying group bonuses for achieving a given level of output can work only if individual team members feel adequately rewarded for their efforts and if there is no perceived free-rider problem. Most of the limited evidence on group incentives is for developed countries and shows that much depends on the production process and the organization of the teams (Ratto, Propper, and Burgess 2002). Group financial incentives tend to be weak, and using other approaches such as team building, better sharing of information, and improved working conditions is probably better.

Influence of System Capacities and Sustainability Issues on Incentives

The theoretical merits and demerits of different incentives are well understood, but system capacities and financial constraints may limit their applicability. Few developing countries have health systems that are capable of effectively implementing and operating some of the payment systems shown in table 71.5. The overall funding for the health sector may be too low to pay providers more. Also, the skills and expertise needed to design and implement contract- and case-based payment methods may be inadequate, and the country may lack the information technology needed to capture relevant data to support such contract- or case-based payment methods. Most health workers in developing countries are civil servants, and the particular needs of health workers may be lost in a general public service. Some countries are considering delinking health workers from public service commissions and setting up independent health commissions to run the health sector. In Zambia, however, delinking failed because of a lack of capacity at both the national and the local levels to implement the necessary HR changes (Martineau and Buchan 2000). Evidence from Trinidad and Tobago suggests that insufficient government commitment impeded the transfer of staff members

Box 71.1

Cambodia's New Deal Experiment: The First Year

The New Deal experiment in Sotnikum district, Siem Reap province, was launched in 2000 by the Ministry of Health, Médicins Sans Frontiéres, and the United Nations Children's Fund. It is an example of a concerted attempt to break the vicious circle of underpayment of health staff members and underuse of public health services by tackling the problem of low official income. The New Deal was developed following wide consultations and consensus building, and locally credible management structures were established to monitor and enforce the new framework.

Staff motivation was a major problem among health workers, as manifested by high levels of absenteeism from work, low time input at work (an average of one to two hours a day), and poor quality of services. Informal charges, drug thefts, and dual practice by public health workers were common, largely because of their low public salaries: government staff received US$10 to US$12 per month, compared with a minimum of US$100 required for a basic standard of living. At the same time, because of informal charges and extensive use of unregulated private services, households spent more than US$30 per inhabitant per year on health services, equivalent to 11 percent of total household expenditure.

The New Deal was seen as a vehicle for improving services by enhancing personal income, and its overall objectives were (a) to improve access to quality health care, (b) to build up the health system, and (c) to act as a catalyst for changes in national health policy. The principle underlying the improvements in the personal income of public health workers was that they would better comply with internal regulations governing (a) job descriptions and working hours; (b) payment of informal fees; (c) misappropriation of drugs, materials, and funds; and (d) diversion of patients to private practice.

The district (referral) hospital, health centers, and operational office were each managed by an elected management committee, and individual contracts were signed between staff members and management committees. The contracts stipulated that a bonus would be paid in exchange for strict adherence to internal regulations. The benchmark bonus level was set at an average of US$60 to US$90 per person per month. The management committee was responsible for enforcing the new framework of accountability. Official fees were also introduced on the assumption that the population would agree to pay for better public service.

The district got its funding from government appropriations, user fees, and external subsidies from various sources; however, given the overall lack of funding available for the scheme, Médicins Sans Frontiéres and the United Nations Children's Fund had to provide an initial injection of funds to support the bonus system.

At the hospital level, individuals signed contracts with the management committees, and compliance with internal regulations improved. The staff was generally present, fees were transparent, emergencies were attended at night, patients received drugs, and informal payments were not demanded. Use of health services increased significantly after the arrangement had been introduced. The number of documented violations was limited, though problems were encountered in sanctioning penalties. Staff members started receiving bonuses that gradually grew beyond the negotiated maximum, creating a hospital debt crisis by midyear, compounded by understaffing and underemployment problems, which meant that most staff members worked overtime. Nevertheless, the quality of services improved significantly, and per capita family expenditures on health fell 40 percent.

Source: Soeters and Griffiths 2003.

---

from the public service, leading to disillusionment among workers and effective opposition from unions (England 2000).

In countries with thriving private sectors, devising strong incentives for public sector workers is difficult. For instance, in Uganda, the private not-for-profit sector used to have better working conditions and pay than the public sector and consequently had better staffing levels. The government had to increase public sector salaries significantly in the 1990s to attract health workers back. The use of fees for service in the private sector when public health workers are paid a salary is likely to encourage private practice among public workers. Thus, the effects of methods and levels of payments are influenced by what is happening in the private sector.

Optimal Combination of Health Worker Compensation and Incentives

Although the optimal mix of provider compensation depends on context and policy objectives, some general policy guidelines on the design of payment methods to achieve organizational and system goals are available. Linking compensation to performance makes intuitive sense, but care is needed in working out the details. Health workers respond to both financial and nonfinancial incentives, but the extent of the effect varies, and the two can interact.

For new payment systems to work well, health workers must be governed by effective managerial authority. Because new payment systems aim to encourage particular behaviors and hold providers accountable, clear responsibility must be delineated within provider organizations. This delineation may be easier to achieve if the management of providers has some autonomy. Evidence from developing countries that have attempted to introduce managerial autonomy and corporatization of health service institutions, such as public hospitals and medical stores, indicates that delinking health workers from government control is politically sensitive. Nevertheless, such organizational or system changes are desirable if new payment methods are to create the right incentives and achieve the desired changes.

Part of the context for incentive systems is what type of disease control activities are best provided through markets or hierarchies. Traditionally, the public sector has been dominant. The economic arguments for government involvement are well understood, but delivery of services within the framework of government policy objectives can be by private (both for-profit and not-for-profit) providers. Thus, the private sector is increasingly involved in the social marketing of condoms and bednets, franchising, and contracting (Bennett, McPake, and Mills 1997).

From an economic viewpoint the only issues are the cost, quality, and sustainability of such arrangements. Emerging evidence on private sector involvement in health services suggests that the private sector is willing to participate in nonclinical disease control activities if the incentive structure is right. Private not-for-profit providers, such as hospitals and clinics associated with churches, have traditionally complemented government health care activities, especially in poor and peripheral populations (Gilson and others 1997). In recent years, Bangladesh has experimented with contracting nongovernmental organizations to provide primary care services in urban areas. Lessons from this experience are still emerging and indicate that, despite many early mistakes, this form of provision can be innovative and can help make a break from bureaucratic traditions. Such contracting depends on having contracting skills in both parties to the contract. A good understanding of context and incentives is also crucial.

In summary, incentive or payment packages should attempt to link payment with individual or group performance and should be assisted by supportive organizational and system changes if the desired provider behavior is to be achieved. No single best combination of payment methods exists.

ADVICE FOR GOVERNMENTS

Governments in developing countries face huge challenges in strengthening their health systems, especially their HR capacity, if cost-effective disease control interventions are to achieve their desired results. Strengthening their systems will entail developing self-sustaining systems for the supply, use, and retention of health workers. The following considerations are important in relation to putting effective policies and incentive structures in place:

- Countries should explicitly link the planned number of each category of staff members to health policy goals and set priorities, taking overall resources into account when planning HR needs.
- Countries should recognize that the salaries necessary to recruit and retain staff members will depend on the opportunities such workers have for other employment within the country and abroad, and planned numbers in each category should be based on this reality.
- Countries should understand both that qualifications that are recognized internationally are likely to attract higher salaries and that such qualifications may only be partially suited to the needs of essential health services in LMICs. They should focus on developing the most important skills by training new types of health workers, taking into account evidence that use of such health workers can be safe when properly trained. Many countries will be unable to prevent the loss of professionals with portable qualifications, because salaries offered will be far below those available elsewhere.
- Countries' training policies should take into account the decline in skills over time and the need to allocate scarce resources between basic training and continuing staff development.
- Countries should adapt and not imitate compensation and incentive structures, given the evidence that effective incentive structures depend on local conditions and traditions as well as on universal principles.
- Policy makers should remember that the availability and cost of suitably qualified human resources will affect feasibility and cost-effectiveness of disease control interventions.
- When developing vertical disease control programs, program managers must avoid introducing powerful incentives that damage existing services by drawing away key personnel.
- Policy makers should identify potentially harmful, unintended consequences when designing regulation and incentive systems. For example, if doctors are allowed to practice in both public and private services, the effects of private practice on incentives in public practice tend to be negative unless carefully monitored.
- Countries should recognize that the use of incentives to improve performance normally requires good regulatory frameworks and skilled managerial resources.

RESEARCH AND DEVELOPMENT AGENDA

New staff categories are emerging in many LMICs, and these workers are an important part of the workforce. Such staff categories are likely to increase, given migration and the high cost of employing people with portable qualifications, but little research is available on the appropriateness and safety of the new sets of skills, and little is known about the range of new professions, the content of and approach to training, the extent of professional supervision, and the outcomes of treatment. Sharing experience of such staff categories would be valuable. Priorities, therefore, include a study to map the different new staff groups in health systems in LMICs and to classify their tasks, roles, and training, and studies to compare the outcomes of conventional and new staff groups.

In addition to gaining a better understanding of the patterns, roles, and performance of new staff groups, data are needed on the length of time such workers remain in their posts, the extent to which their new qualifications are portable, and their migration patterns. Information is also lacking on how best to provide professional supervision for these new staff groups and how to encourage such employees to be professional in their work.

Limited evidence is available on the relationship of different health care compensation methods to individual and organizational behavior in developing countries. The following are possible research areas (and some practical steps) that might help fill information gaps and further understanding of the role of health worker compensation and incentives in disease control in developing countries:

- *Databases.* A useful step would be to set up HR databases for developing countries as the Pan American Health Organization has done for its region.
- *Literature review.* A review of unpublished materials on countries' experiences with using different payment and compensation mechanisms at national or subnational levels would also be useful. Failed experiments are seldom published, but they provide useful lessons.
- *HR supply.* Traditional HR planning models are no longer effective in handling health system dynamics in developing countries. More research is required to develop HR models in health that include the effects of HIV/AIDS, migration, scaling-up of existing interventions, new technology, and reforms. The underlying question should be how HR supply mechanisms can meet health systems' needs in terms of numbers, knowledge, skills mix, and competencies.
- *Demand and utilization.* Getting the size of the health workforce right is important in its own right, but that alone is insufficient for improving health workers' motivation and productivity. Research needs to focus on how to improve the motivation and performance of health workers

in resource-constrained environments and on what is needed to retain professionals in such settings. We know little about how health care workers make decisions about a range of incentives and disincentives generated by organizations and the systems in which they work. For example, what does it take to convince doctors and nurses to work in rural and remote parts of a country? To what extent are financial and nonfinancial incentives important in attracting people into training as health workers, deploying them to needy areas, motivating them, and retaining them in the system?

To a significant extent, current problems in improving access to care, in widening the range of effective services that are provided, and in improving the quality of care depend on better matches of skills to needs, better motivation of staff, and clearer understanding of how improved structures and incentives will work. Perhaps as important is that much of the debate focuses on developments within traditional patterns of staffing of services, but new patterns are increasingly emerging, and the extent of evaluative research is inadequate for drawing strong conclusions on how such developments can alleviate the constraints facing health systems. The development of incentive systems should be coupled with the development of organizational and institutional capacity that supports sustainable HR development in general.

REFERENCES

Adams, O., and V. Hicks. 2000. "Pay and Non-pay Incentives, Performance, and Motivation." Paper prepared for the World Health Organization's December 2000 Global Health Workforce Strategy Group, World Health Organization, Department of Organization of Health Services Delivery, Geneva.

Awases, M., A. Gbary, and R. Chatora. 2003. *Migration of Health Professionals in Six Countries: A Synthesis Report.* Brazzaville: World Health Organization, Regional Office for Africa.

Bach, S. 2000. "Human Resources and New Approaches to Public Sector Management: Improving Human Resource Management (HRM) Capacity." Paper prepared for the World Health Organization's December 2000 Global Health Workforce Strategy Group, World Health Organization, Department of Organization of Health Services Delivery, Geneva.

Balabanova, D., and M. McKee. 2003. "Understanding Informal Payments for Health Care: The Example of Bulgaria." *Health Policy* 62 (3): 243–73.

Barnum, H., J. Kutzin, and H. Saxexian. 1995. "Incentives and Provider Payment Methods." *International Journal of Health Planning and Management* 10 (1): 23–45.

Beith, A., R. Eichler, J. Sanderson, and D. Weil. 2001. "Can Incentives and Enablers Improve Performance of Tuberculosis Control Programs? Analytical Framework, Catalogue of Experiences and Literature Review." Unpublished paper, Management Sciences for Health, Rational Pharmaceutical Management Project Plus, and Stop Tuberculosis Partnership, November, 2004.

Bennett, S., P. McPake, and A. Mills, eds. 1997. *Private Health Providers in Developing Countries: Serving the Public Interest.* London: Zed Books.

Berman, P. A., A. K. Nandakumar, J. J. Frere, H. Salah, M. El-Edawy, S. El-Saharty, and N. Nassar. 1997. *A Reform Strategy for Primary Care in Egypt*. Technical Report 9. Bethesda, MD: Partnership for Health Research, Abt Associates.

Bhat, R. 1996. "Regulation of the Private Health Sector in India." *International Journal of Health Planning and Management* 11 (3): 253–74.

Bir, A., and K. Eggleston. 2003. "Physician Dual Practice: Access Enhancement or Demand Inducement." Working Paper, Tufts University, Department of Economics, Medford, MA.

Bitran, R., and W. C. Yip. 1998. "A Review of Provider Payment Reform in Selected Countries in Asia and Latin America." Major Applied Research 2, Working Paper 1, Partnership for Health Reform, Abt Associates, Bethesda, MD.

Bloom, G., L. Han, and X. Li. 2001. "How Health Workers Earn a Living in China." *Human Resources for Development Journal* 5 (1–3): 25–38.

Buchan, J. M. D., and M. R. Dal Poz. 2003. "Role Definition, Skill Mix, Multi-Skilling, and 'New Workers.'" In *Towards a Global Workforce Strategy: Studies in Health Services Organization and Policy*, vol. 21, ed. P. Ferriho and M. Dal Poz, 275–300. Antwerp, Belgium: ITG Press.

Chakraborty, S., R. Gatti, J. Klugman, and G. Gray-Molina. 2002. "When Is 'Free' Not So Free? Informal Payments for Basic Health Services in Bolivia." Unpublished paper, World Bank, Washington, DC.

Chimbari, M. J. 2003. "A Report on Health Care Providers in Zimbabwe." Disease Control Priorities Project Working Paper.

Corkery, J. 2000. *Public Service Reforms and Their Impact on Health Sector Personnel in Uganda*. Geneva: International Labour Organization and World Health Organization.

England, R. 2000. "Health Sector Reform Experiences: Lessons for Belize from Trinidad and Tobago?" Issues Note, Institute for Health Sector Development, London.

Fenton, P. M., C. J. Whitty, and F. Reynolds. 2003. "Caesarean Section in Malawi: Prospective Study of Early Maternal and Perinatal Mortality." *British Medical Journal* 327 (7415): 587.

Gilson, L., J. Adusei, D. Arhin, C. Hongoro, P. Mujinja, and K. Sagoe. 1997. "Should Governments Contract out Clinical Health Services to Church Hospitals?" In *Private Health Provider in Developing Countries: Serving the Public Interest*, ed. S. Bennett, B. McPake, and A. Mills, 276–302. London: Zed Books.

Gray, A., and V. L. Phillips. 1996. "Labour Turnover in the British National Health Service: A Local Labour Market Analysis." *Health Policy* 36 (3): 273–89.

Hicks, C., and O. Adams. 2001. "Pay and Non-pay Incentives, Performance, and Motivation." Paper prepared for the World Health Organization's December 2001 Global Health Workforce Strategy Group, World Health Organization, Geneva.

Jha, P., and A. Mills. 2002. *Improving Health Outcomes of the Poor: Report on Working Group 5 of the Commission of Macroeconomics and Health*. Geneva: World Health Organization.

Jinadu, M. K., E. O. Olofeitime, and P. Oribador. 2002. "Evaluation of an Innovative Approach to Community-Based Medical Undergraduate Education in Nigeria." *Education for Health* 15 (2): 139–48.

Killingsworth, J. R., N. Hossain, Y. Hedrick-Wong, S. D. Thomas, A. Rahman, and T. Begum. 1999. "Unofficial Fees in Bangladesh: Price, Equity, and Organizational Issues." *Health Policy and Planning* 14 (2): 152–63.

Kurowski, C., K. Wyss, S. Abdulla, N. Yémadji, and A. Mills. 2003. "Human Resources for Health: Requirements and Availability in the Context of Scaling-Up Priority Interventions in Low-Income Countries—Case Studies from Tanzania and Chad." London School of Hygiene and Tropical Medicine, London.

Kyaddondo, D., and S. R. White. 2003. "Working in a Decentralized System: A Threat to Health Workers' Respect and Survival in Uganda." *International Journal of Health Planning and Management* 18 (4): 329–42.

Maceira, D. 1998. "Provider Payment Mechanisms in Health Care: Incentives, Outcomes, and Organizational Impact in Developing Countries." Major Applied Research 2, Working Paper 2, Partnership for Health Reform, Abt Associates, Bethesda, MD.

Martineau, T., and J. Buchan. 2000. *Three Diverse Case Studies on the Importance of Human Resources to Successful Health System Reforms*. Washington, DC: American Public Health Association.

Matomela, N. 2004. "Department Outlines Amended Dental Act." *BuaNews Pretoria*, October 7.

McAuliffe, M. S., and B. Henry. 1995. *Nurse Anaesthesia Worldwide: An Analysis of Practice, Education, and Legislation*. Geneva: World Health Organization.

McPake, B., D. Asiimwe, F. Mwesigye, A. Turinde, M. Ofumbi, L. Ortenblad, and P. Streefland. 1999. "Survival Strategies of Public Health Workers in Uganda: Implications for Quality and Accessibility of Care." *Social Science and Medicine* 49 (7): 849–65.

Normand, C., and C. Thompson. 2000. "Review of the Primary Care Rehabilitation Project in Azerbaijan." Report prepared for the United Nations Children's Fund.

PAHO (Pan American Health Organization). 2003. *Bangladesh Health Labor Market Study*. Washington, DC: PAHO.

Pannarunothai, S., D. Boonpadung, and S. Kittidilokkul. 2001. "Paying Health Personnel in the Government Sector by Fee-for-Service: A Challenge to Productivity and Quality, and a Moral Hazard." *Human Resources for Health Development* (electronic journal) 1 (2)

Phillips, V., A. M. Gray, D. Hermans, and C. Normand. 1994. "Health and Social Service Manpower in the U.K.: A Review of the Research 1986–1992." Public Health and Policy Department Publication 7, London School of Hygiene and Tropical Medicine, London.

Rasheed, S. 1995. "Ethics and Accountability in the African Civil Service." *DPMN Bulletin* 3 (1): 12–14.

Ratto, M., C. Propper, and S. Burgess. 2002. "Using Financial Incentives to Promote Teamwork in Health Care." *Journal of Health Services Research Policy* 7 (2): 69–70.

Soeters, S., and S. Griffiths. 2003. "Improving Government Services through Contract Management: A Case from Cambodia." *Health Policy and Planning* 18 (1): 74–83.

Support for Analysis and Research in Africa. 2003. "The Health Sector Human Resources Crisis: An Issues Paper." Academy for Educational Development, Washington, DC.

Thompson, R., and S. Witter. 2000. "Informal Payments in Transitional Economies: Implications for Health Sector Reform." *International Journal of Health Planning and Management* 15 (3): 169–87.

Venning, P., A. Durie, M. Roland, C. Roberts, and B. Leese. 2000. "Randomised Controlled Trial Comparing Cost-Effectiveness of General Practitioners and Nurse Practitioners in Primary Care." *British Medical Journal* 320 (7241): 1048–53.

WHO (World Health Organization). 2000. *The World Health Report 2000—Health Systems: Improving Performance*. Geneva: WHO.

Wibulpolprasert, S., and P. Pengpaiboon. 2003. "Integrated Strategies to Tackle the Inequitable Distribution of Doctors in Thailand: Four Decades of Experience." *Human Resources for Health* 1: 12.

Zurn, P. 2003. "Incentives for Human Resource Management." Paper presented at the Workshop on Human Resource for Health Development: The Joint Learning Initiative, Veyrier-du-Lac, France, May 8–10.

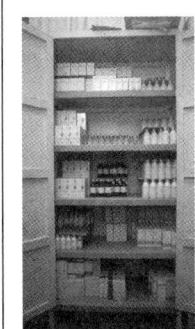

Chapter 72

Ensuring Supplies of Appropriate Drugs and Vaccines

Susan Foster, Richard Laing, Bjørn Melgaard, and Michel Zaffran

In 1988, the World Health Organization (WHO) reported that 30 percent of the world's population, some 1.725 billion people, lacked regular access to essential medicines. By 1999, the 15 percent of the population who lived in high-income countries purchased and consumed 90 percent of all medicines, by value (WHO 2004f). Again as of 1999, a recent WHO report estimates that 30 percent of the world's population, including 47 percent of Africans, 65 percent of people in India, 29 percent of people in the Eastern Mediterranean, and 26 percent of Southeast Asians (excluding those from India), had no access to essential medicines (WHO 2004f). So although access has significantly improved in a number of countries, a large fraction of the world's population still has no effective access to modern medicines or vaccines. The majority of these people are either extremely poor or are living in remote rural areas where the supply of drugs is limited or nonexistent—or both.

Many diseases can be effectively treated, managed, or prevented with pharmaceuticals and vaccines. The WHO figure of 30 percent of the world's population lacking access understates the reality; even within countries with apparently good services, some populations lack access. Similarly, immunization coverage globally has remained static for more than a decade at about 75 percent of children fully immunized, with about 27 million children born every year with no access to immunization services. Some effective vaccines, such as hepatitis B (HepB), are still not in routine use in many countries.

Medicines and vaccines are developed as a result of innovation by researchers and pharmaceutical companies. The global pharmaceutical market was worth more than US$400 billion in 2004, and more than 80 percent of this market is in North America, Europe, and Japan. Lipitor (atorvastatin), a cholesterol-reducing drug and the world's best-selling drug in 2002, had sales of US$8.6 billion, and growth was 20 percent annually. Zocor (simvastatin), another cholesterol reducer and the second-best seller, had sales of US$6.2 billion and was growing at 13 percent (IMS Global Learning Consortium 2003). These figures contrast with the dearth of research on neglected diseases prevalent in developing countries. For example, of the 1,325 new medicines launched between 1975 and 1997, only 11 were specifically for tropical diseases (Trouiller and others 2002). Médecins Sans Frontières (MSF) in 1999 initiated its advocacy program, Drugs for Neglected Diseases, which has highlighted this gap (http://www.accessmed-msf.org/).

Access to effective medicines and vaccines requires a complex and coordinated system. It must encompass production that ensures good quality, selection, procurement, and distribution; correct prescription and dispensing and correct use by patients; adequate financing; and effective monitoring of the system. Multiple delivery systems involving public, private, and nongovernmental organization (NGO) sectors frequently coexist, and patients are very likely to use multiple systems to access these products.

DRUG POLICIES

In any country, many stakeholders are interested in the national policy on pharmaceuticals. In broad terms, they can be characterized as producers, importers, distributors, prescribers, finance providers, and consumers. Each has a different set of interests, which in some cases are contradictory and in other cases congruent. To reconcile these disparate interests, many countries have developed a national drug policy. Managers of disease control programs need to be involved in these discussions at an early stage to prevent policy decisions from adversely affecting their programs. Any national drug policy broadly relates to three key objectives: increasing access, improving and ensuring quality, and ensuring rational prescription and use by providers and patients.

The primary components of a drug policy are selection of essential medicines; assurance of affordability, which includes issues of pricing, taxation, generic competition, and policies related to the Agreement on Trade-Related Aspects of Intellectual Property Rights (WHO 2001a); financing options; supply systems; regulation and quality assurance; rational use; operational research and drug development; clinical research, including clinical trials; human resource development for pharmaceutical policy and program management; and monitoring and evaluation. WHO has developed manuals and has provided technical support to countries to develop such national policies (WHO 2001b, 2003a).

VACCINE POLICIES

Every country has a national vaccine policy, usually laid down in a national health policy or through the establishment of well-defined elements of such a policy. WHO defines global frameworks and produces policy documents to advise developing countries (WHO 2002b). At the national level these guidelines may be adapted to fit national needs and capacities. Standards and norms for vaccines are also set by WHO and are generally adhered to worldwide (WHO 2003b).

WHO's creation of the Expanded Program on Immunization (EPI) in the 1970s established a policy for selection and use of vaccines that the vast majority of developing countries adopted. Only three vaccines—HepB, yellow fever (YF), and *Haemophilus influenzae* type B (Hib)—have been added since then, and the overall program directions remain largely intact.

In recent years, WHO has published a set of policy guidelines for vaccines not included in the global recommendations. These position papers are regularly updated. Three guiding principles provide the pillars for any national vaccine policy:

- Every eligible child must have equal access to nationally adopted vaccines regardless of religion, caste, or economic status.
- Vaccines require active government financial participation to ensure that they are provided and used in adequate quantities, thus ensuring the benefit of their considerable externalities. For example, the benefits to society of an individual's being vaccinated are greater than those to the indi-

vidual, because vaccination prevents transmission. It can also be argued that the elimination or eradication of a disease as a public health problem has public good characteristics: the benefits of the absence of disease are available to everyone, and all persons benefit at the same time. Therefore, governments must take an active role in ensuring that adequate vaccines of assured quality are available for comprehensive immunization programs within the country. The recent flu vaccine shortage and resulting rationing problems in the United States have illustrated this principle clearly.

- Countries should strive toward financial sustainability for the national immunization program.

A vaccine policy normally has six specific objectives:

- To provide a coordinated approach to national vaccines and equipment needs, including national vaccine production where applicable
- To provide criteria for vaccine selection and introduction, including burden-of-disease studies where relevant
- To develop a financial sustainability plan that ensures availability of vaccines in the longer term
- To define guidelines for private-public partnerships, including vaccine research
- To define national research priorities
- To support the implementation of the national immunization programs.

Policy setting is a continuous process that must keep up with global developments and changing national needs. Countries will normally formulate policies that are based on the technical work of a national committee of experts, who meet regularly under the auspices of the ministry of health. Bilateral donors and the Global Alliance for Vaccines and Immunization (GAVI) may influence policy setting, such as the timing for introduction of new vaccines, where they contribute significantly to the national immunization programs.

SELECTION OF DRUGS

Selection of a limited list of essential medicines that should always be available is necessary both for supply officials who work on procurement, storage, and distribution and for clinicians who aim to use medicines most effectively.

In 1977, WHO defined the first Model List of Essential Drugs (WHO 1977); since then it has updated the list 14 times. The latest list defines *essential medicine* as follows:

> Essential medicines are those that satisfy the priority health care needs of the population. They are selected with due regard to public health relevance, evidence on efficacy and safety, and

comparative cost effectiveness. Essential medicines are intended to be available within the context of functioning health systems at all times in adequate amounts, in the appropriate dosage forms, with assured quality and adequate information, and at a price the individual and the community can afford. The implementation of the concept of essential medicines is intended to be flexible and adaptable to many different situations; exactly which medicines are regarded as essential remains a national responsibility.

In 2003, the WHO Expert Committee on Selection and Use of Essential Medicines decided to define the criteria for core and complementary lists, as follows:

> The core list presents a list of minimum medicine needs for a basic health care system, listing the most efficacious, safe, and cost-effective medicine for priority conditions. Priority conditions are selected on the basis of current and estimated future public health relevance, and potential for safe and cost-effective treatment.
>
> The complementary list presents essential medicines for priority diseases, for which specialized diagnostic or monitoring facilities, or specialist medical care, or specialist training, or all three are needed. In case of doubt, medicines may also be listed as complementary because of their consistently higher costs or less attractive cost effectiveness in a variety of settings (WHO 2003d, 28).

At its 2002 meeting, the WHO Expert Committee changed its attitude toward fixed-dose combinations (FDCs). The committee stated that most essential medicines should be formulated as single compounds. Fixed dose combination products are selected only when the combination has a proven advantage over single compounds administered separately in therapeutic effect, safety, adherence or in delaying the development of drug resistance in malaria, tuberculosis and HIV/AIDS (WHO 2002c). This change reflected the interest in preventing the development of resistance and in promoting adherence. Although controversial, these FDC products will very likely be the main form of treatment for AIDS, tuberculosis (TB), and malaria.

The number of medicines on the WHO list has increased over time. The 2003 WHO list has 320 drugs in 559 formulations (Laing and others 2003). At country level, the essential drugs list is used as a guide rather than as a template. A study of 17 national lists of essential drugs showed that 68 percent had fewer than 300 drugs. The number of drugs per list ranged from 108 in Liberia to 389 in Karnataka state, India. Nine of the drugs on the WHO list were not on any of the 17 national drug lists in the study (Laing and others 2003).

At the first stage of identifying common diseases and complaints, managers of disease control programs are in a strong position to provide epidemiological information about the incidence or prevalence of a condition. At the second stage, the

selection of treatments would ideally have already been undertaken on the basis of available evidence or clinical trial data from the country. The medicines identified within these guidelines would thus become the medicines on the essential medicines list. This list would then serve as the basis for procurement, storage, and distribution activities. The evidence-based treatment guidelines would define treatment practices and be the basis of training (including examinations and licensing) and supervision.

SELECTION OF VACCINES

Developing countries select vaccines used in national immunization programs primarily on the basis of WHO policy guidelines. Most countries have adhered strictly to the six original vaccines—Bacillus Calmette-Guérin (BCG), oral polio, diphtheria, pertussis, tetanus, and measles. On the recommendation of the WHO Global Advisory Group on Immunization, HepB vaccine was included in the global guidelines in 1987, and YF vaccine was added in 1988; Hib vaccine was added in 1994. These remain the only vaccines recommended by the WHO for national use, and the recommendation presupposes that a disease burden of public health importance is present (see table 72.1).

A few vaccines, such as YF and Japanese encephalitis (JE), have regional importance in accordance with the prevalence of the disease. These vaccines are used in only a small number of developing countries. WHO has not generally recommended JE, although no evidence indicates that the disease burden of

Table 72.1 Current Vaccines Recommended by the World Health Organization

| Vaccine | Age | | | | |
	Birth	6 weeks	10 weeks	14 weeks	9 months
BCG	X				
Oral polio	X[a]	X	X	X	
Diphtheria-tetanus-pertussis		X	X	X	
Hepatitis B[b]		X	X	X	
Haemophilus influenzae type B[b]		X	X	X	
Yellow fever					X[c]
Measles					X[d]

Source: WHO 2002d, 88.
a. In endemic countries.
b. Only a few African countries have been able to introduce the vaccines to date.
c. In countries where yellow fever poses a risk.
d. In addition, a second opportunity to receive a dose of measles vaccine should be provided for all children.

YF is greater than the JE disease burden. However, a safety issue exists with mouse brain–derived vaccines such as JE.

Oral polio vaccine (OPV) is the vaccine of choice in developing countries, because it is easy to administer and the protective effect spreads to close contacts of vaccinees. It is suitable for mass campaigns, so the vaccine is used in poliomyelitis eradication programs. In 2005, the monovalent type 1 OPV, for which seroconversion rates are substantially higher than for trivalent OPV, has started to be used in areas where only type 1 wild poliovirus remains in circulation.

The selection of the original EPI vaccines was made on programmatic criteria rather than on considerations of disease burden. The need for consistent and standardized regimens determined the strategies selected by EPI. Adaptations over time, as new vaccines came along and local needs changed, were slow, and the uptake of newer vaccines remains a major constraint in most developing countries, although support provided through GAVI has improved the situation.

The term *vaccine gap* is used to describe the phenomenon whereby children in developing countries receive at most eight vaccines, if they are reached by immunization programs at all, whereas children in industrial countries normally receive 10 to 12 antigens, depending on national schedules. Furthermore, two vaccines in the routine schedule in the affluent world are less reactogenic than those given in developing countries: acellular pertussis vaccine (aP) and inactivated polio vaccine (IPV). The combination measles-mumps-rubella (MMR) vaccine is normally given twice, offering long-term protection against measles and rubella, important diseases in the developing world. The vaccine gap therefore consists mainly of three vaccines—aP, IPV, and MMR.

The pneumococcal vaccine, which is currently used in some countries, illustrates an additional aspect of the vaccine gap. Its composition is directed against the most prevalent strains, which cause otitis media in children. At the same time, millions of children die in the developing world from pneumonia caused by other strains of the bacteria, but no vaccine is currently available against those strains.

PROCUREMENT OF DRUGS

After the drugs have been selected, the next step is to decide how much to order. Usually this decision is based in part on past consumption, but it is also based on treatment guidelines and morbidity patterns. Concentrating on larger quantities of fewer drugs and dosage forms simplifies the process of ordering and reduces the chances of running out of stock. Ordering tablets or capsules rather than syrups or injections saves a great deal of money.

In 1997, when the second edition of *Managing Drug Supply* was published (Quick and others 1997), four methods of procurement were recommended under different circumstances. These methods were open tender, restricted tender with performance monitoring, negotiated procurement, and direct procurement. At that time, the World Bank was a major funder, and many countries favored the use of open tender. However, a major shift has taken place to restricted tender based on prequalification and direct procurement from nonprofit suppliers. The World Bank has produced a number of useful documents and resource materials that can be used for national procurement activities (World Bank 2000).

Another method of procurement that has been more widely used has been procurement from nonprofit suppliers, such as the United Nations Children's Fund (UNICEF) or the International Dispensary Association (International Dispensary Association 2004; UNICEF 2004). These organizations produce price lists twice yearly, and products can be ordered directly. Management Sciences for Health (2004) publishes an international drug price indicator guide annually that reports these prices and other procurement prices. Interestingly, the trend in drug prices generally has been downward. Prices of some TB drugs fell by more than 90 percent when procurement managers opened intensive negotiations with suppliers. And since 2000, prices of many important first-line antiretroviral drugs have fallen considerably. This trend is attributable to "advocacy, corporate responsiveness, competition from generic manufacturers, sustained public pressure, and the growing political attention paid to the AIDS epidemic. In addition, originator companies began announcing discount offers for the benefit of the poorest countries or those where the HIV/AIDS prevalence is the highest" (WHO 2004d, 5). The influence of economies of scale, in which unit costs have fallen because of the increased consumption of needed pharmaceuticals, might also have played a role.

Generic drugs obtained in bulk are almost always 10 or more times less expensive than brand-name drugs. Bulk purchase of generic drugs is the single best way to make a given budget go farther to satisfy the drug needs of a population. For price comparison, international prices (ex-factory, free-on-board—that is, not including insurance, freight charges, or taxes) are available online from Management Sciences for Health (2004). Local prices must, of course, include transportation and freight, as well as any applicable local taxes. Organizations that procure drugs in bulk but then sell smaller quantities, usually to nonprofit organizations, can help smaller purchasers obtain the advantages of competitive tendering. Examples include the International Dispensary Association, which is based in the Netherlands, and the Copenhagen office of UNICEF, which is able to supply drugs at very low cost to government-supported institutions.

Recent studies have revealed just how much the local component of drug costs can be, particularly in the private sector. A survey of costs in nine countries found an average markup of 68.6 percent, with retail markups of 16 to 50 percent comprising the largest single component in most cases. In countries that charge a value added tax on drugs, the tax can add 15 to 20 percent to the price of the drug (Levison and Laing 2003). Many of these cost elements are within the control of national policy makers.

Finally, when considering a change of standard therapy, managers of disease control programs need to take into account the long lead time between ordering a particular drug and having it arrive in the country ready for use—which can be a year or more. Time will also be required to prepare, print, and disseminate new guidelines, to train prescribers and dispensers, and to dispose of drugs used in the older therapy (Williams, Durrheim, and Shretta 2004).

PROCUREMENT OF VACCINES

Countries can be grouped into three categories according to the way they procure vaccines: procurement through United Nations (UN) agencies, direct procurement, and local production. Some countries procure their vaccines from a range of sources and may cut across all three categories. Over the past 25 years, UNICEF has been the main bulk procurer of traditional vaccines for most of the developing world, with the Pan American Health Organization Revolving Fund for Vaccine Procurement serving most Latin American countries. Because the fund takes advantage of large volume purchasing, it obtains prices comparable to those of UNICEF, which are available to all participating countries—regardless of their income level or size. The Gulf Cooperation Council also operates a purchasing program for its member states. That program includes 43 different vaccines and sera.

Some countries, where governments take on an increasing share of vaccine financing, purchase the vaccines directly from the producers or their representatives. Unfortunately, procurement is often being undertaken with little recognition that stringent quality assurance procedures must be in place to oversee the entire process. WHO is organizing workshops specifically targeted at vaccine procurement and has developed a vaccine procurement manual to guide such countries (WHO 2005a).

QUALITY ASSURANCE FOR PHARMACEUTICALS AND VACCINES

In an ideal world, all products to be imported into a country would be registered by a fully competent national drug regulatory authority to ensure quality. Unfortunately, this situation is not always the case. A study of antimalarial samples from seven African countries found that failures in ingredient content ranging from 20 percent to 67 percent for chloroquine tablet (CQT) and 5 percent to 38 percent for sulphadoxine/ pyrimethamine tablet (SPT) and dissolution failures ranging from 5 percent to 29 percent for CQT, and 75 percent to 100 percent for SPT (WHO 2003c). Good procurement practices of both brand-name and generic drugs require that suppliers be prequalified through the inspection of dossiers and factory inspections for good manufacturing practice (GMP) and that their performance be monitored.

Counterfeit medicines are a particularly difficult problem. Counterfeit medicines "are deliberately and fraudulently mislabeled with respect to identity and/or source. Counterfeiting can apply to both branded and generic products, and counterfeit medicines may include products with the correct ingredients but fake packaging, with the wrong ingredients, without active ingredients, or with insufficient active ingredients" (WHO 2005b, 1). In industrial countries, the newer brand-name medicines are counterfeited most often; Viagra is the frequent subject of counterfeiters. In poorer developing countries, the most commonly used antimalarials, antibiotics, and now antiretrovirals are the targets of the counterfeiters. The U.S. Food and Drug Administration estimates that up to 25 percent of medicines in developing countries are either counterfeit or otherwise substandard and that earnings from counterfeit drugs are more than US$32 billion per year (WHO 2005b).

THE WHO PREQUALIFICATION SCHEMES

Because undertaking prequalification tasks may be beyond the capabilities of national authorities, WHO has, on behalf of all UN agencies, started a prequalification scheme (WHO 2004d) covering AIDS, TB, and artemisinin-containing malaria drugs. The prequalification process is rigorous but efficient. WHO provides a positive list of prequalified products and manufacturers that have applied for and received favorable product assessments and manufacturing site inspections. Since January 2005, the Global Fund to Fight AIDS, Tuberculosis, and Malaria has required recipients to use WHO-prequalified products.

Ensuring quality is also an important aspect of any immunization program. For countries receiving their vaccines through UN agencies, WHO advises on the quality, efficacy, and safety of vaccines on the market through a prequalification of vaccines that entails the following steps: (a) reliance on a fully functional national regulatory authority (NRA) in the country of production and (b) verification of compliance with specifications through a thorough process of independent dossier reviews, testing of samples, site visits, ongoing monitoring of quality, and follow-up of complaints.

For a successful prequalification process, the NRA of the country of production must be functional and empowered by the government. A set of laws and structures must be in place that guarantee the NRA's authority and independence and that the NRA exercises the following functions: licensing, postmarketing surveillance, lot release, laboratory access, GMP inspections, and evaluation of clinical performance. These functions constitute the prerequisite for vaccines of assured quality and are the focus in vaccine regulation.

LOCAL PRODUCTION OF PHARMACEUTICALS

Large-scale production of pharmaceuticals in the developing world is limited to a few larger countries, most of which export primarily to other developing countries.

Whether local production of pharmaceuticals should be encouraged in low- and middle-income countries is a controversial issue. During the 1980s and early 1990s, the United Nations Industrial Development Organization encouraged the establishment of national production facilities. Recently, the World Bank and the executive board of WHO have reviewed this issue (Kaplan and others 2003; WHO 2004a). The more extensive World Bank report concluded:

> In many parts of the world, there is no reason to produce medicines domestically, since it makes little economic sense. In the local pharmaceutical manufacturing sector, local production is often not reliable and, even if reliable, it does not necessarily mean that medicine prices are reduced for the end user. If local production is adopted by many countries, it may lead to less access to medicines, since there are no economies of scale in having a production facility in each country" (Kaplan and others 2003).

Profit margins on bulk generic drugs are low so that public production must be as efficient as private manufacturing. For many countries, technical expertise, raw materials, quality standards, and production and laboratory equipment all need to be imported, so foreign exchange savings may be small or nonexistent. Few developing countries have the capacity to produce active ingredients for pharmaceutical manufacture. Industrial investment to promote local manufacture of pharmaceuticals in most, but not all, developing countries could be better used to improve health infrastructure (Kaplan and others 2003).

In summary, a manager of a disease control program is likely to obtain quality-assured products by procuring them from prequalified suppliers at the lowest prices without considering whether the products are locally produced.

STORAGE AND DISTRIBUTION OF ESSENTIAL DRUGS AND VACCINES

In the past, essential drugs, vaccines, and contraceptives were for the most part distributed using separate logistics systems. For vaccines and contraceptives, such systems were organized vertically to some extent, and because they were concerned with a far more limited range of products, the task was somewhat simpler.

A push has been made to integrate the distribution systems for drugs, vaccines, and contraceptives, although in most places separate systems are still operating, at least at the national level and often down to provincial levels. Vian and Bates (2003) noted a number of changes to the distribution systems in the past few years. In many countries, health sector reform programs included efforts to reform central medical stores to allow more autonomy and to introduce commercial incentives and improved management methods. In some cases, this reform has led to higher staff productivity, better performance, and more enforcement of payment policies. However, disruption in supply often occurs during central medical store transition phases. Increased integration of commodities, including contraceptives and vaccines, has also been noted. In some cases, it has decreased the amount and reliability of data collected on logistics, creating problems for needs estimation and for tracking of consumption (Vian and Bates 2003).

Another trend is the increasing use of private transporters and contracting out for transportation management; contracting transport can generate cost savings and improve services. Finally, a trend toward computerized systems exists, particularly involving the use of donor-financed software for improved management of logistics as well as a number of comprehensive assessment tools and indicator sets for evaluating drug supply systems. But the proliferation of software systems, with little coordination and not enough support and maintenance of complex and fragile computer systems, can be counterproductive, especially if paper-based systems that are difficult to reintroduce upon failure of the computer system are abandoned (Vian and Bates 2003).

Storage and Stocks Management

Drugs require secure storage in controlled climatic conditions and a reliable method of stock rotation. The FEFO rule (first expiry, first out) helps ensure that older stock is used up first. Security is another major consideration: access to the storehouse must be carefully controlled so that theft and embezzlement are minimized, and the persons who control access must themselves be trustworthy. Proper storage conditions, including minimizing exposure to heat, light, and humidity, are important for some drugs, but most drugs have proved remarkably resistant to poor conditions. Notable exceptions are tetracycline products, which become toxic when exposed to heat, and oxytocin and ergometrine, which lose their potency when exposed to light and heat; all should thus be stored in the refrigerator. The same applies to insulin and, of course, most vaccines. Correct FEFO stock rotation will ensure that exposure to harsh conditions is minimized and that potency is preserved as much as possible. Ensuring good air circulation and preventing direct water contact are most important.

Management of Donated Drugs

Management of donated drugs is a major problem in some areas, particularly if an emergency has precipitated an influx of drug donations. The best strategy is to accept only invited donations of drugs that the facility has specifically asked for (WHO 1999a). Any drug that is neither vital nor essential, that is not labeled clearly with its generic name, that is expired, that is in a package that contains only a few days' dosage, or that is not on the national essential drugs list or on the facility's formulary should be discarded—and the pharmacist should feel no guilt and fear no sanctions about disposing of such materials. They take up space, require tracking like other drugs, and present a risk of being accidentally dispensed to a patient and causing the patient harm—a factor that must also be taken into account. Proper disposal can be a problem. These drugs constitute potential toxic waste, and they should be treated as such and disposed of so that they cannot be retrieved and sold (WHO 1999b).

Vaccine Management

Vaccines are delicate products that are destroyed if handled incorrectly. Vaccine management involves the use and distribution of vaccines, from the manufacturers to the end users. Aspects of vaccine management include inventory and forecasting, stock control, in-country distribution, storage and handling, equipment replacement plans, procedures for the use of the vaccine, monitoring of vaccine storage, transport management, and operational management.

Forecasting of vaccine needs is the first building block of an adequate management system. In 2002, 22 of 82 countries surveyed by UNICEF indicated that they had experienced a vaccine stockout. In addition to lack of resources, the main reasons cited included poor or late forecasting.

In recent years, attention has focused on avoiding heat exposure. The introduction of costly vaccines that are sensitive to freezing has drawn attention to the need to protect vaccines from excessive exposure to cold as well as heat. WHO guidelines for the international transport of vaccines now include specific recommendations for each category of vaccine, including freeze sensitivity. National cold stores are the next critical level of the vaccine management system. A failure there—where vaccines are received, stored, and distributed in bulk—can result in extensive losses. The WHO-UNICEF Effective Cold Store Management Initiative encourages countries to procure equipment and adopt management and training practices that fully protect vaccines in national and intermediate vaccine stores.

At the country level, emphasis is being put on the use of new tools, such as the vaccine vial monitor. This heat-sensitive label is a time-temperature indicator used to ensure that the vaccines have not been damaged by excessive exposure to heat, to identify weaknesses in the cold chain, and to take vaccines beyond the cold chain to children who have no access to fixed health facilities.

Together with the increased use of vaccine vial monitors, the gradual adoption of the multidose vial policy contributes to the reduction of wastage. This policy of using opened multidose vials of vaccine in subsequent immunization sessions applies to all multidose vials of liquid vaccine containing thimerosal (WHO 2000). The policy was formulated in 1996 but its adoption remains limited.

PRESCRIPTION AND RATIONAL USE OF DRUGS

Rational drug use involves the correct drug being given to the correct patient, for the correct indication, in the correct dosage, by the correct route of administration, for the correct duration of treatment. The dispenser must also correctly dispense and label the drug and counsel the patient, and the patient must take the drug correctly or comply with or adhere to treatment. An error at any stage of this complex process can prevent the drug from being effective. Usually, at least half of these errors are attributable to the failure of patients to adhere to treatment, but the other half of the errors occur before the patient actually begins taking the drug. Few of the recommended treatments for common diseases involve more than one or two drugs, yet in actual practice, multiple drugs are often prescribed, even for uncomplicated cases. Such overuse of drugs rapidly consumes stocks, does not add to the quality of care (although patients may believe that more drugs are better), and allows stockpiling by patients.

The use of injections instead of equally effective oral preparations is also common. Not only are risks associated with the injections themselves, but also the cost of these injections is far greater than for the equivalent oral preparations. If all the prescribers at a facility can agree on and adhere to standard treatment guidelines that can be used as the basis for procurement and storage, the problem of overprescription and stockouts can gradually be eliminated. Uncertainties about dosages, particularly pediatric dosages, can also be reduced by the use of standard guidelines by age or weight. Doctors often cite their mistrust or delay of laboratory results as a reason to "cover" the patient for a variety of conditions. Dealing with laboratory efficiency or accuracy issues may be a worthwhile way to improve prescription practices that would also yield great benefits in terms of quality of care. Regularly reviewing a sample of prescriptions or case records and comparing treatments given to the standard treatment guidelines is likely to have a dramatic effect on the improvement of treatment practices (Laing, Hogerzeil, and Ross-Degnan 2001).

DISPENSING

Finally, the last step in the chain of the drug supply system is delivery to the patient. Often, dispensing is done by untrained staff members who know little about the drugs they are dispensing and are unable to communicate effectively with the patient. Anecdotal stories about patients receiving a handful of white pills and throwing them on the ground are discouraging to staff members but demonstrate that patients need explanations about the drugs they are getting. Increasing the use of dispensing materials—paper or plastic bags—may be worthwhile if it improves adherence to treatments. Brief training courses for dispensers can substantially improve the quality of dispensing.

Another major problem is the presence of dispensing doctors. A number of studies in both developed and developing countries have demonstrated that dispensing doctors prescribe more by value and not according to national or accepted guidelines (Trap, Hansen, and Hogerzeil 2002). The higher number of prescriptions is strongly associated with symptomatic treatment (that is, a drug was prescribed for every symptom); general overprescribing of antibiotics; overuse of injections; and prescription of medicines with lower clinical value. From a policy and safety perspective, the functions of prescribing and dispensing should be separated whenever possible (Nizami, Khan, and Bhutta 1996).

ADHERENCE

Delivering the drug to the patient is not the end of the story: the patient must adhere to the therapy. Failure to comply or adhere will result in poorer health outcomes; it may compromise the effectiveness of treatment, decrease the quality of life, increase preventable disability, and lead to premature death. It may also result in increased health care costs, more use of emergency rooms, more and longer hospitalizations, and potentially more use of intensive care units (Sabate 2003).

FINANCING ISSUES

The share of expenditures on health that goes to pharmaceuticals is presented in table 72.2.

Asking patients to pay part or all of the cost of their drugs can aid in holding down costs, reducing overuse, and replenishing the funds for drugs in the system. Drugs are often targeted for such fees because it is felt that patients will pay for them if they have no other choice. A substantial literature now exists on the advantages and disadvantages of user fees. On the one hand, they do raise some revenue, but administrative costs have often taken a large proportion of it. Their net contribution has rarely exceeded 5 percent of a government's recurrent expenditure. On the other hand, they often accounted for as high as 100 percent of nonsalary recurrent expenditures. Moreover, where they have been retained at the facility level, they have allowed for improvements in infrastructure and staff income, as well as ensuring a more regular supply of drugs (Xu and others forthcoming).

However, from a public health perspective, the disadvantages are numerous. They are often applied inequitably, with exemptions provided to richer people—such as government workers, the military, and the police—while poorer people must pay. But the main problem is that user fees discourage some people, particularly the poor, from seeking care at all. And among those who do seek care, the resulting costs can be financially crippling, to the extent that households may sacrifice food, education, or other important purchases to pay for drugs. Some are forced into poverty as a direct result of user fees. A related issue of increasing importance with the advent of effective antiretroviral therapy for AIDS is that user fees discourage adherence to long-term treatment, resulting in treatment failure, increased disease transmission, and the development of drug resistance. Fees are, therefore, particularly problematic for transmissible diseases.

On the basis of similar evidence, Creese (1997, 203) concluded, "A range of policy options other than user fees exists for dealing with situations of both under financing and rapid growth in expenditure. As an instrument of health policy, user fees have proved to be blunt and of limited success and to have potentially serious side effects in terms of equity. They should be prescribed only after alternative interventions have been considered." In this respect, WHO is now advocating that fees should be minimized and that countries should be supported in attempts to channel a high proportion of health expenses through taxes or prepayment mechanisms such as forms of insurance.

Table 72.2 Measured World Pharmaceutical Spending, by per Capita Income Clusters, 1990–2000
(percent)

Income group	Share of world total		Share of expenditure on health	
	1990	2000	1990	2000
High income	80.2	78.7	13.0	13.8
Middle income	17.1	18.8	22.5	24.8
Low income	2.7	2.4	20.8	19.2

Source: WHO 2004f.
Note: Income groups refer to World Bank classifications as of July 2000.

SUSTAINABLE FINANCING OF VACCINES AND IMMUNIZATIONS

Immunization is now generally accepted as representing one of the "best buys" for the health sector that governments must play a lead role in financing, but sustainable financing mechanisms have been largely absent in poor countries (WHO 2004a). The cost of immunizing a child against the six basic diseases hovers between US$15 and US$20 at current levels of coverage, representing no more than US$0.50 per capita, and on average 0.2 percent of the gross domestic product in most low-income countries. These costs suggest that immunizations are affordable for most developing countries from national budgets. However, immunization programs account for only 5 to 10 percent of total government health expenditures in many countries, which often rely heavily on donor funds.

Although the international community has recognized the important reasons that financing of vaccines cannot be left to individuals or households, donor support has often been quite erratic. The result is volatile financing that is vulnerable to shifts in donor priorities. In addition, recipient governments recognize that donors are more likely to fund vaccines than many other services, so they have taken the opportunity to spend their own resources on activities that are important to them but are less attractive to donors. This phenomenon can be seen in the apparent mismatch between data on disease burden, stated government priorities for health, and the allocation of government funds.

The challenge facing governments in poor countries is how best to finance vaccines, taking into account the variety of other health problems and the possible sources of funds. More funds could probably be raised from firms and households for health in general, but user fees for immunization, as for drugs, discourage people from seeking vaccination for their children. However, helping countries move to a system in which more prepayment exists for health services in general—either through taxes or the various possible forms of health insurance—would provide a pool of domestic funds that could be used for vaccines. If these funds were raised progressively, the rich could subsidize the poor.

A number of new issues relevant to immunization financing have arisen recently, including the evolving nature of the world market for vaccines, the growing divergence in vaccination schedules between developed and developing countries, the increasing diversity of products and presentations available to countries, the emergence of developing country manufacturers, and the importance of new global initiatives such as GAVI and the Vaccine Fund. The Vaccine Fund focuses on helping low-income countries introduce newer vaccines, such as HepB and Hib, which are generally more expensive than the older vaccines. In addition, the technology associated with the production of new combination vaccines has increased prices, with the cost per fully immunized child now reaching US$30 if HepB and Hib are included. This increased cost adds to the challenge. Governments in low-income countries and international development partners need to develop long-term strategies to ensure adequate financing for key health programs and interventions, including vaccines.

Since GAVI and the Vaccine Fund were established, renewed attention has been paid to financing issues as they relate to vaccine and immunization financing. GAVI has worked with WHO and countries to consider how much it would require to maintain existing levels of coverage after GAVI funding ends, whereas among the prerequisites for countries to obtain assistance from the Vaccine Fund is preparation of long-term financing plans for immunization programs. However, most low-income countries clearly will be unable to fund even a minimum set of essential interventions in the short to medium term without the assistance of international partners, thereby increasing the need to develop the long-term financing strategies described above. A mix of such strategies would include raising additional domestic funds, ensuring that funds are used effectively and efficiently, moving to greater reliance on prepayment mechanisms, and ensuring increased and stable flows of external funds. Table 72.3 summarizes and compares some recent trends in the financing of essential drugs, vaccines, and contraceptives.

ISSUES FOR THE FUTURE

As the world's population ages, health systems that formerly focused primarily on infectious disease are being asked to deliver new types of care, mostly for chronic illnesses and increasingly for mental illness. By 2020, the major causes of the burden of disease will shift from pneumonia, diarrhea, and perinatal conditions to heart disease, mental illness (particularly depression), and road traffic accidents. Tobacco will kill more people than any other cause of disease, including HIV. Unlike the United States and the countries of Western Europe, China and India will face the challenges of an aging population before they become high-income countries. Most health systems in the developing world are now prepared to deliver acute care, particularly for infectious disease, rather than chronic care. They are ill suited to long-term chronic care and follow-up; in general they lack recordkeeping, demonstrate little development of personal relationships with caregivers, and have little provision for enhancing patient adherence with medication. In many situations, the irregular and intermittent supply of medications for chronic disease means that the chronically ill suffer many interruptions of their treatment. The changing nature of health care will require changes in drug supply, which are only beginning to become visible. The (perceived) difference between "good" and "bad" care is often the availability of

Table 72.3 Trends and Developments in Financing and Procurement of Essential Drugs, Vaccines, and Contraceptives

Commodity	Trends and developments	Implications for logistics
Essential drugs	Use of loans and pooled or "basket" financing arrangements is increasing, leading to increased government involvement in procurement.	In the short term, procurement delays, shortages, emergency procurement requests, higher prices, and greater waste will result while governments develop internal capacity to procure. Also, increasing government involvement can mean less predictable results because of politics and governance issues.
	Procurement models adapted for health reforms such as decentralization and privatization proliferate.	Donors are more concerned about how procurement is done, translating into more technical assistance and emphasis on performance benchmarking. Difficulties in evaluating procurement systems are caused by a proliferation of models.
	Countries are moving toward restrictive tender and prequalification of suppliers.	In the longer term, prequalification may shorten the procurement cycle and lower costs. Similar effects from use of NGO suppliers are possible.
	Role of NGO suppliers continues in some countries as well as role of international NGO suppliers.	
	User fees represent a major trend for essential drugs, with many health facilities operating on a cash-and-carry basis.	Fee systems can decrease demand unless mechanisms exist to ensure service for those unable to pay.
	Private sector role is increasing as it becomes more apparent that public sector and NGO services cannot meet all needs.	Policy makers and managers will need to design and implement programs that promote appropriate use of the private sector
Vaccines	Donor contributions have been decreasing starting in 1990s.	Concerns are similar to those with essential drugs.
	Government financing and procurement of vaccines is increasing; a dependence on external resources persists.	GAVI supplies may require logistics changes because of new vaccines and injection equipment.
	Some shift in financing from grants to loans, and more use of basket financing.	Pressure on governments to finance vaccine purchases may lead to less government funding for EPI operating expenses and other Ministry of Health programs.
	Use of pooled procurement mechanisms and revolving funds or other international financial mechanisms, some based on achievement of outcomes, is increasing.	Outcome-based support requires information systems resistant to manipulation.
	New vaccines and vaccine combinations (new with old) are supplied through GAVI.	
Contraceptives	Donor contributions have been flat or have decreased, starting in 1990s.	Concerns are similar to those with essential drugs.
	Despite efforts to increase government contributions, there is still a major dependence on external resources.	Demand is created without supply keeping up.
	Many governments continue to give contraceptives (as compared with drugs) low priority for procurement with their own funds.	Constraints of Mexico City policy ("global gag rule") have limited funding for contraceptives.
	Financing through loans and basket financing are increasing, and governments are increasingly involved in procurement.	

Source: Adapted from Vian and Bates 2003.

drugs and supplies. Programs and funding agencies that are planning improvements in health care—for example, increasing coverage or case detection rates—often overlook the fact that such improvements will increase drug needs and costs.

Drug Resistance

Although the burden of chronic and noninfectious disease is increasing rapidly in the developing world, infectious diseases still account for nearly half of deaths in low-income countries. Most of these deaths are caused by six diseases: acute respira-

tory infections (mainly pneumonia), diarrheal disease, HIV and AIDS, tuberculosis, malaria, and measles. Drug resistance complicates the effective treatment for nearly all of these acute infections. Furthermore, this trend is expected to accelerate in the coming decades. In the treatment of HIV and AIDS, the increase of retroviral drug resistance is becoming a serious problem, especially in view of the limited number of treatment regimens available to date.

Drug-resistant malaria is now widespread. Chloroquine—once a cheap and reliable first-line treatment for malaria—is no longer effective in most countries. Newer drugs are significantly more expensive. Most recently, the trend has been toward multidrug combinations of products, and the addition of more than one drug is often to "protect" the component drugs from developing resistance as well as to improve the therapeutic effect (WHO 2002a).

Drug resistance in tuberculosis control—in particular, multidrug resistance—is a growing problem. Multidrug-resistant TB has now appeared around the world, and in many places more than 20 percent of resistant new tuberculosis cases are resistant to several drugs. Furthermore, the emergence of multidrug-resistant bacilli means that medication that once cost US$20 must now be replaced with drugs that are significantly more expensive and more difficult to use (WHO 2002a). Another major concern is the use of antimicrobials in farming, because about half of the antimicrobials produced each year are used in farm animals. Some of the new resistant bacteria are transmitted from food of animal origin or through direct contact with farm animals. Some reports indicate that as much as 50 percent of human antimicrobial resistance is caused by growth promoters in livestock, which are added to feed in subtherapeutic antibiotic doses (WHO 2002a).

HIV and AIDS

The HIV epidemic has had a tremendous impact on the pharmaceutical supply situation. First, it has highlighted weaknesses of drug supply and access around the world; the arrival of highly active antiretroviral therapy for the treatment of HIV/AIDS (HAART) means that HIV is to a large extent now a treatable condition, yet treatment is not available to the majority of those who suffer from HIV. Second, it has drawn the world's attention to the growing gap between rich and poor in terms of pharmaceutical provision. Unlike many other highly prevalent illnesses in the developing world, HIV and AIDS are also of major concern in the wealthier countries, and thus significant research has been undertaken and has yielded effective new medications (HAART, in particular).

A recent WHO report highlights the issue of the affordability of medications, pointing out that of the 23 countries that are estimated to make up 80 percent of the 2003 global need for HIV and AIDS treatment—estimated at about US$300 per annum per patient—only 8 have pharmaceutical expenditure levels above US$5 per capita, far short of the level of expenditure needed (WHO 2004c). Prices have fallen dramatically; WHO has continued to monitor the quality of AIDS drugs available on the world market for sale in developing countries and has removed substandard drugs from its list when necessary (WHO 2004e). Many high-profile initiatives to solve this problem have been started, most notably the WHO's "3 × 5" program; the Global Fund to Fight AIDS, Tuberculosis, and Malaria; the Clinton Foundation's efforts to lower prices for

HAART; and President George W. Bush's Emergency Plan for AIDS Relief. A number of issues are raised by the delivery of a complex, lifelong, costly treatment to poorer communities, especially in rural areas, one of which will be how to ensure adequate adherence to treatment in different clinical settings, ranging from district hospitals to health centers or even home settings, for HAART delivery.

Aging and Chronic Diseases

One of the important results of the exercise to estimate the global burden of disease was to highlight the growing importance of chronic disease, particularly in the developing world. A large percentage of chronic illnesses are related to smoking and lifestyle, and thus attempts to reduce smoking—or the lethality of smoking—would have an important effect on the need for medication for chronic disease.

Although many cancers are not yet curable, many are treatable with the goal either of slowing the spread or of palliating the symptoms of the disease. As the burden of cancer increases, palliative care, which involves the treatment of the symptoms and especially the pain that accompanies most cancers, needs to be given much higher priority. At present, the vast majority of the millions of cancer patients in the developing world receive totally inadequate pain control and suffer needless agony, in part because of antiquated laws governing the use of opioid analgesics (particularly morphine) and attitudes of medical and nursing personnel toward pain control (as well as attitudes of family members in some settings). The myths about morphine need to be dispelled. When used appropriately, especially in oral form, morphine does not lead to addiction, tolerance, respiratory depression, cognitive impairment, or premature death. In fact, people live longer when their pain is controlled, and they can eat, sleep, and live normal lives (Merriman and others 2002).

In countries where palliative care is fairly well developed and available, the consumption of morphine per capita averages over 20 milligrams, but in most developing countries it is negligible, and most of the needs for pain relief are unmet (Joranson, Rajagopal, and Gilson 2002). The World Bank recognized the importance of alleviating pain, which it included in its package of "essential clinical services" (World Bank 1993). As the population ages, the ability of the health care system to provide palliative care must grow along with it.

The trend toward more sedentary lifestyles and toward consumption of diets with higher fat and sugar content is leading to a steep increase in the burden of diabetes, with 150 percent increases in prevalence predicted for many countries by 2030; the absolute numbers will grow from 171 million in 2000 to about 366 million in 2030. The greatest increases in diabetes prevalence are predicted for the Middle East, Sub-Saharan Africa, and India (Wild and others 2004). Most of these

Table 72.4 New Vaccines Needed

Priority vaccines	Close to licensure vaccines	Vaccines for neglected diseases	Other vaccines of importance	Vaccines for new threats
HIV, TB, malaria	Meningococcus, streptococcus pneumonia, rotavirus	Shigella, dengue, Japanese encephalitis, leishmaniasis, schistosomiasis, cholera	Human papilloma virus, respiratory syncytial virus, herpes simplex, enterotoxigenic, *Escherichia coli*	SARS, anthrax, smallpox, pandemic influenza

Source: Authors.
SARS = Severe acute respiratory syndrome.

new cases will be type 2 and, thus, most will not be insulin dependent, but they will require oral diabetic medications. For those who do require insulin, given the current state of technology, the main barrier (other than cost) is the need for storage of the insulin in a cold or cool location and for sterile injection equipment. In either case, to meet the predicted rise in cases and to treat them with current drugs, a major expansion of drug supply for diabetes must be anticipated. Many diabetics currently do not receive adequate treatment. The pressure to provide adequate treatment will increase as the population ages and begins to demand treatment of its chronic afflictions—and in that case the increase in demand for diabetes medications would potentially be much more than 150 percent.

Another important finding of the global burden-of-disease exercise was the high number of DALYs lost to mental illness, depression in particular. In 2020, unipolar depression is projected to be the leading cause of morbidity and disability among females worldwide and in developing countries. Whereas in the industrial countries a pharmacological solution is often used, this approach may not be feasible in the developing world, at least not at present price levels. Recent research in the developing world has shown good results with weekly group interpersonal therapy, without the use of antidepressants. Trained laypersons ran the therapy sessions, not psychiatrists or medical personnel (Bolton and others 2003).

VACCINE RESEARCH PRIORITIES

In the past two decades new advances in biotechnology have resulted in the licensure of new vaccines, such as Hib, acellular pertussis, HepB, and attenuated varicella. Research institutions in the public sector have generated most of the basic scientific breakthroughs, whereas the large pharmaceutical companies have borne the cost for clinical development. Because such development requires heavy investments that need to be recouped from profits, new vaccines are expensive and therefore out of reach for poor populations.

Of all the vaccines currently under development, the three most needed today are vaccines to prevent the three big diseases—AIDS, TB, and malaria—which jointly account for more than 5 million deaths per year, or about 50 percent of all infectious disease deaths (see table 72.4). The total investment in vaccine against these diseases is not impressive, and it will probably take at least 5 to 10 years before a vaccine against any of them is available.

GAVI has selected three vaccines for accelerated development: meningococcal meningitis, rotavirus, and pneumococcal vaccines. They have been selected because they are considered close to licensure, or "near term." Other important diseases are considered neglected in terms of vaccine development, among them shigella dysentery and dengue fever.

New diseases emerge and old ones reemerge, influencing priorities in vaccine research. The severe acute respiratory syndrome (SARS) epidemic, the outbreak of avian influenza, and the emergence of bioterrorism threats such as anthrax have led to a new search for vaccines against these infections. The threat of a pandemic of a reassorted influenza virus strain has recently highlighted the need for much greater resources and attention to be devoted to the development and distribution of effective flu vaccines.

New Vaccine Technologies

Alternative routes of administration would improve program safety, avoiding needle transmission of bloodborne pathogens. The ability of nonprofessionals to administer vaccines would also ease vaccine delivery strategies. New administration routes, such as oral, nasal, and transcutaneous routes, are being explored. An interesting project concentrates on the development of a nasal measles vaccine that would greatly enhance the feasibility of eliminating this disease by facilitating the administration during mass campaigns.

The concept of using plant-derived or edible vaccines involves encoding protective antigens from pathogens into transgenic plants. The plants are processed so that they can deliver a uniform dose of vaccines. Human clinical trials have been conducted with, for example, bananas and raw potatoes, which have shown encouraging antibody responses. The potential advantages of this technology could include thermostability, low investment needs, multivalency, and oral administration.

New Immunization Technologies

Priority is given to new delivery technologies that will expand access, improve safety, and cut the cost of immunization programs. They include the following technologies:

- The reuse of disposable syringes and needles is widespread and contributes significantly to the transmission of hepatitis B and C and HIV. The autodisabled syringe prevents reuse, and disposal in safety boxes reduces the risk to health staff and the general public from contaminated syringes and needles.

- Four different technologies are being explored to minimize the risk of infection from accidental exposure to sharps: corrosive disinfectants, thermoprocessing, needle destruction, and plastic melting. However, none of these options will soon be put into use in the field.

- Although the adoption of the multidose vial policy will contribute to the reduction of wastage, the ultimate aim is to provide all immunizations as monodose preparations. Injection devices prefilled with a monodose increase quality and safety at the point of use. UniJect is one such device that has been tested with HepB and tetanus toxoid. Village health workers or traditional birth attendants can use such devices. Currently, the cost of the device and the need for additional cold storage space when multidose presentation is exchanged for monodose pose obstacles to implementation.

- Needle-free injection devices deliver vaccine at high velocity into the skin without penetration of a needle, reducing the risk of transmission of bloodborne pathogens. Technologies are being developed for both mono- and multidose presentations. Available multidose injectors have not been found safe, and new models are under development. However, regulatory obstacles and high cost have rendered the monodose injector models that are currently available infeasible for large-scale programs.

- Vaccine distribution and storage without a cold chain would considerably simplify the delivery system, reduce cost, and allow for an integrated supplies mechanism. Development of vaccines that do not need a cold chain should be the highest priority for technology research. Sugar glass drying is one such technology that has shown great promise. It can be used to produce multivalent vaccines that are completely heat stable except under extreme climatic conditions. The high cost of regulation and licensing and the uncertainty about market prospects in industrial countries have so far impeded the development and use of this technology.

Obstacles to Vaccine Research

A host of obstacles confront vaccine research, the most important being the low level of investment for vaccine development when there are limited market prospects in the industrial world. Only a limited number of research centers have the capacity and experience required to conduct phase 2 and especially phase 3 trials of new vaccines, and they are mainly located in industrial countries. The capacity to conduct phase 3 trials in developing countries needs to be strengthened; the current situation impedes further development of vaccines needed in those countries.

Pilot lot production of vaccines is required for all phases of clinical trials. The global capacity to produce pilot lots is, however, inadequate to meet demand. Close public-private partnerships are necessary to ensure that the production capacity is available.

Manufacturers need markets to provide some assurance that the development cost for new products can be recouped. Such incentives require realistic forecasts of demands. Various mechanisms have recently been put in place to try to guarantee future markets, most notably the Vaccine Fund.

Last, disease burden data are needed for both selections of vaccines for national programs and for estimations of vaccine requirements, including market projections. However, such data are lacking in many countries and regions. Existing data are especially weak for respiratory disease of both bacterial and viral origin.

PRIORITIES FOR PHARMACEUTICAL RESEARCH

The WHO Priority Medicines Project, a recent exercise that used evidence-based methods to outline the priorities for public funding of pharmaceutical research, has recently been published (WHO 2004b). It incorporated data from the burden-of-disease rankings and from the Cochrane Database of Systematic Reviews of data on clinical efficacy. It also incorporated the use of criteria of social justice, social solidarity, and equity, so that neglected diseases and the needs of special patient groups (the elderly, women, and children) were also taken into account. The research identified 20 major diseases that account for 60 percent of the total DALY burden both in Europe and in the rest of the world—diseases that are common to both groups included unipolar depression, ischemic heart disease, cerebrovascular disease, chronic obstructive pulmonary disease, and digestive diseases (excluding diarrheal diseases).

The authors also mention the important contributions of various cancers, lower respiratory tract infections, and diabetes to the burden of disease, which is common to both developed European countries and to the developing world (WHO 2004b). Smoking is clearly a major contributing risk factor, and the authors caution that expenditure on pharmaceuticals for smoking cessation must not divert resources from other efforts to reduce smoking. The priority areas identified by this exercise are presented in table 72.5.

Table 72.5 Preliminary List of 16 Priority Areas for Pharmaceutical Research

Rank	Condition
1	Infections caused by antibacterial resistance
2	Pandemic influenza
3	Cardiovascular disease
4	Diabetes (types 1 and 2)
5	Cancer
6	Acute stroke
7	HIV/AIDS
8	Tuberculosis
9	Neglected diseases[a]
10	Malaria
11	Alzheimer's disease
12	Osteoarthritis
13	Chronic obstructive pulmonary disease
14	Alcohol use disorders: alcoholic liver disease and alcohol dependency
15	Depression in the elderly and adolescents
16	Postpartum hemorrhage

Source: WHO 2004b.

a. Neglected diseases include, but are not limited to, trypanosomiasis (sleeping sickness), Buruli ulcer, leishmaniasis, and Chagas disease.

CONCLUSION

Ensuring that needed essential medicines and vaccines are available is critical for the success of any disease control program. A great deal is known about what works and what does not work. Careful selection, procurement from prequalified suppliers, proper storage and distribution using secure reliable channels, and assurance of rational use and correct dispensing are all critical components of any drug and vaccine supply system. Ensuring that adequate funds are available to pay for the procurement, distribution, and quality assurance of all medicines and vaccines is equally critical. Depending on the circumstances, either the public or the private sector or a combination of both can efficiently deliver quality-assured medicines and vaccines. The experience of a number of countries and programs has demonstrated that essential medicines and vaccines can be reliably delivered to poor people using the approaches described in this chapter.

REFERENCES

Bolton, P., J. Bass, R. Neugebauer, H. Verdeli, K. F. Clougherty, P. Wickramaratne, and others. 2003. "Group Interpersonal Psychotherapy for Depression in Rural Uganda: A Randomized Controlled Trial." *Journal of the American Medical Association* 289: 3117–24.

Creese, A. 1997. "User Fees" (editorial). *British Medical Journal* 315: 202–3.

IMS Global Learning Consortium. 2003. "2002 World Pharma Sales Growth: Slower, but Still Healthy." http://www.ims-global.com/insight/news_story/0302/news_story_030228.htm.

International Dispensary Association. 2004. *E-Catalogue of Products.* http://www.ida.nl/en-us/content.aspx?cid=42.

Joranson, D. E., M. R. Rajagopal, and A. M. Gilson. 2002. "Improving Access to Opioid Analgesics for Palliative Care in India." *Journal of Pain and Symptom Management* 24 (2): 152–59.

Kaplan, W. A., R. O. Laing, B. Waning, L. Levison, and S. D. Foster. 2003. "Is Local Production of Pharmaceuticals a Way to Improve Pharmaceutical Access in Developing and Transitional Countries? Setting a Research Agenda." World Bank, Washington, DC. http://www1.worldbank.org/hnp/hsd/documents/LOCALPRODUCTION.pdf.

Laing, R. O., H. V. Hogerzeil, and D. Ross-Degnan. 2001. "Ten Recommendations to Improve Use of Medicines in Developing Countries." *Health Policy and Planning* 16 (1): 13–20.

Laing, R. O., B. Waning, A. Gray, N. Ford, and E. 't Hoen. 2003. "Twenty-Five Years of the WHO Essential Medicines Lists: Progress and Challenges." *Lancet* 361 (9370): 1723.

Levison, L., and R. O. Laing. 2003. "The Hidden Costs of Essential Medicines." *Essential Drugs Monitor* 33: 20–21.

Management Sciences for Health. 2004. *International Drug Price Indicator Guide.* http://erc.msh.org/mainpage.cfm?file=1.0.htm&module=DMP&language=English.

Merriman, A., adapted from D. Doyle, and T. F. Benson. 2002. *Palliative Medicine: Pain and Symptom Control in the Cancer and/or AIDS Patient in Uganda and Other African Countries.* 3rd ed. Kampala: Hospice Africa Uganda.

Nizami, S. Q., I. A. Khan, and Z. A. Bhutta. 1996. "Drug Prescribing Practices for General Doctors and Paediatricians for Childhood Diarrhoea in Karachi, Pakistan." *Social Science and Medicine* 42 (8): 1133–39.

Quick, J. D., J. R. Rankin, R. O. Laing, R. W. O'Connor, H. V. Hogerzeil, M. N. G. Dukes, and A. Garnett, eds. 1997. *Managing Drug Supply.* 2nd ed. Management Sciences for Health in collaboration with the World Health Organization. West Hartford, CT: Kumarian Press.

Sabate, E., ed. 2003. *Adherence to Long-Term Therapies: Evidence for Action.* Geneva: World Health Organization.

Trap, B., E. H. Hansen, and H. V. Hogerzeil. 2002. "Prescription Habits of Dispensing and Non-Dispensing Doctors in Zimbabwe." *Health Policy and Planning* 17 (3): 288–95.

Trouiller, P., P. Olliaro, E. Torreele, J. Orbinski, R. O. Laing, and N. Ford. 2002. "Drug Development for Neglected Diseases: A Deficient Market and a Public-Health Policy Failure." *Lancet* 359 (9324): 2188–94.

UNICEF (United Nations Children's Fund). 2004. "Supply Catalogue." http://www.supply.unicef.dk/catalogue/index.htm.

Vian, T., and J. Bates. 2003. *Implications and Recommendations for Contraceptive Security.* Vol. 1 of *Commodity Security and Product Availability Issues for Essential Medicines, Vaccines, and Contraceptives.* Arlington, VA: John Snow/U.S. Agency for International Development.

WHO (World Health Organization). 1977. *The Selection of Essential Drugs: Report of a WHO Expert Committee.* WHO Technical Report Series 615. Geneva: World Health Organization.

———. 1999a. *Guidelines for Drug Donations.* 2nd ed. WHO/EDM/PAR/99.4 1999. Geneva: WHO.

———. 1999b. *Guidelines for Safe Disposal of Unwanted Pharmaceuticals in and after Emergencies.* WHO/EDM/PAR/99.2 1999. Geneva: WHO.

———. 2000. *The Use of Opened Multi-dose Vials of Vaccine in Subsequent Immunization Sessions.* WHO/V&B/00.09. Geneva: WHO. http://www.who.int/vaccines-documents/DocsPDF99/www9924.pdf.

———. 2001a. *Globalization, TRIPS and Access to Pharmaceuticals.* WHO Policy Perspectives on Medicine 3. WHO/EDM/2001.2. Geneva: WHO.

———. 2001b. *How to Develop and Implement a National Drug Policy.* 2nd ed. Geneva: WHO. http://whqlibdoc.who.int/publications/924154547X.pdf.

———. 2002a. "Antimicrobial Resistance and Rational Use of Antimicrobial Agents." EM/RC49/8. Geneva: WHO Regional Committee for the Eastern Mediterranean.

———. 2002b. "Core Information for the Development of Immunization Policy: 2002 Update." WHO/V&B/02.28. Department of Vaccines and Biologicals. WHO, Geneva. http://www.who.int/vaccines-documents/DocsPDF02/www557.pdf.

———. 2002c. "Fixed Dose Combinations for HIV/AIDS, Tuberculosis, and Malaria. Current Status and Future Challenges from Clinical, Regulatory, Intellectual Property, and Production Perspectives." WHO, Geneva.

———. 2002d. "State of the World's Vaccines and Immunization."

———. 2003a. *How to Develop and Implement a National Drug Policy.* Policy Perspectives on Medicines. Geneva: WHO. http://www.who.int/medicines/library/general/PPMedicines/PPM_No6-6pg-en.pdf.

———. 2003b. *Vaccines and Biologicals Catalogue 2003.* WHO/V&B/02.06. Geneva: WHO.

———. 2003c. *The Quality of Antimalarials—A Study in Selected African Countries.* Geneva: WHO.

———. 2003d. *Report of the 13th Expert Committee on the Selection and Use of Essential Medicines.* Geneva: WHO. http://whqlibdoc.who.int/trs/WHO_TRS_920.pdf.

———. 2004a. *Economics of Immunization: A Guide to the Literature and Other Resources.* WHO/V&B/04.02. Geneva: WHO. http://www.who.int/vaccines-documents/DocsPDF04/www769.pdf.

———. 2004b. *Priority Medicines for Europe and the World.* WHO/EDM/PAR/2004.7. Geneva: WHO.

———. 2004c. *Sources and Prices of Selected Medicines and Diagnostics for People Living with HIV/AIDS.* A joint UNICEF-UNAIDS Secretariat-WHO-Médecins Sans Frontières project. Geneva: WHO.

———. 2004d. *The WHO Prequalification Project.* Geneva: WHO. http://mednet3.who.int/prequal/.

———. 2004e. "WHO Statement on Removal of Two AIDS Medicines from List of Prequalified Products." WHO, Geneva. http://www.who.int/mediacentre/statements/2004/statement_aidsprequal/en/.

———. 2004f. *World Pharmaceutical Situation Report 2004.* Geneva: WHO.

———. 2005a. *Procurement of Vaccines for Public-Sector Programmes.* WHO/IVB/03.16. Geneva: WHO.

———. 2005b. "Substandard and Counterfeit Medicines." Fact Sheet 275. WHO, Geneva. http://www.who.int/mediacentre/factsheets/fs275/en/.

Wild, S., G. Roglic, A. Green, R. Sicree, and H. King. 2004. "Global Prevalence of Diabetes: Estimates for the Year 2000 and Projections for 2030." *Diabetes Care* 27: 1047–53.

Williams, H. A., D. Durrheim, and R. Shretta. 2004. "The Process of Changing National Malaria Treatment Policy: Lessons from Country-Level Studies." *Health Policy and Planning* 19 (6): 356–70.

World Bank 1993. *World Development Report 1993: Investing in Health.* New York: Oxford University Press.

———. 2000. "Procurement of Health Sector Goods: Technical Note." World Bank, Washington, DC. http://siteresources.worldbank.org/PROCUREMENT/Resources/health-tn-ev2.doc.

Xu, K., D. B. Evans, P. Kadama, J. Nabyonga, P. Ogwang Ogwal, P. Nabukhonzo, and A. M. Aguilar. Forthcoming. "Understanding the Impact of Eliminating User Fees: Utilization and Catastrophic Health Expenditures in Uganda." *Social Science and Medicine.*

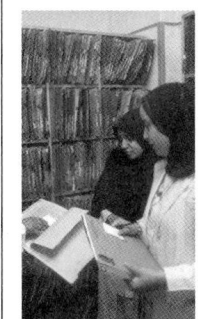

Chapter **73**

Strategic Management of Clinical Services

Alexander S. Preker, Martin McKee, Andrew Mitchell,
and Suwit Wilbulpolprasert

Financial resources alone are insufficient for individuals to benefit from the opportunities presented by modern health care systems. Some countries have achieved much better levels of health than would be expected given their financial resources (Mehotra 2000); many examples of poor-quality care in countries at all levels of development reflect not only scarce resources but also inadequate management of what resources are available (see chapter 70).

Many inputs must come together at the appropriate time and in the appropriate place to achieve maximum health gain. These inputs include human resources (in particular, trained staff); physical resources (such as pharmaceuticals and technology); and intellectual resources (in the form of evidence and the ability to apply it appropriately). This congruence requires that the production, distribution, and combination of these resources be actively managed and that the relations among the various elements that contribute to health care be optimized.

The challenge of bringing these diverse inputs together is becoming increasingly complex. Until the 1950s, providing basic care at low cost to large populations was relatively straightforward, given political will and sufficient resources. Relatively few effective drugs were available; even fewer drugs were effective in managing chronic disease. The available technology was limited to simple x-ray machines and chemistry tests that required few skills to administer. Consequently, scaling up the delivery of basic health care was relatively easy.

The situation in the former Soviet Union illustrates this state of affairs. Beginning in the 1930s, the Soviet Union implemented a vast system to provide basic health care where almost none had existed. The very simple care available was sufficient to produce significant reductions in maternal and childhood mortality rates. What such a system could not do, however, was respond effectively to the possibilities opened up by the explosion in diagnostic and therapeutic knowledge that began in the mid 1960s with the availability of new and easily tolerated treatments for many common chronic disorders. As individuals became able to survive with their chronic diseases, they aged and acquired other conditions, many of which could now be treated effectively, constantly increasing the complexity of the health care required. The inability to manage this increased complexity resulted in persistently high mortality rates from treatable conditions at a time when corresponding mortality rates were falling in Western countries (Andreev and others 2003).

This situation has certain parallels with that faced by many low- and middle-income countries today. Through a variety of mechanisms, a political commitment to the health sector is manifest in the increased availability of funding, such as through the Global Fund for AIDS, Tuberculosis, and Malaria (http://www.theglobalfund.org/en/). Much discussion has focused on one of the elements of health care that these initiatives will support: the supply of drugs that target the microbiological agents responsible for these three diseases. Yet improved outcomes will be achieved only if such agents are linked to the many other elements required to diagnose and treat these patients. Most obviously, the supply of drugs such as antiretroviral agents must be coupled with those used to treat the opportunistic infections that exacerbate AIDS. Care for the acute episode of illness should be linked to general support for patients and family members as well as to activities designed to prevent further spread of the disease. Furthermore, as drugs to combat infections become more widely available, it is probable—unless highly developed prevention systems have been put in place—that drug resistance will increase; this outcome has been evidenced with tuberculosis in those parts of the world where treatment has been available but poorly managed, such as the former Soviet Union and Peru (Farmer, Reichman, and Iseman 1999). The resulting resistant infections are much more complicated and expensive to treat. The rise in antibiotic resistance provides one of the most graphic examples of the consequence of the failure to manage the delivery of health care (see chapter 55).

Yet even where the financial resources and the political will exist to deliver effective health care, many health care systems contain numerous constraints to success (Hanson and others 2003):

- At the first level, that of the community or household, there may be inadequate demand for services or physical, financial, or social obstacles to their use. This situation calls for action to increase access and affordability, including health care financing reforms (see chapter 12). It also requires policies to ensure that services are culturally appropriate, that they address the particular needs of underserved populations, and that they provide dignity and privacy. Moreover, services should be physically accessible, both in terms of distance from population settlements and in terms of their construction—that is, facilities must be responsive to the needs of persons with disabilities.

- At the second level, the delivery of health care, there may be a shortage of resources, such as staff members, drugs, and equipment. However, to bring these resources together would require actions at the third level that anticipate future needs, as well as actions that ensure that the needed drugs and equipment are purchased at the best price possible, are subject to appropriate quality controls, and are distributed where needed.

- The third level includes health sector policy and strategic management. Effective action may be constrained by weak systems of management that are unable to take into account the changing health needs of the population and the changing demands on health care providers. Management weaknesses include inadequate pharmaceutical regulation and supply, ineffective training of health professionals, inability to engage with civil society, and a failure to put in place incentive systems to facilitate effective health care. Constraints at this level may originate outside the country, as governments are faced with demands by donors to follow paths that either undermine their policy goals or remove the flexibility needed to achieve them. Constraints acting at this level also arise when policies in other areas affect the health sector, such as when a weak, overly bureaucratic, and unreformed civil service system implements obsolete regulations; when there are inadequacies in infrastructure, such as poor communication and transportation links; or when there are weaknesses in the banking system.

- The fourth level refers to the environmental and contextual constraints on effective policies. The delivery of effective care may be affected by the physical environment, including climate and population dispersion. However, an equally important constraint is weak governance working within unsupportive policy frameworks, which may be compromised further by corruption, weak rule of law, political instability, weak public accountability, and lack of a free press. For example, de Soto (2000) has shown that, in many middle-income countries, it is almost impossible even to create a simple garment repair business because of a failure of legislative reform, in particular a lack of clearly defined property rights. As a result, much of the economic activity in those countries is informal or even marginally illegal, a response that is of particular concern in health care, given the scope for unlicensed and incompetent providers to endanger the public.

This framework underscores the importance of coordinating action at multiple levels. Health services can operate effectively only if policies are in place at the community level to ensure that those in need have access to services, and only if policies are in place at higher levels to ensure that the resources are available to provide those services.

This analysis of different levels demonstrates the importance of taking a systemwide approach to the management of health services. However, because of limited space, this chapter focuses primarily on the third level, that of strategic management. It first examines the nature of management in general and the specificities of management in the health system. It then explores some issues that arise when managing health services in different settings. It concludes with an exploration of some of the strategies used in low- and middle-income countries to optimize the delivery of care, using a framework developed by Oliveira-Cruz, Hanson, and Mills (2003).

WHAT IS MANAGEMENT?

One of the earliest definitions of management was that of French mining engineer Henri Fayol. Writing at the beginning of the 20th century, he stated, "To manage is to forecast and plan, to organise, to command, to coordinate, and to control" (Fayol 1949). Put simply, managing is about assessing probable future scenarios, deciding how best to respond to them, bringing together the resources needed for that response, and deploying them as effectively as possible. Until relatively recently, most management research was concerned with industrial production, for which outputs could be measured relatively easily. Relatively less attention was given to management of

Box 73.1

Specificities of Health Care Organizations

Health care services differ from many other organizations in many ways:

- Defining and measuring outputs is difficult.
- The work involved is more variable and more complex than in many other organizations.
- Much of the work is of an emergency nature and cannot easily be deferred.
- The consequences of error can be severe.
- Activities by different groups of staff members are highly interdependent, requiring a high level of coordination.

- The work involves a high degree of specialization.
- Workers are highly professional, with a primary loyalty to the profession rather than to the organization.
- There is limited scope for effective organizational or managerial control over clinicians, the group most responsible for generating work and expenditure.
- Dual lines of responsibility often create problems of coordination, accountability, and confusion of roles.

Source: Shortell and Kaluzny 1983.

service industries in general and health care services in particular. As Shortell and Kaluzny (1983) noted, health care services are different from many other organizations. Of course, many of the specificities shown in box 73.1 are differences of degree, with health services sharing many features with other service organizations. Yet important differences exist.

Managing Health Care Services

During the 1970s, health care services in many countries faced growing criticism for their perceived failure to articulate explicit goals or to develop the means to achieve them (Enthoven 1985; Griffiths 1984). This failure was contrasted with the perceived success of the private sector, which was seen as more capable of innovation and more responsive to demand.

These developments gave rise to what has been termed *new public management* (Hood 1991), which is characterized by the following:

- greater role for professional management in the public sector
- closer scrutiny of the work of professionals, involving performance measurement and target setting
- link between resource allocation and measurable outputs
- "unbundling" of previously integrated units, with contracting for previously integrated services
- shift to competition as a key to reducing costs and an emphasis on a private-sector management style
- careful use of resources to drive down the cost of labor and other inputs, where possible.

Recognizing the many reasons for market failure in health care (Arrow 1963), new public management builds on several

concepts that arise from new institutional economics. Included in these is contestability (Baumol, Panzar, and Willig 1982), in which the benefits that competition is thought to bring can arise even when competition is absent, thus ensuring that the barriers to market entry are sufficiently low to allow other providers to emerge. User choice is given priority over most other goals, including equity.

The enthusiasm for new public management was largely ideological, reflecting the contemporary rejection of an expanded role for the state; the extent to which this model was actually able to achieve what was claimed for it remains highly contested (Le Grand and Bartlett 1993; Stewart 1998). In particular, critics drew attention to the high transaction costs involved (Evans 1997) and the lack of evidence that competition can actually bring about the intended improvements in quality of care (Maynard 1998).

One feature of the new public management is its emphasis on general management, with managers possessing skills and expertise that can be applied to any sector. These managerial attributes are considered to be of greater importance than technical or professional knowledge. As a consequence, in some countries, the balance of power has begun to shift away from health professionals and toward general managers. In many places, the initial enthusiasm has given way to disillusionment and subsequently to a more balanced view that, though the precise solution will reflect the particular circumstances of the health care system, what is needed is a partnership between these two groups.

In some countries, this development will mean that managers must assume a greater role in relation to the delivery of clinical care. Such an expanded role will extend from their traditional responsibilities, such as financial controls, hotel services, and payroll management, to active participation in setting and monitoring standards for care delivery, linked to a responsibility for ensuring that the resources needed for care delivery are available.

In other countries, this role may involve stepping back a little. In an analysis of the British National Health Service, in which the degree of managerial control over the delivery of health care has proceeded further than in many other industrial countries, Harrison and Pollitt (1994) note how clinical decision making is increasingly driven by diagnostic and treatment protocols. Although often developed locally, working arrangements are increasingly specified, with the introduction of timetabled job plans for medical specialists and much greater measurement of outcomes. Yet Harrison and Pollitt argue that the growth of managerial control over professional activity is likely to be constrained by the increasing involvement of professionals in management, even if they do not fully adopt the managerial agenda. A further constraint is the persisting ability of professionals, because of their specialized knowledge, to resist managerial control and the related unwillingness of lay managers to extend their control into certain areas in which they do not feel competent.

Managing for Improved Quality of Care

An increasing volume of research in industrial countries has focused specifically on managerial and organizational responses to evidence that health systems often deliver suboptimal care (Institute of Medicine 2001). Quality of care is addressed in more detail in chapter 70. However, some of the key messages from this research are relevant here.

One message is that change must take place at all levels of the system. In this context, Ferlie and Shortell (2001) identify four such levels: the individual, the group or team, the organization, and the larger system or environment. They note the growing evidence that strategies that focus on individuals alone are unlikely to be successful, whereas those that are embedded within broader organizational change are more likely to be effective (Davis and others 1995). A second key message is the importance of teamwork, with evidence that well-functioning, multiprofessional teams provide better quality care (Aiken, Sochalski, and Lake 1997). However, change may be inhibited by barriers at the level of the organization, including lack of a consistent focus on quality, inadequate information, lack of physician involvement, and inadequate managerial support (Shortell, Bennett, and Byck 1998).

MANAGING CLINICAL SERVICES IN DIFFERENT SETTINGS

Clinical services are provided in a variety of settings, from the patient's home to ambulatory care facilities and hospitals providing inpatient care. They include those services that involve direct contact between a patient and a health care professional, as well as indirect contact, such as when a pathologist provides a diagnosis on a biopsy or blood sample. Reflecting the focus of much existing research, this section is structured in terms of different settings of care: ambulatory care, hospitals, and community care. Unfortunately, rather less research transcends these often artificial and arbitrary divisions to look at the more important issue of the patient's journey through the health care system, given that one of the greatest managerial challenges facing those delivering clinical services is how to ensure that the journey is efficiently navigated (McKee and Nolte 2004). Furthermore, available research that focuses on health facilities is often difficult to generalize because of the different meanings attributed to common terms such as *hospital, health center,* or more prosaically, *hospital bed.* For example, a major teaching hospital in a capital city, such as the Kenyatta National Hospital in Nairobi (http://www.kenyattanationalhospital.org/services.html), which offers invasive cardiology, renal transplants, and radiotherapy, is very different from a rural hospital with perhaps 100 beds and a single operating theater that provides only the most basic surgical and obstetric care.

Hospitals

Although hospitals are rarely the first places of contact between patients and health systems, and although hospitals do not provide the greatest share of health care, it is appropriate to begin with them because they often account for the largest share of public health sector expenditure (OECD 2003). They are also particularly difficult to manage for several reasons:

- One reason is the diversity of tasks that a hospital must undertake (Healy and McKee 2002b). Many hospitals fulfill roles that go beyond the delivery of patient care to provide training and research, support to community-based facilities, and even local employment or civic identity symbols.
- A second reason is the blurring of boundaries between hospitals and the rest of the health care system, which has occurred as a result of the emergence of many innovative models of care that cross the boundary between secondary and either primary or social care. A related issue is the shift taking place in many countries to managing patients through a complex combination of short inpatient stays and visits as an outpatient to specialist clinics and diagnostic facilities (McKee and Healy 2001). This approach is vastly more complicated to manage than the traditional model in which patients were admitted to wards from which they were taken to undergo investigations and treatment at a time convenient for the specialist concerned, a process managed by senior nurses. The new model requires new health worker roles, which might be termed *case*

managers. These case managers help patients to navigate the system.

- A third reason is the contrast between the rapidly changing demands on hospitals and the structural rigidities of hospitals themselves (McKee and Healy 2000). The original justification for creating hospitals as institutions was the need to concentrate equipment such as operating theaters, x-ray machines, and laboratories, and expertise such as medical specialists. Yet changes in the nature of health care are raising questions about how hospitals of the future should be configured. Many laboratory functions are being replaced by testing kits that can be used at the bedside, diagnostic equipment such as ultrasound scanners is being used in primary care, and a new generation of primary care workers are acquiring greatly augmented skills. In this rapidly changing environment, managers may be faced with aging hospital buildings that may lack sufficient electrical sockets for the greatly increased amount of equipment now available, or managers may have staff members with deeply ingrained ways of working who pose a particularly acute managerial problem.

These issues can be seen in the Kenyatta National Hospital in Nairobi, where a new managerial approach was developed but faced problems because of an unclear understanding of the kind of services to be provided, weak managerial capacity, and a lack of focus in targeting services (Collins and others 1999). In Zambia, financial management and accountability improved when the hiring of hospital staff was delinked from the national civil service, yet the process has been derailed on a wider scale because of trade unions' resistance to the changes (Hanson and others 2002).

Ambulatory Care

Ambulatory care, delivered on an outpatient basis, is the commonest form of contact between patients and health care providers. Although it often receives relatively little attention from policy makers compared with the more resource-intensive inpatient hospital care, ambulatory care contributes substantially to health care system performance (Berman 2000). Good management of ambulatory services is essential because these services are often the entry and exit points for consumers; however, these services can be difficult to manage effectively (Waghorn and McKee 2000).

Effective coordination of ambulatory and inpatient services is needed to ensure that patients are cared for in the most appropriate settings, thereby reducing inefficiencies such as the overuse of hospitals for nonemergency care. Such coordination often involves developing shared protocols for referral and management. In Benin and Guinea, for example, diagnostic and treatment decision trees were developed collaboratively with the local staff, leading to more efficient use of resources (Levy-Bruhl and others 1997). In Zambia and Tanzania, strengthening of management capacities in primary care facilities through a team-based approach to decision making that linked planning to budgeted action plans led to improved client perceptions of facilities and to a marked increase in utilization (Few and Harpham 2003). However, the challenges of management in the ambulatory care sector are great in many countries; this sector is often highly fragmented, with extensive and largely unregulated private provision and few levers to exert pressure for change.

Community and Social Care

A particular challenge is how best to link long-term management of medical conditions with community and social care in those cases in which an effective response to health needs spans the interface. Management of chronic physical or mental illness in the elderly, for example, can fall under the responsibility of home care and volunteer agencies, day centers, day hospitals, rehabilitation hospitals, and long-term care institutions, as well as community-based health teams (Bergman, Beland, and Perrault 2002). A systematic review of community-based care for elderly people in industrial countries concluded that such schemes can favorably affect rates of institutionalization and costs. However, comprehensive approaches involving program restructuring are often necessary, and cost-effectiveness depends on the characteristics of the health and social care systems. The review's authors identified as a critical challenge the expansion of those programs considered to be successful (Johri, Beland, and Bergman 2003).

Low-income countries face particular obstacles because they often lack effective alternatives to hospital care. As a result, patients are frequently cared for by their families but with little support, or they are consigned to large, poorly equipped, and poorly staffed institutions. This situation has stimulated the development of models of "community care," in which health care providers work with communities to deliver services. In the area of mental health, for example, the World Health Organization (WHO) has developed models of care that cover a range of care settings, including community centers and outreach services and residential homes, backed up by access to hospital outpatient and emergency care (WHO 2001). Similarly, the complexities of caring for people with disabilities in low-income countries have led to internationally developed guidelines that advocate a shared role for heath care providers and local communities (Helander 2000). Accordingly, effective coordination of those services clearly depends in large part on effective management. Shifting from hospital-focused care to community care introduces many managerial challenges. One element of an effective response should be to heighten the autonomy of patients in managing their diseases, but this response requires attitudinal changes among providers, who must commit to a real shift of power to patients, supported by effective information systems and safeguards for vulnerable patients (Litwin and Lightman 1996).

Health care systems are generally poor at addressing long-term illnesses, especially when those illnesses require integrated care spanning primary, secondary, and community providers (McKee and Nolte 2004; WHO 2001). The often low status accorded to these conditions in the hierarchy of priorities, coupled with fragmentation between health and social sectors (WHO 2002), will require greater commitment to managerial reforms that can improve the delivery of appropriate services.

THE SPECIFICS: WHAT WORKS?

This section turns to those policies that are designed to enhance the resources available to deliver health care and to combine them in ways that optimize the potential benefits. It looks, in turn, at the different elements required to deliver effective care: human resources, physical resources, intellectual resources, and the organizational or social resources that bind them together. The section begins with the most important resources for health care systems: the people who provide care.

Developing Human Resources

A key element in the delivery of effective health care is how to provide staff members with the appropriate combination of skills to do their jobs effectively.

Increasing Skills. In their review undertaken to inform the Commission on Macroeconomics and Health, Oliveira-Cruz, Hanson, and Mills (2003) identified 13 studies that assessed the effects of training to enhance skills. Though the results were mixed, training programs were overall more likely to have positive rather than negative effects. Several studies focused on communication and counseling skills, which often lead to improved client satisfaction. A study from Zambia showed that training must be linked to other resources; although training was associated with improved transmission of information, there was no decline in the number of complaints from clients who remained unhappy about long waits and short contact time (Faxelid and others 1997).

Changing Skill Mix. The division of tasks among different health care workers reflects many considerations, but evidence about who would be best at doing these tasks is rarely considered. There may be regulations restricting tasks to one professional group, such as the right to prescribe, or there may be cultural norms, which while unwritten have just as great an effect. Underlying these factors is a set of issues that includes a difference in the power of different professions, itself often a reflection of gender relationships in society, with a predominantly male medical profession controlling a predominantly female nursing profession. However, increasing evidence suggests that traditional demarcations do not support the optimal ways to provide care, and there is considerable scope for changing the mix of skills involved in delivering many aspects of health care.

This topic has recently been reviewed systematically by Sibbald, Shen, and McBride (2004), who have developed a taxonomy of the types of change in skill mixes that are possible (table 73.1). Their review shows that many tasks undertaken by one professional group can yield comparable and often better results when performed by another group. In particular, they show how nurse-led clinics often achieve better outcomes than traditional doctor-led service (Connor, Wright, and Fegan 2002; Stromberg and others 2003; Vrijhoef, Diederiks, and Spreeuwenberg 2000; Vrijhoef and others 2001, 2003).

Table 73.1 A Taxonomy of Changes in Skill Mix in Health Care

Changing roles	
Enhancement	Increasing the depth of a job by extending the role or skills of a particular group of workers
Substitution	Expanding the breadth of a job, in particular by working across professional divides or exchanging one type of worker for another
Delegation	Moving a task down a traditional unidisciplinary ladder
Innovation	Creating new jobs by introducing a new type of worker
Changing the interface between services	
Transfer	Moving the provision of a service from one health care setting to another (for example, substituting community for hospital care)
Relocation	Shifting the venue from which a service is provided from one health care sector to another without changing the people who provide it (for example, running a hospital clinic in a primary care facility)
Liaison	Using specialists in one health care sector to educate and support staff members working in another (for example, hospital outreach facilitators in primary care)

Source: Sibbald, Shen, and McBride 2004.

Although Sibbald, Shen, and McBride focus their review on experience in industrial countries, by challenging many deeply held beliefs they indicate what could be done in other settings around the world, after taking into account local circumstances such as the skills and expertise of those involved, as well as any salient regulatory or training issues.

Strengthening Management

In their review of constraints to health service delivery, Oliveira-Cruz, Hanson, and Mills (2003) identified 10 studies that evaluated the effect of management strengthening. The activities in those studies included the following:

- workshops for identifying and prioritizing managerial programs
- introduction of regular planning and evaluation cycles
- quality assurance methods
- establishment of routine communication systems
- training activities.

They concluded that the results were generally positive, with more rational use of funds; greater availability of funds as a consequence of better planning; improved coordination and integration of programs; improved methods of working; better staff morale; enhanced data collection, reporting, and use; and increased community participation. WHO has developed an approach to strengthening management that has been successful in a variety of settings (Cassels and Janovsky 1995).

It is important to identify where specific managerial skills are lacking and to explore different ways of obtaining them, whether through training, recruitment, or links with related organizations. For example, improved financial management in district health teams in Ghana was made possible by integrating staff members from local government accounts offices (Kanlisi 1991); a similar initiative was successful in The Gambia (Conn, Jenkins, and Touray 1996). However, a word of caution is required. Although a management strengthening exercise undertaken in Tanzania was successful when implemented at the local level, it failed when scaled up because the same degree of involvement by the originating team was no longer possible (Barnett and Ndeki 1992).

Managing Physical Resources

Managing infrastructure and other capital assets such as hospitals and health centers requires investment planning in both the short term (for example, maintenance) and the long term (for example, new acquisitions). Historically, however, costs associated with capital consumption and maintenance have not been met through operating budgets, resulting in few incentives for public sector health planners to efficiently manage infrastructure or to respond to market demand and consumer

needs (England 2000; Preker, Harding, and Travis 2000). Capital charging—requiring managers to explicitly account for the value of physical assets out of funding allocation or contract revenues—has been developed as a response, successfully heightening public sector management of capital investments in the United Kingdom and New Zealand (Heald and Scott 1996). Capital charging has been proposed as a strategy to stimulate better capital management in developing countries as well. For example, in Malaysia a corporatized hospital has been required to reimburse invested capital through dividends, with the Malaysian government recouping one-third of its original investment within five years (Hussein and Al-Junid 2003). Similarly, the Kenyatta National Hospital in Nairobi was obliged to account for all accruals (for example, property and depreciation) when it was given greater autonomy. Though changes in accounting management have experienced some shortcomings, improvements have been seen in financial transparency, timeliness of reporting, donor satisfaction, and revenue collection (Collins and others 1999).

Within the public sector, changes in line management have facilitated the incorporation of more explicit infrastructure concerns into the planning process. The central authority in Hong Kong (China) has made capital acquisition decisions jointly with hospitals during annual planning processes (Yip and Hsiao 2003). The introduction of business planning to district-level planning in Turkmenistan heightened accountability for maintaining physical infrastructure: use of a global budgeting model (that is, increased autonomy in line management as well as performance monitoring) led to reduced resource allocation to personnel and a greater than fivefold increase in maintenance expenditures (Ensor and Amannyazova 2000). Explicitly managing capital investments in both the short and the long term may facilitate efficient resource allocation.

Although capital charging is a relatively straightforward technical solution, capital investment can be particularly susceptible to political derailment (Anell and Barnum 1998). In the hospital sector, for instance, many transition economy countries have had difficulty downsizing infrastructure because those with decision rights to manage capital (that is, local governments) are different from those who have incentives to do so, such as hospital managers (Jakab and Preker 2003).

Strengthening Drug Procurement, Regulation, and Distribution

Managing pharmaceutical resources is crucial for ensuring access to essential drugs and promoting their rational use (Mossialos, Mrazek, and Walley 2004). WHO defines the goals of rational use of drugs as delivering medications effectively—appropriate to patients' clinical needs and at dose levels and durations appropriate to their individual requirements—and at an affordable cost (WHO 1985). The public sector plays a key role in providing the framework for rational use of drugs (Quick 1997) through measures ranging from drug regulation to clinical practice guidelines.

National drug policies (NDPs) can be effective in regulating private and public sector provision of essential medicines. The Lao People's Democratic Republic's NDP has been important in improving private pharmacy service quality (Stenson, Tomson, and Syhakhang 1997). In Burkina Faso, an NDP has enhanced the performance of rural pharmacies (Krause and others 1998). At the local and facility levels, increasing accountability can also lead to a more rational use of drugs. A simulation exercise in Tunisia that required physicians to relate pharmaceutical budgeting to involvement in the procurement process improved prescribing practices by containing costs while increasing the use of essential drugs (Garraoui, Le Feuvre, and Ledoux 1999). Enhanced management information systems, with corresponding supervision, monitoring, and top-level support, have improved contraceptive management in several countries (Kinzett and Bates 2000). The introduction of standard treatment guidelines and formularies has reduced overprescribing in several countries, and educational materials for consumers in Cameroon increased compliance with antibiotic regimens (Nabiswa, Makokha, and Godfrey 1993).

A comprehensive review of interventions used in Sub-Saharan Africa, where health systems are plagued by shortages of supplies, high costs, large-scale use of proprietary drugs, waste, and theft, provided considerable evidence to suggest what works in those countries (Foster 1991). Successful interventions included the following:

- selection and precise quantification of drug needs—in particular, the creation of essential drug lists
- improved procurement, with greater use of generics, competitive bidding, and international procurement agencies
- improved storage and distribution, with better storage conditions, inventory controls, security systems, and use of prepacked kits.

At the same time, several factors constrain better management of pharmaceuticals. Considerable resources are needed to adequately monitor NDPs, and implementation can be difficult (Petrova 2002). Furthermore, much of the pharmaceutical use is outside the control of the public sector: two-thirds or more of health problems are self-medicated. Though the public sector may strive to inform consumers, patients' nonadherence remains high (Le Grand, Hogerzeil, and Haaijer-Ruskamp 1999). As in management of other inputs, political considerations can thwart managerial responses. The Republic of Korea decided to divide its prescribing and dispensing functions precisely to address high levels of pharmaceutical overuse and misuse, but it subsequently faced strikes and stiff opposition

from those same stakeholders (Kwon 2003). Management of pharmaceuticals thus presents a complicated challenge, requiring significant investment and flexible responses.

Using Intellectual Resources

The process of generating, disseminating, and using knowledge is frequently imperfect. Pang and others (2003) have argued that a well-functioning health care system must have in place mechanisms that allow it to access and use research and the products of research. They highlight the weaknesses of much of the existing health care research, including fragmentation, overspecialization, and damaging competition among researchers, who are frequently isolated from other researchers and from the policy-making community. Drawing on concepts of the functions of a health system, they identify a series of four roles for a health *research* system:

- *stewardship*, which includes defining and articulating a vision for a national research system, identifying appropriate priorities, and setting and monitoring ethical standards
- *financing*, which includes obtaining research funds and allocating them accountably
- *creating and sustaining resources*, which includes the physical and human capacity to conduct, absorb, and use research
- *producing and using research*, which includes generating valid research outputs; translating research into formats that inform health policy, practices, and public opinion; and promoting the use of research to support innovation.

Such a system must be able to answer the many different questions requiring research, from basic laboratory science, such as new drug development, through health services research, such as comparisons of the cost-effectiveness of different drug regimens, to organizational research, such as the best way of delivering the most cost-effective drug regimen. Although the majority of health systems and services research continues to be undertaken in the industrial countries, a growing volume of research addresses the needs of low- and middle-income countries, such as that by the participants in the Effective Health Care Alliance Programme (EHCAP), an international research network that is undertaking systematic research within the framework of the Cochrane Collaboration (http://www.liv.ac.uk/lstm/ehcap/introduction.htm).

Establishing Relationships

The debate about the relative benefits of vertical (in which a single disorder is tackled by a program managed across levels from the Ministry of Health to the health care provider) and horizontal (in which health care for a wide range of disorders is delivered through a system that is integrated at each level) systems of health care delivery has been examined in detail in a major review of relevant literature by Oliveira-Cruz, Kurowski, and Mills (2003). They note how many activities lie on a continuum between the two extremes, with the Global Polio Eradication Initiative more vertical than the Expanded Programme on Immunization, which in turn is more vertical than the integrated management of childhood illness approach. They identify certain features that are often associated with vertical programs and that promote success: specific objectives, clear work schedules, well-defined techniques, and frequent supervision. They also identify characteristics that are often associated with horizontal programs and that can hamper effectiveness: shortage of essential drugs, lack of adequate staff training, intermittent supervision, and limited backup. However, they note that horizontal programs have considerable potential to deliver effective services if they are adequately funded, staffed, and managed, largely because of their economies of scale and scope.

To some extent, the approach is determined by the nature of the program. Vertical programs are most effective when the technology involved is very sophisticated or when it includes procedures different from the usual tasks and thus requires specialist skills. Vertical programs may be more appropriate when there is a need to rapidly achieve major reductions in the burden of a disease, although this situation does not preclude embedding the management of the program within existing organizations. These programs are often a response to weak management capacity in the existing system, although it is argued that they can perpetuate this problem or even undermine what does exist, diverting the attention of staff members from their usual tasks. Such programs often have a short time horizon, either being absorbed into existing systems or brought to an end. In part, their duration is linked to the source of their funding, which is often from donors who themselves have a short time horizon.

Integrating previously vertical programs into mainstream systems can be successful, as with schistosomiasis programs in Saudi Arabia (Ageel and Amin 1997) and Brazil (Coura Filho and others 1992). However, a systematic review of integration failed to identify consistent benefits, largely because of the very limited extent of the evidence available and the context-specific nature of this process (Briggs, Capdegelle, and Garner 2001). The authors of that review concluded that the question facing policy makers is not whether one approach is invariably better than the other; rather, it is how best to build on the synergies among them to maximize overall benefits. They note, for example, how the many successes of the Malaria Eradication Programme in the 1950s and 1960s were not sustained because active case surveillance was not integrated into routine health services (see also Bradley 1998).

Successful vertical programs are likely to involve community participation, but not to the extent that there is overdependence and subsequent attrition of volunteers. The programs' developers will have learned lessons from other similar programs, in relation to both organizational and technical issues. Where several vertical programs coexist, the programs' developers should explore how they can share common elements.

Contracting for Services

The setting of contracts by public agencies to purchase health care services is increasingly common in a number of low- and middle-income countries. The theoretical case for contracting out identifies potential advantages from combining public finance with private provision. However, there may also be difficulties, such as ensuring that competition takes place among potential contractors, that competition leads to efficiency, and that contracts and the process of contracting are effectively managed; consequently, these advantages may not always be realized (McPake and Banda 1994).

Unfortunately, the question of whether the advantages outweigh the disadvantages has been the subject of relatively little empirical study in low- and middle-income countries, and what exists is often highly context specific. For example, in Zimbabwe, a comparison of a hospital owned by a colliery, from which services were purchased by the government, and a nearby government hospital found that the colliery hospital offered services of at least comparable quality at prices lower than the unit costs of the government hospital after capital costs were included (McPake and Hongoro 1995). However, failure to establish policies on thresholds for use meant that growth in expenditure on the colliery hospital was not controlled. The authors argue that contracted facilities can achieve powerful bargaining positions if there are no viable competitors and the government does not retain the ability to offer an alternative service. They also identify a need for specific skills to manage contracts at all levels. Where a policy of contracting is a response to crises arising from civil service retrenchment and public expenditure cuts, these skills are unlikely to be developed.

Another study examined the economic arguments for contracting for district hospital care in South Africa, by using private for-profit providers, and in Zimbabwe, by using nongovernmental (mission) providers (Mills, Hongoro, and Broomberg 1997). In the South African setting, there were no significant differences in quality among three contractor hospitals and three government-run hospitals, but the contractor hospitals provided care at significantly lower unit costs. However, the overall cost to the government was similar for the two options because of the additional cost of contracting, with the efficiency gains captured almost entirely by the contractor. In Zimbabwe, two district-designated mission hospitals delivered similar quality care at lower cost than did two government hospitals. However, the contract between the government and the missions was implicit, rather than explicit, and was of long standing. As in the other Zimbabwean example, the authors identified the importance of developing the government's capacity to design and negotiate contracts that allow the government to derive significant efficiency gains from contractual arrangements.

Increasing Provider Autonomy

A review of cross-country experiences with enhanced autonomy of hospitals found improvements in service delivery. The most successful cases—in Hong Kong (China) and Tunisia—applied private sector management techniques and training, with appropriate performance assessment systems for staff. In countries where reforms were considered less successful, managers had been granted greater autonomy without suitable performance-oriented incentives (New Zealand) or vice versa (Indonesia) (Hawkins and Ham 2003). In the Kenyatta National Hospital, greater autonomy led to the introduction of performance appraisal linked to incentives, enabling the dismissal of poor performers and increased benefits and greater responsibilities for good performers. This change was coupled with clarification of clinical management roles. Complementing increased salaries for staff nurses, these changes helped improve the hospital's strategic management, donor accountability, and performance reporting (Collins and others 1999).

Implementing such management strategies in a coherent fashion is not an easy task. Hospital governance in several Eastern European countries, which has been transferred to local governments to improve responsiveness, has included measures such as performance-based payment mechanisms. Performance did not improve as expected because of an "inconsistent incentive environment"; rewards and sanctions were not linked to performance. Important factors in that failure to improve were weak stewardship functions and an absence of effective governance at the regional level, which made it difficult to change the initial configuration of the hospital system. Instead, increased hospital autonomy was used to ensure the survival of the institution rather than to meet the needs of the population. Thus, a continuing excess of capacity, inefficiency, and poor responsiveness to patient expectations remains (Healy and McKee 2002a). A review of experience with programs that increased autonomy in Sub-Saharan Africa also identified only modest success in achieving the stated goals (McPake 1996).

Public or Private Provision?

Although there has been considerable enthusiasm for privatizing state facilities because of the supposed efficiency gains achieved in the private sector, in reality the evidence is somewhat mixed. Thus, a study of dispensaries run by the government and by nongovernmental organizations in Tanzania found considerable variation in both sectors (Gilson 1995). This finding was consistent with another study in Tanzania of primary care providers in Dar es Salaam. In the latter, although the quality of care offered by private providers was, on average, better, much low-quality care was found in both types of facilities (Kanji and others 1995). Considerable variation in providers of both types, although with overall better quality in the private sector, was also reported in a study in Senegal (Bitran 1995). In summary, there is very little evidence to support the contention that private provision is better than public provision, and what evidence exists indicates considerable variations in both.

Strategic Purchasing

The quest to deliver effective health care is a dynamic process, adapting continually to changing health needs and the opportunities that arise that make it possible to respond in new and better ways. However, health systems that have failed in the past to respond to these changing circumstances face even greater problems. The pace of change is constantly increasing, with factors such as greater population mobility contributing to the reemergence of infectious diseases and with demographic changes and lifestyle changes giving rise to a new burden of chronic diseases.

Health care providers have faced difficulties in responding to this challenge on their own. Although they may possess a great deal of information about the patient sitting in front of them and, on the basis of their training and accumulated experience, about what might be done to help that patient, health care providers confront several important information gaps:

- First, they may know little about those who, despite being in need of health care, do not seek help. These people will often be the most disadvantaged in a society, with few means of making their voices heard.
- Second, they may have inadequate knowledge about newly emerging treatments or more effective ways of providing those treatments, especially if the treatments involve creating multidisciplinary teams with new sets of skills, working in ways outside their experience.
- Third, even if providers introduce changes, they may have inadequate knowledge of whether such changes have been effective.

These knowledge gaps provide the justification for action to improve the delivery of health care at several levels above that of the individual encounter between the patient and the health professional. Strategic purchasing brings together a series of interlinked activities: assessing health needs, using appropriate

Health strategy

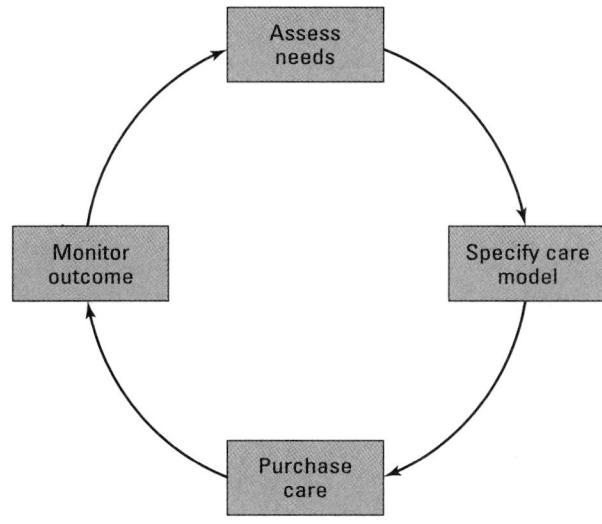

Source: McKee and Brand 2005.

Figure 73.1 A Framework for Strategic Purchasing

evidence to develop models of care that meet priority needs, creating the appropriate combination of regulations and incentives to implement those models, and then evaluating the response and reassessing whether the need remains (Figure 73.1). All of these activities should take place within an overall health strategy that takes into account the goals of a health care system, such as those defined by WHO (2000), of increasing health attainment, providing services responsive to the population's needs and expectations, and financing those services equitably.

The development of a strategic purchasing function is complicated, requiring high levels of information resources, both on health needs and on effectiveness. Strategic purchasing involves using technical and political skills, determining the needs of the population, identifying evidence of the effectiveness of different care packages, and setting priorities within limited resources. The last of these components is arguably the most difficult, given the high level of need and the scarcity of resources in many places. This list of components highlights why, in addition to having skills in financial and personnel management, the effective health service manager needs at least a working knowledge of clinical epidemiology and economic evaluation.

Even in industrial countries, the strategic purchasing function is often poorly developed. Given its many interlinked components and the problem of isolating any benefits from wider changes in the health system, this function is very difficult to evaluate. Nonetheless, it is included here as a model from which concepts may be adopted in low- and middle-income settings.

SUMMARY

Health systems worldwide face unprecedented challenges in responding to the increasing complexity of health care. Systems that were capable of providing basic care to populations for whom diseases were either simple or complex but self-limiting confront a fatal struggle to keep up with the increasing opportunities that modern science has provided. The challenge is especially great for health systems in low- and middle-income countries because the global community is no longer willing to sit back while millions of people die from treatable diseases such as malaria and tuberculosis and fail to receive life-prolonging therapies for AIDS. As a consequence, some of the resources, primarily pharmaceuticals, are being made available to those who need them. However, the challenge that health systems face is not simply a lack of money to purchase pharmaceuticals; effective management systems are requisite as well to create the infrastructure to identify those in need, establish appropriate treatments, and ensure provision of these treatments as long as necessary. Emerging challenges must be identified, and the necessary resources to deal with them must be brought together and applied effectively.

Many countries have a clear need to invest in the development of human resources. Although in many cases this investment will require new and wide-ranging human resource strategies involving training, career progression, and retention, there seems to be scope for rapid gains from some shorter forms of training, particularly, in communications skills. Although the evidence for the effectiveness of current models of management strengthening is somewhat mixed, gains may be realized by identifying and filling key gaps, such as those in financial expertise. Changing the skill mix can do much to match available skills to tasks.

Much also can be done to manage the capital stock better or, in most cases, to manage it at all. For example, mechanisms such as capital charging can focus greater management attention on this issue, although this will work only if sufficient capacity can be focused. Important gains can be made from better management of pharmaceuticals, an issue of increasing importance because of the new funds made available for their purchase.

Modern health care is based on the growth of knowledge, and it is as important to manage intellectual resources as it is to manage people and equipment. Doing so means investing in a health research strategy that includes the generation, synthesis, and adoption of knowledge.

Finally, it is necessary to bring these resources together optimally, which raises issues of relationships between different levels of the system, between the public and private sectors, and between vertical and horizontal programs. Unfortunately, despite the large amount of rhetoric on these often highly ideological issues, there is surprisingly little research to inform policy. More than ever, the issue of context specificity reemerges, leading once more to the answer "it depends."

The delivery of optimal health care requires well-developed managerial skills to apply methods that are appropriate for the setting in which they are being applied. However, it also requires governments to provide oversight of their health systems and to anticipate changes and give managers the tools with which to respond to those changes.

REFERENCES

Ageel, A. R., and M. A. Amin. 1997. "Integration of Schistosomiasis-Control Activities into the Primary-Health-Care System in the Gizan Region, Saudi Arabia." *Annals of Tropical Medicine and Parasitology* 91: 907–15.

Aiken, L., J. Sochalski, and E. Lake. 1997. "Studying Outcomes of Organizational Change in Health Services." *Medical Care* 35 (11 Suppl.): NS6–18.

Andreev, E. M., E. Nolte, V. M. Shkolnikov, E. Varavikova, and M. McKee. 2003. "The Evolving Pattern of Avoidable Mortality in Russia." *International Journal of Epidemiology* 32: 437–46.

Anell, A., and H. Barnum. 1998. "The Allocation of Capital and Health Sector Reform." In *Critical Challenges for Health Care Reform in Europe*, ed. R. B. Saltman, J. Figueras, and C. Sakellarides, 179–96. Buckingham, U.K.: Open University Press.

Arrow, K. 1963. "Uncertainty and the Welfare Economics of Medical Care." *American Economic Review* 53: 941–73.

Barnett, E., and S. Ndeki. 1992. "Action-Based Learning to Improve District Management: A Case Study from Tanzania." *International Journal of Health Plan Management* 7: 299–308.

Baumol, W., J. Panzar, and R. Willig. 1982. *Contestable Markets and the Theory of Industrial Structure.* New York: Harcourt Brace Jovanovich.

Bergman, H., F. Beland, and A. Perrault. 2002. "The Global Challenge of Understanding and Meeting the Needs of the Frail Older Population." *Aging Clinical and Experimental Research* 14: 223–25.

Berman, P. 2000. "Organization of Ambulatory Care Provision: A Critical Determinant of Health System Performance in Developing Countries." *Bulletin of the World Health Organization* 78: 791–802.

Bitran, R. 1995. "Efficiency and Quality in the Public and Private Sectors in Senegal." *Health Policy and Planning* 10: 271–83.

Bradley, D. J. 1998. "The Particular and the General: Issues of Specificity and Verticality in the History of Malaria Control." *Parassitologia* 40: 5–10.

Briggs, C. J., P. Capdegelle, and P. Garner. 2001. "Strategies for Integrating Primary Health Services in Middle- and Low-Income Countries: Effects on Performance, Costs, and Patient Outcomes." *Cochrane Database of Systematic Reviews* (4): CD003318.

Cassels, A., and K. Janovsky. 1995. *Strengthening Health Management in Districts and Provinces.* Geneva: World Health Organization.

Collins, D., G. Njeru, J. Meme, and W. Newbrander. 1999. "Hospital Autonomy: The Experience of Kenyatta National Hospital." *International Journal of Health Planning and Management* 14: 129–53.

Conn, C. P., P. Jenkins, and S. O. Touray. 1996. "Strengthening Health Management: Experience of District Teams in The Gambia." *Health Policy and Planning* 11: 64–71.

Connor, C. A., C. C. Wright, and C. D. Fegan. 2002. "The Safety and Effectiveness of a Nurse-Led Anticoagulant Service." *Journal of Advanced Nursing* 38: 407–15.

Coura Filho, P., R. S. Rocha, E. De Lima, M. F. Costa, and N. Katz. 1992. "A Municipal Level Approach to the Management of Schistosomiasis Control in Peri-Peri, MG, Brazil." *Revisto do Instituto de Medicina Tropical de São Paulo* 34: 543–48.

Davis, D., M. Thomson, A. Oxman, and R. Haynes. 1995. "Changing Physician Performance. A Systematic Review of the Effect of Continuing Medical Education Strategies." *Journal of the American Medical Association* 274: 700–05.

de Soto, H. 2000. *The Mystery of Capital: Why Capitalism Succeeds in the West and Fails Everywhere Else.* Boulder CO: Basic Books.

England, R. 2000. *Contracting and Performance Management in the Health Sector: A Guide for Low and Middle Income Countries.* London: Department for International Development Health Systems Resource Centre.

Ensor, T., and B. Amannyazova. 2000. "Use of Business Planning Methods to Monitor Global Health Budgets in Turkmenistan." *Bulletin of the World Health Organization* 78: 1045–53.

Enthoven, A. C. 1985. *Reflections on the Management of the National Health Service.* London: Nuffield Provincial Hospitals Trust.

Evans, R. G. 1997. "Health Care Reform: Who's Selling the Market, and Why?" *Journal of Public Health Medicine* 19: 45–49.

Farmer, P., L. Reichman, and M. Iseman. 1999. *The Global Impact of Drug Resistant Tuberculosis.* Boston, MA: Harvard Medical School and Open Society Institute.

Faxelid, E., B. M. Ahlberg, S. Freudenthal, J. Ndulo, and I. Krantz. 1997. "Quality of STD Care in Zambia: Impact of Training in STD Management." *International Journal for Quality in Health Care* 9: 361–66.

Fayol, H. 1949. *General and Industrial Management.* Translated from the original, *Administration Industriele et Générale*, 1916. London: Pitman.

Ferlie, E., and S. Shortell. 2001. "Improving the Quality of Health Care in the United Kingdom and the United States: A Framework for Change." *Milbank Quarterly* 79: 281–315.

Few, R., and T. Harpham. 2003. "Urban Primary Health Care in Africa: A Comparative Analysis of City-Wide Public Sector Projects in Lusaka and Dar es Salaam." *Health and Place* 9: 45–53.

Foster, S. 1991. "Supply and Use of Essential Drugs in Sub-Saharan Africa: Some Issues and Possible Solutions." *Social Science and Medicine* 32: 1201–18.

Garraoui, A., P. Le Feuvre, and M. Ledoux. 1999. "Introducing Management Principles into the Supply and Distribution of Medicines in Tunisia." *Bulletin of the World Health Organization* 77: 525–29.

Gilson, L. 1995. "Management and Health Care Reform in Sub-Saharan Africa." *Social Science and Medicine* 40: 695–710.

Griffiths, R. 1984. *National Health Service Management Inquiry Report.* London: Department of Health and Social Security.

Hanson, K., L. Atuyambe, J. Kamwanga, B. McPake, O. Mungule, and F. Ssengooba. 2002. "Towards Improving Hospital Performance in Uganda and Zambia: Reflections and Opportunities for Autonomy." *Health Policy* 61: 73–94.

Hanson, K., M. K. Ranson, V. Oliveira-Cruz, and A. Mills. 2003. "Expanding Access to Priority Health Interventions: A Framework for Understanding the Constraints to Scaling Up." *Journal of International Development* 15: 1–14.

Harrison, S., and C. Pollitt. 1994. *Controlling Health Professionals.* Buckingham, U.K.: Open University Press.

Hawkins, L., and C. Ham. 2003. "Reviewing the Case Studies: Tentative Lessons and Hypotheses for Future Testing." In *Innovations in Health Service Delivery: The Corporatization of Public Hospitals*, ed. A. S. Preker and A. L. Harding. Washington, DC: World Bank.

Heald, D., and D. Scott. 1996. "Assessing Capital Charging in the National Health Service." *Financial Accountability and Management* 12: 225–44.

Healy, J., and M. McKee. 2002a. "Implementing Hospital Reform in Central and Eastern Europe." *Health Policy* 61: 1–19.

————. "The Role and Function of Hospitals." In *Hospitals in a Changing Europe*, ed. M. McKee and J. Healy, 59–80. Buckingham, U.K.: Open University Press.

Helander, E. 2000. "25 Years of Community-Based Rehabilitation." *Asia Pacific Disability Rehabilitation Journal* 11: 4–9.

Hood, C. 1991. "A Public Management for All Seasons." *Public Administration* 69: 3–19.

Hussein, R., and S. Al-Junid. 2003. "Corporatization of a Single Facility: Reforming the Malaysian National Heart Institute." In *Innovations in Health Service Delivery: The Corporatization of Public Hospitals,* ed. A. S. Preker and A. L. Harding. Washington, DC: World Bank.

Institute of Medicine. 2001. *Crossing the Quality Chasm: A New Health System for the 21st Century.* Washington, DC: Institute of Medicine.

Jakab, M., and A. S. Preker. 2003. "The Missing Link? Hospital Reform in Transition Economies." In *Innovations in Health Service Delivery: The Corporatization of Public Hospitals,* ed. A. S. Preker and A. Harding. Washington, DC: World Bank.

Johri, M., F. Beland, and H. Bergman. 2003. "International Experiments in Integrated Care for the Elderly: A Synthesis of the Evidence." *International Journal of Geriatric Psychiatry* 18: 222–35.

Kanji, N., P. Kilima, N. Lorenz, and P. Garner. 1995. "Quality of Primary Outpatient Services in Dar-es-Salaam: A Comparison of Government and Voluntary Providers." *Health Policy and Planning* 10: 186–90.

Kanlisi, N. 1991. "Strengthening District Health Teams in Ghana: The Experience of Ejisu District." *Tropical Doctor* 21: 98–100.

Kinzett, S., and J. Bates. 2000. *Bangladesh: Contraceptive Logistics System, Review of Accomplishments and Lessons Learned.* Arlington, VA: Family Planning Logistics Management and John Snow Inc.

Krause, G., J. Benzler, R. Heinmuller, M. Borchert, E. Koob, K. Ouattara, and H. J. Diesfeld. 1998. "Performance of Village Pharmacies and Patient Compliance after Implementation of Essential Drug Programme in Rural Burkina Faso." *Health Policy and Planning* 13: 159–66.

Kwon, S. 2003. "Pharmaceutical Reform and Physician Strikes in Korea: Separation of Drug Prescribing and Dispensing." *Social Science and Medicine* 57: 529–38.

Le Grand, A., H. V. Hogerzeil, and F. M. Haaijer-Ruskamp. 1999. "Intervention Research in Rational Use of Drugs: A Review." *Health Policy and Planning* 14 (2): 89–102.

Le Grand, J., and W. Bartlett. 1993. *Quasi-Markets and Social Policy.* London: Palgrave Macmillan.

Levy-Bruhl, D., A. Soucat, R. Osseni, J. M. Ndiaye, B. Dieng, X. De Bethune, and others. 1997. "The Bamako Initiative in Benin and Guinea: Improving the Effectiveness of Primary Health Care." *International Journal of Health Planning and Management* 12 (Suppl. 1): S49–79.

Litwin, H., and E. Lightman. 1996. "The Development of Community Care Policy for the Elderly: A Comparative Perspective." *International Journal of Health Services* 26: 691–708.

Maynard, A. 1998. "Competition and Quality: Rhetoric and Reality." *International Journal for Quality in Health Care* 10: 379–84.

McKee, M., and H. Brand. 2005. "Purchasing to Promote Population Health." In *Effective Purchasing for Health Gain,* ed. J. Figueras, R. Robinson, and E. Jakubowski, 140–63. Buckingham, U.K.: Open University Press.

McKee, M., and J. Healy. 2000. "The Role of the Hospital in a Changing Environment." *Bulletin of the World Health Organization* 78: 803–10.

————. 2001. "The Changing Role of the Hospital in Europe: Causes and Consequences." *Clinical Medicine,* 1: 299–304.

McKee, M., and E. Nolte. 2004. "Responding to the Challenge of Chronic Disease: Ideas from Europe." *Clinical Medicine* 4: 336–42.

McPake, B. 1996. "Public Autonomous Hospitals in Sub-Saharan Africa: Trends and Issues." *Health Policy* 35: 155–77.

McPake, B., and E. E. Banda. 1994. "Contracting Out of Health Services in Developing Countries." *Health Policy and Planning* 9: 25–30.

McPake, B., and C. Hongoro. 1995. "Contracting Out of Clinical Services in Zimbabwe." *Social Science and Medicine* 41: 13–24.

Mehotra, S. 2000. "Integrating Economic and Social Policy: Good Practices from High Achieving Countries." Innocenti Working Paper 80, UNICEF Innocenti Research Centre, Florence, Italy.

Mills, A., C. Hongoro, and J. Broomberg. 1997. "Improving the Efficiency of District Hospitals: Is Contracting an Option?" *Tropical Medicine and International Health* 2: 116–26.

Mossialos, E., M. Mrazek, and T. Walley. 2004. *Regulating Pharmaceuticals in Europe: Striving for Efficiency, Equity, and Quality.* Buckingham, U.K.: Open University Press.

Nabiswa, A. K., J. D. Makokha, and R. C. Godfrey. 1993. "Malaria: Impact of a Standardized Protocol on Inpatient Management." *Tropical Doctor* 23: 25–26.

OECD (Organisation for Economic Co-Operation and Development). 2003. *OECD Health Data.* Paris: OECD.

Oliveira-Cruz, V., K. Hanson, and A. Mills. 2003. "Approaches to Overcoming Constraints to Effective Health Service Delivery: A Review of the Evidence." *Journal of International Development* 15: 41–65.

Oliveira-Cruz, V., C. Kurowski, and A. Mills. 2003. "Delivery of Priority Health Services: Searching for Synergies with the Vertical versus Horizontal Debate." *Journal of International Development* 15: 67–86.

Pang, T., R. Sadana, S. Hanney, Z. A. Bhutta, A. A. Hyder, and J. Simon. 2003. "Knowledge for Better Health: A Conceptual Framework and Foundation for Health Research Systems." *Bulletin of the World Health Organization* 81: 815–20.

Petrova, G. I. 2002. "Prescription Patterns Analysis—Variations among Bulgaria, Romania, Macedonia, and Bosnia Herzegovina." *Central European Journal of Public Health* 10 (3): 100–03.

Preker, A. S., A. Harding, and P. Travis. 2000. "'Make or Buy' Decisions in the Production of Health Care Goods and Services: New Insights from Institutional Economics and Organizational Theory." *Bulletin of the World Health Organization* 78: 779–90.

Quick, J. D. 1997. *Managing Drug Supply: The Selection, Procurement, Distribution, and Use of Pharmaceuticals.* West Hartford, CT: Kumarian Press.

Shortell, S., C. Bennett, and G. Byck. 1998. "Assessing the Impact of Continuous Quality Improvement on Clinical Practice: What It Will Take to Accelerate Progress." *Milbank Quarterly* 76: 593–624.

Shortell, S. M., and A. D. Kaluzny. 1983. *Health Care Management: A Text in Organisation Theory and Behaviour.* New York: Wiley.

Sibbald, B., J. Shen, and A. McBride. 2004. "Changing the Skill-Mix of the Health Care Workforce." *Journal of Health Services Research and Policy 2004* 9: 28–38.

Stenson, B., G. Tomson, and L. Syhakhang. 1997. "Pharmaceutical Regulation in Context: The Case of Lao People's Democratic Republic." *Health Policy and Planning* 12: 329–40.

Stewart, J. 1998. "Advance or Retreat: From the Traditions of Public Administration to the New Public Management and Beyond." *Public Policy and Administration* 13: 27.

Stromberg, A., J. Martensson, B. Fridlund, L. A. Levin, J. E. Karlsson, and U. Dahlstrom. 2003. "Nurse-Led Heart Failure Clinics Improve Survival and Self-Care Behaviour in Patients with Heart Failure: Results from a Prospective, Randomised Trial." *European Heart Journal* 24: 1014–23.

Vrijhoef, H. J., J. P. Diederiks, and C. Spreeuwenberg. 2000. "Effects on Quality of Care for Patients with NIDDM or COPD When the Specialised Nurse Has a Central Role: A Literature Review." *Patient Education and Counseling* 41: 243–50.

Vrijhoef, H. J., J. P. Diederiks, C. Spreeuwenberg, and B. H. Wolffenbuttel. 2001. "Substitution Model with Central Role for Nurse Specialist Is Justified in the Care for Stable Type 2 Diabetic Outpatients." *Journal of Advanced Nursing* 36 (4): 546–55.

Vrijhoef, H. J., J. P. Diederiks, G. J. Wesseling, C. P. Van Schayck, and C. Spreeuwenberg. 2003. "Undiagnosed Patients and Patients at Risk for COPD in Primary Health Care: Early Detection with the Support of Non-Physicians." *Journal of Clinical Nursing* 12: 366–73.

Waghorn, A., and M. McKee. 2000. "Why Is It So Difficult to Organise an Outpatient Clinic?" *Journal of Health Services Research and Policy* 5: 140–47.

WHO (World Health Organization). 1985. "The Rational Use of Drugs: Review of Major Issues." Paper prepared for the Conference of Experts on the Rational Use of Drugs, Nairobi, Kenya, November 25–29.

———. 2000. *World Health Report 2000: Health Systems: Improving Performance.* Geneva: WHO.

———. 2001. *Innovative Care for Chronic Conditions.* Geneva: WHO.

———. 2002. *Community Home-Based Care in Resource-Limited Settings: A Framework for Action.* Geneva: WHO.

Yip, W., and W. Hsiao. 2003. "Autonomizing a Hospital System: Corporate Control by Central Authorities in Hong Kong." In *Innovations in Health Service Delivery: The Corporatization of Public Hospitals,* ed. A. S. Preker and A. L. Harding. Washington, DC: World Bank.

Glossary

Age-standardized rate An age-standardized rate is a weighted average of the age-specific rates, where the weights are the proportions of a standard population in the corresponding age groups (q.v.). The potential confounding effect of age is removed when comparing age-standardized rates computed using the same standard population.

Age weights Factor specifying the relative value of a year of healthy life lived at different ages. The DALY can incorporate non-uniform age weights which give less weight to years of life lived in early childhood and at older ages (see Chapter 5).

AIDS: Acquired Immunodeficiency Syndrome Disease due to infection with the human immunodeficiency virus (HIV).

BMI: Body mass index A measure of underweight and overweight calculated as weight (kg) divided by height squared (m^2).

Case Fatality Rate The proportion of cases of a disease or injury that die as a result of their disease or injury over a specified time period.

CHD: Coronary heart disease Synonymous with ischemic heart disease (q.v.).

Childhood-cluster diseases GBD (q.v.) cause group including the following vaccine-preventable diseases of childhood: pertussis, poliomyelitis, diphtheria, measles and tetanus.

CODMOD: Cause of death model A statistical model for the prediction of the broad distribution of causes of death based on observed historical data on the relationships between cause distributions, and overall levels of mortality and per-capita income.

Comorbidity Presence of more than one disease or health condition in an individual at a given time.

COPD: Chronic obstructive pulmonary disease Lung diseases that persistently obstruct bronchial airflow. COPD mainly involves two related diseases—chronic bronchitis and emphysema. COPD is also called chronic obstructive lung disease. Asthma is not included in COPD, as the obstruction to bronchial airflow is usually reversible and between asthma episodes the flow of air through the airways is usually good.

CVD: Cardiovascular disease Cardiovascular disease covers a wide array of disorders, including diseases of the cardiac muscle and of the vascular system supplying the heart, brain, and other vital organs. The most common manifestations of CVD are ischemic heart disease, congestive heart failure, and stroke. CVD is used here as an abbreviation for cardiovascular disease, not cerebrovascular disease (q.v.)

DALY: Disability Adjusted Life Year A measure of the gap in healthy years of life lived by a population as compared with a normative standard. More formally, DALYs are a time based measure which adds together years of life lost due to premature mortality with the equivalent number of years of life lived with disability or illness.

DFLE: Disability-free life expectancy A form of HE (q.v.) which gives a weight of 1 to states of health with no disability above an explicit or implicit threshold and a weight of 0 to states of health with any level of disability above that threshold.

DBP: Diastolic blood pressure

Demography The study of population size, growth and age structure, and of the forces (fertility, mortality, migration) that lead to population change.

Disability Restriction or lack of ability (resulting from an impairment or health condition) to perform an activity in the manner or within the range considered normal. Although the word "disability" is widely used, the ICF (q.v.) uses this term only as a broad umbrella term for capacity and performance in activity/participation domains. The GBD (q.v.) used the term disability, as in the DALY (q.v.), as a synonym for health states (q.v.) less than full health (q.v.). Disability is also commonly used to refer only to long-standing limitations in carrying out activities of daily living.

Disability weight Measure of the relative valuations of a health state on an interval scale. In the GBD (q.v.), health state valuations lie between 0 (full health q.v.) and 1 (states equivalent to death). The disability weight quantifies judgments about overall levels of health associated with different health states (q.v.), not judgments on the relative values of lives lived, persons, or of overall well-being, quality of life or utility. The GBD disability weights are intended to reflect average global valuations.

Discounting Process applied to costs, benefits, and outcomes based on the concept that there is preference for money or health in the present relative to the future.

DisMod An epidemiological disease model linking populations exposed to risk of disease with incident cases, prevalent cases, case fatality and the duration of time lived with a disease or injury, including its sequelae.

DSP Disease Surveillance Points System run by the Chinese Centre for Disease Control and Prevention for the surveillance of mortality and morbidity.

Epidemiological transition The process whereby major communicable diseases and conditions of poverty (e.g. malnutrition) are progressively replaced by non-communicable diseases such as cancers and CVD.

Epidemiology The study of the occurrence and causes of disease and injury in populations.

Full health Health state (q.v.) characterized by optimal levels of functioning or capacity in all the important domains of health, and freedom from any type of illness or disease. The "optimal" levels of functioning are defined as those levels above which further gains would not (in general) be regarded as improvements in health. States of exceptional functioning above these levels are thus considered to be talents or exceptional abilities, not higher states of health.

Garbage codes ICD codes (q.v.) for ill-defined or residual categories of major disease groups (e.g. cardiovascular diseases) that do not provide meaningful information on underlying disease or injury causes of death. Examples include ill-defined primary site of cancer and atherosclerosis.

GBD: Global burden of disease A comprehensive demographic and epidemiological framework to estimate health gaps (q.v.) for an extensive set of disease and injury causes, and for major risk factors, using all available mortality and health data and methods to ensure internal consistency and comparability of estimates. In the first global burden of disease study, Murray and Lopez estimated health gaps using DALYs (q.v.) for eight regions of the world in 1990. This book presents updated estimates for the year 2001 for the world and for World Bank regions.

Group I causes Major disease and injury cause group used in GBD (q.v.). Includes communicable, maternal, perinatal and nutritional conditions. These are causes which are characteristically common in populations who have not yet completed the epidemiological transition (q.v.).

Group II causes Major disease and injury cause group used in GBD (q.v.). Comprises non-communicable diseases, including malignant neoplasms, cardiovascular diseases, chronic respiratory diseases, digestive, musculoskeletal and genitourinary conditions, as well as mental disorders and neurological conditions.

Group III causes Major disease and injury cause group used in GBD (q.v.). Includes unintentional and intentional injuries.

HALE: Health-adjusted life expectancy Any of a number of summary measures which use explicit weights to combine health expectancies for a set of discrete health states into a single indicator of the expectation of equivalent years of good health. Also referred to as 'Healthy life expectancy'.

HE: Health expectancy Generic term for summary measures of population health which estimate the expectation of years of life lived in various health states.

Healthy life expectancy Synonym for HALE (q.v.) or Health-adjusted life expectancy.

Health state Health state refers to an individual's levels of functioning within a set of health domains such as mobility, cognition, pain, emotional functioning, self-care, etc. More specifically, in terms of ICF (q.v.) concepts, health state is defined as the capacities of an individual in all important domains of health, where such domains may include domains of body structure and function, and domains of activities/participation. Health states do not include risk factors, diseases, prognosis or the impact of health states on overall quality of life, well-being or satisfaction.

Health status A general term referring to all aspects of the health of individuals or populations. Usually understood to include mortality risks, diseases, health states (q.v.), impairments and disability. May also include some risk factors or prognosis information.

High income Category in the World Bank income grouping of countries used for countries with Gross National Income (GNI) per capita of US$9,206 or more (exchange rate adjusted currencies) in 2001. See Table 3A-3 for list of countries included.

HIV Acronym for the Human Immunodeficiency Virus, the cause of AIDS (acquired immunodeficiency syndrome).

Ideal health Synonymous with full health (q.v.).

Incidence New cases of disease or injury occurring in a specified population in a given time period.

Incidence rate New cases of disease or injury occurring per unit of population, per unit time.

ICD: International Statistical Classification of Diseases and Related Health Problems A classification of diseases and other causes of mortality prepared by the World Health

Organization since 1948, periodically revised as necessary. The current tenth revision was issued in 1992 to come into effect on 1 January 1993. The ICD is a member of the WHO family of international classifications.

ICF: International Classification of Functioning, Disability and Health A classification of body structures and functions (impairments) and activities/participation domains (performance and capacity). The ICF was endorsed by the WHO World Health Assembly in 2001 as a successor to the 1980 International Classification of Impairment, Disability and Handicap (ICIDH). The ICF is a member of the WHO family of international classifications.

IHD: Ischemic heart disease Any of a number of heart conditions in which heart muscle is damaged or works inefficiently because of an absence or relative deficiency of its blood supply; most often caused by atherosclerosis, it includes angina pectoris, acute myocardial infarction (heart attack), chronic ischemic heart disease and sudden death. The term coronary heart disease is synonymous with IHD.

Life expectancy The average number of years of life expected to be lived by individuals who survive to a specific age. See also: Period life expectancy.

Logit transformation A mathematical function that transforms a variable such as probability of death into another functional form, characterized by asymptotic values.

Low- and middle-income Category in the World Bank income grouping of countries used for countries with Gross National Income (GNI) per capita of less than US$9,206 in 2001 (exchange rate adjusted currencies). See Table 3A-3 for list of countries included.

MONICA Study The MONICA (MONItoring CArdiovascular disease) Study was an international research project coordinated by the World Health Organization from the mid-1980s to the mid-1990s in which teams from 38 populations in 21 countries studied heart disease, stroke and risk factors in their populations.

Neonatal period Persons under the age of 28 days are in the neonatal period. The neonatal period is itself divided into the early neonatal period, age less than 7 days, and the remaining late neonatal period.

PAF: population attributable fraction Proportional reduction in disease or injury that would occur if population exposure to a risk factor or group of risk factors were reduced to an alternative distribution.

Perinatal deaths Includes stillbirths and neonatal deaths from any cause, including tetanus and congenital malformations. The perinatal period includes the period from 27 weeks of gestation to 28 days of life.

Perinatal causes or conditions The cause category *Perinatal causes* refers to the ICD cause group "Conditions arising in the perinatal period". Deaths from these causes (primarily low birth weight and birth trauma/ asphyxia) may occur at any age, but are largely confined to the perinatal period.

Period life expectancy A summary measure of a population's mortality that measures the expectation of years of life lived by a fictitious birth cohort assuming that at each age the cohort experiences the age-specific mortality rates observed in the real population during a specified time period (such as a given calendar year). See also: life expectancy.

Postneonatal period Persons between the age of 28 days and 1 year are in the postneonatal period.

Prevalence Actual number of cases of disease or injury present in a population at any particular moment in time.

Probability of death The chance that an individual, alive at age x, will be dead before his or her $(x + n)^{th}$ birthday, usually written as $_nq_x$. $_5q_0$ denotes the probability that a newborn infant will die before his or her fifth birthday.

PTO: person trade-off A method for valuation of health states that asks respondents to choose between hypothetical interventions that offer health benefits to groups of individuals in different health states.

QALY: Quality-adjusted life year A measure of years of life lived (or gained through an intervention) adjusted for quality of life using health state preferences ranging between 0 (states equivalent to death) through to 1 (full health). QALYs were developed for the assessment of the cost-effectiveness of interventions in health economics. QALYs gained and DALYs averted through an intervention are calculated in very similar ways, and the main differences relate to the interpretation of the weights. Whereas the disability weights in the DALY quantify loss of health, the corresponding QALY weights are often interpreted in terms of well-being, quality of life, or utility.

Risk Factor A risk factor is an attribute or exposure which is causally associated with an increased probability of a disease or injury.

RR: Relative risk Relative risk is a measure of the strength of an association. It is calculated as a ratio of the risk of occurrence of a disease or death among two population groups, such as those exposed to a risk factor and those not exposed.

SD: Standard deviation A measure of the dispersion or spread of values of a variable (e.g. body weight) around a population mean value.

Sensitivity analysis Systematic investigation of the effects on estimates or outcomes of changes in data or parameter inputs or assumptions.

Sequelae The medical conditions that can occur among people who contract a disease or suffer an injury. The GBD (q.v.) focuses on disabling sequelae of diseases and injuries; these may remain present long after the initiating disease episode or injury event.

Standard gamble (SG) A method for valuation of health states based on the axioms of expected utility theory. The standard gamble asks respondents to make choices that weigh improvements in health against mortality risks.

Standard Population A population structure that is used to provide a constant age or covariate distribution, so that the age- and sex-specific rates within different populations can be applied to it and can be compared without confounding by the different age or covariate distributions of the populations.

STD: Sexually transmitted disease See: STI.

STI: Sexually transmitted infection An infection that can be transferred from one person to another through sexual contact. Among the sexually transmitted infections (STIs) are HIV/AIDS, chlamydia, genital herpes, gonorrhea and syphilis. The term "sexually transmitted infection (STI)" corresponds to the older term "sexually transmitted disease (STD)".

SMPH: Summary measures of population health Indicators that summarize the health of a population into a single number. SMPH combine information about mortality and population health states. They may summarize either the average health level or health inequality for a population. The two main classes of summary measures are health expectancies (q.v.) and health gap measures, of which the DALY (q.v.) is the best-known example.

Stillbirth Stillbirth refers to the birth of a dead fetus weighing more than 1,000 grams up to 0.25 years (13 weeks) prior to the expected time of birth (corresponding to 27 weeks of gestational age).

Stroke Stroke is defined as a condition that results in a disruption of blood flow to a region of the brain causing irreversible "death" of brain tissue. There are two main types of stroke: hemorrhagic and ischemic stroke. Stroke is the main cause of mortality and burden for cerebrovascular disease (q.v.).

Sullivan's method A method of calculating health expectancies using data on the current prevalence of health states in a population together with a period life table for the population.

Theoretical-minimum-risk exposure distribution The population distribution of exposure to a risk factor that would result in the lowest population disease burden.

TTO: time trade-off A method for valuation of health states that asks respondents to make hypothetical choices that weigh improvements in health against reduced longevity.

Uncertainty analysis Estimation of range or distribution of uncertainty in estimates based on an assessment of the uncertainty or confidence intervals for all data and parameter inputs. Uncertainty intervals should ideally include all sources of uncertainty, including those arising from systematic biases and measurement error. In contrast, generally reported confidence intervals are based solely on the variation observed in sample data.

Visual analogue scale A method for valuation of health states in which respondents are asked to directly assess health levels associated with different health states. Individuals place these on a 0 to 1 scale representing a continuum from health states considered equivalent to death through to full health (q.v.)

Verbal autopsy A method of inquiry to ascertain the likely cause of death in populations where vital registration of deaths is incomplete and unreliable. Relatives of the deceased are interviewed about symptoms and signs experienced by the deceased prior to death, from which a diagnosis of the probable cause of death is made.

Vital registration A system for the registration of vital events in a population, including births and deaths, with medical certification of the cause of death according to the rules and procedures of the ICD.

YLD: Years Lived With Disability The component of the DALY (q.v.) that measures lost years of healthy life through living in health states of less than full health (q.v.).

YLL: Years of Life Lost The component of the DALY (q.v.) that measures years of life lost due to premature mortality.

Index

Boxes, figures, notes, and tables are indicated by b, f, n, and t following the page number.

combination of high blood pressure,
cholesterol, and obesity in,
853–854, 856
contraceptive use in, 1080
dengue in, 452
diabetes in, 593
diarrheal diseases in, 374, 377
drug addiction in, 908, 916
fall-related injuries in, 748–749
folic acid deficiency in, 836
food manufacture in, 845
food taxes in, 219
hemoglobinopathies in, 668, 670
hypertension in, 835
incentive pay to doctors in, 94–95,
95b, 170
indoor air quality and energy programs
in, 190, 795, 809, 810b
influenza in, 684
kidney and urinary system diseases in,
702, 703
lung cancer in, 795
lymphatic filariasis in, 436
malaria in, 421, 425
mental disorders in, 620
milk fluoridation in, 726
neonatal deaths in, 531
neonatal resuscitation program in, 539b
neurological disorders in, 628
oral and craniofacial diseases and
disorders in, 723
oral health and education program
in, 726
road traffic injuries in, 740, 747, 839
rotavirus vaccine in, 377
salt iodination program in, 168, 173
SARS in, 997, 1005
school-based physical activity in, 838
stomach cancer in, 573
strokes in, 633
TB control program in, 36b, 94–95,
168–169, 174, 247
tobacco use in, 871, 1128
transportation choices in, 839–840
vital events registration in, 1021
water pollution in, 829
women in, 195
chiropractic medicine, 1282, 1286, 1288
chlamydia, 203, 312, 314–315, 316
See also sexually transmitted
infections (STIs)
chlorination, 821
chloroquine, 414, 418, 420f, 423, 1035f,
1043f, 1327
CHNPs. *See* community health and
nutrition programs
cholera, 120, 377, 379, 774, 777, 778

cholesterol levels
in combination with high blood pressure
and obesity, 851–868
See also cardiovascular disease (CVD)
CVD and, 15
diabetes and, 598
drugs to control, 857, 1323
modeling of interventions for lifestyle diseases, 844–845
chronic diseases, 833–850
See also specific diseases
advances in treatment of, 123
alcohol use and, 890
burden of, 107, 1333
community-based interventions, 842, 846
cost-effectiveness of interventions,
844–846
diet and lifestyle changes to prevent,
833–836, 847
evidence of effectiveness, 836–837
educational interventions, 837–838
health care providers modifying
unhealthy behaviors, 838
interventions, 837–844
recommended priority interventions,
846–848
malnutrition in childhood associated
with, 563
medications for, 1331
modeling of likely interventions,
844–846
physical activity interventions, 835, 838,
841b, 842, 846, 847
research and development agenda, 846
surveillance and, 1009–1010
transportation policy and environmental
design as intervention, 839–840
worksite interventions, 838, 838b
chronic kidney disease (CKD). *See* kidney
and urinary system diseases
**chronic obstructive pulmonary disease
(COPD) and asthma,** 684–689,
685f, 687t
See also respiratory diseases of adults
air pollution and asthma in
children, 820
cigarette smoking. *See* tobacco use and
control
**circumcision to protect against sexually
transmitted infections,** 320,
322, 360b
civil service reform, 96
CKD (chronic kidney disease). *See* kidney
and urinary system diseases
Clean Air Act of 1970 (U.S.), 828, 829t
clean drinking water. *See* water supply
cleft lip and palate, 731

climate
See also global warming
health systems' efficacy and, 1340
helminth infections and, 470
Clinton Foundation, 359, 1333
cocaine. *See* drug dependence
cognitive function
cannabis and, 918
malnutrition's effect on, 562
of school-age children. *See* school
health programs
COHRED. *See* Council on Health Research
for Development
collaboration for research. *See* research
and development
collective efficacy, 1067
Colombia
ambulatory surgery in, 1256
contraception, access to, 1076
interpersonal violence in, 756, 763
stomach cancer in, 573
universal coverage approach of, 237
volcanic eruptions in, 1150
colorectal cancer, 570, 574, 575, 575t,
581, 836
**Commission on Health Research in
Development,** 106
**Commission on Macroeconomics and
Health (WHO)**
on close-to-client services, 521
on constraints of low-income countries to
improve health care, 98
on cost-effective analyses, 234, 261
on district hospitals, 1214
on external financing for health, 245
on HIV/AIDS, 9
on mobilizing skills and resources, 134
on primary care interventions, 246,
1194, 1200
on scaling up health coverage, 190
on training to enhance skills of medical
workers, 1344
**Common Rule of Conduct of U.S. Code of
Federal Regulations,** 266
communicable diseases. *See* infectious and
communicable diseases
**communication for emergency medical
services,** 1267
**community-based health insurance
(CBHI),** 231, 236
**community-based programs
and treatment**
breastfeeding, programs to promote, 559
central government transfers to local
authorities for, 253
community health and nutrition
programs, 1053–1074

research and development agenda,
1159–1160
resources for emergency response, 1158
search and rescue, 1157
shelters, 1157
strategic approach to, 1160–1161
water systems, repair of, 1156
disasters, 1147–1162
See also disaster relief
age and, 1149
classification of, 1147
climatic disasters, 1151
communicable diseases and, 1151, 1154
earthquakes, 1149–1150, 1150t
economic valuation of, 1151–1152
environmental health and, 1154
gender and, 1149
hazards, defined, 1148
health and economic losses from,
1148, 1148f
hospitals and health installations,
damage to, 1153
hurricanes, 1151
interventions, 1153–1156
long-term impact, 1151–1153, 1152t
mass casualties, treatment of, 1154
poverty and, 1149
as public health condition, 1147–1153
response and rehabilitation, 1153–1154
risk
defined, 1148
geographic distribution of, 1148–1149
short-term health burden of, 1149–1151
surveillance in, 1008, 1154
terminology for, 1147–1148
tsunamis, 1150
volcanic eruptions, 1150
vulnerability
defined, 1148
factors affecting, 1149
water and sewage systems, damage to,
1153, 1156
discount rate, 262, 278
discrimination
against HIV positive individuals, 109
against persons with disabilities, 264–265
social exclusion and public health,
1072n1
*Disease Control Priorities in Developing
Countries (DCP)* **(Jamison
et al., 1993)**
burden of disease estimates, 279
estimates of deaths by causes, 28
intervention focus of, 16
Disease Control Priorities Project (DCPP)
death estimates for, 11b
on diarrheal diseases, 378–379

focus on most cost-effective interventions
for developing countries, 165
on suicides, 607
on tuberculosis, 295–296
district hospitals, 1211–1228
central financing of, 1220–1221
changing disease spectrum, implications
of, 1226
clinical management of, 1223
clinical services provided by, 1214–1215
cost-effectiveness of services, 1216,
1219, 1220t
costs of care in, 1218–1219, 1218t
cross-cutting services and, 1215,
1222–1226
defined, 1212
demand for services, 1221–1222
economics of, 1216–1219
economics of scale and, 1213, 1213f
efficiency and, 1213, 1217–1218, 1219t,
1224–1225
equity issues and, 1214
factors influencing performance of,
1219–1222
framework for delivery of services
by, 1212f
health information systems and, 1216
hospital-acquired diseases in, 1224
human resources and, 1223
integration with other local health-related
services, 1215
levels of care, 1217
national level and costs, 1217
private sector and, 1217
quality improvements and accreditation
of, 1223–1224, 1224f, 1226
research and development agenda, 1226
services provided by, 1214
supervision and, 1216
supply of services, 1222
surgery and, 5b, 27, 1249, 1253–1255,
1253t, 1254t, 1256f
technology, information, and integration
in, 1223, 1226
training and, 1215–1216
DNA markers, study of. *See* genomics
**Doctors without Borders' Drugs for
Neglected Diseases,** 1323
Doha Declaration, 151
domestic violence, 48–49, 202, 756, 760
See also interpersonal violence
Dominican Republic
contraceptive use in, 1081
sexual risk behaviors in, 312
DOTS. *See* directly observed therapy
short course
Down syndrome, 941–945, 944t

dracunucliasis. *See* guinea worm
eradication
drinking water. *See* water supply
driving injuries. *See* traffic injuries
drowning. *See* unintentional injuries
drug dependence, 907–931
abstinence-oriented treatments, 910–911
adolescents and, 1111
amphetamines, 922–923
interventions, 923
burden of disease associated with, 909,
914–916, 915t
cannabis, 917–919
interventions, 919
causes and health consequences of,
907–909
cocaine, 919–922
interventions, 921–922
cost-effectiveness of interventions,
912–913, 915t
comparing different interventions,
913–914
criminal justice interventions, 911–912
detoxification, 910, 912, 913
in developing countries, 916
drug-free treatment, 912–913
cost-effectiveness of, 913–914
ecstasy (MDMA), 923–924
heroin use
antecedents of, 907–908
health consequences of, 908–909
HIV infection and, 909
mortality and morbidity, 909
prevention of, 909–910
reducing heroin-related harm, 910
interventions, 909–916
methadone maintenance, 910, 911, 913
research and development agenda, 916
self-help groups, 911, 913
drug resistance, 1031–1051, 1332–1333
agenda for action and, 1045–1046, 1340
anthelmintic, 479
antibiotic use and. *See* antibiotics,
indiscriminate use of
containing spread of resistant
micro-organisms, 1041–1042, 1340
diagnostic tests and, 1040
diarrheal diseases and, 378
disease burden and, 1033–1036, 1033t,
1034t, 1340
DOTS and. *See* directly observed therapy
short course (DOTS)
drug quality and, 1040
drug treatment strategies and, 1037–1039
economic burden of, 1036–1037
global coordination and, 1042–1043
gonorrhea and, 1036

stunting, wasting, and micronutrient deficiency disorders, 562–563
WB projections for 2000–15, 183
economic policies to encourage healthy behavior choices, 842–844
ecstasy. *See* drug dependence
eczema, 708
education
See also training of medical personnel
adolescents and, 1115
on alcohol abuse, 893
on diabetes, 598
early childhood education, 221
of girls, 1095
on helminth infections, 472, 475
HIV/AIDS education campaigns, 344, 344b, 1105
on illegal drug use, 910
information, education, and communication campaigns, 176
life-skills and health education, 1115
on lifestyle changes for health, 837–838, 842, 859
on malaria, 422
malnutrition and school performance, 563
on osteoarthritis, 972
patient education, effect of, 98
peer education programs, 1115
referral hospitals' role in, 1233–1234, 1234t
on risk factors, 121
sex education, 344, 344b, 1121
Egypt
diarrheal diseases in, 167, 176, 374, 378
food subsidy programs in, 216
health sector reform in, 1315
kidney and urinary system diseases and, 697
schistosomiasis in, 479
school health insurance program in, 187
El Salvador
contracting for health care services in, 189
interpersonal violence in, 766
occupational health risks in, 1136b
elder abuse, 756
See also interpersonal violence
electrification, 795, 803–804, 810
electronic medical records (EMRs), 1300
ELISA. *See* enzyme-linked immunosorbent assay
embryonic stem cells, 130
emergency medical services, 1261–1279
absence of ambulance system and, 1273b
ambulances, 1267–1271, 1269t, 1270t
burden of disease, 1262–1263, 1263t, 1274f

communication systems for, 1267
costs and cost-effectiveness of interventions, 49, 1265–1266, 1266t, 1267t, 1268, 1270t
deaths from trauma, 1278n1
defined, 1262
description of, 1261, 1262t
disaster relief. *See* disaster relief
documentation and quality assurance, 1272
equipment and supplies, 1266–1267, 1271–1272, 1275–1278t
financing for, 1272
first aid, 1264
future challenges for, 1274
health facility-based system, 1271–1272
helicopter ambulances, 1268
interventions, 1263–1272
lay responders, 1264, 1267t, 1270t
legislation on, 1272
lessons learned, 1272
malaria and, 1262
for newborns, 540–541
paramedical personnel, 1264–1265, 1270t
cost-effectiveness of combining with lay responders, 1267t
defined, 1262
planning and implementation of, 1272
prehospital care, 1264–1271
research and development agenda, 1272–1274
response time, 1265
training for hospital emergency workers, 1271, 1273b
triage, defined, 1262
universal emergency care, 1271
emphysema. *See* chronic obstructive pulmonary disease (COPD) and asthma
EMRs (electronic medical records), 1300
end-of-life care for HIV/AIDS patients, 351–353
end stage renal disease (ESRD). *See* kidney and urinary system diseases
endangered species and traditional medicine, 1286
endemic treponematoses, 709
endoscopic surgery, 130
energy medicine, 1282
See also complementary and alternative medicine (CAM)
Energy Sector Management Assistance Programme, 811
England. *See* United Kingdom
environmental risk factors
air and water pollution, 817–832
clinical epidemiology and, 120

diarrheal diseases and, 373
in disasters, 1154
health systems' efficacy and, 1340
indoor air pollution and, 797–798
interventions for environmental control, 177–179
learning and developmental disabilities and, 936b
mental disorders and, 605
posttraumatic stress disorder (PTSD), 605
respiratory diseases of adults and, 690
surveillance, 1006–1007
enzyme-linked immunosorbent assay (ELISA)
African trypanosomiasis and, 462
leishmaniasis and, 457
EPI. *See* Expanded Program on Immunization
Epidemic Intelligence Service (U.S.), 1002
epidemics
flu. *See* influenza pandemic, possibility of
HIV/AIDS. *See* HIV/AIDS
surveillance for outbreaks, 1005–1006
epidemiological trends, 6–7
modern epidemiology, 120–124, 125
epidemiologists
field epidemiologists providing evidence, 1001–1002
training of, 1002
epilepsy, 629–631
childbirth and, 948
community-based treatment of, 110
costs and cost-effectiveness of interventions, 47
in developing countries, 637, 638t
faith healers and, 630
onchocerciasis and, 435
patient compliance, 630
prevalence, incidence rate, remission, and mortality, 630
recommendations, 640
risk factors, 630
stigma of, 631
treatment gap for, 630, 641
epistemology, defined, 110
equalization funds, 228
equity issues, 259–260
contraception and, 1086
cost-effectiveness analysis and, 272
CVD interventions and, 863
district hospitals and, 1214
Down syndrome and, 944–945
drug accessibility and, 1323
health improvements and, 4b, 7, 104b
helminth infection interventions and, 476
IMCI and, 1184

private health insurance, 238
single pool vs. virtual single pool, 238
sources of financing, 238
universal coverage initiatives, 236,
237–238, 237t
mobilizing government revenues,
229–231
models of, 226
national health service (NHS) model, 226,
238
for new product development, 146–150
pharmaceutical firms in developing
countries, 150
private sector, 146–147
public-private partnerships,
147–150, 149t
public sector, 146
Poverty Reduction Strategy Papers
(PRSPs) and, 235–236
for primary care, 1199–1200, 1200t
private foundations, role of, 182, 253–255
See also specific foundations
private insurance model, 226, 238
project support vs. budget support, 23
purchasing, 226
reallocation based on cost-effective
criteria, 5b, 186
revenue sources, 226, 227, 231t, 240n2
risk pooling, 226, 227–232, 236–238
social insurance model, 226
SWaps, 234–235
trends by country income level,
231–232, 231f
for vaccines, 406–407, 1331, 1332t
Finland
CVD and lifestyle changes in, 837, 837b
diabetes and lifestyle changes in, 593
rheumatoid arthritis in, 974
tobacco taxes in, 882
firearms and violence, 760, 763, 765
See also interpersonal violence
first aid, 1264
fiscal policies to promote health,
211–223
family care leave, 221
lessons in using, 222t
in low-income countries, 211–212
maternity leave, 221
sick leave, 221
subsidies for health and health-related
products, 212–218, 212t,
213–214t
consumer subsidies, 212–218
producer subsidies, 218
taxes. *See* taxation
workplace health, 220–221
fiscal sustainability, 233

fluoridation, 972
dental caries. *See* dental caries
negative health effects of, 821
FOCUS on Young Adults, 1114, 1115t
**Focusing Resources on Effective School
Health (FRESH),** 784, 1096, 1096t,
1097, 1098b, 1099, 1101, 1102–1103t
folic acid, 836, 842, 939, 940–941, 948
folklore and alternative medicine, 1282
food. *See* nutrition
food manufacture, 841–842, 856
foot problems and diabetes, 597
**foreign direct investment and health
gains,** 8
**Framework Convention on Tobacco
Control,** 882
**Framingham, Massachusetts, study of
males and heart disease,** 120, 855
France
homeopathic products, use in, 1282
skin diseases in, 714
free trade agreements, 1141
FRESH. *See* Focusing Resources on Effective
School Health
fuel choice and air quality. *See* indoor air
pollution
full income, 8–9, 9f
defined, 4b, 8
fungal infections of skin, 713–715

Gambia
malaria in, 418
respiratory diseases of children in, 492
GATB. *See* Global Alliance for TB Drug
Development
GAVI. *See* Global Alliance for Vaccines and
Immunization
gender differences, 195–210
See also women
African trypanosomiasis and, 456
background, 195–197
burden of disease and, 197–198
disasters and, 1149
hearing loss and, 958
leishmaniasis and, 455
mental disorders and, 605
research agenda, 206–207
sex distinguished from gender, 196
sexually transmitted infections
and, 318
vision impairment and, 955
general primary care. *See* primary care
generic drugs, 1326, 1328
genetic disorders
hemoglobinopathies and, 669–670, 671,
672, 678
See also hemoglobinopathies

kidney disease and, 696
mental disorders and, 605
genetically modified crops, 131–132
genetics
diabetes and, 593
helminth infections and, 470
hemoglobinopathies and, 673
insulin resistance syndrome and, 834b
genital herpes, 312
See also sexually transmitted
infections (STIs)
genital mutilation, 761, 763
genomics, 107–109, 126–130, 128b, 133, 135
Genomics and World Health (WHO
report), 127, 133, 135
Germany
homeopathic products, use in, 1282
influenza in, 684
transportation choices in, 840
universal coverage approach of, 237
GFHR. *See* Global Forum for Health
Research
Ghana
breastfeeding programs in, 559, 561
deworming programs in, 478
emergency transport to hospital in, 1264
food fortification in, 558
health sector support program in, 251
malaria in, 1092
medical workers in, 1309
newborn survival rates in, 540
organizational structure of health systems
in, 93, 1345
road traffic injuries in, 746–747
sexually transmitted infections in,
323, 325
traditional medicine in, 1283–1284
gingivitis, 729–730
See also oral and craniofacial diseases and
disorders
Global Alliance for Improved Nutrition,
182, 254
**Global Alliance for TB Drug Development
(GATB),** 140, 142
Global Alliance for Tuberculosis, 182
**Global Alliance for Vaccines and
Immunization (GAVI),** 24, 182, 234,
244, 245, 253, 389, 397, 406, 491,
492, 493
**Global Burden of Diseases 2000 study
(World Health Organization),** 613
Global Campaign against Epilepsy, 631
**Global Forum for Health Research
(GFHR),** 106, 114, 157, 161, 749
**Global Fund to Fight AIDS, Tuberculosis
and Malaria,** 110, 147, 182, 234, 243,
245, 305, 332, 425, 1333

improved health
    See also health gains
    lessons of experience, 165–179
    value of, 158–160
incentive pay to medical providers, 4b,
        94–95, 95b, 170, 1299, 1310–1311,
        1313–1320
    community workers, 1063
income levels and health gains, 6
**INDEPTH (International Network of Field
        Sites with Continuous
        Demographic Evaluation of
        Populations and Their Health in
        Developing Countries),** 1021
India
    ambulances in, 1268
    arsenic contamination of water in, 821
    asthma in, 688
    Bhopal catastrophe, 819, 819b, 1133, 1149
    breast cancer in, 578, 584
    burn-related injuries in, 741
    cardiovascular disease in, 658, 659,
        861, 863t
    cataract surgery in, 1258b
    child survival in, 1068
    combination of high blood pressure,
        cholesterol, and obesity in, 853–854,
        861, 863t
    community-based programs in,
        1064, 1066
    dengue in, 452
    dental treatment in, 729
    development assistance for health to, 245
    diabetes in, 597, 1333
    diarrheal diseases in, 372, 377, 378
    district hospitals in, 1217
    drug addiction in, 908
    emergency medical care in, 1273b
    epilepsy in, 630
    food fortification in, 558
    food subsidies in, 216
    hemoglobinopathies in, 664, 665,
        668, 670
    HIV/AIDS in, 254, 358
    immunization services in, 404b
    indoor air quality and energy programs
        in, 190, 809, 809b
    Integrated Child Development Services
        Program, 556
    Kaposi's sarcoma in, 730
    kidney and urinary system diseases in,
        695, 697, 700, 702, 703
    leishmaniasis in, 452, 459, 461
    leprosy in, 437, 445
    lymphatic filariasis in, 436, 439, 440,
        442, 443

    malaria in, 414, 418
    morphine use in, 990–991
    National Cancer Registry program, 1009
    neonatal deaths in, 531, 545, 545b
    neurological disorders in, 628
    occupational risks of silica dust in,
        1137, 1138b
    performance-based contracts with NGOs
        in, 253
    quality of care in, 1298
    rotavirus vaccine in, 377
    skin diseases in, 714, 715
    smallpox eradication in, 1163, 1170
    strokes in, 633
    TB in, 253, 291
    training for emergency medical
        personnel, 1273b
    vaccine-preventable diseases in, 404b, 406
    vital events registration in, 1021
    water pollution in, 821, 825b, 828
    water supply in, 773–774
    women in, 195
Indonesia
    avian influenza in, 682b
    community-based programs in, 1064
    dengue in, 459
    dental caries in, 725
    diarrheal disease in, 1303
    kidney and urinary system diseases
        and, 697
    leprosy in, 441
    maternal deaths in, 533
    mental disorders in, 621
    neonatal deaths in, 533
    polio in, 1170
    rice subsidy in, 216
    skin diseases in, 708, 715
    smallpox in, 1163
    TB in, 291, 295, 296
    tsunami in, 1149
indoor air pollution, 190, 793–815
    causes and burden of, 793–799
    COPD and, 688, 690, 691–692, 804, 805
    costs and cost-effectiveness of
        interventions, 799–808, 801b, 802b
        cost assumptions, 804
        cost-benefit analysis, 807–808, 808t
        cost-effectiveness analysis, 804–807,
            806t, 812
        effectiveness assumptions, 804–805
        implementation period, 805
    DALYs and deaths due to, 797, 798t
    economic effects of fuel collection, 797
    electrification in rural areas, 795,
        803–804, 810
    environmental consequences of, 797–798

    fuel subsidy programs to control, 217
    health impacts of, 795–796, 796t, 797t
    interventions and policy, 799, 800–801t
    kerosene and LPG as cleaner fuels, 803,
        805, 810, 811b
    lack of lighting and, 797
    lessons learned, 808–811
    levels of pollution and exposure, 795
    MDGs on poverty reduction and,
        799, 812
    method used for determining attributable
        disease burden, 796
    research and development agenda,
        811–812
    solid fuel use, 797
infant care. *See* perinatal conditions
infant mortality. *See* child mortality rates
infectious and communicable diseases
    See also specific diseases
    burden of, 105
    colonization efforts and control of, 120
    control of
        defined, 1164–1165
        distinguished from eradication, 1165
    cost-effective interventions for, 53
    disasters and, 1151, 1154
    elimination of, defined, 1165
    eradication of, 1163–1176
        See also specific diseases
        certification process for, 1167
        defined, 1164
        distinguished from control, 1165
        economic considerations, 1167–1169
        frameworks for, 1165–1169
        geographic and environmental factors,
            1165–1166
        interventions to block transmission,
            1166–1167
        laboratory containment and, 1166
        local vs. international net benefits,
            1167–1168
        natural resistance to reinfection
            and, 1166
        operational considerations, 1166–1167
        potential reservoirs and, 1166
        private vs. social net benefits, 1167
        scientific considerations, 1165–1166
        short-term vs. long-term net
            benefits, 1167
        surveillance and, 1166
        transmissibility and, 1166
        vertical vs. horizontal programs,
            1168–1169
    extinction of, defined, 1165
    gene therapy and, 127
    kidney disease and, 697

International League against Epilepsy, 631
International Monetary Fund (IMF)
 on AIDS impact on full income, 9
 criticisms of structural adjustment
  programs and fiscal ceilings of, 233
 Poverty Reduction Strategy Papers
  (PRSPs), 235–236
International Network of Field Sites with
 Continuous Demographic
 Evaluation of Populations and
 Their Health in Developing
 Countries (INDEPTH), 1021
International Partnership for
 Microbicides, 244
International Society of Nephrology,
 700, 703
International Strategy for Disaster
 Reduction (ISDR), 1147
International Trachoma Initiative, 182
International Union against Tuberculosis
 and Lung Disease (IUATLD), 691
International Zinc Nutrition Consultative
 Group, 554, 565
Internet access, 1022
interpersonal violence
 adolescents and, 1111
 burden and causes of, 756–759
 collecting and managing data on, 765
 cost-effectiveness of interventions,
  764–765
 cost of, 760
 data on, 756–757
  cost-benefit data needed, 765
 deaths resulting from, 757, 757f, 757t, 758t
 in developing countries, 758
 economic impact of, 760–761
 effects on public finance, 761
 firearm registration, 765
 future challenges for, 766–767
 interventions, 761–764
 legislation and shelter for abused women,
  764–765
 parent training and home
  visitation, 765
 prevention
  implementation of, 765–766
  primary, 761, 763–764, 766
  secondary and tertiary, 764
  strategies, 761–764, 762–763t
 research and development agenda,
  765–766
 risk factors, 759, 759t, 760
 support services for victims, 766
 youth intervention, 765
interventions
 See also specific diseases and conditions

categories and pertinent policy
 instruments of, 59, 274b, 275
child mortality and, 11–13
community level of care.
 See community-based programs and
 treatment
cost-effectiveness of. See cost-effective
 interventions
costs of
 amount of health (by service or
  intervention) US$1 million
  will buy, 25t
 determination of, 280–281
defined, 273–277
distribution by cost-effectiveness ratio, 53f
district hospitals. See district hospitals
drugs. See drugs
general primary care. See primary care
for MDGs, 183–185, 184t
packaging of, 49–50
personal. See personal interventions
population-based. See population-based
 interventions
quality as determinant of
 cost-effectiveness, 50
referral hospitals. See referral hospitals
intrauterine devices, 1080
intussusception and rotavirus vaccine, 376
iodine deficiency
 in children, 554, 558–559
 costs and cost-effectiveness of
  interventions, 561
 interventions, 558–559
 lessons learned, 563
 mental retardation and, 562
 during pregnancy, 936b
 salt iodination program to combat,
  168, 173
 in school-age children, 1094
IOM. See Institute of Medicine
IQ. See cognitive function
Iran. See Islamic Republic of Iran
Ireland
 development assistance for health
  from, 244
 fluoridation of water in, 725
iron deficiency. See anemia
ischemic heart disease (IHD), 645–646
 burden of, 649–650, 1278n2
 cost-effectiveness of interventions,
  650–654, 655t, 656t, 658
 epidemiological transition and, 647, 648t
 linking costs and effectiveness
  in developing countries, 653–654,
   655t, 656t
  in high-income countries, 658

long-term management of existing
 vascular disease, 651–652
invasive interventions, 651
nonpharmacological
 interventions, 652
pharmacological interventions,
 651–652
secondary prevention, 654
ISDR (International Strategy for Disaster
 Reduction), 1147
Islamic Republic of Iran
 earthquake in, 1149
 hemoglobinopathies in, 669, 670
 Isfahan Healthy Heart Program in, 842
 kidney and urinary system diseases in,
  697, 698
ITNs. See insecticide-treated nets (ITNs)
 for malaria prevention
IUATLD (International Union against
 Tuberculosis and Lung
 Disease), 691
IUDs, 1080
ivermectin
 distribution in Africa, 168, 172
 lymphatic filariasis and, 439
 onchocerciasis and, 109, 110, 168, 172,
  440–441, 444, 957

Jamaica
 community-based programs in, 1065,
  1066, 1067
 hemoglobinopathies in, 664, 668, 676
 quality of health care in, 1295–1296
 salt fluoridation in, 168, 173, 726
Japan
 cleft lip and palate in, 731
 dengue in, 452
 kidney and urinary system diseases
  in, 695
 strokes in, 633
 water pollution in, 829
Japanese encephalitis
 vaccine for, 406, 1325–1326
 See also vaccine-preventable diseases
Johns Hopkins School of Public Health on
 development of pneumococcal
 vaccines, 493
Joint Learning Initiative, 26b
Joint United Nations Programme on
 HIV/AIDS. See United Nations
 Programme on HIV/AIDS
 (UNAIDS)
justice and special concern for the worst
 off, 262
juvenile violence, 760
 See also interpersonal violence

research and development agenda,
977–978
risk factors for, 966, 966t
screening for, 971
surgery for, 968
symptomatic treatments for,
966–967, 967t
women and, 201, 206
Myanmar
dengue in, 454
kidney and urinary system diseases
and, 697
as opium producer, 908
oral precancer and cancer in, 730
myocardial infarction. *See* acute myocardial
infarction (AMI)

NAFTA (North American Free Trade
Agreement), 1141
NAP. *See* schizophrenia and nonaffective
psychoses
Narcotics Anonymous, 911
National Academy of Sciences (U.S.), 9
National Center for Complementary and
Alternative Medicine
(NCCAM), 1289
National Center for Policy Analysis
(Harvard University) study of
life-saving interventions, 39b
National Commission for the Protection of
Human Subjects, 266, 267
National Crime Prevention Council, 760
National Evaluation of Pharmacother
apies for Opioid Dependence
Project, 913
National Institute for Occupational Safety
and Health (NIOSH; U.S.), 1134
National Institute of Allergy and Infectious
Diseases, 114, 115
National Institutes of Health (U.S.)
on complementary and alternative
medicine, 1281–1282
on COPD, 684
on eradication of infectious
diseases, 1164
research fund allocation assessments, 161
national statistics office, role of, 1018
natural disasters, 1147–1162
See also disasters
NCCAM (National Center for
Complementary and Alternative
Medicine), 1289
neonatal conditions. *See* child mortality
rates; childbirth conditions; perinatal
conditions
neoplasms. *See* cancer

Nepal
arsenic contamination of water in, 821
leishmaniasis in, 452, 459
leprosy in, 437
maternal mortality in, 510
newborn care in, 535
oral health program in, 733–734
reproductive health in, 474
respiratory diseases of adults in, 691
respiratory diseases of children in, 492
sexually transmitted infections in, 323
TB in, 295
tobacco taxes in, 882
Netherlands
breast cancer in, 584
COPD and asthma in, 686
development assistance for health
from, 244, 254
food manufacture to reduce fat
content, 845
hospitals in, 1224–1225
transportation choices in, 840
universal coverage approach of, 237
neural tube defects during pregnancy,
939–940
neurological disorders, 627–662
Alzheimer's disease (AD) and other
dementias, 627–629
burden of, 628, 629t, 632
in children with HIV/AIDS, 935b
costs and cost-effectiveness of
interventions, 47
in developing countries, 635–640, 635t,
636t, 638t, 639t
epilepsy, 629–631
See also epilepsy
learning disabilities and, 935–936b
See also learning and developmental
disabilities (LDDs)
malaria and. *See* malaria
Parkinson's disease, 632–633
See also Parkinson's disease (PD)
recommendations, 640
research and development agenda,
640–641
stroke, 633–635
burden of disease, 634
cost-effectiveness of interventions in
developing countries, 638t,
639t, 640
frequency of types, prevalence,
incidence rates, mortality, and
disability after stroke, 633
interventions, 634–635
recommendations, 640
risk factors, 633–634

neuropsychiatric diseases
research and development agenda, 109
technological advances and, 131
new product development. *See* research and
development
new public management, 92, 1341–1342
New Zealand
capital charging and management of
physical resources in, 1345
combination of high blood pressure,
cholesterol, and obesity in, 855, 859
fluoridation of water in, 725
interpersonal violence in, 765
suicide prevention for youth in, 1121
universal coverage approach of, 237
newborns. *See* child mortality rates;
perinatal conditions
disorders of. *See* congenital and
developmental disorders
NGOs. *See* nongovernmental organizations
Nicaragua
community-based programs in,
1066, 1067
injury surveillance system of, 168
interpersonal violence in, 760, 766
kidney and urinary system diseases
in, 702
occupational health risks in, 1136b
performance-based remuneration for
health workers in, 1299
pesticide poisoning prevention measures
in, 1139
nicotine. *See* tobacco use and control
Niger
doctor visits for sick children in, 89
IMCI program in, 1187
Nigeria
hemoglobinopathies in, 664
IMCI program in, 1180
insecticide-treated nets (ITNs) for
malaria prevention in, 217
lymphatic filariasis in, 439
malaria in, 426
neonatal deaths in, 531
neurological disorders in, 628
polio in, 254b, 1168
refugee populations and surveillance, 1008
nonaffective psychoses and schizophrenia.
See schizophrenia and nonaffective
psychoses (NAP)
noncommunicable diseases, 15–16
See also specific diseases and conditions
burden of, 105, 1331
cost-effective interventions for, 53
increase in, 4b, 6
research priorities for, 115–116, 132

oral precancer and cancer, 572, 730
oral rehydration therapy (ORT), 374, 378, 1059, 1180, 1303
cost-effectiveness of, 379, 383t
Oregon Health Services Commission, 263
Organisation for Economic Co-operation and Development (OECD) on development assistance for health, 243, 244
orphan drug acts, 147
osteoarthritis. *See* musculoskeletal disorders
osteopathic medicine, 1282, 1288
osteoporosis. *See* musculoskeletal disorders
out-of-school children and youth, 1098, 1121–1122
outpatient treatment
See also primary care
TB, quality of care and treatment of, 295
outreach and referral programs, 174, 1186, 1194–1195
outsourcing of health care services, 93–94, 93b, 96b, 1320, 1347–1348
quality of care, 188–189

Pacific islands. *See* East Asia and Pacific
Packard Foundation, 182
PAHO. *See* Pan American Health Organization
pain control. *See* palliation
Pakistan
diarrheal diseases in, 217, 372, 378
drug addiction in, 908
hemoglobinopathies in, 670
interpersonal violence in, 756
kidney and urinary system diseases in, 697, 702, 703
leprosy in, 444
neonatal deaths in, 531
polio in, 254b
refugee populations and surveillance, 1009
respiratory diseases of children in, 493
road traffic injuries in, 749b
TB in, 291
PAL. *See* Practical Approach to Lung Health
palliation, 981–993
adequacy of and barriers to pain control in developing countries, 984–985
burden of pain from cancer and AIDS, 981–982
cancer and, 572, 581–582, 983–984t, 1333
classification of pain, 982b
costs and cost-effectiveness of morphine and drugs, 987–989, 988t
defined, 59
effects of pain, 981
HIV/AIDS and, 351–353, 981–982

implementation of strategies to improve, 989–991
interventions for pain relief, 982–987
legal controls on opioid drugs, 986–987
measurement of pain, 981
morphine use, 984–985, 986f, 987b, 1333
pain in patients with cancer and AIDS, 982
research and development agenda, 991–992
resources available to countries for developing national palliative care programs, 991b
three-step analgesic ladder, 984, 984f
Pan African Initiative, 462
Pan American Health Organization (PAHO)
campaign to eliminate polio, 168
Chagas disease campaign. *See* Southern Cone Initiative on Chagas disease
injury surveillance system of, 1007
Regional Core Health Data Initiative of, 1019
revolving fund for drugs, 1327
Safe Water System Initiative of, 216
Panama
scabies in, 710
universal coverage approach of, 237
yellow fever in, 396–397
panic disorder, 47, 611, 612–613
Pap smear, 575
Papua New Guinea
lymphatic filariasis in, 439
malaria in, 413, 414
newborn survival rates in, 540
quality of health care in, 1293
skin diseases in, 715, 718
water supply in, 777
Paraguay
Chagas disease in, 438
out-of-school youth in, 1122
paramedical personnel, 1262, 1264–1265
parasites. *See* helminth infections
Parkinson's disease (PD), 632–633
burden of, 632
costs and cost-effectiveness of interventions, 47, 637, 638t
interventions, 632–633
personal intervention, 632–633
prevalence, incidence rate, and mortality, 632
recommendations, 640
technological treatment of, 131
Partnership for Child Development (PCD), 478, 1095
Partnership in Statistics for Development in the 21st Century, 1028

Pasteur, Louis, 119, 1163
patent system and drugs, 150–152
pathophysiology, 122–124
PCD. *See* Partnership for Child Development
PD. *See* Parkinson's disease
pediculosis, 708
peer education programs, 344–345, 1115
peer review in medical profession, 1296–1297, 1299
pelvic inflammatory disease, 312
See also sexually transmitted infections (STIs)
penicillin
See also antibiotics, indiscriminate use of
development of, 122
resistance to, 122, 1033–1034
penicillin prophylaxis for newborns with sickle cell anemia, 670, 676–677
performance-based professional recognition for providers, 1299–1300
performance-based remuneration for providers, 1299, 1348
perinatal conditions, 499–529
breastfeeding. *See* breastfeeding
burden of, 508
Chagas disease and, 434
comparison of alternative intervention packages, 514–517, 518–519t
complementary feeding practices and, 376
costs and cost-effectiveness of interventions, 46, 513–522, 520t
cost-effectiveness ratios, 517, 521–522
model assumptions, 525, 525t, 526t
DALYs for, 508
defined, 500
economic benefits of intervention, 522
epidemiology of, 499–508
fetal alcohol syndrome, 936b
focus conditions and their risk factors, 501–504t
interventions, 508–513, 536–537t
lessons learned, 522–524
levels, trends, and differentials of deaths, 505–508
MDGs on, 499
policy considerations and approaches, 513
research and development agenda, 524
resource use and costs, 517
retinopathy, 954–955
sexually transmitted infections of mother and, 315
tetanus and, 394
transmission of HIV/AIDS, 335–336

periodontal diseases, 729–730
  See also oral and craniofacial diseases and
    disorders
personal interventions
  Alzheimer's disease, 629
  "boutique medicine" resulting from
    genomics, 108
  combination of high blood pressure,
    cholesterol, and obesity,
    856–860, 861t
    in developed countries, 859–860
    in developing countries, 860–863
  CVD, 48, 856–858
  defined, 59, 274b
  hearing loss, 959–960
  maternal conditions, 510–513
  Parkinson's disease, 632–633
  population-based interventions vs., 50
  stroke, 634–635
  summary of, 60–69t
  using measures other than $/DALY
    averted, 78–82t
pertussis. *See* diphtheria, pertussis, tetanus
Peru
  collaborative improvement model
    in, 1298
  contracting for health care services in, 189
  household fuel use in, 793, 794f
  IMCI program in, 1181, 1186, 1187
  immunization in, 405b
  maternal and child mortality in, 1225b
  quality of health services in, 1225b
  sexually transmitted infections in, 323
  TB control program in, 168–169, 175
pesticides, 821, 822
pharmaceuticals. *See* drugs
pharmacogenomics, 129, 129t
Philippine National Epidemic Surveillance
    System, 1004, 1004t
Philippines
  childbirth in, 20, 21f
  community-based programs in,
    1064, 1066
  diarrheal diseases in, 374, 378
  immunization in, 20, 21f
  kidney and urinary system diseases in,
    697, 702
  quality of health care in, 1296
  surveillance in, 1004, 1004t
  universal coverage approach of, 237
  volcanic eruptions in, 1150
  water pollution in, 829
phobias, 612
  See also anxiety disorders
physical activity interventions, 652, 835,
    838, 841b, 842, 846, 847, 970,
    972–973, 1112

physicians, 94
  See also medical workers
pigmentary skin disorders, 708,
    717–718
PLACE (Priorities for Local AIDS Control
    Effort), 324–325, 326
placebo controls and ethics, 268
Planet Health program, 838b
Planned Parenthood Association of South
    Africa, 203
pneumoconiosis. *See* occupational lung
    diseases
pneumonia and HIV/AIDS, 354
pneumonia and influenza, 484–485,
    681–684, 682–683b
  See also respiratory diseases of adults;
    respiratory diseases of children
  drug resistance and, 1033–1034, 1045
  IMCI and, 1180
  improved quality of treatment for
    children with, 1303
Poland
  cardiovascular disease in, 649, 844b
  food price policies in, 219
  tobacco-related legislation in, 168
policy instruments
  See also legislation
  defined, 59
  ensuring use of resources for greatest
    effect, 97–98
polio
  burden of, 395
  elimination, goal of, 121, 168, 172, 1164,
    1170–1173
    costs of, 1171–1173, 1172t
    IDA credit buy-downs for, 253, 254b
  vaccine for, 172, 395, 406, 1164, 1171,
    1325, 1326
  See also vaccine-preventable diseases
pollution. *See* air and water pollution;
    environmental risk factors; indoor
    air pollution
polypill
  cost-effectiveness analysis of, 275, 598
  preventing CVD, 598, 860–861, 863t
pooling. *See* risk pooling
population-based interventions
  alcohol use and control, 896–899, 897t
  Alzheimer's disease, 628–629
  combination of high blood pressure,
    cholesterol, and obesity,
    855–856, 859
  CVD and, 47–48
  defined, 59, 274b
  hearing loss, 959
  maternal conditions, 510
  personal interventions vs., 50

research, 109
  summary of, 70–77t
  surgery, 1248–1249
  using measures other than $/DALY
    averted, 83–85t
population growth as concern, 104b,
    1075–1076, 1086
posttraumatic stress disorder (PTSD), 605,
    610, 621
  See also anxiety disorders
Poverty Reduction Strategy Papers
    (PRSPs), 235–236
poverty reduction support credits (PRSCs),
    248, 250–251
Practical Approach to Lung Health (PAL),
    295, 691
pregnancy. *See* abortions; family planning;
    maternal conditions; prenatal care
    programs
prehospital care, 1264–1271
premature births. *See* childbirth conditions;
    low birthweight
prenatal care programs
  See also maternal conditions
  community health and nutrition
    programs, 1058
  costs and cost-effectiveness of, 203
  failure of women to participate in, 184
  medical advances in, 123
  routine prenatal care, 511–512,
    514–517
prescriptions. *See* drugs
prevention
  See also specific diseases and conditions
  prevention fatigue, 312
  primary. *See* primary prevention
  research and development in preventive
    medicine, 107–109
  secondary. *See* secondary prevention
price increases to deter high-risk
    behaviors. *See specific behavior
    (e.g., tobacco use)*
primary care, 1193–1209
  antiretroviral therapy for HIV/AIDS
    and, 1204
  community-oriented, 1202, 1204
  comparison of proposed basic packages of
    interventions, 1206–1207t
  comprehensive vs. selective care,
    1193–1194, 1195t
  cost-effectiveness of interventions,
    1199, 1199t
  defined, 1193
  district health system and, 1202–1203
  effectiveness of, 1196–1198, 1198b
  equity goals and, 1198
  expenditures for, 1199–1200, 1200t

air pollution and, 820
bronchiolitis, 485
case management of, 487–489, 490t,
    492–493, 494
causes and burden of, 483–485
cost-effectiveness of interventions,
    489–491, 490t, 491t
HIV/AIDS and, 485, 489
hypoxemia diagnosis, 488
influenza, 485
interventions, 485–489
lessons learned on control strategies,
    491–493
lower respiratory tract infections
    (LRIs), 484–485
newborns and resuscitation, 539–540,
    539b, 545
pneumonia, 484–485
    diagnosis of, 487
    intramuscular antibiotics for, 488
    oral treatment of, 488
    treatment guidelines for, 488–489
research and development agenda,
    493–494
school-age children, 1093
upper respiratory tract infections
    (URIs), 483–484
vaccine strategies, 491–492
retinopathy of prematurity, 954–955
rheumatic heart disease (RHD), 647
    See also cardiovascular disease (CVD)
    burden of, 650
    cost-effectiveness of interventions, 653,
        656, 657t, 658
    epidemiological transition and, 648t
    strokes and, 634
rheumatoid arthritis. *See* musculoskeletal
    disorders
rickets, 965
risk factors
    *See also specific risks
        (e.g., cholesterol levels, obesity)*
    behavioral risk factor surveillance system,
        defined, 998
    CVD and, 15, 851–868, 854t
    development of concept of, 120
    diabetes and, 593, 851
    drug resistance and, 1031–1036
    education about, 121
    genomics and, 108, 108b
    helminth infections and, 470
    lifelong medical management of, 4b
    multiple risks in combination, effect of,
        109, 851–862
    musculoskeletal disorders and,
        966, 966t
    TB and, 304

risk pooling, 226, 227–232, 236–238
river blindness. *See* onchocerciasis
road traffic injuries. *See* traffic injuries
Rockefeller Foundation
    funding commitment for disease control
        in developing countries, 147
    International AIDS Vaccine Initiative
        (IAVI) support from, 255b
    MDGs and, 182
    on sanitation and hygiene, 783
    stimulating growth of public-private part-
        nerships, 147
    vaccine-preventable diseases and, 397
    on yellow fever eradication, 1163
Roll Back Malaria Partnership, 182, 234,
    418, 419b
Romania
    cardiovascular disease in, 649, 649t
    pain control in, 987b
Rotary International, 254b, 1171
rotavirus, 371, 376–377
    See also diarrheal diseases
rubella
    See also vaccine-preventable diseases
    congenital rubella, 935b, 937
    vaccination, 406
    vaccine gap and, 1326
Russian Federation
    cardiovascular disease in, 649, 1298
    collaborative improvement model
        in, 1298
    interpersonal violence in, 766
    milk fluoridation in, 726
    sexually transmitted infections in, 318
Rwanda
    government reform and health care
        delivery in, 91

**SAFE (surgery, antibiotics, face washing,
    environmental change) strategy to
    combat trachoma,** 168, 170, 174,
    178, 956
Safe Motherhood Initiative, 499, 1215
Safe Routes to School program, 840b
Safe Water System Initiative, 216
St. John's wort, 1283
**sales tax exemptions on healthy foods and
    medicines,** 220
Salmonella, 371
    See also diarrheal diseases
salt
    fluoridation, 168, 173
    iodination, 168, 559
    reduction in food content of, 836,
        845–846, 846t
sanitation improvements, 187,
    189–190, 377

See also water supply
    disaster damage to, 1153
    effect on burden of diseases,
        786–791, 1163
    epilepsy and, 631
    excreta disposal, 779–784
        calculation of burden of diseases,
            788–789, 788t
        costs of promotion, 782
        diarrheal disease and, 384,
            782–783, 782t
        direct health benefits, 782–784
        effect on burden of diseases,
            786–791
        effect on other disease categories,
            783–784
        hygiene promotion and, 786
        levels of service, technologies, and
            costs, 779–780, 780f
        policy implications, 781–782
        reduction in diarrheal disease, 786–791,
            786t, 787f, 789t,
            790t, 791t
        social benefits, 780, 780t
        water supply and, 783
        willingness to pay, 781
    helminth infections and, 470, 472
    promotion of hygiene, 784–786
        calculation of burden of diseases,
            788–789, 788t
        costs of, 785
        effect on burden of diseases, 786–791
        effect on diarrheal diseases, 785
        effect on respiratory infections,
            785–786
        evidence and, 784
        reduction in diarrheal disease, 786–791,
            786t, 787f, 789t,
            790t, 791t
        sustainability of, 784–785
    subsidy for, 217
SARS (severe acute respiratory syndrome),
    112b, 122, 682–683, 683t
    economic effect of, 1010
    surveillance and, 997, 1005
Saudi Arabia
    cardiovascular disease in, 650
    hemoglobinopathies in, 664
    kidney and urinary system diseases
        and, 697
    polio in, 1170
scabies, 708, 709–710, 711t, 719t
    See also skin diseases
Scandinavia
    See also specific countries
    alcohol use and control in, 893
    dental treatment in, 729

for epilepsy, 631, 637

for hearing improvement, 959

high volume of care and quality
of, 1299

hip replacement surgery, 973

human resources and, 1256

interventions, 1248–1251

for kidney disease, 701–702

knee replacement surgery, 973

minimally invasive, 130–131

for musculoskeletal disorders, 968

for Parkinson's disease, 632–633, 637

population-based interventions,
1248–1249

research and development agenda,
1255–1257

resource requirements for services and
level of care, 1250–1251t

SAFE strategy to combat trachoma.
See SAFE (surgery, antibiotics, face
washing, environmental change)
strategy to combat trachoma

single-shot surgical services, successful
programs involving, 174

at tertiary hospitals, 1249–1250

surveillance, 997–1015

active surveillance, defined, 998, 1021

analysis and dissemination of surveillance
data, 999–1000

avian influenza and, 1005–1006

as basis for evidence-based
decisions, 1001

behavioral risk factor surveillance system,
defined, 998

biologic terrorism and, 998, 1008

categorical surveillance, defined, 998

chronic disease and, 1009–1010

disaster situations and, 1008, 1154

drug resistance and, 1042–1043

Ebola and, 1006

economics of, 1010–1011, 1010t

emergency surveillance, 1008

environmental public health surveillance,
1006–1007, 1006f

eradication of infectious diseases
and, 1166

establishing and maintaining system for,
999, 1000b

field epidemiologists providing evidence,
1001–1002

future of, 1011

global surveillance networks, 1011–1012,
1012f

health information and management
system, defined, 998

indicator, defined, 997

informal networks as elements of,
1004–1005

injury surveillance, 1007–1008

Integrated Disease Surveillance and
Response (IDSR), 1003–1004

integrated surveillance, defined, 998

laboratory-based surveillance,
1002–1003, 1003f

objectives of, 998–999, 999b

occupational health, 1133, 1143

as part of national public health
systems, 1000

passive surveillance, defined, 998, 1021

population-based surveys used
in, 1002

principles and uses of, 999, 999t, 1021

refugee populations and, 1008–1009

research agenda for, 1012–1013

routine health information system,
defined, 998

SARS and, 1005

sentinel surveillance, 1002, 1021

strategies for, 1002–1005

syndromic surveillance, defined,
998, 1008

as tool to improve public health,
1001–1002

training for, 117

SWaps (finance instruments), 234–235

Sweden

development assistance for health
from, 244

diabetes and lifestyle changes in, 593

fluoridation programs in, 729

oral health programs in, 729, 733

oral precancer and cancer in, 730

Switzerland

iodine fortification program in, 554

salt fluoridation in, 725–726

synovial fluid replacement, 973

syphilis. *See* sexually transmitted
infections (STIs)

T. vaginalis, 315

tacit knowledge, 110

Taiwan

arsenic contamination of water
in, 821

strokes in, 633

universal coverage approach of, 237

tamoxifen, 574, 580

Tanzania

adolescents in, 1116

African trypanosomiasis in, 458

community-based programs in,
1066, 1068

deworming programs in, 478

DOTS development in, 111

drug shops, regulation in, 92b

HIV/AIDS in, 320, 331, 352

hospitals in, 1218

IMCI program in, 1181–1183, 1183b,
1184, 1184f, 1185b, 1186, 1187

kidney and urinary system diseases
in, 702

leprosy in, 437

lymphatic filariasis in, 440

malaria in, 421, 425

malnutrition in, 1068

management of health care in,
1345, 1348

mental disorders in, 620

Multi-Country Evaluation of IMCI
Effectiveness, Cost, and Impact
(MCE) in, 1181–1183, 1183b

oral health and education program
in, 726

primary care in, 1343, 1348

regulation of health care in, 1296

road traffic injuries in, 749b

sexually transmitted infections in,
320, 322

skin diseases in, 708, 720

strokes in, 633

training of medical staff on acute
respiratory infections of children
in, 1297

vital events registration in, 1021

water supply in, 773

**Tanzania Essential Health Intervention
Program (TEHIP),** 1024,
1026–1027, 1026b, 1202, 1208n2

targeting of interventions. *See specific
diseases and conditions*

taxation

on alcohol, 218, 893, 895t

consumer taxes, 218–220, 219b

discouraging high-risk behaviors by, 177,
213–215t

on drugs, 1327

as method of revenue collection,
227, 229

producer taxes, 220

promoting health policies, 213–215t,
218–220

sales tax exemptions on healthy foods and
medicines, 220

on tobacco, 177, 218, 874–875, 875f,
879f, 882

on unhealthy foods, 219–220

TDR. *See* Special Programme for Research
and Training in Tropical Diseases

motorcycle helmet legislation and
enforcement, 747
risk factors for, 739–740
safer roads and, 743–744
speed and safety regulations, 745–746, 746t
speed bumps, 746–747, 747t
training of medical personnel
alternative medicine and, 1286, 1287
changes needed in medical education for
global perspective, 134–135
for childbirth and newborn care, 545
community workers, 1063
continuing skill development, 1312, 1344
dissemination and use of health information for, 1023
district hospitals' role in, 1215–1216
epidemiologists, 1002
for hospital emergency workers,
1271, 1273b
nurses, 94
for occupational health, 1134–1135, 1142
professional retraining to improve quality
of care, 1297
for surgery, 1256–1257
for surveillance purposes, 117
traditional healers, 1286
transplant surgery, 130, 131
transportation
See also traffic injuries
automobile use, 839, 843
costs of unreliable systems, 187
for emergency medical services, 1264,
1267–1271
See also ambulances
intersectoral action for improvements
in, 189
policy and environmental design,
839–840
walking and bicycle use, 839–840, 840b,
843–844
trauma care. *See* emergency medical services
Trichomonas vaginalis, 315
Trinidad and Tobago
health service agency reform in, 93,
1318–1319
**TRIPS (Agreement on Trade-Related
Aspects of Intellectual Property
Rights),** 150–152, 351, 1324
tropical diseases, 433–466
See also specific types
burden of, 436–438, 454–456
characteristics and transmission, 433–436,
451–454, 454t
costs and cost-effectiveness of
interventions, 442–445, 445t,
459–460

DALY estimates for, 437–438, 438t
interventions and effectiveness of, 45–46,
438–442, 460–463
kidney disease and, 697
management and control strategies of,
457–458, 463t
research needs and priorities, 115,
445–446, 446t
skin diseases, 709
See also skin diseases
tropical ulcers, 709, 715, 717, 718
See also skin diseases
tsetse flies, 453, 456, 458, 462, 464
tsunamis, 1150
tubal ligation, 1080
tuberculosis (TB), 289–309
alternative approaches to diagnosis and
treatment, 294–295
burden and trends, 291–292
averted and avertable burden, 302,
302f, 303f
children and, 293
complementary strategies, 304
cost-effectiveness of interventions,
40–43, 295–297, 296t, 297t,
301–303, 301b
managing endemic TB, 297–299, 298f
managing TB outbreaks, 299–301, 300f
cost per case prevented, 297–299
cost per death prevented and DALY
gained, 299
deaths due to in low- and middle-income
countries, 290–291
cost per death prevented and DALY
gained, 299
development assistance and, 244
diagnostics development for, 144,
145, 145t
DOTS strategy for treatment. *See* directly
observed therapy short course
(DOTS)
drug resistance and, 294, 304–305, 1036,
1045–1046
drugs for, 304, 1326
economic benefits of interventions,
302–303
HIV/AIDS and, 291, 292–293, 294, 301,
302, 304–305
impact and targets, 304
infection, disease, and death, 290–291
integrated management of, 295
interventions, 292–294
kidney and urinary system diseases
and, 697
latent infection, treatment of, 292–293
MDGs and, 290, 305

outpatient and community-based
treatment, 295
private sector treatment, 295
quality of care and treatment of, 27,
292–299
research and development agenda,
303–304
risk factors, 304
service delivery, 304
silicosis and, 689
successful programs in controlling, 94–95,
168–169, 174, 175
targeting poor in allocation of health
resources to fight, 5b
tobacco use and, 289, 304
vaccination, 292, 304
See also vaccine-preventable diseases
Turkey
ambulances in, 1268
condom program in, 216
epilepsy in, 630
kidney and urinary system diseases in,
698, 702, 703
leishmaniasis in, 459
mental disorders in, 621
universal coverage approach of, 237
typhoid, 775t, 776t, 777, 778

Uganda
African trypanosomiasis in, 454, 456, 460
Ebola in, 1006
government reform and health care
delivery in, 91, 247, 1315
HIV/AIDS in, 13, 106, 320, 348b, 354, 358
Hospice Uganda, 990
IMCI program in, 1181, 1185b,
1186, 1187
interpersonal violence in, 756, 757, 763
malaria in, 418, 421
medical workers in, 94, 1312
primary care and removal of fees for
health services in, 97b
road traffic injuries in, 749b
sexually transmitted infections in,
312, 320
training of medical personnel in, 94
water supply in, 773
**U.K. National Institute for Clinical
Excellence,** 1297
UNAIDS. *See* United Nations Programme
on HIV/AIDS
**UNESCO (United Nations Education,
Scientific, and Cultural
Organization),** 1095
UNICEF. *See* United Nations Children's
Fund

Credits

Cover and Interior Design
Naylor Design, Washington, D.C.

Part One Photographs
Chapter 1: Curt Carnemark/The World Bank; chapter 2: Sebastian Szyd/The World Bank; chapter 3: Richard Lord, www.rlordphoto.com; chapter 4: Richard Lord, www.rlordphoto.com; chapter 5: Micheal Simpson/Getty Images; chapter 6: Richard Lord, www.rlordphoto.com; chapter 7: Royalty-Free/Corbis; chapter 8: Richard Lord, www.rlordphoto.com; chapter 9: Richard Lord, www.rlordphoto.com; chapter 10: Shehzad Noorani/The World Bank; chapter 11: Royalty-Free/Corbis; chapter 12: Royalty-Free/Corbis; chapter 13: Richard Lord, www.rlordphoto.com; chapter 14: Royalty-Free/Corbis; chapter 15: Naylor Design Inc.

Part Two Photographs
Chapter 16: CDC; chapter 17: Richard Lord, www.rlordphoto.com; chapter 18: Pep Bonet/PANOS; chapter 19: Richard Lord, www.rlordphoto.com; chapter 20: Richard Lord, www.rlordphoto.com; chapter 21: CDC/PHIL/Corbis; chapter 22: Pan American Health Organization; chapter 23: Dr. Dennis Kunkel/Getty Images; chapter 24: Richard Lord, www.rlordphoto.com; chapter 25: Richard Lord, www.rlordphoto.com; chapter 26: Richard Lord, www.rlordphoto.com; chapter 27: Richard Lord, www.rlordphoto.com; chapter 28: Richard Lord, www.rlordphoto.com; chapter 29: David Becker/Getty Images; chapter 30: Royalty-Free/Corbis; chapter 31: Royalty-Free/Corbis; chapter 32: 3D4Medical.com/Getty Images; chapter 33: Richard Lord, www.rlordphoto.com; chapter 34: Spike Walker/Getty Images; chapter 35: Richard Lord, www.rlordphoto.com; chapter 36: SIU/Visuals Unlimited/Getty Images; chapter 37: CDC/Joe Miller/Reed and Crnrick Pharmaceuticals; chapter 38: Richard Lord, www.rlordphoto.com; chapter 39: Richard Lord, www.rlordphoto.com; chapter 40: Gabe Palmer/Corbis; chapter 41: Richard Lord, www.rlordphoto.com; chapter 42: Richard Lord, www.rlordphoto.com; chapter 43: Richard Lord, www.rlordphoto.com; chapter 44: Richard Lord, www.rlordphoto.com; chapter 45: Richard Lord, www.rlordphoto.com; chapter 46: Richard Lord, www.rlordphoto.com; chapter 47: Royalty-Free/Corbis; chapter 48: Royalty-Free/Corbis; chapter 49: Richard Lord, www.rlordphoto.com; chapter 50: Ray Witlin/The World Bank; chapter 51: Richard Lord, www.rlordphoto.com; chapter 52: Royalty-Free/Corbis

Part Three Photographs
Chapter 53: Richard Lord, www.rlordphoto.com; chapter 54: Richard Lord, www.rlordphoto.com; chapter 55: Shehzad Noorani/The World Bank; chapter 56: Richard Lord, www.rlordphoto.com; chapter 57: Richard Lord, www.rlordphoto.com; chapter 58: Richard Lord, www.rlordphoto.com; chapter 59: Richard Lord, www.rlordphoto.com; chapter 60: Richard Lord, www.rlordphoto.com; chapter 61: Richard Lord, www.rlordphoto.com; chapter 62: Ray Witlin/The World Bank; chapter 63: Gideon Mendel/Corbis; chapter 64: Richard Lord, www.rlordphoto.com; chapter 65: Richard Lord, www.rlordphoto.com; chapter 66: Richard Lord, www.rlordphoto.com; chapter 67: Richard Lord, www.rlordphoto.com; chapter 68: Curt Carnemark/The World Bank; chapter 69: Royalty-Free/Corbis; chapter 70: Richard Lord, www.rlordphoto.com; chapter 71: Richard Lord, www.rlordphoto.com; chapter 72: Richard Lord, www.rlordphoto.com; chapter 73: Richard Lord, www.rlordphoto.com.

Rate of Decline in Under-Five Mortality 1990-2001

Note: Meeting the Millenium Development Goal No.4, to reduce under-5 mortality by 2/3 between 1990 and 2015, requi

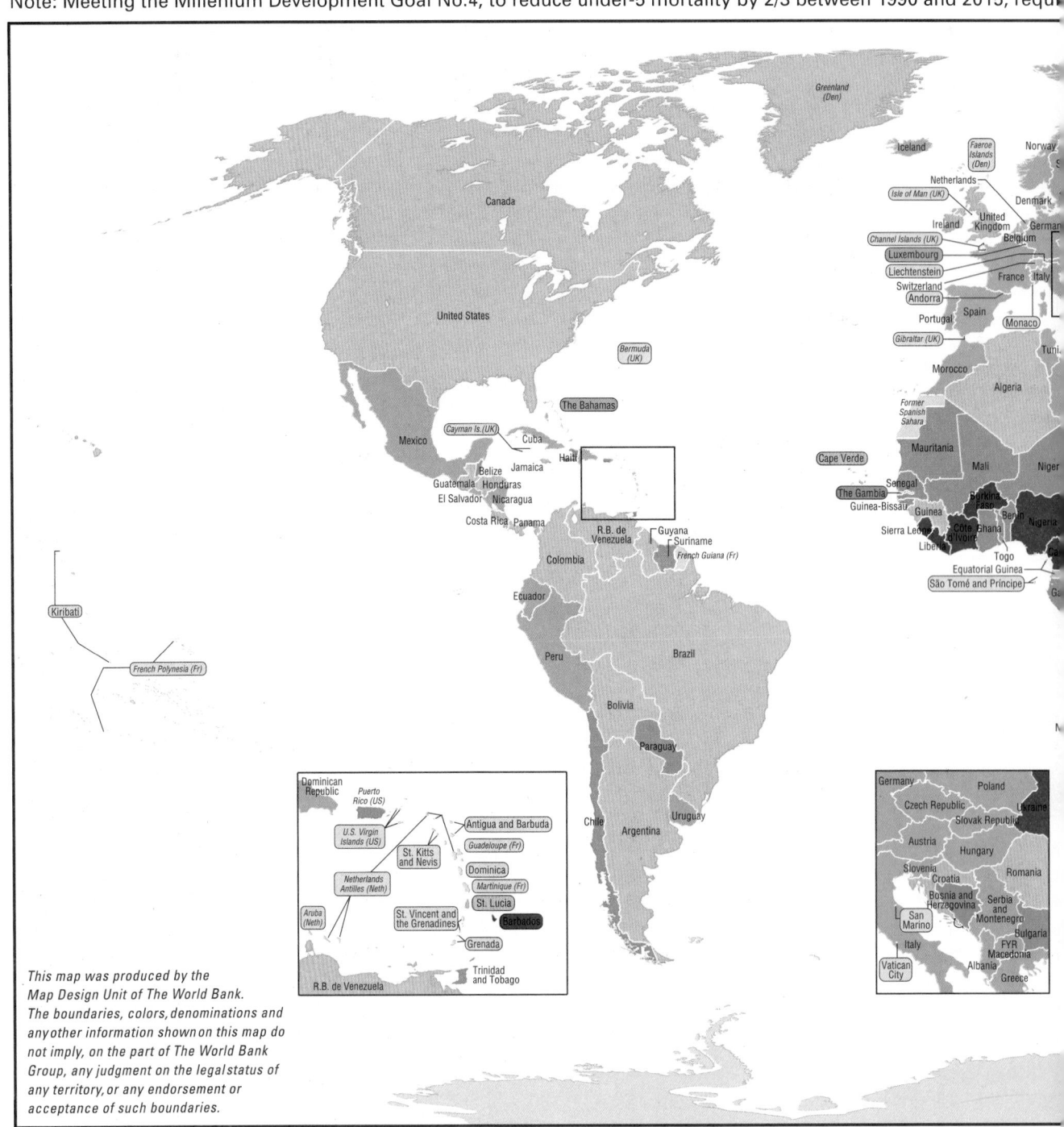

This map was produced by the
Map Design Unit of The World Bank.
The boundaries, colors, denominations and
any other information shown on this map do
not imply, on the part of The World Bank
Group, any judgment on the legal status of
any territory, or any endorsement or
acceptance of such boundaries.